SCHALM'S

VETERINARY HEMATOLOGY

SCHALM'S

VETERINARY HEMATOLOGY

FIFTH EDITION

EDITORS
• • •

BERNARD F. FELDMAN, DVM, PhD
Department of Biomedical Sciences and Pathobiology
Virginia-Maryland Regional College of Veterinary Medicine
Virginia-Polytechnic Institute and State University
Blacksburg, Virginia

JOSEPH G. ZINKL, DVM, PhD
Department of Microbiology, Immunology, and Pathology
School of Veterinary Medicine
University of California, Davis
Davis, California

NEMI C. JAIN, BVSc and AH, MVSc, PhD
Department of Microbiology, Immunology, and Pathology
School of Veterinary Medicine
University of California, Davis
Davis, California

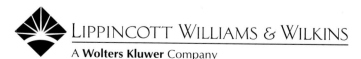

LIPPINCOTT WILLIAMS & WILKINS
A **Wolters Kluwer** Company
Philadelphia • Baltimore • New York • London
Buenos Aires • Hong Kong • Sydney • Tokyo

Editor: Donna Balado
Managing Editor: Dana Battaglia
Marketing Manager: Anne Smith
Production Editor: Jennifer D. Weir

351 West Camden Street
Baltimore, Maryland 21201-2436 USA

530 Walnut Street
Philadelphia, Pennsylvania 19106-3621 USA

Library of Congress Cataloging-in-Publication Data

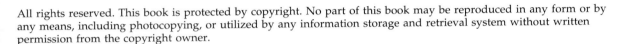

Schalm's veterinary hematology / editors, Bernard V. Feldman, Joseph G. Zinkl, Nemi C. Jain.—5th ed.
   p. cm.
  Rev. ed. of: Schalm's veterinary hematology. 4th ed. / Nemi C. Jain. 1986.
  Includes bibliographical references.
  ISBN 0-683-30692-8
   1. Veterinary hematology. I. Title: Veterinary hematology. II. Feldman, Bernard F. III. Zinkl, Joseph G. IV. Jain, Nemi C. (Nemi Chand), 1936- V. Schalm, O. W. (Oscar William), 1909-1982 Schalm's veterinary hematology.
  SF769.5 .S3 2000
  636.089'615—dc21

                                                    99-089116

To purchase additional copies of this book call our customer service department at **(800) 638-3030** or fax orders to **(301) 824-7390**. International customers should call **(301) 714-2324**.

Visit Lippincott Williams & Wilkins on the Internet: **http://www.lww.com.** Lippincott Williams & Wilkins customer service representatives are available from 8:30 am to 6:00 pm, EST, Monday through Friday, for telephone access.

00 01 02 03 04

Printed in Canada

1 2 3 4 5 6 7 8 9 10

To the memory of my parents, Lucienne and Eli, who constantly encouraged and stood with me.

To Karen Jeanne Thomason, DVM, the love of my life, and to Jay Porter Thomason Feldman who is and always will be our joy.

Also, dedicated to my brother Edward Charles Feldman, DVM, always the consummate professional.

Bernard F. Feldman

To the memory of my parents, Louise and Andy, who encouraged me to pursue a profession I would enjoy for a lifetime.

To my wife, Joanie, and sons, Matt and Andy, who bring me great happiness.

Also dedicated to the many technologists, residents, and graduate students who have taught me more than I taught them.

Joseph G. Zinkl

To all of the veterinary professionals who have continually nurtured the field of veterinary clinical hematology and who have made it a distinct and invaluable discipline.

Also dedicated to all of our grandchildren, Saahil, Shaina, Shivani, and Maya, for the immense joy they have infused in my and Javitri's lives.

Nemi Chand Jain

PREFACE TO THE FIFTH EDITION

From the first edition, published in 1961, and with each subsequent edition, *Schalm's Veterinary Hematology* has been universally recognized as an invaluable reference text for veterinary clinical hematologists, internists, undergraduate and graduate veterinary students, veterinary practitioners, veterinary technologists, veterinarians engaged in teaching and research, and other scientists interested in comparative hematology. From the yeoman work first accomplished by Oscar W. Schalm, later with Edward J. Carroll and Nemi Chand Jain, and then continued so eloquently through the work of Nemi Chand Jain, this fifth edition reflects the growth in the field of veterinary hematology. Almost 15 years have sped by since the publication of the fourth edition. It was with some trepidation that this new edition's editors developed the concept of this project, shared the mantle of responsibility, and appointed many new associate editors who, in turn, sought the help of numerous expert authors.

This fifth edition is a reflection of our knowledge of veterinary hematology as we begin the twenty-first century. The essence of *Schalm's Veterinary Hematology*, the fifth edition, is the information contained in 190 chapters with 174 authors. We thank the associate editors and many authors. As authors ourselves, we recognize the difficulties in working on a project as new as this edition is considering the scope of the project and use of a completely new concept. No author wants an editor to change her or his message or journalistic style or to insist on a specific numbers of pages. To a large extent, we have tried to allow individual authors some freedoms in their journalistic style, thinking that in so doing, their subject would be more readable. We believe that this coordinated effort between editors, associate editors, and authors has produced a book that will serve as an essential veterinary hematology reference text for the present and future.

The success of any book depends on concept and timely publication. We thank the many people who have been involved in the initiation and culmination of this project. First we want to thank Carroll C. Cann who fostered the idea and worked so hard to bring this book into being and Dr. M. Renee Prater who so capably organized, cajoled, and pleaded with everybody to maintain our time lines. We also wish to thank Donna Balado, Senior Acquisitions Editor, for providing so much help and Dana Battaglia, Managing Editor, for accomplishing the huge amount of work and keeping us on track, despite the book's size and diversity.

Finally, we hope the users of the fifth edition of *Schalm's Veterinary Hematology* will find the tradition of excellence has been maintained in this edition. Accomplishing this will be the most satisfying thank you for all who have worked hard in creating this text.

BERNARD F. FELDMAN
JOSEPH G. ZINKL
NEMI C. JAIN

PREFACE TO THE FOURTH EDITION

Eleven years have passed since the publication of the third edition of *Veterinary Hematology*. Great expansion in the fields of veterinary and human hematology and immunology during this period necessitated an extensive revision and expansion of this book. The current edition is titled *Schalm's Veterinary Hematology*, honoring the immense contributions of the late Dr. Oscar W. Schalm to veterinary hematology and his establishing it as a vital discipline of veterinary medicine. Because of the untimely demise of Drs. Schalm and Carroll, the fourth edition has evolved primarily as a single-author text.

The text has been extensively reorganized, revised, and expanded. The use of color plates has been expanded from 20 to 25 plates containing 202 individual figures; some old plates have been replaced. The number of black and while illustrations has been increased from 230 to 286. Extensive use has been made of scanning and transmission electron photomicrographs to depict the ultrastructure of leukocytes, erythrocytes, and platelets.

Two new chapters have been added: Chapter 1, concerning examination of the blood and bone marrow in general, and Chapter 11, concerning avian hematology. The normal hematology of common domestic animals is presented separately for each species in Chapters 4 through 10. The information on platelets, normal erythrocytes, erythrocytes in disease, and leukocytes, which composed one chapter each in the third edition, has been greatly expanded and is now presented in several individual chapters. Thus, Chapters 15 to 17 concern platelet production, structure, function, and abnormalities; Chapters 18 through 25, erythrocytes and their abnormalities, including anemias; and Chapters 26 through 31, various leukocytes and their abnormalities and responses to disease. The comparative cytochemistry of normal and leukemic human and animal leukocytes is presented separately in Chapter 33, in view of the increasing use of cytochemistry in the diagnosis of leukemia. Other chapters have been revised, updated, and expanded.

This book is aimed at undergraduate and graduate veterinary students, veterinary practitioners, veterinarians engaged in teaching and research, and other scientists interested in comparative hematology. The subject has been presented primarily from the point of view of its application to clinical veterinary medicine, yet provides some in-depth information about the fundamentals of hematology necessary to understand the pathophysiology of hematopoietic disorders. Up-to-date references have been incorporated wherever possible. Although an extensive literature search was made for all the chapters, it was impossible to cite all references. Selection of reference citations has not been an easy task, and I apologize for omission of a particular reference deemed important by the reader.

I am thankful to Dr. Joseph G. Zinkl for contributing the chapter on avian hematology and to Dr. Bernard F. Feldman for his contributions to the chapter on blood coagulation. The assistance of Dr. John W. Switzer in preparing the chapter on immunohematology and of Dr. Prem Handagama in preparing several photographs to illustrate cell morphology is acknowledged. The courtesy of various investigators and colleagues in supplying their published and unpublished photographs for inclusion in the book is highly appreciated. I express my sincere gratitude to Mrs. Constance S. Kono for her painstaking efforts in overseeing the minute details necessary to publication of this book and my thanks to Rosanna Ullrich for skillfully word processing some challenging tables and parts of the manuscript and to Mrs. Carroll for typing some references. I am thankful to the staff of Lea & Febiger for preparing this fourth edition for publication.

Finally, my deepest gratitude is caused by my entire family, without whose unceasing moral support this book would have not come to fruition. My lovely children Kamal, Madhu, and Anant gave their untiring help in searching the literature, typing and cross-checking references, and typing parts of the manuscript. Special thanks and indebtedness are due to my wife, Javitri, and my mother, Shrimati Manfulbai, for their understanding and perseverance in making the dream of publication of this book come true.

NEMI C. JAIN

Anthony C.G. Abrams-Ogg, DVM, DVSc
Diplomate ACVIM
Associate Professor
Department of Clinical Studies
Ontario Veterinary College
University of Guelph
Guelph, Ontario, Canada

Mark R. Ackermann, DVM, PhD
Diplomate ACVP
Associate Professor
Department of Veterinary Pathology
Iowa State University
Ames, Iowa

Betsy Aird, DVM, PhD
Diplomate ACVP
Assistant Professor of Clinical Pathology
College of Veterinary Medicine
University of Minnesota
St. Paul, Minnesota

Claire B. Andreasen, DVM, PhD
Diplomate ACVP
Department of Veterinary Pathology
College of Veterinary Medicine
Iowa State University
Ames, Iowa

Gordon A. Andrews, DVM, PhD
Diplomate ACVP
Associate Professor
Department of Diagnostic Medicine/Pathobiology
College of Veterinary Medicine
Veterinary Medical Center
Kansas State University
Manhattan, Kansas

Janice M. Andrews, DVM, PhD
Diplomate ACVP
Veterinary Laboratory Director
Veterinary Laboratory Services of Rex Healthcare
Raleigh, North Carolina

Anne M. Barger, MS, DVM
Department of Microbiology, Pathology, and Parasitology
College of Veterinary Medicine
North Carolina State University
Raleigh, North Carolina

Robert N. Barker, BSc, BVSc, PhD, MRCVS
Lecturer in Immunology
University of Aberdeen
Foresterhill, Aberdeen, United Kingdom

Holly Bender, DVM, PhD
Diplomate ACVP
Department of Biomedical Sciences and Pathobiology
Virginia-Maryland Regional College of Veterinary Medicine
Virginia-Polytechnic Institute and State University
Blacksburg, Virgina

Dorothee Bienzle, DVM, MSc, PhD
Diplomate ACVP
Department of Pathobiology, University of Guelph
Guelph, Ontario, Canada
(Formerly Assistant Professor, Department of Pathology
College of Veterinary Medicine, The University of Georgia
Athens, Georgia)

Julia T. Blue, DVM, PhD
Diplomate ACVP
Associate Professor of Clinical Pathology
Department of Population Medicine and Diagnostic Services
College of Veterinary Medicine
Cornell University
Ithaca, New York

Alice Blue-McLendon, BS, DVM
Veterinary Clinical Associate
Department of Veterinary Physiology
  and Pharmacology
Texas A & M University
College Station, Texas

Laura I. Boone, DVM
Senior Pathologist
Lilly Research Laboratories
Greenfield, Indiana

Mary K. Boudreaux, DVM, PhD
Associate Professor
Department of Pathobiology
College of Veterinary Medicine
Auburn University
Auburn, Alabama

Denise I. Bounous, DVM, PhD
Diplomate ACVP
Professor
Department of Pathology
College of Veterinary Medicine
University of Georgia
Athens, Georgia

Ann Bowling, PhD
Adjunct Professor
Department of Population Health and Reproduction
School of Veterinary Medicine
Executive Associate Director
Veterinary Genetics Laboratory
University of California, Davis
Davis, California

Marjory Brooks, DVM
Diplomate ACVIM
Associate Section Director—Comparative Coagulation
  Section
Diagnostic Laboratory, College of Veterinary Medicine
Cornell University
Ithaca, New York

Mary Beth Callan, VMD
Diplomate ACVIM
Assistant Professor of Medicine
Department of Clinical Studies
School of Veterinary Medicine
University of Pennsylvania
Philadelphia, Pennsylvania

Terry W. Campbell, MS, DVM, PhD
Associate Professor
Zoological Medicine
Service Chief, Veterinary Teaching Hospital
Colorado State University
College of Veterinary Medicine and Biomedical Sciences
Fort Collins, Colorado

**Paul John Canfield, BVSc, PhD,
  FRCPath, FACVSc, MRCVS**
Department of Veterinary Anatomy and Pathology
The University of Sydney
New South Wales, Australia

Charles C. Capen, DVM, PhD
Diplomate ACVP
Professor and Chairperson
Department of Veterinary Biosciences
College of Veterinary Medicine
The Ohio State University
Columbus, Ohio

Bruce D. Car, BVSc, MVS, PhD
Diplomate ACVP, DABT
Director of Discovery Toxicology
The Dupont Pharmaceuticals Company
Stine-Haskell Research Center
Newark, Delaware

James L. Catalfamo, MS, PhD
Director, Comparative Coagulation Section
Diagnostic Laboratory
College of Veterinary Medicine
Cornell University
Ithaca, New York

John A. Christian, DVM, PhD
Associate Professor
Veterinary Clinical Pathology
Purdue University School of Veterinary Medicine
West Lafayette, Indiana

Kenneth D. Clinkenbeard, PhD, DVM
Professor
Department of Anatomy, Pathology, and Pharmacology
College of Veterinary Medicine
Oklahoma State University
Stillwater, Oklahoma

Joan R. Coates, DVM, MS
Diplomate ACVIM (Neurology)
Assistant Professor Neurology/Neurosurgery
Department of Small Animal Medicine and Surgery
College of Veterinary Medicine
Texas A&M University
College Station, Texas

Gary L. Cockerell, DVM, PhD
Diplomate ACVP
Director, Predictive and Mechanistic Toxicology
Pharmacia & Upjohn, Incorporated
Kalamazoo, Michigan

C. Guillermo Couto, DVM
Diplomate ACVIM (Oncology and Internal Medicine)
Professor
Department of Veterinary Clinical Sciences
College of Veterinary Medicine
The Ohio State University
Columbus, Ohio

Rick L. Cowell, DVM, MS
Diplomate ACVP
Professor, Veterinary Clinical Pathology
Director, Clinical Pathology Laboratory
Department of Anatomy, Pathology, and Pharmacology
College of Veterinary Medicine
Oklahoma State University
Stillwater, Oklahoma

Benjamin J. Darien, DVM, MS
Diplomate ACVIM
Associate Professor of Internal Medicine
Department of Medical Sciences
School of Veterinary Medicine
University of Wisconsin-Madison
Madison, Wisconsin

Michael J. Day, BSc, BVMS(Hons), PhD, FASM
Diplomate ECVP, MRCPath, FRCVS
Reader in Veterinary Pathology
Department of Pathology and Microbiology
University of Bristol
Langford, United Kingdom

Gregg A. Dean, DVM, PhD
Diplomate ACVP
Assistant Professor
Department of Microbiology, Pathology, and Parasitology
College of Veterinary Medicine
North Carolina State University
Raleigh, North Carolina

Lilli S. Decker, DVM
Resident, Clinical Pathology
Department of Anatomy, Pathology, and Pharmacology
College of Veterinary Medicine
Oklahoma State University
Stillwater, Oklahoma

Heather Leigh DeHeer, DVM
Clinical Pathology Instructor
Department of Microbiology,
    Pathology, and Parasitology
College of Veterinary Medicine
North Carolina State University
Raleigh, North Carolina

Michel Desnoyers, DVM, IPSAV, MVSC
Diplomate ACVP
Associate Professor
Department of Pathology and Microbiology
College of Veterinary Medicine
University of Montreal
St. Hyacinthe, Quebec, Canada

W. Jean Dodds, DVM
President, Hemopet
Santa Monica, California
Adjunct Professor, Department of Clinical Sciences
University of Pennsylvania School of Veterinary Medicine
Philadelphia, Pennsylvania

Deborah Duffield, PhD
Professor of Biology
Portland State University
Portland, Oregon

Yvonne Espada, DVM, PhD
Associate Professor of Internal Medicine
Department of Pathology and Animal Production
Faculty of Veterinary Medicine
Universitat Autonoma de Barcelona
Badalona (Barcelona), Spain

Ellen W. Evans, DVM, PhD
Diplomate ACVP
Senior Associate Director
Diagnostic and Veterinary Services
Schering-Plough Research Institute
Lafayette, New Jersey

Peter J. Felsburg, VMD, PhD
Trustee Professor of Clinical Immunology
Department of Clinical Studies
School of Veterinary Medicine
University of Pennsylvania
Philadelphia, Pennsylvania

Fidelia R. Fernandez, DVM, MS
Diplomate ACVP
Antech Diagnostics
Chapel Hill, North Carolina

Francisco Fernández, MD
Hematologist
Hematology Department
Hospital Universitari Germans Trias i Pujol
Universitat Autonoma de Barcelona
Badalona (Barcelona), Spain

S. Dru Forrester, DVM, MS
Diplomate ACVIM (Internal Medicine)
Associate Professor
Department of Small Animal Clinical Sciences
Virginia-Maryland Regional College of Veterinary Medicine
Virginia-Polytechnic Institute and State University
Blacksburg, Virginia

Kathleen P. Freeman, DVM, MS, PhD
Head, Clinical Pathology and Diagnostic Laboratory
    Services
Animal Health Trust, Lanwades Park
Kentford, Newmarket, Suffolk, United Kingdom

John C. Fyfe, DVM, PhD
Assistant Professor of Microbiology and
    Small Animal Clinical Sciences
College of Veterinary Medicine
Michigan State University
East Lansing, Michigan

Rance M. Gamblin, DVM
Diplomate ACVIM, Specialty of Oncology
Staff Oncologist
Akron Veterinary Referral and Emergency Center
Akron, Ohio

Peter W. Gasper, DVM, PhD
Hematopathologist
Avrum Gudelksy Veterinary Center
University of Maryland
College Park, Maryland

Stephen D. Gaunt, DVM, PhD
Diplomate ACVP
Department of Veterinary Pathology
School of Veterinary Medicine
Louisiana State University
Baton Rouge, Louisiana

Nazareth Gengozian, PhD
Professor and Director
Stem Cell Transplant Laboratory
Thompson Cancer Survival Center
Department of Pediatrics
University of Tennessee Medical Center
Knoxville, Tennessee

Patricia A. Gentry, PhD
Professor
Department of Biomedical Sciences
Ontario Veterinary College
University of Guelph
Guelph, Ontario, Canada

John A. Gerlach, PhD
Diplomate ABHI
Laboratory Director
Immunohematology and Serology Laboratory
Associate Professor
Medical Technology Program and Department of Medicine
Michigan State University
East Lansing, Michigan

Urs Giger, PD Dr. Med. Vet. MS, FVH
Diplomate ACVIM, Diplomate ECVIM-CA
Charlotte Newton Sheppard Professor of Medicine
Chief, Section of Medical Genetics
Department of Clinical Studies
School of Veterinary Medicine
University of Pennsylvania
Philadelphia, Pennsylvania

Robert O. Gilbert, BVSc, MmedVet
Diplomate ACT, MRCVS
Associate Dean
College of Veterinary Medicine
Cornell University
Ithaca, New York

Elizabeth E. Goldman, DVM
Adjunct Instructor
College of Veterinary Medicine
Iowa State University
Ames, Iowa

Kent A. Gossett, DVM, PhD
Director, Scientific Licensing
SmithKline Beecham Pharmaceuticals
King of Prussia, Pennsylvania

Joanne C. Graham, DVM, MS
Diplomate ACVIM (Oncology)
Assistant Professor/Staff Oncologist
Veterinary Teaching Hospital
College of Veterinary Medicine
Iowa State University
Ames, Iowa

Robert A. Green, DVM, PhD
Diplomate ACVP
Professor
Department of Veterinary Pathobiology
Texas A&M University
College Station, Texas

Carol B. Grindem, DVM, PhD
Diplomate ACVP
Professor of Clinical Pathology
Department of Microbiology, Pathology, and Parasitology
College of Veterinary Medicine
North Carolina State University
Raleigh, North Carolina

Timothy Hackett, DVM, MS
Diplomate ACVECC
Assistant Professor
Department of Clinical Sciences
College of Veterinary Medicine and
    Biomedical Sciences
Colorado State University
Fort Collins, Colorado

Anne S. Hale, DVM
Research Associate
MSU Immunohematology and Serology Laboratory
East Lansing, Michigan
Director, Midwest Animal Blood Services, Inc.
Stockbridge, Michigan

Shimon Harrus, DVM, PhD
Lecturer at the School of Veterinary Medicine
Hebrew University of Jerusalem, Israel

John W. Harvey, DVM, PhD
Diplomate ACVP
Professor and Chair
Department of Physiological Sciences
College of Veterinary Medicine
University of Florida
Gainesville, Florida

Stuart C. Helfand, DVM
Diplomate ACVIM (Oncology and Internal Medicine)
Associate Professor
School of Veterinary Medicine
University of Wisconsin-Madison
Madison, Wisconsin

Kurt A. Henkel, DVM
President
Charlevoix Veterinary Hospital, P.C.
Charlevoix, Michigan

Paula S. Henthorn, PhD
Associate Professor of Medical Genetics
Department of Clinical Studies
School of Veterinary Medicine
University of Pennsylvania
Philadelphia, Pennsylvania

Ann Hohenhaus, DVM
Diplomate ACVIM (Oncology and Internal Medicine)
Chairman, Department of Medicine
Animal Medical Center
Head, George Jaqua Transfusion Medicine Service
New York, New York

Terry C. Hrubec, DVM, PhD
Department of Biomedical Sciences and Pathobiology
Virginia-Maryland Regional College of Veterinary Medicine
Virginia-Polytechnic Institute and State University
Blacksburg, Virginia

Mutsumi Inaba, MS, DVM, PhD
Associate Professor
Laboratory of Veterinary Clinical Pathobiology
Department of Veterinary Medical Sciences
Graduate School of Agricultural and Life Sciences
University of Tokyo
Bunko-ku, Tokyo, Japan

Robert M. Jacobs, DVM, PhD
Diplomate ACVP
Professor
Department of Pathobiology
Ontario Veterinary College
University of Guelph
Guelph, Ontario, Canada

Asger Lundorff Jensen, DVM, PhD, DVS
Diplomate ECVIM-CA
Professor
Central Laboratory
Department of Clinical Studies
The Royal Veterinary and Agricultural University
Frederiksberg, Denmark

Carmen Jiménez, MD
Hematologist
Hematology Department
Hospital Universitari Germans Trias i Pujol
Universitat Autonoma de Barcelona
Badalona (Barcelona), Spain

Ian B. Johnstone, DVM, MSc, PhD
Associate Professor
Department of Biomedical Sciences
Ontario Veterinary College
University of Guelph
Guelph, Ontario, Canada

Holly Jordan, PhD, DVM
Diplomate ACVP
Research Assistant Professor
Department of Medicine
Division of Infectious Diseases
University of North Carolina at Chapel Hill
Chapel Hill, North Carolina

Marc J. Kahn, MD
Associate Professor of Medicine
Department of Medicine
Tulane University School of Medicine
New Orleans, Louisiana

J. Jerry Kaneko, DVM, PhD, DVSc(hc)
Professor Emeritus
Department of Pathology, Microbiology, and Immunology
School of Veterinary Medicine
University of California, Davis
Davis, California

Markus E. Kehrli, Jr, DVM, PhD
Formerly, Veterinary Medical Officer
National Animal Disease Center-USDA-ARS
Ames, Iowa
Currently, Principal Research Investigator
Animal Health Discovery Research
Pfizer, Inc.
Terre Haute, Indiana

Rebecca Kirby, DVM
Diplomate ACVIM, Charter Diplomate ACVECC
Executive Director, Animal Emergency Center
Milwaukee, Wisconsin

Joyce S. Knoll, VMD, PhD
Diplomate ACVP (Clinical Pathology)
Associate Professor
Department of Biomedical Sciences
Tufts School of Veterinary Medicine
Tufts University
North Grafton, Massachusetts

Gary J. Kociba, DVM, PhD
Professor of Clinical Pathology
Department of Veterinary Biosciences
Ohio State University Veterinary Teaching Hospital
The Ohio State University
Columbus, Ohio

John W. Kramer, DVM, PhD
Professor
Veterinary Clinical Pathologist
Department Of Veterinary Clinical Sciences
College of Veterinary Medicine
Washington State University
Pullman, Washington

Annemarie T. Kristensen, DVM, PhD
Diplomate ACVIM
Principal Scientist
Health Care Discovery
Novo Nordisk A/S
Maaloev, Denmark

Kenneth S. Latimer, DVM, PhD
Diplomate ACVP
Professor of Pathology
College of Veterinary Medicine
The University of Georgia
Athens, Georgia

Robert M. Leven, PhD
Assistant Professor of Anatomy
Director of Specialized Student Services
Rush Medical College
Chicago, Illinois

David C. Lewis, BVSc, PhD
Diplomate ACVIM
Director, Consultation Services
Internal Medicine Consultant
Antech Diagnostics
Portland, Oregon

Clinton D. Lothrop, Jr, DVM, PhD
Diplomate ACVIM
Alumni Professor of Medicine
Scott-Ritchey Research Center
Department of Small Animal Surgery and Medicine
College of Veterinary Medicine
Auburn University
Auburn, Alabama

John H. Lumsden, DVM, MSc, Diploma in Clin Path
Diplomate ACVP
Department of Pathobiology
University of Guelph
Guelph, Ontario, Canada

John E. Lund, DVM, PhD
Distinguished Research Veterinary Pathologist
Pharmacia and Upjohn
Kalamazoo, Michigan

E. Gregory MacEwen, VMD
Diplomate ACVIM
Professor
Department of Medical Sciences
School of Veterinary Medicine
Member, University of Wisconsin Comprehensive Cancer Center
University of Wisconsin-Madison
Madison, Wisconsin

Peter S. MacWilliams, DVM, PhD
Diplomate ACVP
Professor of Clinical Pathology
University of Wisconsin-Madison
Madison, Wisconsin

Douglas R. Mader, MS, DVM
Diplomate ABVP
Owner, Marathon Veterinary Hospital
Marathon, Florida

Carol P. Mandell, DVM, PhD
Department of Veterinary Pathology, Microbiology, and Immunology
School of Veterinary Medicine
University of California, Davis
Davis, California

Peter Mansell, BVSc, PhD, MACVSc
Lecturer
Department of Veterinary Science
University of Melbourne
Werribee, Victoria, Australia

Maron B. Calderwood Mays, VMD, PhD
Diplomate ACVP
Veterinary Pathologist
Florida Vet Path, Incorporated
Bushnell and Gainesville, Florida

James McBain, DVM
Vice President/Corporate Veterinary Service
AnheuserBusch Theme Parks
San Diego, California

James H. Meinkoth, DVM, PhD
Diplomate ACVP
Associate Professor
Department of Anatomy, Pathology, and Pharmacology
College of Veterinary Medicine
Oklahoma State University
Stillwater, Oklahoma

Joanne B. Messick, VMD, PhD
Diplomate ACVP
Assistant Professor
Department of Veterinary Pathobiology
University of Illinois at Urbana-Champaign
Urbana, Illinois

Kenneth M. Meyers, PhD
Professor and Associate Dean of Student
  Services and Academic Affairs
Washington State University
College of Veterinary Medicine
Pullman, Washington

Susan K. Mikota, DVM
Director of Veterinary Research and Animal Health
Audubon Center for Research of Endangered Species
Audubon Institute
New Orleans, Louisiana

Reinhard Mischke, DVM, PO
Diplomate ECVIM-CA
Klinik für kleine Haustiere
Tierärztlichen Hochschule
Hannover, Germany

Jaime F. Modiano, VMD, PhD
Center for Cancer Causation and Prevention
AMC Cancer Research Center
Denver, Colorado

Luis Monreal, DVM, PhD
Associate Professor
Head of the Equine Internal Medicine Service
Large Animal Teaching Hospital
Member of the Experimental Unit of Thrombosis
Faculty of Veterinary Medicine
Universitat Autonoma de Barcelona
Badalona (Barcelona), Spain

David M. Moore, MS, DVM
Diplomate ACLAM
University Veterinarian and Director
Office of Animal Resources
Virginia Polytechnic Institute and State University
Associate Professor
Department of Biomedical Sciences and Pathobiology
Virginia-Maryland Regional College of Veterinary Medicine
Virginia-Polytechnic Institute and State University
Blacksburg, Virginia

Frances M. Moore, DVM
Diplomate ACVP
Marshfield Laboratories
Veterinary Division
Marshfield, Wisconsin

Peter F. Moore, BVSc, PhD
Professor
Department of Pathology, Microbiology, and Immunology
School of Veterinary Medicine
University of California, Davis
Davis, California

Karen A. Moriello, DVM
Diplomate ACVD
Clinical Associate Professor of Dermatology
School of Veterinary Medicine
University of Wisconsin-Madison
Madison, Wisconsin

James K. Morrisey, DVM
Diplomate ABCP (Avian)
Avian and Exotic Animal Medicine
Animal Medical Center
New York, New York

Tomás Navarro, MD
Hematologist
Hematology Department
Hospital Universitari Germans Trias i Pujol
Universitat Autonoma de Barcelona
Badalona (Barcelona), Spain

Shelley J. Newman, DVM, DVSc
Diplomate ACVP
Animal Health Laboratory
Ontario Veterinary College
University of Guelph
Guelph, Ontario, Canada

Glenn P. Niemeyer, PhD
Scott-Ritchey Research Center
College of Veterinary Medicine
Auburn University
Auburn, Alabama

Edward J. Noga, MS, DVM
Professor of Aquatic Medicine
College of Veterinary Medicine
North Carolina State University
Raleigh, North Carolina

Ingo J.A. Nolte, DVM
Diplomate ECVIM-CA
Professor
Klinik für kleine Haustiere
Tierärztlichen Hochschule
Hannover, Germany

Kwasi Nyarko, PhD
Department of Biomedical Sciences
Ontario Veterinary College
University of Guelph
Guelph, Ontario, Canada

Gregory K. Ogilvie, DVM
Diplomate ACVIM
Specialties of Internal Medicine/Oncology
Professor
Colorado State University
College of Veterinary Medicine and Biomedical Sciences
Animal Cancer Center, Veterinary Teaching Hospital
Fort Collins, Colorado

Maria Cecilia T. Penedo, PhD
Veterinary Genetics Laboratory
School of Veterinary Medicine
University of California, Davis
Davis, California

Paula Perkins, DVM
Diplomate ACVP
Clinical Pathologist
Heska Corporation
Fort Collins, Colorado

Lance E. Perryman, MS, DVM, PhD
Diplomate ACVP
Professor and Head
Department of Microbiology, Pathology, and Parasitology
College of Veterinary Medicine
North Carolina State University
Raleigh, North Carolina

F. William Pierson, MS, DVM, PhD
Diplomate ACPV
Associate Professor
Avian Medicine
Center for Molecular Medicine and Infectious Diseases
Virginia-Maryland Regional College of Veterinary Medicine
Virginia-Polytechnic Institute and State University
Blacksburg, Virginia

Michelle Plier, DVM
Diplomate ACVP
(Formerly Clinical Instructor, Clinical Pathology
School of Veterinary Medicine
University of Wisconsin-Madison
Madison, Wisconsin)

Gerald S. Post, DVM
Diplomate ACVIM (Oncology)
Veterinary Oncology and Hematology Center
Norwalk, Connecticut
New York, New York
Plainview, New York

M. Renee Prater, DVM, MS
Senior Resident, Clinical Pathology
Virginia-Maryland Regional College of Veterinary Medicine
Virginia-Polytechnic Institute and State University
Blacksburg, Virginia

Rose E. Raskin, DVM, PhD
Diplomate ACVP
Associate Professor and Service Chief of Clinical Pathology
Department of Physiological Sciences
University of Florida
College of Veterinary Medicine
Gainesville, Florida

Thomas H. Reidarson, DVM
Diplomate ACZM
Senior Veterinarian
SeaWorld of California
San Diego, California

Brandon P. Reines, DVM
Graduate Teaching Associate
Graduate Program in Veterinary Medical Sciences
Virginia-Maryland Regional College of Veterinary Medicine
College Park, Maryland

Roberta Relford, DVM, MS, PhD
Diplomate ACVIM (Internal Medicine), Diplomate ACVP
Head of Clinical Pathology
IDEXX Veterinary Services
Dallas, Texas

Virginia T. Rentko, VMD
Diplomate ACVIM
Director, Veterinary Medicine
Biopure Corporation
Clinical Assistant Professor
School of Veterinary Medicine
Tufts University
North Grafton, Massachusetts

Richard A. Reyes, MS, DVM, PhD
The Center for Comparative Medicine
School of Veterinary Medicine
University of California, Davis
Davis, California

Michelle G. Ritt, DVM
Diplomate ACVIM
Animal Hospital Center
Highlands Ranch, Colorado

John L. Robertson, VMD, PhD
Professor Veterinary Pathology
Chief, Anatomic Pathology Services
Virginia-Maryland Regional College of Veterinary Medicine
Virginia-Polytechnic Institute and State University
Blacksburg, Virginia

Kenita S. Rogers, DVM, MS
Diplomate ACVIM (Internal Medicine and Oncology)
Associate Professor, Chief of Medicine
Department of Small Animal Medicine and Surgery
Staff Oncologist, Texas Veterinary Medical Center
College of Veterinary Medicine
Texas A&M University
College Station, Texas

Francisco J. Roncalés, MD, PhD
Hematologist
Thrombosis and Hemostasis Laboratory
Hospital Universitari Germans Trias i Pujol
Universitat Autonoma de Barcelona
Badalona (Barcelona), Spain

Thomas J. Rosol, DVM, PhD
Diplomate ACVP
Professor, Department of Veterinary Biosciences
College of Veterinary Medicine
The Ohio State University
Columbus, Ohio

James A. Roth, DVM, PhD
Diplomate ACVM
Distinguished Professor
Iowa State University
College of Veterinary Medicine
Ames, Iowa

Elke Rudloff, DVM
Clinical Instructor
Director of Medical Services
Animal Emergency Center
Milwaukee, Wisconsin

Rafael Ruiz de Gopegui, DVM, PhD
Diplomate ECVIM
Associate Professor of Internal Medicine
Department of Pathology and Animal Production
Faculty of Veterinary Medicine
Universitat Autonoma de Barcelona
Badalona (Barcelona), Spain

Karen E. Russell, DVM, PhD
Diplomate ACVP
Assistant Professor, Clinical Pathology
Department of Veterinary Pathobiology
College of Veterinary Medicine
Texas A & M University
College Station, Texas

Juan M. Sancho, MD
Hematologist
Hematology Department
Hospital Universitari Germans Trias i Pujol
Universitat Autonoma de Barcelona
Badalona (Barcelona), Spain

Ann Schneider, DVM
Director
Eastern Veterinary Blood Bank, Inc.
Annapolis, Maryland

A. Eric Schultze, MT(ASCP), DVM, PhD
Diplomate ACVP
Assistant Professor of Clinical Pathology
College of Veterinary Medicine
University of Tennessee
Knoxville, Tennessee

Michael A. Scott, DVM, PhD
Diplomate ACVP
Assistant Professor
Department of Veterinary Pathobiology and
   Veterinary Medical Diagnostic Laboratory
University of Missouri-Columbia
Columbia, Missouri

Debra C. Sellon, DVM, PhD
Diplomate ACVIM
Associate Professor
Equine Medicine
College of Veterinary Medicine
Washington State University
Pullman, Washington

Terrilyn A. Sharpe, BS
Clinical Research and Education Manager
Biopure Corporation
Cambridge, Massachusetts

Dale E. Shuster, PhD
Manager, Drug Discovery
Schering-Plough Animal Health
Union, New Jersey

Graham S. Smith, BVMS, MRCVS, MSc
Diplomate ACVP
Senior Division Manager
Milestone Biomedical Associates
Milton, Ontario, Canada

Joseph E. Smith, DVM, PhD
Diplomate ACVP
Professor
Department of Diagnostic Medicine/Pathobiology
College of Veterinary Medicine, Veterinary Medical Center
Manhattan, Kansas

Stephen A. Smith, DVM, PhD
Director, Aquatic Medicine Laboratory
Associate Professor
Aquatic Medicine/Fish Health
Department of Biomedical Sciences and Pathobiology
Virginia-Maryland Regional College of Veterinary Medicine
Virginia-Polytechnic Institute and State University
Blacksburg, Virginia

Nancy L. Stedman, DVM
Diplomate ACPV
Resident Pathologist
Department of Pathology
College of Veterinary Medicine
University of Georgia

W.L. Steffens III, PhD
Director, Electron Microscopy Laboratory
Department of Pathology
College of Veterinary Medicine
University of Georgia
Athens, Georgia

Steven L. Stockham, DVM, MS
Diplomate ACVP
Associate Professor
Department of Veterinary Pathobiology and
  Veterinary Medical Diagnostic Laboratory
College of Veterinary Medicine
University of Missouri-Columbia
Columbia, Missouri

Michael K. Stoskopf, DVM, PhD
Diplomate ACZM
Professor of Aquatic and Wildlife Medicine and Toxicology
Coordinator of Environmental Medicine Consortium and
  Chair of Marine Sciences Council
Department of Clinical Sciences
College of Veterinary Medicine
Department of Toxicology
College of Agriculture and Life Sciences
North Carolina State University
Raleigh, North Carolina

Fern Tablin, VMD, PhD
Professor
Department of Anatomy, Physiology, and Cell Biology
School of Veterinary Medicine
University of California, Davis
Davis, California

Judith A. Taylor, DVM, DVSc
Staff Clinical Pathologist
Department of Pathobiology
Ontario Veterinary College
University of Guelph
Guelph, Ontario, Canada

Erik Teske, DVM, PhD
Diplomate ECVIM-CA
Department of Clinical Sciences—Companion Animals
Faculty of Veterinary Medicine
Utrecht University
Utrecht, The Netherlands

Douglas H. Thamm, VMD
Diplomate ACVIM (Oncology)
Oncology/Gene Therapy Fellow
Department of Medical Sciences
School of Veterinary Medicine
University of Wisconsin-Madison
Madison, Wisconsin

Jennifer S. Thomas, DVM, PhD
Diplomate ACVP
Associate Professor
Department of Veterinary Pathobiology
College of Veterinary Medicine
Texas A&M University
College Station, Texas

Catherine E. Thorn, DVM, DVSc, MSc
Diplomate ACVP
Clinical Pathologist
Antech Diagnostics
Atlanta, Georgia

Mary Anna Thrall, DVM, MS
Diplomate ACVP
Professor
Department of Pathology
College of Veterinary Medicine & Biomedical Sciences
Colorado State University
Fort Collins, Colorado

Mary B. Tompkins, DVM, PhD
Professor
Department of Microbiology, Pathology, and Parasitology
College of Veterinary Medicine
North Carolina State University
Raleigh, North Carolina

Wayne A.F. Tompkins, PhD
Director of Graduate Programs
Immunology
North Carolina State University
Raleigh, North Carolina

Harold Tvedten, DVM, PhD
Diplomate ACVP
Professor of Pathology
Veterinary Medical Teaching Hospital
Michigan State University
East Lansing, Michigan

David M. Vail, DVM, MS
Diplomate ACVIM (Oncology)
Associate Professor of Oncology
Department of Medical Sciences
School of Veterinary Medicine and
The Comprehensive Cancer Center
University of Wisconsin-Madison
Madison, Wisconsin

Amy Valenciano
Department of Microbiology, Pathology, and Parasitology
College of Veterinary Medicine
North Carolina State University
Raleigh, North Carolina

Victor E.O. Valli, DVM, MSc, PhD
Diplomate ACVP Anatomic and Clinical Pathology
Professor of Pathology
College of Veterinary Medicine
University of Illinois
Urbana, Illinois

Jawahar Lal Vegad, BVSc, MVSc, PhD (New Zealand)
President, Indian Association of Veterinary Pathologists
Professor Emeritus
Department of Pathology
College of Veterinary Science and Animal Husbandry
Jabalpur, India

William Vernau, BSc, BVMS, DVSc
Diplomate ACVP
Department of Pathology, Microbiology, and Immunology
School of Veterinary Medicine
University of California, Davis
Davis, California

Trevor Waner, BVSc, MSc
Director of Animal Facilities
Israel Institute for Biological Research
Ness Ziona, Israel

K. Jane Wardrop, DVM, MS
Diplomate ACVP
Associate Professor
Department Veterinary Clinical Sciences
College of Veterinary Medicine
Washington State University
Pullman, Washington

A.D.J. Watson, BVSc, PhD, FRCVS, FAAVPT, MACVSc
Associate Professor in Veterinary Medicine
Specialist Consultant, University Veterinary Center, Sydney
Department of Veterinary Clinical Sciences
The University of Sydney
New South Wales, Australia

Douglas J. Weiss, DVM, PhD
Diplomate ACVP
Professor
Department of Veterinary PathoBiology
College of Veterinary Medicine
University of Minnesota
St. Paul, Minnesota

Elizabeth G. Welles, DVM, PhD
Diplomate ACVP
Associate Professor, Pathobiology
Department of Pathobiology
Auburn University
Auburn, Alabama

Maxey L. Wellman, DVM, PhD
Diplomate ACVP
Associate Professor
Department of Veterinary Biosciences
College of Veterinary Medicine
The Ohio State University
Columbus, Ohio

Randall S. Wells, PhD
Conservation Biologist, Chicago Zoological Society
Director for Marine Mammal and Sea Turtle Research
Mote Marine Laboratory
Sarasota, Florida

M.D. Willard, DVM, MS
Diplomate ACVIM
Professor
Department of Small Animal Medicine and Surgery
College of Veterinary Medicine
Texas A&M University
College Station, Texas

Karen M. Young, VMD, PhD
Clinical Associate Professor of Clinical Pathology
Department of Pathobiological Sciences
School of Veterinary Medicine
University of Wisconsin-Madison
Madison, Wisconsin

Kurt L. Zimmerman, DVM
Clinical Pathology Resident and PhD Candidate
Virginia-Maryland Regional College of Veterinary Medicine
Virginia-Polytechnic Institute and State University
Blacksburg, Virginia

Debra Zoran, DVM, MS, PhD
Diplomate ACVIM (Internal Medicine)
Clinical Assistant Professor
Department of Small Animal Medicine and Surgery
College of Veterinary Medicine
Texas A&M University
College Station, Texas

CONTENTS

SECTION I
Essential Hematologic Concepts
Harold Tvedten

CHAPTER 1

Clinical Automated Hematology Systems

• JOYCE S. KNOLL

Hematology testing of veterinary samples has become a routine part of a diagnostic evaluation, food and drug safety assessment, and research studies. Complete blood counts (CBC) are commonly performed by veterinarians as part of a presurgical screen, and, increasingly, as part of well-animal care. Traditionally, these samples were sent to large diagnostic laboratories or were performed in the office with time-consuming, labor-intensive manual methods. The increasing availability of semi-automated and automated hematology instrumentation offers pharmaceutical companies, research facilities, and veterinary practitioners more efficient, precise testing than can be achieved through manual methods. In a veterinary practice, these instruments provide fast turnaround of results, potentially improving patient care and client satisfaction. In a research setting, more sophisticated analyzers can rapidly process many samples and can be used to identify cell population shifts or to quantify subtle changes in cell size.

The decision about the type of system to be used should depend on various factors, including the number of samples to be analyzed, the species types in question, and the availability of trained personnel to operate and maintain an instrument. Manual methods or a semi-automated system may be adequate in a veterinary practice in which only emergency or off-hours testing is performed in-house, whereas a fully automated system is more efficient and cost effective for a diagnostic laboratory or a pharmaceutical company. Adherence to a routine quality-control program is essential to ensure accuracy of results as well as an understanding of the technology and factors that affect results.

AUTOMATED SYSTEMS

Because thousands of cells are evaluated from each sample, automated cell counters generally have better precision and accuracy than manual techniques. A wide variety of instruments, most of which are specifically designed for analysis of human blood, are available. Methods for analysis include aperture-resistance measurements, buffy coat analysis, light scatter, cell staining and light absorption, or a combination of these. When analyzing nonhuman hematology specimens, it is essential that the selected instrument be designed and validated for multispecies analysis. Instruments designed for analysis of human samples require modification to provide more accurate red blood cell (RBC) and leukocyte counts.[1] More recently, instruments have become available with multiple preprogrammed settings for the more common types of domestic animals. Instruments vary in their degree of sophistication and cost, and they range in price from approximately $10,000–$200,000. Instruments with veterinary applications are described below and include the Coulter Z1 or ZBI, QBC® VetAutoread™ Hematology System, Baker 9110, Vet ABC, CDC Hemovet, Bayer H1, and Cell-Dyn 3500. The simplest models provide only cell counts (RBC, white blood cell [WBC], and platelets), whereas instruments in which newer technologic advances are used provide a far greater amount of information, including some traditionally obtained only through a microscopic examination of a blood smear. Semiautomated instruments are more labor intensive, requiring some sample preparation prior to analysis (e.g., sample dilution). Fully automated instruments dilute the sample, add lyse solution, perform cell counts, and print test results. With all the analyzers discussed in this chapter, microscopic blood smear evaluation is recommended to confirm WBC abnormalities and to rule out the presence of platelet clumps. A microscopic examination is also needed to identify additional important abnormalities such as spherocytosis, Heinz bodies or the presence of blasts, mast cells, microfilaria, or RBC parasites.

QBC VetAutoread Hematology System (IDEXX, Inc., Westbrook, ME) is an automated version of the quantitative buffy coat technology specifically optimized for veterinary samples. Quantitative buffy coat analysis[2] (QBC) was developed in the early 1980s as a tool to screen blood samples without performing the individual assays required in a traditional blood count. The system is based on the fact that variable cell density causes blood

---

QBC and VetAutoread are trademarks of Becton Dickinson and Company.

cells to sort into individual layers when blood is spun in a hematocrit tube. A molded cylindrical float is used to expand the white-cell and platelet layers of the buffy coat and the width of each band reflects the number of cells present in each population. In addition, acridine orange, which coats the tube, stains nucleoproteins, lipoproteins, glycosamines, and other cellular substances. These cellular components fluoresce when subjected to blue-violet light, and differential fluorescence is used to further distinguish cellular subtypes. The QBC VetAutoread Analyzer automatically delimits the various layers and quantifies blood components, with calculated results appearing as both a digital readout and a printout. Parameters available include a packed cell volume (PCV), hemoglobin (Hgb) concentration, RBC and WBC counts, total granulocyte count, neutrophil count, lymphocyte and monocyte count, eosinophil count (canine and bovine only), platelets, mean corpuscular Hgb concentration (MCHC), and reticulocyte percentage. The printout includes flags to alert the operator of potential problems such as the presence of unusual cell types or uneven separation of cellular layers. In addition, the instrument graphs the output of the scan. Through inspection of this graph, a trained individual can often discern the cause of the flagged results (Fig. 1.1).

With the addition of a 57°C block heater, the heat precipitation method can be used to quantify fibrinogen. After the initial scan, the hematocrit tube is incubated and again centrifuged, resulting in a band of fibrinogen resting on top of the float. The QBC VetAutoread Analyzer can measure the width of this band and determine the fibrinogen level of the sample. This method is primarily useful for detecting increased levels of fibrinogen and can be a useful adjunct for detecting an inflammatory process. It is not sufficiently sensitive to detect the decreased fibrinogen levels associated with some coagulopathies (e.g., disseminated intravascular coagulation [DIC]).

This instrument is easy to operate and appears to be a reasonable screening tool for use in the more common domestic species (dog, cat, horse, cow).[3] A sample volume of 111 mL is required, with results available in approximately 7 minutes, although longer incubation times and additional centrifugation steps may be required for improving separation of cell layers, especially in cats.[4] Hematocrit (HCT), Hgb, and WBC counts correlate well with reference methods with unexpectedly accurate platelet counts even in cats and horses.[4] Aggregated platelets stuck on the end of the float may lead to underestimation of the platelet count, but they can be recognized through visual inspection of the graphed buffy coat profile. This problem warrants a second centrifugation step. Reticulocytes were identified in most feline and canine samples with a regenerative anemia, although the actual counts correlated poorly with reference methods.[4] The QBC VetAutoread System works best, however, on samples from hematologically normal animals. In one study,[4] the QBC VetAutoread Analyzer accurately identified most cases of leukocytosis; however, it correctly identified only 57% of leukopenias. Identification of canine eosinophils was also noted to be inconsistent, with a tendency to include lymphocytes or monocytes in the eosinophil count. Hemoglobin determinations from horses with colic were often abnormal. This may have been caused by effects of an increased RBC sedimentation rate on Hgb determination that is based on the draft of the float in the plasma.[4] Abnormalities such as microcytosis, hypochromasia, or cell immaturity can also invalidate results.

This instrument has limited applications and can be

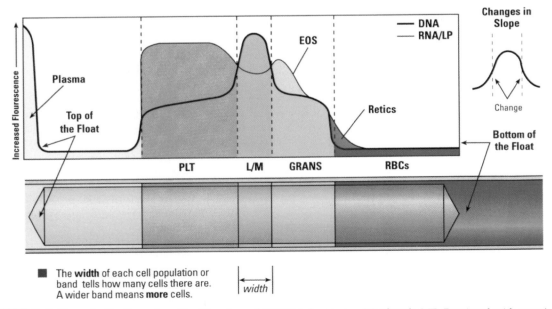

The **width** of each cell population or band tells how many cells there are. A wider band means **more** cells.

FIGURE 1.1 Expanded buffy coat profile. (Courtesy of IDEXX Laboratories, Westbrook, ME. Reprinted with permission.)

used only for analysis of whole blood from the species indicated. The algorithms used to calculate RBC and WBC counts assume a normal cell size and structure. These assumptions may not be valid for exotic species such as ferrets or rabbits, and parameters have not be established for avian and reptile specimens.

IMPEDANCE ANALYZERS

Currently on the market are several analyzers that rely on a conductivity or resistance measurement (impedance) to count and size cells. This technology uses the principle that cells are poor electrical conductors. In these instruments, blood diluted in an electrically conducting diluent is passed through a small aperture between two electrodes. Each cell produces a change in electrical impedance and a measurable voltage pulse, with cell size proportional to the magnitude of the change in resistance or height of each voltage pulse. Erythrocytes and platelets are separated on the basis of size. WBCs may be included in the RBC count, but they generally cause an insignificant problem unless the animal is leukemic and anemic. WBC counts are determined after lysis of RBCs with a few drops of saponin solution. A precise quantity of suspension is drawn through the aperture, and several thousand cells per second are counted and sized, generally making these results more accurate than those obtained with manual methods.

The impedance principle (Fig. 1.2) was first used in Coulter particle counters (Models FN, ZBI; Coulter Corporation, Miami, FL) and subsequent hematology analyzers (Models S770, S880, S-Senior). The ZBI, and newer Z1, semi-automated instruments continue to be the accepted reference method for cell and particle counting. These instruments are somewhat inexpensive and can be readily used to determine RBC and WBC counts in veterinary samples. Refurbished ZBI models continue to be available, with prices that vary depending on the age and condition of the instrument. Compared with other, more automated, impedance analyzers, these in-

struments are time consuming and labor intensive because RBC and WBC counts are performed separately, and samples must be manually diluted prior to analysis. Results are available within approximately 5 minutes. It is important that dilution be sufficient to minimize the coincidence of two or more cells simultaneously entering the aperture. For accuracy to be ensured, counts should be <80,000/μL. Most whole blood samples are diluted 1:500 for WBC counts (40 μL whole blood/20 mL isotonic saline) and 1:250,000 for RBC counts (40 μL of the first dilution/20 mL isotonic saline), but other dilutions may be needed to compensate for species variation or for the effects of disease. A separate automatic dilutor unit (Dual Dilutor III, Coulter Corporation, Miami, FL 33116) is available for this purpose, or manual dilutions can be made. Platelet counts can also be determined, but only after manual installation of a smaller aperture.

The ZBI and Z1 models have the advantage of easily adjustable threshold settings, making these extremely versatile instruments that can be used to analyze blood from a wide diversity of species or determine cell counts on various other fluids or research specimens. Single- or dual-threshold models are available. It is particularly important to adjust the lower threshold to accommodate the smaller RBCs present in some species, whereas an adjustable upper threshold setting minimizes interference associated with elevated WBC counts. Upper and lower thresholds should be determined for each new species analyzed. Once established, the Z1 allows threshold settings for as many as five species (or cell types) to be stored for later recall. Calibration settings often vary from instrument to instrument, but the Z1 offers automated calibration with correct settings computed and set automatically. The older ZBI model requires a more extensive calibration process than does the newer Z1 model. Unlike previous models, the Z1 does not generally require manual adjustment of either current or gain settings. The Coulter Model Z2 is similar to the Z1 but further performs channelization of particle data in as many as 256 channels, displaying size distribution data along with count information. This function is primarily useful as a research tool.

Fully automated, impedance instruments with veterinary applications include the Baker 9000 series (Bio-Chem ImmunoSystems [U.S.] Inc, Allentown, PA), and the new Vet ABC animal blood counter (ABX Hematology Inc., Garden Grove, CA) These instruments simultaneously perform RBC, WBC, and platelet counts; determine mean corpuscular volume (MCV) and colorimetric Hgb; and then calculate HCT, MCHC, and mean corpuscular Hgb (MCH). These instruments are moderately priced and both can process as many as 45 samples per hour. Several Coulter instruments (Models S770, S880, S-Senior) were previously used to analyze veterinary samples. These instruments, however are calibrated for human blood and require voltage adjustments prior to use on animal samples. Because of the need for instrument modification, the manufacturer no longer supports veterinary applications.

Baker 9000 analyzers have been in the field for many

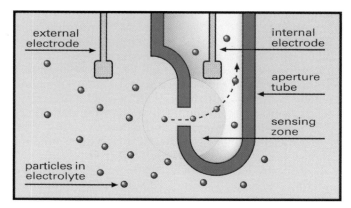

FIGURE 1.2 Illustration of the impedance principle. (Courtesy of Coulter International Reprinted with permission.)

years, with a well-established level of performance. As a new instrument, field trials assessing the accuracy of the Vet ABC are not currently available. In the Baker 9110 model, which is designed specifically for veterinary samples, the stronger lysing agent needed for feline and bovine RBCs is used. Its sample requirement depends on the sampling mode used and ranges from 110 μL of blood to a predilute option requiring only 40 μL of sample. Convenient prefilled dilution reservoirs and calibrated pipettes are available to facilitate accurate sample dilution. The Vet ABC needs only 12 μL of blood, a decided advantage when processing rodent samples.

With the Baker 9110, thresholds can be readily adjusted and preprogrammed to facilitate analysis of blood from as many as 10 species. Specific threshold definitions are available for some species, or settings can be manually adjusted for analysis of new species. Thresholds on the Vet ABC are adjusted for each species by insertion of species-specific smart cards with parameters available for cats, horses, dogs, rats, mice, guinea pigs, and cows. Thresholds cannot be manually adjusted. The stated linearity of Baker MCV determinations is between 50 and 150 fL, with some problems evident in detecting the smaller RBCs present in some species such as sheep and goats. Because of the overlap in size, the Baker 9110 can have some problems differentiating feline large platelets from their small RBCs. The Vet ABC has a stated MCV linearity range of 25 to 300. This expanded range may eliminate the problems with small RBCs noted with use of the Baker. The Vet ABC further uses a sophisticated impulse sorting system to separate RBCs and platelets. Any impulse not having the typical platelet shape is rejected from the platelet count. It is unclear how this system handles the large, fluffy platelets often seen in cats. Both instruments can provide RBC and platelet histograms. Although both analyzers perform a three-part leukocyte differential count (monocytes, lymphocytes, granulocytes), these results on the Baker have not proved accurate in animal samples, and further field studies are needed to determine the accuracy of the Vet ABC's results. Both systems include a diagnostic program that signals the presence of abnormal cells or instrument problems. Any signaled cellular abnormalities must be verified manually. The Vet ABC's option for programmable startup and automatic cleaning minimizes maintenance time.

The Mascot multispecies hematology system (CDC Technologies, Inc., Oxford, CT) was the first hematology analyzer designed specifically for veterinary applications and use in a veterinary practice. The newer Hemavet series (CDC Technologies, Inc.) is composed of several modular, fully upgradable systems that allow a practice to choose between variably priced models that provide from as few as six to as many as 27 parameters of patient data, including a five-part leukocyte differential count and flags for nucleated RBC (NRBC) and reticulocytes. Species-specific parameters are preprogrammed into each analyzer; with a wide variety of species options available, including the common domestic species, ferrets, goats, guinea pigs, llamas, monkeys, mice, pigs, rabbits, rats, and sheep. The choice of species can be tailored to suit the type of samples most commonly analyzed by the practice. Only 20 μL of blood is required for sample analysis. The sample is automatically diluted, with WBC and RBC counts performed sequentially rather than simultaneously, and results are available within approximately 5 minutes. These instruments are significantly slower than the impedance instruments described above, but they require only approximately 10 to 15 seconds hands on per test. The more expensive model includes an option for programmed startup and automated cleanup cycles that minimizes maintenance time.

The flow system used by these analyzers is designed to minimize cell distortion and prevent probe clogging, and they use a proprietary technique that characterizes cells on the basis of both size and intracellular complexity. This allows these instruments to distinguish more readily between small RBCs and platelets. The extended linearity of MCV (10 to 600 fL) and RBC (0.01 $\times$ $10^6/\mu$L) determinations facilitates accurate RBC and WBC counts from a wide variety of species, including goats and llamas, with few of the RBC problems noted with the Baker. Species-specific programmed settings result in both threshold adjustments as well as optimization of the reagent mixture to accommodate physiologic differences inherent in the cells of various species. Unlike most impedance systems, the lysing reagent used in this system does not strip away the leukocyte membrane, leaving a bare nucleus. Because leukocytes remain intact, their size and intracellular complexity can be measured. A patented software program (Expectation Maximization) uses floating thresholds to identify populations of both normal or abnormal cells and, in some species, to determine a differential leukocyte count. The most sophisticated model displays a three-dimensional (3-D) triaxial display of RBC, platelet, and WBC subpopulations and flags abnormal results. Further field trials are needed to assess the accuracy of these differential counts and the reliability of the flagging system.

FLOW CYTOMETER

Two of the more advanced, hematology systems, the Bayer H1 (formerly Technicon H-1; Bayer, Tarrytown, NY) and the Cell-Dyn 3500 (Abbott Laboratories, North Chicago, IL) use flow cytometry to count and identify blood cells in veterinary samples. As cells pass through a laser beam they absorb and scatter light. Interruptions in the light beam can be used to determine cell counts, whereas changes in light scatter are used to determine cell size and internal complexity or density. Both instruments are fully automated and determine RBC, WBC, and platelet counts; a cytochemical Hgb determination; and a leukocyte differential count on approximately 100 μL of blood. The Cell-Dyn 3500 is somewhat easier to operate and slightly faster, with results available in 45 seconds compared with 60 seconds with the H1. Unlike other advanced instruments, such as the Coulter STKS, both the H1 and the Cell-Dyn 3500 have established

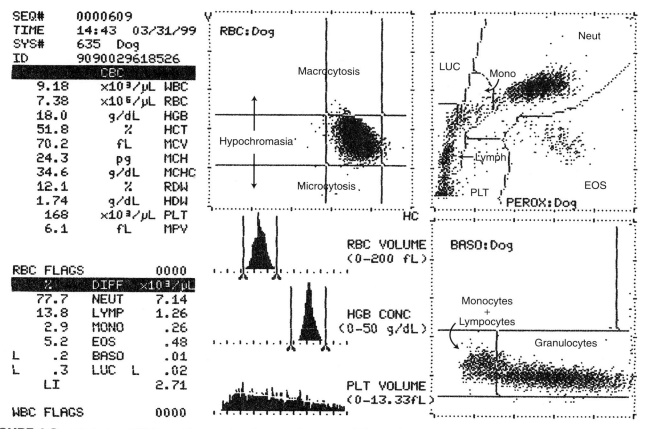

FIGURE 1.3 A Technicon H1E hematology analyzer's report for a normal dog, including red blood cell (RBC), hemoglobin (HgB), and platelet (PLT) histograms and RBC and white blood cell (WBC) cytograms. The RBC cytogram (top left box) is divided into nine boxes based on RBC volume (vertical axis) and hemoglobin concentration (horizontal axis), allowing rapid identification of macrocytic, microcytic, or hypochromic RBC. WBCs in the Peroxidase (PEROX) cytogram (top right corner) are separated according to size (vertical axis) and cell myeloperoxidase activity (horizontal axis). Neutrophils (Neut) and Eosinophils (EOS) in most species have strong peroxidase staining and cluster to the right side of the cytogram. The weak peroxidase reaction in monocytes (Mono) causes them to cluster to the left of neutrophils. Lymphocytes have no peroxidase staining and these small cells all just above platelets on the far left of the cytogram. Large, unstained cells (LUC) include a mixture of monocytes, large lymphocytes, and blasts, which fall in the upper left corner, merging with monocytes and lymphocytes on the cytogram. The Basophil (BASO) cytogram separates most leukocytes after the cytoplasm has been stripped away. Nuclei are plotted by size (vertical axis) and density (horizontal axis). The resulting cytogram typically resembles a worm, with monocytes and lymphocytes in the head and neutrophils and eosinophils comprising the elongated body. Cells found in the upper box are counted as basophils, but may include blasts, nucleated RBC. (Illustration provided by Dr. Harold Tvedten, Department of Pathology, Michigan State University.)

veterinary applications, with manufacturer support for these applications.

The H1 has been used for analysis of veterinary samples for several years, with initial validation work published in 1991 (5). Species-specific parameters for 9 species (human, rat, mouse, dog, rabbit, cynomolgus monkey, rhesus monkey, cat, and horse) are preprogrammed into a multi-species software package. Any other species must be run using the most appropriate set of parameters. Accurate results cannot be determined on samples from species with unusual RBC, such as goats and llamas. The Cell-Dyn 3500 software contains a set of baseline parameters established for humans. Gain settings for the laser can be readily modified, allowing the user to customize and store parameters for a large number of species, making this an ex-

tremely flexible analyzer. Parameters for each new species must be verified, however, by processing a minimum of 5 samples from healthy individuals on the Cell-Dyn in parallel with a reference method. Since settings can differ significantly from instrument to instrument, this calibration process is required for all species run on a new instrument.

Although both instruments use flow cytometry, they differ in their applications of this technology. The H1 is unique in its use of two-angle light scatter to count and size RBCs and platelets, as well as to determine the Hgb concentration of individual RBCs. RBCs are first sphered and fixed; this reduces orientational artifacts as they pass through the flow path. As RBCs and platelets pass through the laser beam, individual measurements are made on each cell. Low-angle (forward) deflection of light correlates with cell size, whereas right- or high-angle light scatter correlates with the internal granularity or the density of the cell, with intracellular Hgb concentration linearly related to the RBC's refractive index (high-angle light scatter). This process provides an improved separation of RBCs and platelets, which have significantly different refractive indices, as well as enhanced information about abnormal RBC populations. RBC volume and Hgb concentration histograms are generated, with red cell morphology flags triggered when a significant proportion of RBCs fall outside the programed normal limits. Normal ranges can be adjusted for each species. Based on size and Hgb concentration, each RBC is classified into one of nine categories, and the percentages of macrocytic, microcytic, hypochromic, and hyperchromic RBCs are determined. This feature provides quantitative information about changes in RBC populations that can be particularly useful for research and diagnostic purposes. By contrast, the Cell-Dyn 3500 uses traditional impedance technology to determine RBC and platelet counts. Flags for abnormal RBC populations are not available.

The H1 and Cell-Dyn 3500 also differ in the way WBC counts and leukocyte differential counts are determined. The Cell-Dyn 3500 compares an impedance WBC count (WIC) with an optical WBC count (WOC) determined with flow cytometry. WBCs are identified with a novel approach referred to as Multi Angle Polarized Scatter Separation. As cells are passed through a laser beam, light scatter measurements are taken at three different angles. In addition, a portion of the light beam is depolarized, and light scatter is measured as cells pass through this beam. This information is used to count WBCs and to classify them on the basis of size, nuclear lobularity, and granularity. Eosinophils can be distinguished from other leukocytes by the tendency of their unique granules to scatter polarized light. Because of the water-soluble nature of basophil granules, these cells fall with mononuclear cells on the scattergram. Dynamic thresholds are used to determine the best separations between the main leukocyte populations. Significant differences between WIC and WOC can be caused by fragile WBCs, NRBCs, platelet clumps, or lyse-resistant RBCs. This system analyzes the data to determine which count is more appropriate, but a discrepancy in counts can be an indication that the operator needs to screen a blood smear. In one study,[6] some equine samples were noted to have higher WOC than WIC because of the presence of a population of lyse-resistant RBC. In some cases the discrepancy was large enough to trigger an instrument alert, and the WIC was correctly reported. For the remaining samples, the system reported the higher WOC, with the lyse-resistant RBC likely interpreted as lymphocytes. The Resistant Red Cell Mode, with an extended lyse time, was found to alleviate this problem.

After lysis of RBC, the H1 also uses two different techniques to determine a total WBC count. In the peroxidase channel, flow cytometry is combined with automated cytochemistry to count WBCs and to provide a six-part leukocyte differential count. In this flow cell,

leukocytes are distinguished from one another by a combination of size and variable levels of granular peroxidase activity. In most species, eosinophils are characterized by the strongest peroxidase activity, whereas lymphocytes lack activity. In a second flow cell, cytoplasm is stripped away, and the resulting bare nuclei are classified as polymorphonuclear or mononuclear, with cell types further separated by size. Basophils are distinguished from other leukocytes because their membranes are resistant to the lytic effects of surfactants. Discrepancies between the outputs of these two channels is used to generate flags for immature granulocytes (including bands), blasts, and NRBCs. A guide to interpretation of red cell and leukocyte cytograms has been published.[7] Past problems caused by frequently plugged tubing has been corrected by the addition of a clot filter.

Bayer recently introduced the Advia 120 for analysis of human samples with veterinary applications for 13 species (with the addition of guinea pigs, goats, cows, and sheep). Although based on similar technology, this system promises significant improvement over the H1. This analyzer is significantly faster than either the H1 or the Cell-Dyn 3500, processing 120 samples per hour. Its UnFluidics technology greatly reduces tubing and the problems associated with this aspect of the H1. After collecting information on RBCs, the Advia 120 makes a second measurement, with amplified low- and high-angle scattering signals. This increases platelet resolution, allowing more accurate platelet counts, with improved determination of mean platelet volume (MPV) and mean platelet component determination (MPC).[8] This may have important research applications, because MPC, in particular, is thought to be useful in determining platelet activation state in humans[9] and is less expensive and less labor intensive than fluorescence flow-cytometry or density-gradient analysis. In addition, the Advia 120 performs automated reticulocyte counts, along with the other parameters provided by the H1. Validation of this system and its use for veterinary samples is currently in progress.

Leukocyte differential counts from these instruments should be viewed cautiously. The H1 cannot reliably identify feline eosinophils owing to their weak peroxidase activity, with both false-positive and false-negative results seen. Problems identifying basophils and monocytes in both dogs and cats have also been noted. A high basophil count usually indicates an error. Alternatively, the Cell-Dyn 3500 often misses canine eosinophils and also has problems identifying monocytes in some dogs and horses.[6] The reliability of the Cell-Dyn 3500 basophil count in dogs and cats is unclear. Although the H1 flags various abnormal cells, these flags have proved of minimal use in veterinary samples, and some abnormal samples may produce no flags. Such flags have been eliminated from the Cell-Dyn 3500 software because of similar reliability problems. With both instruments, examination of leukocyte cytograms can be useful for identifying abnormal cell populations. Criteria should be established for blood smear review. A quick scan often detects problems with the automated differential count, with a more detailed microscopic examina-

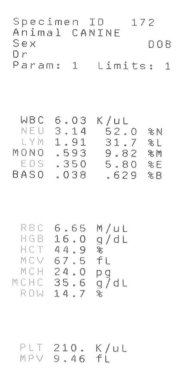
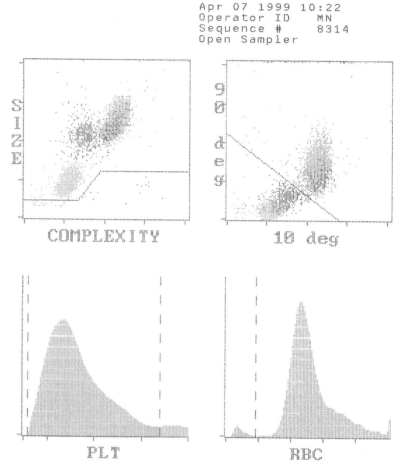

```
Specimen ID    172                          Apr 07 1999 10:22
Animal CANINE                               Operator ID    MN
Sex                DOB                       Sequence #     8314
Dr                                           Open Sampler
Param: 1  Limits: 1
```

```
WBC  6.03  K/uL
NEU  3.14    52.0  %N
LYM  1.91    31.7  %L
MONO .593   9.82  %M
EOS  .350   5.80  %E
BASO .038   .629  %B


RBC  6.65  M/uL
HGB  16.0  g/dL
HCT  44.9  %
MCV  67.5  fL
MCH  24.0  pg
MCHC 35.6  g/dL
RDW  14.7  %


PLT  210.  K/uL
MPV  9.46  fL
```

FIGURE 1.4 Cell-Dyn 3500 hematology analyzer's report for a normal dog, including red blood cell (RBC), and platelet (PLT) histograms and white blood cell (WBC) cytograms. The instrument records information from four different light scatter measurements and combines them in the form of three different scattergrams, two illustrated here. The leukocyte cytogram on the left separates cells on the basis of size (forward angle light scatter) and complexity (narrow angle light scatter; 10°). Lymphocytes fall in the lowest, large cluster, with basophils, when present, slightly to the right. Monocytes fall in the cluster above lymphocytes. Orthogonal light scatter (90°) is used to further separate neutrophils from mononuclear cells, with eosinophils identified by their scatter pattern in response to 90° depolarized light (scattergram not shown). (Illustration provided by Dr. Lois Roth, Department of Pathology, Angell Memorial Animal Hospital.)

tion needed to identity additional important abnormalities such as a left shift, neutrophil toxicity, spherocytosis, Heinz bodies, or the presence of blasts, mast cells, microfilaria, or RBC parasites.

MANUAL TECHNIQUES

In an emergency setting, determination of an animal's hematologic status can be practically and economically assessed through microscopic examination of a blood smear in conjunction with determination of a PCV and a manual WBC count. These techniques, which require only a microhematocrit centrifuge, a hemacytometer and a good quality microscope, have been described in detail elsewhere.[10,11] A hemacytometer is an extremely flexible tool that can be used to count not only peripheral blood cells but also cells in serous cavity effusions, cerebrospinal fluid, and various other cell suspensions. The Unopette System (Becton Dickinson, Rutherford, NJ) provides a convenient method for diluting a specimen and lysing RBC prior to WBC and platelet counting. Unopettes containing phloxin B dye are widely used for performing avian WBC counts. PCV, as determined with a microhematocrit, is determined by both the number and the size of RBC. The presence of many macrocytic RBCs increases the PCV. Knowledge of both the PCV and the RBC count can be used to calculate RBC MCV with the equation: $(PCV \times 10)/RBC = MCV$ (fL). This parameter can be useful in classifying types of anemia.

Hgb concentration can also provide a sensitive and consistent means of identifying anemia and can also be used to calculate MCH (Hgb/RBC $\times$ 10) and MCHC (Hgb/PCV $\times$ 100). These parameters are particularly useful in documenting hypochromasia caused by iron deficiency. Historically, manual Hgb determinations were rarely performed in the veterinary clinic because of the cumbersome nature of the assay. The introduction of hand-held hemoglobinometers has simplified this assay, allowing screening to be performed in either the office or the field. This is particularly useful for mobile veterinarians and large-animal practitioners. Accurate Hgb levels can be determined with the HemoCue (HemoCue, Inc., Mission Viejo, CA). This instrument uses a modified azide methemoglobin reaction. Capillary action is used to draw 10 μL of whole blood into a microcuvette containing dry reagents with which blood is spontaneously mixed. The microcuvette is then placed into the photometer, and absorbance values are measured at two wavelengths (565 and 880 nm). The second absorbance measurement is used to compensate for any sample turbidity. Results are calculated and digitally displayed within 30 to 60 seconds. Results have been shown to be comparable, and even superior, to those obtained with the traditional cyanmethemoglobin method because of the ability to correct for the effects of sample turbidity.[12,13] Instrument precision is good, although filled cuvettes must be closely inspected for air bubbles; the presence of these air bubbles leads to erroneous results. A control cuvette is provided for checking photometer function daily. Abnormal patient results justify a full CBC to better define the nature of the problem.

Hand-held point-of-care (primarily clinical chemistry) analyzers such as the I-Stat (Sensor Devices, Inc., Waukesha, WI) and the IRMA Blood Analysis System (Diametrics Medical, Saint Paul, MN) use electrochemical sensors to measure both various chemical analytes in a whole blood sample, as well as HCT (%RBC). From this value, Hgb is calculated. This calculation assumes RBC indices are normal. These instruments use cartridges, each designed to perform a battery of assays on a small volume of whole blood. Individual assays are not possible.

Systematic microscopic examination of a blood smear includes estimated WBC and platelet counts, a differential leukocyte count, and evaluation of RBC and WBC morphologic features. The accuracy of the differential count depends on the quality of the smear, and the technologist's skill and is further influenced by the area of the smear examined, the number of cells counted, and the number of each cell type present. A significant amount of practice and a familiarity with species differences is needed to develop expertise and an ability to identify the wide range of abnormalities that can appear. Detailed information on blood smear evaluation is published elsewhere[10] and atlases are available that illustrate normal and abnormal blood cells in various species.[14,15]

LABORATORY ERROR

Some of the smaller, automated instruments available require few technical skills to obtain patient results, whereas the more sophisticated instruments require a greater level of technical expertise to ensure optimal instrument function and to analyze instrument flags on samples. In both cases, the accuracy and clinical relevance of tests results depend on the quality of both the specimen and the analytic method, and it is important to understand the factors that can lead to inaccuracies in patient results. Test result variation can be caused by either preanalytical or analytical sources of error. Preanalysis errors occur during sample collection, separation, and storage and can be caused by factors such as excess ethylenediamine tetra-acetic acid (EDTA) and in vitro hemolysis. Errors can also be caused by the choice of anticoagulant. Heparin is generally less useful for hematologic testing because it does not prevent platelet aggregation and can alter leukocyte morphologic features on a blood smear. EDTA, however, causes severe hemolysis and lysis of some WBC types in some species of reptiles (e.g., turtles, tortoises) and birds (e.g., ostriches, emus, jays, raptors); heparin is the preferred anticoagulant in these species. In some mammalian samples the anticoagulant, especially EDTA, induces clumping of platelets, RBCs, and WBCs, resulting in artificially decreased counts. Results are also affected by sample deterioration caused by a delay in analysis. Because of their short life span, platelet counts are most accurate when determined within 4 to 6 hours after collection. In addition, platelets have a tendency to clump over time, in spite of the presence of an anticoagulant, further invalidating the platelet count. Leukocyte morphologic features are also affected by sample age, with nuclear pyknosis and fragmentation the most obvious change. EDTA-induced nuclear swelling can result in an increased percentage of bands on a microscopic differential count or an instrument flag, suggesting the presence of immature cells. These changes may prevent accurate identification of leukocytes with either manual or automated methods.

Analysis errors can be the result of operator error or instrument malfunction and can occur randomly or consistently. Operator errors are more common with manual methods, and it is important that analysts are well trained in the techniques used. Examples of operator errors that can occur with automated hematology systems include improper sample dilution, use of outdated reagents or control material, and improper instrument calibration.

Errors can also be caused by problems inherent to the sample. Most Hgb assays are falsely elevated by increased sample turbidity. This includes factors such as hemolysis, lipemia, increased plasma proteins, or cell stroma caused by severe leukocytosis or the presence of numerous large Heinz bodies.[16] Lipemia, when severe, can also increase the platelet count or, occasionally, the WBC count.

As mentioned above, instruments optimized for human samples, particularly those with electronic resistance (impedance) technology, may fail to identify the smaller RBCs present in many domestic species (cats, cows, horses, sheep), falsely reporting anemia. With impedance counters, the overlap in size between RBC and platelets can result in an overestimated RBC count and an inaccurate platelet count. This is a particular problem in cats because of their unusually large platelets and small RBCs. Alternatively, the presence of abnormally small RBCs can result in falsely elevated platelet counts.[17] These problems can often be detected through examination of the platelet histogram, which shows a shoulder extending into the RBC compartment. Comparison of PCV and HCT can serve as a simple quality-control check for hematology analyzers. Automated instruments measure MCV and calculate the HCT by multiplying the RBC count by the MCV. Differences between PCV and HCT may signal inaccuracies in the RBC count or in the MCV.[18]

WBC counts can be falsely increased by lipemia or by the presence of NRBC. The RBC of some animals are resistant to the lysing solutions used before WBC counts. Residual RBC stroma may be included in the subsequent WBC count, causing it to be falsely increased. This has been reported to be a particular problem with bovine, feline[1] and some rodent (personal observation) samples. This problem can be exacerbated by the presence of increased numbers of polychromatophilic RBCs.

Platelet clumping is a common cause of falsely decreased platelet counts. Because of the frequency of this problem in cats and cows, automated platelet counts should be viewed with suspicion in these species. The presence of platelet clumps can also interfere with the WBC count. Large clumps may be included in the WBC count, causing a false increase, whereas platelet trapping of leukocytes may cause the WBC count to be decreased.[19] In some cases, platelet clumping appears to be triggered by EDTA, and collecting the sample into sodium citrate can alleviate the problem.[20] Platelet clumping can also be a problem with heparin and, to a lesser extent, other anticoagulants.

Regardless of the hematology system used, microscopic blood smear evaluation remains essential as a quality-control check. Platelets and WBCs should be evaluated for any tendency to clump, and estimated counts should be compared with automated values. Automated differential leukocyte counts vary in accuracy, depending on the sophistication of the instrument, but even the most sophisticated systems remain unable to detect abnormalities such as bands, toxic granulocyte, atypical cells (blasts, mast cells), microfilaria, or NRBCs accurately. Although many hematology instruments attempt to signal the presence of abnormal cells, these flags are imperfect and should only be used to indicate the need for further investigation. Abnormal RBCs findings such as spherocytes, Heinz bodies, or blood-cell parasites also go undetected. These problems can often be ruled out by brief microscopic examination of a blood smear.

IN-CLINIC USE OF AUTOMATED HEMATOLOGY INSTRUMENTS

Purchasing an automated blood counting system is a large capital expense that carries with it maintenance, supply, and personnel costs. One should carefully review all of these factors before purchasing any type of laboratory equipment. It is important to look beyond the cost of the instrument and to consider the costs of personnel, supplies, quality control, and maintenance. Calculation of replacement labor should be included because purchase of equipment often requires a shift of available personnel and possibly new hires to accommodate the increased in-house workload. As with any instrumentation, trained operators are required regardless of the simplicity of operation. It is important that a trained clinician or experienced technologist be responsible for supervising all aspects of in-house laboratory testing. Hematology analyzers require rigorous quality control to assure that results are accurate and consistent, and a working knowledge of quality-assurance and quality-control procedures is necessary to ensure correct results (see Chapter 3, Quality Control). Use of any of these instruments also requires a person competent to prepare and read stained blood smears. When an operator uses an instrument that provides differential leukocyte counts, a procedure should be established determining which blood smears need review. The laboratory arrangement must provide results that are accurate and consistent. Any of these instruments readily provide numbers. The key is to ensure that the numbers are also values that can be relied upon to make good clinical diagnoses.

REFERENCES

1. **Weiser MG.** Modification and evaluation of a multichannel blood cell counting system for blood analysis in veterinary medicine. J Am Vet Med Assoc 1987;190:411–415.
2. **Wardlaw SC, Levine RA.** Quantitative buffy coat analysis. JAMA 1983;249:617–620, 1983.
3. **Levine RA, Hart AH, Wardlaw SC.** Quantitative buffy coat analysis of blood collected from dogs, cats, and horses. J Am Vet Med Assoc 1986;189:670–673.
4. **Hofmann-Lehmann R, Wegmann D, Winkler GC, Lutz H.** Evaluation of the QBC-Vet Autoread haematology system for domestic and pet animal species. Comp Haematol Int 1998;8:108–116.
5. **Davies DT, Fisher GV.** The validation and application of the Technicon H-1 for the complete automated evaluation of laboratory animal haematology. Comp Haem International 1991;1:91–105.
6. **Hennessy M, Buckley TC, Leadon DP, Scott CS.** Automated analysis of blood samples from thoroughbred horses with the Abbott Cell Dyn 3500 (CD3500) haematology analyser. Comp Haematol Int 1998;8:150–158.
7. **Tvedten H.** Multi-species hematology atlas: Technicon H 1e system interpretation of results. Tarrytown, New York: Miles, Inc, 1993a.
8. **Zelmanovic D, Hetherington EJ.** Automated analysis of feline platelets in whole blood, including platelet count, mean platelet volume, and activation state. Vet Clin Pathol 1998;27:2–9.
9. **Chapman ES, Hetherington EJ, Zelmanovic D.** A simple automated method for determining ex-vivo platelet activation status. Blood 1996;88:2929.
10. **Jain NC.** Hematologic techniques. In: Schalm's veterinary hematology. 4th ed. Philadelphia: Lea & Febiger, 1986;46–51.
11. **Knoll JS, Rowell SL.** Clinical hematology: in-clinic analysis, quality control, reference values, and system selection. Vet Clin North Am 1996;26:981–1002.
12. **Nicholls P.** An evaluation of the HemoCue™ for correcting the haemoglobin value of lipaemic samples. Med Lab Sci 1990;47:226–229.
13. **Von Schenck H, Falkensson M, Lundberg B.** Evaluation of "HemoCue," a new device for determining hemoglobin. Clin Chem 1986;32:526–529.
14. **Hawkey CM, Dennett TB.** Color atlas of comparative veterinary hematology, Ames, Iowa: Iowa State University Press, 1989.
15. **Reagan WJ, Sanders TG, DeNicola DB.** Veterinary hematology: atlas of common domestic species. Ames, Iowa: Iowa Sate University Press, 1998.
16. **Creer MH, Ladenson J.** Analytical errors due to lipemia. Lab Med 1983;14:351–355.
17. **Tvedten H.** Advanced hematology analyzers. Interpretation of results. Vet Clin Pathol 1993b;22:72–80.
18. **Crawford JM, Lau YR, Bull B.** Calibration of hematology analyzers. Role of the microhematocrit. Arch Pathol Lab Med 1987;11:324–327.
19. **Schalm O, Tvedten HW, Wilkins RJ.** Automated blood cell counting systems: a comparison of the Coulter S-Plus IV, OrthoELT-8/DS, Ortho ELT-8/WS, Technicon H-1, and Sysmex E-5,000. Vet Clin Path 1988;17:47–54.
20. **Hillyer CD, Knopf AN, Berkman EM.** EDTA-dependent leukoagglutination. Am J Clin Pathol 1990;94:458–461.

CHAPTER 2

Reference Values

• JOHN H. LUMSDEN

Patient observations (test results) are interpreted in relation to observations predetermined for individuals that have specific diseases or disorders[1,2] or alternatively, to clinically healthy individuals.[3] When observations made for individuals that have a confirmed disease or disorder are examined at defined cut points or decision limits, predictive values of a positive or negative test, or likelihood ratios, can be calculated. These cut points can then be used to assist clinical interpretation and diagnosis of patients that have similar signalment and differential diagnoses.[1,2] When such predictive values or likelihood ratios have not been predetermined for a suspected disease or disorder, the clinician must compare the patient observations with the lower and upper limits expected from healthy individuals, traditionally called normal values. Because the influence of analytical methods and the patient demographics can be significant, the appropriateness of recommended limits for normal values must be validated within each laboratory.

TERMINOLOGY

Use of terminology is not uniform at this time. The definition of normal is frequently misunderstood.[1,2,4] The guidelines developed and proposed by the International Federation of Clinical Chemists (IFCC) are recommended.[5] Reference observations (test results) are determined for samples collected from healthy individuals (reference individuals) with described procedures for sample collection, handling, and analytical and statistical methods. The reference interval as defined by the lower and the upper reference limits is calculated to include a desired percentage of reference observations, usually the central 95%, as expected limits for clinically healthy individuals. These calculated or observed lower and upper limits may be reliable estimates for the population. If the data allows, which depends on the distribution as well as the number of observations, a confidence interval may be calculated for these limits, e.g., 0.90 confidence interval. The 0.90 confidence interval indicates the range in estimated limits that might be expected if another group of similar reference individuals

were sampled and the lower and the upper reference limits determined with 0.90 probability. Use of the term reference range is discouraged because range in statistical terminology is a single number, i.e., 6 is the range between 8 and 14. Reference values is used as a collective term to include all reference data.

REFERENCE INDIVIDUALS

Individuals used for reference should approximate as closely as possible the demographics of the patient case load presented to the clinical laboratory. Ideally, subsets of individuals that have a defined state of health are selected to provide representation for species, age, sex, dietary, and management and production factors. For some species breed must be considered, e.g., hot- and cold-blooded horses. Neonates, maturing, mature, and geriatric individuals may have differences of clinical significance for one or more variables. Practically, at least one, but preferably more than one, defined subset is chosen for study for each species. Either, an attempt is made to include individuals to represent all subjects of interest, or, individuals are chosen from a selected subgroup. For example, warm-blooded horses might include several breeds, age, sex, training condition, and so forth, or this category might be restricted to standardbred horses in racing condition. Clinically healthy animals from one breeding colony or dairy are not ideal, but, if informed, the clinician can consider possible bias. If reference observations are obtained from healthy animals presented for routine vaccination or neutering, age-related factors must be considered. Compared with adult animals, dogs less than 1 year of age have lower erythrocytes, hemoglobin concentration, and erythrocyte indices; a possible increase in absolute lymphocyte count that results in a decreased neutrophil to lymphocyte ratio; and an increase in serum alkaline phosphatase activity and phosphorus concentration. If the source of reference individuals is described, the clinician can make allowance for potential influences on the lower and the upper reference limits provided by the laboratory.

SAMPLE SIZE

How many observations must be obtained? There are some basic principles involved. Many more observations are needed to estimate the true lower and upper reference limits than are needed to estimate the population mean with the same degree of confidence.[3,5-9] The observed range appears to be the best estimate of the lower and the upper reference limits until the observations exceed 40.[3] The IFCC[5] and the National Committee for Clinical Laboratory Standards[10] (NCCLS) recommend sample sizes of at least 100 to 120, especially if the data is examined with nonparametric analysis. As the sample size increases to more than $n = 120$, there is decreasing improvement in the reliability of the estimated lower and upper limits. When the reference observations do not have a Gaussian distribution, nonparametric analysis must be used to estimate the 2.5 and the 97.5 percentiles, which define the central 95% reference interval.[3,5] If the reference observations have a Gaussian distribution, parametric analysis can be used to determine the reference limits, where the mean $+/-2$ SD includes the central 95%. The 0.90 confidence intervals for the lower and the upper reference limits are approximately similar for 60 observations with a Gaussian distribution allowing parametric analysis as would be expected for 100 to 120 observations if data are skewed and require use of nonparametric analysis.[7,11]

Practically, the number of reference observations must be sufficiently large before the 0.90 confidence interval can be readily determined for the lower and upper limit.[3,5,11] Size requirement varies with the distribution of the data.[3,5,9] Confidence intervals for the central 95% reference lower and upper limits are seldom reported. When determined, they do provide insight into the expected reliability of the reference limits for that subset of reference individuals. Patient observations within the confidence interval may suggest disorder or disease. Access to expected reliability of the reference limits is especially useful when a new method is introduced or assessed in a teaching environment and when data are interpreted from a new laboratory.

Obtaining the recommended number of observations is both challenging and expensive,[12] especially for veterinary laboratories. Initially, effort should be concentrated on determining adequate observations for one defined subset of primary clinical interest for each species. Trends caused by age, stage of lactation, training, and so forth can be extrapolated from the scientific literature or obtained from the mean values observed for smaller studies. If the observations available are limited, e.g., 30, the low number of reference observations should not lead to misinterpretation of laboratory results for most disorders or diseases, providing the clinician is informed about the potential reliability of the reference limits and the source of reference individuals. Conversely, when the reliability of reference limits either is not provided or is overestimated, there is increasing potential for misinterpretation and risk to the patient.

ANALYTICAL METHODS

Reference observations, i.e., test values, can be affected by method, instrument, and reagent source, as well as by source of reference individuals. Description of the sample collection and handling procedures, instrumentation, and methodology should be provided on request to users or should, preferably, be published with the laboratory reference values. For example, were all monogastric reference individuals fasted overnight? What was the minimum and the maximum time interval between collection and testing? For hematology tests, calculated hematocrit often differs from packed cell volume, depending on the calibration of multichannel instruments; manual leukocyte values differ from automated differentials and between instruments.

STATISTICAL ANALYSES

Guidelines are published by the IFCC[3,5] and the NCCLS[10] for establishing reference intervals in laboratory medicine. Most statistical procedures described in the scientific literature are feasible with available computer programs.

A simple approach is outlined. The initial step is to order and examine all observed absolute values, including a histogram, for kurtosis, skewness, and outliers.[3] The handling of outliers remains controversial.[3,5,12] If an outlier is suspected at the time of initial recording of hematology analyte observations, the analysis can be repeated immediately on the same sample to rule out analytical error. Many mathematical tests for outliers have low sensitivity. If an outlier is observed, data should be reviewed to exclude a reporting error, undetected clinical disease, and so forth. Removal of outliers should be noted, including whether one data point, or all data, from the reference individual is removed. If during examination of the reference observations some variables are suggestive of subclinical disorder or disease, a decision must be made to remove either all observations from that individual or only those variables that are unexpected. For example, an unexpected increase in globulin may be observed in clinically healthy research cats. The decisions made and actions taken should be recorded and accessible to users.

With 40 or fewer reference observations, the lowest and the highest observed values are often the best estimations of the central 95% reference interval.[3] A method has been proposed, including robust transformation, for the estimation of reference intervals for data sets with small numbers of observations of where outliers are present.[12]

With 50 to 60 or more reference observations, the data set is examined for Gaussian distribution.[3,5,7] If the data are Gaussian, parametric analysis is used to calculate the lower and the upper reference limits and, if possible, 0.90 confidence intervals. If the data is non-Gaussian, various transformations can be examined. If Gaussian distribution is attained by transformation, parametric

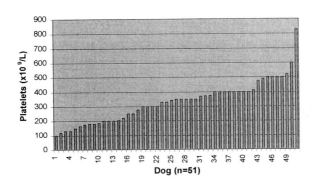

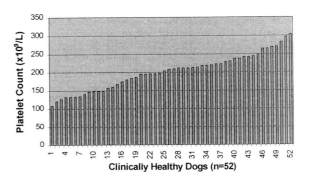

CANINE PLATELET LOWER REFERENCE LIMITS			
Platelet Count (x10 9/L)	n	Lower Limit	Confidence Interval (p 0.90)
Manual[1]	51[3]		
Non-parametric		106	***_***[5]
Parametric		102	71-138
Bootstrap		112	93-131
Technicon H-1[2]	52[4]		
Non-parametric		113	***_***
Parametric		115	103-127
Bootstrap		116	105-128

1 Conditioned dogs (Can J Comp Med 1979; 43: 125-131)
2 Clinically healthy dogs used to determined Reference Values for Animal Health Laboratory, University of Guelph, 1998.
3 All 51 observations included.
4 An observation of 61 removed based upon evidence for clumping visible during microscopic examination of tip of blood film.
5 Unable to estimate.

FIGURE 2.1 Manual and Technicon H-1 platelet counts of clinically healthy dogs.

analysis can be used and the calculated limits of the transformed data retransformed to initial units. If there are sufficient observations, percentiles can be calculated without concern for data distribution. Similarly, if the number of observations is sufficient and if the data allow, confidence intervals are calculated to indicate the expected variation in reference limits that might be expected if another group of individuals were examined.

Bootstrapping and additional methods for examination of the data increase the precision for estimating reference limits and the 0.90 confidence intervals.[3] A DOS-based program is available that incorporates the IFCC-recommended procedures, particularly the use of bootstrapping and the calculation of 0.90 confidence intervals for the central 95% reference limits.[13] The Analyse-it Clinical Laboratory statistics module for Microsoft Excel (http://www.analyse-it.com) includes statistical programs for method comparison and evalua-

tion, as well as parametric and non-parametric methods for calculating reference intervals. Figure 2.1 illustrates platelet counts observed from clinically healthy dogs. Blood samples were collected by experienced veterinarians and preserved in ethylenediamine tetra-acetic acid (EDTA), and platelet counts were determined within 2 hours. Manual counts were determined in duplicate with a hemocytometer calibrated by the Dominion Bureau of Standards.[14] Examination was made for gross or microscopic evidence for platelet clumping. One observation of 61×10^9/L was rejected on the basis of microscopic evidence for platelet clumping.

REFERENCE VALUES FOR NEW METHODS

The initial development and upgrading of reference values are a continuous requirement in a clinical diagnostic laboratory. New instruments and reagents are routinely introduced. Patient demographics may change. The source of the reference individuals; sample size; what the limits describe, i.e., central 90% or 95%; and the statistical analyses used for determining reference limits should be examined carefully for manufacturers' suggested normals. If there is an opportunity, use least-squares and orthogonal regression[15] (see Chapter 4, Validation of Diagnostic Tests in Hematology Laboratories) to compare the new method with the old. After regression analysis of paired observations, the estimated lower and upper limits for the new method can be used as temporary reference limits to assist in interpretation of patient observations until de novo reference intervals are determined. Use of regression is practical and often necessary to facilitate introduction of a new method. Confirmation of the reliability of the estimated lower and upper reference limits is necessary. Application of this comparative approach is of concern when the clinician is uninformed or if subsequent effort is not made to validate appropriate reference limits for the new method.

USE OF HOSPITAL DATABASE FOR ESTIMATING REFERENCE LIMITS

Alternative approaches are proposed for establishing reference values with the hospital database.[16-18] Further validation of these procedures is needed. An alternative to establishing reference limits has been proposed and is used in one teaching institution. Patient values are reported as a percentile of previous patient observations.[19]

ADDITIONAL INFLUENCES

An experienced clinician considers additional sources of variation in reported patient values. These include physiologic factors, caused by excitement of the patient, and sampling errors, such as lipidemia resulting from collection during the postprandial period. The interferences caused by bilirubinemia, hemoglobinemia, medication, and the like are not documented for hematologic methods to the extent that they have been for clinical chemistry methods.[20]

If a clinician assumes that the laboratory reference limits are an approximation, there is a low probability for overinterpretation of small increases or decreases in patient test results. Less-experienced clinicians may interpret small changes as significant when observation is still within the 0.90 confidence interval for the central 90% or 95% reference limits unless they are informed

and understand how the reference intervals were established. Also, the clinician must consider the probability of an additional small increase or decrease caused by chance, i.e., 5 % probability of any value from a clinically healthy individual to be an additional one standard deviation above or below the reported reference limits.[4] Conversely, if the reference interval has been carefully determined, small changes, especially for related variables, should be considered if not otherwise explained. In addition, the reliability of reference limits influences the results of retrospective studies of patient records, especially in relation to prevalence of either increase or decrease, in analyte values with specific disorders or diseases.

REFERENCES

1. **Kraemer HC.** Evaluating medical tests: objective and quantitative guidelines. Newbury Park, California: SAGE Publications, 1992.
2. **Sackett DL, Haynes RB, Guyatt GH, Tugwell P.** Clinical epidemiology: a basic science for clinical medicine. 2nd ed. London: Little, Brown and Company, 1991.
3. **Solberg HE.** Establishment and use of reference values. In: Burtis CA, Ashwood ER, eds. Tietz textbook of cinical chemistry. 2nd ed. London: W.B. Saunders, 1994;454–484.
4. **Galen RS.** Statistics. In: Sonnenwirth AC, Jarett L, eds. Gradwohl's clinical laboratory methods and diagnosis. 8th ed. St Louis: C.V. Mosby, 1980;41–68.
5. **Solberg HE.** The theory of reference values. Part 5. Statistical treatment of collected reference values–determination of reference limits. J Clin Chem Clin Biochem 1983;21:749–760.
6. **Lott JA, Mitchell LC, Moeschberger ML, Sutherland DE.** Estimation of reference ranges: how many subjects are needed? Clin Chem 1992;38:648–650.
7. **Lumsden JH, Mullen K.** On establishing reference values. Can J Comp Med 1978;42:293–301.
8. **Altman DG.** Practical statistics for medical researchers. London: Chapman & Hall, 1991.
9. **Harris EK, Boyd JC.** Statistical bases of reference values in laboratory medicine. New York: Marcel Dekker, 1995;35–39.
10. **National Committee for Clinical Laboratory Standards.** How to define, determine, and utilize reference intervals in the clinical laboratory. NCCLS Document C28-P. ISBN 1-56238-143-1, 1992.
11. **Gardner MJ, Altman DG.** Statistics with confidence–confidence intervals and statistical guidelines. Belfast: University Press, 1989.
12. **Horn PS, Pesce AJ, Copeland BE.** A robust approach to reference interval estimation and evaluation. Clin Chem 1998;44:622–631.
13. **Solberg HE.** RefVal: a program implementing the recommendations of the International Federation of Clinical Chemistry on the statistical treatment of reference values. Comp Methods Programs Biomed 1995;48:247–250.
14. **Lumsden JH, Mullen K, McSherry BJ.** Canine hematology and biochemistry references values. Can J Comp Med 1979;43:125–131.
15. **Altman DG, Bland JM.** Measurements in medicine: the analysis of method comparison studies. The Statistician 1983;32:307–317.
16. **Baadenhuijsen H, Smit JC.** Indirect estimation of clinical chemical reference intervals from total hospital patient data: application of a modified Bhattacharya procedure. J Clin Chem Clin Biochem 1985;23:829–839.
17. **Kouri T, Kairisto V, Virtanen A, Uusipaikka E, Rajamaki A, Finneman H, Juva K, Koivula T, Nanto V.** Reference intervals developed from data for hospitalized patients: computerized method based upon combination of laboratory and diagnostic data. Clin Chem 1994;40:2209–2215.
18. **Solberg HE.** Using a hospitalized population to establish reference intervals: pros and cons. Clin Chem 1994;40:2205–2206.
19. **Little CJL, Gettinby G, Irvine D.** Rarity indices for clinical chemistry data based upon distributions found in a large veterinary hospital database. In: Lumsden JH, ed. Proceedings of the Fifth Congress of the International Society for Animal Clinical Biochemistry. Ontario: University of Guelph, 1994.
20. **Jacobs RM, Lumsden JH, Grift E.** Effects of bilirubinemia, hemolysis, and lipemia on clinical chemistry analytes in bovine, equine, and feline sera. Can Vet J 1992;33:605–608.

CHAPTER 3

Quality Control

• JOHN H. LUMSDEN

Every laboratory test should provide the clinician with trustworthy answers that assist in diagnosis or management of a patient. Quality-control procedures are designed (a) to eliminate errors and resulting consequences, (b) to eliminate repeat analyses and wasted resources, and (c) to assist in achieving these goals at the lowest possible cost.[1] Traditional quality-control methods are effective for detecting systematic error caused by instrument calibration or reagents but are ineffective for detecting other errors, such as sporadic errors, especially those encountered in low-volume laboratories.[1-3] Quality-assurance or total quality management programs are needed to reduce and to monitor other preanalytical, postanalytical, and analytical errors.[1,4-6] A major source of laboratory error occurs owing to mistakes[1] that may be detected by use of traditional quality-control and quality-assurance protocols.[1,3] A conscientious effort is required by each participant to prevent, or detect, all sources of laboratory error.[1] This includes laboratory persons indicating when errors may be suspect because of sample quality or the presence of potential interferences, such as hemolysis and, conversely, clinicians providing immediate feedback when errors are suspected.

Veterinary clinical diagnostic laboratories are not subjected to the legislative and the licensing requirements that apply to medical diagnostic laboratories, although the requirement for quality results is similar. In some aspects, quality results may be more difficult to attain in a veterinary diagnostic laboratory owing to the significant species differences and the use of instrumentation designed for human blood. Consultative and legislated management and quality-control protocols have been developed for medical diagnostic laboratories.[5,7] Similar standard operating procedures should be used throughout veterinary diagnostic laboratories. Although it has been suggested that clinical laboratory quality control is a costly process now out of control,[8] veterinary diagnostic laboratories currently can choose to use those aspects of quality control that are most cost beneficial to the needs of a particular laboratory. The minimum objective is to do whatever is necessary to assure that results reported to the clinician are useful and reliable.

Routine cellular hematology analyses use manual techniques, single or multichannel instruments based on the principle of impedance, multichannel instruments in which flow cytometry is used, or centrifugation with buffy coat analysis.[9] Cellular hematology includes those procedures used for the counting and sizing of blood cells and the determining of hemoglobin concentration, hematocrit, and erythrocyte indices. Cytohematology has been designated as the procedure used to characterize blood cell morphology, particularly in respect to automated leukocyte differentiation.[10] Cellular hematology quality-control protocols, and reagent sources, are better developed than those available for cytohematology.

QUALITY ASSURANCE

The basic principles of laboratory operation are similar in small offices and in large diagnostic laboratories.[2,4] Standard operating procedures should be written and available in a format that is understood by the least-qualified or least-experienced technologist or clinician. Instrument calibration and maintenance, as defined by the manufacturer, should be followed closely. When new instruments are introduced, the methods and reagents must be validated for each animal species (see Chapter 4, Validation of Diagnostic Tests in Hematology Laboratories). Quality assurance within a diagnostic laboratory includes the development and publication of guidelines that describe the procedures used to monitor all aspects of collecting, submitting, and identifying samples; of operating procedures, including instrument maintenance, reagent source, sample analysis; and of recording and reporting results.[5,7]

Because sample quality is a major contributor to analytical errors, directions for sample collection, submission, and storage must be provided to clinicians. Within the laboratory, sample hemolysis is sometimes visible when manual is used, but not during multichannel instrumentation. If severe, the clinician may detect microclotting by visually examining the whole blood sample, but if mild, microscopic examination of a prepared slide or a wet-mount preparation is required for confirmation.[9] The fibrin aggregates that form during microclotting can lead to many errors. For example, fibrin plugs, with or without platelet aggregation, may create tube or aperture obstruction that can cause false high or low counts, depending on the method used. Platelet microclumping can create error in cell counts and in altered erythrocyte indices. Protocols should be established within each laboratory describing the criteria for addressing and reporting potential influence of sample quality on reliability of reported values.

QUALITY CONTROL

Quality-control is used to address those procedures used to monitor analytical accuracy and precision[11] (imprecision or repeatability; see Chapter 4). Accuracy, the true value, depends primarily on instrument calibration, providing the method has been validated for the species. The clinician determines method precision, or repeatability, by examination of the observations obtained from repeated analyses of representative samples. The repeatability is expressed in absolute values as standard deviation (SD) or as a percentage related to the mean value by the coefficient of variation (CV) [where CV = mean/SD × 100]. As the mean concentration increases, the absolute variation or SD usually increases while the CV decreases. By repeated analyses of control samples within-run, between-run, and between-day precision may be determined (see Chapter 4) and provided to users as the method CV at low, normal, or high mean concentrations. Also, the method CV varies with the method and instrumentation. The acceptable CV for manual methods or single-cell counters is significantly higher than for state-of-the art, multichannel hematology instruments. For erythrocyte counts an acceptable CV may be 10% for manual counts or single-cell counters but 3% to 5% for multichannel instruments. For leukocyte counts the CV may be 20% for manual methods, 10% for single-cell counters, and an expected 3% to 5% for multichannel instruments, again depending on the mean concentration. The acceptable 1% to 2% CV for packed cell volume is much lower than the CV expected for calculated hematocrit that is influenced by precision of both the erythrocyte count and the mean corpuscular volume (MCV). Conversely, the CV for MCV is much higher when calculated from manual or single-cell counter erythrocyte determinations than if determined directly with multichannel instrumentation.

Within the laboratory, cellular hematology quality control relies primarily on the use of the manufacturer's assayed or known controls.[9] Proprietary methods are used to prepare specimens that simulate blood cells but have increased storage life. Low, intermediate, and high concentrations of each blood component of interest are prepared. The assayed values are predetermined by the manufacturer. Multiple reference laboratories that use similar instrument models and reagent sources may develop the observations used for determining the assayed values. Because of the different principles used for counting, sizing, and differentiating blood cells, assayed controls are valid only for use in similar specific instruments. The assayed values may differ between instrument models from the same manufacturer.

Assayed controls are analyzed prior to patient samples.[9,12] The assayed mean +/−2 SD are the most commonly accepted limits for within laboratory variation, i.e., 95% of observations are expected to occur within these limits. The observed mean value must approximate the assayed mean. At least two concentrations of controls are used daily.[4,9] If assayed control values are within expected limits, it is assumed that the instrument is calibrated correctly and the reagents, instrument, and technologist are functioning as expected. If control values are outside of acceptable limits, patient values are not reported until there is resolution. If no bias exists, there is equal chance of observed control values falling below or above the assayed mean value. The probability that there is bias within a method, i.e., an error in accuracy, increases with each day that there is a consistent increase or decrease in the observed values. This is apparent immediately if multiple controls at one or more level are examined daily but may only become apparent after 4 to 5 days if only one level of control is examined daily.[1,12–15] Various rules are described for detecting unacceptable control values.[11,16,17] When control observations are unacceptable, potential causes must be investigated and resolved. This may require instrument recalibration and verification before patient values are determined and reported.

Charting and statistical analysis of within laboratory observations for control reagents is done manually or is incorporated into software programs for computer-controlled instruments.[18] Levey-Jennings or Cusum charting provides technologists and supervisors immediate visual assessment of within-run and between-day repeatability for each level of control.[19] Historical performance is documented after 20 to 30 control observations are made. If too many observations are included, a false low estimation of method CV is obtained. An increase in the method CV is an indicator for review of possible sources of variation.

To interpret whether there is a biological variation in sequential patient values rather than just changes associated with analytical variation, the clinician must be aware of the method CV at different control levels. One simple guideline suggests that the difference between sequential patient values should be greater than 3 SD before analytical variation is ruled out as the potential source of the difference. Counting and morphological differentiation are additive sources of variation in leukocyte concentration.

Retained patient specimens, in many respects, are an ideal source of control material.[14] Control rules for use of one retained patient specimen, appropriate for use by smaller laboratories, have been described.[14] Shared patient specimens can be used as control samples for satellite instruments.[14] Aliquots of refrigerated bovine and canine ethylenediamine tetra-acetic acid (EDTA) blood have been used, for as long as 1 month, as an independent additional species control for assessing changes in instrument calibration for hemoglobin, erythrocyte count, and MCV. These independent controls were useful for assessing changes observed after recalibration of earlier models of multichannel instruments and after introduction of a new batch of reagents or controls (personal observation).

Each hematology instrument requires specific procedures for calibration as outlined by the manufacturer.[9] Some manufacturers provide preserved blood cell specimens as calibrators, whereas other manufacturers expect the assayed control reagents to be used for instrument calibration. Shelf life is short, often 1 month for control reagents but may be as long as 2 months for calibration reagents. The short shelf life of calibrators, or controls, for hematology methods dictate significant differences in protocols for calibration and quality control compared with clinical chemistry procedures for which standards and lyophilized quality-control reagents with stability for at least 1 year are available. Reliability depends on the manufacturer. Different lot numbers, or source, of assayed controls should be used for daily quality control than are used for calibration. Controls are not interchangeable between instruments owing to the different principles for the methods used by different manufacturers. The mean value obtained from replicate analyses is compared with expected values as an indicator of accuracy for instrument calibration. Background counts are examined as part of the calibration procedure.

Instrument settings may be altered for single-channel or multichannel instruments to accommodate blood cells from certain animal species. Instrument settings can be changed manually for single-channel instruments or by specific software computer programs for multichannel instruments. If the instruments are calibrated with the manufacturer's calibrators or controls, method accuracy for blood cells from each animal species must be confirmed. With new and older validated methods, e.g., hemocytometer, hemoglobinometer, and packed cell volume, fresh blood is used to determine mean observations for each analyte.

Proficiency testing procedures are used to provide independent assessment of within laboratory quality control by use of unknown samples distributed to many laboratories.[9,17,20] Proficiency testing is a component of the accreditation procedure for medical laboratories but is usually voluntary in veterinary hematology laboratories. The values for the unknowns from each participating laboratory controls are forwarded to a central location for statistical analyses and graphical presentation. The mean and range of values are reported for each variable for all methods and according to method or instrumentation. Only the observations from the submitting laboratory are identified as to laboratory origin. These observations provide an unbiased assessment of analytical performance, albeit retrospective. Increasingly, instrument companies provide a similar retrospective analysis of observations for the assayed control reagents observed within a laboratory.[20] Animal source blood distributed by the Veterinary Laboratory Association Quality Assurance Program has been used with varying degrees of performance in veterinary diagnostic laboratories.[21] The control material is of animal origin in the form of a stabilized cell preparation, thus enabling increased stability and shelf life to endure shipping and handling. These controls are not to be used for calibration or internal quality control. Participation in external quality-control programs is voluntary. Cost is a consideration. The cost benefit must be assessed in light of the detection rate and the perceived improvement in quality of patient values.

CYTOHEMATOLOGY

Multichannel instruments use flow-cytometry principles, including impedance, light scatter, and staining, to count and size human blood cells and to differentiate human leukocytes. The high number of cells examined, e.g., 10,000, produce repeatable leukocyte differentials and absolute counts.[22] Software programs have been developed that attempt to allow differentiation of domestic animal leukocytes by use of similar technology. Varying degrees of success are reported.[9] The correlation between automated and microscopic differentiation varies with the instrumentation. Good correlation is reported for some instruments when hematologic values are within reference limits for certain species. The accuracy of abnormal values is less dependable. Instrument graphics, i.e., flagging of one or more analyte values, scattergrams, or buffy coat diagrams for the quantitative buffy coat (QBC) with centrifugation principles, or histograms for flow cytometry instruments must be examined carefully by an experienced technologist or hematologist.[9,23] For the current state-of-the-art instrumentation, if there is any suspicion in regards to cell differentiation, microscopic examination of a stained blood slide should be used for confirmation or correction of patient values. Also, the laboratory management should establish protocols for routine microscopic examination of a predetermined percentage of samples that have no apparent abnormality as part of the quality-assurance program.

In each, laboratory protocols must be established for reporting of automated leukocyte differentials. This will be based on the type of instrumentation, the species involved, experience, and discussion with clinicians. In some laboratories, clinicians are provided with an option for receiving only the automated leukocyte differential, but at a reduced fee. If automated leukocyte values are reported, instrument-specific leukocyte reference limits must be determined for each animal species, preferably in parallel with reference methods, so that clinicians can be informed of the method bias expected for blood cells from both clinically healthy and sick animals.

Conventional methods of quality control cannot be used for multichannel instruments, especially for the automated differential leukocyte counts resulting from lack of standards and generally accepted reference methods for cell enumeration. The instrument graphics output for commercial controls indicates cell distribution. This provides indication of instrument performance, but not necessarily reliability, for the animal species involved. Performance goals have been studied and used to assess performance and cost effectiveness of various quality-control strategies,[7,10,24] Unit-testing devices, such as used for buffy coat analyses, create an additional quality-control challenge.[25]

RETICULOCYTES

Microscopic examination is used to count vitally stained erythrocytes that are then expressed as a percentage or as an absolute concentration. Repeatability is poor unless adequate cells are examined, e.g., >2000 erythrocytes. Technical time and thus cost becomes a limiting factor. Flow-cytometry methods count and differentiate large numbers of erythrocytes and reticulocytes, leading to the precision necessary for reliable monitoring of daily changes in a patient.[26] Use of flow-cytometry methods must be validated in each laboratory, including the establishment of reference limits for a defined population.

BLOOD SLIDE REVIEW

Hematology quality control includes the review of patient hematology reports and the microscopic examination of stained blood slides.[9,23,27] Ideally, all slides are reviewed by another experienced microscopist. Practically, a random selection of slides from individuals that have no apparent abnormalities and all slides from patients that have abnormalities should be reviewed. The standard operating procedures for the laboratory should include criteria for the classification and reporting of cell types and abnormalities. The more common uncertainties include criteria for differentiating maturity of neutrophils and for classifying neutrophil toxic changes and erythrocyte morphologic changes such as acanthocytes. Regular training sessions increase uniformity for reporting, especially for new staff.

REFERENCES

1. **Hinckley MC.** Defining the best quality-control systems by design and inspection. Clin Chem 1997;4:873–879.
2. **Baer DM, Belsey RE.** Limitations of quality control in physicians' offices and other decentralized testing situations: the challenge to develop new methods of test validation. Clin Chem 1993;39:9–12.
3. **Hurst J, Nickel K, Hilborne LH.** Are physicians' office laboratory results of comparable quality to those produced in other laboratory settings? JAMA 1998;279:468–471.
4. **Laessig RH, Ehrmeyer SS, Hassemer DJ.** Quality control and quality assurance. Clin Lab Med 1986;6:317–327.
5. NCCLS GP22-P. Continuous quality improvement: essential management approaches and their use in proficiency testing; proposed guideline. National Committee for Clinical Laboratory Standards, 1997;ISBN 1-56238-324-8 (http://www.nccls.org).
6. **Laessig RH, Ehrmeyer SS.** Quality: the next six months. Clin Chem 1997;43:903–907.
7. **Bachner P, Hamlin W.** Federal regulation of clinical laboratories and the Clinical Laboratory Improvement Amendments of 1988—Part 1. Clin Lab Med 1993;13:739–752.
8. **Howanitz PJ, Tetrault GA, Steindel SJ.** Clinical laboratory quality control: a costly process now out of control. Clin Chim Acta 1997;260:163–174.
9. **Knoll JS, Rowell SL.** Clinical hematology. In-clinic analysis, quality control, reference values, and system selection. Vet Clin North Am Small Anim Pract 1996;26:981–1002.
10. NCCLS H26-A. Performance goals for the internal quality control of multichannel hematology analyzers; approved standard. National Committee for Clinical Laboratory Standards, 1996;ISBN 1-56238-312-4 (http://www.nccls.org).
11. **Williams GW, Schork MA.** Basic statistics for quality control in the clinical laboratory. Crit Rev Clin Lab Sci 1982;17:171–199.
12. **Gulati GL, Hyun BH.** Quality control in hematology. Clin Lab Med 1986;6:675–688.
13. **Koepke JA.** Current practices for quality assurance in laboratory haematology. Clin Lab Haematol 1990;12 Suppl 1:75–81.
14. **Hackney JR, Cembrowski GS.** The use of retained specimens for haematology quality control. Clin Lab Haematol 1990;12 Suppl 1:83–89.
15. **Klee GG.** Performance goals for internal quality control of multichannel haematology analysers. Clin Lab Haematol 1990;Suppl 1:65–74.
16. **Westgard JO, Groth T.** Design and evaluation of statistical control procedures: applications of a computer "quality control simulator" program. Clin Chem 1981;27:1536–1545.
17. **Westgard JO, Bawa N, Ross JW, Lawson NS.** Laboratory precision performance: state of the art versus operating specifications that assure the analytical quality required by clinical laboratory improvement amendments proficiency testing. Arch Pathol Lab Med 1996;120:621–625.
18. **Westgard JO, Stein B, Westgard SA, Kennedy R.** QC Validator 2.0: a computer program for automatic selection of statistical QC procedures for applications in healthcare laboratories. Comput Methods Programs Biomed 1997;53:175–186.
19. **Allison FS.** An historical review of quality control in hematology. Am J Med Technol 1983;49:625–632.
20. **Anderson FC.** Interlaboratory quality assurance program. Clin Lab Haematol 1990;12 Suppl 1:111–116.
21. **Veterinary Laboratory Association Quality Assurance Program.** West Royalty Industrial Park, Charlottetown, PE, Canada C1E 1B0 (http://www.dclchem.com).
22. **Krause JR.** The automated white blood cell differential. A current perspective. Hematol Oncol Clin North Am 1994;8:605–616.
23. **Lewis SM.** Blood film evaluations as a quality control activity. Clin Lab Haematol 1990;12 Suppl 1:119–127.
24. **O'Sullivan MB.** Quality control of multichannel haematology analysers: critique of current methods and the need for performance goals. Clin Lab Haematol 1990;12 Suppl 1:3–12.
25. **Phillips DL.** Quality systems for unit-testing devices. Clin Chem 1997;443:893–896.
26. NCCLS H44-A Methods for reticulocyte counting (flow cytometry and supravital dyes); approved guideline. National Committee for Clinical Laboratory Standards, 1997;H44:ISBN 1-56238-302-7 (http://www.nccls.org).
27. **Koepke JA.** Future directions for quality assurance in laboratory haematology. Clin Lab Haematol 1990;12 Suppl 1:171–176.

CHAPTER 4

Validation of Diagnostic Tests in Hematology Laboratories

• ASGER LUNDORFF JENSEN

A fundamental requirement to a laboratory test is that the test results reflect the status of the animal more than they reflect the variation caused by the laboratory test itself. To investigate, differentiate, grade and/or correct for this, various somewhat complicated procedures and statistical analyses can be used. Here a panel of practical procedures and statistical tests useful for solving problems in hematology laboratories with minimal emphasis on mathematical and statistical details and calculations is presented. Readers interested in the latter are directed to textbook coverage of these aspects.[1,2] In this chapter, strategies useful for investigating technical features of the analysis, such as imprecision, inaccuracy, method comparison, detection limit, and interference, are considered. Second, strategies for investigating how the test works when it is applied to healthy and to sick animals (e.g., reference intervals, sensitivity, specificity, predictive values, and receiver-operating-characteristic [ROC] curves) are outlined. Finally, a description is given of how to generate and to use data on biologic variation (i.e., within- and between-animal variation), for example, to assess the usefulness of population-based reference intervals, to set desirable goals for analytical performance, and to estimate the difference needed between two serial test results to be significant. Several commercial computer programs that assist in the statistical analyses are available. This author most frequently uses GraphPad Prism (GraphPad Software, Inc., USA, http://www.graphpad.com), MedCalc for Windows (MedCalc Software, Belgium, http://www.medcalc.be), GraphROC for Windows (Veli Kairisto and Allan Poola, Finland, http://www.netti.fi/~maxiw/index.html), and Analyse-It (for Microsoft Excel [Analyse-It Software Ltd. UK, http://www.analyse-it.com]).

Validation of a laboratory test is a common task in clinical laboratories, for instance, when a new test or a new analyzer is introduced. In either case, it is necessary to know whether there might be changes (e.g., in imprecision and inaccuracy) that would likely affect clinical interpretation. In veterinary laboratory medicine, standardized guidelines for test validation are generally lacking; this lack has lead laboratory professionals to use parts of the guidelines used in human laboratory medicine (e.g., the National Committee for Clinical Laboratory Standards [NCCLS; http://www.nccls.org]) or to use guidelines listed in various scientific journals (e.g., Clinical Chemistry—Instructions for Authors; http://www.aacc.org).

In practice, validation is performed by considering analytical performance first and then by observing how the test behaves when it is used on patients (overlap and clinical performance). Prior to the validation procedure, it is important that one is familiar with the test, both theoretically and practically.

Phase 1—Analytical Performance

Assessment of analytical performance should minimally include a description of the test and estimates of imprecision, inaccuracy, and detection limit.

Description of the Laboratory Test

Here a description of the analytical procedure, materials, and equipment necessary for an experienced analyst to obtain a test result is listed. As a minimum the following information should be considered:

- Intended use of the test—e.g., diagnosing a specific disease among sick animals, monitoring therapy, or screening for a specific disease among healthy animals
- Outline of the analytical principle—preferably with references to the literature.
- System requirements—specifications of the analytical instruments and equipment.
- List of reagents—source, brand name, and concentrations in appropriate SI units.
- Specimen requirements—e.g., volume, anticoagulants, and storage.
- Description—complete delineation of all steps in the analytical procedure.

- Process—calibrating procedure and method for calculating test results.
- Control material—source, brand name, concentrations in appropriate SI units, control rules applied together with the probability of error detection and probability of false rejection.
- Safety precautions—e.g., when preparing reagents and disposing of waste.
- Practicability—e.g., time needed for analysis of one specimen when the analyst is not prepared for it, costs, and technical skill requirement.

Imprecision

Imprecision is a measure of the closeness of a series of measurements of the same material (Fig. 4.1). Imprecision is most often expressed in percent as a coefficient of variation (CV) and it is calculated as within-run (within-day; intra-assay) and between-run (between-day; interassay) imprecision. Because imprecision varies with analyte concentration, patient samples with analyte concentrations spanning the analytical range are preferred. Control material can also be used, especially when assessing the between-run imprecision in cases in which the analyte is unstable.

Within-run imprecision can be assessed in two ways, either from the differences between duplicate measurements obtained with several different samples or from the results of several replicate measurements made on the same specimen. A practical approach is to select patient specimens (e.g., 30 to 100) and analyze these in duplicate. The specimens are then divided into three groups (lower, middle, and higher end of the analytical

range) according to their analyte concentration. The mean value and the number of duplicate pairs in each group are recorded. The differences between the duplicates are used to calculate the standard deviation (SD) for each group and eventually, with the mean value of each group, the CV of each group is calculated. An F-test can be used to test whether the SDs differ significantly between the groups. Alternatively, three patient samples with low, middle and high analyte concentrations are measured (e.g., 10 to 30 times) in the same analytical run, and the mean value, the SD, and the CV for each patient sample are calculated. A graphical picture of the imprecision (a precision profile) with the CVs on the y axis plotted against the analyte concentration on the x axis can be constructed after enough samples have been analyzed.

Between-run imprecision is assessed by selection of no less than three patient samples with low, intermediate and high analyte concentrations. The samples are analyzed daily for several days (e.g., 5 to 20 days). The number of replicate measurements is recorded and the mean value, the SD, and the CV for each sample are calculated. During the investigation period, the samples should be stored appropriately, e.g., at 4°C. If the analyte is unstable, control material can be used instead.

Inaccuracy

Inaccuracy (also referred to as bias or accuracy) is generally defined as the agreement between the mean value of a series of measurements on the same material and the true value (Fig. 4.1). It may be difficult to obtain a species-specific specimen with a universally recognized true value, and in practice, inaccuracy is often assessed with spiking recovery, linearity check, control material, or comparison of analytical methods.

Spiking Recovery and Linearity Check

In spiking recovery, the analyte concentration is measured in duplicate in patient samples before and after the addition of known amounts of the analyte. Alternatively, patient samples with known analyte concentrations are mixed in various ratios, and the analyte concentration in the mixtures is measured in duplicate. In linearity check, the analyte concentration is measured in duplicate in patient samples before and after dilutions with an appropriate diluent (e.g., physiologic saline or zero calibrator).

The percentages of the measured analyte concentrations compared to the expected analyte concentrations are then calculated. Ideally, these percentages should be approximately 100%. The relation between the measured and the expected analyte concentrations can also be investigated by means of regression analysis of both the untransformed and the logarithmically transformed data. The confidence interval of the slope of the linear regression equation should include 1, thus indicating that recovery is 100%. When necessary, data are logarithmically transformed to achieve homogeneity of the vari-

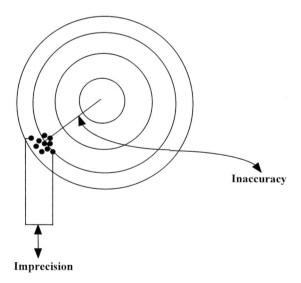

FIGURE 4.1 Imprecision and inaccuracy. The single points represent repeated measurements and the bull's-eye represents the true value. Imprecision is the closeness of a series of measurements on the same material, whereas inaccuracy is the difference between the true value and the mean of a series of measurements of the same material.

ances. The confidence interval of the slope of the logarithmic regression equation should include 1, thereby indicating that recovery is proportional. It is also worthwhile to examine, by use of either the simple Runs-test or the more complex Lack-of-Fit (LOF) test, whether the data follow a straight line.

Control Material

Inaccuracy can be assessed with control material having a value assigned by the manufacturer. Alternatively, one can use the mean of values assayed in specimens by participants in an external quality-assurance scheme. Basically, the control material or the quality-assurance specimens are subjected to replicate (e.g., 20 to 40) measurements. Using a one-sample t test or Wilcoxon Signed Rank test, depending on whether the data are normally distributed, it is tested whether the measured mean (or median) analyte concentration differs from the expected value. The difference between the observed mean (or median) value and the expected mean value is the bias of the analytical method, and it can be expressed in percentages of the expected value.

Comparison of Methods

Essentially, patient samples (e.g., 30 to 100) with analyte concentrations spanning the analytical range are analyzed by two methods, e.g., an automatic lymphocyte or a manual count. Duplicate measurements are preferred because outlying values are more easily identified and because the data set can be used to calculate imprecision also. Initially, a plot of the results (or the means of the duplicate measurements) by one method against the other method together with a line of equality is inspected (Fig. 4.2). This allows for an intuitive assessment of inaccuracy (the eyeball test). If the plot shows a higher degree of scatter at higher values, it may be advisable to transform the data logarithmically. Next, one can construct a difference plot (Altman & Bland plot) by plotting the difference between the methods (A-B) on

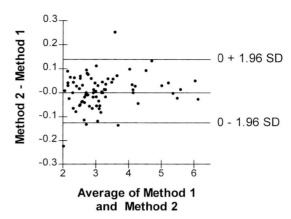

FIGURE 4.3 Method of comparison—difference plot. Several patient specimens with analyte concentrations covering the analytical range are measured by two methods. The difference between the methods on the y axis is plotted against the mean of the methods on the x axis.

the y axis against the mean of the methods ([A+B]/2) on the x axis (Fig. 4.3). If one method is considered a reference method, the differences are plotted against test results yielded by this method. Ideally, the two methods should yield identical results, that is, the difference between the methods should on average be zero, a hypothesis that can easily be tested by means of a paired t-test or a Wilcoxon Signed Rank test. To test whether the differences change with analyte concentration, apply linear regression analysis of the differences. With these tests and by inspection of the plot, two common types of inaccuracy (absolute and proportional) can be detected (Figs. 4.4A and 4.4B). Absolute inaccuracy exists when the differences lie at a similar distance above or below the horizontal zero line. Proportional inaccuracy is present when the differences change with analyte concentration. Combined absolute and proportional inaccuracy is also possible (Fig. 4.4C).

Additional analysis of the differences, e.g., after logarithmic transformation of the data or by one's plotting the percentage differences, can be used to study the relation between the two methods further, but frequently, a simple difference plot suffices. Comparing laboratory methods by use of regression and correlation analysis (e.g., least-squares regression, Deming regression, Passing–Bablok regression) may not be useful for assessing inaccuracy because regression and correlation analysis describes the relation (association) between the methods more than it describes the agreement between the methods.[3]

Analytical goals

Acceptable goals for imprecision and inaccuracy are difficult to specify. In many cases, the obtained imprecision CVs are compared to the CVs reported by the manufacturer or the CVs found in scientific literature. A common rule of thumb is that imprecision CV should be below 5%. Tonks[4] suggested that imprecision CV should not

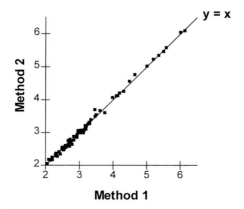

FIGURE 4.2 Method comparison—conventional plot. Several patient specimens with analyte concentrations covering the analytical range are measured by two methods, and the results are displayed in a conventional plot. The line ($y = x$) represents the line of equality.

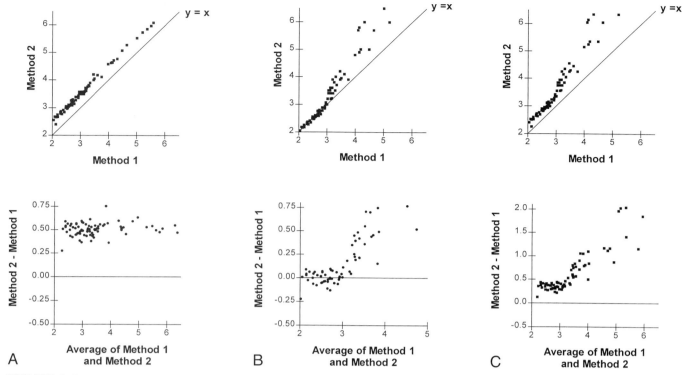

FIGURE 4.4 **(A)** Absolute inaccuracy (bias) is present when the points lie at a similar distance to one side of the line of equality in a conventional plot or at a similar distance below or above the horizontal zero line in the difference plot. **(B)** Proportional inaccuracy (bias) is present when the distance between the points and the line of equality or the horizontal zero line increases with measured values but is negligible at 0. **(C)** Combined inaccuracy (bias) is a mixture of absolute and proportional inaccuracy (bias).

exceed one-eighth of the width of the reference interval expressed as a percentage of the mean of the range. For inaccuracy, it has been suggested that the maximum deviation from a true value should be less than one-sixteenth of the reference interval.[5] If inaccuracy is tested by recovery studies, the percentage recovery should be close to 100%, and the slope of the linear and the logarithmic regression equations should not differ from 1, thereby indicating that the test has linear and proportional recovery. In method comparison studies, the usual goals are that the differences between the two methods do not differ from 0 and that the distribution of the differences (i.e., their mean $\pm 2 \times$ SD) is clinically unimportant, which, to some degree, depends on a subjective decision (see "Generation and Use of Data on Biological Variation" in this chapter). As is described below, more objective goals for imprecision and inaccuracy have also been derived with data on biological variation.[5] Another way of judging whether imprecision and inaccuracy are acceptable is to use total error criteria. This can be accomplished by means of the MEDx chart[6] that provides a simple graphical tool for comparing imprecision and inaccuracy observed for a test with an analytical quality requirement that is stated in form of an allowable total error (Figs. 4.5A and 4.5B). The size of allowable total errors can be derived from data on biologic variation. In many cases, however, a reasonable estimate of the maximum allowable total error can be obtained from

the Clinical Laboratory Improvement Amendments of 1998 (CLIA) proficiency testing criteria.[7]

Detection Limit

The detection limit can be defined as the smallest concentration that the laboratory test, with a stated probability, can distinguish from a suitable blank. A practical approach is to measure a sample with no or with a low content of the analyte (e.g., physiologic saline or a serum sample during investigation of an automated blood cell counter) 20 to 30 times, calculate the mean value and the SD, and estimate the detection limit as mean value (or 0) + 2 (or 3) $\times$ SD. More precise or rigorous calculations are rarely necessary, bearing in mind that the detection limit should serve as a warning limit rather than as a justification for continual use of the test at its lowest analytical level.

Additional Analysis of Analytical Performance

High levels of usual blood contents (e.g., lipids, bilirubin, hemoglobin, and glucose[8] may interfere with the laboratory test, and it may be useful to examine the effects of such substances in greater detail, for instance,

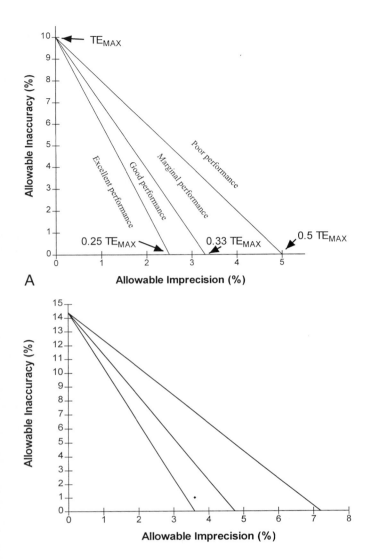

B   • Observed imprecision and inaccuracy

FIGURE 4.5 MEDx chart for assessing analytical performance. **(A)** Shows a MEDx chart for a test with a maximum allowable total error (TE_MAX) of 10%. The lines represent different currently accepted total error criteria (for references, see Westgard 1995): Line marked 0.5 (TE_MAX) represents the total error criterion TE_MAX = Inaccuracy (bias) + 2SD. Line marked 0.33 (TE_MAX) represents the total error criterion TE_MAX = Inaccuracy (bias) + 3SD. Line marked 0.25 (TE_MAX) represents the total error criterion TE_MAX = Inaccuracy + 4SD. TE_MAX can be calculated from data on biologic variation or can be estimated from CLIA proficiency testing criteria. By plotting the observed inaccuracy and imprecision of a test into its MEDx chart, one can classify the analytical performance of the assay as poor, marginal, good, or excellent. **(B)** Displays the MEDx chart for WBC with TE_MAX being calculated as 14.4% (see details in "Generation and Use of Data on Biologic Variation" in this chapter). Inaccuracy and imprecision were estimated for WBC on an automated hematology analyzer as 1% and 3.6%, respectively, and with the MEDx chart, it is concluded that the test has good analytical performance.

by comparing the analyte concentration in patient samples before and after addition of the different amounts of the substances. Unconjugated bilirubin and glucose can be purchased as dry matter, hemoglobin can be obtained by freezing of washed erythrocytes, and lipids can be obtained from human parenteral nutrition prescriptions. Displacement of the analyte from its carrier proteins or the binding of important cofactors are examples of the way in which different medications and diseases may also interfere in the test. In most cases, it is very complicated to examine for potential interference, but significant information can be derived from sources, e.g., Young.[9]

Although not a topic related to analytical performance per se, sources of preanalytical variation such as storage, type of anticoagulants, medication, venous site of blood sampling, and so on may significantly affect test results. Often, investigation of this is valuable.[10,11]

PHASE 2—OVERLAP PERFORMANCE

Initial Test Application

The aim here is to compare test results in healthy animals to various groups of diseased animals. Approximately 20 to 30 animals in each group are tested, and the number of animals in each group together with the mean value (or median value), the SD (or 25 to 75 percentiles), and the minimum and the maximum values are recorded. A plot of the data, e.g., in a dot diagram, allows for an initial visual assessment of the degree of overlap between the groups. Unpaired t-tests or a Mann–Whitney U-test for unpaired observations can be used to test statistically whether test results differ between groups. If a great overlap is detected, the diagnostic value of the assay is usually so low that further evaluation is unnecessary.

It is important to remember that at this initial stage, the prevalence of the disease frequently is unrealistically high and that animals with the disease in question may be in advanced disease stages that are more easy to recognize and, thus, to include in the study. Furthermore, if the group of animals without the disease in question consists of healthy animals only, then the overlap of test values between animals with and without the disease in question is often further minimized.

Reference Intervals

The next step is then to calculate a reference interval. The ideal approach to this task calls for each laboratory to establish reference intervals locally by sampling healthy animals from the population it serves. Traditionally, the reference interval contains the central 95% of test results from an appropriate reference population. Obtaining an appropriate reference population can be difficult because the reference population can be subdivided in many subsets according to sex, age, breed, pregnancy status, lactation, environment, herd, country, health status, laboratory test, and so forth.[12] Usually, however, the reference population consists of a collection of clinically healthy animals of different sexes, ages, breeds etc. that are often selected to encompass the spectrum of the types of animals normally presented in a hospital setting. Thus, when reporting reference intervals, it is important that the number of animals, their characteristics, and the method of calculating the reference interval or intervals are given and that it is understood that a reference interval only serves as a basis for a somewhat intuitive assessment of the biologic information given by the test.

Guidelines for establishing reference intervals in human laboratory medicine have been proposed by the NCCLS and the International Federation of Clinical Chemists[13,14] (IFCC). According to these guidelines, a reference sample group of at least 120 individuals (animals) belonging to the selected reference population should be tested. The reference interval is then calculated so that it contains 95% of the test results. In practice, the reference interval is calculated as the mean value $\pm 1.96 \times SD$. Depending on sample size, skewness of the data, and so on, other ways of calculating the reference interval may be more appropriate, for instance use of the 2.5 to 97.5 percentiles or calculations based on logarithmically transformed data, and one may even calculate confidence intervals for the limits of the reference interval. Another simple way to obtain a reference interval after having collected and analyzed more than 120 samples is to rank the test results from the lowest to the highest value. Outliers are then identified with Reed's criterion,[15] which considers the difference between the extreme value and the next highest (or lowest) value, rejecting the extreme value if this difference exceeds one third the range of all values. Then, values less than 2.5% and greater than 97.5% of the test results are removed.

Because the reference interval is based on the central 95% of the distribution of test results, 5% (or one of 20 tests in a laboratory panel), as a rule of thumb, falls out of the reference interval by chance alone and hence is considered abnormal when the animal may in fact be free of disease. This must be remembered when multiple tests are performed. Also, when test results from a single animal are compared with population-based reference intervals, it is to some degree assumed that the analyte variation in the single animal is equal to the analyte variation in the population. The validity of this assumption can be assessed with data on biologic variation as described later (see "Generation and Use of Data on Biological Variation" in this chapter).

PHASE 3—CLINICAL PERFORMANCE

In phase 3, the clinical usefulness of the laboratory test is investigated. The outcome of this investigation can be seriously biased, e.g., by incorporation of the test under investigation into the evidence used to diagnose the disease in question. Potential sources of bias have been described by Ransohoff and Feinstein.[16] To avoid biasing the outcome of this investigation as much as

| | | Disease | |
		Present	Absent
Test	Positive	A	B
	Negative	C	D

possible, a blind, prospective, and controlled investigation fulfilling the following criteria should be used:

1. Selection of appropriate animals: The clinical usefulness must be evaluated in the relevant clinical target population, i.e., the spectrum of animals for which the disease in question is a possible differential diagnosis and to which the laboratory test is most likely to be applied later. The total number of animals should at least be greater than 40. It is important to specify the criteria for including animals, especially because animals without the disease in question may have diseases that other users of the test do not consider appropriate differential diagnoses.
2. Independent classification of the selected animals: The animals in the clinical target population must be classified as being with or without the disease in question independently of the laboratory test being evaluated. Criteria for establishing the diagnosis in question should be specified.
3. Applying the test to all animals in the study population: Ideally, but rarely practical, the test should be applied at the same point in the animals clinical course.

Sensitivity and Specificity

The test results are then divided into positives and negatives, depending on whether they exceed a predefined limit, usually the upper or the lower limit of the reference interval. The number of positives and negatives for each patient group (with and without the disease) is then arranged in a two-by-two table and sensitivity (SE) (the proportion of patients that have the disease that tests positive) and specificity (SP) (the proportion of patients that do not have the disease that tests negative) are calculated as follows[17]:

$$SE = A/(A + C) \text{ and } SP = D/(B + D).$$

The reliability of SE and SP depends on the size of the chosen population, and it is therefore necessary to provide 95% confidence intervals for SE and SP. These intervals can be calculated with the normal approximation to the binomial distribution or by a computer software, or they can simply be obtained from tables of the binomial distribution.

Further, a first-line assessment of the test can be performed by calculation of Youdens index (Y = SE + SP − 1). Generally, the closer this value is to 1, the better the test is.

Predictive Values

For diagnostic purposes, it is more of interest to know how likely the disease is when the test is positive and how unlikely the disease is when the test is negative. This information is provided by the positive predictive value (PPV) (or predictive value of a positive test or posttest probability of disease after a positive test result) and the negative predictive value (NPV) (or predictive value of a negative test or posttest probability of no disease after a negative test result).[18] PPV and NPV can be calculated with the same two-by-two table used for calculation of SE and SP, if the proportion of diseased animals reflects the disease prevalence in the group of animals to which the test is to be applied. PPV is calculated as [A/(A + B)], NPV is calculated as [D/(D + C)], and 95% confidence limits can be calculated as for SE and SP. In many cases, the proportion of diseased animals in the two-by-two table does not reflect the prevalence of the disease in the target animal population and therefore, PPV and NPV are calculated for disease prevalences (P) varying from 0 to 1 with the following formulas:

$$PPV = (SE{\times}P)/\{(SE{\times}P) + [(1 - P){\times}(1 - SP)]\}$$

$$NPV = [SP{\times}(1 - P)]/\{[SP{\times}(1 - P)] + [(1 - SE){\times}P]\}.$$

PPV and NPV can then be plotted in a graph with PPV and NPV on the y axis and P on the x axis (Fig. 4.6). At low disease prevalences, PPV is low, and at high disease prevalences, PPV is high. The clinical approach to increasing disease prevalence of the suspected disease is to obtain a history and to perform a clinical examination before applying the test. In contrast, NPV is maximal at low disease prevalences, and a negative test result therefore appears to be most useful for ruling out the disease at low disease prevalences.

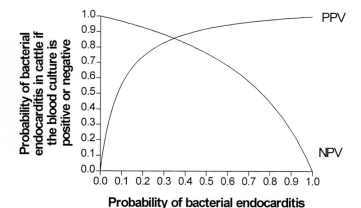

FIGURE 4.6 Positive and negative predictive values. The x axis is the probability of disease if the test is positive (PPV) or the probability that the patient does not have the disease when the test is negative (NPV). In the plot, blood culture is used as a test for bacterial endocarditis in cattle. SE of the test is 0.707, and SP is 0.938 (Houe H, Eriksen L, Jungersen G, et al. Sensitivity, specificity, and predictive value of blood cultures from cattle clinically suspected of bacterial endocarditis. Vet Rec 1993;133:263–266).

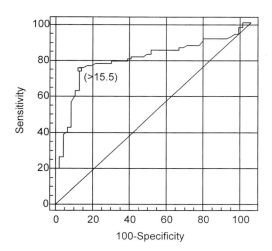

FIGURE 4.7 ROC curve. One constructs a ROC curve by plotting sensitivity as a function of (1-SP) over the range of selected cutoff values. Tests with poor performance tend toward the diagonal line. Tests with good performance tend upward and leftward. The highest SE and SP is the top-leftmost point, and the cutoff value that gives this point is, in this plot, 15.5.

Receiver-Operating-Characteristic Curves

By changing the cutoff value by which test results are divided into negatives and positives, SE and SP changes so that when SE increases, SP decreases and vise versa. The cutoff value is varied over the spectrum of test results, and the resulting pairs of SE and SP are plotted in a graph (a ROC curve) with SE on the y axis and $(1 - SP)$ on the x axis (Fig. 4.7).[19]

The ROC curve is used to assess the overall diagnostic accuracy of the test. This can be done visually because the better a test discriminates between the two patient groups, the closer to the upper left-hand corner of the graph is its ROC curve situated. More formally, the area under the ROC curve (W) and the standard error of the area (se_W) are calculated with the trapezoidal rule or a computer program. The area is then compared with 0.5, which is the area under the ROC curve of a worthless test that does not discriminate between the two patient groups, by calculation of a z value ($z = (W{-}0.5)/se_W$). Values of z greater than 1.96 indicate that the area under the ROC curve is significantly different from 0.5 and that the test is different from a worthless test. Two or more tests used to discriminate between two patient groups can also be compared by use of their ROC curves. Again, a visual assessment can be used, or the areas under the ROC curves can be compared statistically. The latter is most often done with a computer program. For further information, see Hanley and McNiel[20] and Zweig.[19]

The ROC curve is a plot of SE and SP pairs for different cutoff values. From the list of SE and SP corresponding to each cutoff value, it is possible to identify the cutoff value associated with the highest SE and SP simply by calculation of the differential positive rate (DPR) for each cutoff value from the following formula:

$$DPR = [SE - (1 - SP)].$$

The cutoff value with the highest DPR is also the cutoff value associated with the highest SE and SP.

Likelihood Ratio

The ROC curve is a plot of the effect of changing the cutoff value on SE and SP. This dynamism can be described by the slope (or tangent) of the ROC curve at any single, defined, point corresponding to the cutoff value of interest. Two slopes have been defined [SE/ (1 − SP)] and [(1 − SE)/SP]. The former is called the likelihood ratio of a positive test result (LR+), and the latter is called the likelihood ratio of a negative test result (LR−). Another definition for LR+ is the probability of obtaining a positive test result in an animal that has the disease divided by the probability of obtaining a positive test result in an animal that does not have the disease. In other words, a LR+ of 4 means that a positive test result is four times as likely to occur in a diseased animal as in a nondiseased animal. Likewise, LR- is defined as the probability of obtaining a negative test result in an animal that has the disease divided by the probability of obtaining a negative test result in an animal that does not have the disease. Generally, a good LR+ exceeds two, whereas a good LR- is near zero. Because likelihood ratios are derived from SE and SP, it is necessary to determine the confidence intervals of the ratio, which is a somewhat complicated procedure involving X^2 statistics as described by Miettinen.[21]

Generation and Use of Data on Biologic Variation

Biologic variation concerns the variation within and between animals.[22] Data on biologic variation have important applications, e.g., in assessing the usefulness of population-based reference intervals, setting desirable goals for analytical performance, and in estimating the difference needed between two serial test results to be significant. An in-depth description of the generation and application of data on biologic variation has been given by Fraser and Harris.[23]

The task during generation of data on biologic variation is to split the total variation into variation within and between animals and analytical variation. Studies in humans have indicated that biologic variation in health and stable disease is of the same order, irrespective of whether the analyte is within or outside reference intervals and therefore, data on biologic variation are usually derived from healthy subjects. Furthermore, estimates of biologic variation appear to be independent of study design, location of the study, number of subjects studied, and methodology.

A simple procedure to obtain data on biologic variation is to use 8 to 10 clinically healthy animals and to obtain blood samples from these 5 to 10 times on a daily, weekly, or monthly basis. If the analyte is stable, the samples are stored until analysis for all samples are analyzed in duplicate. Otherwise, the samples are analyzed immediately. When all samples have been analyzed, the results are subjected to nested analysis of variance that splits the total variation into between-animal, within-animal, and analytical variance. With the overall mean value, these variances are transformed into coefficients of variance [i.e., between-animal coefficient of variation (CV_G), the within-animal coefficient of variation (CV_I), and the analytical coefficient of variation (CV_A)]. With the obtained values for CV_G, CV_I, and CV_A, the following can be calculated:

Desirable Standards for Analytical Performance

- Maximum allowable analytical imprecision (CV_{MAX}): $1/2(CV_I)$.[23]
- Maximum allowable analytical inaccuracy (percent maximum allowable deviation) (B_{MAX}): $1/4(CV_G^2 + CV_I^2)^{1/2}$.[5]
- Maximum allowable difference between two methods: $1/3(CV_I)$.[5]
- Maximum allowable total error (TE_{MAX}): $1.65 (CV_{MAX}) + B_{MAX}$.[24]

Usefulness of Population-Based Reference Intervals

The index of individuality (R) is calculated $[(CV_I^2 + CV_A^2)/CV_G^2]^{1/2}$.[25] If R is more than 1.4, test results can be compared usefully with the population-based reference interval (i.e., the single animal resembles the group of animals). If R is less than 0.6, then reference intervals are of limited values in detecting small, but important changes in a single animal (i.e., the single animal resembles itself more than it resembles other animals), and it may be necessary to subdivide the reference interval, e.g., according to sex, age, and breed.

Number of Samples Needed to Estimate the True Mean Value in a Single Animal

The number of samples ($N_{samples}$) needed to estimate the true mean value in a single animal is estimated from the formula

$$N_{samples} = (\{Z[(CV_I^2 + CV_A^2)^{1/2}]\}/D)^2,$$

where D is the desired percentage closeness to the true mean value, usually 5%; and Z is the standard deviate for the appropriate probability, usually 1.96.[23]

Critical Difference

The change needed between two serial results to be significant, or the critical difference, is calculated with the formula

$$1.96\{2[(CV_I^2 + CV_A^2)^{1/2}]\}.[23]$$

Example

EDTA-stabilized blood was collected at monthly intervals for 10 months from 23 clinically healthy Beagle male and female dogs, aged 1 to 7 years.[26] Immediately after collection of the blood, total white blood cell count (WBC) was determined in duplicate with the Model

S560 Coulter Counter. Preliminary studies had shown that interassay and intra-assay variation of the measurements generally were of the same magnitude (3.7%); therefore, the CV_A calculated by the nested analysis of variance is used. Subjecting all the data to nested analysis of variance resulted in a between-dog variance of 1.203, a within-dog variance of 1.1649, and an analytical variance of 0.1089. The overall mean value was 8.92×10^9/L.

The between-dog coefficient of variance is then 12.3%, the within-dog coefficient of variance is 12.1%, and the analytical coefficient of variance is 3.7%. With these estimates, the following indices are calculated:

- $CV_{Max} = 6.1\%$
- $B_{Max} = 4.3\%$
- Maximum difference between methods = 4.0%
- $TE_{Max} = 14.4\%$
- $R = 1.0$
- Critical difference = 35%
- $N = 25$

This means that analytical imprecision should be less than 6.1%, that the maximum deviation from a known WBC value should be less than 4.3%, that the difference between two methods designed to measure WBC should be less than 4%, that the total error should be less than 14.4%, that the reference interval may be too wide to detect small but important changes in WBC, that the difference between two serial WBC determinations should be more than 35% if the difference is to be considered significant, and that 25 samples are needed to estimate the true mean WBC value ±5% in a single dog.

References

1. **Altman DG.** Practical statistics for medical researchers. London: Chapman & Hall, 1991.
2. **Armitage P, Berry G.** Statistical methods in medical research. 2nd ed. Oxford: Blackwell Scientific Publications, 1987.
3. **Altman DG, Bland JM.** Measurements in medicine: the analysis of method comparison studies. The Statistician 1983;32:307–317.
4. **Tonks DB.** A study of the accuracy and precision of clinical chemistry determinations in 170 Canadian laboratories. Clin Chem 1963;9:217–233.
5. **Fraser CG, Petersen PH, Ricos C, Haeckel R.** Proposed quality specifications for imprecision and inaccuracy of analytical systems for clinical chemistry. Eur J Clin Chem Clin Biochem 1992;30:311–317.
6. **Westgard JO.** A method evaluation decision chart (MEDx chart) for judging method performance. Clin Lab Sci 1995;8:277–283.
7. US Dept. of Health and Social Services. Medicare, medicaid, and CLIA programs: regulations implementing the Clinical Laboratory Improvement Amendments of 1998 (CLIA). Final rule. Federal Register 1992; 57:7002–7186.
8. **van Duijnhoven HL, Treskes M.** Marked interference of hyperglycemia in measurements of mean (red) cell volume by Technicon H analyzers. Clin Chem 1996;42:76–80.
9. **Young DS.** Effects of drugs on clinical laboratory tests. 3rd ed. Washington, DC: American Association of Clinical Chemists, 1990.
10. **Jensen AL, Wenck A, Koch J, Poulsen JSD.** Comparison of results of haematological and clinical chemical analyses on blood samples obtained from the cephalic and external jugular vein in dogs. Res Vet Sci 1994;56:24–29.
11. **Thoresen SI, Tverdal A, Havre G, Morberg H.** Effects of storage time and freezing on clinical chemical parameters from canine serum and heparinized plasma. Vet Clin Pathol 1995;24:129–133.
12. **Mbassa GK, Poulsen JSD.** Influence of pregnancy, lactation and environment on haematological profiles in Danish landrace dairy goats (Capra hircus) of different parity. Compendium Biochem Physiol B 1991;100:403–412.
13. **National Committee for Clinical Laboratory Standards.** How to define, determine, and utilize reference intervals in the clinical laboratory. NCCLS Document C28-P, Wayne, PA. ISBN 1-56238-143-1, 1992.
14. **Solberg HE.** The theory of reference values. Part 5. Statistical treatment of collected reference values–determination of reference limits. J Clin Chem Clin Biochem 1983;21:749–760.
15. **Reed AH, Henry RJ, Mason WB.** Influence of statistical method used on the resulting estimate of normal range. Clin Chem 1971;17:275–284.
16. **Ransohoff DF, Feinstein AR.** Problems of spectrum and bias in evaluating the efficacy of diagnostic tests. N Engl J Med 1978;299:926–930.
17. **Youden WJ.** Index for rating diagnostic tests. Cancer 1950;3:32–35.
18. **Vecchio TJ.** Predictive value of a single diagnostic test in unselected populations. N Engl J Med 1966;274:1171–1173.
19. **Zweig MH, Campbell G.** Receiver-operating characteristic (ROC) plots: a fundamental evaluation tool in clinical medicine. Clin Chem 1993;39:561–577.
20. **Hanley JA, McNeil BJ.** A method of comparing the areas under receiver operating characteristic curves derived from the same cases. Radiology 1983;148:839–843.
21. **Miettinen OS.** Estimability and estimation in case-referent studies. Am J Epidemiol 1976;103:226–235.
22. **Jensen AL, Aaes H.** Critical differences of clinical chemical parameters in blood from dogs. Res Vet Sci 1993;54:10–14.
23. **Fraser CG, Harris EK.** Generation and application of data on biological variation in clinical chemistry. Crit Rev Clin Lab Sci 1989;29:409–430.
24. **Petersen PH, Ricos C, Stoeckl D, Libeer JC, Baadenhuijsen H, Fraser C, Thienpont L.** Proposed guidelines for the internal quality control of analytical results in the medical laboratory. Eur J Clin Chem Clin Biochem 1996;34:983–999.
25. **Harris EK.** Effects of intra- and interindividual variation on the appropriate use of normal ranges. Clin Chem 1974;12:1535–1542.
26. **Jensen AL, Iversen L, Petersen TK.** Study on biological variability of haematological components in dogs. Comp Haemat Internat 1998;8:202–204.

CHAPTER 6

Approaches to Evaluation of Bone Marrow Function

• BRUCE D. CAR and JULIA T. BLUE

Bone marrow function is studied both to gain insight into the basic mechanisms of and to better understand disorders of hemopoiesis. The tremendous advancement in sophistication of research tools used to evaluate bone marrow function, particularly those molecular approaches used to identify hemopoietic cytokines, growth factors, and their in vivo roles in gene-deleted mice, have resulted in a heightened understanding of hemopoiesis and bone marrow disease.

PERIPHERAL BLOOD STUDIES: SPECIAL CONSIDERATIONS

A thorough assessment of the products of hemopoiesis is central to the evaluation of bone marrow function and is essentially similar to that used in routine clinical diagnostics. Close attention is paid to parameters in a complete blood count that are influenced by the rate of hemopoiesis. The absolute reticulocyte count, mean cell volume (MCV) and red cell distribution width (RDW) collectively provide an overview of the rate of erythropoiesis. Because of their long life span relative to other blood cells, changes in numbers of mature erythrocytes occur only gradually after events that inhibit or promote erythropoiesis. Complete inhibition of erythropoiesis for 5 days in the mouse, rat, or dog would theoretically result only in a 20, 10, or 5% drop in count, assuming erythrocyte life spans of 25, 55, and 100 days.[1] Short-term inhibition of erythropoiesis may not lower the erythrocyte count below the reference interval, but the absolute reticulocyte count will be significantly reduced. A transient effect on the erythron, such as that induced by a single dose of 5-fluorouracil, can be compensated by accelerated erythropoiesis, resulting in minimal change in the total erythrocyte count but significant increase in the proportion of reticulocytes.

Owing to the somewhat precarious energy metabolism of the bone marrow erythroblast, which results from the halving of mitochondrial numbers with each of the approximate five to six cell divisions, the erythroid lineage is particularly sensitive to agents that alter mitochondrial function, such as chloramphenicol.[2,3] Depression of absolute numbers of reticulocytes is frequently an early manifestation of the deleterious effects of xenobiotics on bone marrow function. The short (approximately 24 hours) life span of the neutrophil also renders it a sensitive indicator of altered bone marrow function. Quantification of immature neutrophils in peripheral blood smears permits the evaluation of the rate of granulocytopoiesis. Platelet counts alter more slowly with myelosuppression because of their longer life span (approximately 10 days), however, changes in mean platelet volume (MPV) may be indicative of a subset of less mature platelets.

Gene-deleted and transgenic mice provide a special challenge to the hematologist. These mice are frequently nonviable, dying during the embryonic, fetal, or early neonatal period. Peripheral blood examinations may still provide invaluable information on such mice. A 3-μL volume of heart blood obtained with a fine-gauge needle is sufficient to prepare a blood smear; as little as 20 μL of heart blood may be diluted with 2 mg/mL of ethylenediamine tetra-acetic acid (EDTA) saline and analyzed with an electronic counter. Potential artefacts of linearity with dilutions of small quantities can be overcome by comparison of results from treated or genetically altered mice with similarly diluted volumes from control or wild-type mice, permitting valid conclusions.

BONE MARROW ASPIRATION AND BIOPSY

Direct examination of bone marrow is needed to complement information collected from assessment of blood. Bone marrow aspirates or core biopsies are readily obtained from all domestic and research animal species. Careful preparation of evenly spread smears with allogeneic sera, rapid fixation in methanol, and routine staining with Wright or May-Grünwald-Giemsa provide optimal specimens for cytologic evaluation. Morphologically identifiable myeloid and erythroid precursors and other cells may be quantitated in 200- to 500-cell differential counts. In the mouse this technique can provide highly quantitative information. The femur of a destroyed mouse can be removed intact, the distal physis carefully removed, and a fine-gauge needle inserted to create an exit port. The entire contents of the femur can be flushed into a collection tube after the femoral neck is cut and the tip of a needle attached to a tuberculin syringe filled with approximately 1 mL of saline is inserted. After gentle resuspension of the extruded bone marrow and filtration through a 70-μm mesh, samples may be counted accurately with a hematology analyzer or a hemocytometer. The number of bone marrow cells per femur (referred to as cellularity in this experimental field) is highly consistent for a mouse strain of a given age range. A typical 8-week-old mouse has approximately 15 to 20 million cells per femur. Two days after a single dose of 150 mg/kg 5-fluorouracil this number is reduced to 2 to 5 million cells per femur. With differential and total counts to calculate absolute counts of precursors, a great deal of valuable information may be obtained per mouse.[4] In fetal mice, which lack well-developed medullary hemopoiesis, the cytologic examination of liver imprints for hemopoietic precursors is useful for assessing early hemopoietic function.

Altered bone marrow function, whether associated with neoplasia or in response to administration of cytotoxicants or cytokines, may profoundly alter the appearance of normal bone marrow elements. The use of enzyme histochemistry to differentiate these elements is described under Section V, Chapter 51, Cytochemistry of Normal Leukocytes.

The histologic examination of decalcified or undecalcified bone marrow sections provides a better overview of bone marrow cellularity, iron storage, and bone marrow stromal alterations such as myelofibrosis. Ultrastructural or immunohistochemical analyses of bone marrow may provide an additional dimension of resolution.

FLOW CYTOMETRY OF BONE MARROW

Potential limitations to the cytologic examination of bone marrow are the expertise and time needed to perform differential analyses. The recent development of monoclonal antibodies specific for individual hemopoietic lineages has simplified the assessment of the bone marrow of rodents and is applicable to larger species when specific reagents are available. In mice, the antibodies Gr-1 (Ly-6G) and Ter-119 (Ly-76) adequately differentiate granulocyte and erythrocyte precursors, respectively.[5,6] The availability of different fluorescent indicators for both of these lineages allows the simultaneous generation of a usable myeloid cell relative to erythroid cells (M:E ratio). Additional antibody markers may be used to identify monocytic and megakaryocytic lineages. Subset analyses of bone marrow lymphocytes (CD3-pan T, CD4-T helper, CD8-T cytotoxic, CD56-NK, and B220-B cells) can readily be performed in mice. Many reagents for detection of lymphocyte and leukocyte subpopulations in domestic animal species are currently available.[7-9] When flowcytometric analyses are of insufficient sensitivity to detect target antigens, such as hemopoietic cytokines or their receptors, the quantitative reverse-transcriptase polymerase chain reaction (RT-PCR) may be used to amplify messenger RNA (mRNA) to detectable quantities of complementary DNA (cDNA) and thereby establish expression levels in species for which specific gene sequences have been obtained.

BONE MARROW CULTURE

Hematopoietic interactions are best dissected in vitro where culture systems permit the evaluation of effects of individual cytokines, growth factors, or regulators, and combinations of factors. Target gene expression may be transiently induced by gene transfection or inhibited by transfection with antisense RNA. The significance of functions assessed in vitro must be confirmed as far as possible in vivo. Deficiency of hemopoietic cytokines or growth factors that would predictably have severe phenotypes based on in vitro work, such as interleukin-2 (IL-2) and granulocyte-macrophage-colony stimulating factor (GM-CSF), have much milder hematologic phenotypes than expected (i.e., failure to develop lymphopenia and neutropenia), underscoring the redundancy and pleiotropy that characterize many of these factors.[10-12]

Bone marrow cells can be cultured from aspirates or core samples obtained from diseased or healthy animals. Generally these cells are cultured in semisolid methylcellulose-based media with cocktails of cytokines, erythropoietin, transferrin, bovine fetal serum, and albumin. Whereas erythropoietin is highly reactive across species and has been cloned from a variety of species, other cytokines have more limited cross-species effects. When a species-specific cytokine is unavailable, conditioned spleen cell media (obtained from phytohemagglutinin, endotoxin, or phorbol ester-stimulated cells) may serve as a useful source. Conditions for the culture of bone marrow progenitors from dogs,[13] cats,[14] sheep,[15] cattle,[16,17] horses,[18] and chickens[19] have been described.

Cultured colonies are morphologically identified and enumerated. Most species examined exhibit early development of colony-forming units-erythroid (CFU-E), blast forming units-erythroid (BFU-E), and CFU-granulocyte-macrophage (CFU-GM). The optimum time for counting of colonies varies significantly between species and should be determined in pilot experiments. For example, CFU-E are detected at 2 days in mice, 6 days in dogs, and 7 to 10 days in man. These colonies are generally single and small (approximately 50 to 100 cells). BFU-E are much larger colonies surrounded by multiple daughter colonies in a burst formation and may contain hundreds to thousands of cells per colony. Colonies tend to achieve an optimal appearance during restricted periods of culture characteristic of an individual species and to degenerate rapidly thereafter. Conditions may need to be optimized separately for each of the hemopoietic lineages. Murine spleen cells can also be cultured under the same conditions as those for bone marrow. Criteria for evaluation of colonies and designation of lineage include cell size, which allow simple recognition of colonies containing megakaryocytes. Granulocyte-macrophage colonies usually exhibit chemokinesis of mature cells, with granulocytes and macrophages migrating away from colony borders (Fig. 6.1). Hemoglobinization of erythroid colonies imparts a red-brown hue. Colony designation must periodically be confirmed by manual selection of individual colonies, by preparation of smears, and by confirmation of cell identity by morphologic features in Wright-Giemsa-stained specimens. Although numerous bizarre forms and inclusions may be observed, hemopoietic cell precursors, and thus specific colony types, are readily identified by the trained cytologist.

Alterations in numbers of individual lineage-restricted progenitors as determined by colony assay from diseased or healthy animals, reflect corresponding alterations in hemopoietic progenitor pools. Given the ability to quantify bone marrow cells per femur in mice, and assuming femoral marrow to represent a relatively stable proportion of all hemopoietic tissue, numbers of individual lineage-restricted progenitors per femur or per 10^5 cells provide an accurate picture of murine progenitor cell pools. In larger species, relative progenitor cell counts are generated in vitro and cellularity is assessed by histologic evaluation. Short-term bone marrow cultures from mice, rats, and dogs are routinely performed to assess the potential toxicity of xenobiotics[20,21] and to define hemopoietic phenotypes of genetically altered animals.

Bone marrow culture systems may be used to study hemopoiesis by the addition of individual cytokines, growth factors or their regulators, or combinations thereof. Alternatively, neutralizing antibodies to these components or small molecules can be used to dissect regulatory pathways. Similarly, the hemopoietic progenitors of clinical cases can be studied in vitro by direct culture after aspiration biopsy. Alternatively, whole plasma or plasma components from animals with bone marrow disorders may be added to the bone marrow cells of clinically normal animals to study the nature of potential humoral myelosuppressive activities.

Long-term cultures of hemopoietic cells on established stromal cell layers (Dexter cultures) more closely recapitulate the hemopoietic microenvironment and allow long-term survival of pluripotent hemopoietic stem cells.[22] These culture systems were used to identify and study the stromal-cell defect (defective c-kit or stem cell factor receptor) in Sl/Sl[d] (Steel anemia) and the complementary defect in W/W[v] (white-spotted) mice (kit-ligand or stem cell factor deficiency).[23,24] Long-term culture of bone marrow has been described for dogs[25] and sheep.[26]

LETHAL IRRADIATION AND BONE MARROW TRANSPLANTATION

Lethally irradiated mice receiving bone marrow or hemopoietic cells with a capacity for partial or complete renewal of hemopoiesis develop large splenic foci of extramedullary hemopoiesis thought to be initiated by a single pluripotent stem cell. These colonies are grossly visible after 8 to 14 days, creating hemispherical distortions of the splenic contour that may be visually enumerated.[22,27,28] These colonies were designated the CFU-spleen (CFU-S) and have since been found to represent a multipotent committed progenitor cell rather than the pluripotent stem cell as originally hypothesized. By using female Safari cats (Geoffroy × domestic F1) heterozygous for glucose 6-phosphate dehydrogenase as autologous transplant recipients after lethal irradiation, Abkowitz et al.[29] defined the stochastic or random nature

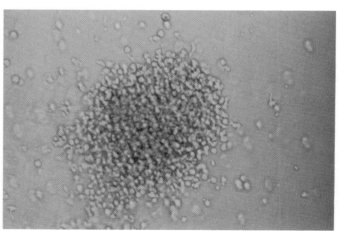
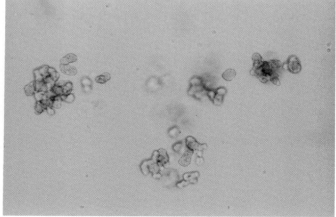

FIGURE 6.1 Hemopoietic colonies in semisolid culture. On the left is a CFU-GM cultured from mouse bone marrow. Notable are wandering leukocytes around the margin. Original magnification 100×. On the right are small erythroid colonies. Mature hemoglobinization of cytoplasm imparts a red-brown hue to cells. Original magnification 200×.

of lineage commitment of pluripotential stem cells and the frequency of hemopoietic stem cells in cats (6 per 10^7 nucleated marrow cells). This frequency is less than that of mice or man (10^{-4} to 10^{-5}). The roles of cytokines in the recovery of normal hemopoiesis after lethal irradiation has been studied extensively in the dog.[30,31]

GENETICALLY ALTERED MICE

Through the technology that permits homologous recombination of partially homologous generally noncoding, genetic sequences in cultured murine stem cells, mice deficient in the protein product of specific target genes can be created. This technology has been extensively exploited in the study of function of individual hemopoietic cytokines, growth factors and their cognate receptors, and hemopoietic transcription factors.[32] Without this technology, the study of transcription factors associated with primitive multipotent progenitors (SCL/TAL, GATA-2, Pu-1, Ikaros), erythropoiesis (GATA-1, GATA-2, tal-1, rbtn-1), megakaryocytopoiesis (NF-E2, p45), and myelopoiesis (Pu-1) would not have been possible.[33,34] The hematologic evaluation of mouse embryos or fetuses is a critical part of the phenotypic assessment of knockout mice. By rendering gene-deleted mice ($-/-$) transgenic ($+/+$) for a deficient gene under the control of an inducible or repressible tissue-specific promoter, the function(s) of a gene in adults, for which deletion otherwise results in nonviable fetuses, can be examined. Using the Cre-loxP system,[35] genes may be removed or reactivated in a tissue-specific manner in the adult mouse[36]

The development of methods to transplant human hemopoietic cells into immunodeficient severe combined immunodeficiency (SCID) mice (SCID-hu) has provided an experimental tool with potential use in modeling leukemias, infectious diseases, autoimmune diseases, and various primary nonneoplastic bone marrow disorders[37] Potential deficiencies of this model include incomplete cross-species functionality between murine cytokines or cytokine receptors and human receptors or ligands since the absence of human bone marrow stroma in mice transplanted with human hemopoietic cells creates a chimeric hemopoietic microenvironment. Impaired passage of mature cells into and out of the bone marrow or circulation may occur when adhesion molecules and their receptors on leukocytes, platelets, and endothelial cells fail to recognize their respective murine or human counterparts.

MODELS OF ACCELERATED HEMOPOIESIS

The intraperitoneal administration of a single 150-mg/kg dose of 5-fluorouracil or appropriate dosing regimen of cyclophosphamide completely depopulates murine bone marrow. Treatment with 5-fluorouracil spares the slowly cycling or noncycling stem cells.[38] Recovery of hematologic parameters is first detectable 5 days post-

treatment with complete recovery occurring after 15 to 20 days. This model has been used extensively to study accelerated hemopoiesis in gene-deleted mice with apparently normal basal hemopoiesis or in mice treated with agents that do not alter basal hemopoietic function. In this manner, the immunosuppressant rapamycin was shown, by virtue of its ability to inhibit signal transduction of various proliferation-inducing cytokines, to have a potential liability when administered in concert with cytotoxic agents.[39] Accelerated erythropoiesis without marrow depletion is readily induced in rodents after a single 60-mg/kg intraperitoneal injection of phenylhydrazine. This regimen produces a Heinz body hemolytic anemia with approximately 30% decrease in hematocrit after 2 days and a robust reticulocytosis by 5 days post-treatment.[40] Alternatively, a fixed volume of blood (to 3% of body weight) may be removed from a rodent and replaced with intraperitoneal saline, stimulating erythropoiesis. Bacto-tryptone (a potent chemotactic casein digest, 1 mL of 10% solution) is administered intraperitoneally to mobilize granulocytes and to accelerate granulopoiesis. A similar effect is achieved with intravenous dosing of granulocyte-colony stimulating factor (G-CSF) (generally species cross reactive) at a dose of 5 μg/kg.[41]

Lessons learned from the evaluation of bone marrow function in genetically altered rodents may be extended to the study of hemopoiesis in domestic species and provide a better understanding of dysregulation in primary diseases of bone marrow. The availability of specific reagents for domestic species and accessibility to bone marrow culture, flowcytometry, and polymerase chain reaction (PCR) technologies permit the increasingly sophisticated examination of bone marrow function, thus providing greater insight into abnormalities of bone marrow function recognized by traditional hematologic methods.

REFERENCES

1. **Harvey JW.** Erythrocyte metabolism. Table 1. In: Kaneko JJ, ed. Clinical biochemistry of domestic animals. 4th ed. San Diego: Academic Press, 1989;196–197.
2. **Martelo OJ, Manyan DR, Smith US, Yunis AA.** Chloramphenicol and bone marrow mitochondria. J Lab Clin Med 1969;74:927–940.
3. **Firkin FC.** Mitochondrial lesions in reversible erythropoietic depression due to chloramphenicol. J Clin Invest 1972;51:2085–2092.
4. **Eng VM, Car BD, Schnyder B, Lorenz M, Lugli S, Aguet M, Anderson TD, Ryffel B, Quesniaux VFJ.** The stimulatory effects of interleukin (IL)-12 on hematopoiesis are antagonized by IL-12-induced interferon-γ in vivo. J Exp Med 1995;181:1893–1898.
5. **Randall TD, Lund FE, Howard MC, Weissman IL.** Expression of murine CD38 defines a population of long-term reconstituting hematopoietic stem cells. Blood 1996;87:4057–4067.
6. **Rudin W, Quesniaux V, Favre N, Bordmann G.** Malaria toxins from *P. chabaudi chabaudi* AS and *P. berghei* ANKA cause dyserythropoiesis in C57BL/6 mice. Parasitology 1997;115:467–474.
7. **Cobbold S, Metcalfe S.** Monoclonal antibodies that define canine homologues of human CD antigens: summary of the First International Canine Leukocyte Antigen Workshop (CLAW). Tissue Antigens 1994;43:137–154.
8. **Cobbold S, Holmes M, Willett B.** The immunology of companion animals: reagents and therapeutic strategies with potential veterinary and human clinical applications. Immunol Today 1994;15:347–353.
9. **Saalmüller A.** Characterization of swine leukocyte differentiation antigens. Immunol Today 1996;17:352–356.
10. **Lohler J, Sadlack B, Schorle H, Klebb G, Haber H, Horak I.** Generalisierte autoimmunkrankheit in BALB/c-Mäusen mit genetisch bedingtem Interleukin-2-Mangel. Verh Dtsch Ges Pathol 1996;80:293–296.
11. **Thèze J, Alzari PM, Bertoglio J.** Interleukin 2 and its receptors: recent advances and new immunological functions. Immunol Today 1996;17:481–486.

12. Dranoff G, Crawford AD, Sadelain M, Ream B, Rashid A, Bronson RT, Dickerin GR, Bachurski CJ, Mark EL, Whitsett JA, Mulligan RC. Involvement of granulocyte-macrophage colony stimulating factor in pulmonary homeostasis. Science 1994;264:713–716.

13. Kreja L, Baltschukat K, Nothdurft W. In vitro studies of the sensitivity of canine bone-marrow erythroid burst-forming units (BFU-E) and fibroblast colony-forming units (CFU-F) to X-irradiation. Int J Radiat 1989;55:435–444.

14. Khan KN, Kociba GJ, Wellman ML, Reiter JA. Effects of tumor necrosis factor-# on normal feline hematopoietic progenitor cells. Exp Hematol 1992;20:900–903.

15. Haig DM, Thomson J, Percival A. The in-vitro detection and quantitation of ovine bone marrow precursors of colony-forming cells. J Comp Pathol 1994;111:73–85.

16. Fritsch G, Nelson RT. Bovine erythroid (CFU-E, BFU-E) and granulocyte-macrophage colony formation in culture. Exp Hematol 1990;18:195–200.

17. Fritsch G, Nelson RT, Muiya P, Naessens J, Black SJ. Characterization of bovine haemopoietic progenitor cells using monoclonal and fluorocytometry. Vet Immunol Immunopathol 1991;27:277–292.

18. Swardson CJ, Kociba GJ, Perryman LE. Effects of equine infectious anemia virus on hematopoietic progenitors in vitro. Am J Vet Res 1992;53:1176–1179.

19. Beug H, Steinlein P, Bartunek P, Hayman MJ. Avian hematopoietic cell culture: in vitro model systems to study oncogenic transformation of hematopoietic cells. Methods Enzymol 1995;254:41–76.

20. Deldar A, Stevens CE. Development and application of in vitro models of hematopoiesis to drug development. Tox Pathol 1993;21:231–240.

21. Parchment RE, Huang M, Erickson-Miller CL. Roles for in vitro myelotoxicity tests in preclinical drug development and clinical trial planning. Tox Pathol 1993;21:241–250.

22. Quesenberry PJ, Temples D, McGrath H, Lowry P, Meyer D, Kittler E, Deacon D, Kister K, Crittenden R, Srikumar K. Stroma-dependent hematolymphopoietic stem cells. Curr Top Micro Immunol 1992;177:151–166.

23. Dexter TM, Moore MAS. In vitro duplication and "cure" of haematopoietic defects in genetically anaemic mice. Nature 1977;269:412–414.

24. Huang E, Nocka K, Beier DR, Chu T-Y, Buck J, Lahm H-W, Wellner D, Leder P, Besmer P. The hematopoietic growth factor KL is encoded by the SL locus and is the ligand of the c-kit receptor, the gene product of the W locus. Cell 1990;63:225–233.

25. Schuening FG, Storb R, Meyer J, Goehle S. Long-term culture of canine bone marrow cells. Exp Hematol 1989;17:411–417.

26. Marsicano G, Shehu D, Galli C. Factors controlling haemopoiesis in ovine long-term bone marrow cultures. Vet Immunol Immunopathol 1997;55:291–301.

27. Ross EAM, Anderson N, Micklem HS. Serial depletion and regeneration of the murine hematopoietic system: implications for hematopoietic organization and the study of cellular aging. J Exp Med 1982;155:332–344.

28. Quesenberry PJ. Long-term marrow cultures: human and murine systems. J Cell Biochem 1991;45:273–278.

29. Abkowitz JL, Catlin SN, Guttorp P. Evidence that hematopoiesis may be a stochastic process in vivo. Nature Medicine 1996;2:190–197.

30. Schuening FG, Nemunaitis J, Appelbaum FR, Storb R. Hematopoietic growth factors after allogeneic marrow transplantation in animal studies and clinical trials. Bone Marrow Transplant 1994;14:S74–S79.

31. Schuening FG, Appelbaum FR, Deeg HJ, Sullivan-Pepe M, Graham TC, Hackman R, Zsebo KM, Storb R. Effects of recombinant canine stem cell factor, a c-kit ligand, and recombinant granulocyte colony-stimulating factor on hematopoietic recovery after otherwise lethal total body irradiation. Blood 1993;81:20–26.

32. Pandolfi PP. Knocking in and out genes and trans genes: the use of the engineered mouse to study normal and aberrant hemopoiesis. Semin Hematol 1998;35:136–148.

33. Shivdasani RA, Orkin SH. Review: the transcriptional control of hematopoiesis. Blood 1996;87:4025–4039.

34. Silver L, Palis J. Initiation of murine embryonic erythropoiesis: a spatial analysis. Blood 1997;89:1154–1164.

35. Sternberg N. Bacteriophage P1 cloning system for the isolation, amplification, and recovery of DNA fragments as large as 100 kilobase pairs. Proc Natl Acad Sci USA 1990;87:103–107.

36. Marth JD. Recent advances in gene mutagenesis by site-directed recombination. J Clin Invest 1996;97:1999–2002.

37. Lapidot T, Pflumio F, Dick JE. Modeling human hematopoiesis in immunodeficient mice. Lab Anim Sci 1993;43:147–150.

38. Yeager AM, Levin J, Levin F. The effects of 5-fluorouracil on hematopoiesis: studies of murine megakaryocyte-CFC, granulocyte-macrophage CFC and peripheral blood cell levels. Exp Hematol 1983;11:944–952.

39. Quesniaux VFJ, Wehrli S, Steiner C, Joergensen J, Schuurman H-J, Herrmann P, Schreier MH, Schuler W. The immunosuppressant rapamycin blocks in vitro responses to hematopoietic cytokines and inhibits recovering but not steady-state hematopoiesis in vivo. Blood 1994;84:1543–1552.

40. Tambourin PE, Wendling F, Gallien-Lartigue O, Huaulme D. Production of high plasma levels of erythropoietin in mice. Biomedicine 1973;19:112–116.

41. Benestad HB, Strøm-Gundersen I, Iversen PO, Haug E, Njå A. No neuronal regulation of murine bone marrow function. Blood 1998;91:1280–1287.

CHAPTER 7

Hematologic Changes Due to Bacterial Infections

• STEVEN L. STOCKHAM

Hematologic changes caused by bacterial infections are usually first detected during a routine complete blood cell count (CBC). The CBC results provide a veterinarian with a snapshot picture of the cells that are circulating in an animal's blood; the CBC is a hemopoietic system biopsy. Most hematologic changes are caused by the animal's response to the infection and are not directly caused by the infectious agent. However, an animal's defensive mechanisms can react quite differently to various infective bacteria, including cocci, bacilli, spirochetes, and rickettsial species (*Ehrlichia spp., Hemobartonella spp., Eperythrozoon spp.,* and *Anaplasma spp.*). Therefore, there is no singular pattern in CBC changes that indicates a bacterial infection. But a few abnormalities exist that are suggestive of bacterial infections (see Major Complete Blood Cell Count Abnormalities Related to Bacterial Infections); these abnormalities are described later.

It may be helpful when considering the hematologic changes caused by bacterial infections to remember that less than 5% of neutrophils in a body circulate in peripheral blood, and approximately three new populations of neutrophils in peripheral blood[1] each day. Blood lymphocytes are part of a complex lymphoid system in which lymphocytes are constantly leaving blood, entering lymphoid and other tissues, and then returning to blood to start another cycle. Blood monocytes are destined to be part of an extensive mononuclear phagocytic system. Eosinophils and basophils are typically uncommon cells in peripheral blood but play vital roles in inflammatory responses in tissues. Mast cells, which rarely are found in peripheral blood of domestic mammals, play critical roles in common and unique inflammatory reactions. Also, changes occur to both erythrocytes and platelets during many bacterial diseases.

EFFECTS OF VIRULENCE FACTORS ON HEMIC SYSTEM

Pathogenicity and virulence of organisms partially determine how the hemic system becomes involved in the response to the infection; another determinant is the tissue infected. Virulence factors include adherence, invasion of host cells, production of exotoxins and endotoxins, production of enzymes, prevention of phagocytosis, ability to inhibit phagolysosome formation, antigenic heterogeneity, competition for nutrients, and promotion of immunologic injury to tissues.[2] The following sections highlight how some virulence factors either directly or indirectly create hematologic changes.

Adherence

Once bacteria invade an animal, they must adhere to cells to establish microcolonies and begin the complex events related to the pathogenesis of the infection. Adherence alone does not lead to hematologic changes but it may allow invasion of host cells or initiate immunologic reactions (see Invasion of Host Cells and Promotion of Immunologic Injury).

Invasion of Host Cells

For some bacteria, invasion of host cells may lead to activation of inflammatory cells and systems or may lead to cell death. Once bacteria are in tissues and are recognized by the immune system, activated macrophages release cytokines, digestive enzymes, and arachidonic acid metabolites to promote emigration of leukocytes to the inflamed tissue and the production and release of leukocytes from marrow. After processing, macrophages may present antigens to T-lymphocytes or B-lymphocytes to initiate cellular and humoral immune responses. Also, antigen-bound antibodies, components of bacterial and viral membranes, plasmin, and other factors may activate the classical or alternative complement pathway and the generation of complement components that are leukocyte chemotaxins (C3a, C5a, C567, Bb), promoters of leukocytosis (C3e), and cause mast cell degranulation (C3a, C5a).

For most bacteria and through the processes just mentioned, cell invasion leads to destruction of cells or the invading organisms. But for other bacteria such as ehrlichial and mycobacterial species, entry of an organism and the resulting formation of a phagosome establishes a protective environment (see Inhibition of Phagolysosome Formation).

Production of Exotoxins

Many bacteria produce exotoxins, which are polypeptides that typically bind to specific receptors on cells. The exotoxins of *Clostridium perfringens* Type A, *Clostridium haemolyticum, Clostridium novyi* Type D, and *Corynebacterium pseudotuberculosis* are phospholipases that cause hemolytic anemias by catalyzing the breakdown of erythrocyte membrane lipids. (See Chapter 28, Anemia Associated with Bacterial and Viral Infections.) The (toxin of *C. perfringens* Type A also damages leukocyte, platelet, and endothelial cell membranes and causes leukopenia, thrombocytopenia, hemorrhage, and thrombi formation. The rapid extravasation of plasma through the damaged vessels can cause shock, erythrocytosis caused by hemoconcentration, and death.[3]

Another exotoxin is a leukotoxin that is produced by *Pasteurella haemolytica* and binds to bovine neutrophils to cause release of inflammatory mediators and eventually apoptotic neutrophil death.[4] Also, the leukotoxin's binding to macrophages causes the release of interleukin-1 (IL-1) and tumor necrosis factor (TNF or cachectin) that decreases erythropoiesis and initiates changes in leukocyte kinetics that alter leukocyte concentrations in blood.[5] The leukotoxin is also a platelet agonist and promotes the formation of pulmonary microvascular thrombi.[6,7]

Production of Endotoxins

Perhaps no virulence factor has been studied as much as endotoxin, the membrane lipopolysaccharide (LPS) of gram-negative bacteria. When LPS is released from dying gram-negative bacteria, enters the blood, and binds to LPS-binding protein or high-density lipoproteins, it activates cells (monocytes, macrophages, endothelial cells, platelets, and other hemic cells) and complement, coagulation, or bradykinin–kinin systems. The activation of the cells or systems can result in an initial neutropenia followed by a neutrophilia, lymphopenia, thrombocytopenia, microvascular disease, and disseminated intravascular coagulation (DIC).[8–11] Many of the inflammatory responses in the leukocytes are promoted by the LPS-stimulated release of TNF, IL-1, IL-6, IL-8, and nitrous oxide from macrophages.[10,12–16] The TNF also promotes the development of the anemia of inflammatory disease by shortening erythrocyte life span and decreasing erythropoiesis.[17]

Production of Proteases

Besides the exotoxins that have phospholipase activity, the virulence of some bacteria is mediated through the action of proteases. The actions of the proteases include inactivation of plasma protein protease inhibitors (such as α_1-protease inhibitor and α_2-macroglobulin); activation of bradykinin-generating cascade; activation of coagulation cascade; cleavage of immunoglobulin, fibronectin, complement, and bacterial chemotactic factors (such as formyl-methionyl-leucyl-phenylalanine); degradation of transferrin; activation of plasminogen; and destruction of tissues.[18] With this broad range of protease activity, it is easy to see how the bacterial infections cause changes in leukocytes, erythrocytes, platelets, and coagulation factors.

Inhibition of Phagolysosome Formation

Survival of some organisms in phagocytes depends on the inhibition of phagolysosome formation. This is especially true for the ehrlichial species that infect neutrophils, eosinophils, and monocytes.[19] Such ability allows for the replication of organisms in the phagosome and thus the formation of the morula that can be identified in infected leukocytes. Similar processes allow for the multiplication of mycobacterial species in monocytes or macrophages and leads to the macrophages and neutrophils laden with mycobacterial bacilli.

Competition for Nutrients

Survival of bacteria in tissues depends on their ability to compete for needed nutrients. In the context of this chapter, bacterial competition for iron plays a role in the development of the anemia of inflammation. Some bacteria contain siderophores, which are ligands with a high affinity for ferric iron. The siderophores capture free iron or can even remove iron from transferrin.[2] As part of the bacteriostatic mechanisms in animals, inflammatory mediators such as TNF upregulate ferritin and transferrin macrophage receptors and thus promote iron storage in the mononuclear phagocytic system.[20] The shifting of iron to storage plus the use of iron by bacteria makes less iron available to erythroid precursors. Such limited access to iron is a classic component of the pathogenesis of the anemia of inflammatory disease.

Promotion of Immunologic Injury

Bacterial infections can directly or indirectly lead to immune-mediated damage of blood cells. For example, the binding or infection of *Hemobartonella spp., Eperythrozoon spp.*, and *Anaplasma spp.* leads to antibody-mediated destruction of erythrocytes (see Chapter 27, Hemolytic Anemias Caused by Blood Rickettsial Agents and Protozoa). Also, the hemolytic anemia of leptospirosis in lambs may be immune mediated.[21,22] In people who have *Hemophilus influenzae* infections, an anemia may result from the immune-mediated hemolysis after the organism's capsular polysaccharide binds to erythrocytes.[23] The inflammatory response itself may cause oxidative and proteolytic damage to erythrocytes and result in the production of immunoglobulins that bind to the damaged cells.[24]

Besides the thrombocytopenia that may result from damage caused by exotoxins and endotoxins, bacterial infections may lead to thrombocytopenia through immunologic injury. Either the binding of bacteria to platelets or the development of increased platelet-associated immunoglobulins can lead to platelet destruction. Also, antiplatelet antibodies play a role in the development of thrombocytopenia and thrombopathy in dogs infected with *Ehrlichia canis*.[25,26] The cyclic nature of the parasitemia and thrombocytopenia of an *Ehrlichia platys* infection suggests an immunologic basis of the thrombocytopenia.

MAJOR COMPLETE BLOOD CELL COUNT ABNORMALITIES RELATED TO BACTERIAL INFECTIONS

Diagnostic value of CBC results depends on a person's ability to relate historical and physical findings with abnormal concentrations or structure of blood cells. No one pattern is unique to any infection, and no agent consistently produces unique hematologic changes. As is addressed in later chapters on individual blood cells, many factors can cause abnormal CBC results other than bacterial infections.

Before highlighting the major CBC changes, the meaning of terms used to describe or classify inflammatory responses needs to be considered. No classification system for describing or characterizing inflammatory responses is both complete and simple. Abnormal leukogram results might be classified as acute, acute purulent, acute severe, acute overwhelming, chronic, chronic active, established purulent, chronic suppurative or chronic pyogranulomatous. Such classifications may help a group from one school communicate effectively, but can lead to confusion when colleagues from another school are not well versed in applying the same classification criteria.

Neutrophilia With a Left Shift, Frequently With a Lymphopenia, May Be Accompanied by a Monocytosis

Neutrophilia with a left shift is the hallmark of acute inflammation. In this context, it is important to recognize that acute refers to the type of inflammatory reaction and not the duration of the disease or inflammatory process. The active bacterial infection of several weeks duration that still promotes release of immature neutrophils from marrow is still promoting an acute inflammatory response. In people and probably in domestic animals, a left shift has high diagnostic specificity for inflammatory disease, whereas toxic changes have high diagnostic sensitivity.[27] Bacterial, nonbacterial, and noninfectious inflammatory disorders can initiate similar changes in blood.

With persistence of an infection, cytokines may stimulate neutropoiesis sufficiently to allow time for cell maturation before marrow release. Accordingly, the left shift diminishes, and a mature neutrophilia is created.

Lymphopenia is common in an acute inflammatory response because inflammatory mediators that stimulate movement of neutrophils during acute inflammation also stimulate movement of lymphocytes from blood to the inflamed tissue and lymphoid tissues.[28] The severity of the lymphopenia somewhat reflects the severity of the systemic inflammatory response.

Monocytosis may occur early or late in an inflammatory response. It is commonly associated with necrosis caused by infectious and noninfectious disorders.

Neutrophils With Toxic Changes

Toxic changes in neutrophils include diffuse cytoplasmic basophilia, focal cytoplasmic basophilia or Döhle bodies, cytoplasmic foaminess or vacuolization, asynchronous nuclear maturation, and, rarely, toxic granulation. Abnormally large neutrophils (giant neutrophils) are considered to represent toxic change. These structural changes in neutrophils represent degenerative changes or maturation defects that occur during rapid neutropoiesis. Neutrophils with toxic changes are commonly associated with severe bacterial infections but can be found in other inflammatory disorders, after granulocyte-colony stimulating factor (G-CSF) administration, in turpentine-induced inflammation,[29] and in dyscrasias induced by cefonicid and cefazedone.[30]

The origin of the term "toxic change" is uncertain but has been associated with the endotoxemia.[31] Although toxic change is not specific for bacterial infections or endotoxemia, toxic change usually indicates that an animal has a severe inflammatory disorder that commonly is bacterial. In one study with people as subjects, 85.9% of patients who had vacuolated neutrophils (with or without other toxic changes) had positive cultures from blood, urine, sputum, or stool, and 51.3% had positive blood cultures. Several organisms were cultured, including gram-positive cocci, gram-negative bacilli, and *Candida*.[32]

Neutropenia, With or Without a Left Shift

Severe inflammatory diseases, regardless of the inciting agent, can create a neutropenia if neutrophil margination and emigration into inflamed tissues exceeds the release of neutrophils from marrow. Classic examples of such a response are salmonellosis in horses and coliform mastitis in cattle, but similar patterns can be seen with parvovirus enteritis in dogs and cats.

Because of a small storage pool of segmented neutrophils in bovine marrow, it is common for cattle with acute bacterial infections to have a neutropenia. Within days, increased neutrophil production and release may result in a neutrophilia.

Lymphocytosis

When seen in association with infectious diseases, a lymphocytosis typically reflects a generalized state of lymphoid hyperplasia. Accordingly, there may be enlargement of spleen or lymph nodes. For lymphocytosis to develop, the infectious process must persist for weeks to months and thus is associated with chronic infections. Typically, the magnitude of the inflammatory lymphocytosis is not more than double the upper limit of a species normal lymphocyte concentration. However, the author has seen a lymphocytosis of $35,000/\mu L$ in a dog that had an *Ehrlichia canis* infection.

Reactive Lymphocytes

Reactive lymphocytes (or immunocytes, virocytes) represent either stimulated T- or B-lymphocytes and can be found in blood of animals that have various acute and chronic infectious diseases. Reactive lymphocytes may have several structural features that are considered reactive changes: enhanced cytoplasmic basophilia; perinuclear halo; prominent Golgi zone; and eccentric, enlarged, cleaved, convoluted, lobulated, or bilobed nuclei. In some bacterial infections (e.g., ehrlichial infections in dogs), reactive hyperplasia can result in lymphoblasts and other lymphoid cells with mitotic nuclei in the peripheral blood.

Eosinophilia

Eosinophilia is an occasional finding in bacterial infections. If seen, it may represent a hypersensitivity to an agent (for example, staphylococcal hypersensitivity) or involvement of mast cells or basophils in a tissue's inflammatory response.

Mastocytemia

Transient mastocytemia is occasionally seen in dogs that have acute inflammatory diseases, including bacterial infections (see Chapter 48, Basophil and Mast Cell).

Anemia

The most common anemia seen in domestic mammals is the anemia of inflammatory disease; many of these diseases are caused by bacterial infections. This anemia is classically mild to moderate, normocytic, normochromic, and nonregenerative and results from both decreased erythrocyte production and decreased erythrocyte survival (see Chapter 35, Anemia of Inflammatory and Neoplastic Disease).

The erythrocytic bacterial parasites (*Hemobartonella, Eperythrozoon,* and *Anaplasma*) must be considered potential causes of hemolytic regenerative anemias in the appropriate species of animals. As mentioned previously, bacterial exotoxins also can cause hemolytic disorders such as bacillary hemoglobinuria and yellow lamb disease.

Thrombocytopenia

Thrombocytopenia develops as a result of decreased platelet survival or decreased platelet production. Both processes may be present in animals that have bacterial infections. Thrombocytopenia has long been recognized as the most common hematologic abnormality in animals that have rickettsial and especially ehrlichial infections.[33-36]

ESTABLISHING RELATIONSHIP BETWEEN DISEASE AND BACTERIAL INFECTION

Proving the relation between an organism and a disease is the basis of Koch's Rules or Postulates.[37]

1. The organism must be found in each case of the disease.
2. The organism must be isolated and grown in pure culture.
3. The organism must experimentally reproduce the disease in susceptible animals.
4. The organism must be isolated from the experimentally infected animals.

The need to fulfill Koch's Postulates varies considerably in clinical medicine. A presumptive clinical diagnosis is frequently sufficient to initiate antimicrobial therapy, and the diagnosis is often thought to be confirmed if an animal responds to treatment. However, fulfilling Koch's Postulates should still be our goal for establishing the relation between an organism and a disease, especially when new organisms are discovered or a new clinical manifestation of an infection is suspected.

Detecting and Identifying Infective Agents

Detecting and identifying an infective agent in an animal is an essential step in confirming a diagnosis of cause. However, methods available to veterinarians vary greatly in their diagnostic sensitivity and specificity and thus in their diagnostic accuracy and predictive value.

Microscopic analysis of inflammatory exudates or inflamed tissues may allow a diagnostician to detect the presence of bacteria but not allow the identification of the specific organisms. Microscopic detection of the rickettsial agents is possible but the diagnostic sensitivity may be high or low. For example, the granulocytic ehrlichial species of dogs (*E. ewingii* and other species) and horses (*E. equi*) are readily detected in blood neutrophils and eosinophils during early stages of the infection, but the monocytic ehrlichial species of dogs (*E. canis*) and horses (*E. risticii*) are rarely detected in peripheral blood. Blood buffy coat preparations increase the chances of finding infected cells because more leukocytes can be examined in a given time period.

Other bacteria (bacilli, cocci, spirochetes) are rarely detected by direct microscopic examinations of Gram-stained blood films as the number of bacteria are much lower than the reported 10^5 organisms/mL needed for detection. The sensitivity on Wright-stained and Acridine Orange-stained smears may be better because of the better differential staining.

Blood culturing is more sensitive than microscopic examination for detecting a bacteremia, but false-negative results are still common because of timing of sampling, inappropriate sample volumes, and inadequate processing. However, blood culture results can be positive when there are less than 5 organisms/mL of blood.[38]

Culturing of rickettsial species require cell cultures that support the growth and multiplication of the agents. For some agents (e.g., *E. canis*), several monocytic cultures have been used successfully, whereas a cell line to propagate *E. ewingii* has not been established.

During the 1990s, molecular biologic techniques (such as polymerase chain reaction [PCR]) have been developed and they have extremely high analytical sensitivity but varying degrees of analytical specificity and accuracy. For example, PCR assays for *E. canis* may generate positive results with a minute number of organisms, but the assay might detect ehrlichial species other than *E. canis*. The issue is complicated further because some ehrlichial isolates have been considered of the same species but have been shown to vary in nucleotide sequences. Are they unique species or separate strains within a species?

Establishing Serologic Evidence of Bacterial Infections

Establishing that an animal has a serologic titer to an infectious agent has long been a method of providing circumstantial evidence of a clinical infection. Although methods of detecting antibodies have improved, results still must be interpreted with caution. A single positive titer means that an animal has an antibody that reacts with the antigen in the serologic assay. A low titer might reflect a convalescent titer and not an active infection. Therefore, at least a fourfold elevation in a convalescent titer compared with the initial titer is recommended for a serologic diagnosis. An extremely high initial titer generally indicates an active infection.

Assuming that a titer indicates an active infection with a specific organism has led to much confusion in the past two decades. For many years, a dog that had a titer to *E. canis* was considered to have canine ehrlichiosis, and just about any clinical illness present in the tested animal was attributed to an *E. canis* infection. However these conclusions were reconsidered when it was learned that such titers could represent cross-reactive antibodies and that dogs could have such antibodies and not have a clinical illness. Similar presumptive conclusions resulting from animals that had titers against *Borrellia burgdorferi* have led to erroneous diagnoses of Lyme disease.

Fulfilling Koch's Postulates

Microscopic examinations, cultures, molecular techniques, and serologic assays either directly or indirectly help fulfill the first two Koch's Postulates. The last two postulates involving experimental infections are rarely fulfilled in clinical medicine. However, the difficulty in justifying experimental infections should not exclude the need for such research to establish firmly the relation between an infective agent and a disease. Also, experimental infections may be necessary to control sufficient factors so that a pathogenesis of the disease can be studied.

REFERENCES

1. **Dale DC, Liles C.** How many neutrophils are enough? Lancet 1998;351: 1752–1753.
2. **Brooks GF, Butel JS, Ornston LN, Jawetz E, Melnick JL, Adelberg EA.** Pathogenesis of bacterial infection & host resistance to infection. In: Brooks GF, Butel JS, Ornston LN, Jawetz E, Melnick JL, Adelberg EA, eds. Jawetz, Melnick & Adelberg's medical microbiology. 19th ed. Norwalk: Appleton & Lange, 1991;130–147.
3. **Rutter JM.** Bacterial toxins as virulence determinants of veterinary pathogens: an overview. In: Roth JA, ed. Virulence mechanisms of bacterial pathogens. Washington, DC: American Society for Microbiology, 1988;213–227.
4. **Brown JF, Leite F, Czuprynski CJ.** Binding of *Pasteurella haemolytica* leukotoxin to bovine leukocytes. Infect Immun 1997;65:3719–3724.
5. **Stevens PK, Czuprynski CJ.** *Pasteurella haemolytica* leukotoxin induces bovine leukocytes to undergo morphologic changes consistent with apoptosis in vitro. Infect Immun 1996;64:2687–2694.
6. **Cheryk LA, Hooper-McGrevy KE, Gentry PA.** Alterations in bovine platelet function and acute phase proteins induced by *Pasteurella haemolytica* A1. Can J Vet Res 1998;62:1–8.
7. **Nyarko KA, Coomber BL, Mellors A, Gentry PA.** Bovine platelet adhesion is enhanced by leukotoxin and sialoglycoprotease isolated from *Pasteurella haemolytica* A1 cultures. Vet Microbiol 1998;61:81–91.
8. **Weiss DJ, Rashid J.** The sepsis-coagulant axis: a review. J Vet Intern Med 1998;12:317–324.
9. **McCuskey RS, Urbaschek R, Urbaschek B.** The microcirculation during endotoxemia. Cardiovasc Res 1996;32:752–763.
10. **Kitajima S, Tsuda M, Eshita N, Matsushima Y, Saitoh M, Momma J, Kurokawa Y.** Lipopolysaccharide-associated elevation of serum and urinary nitrite/nitrate levels and hematological changes in rats. Toxicol Lett 1995; 78:135–140.
11. **Wachowicz B, Saluk J, Kaca W.** Response of blood platelets to *Proteus mirabilis* lipopolysaccharide. Microbiol Immunol 1998;42:47–49.
12. **Otto CM, Rawlings CA.** Tumor necrosis factor production in cats in response to lipopolysaccharide: an in vivo and in vitro study. Vet Immuno Immunopathol 1995;49:183–188.
13. **Michie HR, Manogue KR, Spriggs DR, Revhaug A, O'Dwyer S, Dinarello CA, Cerami A, Wolff SM, Wilmore DW.** Detection of circulating tumor necrosis factor after endotoxin administration. N Engl J Med 1988;318:1481–1486.
14. **Kreutz M, Ackermann U, Hauschildt S, Krause SW, Riedel D, Bessler W, Andreesen R.** A comparative analysis of cytokine production and tolerance induction by bacterial lipopeptides, lipopolysaccharides and *Staphyloccous aureus* in human monocytes. Immunology 1997;92:396–401.
15. **Heinrich PC, Castell JV, Andus T.** Interleukin-6 and the acute phase response. Biochem J 1990;265:621–636.
16. **Horn KD.** Evolving strategies in the treatment of sepsis and systemic inflammatory response syndrome (SIRS). QJM 1998;91:265–277.
17. **Moldawer LL, Marano MA, Wei H, Fong Y, Silen ML, Kuo G, Manogue KR, Vlassara H, Cohen H, Cerami A, Lowry SF.** Cachectin/tumor necrosis factor-α alters red blood cell kinetics and induces anemia in vivo. FASEB J 1989;3:1637–1643.
18. **Maeda H.** Role of microbial proteases in pathogenesis. Microbiol Immunol 1996;40:685–699.
19. **Rikihisa Y.** Ultrastructure of *Rickettsiae* with special emphasis on *Ehrlichiae*. In: Williams JC, Kakoma I, eds. Ehrlichiosis. Boston: Kluwer Academic Publisher, 1990;22–31.
20. **Silver BJ, Hamilton BD, Toossi Z.** Suppression of TNF-α gene expression by hemin: implications for the role of iron homeostasis in host inflammatory responses. J Leukoc Biol 1997;62:547–552.
21. **Decker MJ, Freeman MJ, Morter RL.** Evaluation of mechanisms of leptospiral hemolytic anemia. Am J Vet Res 1970;31:873–878.
22. **Bhasin JL, Freeman MJ, Morter RL.** Properties of a cold hemagglutinin

associated with leptospiral hemolytic anemia of sheep. Infect Immun 1971;3:398–404.

23. **Shurin SB, Anderson P, Zollinger J, Rathbun RK.** Pathophysiology of hemolysis in infections with *Hemophilus influenzae* type b. J Clin Invest 1986;77:1340–1348.

24. **Weiss DJ, Aird B, Murtaugh MP.** Neutrophil-induced immunoglobulin binding to erythrocytes involves proteolytic and oxidative injury. J Leukoc Biol 1992;51:19–23.

25. **Harrus S, Waner T, Weiss DJ, Keysary A, Bark H.** Kinetics of serum antiplatelet antibodies in experimental acute canine ehrlichiosis. Vet Immuno Immunopathol 1996;51:13–20.

26. **Harrus S, Waner T, Eldor A, Zwang E, Bark H.** Platelet dysfunction associated with experimental acute canine ehrlichiosis. Vet Record 1996;139:290–293.

27. **Seebach JD, Morant R, Ruegg R, Seifer B, Fehr J.** The diagnostic value of the neutrophil left shift in predicting inflammatory and infectious disease. Am J Clin Pathol 1997;107:582–591.

28. **Imhof BA, Dunon D.** Leukocyte migration and adhesion. Adv Immunol 1995;58:345–416.

29. **Gossett KA, MacWilliams PS.** Ultrastructure of canine toxic neutrophils. Am J Vet Res 1982;43:1634–1637.

30. **Bloom JC, Lewis HB, Sellers TS, Deldar A, Morgan DG.** The hematopathology of cefonicid- and cefazedone-induced blood dyscrasias in the dog. Toxicol Appl Pharmacol 1987;90:143–155.

31. **Deldar A, Naylor JM, Bloom JC.** Effects of *Escherichia coli* endotoxin on leukocyte and platelet counts, fibrinogen concentrations, and blood clotting in colostrum-fed and colostrum-deficient neonatal calves. Am J Vet Res 1984;45:670–677.

32. **Jafri AK, Kass L.** Vacuolated neutrophils can predict serious infection. Lab Med 1998;29:633–636.

33. **Troy GC, Vulgamott JC, Turnwald GH.** Canine ehrlichiosis: a retrospective study of 30 naturally occurring cases. J Am Anim Hosp Assoc 1980;16:181–187.

34. **Stockham SL, Schmidt DA, Curtis KS, Schauf BG, Tyler JW, Simpson ST.** Evaluation of granulocytic ehrlichiosis in dogs of Missouri, including serologic status in dogs of Missouri, including serologic status to *Ehrlichia canis, Ehrlichia equi* and *Borrelia burgdorferi*. Am J Vet Res 1992;53:63–68.

35. **Harrus S, Kass PH, Klement E, Waner T.** Canine monocytic ehrlichiosis: a retrospective study of 100 cases, and an epidemiological investigation of prognostic indicators for the disease. Vet Record 1997;141:360–363.

36. **Gribble DH.** Equine ehrlichiosis. J Am Vet Med Assoc 1969;155:462–469.

37. **Merchant IA, Packer RA.** The mechanism of infection. In: Merchant IA, Packer RA, eds. Veterinary bacteriology and virology. 7th ed. Ames: The Iowa State University Press, 1967;117–128.

38. **Calvert CA.** Cardiovascular infections: bacteremia and endocarditis. In: Greene CE, ed. Infectious diseases of the dog and cat. 2nd ed. Philadelphia: W.B. Saunders, 1998;567–582.

CHAPTER 8

Toxicologic Effects on Blood and Bone Marrow

• JOHN E. LUND

The presence or absence of hematologic changes in laboratory animals exposed to environmental chemicals or new pharmaceutical agents is an important element in the overall assessment of the risks and hazards of potential human or animal exposure. Blood and bone marrow are a complex mixture of cells that respond in different ways to various toxicologic insults. Chemically induced anemia, for example, may result from direct myelotoxicity, hypoproliferative bone marrow effects, oxidative stress, nonoxidative destruction, immune hemolysis, megaloblastic change, ineffective erythropoiesis, or blood loss. The effects of chemicals on blood cells are not restricted to the blood cell destruction or the inhibition of hemopoiesis. Some agents stimulate hemopoiesis. Others affect the function of blood cells, resulting in depressed or enhanced function. This chapter summarizes the basic principles of toxicologic hematology and presents some of the potential hematologic effects that can be anticipated in animals exposed to xenobiotics. The broad topic of chemically induced hemopoietic neoplasia is not discussed.

TOXICOLOGY STUDY METHODS

The core group of tests that has been recommended for the hematologic evaluation of toxicity in study animals includes white blood cell (WBC), red blood cell (RBC), platelet (PLT), differential leukocyte count, hemoglobin (Hgb), hematocrit (HCT), mean corpuscular volume (MCV), mean corpuscular hemoglobin (MCH), MCH concentration (MCHC), activated partial thromboplastin time (APTT), and prothrombin time (PT).[1-3] Some laboratories include fibrinogen levels in the core group. Reticulocyte counts and bone marrow cytology were not included; however, if the counting instrument that is used has the capability for automated reticulocyte counts, they should be included in the core group. If the counting instrument does not have the capability for automated reticulocyte counts, air-dried blood slides stained for reticulocytes should be prepared and saved for evaluation if needed. Similarly, bone marrow slides should be prepared for each animal and should be evalu-

ated if the hematology results indicate the need for such an evaluation. Bone marrow smears are used for evaluation of cytologic detail. Sections of bone marrow from the sternum or another active bone marrow site are used to assess bone marrow cellularity. The minimum cytologic examination should include a myeloid relative to erythroid cell ratio (M:E ratio) and a morphologic assessment of the precursor cells. Bone marrow toxicity can be assessed directly with in vitro bone marrow culture methods.

Blood samples for hematology tests are commonly taken from the jugular vein in dogs, the femoral vein in monkeys, and the heart, vena cava, abdominal aorta, or orbital venous plexus in rats and mice. Interim hematology tests are performed on studies of 30 days' duration or more to determine the time of onset and the progression of hematologic changes. In rodent studies, interim blood samples can be obtained from the orbital venous plexus, by clipping the tail or piercing a lateral tail vein. However, test results from samples obtained by these methods are not comparable with results obtained from aortic or cardiac blood samples.[4] Because of the large volume of blood required, interim coagulation tests are normally only performed on nonrodent species. However, coagulation tests can be performed in rat studies if there are animals specifically designated for removal from the study for interim sampling. A 12- to 18-hour overnight fast is recommended for both rodent and nonrodent species prior to collection of blood samples since the samples are also used for serum chemistry tests. Fasting of dogs and rats for 16 hours does not appear to affect the hematology results.[5] However, fasting rats for 24 hours may result in a slightly increased RBC, Hgb, HCT, and platelet count as a result of decreased water intake during the period of food deprivation.[6]

GOOD LABORATORY PRACTICE REGULATIONS

Hematology tests performed in preclinical toxicity studies or chemical toxicity studies that are to be used for submissions to governmental regulatory agencies are subject to the Good Laboratory Practice (GLP) regulations and guidelines issued separately by the governments of Japan, the United States, and the European Community. The regulations require that the clinical laboratory have standard operating procedures (SOP) for the assays conducted and that laboratory personnel be properly trained. Routine quality-assurance inspections must be performed to ensure adherence to the SOPs. In addition, the regulations require that the laboratories retain training records for laboratory personnel and records of equipment maintenance and repair, assay validation, and validation of electronic systems (including data output and transfer). The regulations also require that the raw data from the laboratory tests be retained for a specified period.

SECONDARY HEMATOLOGIC CHANGES

The animals used in toxicity studies, with the exception of primates, are purposely bred with a known genetic background. They have been sheltered from common pathogens, are housed in a controlled environment, and have a common diet with a comparable caloric intake. In rodent studies, the combination of a controlled animal population and a relatively large number of animals per treatment group results in test results that are fairly uniform. Small differences in the group mean values for the treated animals compared with the control group values are often statistically significant. However, not all of the small group differences detectable in this setting are directly related to the toxicologic effects of the compound being studied. Some of the small differences result from chance variation or are the result of secondary changes related to effects of the agent on fluid balance or food intake. Some differences also result from blood loss as a consequence of drawing frequent blood samples for hematology tests and pharmacokinetic determinations. One example of a secondary change is the observation of bone marrow hypocellularity in rats dosed with agents or formulations that produce diarrhea. The fluid loss and hemoconcentration result in a feedback inhibition of erythropoiesis and a decrease in the number of erythrocytic precursors in the bone marrow. [7,8] It is important to recognize secondary effects. In the above example, a potential new drug could be dropped from further development or the risk of exposure to a chemical could be overestimated because of a false assumption of bone marrow toxicity. In studies with dogs and primates, the treatment group size is smaller, and there is more variation among animals. It is often difficult to demonstrate statistical significance for hematologic changes because of the small group size.

CHEMICALLY INDUCED CHANGES IN CELLULAR FUNCTION

Altered cellular function is an important hematologic consequence of exposure of laboratory animals to xeno-

biotics. Altered erythrocyte function results in a decreased capacity to carry oxygen to the tissues. Methemoglobin, sulfhemoglobin, and carboxyhemoglobin are chemically induced hemoglobin variants that are ineffective for the transport of oxygen. Methemoglobin is the most commonly encountered hemoglobin variant in toxicity study animals. Substances that are capable of oxidizing hemoglobin, resulting in methemoglobin formation, include nitrites, nitrates, chlorates, quinones, and various pharmaceutical products. The presence of Heinz bodies is an indication of oxidized hemoglobin. Hemoglobin variants are detected and quantitated by spectrophotometric methods (see Chapter 31, Anemias Associated With Drugs and Chemicals). Altered erythrocyte function can also result from changes in the affinity of hemoglobin for oxygen not associated with hemoglobin variants. Salicylate poisoning and cobalt toxicity are two examples.[9,10] Increased affinity of hemoglobin for oxygen can be inferred by increased venous oxygen saturation and can be confirmed by demonstration of a shift in the oxygen dissociation curve. Erythrocyte shape changes have been reported after exposure of erythrocytes to various drugs. Echinocytes are produced when blood is incubated with anionic amphipathic drugs, and stomatocytes are produced when blood is incubated with cationic amphipathic drugs.[11] Adverse effects of chemicals on neutrophil function are usually detected by the presence of abscesses, inflammatory lesions, or early death of animals on longer-term toxicity studies. When impairment of neutrophil function is suspected, there are several in vitro tests that can be used for confirmation.[12] In vitro tests are not recommended as a screen to detect functional deficits in the absence of clinical evidence of impaired function. In vitro assessment of neutrophil function should not be attempted if an animal is ill or debilitated since the results are influenced by the general condition of the animal.[12] Activation of neutrophils resulting in liver injury was observed in rats given alpha-naphthylisothiocyanate.[13] The hepatocellular injury was considered the result of the release of cathepsin G and elastase from the activated neutrophils. Aggregates of histiocytes in various tissues, indicating possible altered monocyte or macrophage function, have been reported in several toxicity studies in dogs.[14,15]

Altered lymphocyte function may be nonspecific, secondary to generalized toxicity, or the result of specific targeting of lymphocytes by the chemical under evaluation.[16] The changes can be divided into those in which immune function is impaired and those in which tissue-damaging allergic or autoimmune responses are initiated.[17,18] The animals that have impaired function are often lymphocytopenic.[19] Both in vivo and in vitro tests are available to document altered lymphocyte function.[19-22] Alterations in host resistance provide the best prediction for potential health-threatening immune dysfunction.[16]

Platelet function can be altered by various chemicals and drugs either by inhibition of platelet aggregation or by activation of platelets. Activation of platelets may result in the formation of intravascular thrombi and subsequent vascular damage.[23,24] Platelet function can be assessed by in vitro, in vivo, and ex vivo methods.[25]

INCREASED BLOOD CELL COUNTS

An increase in the number of peripheral blood cells after exposure to a xenobiotic may be the result of altered distribution, increased rate of production and release, or longer residence time in the blood. The neutrophilia observed after the administration of glucocorticoids is the result of both an increased release of neutrophils from the bone marrow and a delay in the egress of neutrophils from the blood into the tissues. Cytokines are polypeptide cell regulators that are produced by many different cell types in the body (see Chapter 15, Cytokine Regulation of Hemopoiesis, and Chapter 42, Cytokines). The toxicologic effects of large doses of recombinant cytokines on blood and bone marrow include stimulation or depression of bone marrow cell proliferation, enhanced differentiation, enhanced endothelial adhesion, enhanced migration, and enhanced activation.[26] The hematologic response to a particular cytokine can be variable, depending on the blood cell type examined and the time of evaluation in relation to the time of cytokine administration.[26,27] Some cytokines, for example, erythropoietin and granulocyte colony-stimulating factor (CSF) are somewhat cell line specific, and their administration to laboratory animals at pharmacologic and toxicologic doses results in enhanced cell proliferation and differentiation of the target cell population, with an absolute increase in the number of circulating cells.[28] However, if a heterologous cytokine is administered to laboratory animals, antibodies produced against the protein may cross react with the host cytokine. Dogs and rabbits treated with heterologous recombinant CSF developed neutropenia, which persisted after the administration of CSF was terminated.[29,30] Chemicals unrelated to cytokines can also stimulate bone marrow cell production. Cobalt stimulates erythropoiesis through an effect on oxygen affinity, resulting in increased levels of erythropoietin.[31] Lithium stimulates granulocytopoiesis by stimulating increased stem cell differentiation into the granulopoietic pathway.[32] Thrombocytosis was observed in dogs after dietary administration of N-methylpyrrolidone.[33] Secondary polycythemia in toxicity studies is most often the result of decreased fluid volume. Increased neutrophil counts, secondary to release of cells from the bone marrow storage pool or demargination of cells from the blood vessel walls, are not often observed with standard toxicity study protocols because blood samples are not routinely taken immediately or shortly after dosing.

DIRECT MYELOTOXICITY

Bone marrow is a complex mixture of cells with a high rate of reproduction and is vulnerable to the harmful effects of many chemicals. Bone marrow appears to react uniformly in all the scattered parts. It is capable of ex-

panding output by 5 to 10 times the normal rate if demand is increased. However, if the pluripotent stem cell input is reduced below 10% of normal, the ability to compensate fails and pancytopenia results. Direct myelotoxicity is a serious dose-limiting toxicologic effect that generally affects all hemopoietic cell lines but may have some degree of preferential toxicity, depending on the agent involved. Direct myelotoxicity is observed in animals dosed with antineoplastic agents but is also observed after exposure to some antibiotics and other unrelated compounds. The sequence of declining blood cell counts is related to the residence time of the cells in the blood. Because of the short half-life of the neutrophil, neutropenia is observed first, followed by thrombocytopenia, and then anemia. There is a large reserve of mature neutrophils in the bone marrow. The reserve pool in the dog is approximately 7.5 times the number of cells in circulation and represents a 3- to 4-day supply of neutrophils. In addition, there are enough maturing postmitotic cells to supply the daily neutrophil requirement for approximately 1 week. After exposure to a myelotoxic agent, the number of circulating neutrophils does not decline until the bone marrow storage pool is depleted and the rate of neutrophil production and maturation is insufficient to keep up with demand. Erythrocytes and platelets have a longer residence time in the blood. Declining platelet counts are observed after a 2- to 4-week period, and erythrocyte decline is observed after a longer period, depending on the extent of bone marrow damage. The decline in erythrocytes and platelets does not depend on depletion of a reserve population. There is only a small reserve of reticulocytes that is rapidly released,[34] and no platelet reserve. Immune-mediated cytotoxicity has a similar clinical presentation when the effect is confined to bone marrow cells. However, unlike direct bone marrow toxicity, the incidence of immune bone marrow cell damage is not dose dependent, and not all animals in a particular dose group are affected. To a large extent, bone marrow toxicity can be assessed by the changes observed in the peripheral blood and is confirmed by examination of the bone marrow. Histologically, the initial loss of cells in the bone marrow is most evident in the central portion of the medullary cavity. With the loss of bone marrow parenchymal cells, the vascular sinusoids are enlarged, dilated, and engorged with RBCs.

HYPOPROLIFERATIVE RESPONSE

Minimal to mild normocytic normochromic anemia with a poor reticulocyte response is often observed in toxicity study animals. Production of neither WBCs nor platelets is impaired. The histologic and cytologic appearance of the bone marrow is usually within normal limits. The pathogenesis of this hypoproliferative anemia is probably secondary to inanition associated with inappetence, endocrine dysfunction, renal toxicity, or other systemic toxicologic effects. A similar hypoproliferative anemia, secondary to decreased availability of iron, has been induced by the chronic administration of tumor necrosis factor or the administration of agents that produce chronic inflammatory changes.[35,36] Diagnostic features of anemia secondary to inflammation are presented in Chapter 35. Chloramphenicol in concentrations within the therapeutic range suppressed the activity of bone marrow mitochondrial ferrochelatase activity in dogs, which resulted in a block in the final step of heme synthesis and a significant reticulocytopenia.[37] Hypoproliferative anemia resulting from decreased levels of erythropoietin secondary to chronic renal toxicity has been observed after the long-term administration of cadmium.[38] Hypoplastic granulocytopenia is not often observed in toxicity studies but has been reported in rats and dogs exposed to an antihypertensive agent.[39] Hypoproliferative thrombocytopenia has been reported in dogs given a single dose of estrogen.[40] The dogs exhibited slight granulocytosis, a slight decline in the HCT, and a significant thrombocytopenia with few megakaryocytes in the bone marrow.

MACROCYTIC RESPONSE

Macrocytic anemia observed in toxicity studies is usually the result of a regenerative bone marrow response to erythrocyte loss or destruction. Nonregenerative macrocytic anemia has been reported in mice exposed to 3'-azido'3-deoxythymidine (AZT), isoprene, and 1,3-butadiene.[41,42] The cellularity of the bone marrow in the AZT-treated mice was decreased. Bone marrow cellularity was not altered in the mice exposed to the other two chemicals. All three chemicals interacted with DNA; however, the mechanism for macrocytosis in these refractory anemias was not determined. Rats treated with AZT also developed nonregenerative macrocytic anemia; however, erythroid hyperplasia was observed in the bone marrow, and this led to the diagnosis of ineffective erythropoiesis.[43] Megaloblasts were not observed in the blood or in the bone marrow. Megaloblastic anemia with ineffective erythropoiesis is the clinical expression of impaired DNA synthesis in bone marrow cells caused by a deficiency of folate or cobalamin, the two vitamins necessary for normal production of DNA. Megaloblastic anemia has been observed in human patients who have drug-induced folate or cobalamin deficiency but has not been reported in toxicity study animals. The presence of ring sideroblasts in the bone marrow is an indication of impaired heme synthesis. Ring sideroblasts have been reported in dogs treated with an antibiotic that suppressed bacterial protein synthesis.[44] The dogs were not anemic, and the significance of the ring sideroblasts was not known.

DECREASED PERIPHERAL LIFESPAN

Drugs or chemicals that cause anemia by decreasing the life span of the erythrocyte are classified as oxidants, nonoxidants, or agents that provoke an immune response. Erythrocytes have several defense mechanisms that protect against the harmful effects of activated oxygen. Inherited antioxidant deficiencies, such as glucose-6-phosphate dehydrogenase deficiency or unstable hemoglobins are present in the human population but have not been observed in purpose-bred laboratory animals. As a result, animals that have increased sensitivity to oxidative agents are not encountered in toxicity studies. However, many oxidant compounds exist that can overwhelm the intact antioxidative defenses of the erythrocytes in normal animals if given in sufficient amounts, resulting in the formation of denatured hemoglobin and damage to other cellular structures. Nonoxidant mechanisms of hemolysis may involve inhibition of enzymes of the pentose-phosphate and glycolytic pathways or damage to the cellular membrane. In many cases the mechanism by which these hematotoxic chemicals shorten the life span of erythrocytes is not completely understood. Hemolysis can be inferred by the rapidity of the onset of anemia and the presence of increased reticulocytes (polychromasia), nucleated erythrocytes, Howell–Jolly bodies, increased anisocytosis (increased RBC distribution width), or increased RBC volume. Heinz bodies, eccentrocytes, and the presence of increased methemoglobin are more definitive findings that would indicate an oxidant mechanism of erythrocyte destruction. Persistence of Howell–Jolly bodies without anemia is an indication of DNA damage.[45] To determine if the erythrocyte life span has been shortened by the agent under study, random-labeling methods rather than cohort methods are used because the results are available in a relatively short time. In a random-label study, erythrocytes in a small sample of blood from the study animal or a donor animal, depending on the purpose of the study, are labeled and are infused into the study animal. Because the ages of the erythrocytes in the labeled sample range from newly released to senescent erythrocytes, the decrease in the number of labeled cells over time is exponential, and the result is expressed as the half-life of the erythrocytes. Cohort methods label a cohort of precursor cells in the bone marrow and the appearance and loss of labeled cells in the blood is monitored to determine the life span of the erythrocytes. The animals have to be sampled for a time period encompassing the normal life span of their erythrocytes. When hemolysis is observed in intravenous studies, the formulation should be evaluated for compatibility with blood using in vitro assays.[46,47] Hemosiderin can be demonstrated in Prussian blue-stained kidney sections if the hemolysis was intravascular.[48]

Neutropenia and thrombocytopenia resulting from non-immune-mediated increased utilization, destruction, or sequestration have also been reported.[49,50] A slight to mild neutropenia, with no evidence of direct myelotoxicity, is often observed in animals administered antibiotics. The neutropenia, along with reduced globulin levels, has been attributed to a reduced demand on normal host defense mechanisms as the result of antibiotic treatment.[51] Decreased demand as the mechanism for neutropenia in animals treated with antibiotics can be differentiated from direct myelotoxicity by the presence of normal bone marrow cellularity, with no depletion of the neutrophil reserve. Endotoxin contamination of intravenous formulations should be considered if neutropenia is observed shortly after the administration of intravenous formulations.

Slight to mild lymphocytopenia is often observed in toxicity study animals that have clinical and physical evidence of toxicity and is assumed to be a nonspecific stress response. Glucocorticoids produce a significant lymphocytopenia in corticosteroid-sensitive species secondary to lysis or redistribution of lymphocytes out of the circulation to other lymphoid compartments.[52] Lymphocytopenia is also observed after treatment with the same agents that are associated with neutropenia, thrombocytopenia, and anemia as the result of direct myelotoxicity.

IMMUNE-MEDIATED CYTOPENIAS

The occurrence of immune-mediated cytopenias is observed more frequently in dogs and monkeys than in rodents. Study animals may have immune-mediated destruction of all peripheral blood cells or only of neutrophils, erythrocytes, platelets, or a combination of any two.[53] Not all animals in a treatment group are affected, and the incidence of affected animals may not have a positive dose-response relation, although frequently the incidence is higher in the high-dose groups.[53] The onset of decreased blood cell counts is delayed compared with direct bone marrow cell toxicity, and the time of onset is shorter on reexposure. When dosing is stopped, the restoration of normal blood cell counts usually takes a matter of days but may be delayed if the agent or metabolite(s) have a long clearance time. Direct antiglobulin assays and tests for antierythrocyte, antineutrophil, and antiplatelet antibodies in serum are used to confirm immune-mediated cell destruction. The assays do not always confirm the presence of antibodies[53] and within dose groups the test results are not always positive for cytopenic animals or negative for animals with normal cell counts. The bone marrow is normally very cellular, with a large population of proliferating cells. If the animals are neutropenic, the storage pool of mature neutrophils and band cells is virtually absent. This very cellular bone marrow, with no band or mature neutrophils, has been referred to as a maturation arrest by some investigators but the lack of mature cells is the result of increased utilization, not arrested maturation. When dosing is stopped and the agent or metabolite(s) is cleared from the blood, the number of neutrophils in the blood rapidly increases. As the number of neutrophils in the circulation approaches the normal level, the bone marrow storage pool is replenished.

BLOOD LOSS

Anemia in toxicity study animals as the result of blood loss, with the exception of altered hemostasis, is most often the result of gastrointestinal lesions.[54-56] The clinical presentation of hemorrhagic anemia is variable and depends on the extent and duration of blood loss.[48] Detection of anemia secondary to blood loss requires a careful search for the site of hemorrhage, particularly in the gastrointestinal tract. Gastrointestinal blood loss can be quantitated with radioisotope-tagged erythrocytes.

EFFECTS ON HEMOSTASIS

Hemostasis is accomplished by a combination of three factors: contraction of injured blood vessels, adhesion of platelets at the site of injury, and blood coagulation. Chemicals and drugs may enhance or depress hemostasis by effects on any of these three factors. Promotion of thrombosis is observed after vascular endothelial damage or induction of a hypercoagulable state. There are two cell types in blood vessels that are the principal targets of chemical injury: endothelial cells of the intima and smooth muscle cells of the media.[57] Endothelial cell injury with thrombus formation is most often observed after the intravascular administration of irritating formulations. In addition, there are compounds that cause generalized endothelial damage when administered intravenously.[57,58] A hypercoagulable state may result from platelet activation,[23] procoagulant effects,[59] or decreased fibrinolysis.[60] Administration of recombinant interleukin-1α to monkeys resulted in increased vascular procoagulant activity and microvascular deposits of fibrin strands without evidence of endothelial cell injury.[61] Intravascular thrombogenesis can be diagnosed by the microscopic observation of fibrin deposits in the capillaries of the lungs and glomeruli of the kidneys, but the animals must be examined as early as possible, since the microthrombi are often dissolved rapidly by fibrinolytic proteases.[60,61] Administration of ϵ-aminocaproic acid along with the agent being examined preserves the microthrombi from lysis.[62] The clinical toxicologist can obtain indirect evidence for thrombus formation from decreased platelet counts, assays for the presence of specific platelet factors, and the presence of fibrinogen and fibrin degradation products.[60] Ex vivo and in vitro methods are also available for the evaluation of potential thrombogenic substances.[60]

Chemically induced vascular injury as a cause of spontaneous or excessive bleeding in toxicity study animals is uncommon.[48] Clotting problems after hepatocellular necrosis occur only when there is substantial impairment of the synthetic ability of the liver since most of the clotting factors are produced in excess of the amount required in the plasma for hemostasis.[3] However, prolongation of the PT and APTT has been observed in rats as the result of chronic hepatotoxicity.[63] Depression of hepatocellular protein synthesis or inhibition of the synthesis of the vitamin-K-dependent clotting factors is frequently observed in toxicity study animals. Of particular interest was the inhibition of vitamin K synthesis by estrogen treatment in rats.[64] This finding was unexpected because oral estrogen contraceptive use in women was associated with an increased tendency for thrombosis and other circulatory disorders. A decrease in vitamin-K-dependent clotting factors has also been observed as the result of an effect of butylated hydroxytoluene on intestinal absorption and excretion of vitamin K.[65] Specific inhibitory effects on the hemostatic cascade have been reported after the administration of recombinant tissue-type plasminogen activator, recombinant hirudin, low-molecular-weight heparins, and dermatin sulfate.[62–68] In determining the cause of hemorrhage in toxicity study animals, both clinical findings and laboratory tests are important.[48]

BONE MARROW STROMAL REACTIONS

The bone marrow stroma consists of blood vessels, branching fibroblasts, adipose cells, macrophages, and myelinated and nonmyelinated nerve fibers supported by a delicate reticulin fiber network. The stromal macrophages and fibroblasts have an important role in the regulation of hemopoiesis, and chemicals that damage the stromal cells can adversely affect hemopoiesis.[41,67,69,70] Toxicologic stromal changes include fibrosis, several distinct types of necrosis, and increased fat cells. Primary myelofibrosis has not been reported in laboratory animals. However, myelofibrosis has been produced experimentally with various agents,[71–73] and there are reports of myelofibrosis in toxicity study animals.[74,75] Small foci of bone marrow necrosis, presumably the result of focal stromal cell toxicity, have been occasionally observed in animals dosed with noncyototoxic compounds (unpublished observation). The focal bone marrow necrosis was not associated with decreased blood cell counts. Focal to diffuse areas of fibrinoid necrosis may be observed after treatment with cytotoxic agents.[76] Treatment of rats with thiazolidinedione antidiabetic agents resulted in an increase in the size of the subcutaneous, intra-abdominal and, intrathoracic adipose tissue deposits and an increased number of fat cells in the bone marrow (unpublished observation). The increased number of fat cells was attributed to the pharmacologic action of the agent and was not considered an indication of bone marrow damage. Evaluation of the bone marrow stroma must be performed on bone marrow sections.

REFERENCES

1. **Thompson MB.** Clinical pathology in the National Toxicology Program. Tox Pathol 1992;20:484–489.
2. **Weingand K, Bloom J, Carakostas M, Hall R, Helfrich M, Latimer K, Levine B, Neptun D, Rebar A, Stitzel K, Troup C.** Clinical pathology testing recommendations for nonclinical toxicity and safety studies. Tox Pathol 1992;20:539–543.
3. **Boon GD.** An overview of hemostasis. Tox Pathol 1993;21:170–179.
4. **Suber RL, Kodell RL.** The effect of three phlebotomy techniques on hematological and clinical chemical evaluation in Sprague-Dawley rats. Vet Clin Pathol 1985;14:23–30.
5. **Matsuzawa T, Sakazume M.** Effects of fasting on hematology and clinical-chemistry values in the rat and dog. Comp Haematol Int 1994;4:152–156.
6. **Maejima K, Nagase S.** Effect of starvation and refeeding on the circadian rhythms of hematological and clinico-biochemical values and water intake of rats. Exp Anim 1991;40:389–393.
7. **Glader BE, Rambach WA, Howard HL.** Observations on the effect of testosterone and hydrocortisone on erythropoiesis. Ann N Y Acad Sci 1968;149:383–388.
8. **Dunn CDR.** Effect of dehydration on erythropoiesis in mice: relevance to the "anemia" of space flight. Av Space and Environ Med 1978;49:990–993.
9. **Miller ME, Howard D, Stohlman F Jr, Flanagan P.** Mechanism of erythropoietin production by cobaltous chloride. Blood 1974;44:339–346.
10. **Kravath RE, Abel G, Colli A, McNamara H, Cohen MJ.** Salicylate poisoning—effect on 2,3-diphosphoglycerate levels in the rat. Biochem Pharmacol 1972;21:2656–2658.
11. **Smith JE.** Erythrocyte membrane: structure, function, and pathophysiology. Vet Pathol 1987;24:471–476.
12. **Roth JA.** Evaluation of the influence of potential toxins on neutrophil function. Tox Pathol 1993;21:141–146.
13. **Hill DA, Roth RA.** Alpha-naphthylisothiocyanate causes neutrophils to release factors that are cytotoxic to hepatocytes. Toxicol Appl Physiol 1998;148:169–175.
14. **Kerry PJ, Wakefield ID, Evans JG.** Ocular changes induced in the beagle dog by intravenous infusion of a novel dopaminergic compound, FLP 65447. Tox Pathol 1993;21:274–282.
15. **Westwood FR, Duffy PA, Malpass DA, Jones HB, Topham JC.** Disturbance of macrophage and monocyte function in the dog by a thromboxane receptor antagonist: ICI 185,282. Tox Pathol 1995;23:373–384.
16. **Dean JH, Luster MI, Boorman GA, Lauer LD.** Procedures available to examine the immunotoxicity of chemicals and drugs. Pharmacol Rev 1982;34:137–148.
17. **Gleichmann E, Kimber I, Purchase IFH.** Immunotoxicology: suppressive and stimulatory effects of drugs and environmental chemicals on the immune system. Arch Toxicol 1989;63:257–273.
18. **Dean JH, Hincks J, Luster MI, Gerberick GF, Neumann DA, Hastings KL.** Safety evaluation and risk assessment using immunotoxicology methods. Int J Toxicol 1998;17:277–296.
19. **Houben GF, Penninks AH, Seinen W, Vos JG, van Loveren H.** Immunotoxic Effects of the color additive carmel color III: immune function studies in rats. Fund Appl Toxicol 1993;20:30–37.
20. **Garssen J, Van der Vliet H, De Klerk A, Goettsch W, Dormans JAMA, Bruggeman CA, Osterhaus ADME, van Loveren H.** A rat cytomegalovirus infection model as a tool for immunotoxicity testing. Eur J Pharmacol 1995;292:223–231.
21. **Burchiel SW, Kerkvliet NL, Gerberick GF, Lawrence DA, Ladics GS.** Assessment of immunotoxicity by multiparameter flow cytometry. Fund Appl Toxicol 1997;38:38–54.
22. **Vos JG, Smialowicz RJ, van Loveren H.** Animal models for assessment. In: Dean JH, Luster MI, Munson AE, Kimber I, eds. Immunotoxicology and immunopharmacology. New York: Raven Press, 1994.
23. **Bernat A, Herbert J-M.** Effect of various drugs on adriamycin-enhanced venous thrombosis in the rat: importance of PAF. Thromb Res 1994;75:91–97.
24. **Wang D, Chou C-L, Hsu K, Chen HI.** Cyclooxygenase pathway mediates lung injury induced by phorbol and platelets. J Appl Physiol 1991;70:2417–2421.
25. **Shebuski RJ.** Interruption of thrombosis and hemostasis by anti-platelet agents. Tox Pathol 1993;21:180–189.
26. **Anderson TD.** Cytokine-induced changes in the leukon. Tox Pathol 1993;21:147–157.
27. **Ulrich TR, del Castillo J, Yi ES, Yin S, McNiece I, Yung YP, Zsebo KM.** Hematologic effects of stem cell factor in vivo and in vitro in rodents. Blood 1991;78:645–650.
28. **Zinkl JG, Cain G, Jain NC, Sousa LM.** Haematological response of dogs to canine recombinant granulocyte colony stimulating factor (rcG-CSF). Comp Haematol Int 1992;2:151–156.
29. **Hammond WP, Csiba E, Canin A, Hockman H, Souza LM, Layton JE, Dale DC.** Chronic neutropenia. A new canine model induced by human granulocyte colony-stimulating factor. J Clin Invest 1991;87:704–710.
30. **Reagan WJ, Murphy D, Battaglino M, Bonney P, Boone TC.** Antibodies to canine granulocyte colony-stimulating factor induce persistent neutropenia. Vet Pathol 1995;32:374–378.
31. **Rakusan K, Rajhathy J.** Oxygen affinity of blood during cobalt-induced erythrocytic polycythemia and after its correction. Life Sci 1974;15:23–28.
32. **Gallicchio VS, Chen MG.** Modulation of murine pluripotential stem cell proliferation in vivo by lithium carbonate. Blood 1980;56:1150–1152.
33. **Becci PJ, Gephart LA, Koschier FJ, Johnson WD, Burnette LW.** Subchronic feeding study in beagle dogs of N-methylpyrrolidone. J Appl Toxicol 1983;3:83–86.
34. **Tavassoli M, Yoffey JM.** Bone marrow: structure and function. New York: Alan R. Liss, 1983:137.
35. **Johnson RA, Waddelow TA, Caro J, Oliff A, Roodman GD.** Chronic exposure to tumor necrosis factor in vivo preferentially inhibits erythropoiesis in nude mice. Blood 1989;74:130–138.
36. **Sartor RB, Anderle SK, Rifai N, Goo DAT, Comartie WJ, Schwab JH.** Protracted anemia associated with chronic, relapsing systemic inflammation induced by arthropathic peptidoglycan-polysaccharide polymers in rats. Infect Immun 1989;57:1177–1185.
37. **Manyan DR, Arimura GK, Yunis AA.** Chloramphenicol-induced erythroid suppression and bone marrow ferrochelatase activity in dogs. J Lab Clin Med 1972;79:137–144.
38. **Hiratsuka H, Katsuta O, Toyota N, Tsuchitani M, Umemura T, Marumo F.** Chronic cadmium exposure-induced renal anemia in ovariectomized rats. Toxicol Appl Pharmacol 1996;137:228–236.

39. **Martin RA, Barsoum NJ, Sturgess JM, de la Iglesia FA.** Leukocyte and bone marrow effects of a thiomorpholine quinazosin antihypertensive agent. Toxicol Appl Pharmacol 1985;81:166–173.

40. **Aranda E, Pizarro M, Pereira J, Mezzano D.** Accumulation of 5-hydroxy-tryptamine by aging platelets: studies in a model of suppressed thrombopoiesis in dogs. Thromb Haemostasis 1994;71:488–492.

41. **Luster MI, Germolec DR, White KL, Fuchs BA, Fort MM, Tomaszewski JE, Thompson M, Blair PC, McCay A, Munson AE, Rosenthal GJ.** A comparison of three nucleoside analogs with anti-retroviral activity on immune and hematopoietic functions in mice: in vitro toxicity to precursor cells and microstromal environment. Toxicol Appl Pharmacol 1989;101:328–339.

42. **Melnick RL, Sills RC, Roycroft JH, Chou BJ, Ragan HA, Miller RA.** Inhalation toxicity and carcinogenicity of isoprene in rats and mice: comparisons with 1,3-butadiene. Toxicol 1996;113:247–252.

43. **Thompson MB, Dunnick JK, Sutphin ME, Giles HD, Irwin RD, Prejean JD.** Hematologic toxicity of AZT and ddc administered as single agents and in combination to rats and mice. Fund Appl Toxicol 1991;17:159–176.

44. **Lund JE, Brown PK.** Hypersegmented megakaryocytes and megakaryocytes with multiple separate nuclei in dogs treated with PNU-100592, an oxazolidinone antibiotic. Tox Pathol 1997;25:339–343.

45. **Bailie NC, Osborne CA, Leininger JR, Fletcher TF, Johnston SD, Ogburn PN Griffith DP.** Teratogenic effect of acetohydroxamic acid in clinically normal beagles. Am J Vet Res 1986;47:2604–2611.

46. **Salauze D, Decouvetaere D.** In vitro assessment of the haemolytic potential of candidate drugs. Comp Haematol Int 1994;4:34–36.

47. **Jones HB, Reid DG, Luke JSH.** Evolution of structural changes leading to haemolysis in human erythrocytes treated with SF&F 95018, an antihypertensive compound with combined vasodilator and β-adrenoceptor antagonist properties. Toxicol In Vitro 1989;3:299–309.

48. **McGrath JP.** Assessment of hemolytic and hemorrhagic anemias in preclinical safety assessment studies. Tox Pathol 1993;21:158–163.

49. **Okada Y, Kawagishi M, Kusaka M.** Neutrophil kinetics of recombinant human granulocyte colony-stimulating factor-induced neutropenia in rats. Life Sci 1990;47:PL65–PL70.

50. **Yarrington JT, Kociba GJ, Gibson JP.** Thrombocytopenia in rats and dogs administered the antidepressant compound MDL-19,660. Toxicol Lett 1991;56:1–2.

51. **Spurling NW, Harcourt RA, Hyde JJ.** An evaluation of the safety of cefuroxime axetil during six months oral administration to beagle dogs. J Toxicol Sci 1986;11:237–277.

52. **Parrillo JE, Fauci AS.** Mechanisms of glucocorticoid action on immune processes. Ann Rev Pharmacol Toxicol 1979;19:179–201.

53. **Bloom JC, Thiem PA, Sellers TS, Deldar A, Lewis HB.** Cephalosporin-induced immune cytopenia in the dog: demonstration of erythrocyte-, neutrophil-, and platelet-associated IgG following treatment with cefazedone. Am J Hematol 1988;28:71–78.

54. **Okamura T, Garland EM, Cohen SM.** Glandular stomach hemorrhage induced by high dose saccharin in young rodents. Toxicol Lett 1994;74:129–140.

55. **Anthony A, Dhillon AP, Sim R, Nygard G, Pounder RE, Wakefield AJ.** Ulceration, fibrosis and diaphragm-like lesions in the caecum of rats treated with indomethacin. Aliment Pharmacol Ther 1994;8:417–424.

56. **Rodman LE, Farnell DR, Coyne JM, Allan PW, Hill DL, Duncan KLK, Tomaszewski JE, Smith AC, Page JG.** Toxicity of cordycepin in combination with the adenosine deaminase inhibitor 2'-deoxycoformycin in beagle dogs. Toxicol Appl Pharmacol 1997;147;39–45.

57. **Boor PJ, Gotlieb AI, Joseph EC, Kerns WD, Roth RA, Tomaszewski KE.** Chemical-induced vascular injury. Toxicol Appl Pharmacol 1995;132:177–195.

58. **Zbinden G, Grimm L.** Thrombogenic effects of xenobiotics. Arch Toxicol 1985;Suppl 8:131–141.

59. **Kanfer A, de Prost D, Guettier C, Nochy D, Le Floch V, Hinglais N, Druet P.** Enhanced glomerular procoagulant activity and fibrin deposition in rats with mercuric chloride-induced autoimmune nephritis. Lab Invest 1987;57:138–143.

60. **Schultz AE, Roth RA.** Fibrinolytic activity in blood and lungs of rats treated with monocrotaline pyrrole. Toxicol Appl Pharmacol 1993;121:129–137.

61. **Anderson TD, Arceo R, Hayes TJ.** Comparative toxicity and pathology associated with administration of recombinant HuIL-1α to animals. Int Rev Exp Pathol 1993;34A:9–36.

62. **Muller-Berghaus G, Reuter C.** Disseminated intravascular coagulation in galactosamine-induced experimental hepatitis. Thromb Res 1972;1:473–486.

63. **Lox CD, Davis JR.** The effects of long-term malathion or diazinon ingestion on the activity of hepatic synthesized clotting factors. Ectotoxicol Environ Saf 1983;7:546–551.

64. **Hart JE.** Vitamin K-dependent blood clotting changes in female rats treated with oestrogens. Thromb Haemost 1987;57:273–277.

65. **Suzuki H, Nako T, Hiraga K.** Vitamin K content of liver and feces from vitamin K-deficient and butylated hydroxytoluene (BHT)-treated male rats. Toxicol Appl Pharmacol 1983;67:152–155.

66. **Bloom JC, Sellers TS, Gries GC, Wheeldon EB, O'Rrien SR, Lewis HB.** The effect of human recombinant tissue-type plasminogen activator on clinical and laboratory parameters of hemostasis and systemic plasmogen activation in the dog and rat. Thromb Haemost 1988;60:271–279.

67. **Matthiasson SE, Lindblad B, Stjernquist U, Berggvist D.** The haemorrhagic effect of low molecular weight heparins, dermatin and hirudin. Haemostasis 1995;25:203–211.

68. **Lojewski B, Bacher P, Iqbal O, Walenga JM, Hoppensteadt D, Leya F, Fareed J.** Evaluation of hemostatic and fibrinolytic alterations associated with daily administration of low-molecular-weight heparin for a 12-week period. Sem Thromb Hemost 1995;21:228–239.

69. **Nikkels PG, de Jong JP, Ploemacher RE.** Effects of cis-diamminedichloroplatinum (II) upon haemopoietic progenitors and the haemopoietic microenvironment in mice. Br J Haematol 1988;68:3–9.

70. **Abraham NG.** Hematopoietic effects of benzene inhalation assessed by long-term bone marrow culture. Environ Health Perspect 1996;104 Suppl 6:1277–1282.

71. **Reagan WJ.** A review of myelofibrosis in dogs. Tox Pathol 1993;21:164–169.

72. **Argano SA, Marasa L, Daniele E, Pitre V, Morello V, Lampsona G, Tomasino RM.** Experimental myelofibrosis. Problems related to histogenesis and to spontaneous and therapeutic reversibility of the lesions. Haemologica 1977;62:590–602.

73. **Hunstein W.** Experimental myelofibrosis. Clin Haematol 1975;4:457–478.

74. **Poon R, Chu I, Davis H, Yagminas AP, Valli VE.** Systemic toxicity of a bitumen upgrading product in the rat following subchronic dermal exposure. Toxicol 1996;109:129–146.

75. **Graziano MJ, Pilcher GD, Walsh KM, Kasali OB, Radulovic L.** Preclinical toxicity of a new oral anticancer drug, CI-994 (acetyldinaline), in rats and dogs. Invest New Drug 1997;15:295–310.

76. **Foucar K.** Bone marrow pathology. Chicago: ASCP Press, 1995;532.

CHAPTER 9

The Hematologic Effects of Immunologic Diseases

• MICHAEL A. SCOTT

Hematologic abnormalities accompany immunologic involvement in numerous diseases, but most are indirect effects related to the generation of inflammatory mediators. These include inflammatory leukocyte patterns, reactive thrombocytosis, the anemia of chronic inflammation, and dysproteinemias. Hematologic abnormalities may also occur with diseases of the immune system itself, including: congenital abnormalities of the immune system, infectious diseases that target and damage the immune system, and immune-mediated diseases that injure hemic cells and lead to hemocytopenias (Table 9.1). Immune-mediated hemocytopenias are discussed in this chapter because hemic changes are central to their pathogenesis, clinical signs, and diagnosis.

Cytopenias may develop from immune or nonimmune mechanisms, and these sometimes develop multifactorially with components of each. The immune-mediated cytopenias may be primary autoimmune (idiopathic) diseases, alloimmune diseases caused by alloantibodies from another member of the same species, secondary to systemic immune-mediated diseases, or secondary to infections, neoplasia, or drug exposure. Failure to identify an underlying condition does not exclude the possibility that one exists, so primary disease is not a certainty. The term "autoimmune" should be applied only after special testing has confirmed specific antibody reactivity with autoantigens. Autoimmune mechanisms of cytopenias are rarely established in veterinary medicine, although many anemias and thrombocytopenias appear to be immune-mediated.

Immune-mediated cytopenias are usually the result of humoral immune responses that lead to accelerated destruction of circulating hemic cells or their bone marrow precursors. Cell destruction occurs by means of complement-mediated lysis or phagocytosis of opsonized cells by the mononuclear phagocyte system. Circulating cells are usually the primary targets of the destructive processes, and the resulting cytopenias are typically accompanied by secondary hemopoietic hyperplasia. However, when bone marrow precursor cells are a major target, the result may be aplastic anemia (pancytopenia), bicytopenia, pure red- or pure white-cell aplasia, amegakaryocytic thrombocytopenia, or maturation arrest of the affected cell line(s). Rarely, production failure cytopenias have resulted from antibodies reactive with hemopoietic cytokines rather than with cells.[1] The potential for cell-mediated destruction is also recognized.[2]

The opsonization of hemic cells with antibody or complement can occur in several ways (Fig. 9.1). Fab-mediated binding refers to the specific binding of an antibody by its antigen-binding (Fab) end. This occurs in the case of autoantibodies, alloantibodies, some drug-induced antibodies and with binding to adsorbed antigens from infectious agents or neoplasms.[3-5] Immunoglobulins may also be bound to cells by means of Fc receptors, which bind the Fc end (crystallizable fragment) of immunoglobulins, complement receptors,[6] and possibly, integrins in the form of immune complexes or antibody aggregates.[7,8] Complement proteins may be present with or without detectable immunoglobulins. In each case, cell-associated antibody or complement may lead to decreased cell survival because of cell lysis or receptor-mediated phagocytosis. When hemopoiesis does not compensate adequately for accelerated cell destruction, which is usually the case, cytopenias ensue. When the cytopenias are severe, clinical signs of anemia (pallor and lethargy), thrombocytopenia (petechiae and mucosal hemorrhage), or neutropenia (depression and pyrexia) may become apparent, thus prompting diagnostic and therapeutic intervention.

Specific tests for immune-mediated destruction have been sought because immune-mediated and nonimmunologic cytopenias may produce the same constellation of signs despite requiring different therapies. However, even after decades of assay development in human medicine, the diagnoses of primary immune-mediated cytopenias remain largely diagnoses of exclusion.[9] Assay results may support clinical suspicions, but diagnostic and therapeutic plans may be unaffected. Human assays are important, however, in diagnosing drug-induced immune-mediated cytopenias, neonatal alloimmune cytopenias, posttransfusion purpura, and refractoriness to

TABLE 9.1	Diseases of the Immune System and Their Associated Hematologic Abnormalities	

Disease	Major Hematologic Abnormalities
Congenital	
Combined immunodeficiencies	Lymphopenia
Chediak–Higashi syndrome	Abnormal leukocyte granulation
Pelger–Huët anomaly	Hyposegmented granulocyte nuclei
Leukocyte adhesion deficiencies	Significant leukocytosis/neutrophilia
Cyclic hemopoiesis	Cyclic neutropenia
Acquired	
Immune-mediated anemia*	Anemia, spherocytosis, erythroagglutination, ghost cells, erythrophagocytosis, sideroleukocytes, inflammatory leukogram, hemoglobin(emia/uria)
Immune-mediated thrombocytopenia*	Thrombocytopenia
Immune-mediated neutropenia*	Neutropenia
Viral infections causing lymphoid depletion	Lymphopenia
Anaphylaxis	Thrombocytopenia
Neoplasia with paraproteinemia	Hyperproteinemia and rouleaux

*May occur independently or multiply (e.g., Evans' syndrome, systemic lupus erythematosus).

transfusions, in which case they can also be used to screen potential donors for cell compatibility and to define important alloantigens.[5,10] Assays are also important research tools to understand the contributions of immune-mediated cell destruction to cytopenic patients who have various diseases. It is to these ends that the evolution of veterinary assays for immune-mediated cytopenias continues.

ANTIBODY ASSAYS

There are two general classes of assays for investigating immune-mediated cell destruction: (1) direct assays that detect patient immunoglobulin or complement already bound to patient cells, and (2) indirect assays that assess patient serum or plasma for immunoglobulins that can bind to test cells or antigens. It is important to differentiate direct assays from indirect assays. Direct assays require patient cells as the test sample, and when truly positive, they provide direct evidence of cell-associated immunoglobulin or complement. Indirect assays have the advantage of requiring only patient serum or plasma as the test sample. However, antibody titers may be undetectably low when cell-associated antibodies are still detectable, and misleading results are more likely because autoreactive antibodies may be indistinguishable from alloantibodies, circulating immune complexes, aggregates of normal immunoglobulin G (IgG), or nonpathologic cold-reacting antibodies.[11]

Platelet Antibody Assays

The development of direct and indirect assays for platelet antibodies has gone through three phases.[12] Phase I

assays are indirect assays that use platelet activation as indirect evidence of platelet-reactive antibodies. The platelet factor 3 (PF3) assay, for example, used increased platelet procoagulant activity as a marker of platelet stimulation by antibodies. Except for the use of serotonin release and aggregation testing for heparin-induced thrombocytopenia in human patients, phase I tests, including the PF3 test, are too insensitive and nonspecific to be of much value.

Phase II assays use labeled antiglobulin and are designed to measure antibody bound to platelets or megakaryocytes. They include direct and indirect techniques and can be modified to detect cell-associated complement. Some assays have detected total platelet-associated immunoglobulin, 99% of which is within α-granules at concentrations proportional to those in plasma.[13] More useful assays measure only surface-associated immunoglobulin. These latter assays appear to be accurate, repeatable, and sensitive tests, but they are not specific for diagnosing primary immune-mediated thrombocytopenia.[12] Several phase II platelet antibody assays have been developed in veterinary medicine, but they have undergone somewhat limited testing. The direct and indirect megakaryocyte immunofluorescence tests assess antibody reactivity with precursor cells instead of with mature, circulating cells. Results must be interpreted in light of incomplete antigenic homology between megakaryocytes and platelets.[14] False-positive reactivity caused by cytosolic immunoglobulins exposed by megakaryocyte damage during smearing is an additional concern with air-dried smear techniques.[15]

Immunoblotting, immunoprecipitation, or specific antigen capture techniques are used in phase III assays, which detect the binding of antibodies to specific membrane glycoproteins. Antigen-capture assays have not been used in veterinary medicine, but they have been

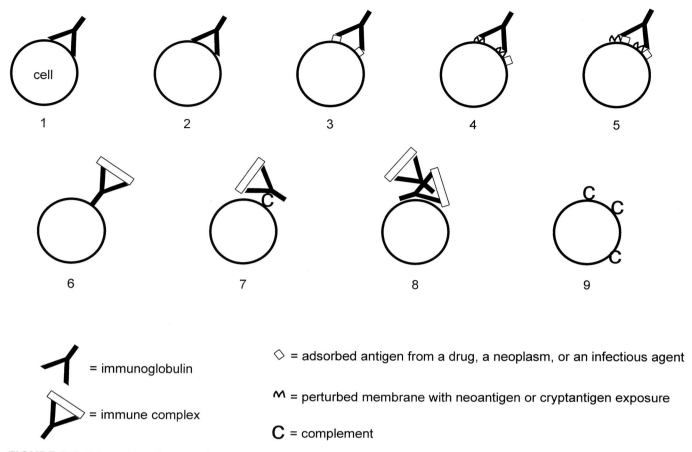

FIGURE 9.1 Schematic mechanisms of immunoglobulin and complement binding to hemic cells. **1.** Autoantibodies (Fab-mediated), ±complement—usually idiopathic; may be drug-induced or secondary to neoplasia and infection.[3,5] **2.** Alloantibodies (Fab-mediated), ±complement—related to transfusions or placental or colostral transfer of alloantibodies; the antibody and cell are from different individuals. **3.** Fab-mediated binding to adsorbed antigens (the antigen could be complexed with a plasma protein that is also part of the reactive epitope), ±complement. **4.** Fab-mediated binding to a perturbed surface site, ±complement; cause of perturbation not part of reactive epitope, but may be needed to maintain epitope exposure. **5.** Fab-mediated binding to a combination of perturbed membrane and adsorbed antigen, ±complement; may be drug-induced. **6.** Fc-mediated binding of immune complexes to Fc receptors on neutrophils or to Fc receptors on platelets and megakaryocytes of some species, ±complement. **7.** Complement-mediated attachment of immune complexes to cells with complement receptors (immune adherence)—species differences exist. **8.** Nonspecific association, possibly integrin mediated—may be seen as an in vitro storage artifact when immunoglobulins aggregate during freezing. **9.** Complement deposition as an innocent bystander phenomenon or with cold-reacting antibodies that dissociate from the cells before testing. In each case, the cell may be (1) a mature circulating cell, (2) a precursor in the bone marrow, or (3) mature and precursor cells of one or more cell lines. The antibody may (1) be IgG, IgM, IgA, or combinations thereof, (2) activate complement and cause complement deposition on the cell, or (3) have varying thermal reactivity; cold RBC agglutinin disease may cause ischemic necrosis of extremities.

widely used as clinical assays in human medicine. Monoclonal antibodies affixed to wells or beads are incubated with disrupted test platelets to capture specific membrane glycoproteins known to be involved in many cases of immune-mediated thrombocytopenia. In the direct assay, labeled antiglobulin reagents are then used to determine if antibodies are bound to the patient's captured glycoproteins. In the indirect assay, patient serum is first incubated with the captured glycoproteins before the addition of antiglobulin reagent. A panel of capture monoclonal antibodies is required for reducing false-negative reactions that occur when the capture antibodies and pathogenic antibodies compete for the same or neighboring target epitopes. These assays are expensive and can detect reactivity only to the glycoproteins that are captured. However, they have been shown to be more sensitive and reproducible for alloantibody detection than are phase II assays. Immunoprecipitation and immunoblotting have been used to identify the targets of platelet-reactive antibodies in dogs.[16,17]

Neutrophil Antibody Assays

The development of assays to detect antibodies reactive with neutrophils parallels, but lags behind, that of platelet antibody assays.[18,19] Slower progress is partially a reflection of less frequent recognition of immune-mediated neutropenias. Some of the assays are indirect functional tests like phase I platelet assays that detect antibody effects such as aggregation or opsonization. Others, like phase II platelet assays, detect cell-associated immunoglobulins, including immune complexes, autoantibodies, alloantibodies, and nonspecific binding. Antigen-capture methods have also been developed, but they are not yet as useful as their platelet counterparts. This is partly because of limited knowledge about the location of common antigenic epitopes and the resulting lack of appropriate monoclonal antibodies for antigen capture. None of the human neutrophil antibody assays can detect all neutrophil antibodies, and none has clinical usefulness for diagnosing primary immune-mediated neutropenia.[20] The few veterinary assays developed to detect neutrophil antibodies have undergone little testing and use.[21–23]

Erythrocyte Antibody Assays

The mainstay of erythrocyte antibody assays has been the Coombs' test. It can be used as a direct test for erythrocyte-associated antibodies or as an indirect assay for erythrocyte-bindable immunoglobulins. Passive erythrocyte agglutination is the end point of a positive reaction. It occurs when antibodies in a species-specific Coombs' reagent bind to erythrocyte-associated immunoglobulins or complement and bridge the cells together. The Coombs' test suffers from suboptimal sensitivity, subjective interpretation, and, in veterinary medicine, a lack of standardization. There are great inter-laboratory variations in reagents, assay temperatures, sample dilutions, and test end points. Proof of clinical usefulness and predictive value for diagnosing immune-mediated hemolytic anemia are lacking.[24] Negative Coombs' test results have been repeatedly noted in samples from dogs that appear to have immune-mediated hemolytic anemia based on other clinical and laboratory findings. Positive results, primarily caused by complement, have occurred commonly in the absence of significant hemolytic disease.[25] Improvements of the Coombs' test have been sought, and other direct antiglobulin tests have been developed with enzyme-conjugated or radiolabeled antiglobulin reagents to detect antibodies on test cells. These assays have generally been more sensitive than the agglutination test, but they have not received widespread use and clinical testing in veterinary medicine.

INTERPRETATION OF ASSAY RESULTS

Positive results of antibody assays suggest immune-mediated disease. However, they do not differentiate primary from secondary disease, or an autoimmune pathogenesis from the many other possible immune-mediated pathogeneses (Fig. 9.1). Sound clinical diagnoses are generally considered to take precedence over assay results and have been the standard for determining the sensitivity and specificity of antibody assays in the detection of primary immune-mediated cytopenias. Differentiation of primary disease from secondary, and determination of the underlying cause of secondary cytopenias, rely on thorough clinical and laboratory diagnostics.

The search for underlying disease involves assessment of the patient's history, physical examination findings, and other clinical and laboratory data. Diagnostics that may detect or help exclude causes of nonimmune or secondary immune cytopenias include complete blood cell counts (CBCs), routine chemistries, urinalyses, hemostasis profiles, radiographs, ultrasound imaging, serology, polymerase chain reaction (PCR) tests, and blood cultures. Single or serial bone marrow aspirates or core biopsies may be indicated for atypical or unresponsive cases. These samples may reveal infiltrative marrow disease or destruction of early precursors. Evidence of systemic immune-mediated disease may be obtained from antinuclear antibody (ANA) and lupus erythematosus (LE) cell tests.

A careful blood smear review is essential, especially during evaluation for immune-mediated hemolytic anemia. The anemia can be classified as regenerative or nonregenerative, and the erythrocytes and leukoocytes can be inspected for hemoparasites, Heinz bodies, eccentrocytes, fragmentation, hypochromasia, neoplasia, and other changes suggestive of nonimmune cytopenias or immune-mediated cytopenias secondary to underlying disease. Direct evidence of immune-mediated anemia may also be detected, including spherocytosis, erythroagglutination, ghost cells, and, rarely, erythrophagocytosis or sideroleukocytes.

Laboratory data are also important to confirm the presence of a cytopenia before special testing is even considered. Antibody assay results are sometimes generated in noncytopenic patients that were thought to be cytopenic but should not have been tested. This occurs with greyhounds when their normally lower platelet concentrations,[26] and perhaps neutrophil concentrations in some populations, are compared with general canine reference intervals instead of breed-specific values. It also occurs when the low results of automated instruments are not confirmed by direct examination of blood smears. Smear reviews should minimize the reporting of pseudothrombocytopenia caused by platelet activation and clumping, pseudothrombocytopenias and pseudoleukopenias caused by anticoagulant-induced agglutination, and falsely low platelet concentrations in patients that have abnormally large platelets that may be undetected by automated analyzers, e.g., cavalier King Charles spaniels.[27]

When assay results and clinical diagnoses differ, one should reassess the clinical diagnosis and also consider potential reasons for false assay results. Misleading assay results may occur for many reasons that vary with the type of assay used (Table 9.2). Truly positive results suggest that there is an immune-mediated component to the cytopenia and that immunosuppressive therapy may be indicated. Positive results in patients presumed to have nonimmune cytopenias may reflect an unsuspected immune component, an unsuspected technical

TABLE 9.2   Potential Reasons for False-Positive and False-Negative Results of Direct and Indirect Antibody Assays

Potential Causes of False-Positive Results		Potential Causes of False-Negative Results	
Direct Assays	**Indirect Assays**	**Direct Assays**	**Indirect Assays**
Nonspecifically adsorbed surface immunoglobulins	Nonspecifically adsorbed surface immunoglobulins	Limited reactivity of antiglobulin reagent (cannot detect all immunoglobulin classes/subclasses)	Limited reactivity of antiglobulin reagent (cannot detect all immunoglobulin classes/subclasses)
Nonpathologic cold-reacting antibody[a]	Nonpathologic cold-reacting antibody[a]	Assay too insensitive to detect low numbers of cell-bound antibodies	Assay too insensitive to detect low titers (titers may be undetectable even with optimized assays)
Nonpathologic antibodies bound to epitopes induced by anticoagulation or cell activation[a]	Nonpathologic antibody binding to epitopes induced by anticoagulation, fixation, enzymes, cell activation, sample heating, sample freezing[a]	Low-affinity antibodies removed during washing	Low-affinity antibodies removed during washing
Binding of antiglobulin reagent to test cell Fc receptors	Binding of antiglobulin reagent to test cell Fc receptors	Drug not present in assay fluids to maintain binding of drug-dependent antibodies	Drug not present in assay fluids to maintain binding of drug-dependent antibodies
Contamination of test cells with other antibody-coated cells (e.g., platelets with RBCs[b])	Contamination of test cells with other positively reacting cell types	Inappropriate antigen–antibody ratios in agglutination tests (prozone effect)	Inappropriate antigen–antibody ratios in agglutination tests (prozone effect)
Internal rather than surface-bound immunoglobulin detected (platelets/megakaryocytes)	Nonpathologic reactivity to exposed cytosolic epitopes (especially with some antigen capture methods)	Steric hindrance prevents antigen capture (capture antibodies cannot bind to site already bound by pathologic antibody)	Reactive epitopes altered by anticoagulant, fixative, enzymes, or other treatment
Inappropriate cut-off value for positivity	Inappropriate cut-off value for positivity	Inappropriate cut-off value for positivity	Inappropriate cut-off value for positivity
Inconsistent results due to inappropriate standarization or controls	Inconsistent results due to inappropriate standardization or controls	Inconsistent results due to inappropriate standardization or controls	Inconsistent results due to inappropriate standardization or controls
Positivity induced by recent transfusion[a]	Nonpathologic alloantibody (naturally occurring or secondary to transfusion or pregnancy)[a]	Cytopenia is immune-mediated but caused by anticytokine rather than anti-cell antibody[a]	Cytopenia is immune-mediated but caused by anticytokine rather than anti-cell antibody[a]
		Antibody is directed at precursor, not circulating cell, or vice versa for megakaryocyte testing[a]	Antibody is directed at precursor, not circulating cell, or vice versa for megakaryocyte testing[a]
		Cytopenia is cell-mediated, not humorally mediated[a]	Cytopenia is cell-mediated, not humorally mediated[a]
			Test cells/antigens lack the reactive epitope

[a]Accurate results but can be considered false reactions because they do not reflect the true presence or absence of an immune-mediated cytopenia.
[b]RBC, red blood cell.

problem, or nonpathogenic increases in cell-associated immunoglobulin induced by the underlying disease state. Positive results for cell-associated immunoglobulin in the absence of cytopenias should be questioned, but they may be explained by adequate bone marrow compensation for the accelerated destruction,[28] by a defect in the mononuclear phagocyte system such that coated cells are not removed,[29] by nonspecific immunoglobulin binding, or by unsuspected technical problems.

Veterinary assays for cell-associated or cell-bindable immunoglobulin are still in the developmental and testing stages, especially those for immune-mediated neutropenia. Widespread standardization and controlled clinical studies of usefulness and predictive value are lacking. Therefore, assay results should be carefully interpreted in light of all other clinical and laboratory findings.

REFERENCES

1. **Hoffman R, Briddell RA, van Besien K, Srour EF, Guscar T, Hudson NW, Ganser A.** Acquired cyclic amegakaryocytic thrombocytopenia associated with an immunoglobulin blocking the action of granulocyte-macrophage colony-stimulating factor. N Engl J Med 1989;321:97–102.
2. **Gewirtz AM, Keefer Sacchetti M, Bien R, Barry WE.** Cell-mediated suppression of megakaryocytopoiesis in acquired amegakaryocytic thrombocytopenic purpura. Blood 1986;68:619–626.
3. **Warkentin TE, Trimble MS, Kelton JG.** Thrombocytopenia due to platelet destruction and hypersplenism. In: Hoffman R, Benz EJ, Jr, Shattil SJ, Furie B, Cohen HJ, Silberstein LE, eds. Hematology: Basic principles and practice. 2nd ed. New York: Churchill Livingstone, 1995;1889–1908.

4. **Coates TD, Baehner R.** Leukocytosis and leukopenia. In: Hoffman R, Benz EJ, Jr, Shattil SJ, Furie B, Cohen HJ, Silberstein LE, eds. Hematology: basic principles and practice. 2nd ed. New York: Churchill Livingstone, 1995;769–783.

5. **Lalezari P.** Leukocyte antigens and antibodies. In: Hoffman R, Furie B, Shattil SJ, Benz EJ, Jr, Cohen HJ, Silberstein LE, eds. Hematology: basic principles and practice. 2nd ed. New York: Churchill Livingstone, 1995;1974–1980.

6. **Nelson DS.** Immune adherence. In: Dixon FJ, Humphrey JH, eds. Advances in immunology. New York: Academic Press, 1963;3:131–180.

7. **George JN.** The origin and significance of platelet IgG. In: Kunicki TJ, George JN, eds. Platelet immunobiology: molecular and clinical aspects. Philadelphia: JB Lippincott, 1989;305–336.

8. **Karpatkin S, Xia J, Patel J, Thorbecke GJ.** Serum platelet-reactive IgG of autoimmune thrombocytopenic purpura patients is not F(ab′)$_2$ mediated and a function of storage. Blood 1992;80:3164–3172.

9. **George JN, Raskob GE.** Idiopathic thrombocytopenic purpura: a concise summary of the pathophysiology and diagnosis in children and adults. Semin Hematol 1998;35:5–8.

10. **Mueller-Eckhardt C, Kiefel V.** Laboratory methods for the detection of platelet antibodies and identification of antigens. In: Kunicki TJ, George JN, eds. Platelet immunobiology: molecular and clinical aspects. Philadelphia: JB Lippincott, 1989;436–453.

11. **Aster RH.** The immunologic thrombocytopenias. In: Kunicki TJ, George JN, eds. Platelet immunobiology: molecular and clinical aspects. Philadelphia: JB Lippincott, 1989;387–435.

12. **Warner M, Kelton JG.** Laboratory investigation of immune thrombocytopenia. J Clin Pathol 1997;50:5–12.

13. **George JN.** Platelet immunoglobulin G: its significance for the evaluation of thrombocytopenia and for understanding the origin of α-granule proteins. Blood 1990;76:859–870.

14. **Stahl CP, Zucker-Franklin D, McDonald TP.** Incomplete antigenic cross-reactivity between platelets and megakaryocytes: relevance to ITP. Blood 1986;67:426–428.

15. **Hyde P, Zucker-Franklin D.** Antigenic differences between human platelets and megakaryocytes. Am J Pathol 1987;127:349–357.

16. **Lewis DC, Meyers KM.** Studies of platelet-bound and serum platelet-bindable immunoglobulins in dogs with idiopathic thrombocytopenic purpura. Exp Hematol 1996;24:696–701.

17. **Scott MA.** Canine immune-mediated thrombocytopenia: assay development, a role for complement, and assessment in a toxicologic study. Michigan State University, PhD, 1995; p 451.

18. **Bux J, Chapman J.** Report on the Second International Granulocyte Serology Workshop. Transfusion 1997;37:977–983.

19. **Madyastha PR, Glassman AB.** Neutrophil antigens and antibodies in the diagnosis of immune neutropenias. Ann Clin Lab Sci 1989;19:146–154.

20. **Shastri KA, Logue GL.** Autoimmune neutropenia. Blood 1993;81:1984–1995.

21. **Bloom JC, Thiem PA, Sellers TS, Deldar A, Lewis HB.** Cephalosporin-induced immune cytopenia in the dog: demonstration of erythrocyte-, neutrophil-, and platelet-associated IgG following treatment with cefazedone. Am J Hematol 1988;28:71–78.

22. **Jain NC, Vegad JL, Kono CS.** Methods for detection of immune-mediated neutropenia in horses, using antineutrophil serum of rabbit origin. Am J Vet Res 1990;51:1026–1031.

23. **Chickering WR, Prasse KW, Dawe DL.** Development and clinical application of methods for detection of antineutrophil antibody in serum of the cat. Am J Vet Res 1985;46:1809–1814.

24. **Weiser MG.** Diagnosis of immunohemolytic disease. Semin Vet Med Surg (Small Anim) 1992;7:311–314.

25. **Slappendel RJ.** The diagnostic significance of the direct antiglobulin test (DAT) in anemic dogs. Vet Immunol Immunopathol 1979;1:49–59.

26. **Sullivan PS, Evans HL, McDonald TP.** Platelet concentration and hemoglobin function in greyhounds. J Am Vet Med Assoc 1994;205:838–841.

27. **Smedile LE, Houston DM, Taylor SM, Post K, Searcy GP.** Idiopathic, asymptomatic thrombocytopenia in Cavalier King Charles Spaniels: 11 cases (1983–1993). J Am Anim Hosp Assoc 1997;33:411–415.

28. **Mills JN.** Compensated immune mediated haemolytic anaemia in a dog. Aust Vet J 1997;75:24–26.

29. **Kelton JG, Carter CJ, Rodger C, Bebenek G, Gauldie J, Sheridan D, Kassam Y, Kean WF, Buchanan WW, Rooney PJ, Bianchi F, Denburg J.** The relationship among platelet-associated IgG, platelet lifespan, and reticuloendothelial cell function. Blood 1984;63:1434–1438.

CHAPTER 10

Clinical Hemorrheology

• DOUGLAS J. WEISS

Hemorrheology is a study of the flow properties of blood. The resistance of blood to flow is defined as blood viscosity.[1] Blood viscosity is determined by hematocrit, red blood cell (RBC) deformability, RBC aggregation, and to a lesser extent by plasma viscosity and leukocyte and platelet numbers. The major determinant of blood viscosity in arteries and veins (i.e., macrocirculation) is hematocrit. The relation between hematocrit and viscosity is logarithmic; therefore, slight increases in hematocrit can result in significant increases in blood viscosity. In the microcirculation, individual cells must deform in passage through capillaries. Therefore, RBC deformability and RBC aggregation are major determinants of blood viscosity in the microvasculature. Flow resistance in the microcirculation is best predicted by determining filterability of blood through membranes with capillary-sized pores. In certain pathologic conditions leukocytes or platelets may contribute significantly to blood viscosity in the microvasculature. These pathologic conditions include leukocytosis, thrombocytosis, leukemia, systemic neutrophil activation, adhesion of leukocytes or platelets to endothelium, or formation of leukocyte–leukocyte or platelet–leukocyte aggregates.

HEMORRHEOLOGIC MEASUREMENTS

Blood Viscosity

Viscosity is a measure of the internal friction of a fluid.[2] The greater the friction, the greater the force needed to cause a layer of fluid to move in relation to another layer of fluid. In rheologic terms, viscosity is defined as the ratio of shear stress to shear rate. Shear rate is the velocity gradient between flowing layers of blood, whereas shear stress is the tangential force per unit area exerted on the vessel wall. The effect of hematocrit on blood viscosity varies with shear rate. Unlike simple liquids, the viscosity of blood decreases as shear rate increases. This is in part caused by aggregation of RBC at low shear rates and deformation of RBC at higher shear rates (Fig. 10.1). Therefore, at low shear rates, the viscosity of equine blood with a packed cell volume

(PCV) of 60 is fourfold to fivefold greater than blood with a PCV of 40, but it is only twofold greater at high shear rates.

Blood viscosity has been measured with rotational, cone-plate-type, viscometers.[2–4] Rotational viscometers have the advantage of measuring viscosity at different shear rates, thereby, defining the non-Newtonian properties of blood. These instruments provide accurate and repeatable measurements of blood viscosity at high shear rates but lack precision at lower shear rates. Rotation of the cone produces a torque that depends on the viscosity of the fluid between the cone and the plate. Cone-plate viscometers measure the bulk flow properties of blood and predict flow properties within large blood vessels.[1]

Red Blood Cell Deformability

Deformability of RBC is determined by the viscoelastic properties of the cell membrane, cell geometry, and cytoplasmic viscosity.[5,6] Deformation occurs through a combination of shearing (i.e., elongation) and bending of the plasma membrane. Geometric factors that affect RBC deformability include cell size, shape, and surface area to volume ratio.[7] RBC cytoplasmic viscosity is primarily dependent on hemoglobin concentration.

Methods to quantify RBC deformability include ectacytometry, RBC filterability, and individual cell deformability as studied by micropipette aspiration.[5,7,8] Elongation of RBCs subjected to rotational shear is measured with ectacytometers. RBC filterability evaluates the filtration of RBC suspensions through membranes with pores 3 or 5 μm in diameter (Fig. 10.2). Simple filtrometers evaluate the initial pressure increment that develops when a suspension of RBC is pumped through membranes at a constant rate. Most commercial filtrometers evaluate the initial flow rate and calculate pore transit time, which is expressed as the ratio of the flow rate of cell suspensions to the flow rate of buffer alone. Deformability of individual cells can be determined by means of measuring the pressure required for entry of RBC into a glass pipette with an internal diameter of approximately 3 μm.[9] Smaller-diameter pipettes can be used to

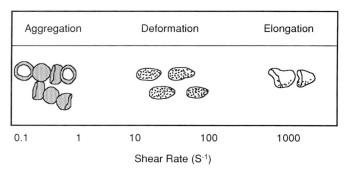

FIGURE 10.1 Schematic drawing showing the effect of shear rate on RBC flow behavior. At low shear rates, RBCs aggregate, resulting in a significant increase in blood viscosity. As shear rate increases, RBCs disaggregate, deform, and elongate decreasing the apparent viscosity of blood. Therefore, as shear rate increases, the apparent viscosity of blood decreases.

aspirate a portion of RBC membrane into the pipette. This procedure defines the elastic properties of the cell membrane.

Red Blood Cell Volume and Hemoglobin Concentration

Large cells must undergo greater deformation to pass through capillaries, and therefore have a greater effect on resistance to flow in the microvasculature.[5] Hemoglobin concentration within RBC is the major determinant of RBC cytoplasmic viscosity and RBC density.[5] Because this is an exponential relation, small increases in mean cell hemoglobin concentration result in large increases in cytoplasmic viscosity. Llamas have high mean cell hemoglobin concentration with a resultant decrease in RBC deformability. The flattened elliptical shape of

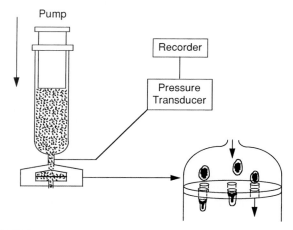

FIGURE 10.2 Schematic of the principal of RBC filtrometry that simulates flow of RBC through the microvasculature. An RBC suspension is pumped at constant rate through a filter with capillary-sized pores. Initial pressure increases, and initial flow rates are affected by RBC size and deformability.

llama RBC apparently permits RBC to pass through the microvasculature without the need to deform.

RBC Density

Density-gradient centrifugation can be used to define changes in RBC density and identify subpopulations of RBC within blood. Changes in RBC density can be determined by quantification of the location of RBC layers within discontinuous stractan density gradients and by determination of the percentage of cells within each band (Fig. 10.3). Other rheologic tests can be used to analyze RBC within each layer.[10,11]

RBC Sedimentation Rate

RBC erythrocyte sedimentation rate (ESR) varies with hematocrit and RBC aggregation.[8,10] Therefore, if ESR is to be used as a measure of RBC aggregation, hematocrit must be standardized or a correction table used. ESR varies significantly among domestic species. Horses and

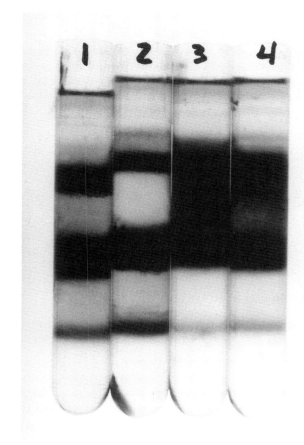

FIGURE 10.3 RBC density gradients for a thoroughbred before exercise,[1] during treadmill exercise at 9 (Ref. 2) and 13 m/s (Ref. 3), and 20 minutes after exercise.[4] Notice an upward shift of RBC in the density gradient during exercise, indicating that RBCs become less dense during exercise.

ponies have rapid ESR (caused by extensive rouleaux formation), ESR is intermediate in dogs and cats, and ruminants have slow ESR. Variation in ESR within species primarily depends on the concentration of fibrinogen and immunoglobulin. Therefore, animals that have inflammatory diseases or chronic immunologic stimulation have increased ESR.

The Wintrobe method has been used most extensively to determine ESR.[12] Some veterinary practices use a capillary-tube ESR technique to screen for the prodromal stages of infectious disease in dogs.

Plasma Viscosity

Plasma viscosity can be measured by use of cone-plate-type rotational viscometers and various simple devices that measure flow of plasma through capillary tubes. Both plasma protein concentration and composition contributes to plasma viscosity. Total plasma protein concentration is the major determinant of plasma viscosity, however, some proteins contribute proportionately more to viscosity than others.[5] Fibrinogen has the highest intrinsic viscosity of all plasma proteins. Immunoglobulin-M, because of its large size, has higher intrinsic viscosity than do other immunoglobulins. Clinically significant plasma hyperviscosity results from overproduction of immunoglobulin and is seen with multiple myeloma, immunoglobulin-secreting lymphosarcoma, and certain chronic inflammatory diseases, including canine ehrlichiosis and feline infectious peritonitis.

HEMORRHEOLOGIC ALTERATIONS ASSOCIATED WITH EXERCISE

Significant changes in the flow properties of blood occur during strenuous exercise in horses.[2,3,10,13] During competitive racing activity, equine whole blood viscosity increases twofold to fivefold.[2] The major factor in exercise-induced hyperviscosity is an increase in hematocrit that results from splenic contraction and decreased plasma volume. Hematocrits typically increase from baseline values of 32 to 38% to 58 to 72% during competitive racing activity.[2] Other factors that contribute to increased blood viscosity include increased plasma protein concentration, increased neutrophil and lymphocyte numbers, and increased RBC hemoglobin concentration.[2]

A transient decrease in RBC filterability (i.e., decreased RBC deformability) occurs during submaximal treadmill exercise (Fig. 10.3).[10] This decrease in filterability is associated with increases in RBC size and RBC sodium, potassium, and chloride concentrations. Therefore, decreased filterability may have resulted from transient uptake of fluid and electrolytes, resulting in RBC swelling. Another possible explanation for decreased RBC filterability during exercise could be release of less deformable RBC from the spleen.[14] However, the percentage of dense RBC in density-gradient profiles from horses undergoing submaximal treadmill exercise was decreased compared with preexercise samples (Fig. 10.3).[6]

PATHOLOGIC ALTERATION IN BLOOD FLOW

Exercise-Induced Pulmonary Hemorrhage

Pulmonary hemorrhage of variable severity occurs in most, if not all, horses undergoing competitive racing activity.[15] Pulmonary hemorrhage probably results from high shear stress within lung septal capillaries; this stress causes vessel rupture.[16] Pulmonary capillary pressures in racehorses exercising on a treadmill has been estimated to be 72.5 and 92.5 mm Hg.[17,18] These extremely high pressures within lung capillaries may result from a combination of increased cardiac output and increased blood viscosity.

Polycythemia

Both absolute and relative polycythemia result in hyperviscosity of blood.[19] Hyperviscosity of blood causes reduced blood flow through the microvasculature and may induce ischemic tissue injury. Reduced blood flow through dilated cutaneous vessels is responsible for the brick-red appearance of mucous membranes and excessive deoxygenation of blood induces cyanosis.

Paraproteinemia

Excessive production of immunoglobulin results in plasma hyperviscosity. Hyperglobulemias have been associated with multiple myeloma in dogs, cats, and horses and with chronic lymphocytic leukemia and ehrlichiosis in dogs.[20] The significantly increased plasma viscosity may impair microvascular blood flow and induce RBC aggregation.

Red Blood Cell Aggregation

RBC aggregation (i.e., rouleaux formation) is defined as reversible adhesion induced by the bridging of adjacent RBC by globular proteins or fibrinogen.[1] RBC aggregates form at low shear rates that commonly occur in the venous circulation (Fig. 10.1). In the arterial circulation, where shear rates are high, RBC aggregates dissociate. RBC aggregation can be measured by determination of the ESR and is directly related to the plasma concentrations of fibrinogen and immunoglobulins.

Clinically, RBC aggregation is most important in dysproteinemias and paraproteinemias. RBC aggregation contributes to elevated capillary pressure, tissue ischemia, and capillary rupture associated with multiple myeloma and Waldenstrom's-type macroglobulinemia.

Platelet–Neutrophil Aggregation

Platelet–neutrophil aggregates have been identified in horses undergoing intense treadmill exercise and in ponies that have experimental laminitis.[21,22] Platelet–neutrophil aggregates probably occur secondary to intravascular platelet activation. Activated platelets express the alpha granule-derived glycoprotein P-selectin that binds to P-selectin glycoprotein ligand-1 (PSGL-1) which is constitutively expressed on neutrophils and monocytes. Platelet–neutrophil aggregates are large and poorly deformable and have a tendency to be retained in filters with 5 μm pores. Larger aggregates, which contain more than one neutrophil, readily obstruct 5 μm pores, whereas, aggregates containing only one neutrophil require considerably greater pressure to pass through 5 μm pores.[24]

Activated platelets or platelet–neutrophil aggregates may play a central role in the pathogenesis of alimentary laminitis. Platelet–neutrophil aggregates were detected early in the prodromal stages of carbohydrate-induced laminitis. Their role in causing laminitis is inferred by the capacity of a platelet aggregation-inhibiting compound to prevent onset of clinical laminitis.[21,23]

Platelet activation during exercise probably results from shear-induced platelet activation.[25] Increased shear forces during exercise probably result from a combination of increased heart rate and cardiac output and increased blood viscosity. The clinical significance of platelet–neutrophil aggregates in horses undergoing intense exercise is unknown.

References

1. **Somer T, Meiselman HJ.** Disorders of blood viscosity. Ann Med 1993;25:31–39.
2. **McClay CB, Weiss DJ, Smith CM, Gordon B.** Evaluation of hemorheologic variables as implications for exercise-induced pulmonary hemorrhage in racing thoroughbreds. Am J Vet Res 1992;53:1380–1385.
3. **Coyne CP, Carlson GP, Spensley MS.** Preliminary investigation of alterations in blood viscosity, cellular composition, and electrophoresis plasma protein fractions profile after competitive racing activity in thoroughbred horses. Am J Vet Res 1990;51:1956–1963.
4. **Andrews FM, Korenek NL, Sanders WL.** Viscosity and rheologic properties of blood from clinically normal horses. Am J Vet Res 1992;53:966–970.
5. **Stuart J, Nash GB.** Red cell deformability and haematological disorders. Blood Rev 1993;23:141–147.
6. **Weiss DJ, Evanson O, Geor RJ.** Filterability of equine erythrocytes and whole blood: effects of haematocrit, pore size, and flow rate. Compar Haematol Int 1994;4:11–16.
7. **Chien S.** Red cell deformability and its relevance to blood flow. Ann Rev Physiol 1987;49:177–192.
8. **Stuart J, Nash GB.** Technological advances in blood rheology. Critical Rev Clin Lab Sci 1990;28:61–93.
9. **Waugh RE, Agre P.** Reduction of erythrocyte membrane viscoelastic coefficients reflect spectrin deficiencies in hereditary spherocytosis. J Clin Invest 1988;81:133–141.
10. **Geor RJ, Weiss DJ, Smith CM.** Hemorheologic alterations induced by incremental treadmill exercise in thoroughbreds. Am J Vet Res 1994;55:854–861.
11. **Weiss DJ, Geor RJ, Smith CM.** Effects of echinocytosis on hemorheologic values and exercise performance. Am J Vet Res 1994;55:204–210.
12. **Archer RK.** Technical methods. In: Archer RK, Jeffcott LB, eds. Comparative clinical haematology. Oxford, England: Blackwell Scientific Publications, 1977;537–610.
13. **Fedde MR, Ho HH, Wood SC.** Oxygen transport in exercising horses: importance of rheological properties of blood. In: Eduardo J, Bicudo PW, eds. The vertebrate gas transport cascade. Ann Arbor, MI: CRC Press, 1993;200–207.
14. **Boucher JH, Ferguson EW, Wilhemsen CL.** Erythrocyte alterations during endurance exercise in horses. J Appl Physiol 1981;1;131–134.
15. **Lapointe JM, Vrins A, McCarvill E.** A survey of exercise-induced pulmonary haemorrhage in Quebec standardbred racehorses. Equine Vet J 1995;26:482–485.
16. **West JB, Mathieu-Costello O, Jones JH, Birks EK, Logemann RB, Pascoe JR, Tyler WS.** Stress failure of pulmonary capillaries in racehorses with exercise-induced pulmonary hemorrhage. J Appl Physiol 1993;75:1097–1109.
17. **Manohar M.** Pulmonary artery wedge pressure increases with high-intensity exercise in horses. Am J Vet Res 1993;54:142–146.
18. **Jones JH, Smith BL, Birks EK, Pascoe JR, Hughes TR.** Left atrial and pulmonary artery pressures in exercising horses. FASEB J 1992;6:A2020.
19. **Cambell K.** Diagnosis and management of polycythemia in dogs. Compend Contin Educ 1992;12:543–550.
20. **Williams DA.** Gammopathies. Compend Contin Educ 1981;3:815–822.
21. **Weiss DJ, Evanson OA, McClenahan D, Fagliari JJ.** Evaulation of platelet activation and platelet-neutrophil aggregates in ponies with alimentary laminitis. Am J Vet Res 1997;58:1376–1380.
22. **Weiss DJ, Evanson OA, Fagliari JJ, Valberg S.** Evaluation of platelet activation and platelet-neutrophil aggregates in thoroughbreds undergoing near-maximal treadmill exercise. Am J Vet Res 1998;59:393–396.
23. **Weiss DJ, Evanson OA, McClenahan D, Fagliari JJ, Dunnwiddie CT, Wells RE.** Effects of a competitive inhibitor of platelet aggregation on experimentally induced laminitis in ponies. Am J Vet Res 1998;59:814–817.
24. **Weiss DJ, Evanson OA, McClenahan D, Fagliari JJ.** Haemorrheology of equine platelet-neutrophil aggregates. Compar Haematol Int 1999;9:55–59.
25. **Weiss DJ, Evanson OA, McClenahan D, Fagliari J, Walcheck B.** Shear-induced platelet activation and platelet-neutrophil aggregate formation by equine platelets. Am J Vet Res 1998;59:1243–1246.

SECTION II

Hemopoiesis
Peter W. Gasper

CHAPTER 11

The Hemopoietic System

• PETER W. GASPER

Blood is the life-sustaining medium for each of the estimated 30 to 40 trillion cells in a mammal's body. This vital fluid courses to within roughly 5 μm of most every cell, providing it with nutrients and oxygen and carrying away its CO_2 and other products of metabolism or protein synthesis. The cellular and molecular components necessary for immunologic surveillance and defense, hemostasis, and systemic homeostasis reside and function in the blood. Hemopoiesis (*hemo* or *hemato* means blood, *poiesis* means to make) literally means blood formation. However, hemopoiesis (or *hemopoiesis*) is used to denote only the formation of mature blood cells: erythrocytes, granulocytes, monocytes, lymphocytes, and platelets. The student of hematology should note that the formation and maintenance of the plasma portion of blood occurs through an analogous dynamic physiology orchestrated by a multiplicity of widely dispersed cells located in hepatic, digestive, renal, endocrine, and other tissues. Plasma production unites with erythropoiesis, myelopoiesis, lymphopoiesis, and thrombopoiesis to keep a mammal's blood pure and eloquent.[1] The hemopoietic system, therefore, consists of the functional formed elements of blood, the progenitor and stem cells that give rise to them, and the hemopoietic tissues (termed the *hemopoietic microenvironment*) that are dispersed in varying amounts in marrow cavities of flat and long bones, spleen, liver, lymph nodes, and thymus. This system is an integrated network of cells that initiates and facilitates continuous cycles of differentiation of a small population of self-renewing germ cells (hemopoietic stem cells [HSCs]).

Four characteristics of the hemopoietic system and hemopoiesis are unique and serve as keystones to one's understanding and practice of hematology.

1. Hemopoietic cells are the most proliferative, mitotically active, cells in an animal. Within a mammal's lifetime, the estimated basal production rates for these cells are 2.5 billion red cells, 2.5 billion platelets, and 1.0 billion granulocytes per kilogram per day.[2]
2. The life span of blood cells is short (from hours to weeks) with the exception of erythrocytes and certain lymphocytes.
3. Pluripotent HSCs give rise to all the billions of heterogeneous functional cells of the blood and the immune system. This phenomenon is referred to as the monophyletic origin of blood (reviewed in Chapter 12 [stem cell biology is monophyletic]).
4. Hemopoiesis invokes a rapid response. It involves a requirement for both direct cell-to-cell contacts in hemopoietic microenvironments and specific inductive and regulatory molecules elaborated by many different cells distributed throughout the body.

This chapter provides a conceptual overview and resource for understanding the terminology used in the remaining chapters on hemopoiesis. The following is a discussion of the hemopoietic compartments and an introduction to the methods that investigators working within the field of experimental hematology have employed to delineate the features of this complex system. The biology of HSCs, anatomy of the microenvironment, ontogeny of the hemopoietic system, cytokine regulation of hemopoiesis, identification and purification of hemopoietic cells, and hemopoietic stem cell transplantation are discussed in the subsequent chapters of this section.

HEMOPOIETIC COMPARTMENTS

The hemopoietic system is usually described as a connected continuum of three functional extravascular compartments—the stem cell compartment, the progenitor-cell compartment, and the precursor-cell compartment—within these, hemopoietic cells arise and differentiate before release into circulation. It is important to remember that this is a conceptual framework that aids in visualizing the production of blood cells and not an anatomic description. Hemopoiesis actually occurs in the form of multifocal three-dimensional extravascular colonies of cells in which mature precursor cells predominate. Figure 11.1 illustrates the progression of expanding differentiation and introduces the current terminology that is used to describe cells at various stages. Characterization of hemopoietic cells in vitro resulted in the various colony-forming unit (CFU) designations that are at the root of the names of hemopoietic growth factors, e.g., granulocyte-colony stimulating factor, (G-CSF). The in vivo and in vitro methods for studying hemopoiesis are described below.

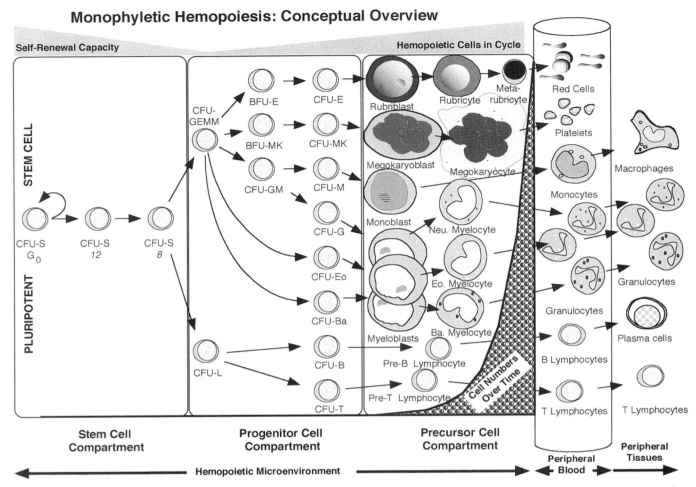

FIGURE 11.1 Monophylitic origin of all blood and immune cells. Single hemopoietic stem cells differentiate through three conceptual compartments or "pools"—(reading left to right) the stem cell, progenitor cell, and precursor cell compartments—before mature blood cells are released into peripheral blood. In the development from stem cells to mature differentiated blood cells, self-renewal capacity declines, and the proportion of mitotic cells and total number of cells increase.

Stem Cell Compartment

These rare cells can be thought of as a cache of seeds that retain the capacity for self-renewal and can establish and maintain the entirety of hemopoiesis and peripheral blood and immune cells by clonal proliferation. As few as 30 purified HSCs have been used to repopulate the entire lymphohemopoietic system of lethally irradiated mice.[4] The incidence of such reconsituting HSCs is estimated at 1 to 2.5 per 100,000 injected nucleated cells or 1 per 10,000 transplanted cells.[5] Few mitotically active cells are in this compartment. Most HSCs are in a resting (G_0) state. Morphologically, these cells resemble and cannot be distinguished from small lymphocytes, cells with a high nuclear to cytoplasmic ratio, prominent nucleoli, and basophilic cytoplasm devoid of granules. The biology of HSCs is discussed in the Chapter 12.

Progenitor Cell Compartment

Progenitor cells can be separated from HSCs on the basis of some restriction in differentiation and proliferative

capacity. All are derived from HSCs. There are rare multipotent (capable of differentiating along several cell lineages) progenitor cells that are capable of limited self-renewal and some bipotent progenitors, whereas most are unipotent progenitor cells even less capable of self-renewal and more restricted in differentiation (see Fig. 11.1). Progenitor cells are more likely to be in a cell cycle than HSCs. One can identify these cells by specific cell-surface differentiation antigens and can enumerate them by counting the colonies that can be grown in a semisolid medium (see below). Like HSCs, these cells resemble and cannot be distinguished from small lymphocytes without special stains.

Precursor Cell Compartment

Precursor cells include lineage-specific blast cells and their progeny. The divergence from pluripotent to unipotent hemopoiesis, i.e., erythropoiesis, myelopoiesis, lymphopoiesis, and thrombopoiesis, commences in the progenitor-cell compartment. Precursor cells make up the majority of cells seen in marrow aspirate pull films (see Fig 11.1.) These cells exhibit well-described nuclear and cytoplasmic morphologic features of differentiation progressing to the functional blood and immune cells found in circulation and extravascularly. They have no self-renewal capacity and are unipotent. Almost all precursor cells are in an active phase of the cell cycle. This compartment contains more or less equal percentages of myeloid and erythroid precursors with the remaining cells (approximately 10%) composed of lymphocytes, plasma cells, and macrophages.

The precursor-cell compartment is divided further into three additional functional groups, the proliferation (mitotic), maturation, and storage pools. The kinetics of neutrophil production can be used to illustrate these divisions. Approximately five cell divisions occur between the myeloblast and the myelocyte stages. There are four times as many myelocytes on marrow films as promyelocytes; therefore myelocytes are thought to undergo three cycles of cell division. The major expansion of neutrophils probably occurs through cell division at the myelocyte stage. The size of the proliferation pool (myeloblasts, promyelocytes, and myelocytes) is estimated to be 2.0 to 2.6 billion cells/kg, whereas the maturation-storage (postmitotic) pool (metamyelocytes, bands, and segmented neutrophils) is approximately 6.6 to 13.0 billion cells/kg.[6] Radionuclide studies suggest that cells spend 134.4 hours (5.6 days) in differentiation in the proliferation pool, 14 hours at the myeloblast stage, 19 hours as a promyelocyte, and 102 hours (4.25 days) as a myelocyte. Transit from myelocytes to mature blood neutrophil is estimated to be 130.8 to 157.9 hours (5.45 to 6.58 days), 30 hours (1.25 days) as a metamyelocyte, 50 hours (2.08 days) as a band neutrophil, and 72 hours (3 days) as a segmented neutrophil. Thus, under normal conditions it is thought to take 264 to 288 hours (11 to 12 days) for the mature neutrophil to traverse the precursor compartment.[7] The reserve of mature neutrophils in the hemopoietic microenvironment greatly exceeds the number of neutrophils circulating in the blood, and release of these cells from the storage pool is the mechanism used to respond immediately to a need for additional circulating neutrophils.[8] Under stress conditions, the number of myeloid progenitors increases, and maturation times are shortened. In the presence of active infection the myelocyte-to-neutrophil transit may require only 48 hours (2 days).[9]

As discussed in the chapter on the hemopoietic microenvironment, there are no discrete anatomic sites correlating with the stem-, progenitor-, and precursor-cell compartments or the mitotic and postmitotic pools. However, once neutrophils leave the hemopoietic storage pool, the total neutrophil population can be divided into two further populations that do have anatomic correlates. Total blood neutrophils consist of cells that circulate freely and cells that adhere to the endothelium of capillaries and postcapillary venules, referred to as the circulating neutrophil pool and the marginated neutrophil pool, respectively.[8,9]

METHODS FOR INVESTIGATING HEMOPOIESIS

Development of the techniques for and the disciplined examination of the morphologic features of stained cells from bone marrow and peripheral blood over the past 50 years has resulted in a clear characterization of the maturational sequence during precursor-cell differentiation. The introduction of the paradigm of the monophyletic origin of lymphohemopoietic cells and our current understanding of growth factor and stomal-cell requirements for hemopoiesis arose primarily from three experimental methods; an in vivo HSC assay system [the colony-forming unit-spleen (CFU-S) assay], in vitro clonogenic culture systems, and in vitro long-term bone marrow culture systems. A short discussion of these three methods provide a background for understanding the origins of the terminology of hemopoiesis.

In Vivo Hemopoietic Stem Cell Assay

In 1949, Jacobson and colleagues[10] showed that mice could be protected from the effects of whole-body irradiation if the spleen–a site of hemopoiesis in mice–was exteriorized and excluded from the radiation field. They also showed that the continued presence of the unirradiated spleen was unnecessary, it could be removed 1 hour after irradiation and still provide survival from a lethal dosage of irradiation. Further work showing injected spleen cells could initiate recovery and reestablish hemopoiesis demonstrated that this protective effect was cellular rather than noncellular in origin.[11] These studies unveiled two of the keystones of hemopoiesis: hemopoietic cells are the most proliferative, mitotically active, cells in an animal (titration of a lethal dose of whole-body irradiation indicated one can spare rapidly dividing gastrointestinal cells while irreversibly damaging the even more rapidly dividing hemopoietic cells) and select cells can repopulate both the immune and the hemopoietic lineages.

In 1961, Till and McCulloch[12] described how the colonies that form in the spleens of lethally irradiated mice after injection of bone marrow cells were stem cell derived. Thus the origin of the name, CFU-S assay, and a method for quantitating stem cells. CFU-S colonies are obtained by injection of a limited number of bone marrow cells intravenously into a lethally irradiated, syngeneic recipient mouse.[13] After 8 to 14 days, the mice are euthanized. The spleens are harvested and fixed (or counting or histologic analysis), or the individual spleen colonies can be dissected and analyzed further. A CFU-S, therefore, is a cell that gives rise to a spleen colony. The splenic colonies contain clonogenic populations of erythroid, myeloid, or megakaryocyte precursor cells. The CFU-Ss that appear late (day 14 or CFU-S$_{14}$) also contain cells capable of self-renewal, i.e. they form additional CFU-Ss of differentiated progeny when infused into a second lethally irradiated mouse.[14] After a 3-hour exposure to high-dose ^{3}H-thymidine or hydroxy-

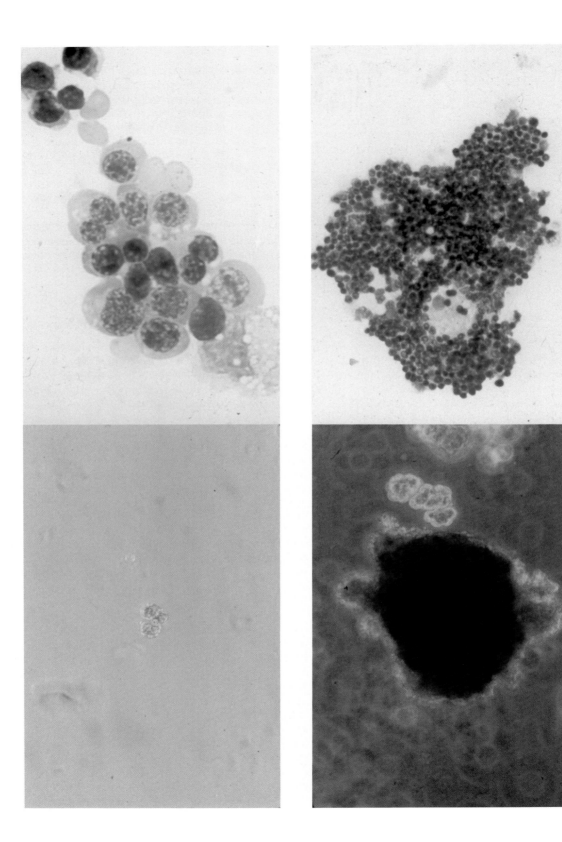

FIGURE 11.2 Erythroid hemopoietic colony forming units. The colony forming unit erythroid (CFU-e) in the upper left panel is the appearance of a single feline CFU-e at day five in situ in methylcellulose culture. The upper right panel is a Wright-Giemsa stained day five feline CFU-e. The lower left panel is a single feline burst forming unit erythroid (BFU-e) at day eleven in situ in methylcellulose culture. The lower right panel is a Wright-Giemsa stained day eleven feline BFU-e.

urea, no more than 20% to 30% of CFU-Ss are in cell cycle.[15]

In Vitro Clonogenic Culture Systems

Most of the fundamentals of hemopoiesis have been learned in semisolid cell-culture systems in which fetal calf serum, conditioned medium, and unfractioned bone marrow cells are used. Some of the early cultures were performed in plasma clots.[16] Only particular lots of fetal calf serum succeeded in supporting the growth of particular hemopoietic progenitor cells. Conditioned medium was poorly characterized medium supernatants, or certain fractions thereof, obtained from cells of various lineages. In recent years, the availability of pure recombinant growth factors, various means to enrich the targeted progenitor cells (Chapter 16), and the use of defined serum-free culture conditions have provided insights into the role of these factors during hemopoiesis.[17] Semisolid systems, agar, or methylcellulose, are still used to provide a sol-gel matrix that facilitates the growth of hemopoietic progenitor cells and assures that individual cells do not migrate together. A more fluid medium would preclude the enumeration of the resultant colonies is similar to the way individual colonies of bacteria are counted so that the number of original bacteria plated in a particular sample can be quantitated.

The kinetics of hemopoietic cell growth in vitro is counterintuitive at first glance. The most mature progenitor cells arise in culture first, and the immature cells appear days later. For example, 3 to 5 days after mononuclear cells separated from feline bone marrow are placed in culture, small colonies (8 to 50 cells) of hemoglobinizing red blood cells (RBCs) can be seen (Fig. 11.2). These are termed CFU-erythroid (CFU-e). Each colony represents a single CFU-e progenitor cell present in the original mononuclear cells that were placed in culture. Near day 11 of culture, fewer, large colonies (100 to 1000 cells) of hemoglobinizing RBCs appear. The remarkable appearance of these colonies led to the term burst-forming units-erythroid (BFU-e) (see Fig. 11.2). Each colony represents the clonal differentiation of a BFU-e progenitor cell. Of course this phenomenon of the more immature cells arising later is consistent with the distance that cells must differentiate along the monophyletic continuum before producing mature hemoglobinized RBCs.

In Vitro Long-Term Bone Marrow Culture Systems

Insights regarding the complex physiology of hemopoiesis and cell interactions occurring in the hemopoietic microenvironment were made possible by an in vitro culture system developed by Dexter.[18] In contrast to the semisolid systems that allows the characterization of clonogenic differentiation of select progenitor cells, this is a liquid system that can be considered an organ culture. The cultures are made up of an elaborate variety of adherent cells, which include endothelial cells, fibroblasts, macrophages, and preadipocytes. One creates the cultures by seeding a large inoculum of unseparated marrow cells into flasks with media containing prescreened horse serum and hydrocortisone. They are maintained in high CO_2, at low temperature (33°C) and depopulated of 50% to 70% of nonadherent cells and fed fresh media at weekly intervals. Handling marrow cells in this manner encourages the growth of a characteristic adherent cell population, which matures in approximately 3 weeks.

Long-term cultures facilitate continuous proliferation and differentiation of hemopoietic cells. Hemopoiesis occurs within, and on the surface of, the adherent cell population. Hemopoietic progenitor cells are continuously shed into the overlying media. Remarkably, HSCs can be maintained for several months in vitro with this method. Furthermore, HSCs collected from such cultures maintain the ability to completely reconstitute the lymphohemopoietic systems of lethally irradiated recipients. The HSCs and progenitor cells are found in large groups of round, refractile cells, termed hemopoietic islands or cobblestone areas, located within the adherent cell population. Maintenance of the stem cell population in such cultures appears to require direct stem cell–stromal-cell contact.[19] The contribution of individual cell types in long-term cultures to this maintenance is not fully known and is the focus of active research. Investigators are striving to develop systems that can be used to maintain HSCs without direct contact with stromal cells.

REFERENCES

1. **Wintrobe MM, ed.** Blood, pure and eloquent: a story of discovery, of people, and of ideas. New York: McGraw-Hill, 1980.
2. **Finch CA, Harker LA, and Cook JD.** Kinetics of the formed elements of human blood. Blood 1977;50:699–713.
3. **Sieff CA, Williams DA.** Hematopoiesis. In: Handin RI, Lus SE, Stossel TP, eds. Blood: principles & practice of hematology. Philadelphia: JB Lippincott, 1995:171–224.
4. **Spangrude GJ, Heimfeld S, Weissman IL.** Purification and characterization of mouse hematopoietic cells. Science 1988;241:58–62.
5. **Micklem Hs, Lennon, JE, Ansell, JD, Gray RA.** Numbers and dispersion of repopulating chimeras as functions of cell dose. Exp. Hematol 1987;15:251–257.
6. **Cronkite EP, Vincent PC.** Granulocytopoiesis. Ser Haematol II 1969;4:3–40.
7. **Bintom DF, Ullyot JL, Farquhar MG.** The development of neurophilic polymorphonuclear leukocytes in human bone marrow. J Exp Med 1971;134:907–915.
8. **Price TH, Chatta GS, Dale DC.** Effect of recombinant granulocyte colony-stimulating factor on neutrophil kinetics in normal young and elderly humans. Blood 1996;88:335–340.
9. **Terashima T, Wiggs B, English D, Hogg JC, van Eeden SF.** Polymorphonuclear leukocyte transit times in bone marrow during streptococcal pneumonia. Am J Physiol 1996;271:587–592.
10. **Jacobson LO, Marks EK, Gaston EO, Robson MJ, Zirkle RE.** Role of the spleen in radiation injury. Roc Soc Exp Biol Med 1949;70:7440–7448.
11. **Jacobson LO, Simmons EL, Marks EK, Gaston EO, Robson MJ, Eldredge JH.** Further studies on recovery from radiation injury. J Lab Clin Med 1951;37:683–689.
12. **Till JE, McCulloch EA.** A direct measurement of the radiation sensitivity of normal mouse bone marrow cells. Rad Res 1961;14:213–219.
13. **Curry JL, Trentin JJ.** Hemopoietic spleen colony studies. I. Growth and differentiation. Dev Bio 1967;15:395–410.
14. **Harrison DE, Astle CM.** Loss of stem cell repopulating ability upon transplantation: effects of donor age, cell number, and transplantation procedure. J Exp Med 1982;156:1767–1777.

15. **Necas E, Znajil V, Frindel E.** Thymidine suicide and hydroxyurea kill ratios accurately reflect the proliferative status of stem cells (CFU-S). Exp Hematol 1989;17:53–60.

16. **Stephenson JR, Axelrad AA, McLeod DL, Shreeve MM.** Induction of colonies of hemoglobin-synthesizing cells by erythropoietin in vitro. Proc Natl Acad Sci 1971;68:1542–1550.

17. **Kawamura M, Hisha H, Li Y, Fukuhara S, Ikehara S.** Distinct qualitative differences between normal and abnormal hemopoietic stem cells in vivo and in vitro. Stem Cells 1997;15:56–62.

18. **Dexter TM, Allen TD, Lajtha LG.** Conditions controlling the proliferation of haemopoietic stem cells in vitro. J Cell Physiol 1977;91:335–343.

19. **Mauch P, Greenberger JS, Botnick L, Hannon E, Hellman S.** Evidence for structured variation in self-renewal capacity within long-term bone marrow cultures. Proc Natl. Acad Sci 1980;77:2927–2936.

CHAPTER 12

Stem Cell Biology

• PETER W. GASPER

Interest in stem cells is increasing because embryonic stem cells may potentially lead to in vitro or ex vivo production of almost any tissue and perhaps organ. In addition, stem cells will likely be increasingly employed in novel gene therapy.[1] Stem cells are defined as formative cells whose daughter cells may give rise to other cell types. A fertilized egg might be thought of as the ultimate stem cell. For most tissues, multilineage potentiality declines as gestation proceeds, and it is functionally irreversible at birth. However, hemopoietic stem cells (HSC) are unique cells found in hemopoietic tissues that exhibit extensive proliferative potential and a capacity to differentiate into all the cells of lympho-hemopoietic lineages continuously until death. The multitude of cells that can arise from a single pluripotent hemopoietic stem cell (PHSC) is surpassed in complexity only by the logarithmic expansion of cells after the union of a sperm and ova.

Current knowledge of HSCs arose from bone marrow transplantation studies, in vivo and in vitro assay systems, characterization of hemopoietic growth factors, and the development of methods to enrich subpopulations of hemopoietic cells. This chapter provides a survey of the biology of HSCs through a discussion of the divergency and growth kinetics of HSCs and hemopoietic growth factors.

DIVERGENCY OF HEMOPOIETIC STEM CELLS

HSCs are now considered a heterogeneous population of cells with varying self-renewal capacities. At the most proximal end of the stem cell compartment are the PHSCs and at the distal margin, next to the progenitor-cell compartment, are HSCs with less self-renewal capacity and more surface antigens (see Fig. 11.1). It becomes more difficult to establish strict criteria for what constitutes an HSC as one approaches the progenitor-cell compartment. Orlic and Bodine[2] proposed the following in a review titled *What Defines a Pluripotent Hemopoietic Stem Cell (PHSC): Will the Real PHSC Please Stand Up!* The term PHSC would then be reserved for cells that have an in vivo capacity of long-term repopulation of all blood cell lineages. Progress has been made in isolating and separating hemopoietic cells from various sources, including bone marrow, peripheral blood, umbilical cord blood, and fetal liver tissue, using combinations of monoclonal antibodies to cell surface antigens, flow cytometry, and counterflow centrifugal elutriation (see Chapter 16, Identification and Isolation of Hemopoietic Progenitors). A shared goal of these investigations is to select and purify PHSCs for use in therapeutic bone marrow transplants or HSC gene-therapy trials (see Chapter 17, Hemopoietic Stem-Cell Transplantation). There is a danger in concluding that one has successfully isolated PHSCs in enriched subpopulations if one has performed the evaluations in short-term in vivo colony-forming unit-spleen(CFU-S) or in vitro (clonogenic hemopoietic cell) assays (methods described in Chapter 11, The Hemopoietic System). For example, serial transplantations of separated cells believed to be PHSCs exhibited multipotentiality in vitro and in short-term (30-day) CFU-S studies. However, the putative PHSCs were unable to repopulate secondary irradiated recipients because the separated cells actually contained many short-term repopulating cells.[3]

Botnick and coworkers[4,5] suggest a continuum of three broad classes of HSCs with respect to self-renewal and proliferative potential. PHSCs are the most primitive and are present in the lowest number. As few as 30 purified PHSCs have been used to repopulate the entire lymphohemopoietic system of lethally irradiated mice.[6] The incidence of such reconsituting HSC is estimated at 1 to 2.5/100,000 injected nucleated cells or 1/10,000 transplanted cells.[7] Next are more divergent HSC that give rise to spleen colonies 12 to 14 days after injection into irradiated mice (CFU-S_{12}) followed by HSC that give rise to spleen colonies 6 to 8 days after transplantation (CFU-S_8) (see Fig. 11.1).[4,5] The distinction between the PHSC and the short-term repopulating cells was demonstrated in studies with 5-fluorouracil (5-FU). Within 1 to 2 days after a single injection of 5-FU, which is toxic for dividing cells, 99.5% of all CFU-S (the CFU-S_{12} and CFU-S_8 cells) were killed, whereas the long-term repopulating PHSCs survived the 5-FU treatment.[8-9] This showed that PHSC, but not divergent CFU-S, were in G_0 of the cell cycle and therefore resistant to 5-FU. As convenient as short-term CFU-S assays may be, it is now clear that only long-term in vivo studies (months to years), documenting whether a complete and stable reconstitution has occurred, can be used to determine if one has successfully isolated PHSC. Furthermore, some contend that an animal model larger than the mouse is needed to extrapolate results of the many investigations of murine hemopoiesis to understand the HSC biology of larger mammals, particularly humans.[10,11]

The science of HSC will advance when PHSC can be examined ex vivo. Colonies have been detected in vitro that give rise to mixed lineage hemopoietic colonies (colony-forming unit-granulocyte, erythrocyte, monocyte, and megakaryocyte [CFU-GEMM] or CFU-Mix). Treatment of bone marrow ex vivo with 4-hydroperoxy-cyclophosphamide eliminates the ability to grow CFU-GEMM in culture, yet does not interfere with reconstitution of hemopoiesis and detection of CFU-S-derived spleen colonies in vivo.[12] Hemopoietic cells with short-term HSC-like abilities have been found to give rise to colonies with high proliferative potential (HPP-CFUs) and blast-cell colonies, but none have been isolated that have the capacity for stable long-term repopulation of the lymphohemopoietic lineages.[13,14]

Using the liquid long-term marrow cultures to assay HSCs and progenitor cells growing on an adherent stromal layer, a long-term culture-initiating cell (LTC-IC) has been described.[15] These cells give rise to multipotent and unipotent progenitor cells for as long at 5 to 8 weeks in culture. The frequency of LTC-ICs in unfractionated marrow is approximately 1 to $2/10^4$ cells. Each LTC-IC can produce several progenitor cells. It was hoped that LTC-ICs represented actual PHSCs. However, when adherent and nonadherent cells from long-term cultures were compared with cultures of equivalent numbers of cells from fresh marrow, their ability to repopulate the erythron of recipient mice was consistently lower than the fresh marrow cells for the adherent cells, and the nonadherent cells failed to show any signs of engraftment.[16] These results suggest that PHSC activity decreases after long-term culture and highlights a recurrent theme and a challenge in studying HSC biology: direct stem cell contact with stromal cells appears to be necessary for HSC survival (see Chapter 13, Hemopoietic Microenvironment). The physical act of separating and isolating a PHSC may initiate its differentiation.

GROWTH KINETICS OF HEMOPOIETIC STEM CELLS

Hemopoietic cells are the most proliferative, mitotically active, cells in an animal. Steady-state peripheral blood cell numbers are maintained within narrow ranges and yet the system is capable of massive rapid production when needed. The capacity of PHSC for concomitant continuous and responsive production of cells raises questions regarding how PHSC are governed; what mechanisms determine whether they remain in G_0, self-renew, undergo apoptosis, or commit to a differentiation pathway? Answering these questions is of immediate practical importance for developing new therapies for

proliferative (neoplastic) or degenerative (aplastic) conditions and will contribute to designing and anticipating possible pitfalls of gene-therapy strategies. Once a PHSC commences differentiation the mechanisms involved are better characterized. In general, there are several direct-acting and circulating growth factors and cytokines that encourage the production of particular lineages of blood or immune cells, depending on the animal's homeostatic needs at that time (see Hemopoietic Growth Factors below and Chapter 15, Cytokine Regulation of Hemopoiesis).

In attempting to explain how few PHSC maintain lymphohemopoiesis, Kay[17] advanced a hypothesis of clonal succession; that is, a series of PHSC advance to populate the peripheral circulation sequentially. There is limited evidence for this thesis.[18,19] It was suggested after an evaluation of studies that many HSC clones exhibit concurrent continuous proliferation when retroviral-mediated gene transfer was used to mark HSCs.[20] Progeny of HSC transplanted into mice show unstable integration patterns initially, then they stabilize and maintain a consistent pattern over many months. It appears the latter hypothesis better fits what is observed in larger mammals. Abkowitz and colleagues[10] performed autologous marrow transplantation studies of glucose 6-phosphate dehydrogenase (G6PD) heterozygous female Safari cats. This model system exploits the female exhibition of a random mosaic expression of traits, such as different isotypes of G6PD, located on the X chromosome. After transplantation, the peripheral blood counts, marrow morphologies, frequencies of progenitors, and progenitor-cell cycle kinetics returned to normal. However, abrupt and significant fluctuations were seen in the G6PD type of progenitors from each cat during the 1 to 1.5 years of observation. Abkowitz and colleagues[10] felt their data could not be explained if there were either a large or constant population of active stem cells and thus initially thought hemopoiesis was maintained through clonal succession.[10] In examining these cats repeatedly for 3.5 to 6 years after transplantation, they characterized two phases of stem cell kinetics. The first phase was as per their first report noting significant fluctuations in contributions of stem cell clones. Later clonal contributions to hemopoiesis stabilized. The initial phase of clonal disequilibrium extended for 1 to 4.5 years. After this subsided, all progenitor cells from some animals expressed a single parental G6PD phenotype, suggesting that blood-cell production could be stably maintained by the progeny of one (or a few) cells. They concluded that, as the hemopoietic demand of a cat (i.e., number of blood cells produced per lifetime) is more than 600 times that of a mouse. This provides evidence that an individual hemopoietic stem cell has a vast self-renewal or proliferative capacity. The long phase of clonal instability may reflect the time required for stem cells to replicate sufficiently to reconstitute a large stem cell reserve.[22] In computer simulation models in which data from the above-mentioned transplants of G6PD heterozygous female Safari cats were used, it was concluded that the entrance of a PHSC to a particular pathway (self-renewal, apoptosis, or initiation of a differentiation or a maturation sequence) is compatible with a stochastic (random) process.[23] The question of clonal succession versus continuous proliferation of PHSCs is further resolved by studies that suggest hemopoiesis is mitotically asymmetric.[24] In this process, one daughter cell becomes quiescent and returns to G_0 and the other daughter cell becomes committed to differentiation. Asymmetric division of PHSC is more consistent with the continuous-proliferation hypothesis. In contrast, symmetric differentiation of PHSC, i.e., mitosis producing two daughter cells that both differentiate or both regenerate PHSC, would be more consistent with a clonal succession model. It is important to remember, however, that steady-state hemopoiesis may manifest different kinetics than what is witnessed during the profound proliferative pressures that accompany transplantation and the reconstitution of the entire lympho-hemopoietic systems.[25]

HEMOPOIETIC GROWTH FACTORS

A family of glycoproteins conducts the orchestration of hemopoietic differentiation once a PHSC commits. The specific hemopoietic growth factors that influence immature hemopoietic cells are considered here. Cytokine regulation of hemopoiesis is discussed in Chapter 15, Cytokine Regulation of Hemopoiesis. Figure 15.1 illustrates the multiplicity of factors and the overlapping sites along the continuum of differentiation where cytokines and hemopoietic growth factors exert an effect. The growth factor or cytokine to progenitor cell (ligand to receptor) relations have mostly been established in in vitro investigations. As is discussed in Chapter 13, stromal cells play an essential role in hemopoiesis in vivo. It is incorrect to envision hemopoietic differentiation as a process in which soluble growth factors in blood bathe suspended lymphocytelike cells, thereby encouraging them to develop along a particular blood-cell lineage. Cloned hemopoietic growth factors and cytokines have allowed us to expose progenitor cells to these factors in such a fashion in vitro, whereas, extravascular cell-to-cell contact or stromal-cell niches are vital to HSC survival and differentiation in vivo.

It is likely that a unifying paradigm will emerge from the rapid advancements and seemingly ever-increasing complexity of the biology of hemopoietic growth factors and cytokines. Biological principles predict that there are a finite number of molecular means to initiate the expression of cell-lineage-specific genes. Many of the genes for these molecules have been mapped to the same chromosome (in humans, the long arm of chromosome 5), and there are structural homologies in a group of gonadotropin-releasing hormone (GRH)-like cytokines that include GRH, prolactin, erythropoietin, interleukin (IL)-6, and granulocyte-colony-stimulating factor (G-CSF).[26–28] Interestingly, deletions in the long arm of chromosome 5 are common in humans who have myelodysplastic syndromes and other hemopoietic diseases.[29]

TABLE 12.1   Hemopoietic Stem-Cell Biology

Hemopoietic Growth Factor	Synonym	Size (kD)	Source
Stem-Cell Factor (SCF)	Steel factor, mast cell growth factor.	37–42	Marrow stromal cells Fetal tissues
Granulocyte-macrophage-colony-stimulating factor (GM-CSF)	CSF α	18–30	T Lymphocytes Monocytes Endothelial cells Fibroblasts Macrophages
Granulocyte-colony-stimulating factor (G-CSF)	CSF β	19.6	Monocytes Macrophages Endothelial cells Fibroblasts Neutrophils
Macrophage-colony-stimulating factor (M-CSF)	CSF-1	90*	Monocytes Macrophages Endothelial cells Placenta Urine
Erythropoietin (EPO)	—	38	Kidney
Thrombopoietin (TPO)	—	35–70	Kidney Liver

*Alternate splicing of the messenger RNA (mRNA) produces two forms of the mature protein. The shorter mRNA produces a 26-kD polypeptide expressed on cell surfaces. The larger transcript encodes a 61-kD protein that is heavily glycosylated and initially appears on the cell membrane. Subsequent cleavage and dimerization yields the mature soluble factor of 90 kD.

The nomenclature of the hemopoietic growth factors originated from the in vitro investigations of hemopoietic cells. The first factors characterized were ones that stimulated hemopoietic colony proliferation, hence the designation CSF. For example, GM-CSF was the factor that stimulated progenitor cells to form colonies of recognizable granulocytes and macrophages in culture dishes. Table 12.1 outlines the key details of the CSFs that are briefly discussed herein. See the excellent review by Alexander[30] for a more detailed treatise of both hemopoietic growth factors and cytokines.

Stem-Cell Factor

The isolation of stem cell factor (SCF), originally known as c-kit ligand, illustrates how direct stem cell contact with stromal cells appears to be necessary for HSC survival in vivo. For years, two particular mutant strains of mice have been the subject of various investigations of hemopoiesis. Affected dominant white-spotting (W) and Steel (Sl) mice have fatal heritable defects of HSCs and of the hemopoietic microenvironment respectively. Transplantation of normal HSCs into affected W/W^v recipients results in functional hemopoiesis, whereas transplantation of HSCs from W/W^v-affected mice fails to establish hemopoiesis in lethally irradiated normal mice. In contrast, HSCs of Sl/Sl^d mice are capable of reconstituting hemopoiesis in irradiated normal mice, whereas transplantation of normal HSCs into Sl/Sl^d-affected mice fail because of their malfunctioning hemopoietic microenviroment.[31] Investigations of the mice that have the HSC defect revealed that the W gene mutation is of a gene allelic with product of the c-kit protooncogene. The c-kit protooncogene product was known to be a member of the tyrosine kinase receptor family.[32] Purification of a factor present on mast cells and mouse marrow cells that had been treated with 5-FU led to the demonstration that this factor is the ligand for the c-kit receptor.[33] Administration of this purified factor, c-kit ligand (SCF), to Sl/Sl^d mice corrected their microenvironmental defect and resultant fatal macrocytic anemia and repaired their mast cell deficiency.

Many studies that examine the structure of SCF, the sites of its production, its role in ontogeny, and its role in hemopoiesis are being conducted.[34] In short, there are two biologically active forms of SCF, a soluble and a transmembrane gene product. SCF is produced by fetal cells and influences the migration of germ cells, melanocytes, and HSCs to their ultimate destinations during development. It is produced constitutively by marrow stromal cells and directly stimulates HSC to enter the cell cycle. Alone, it has a limited effect on hemopoiesis in vitro; however, in the presence of other cytokines, SCF increases both the size and the number of colonies. Treatment of adult mice that have a neutralizing c-kit receptor monoclonal antibody causes pancytopenia and significant decreases in bone marrow cellularity. Studies of humans who have aplastic anemia, myelodysplasia, and several other types of chronic anemia have shown no increase in serum SCF levels, nor have they shown that levels of SCF increase during the period of profound pancytopenia after marrow ablative chemoradiotherapy. Canine SCF has been isolated, cloned, and used in many investigations.[35-37] Clinical uses of hemopoietic growth factors in veterinary medicine are discussed in Chapter 133.

Granulocyte-Macrophage Colony-Stimulating Factor

Granulocyte-macrophage CSF (GM-CSF) is produced by activated T lymphocytes, macrophages, endothelial cells, and fibroblasts in response to other cytokines and endotoxin. Its cellular receptor is a dimer. Although the α–subunit binds GM-CSF, the presence of the β–subunit significantly increases its affinity. Receptor density increases with differentiation, and most are dense on mature neutrophils. The primary progenitors stimulated by GM-CSF are colony-forming unit granulocyte-macrophage (CFU-GM) that proceed to produce mature neutrophils and monocytes and CFU-E$_O$ that produce mature eosinophils. It has a weak synergistic effect with other growth factors and cytokines in stimulating earlier progenitor cells. Mature neutrophils and macrophages

exhibit increased motility and cytotoxicity after exposure to GM-CSF.[30]

Granulocyte-Colony-Stimulating Factor

G-CSF is produced by monocytes, endothelial cells, fibroblasts, neutrophils, and various tumor cells in response to various stimuli, including IL-1, tumor necrosis factor (TNF), interferon-g, other CSFs, and endotoxin. Because there is no storage form of G-CSF, these stimuli promote gene transcription. Its cellular receptors are present on granulocyte precursor cells with the greatest concentration on mature neutrophils. Receptors for G-CSF have also been identified in the placenta, endothelium, and cell lines of pulmonary small cell tumors. G-CSF acts to accelerate differentiation of neutrophil precursors and shortens neutrophil maturation time. It also stimulates the cytotoxic functions of neutrophils.[30]

Macrophage-Colony-Stimulating Factor

Macrophage-CSF (M-CSF) is produced by monocytes and macrophages, endothelial cells, and the placenta. The receptor of M-CSF is a transmembrane glycoprotein tyrosine kinase, which phosphorylates the guanosine triphosphatase (GTP-ase)-activating protein associated with H-ras. M-CSF stimulates the maturation of monocyte and macrophage precursor cells and enhances opsonization.

Erythropoietin

Erythropoietin (EPO) is produced primarily by the juxaglomerular cells in the kidney. A small fraction of total EPO is produced by hepatic Kupffer's cells and other macrophages. Hypoxemia stimulates the production of EPO, the levels of which can increase 100-fold. There are approximately 1000 EPO receptors per erythroid progenitor cell. Once EPO binds the receptor, differentiation of erythroid progenitors proceeds to precursors and mature RBCs. If EPO is not present, these cells undergo apoptosis.[30]

Thrombopoietin

The most recently characterized hemopoietic growth factor, thrombopoietin (TPO), was discovered in a fashion similar to the discovery of SCF. Souyri and colleagues[38,39] identified the gene for the TPO receptor, a cellular oncogene called c-mpl. Others determined that c-mpl is expressed on HSCs, megakaryocytes, and platelets Finally, several groups identified TPO as the c-mpl ligand.[39] Synthesized in the kidney and the liver, TPO levels are regulated by mature platelets. They bind and metabolize TPO during unperturbed conditions but do not clear TPO during thrombocytopenic episodes. This makes it available to circulation and the hemopoietic microenvironments. Thrombopoietin stimulates burst-forming unit megakaryocyte (BFU-MK) progenitor cells to proliferate and to differentiate. Continued presence of TPO induces megakaryocytes to enlarge, undergo endoreduplication and release proplatelets that fragment into platelets.

Although much remains to be determined about the biology of HSCs, one can see how the dynamic proliferative potential of these cells effects every other organ system and vice versa, thereby placing the hematologist in a position to contribute to the improved health of almost any patient.

REFERENCES

1. **Marshall E**. A versatile cell line raises scientific hopes, legal questions. Science 1998;282:1014–1015.
2. **Orlic D, Bodine DM**. What defines a pluripotent hematopoietic stem cell (PHSC): will the real PHSC please stand up! Blood 1994;84:3991–3994.
3. **Jones RJ, Celano P, Sharkis SJ, Sensenbrenner LL**. Two phases of engraftment established by serial bone marrow transplantation in mice. Blood;73:397–401.
4. **Botnick LE, Hannon EC, Hellman S**. Nature of the hemopoietic stem cell compartment and its proliferative potential. Blood Cells 1979;5:195–210.
5. **Botnick LE, Hannon EC, Obbagy J, Hellman S**. The variation of hematopoietic stem cell self-renewal capacity as a function of age: further evidence for heterogenicity of the stem cell compartment. Blood 1982;60:268–271.
6. **Spangrude GJ, Heimfeld S, Weissman IL**. Purification and characterization of mouse hematopoietic cells. Science 1988;241:58–62.
7. **Micklem HS, Lennon JE, Ansell JD, Gray RA**. Numbers and dispersion of repopulating chimeras as functions of cell dose. Exp Hematol 1987;15:251–257.
8. **Bradley TR, Hodgson GS**. Detection of primitive macrophage progenitor cells in mouse bone marrow. Blood 1979;54:1446–1450.
9. **Van Zant G**. Studies of hematopoietic stem cells spared by 5-fluorouracil. J Exp Med 1984;159:679–690.
10. **Abkowitz JL, Persik MT, Shelton GH, Ott RL, Kiklevich JV, Catlin SN, Guttorp P**. Behavior of hematopoietic stem cells in a large animal. Proc Natl Acad Sci U S A 1995;92:2031–2035.
11. **Abkowitz JL, Taboada MR, Sabo KM, Shelton GH**. The *ex vivo* expansion of feline marrow cells leads to increased numbers of BFU-E and CFU-GM but a loss of reconstituting ability. Stem Cells 1998;288–293.
12. **Porcellini A, Manna A, Talevi N, Sparaventi G, Marchetti-Rossi MT, Baronciani D, De Biagi M**. Effect of two cyclophosphamide derivatives on hemopoietic progenitor cells and pluripotential stem cells. Exp Hematol 1984;:863–866.
13. **McNiece IK, Bertoncello I, Kriegler AB, Quesenberry PJ**. Colony-forming cells with high proliferative potential (HPP-CFC). Int J Cell Cloning 1990;8:146–160.
14. **Leary AG, Ogawa M**. Blast cell colony assay for umbilical cord blood and adult bone marrow progenitors. Blood 1987;69:953–956.
15. **Sutherland HJ, Lansdorp PM, Henkelman DH, Eaves AC, Eaves CJ**. Functional characterization of individual human hematopoietic stem cells cultured at limiting dilution on supportive marrow stromal layers. Proc Natl Acad Sci U S A 1990;87:3584–3588.
16. **Harrison DE, Lerner CP, Spooncer E**. Erythropoietic repopulating ability of stem cells from long-term marrow culture. Blood 1987;69:1021–1025.
17. **Kay HEM**. Hypothesis: How many cell-generations? Lancet 1965;1:418–420.
18. **Brecher G, Beal SL, Schneiderman M**. Renewal and release of hemopoietic stem cells: does clonal succession exist? Blood Cells 1986;12(1):103–127.
19. **Prchal JT, Prchal JF, Belickova M, Chen S, Guan Y, Gartland GL, Cooper MD**. Clonal stability of blood cell lineages indicated by X-chromosomal transcriptional polymorphism. J Exp Med 1996;183:561–567.
20. **Harrison DE, Astle CM, Lerner C**. Number and continuous proliferative pattern of transplanted primitive immunohematopoietic stem cells. Proc Natl Acad Sci U S A 1988;85:822–826.
21. **Lemischka IR**. What we have learned from retroviral marking of hematopoietic stem cells. Curr Top Microbiol Immunol 1992;177:59–71.
22. **Abkowitz JL, Linenberger ML, Newton MA, Shelton GH, Ott RL, Guttorp P**. Evidence for the maintenance of hematopoiesis in a large animal by the sequential activation of stem cell clones. Proc Natl Acad Sci U S A 1990;87:9062–9066.
23. **Abkowitz JL, Catlin SN, Guttorp P**. Evidence that hematopoiesis may be a stochastic process in vivo. Nat Med 1996;2:190–197.
24. **Brummendorf TH, Dragowska W, Zijlmans JMJM, Thornbury G, Lansdorp PM**. Asymmetric cell divisions sustain long-term hematopoiesis from single-sorted human fetal liver cells. J Exp Med 1998;188(6):1117–1124.
25. **Abkowitz JL, Catlin SN, Guttorp P**. Strategies for hematopoietic stem cell gene therapy: insights from computer simulation studies. Blood 1997;89:3192–3198.
26. **Pettenati MJ, Le Beau MM, Lemons RS, Shima EA, Kawasaki ES, Larson RA, Sherr CJ, Diaz MO, Rowley JD**. Assignment of CSF-1 to 5q33.1: evidence for clustering of genes regulating hematopoiesis and for their involvement in the deletion of the long arm of chromosome 5 in myeloid disorders. Proc Natl Acad Sci U S A 1987;84:2970–2974.
27. **Bazan JF**. Structural design and molecular evolution of a cytokine receptor superfamily. Proc Natl Acad Sci U S A 1990;87:6934–6938.
28. **Kirken RA, Evans GA, Duhe RJ, DaSilva L, Malabarba MG, Erwin RA, Farrar WL**. Mechanisms of cytokine signal transduction: IL-2, IL-4 and prolactin as hematopoietin receptor models. Vet Immunol Immunopathol 1998;63:27–36.
29. **Lewis S, Oscier D, Boultwood J, Ross F, Fitchett M, Rack K, Abrahamson G, Buckle V, Wainscoat JS**. Hematological features of patients with myelodysplastic syndromes associated with a chromosome 5q deletion. Am J Hematol 1995;49:194–200.
30. **Alexander WS**. Cytokines in hematopoiesis. Int Rev Immunol 1998;16:651–682.
31. **Russell ES**. Hereditary anemias of the mouse: a review for geneticists. Adv Genet 1979;20:357–367.
32. **Chabot B, Stephenson DA, Chapman VM, Besmer P, Bernstein A**. The protooncogene c-kit encoding a transmembrane tyrosine kinase receptor maps to the mouse W locus. Nature 1988;335:88–89.
33. **Williams DE, Eisenman J, Baird A, Rauch C, Van Ness K, March CJ, Park LS, Martin U, Mochizuki DY, Boswell HS**. Identification of a ligand for the c-kit proto-oncogene. Cell 1990;63:167–174.
34. **Broudy VC**. Stem cell factor and hematopoiesis. Blood 1997;90:1345–1364.
35. **Shull RM, Suggs SV, Langley KE, Okino KH, Jacobsen FW, Martin FH**. Canine stem cell factor (c-kit ligand) supports the survival of hematopoietic progenitors in long-term canine marrow culture. Exp Hematol 1992;20:1118–1124.
36. **Sandmaier BM, Storb R, Santos EB, Krizanac-Bengez L, Lian T, McSweeney PA, Yu C, Schuening FG, Deeg HJ, Graham T**. Allogenic transplant of canine peripheral blood stem cells mobilized by recombinant canine hematopoietic growth factors. Blood 1996;87:3508–3513.
37. **Whitwam T, Haskins ME, Henthorn PS, Kraszewski JN, Kleiman SE, Seidel NE, Bodine DM, Puck JM**. Retroviral marking of canine bone marrow: long-term, high-level expression of human interleukin-2 receptor common gamma chain in canine lymphocytes. Blood 1998;92:1565–1575.
38. **Souyri M, Vigon I, Penciolelli JF, Heard JM, Tambourin P, Wendling F**. A putative truncated cytokine receptor gene transduced by the myeloproliferative leukemia virus immortalizes hematopoietic progenitors. Cell 1990;63(6):1137–1147.
39. **Souyri M**. Mpl: from an acute myeloproliferative virus to the isolation of the long sought thrombopoietin. Semin Hematol 1998;35:222–231.

CHAPTER 13

Hemopoietic Microenvironment

• PETER W. GASPER

Hemopoiesis occurs in three-dimensional extra-vascular niches, where sustentacular cells and an extracellular matrix create a microenviron-ment that shelters and regulates hemopoietic stem cells (HSC) as they differentiate, proliferate, and mature be-fore their blood-cell progeny are permitted to enter cir-culation. In adult mammals, bone marrow is the primary site of hemopoiesis, and it is estimated that marrow is 1.9 to 2.5% of an animal's body weight, making it second to the liver in organ size.[1] Four phenomena can be used to illustrate how hemopoietic tissues are unique in serv-ing as nomadic nurseries for mobilized HSCs: HSC transplantation, the ontogeny of the hemopoietic sys-tem, bone-matrix explants, and myelolipomas. A HSC transplantation is an intravenous injection of cells (see Chapter 17, Hemopoietic Stem-Cell Transplantation). Although these injected cells, which include HSCs, cir-culate through all the organs of the body, they only become established and proliferate in those anatomic sites conducive to and capable of supporting hemopoie-sis. In most animals, these sites of engraftment are in the marrow. In others, most notably mice, the trans-planted cells also seed and grow in the spleen. During ontogeny, hemopoiesis commences in the yolk sac, pro-ceeds to the liver, and then relocates to bone marrow (see Chapter 14, Ontogeny of the Hemopoietic System). Several studies performed primarily in adult mice, have shown that bone matrix implanted under the capsule of the kidney, subcutaneously, or on various membranes in the peritoneal cavity, leads to hemopoiesis in these sites in a period of weeks.[2–6] Myelolipomas are benign tumors composed of well-differentiated adipose tissue that supports the growth of hemopoietic cells. The tu-mors are usually found associated with the adrenal gland, but have been described in the mediastium, liver, spleen, and intracranial space in various species.[7–13] In each of these examples, hemopoiesis occurs when HSCs encounter a supportive site. The specific cells of the hemopoietic microenvironment include adventitial re-ticular cells, endothelial cells, adipocytes, and, perhaps, osteoblasts. The necessary extracelluar matrix elements and blood flow dynamics have yet to be definitively described. The hemopoietic microenvironment facili-tates hemopoietic differentiation and proliferation. In addition, it performs a gatekeeper function, overseeing the release of mature but not immature blood cells into peripheral blood. The anatomy and physiology of the hemopoietic microenvironment are discussed herein. The work of Tavassoli[14] provides a complete treatise on and history of the characterization of the hemopoietic microenvironment.

ANATOMY OF THE HEMOPOIETIC MICROENVIRONMENT

A clinical pathologist arrives at a morphologic or a causal diagnosis after the thoughtful microscopic evalu-ation of individual marrow precursor cells that are pres-ent on a pull film. Figure 13.1 illustrates the long-known difference between how erythropoiesis appears in vivo and how it looks on a smear.[15] As was introduced in Chapters 11 and 12, The Hemopoietic System and Stem-Cell Biology, respectively, all blood cells arise in lineage-specific colony-forming units (CFUs) consisting of clones of hemopoietic progenitor cells. Active hemopoi-etic tissue, red marrow for instance, consists of two parts: a latticelike cellular and extracellular scaffolding and CFUs that are aggregates of different types of lympho-hemopoietic cells wherein cells of the precursor com-partment predominate (Fig. 13.2). Investigators at-tempting ex vivo reconstitution of human hemopoiesis have suggested evaluation of a CFUs:mesenchymal cell ratio referred to as the parenchymal:stromal cell ratio.[16]

Marrow stromal cells can be isolated from other mar-row cells by their tendency to adhere to plastic tissue culture flasks in long-term bone marrow culture sys-tems. In vitro, the stromal cells exhibit many of the characteristics of germ cells for tissues that can roughly be defined as mesenchymal, because they can be stimu-lated to differentiate into osteoblasts, chondrocytes, adi-pocytes, and even myoblasts.[17] The plasticity of stromal-cell differentiation likely contributes to the ability of the hemopoietic system to respond rapidly to varying demands for different blood cells of different lineages. It is important, therefore, that the young hematologist appreciate the multipotentiality of both the HSCs and the cells that support them.

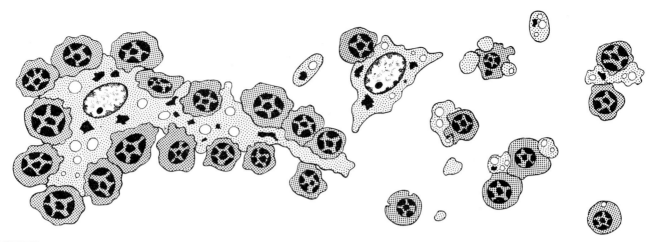

FIGURE 13.1 Disruption of an rubriblastic colony or "islet" at the moment of marrow smear preparation. On the left is an intact colony of developing erythroid precursor cells as they appear in vivo or in in vitro colony forming assays. On the right are the cells disrupted as they appear on a marrow smear. (Reprinted with permission from Bessis M. Living Blood Cells and their Ultrastructure. New York: Springer-Verlag, 1973:87)

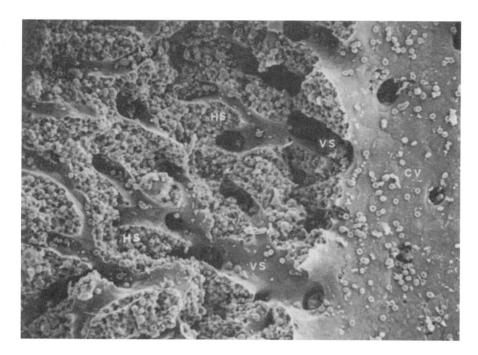

FIGURE 13.2 Scanning electron micrograph of a rat bone marrow showing developing cells in hemopoietic spaces (HSs), anastomosing venous sinusoids (VS), and central vein (CV). X290 (prepared with assistance of Dr. Prem Handagama.)

Structural Components of the Hemopoietic Microenvironment

Adventitial reticular cells are large fibroblastic cells that branch out from the abluminal side of vascular sinuses into the perivascular space and provide the scaffolding that harbors the growing hemopoietic colonies (Fig. 13.3).[17] Ultrastructurally, these cells have many pseudopods that may completely encircle developing precursor cells (see Fig. 13.1).[15,17] It is thought that these cells, in concert with others, play an active role in the epigenetic regulation of hemopoiesis by direct cell contact or local secretion of growth-regulating glycoproteins (see "Physiology of Hemopoietic Microenvironment" below). The cells may cover the majority of the adventitial surface of the sinuses where they appear to control access to the wall of the sinus for cells seeking circulation; however, in cases of massive demand for peripheral blood cells, the amount of surface the cell covers is considerably reduced. Adventitial cells may accumulate fat droplets, thereby reducing the space available for hemopoietic CFUs.[17]

There is a heterogeneity of endothelial cells throughout the body. Those of the marrow microvasculature

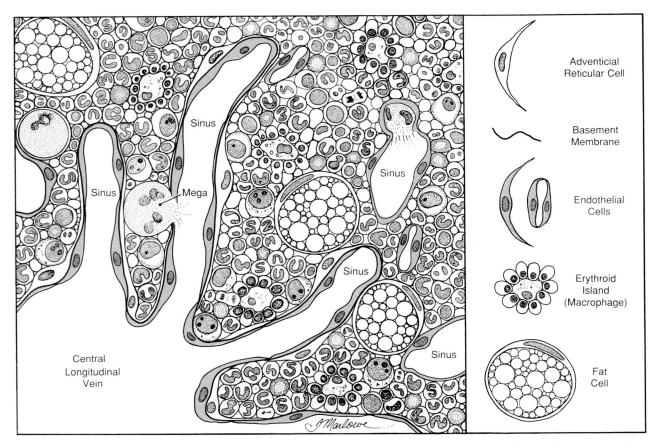

FIGURE 13.3 Diagram of the hemopoietic microenvironment. Numerous granulocytic precursors cells, megakaryocytes, and erythroid colonies ("islands"), are shown in relationship to the structural components of the microenvironment, adventitial cells, endothelial cells, and fat cells. (From Sieff C, Williams D. Hemopoiesis. In: Handin R, Lux S, Stossel T. Blood: Principles & Practice of Hematology. Philadelphia: J.B. Lippincott, 1995)

are considered highly specialized.[18] Figure 13.4 depicts a segment of the wall of a vascular sinus. Weiss,[19] on the basis of extensive ultrastructural examination of the rat marrow, described a single layer of endothelial cells of variable thickness that exhibited active pinocytosis with a moderate number of lysosomes and mitochondria. He noted an attenuated and discontinuous basement membrane with a degree of granularity.[19] Mature blood cells traverse transcellularly through the cytoplasm of endothelial cells to enter circulation (see "Physiology of Hemopoietic Microenvironment" below).[20]

Adipocytes are a major constituent of marrow tissue, occupying approximately half the potential marrow volume in most adult mammals. Severe hemolytic anemias or chronic exposure to hypoxia results in a reduction of marrow fat content.[21] In contrast, there is extensive infiltration of yellow marrow after aplastic anemia and in mice after long-term RBC transfusions.[22] Additional cells of the hemopoietic microenvironment include macrophages and osteoblasts.[20] Extracellular matrix molecules such as fibronectin (FN), collagens, and laminin are present and contribute to the upregulation or the downregulation of hemopoiesis, some of aspects of this

regulation are currently being determined in vitro (see "Physiology of Hemopoietic Microenvironment" below).

Hemopoietic Macroenvironments

Bone marrow of all flat bones supports a lifetime of active hemopoiesis. Extramedullary hemopoiesis is seen occasionally in several species, usually in the spleen and in response to severe anemia and or myelofibrosis.[1] The mouse is a notable exception in that the spleen normally serves as a hemopoietic organ. Bone provides protection for the rapidly dividing blood cell, and its slow, low-pressure, venous sinusoidal microcirculation flowing among fingerlike extensions of hemopoietic cords allows exquisite control of the egress of mature elements from the nurturing microenvironments into the peripheral blood (Fig. 13.5). De Bruyn and colleagues[23] demonstrated that the vascular system of mammalian marrow could be classified as a portal system. The major blood supply to the sinusoids is contained in the vessels that perforate cortical bone through osteal canals. Long

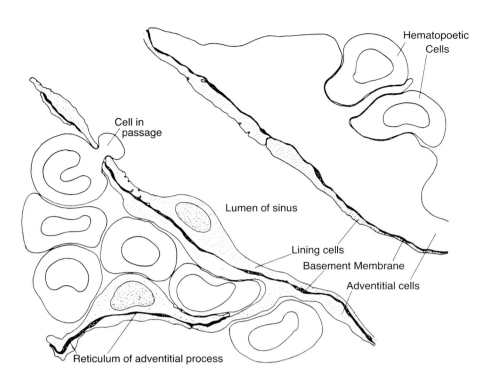

FIGURE 13.4 Segment of the wall of a vascular sinus, including an adventitial process. The sinus wall is trilaminar in most places, consisting of a lining (or endothelial) cell, a basement membrane, and an adventitial cell. In places apertures may occur in the wall, and free cells may pass through such apertures. Elsewhere, the basement membrane or the adventitial layer may be absent, resulting in a wall of one or two layers. The adventitial cells are commonly voluminous and rarefied, extending deeply into the contiguous HS and displacing hemopoietic cells. (The upper labeled adventitial cell exemplifies this.) An adventitial process is of the same structure as the sinus wall.

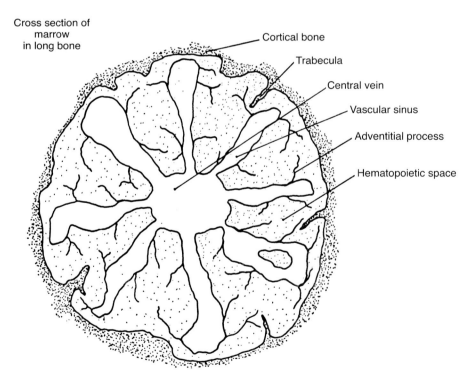

FIGURE 13.5 Organization of the venous vasculature of the marrow of a long bone. Thin-walled vascular sinuses originate at the periphery from termination of transverse branches of the nutrient artery (not shown). The vascular sinuses run transversely toward the center to join the CV. Hemopoiesis takes place in the space between the vascular sinuses. Adventitial processes project into the HS, producing partial compartmentalization.

bones stripped of their periosteum are pitted by numerous small holes, some 100 μm apart. The periosteal capillary network sends small branches, the transosteal vessels, through these foramina. The transosteal vessels are composed of a single layer of endothelium and their diameters are on average, three times larger than the periosteal capillaries. These vessels widen at the osteomyeloid junction to form the sinusoids whose lumen is now twice that of the transosteal vessel. Perhaps associated with this unique blood supply is the observation that quiescent, less proliferative HSCs reside at the periphery of the hemopoietic cords in the subcortical, endosteal space, whereas stem cells with higher proliferative rates are observed toward the middle of the vascular sinus.[24,25] In addition, it has been observed in vitro that osteoblasts induced a threefold to fourfold increase in the number of long-term culture-initiating cells.[26]

Physiology of Hemopoietic Microenvironment

It has been proposed that the hemopoietic microenvironment is a translator of peripheral signals for HSCs.[27] Thus, stromal cells can be viewed as tools to analyze the physiologic conditions that regulate stem cells. The combination of long-term marrow cultures and an ever-increasing number of immortalized stromal-cell lines demonstrates that there are unique clones of cells that elaborate unique combinations of glycoproteins. These molecules are such that they support the growth of some progenitor cells while inhibiting the growth of others.[28,29]

Adipocytes might seem to be the least complex portion of the cells responsible for regulation of hemopoiesis in that they act only as a passive storage site for energy. Medullary adipocytes exhibit characteristics similar to both white and brown adipocytes.[30] After calorie depravation, white adipocyte tissue is rapidly depleted, whereas marrow fat is spared.[31] White adipocytes are lipogenic in response to insulin, whereas marrow adipocytes differentiate in response to glucocorticoids and do not respond to insulin treatment.[32] Recent work suggests that marrow adipocytes are unique in their production of leptin.[33] In a recent review of the role of adipocytes, marrow adipocyte morphology and physiology, the transcriptional and cytokine mechanisms regulating their differentiation, and the interrelations among bone marrow adipocytes, hemopoiesis, and osteogenesis were discussed. The authors concluded with the following statement: "Overall, these data lend support to a "plastic" model of bone marrow stromal cell differentiation; adipocytes may share common functions with stromal stem cells, osteoblasts, and hemopoietic supportive cells."[30]

Extracellular matrix components of the adherent cell layer are shared by many stromal-cell lines capable of supporting the proliferation of myeloid progenitors. These cells produce laminin and type IV collagen as well as FN. The binding of hemopoietic growth factors with matrix components, as well as the positive and negative feedback regulatory role of hemopoietic stem cells bound to the microenvironment, represents the number of possible variables to be considered during assessment of the physiologic role of the extracelluar matrix proteins. Furthermore, receptors responsible for this interaction may be important in the homing of primitive progenitors to the bone marrow.

REFERENCES

1. **Jain NC**. Schalm's Veterinary Hematology. 4th ed. Philadelphia: Lea & Febiger, 1986:362.
2. **Reddi AH, Gay R, Gay S, Miller EJ**. Transitions in collagen types during matrix-induced cartilage, bone, and bone marrow formation. Proc Natl Acad Sci U S A 1977;74:5589–5592.
3. **Knospe WH, Husseini SG, Adler SS, Reddi AH**. Hematopoiesis on cellulose ester membranes (CEM). V. Enrichment of CEM by demineralized mouse bone matrix powder. Exp Hematol 1983;11(10):1021–1026.
4. **Knospe WH, Husseini SG, Adler SS, Reddi AH**. Decalcified tooth matrix powder induces new bone formation and hematopoietic microenvironment in the mouse. Int J Cell Cloning 1985;3(5):320–329.
5. **Knospe WH, Husseini SG, Fried W**. Hematopoiesis on cellulose ester membranes. XI. Induction of new bone and a hematopoietic microenvironment by matrix factors secreted by marrow stromal cells. Blood 1989;74(1):66–70.
6. **Gurevitch O, Fabian I**. Ability of the hemopoietic microenvironment in the induced bone to maintain the proliferative potential of early hemopoietic precursors. Stem Cells 1993;11:56–61.
7. **Rao P, Kenney PJ, Wagner BJ, Davidson AJ**. Imaging and pathologic features of myelolipoma. Radiographics 1997;17(6):1373–1385.
8. **Latimer KS, Rakich PM**. Subcutaneous and hepatic myelolipomas in four exotic birds. Vet Pathol 1995;32:84–87.
9. **Sander CH, Langham RF**. Myelolipoma of the spleen in a cat. J Am Vet Med Assoc 1972;160(8):1101–1103.
10. **McCaw DL, da Silva Curiel JM, Shaw DP**. Hepatic myelolipomas in a cat. J Am Vet Med Assoc 1990;197:243–244.
11. **Li X, Fox JG, Erdman SE**. Multiple splenic myelolipomas in a ferret (Mustela putorius furo). Lab Anim Sci 1996;46(1):101–103.
12. **Spangler WL, Culbertson MR, Kass PH**. Primary mesenchymal (nonangiomatous/nonlymphomatous) neoplasms occurring in the canine spleen: anatomic classification, immunohistochemistry, and mitotic activity correlated with patient survival. Vet Pathol 1994;31:37–47.
13. **Kakinuma C, Harada T, Watanabe M, Shibutani Y**. Spontaneous adrenal and hepatic myelolipomas in the common marmoset. Toxicol Pathol 1994;22(4):440–445.
14. **Tavassoli M**, ed. Handbook of the hemopoietic microenvironment. Clifton, NJ: Humana Press, 1989.
15. **Bessis M**. Living blood cells and their ultrastructure. New York: Springer-Verlag, 1973;87.
16. **Koller MR, Manchel I, Palsson BO**. Importance of parenchymal:stromal cell ratio for the ex vivo reconstitution of human hematopoiesis. Stem Cells 1997;15(4):305–313.
17. **Prockop DJ**. Marrow stromal cells as stem cells for nonhematopoietic tissues. Science 1997;276:71–74.
18. **Garlanda C, Dejana E**. Heterogeneity of endothelial cells. Specific markers. Arterioscler Thromb Vasc Biol 1997;17(7):1193–1202.
19. **Weiss LP**. The structure of hematopoietic tissues. In: Handin RI, Lus SE, Stossel TP, eds. Blood: principles & practice of hematology. Philadelphia: JB Lippincott, 1995;155–169.
20. **Weiss L**. The histophysiology of bone marrow. Clin Orthop 1967;52:13–23.
21. **Weiss L**. The structure of bone marrow: functional interrelationships of vascular hematopoietic compartments in experimental hemolytic anemia. J Morphol 1965;117:127.
22. **Brookoff D, Weiss L**. Adipocyte development and the loss of erythropoietic capacity in the bone marrow of mice after sustained transfusion. Blood 1982;60:1337–1343.
23. **De Bruyn PPH, Breen PC, Thomas TB**. The microcirculation of the bone marrow. Anat Rec 1970;168;55–65.
24. **Lord BI, Testa NG, Hendry JH**. The relative spatial distributions of CFUs and CFUc in the normal mouse femur. Blood 1975;46:65–72.
25. **Lambertsen RH, Weiss L**. A model of intramedullary hematopoietic microenvironments based on stereologic study of the distribution of endocloned marrow colonies. Blood 1984;63:287–297.
26. **Taichman RS, Reilly MJ, Emerson SG**. Human osteoblasts support human hematopoietic progenitor cells in vitro bone marrow cultures. Blood 1996;87:518–524.
27. **Muller-Sieburg CE, Deryugina E**. The stromal cells' guide to the stem cell universe. Stem Cells 1995;13:477–486.
28. **Aiuti A, Friedrich C, Sieff CA, Gutierrez-Ramos JC**. Identification of distinct elements of the stromal microenvironment that control human hematopoietic stem/progenitor cell growth and differentiation. Exp Hematol 1998;26:143–157.
29. **Issaad C, Croisille L, Katz A, Vainchenker W, Coulombel L**. A murine stromal cell line allows the proliferation of very primitive human CD34++/CD38– progenitor cells in long-term cultures and semisolid assays. Blood 1993;81:2916–2924.
30. **Gimble JM, Robinson CE, Wu X, Kelly KA**. The function of adipocytes in the bone marrow stroma: an update. Bone 1996;19:421–428.
31. **Bathija A, Davis S, Trubowitz S**. Bone marrow adipose tissue: response to acute starvation. Am J Hematol 1979;6:191–198.
32. **Greenberger JS**. Sensitivity of corticosteroid-dependent insulin-resistant lipogenesis in marrow preadipocytes of obese-diabetic (db/db) mice. Nature 1978;275(5682):752–754.
33. **Weigle DS**. Leptin and other secretory products of adipocytes modulate multiple physiological functions. Ann Endocrinol 1997;58:132–136.
34. **Verfaillie CM, McCarthy JB, McGlave PB**. Differentiation of primitive human multipotent hematopoietic progenitors into single lineage clonogenic progenitors is accompanied by alterations in their interaction with fibronectin. J Exp Med 1991;174:693–703.

CHAPTER 14

Ontogeny of the Hemopoietic System

• BRANDON P. REINES

Ontogeny refers to development of an individual animal. Such development occurs only once for each organism and proceeds inexorably from zygote formation to old age. In contrast, the hemopoietic system can be completely destroyed and reconstituted repeatedly by transplantation of blood cell progenitors.[1] This is because the hemopoietic system derives from stem cells that exhibit the free-living property of independence.[2-4] Blood stem cells are uniquely capable of adapting to and evolving in a completely foreign host. Conceptually, the hemopoietic system results in a dynamic phylogeny of blood-cell populations. This successful means of continual cell production involves certain predictable embryologic and postnatal events in hemopoietic development. An understanding of the significance of such events is facilitated by analysis of the evolutionary history of the hemopoietic systems of higher vertebrates.

EVOLUTION OF THE VERTEBRATE HEMOPOIETIC SYSTEM

Molded largely by the shift from aquatic to terrestrial life, the immunohemopoietic system of adult higher vertebrates exhibits an anatomic dichotomy: localized production sites in the marrow with body-wide dissemination of all blood cells, including immune-competent cells.[5] This anatomic arrangement seems to have been driven by intense selection pressure to protect and nourish blood-cell progenitors,[6] while simultaneously assuring the widest possible dispersal of cells capable of transporting oxygen and orchestrating immunologic functions in terrestrial animals of increasingly large size. The somewhat benign and stable aquatic environment allows fish to conduct hemopoiesis in a moderately unprotected parenchymatous organ such as the spleen. This site of production is sufficient to ensure survival of progenitors and to produce immune-competent cells against antigens in ingested food. The ocean serves to filter or dilute many potentially-hazardous agents including viruses, bacteria, waste products, cosmic X-rays and ultraviolet radiation from the sun.

With the shift to land dwelling, however, such environmental hazards selected for new, more protected, tissue and organ systems, including a lymphohemopoietic system capable of replacing much of the homeostatic stability originally supplied by the sea. In land animals, splenic hemopoiesis was no longer sufficient and the bone marrow became the primary production site with secondary lymphoid organs, including thymus and lymph nodes that assure maturation and dissemination of immune-competent cells. In a series of reviews, Manning[7-9] outlines six principal changes in vertebrate hemopoiesis selected by land dwelling. Particularly intriguing is his notion that stem cells hidden behind radiation-shielding bone in the marrow protects them from mutagenic and aging effects of radiation. There is abundant epidemiologic evidence consistent with Manning's hypothesis: lymphatic leukemias are rarely induced by radiation, whereas bone-marrow-derived (myeloid) leukemias are highly radiogenic at most doses.[10,11] In addition, the evolutionary origins of the various blood cells types has become clearer in recent years. Macrophages are thought most primitive and may have evolved into natural killer (NK) cells to extrathymic T cells to thymus-derived T cells and perhaps B cells.[12-14] Largely non-MHC-restricted cytotoxicity by macrophages and NK cells is most prevalent in fish and amphibians. In terrestrial animals, nonspecific immunity is supplemented by MHC-restricted or adaptive antimicrobial immunity by B cells and thymus-derived T cells in birds and mammals. The purported advantage of the adaptive immune system is to distinguish self from non-self.

PROGENITOR MOBILIZATION AND HOMING IN EMBRYONIC, FETAL, AND ADULT LIFE

Stem-Cell Ontogeny and Movements Among Anatomic Sites in Embryo and Fetus

During prenatal development of birds and mammals, hemopoietic stem cells (HSC) move from blood islands

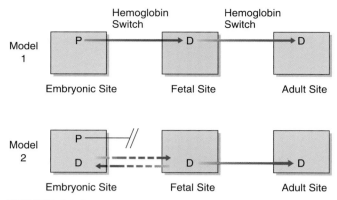

FIGURE 14.1 The mysterious changes in site of blood-forming HSCs from embryo to fetal liver to fetal bone marrow have been explained differently. Two main theories or models now dominate discussion. Adherents of Model I contend that HSCs in yolk sac produce primitive-type erythrocytes and then those same HSCs move to fetal liver and bone marrow where they produce mature definitive erythrocytes. Adherents of Model II postulate that HSCs in the yolk sac produce primitive-type erythrocytes and then die by apoptosis; then, a distinct population of HSCs in the embryo (possibly in the aorta-gonad-mesonephros region), which already has the capacity to produce mature definitive-type RBCs, travels to fetal liver and then bone marrow. P, HSCs producing primitive-type erythrocytes; D, HSCs producing mature definitive-type erythrocytes.

in the yolk sac to organs within the embryo and fetus. The mechanisms involved, however, are much debated (Fig. 14.1). At issue are

1. Do HSCs producing primitive-type red blood cells (RBCs) in the yolk sac move to internal organs and produce fetal or adult definitive erythrocytes or do the yolk-sac HSCs undergo apoptosis and a new population of HSC arise?[15]
2. Is the apparently distinct population of HSCs recently uncovered in the aorta-gonad-mesonephros (AGM) region of the avian and the mammalian embryo the actual source of HSCs seeding the marrow in birds and liver and then marrow in mammals?[16]
3. Is there only one source population of HSCs that begins in the yolk sac and disseminates to internal organs, or is the new organic microenvironment or genetic programming more important in the ability of HSCs to produce definitive fetal or adult erythrocytes?
4. Do HSCs age in the sense that they pass through ontogenetic stages, losing certain capacities and gaining others irreversibly?

Despite such ambiguities, it is nonetheless clear that most HSCs and erythyrocytes do change both prenatally and postnatally in many ways that reflect the demands of intrauterine and extrauterine life. In mammals, the primitive yolk-sac HSCs and RBCs are more easily distinguished from fetal or adult definitive-type HSCs and RBCs.[6] Embryonic HSCs are constantly dividing during development and rarely pause long enough to differentiate; fetal and adult HSCs are usually in G_0 and rarely

cycle. Challenging the view that HSCs do not age, Lansdorp[17] has shown that human HSCs not only lose the ability to produce fetal globins but undergo progressive reduction in telomere length and proliferative potential. Such changes are not, however, absolute as a low level of fetal globin production continues throughout life[18] and may increase under hemopoietic stress (e.g., anemia).

With regard to erythrocyte ontogeny, primitive RBCs are nucleated, formed intravascularly in the yolk sac, erythropoietin-insensitive, produce embryonic hemoglobin (Hgb), differentiate in a cohort, and are expelled to the circulation almost synchronously. In addition, primitive RBCs have a shorter life span and are macrocytic. At approximately 10 days postcoitus in mice and 6 weeks in humans, the blood islands begin to regress and the liver becomes the main site of hemopoiesis. Whereas still predominantly erythropoietic, the liver HSCs produce definitive-type RBCs that secrete fetal globin chains in humans. In mice, the shift to fetal liver hemopoiesis is accompanied by a change from fetal globins (EI, EII, EIII) to adult ($\alpha2\alpha2$) globins.[44] In humans, by the end of the first trimester, the major Hgb produced in fetal RBCs is Hgb F. Such definitive RBCs are smaller; erythropoietin-sensitive; express i surface antigen and low levels of carbonic anhydrase, formed extravascularly; and have a nuclear structure that more closely resembles normoblasts of adult bone marrow.[45] After birth, hemopoiesis increasingly occurs principally in the warm, thick flat bones of the skull, pelvis, and sternum. In later life, if demand for blood cells is sufficiently great, hemopoiesis may again occur in the long bones and viscera. In most animals, including humans, erythropoietic activity declines rapidly at birth, leading to a physiologic Hgb nadir that is coincident with a gradual shift in the oxygen dissociation curve. This shift results both from gradual replacement of fetal Hgb with adult Hgb and from increased RBC 2,3-DPG; the ease of release of O2 from adult RBCs may be related to the low Hb concentration and need for rapid oxygenation of tissues postnatally.

Mechanisms of Mobilization and Homing of Hemopoietic Stem Cells

Although the mechanisms accounting for the sudden movement of HSC en masse from one site to another remain obscure, the pattern yolk sac or AGM to liver or spleen to bone marrow is at least temporally related to the concomitant embryologic development of these anatomic sites in mammals. HSC cannot home from AGM to liver until it is formed, and it cannot home to bone marrow until bone formation is nearly complete. However, the rapidity and specificity of HSC dissemination to the liver, spleen, and then bone marrow has remained enigmatic until recently. It is increasingly clear that HSCs leave the liver both because its environment becomes somewhat stressful for the HSCs and because they actively home to the more hospitable marrow. Fukumoto's[19] immunocytochemical, ultrastructural, and histologic analyses of the ontogeny of fetal rat hepatocyte–HSC interaction have suggested that the HSCs leave the liver after day 19 because its microenvironment ceases to be conducive to hemopoiesis (Fig. 14.2). Specifically, fetal hepatocytes undergo morphologic changes near day 19 such that they lose their ability to foster hemopoiesis. Before day 19, when the liver is composed of loosely associated, rounded hepatocytes and HSCs, hemopoiesis is intense. Fetal hepatocytes are characterized by a surface antigen designated UB-12 and are more highly proliferative than adult hepatocytes; UB-12 may be involved in adhesion or communication

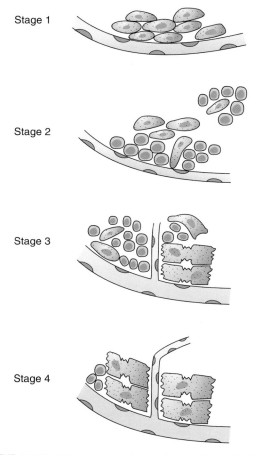

Stage 1

Stage 2

Stage 3

Stage 4

FIGURE 14.2 Schematic drawing of changes in rat fetal liver cells (hepatocytes) relative to numbers of infiltrating blood-forming cells during early (0 to 12 days), mid (13 to 18 days), and late (19 to 20) gestation. During early gestation (Stage 1), hepatocytes are morphologically and functionally immature as depicted by their oblong shape and somewhat loose association; blood-forming cells are confined to embryonic sites during early gestation. In mid gestation, however, blood-forming cells multiply and produce blood cells among the loosely associated immature hepatocytes (Stages 2 and 3). Once the hepatocytes mature in late gestation (Stage 4) and become somewhat polarized and tightly conjoined, blood-forming cells leave the liver and travel to the bone marrow. That abrupt movement from liver to marrow may be partly caused by loss of the more conducive microenvironment provided by immature hepatocytes and a squeezing out of blood-forming cells by more rigid adult-type hepatocytes.

between fetal hepatocytes and HSCs. Adult hepatocytes, in contrast, lack an ability for autocrine cell growth, are rectangular and polarized, with each face expressing distinctive membrane antigens. Most important, from the standpoint of hemopoietic microenvironment, adult hepatocytes are tightly bound together and have junctional complexes for intercellular communication. Such rigid intercellular geometry prevents effective HSC–hepatocyte cohabitation and communication. Fukumoto[19] postulates that fetal hepatocytes may function as stromal cells for HSC growth (and differentiation) and that HSC–hepatocyte interaction may be necessary to stimulate the stromal function of fetal hepatocyes. Like fetal hepatocytes, macrophagelike cells play a role in fostering erythroblast differentiation into RBCs in the erythroblastic islets of bone marrow.[20,21] Fukumoto's[19] findings indirectly corroborate Bessis'[20] hypothesis and suggest that loose association between hemopoietic progenitor cells and other cells that function as nurse stromal cells are necessary for maintenance of normal hemopoiesis. In attempting to explain reasons for the shift from liver to bone marrow, Fukumoto[19] contends that HSCs do not so much home to bone marrow, but are effectively exiled from the hepatic parenchyma. Free in the circulation, once bone marrow has been formed near day 18, HSCs are essentially trapped in it by adhesion molecules. As bone marrow HSCs provide more and more blood cells to the circulation, demand for such cells from the liver may be lowered by a lessening of feedback inhibition; as fewer and fewer HSCs remain in the liver to stimulate hepatocyte stromal function, hemopoiesis rapidly declines in the liver and bone marrow hemopoiesis gradually takes over. Fukumoto[19] contends that the intrauterine shift from one focus of hemopoiesis to another can be explained in this way. Fukumoto's[19] model suggests that gestational length is not the only variable that influences the spatiotemporal pattern of intrauterine hemopoiesis in different species. In the cat, for instance, in which intraembryonic liver hemopoiesis is unusually prolonged, it may be that hepatocytes remain in a fetal state longer than in other species.[22] However, the mature liver parenchyma is not so hostile to HSCs that they will not home to liver during periods of severe marrow stress in adult life (e.g., aplasia or leukemia). There is some evidence that small populations of HSCs may be present in adult liver of certain individuals.[23] This suggests that, intraembryonically, HSCs are not simply squeezed out by maturing hepatocyes, as Fukumoto's[19] model implies. Near day 19, HSCs somehow discover that the maturing liver provides less sure stromal support than the developing bone marrow stroma and travel to it en masse.

How HSCs mobilize from liver and home to bone marrow is enigmatic as is mobilization or homing of HSCs during adulthood. Most research on these topics has focused at the molecular level and answers have been sought in identification of adhesion molecules or chemoattractants. Tavossoli and Hardy[24] have identified a lectin on the surface of HSCs that binds to a glycoconjugate on the surface of stromal cells in a long-term culture. This homing protein is believed to mediate

T-Cell selection in normal thymus

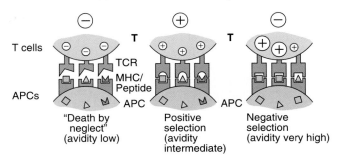

FIGURE 14.3 How pre-T-cells from bone marrow are educated in the thymus gland during development is much debated. It is currently suggested that selection of pre-T-cells for elimination (negative selection) or maturation to T cells (positive selection) depends on the strength of the intracellular signal within pre-T-cells induced by a binding between pre-T-cell TCRs and a given self-antigen/MHC complex. In this model, pre-T-cells experiencing the strongest signals undergo negative selection (clonal deletion), whereas those having intermediate-strength signals are positively selected; pre-T-cells with weak intracellular signals from surface TCR interactions with self-antigen/MHC complexes succumb to apoptosis.

initial recognition between HSCs and stromal cells in the bone marrow. Zanjani et al[25] undertook in utero transplantation of allogeneic or xenogeneic HSC into sheep fetuses and found that HSCs preferentially migrate to bone marrow once it is formed. Similarly, Blair and Thomas[26] have shown that fetal liver HSCs do adhere selectively to bone marrow stroma in long-term cultures. These studies do not seem to address the issue of homing per se so much as adhesion of HSCs to marrow once the HSCs are close enough for binding to occur. Continued analysis of adhesion molecules and other receptor-ligand-type interactions may not clarify homing per se. The binding of HSC ligand by a bone marrow stromal cell receptor would seem to be the final event in a long journey governed by both biophysical and cellular processes.[27,28]

Insights into homing may arise from investigations into the role of chemoattractants for HSCs. For instance, Kim and Broxmeyer[29] recently studied the migratory behavior of HSCs in a two-chamber in vitro system in response to various chemoattractants. They found that stromal-cell-derived factor-1, Steel factor, and plasma from bone marrow aspirates may cooperatively act to induce homing to marrow. Current theory suggests that HSCs may somehow follow a concentration gradient of chemoattractants to the bone marrow. In situations of marrow stress (e.g., myeloablation prior to marrow transplant), stromal cells might produce high concentrations of chemoattractants to mobilize any HSC from peripheral blood. It remains to be seen whether chemoattracts might affect cytoskeletal reorganization and cell movement through receptor-ligand-type interactions. A wide variety of growth factors and toxic chemotherapeutic agents have been shown to mobilize HSCs from peripheral blood to marrow or vice versa.

Aguila et al.[30] contend that embryonic or fetal movements of HSC are mediated by changes in adhesive properties of HSCs and explain adult mobilization as being stress-induced changes in HSC adhesive properties. They suggest that pancytopenia and cytokines may induce such changes in adhesive properties, implying that both cytokines and chemotherapeutic agents are perceived by the HSCs as stressful. Further evidence for the view that HSC mobilizing agents cause HSC movement en masse through a stress mechanism is the recent observation by Eddleman et al[31] that intravascular transfusion of fetuses triggered a massive release of HSC from the marrow. This suggests that marrow HSC could somehow sense that HSC concentration in the peripheral blood had been decreased by transfusion. How various stressors might induce changes in stem cells such that their adhesivity is changed is unclear. Though mechanisms of homing or mobilization remain unclear, homing of T-cell progenitors to the fetal thymus is among the signal events in the ontogeny of the lymphohemopoietic system.

T-CELL ONTOGENY IN THYMIC AND EXTRATHYMIC SITES

Intrathymic Education of αβ T Cells

Lymphocyte progenitors clearly home to the fetal thymus in successive waves during gestation in mammals. In humans, the first wave of pre-T-cells enters the thymic rudiment at approximately 7 weeks of gestation. However, the precise effects of the thymic microenvironment on pre-T-cell ontogeny are still debated. Accumulating knowledge about the molecular structure of the T-cell receptor (TCR) complexes on the T-cell surface and their interactions with various ligands in the thymus in various species has not resolved the controversy. The complex multimeric structure of the TCR seems to have evolved to provide the flexibility necessary to mediate both early intrathymic selection events and later interactions of mature T cells with antigen.[32] In spite of the early interest in negative selection or clonal deletion of self-reactive thymocytes, however, recent TCR studies highlight the significance of the opposite process: positive selection of thymocytes bearing pre-TCRs that recognize antigen in the context of self-MHC.[33,34]

Nonetheless, current theory suggests that positive and negative thymic selection of pre-T-cells depends principally on the strength of the intracellular signal induced by binding between pre-T-cell TCRs and a given self-antigen or MHC complex[35] (Fig. 14.3). In this model, pre-T-cells experiencing the strongest signals undergo negative selection (clonal deletion), whereas those having intermediate-strength signals are positively selected; pre-T-cells with weak intracellular signals from surface TCR interactions with self-antigen or MHC complexes succumb to apoptosis (Fig. 14.3). This simple model is increasingly complicated, however, by a growing list of factors that may affect the strength of the intracellular signal created by TCR–self-antigen–MHC

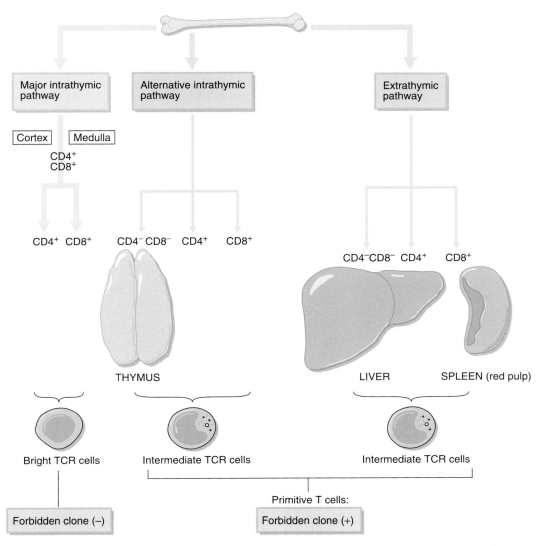

FIGURE 14.4 The persistence of T cells that are capable of reacting with self-cells during adulthood is increasingly recognized. T cells bearing TCRs composed of $\gamma\delta$ subunits are self-reactive, increase in numbers during adulthood, but develop in intestinal rather than thymic epithelium; self-reactive $\gamma\delta$ T cells would not, therefore, be expected to be eliminated. On the other hand, $\alpha\beta$ T cells do undergo thymic education, and the finding of self-reactive $\alpha\beta$ T cells has been difficult to explain. Abo, Watanabe, Sato et al[14] postulate that such $\alpha\beta$ T cells survive thymic education because they encounter thymic epithelial cells that do not prominently display certain major histocompatibility complex antigens (alternate pathway) and so are not clearly marked as self-cells. Self-reactive $\alpha\beta$ T cells are referred to as forbidden clones because they had once been thought to be completely eliminated during thymic education. Their occurrence had been thought to cause pathologic autoimmunity.

coupling. Modulating factors identified in recent studies include the number of TCRs on the cell surface, the avidity or efficacy of binding, the agonist versus antagonist effects of various self-ligands, the nature of the various self-peptides, and the density of peptide-MHC complexes presented. Williams et al.[34] contend that a given thymocyte's TCRs may bind many different self-peptides in the thymus with varying agonist or antagonist properties; the summation of the effects of those antigens determines whether a pre-T-cell is positively or negatively affected. Hence, many self-reacting T-cell clones may be positively selected. An emerging theme from such investigations is that mature $\alpha\beta$ T cells retain

a surprising degree of self-reactivity.[34] In view of such findings, some authors question whether thymic education functions principally to teach T cells how to distinguish self from nonself.[36,37]

Extrathymic T Cells in Neonatal and Adult Life

In many model systems, the most strongly self-reactive T-cell clones are nonetheless usually eliminated during fetal ontogeny.[38] Attempting to explain why certain strongly self-reactive $\alpha\beta$ T cells may survive thymic

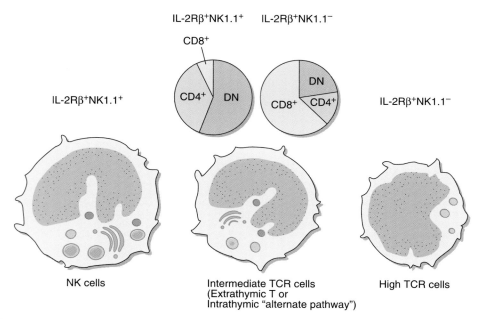

FIGURE 14.5 We now know that there is a spectrum of T cell and T-cell-like cells with different functions in the animal body, many of which are self-reactive under physiologic conditions. These cells may be distinguished by the density of TCRs on the cell surface. NK cells are large T-cell-like cells that lack TCRs but have abundant cytoplasmic granules and organelles that function in surveillance against leukemias, lymphomas, and perhaps other tumors. Alternate-thymic-pathway-derived $\alpha\beta$ T cells as well as $\gamma\delta$ T cells increase in number during adulthood and display an intermediate density of TCRs on their surface; such T cells may be involved in autoimmune surveillance and may attack self-cells that are stressed or are transforming into cancer cells. T cells with a high density of TCRs on their surface are most likely the product of thymic eduation of marrow-derived pre-T-cells that are positively selected because of intermediate-binding affinity with the self-antigen / MHC complex.

education, Abo et al[39] postulate the existence of an alternative pathway of pre-T-cell interactions with self-antigens that do not prominently display class II MHC antigens (Fig. 14.4). They further contend that such primitive T cells are phenotypically indistinguishable from extrathymic $\gamma\delta$ T cells in gut epithelium (Fig. 14.5). After birth, in parallel with thymic involution, $\gamma\delta$ T cells increase in number in the intestine. In aging individuals, $\gamma\delta$ T cells are often the predominant T-cell-type infiltrating target tissues in malignancy, intracellular infections and, autoimmune diseases.[39] Abo et al[39] argue that such extrathymic T cells and intrathymic T cells generated by the alternative pathway may function to conduct surveillance of abnormal self-cells that increasingly arise during the aging process. An implication of their model is that target tissue cells in organ-specific autoimmune diseases may be pathologic and the immune response physiologic and appropriate. In the author's view, some autoimmune disease may actually constitute chronic hypersensitivity syndromes due to unusually strong antineoplastic immunity in individuals predisposed to tumor formation (B. R., unpublished data, 1998). The fact that target cells in many autoimmune diseases have neoplastic features, including atypia and clonality in aplastic anemia,[40] insulinomalike cells in type I diabetic pancreas,[41] and invasive synoviocytes in rheumatoid arthritis,[42] is consistent with this idea. Immunosuppression of both aplastic anemia and autoimmune liver disease does convert certain patients to overt malignancy of

target cells.[40,43] Hence, hemopoietic cells continue to undergo extensive intraspecific evolution in the blood ocean of the vertebrate body.

REFERENCES

1. **Storek J, Ferrara S, Ku N, Georgi JV, Champlin RE, Saxon A.** B cell reconstitution after human bone marrow transplantation:recapitulation of ontogeny? Bone Marrow Trans 1993;2:387–398.
2. **Till J, McCulloch E.** Hemopoietic stem cell differentiation. Biochem Biophys Acta 1980;605:431–459, 1980.
3. **Margulis L.** Origins of species: acquired genomes and individuality. Biosystems 1993;31(2–3):121–125.
4. **Hochman A.** Programmed cell death in prokaryotes. Crit Rev Microbiol 1997;23(3):207–214.
5. **Jonsson V.** Comparison and definition of spleen and lymph node: a phylogenetic analysis. J Theor Biol 1985;117:691–699.
6. **Tavassoli M.** Embryonic and fetal hemopoiesis: an overview. Blood Cells 1991;1:269–281.
7. **Manning MJ.** The phylogeny of thymic dependence. Amer Zool 1975; 15:63–71.
8. **Manning MJ.** The evolution of the vertebrate immune system. J R Soc Med 1979;72:683–688.
9. **Manning MJ.** The evolution of vertebrate lymphoid organs. In: Solomon JB, ed. Aspects of developmental and comparative immunology. Oxford, England: Pergamon Press, 1980.
10. **Bertell R.** X-ray exposure and premature aging. J Surg Oncol 1977;9(4): 379–391.
11. **Andersson M, Storm H, Mouridsen H.** Incidence of new primary cancers after adjuvant tamoxifen therapy and radiotherapy for early breast cancer. J Natl Cancer Inst 1991;83(14):1013–1017.
12. **Millar D, Ratcliffe N.** The evolution of blood cells: facts and enigmas. Endeavour 1989;13(2):72–77.
13. **Rast JP, Litman GW.** T-cell receptor gene homologs are present in the most primitive jawed vertebrates. Proc Natl Acad Sci USA 1994;91(20):9248–9252.
14. **Abo T, Watanabe H, Sato K et al.** Extrathymic T cells stand at an intermediate phylogenetic position between natural killer cells and thymus-derived T cells. Nat Immun 1995;14(4):173–187.

15. **Zon L.** Developmental biology of hematopoiesis. Blood 1995;86(8):2876–2891.
16. **Dieterlen-Lievre F, Godin I, Pardanaud L, et al.** Sites of hemopoietic stem cell production in early embryogenesis. In: Gluckman E, Coulombel L, eds. Ontogeny of hematopoiesis: aplastic anemia (Colloque INSERM). France: John Libbey Eurotext Ltd, 1995;235:5–11.
17. **Lansdorp P.** Developmental changes in the function of hematopoietic stem cells. Exp Hematol 1995;23:187–191.
18. **Huehna E, Beaven G.** Developmental changes in human hemoblogins. Clin Dev Med 1971;37:175.
19. **Fukumoto T.** Possible developmental interactions of hematopoietic cells and hepatocytes in fetal rat liver. Biomed Res 1992;13(6):385–413.
20. **Bessis M.** L'Ilot erythroblastique. Unite fonctionelle de la moelle osseuse. Rev Hematol 1958;13:8–11.
21. **Mohandas N.** Cell–cell interactions and erythropoiesis. Blood Cells 1991;17:59–64.
22. **Tiedemann K, van Ooyen B.** Prenatal hematopoiesis and blood characteristics of the cat. Anat Embryol 1978;153:243–267.
23. **Taniguchi H, Toyoshima T, Fukao K, Nakauchi H.** Presence of hematopoietic stem cells in the adult liver. Nature Med 1996;2(2):198–201.
24. **Tavassoli M, Hardy CL.** Molecular basis of homing of intravenously transplanted stem cells to the marrow. Blood 1990;76:1059–1070.
25. **Zanjani E, Ascensao J, Tavassoli M.** Liver-derived fetal hematopoietic stem cells selectively and preferentially home to the fetal bone marrow. Blood 1993;81(2):399–404.
26. **Blair A, Thomas DB.** Preferential adhesion of fetal liver derived primitive haemopoietic progenitor cells to bone marrow stroma. Br J Haematol 1997;99(4):726–731.
27. **Graner F.** Can surface adhesion drive cell-rearrangement? Part I: Biological cell sorting. J Theor Biol 1993;164:455–476.
28. **Graner F, Sawada Y.** Can surface adhesion drive cell rearrangement? Part II: A geometrical model. J Theor Biol 1993;164:477–506.
29. **Kim C, Broxmeyer HE.** In vitro behavior of hematopoietic progenitor cells under the influence of chemoattractants:stromal cell-derived factor-1, steel factor, and the bone marrow environment. Blood 1998;91(1):100–110.
30. **Aguila H, Akashi K, Domen J, et al.** From stem cells to lymphocytes: biology and transplantation. Immunol Rev 1997;157:13–40.
31. **Eddleman K, Chervenak F, George-Siegel P, et al.** Circulating hematopietic stem cell populations in human fetuses: implications for fetal gene therapy and alterations with in utero red cell transfusion. Fetal Diagn Ther 1996;11:231–240.
32. **Shores E, Love P.** TCR z chain in T cell development and selection. Curr Opin Immunol 1997;9:380–389.
33. **Spits H, Touraine J, Yssel H, et al.** Presence of host-reactive and MHC-restricted T cells in a transplanted severe combined immunodeficient (SCID) patient suggest positive selection and absence of clonal deletion. Immunol Rev 1990;116:101–116.
34. **Williams O, Tanaka Y, Tarazona R, Kioussis D.** The agonist-antagonist balance in positive selection. Immunol Today 1997;18(3):121–126.
35. **Muller-Hermelink HK, Wilisch A, Schultz A, Marx A.** Characterization of the human thymic microenvironment: lymphoepithelial interaction in normal thymus and thymoma. Arch Histol Cytol 1997;60(1):9–28.
37. **Silverstein AM, Rose NR.** On the mystique of the immunological self. Immunol Rev 1997;159:197–206.
38. **Spits H, Lanier L, Phillips J.** Development of human T and natural killer cells. Blood 1995;85(10):2654–2670.
40. **Young NS.** The problem of clonality in aplastic anemia: Dr. Dameshek's riddle revisited. Blood 1992;79(6):1385–1392.
41. **Gepts W.** Islet cell survival determined by morphology: an immunocytochemical study of the islets of langerhans in juvenile diabetes mellitus. Diabetes 1978;27 (Supplement 1):251–266.
42. **Harris E.** Rheumatoid arthritis: pathophysiology and implications for therapy. New Engl J Med 1990;322(18):1277–1288.
43. **Imai H, Nakano Y, Kiyosawa K, Tan E.** Increasing titers and changing specificities of antinuclear antibodies in patients with chronic liver disease who develop hepatocellular carcinoma. Cancer 1993;71:26–35.
44. **Tavian M, Charbord P, Humeau L, et al.** Embryonic and early fetal development of the human hematopoietic system in the yolk sac, dorsal aorta, liver and bone marrow. In: Gluckman E, Coulombel L, eds. Ontogeny of hematopoiesis: aplastic anemia (Colloque INSERM). France: John Libbey Eurotext Ltd, 1995;235:37–42.
45. **Kelemen E, Calvo W.** Prenatal hematopoiesis in human bone marrow and its developmental antecedents. In: Trubowitz S, Davis S, eds. The human bone marrow: anatomy, physiology and pathophysiology. Boca Raton, FL: CRC Press, 1982;1:3–41.

CHAPTER 15

Cytokine Regulation of Hemopoiesis

• GREGG A. DEAN

Regulation of hemopoiesis by soluble factors is not a recent concept. In 1906 two French scientists, Carnot and Deflandre, observed that serum transfused from anemic rabbits into normal rabbits resulted in an increase in hematocrit. They concluded that a soluble factor was present that induced the production of red blood cells. From this initial observation, it was not until 1948 that erythropoietin (EPO) was identified. Today several soluble factors that directly influence hematopoiesis have been identified. After a decades-long search, thrombopoietin (TPO) was cloned in 1994 as the EPO homologue for thrombopoiesis. Stem-cell factor [(SCF), also called Steel factor and c-kit ligand] was identified in 1990 and was an important breakthrough in the study and therapeutic manipulation of pluripotent stem cells. Several colony-stimulating factors (CSF), including granulocyte-macrophage-CSF (GM-CSF), granulocyte-CSF (G-CSF), and macrophage-CSF (M-CSF) have been exploited clinically for their ability to stimulate lineage-committed stem cells. The above-mentioned cytokines exert their effects on a narrow target cell range (hemopoietic precursors) and are discussed in more detail in other chapters on stem cell biology, erythropoiesis, thrombopoiesis, and clinical applications of cytokines. In this chapter, the interleukins (IL), interferons (IFN), tumor necrosis factors (TNF), tumor growth factor-β (TGF-β), chemokines, and neurokinins are discussed. These cytokines, in general, have pleiotropic effects on numerous cell types, but are discussed only with respect to their role in hemopoiesis.

There are several mechanisms by which cytokines have been shown to influence hemopoiesis (Fig. 15.1). First, quiescent primitive cells may be induced to begin cycling. Second, cell cycle time of actively dividing progenitor cells may be increased or decreased. Third, transit time, that is the time needed for a cell to enter and leave a defined compartment, may be affected by cytokines. Fourth, preventing or inducing apoptosis is an important means of regulation by cytokines. Fifth and last, some cytokines are known to influence the migration of medullary hemopoietic progenitors to extramedullary sites.

Studying and understanding the role of soluble factors in hemopoiesis has been difficult because of the fundamental characteristics of individual cytokines and the cytokine network. These fundamental characteristics are synergy, pleiotropy, and redundancy.[1] Synergy occurs when two cytokines simultaneously act on different parameters. Pleiotropy is the ability of a cytokine to affect more than one parameter. Redundancy is the ability of multiple cytokines to affect the same parameter and is prevalent in the cytokine network.

Our knowledge of the role cytokines play in hemopoiesis comes predominantly from studies of the human and murine systems. It is these two species for which cytokine sequences and chromosomal locations have been determined and for which recombinant cytokines are readily available. Furthermore, in vitro techniques to sort and culture hemopoietic progenitors have been well developed for mice and humans. Therefore, the discussion of each cytokine that follows is drawn predominantly from studies of mice and humans. In vitro studies are most useful to determine the effect of cytokines individually or in combination on mixed hemopoietic cultures, purified hemopoietic progenitors, or bone marrow origin cell lines. In vivo data is derived from treatment with recombinant cytokines, treatment with anticytokine antibodies, or treatment with cytokine inhibitors. Transgenic mice that do not produce a specific cytokine, overproduce a cytokine, or do not express cellular receptors for a cytokine have also provided valuable data. Presented here is a summary of consensus data from this variety of experimental systems. This is a rapidly evolving field of study, and it is certain that our current understanding of cytokines and hemopoiesis is superficial.

INTERLEUKIN-1

IL-1 is perhaps the most pleiotropic cytokine and this is likely caused by stimulation of secondary cytokine production. It is known that IL-1 stimulates production of GM-CSF, G-CSF, M-CSF, and IL-3. A cofactor, termed haemopoietin-1, necessary for myeloid colony formation after toxic bone marrow insult was ultimately cloned and identified as IL-1a. It acts synergistically with GM-CSF, G-CSF, M-CSF, IL-3, and IL-6 to stimulate myelopoiesis at the committed stem cell level. IL-1 negatively effects erythropoiesis through suppression of ery-

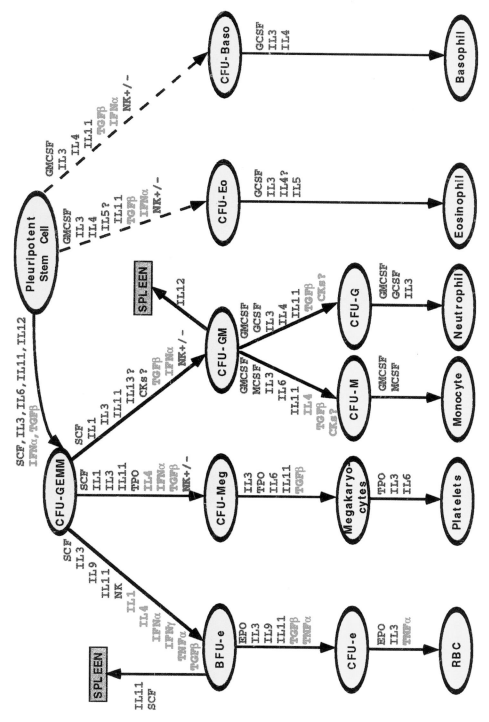

FIGURE 15.1 Cytokine regulation of hemopoiesis. Cytokines in green are stimulatory, whereas those in red are inhibitory. Cytokines in blue have either variable effects or different members of the cytokine group have different effects. CK = chemokines; NK = neurokinins. See text for other abbreviations.

throid precursors. It is clear that elevated blood levels of IL-1 contribute to poorly regenerative or nonregenerative anemia associated with chronic disease and inflammatory conditions.[2]

INTERLEUKIN-3

The target cell range of IL-3 includes every derivative from the hemopoietic pluripotent stem cell except lymphoid progenitors. IL-3 acts at multiple stages of differentiation to both inhibit cell death and induce proliferation. Particularly strong synergistic effects are observed with IL-3 and other cytokines, including CSF-1, G-CSF, GM-CSF, IL-1, IL-4, IL-5, IL-9, IL-10, and IL-11.[3,4] The apparent redundancy in IL-3 function is demonstrated by the normal hemopoietic development of IL-3 or IL-3-receptor knockout mice.[4] What then is the role or need for IL-3 in hemopoiesis? In vitro data show cells induced to proliferate under the influence of IL-3 are then IL-3 dependent. Thus, when IL-3 is withdrawn, the cells undergo apoptosis. This may be a useful function in times of crisis to induce hemopoiesis by upregulation of IL-3 expression until the crisis is resolved, after which the expanded proliferative pool is reduced in the IL-3 downregulated environment.

INTERLEUKIN-4

The pleiotropic effects of IL-4 have resulted in contradictory reports on this IL's modulation of myelopoiesis. Now it is clear that IL-4 acts synergistically with G-CSF to promote colony-forming unit-granulocyte (CFU-G) colonies while inhibiting CFU-macrophage (CFU-M).[5,6] The synergistic effects of IL-4 with G-CSF appears to be caused, at least in part, by IL-4-induced upregulation of G-CSF receptors and downregulation of M-CSF receptors.[7] Basophil and possibly eosinophil production are positively influenced by IL-4.[8] IL-4 is a negative regulator of erythropoiesis through the inhibition of GM-CSF production by mononuclear accessory cells.[9] Megakaryocytic colony formation is also inhibited by IL-4 in vitro.

INTERLEUKIN-5

In contrast to the broad effects of IL-4, the effects of IL-5 are focused on the eosinophil lineage. In vitro studies indicate IL-5 is active only at a late stage of differentiation.[10] However, transgenic mice that overexpress IL-5 show a profound and lifelong eosinophilia.[11] This suggests IL-5 is capable of inducing the full pathway of eosinophil production. The in vitro results indicate other cytokines may be involved in eosinophil generation, but the in vivo results indicate that if this is true, those cytokines must be constitutively expressed.

INTERLEUKIN-6

Pluripotent hemopoietic progenitors are stimulated to proliferate under the synergistic influence of IL-6 and IL-3.[12] IL-6 induces dormant progenitor cells to leave G_0 and enter the cell cycle, whereas IL-3 supports continued proliferation of the progenitors after they begin cycling .[13] IL-6 also synergizes with M-CSF to stimulate CFU-M.[14] The combination of IL-6 and IL-3 also induce maturation of megakaryocytes.[15] Megakaryocytes express IL-6 receptors, and transgenic mice overexpressing IL-6 have increased numbers of megakaryocytes.[16]

INTERLEUKIN-9

Initially, IL-9 was identified by its ability to stimulate mast cell differentiation from bone marrow hemopoietic progenitors.[17] This effect was determined to be a result of synergism with IL-3 and IL-4.[17,18] IL-9 seems to provide direct support of erythroid colony formation in combination with erythropoietin.[19] This effect is more profound on fetal progenitors compared with adult hematopoietic progenitors possibly because it is more stimulatory on less differentiated progenitors.

INTERLEUKIN-11

IL-11 acts synergistically with IL3, IL-4, IL-12, IL-13, SCF, and GM-CSF to stimulate various stages and lineages of hemopoietic progenitors. IL-11 stimulates proliferation of primitive stem cells and multipotential and committed progenitors cells by initiating cell cycling of quiescent G_0 populations.[20] In addition, IL-11 may shorten the cycling time of some cell types.[21] IL-11 can induce the commitment of primitive stem cells into the multilineage compartment and stimulate the differentiation of committed progenitors, depending on which other cytokines are also present. In combination with IL-3 and TPO or SCF, IL-11 stimulates megakaryocytopoiesis and thrombopoiesis.[22,23] This is also observed when exogenous IL-11 is administered to animals.[24] IL-11 alone or with IL-3, SCF, or EPO stimulates multiple stages of erythropoiesis.[24] This appears to be a direct effect of IL-11, as treatment with antibody against other cytokines does not abrogate this activity.[25] With SCF, IL-11 leads to a redistribution of erythroid cells from bone marrow to spleen.[26] IL-11 in combination with SCF, G-CSF, IL-13, and IL-4 modulates the differentiation and maturation of myeloid progenitors. Depending on the combination of cytokines, maturation can be skewed toward macrophage or granulocyte predominance.

INTERLEUKIN-12

IL-12 is a heterodimeric cytokine that is known primarily for its effects on growth and function of T cells and natural killer cells. However, IL-12 has been shown to synergize with SCF, IL-3, and IL-11 to stimulate the proliferation and differentiation of early hemopoietic progenitors in vitro.[27–29] In vivo, treatment of mice with IL-12 results in decreased CFU-GM in the bone marrow. In contrast, CFU-GM in the spleen increases.[30] Long-term therapy with IL-12 results in bone marrow depletion, splenic hyperplasia, and increased circulating progenitor cells. Thus, it appears IL-12 is important for hemopoietic mobilization and induction of extramedullary hemopoiesis.

INTERLEUKIN-13

IL-13 is clustered with IL-3, IL-4, IL-5, and GM-CSF on murine chromosome 11 and human chromosome 5. This suggests it is part of a cytokine family that most likely has arisen by gene duplication. IL-13 shares many of the same activities of IL-4, but its effects on hemopoiesis are not well characterized. IL-13 does seem to have stimulatory effects on myeloid progenitors.[31]

TYPE I INTERFERONS (INTERFERON-α AND INTERFERON-β)

Although used therapeutically for their antiviral, antitumor, and immunity-enhancing properties, Type I interferons produce leukopenia, an undesirable side effect caused by myelosuppression. IFN-α has been shown to inhibit production of GM-CSF, IL-3, IL-5, IL-6, and IL-11, thereby explaining the in vivo results.[32,33]

TUMOR NECROSIS FACTOR-α AND INTERFERON-γ

TNF-α and IFN-γ have been identified as negative regulators of hemopoiesis and as such play a role in the development of the anemia of chronic disease.[34] Administration of TNF-α results in a reduced hematocrit owing to suppressed hemopoiesis and increased red blood cell degradation.[35] It has been shown that TNF-α and IFN-γ can induce apoptosis in committed and uncommitted progenitors and that this may be mediated by nitric oxide (NO).[36,37]

TUMOR GROWTH FACTOR-β

The transforming growth factors (TGF-β1, TGF-β2, and TGF-β3) are growth-inhibitory cytokines with multiple actions. TGF-β has been shown to be a bifunctional regulator of hemopoietic progenitor growth. Whether TGF-β is stimulatory or inhibitory depends on the maturation stage of the target population and the existing cytokine milieu. It has been shown to be inhibitory to all precursors expressing CD34, which includes every hemopoietic lineage. More mature elements such as CFU-erythroid (CFU-E) that do not express CD34 appear to be unaffected by TGF-β. Interestingly, TGF-β production by stems cells may act in an autocrine manner to maintain these early stem cells in a quiescent state. There is some evidence that overproduction of TGF-β by megakaryocytes and platelets may promote myelofibrosis.[38]

CHEMOKINES

The chemokine family is a large group of more than 25 structurally related proteins. Within this group, the macrophage inhibitory proteins (MIP) 1 and 2 have been reported to have activity on hemopoietic precursor cells. Their activity is synergistic with GM-CSF and M-CSF to enhance CFU-GM formation.[39] MIP-1α is inhibitory to less differentiated stem cells and myeloid progenitors apparently because of decreased cycling rates induced by this chemokine.[40] Several other chemokines are also reported to have an inhibitory effect on immature myeloid progenitors, including MIP-2α, platelet factor 4, IL-8, and monocyte chemotactic protein-1.[41]

NEUROKININS

Innervation of the bone marrow provides close contact between nerve endings and hemopoietic cells. This allows bidirectional crosstalk in the neurohemopoietic axis that is mediated by cytokines. Neuropeptides are derived from neural and nonneural sources and may be transported in the circulation or released locally by nerve fibers. The neurokinins, neurokinin-A, neurokinin-B, and substance P (NK-A, NK-B, and SP, respectively) are structurally related peptides that are widely distributed and mediate a broad spectrum of biological responses. NK receptors are present on bone marrow stromal cells as well as CD34+ hemopoietic progenitors and stem cells. SP induces production of IL-1, IL-3, IL-6, GM-CSF, and SCF and as a result has potent stimulatory effects on myeloid and erythroid progenitors. NK-A is inhibitory on myeloid progenitors and is weakly stimulatory to erythroid progenitors. Part of the inhibitory activity of NK-A is mediated by its induction of TGF-β and MIP-1α.[42]

REFERENCES

1. **de Haan G, Dontje B, Nijhof W.** Concepts of hemopoietic cell amplification. Synergy, redundancy and pleiotropy of cytokines affecting the regulation of erythropoiesis. Leuk Lymphoma 1996;22:385–394.
2. **Dinarello CA.** Interleukin-1. In: Thomson AW, ed. The cytokine handbook. London: Academic Press Limited, 1994;31–56.
3. **Schrader JW.** Interleukin-3. In: Thomson AW, ed. The cytokine handbook. London: Academic Press Limited, 1994;81–98.
4. **Nishinakamura R, Mijajima A, Mee PJ, Tybulewicz VL, Murray R.** Hematopoiesis in mice lacking the entire granulocyte-macrophage colony-stimulating factor/interleukin-3/interleukin-5 functions. Blood 1996;88:2458–2464.
5. **Sonoda Y, Okuda T, Yokota S, Maekawa T, Shizumi Y, Nishigaki H, Misawa S, Fujii H, Abe T.** Actions of human interleukin-4/B-cell stimulatory factor-1 on proliferation and differentiation of enriched hematopoietic progenitor cells in culture. Blood 1990;75:1615–1621.
6. **Snoeck HW, Lardon F, Van BD, Peetermans ME.** Effects of interleukin-4 on myelopoiesis: localization of the action of IL-4 in the CD34+HLA-DR+

subset and distinction between direct and indirect effects of IL-4. Exp Hematol 1993;21:635–639.

7. **Ferrajoli A, Zipf TF, Talpaz M, Felix EA, Estrov Z.** Growth factors controlling interleukin-4 action on hematopoietic progenitors. Ann Hematol 1993;67:277–284.

8. **Favre C, Saeland S, Caux C, Duvert V, De VJ.** Interleukin-4 has basophilic and eosinophilic cell growth-promoting activity on cord blood cells. Blood 1990;75:67–73.

9. **Sawada K, Sato N, Koike T.** Inhibition of GM-CSF production by recombinant human interleukin-4: negative regulator of hematopoiesis. Leuk Lymphoma 1995;19:33–42.

10. **Yamaguchi Y, Suda T, Suda J, Eguchi M, Miura Y, Harada N, Tominaga A, Takatsu K.** Purified interleukin 5 supports the terminal differentiation and proliferation of murine eosinophilic precursors. J Exp Med 1998;167:43–56.

11. **Dent LA, Strath M, Mellor AL, Sanderson CJ.** Eosinophilia in transgenic mice expressing interleukin 5. J Exp Med 1990;172:1425–1431.

12. **Ikebuchi K, Clark SC, Ihle JN, Souza LM, Ogawa M.** Granulocyte colony-stimulating factor enhances interleukin 3-dependent proliferation of multipotential hemopoietic progenitors. Proc Natl Acad Sci U S A 1988;85:3445–3449.

13. **Ogawa M.** IL6 and haematopoietic stem cells. Res Immunol. 1992;143:749–751.

14. **Bot FJ, Van EL, Broeders L, Aarden LA, Lowenberg B.** Interleukin-6 synergizes with M-CSF in the formation of macrophage colonies from purified human marrow progenitor cells. Blood 1989;73:435–437.

15. **Hegyi E, Navarro S, Debili N, Mouthon MA, Katz A, Breton GJ, Vainchenker W.** Regulation of human megakaryocytopoiesis: analysis of proliferation, ploidy and maturation in liquid cultures. Int J Cell Cloning 1990;8:236–244.

16. **Suematsu S, Matsuda T, Aozasa K, Akira S, Nakano N, Ohno S, Miyazaki J, Yamamura K, Hirano T, Kishimoto T.** IgG1 plasmacytosis in interleukin 6 transgenic mice. Proc Natl Acad Sci U S A 1989;86:7547–7551.

17. **Hultner L, Moeller J.** 1990. Mast cell growth-enhancing activity (MEA) stimulates interleukin 6 production in a mouse bone marrow-derived mast cell line and a malignant subline. Exp Hematol 1990;18:873–877.

18. **Mosmann TR, Bond MW, Coffman RL, Ohara J, Paul WE.** T-cell and mast cell lines respond to B-cell stimulatory factor 1. Proc Natl Acad Sci U S A 1986;83:5654–5658.

19. **Donahue RE, Yang YC, Clark SC.** 1990. Human P40 T-cell growth factor (interleukin-9) supports erythroid colony formation. Blood 1990;75:2271–2275.

20. **Leary AG, Zeng HQ, Clark SC, Ogawa M.** Growth factor requirements for survival in G0 and entry into the cell cycle of primitive human hemopoietic progenitors. Proc Natl Acad Sci U S A 1992;89:4013–4017.

21. **Tanaka R, Katayama N, Ohishi K, Mahmud N, Itoh R, Tanaka Y, Komada Y, Minami, N, Sakurai M, Shirakawa S, Shiku H.** Accelerated cell-cycling of hematopoietic progenitor cells by growth factors. Blood 1995;86:73–79.

22. **Kaushansky K, Broudy VC, Lin N, Jorgensen MJ, McCarty J, Fox N, Zucker FD, Lofton DC.** Thrombopoietin, the Mp1 ligand, is essential for full megakaryocyte development. Proc Natl Acad Sci U S A 1995;92:3234–3238.

23. **Broudy VC, Lin NL, Kaushansky K.** Thrombopoietin (c-mpl ligand) acts synergistically with erythropoietin, stem cell factor, and interleukin-11 to enhance murine megakaryocyte colony growth and increases megakaryocyte ploidy in vitro. Blood 1995;85:1719–1726.

24. **Du X, Williams DA.** Interleukin-11: review of molecular, cell biology, and clinical use. Blood 1997;89:3897–3908.

25. **Rodriguez MH, Arnaud S, Blanchet JP.** IL-11 directly stimulates murine and human erythroid burst formation in semisolid cultures. Exp Hematol. 1995;23:545–550.

26. **de Haan G, Dontje B, Engel C, Loeffler M, Nijhof W.** In vivo effects of interleukin-11 and stem cell factor in combination with erythropoietin in the regulation of erythropoiesis. Br J Haematol 1995;90:783–790.

27. **Jacobsen SE, Veiby OP, Smeland EB.** Cytotoxic lymphocyte maturation factor (interleukin 12) is a synergistic growth factor for hematopoietic stem cells. J Exp Med 1993;178:413–418.

28. **Ploemacher RE, Van SP, Boudewijn A, Neben S.** Interleukin-12 enhances interleukin-3 dependent multilineage hematopoietic colony formation stimulated by interleukin-11 or steel factor. Leukemia 1993;7:1374–1380.

29. **Ploemacher RE, Van SP, Voorwinden H, Boudewijn A.** Interleukin-12 synergizes with interleukin-3 and steel factor to enhance recovery of murine hemopoietic stem cells in liquid culture. Leukemia 1993;7:1381–1388.

30. **Jackson JD, Yan Y, Brunda MJ, Kelsey LS, Talmadge JE.** Interleukin-12 enhances peripheral hematopoiesis in vivo. Blood 1995;85:2371–2376.

31. **Thomson AW, Lotze MT.** Interleukins 13, 14, and 15. In: Thomson AW, ed. The cytokine handbook. London: Academic Press Limited, 1994;257–264.

32. **Lu L, Welte K, Gabrilove JL, Hangoc G, Bruno E, Hoffman R, Broxmeyer HE.** Effects of recombinant human tumor necrosis factor alpha, recombinant human gamma-interferon, and prostaglandin E on colony formation of human hematopoietic progenitor cells stimulated by natural human pluripotent colony-stimulating factor, pluripoietin alpha, and recombinant erythropoietin in serum-free cultures. Cancer Res. 1986;46:4357–4361.

33. **Pretnar G, Steindl F, Meager A, Thorpe R, Borth N, Schmatz C, Metzger R, Katinger HW, Ferlan I.** Interferon alpha primes early proliferative response of bone marrow cells in vivo. Cytokine 1998;10:185–191.

34. **Tracey KJ, Wei H, Manogue KR, Fong Y, Hesse DG, Nguyen HT, Kuo GC, Beutler B, Cotran RS, Cerami A, Lowry SF.** Cachectin/tumor necrosis factor induces cachexia, anemia, and inflammation. J Exp Med 1988;167:1211–1227.

35. **Moldawer LL, Marano MA, Wei H, Fong Y, Silen ML, Kuo G, Manogue KR, Vlassara H, Cohen H, Cerami A, Lowry SF.** Cachectin/tumor necrosis factor-alpha alters red blood cell kinetics and induces anemia in vivo. Faseb J 1989;3:1637–1643.

36. **Maciejewski JP, Selleri C, Sato T, Cho HJ, Keefer LK, Nathan CF, Young NS.** Nitric oxide suppression of human hematopoiesis in vitro. Contribution to inhibitory action of interferon-gamma and tumor necrosis factor-alpha. J Clin Invest 1995;96:1085–1092.

37. **Selleri C, Sato T, Anderson S, Young NS, Maciejewski JP.** Interferon-gamma and tumor necrosis factor-alpha suppress both early and late stages of hematopoiesis and induce programmed cell death. J Cell Physiol 1995;165:538–546.

38. **Dybedal I, Jacobsen SE.** Transforming growth factor beta (TGF-beta), a potent inhibitor of erythropoiesis: neutralizing TGF-beta antibodies show erythropoietin as a potent stimulator of murine burst-forming unit erythroid colony formation in the absence of a burst-promoting activity. Blood 1995;86:949–957.

39. **Broxmeyer HE, Sherry B, Lu L, Cooper S, Carow C, Wolpe SD, Cerami A.** Myelopoietic enhancing effects of murine macrophage inflammatory proteins 1 and 2 on colony formation in vitro by murine and human bone marrow granulocyte/macrophage progenitor cells. J Exp Med 1989;170:1583–1594.

40. **Quesniaux VF, Graham GJ, Pragnell I, Donaldson D, Wolpe SD, Iscove NN, Fagg B.** Use of 5-fluorouracil to analyze the effect of macrophage inflammatory protein-1 alpha on long-term reconstituting stem cells in vivo. Blood 1993;81:1497–1504.

41. **Broxmeyer HE, Sherry B, Cooper S, Lu L, Maze R, Beckmann MP, Cerami A, Ralph P.** Comparative analysis of the human macrophage inflammatory protein family of cytokines (chemokines) on proliferation of human myeloid progenitor cells. Interacting effects involving suppression, synergistic suppression, and blocking of suppression. J Immunol 1993;3448–3458.

42. **Rameshwar P, Poddar A, Gascon P.** Hematopoietic regulation mediated by interactions among the neurokinins and cytokines. Leuk Lymphoma 1997;28:1–10.

CHAPTER 16

Identification and Isolation of Hemopoietic Progenitors

• NAZARETH GENGOZIAN

Bone marrow transplantation as a therapeutic modality for hematologic dyscrasias in man was first attempted in 1957 by Thomas et al[1]; although largely unsuccessful with only two transient grafts in six patients, the procedure demonstrated that large amounts of marrow could be infused intravenously without ill effect. This clinical effort was predated by the earlier spleen-shielding experiments of Jacobson et al[2] and the bone marrow inoculation studies of Lorenz et al[3] in mice, each demonstrating the survival value of these hemopoietic tissues in lethally irradiated recipients. Although humoral factors were at first considered responsible for the observed effects, subsequent studies in mice, dogs, and primates performed in the 1950s–1960s unequivocally showed a transplantation of donor hemopoietic elements in animals receiving intensive chemotherapy or irradiation.[4] The clinical benefits to be derived from this biology of marrow transplantation are now well documented with more than 30,000 autologous and allogeneic transplants of bone marrow or bloodstem cells being performed yearly worldwide (1998) for treatment of hematologic malignancies in man.[5] Only in the past decade have there been attempts to use bone marrow transplantation as a therapeutic intervention for malignant diseases in veterinary medicine. The initial study of Haskins et al[6] in 1984 demonstrating the feasibility of allogeneic marrow transplants in cats prompted clinical trials in this species. Correction of inborn errors of metabolism,[7–9] e.g., multisystemic lysosomal storage diseases, as well as a favorable outcome for the treatment of acute myeloid leukemia by bone marrow transplantation,[10] has been reported. The discovery of the feline immunodeficiency virus (FIV) by Pedersen et al[11] in 1987 has led to acceptance of this species as an excellent animal model to study the pathogenesis and therapy of human AIDS. The potential for marrow transplants to alleviate immune dysfunctions in FIV- and feline-leukemia-virus (FeLV)-infected animals has been suggested in preliminary studies by Yamamoto et al[12] and Gasper et al.[13] In contrast to the limited marrow transplant studies reported for the cat, there is extensive literature on transplantation of this tissue in the dog; indeed, the canine has served as an excellent random-bred animal model, providing a basis for many of the principles and techniques of marrow transplantation shown to be applicable to man.[14] Correction of potentially lethal enzymatic deficiencies and treatment of malignant lymphomas have also been attempted in this species by bone marrow transplants.[15,16]

The majority of clinical marrow transplants in veterinary medicine have been allogeneic, with siblings or unrelated donors. A primary complication of allogeneic marrow has been graft-versus-host disease (GVHD), this occurring in varying frequency and severity even when genetic matching at the major histocompatibility complex (MHC) is available. Dog leukocyte antigen (DLA) matching in dogs (three recognized loci, DLA–A, DLA–B, and DLA–D) has largely mitigated GVHD, but even here severe GVHD can be encountered, suggesting the presence of minor transplantation antigens as targets of histoincompatibility. Although MHC antigens have also been identified for the feline (feline leukocyte antigen [FLA], classes I and II[17]), the mixed leukocyte reaction is frequently used as an adjunct to minimize incompatibility. Autologous marrow transplants, on the other hand, avoid host-graft complications and have been used in these species[12,15,18]; as a therapeutic measure, however, this can be limiting in situations in which contamination of marrow with viral-infected or clonogenic malignant cells may occur. In humans, autologous transplants are performed for many solid-tumor malignancies, and the potential for marrow contamination has led to chemical or biological purging of this tissue with tumor-specific monoclonal antibodies (mAbs).[19] An alternative method to cleanse the marrow of undesirable cells has been the use of a fractionation scheme wherein an enriched population of hemopoietic progenitors can be realized. For example, in the feline AIDS model, select marrow fractions obtained by counterflow centrifugal elutriation and subsequently treated with soybean agglutinin lectin have been found to be free of viral-infected cells.[18,20] An approach with broader applicability would be the use of a mAb for a positive selection of hemopoietic progenitors: because of the elimination of nascent T cells in the marrow as well as the purification of the hemopoietic stem cell population, success in this direction would preclude any GVHD potential.

HUMAN CD34 ANTIGEN

CD34 is a transmembrane glycoprotein (MW 105–120 kDs) expressed on lymphohemopoietic stem and progenitor cells.[21,22] Several mAbs have been developed against different epitopes of this antigen with a division of the antibodies into three classes based on the sensitivity of the epitopes to enzymatic cleavage: class I antibodies (My10, BI.3C5, 12.8, ICH3, I4G3) are sensitive to neuraminidase (NA), chymopapain (CP), and the glycoprotease from Pasteurella hemolytica (GP); class II antibodies (QBen10, 43A1, MD34.1, MD34.2 MD34.3, 4A1, 9044, 9049) are sensitive to only NA; and class III antibodies (TUK3, 9F2, 115.2, HPCA2) are resistant to NA, CP, and GP.[21,22] Cells contained within this CD34 cluster of antigens have been shown to reconstitute hemopoiesis after myeloablative chemical or radiation therapy.[23] Purification of CD34 cells from marrow, which normally contains 1 to 3% of these cells and peripheral blood with frequencies less than 1%, has been realized with these antibodies when used singly or in combination for research purposes by means of (a) sorting with FACS (fluorescence-activated cell sorting) analyzers, (b) immunomagnetic beads, and (c) immunoadsorption on affinity columns. Adaptation of the latter two methods for separations on a large scale suitable for transplantation has yielded purities ranging from 50 to 90%; such CD34+ cell enrichment has led to 3 to 4 log depletions of tumor cells from bone marrow or peripheral blood and more than 3 log depletions of T cells from the latter tissue, which is clinically important for allogeneic blood-stem cell transplants.[24–26]

A literature search failed to reveal any systematic study of the cross reactivity of human CD34 mAbs to any grouping of domestic animals. Joling et al[27] tested 95 antibodies (monoclonal and polyclonal) directed against human antigens on cryostat tissue sections (tonsil, lymph node, thymus, intestine, spleen) of the cat. Only 25 showed reactivity toward the feline comparable with that observed with human tissues; a few, including a CD34 antibody (DAKO, BIRMA–K3), gave miscellaneous reactivities, i.e., insufficient to use as a definition of cells in this species. Brodersen et al[28] examined the reactivities of 213 mAbs raised against leukocyte surface antigens of humans toward blood leukocytes of 15 different animal species. Seventy-seven (36%) were found to cross react in a manner that suggested their potential applicability to the species in question; because hemopoietic tissues were not included in this screening, CD34 mAbs were not tested. This reference also cites earlier surveys of human-directed antibodies to MHC antigens of ruminants and other domestic animals; although cross reactivities following the accepted evolutionary pattern were found toward classes I and II MHC antigens, specificities allowing selection of hemopoietic progenitors were not discerned.

As may be anticipated, excellent cross reactivity of human CD34 antibodies to primate bone marrow has been reported. An enriched population (65 to 81%) of CD34+ cells from baboon marrow was obtained with mAb 12.8 (class I) by affinity column fractionation.[29] Infusion of only $2.7–3.5 \times 10^6$/kg autologous CD34+ selected cells into lethally irradiated (9.2 Gy) baboons led to survival with trilineage hemopoietic engraftment comparable with that observed with $200–270 \times 10^6$ cells/kg of unprocessed marrow. Animals receiving marrow (184 and 285×10^6 cells/kg) depleted of CD34+ cells failed to engraft. In vitro clonogenic assays showed a significant enrichment of colony-forming unit-granulocyte-macrophage (CFU–GM), blast-forming units-erythroid (BFU–E) and CFU–Mix colonies in the CD34 positively selected populations, whereas the depleted marrow was essentially devoid of these progenitors. Allogeneic transplants of highly purified CD34+ cells (95 to 97%; $0.6–2.1 \times 10^6$/kg) into lethally irradiated baboons was also reported by these investigators; in this instance, stable mixed chimerism (host and donor cells) in both the myelopoietic and the lymphopoietic cell lineages was observed 51 weeks posttransplant.[30] Comparable studies have been reported for the rhesus monkey; in these studies autologous and allogeneic transplants of CD34-selected cells (mAb ICH3, class I) in numbers 40- to 140-fold less than with unfractionated marrow were achieved.[31]

CANINE CD34 PROGENITORS

The canine has long served as an excellent animal model for the translation of hemopoietic transplant technology to man. It is not surprising therefore that among domestic laboratory animals, identification of hemopoietic progenitors in this species has been accomplished with mAbs. Studies by McSweeney et al[32] illustrate a systematic approach to this problem. A complementary DNA (cDNA) library made from the canine myelomonocytic leukemia (ML) cell line ML2 was used to clone a cDNA for the canine homologue to CD34. The genomic structure of the canine CD34 was found to be similar to that of the human and murine CD34 genes, and the resulting proteins from all three species showed significant amino acid homology in the cytoplasmic and transmembrane domains of the protein. A polyclonal antiserum to a recombinant fusion protein, caCD34–Ig, was produced in the rabbit. This antiserum reacted with canine leukemic cell lines and approximately 1% of marrow cells. Sorting of marrow cells with this antiserum yielded a 25- to 50-fold enrichment of CFU–GM colonies. Because this antiserum did not lend itself to precise FACS sorting owing to the presence of some nonspecific staining of monocytes and granulocytes, mAbs to the same caCD34–Ig protein were developed and characterized.[33] Of ten hybridomas cloned that produced antibody to the CD34 antigen, two with high-affinity antibodies showing intense staining of a homogenous population of cells were used in in vitro and in vivo studies to establish their specificities for canine hemopoietic pro-

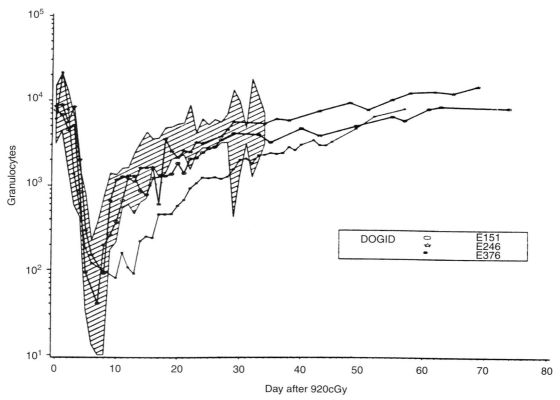

FIGURE 16.1 Peripheral blood granulocyte counts in three dogs that received 9.2 Gy total body irradiation followed by infusion of CD34-selected marrow cells in doses ranging from 1.2 to 3.4 × 10⁶ cells/kg. The hatch-marked portion shows the range of counts from 16 control dogs receiving unmodified bone marrow. (Adapted from McSweeney P, Rouleau K, Wallace P, et al. Characterization of monoclonal antibodies that recognize canine CD34. Blood 1998; 91(6):1977–1986).

genitors. In ten samples of unfractionated marrow, the mAbs detected 2.1% (SD ± 1.0%) CD34+ cells and less than 0.1% CD34+ cells in peripheral blood. Marrow cells positively selected by sorting with purities greater than 95% showed an enriched population of CFU–GM colony–forming cells; those negatively selected contained a paucity of these cells. Marrow cells to be used for transplantation were obtained with positive immunomagnetic selection for a more quantitative isolation of cells. Purities of 29%, 60%, and 70% CD34+ cells were achieved, and autologous transplants into three lethally irradiated (9.2 Gy) recipients led to hemopoietic engraftment similar to that of control dogs receiving unfractionated marrow (Fig. 16.1). The number of CD34+ cells used in the transplants ranged from 1.2 to 3.4 × 10⁶/kg body weight, comparable with that of the baboon studies cited above.

HEMOPOIETIC PROGENITORS OF THE CAT

The potential value of the feline as an animal model for veterinary medicine in the treatment of hematologic and enzymatic diseases correctable by bone marrow transplantation is yet to be realized. Allogeneic transplants,

even when performed with our current understanding of MHC antigens in this species, are compromised by the preemptive steps taken to mitigate graft-versus-host (GVH) reactions and preconditioning regimens to minimize GVH problems.[34,35] Autologous transplants, although free of such complications, have yet to receive serious attention because of insufficient information on stem cell purification or means of isolating CD34-equivalent stem cells in this species, methodologies that would provide hemopoietic progenitors free of contaminating diseased cells. Recent application of a sophisticated marrow fractionation and lectin treatment scheme has yielded hemopoietic cells free of viral-infected cells when these were obtained from FIV-infected animals. Thus, select fractions of marrow obtained with counterflow centrifugal elutriation (CCE) were found to contain hemopoietic cells early in lineage development[36]; treatment of the fractions with the soybean agglutinin (SBA) lectin yielded a population [SBA(−) fraction] enriched for BFU–E progenitors and essentially devoid of T lymphocytes and immature myeloid cells that are candidates for FIV infectivity.[18] Proviral polymerase chain reaction (PCR) analyses of these CCE/SBA(−) fractions revealed little or no evidence of viral-infected cells.[20] Germane to the present discussion, it was subsequently shown that the CCE/SBA(−)

FIGURE 16.2 Schematics of immunomagnetic procedure used for a negative and a positive collection of cells. Antibody-labeled cells bound to ferromagnetic beads are passed through a magnetizable iron matrix attached to a strong magnetic field. The depleted population, i.e., lacking cells reactive with the antibody, pass through the column; the antibody-labeled cells are retained and collected as positively selected cells after removal of the column from the magnetic field. (Adapted from Miltenyi Biotech Inc., Auburn, CA.)

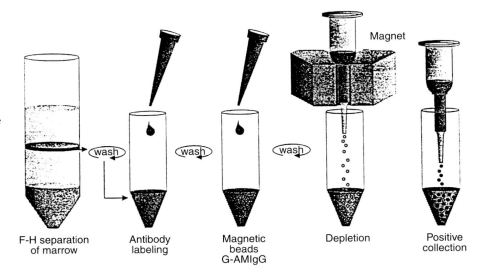

populations contained cells capable of providing hemopoietic reconstitution of autologous, lethally irradiated cats.[18] The therapeutic value of such cells, in an autologous or allogeneic setting, in combination with any antiretroviral drug treatment for immunologic reconstitution of FIV-infected animals, has not yet been determined.

The apparent presence of self-renewing hemopoietic progenitors in the CCE/SBA(−) fractions prompted immunization of mice with these cells to develop mAbs that would identify either erythroid or myeloid progenitors. In a screening of 400 hybridomas, 3 were found reactive with erythroid lineage cells.[37] Although FACScan analyses with whole marrow and CCE fractions were used in the initial screening, the final methodologies used to identify the cellular specificity of the mAbs were immunomagnetic depletions followed by colony-forming assays. Figure 16.2 shows the schematics of the immunomagnetic procedure, allowing for a negative collection, a population depleted of cells reactive with the antibody, and, alternatively, a positive collection, cells reactive with the antibody. Three hybridomas, K-1, K-7, and Q-3, having an apparent specificity for erythroid lineage cells as indicated by immunofluorescent staining of a high percentage (>70%) of SBA(−) cells were subcloned, and the resulting mAbs tested in the depletion or the colony-forming assays. K-1 and Q-3 mAbs were found to be specific for BFU−E progenitors, i.e., immunomagnetic depletions led to an almost complete loss of BFU−E colonies in the CCE/SBA(−) fractions and an increase of CFU−GM colonies (Fig. 6.3; data for Q-3 not shown). In contrast, depletions with mAb K-7 led to a significant enrichment, fivefold to eightfold, of both BFU−E and CFU−GM progenitors (Fig. 16.3), suggesting that this antibody was reacting not with BFU−E progenitors but with nonclonogenic, late-developing erythroid lineage cells. K-1 stained 11.9 ± 1.1% of bone marrow cells and Q-3 12.8 ± 1.1% (*n* = 6); dual immunofluorescent staining was not addi-

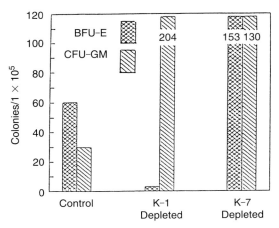

FIGURE 16.3 CFU-GM and BFU-E colony-forming assays of an SBA(−) population of feline marrow after immunomagnetic depletions with mAbs K-1 and K-7. K-1 removed only BFU-E progenitors from the cell suspension, resulting in an enriched population of CFU-GM progenitors. Depletion with mAb K-7 leads to a significant enrichment of both BFU-E and CFU-GM progenitors. (Adapted from Gengozian N. Development of monoclonal antibodies to erythroid progenitors in feline bone marrow. J Vet Immunol Immunopathol 1998;64(4):299–312).

tive, indicating that they were detecting the same population of cells. K-7 stained 8.3 ± 0.7% of whole marrow, and additive tests indicated that cells recognized by this antibody were contained within that population identified by mAbs K-1 and Q-3.

Three mAbs, CH-152, CH-755, and CH-799, derived from another group of more than 800 hybridomas showed reactivity toward both BFU−E and CFU−GM progenitors in feline bone marrow as revealed in the immunomagnetic depletion or colony-forming assays (Fig. 16.4). The percentage of marrow cells stained with these antibodies was CH-152, 3.1 ± 0.5%; CH-799,

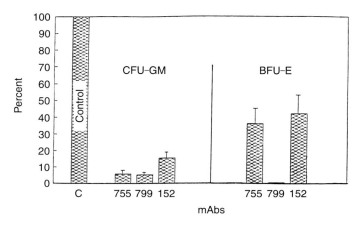

FIGURE 16.4 Removal of CFU-GM and BFU-E progenitors from feline bone marrow by immunomagnetic depletions with mAbs CH-152, CH-755, and CH-799. Treatment with mAb CH-799 resulted in almost complete depletions of both progenitors (N.G., unpublished,).

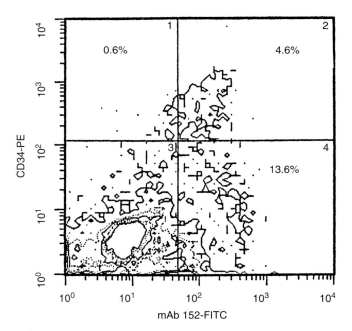

FIGURE 16.5 Dual immunofluorescent staining of human bone marrow cells with mAb CH-152 (secondarily labeled with FITC) and the human CD34 antibody, HPCA-2 (PE-conjugated) (N.G., unpublished).

9.9 ± 1.0%; CH-755, 10.3 ± 2.3% (n = 5) (N.G., unpublished). Of interest, CH-152 also stained human bone marrow, 9.8 ± 1.5%, and cord blood cells, 6.7 ± 1.3% (n = 5). Dual immunofluorescent staining of human marrow with this antibody and a human CD34 mAb (Becton-Dickinson, hemopoietic progenitor cell antigen-2 [HPCA-2] 8G 12; phycoerythrin [PE]) is shown in Figure 16.5. CH-152, although reacting with approximately 14% of the marrow cells, stained 90% of the CD34+

population detected by HPCA-2. Immunomagnetic depletion studies with this antibody on human marrow and cord blood cells eliminated greater than 90% of the CFU-GM and BFU-E progenitors in these tissues; this is comparable with depletions obtained with the control human CD34 mAbs, HPCA-1 (My10) and HPCA-2 (Becton-Dickinson). Whether these antibodies are detecting committed as opposed to earlier progenitors (or both) of CD34-equivalent cells in feline marrow is not known. The large percentage of marrow cells stained with mAbs CH-799 and CH-755 would suggest reactivities with later-developing progenitors, although this would not exclude containment also of earlier self-renewing cells in the populations detected. Transplantation of marrow cells isolated with these mAbs is needed to answer this question. Positive selection of marrow cells with affinity-columns and immunomagnetic beads have yielded purities of 85 to 95% with mAb CH-755 and 60 to 70% with mAbs CH-152 and CH-799, predicating future autologous and allogeneic transplants.

REFERENCES

1. **Thomas ED, Lochte H, Lu WC, Ferrebee JW.** Intravenous infusion of bone marrow in patients receiving radiation and chemotherapy. N Engl J Med 1957; 257(11):491–496.
2. **Jacobson LO, Marks EK, Robson MJ, Gaston EO, Zirkle RE.** Effect of spleen protection on mortality following X-irradiation. J Lab Clin Med 1949;34:1538–1543.
3. **Lorenz E, Congdon CC, Uphoff DE.** Modification of acute irradiation injury in mice and guinea pigs by bone marrow injections. Radiology 1952;58: 863–877.
4. **Van Bekkum DW, De Vries MJ.** Radiation chimaeras. New York: Academic Press, 1967.
5. **Horowitz MM.** IBMTR/ABMTR Newsletter. Milwaukee, WI: Medical College of Wisconsin, 1998;5:1–12.
6. **Haskins ME, Wortman JA, Wilson S, Wolfe JH.** Bone marrow transplantation in the cat. Transplantation 1984;37:634–636.
7. **Gasper PW, Thrall MA, Wenger DA, et al.** Correction of feline arylsulfatase B deficiency (mucopolysaccharidosis VI) by bone marrow transplantation. Nature 1984;312:467–469.
8. **Colgan SP, Hull-Thrall MA, Gasper PW, et al.** Restoration of neutrophil and platelet function in feline Chediak–Higashi syndrome by bone marrow transplantation. Bone Marrow Transplant 1991;7:365–374.
9. **Walkley SU, Thrall MA, Dobrenis K, et al.** Bone marrow transplantation corrects the enzyme defect in neurons of the central nervous system in a lysosomal storage disease. Proc Natl Acad Sci U S A 1994;91:2970–2975.
10. **Gasper PW, Rosen DK, Fulton R.** Allogeneic marrow transplantation in a cat with acute myeloid leukemia:M6-ER. J Am Vet Med Assoc 1996;208: 1280–1284.
11. **Pedersen NC, Ho EW, Brown ML, Yamamoto JK.** Isolation of a T-lymphotropic virus from domestic cats with an immunodeficiency-like syndrome. Science 1987;235:790–793.
12. **Yamamoto JK, Pu R, Arai M, et al.** Feline bone marrow transplantation; its use in FIV-infected cats. J Vet Immunol Immunopathol 1998;65:323–351.
13. **Gasper PW, Fulton R, Thrall MA, et al.** Marrow transplant therapy for retrovirus-infected cats. Blood 1992;80:239a.
14. **Thomas ED, Storb R.** The development of the scientific foundation of hematopoietic cell transplantation based on animal and human studies. In: Thomas ED, Blume KG, Forman SJ, eds. Hematopoietic Cell Transplantation. Oxford, England: Blackwell Scientific Publications, 1999.
15. **Weiden P, Storb R, Deeg HJ, Graham TC, Thomas ED.** Prolonged disease-free survival in dogs with lymphoma after total-body irradiation and autologous marrow transplantation consolidation of combination-chemotherapy-induced remissions. Blood 1979;54:1039–1049.
16. **Breider MA, Shull RM, Constantopoulos GC.** Long term effects of bone marrow transplantation in dogs with mucopolysaccharidosis. Am J Pathol 1989;134:677–692.
17. **Winkler C, Schultz A, Cevario S, O'Brien S.** Genetic characterization of FLA, the cat major histocompatibility complex. Proc Natl Acad Sci U S A 1989;86:943–947.
18. **Gengozian N, Reyes L, Pu R, et al.** Fractionation of feline bone marrow with the soybean agglutinin lectin yields populations enriched for erythroid and myeloid elements: transplantation of soybean agglutinin-negative cells into lethally irradiated recipients. Transplantation 1997;64(3):510–518.

19. **Gee AP, Gross S, Worthington-White DA, eds.** Advances in bone marrow purging. New York, NY: Wiley-Liss, 1994.
20. **Gengozian N, Okada S, Yamamoto JK.** Procurement of presumptive hematopoietic stem cells free of the feline immunodeficiency virus from bone marrow of infected animals. FASEB J 1996;10(6):A1062.
21. **Stella CC, Cazzola M, De Fabritiis P, et al.** CD34-positive cells: biology and clinical relevance. Haematologica 1995;80:367–387.
22. **Krause D, Fackler MJ, Civin C, May WS.** CD34: structure, biology, and clinical utility. J Am Soc Hematol 1996;87(1):1–13.
23. **Shpall E, Jones R, Bearman S, et al.** Transplantation of enriched CD34-positive autologous marrow into breast cancer patients following high-dose chemotherapy: influence of CD34-positive peripheral-blood progenitors and growth factors on engraftment. J Clin Oncol 1994;12(1):28–36.
24. **Farley T, Ahmed T, Fitzgerald M, Preti RA.** Optimization of CD34+ cell selection using immunomagnetic beads: implications for use in cryopreserved peripheral blood stem cell collections. J Hematother 1997;6:53–60.
25. **McNiece I, Briddle R, Stoney G, et al.** Large-scale isolation of CD34+ cells using the Amgen cell selection device results in high levels of purity and recovery. J Hematother 1997;6:5–11.
26. **Stainer CJ, Miflin G, Anderson S, et al.** A comparison of two different systems for CD34+ selection of autologous or allogeneic PBSC collections. J Hematother 1998;7:375–383.
27. **Joling P, Broekhuizen R, de Weger R, Rottier PJM, Egberink H.** Immunohistochemical demonstration of cellular antigens of the cat defined by anti-human antibodies. J Vet Immunol Immunopathol 1996;53:115–127.
28. **Brodersen R, Bijlsma F, Gori K, et al.** Analysis of the immunological cross reactivities of 213 well characterized monoclonal antibodies with specificities against various leucocyte surface antigens of human and 11 animal species. J Vet Immunol Immunopathol 1998;64:1–13.
29. **Berenson R, Andrews R, Bensinger W, et al.** Antigen CD34+ marrow cells engraft lethally irradiated baboons. J Clin Invest 1988;81:951–955.
30. **Andrews R, Bryant E, Bartelmez S, et al.** CD34+ marrow cells, devoid of T and B lymphocytes, reconstitute stable lymphopoiesis and myelopoiesis in lethally irradiated allogeneic baboons. Blood 1992;80(7):1693–1701.
31. **Wagemaker G, Van Gils F, Bart-Baumeister J, Wielenga JJ, Levinsky RJ.** Sustained engraftment of allogeneic CD34 positive hemopoietic stem cells in rhesus monkeys. Exp Hematol 1990;18:704.
32. **McSweeney P, Rouleau K, Storb R, et al.** Canine CD34: cloning of the cDNA and evaluation of an antiserum to recombinant protein. Blood 1996;88(6):1992–2003.
33. **McSweeney P, Rouleau K, Wallace P, et al.** Characterization of monoclonal antibodies that recognize canine CD34. Blood 1998;91(6):1977–1986.
34. **Gasper PW.** Bone marrow transplantation. In: Kirk RW, ed. Current veterinary therapy, 10th ed. Philadelphia: WB Saunders, 1989:515–521.
35. **Thrall MA, Haskins ME.** Bone marrow transplantation. In: August JR, ed. Consultation in feline internal medicine, Vol 3. Philadelphia, PA: WB Saunders, 1997.
36. **Gengozian N, Legendre AM.** Separation of feline bone marrow cells by counterflow centrifugal elutriation. Identification and isolation of presumptive early and late myeloid/erythroid progenitors. Transplantation 1995;60(8):836–841.
37. **Gengozian N.** Development of monoclonal antibodies to erythroid progenitors in feline bone marrow. J Vet Immunol Immunopathol 1998;64(4):299–312.

CHAPTER 17

Hemopoietic Stem Cell Transplantation

• PETER W. GASPER and MARY ANNA THRALL

Dr. E. Donnall Thomas said the following when he received the Nobel Prize in 1990 for establishing bone marrow transplantation (BMT) as a life-saving treatment for various diseases: "It should be noted that marrow grafting could not have reached clinical application without animal research, first in inbred rodents and then in outbred species, particularly the dog."[1] Because significant progress has been made in isolating and using hemopoietic stem cells (HSCs) from marrow and peripheral and umbilical cord blood, the more inclusive title HSC transplantation (HSCT) is warranted. Just as the hemopoietic system differs from the other organ systems, so differs HSCT from solid organ transplantation in two conspicuous ways. First, a HSCT requires no surgery. It is simply an intravenous injection of cells. Once injected, HSCs seed and grow in specialized microenvironments (Chapter 13, Hemopoietic Microenvironment) that shelter and regulate HSCs as they differentiate, proliferate, and mature before their many blood-cell progeny are permitted to enter circulation. Second, because engraftment of donor-origin HSC endows the recipient with new immune cells, HSCT does not require the lifelong administration of immune-suppressive drugs to prevent organ rejection but may result in graft (new lymphohemopoietic system)-versus-host (recipient somatic organs and cells) disease (GVHD).

Our understanding of hemopoiesis emerges from and contributes to the science of HSCT. As few as 30 purified HSCs have been used to repopulate the entire lympho-hemopoietic system of lethally irradiated mice.[2] After examining the clonal stability of hemopoiesis for 2.5 years, Prchal and coworkers[3] concluded that the progeny of approximately eight original embryonic hemopoietic stem cells contribute to the sustained production of all types of blood cells in healthy individuals. The possibility that one could transplant so few cells to provide a lifelong source of healthy, or new gene-bearing cells, portends the potential that HSCT has for treating a wide range of heretofore fatal conditions. In this chapter, the types, methods, and applications of HSCT are discussed. Readers are referred to the texts of Forman et al,[4] Reiffers et al,[5] and Thomas et al[6] for in-depth and historical discussions of the growing field of HSCT and to Gasper,[7] Gasper et al,[8] and Thrall and Haskins[9] for reviews of HSCT in veterinary medicine.

TYPES OF HEMOPOIETIC STEM CELL TRANSPLANTATIONS

Autologous and allogeneic are the two types of HSCTs performed in a clinical setting in veterinary medicine. Autologous (*auto* = self, *legein* = to gather) transplants involve temporary removal of HSCs followed by myeloablation–permanent chemical or radiologic obliteration of the hemopoietic cells remaining in the mitotically active HSC progenitor compartment (Chapter 11, The Hemopoietic System)–and reinfusion of the premyeloablation-harvested HSCs. Allogeneic (*allo* = other, *geneic* = origin) transplants involve infusion of HSCs from an individual of the same species with a different genome (Fig. 17.1). Syngeneic (*syn* = identical) transplants refer to grafts between monozygotic twins or between animals, usually mouse strains, with the same genotype. Xenogeneic (*xeno* = foreign) transplants refer to grafts between animals of different species.

Table 17.1 lists the pros and cons for autologous versus allogeneic HSCTs. Autologous (and syngeneic) HSCTs are easier to perform and have fewer complications because there are no immunologic barriers between donor and recipient and therefore no resistance to engraftment (no host versus graft disease) and no GVHD. Allogeneic (and xenogeneic) HSCTs are much more difficult to perform because of both immunologic resistance to engraftment and GVHD after engraftment. Allogeneic transplants are divided into other categories depending on whether the donor is related or unrelated or histocompatible or nonhistocompatible (i.e., a donor could be unrelated but histocompatible with the recipient, or related but nonhistocompatible and so forth).

HEMOPOIETIC STEM CELL TRANSPLANTATION METHODOLOGY

The technique of HSCT can be divided into five distinct steps (Fig. 17.2). Step one is to select the best possible donor. In the case of an autologous or a syngeneic HSCT the donor is the recipient or an individual with the same genotype, respectively. Large litter sizes and the short gestation times of dogs and cats allow for more donor–

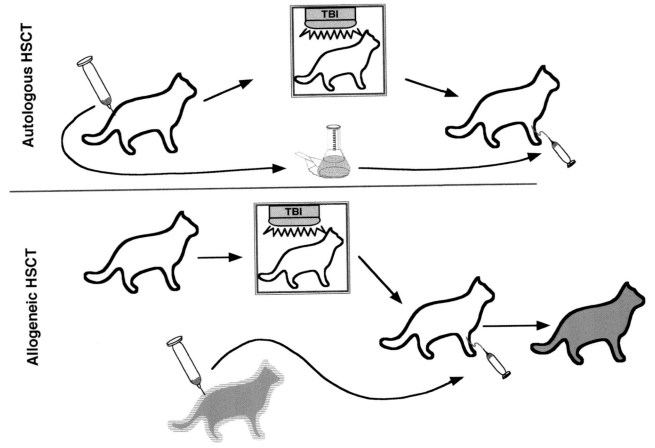

FIGURE 17.1 Autologous and allogeneic types of HSCTs. Autologous transplants involve temporary removal of HSC followed by myeloablation. Allogeneic transplants involve infusion of HSCs from an individual of the same species with a different genome.

recipient alternatives than are generally available in human medicine. Step two is to prepare the patient for its transplant—a euphemism for pretransplant antibiotic therapy and myeloablation. How one proceeds at this step varies according to the disease being treated (discussed two paragraphs below). Step three is the actual HSCT in which a cell suspension containing enough stem cells to beget a complete population of functional peripheral blood cells is infused intravenously. Hematologic engraftment occurs with donor-origin end cells appearing in the recipient's circulation within 14 to 21 days. Step four is the prevention of host-versus-graft disease. Like solid organ transplantation, one must immune suppress the patient after transplantation to avoid rejection of allogeneic marrow. Alert medical skills are needed during the transition period between myeloablation and lymphohemopoietic engraftment of donor cells. Step five is the prevention of GVHD. As soon as donor lymphohemopoiesis can be demonstrated, the clinician must focus on the possible development of and complications arising from graft-versus-host reactivity. The final result is a patient endowed with a donor-origin

TABLE 17.1	Allogenic Versus Autologous HSCTs	
	Allogenic	**Autologous**
Pro	Graft vs leukemia	None of the allogenic "cons" apply
Con	Donor selection/matching	Tumor purging
	Graft rejection	No graft vs leukemia
	Myeloablation required	
	Graft vs host disease	
	Post-HSCT immunosuppression	
	MHC restriction	

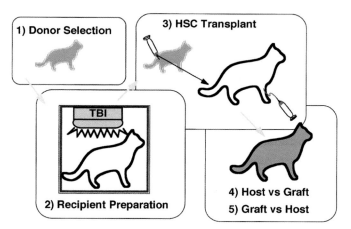

FIGURE 17.2 The five steps involved in the HSCT technique.

lymphohemopoietic system or in the case of autologous HSCT, a reconstituted system.

Selecting of the donor for autologous HSCTs is synonymous with deciding whether the individual is a candidate for an autologous HSCT. In allogeneic HSCTs, the current focus for donor selection is on identification of a histocompatible donor because the incidence of graft rejection and GVHD rises rapidly if the donor and recipient are immunologically mismatched.[4-9] Before our current knowledge of the histocompatibility complex, dogs were used in initial studies in which myeloablation with total body irradiation was induced and in which allogeneic transplants with unseparated marrow were performed. These investigations resulted in some long-term canine chimeras that survived in good health for several years while also experiencing and characterizing the complications of graft rejection and GVHD.[10,11] The dog was the first animal in which the predictive value of in vitro histocompatibility testing for the outcome of marrow grafts was demonstrated.[12] The information learned in canine studies was rapidly applied to matching human donor–recipient pairs. Less is known about the feline histocompatibility system than is known about the human and the canine systems, although our understanding is increasing.[9,13]

Hemopoietic transplant recipients are prepared for BMT in two ways. One set of procedures is performed regardless of the condition treated or the type of HSCT. The objective here is to have the patient in the best possible physical condition at the commencement of the transplant. One examines the patient for potential sources of complications, including removal of dental calculi, bacterial analysis, and parasitologic analysis of feces, and collects baseline clinical data such as complete blood count, platelet count, and serum chemistry profile. As discussed in Chapter 11, hemopoietic cells are the most proliferative, mitotically active, cells in an animal. The cells of the gastrointestinal (GI) tract are among the next most mitotically active cells. More so than total GI decontamination, which leaves the patient susceptible to rapid colonization of the intestine if microorganisms are inadvertently introduced, selective GI decontamination through pre-HSCT antibiotic therapy has been shown to be helpful in decreasing the incidence of infections during the critical period of post-HSCT immune suppression.[4-9] Myeloablation differs in accordance with the disease treated. Here one addresses three concerns: marrow space, host resistance to donor lymphohemopoietic stem cells, and tumor cell elimination. Table 17.2 illustrates how the strategy of patient conditioning varies in four representative indications for HSCT: severe combined immune deficiency (SCID), aplastic anemia (AA), leukemia, and gene therapy. Marrow space is a conceptual, rather than anatomic concern. It has been found that replication and differentiation of stem cells can proceed only if a proper microenvironment is available in the new host (see Chapter 13). Patients who have AA apparently have sufficient space in the marrow to support donor-origin hemopoiesis, whereas leukemic or SCID patients do not. Host resistance to donor cells must be blunted for the graft to seed and grow. Resistance does not occur in SCID patients, who lack a functioning immune system, whereas AA and leukemic patients must be immune suppressed so that they will not reject the graft. If the patient has ever received blood transfusions, the potential for host resistance is increased. Ablation of tumor cells is relevant during use of HSCT to treat patients who have neoplasms. Replacement of malignant lymph or hemopoietic systems by newly transplanted systems will be of lasting usefulness only if all clonogenic leukemia cells in the host can be eliminated. As noted in Table 17.1, a positive aspect of allogeneic HSCT is a graft-versus-leukemia effect that does not occur if an autologous HSCT is performed.

The variable myeloablative conditioning strategies for HSC gene therapy highlights the possibility that this therapy can offer hope for heretofore fatal nonmalignant

TABLE 17.2	Myeloablative Conditioning Considerations		
Reason for HSCT	Provide Space for HSC?	Decrease Resistance to HSC?	Eliminate Neoplastic Cells?
Severe combined immune deficiency	No	No	No
Aplastic anemia	Yes	Yes	No
Acute leukemia	Yes	Yes	Yes
Gene therapy	Maybe	Maybe	Maybe

and malignant diseases. These strategies are discussed in the section, "Therapeutic Applications of HSC Transplantation." High-dose radiotherapy or chemotherapy or combinations of the two are the most commonly used conditioning regimes. Total body irradiation (TBI) has the advantage of killing noncycling tumor cells as effectively as killing cycling cells; this is especially pertinent to the treatment of lymphoid malignancies. Radiation penetrates privileged sites such as the central nervous system (CNS) and testicle that are not accessible by most chemotherapeutic agents. Consistent and sustained engraftment of allogeneic marrow in the dog was achieved above 12.0 gray (Gy) midline air exposure (9.0 to −10.0 Gy midline tissue) dose. Dogs grafted after 12.0 Gy usually achieved stable complete chimerism, that is, all cells analyzed in marrow, lymph nodes, and peripheral blood are determined to be of donor origin. Dogs conditioned with a single TBI dose of 12.0 Gy manifest signs of GI toxicity within 60 hours of treatment. Vomiting, diarrhea, and polydipsia are observed. Within 7 days of TBI, untreated dogs die of extreme dehydration and electrolyte loss. One can prevent this by stopping oral intake for 5 days after TBI and by aggressive fluid therapy. However, a fractionated TBI dose allows one to increase the total radiation dose while decreasing the severity of acute GI toxicity and respiratory late effects (pulmonary interstitial fibrosis). Cats conditioned with a fractionated dose of 10 Gy (6 × 1.67 Gy fractions over 3 days) show no signs of GI toxicity; moreover they continue to eat and drink post TBI. Conditioning with a combination of agents is effective and enough HSCTs have been performed to conduct analyses of the long-term effects of these combinations.[4–9]

HSCs can be thought of as a renewable resource. Collection of HSCs from a suitable donor or from the patient receiving an autologous transplant may be as pain-free as donating blood. The process can be now automated by connecting the donor to an apheresis ma-chine and performing a modified leukoapheresis procedure. If marrow is the source of HSCs, bone marrow is collected aseptically from a histocompatible donor under general anesthesia, but again, has no lasting effect on donors' health and life expectancy. In dogs and humans marrow aspiration is performed with a suction apparatus that draws marrow into a flask containing anticoagulant. Multiple aspirations of the pelvis and long bones with large-bore (15 gauge) needles yield approximately 300 ml of hemodiluted marrow. In cats, it has been found that aspiration of 3 to 4 ml of marrow from each of the donor cat's long bones (humeri, femurs, and tibias) with 18-gauge marrow biopsy needles into anticoagulant-containing syringes yields approximately 20 ml of marrow. This difference in collection procedures may be responsible for the decreased incidence of GVHD seen in feline HSCT, i.e., hemodilution increased the number of donor-origin effector T lymphocytes. Originally, and in a few species still, the only processing was centrifugation, to remove fat, and passage of the marrow through a sterile sieve to remove large particulate material—bone spickules and any clotted material—before intravenous administration of suspended cells to the recipient. As techniques have improved identification and isolation of HSC (Chapter 16, Identification and Isolation of Hemopoietic Progenitors), the relative importance and role of the various cell populations are being determined. Figure 17.3 illustrates the general kinetics of TBI-induced destruction of host blood cells followed by donor-origin lymphohemopoiesis. The declines in the cell lineages reflect their respective life span in peripheral circulation (with the exception being lymphocytes that are killed in interphase by irradiation). Because of the long half-life of erythrocytes, a decline in hematocrit is not usually observed. Progeny of donor stem cells generally begin to appear in the marrow and blood of the recipient between 2 and 3 weeks after transplantation. Engraftment can be accelerated by use of combinations

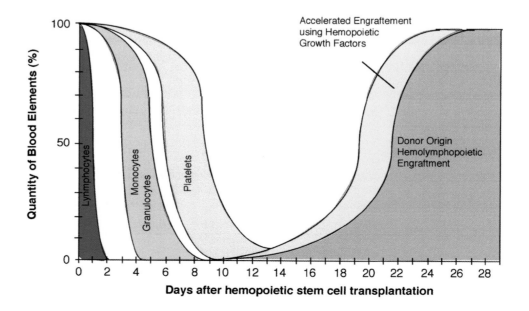

FIGURE 17.3 An illustration of the general kinetics of TBI-induced destruction of host blood cells followed by donor-origin lymphohemopoiesis.

of hemopoietic growth factors and cytokines (Chapters 12, Stem-Cell Biology and 14, Ontogeny of Hemopoietic System). In successful HSCTs, hemopoiesis appears entirely normal and persists indefinitely. Because chemotherapy and TBI given in preparation for marrow transplantation cause extensive ablation of cellular and humoral immunity, it takes time to reestablish a reserve of HSCs.[14] The extensive issues of medical management preceding and documenting engraftment and the various possible complications of performing a HSCT are reviewed in References 4 to 9.

THERAPEUTIC APPLICATIONS OF HEMOPOIETIC STEM-CELL TRANSPLANTATION

Most HSCTs performed in animals have been in studies designed to develop new techniques and new therapies for certain inherited and acquired diseases for which there are human analogs. Examples of past and present studies include HSCT therapy for cyclic neutropenia, pyruvate kinase deficiency and, mucopolysaccharidosis I in dogs and BMT therapy for Chédiak–Higashi Syndrome, mucopolysaccharidosis VI, mucopolysaccharidosis I, alpha mannosidosis, G_{M1} gangliosidosis, and retrovirus infections in cats. In addition to the stated objectives of HSCT studies, insight is gained into the basic science of each condition, and techniques are learned that can be applied to performing HSCT for client-owned animals. Ironically, the explosive developments in HSCT in human medicine will lead the way for some exciting new therapies for animals, e.g., gene therapy, fetal HSC transplantation, use of nonhistocompatibility matched marrow donors and intrauterine HSCT therapy.

Marrow transplantation offers a potential cure for many conditions of dogs and cats that have heretofore been considered fatal diseases. It is a simple procedure that requires state-of-the-art patient management. Evaluating the meaning of the victorious conclusion of the North African campaign during WW II, Winston Churchill stated, "It is not the end of the war, nor is it the beginning of its end, but perhaps it is the end of the beginning." HSC transplantation is currently not a practical therapy for most veterinary patients; however, we may be near the end of considering HSCT a solely experimental procedure.

REFERENCES

1. **Thomas ED.** The Nobel Prizes, 1990. In: Tryckeri AB, ed. Les Prix Nobel. Stockholm: Norstedts, 1991;227.
2. **Spangrude GJ, Heimfeld S, Weissman IL.** Purification and characterization of mouse hematopoietic cells. Science 1988;241:58–62.
3. **Prchal JT, Prchal JF, Belickova M, Chen S, Guan Y, Gartland GL, Cooper MD.** Clonal stability of blood cell lineages indicated by X-chromosomal transcriptional polymorphism. J Exp Med 1996;183:561–567.
4. **Forman SJ, Blume KG, Thomas ED, eds.** Bone marrow transplantation. Boston: Blackwell Scientific Publications, 1994.
5. **Reiffers J, Goldman JM, Armitage JO, eds.** Blood stem cell transplantation. St. Louis: Mosby, 1998.
6. **Thomas ED, Blume KG, Forman SJ, eds.** Hematopoietic cell transplantation. 2nd ed. Boston: Blackwell Scientific Publications, 1998.
7. **Gasper PW.** Bone marrow transplantation. In: Kirk RW, ed. Current veterinary therapy. 10th ed. Philadelphia: W.B. Saunders, 1989;515–521.
8. **Gasper PW, Fulton R, Thrall MA.** Bone marrow transplantation: update and current considerations. In: Kirk RW, ed. Current veterinary therapy. 11th ed. Philadelphia: W.B. Saunders, 1992;493–496
9. **Thrall MA, Haskins MD.** Bone marrow transplantation. In: August JR, ed. Consultation in feline internal medicine Vol. 3. Philadelphia: W.B. Saunders, 1997;3:514–524.
10. **Thomas ED, Collins JA, Herman ED Jr, Ferrebee JW.** Marrow transplants in lethally irradiated dogs given methotrexate. Blood 1962;19:217–228.
11. **Epstein RB, Bryant J, Thomas ED.** Cytogenetic demonstration of permanent tolerance in adult outbred dogs. Transplantation 1967;5:267–272.
12. **Epstein RB, Storb R, Ragde H, Thomas ED.** Cytotoxic typing antisera for marrow grafting in littermate dogs. Transplantation 1968;6:45–58.
13. **O'Brien SJ, Yujki N.** Comparative genome organization of major histocompatibility complex: Lessons from the Felidae. Immun Rev 1998;167:423–432.
14. **Abkowitz JL, Persik MT, Shelton GH, Ott RL, Kiklevich JV, Catlin SN, Guttorp P.** Behavior of hematopoietic stem cells in a large animal. Proc Natl Acad Sci U S A 1995;92:2031–2035.

SECTION III
The Erythrocytes
Douglas J. Weiss

CHAPTER 18

Erythropoiesis and Erythrokinetics

• BRUCE D. CAR

Erythropoiesis is the process by which committed hemopoietic progenitor cells develop into reticulocytes and erythrocytes. These cells egress from bone marrow into bone marrow sinuses and then pass into the peripheral blood. The regulation or dysregulation of this process must be considered within the framework of erythrokinetics or the dynamic maintenance of the peripheral red cell mass. Erythrokinetics are determined by the cellular kinetics of four distinct compartments that make up the erythron: the stem cells, progenitor cells, precursor cells, and mature erythrocytes.[1]

ERYTHROPOIESIS

Primitive hemopoietic stem cells are characterized by a capacity for self-renewal, expression of CD34, absence of lineage-specific markers, and low mitochrondrial uptake of rhodamine123, and they become committed to differentiate into the various hemopoietic lineages in a process thought to be largely stochastic (random).[2] Erythropoiesis is controlled by the combined effects of growth factors that permit cellular survival and proliferation and by nuclear regulators (transcription factors) that activate lineage-specific genes.[3] Multipotent, committed progenitor cells, also referred to as colony-forming unit-granulocyte, erythroid, monocyte, megakaryocyte (CFU-GEMM), differ from stem cells committed to lymphoid development by expression of the transcription factor tal-1/SCL and by an absence of ikaros transcription factor induction. The CFU-GEMM differentiates into early blast-forming unit-erythroid (BFU-E) in a continuous spectrum of maturation that extends to more mature CFU-erythroid (CFU-E) cells (Fig. 18.1). These names derive from the appearance of progenitor cells cultured in semisolid media (see Approaches to Evaluation of Bone Marrow Function, Chapter 6).

A list of growth factors and transcription factors currently known to regulate erythropoiesis is shown in Table 18.1. The erythropoietic roles of most of these individual cytokines, inhibitory factors, and all transcription factors have been examined both in cell culture and in mice rendered deficient in individual genes. The redundancy and pleiotropism of the individual erythro-poietic growth factors is extensive. Most of these growth factors synergize with erythropoietin (Epo) but are not capable of inducing significant in vitro erythropoiesis per se. The deficiency of Epo or the Epo receptor results in murine fetal death on approximately day 13 of gestation.[4] Lineage commitment in these mice is normal, and numbers of BFU-Es are only slightly reduced, but there is a failure of maturation beyond immature CFU-Es. The naturally occurring murine mutants of kit ligand (KL), (Steel; Sl/Sl^d) and its receptor c-kit (White-spotting; W/W^v) have severe macrocytic anemia,[5,6] thus, KL is considered nonredundant in erythropoiesis. KL is expressed as a membrane bound form on marrow stromal cells where it has significantly more growth-promoting activity than its soluble form.

Mice rendered deficient in the transcription factors of the GATA family, tal-1/SCL and rbtn-2, generally fail to develop primitive and definitive embryonic erythropoiesis.[3,7-9] A failure to establish primitive erythropoiesis is generally lethal in the embryonic period. The STAT (signal-transducing and activating factors) peptides 1 and 5 transduce the cytoplasmic signal of Epo after tyrosine phosphorylation by Jak-2 kinase, which is associated with the cytoplasmic domain of the Epo receptor.

Evidence for the regulatory roles of the inhibitory factors listed in Table 18.1 come from many in vitro studies, overexpression in transgenic mice, preclinical studies and clinical trials in which pharmacologic doses of these factors are administered (generally by the subcutaneous route), and compelling disease associations characterized by high levels of tumor necrosis factor alpha (TNFα), interferon gamma (IFNγ), interleukin-1 beta (IL-1β), or cortisol and the development of anemia.[10-14]

Erythropoietin

Normal tissue oxygenation is largely determined by the concentration of erythrocytes in the blood and relies on the low-affinity interaction of O_2 with hemoglobin. Epo is the hormone that is primarily responsible for regulating the production of red blood cells and thus ensuring

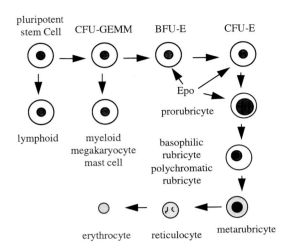

FIGURE 18.1 Schematic presentation of the various stages of erythroid differentiation.

adequate oxygenation of tissues. In the fetal rodent, Epo is first produced in the liver, with production shifting to the kidney toward the end of gestation.[15] In the fetal sheep, higher expression of Epo messenger ribonucleic acid (mRNA) has been found in the mesonephros and the metanephros than the hepatic anlage.[16] Epo is not stored in the adult kidney or liver and when secreted has a half-life of 6 to 10 hours. In the adult, the kidney is the major site of Epo synthesis although the liver may account for as much as 10% to 15% of plasma Epo. Although the exact sites of Epo synthesis have not been definitively determined, in situ hybridization studies suggest that Epo is produced in peritubular interstitial cells of the renal inner cortex and outer medulla and to a lesser extent by the centriacinar hepatocytes and Ito cells of the liver.[15–17] Epo is a highly glycosylated glycoprotein with a peptide core of approximately 18 kDa and a mature molecular weight of 30 kDa. The posttranslational modifications of Epo are essential for its export and activity. The genetic coding sequences for the Epo gene have now been elucidated for at least 10 mamma-

lian species, including humans, two nonhuman primate species, rats, mice, cats, dogs, sheep, and pigs.[18–21]

There is a direct inverse correlation between plasma Epo concentration and the red cell mass, with hypoxia (low arterial pO_2) serving as the specific stimulus for Epo synthesis. The transcription of Epo is mediated by hypoxia-inducible factor-1, (HIF-1), which is responsive to low oxygen concentrations[22]; the nature of the oxygen sensor, which upregulates HIF-1, is presently unknown. HIF-1 binds a regulatory element in the 3' noncoding DNA adjacent to the Epo gene. In response to hypoxia or severe anemia, Epo mRNA levels in the kidney and the liver increase significantly.[23] Severe reductions in renal blood flow result in only slight changes in Epo production when compared with the induction observed in response to anemia.[24] It is hypothesized that the decrease in glomerular filtration rate after reduction in renal blood flow and consequent decrease in sodium reabsorption in the proximal tubules reduces oxygen consumption in the kidneys, thus minimizing oxygen depletion in the vicinity of the putative oxygen sensor. In addition to hypoxia, cobalt, and nickel have been shown in vivo and in vitro to enhance Epo synthesis in an HIF-1-dependent manner. In response to hypoxia or anemia, Epo is formed within minutes or hours and reaches maximum production within 24 hours, yet few red blood cells appear in the circulating blood until approximately 5 days later. This is consistent with the role of Epo-facilitating expansion of the CFU-E and numbers or prorubricytes entering the maturation pool and the approximate time (3 to 4 days) for the maturation of prorubricytes to reticulocytes.

The principal function of Epo, once released in the circulation and transported to bone marrow or spleen (an important erythropoietic site in rodents), appears to be that of a survival factor. Epo inhibits the apoptosis of newly formed progenitor cells and prorubricytes and thereby allows them to differentiate to mature erythrocytes.[15] Epo induces the Bcl-2 family member, Bcl-X_L, to reach maximal transcript and protein levels at the time of maximal hemoglobin synthesis. This protein, located in the inner mitochrondrial membrane, exerts a protec-

TABLE 18.1	Erythropoietic Growth Factors, Inhibitory Factors, and Transcription Factors	
Stimulatory Growth Factor	**Inhibitory Factors**	**Transcription Factors**
Erythropoietin (epo)	TNFα	GATA-1
Kit ligand (KL, stem cell factor)	IL-1β	GATA-2
Interleukin-3	IFNγ	GATA-3
GM CSF	TGFβ	tal-1/SCL
IL-6, IL-11	MIP-1α	rbtn2
Insulin-like growth factor-1	IL-2	Stat 1 (epo signaling)
Hepatocyte growth factor	glucocorticoid	Stat 5 (epo signaling)
Thrombopoietin		
Testosterone		

The roles of stimulatory and inhibitory proteins or transcription factors in erythropoiesis have been identified in diseases associated with the deficiency or excess of these factors, through phenotypes of gene-deleted mice and by the exogenous administration to animals and man.

tive effect akin to Bcl-2 in promoting survival of cells exposed to apoptosis-inducing agents.[25]

Morphology of Erythropoiesis

Erythropoiesis is initiated in the primitive yolk sac, relocating to the liver and ultimately to the bone marrow in adult animals.[26] In rodents, both the spleen and the bone marrow are significant erythropoietic tissues. Erythropoiesis occurs in distinct microanatomic units called erythroblastic islands that consist of a central macrophage surrounded by a ring of developing rubriblasts.[27,28] The macrophage has been hypothesized to contribute important signals to developing rubriblasts. Adhesion molecules mediating important structural and functional interactions between developing erythroblasts and central macrophage include vascular cell adhesion molecule-1 (VCAM-1)/very late antigen-4 (VLA-4) ($\alpha4\beta1$ integrin) and E-cadherin. VLA-4 and VLA-5 are involved in the binding of BFU-E to hemopoietic stromal cells. The expression of these adhesion molecules is generally highest on BFU-E and CFU-E and is progressively lost during erythroid maturation. Hemonectin and collagen type I have been shown to support binding of BFU-E in vitro, and a role for tenascin-C has been inferred from the knockout mouse of that gene.[29] Hemonectin is absent from anemic mice with KL or c-kit deficiency. The surface antigen CD44 is highly expressed on almost all hemopoietic cells in the bone marrow and is responsible for interaction of cells with both collagen type I and IV, fibronectin, and hyaluronate (reviewed in Chapter 30). Reticulocytes express only low levels of a few surface adhesion receptors, such a CD36 (thrombospondin receptor) and VLA-4. Thrombospondin serves as an adhesive ligand for committed progenitors, including CFU-GEMM and BFU-E. Adhesion molecule interactions of reticulocytes with bone marrow stromal cells and extracellular matrix may facilitate their egress into bone marrow sinuses. Mature erythrocytes do not express adhesion molecules under normal conditions and are nonadherent.

The earliest recognizable erythroid precursor is the rubriblast. Progressive maturation, from prorubricyte, to basophilic, and polychromatic rubricytes, which, in turn, are capable of division to postmitotic metarubricytes, involves the progressive loss of nucleoli, cytoplasmic golgi apparatus, mitochondria and ribosomes, progressive synthesis of hemoglobin, reduction in cell volume, and ultimate expulsion of the pyknotic nucleus to form the reticulocyte. The central macrophage of the erythropoietic island (Fig. 18.2) is important in the removal of this nucleus. The ultrastructural morphology of steady-state erythropoiesis is described in detail in the fourth edition of Schalm's Veterinary Hematology,[31] by Bessis et al (32) and for disorders of erythropoiesis, by Fresco (33). The ultrastructure of *in vitro* erythropoiesis has been reported by Koury et al.[34] Hemoglobinization of developing erythrocyte precursors occurs in cells expressing the transferrin receptor, which represents the sole portal for ferric iron entry into the cell. The matura-

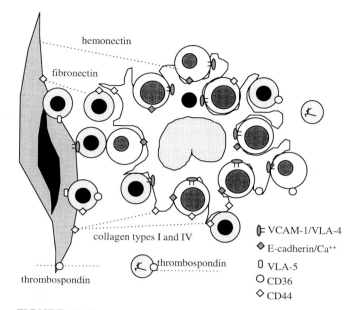

FIGURE 18.2 Erythropoietic microenvironment. An erythroblastic island is depicted with central macrophage surrounded by developing erythroblasts and adjacent reticular cell (left). Important adhesion molecules and adhesion receptors are indicated.

tion of rubricytes is intimately linked to hemoglobinization and erythrocyte metabolism, which are discussed elsewhere in this section (Chapter 21, Erythrocyte Metabolism and Chapter 23, Hemoglobin Synthesis and Destruction). DNA-histone binding of nuclear heme is hypothesized to inhibit further DNA synthesis once exceeding a certain threshold (20 μg/dL).[35] In health, reticulocyte maturation occurs entirely within the bone marrow (cattle, sheep, goats, and horses) or partially in peripheral blood (man, dogs, cats, rabbits, and rodents). In the latter species, the pitting function of splenic macrophages assists in the final removal of cytoplasmic organelles and nuclear fragments from the maturing erythrocyte. The mature erythrocyte must be organelle-free for optimal plasticity of shape in its passage through capillary beds.

ERYTHROKINETICS

The maintenance of the size of the red blood cell mass is determined by the cellular kinetics of four distinct compartments that make up the erythron, the stem cells, the progenitor cells, the precursor cells, and the mature erythrocytes.[1] Under pathologic conditions, the kinetics of each of the compartments may affect the size of the red cell mass, resulting in anemia or erythrocytosis. Specifically, anemia is defined as a reduction in the hemoglobin concentration and erythocytosis as an increase in the hematocrit percentage.

The maintenance, differentiation and self-renewal of

stem cells are poorly understood. Since differentiation of stem cells into committed progenitor cells occurs at random and is not affected by the demands for red blood cells in the circulation, this compartment has little capacity for altering the rate of erythropoiesis. However, small, apparently compensatory increases in the rate of stem cell differentiation occur in severe anemia.[36] Idiopathic aplastic anemia may be associated with a decrease in the differentiation of stem cells to all lineage-specific progenitor cells.[1]

The kinetics of the progenitor-cell compartment (BFU-E and CFU-E) normally determines the size of the red cell mass. Proliferation in the progenitor-cell pool appears to depend entirely on the apoptosis-sparing effect of Epo. In the event of nephrectomy, chronic renal disease associated with substantial reduction in renal mass, various inflammatory diseases (anemia of chronic disease), malignancy and prematurity, the steady-state production of Epo, and the erythropoietic response to hypoxia is reduced, resulting in anemia.[13,37-39] The liver is unable to compensate for deficient renal production of Epo. Absolute erythrocytosis may result from inappropriate tumor production of Epo or from excessive erythroid proliferation, which is characterized by either inappropriate hypersensitivity to Epo or resistance to Epo.[40,41]

The maturation and proliferation of precursor cells (rubriblasts) are not controlled by specific growth factors but proceed at a steady pace. Approximately 16 to 32 reticulocytes are produced from each prorubricyte. Deficiency in B_{12} or folic acid and genetic disorders characterized by mutations in hemoglobin or erythrocyte cytoskeleton reduce this number and result in ineffective erythropoiesis. Under normal conditions, 70% to 90% of iron is used in hemoglobin synthesis. Decreased use of iron (<70%) suggests the presence of ineffective erythropoiesis. Ferrokinetic techniques based on the uptake and use of a probe of radioactive iron (^{59}Fe) have been widely used to measure both ineffective and effective erythrocyte production.[42,43]

The kinetic changes of the mature erythrocyte compartment are induced by a shortening of red cell life span caused by blood loss or hemolysis. The red cell mass can be accurately determined by infusion of a known volume of autologous red cells labeled with an isotope such as ^{51}Cr or [^{14}C]cyanate and by measurement of the degree of dilution by unlabeled red cells. Plasma volume contraction observed with dehydration or with the expansion noted in pregnancy, in highly trained athletes, with gammopathies, or after treatment with certain xenobiotics result in relative concentration or dilution of the red cell concentration without altering the red cell mass.[1] Similarly, ^{51}Cr or [^{14}C]cyanate can be used to determine red cell survival.[44]

REFERENCES

1. **Erslev AJ.** Clinical erythrokinetics: a critical review. Blood Rev 1997;11: 160–167.
2. **Abkowitz JL, Catlin SN, Guttorp P.** Evidence that hematopoiesis may be a stochastic process in vivo. Nature Medicine 1996;2:190–197.
3. **Orkin SH.** Transcription factors and hematopoietic development. J Biol Chem 1995;270:4955–4958.
4. **Wu H, Liu X, Jaenisch R, Lodish HF.** Generation of committed erythroid BFU-E and CFU-E progenitors does not require erythropoietin or the erythropoietin receptor. Cell 1995;83:59–67.
5. **Dexter TM, Moore MAS.** In vitro duplication and "cure" of haematopoietic defects in genetically anaemic mice. Nature 1977;269:412–414.
6. **Huang E, Nocka K, Beier DR, Chu T-Y, Buck J, Lahm H-W, Wellner D, Leder P, Besmer P.** The hematopoietic growth factor KL is encoded by the SL locus and is the ligand of the c-kit receptor, the gene product of the W locus. Cell 1990;63:225–233.
7. **Green T.** Master regulator unmasked. [editorial] Nature 1996;383:575–577.
8. **Shivdasani RA, Orkin SH.** Review: the transcriptional control of hematopoiesis. Blood 1996;87:4025–4039.
9. **Silver L, Palis J.** Initiation of murine embryonic erythropoiesis: a spatial analysis. Blood 1997;89:1154–1164.
10. **Anderson TD, Powers GD, Gately MK, Tudor R, Rushton A, Hayes TJ.** Comparative toxicity and pathology associated with administration of recombinant IL-2 to animals. Intern Rev Exp Pathol 1993;34A:58–72.
11. **Broxmeyer HE, Williams DE, Lu L, Cooper S, Anderson SL, Beyer GS, Hoffman R, Rubin BY.** The suppressive influences of human tumor necrosis factors on bone marrow hematopoietic progenitor cells from normal donors and patients with leukemia: synergism of tumor necrosis factor and interferon-γ. J Immunol 1986;136:4487–4495.
12. **Kurzrock R, Rosenblum MG, Sherwin SA, Rios A, Talpaz M, Quesada JR, Gutterman JU.** Pharmacokinetics, single-dose tolerance, and biological activity of recombinant gamma-interferon in cancer patients. Cancer Res 1985;45:2866–2872.
13. **Maury CP, Andersson LC, Teppo AM, Partanen S, Juvonen E.** Mechanisms of anemia in rheumatoid arthritis: demonstration of raised interleukin-1 beta concentrations in anaemic patients and of interleukin-1 mediated suppression of normal erythropoiesis and proliferation of human erythroleukaemia (HEL) cells in vitro. Ann Rheum Dis 1988;47:972–978.
14. **Terrell TG, Green JD.** Comparative pathology of recombinant murine interferon-γ in mice and recombinant human interferon-γ in cynomolgus monkeys. Intern Rev Exp Pathol 1993;34B:73–101.
15. **Semenza GL.** Regulation of erythropoietin production: new insights into molecular mechanism of oxygen homeostasis. Hematol/Oncol Clin North Am 1994;8:863–884.
16. **Moritz KM, Lim GB, Wintour EM.** Developmental regulation of erythropoietin and erythropoiesis. Am J Physiol 1997;273:R1829–R1844.
17. **Porter DL, Goldberg MA.** Physiology of erythropoietin production. Seminars Hematol 1994;31:112–121.
18. **Fu P, Evans B, Lim GB, Moritz KM, Wintour EM.** The sheep erythropoietin gene: molecular cloning and effect of hemorrhage on plasma erythropoietin and renal/liver messenger RNA in adult sheep. Mol Cell Endocrinol 1993; 93:107–116.
19. **Lin FK, Lin C-H, Lai P-H, Browne JK, Egrie JC, Smalling R, Fox GM, Chen KK, Castro M, Suggs S.** Monkey erythropoietin gene: cloning expression and comparison with the human erythropoietin gene. Gene 1986;44: 201–209.
20. **Jacobs K, Shoemaker C, Rudersdorf R, Neill DS, Kaufmann RJ, Mufson A, Seehra J, Jones SS, Hewick R, Fritsch EF, Kawakite M, Shimizu T, Miyake T.** Isolation and characterization of genomic and cDNA clones of human erythropoietin. Nature 1985;313:806–810.
21. **Wen D, Boissel JPR, Tracey TE, Gruninger RH, Mulcahy LS, Czelusniak J, Goddman M, Bunn HF.** Erythropoietin structure-function relationships: high degree of sequence homology among mammals. Blood 1993;82:1507–1516.
22. **Wenger RH, Gassmann M.** Oxygen(es) and the hypoxia-inducible factor-1. Biol Chem 1997;378:609–616.
23. **Beru N, McDonald J, Lacombe C, Goldwasser E.** Expression of the erythropoietin gene. Mol Cell Biol 1986;6: 2571–2575.
24. **Pagel H, Jelkmann W, Weiss C.** A comparison of the effects of renal artery constriction and anemia on the production of erythropoietin. Pflugers Arch 1988;413:62–66.
25. **Gregoli PA, Bondurant MC.** The role of Bcl-X_L and apopain in the control of erythropoiesis by erythropoietin. Blood 1997;90:630–640.
26. **Zon L.** Developmental biology of hematopoiesis. Blood 1995;86:2876–2981.
27. **Bessis M.** Living blood cells and their ultrastructure. Springer-Verlag, New York, 1973.
28. **Hanspal M.** Importance of cell-cell interactions in regulation of erythropoiesis. Curr Op Hematol 1997;4:142–147.
29. **Ohta M, Sakai T, Saga Y, Aizawa S-I, Saito M.** Suppression of hematopoietic activity in tenascin-C-deficient mice. Blood 1998;91:4074–4083.
30. **Verfaillie C, Hurley R, Bhatia R, McCarthy JB.** Role of bone marrow matrix in normal and abnormal hematopoiesis. Crit Rev Oncology/Hematology 1994;16:201–224.
31. **Jain NC.** Erythropoiesis and its regulation. In: Schalm's veterinary hematology, 4th ed. Philadelphia: Lea & Febiger, 1986;487–513.
32. **Bessis M, Lessin LS, Beutler E.** Morphology of the erythron. In: Williams WJ, Beutler E., Erslev A, Lichtman MA, eds. Hematology. New York: McGraw-Hill, 1983;257–279.
33. **Fresco R.** Electron microscopy in the diagnosis of the bone marrow disorders of the erythroid series. Seminars Hematol 1981;18:279–292.

34. **Koury ST, Koury MJ, Bondurant MC.** Morphological changes in erythroblasts during erythropoietin-induced terminal differentiation in vitro. Exp Hematol 1988;16:758–763.
35. **Stohlman F Jr.** Some aspects of erythrokinetics. Semin Hematol 1967;4:304–314.
36. **Fukamachi H, Urabe A, Saito T, Takaku F, Kubota M.** Burst promoting activity in anemia and polycythemia. Int J Cell Cloning 1986;4:74–81.
37. **Means RT Jr, Krantz SB.** Progress in understanding the pathogenesis of the anemia of chronic disease. Blood 1992;80:1639–1647.
38. **Faquin WC, Schneider TJ, Goldberg MA.** Effect of inflammatory cytokines on hypoxia-induced erythropoietin production. Blood 1992;79:1987–1994.
39. **Ludwig H, Fritz E, Leitgeb C, Pecherstorfer M, Samonigg H, Schuster J.** Prediction of response to erythropoietin treatment in chronic anemia of cancer. Blood 1994;84:1056–1063.
40. **de la Chapelle A, Traskelin AL, Juconen E.** Truncated erythropoietin receptor causes dominantly inherited benign human erythropoiesis. Proc Natl Acad Sci USA 1993;90:4495–4499.
41. **Partanen S, Juvonen E, Ikkala E, Ruutu T.** Spontaneous erythroid colony formation in the differential diagnosis of erythrocytosis. Eur J Haematol 1989;42:327–330.
42. **Kaneko JJ, Mattheeuws DRG.** Iron metabolism in normal and porphyric calves. Amer J Vet Res. 1966;27:923–929.
43. **Kaneko JJ, Zinkl JG, Keeton KS.** Erythrocyte porphyrin and erythrocyte survival in bovine erythropoietic porphyria. Am J Vet Res 1971;32:1981–1985.
44. **Mock DM, Lankford GL, Burmeister LF, Strauss RG.** Circulating red cell volume and red cell survival can be accurately determined in sheep using the [14C]cyanate label. Pediatr Res 1997;41:916–921.

CHAPTER 19

Reticulocyte Response

• FIDELIA R. FERNANDEZ and CAROL B. GRINDEM

Reticulocytes are immature red blood cells (RBC) that demonstrate the characteristic reticulum of precipitated ribonucleic acid (RNA), mitochondria, and organelles with supravital stains such as new methylene blue (NMB) or brilliant cresyl blue (Fig. 19.1). Two types of reticulocytes are recognizable: aggregate and punctate. Aggregate reticulocytes are larger cells with coarsely clumped reticulum. Punctate reticulocytes are the more mature cells that have dots and granules of residual RNA. On Wright's stain, aggregate reticulocytes are bluish pink and are therefore called polychromatic or polychromatophilic red cells, polychromatophils, or polychromatocytes,[1-3] and their presence is referred to as polychromasia. Reticulocytes are often larger than mature red cells, accounting for macrocytosis and anisocytosis on blood smears. They usually appear as target cells or knizocytes and may contain nuclear remnants called Howell–Jolly bodies. Reticulocytes are metabolically more active than mature red cells, having more mitochondria and glycolytic enzyme activity to produce energy.[1]

Reticulocytes are released from the bone marrow (BM) through the action of erythropoietin in response to tissue hypoxia. They may remain in the BM 2 to 3 days before entering the blood by diapedesis through marrow sinusoids. During intense erythropoiesis, large (stress or shift) reticulocytes are prematurely released into the circulation with a small number of nucleated RBCs (nRBC). They mature to erythrocytes within 24 to 48 hours in circulation or in the spleen, where they may remain temporarily. As these cells mature, they generally become smaller; lose some surface membrane, transferrin, and fibronectin receptors and other organelles; show diminished erythrocytic enzyme activity; and attain complete hemoglobinization (Fig. 19.2).[1]

Reticulocytosis or polychromasia is the hallmark and best single indicator of intensified erythropoiesis, allowing classification of anemias into regenerative or nonregenerative types based on BM response. Its presence precludes the need for BM examination. Polychromasia may be accompanied by anisocytosis, macrocytosis, nRBCs (normoblastemia), Howell–Jolly bodies, and in ruminants, basophilic stippling. Presence of normoblastemia and Howell–Jolly bodies without adequate polychromasia indicates an underlying BM injury or disease, splenic hypofunction, myeloproliferative disease, or lead poisoning. Normoblastemia may be seen in asymptomatic miniature schnauzers and dachshunds, in various organ disorders or as a component of leukoerythroblastic reaction.[4] Basophilic stippling without accompanying polychromasia may denote dyserythropoiesis and occasionally, lead toxicity. Iron-containing Pappenheimer bodies in dyserythropoiesis appear as blue-black granules on Wright-stained RBCs and may be mistaken for retained RNA unless stained with Prussian blue. Additionally, macrocytosis without polychromasia may be an ethylenediamine tetra acetic acid (EDTA)-induced storage artifact, a feature in some poodles and miniature schnauzers that have stomatocytosis, or a manifestation of feline leukemia virus.[5]

CONDITIONS ASSOCIATED WITH RETICULOCYTOSIS OR POLYCHROMASIA

Regenerative response evidenced by polychromasia is expected in acute blood loss and hemolysis and may occur in early iron deficiency anemia, especially in young animals. Early-stage responsive anemia, however, presents as normocytic and normochromic until reticulocytes from increased erythropoiesis appear in circulation. Reticulocytosis is initially observed 2 to 4 days after sufficient insult, usually peaks at 4 to 7 days, and gradually declines in 2 to 3 weeks.[1,2,7] During peak response, red cell indices tend toward increased mean corpuscular volume (MCV) and red cell distribution width (RDW) and decreased mean corpuscular hemoglobin concentration (MCHC) because of polychromatic macrocytes.

Hemolysis elicits a greater regenerative response than blood loss probably owing to a readily available source of iron and protein for erythropoiesis. Severe hemolytic anemia of rapid onset as in intravascular hemolysis, leads to more prominent shift reticulocytosis developing in 1 to 2 days followed by significant polychromasia. Intense regenerative response has been reported in phenylhydrazine-induced Heinz body hemolytic anemia (6 to 55%), enzyme deficiencies such as phosphofructokinase (7 to 23% reticulocytes) and pyruvate kinase (15 to 50%), some hereditary membrane defects,

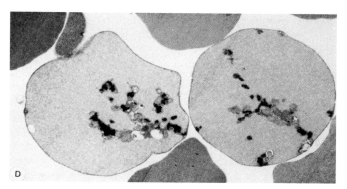

FIGURE 19.1 Aggregate reticulocytes, electron photomicrograph (EM). The characteristic reticulum consists of precipitated ribosomes (dark aggregates) and mitochondria (pale-staining structures). On NMB or other supravital stains, this reticulum appears as a dark blue network of strings or clumps of nucleoprotein. (Reprinted with permission from **Jain NC.** Schalm's Veterinary Hematology, 4th ed. Philadelphia: Lea & Febiger, 1986:497.)

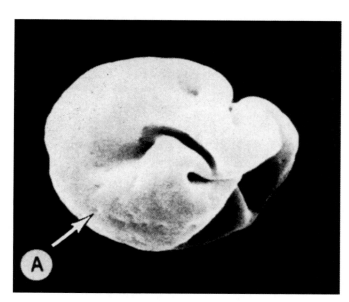

FIGURE 19.2 Reticulocyte, scanning electron microscope (SEM). This immature red cell is anucleate and irregularly shaped with numerous small pits (exemplified by **A**), infolding, and depressions on the cell surface. (Reprinted with permission from **Jain NC.** Schalm's Veterinary Hematology, 4th ed. Philadelphia: Lea & Febiger, 1986:498.)

immune-mediated anemias, zinc and copper poisoning, and hemoparasites such as *Babesia*.[1]

Internal blood loss, where breakdown products of red cells are conserved, may simulate the strong regenerative response of acute hemolytic anemia. Some red cells lost within body cavities may actually recirculate via lymphatics.[5]

Reticulocytosis, polychromasia, and normoblastemia are prominent in the neonate because of rapid replacement of fetal red cells and the demand of rapid growth.[1]

Erythropoietin-induced reticulocytosis without anemia may occur in hypoxic conditions caused by reduced oxygenation of blood or diminished tissue perfusion. Mild reticulocytosis without anemia may be seen in healthy dogs recovering from an acute hemorrhagic episode.

CONDITIONS ASSOCIATED WITH DECREASED PRODUCTION OR MATURATION OF RETICULOCYTES

In nonregenerative anemia, polychromasia is either lacking or inadequate for the degree of anemia, requiring BM examination to assess red cell production and explore possible etiologies. Anemia of chronic disease is the most common cause of nonregenerative anemia. Specific causes of nonregenerative anemia include inflammatory disease, renal disease, neoplasia, liver disease, chronic blood loss, BM depression or failure, nutritional deficiencies (Vitamins B_6, B_{12}, C, folic acid, and iron), toxicities (lead), and endocrinopathies. Early- or late-stage regenerative anemias may manifest as nonregenerative so that sequential hemograms are needed for accurate interpretation.

Whole blood transfusion may rapidly suppress reticulocyte release in circulation. This is probably because of inhibition of erythropoietin synthesis with resolution of tissue hypoxia in an anemic patient.[1]

RETICULOCYTE ENUMERATION

Reticulocyte counts can be derived manually from NMB or Wright-stained smears, or flow cytometrically and correspond to percentage of polychromasia on Wright-stained smears. Dog, cat, swine, rabbit, mouse, and rat reticulocytes are quickly and easily enumerated by flow cytometry (FCM), the current gold standard for reticulocyte enumeration in humans.[4,7–9] The reticulocyte percentage can then be multiplied by the RBC count to obtain the absolute reticulocyte count/μL of blood that allows a more accurate interpretation of response to anemia. Technique-related problems with reticulocyte counts include lack of precision and uneven distribution of reticulocytes on smears (reticulocytes tend to aggregate on the feathered edge, falsely lowering counts) and falsely elevated FCM counts caused by immature platelets, Heinz bodies, nRBCs, and hemic parasites. In cats, excitement or struggling during blood sampling can also elevate the reticulocyte counts because of the release of previously entrapped reticulocytes in the capillaries and spleen.[1] One can correct the reticulocyte count for the degree of anemia by use of the formula extrapolated from humans:

$$\text{Corrected reticulocyte } \% =$$

$$\text{reported } \% \text{ reticulocyte} \times \frac{\text{patient's reported PCV}}{\text{patient's normal PCV}}$$

If the patient's normal PCV is unknown, 45% and 37% may be used as the normal PCV for the dog and cat, respectively.

The reticulocyte production index (RPI) can also be calculated for the dog to correct for the premature release of shift reticulocytes, which require a longer time to mature in circulation. The corrected reticulocyte count is divided by the reticulocyte maturation time, which varies with the degree of anemia: PCV 45% = 1 day; 35% = 1.5 days; 25% = 2 days and 15% = 2.5 days. In the dog, an RPI of ≤1 indicates nonregenerative anemia; between 1 and 2, an active marrow with some response to anemia; >2, accelerated erythropoiesis; and ≥3, significant regenerative response as seen in hemolysis.[1,5]

SPECIES VARIATION IN RETICULOCYTE RESPONSE

Reticulocyte response varies with the degree of anemia, type, severity and duration of stimulus, species involved, and presence of concurrent disease. In general, dogs, cats, and pigs normally have few reticulocytes in circulation, whereas cattle, sheep, and goats rarely have any, and horses, none at all. Laboratory animals and other small-sized mammals, birds, and fish normally have slight to moderate polychromasia, reflecting shorter red cell survival and therefore more active erythropoiesis.[3,10] Tables 19.1 and 19.2 summarize the normal reticulocyte counts and morphology in domestic, exotic, and laboratory animals.

Dogs

Like humans, dogs respond vigorously with aggregate reticulocytosis in regenerative anemias. Punctate reticulocytes are also observed in the dog, but numbers are too few to require separate enumeration.[1,5] Basophilic stippling may occur during intense erythropoiesis and should be differentiated from lead toxicity.[1] Plumbism is suspected if polychromatic red cells and nRBCs are out of proportion to the PCV, which may remain normal. Presence of 15 RBCs with basophilic stippling/10,000 RBCs examined is suspicious and 40 RBCs with basophilic stippling/10,000 RBCs is almost pathognomonic of lead poisoning.[1] A reticulocyte count of >1% or >60,000/μL blood in the dog indicates regenerative anemia.[5] Polychromasia or reticulocytosis may be graded as

	%	Reticulocytes/μL
Slight	1–4	150,000
Moderate	5–20	300,000
Marked	>20	>500,000

Cats

Presence of both aggregate and punctate reticulocytes complicates reticulocyte enumeration and interpretation

in this species (Fig. 19.3, 19.4). Aggregate reticulocytes mature into punctate reticulocytes within 12 hours, and the latter mature into erythrocytes in approximately 10 days, thus persisting longer in circulation.[6] Aggregate reticulocytes are observed in circulation within 24 to 48 hours after blood loss or hemolysis, peak by day 4 to 6 and then return to normal by day 9 to 13.[2,7] Punctate reticulocytes, on the other hand, increase above reference range in approximately 1 week, peak on day 9 to 13, remain high until day 15, and gradually decline.[2,7] In the cat, increased aggregate reticulocyte count is interpreted as evidence of recent BM stimulation, whereas a high punctate count implies a regenerative response 2 to 4 weeks earlier.[2] As in dogs, basophilic stippling may be seen in intense regenerative anemia.[1] Reticulocyte response may be graded as

	%	Aggregate/μL	Punctate/μL
Slight	0.5–2	50,000	500,000
Moderate	3–4	100,000	1,000,000
Marked	>4	200,000	1,500,000

Horses

The horse does not respond with polychromasia even with significant blood loss or hemolysis. Sometimes the only evidence of responsive anemia is moderate to significant anisocytosis or rarely, macrocytosis based on MCV. Red cell distribution width and the RBC histogram may be used to detect regenerative response to blood loss or hemolytic anemia. There is an increase in RDW and MCV 2 weeks after the insult and lasts for 4 to 6 weeks.[11] Evaluation of the BM is necessary for accurate assessment of regenerative response. Erythroid hyperplasia and reticulocyte counts >5% indicate increased erythropoiesis.[1]

Pigs

Reticulocytosis, accompanied by nRBCs and anisocytosis with macrocytosis, characterizes regenerative anemias secondary to blood loss or hemolysis in this species.[1] Conditions associated with this response include gastric ulcers, enteric and hemic parasites, gastroenteritis, and coagulopathies (warfarin poisoning) among others. Inadequate source of dietary iron in growing pigs and chronic blood loss may lead to nonregenerative anemia.

Ruminants

Magnitude of reticulocyte response is less than in the dog or cat; therefore, observation of some reticulocytes in blood is sufficient evidence of regenerative response in this species.[1] The usual morphologic feature of regenerative anemia is macrocytic and hypochromic as in dogs and cats. Basophilic stippling (punctate basophilia), evident as variably sized dark blue dots in the

TABLE 19.1	Normal Reticulocyte Count and Morphology in Domestic and Exotic Animals	

Species/ Reference	Normal Reticulocyte Count (% or Absolute/μL)	Remarks
Dog 1, 8, 9, 24	Adults: 0–1.5 *Beagles:* <1 year Male: 0.5 ± 0.46 Female: 0.7 ± 0.47 >1 year Male: 0.5 ± 0.43 Female: 0.5 ± 0.60 Flow cytometric counts: Retic-Count®: 1.9 ± 0.9 (133,000 ± 41,000 μL) Sysmex R-1000: 0.62 ± 0.25 (45,000 ± 18,550/μL)	Reticulocytes are periodically released into the blood stream every 14 days and mature in approximately 30 hours (19–43 hrs) once in circulation. Puppies can have reticulocyte counts as high as 7%. Manual counts are based on aggregate reticulocytes only. Flow cytometric counts are always higher. There are no "0" counts with this procedure.
Cat 1, 7	Aggregate: 0.2–1.6 Punctate: 1.4–10.8 Flow cytometric counts: Aggregate: 0.1–0.5 (8,487–42,120/μL) Punctate: 2–17 (225,400–1,268,584/μL)	A continuum of maturation occurs in circulation. Punctate reticulocytes are the predominant and more mature form. Aggregate and punctate reticulocytes are enumerated separately. Polychromasia on Wright's stain correlates only with the aggregate reticulocytes.
Horse 1, 11	0 in peripheral blood BM film: average (ave.) of 0.5/100× objective oil immersion field (OIF)	Macrocytic red cells, anisocytosis and increased RDW may be observed in blood smears and CBC[a] of horses that have responsive anemia. Reticulocyte maturation is completed in the BM.
Cow 1	0 to rare	Basophilic stippling is part of the regenerative response and accompanies polychromasia or reticulocytosis
Goat 1, 25	Adults: 0 *Dwarf* 0–7 days: 0.6 ± 0.36 7–30 days: 0.2 ± 0.05 *Danish landrace* 0–7 days: 1.0 ± 0.56 7–30 days: 0.4 ± 0.24	Polychromasia, anisocytosis, and reticulocytosis (aggregate and punctate present on NMB smears) are common in neonates but diminish with age. Breed and sex affect counts. Rare to see reticulocytosis caused by anemia in adult goats.
Sheep 1	<1.0 may be found at birth Adults: 0	Basophilic stippling accompanies polychromasia or reticulocytosis as part of regenerative response. As much as 9%, including punctate reticulocytes, are seen in lambs 2–7 days of age.
Pig 1, 9	0–1 Sysmex R-1000: 1.65 ± 0.40 (121,010 ± 28,810/μL)	Red cell production is active during the suckling stage. Polychromatophils accompanied by nRBCs and Howell–Jolly bodies are normally seen in circulation from birth to 3 months of age.
Llama 1, 14	<1/OIF in peripheral blood 1–15 (ave. 5)/OIF in BM All ages: 0–2.4 1 month: 0–7.5 Juvenile: (6–18 mos) and adults: 0–0.4	Polychromatic red cells are round but elongate and lose polychromasia as they mature.
Reptile 26	*Desert tortoise:* <1	Polychromatophils are round, smaller, and more basophilic than mature RBCs; they have large nuclei and may appear folded. Reticulum forms a ring around the nucleus on NMB.
Bird 1, 19	Slight polychromasia is typical *Chicken (Gallus gallus domesticus):* 0–0.6 (ave. of 0)	Polychromatophils are round to oval with more basophilic cytoplasm and less coarse nuclear chromatin than mature red cells. At least five clumps of reticulum or a complete ring of reticulum around the nucleus should be seen to call it a reticulocyte.
Fish 20	Slight to moderate amount of anisocytosis and polychromasia is normal in many species.	Polychromasia is indicated by rounder RBCs with pale blue cytoplasm and more vesicular nuclear chromatin.

[a] CBC, complete blood count.

cytoplasm of Wright-stained RBCs, is typical in ruminants during vigorous erythropoiesis and represents retained RNA (Fig. 19.5). Both polychromatophils and red cells with basophilic stippling are enumerated to assess regenerative response. Peripheral polychromasia or reticulocytosis is notable after acute hemorrhage or hemolytic injury, and varies with the degree of insult and age of the animal. Howell–Jolly bodies and normoblastemia may also be seen. Goats are reported to have as much as 5 to 6% reticulocyte count in response to acute blood loss.[1] While most hemoparasites elicit a responsive anemia because of hemolysis, *Typanosoma vivax, T. congolense,* and *T. brucei* induce little to no reticulocyte response in sheep, calves, and goats.[12,13] Dyserythropoiesis and macrophage destruction of early red cell precursors may be partly responsible.[12]

TABLE 19.2   Normal Reticulocyte Counts in Laboratory Animals

Species/Reference	Normal Reticulocyte Count (% or Absolute/μL)	Remarks
Rats 1, 8, 9, 22, 24, 27	*Rattus norvegicus* <6 months Male: 2 ± 1.23 Female: 1.6 ± 0.87 6–18 months Male: 1.7 ± 1.29 Female: 1.9 ± 3.55 *Long-Evans rats* both sexes, 7–12 months: 2.4 ± 1.5 *Sprague-Dawley rats* both sexes, 7–12 months: 2.2 ± 1.2 *Fischer 344* rats 2 weeks: 16.5 ± 6.1 8 weeks: 1.4 ± 1.1 121 weeks: 5.3 ± 3.7 *Wistar* 3 days: 90 15 days: 35 30 days: 14 90–180 days: 8–9 *Wistar* flow cytometric counts: Retic-Count®, 6–12 weeks: 4.8 ± 1.6 (352,000 ± 128,000/μL) Sysmex R-1000: 2.52 ± 0.34 (205,460 ± 37,440/μL)	Albino rats at birth have reticulocyte count approaching 99%, decreasing to 25% at weaning (21 days) and to 3% by 70 days of age. 6–40% reticulocytes are seen in the youngest Long–Evans (L–E) and Sprague–Dawley (S–D) strains with highest counts at 6 weeks, reaching a plateau at 3 months. Adult L–E females have greater reticulocyte counts (4.3 ± 1.4%) than adult males (2 ± 1%). <2 week-old F344 rats show a high degree of anisocytosis, poikilocytosis, and polychromasia with some nRBCs. Values up to 10% are normal in Wistar rats and daily fluctuations up to 5% in the same rat is usual.
Hamster (Syrian) 24	All ages: Male: 1.7 ± 1.18 Female: 1.8 ± 1.24	Newborn hamsters have prominent polychromasia accompanied by 10–30% normoblastemia. Polychromasia is also seen in adults but normoblastemia is <2%.
Rabbits 1, 9, 24	*New Zealand White* all ages: Male: 1.9 ± 1.02 Female: 2.1 ± 0.88 *Wild jack rabbits* Both sexes, <1 year: 0.3 ± 0.74 Flow cytometric counts: Sysmex R-1000: 2.63 ± 1 (169,490 ± 58,820)	Significant variation in normal values influenced by breed. Some polychromasia occurs in peripheral blood.
Guinea pigs 1, 22	7–12 months both sexes: 2.3 ± 1.9 *Mixed strain* adult: 1.8 ± 2.2 *Albino* adult: 2.3 ± 0.3	Reticulocyte values are highest in the neonate and immature animals, decreasing to normal values between 2 and 3 months of age.
Mice 24	*Regular yellow* 7–12 months both sexes: 4.7 ± 3.3 *Mus musculus* <1 year Male: 3.3 ± 1.29 Female: 2.7 ± 1.05 *Parkes strain* 7–12 months both sexes: 6.7 ± 4.0 >1 year Male: 3.4 ± 1.14 Female: 3.5 ± 1.51	Some amount of polychromasia and a moderate anisocytosis are normally seen in blood smears. Up to 90% reticulocytes are seen in the newborn, decreasing to 2–4% in the adult mouse. Normal counts vary among strains of mice.
Wooly opossum 28	*Caluromys derbianus*: 5.9 (1.2–11.6) 0–2/high power field (hpf) to 5–10/hpf	Polychromatic RBCs are a consistent finding along with occasional nRBCs (0–0.5/100 RBC); blood cell morphology resembles human and a variety of monkeys.
Nonhuman primates 22, 24	*Cynomolgus monkey* all ages: Male: 0.5 ± 0.48 Female: 0.5 ± 0.62 Rhesus monkey (*Macaca mulata*): 0.1–2 Bushbaby (*Galago sp*): 1–2 Lemur: <1 Marmosets: 1–1.1 Owl monkey: 2.4 ± 1.7 Squirrel monkey: 0–3.5 (ave. 0.97)	Polychromatophils are rare and nRBCs are not seen in health. In the rhesus monkey, reticulocyte count increases within 24 hours postpartum and continues to rise up to 7 days then returns to normal as the PCV increases.

Llamas

Regenerative response is variable in both natural and experimental iron deficiency and blood loss anemias.[14] Reticulocytosis accompanied by normoblastemia [20/100 white blood cells (WBCs)] may occur within 1 week and rapidly disappear after experimental blood loss. Anemia is regenerative in llamas undergoing repeated phlebotomy but nonregenerative in naturally occurring iron deficiency.[15] Eperythrozoonosis presents with a virtually nonregenerative anemia and may accompany inflammatory disease, hypoproteinemia, chronic weight loss, and iron deficiency.[16]

Birds

All stages of erythrocyte maturation from erythroblasts to mature red cells may be found in circulation; thus,

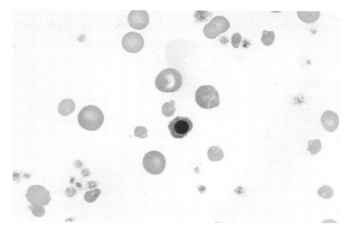

FIGURE 19.3 Cat, Heinz body hemolytic anemia induced by a propylene glycol-containing stool softener, Wright's stain. The large immature polychromatic red cells surround a metarubricyte. Note the anisocytosis, occasional ghost red cell, and several Heinz bodies occurring as pale-staining protrusions along the margins of red cells or free in the background. Excessive Heinz bodies falsely elevate and thus invalidate flow cytometric reticulocyte counts.

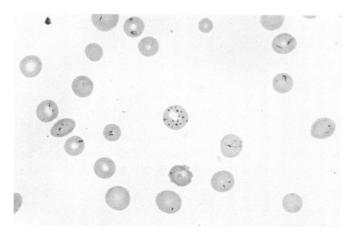

FIGURE 19.5 Bovine theileriosis, Wright's stain. The red cell in the center demonstrates basophilic stippling, which represents retained RNA. Polychromasia and basophilic stippling are both enumerated to assess the ruminant regenerative response to anemia.

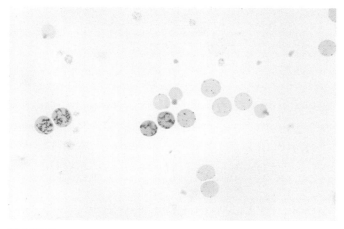

FIGURE 19.4 Cat, Heinz body hemolytic anemia, NMB stain. The aggregate reticulocytes, visible as cells with a dense network of precipitated RNA correlate with the polychromatic red cells on Wright's stain. Punctate reticulocytes, which are the more mature cells, exhibit diffusely scattered dots and are counted separately. The Heinz bodies appear as large, pale blue-staining inclusions on the red cell membrane or free in the background with the platelets.

the presence of an occasional immature red cell cannot be construed as abnormal or pathologic.[17] Because all cells are nucleated and stainable granules may persist in the cytoplasm of most red cells through the maturation stages, the definition of reticulocytes is stricter than in mammals (Table 19.1). Smaller birds, similar to smaller mammals, normally show greater erythropoietic activity than larger ones. Chicken regenerative response is so vigorous, recovery from anemia is attained in approximately 1 week.[17] Regenerative anemia evidenced by basophilic erythroblasts is often found in young birds but

is self-limiting.[3] Polychromasia may be graded, on the basis of numbers of polychromatic RBCs seen per 100× objective oil immersion field, as slight (5 to 10), moderate (approximately 10 to 20), or significant (when 40 to 50% of RBCs are polychromatic).[18] A polychromatophilic index of 1 to 5 may also be used to evaluate erythropoiesis in birds.[19] Blood loss may present with a polychromatophilic index of 3 to 5 (reticulocytes >10%). Regenerative anemia in birds is also associated with hemolysis, bacterial infections, blood parasites such as *Plasmodium*, toxic agents (acute aflatoxicosis), coagulopathies, and recovery phase of nonregenerative anemia.[10] Autoimmune hemolytic anemia has not yet been reported in pet birds.[10] Conversely, nonregenerative anemias, with polychromatophilic index of 1 to 2 (<10% reticulocytes) may be seen in chronic disorders, nutritional deficiency, viral infection, chloramphenicol administration, toxic agents, fasting or starving, and avian leukosis complex.[10,19] Birds develop anemia of chronic disease more easily than mammals because of the short RBC life span. This type of anemia is seen in aspergillosis, tuberculosis, chlamydiosis, and chronic liver disease.[10]

Fish

Numerous immature erythrocytes or increased polychromasia also characterizes regenerative response in the fish.[20] Evaluation of reticulocyte response is difficult for lack of published baseline data even for basic hematologic parameters. Most published material pertains to the food variety of fish. In general, normal fish PCV is lower than mammalian, in the vicinity of 25%; thus a PCV of <20% is interpreted as anemia and 45%, as a sign of hemoconcentration. Species, age, sex, photoperiod, and environmental factors such as water temperature and seasonal variation may alter red cell parameters. Mitotic figures are occasionally noted within red cells in circulation, and immature RBCs have been shown to use tritiated thymidine, suggesting that erythropoiesis can possibly occur in circulation.[20]

Reptiles

The degree of polychromasia is the best indicator of accelerated erythropoiesis. Immature red cells are often seen in reptiles responding to anemia and in the blood films of the young. Often, binucleation and abnormal nuclear division or mitotic activity are seen in RBCs of reptiles with significant regenerative anemia or inflammatory disease or in reptiles awakening from hibernation.[21] As in birds, it is difficult to interpret samples stained for reticulocytes in reptiles because virtually all red cells contain reticular material. By definition, a reptilian reticulocyte has a distinct ring of reticulum surrounding the nucleus.[21] There is little known information about reticulocyte response in reptiles.

Laboratory Animals

Polychromasia is typical in blood films of normal laboratory animals and is related to the shorter life span of their red cells. Reticulocytosis of as much as 98% is observed in rats at birth, and decreases with age.[22] Significant polychromasia in mice has been associated with blood parasites such as *Plasmodium*, which preferentially invades reticulocytes.[22] Red cell longevity in hamsters increases significantly from approximately 60 to 70 days to as many as 160 days during hibernation. Hence the number of circulating reticulocytes greatly decreases during hibernation after which it rises again. Massive blood withdrawal does not elicit reticulocytosis unless hibernation is terminated.[22] The Fisher 344 rats with mononuclear cell leukemia have a severe form of immune-mediated hemolytic anemia characterized by significant polychromasia (occasionally exceeding 80%), normoblastemia, and spherocytosis.[23]

Ferrets

Female ferrets are prone to a nonregenerative anemia from BM aplasia secondary to hyperestrogenism induced by prolonged estrus.[6,7]

REFERENCES

1. **Jain NC.** Erythrocyte physiology and changes in disease. Essentials of veterinary hematology. Philadelphia: Lea & Febiger, 1993.
2. **Alsaker RD, Lober J, Stevens JB, et al.** A comparison of polychromasia and reticulocyte counts in assessing erythrocyte regenerative response in the cat. J Vet Med Assoc 1977;170(1):39–41.
3. **Hawkey CM, Dennett TB.** Color atlas of comparative veterinary hematology. Ames, IA: Iowa State University Press, 1989.
4. **Mandell CP, Jain NC, Farver TB.** The significance of normoblastemia and leukoerythroblastic reaction in the dog. J Am Anim Hosp Assoc 1989; 25:665–672.
5. **Tvedten H.** Erythrocyte Disorders. In: Willard MD, Tvedten H, Turnwald GH,eds. Small animal clinical diagnosis by laboratory methods. 2nd ed. Philadelphia: W.B. Saunders, 1994:31–49.
6. **Reagan WJ, Vap LM, Weiser MG.** Flow cytometric analysis of feline reticulocytes. Vet Pathol 1992;29:503–508.
7. **Perkins PC, Grindem CB, Cullins LD.** Flow cytometric analysis of punctate and aggregate reticulocyte responses in phlebotomized cats. Am J Vet Res 1995;56(12):1564–1569.
8. **Evans GO, Fagg R.** Reticulocyte counts in canine and rat blood made by flow cytometry. J Comp Pathol 1994;111:107–111.
9. **Fuchs A, Eder H.** Zahl und reifegradverteilung der retikulozyten von sechs tierarten. J Vet Med Assoc 1991;38:749–754.
10. **Hoefer HL.** Transfusions in exotic species. Probl Vet Med 1992;4(4):625–635.
11. **Easley JR.** Erythrogram and red cell distribution width of equidae with experimentally induced anemia. Am J Vet Res 1985;46(11):2378–2384.
12. **Anosa VO, Logan-Henfrey LL, Shaw MK.** A light and electron microscopic study of changes in blood and bone marrow in acute hemorrhagic Typanosoma vivax infection in calves. Vet Pathol 1992;29:33–45.
13. **Igbokwe IO, Anosa VO.** Response to anemia in experimental Typanosoma vivax infection of sheep. J Comp Pathol 1989;100:111–118.
14. **Andreasen CB, Gerros TC, Lassen ED.** Evaluation of bone marrow cytology and stainable iron content in healthy adult llamas. Vet Clin Pathol 1994; 23(2):38–42.
15. **Morin DE, Garry FB, Weiser MG.** Hematologic responses in llamas with experimentally-induced iron-deficiency anemia. Vet Clin Pathol 1993; 22(3):81–86.
16. **Reagan WJ, Garry F, Thrall MA, et al.** The clinicopathologic, light, and scanning electron microscopic features of eperythrozoonosis in four naturally infected llamas. Vet Pathol 1990;27:426–431.
17. **Lucas AM, Jamroz C.** Atlas of avian hematology. Washington, DC: US Department of Agriculture, 1961:17–30.
18. **Lane RA.** Avian hematology. Basic cell identification, white blood cell count determinations, and clinical pathology. In: Rosskoff W, Woerpel R, eds. Disease of cage and aviary birds. 3rd ed. Baltimore: Williams and Wilkins, 1996:739–765.
19. **Dein FJ.** Laboratory manual of avian hematology. East Northport, NY: Association of Avian Veterinarians, 1984.
20. **Campbell TW.** Tropical fish medicine. Fish cytology and hematology. Vet Clin North Am Small Anim Pract 1988;18(2):349–364.
21. **Campbell TW.** Clinical Pathology. In: Mader DR, ed. Reptile medicine and surgery. Philadelphia, PA: WB Saunders, 1996:248–257.
22. **Loeb WF, Bannerman RM, Rininger BF and Johnson AJ.** Hematologic disorders. The evaluation of the hemic system. In: Benirschke K, Garner FM, Jones TC, eds. Pathology of laboratory animals. Vol 1. New York: Springer Verlag, 1978:890–978.
23. **Stromberg PC, Vogtsberger LM, Marsh LR, et al.** Pathology of the mononuclear cell leukemia of Fisher rats. II. Hematology. Vet Pathol 1983;20:709–717.
24. **Wolford ST, Schroer RA, Gohs FX, et al.** Reference range data base for serum chemistry and hematology values in laboratory animals. J Toxicol Environ Health 1986;18:161–188.
25. **Mbassa GK, Poulsen JSD.** Erythrocyte maturation in neonatal dwarf and landrace kids. Vet Res Commun 1991;15:239–247.
26. **Alleman AR, Jacobson ER, Raskin RE.** Morphologic and cytochemical characteristics of blood cells from the desert tortoise (Gopherus agassizii). Am J Vet Res 1992;53(9):1645–1651.
27. **Turton JA, Hawkey CM, Hart MG, et al.** Age-related changes in the haematology of the female F344 rats. Lab Anim 1989;23:295–301.
28. **Rothstein R, Hunsaker D II.** Baseline Hematology and blood chemistry of the South American wooly opossum, Caluromys derbianus. Lab Anim Sci 1992;22(2):227–232.

CHAPTER 20

Red Blood Cell Survival and Destruction

• JOHN A. CHRISTIAN

Mammalian red blood cells (RBCs) leave hemopoietic tissues as anuclear, concentrated solutions of hemoglobin contained within protein-stabilized lipid bilayers. Each cell typically circulates through the vascular system thousands of times over a finite period before being dissembled and recycled by the mononuclear phagocyte system found predominantly in the spleen, liver, and bone marrow. The time in circulation (i.e., RBC survival or life span) varies characteristically with species. Although numerous, specific pathologic events are known to decrease RBC survival, it is less clear what factors determine RBC life span in health, why this parameter varies between species, and what events signal the termination of RBC circulation.

COMPARATIVE AND GENERAL ASPECTS OF RBC LIFE SPAN

Comparative studies have demonstrated that RBC life span correlates consistently with several physiologic parameters. For centuries it has been recognized that, across species, increasing size is generally associated with increasing species longevity—larger species of animals live longer than smaller species.[1] (Note: Longevity will be used exclusively to describe the life span of animals.) More recently, studies have illustrated that RBC life span also varies in concert with species size and longevity.[2] For instance, the RBC life span is approximately 140 to 145 days for horses, 130 days for cows, 120 days for humans, 100 to 115 days for dogs, 73 days for cats, and 43 days for mice. The positive correlation between size and longevity has most commonly been attributed to metabolic rate (and its associated rate of oxidative injury), which is inversely proportional to size and longevity. Thus, small species have higher metabolic rate and greater cumulative oxidative stress, leading to more rapid aging and shorter longevity. It is reasonable to hypothesize that the associations among species size, metabolic rate, and oxidative stress could mechanistically help explain the positive correlations between longevity and RBC life span.

Experimental evidence does, in fact, suggest that RBC life span in health may be influenced by RBC antioxidant status and further that this may be influenced by corporal aging. Kurata et al[3] found that RBC potential life span in several mammals correlated significantly with the species RBC levels of superoxide dismutase (SOD), glutathione peroxidase, and glutathione. RBCs from old rats are reported to have lower quantities of several antioxidant enzymes compared with young rat RBCs.[4] Reticulocytes from old rats have lower SOD activity, and increased quantities of catalytically inactive SOD, suggesting an age-associated defect in erythropoiesis.[4] These differences are associated with differences in RBC viability as evidenced by a 40 to 60% shorter RBC life span in old mice and rats versus young animals.[5,6] A similar pattern of shorter RBC life span with age has been reported for the greyhound as well.[7] Limited studies suggest that dogs also experience age-associated changes in oxidation parameters. For example, 9-year-old male, but not female, beagles are reported to have lower levels of glutathione and higher levels of malondialdehyde (an end product of lipid peroxidation) than do 1-year-old beagles.[8] RBC glutathione peroxidase and SOD activities were, however, higher in both male and female 9-year-old dogs (highest in females).

AGING CHANGES IN CIRCULATING RED BLOOD CELLS

RBCs in blood smears from normal animals represent a uniform distribution of cell ages with minimal or no microscopically discernible changes in morphology past the polychromatophilic stage of maturation. In spite of the morphologic similarity of circulating RBCs, senescence-based changes do occur that trigger the removal of old cells while generally sparing young and mature cells. Biochemical, physiologic, physical or structural, and immunologic features of normal RBCs have been scrutinized for decades to characterize RBC senescence and to identify the signal(s) that trigger removal of the oldest cells from circulation. Dozens of alterations have been described in reportedly old RBCs yet a consensus as to which changes are real and, further, which ones are most important in aging and clearance of RBCs remains surprisingly controversial.

Not all circulating RBCs, however, are removed exclusively based on cell age (senescence-based clearance). In most species of mammals, a variable proportion of RBCs leave circulation independently of cell age (random clearance). Although the mechanism for random clearance is mainly speculative, the degree of random clearance does appear to correlate positively with metabolic rate.[2] Higher rates of random loss are therefore found in smaller species (e.g., rabbits and rodents) and, because senescent and random clearance cannot be readily distinguished, its presence confounds studies attempting to characterize mechanisms for senescence-based clearance.

The plethora of alterations reportedly present in senescent RBCs are often difficult to compare critically, largely because researchers use different methodologic approaches, species, and reference cell populations for comparisons. Isolation of the most dense circulating RBCs by density-gradient centrifugation has been the most popular method for collecting presumably senescent RBCs. This has been justified primarily based on early human studies suggesting that as radiolabeled cohorts of young red cells aged, fractionation on density gradients resulted in increasing enrichment of labeled cells in the more dense centrifugation fractions.[9] Although rarely reiterated, the authors also noted a wide variability in the consistency of this observation. Supporting information came from an observation that the most dense fraction of human RBCs had short survival after autologous reinfusion.[10] Nevertheless, the significance of the correlation between the RBC's density and age and the efficacy of density-gradient centrifugation for isolating pure populations of senescent RBCs has remained controversial. A failure to demonstrate quantitatively the relation between cell density and cell age remains a critical caveat for this approach. Straightforward proof that the 1% most dense cells in circulation are the oldest cells is lacking. Furthermore, assuming cell density is a distinguishing feature of old RBCs, the methodologies and protocols employed clearly vary in their efficacy for isolating the targeted dense RBCs.[11,12]

Creative methods for allowing retrievable populations of cells to age for defined periods in circulation have been developed in animal models to help resolve these problems. Serial hypertransfusion of rats, mice, and rabbits, resulting in polycythemic shutdown of erythropoiesis over the life span of circulating erythrocytes, has allowed retrieval of cells clearly at the end of their normal life span.[13–15] Hypertransfused rat RBCs do show increasing cell density (measured by MCHC) early, not late, in the RBC life span, suggesting primarily a maturation rather than a senescence change.[13] Note that in many density-gradient-based studies the processes of maturation and senescence are confounded because of comparison of the most dense RBCs with the least dense (reticulocyte enriched) cells. Hypertransfused mice also showed minimal age-associated changes in RBC density profiles.[14,16]

With a different approach, RBC senescence in rabbits and dogs has been evaluated by covalent linking of biotin to RBC membranes.[17,18] After defined periods of circulation, biotinylated RBCs can be isolated from other cells on the basis of affinity to avidin support and analyzed. The biotinylated cells can also be distinguished from nonlabeled cells by means of a secondary avidin label conjugated to microbeads or a fluorescent probe. This latter approach has been used effectively to measure RBC life span by flow cytometry, circumventing the need for radiolabeling.[18–20]

For the relation between cell age and cell density in rabbits to be critically evaluated, biotinylated RBC cohorts produced by treatment with phenylhydrazine were subjected to density-gradient centrifugation at various intervals of the RBC life span. During the last 10 days of circulation, the percentage of old biotinylated RBCs found in the most dense fractions of Percoll–Hypaque density gradients was only twofold to threefold greater than circulating levels of biotinylated RBCs, and they only composed approximately one third of the RBCs in the dense fraction, as measured by a bead-binding assay.[21] Although rabbit RBCs appear to show some increase in density with cell age, this method of isolation did not appear to provide effective enrichment for old cells. The enrichment would have been even less effective if a random-age population of cells rather than a young cohort had been biotinylated. Conversely, the proportion of biotinylated cells in dense fractions may have been underestimated because the bead-binding assay is somewhat insensitive to biotinylated cells compared with more recently developed flow cytometric methods.[18] The canine biotinylation model has recently demonstrated quantitatively that the 1% most dense RBCs fractionated on arabinogalactan gradients are at least moderately enriched for old RBCs.[22] More than 75% of these dense cells were between 86 to 115 days old with a mean cell age of approximately 101 days. Although clearly enriched for old cells, it is still unclear if critical changes occurring in the last day or so of RBC survival would be well represented in this population.

Although density-gradient centrifugation has been widely used as the preferred approach to the study of RBC senescence, it should be recognized that the correlation between cell density and cell age remains rather equivocal and may vary with species. Also, few studies use carefully validated methods that clearly purify the targeted population for analysis.

MECHANISMS FOR RBC CLEARANCE

Based on evidence that cell density and cell age were positively correlated,[9] early RBC aging studies concentrated heavily on identifying worn-out cells with severely compromised rheologic abilities. Even rather recent, comparative studies have confirmed that some rheologic compromise accompanies cell aging, but the magnitude and significance of these changes in explaining RBC clearance remain equivocal. With ektacytometry, decreases in deformability have been reported for in vivo, aged rabbit biotinylated RBCs; hypertransfused mouse RBCs; and for human dense RBCs fractionated on arabinogalactan or Percoll density gradients.[12,23] Waugh and coworkers[23] showed that decreased deformability was primarily attributed to cellular dehydration. Furthermore, they used micropipette techniques to demonstrate that aged rabbit RBCs have decreased surface area (10.5%), and volume (8.4%) but no change in membrane elasticity. Dense human RBCs (MCHC >37; 0.8% of total RBCs) had slightly greater decreases in surface area (17%) and volume (25%). In both cases, changes in the two parameters were such that surface area / volume ratios (sphericity) remained fairly constant. The authors suggest that the volume loss might occur simultaneously with membrane loss such as occurs with splenic pitting. However, in other conditions in which this occurs, pitting results in a selective loss of membrane with subsequent spherocytosis. Because constant sphericity is maintained in the face of increasing hemoglobin concentration, it would seem that a selective loss of water (and electrolytes) would be necessary to explain the decreased volume in association with these aging models. Further investigations to confirm the mechanisms of surface area and volume losses are needed. Nonetheless, these findings do support common rheologic alterations in RBCs from different species collected by means of in vivo aging and density-gradient centrifugation methodologies. Specifically, it appears that decreased deformability associated with a loss of cell surface area and dehydration are characteristic features of RBC aging in several species of animals.

The relevance of these findings in explaining the ultimate removal mechanism(s) for senescent RBCs remains unclear. Earlier findings of decreased deformability in dense human RBCs provided the basis for reviewing factors that affect RBC deformability and the ability of RBCs to traverse narrow sinusoids.[24] It was concluded that the decrease in deformability associated with dense RBCs is insufficient to prevent passage through sinusoids or to explain RBC removal. These concerns were echoed in the above work by Waugh and coworkers.[23] Calculation of a minimum cylindrical diameter (the smallest opening through which an RBC should be able to pass) for biotinylated rabbit cohorts revealed a similar value for all cell age groups. Furthermore, although human dense RBCs did have decreased deformability, they also have a slight but significantly smaller mean minimum diameter, suggesting they may be uncompromised in their ability to traverse sinusoids. Of related interest, human hereditary ovalocytosis is characterized by RBCs with several-fold greater rigidity than normal RBCs, yet RBC life span is apparently near normal.[25] Therefore, the relation of decreased deformability to the removal of senescent, and even pathologic RBCs, remains equivocal.

In recent years, the general focus of studies has shifted from global, rheologic changes toward identification of sensitive and specific signals that trigger clearance of aging RBCs long before they become effete. This presupposes that the clearance mechanism is initiated early

enough to avoid dilution of the circulating RBC mass with dysfunctional cells. Both immunologic and nonimmunologic pathways of RBC clearance have been identified. The importance in identifying these pathways lies in the fact that many of these mechanisms are foundational for understanding similar pathways of accelerated RBC clearance in various anemias.

Gamma G Immunoglobulin Binding

Autologous immunoglobulin binding to the most dense human RBCs and increased phagocytosis of these RBCs by autologous macrophages was first described by Kay.[26] This study also reported similar gamma-G-immunoglobulin (IgG) [but not gamma M Immunoglobulin (IgM) or gamma A Immunoglobulin (IgA)]-mediated binding and phagocytosis by use of in vitro aged RBCs. Furthermore, Fab-dependent IgG binding and phagocytosis suggested the involvement of specific receptor recognition by the IgG.[27] Kay's[26] findings have support from several other density-gradient centrifugation-based studies that have also reported increased immunoglobulin binding in the most dense RBCs.[6,28] Furthermore, using the mouse hypertransfusion model of in vivo aging, Singer et al[29] identified autologous IgG only in the oldest RBCs and associated it with in vitro phagocytosis.[29] Increased IgG binding to dog RBCs older than 104 days old has been demonstrated with the dog biotinylation model, although the significance of the IgG binding in mediating phagocytosis has not been tested.[30] In contrast, with the rabbit biotinylation model, in vivo aged rabbit RBCs failed to show terminal increases in IgG binding.[31] The authors concluded that IgG accumulation is not a significant factor in the normal senescence process of rabbit RBCs. If this represents species variation in the mechanisms of RBC senescence and removal, it certainly accentuates the need for caution in extrapolating information from different studies and in establishing appropriate models for human studies.

The identity of the epitope responsible for antibody binding to senescent RBCs has been controversial. Although rarely addressed, it is not unreasonable to consider that more than one epitope may develop and that this could vary between species. The anion transport protein (band 3 on polyacrylamide electrophoresis) has received the most support as an important site in the opsonization process, although other sites such as glycophorin A and aminophospholipids have also been proposed. Band 3 reportedly becomes antigenic through either proteolytic cleavage, revealing a 62-kd immunoreactive fragment, or by horizontal redistribution of the transmembrane protein into immunoreactive clusters. Exposure of the cryptic 62-kd antigen by proteolysis is proposed to occur as a consequence of cumulative oxidation injury.[32] Interestingly, cat RBCs exposed to activated neutrophils show evidence of proteolysis and increased IgG binding.[33–35] The changes, which appear to contribute to accelerated clearance of RBCs in the anemia of inflammatory disease, ensued from a combination of oxidation and serine protease activity. Lower level, cumulative injury could conceivably play a role in RBC injury and clearance under normal homeostasis, as described by Kay et al.[32]

The role of band-3 clustering in initiating autologous antibody binding has been well documented in senescent and diseased RBCs.[28,36–42] It is theorized that unclustered band 3 does not sustain antibody binding because the senescent cell IgG binds weakly and requires a two-point attachment to form a stable association. Normally, the distance between band-3 molecules is too great for the binding of both Fab portions of IgG. Clustering of band 3 can be accomplished by several methods, including nucleation of denatured hemoglobin (hemichromes, Heinz bodies, see below) at the cytoplasmic domain of band 3 and by chemical agents such as zinc, mellitin, and acridine orange.[37,43,44] Oxidized, denatured hemoglobin has a specific high-affinity binding site on the cytoplasmic domain of band 3. This binding leads to a horizontal redistribution of band 3 (an integral or transmembrane protein) into a clustered arrangement that is then recognized on the external surface by autologous antibodies. This pathway explains how an early intracellular compromise in maintaining reduced hemoglobin could initiate a morphologic change on the exofacial surface and thus lead to opsonization and phagocytosis. These changes have been identified in various conditions. The most dense human RBCs separated on arabinogalactan density fractions contain membrane aggregates that are highly enriched for hemichrome, band 3, and IgG.[28] Similar, although more pronounced, lesions are present in RBCs with pathologic, denatured hemoglobin resulting from sickle cell disease and thalassemia.[38,41,42] Evidence indicates that it is the clustering of band 3, not the oxidative effects associated with hemichrome formation, that forms the signal for IgG binding. This was demonstrated with chemical agents (acridine orange, Zn^{++}, and melittin) known to cause reversible clustering of band 3, independent of hemoglobin denaturation.[36,44] In each case, autologous antibody binding was induced by the clustered arrangement but was reversed by removal of the clustered distribution. The pathway of hemoglobin denaturation leading to band-3 clustering and opsonization is at least partially supported by in vivo RBC aging studies. Hypertransfused mouse RBCs and dog biotinylated RBCs both show similar changes of increased membrane-bound hemoglobin and increased IgG binding late in the RBC life span, although these changes have not yet been specifically colocalized to band-3 clusters.[14,45]

Opsonization of RBCs secondary to band-3 clustering may play a notable role in the pathogenesis of several hemolytic anemias of significant importance to veterinary medicine. Heinz body hemolytic anemia occurs in several species as a result of exogenous intoxicants and, in the cat, is associated with certain metabolic diseases.[46] Because Heinz bodies represent aggregates of hemichromes, nucleation of the denatured hemoglobin at the cytoplasmic domain of band 3 with subsequent clustering and opsonization is likely. Traditionally, clearance of Heinz-body-containing cells has been explained as a result of compromised deformability with subsequent pitting in the spleen. However, the role of compromised cell deformability in retarding passage of Heinz-body-containing cells through the spleen has been questioned.[47] Induction of discrete Heinz bodies by incubating normal human RBC's with phenylhydrazine led to focal rigidification, but overall RBC deformability was not significantly altered. Not until Heinz bodies covered nearly the entire inner membrane surface was total deformability compromised sufficiently for interference with normal circulatory passage to be expected. Slowed splenic transit and pitting by macrophages based on immunologic recognition of IgG localized on band-3 clusters may be a more plausible explanation for the removal of these cells.

Zinc intoxication in dogs is frequently associated with severe hemolytic anemia. The presence of strong regenerative responses, occasionally with spherocytosis, accompanied by inflammatory leukograms can contribute to the misdiagnosis of zinc intoxication as autoimmune hemolytic anemia.[48–51] However, negative Coomb's test results are consistently reported, possibly raising doubts as to the mechanism of hemolysis. Nevertheless, the well-documented role of zinc in band-3 clustering would suggest that accelerated opsonization by senescent antibody is involved. The negative Coomb's tests are predictable based on the known reversibility of zinc-induced band-3 clustering. Cells are thoroughly washed, removing zinc, prior to running the assay. The return of band 3 to a dispersed distribution would lead to elution of antibodies and a negative test result. Finally, mellitin in bee venom is another band-3 clustering agent. Although other elements in bee venom (e.g., phospholipase A_2) are clearly important in the demise of exposed RBCs, the potential for an immunologic component secondary to band-3 clustering should also be considered in the pathogenesis.

Complement

Another factor likely to be important in the efficient removal of IgG opsonized RBCs is the amplification of the signal by complement binding and activation. Turrini et al.[44] showed that when band 3 in human RBCs was clustered with ZnCl2, a sequence of IgG-binding, complement-binding, and in vitro phagocytosis followed.[44] Phagocytosis was maximal in the presence of clustered band 3, IgG, and complement. Inactivation of complement reduced phagocytosis by 80%, which demonstrated the IgG's rather weak ability to initiate phagocytosis alone, and emphasized complement's importance in amplification. However, phagocytosis was virtually eliminated if IgG or band-3 clustering were removed from the process, showing the absolute requirement for these two steps. Complement's role in the removal of RBCs through amplification of immunologic signals is not new. Decades ago it was shown that surface-bound IgG or IgM on RBCs can fix complement; such a process enhanced RBC removal from circulation.[52,53] However, the potential significance of this phenomenon in RBC senescence has only recently been uncovered. Lutz et al.[54,55] laid much of the groundwork in this area by describing the presence of C3b-IgG complexes on oxidatively stressed[54] and density-gradient-derived senescent human RBCs.[55] Then, by blocking CR1 receptors on RBCs with a monoclonal antibody, they demonstrated that these complexes must be bound by the Fab portion of the antibody. This suggests that, rather than simply representing the adsorption of non-specific immune complexes to CR1, the complexes were bound to a specific, antibody-recognized site. Finally, they liberated IgG from the complexes by ester bond cleavage and found that the released antibody primarily showed antiband-3 reactivity on immunoblots.[56] Interestingly, only low numbers of IgG (an increase of <20 IgG/RBC) were needed to stimulate significant complement deposition.[54] These findings were instructive from at least two aspects. First, band-3 protein was again identified as an antigenic determinant under the conditions described (both studies use conditions that result in hemoglobin oxidation and band-3 clustering). Second, the efficiency of antiband-3 antibodies in stimulating signal amplification through complement deposition was demonstrated. Quantitative studies on antibody binding to dense RBCs have generally reported an increase of only a few hundred IgG/RBC.[27,28] However, with amplification, this degree of antibody binding should be a more than adequate signal to initiate phagocytosis.

Oxidation

Several indications of compromised antioxidant capacity have been observed in dense and in vivo aged RBCs from various species. A few examples include decreases in total free thiol and reduced glutathione and glutathione reductase activity, and increases in methemoglobin, membrane-bound hemichrome, and lipid peroxidation byproducts.[5,28,57–59] Not all results, however, can be taken at face value. Comparisons between light (young) and dense (old) cells may confound processes of maturation versus aging. Further, some parameters (e.g., glutathione) are typically measured based on cell hemoglobin concentration. Because hemoglobin concentration of cells tends to increase, whereas total volume decreases in aging[23], this may artificially deflate values.[60]

Although there has been controversy concerning the significance of decline, if any, in antioxidant defenses,[61] the presence of irreversibly denatured hemoglobin bound to membranes is evidence of antioxidant decline. Conversion of oxyhemoglobin to methemoglobin produces superoxide radicals that, when reacted with hydrogen peroxide, produces the highly reactive hydroxyl radical.[62,63] Further injury to methemoglobin results in the formation of reversible hemichromes, irreversible hemichromes, and eventually of aggregates of irreversible hemichromes called Heinz bodies.[64] Among the numerous reports describing hemoglobin oxidant damage, at least two different effects have been described that potentially implicate different mechanisms of RBC re-

moval. These are hemoglobin-spectrin cross-linking and hemoglobin-band-3 cross-linking.

Sodium dodecyl sulfate-polyacrylamide gel electrophoresis (SDS-PAGE) of membrane samples from the most dense fraction of Percoll or hypaque density-gradient centrifugation-isolated normal human RBCs revealed irreversible spectrin-hemoglobin cross linkages.[65] To further define these changes, Synder et al[66] exposed normal human RBCs to varying concentrations of H_2O_2 (45 to 180 mM). Spectrin-hemoglobin cross-linking was again identified with evidence of increased membrane rigidity and decreased deformability. Preexposure of RBCs to carbon monoxide completely prevented the observed changes. Therefore, the authors suggested that spectrin-hemoglobin cross-linking could contribute to removal of RBCs secondary to increased membrane rigidity and the subsequent inability to traverse sinusoids. Alternatively, because hemichrome binding to the membrane is known to stimulate proteolysis, this could contribute to a cumulative breakdown in membrane integrity that eventually triggers some exofacial signal for RBC removal.

The other primary site of interaction described for oxidant-damaged hemoglobin is the integral membrane protein band 3, as mentioned above.[36,37] Hemichromes or Heinz bodies prepared by treatment with phenylhydrazine were found to have a high affinity for the cytoplasmic domain of band 3 and bind with a defined stoichiometry of approximately 2.5 hemichrome tetramers per band-3 dimer.[37] Furthermore, the cross-linking of hemichromes to band 3 induced clustering of band 3 into aggregates.[36] Pathophysiologic relevance of these in vitro manipulations has been demonstrated by identifying hemichrome-band-3 aggregates in sickle RBCs,[38,41] in thalassemic RBCs,[42] and in the 1% most dense human RBCs isolated on Stractan density gradients.[28] Significantly, clustering of band 3 induces binding of autologous antibodies (discussed above), thus linking an aging mechanism (cumulative oxidative damage to hemoglobin) with a removal mechanism (immunologic).

Peroxidation of membrane lipids could facilitate RBC removal by altering deformability[67] (decreasing the ability to traverse sinusoids) or by increasing recognition by macrophages.[68] Evidence for lipid peroxidation in aged RBCs has mainly been presented in density-gradient, centrifugation-separated RBCs and through in vitro manipulation. In comparing fractions of RBCs separated on discontinuous Stractan density gradients, the most dense cells showed increased fluorescence in RBC lipid extracts and formation of a phospholipid-malondialdehyde adduct.[59] Both of these findings represent cross-linking of membrane components with malondialdehyde, an end product of lipid peroxidation. In vitro treatment of RBCs with malondialdehyde leads to reduced deformability and reduced in vivo survivability.[67,69] In another study, treatment of human erythrocytes with H_2O_2 induced lipid peroxidation (generation of fluorescent immunopropene derivatives), methemoglobin formation, and spectrin-hemoglobin cross-linking resulting in decreased deformability and increased in vitro recognition by monocytes.[66] These authors showed that blocking lipid peroxidation using butylated hydroxytoluene did not prevent the associated alterations in deformability or phagocytosis. However, these changes were prevented by blocking hemoglobin oxidation with carbon monoxide. This suggests that although lipid peroxidation was present, hemoglobin oxidation was primarily responsible for the described membrane alterations.

Aminophospholipid Exposure

The RBC membrane lipid bilayer contains an asymmetric distribution of phospholipids under normal conditions. The outer leaflet is enriched with phosphatidylcholine and sphingomyelin, whereas the inner leaflet is enriched with the aminophospholipids phosphatidylserine (PS) and phosphatidylethanolamine. Loss of asymmetry, especially the exposure of PS at the outer leaflet, has been associated with increased clearance rates for RBCs. In vitro loading of PS in the outer leaflet of mice RBCs causes immediate recognition and phagocytosis by macrophages in vitro and in vivo.[68] In the rabbit biotinylation model, older RBCs were found to expose more PS than younger cells and the increased exposure correlated well with senescence-based removal, but not with random removal of RBCs.[70] This may well be an important mechanism for clearance of senescent RBCs, particularly in the rabbit, in which IgG binding does not appear to be a significant factor in the clearance of old cells.[31]

Desialation

Clearance of old RBCs has also been proposed to occur as a result of sialidases and glycoproteinases that are active at the external surface of the RBC. However, results of many studies in this area have been questioned because investigators have failed to remove leukocytes adequately or to include protease inhibitors during RBC preparation, making it difficult to distinguish in vivo versus in vitro changes.[71] Aminoff[72,73] who has been a strong proponent for sialoglycoconjugates playing a major role in the aging and removal of RBCs, has suggested that both immunologic and nonimmunologic mechanisms contribute to the final demise of RBCs. The working hypothesis proposed that, in addition to a uniform loss of carbohydrate from the surface of RBCs that accompanied aging-related membrane loss, there was specific loss of covalently bound sialic acid residues that occurred precipitously at the end of the RBC life span. The primary desialation reportedly occurred on glycophorin A and unmasked specific beta-galactosyl residues. These residues could be recognized both by an autoimmune, antigalactosyl IgG and by lectinlike receptors on monocytes and macrophages, leading to clearance of these RBCs from circulation, predominantly in the spleen. Others have found specific carbohydrate epitopes (poly-N-acetyllactosaminyl saccharide chains) on band 3 that bind autoantibodies and presumably would provide multivalent epitopes when band 3 is clustered.[74]

Interestingly, these band-3 carbohydrate chains on oxidized RBCs are also recognized by macrophages directly, suggesting both immunologic and nonimmunologic recognition modalities.

Energy and Metabolism

Energy, produced primarily through use of glucose, is critical to RBC stability by maintaining (a) iron in the divalent form, (b) proper electrolyte levels and thus water content, (c) low cytosolic calcium concentration, (d) sulfhydryl groups of RBC enzymes and hemoglobin in the reduced form, and (e) the normal biconcave disc shape, among others.[75] A decrease in the RBCs energy-producing capacity would have dire consequences. Considering that RBCs are subjected to repeated passages through the spleen where more harsh conditions such as mild hypoxia and lower pH exist, progressive depletion of metabolic resources (such as glycolytic enzymes) could easily be expected. For the change to be severe enough to effect RBC removal routinely, consistent decreases in adenosine triphosphate (ATP) should be evident.

Although ATP decreases in high-density RBCs versus low-density RBCs have been reported,[76] this is basically a comparison of reticulocytes versus mature to old RBCs. Based on Kreb's cycle activity being present only in reticulocytes,[75] a maturation associated decrease in ATP would be expected. Similar problems are a concern for studies evaluating activities of glycolytic enzymes.[77,78] Although some studies have shown that total ATP does decrease with increasing RBC density, if the quantity of RBC water loss is considered, the ATP concentration is actually fairly constant.[79] In contrast to studies showing decreased or normal ATP in association with increasing RBC density, a significant increase in ATP was observed during the last 10 days of survival with in vivo, aged, biotinylated rabbit RBCs.[80] This somewhat unexpected finding is attributed to decreased catabolism of adenine nucleotides by adenosine 5′ monophosphate deaminase.[81] Although the degree to which rabbit RBCs are affected may be unique, a similar phenomenon has been observed in children who have old circulating RBCs caused by transient erythroblastopenia.[82] It appears that direct evidence for a fatal depletion of energy as a major cause of RBC senescence and removal is lacking.

REFERENCES

1. **Sacher G.** Relation of lifespan to brain weight and body weight in mammals. In: Wolstenholme G, O'Connor M, eds. The lifespan of animals. Boston: Little, Brown and Company, 1959.
2. **Vacha J.** Red cell life span. In: Agar NS, Board PG, eds. Red blood cells of domestic mammals. New York: Elsevier, 1983;67–132.
3. **Kurata M, Suzuki M, Agar NS.** Antioxidant systems and erythrocyte lifespan in mammals. Comp Biochem Physiol 1993;106B(3):477–487.
4. **Glass GA, Gershon D.** Decreased enzymic protection and increased sensitivity to oxidative damage in erythrocytes as a function of cell and donor aging. Biochem J 1984;218:531–537.
5. **Abraham EC, Taylor JF, Lang CA.** Influence of mouse age and erythrocyte age on glutathione metabolism. Biochem J 1978;174:819–825.
6. **Glass G, Gershon H, Gershon D.** The effect of donor and cell age on several characteristics of rat erythrocytes. Exp Hematol 1983;11:987–995.
7. **Novinger MS, Sullivan PS, McDonald TP.** Determination of the lifespan

of erythrocytes from Greyhounds using an in vitro biotinylation technique. Am J Vet Res 1996;57:739–742.

8. **Gaal T, Speake B, Mezes M, Noble R, Surai P, Vajdovich P.** Antioxidant parameters and ageing in some animal species. Comp Haematol Int 1996; 6:208–213.

9. **Borun ER, Figueroa WG, Perry SM.** The distribution of Fe59 tagged human erythrocytes in centrifuged specimens as a function of cell age. J Clin Invest 1957;36:676–679.

10. **TenBrinke M, Regt JD.** 51Cr-half life of heavy and light human erythrocytes. Scand J Haematol 1970;7:336–341.

11. **Corash L.** Density dependent red cell separation. In: Beutler E, ed. Red cell metabolism. New York: Churchill Livingstone, 1986:90–107.

12. **Lutz HU, Stammler P, Fasler S, Ingold PM, Fehr J.** Density separation of human red blood cells on self forming Percoll gradients: correlation with cell age. Biochim Biophys Acta 1992;1116:1–10.

13. **Ganzoni AM, Oakes R, Hillman RS.** Red cell aging in vivo. J Clin Invest 1971;50:1373–1378.

14. **Morrison M, Jackson CW, Mueller TJ, et al.** Does cell density correlate with red cell age? Biomed Biochim Acta 1983;42(11/12):S107–S111.

15. **Zimran A, Torem S, Beutler E.** The in vivo ageing of red cell enzymes: direct evidence of biphasic decay from polycythaemic rabbits with reticulocytosis. Br J Haematol 1988;69:67–70.

16. **Mueller TJ, Jackson CW, Dockter ME, Morrison M.** Membrane skeletal alterations during in vivo mouse red cell aging. Increase in the 4.1a:4.1b ratio. J Clin Invest 1987;79:492–499.

17. **Suzuki T, Dale GL.** Biotinylated erythrocytes: in vivo survival and in vitro recovery. Blood 1987;70(3):791–795.

18. **Christian JA, Rebar AH, Boon GD, Low PS.** Methodological considerations for the use of canine in vivo biotinylated erythrocytes to study RBC senescence. Exp Hematol 1996;24:82–88.

19. **Russo V, Barker-Gear R, Gates R, Franco R.** Studies with biotinylated rbc: (1) Use of flow cytometry to determine posttransfusion survival and (2) Isolation using streptavidin conjugated magnetic beads. In: Magnani M, DeLoach JR, eds. The use of resealed erythrocytes as carriers and bioreactors: advances in experimental medicine and biology. Vol. 326. New York: Plenum Press, 1992:101–107.

20. **Hoffmann-Fezer G, Mysliwietz J, Mortlbauer W, et al.** Biotin labeling as an alternative nonradioactive approach to determination of red cell survival. Ann Hematol 1993;67:81–87.

21. **Dale GL, Norenberg SL.** Density fractionation of erythrocytes by percoll/hypaque results in only a slight enrichment for aged cells. Biochimi Biophys Acta 1990;1036:183–187.

22. **Christian JA, Wang J, Rettig M, Kiyatkina N, Low PS.** How old are dense RBC? The Dog's Tale. Blood 1998;92:2590–2591.

23. **Waugh RE, Mohandas N, Jackson CW, Mueller TJ, Suzuki T, Dale G.** Rheological properties of senescent erythrocytes: loss of surface area and volume with red cell age. Blood 1992;79(5):1351–1358.

24. **Nash GB, Meiselman HJ.** Red cell ageing: changes in deformability and other possible determinants of in vivo survival. Microcirculation 1981; 1(3):255–284.

25. **Mohandas N, Winardi R, Knowles D, et al.** Molecular basis for membrane rigidity of hereditary ovalocytosis. J Clin Invest 1992;89:686–692.

26. **Kay MMB.** Mechanism of removal of senescent cells by human macrophages in situ. Proc Natl Acad Sci U S A 1975;72(9):3521–3525.

27. **Kay MMB.** Role of physiologic autoantibody in the removal of senescent human red cells. J Supramolecular Structure 1978;9:555–567.

28. **Kannan R, Yuan J, Low PS.** Isolation and partial characterization of antibody and globin-enriched complexes from membranes of dense human erythrocytes. Biochem J 1991;278:57–62.

29. **Singer JA, Jennings LK, Jackson CE, Dockter ME, Morrison M, Walker WS.** Erythrocyte homeostasis: antibody-mediated recognition of the senescent state by macrophages. Proc Natl Acad Sci U S A 1986;83:5498–5501.

30. **Christian JA, Rebar AH, Boon GD, Low PS.** Senescence of canine biotinylated erythrocytes: increased autologous immunoglobulin binding occurs on erythrocytes aged in vivo for 104 to 110 days. Blood 1993;82(11):3469–3473.

31. **Dale GL, Daniels RB.** Quantitation of immunoglobulin associated with senescent erythrocytes from the rabbit. Blood 1991;77(5):1096–1099.

32. **Kay MMB, Bosman GJCGM, Shapiro SS, Bendich A, Bassel PS.** Oxidation as a possible mechanism of cellular aging: vitamin E deficiency causes premature aging and IgG binding to erythrocytes. Proc Natl Acad Sci U S A 1986;83:2463–2467.

33. **Weiss D, Klausner J.** Neutrophil-induced erythrocyte injury: a possible cause of erythrocyte destruction in the anemia associated with inflammatory disease. Vet Pathol 1988;25:450–455.

34. **Weiss DJ, Murtaugh MP.** Activated neutrophils induce erythrocyte immunoglobulin binding and membrane protein degradation. J Leukoc Biol 1990;48:438–443.

35. **Weiss DJ, Aird B, Murtaugh MP.** Neutrophil-induced immunoglobulin binding to erythrocytes involves proteolytic and oxidative injury. J Leukoc Biol 1992;51:19–23.

36. **Low PS, Waugh SM, Zinke K, Drenckhahn D.** The role of hemoglobin denaturation and band 3 clustering in red blood cell aging. Science 1985; 227:531–533.

37. **Waugh SM, Low PS.** Hemichrome binding to band 3: nucleation of Heinz bodies on the erythrocyte membrane. Biochemistry 1985;24:34–39.

38. **Waugh SM, Willardson BM, Kannan R, Labotka RJ, Low PS.** Heinz bodies induce clustering of band 3, glycophorin, and ankyrin in sickle cell erythrocytes. J Clinical Invest 1986;78:1155–1160.

39. **Lutz HU, Stringaro-Wipf G.** Senescent red cell-bound IgG is attached to band 3 protein. Biomed Biochim Acta 1983;42:117–121.

40. **Lutz HU, Bussolino F, Flepp R, et al.** Naturally occurring anti-band-3 antibodies and complement together mediate phagocytosis of oxidatively stressed human erythrocytes. Proc Natl Acad Sci U S A 1987;84:7368–7372.

41. **Kannan R, Labotka R, Low PS.** Isolation and characterization of the hemichrome-stabilized membrane protein aggregates from sickle erythrocytes. The J Biol Chem 1988;263(27):13766–13773.

42. **Yuan J, Kannan R, Shinar E, Rachmilewitz EA, Low PS.** Isolation, characterization, and immunoprecipitation studies of immune complexes from membranes of b-Thalassemic erythrocytes. Blood 1992;79(11):3007–3013.

43. **Clague MJ, Cherry RJ.** A comparative study of band 3 aggregation in erythrocyte membranes by melittin and other cationic agents. Biochim Biophys Acta 1989;980:93–99.

44. **Turrini F, Arese P, Yuan J, Low PS.** Clustering of integral membrane proteins of the human erythrocyte membrane stimulates autologous IgG binding, complement desposition, and phagocytosis. J Biol Chem 1991; 266(35):23611–23617.

45. **Rettig MP, Low PS, Gimm JA, Mohandas N, Wang J, Christian JA.** Evaluation of biochemical changes during in vivo erythrocyte senescence in the dog. Blood 1999;93:376–384.

46. **Harvey JW.** The erythrocyte: physiology, metabolism and biochemical disorders. In: Kaneko J, Harvey J, Bruss M, eds. Clinical biochemistry of domestic animals. 5th ed. San Diego: Academic Press, 1997:157–203.

47. **Reinhart WH, Sung LA, Chien S.** Quantitative relationship between Heinz body formation and red blood cell deformability. Blood 1986;68(6):1376–1383.

48. **Breitschwerdt E, Armstrong P, Robinette C, Dillman R, Karl M.** Three cases of acute zinc toxicosis in dogs. Vet Hum Toxicol 1986;28(2):109–117.

49. **Latimer K, Jain A, Inglesby H, Clarkson W, Johnson G.** Zinc-induced hemolytic anemia caused by ingestion of pennies by a pup. J Am Vet Med Assoc 1989;195(1):77–80.

50. **Luttgen PJ, Whitney MS, Wolf AM, Scruggs DW.** Heinz body hemolytic anemia associated with high plasma zinc concentration in a dog. J Am Vet Med Assoc 1990;197(10):1347–1350.

51. **Robinson F, Mason R.** Zinc toxicosis in a dog. Canine Practice 1991; 16(3):27–31.

52. **Schreiber AD, Frank MM.** Role of antibody and complement in the immune clearance and destruction of erythrocytes 1. In vivo effects of IgG and IgM complement-fixing sites. J Clin Invest 1972;51:575–582.

53. **Schreiber AD, Frank MM.** Role of antibody and complement in the immune clearance and destruction of erythrocytes II. Molecular nature of IgG and IgM complement-fixing sites and effects of their interaction with serum. J Clin Invest 1972;51:583–589.

54. **Lutz HU.** Red cell clearance (a review). Biomed Biochim Acta 1987;46:65–71.

55. **Lutz HU, Fasler S, Stammler P, Bussolino F, Arese P.** Naturally occurring anti-band 3 antibodies and complement in phagocytosis of oxidatively-stressed and in clearance of senescent red cells. Blood Cells 1988;14:175–179.

56. **Lutz HU, Fasler S, Stammler P.** An affinity for complement C3 as a possible reason for the potency of naturally occurring antibodies in mediating tissue homeostasis. Beitr Infusionsther Transfusionsmed 1989;24:193–199.

57. **Imanishi H, Nakai T, Abe T, Takino T.** Glutathione metabolism in red cell aging. Mech Ageing Dev 1985;32:57–62.

58. **Campwala HQ, Desforges JF.** Membrane-bound hemichrome in density-separated cohorts of normal (AA) and sickled (SS) cells. J Lab Clin Med 1982;99:25–28.

59. **Jain SK.** Evidence for membrane lipid peroxidation during the in vivo aging of human erythrocytes. Biochim Biophys Acta 1988;937:205–210.

60. **Piccinini G, Minetti G, Balduini C, Brovelli A.** Oxidation status of glutathione and membrane proteins in human red cells of different age. Mech Ageing Dev 1995;78:15–26.

61. **Clark MR.** Senescence of red blood cells: progress and problems. Physiol Rev 1988;68(2):503–554.

62. **Hebbel RP, Eaton JW.** Pathobiology of heme interaction with the erythrocyte membrane. Semin Hematol 1989;26(2):136–149.

63. **Winterbourn CC.** Oxidative denaturation in congenital hemolytic anemias: the unstable hemoglobins. Semin Hematol 1990;27:41–50.

64. **Winterbourn CC, Carrell RW.** Studies of hemoglobin denaturation and Heinz body formation in the unstable hemoglobins. J Clin Invest 1974; 54:678–689.

65. **Snyder LM, Leb L, Piotrowski J, Sauberman N, Liu SC, Fortier NL.** Irreversible spectrin-haemoglobin crosslinking in vivo: a marker for red cell senescence. Br J Haematol 1983;53:379–384.

66. **Snyder L, Fortier N, Trainor J, et al.** Effect of hydrogen peroxide exposure on normal human erythrocyte deformability, morphology, surface characteristics, and spectrin-hemoglobin cross-linking. J Clin Invest 1985;76:1971–1977.

67. **Pfafferott C, Meiselman HJ, Hochstein P.** The effect of malonyldialdehyde on erythrocyte deformability. Blood 1982;59(1):12–15.

68. **Schroit AJ, Madsen JW, Tanaka Y.** In vivo recognition and clearance of red blood cells containing phosphatidylserine in their plasma membranes. J Biol Chem 1985;260(8):5131–5138.

69. **Jain SK, Mohandas N, Clark MR, Shohet SB.** The effect of malonyldialdehyde, a product of lipid peroxidation, on the deformability, dehydration, and ^{51}Cr-survival of erythrocytes. Br J Haematol 1983;53:247–255.

70. **Boas FE, Forman L, Beutler E.** Phosphatidylserine exposure and red cell viability in red cell aging and in hemolytic anemia. Proc Natl Acad Sci U S A 1998;95:3077–3081.

71. **Beutler E, Kuhl W.** Human erythrocyte membrane enzymes. Blood 1978; 51(2):367–368.

72. **Aminoff D.** The role of sialoglycoconjugates in the aging and sequestration of red cells from circulation. Blood Cells 1988;14:229–247.

73. **Aminoff D.** The molecular basis of aging and sequestration of mammalian erythrocytes. Seventh Ann Arbor Conference: Alan R. Liss, 1989:247–258.

74. **Beppu M, Ando K, Kikugawa K.** Poly-N-acetyllactosaminyl saccharide chains of band 3 as determinants for anti-band 3 autoantibody binding to senescent and oxidized erythrocytes. Cell Mol Biol 1996;41:1007–1024.

75. **Beutler E.** Energy metabolism and maintenance of erythrocytes. Williams hematology. 3rd ed. New York: McGraw Hill, 1983:331–345.

76. **Bartosz G, Grzelinska E, Wagner J.** Aging of the erythrocyte. XIV. ATP content does decrease. Experientia 1982;38:575.

77. **Beutler E.** How do red cell enzymes age? A new perspective. Br J Haematol 1985;61:377–384.

78. **Beutler E.** Biphasic loss of red cell enzyme activity during in vivo aging. Progress in clinical and biological research. Vo.l 195. New York: Alan R. Liss, 1985:317–329.

79. **Kirkpatrick FH, Muhs AG, Kostuk RK, Gabel CW.** Dense (aged) circulating red cells contain normal concentrations of adenosine triphosphate (ATP). Blood 1979;54(4):946–950.

80. **Suzuki T, Dale GL.** Senescent erythrocytes: isolation of in vivo aged cells and their biochemical characteristics. Proc Natl Acad Sci U S A 1988;85:1647–1651.

81. **Dale GL, Norenberg SL.** Time-dependent loss of adenosine 5′-monophosphate deaminase activity may explain elevated adenosine 5′-triphosphate levels in senescent erythrocytes. Blood 1989;74(6):2157–2160.

82. **Paglia D, Valentine W, Nakatani M, Brockway R.** AMP deaminase as a cell-age marker in transient erythroblastopenia of childhood and its role in the adenylate economy of erythrocytes. Blood 1989;74:2161–2165.

CHAPTER 21

Erythrocyte Metabolism

• JOHN W. HARVEY

Erythrocytes provide vital functions of oxygen transport, carbon dioxide transport, and buffering of hydrogen ions. These functions do not require energy per se, but energy in the form of adenosine triphosphate (ATP), reduced nicotine adenine dinucleotide (NADH), and reduced nicotine adenine dinucleotide phosphate (NADPH) is needed to keep the cells circulating for months in a functional state despite repeated exposures to mechanical and metabolic insults.

Mature mammalian erythrocytes do not have nuclei; consequently, they cannot synthesize nucleic acids or proteins. The loss of mitochondria during the maturation of reticulocytes results in a loss of Krebs's cycle and oxidative phosphorylation capabilities and prevents the synthesis of heme or lipids de novo in erythrocytes.

Although metabolic demands are lower than in other blood-cell types, erythrocytes still require energy. ATP is necessary for maintenance of shape, deformability, phosphorylation of membrane phospholipids and proteins, active membrane transport of various molecules, partial synthesis of purine and pyrimidine nucleotides, and synthesis of reduced glutathione (GSH).[1]

MEMBRANE TRANSPORT

The erythrocyte lipid bilayer is impermeable to most molecules. Consequently, various membrane protein transport systems are used for movement of molecules into and out of erythrocytes. Band-3 protein appears to function as an aqueous pore or channel for the movement of anions (e.g., bicarbonate and chloride), water, certain nonelectrolytes, and probably cations to some extent. Defective anion transport and marked spherocytosis with membrane instability occurs in anemic cattle with an inherited deficiency of the band 3.[2]

Major interspecies, and in some cases intraspecies, differences occur in cation transport and subsequently in intracellular Na^+ and K^+ concentrations.[3] Animal species with high intracellular K^+ concentrations, horses, pigs, and some ruminants have an active Na^+, K^+ pump that exchanges intracellular Na^+ for extracellular K^+ with the hydrolysis of ATP. In addition to individuals who have high potassium (HK^+) erythrocytes, some sheep, goats,

buffaloes, and most cattle have low potassium (LK^+) and, consequently, high sodium erythrocytes. These LK^+ erythrocytes have low Na^+, K^+ pump activity and high passive K^+ permeability.

Erythrocytes from cats and most dogs do not have Na^+, K^+ pump activity and have Na^+ and K^+ concentrations near those predicted for the Donnan equilibrium with plasma. However, many clinically normal Japanese and Korean dogs have HK^+ erythrocytes.[4] Erythrocytes from these dogs have substantial Na^+, K^+-adenosine triphosphatase (ATPase) activity, and some of these dogs also have increased glutamate transport, which results in high GSH concentrations.[5] Other pathways of Na^+ and K^+ transport occur to variable degrees in certain species.[1,3]

Excessive intracellular Ca^{2+} is deleterious to erythrocytes; consequently, they actively extrude Ca^{2+} with a calcium pump having Ca^{2+}-activated, Mg^{2+}-dependent ATPase activity. The calcium pump is activated by a calcium-binding protein called calmodulin.[1]

Amino acid transport in erythrocytes provides amino acids for synthesis of GSH. In addition, amino acid transporters may be responsible for efflux of amino acids during reticulocyte maturation.[1]

Species vary in their permeability to glucose, with human erythrocytes being permeable and pig erythrocytes being poorly permeable.[1] Erythrocytes of other domestic animals appear to be intermediate between these extremes. Glucose transportation into erythrocytes occurs by passive diffusion and is not regulated by insulin.[6] Erythrocytes from adult pigs lack a functional glucose transporter and therefore have limited ability to use glucose for energy.

Erythrocyte membranes from most animal species have a nucleoside transporter.[7] Rabbit, pig, and human erythrocytes exhibit substantially more adenosine uptake than those of other species studied. Erythrocytes from dogs exhibit more adenosine uptake than cats, goats, or cattle, and erythrocytes from horses and most sheep appear to be nearly impermeable to adenosine. Although dog erythrocytes are permeable to adenosine, they are impermeable to inosine. Dog and cat erythrocytes exhibit adenine uptake and incorporation into nucleotides, but values are much lower than those of human, rabbit, or rodent erythrocytes.[1]

CARBOHYDRATE METABOLISM

Although substrates such as ribose, fructose, mannose, galactose, dihydroxyacetone, glyceraldehyde, adenosine, and inosine may be metabolized to some extent, depending on the species, glucose is the primary substrate for energy needs of erythrocytes from all species except the pig.[8] Inosine appears to be the major substrate for pig erythrocytes. Its production by the liver is sufficient to meet erythrocyte energy requirements.[9]

Once glucose enters the cell, it is phosphorylated to glucose 6-phosphate (G6P) by means of the hexokinase (HK) enzyme. The G6P is then metabolized through either the Embden-Meyerhof pathway (EMP) or the pentose phosphate pathway (PPP) as shown (Fig. 21.1).

EMBDEN-MEYERHOF PATHWAY AND ADENOSINE TRIPHOSPHATE PRODUCTION

A net of two molecules of ATP is produced for each molecule of glucose metabolized to two molecules of lactate in the EMP. Because mature erythrocytes lack mitochondria, the EMP is the only source of ATP production in these cells. Reactions catalyzed by HK, phosphofructokinase (PFK), and pyruvate kinase (PK) appear to be rate-limiting steps in glycolysis, with the PFK reaction being most important under physiologic steady-state conditions.[1]

At physiologic pH values, high concentrations of inorganic phosphate (P_i) stimulate glycolysis through the EMP by reduction of the ATP inhibition of PFK. Conversely, glycolysis is inhibited by short-term phosphate deficiency, primarily by decreasing intracellular P_i for glyceraldehyde phosphate dehydrogenase (GAPD). Decreased glycolytic rates result in decreased erythrocyte ATP concentrations and hemolytic anemia in experimental dogs made severely hypophosphatemic by hyperalimentation. Hemolytic anemia associated with hypophosphatemia has also been reported in diabetic cats and a diabetic dog after insulin therapy, in a cat that has hepatic lipidosis, and in postparturient cattle in which decreased erythrocyte ATP concentrations have been measured.[1]

Because mature erythrocytes depend solely on anaerobic glycolysis for ATP generation, deficiencies of enzymes involved in glycolysis can have significant effects on erythrocyte survival. PK-deficient dogs and cats have mild to severe regenerative hemolytic anemia, and PFK-deficient dogs have compensated hemolytic anemia, with sporadic episodes of intravascular hemolysis and hemoglobinuria.[10] PFK-deficient dog erythrocytes are alkaline fragile, because 2,3-diphosphoglycerate (2,3DPG) is decreased in these cells. Episodes of intravascular hemolysis occur when PFK-deficient dogs hyperventilate, resulting in increased plasma pH.[10]

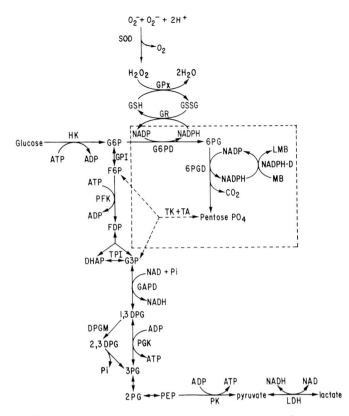

FIGURE 21.1 Metabolic pathways of the mature erythrocyte. HK, hexokinase; GPI, glucose phosphate isomerase; PFK, phosphofructokinase; TPI, triosephosphate isomerase; GAPD, glyceraldehyde-3-phosphate dehydrogenase; PGK, phosphoglycerate kinase: MPGM monophosphoglycerate mutase; DPGM, diphosphoglycerate mutase; PK, pyruvate kinase; G6PD, glucose-6-phosphate dehydrogenase; 6PGD, 6-phosphogluconate dehydrogenase; LDH, lactate dehydrogenase; GR, glutathione reductase; GPx, glutathione peroxidase; TK, transketolase; TA, transaldolase; GSSG, oxidized glutathione; G6P, glucose 6-phosphate; F6P, fructose 6-phosphate; FDP, fructose 1,6-diphosphate; DHAP, dihydroxyacetone phosphate; GAP, glyceraldehyde 3-phosphate; 1,3DPG, 1,3-diphosphoglycerate; 2,3DPG, 2,3-diphosphoglycerate; 3PG, 3-phosphoglycerate; 2PG, 2-phosphoglycerate; PEP, phosphoenolpyruvate; ADP, adenosine diphosphate; ATP, adenosine triphosphate; NAD, nicotinamide adenine dinucleotide; NADH, reduced nicotinamide adenine dinucleotide; NADP, nicotinamide adenine dinucleotide phosphate; NADPH, reduced nicotinamide adenine dinucleotide phosphate; GSH, reduced glutathione; P_i, inorganic phosphate; SOD, superoxide dismutase (**Harvey JW**. The erythrocyte: physiology, metabolism and biochemical disorders. In: Kaneko JJ, Harvey JW, Bruss ML, eds. Clinical biochemistry of domestic animals. 5th ed. San Diego: Academic Press, 1997;157–203, with permission).

DIPHOSPHOGLYCERATE PATHWAY AND OXYGEN AFFINITY OF HEMOGLOBIN

Molecules of 1,3-diphosphoglycerate (1,3DPG), produced by the GAPD reaction, may be used by the phosphoglycerate kinase (PGK) reaction in the EMP or may be converted to 2,3DPG by the diphosphoglycerate mutase (DPGM) reaction (Fig. 21.1). 2,3DPG degradation to 3- phosphoglycerate (3PG) is catalyzed by diphosphoglycerate phosphatase activity (DPGP). The DPG pathway or shunt (Rapoport–Luebering cycle) bypasses the ATP-generating PGK step in glycolysis; consequently, no net ATP is generated when glucose is metabolized through this pathway.

Erythrocytes of dogs, horses, pigs, and humans normally contain high concentrations of 2,3DPG, whereas those of cats and domestic ruminants have low concentrations. In erythrocytes from most mammalian species, 2,3DPG decreases the oxygen affinity of hemoglobin. When the oxygen affinity of hemoglobin is studied in hemolysates dialyzed to remove 2,3DPG and ATP, the stripped hemoglobins from species with low 2,3DPG erythrocytes have considerably lower oxygen affinities than stripped hemoglobin from species with high 2,3DPG erythrocytes. Because stripped hemoglobins from species with high 2,3DPG erythrocytes have high oxygen affinities, it appears that 2,3DPG is needed within erythrocytes of these species to maintain hemoglobin oxygen affinity within a physiologically useful range.[1]

PENTOSE PHOSPHATE PATHWAY AND PROTECTION AGAINST OXIDANTS

Normally only approximately 5 to 13% of glucose metabolized by erythrocytes flows through the PPP (Fig. 21.1), but this flow can be accelerated significantly by oxidants.[1]

Circulating erythrocytes are exposed to endogenously generated oxidants, including superoxide (O_2^-) and hydrogen peroxide. As a result, the damage from these oxidants may play an important role in the natural aging and ultimate removal of these cells from the circulation by mononuclear phagocytes.[11]

Superoxide dismutase (SOD) is a copper- and zinc-containing enzyme that catalyzes the dismutation of two O_2^- molecules to H_2O_2 and O_2 (Fig. 21.1). The importance of SOD as an oxidant defense in erythrocytes is unclear. Although generally considered protective, SOD may actually increase oxidant injury in conditions for instances in which H_2O_2 catabolism is compromised.[1]

NADPH generated in the PPP is important in protecting against these oxidants. It is needed to maintain glutathione in the reduced state and is important in maintaining catalase in a functional form.[12] Defects in the PPP can render erythrocytes susceptible to endogenous and exogenous oxidant injury. G6P dehydrogenase (G6PD) is the rate-controlling enzyme in the PPP. A persistent hemolytic anemia has been described in an American saddlebred colt with <1% of normal G6PD activity.[13]

GSH is a tripeptide of glutamic acid, cysteine, and glycine that is synthesized de novo in erythrocytes of animals from constituent amino acids by means of two ATP-requiring reactions. GSH has a highly reactive (easily oxidizable) sulfhydryl group that, like other thiols, may act nonenzymatically as a free-radical acceptor to counteract oxidant damage.

GSH deficiency occurs in some sheep because of a deficiency of γ-glutamylcysteine synthetase, the first enzyme involved in GSH synthesis. GSH deficiency occurs in other sheep deficient in the amino acid transporter responsible for cysteine transport into erythrocytes, thereby limiting cysteine uptake and restricting GSH synthesis.[1]

Glutathione peroxidase (GPx) catalyzes the conversion of H_2O_2 to H_2O (Fig. 21.1) and participates in the disposal of organic peroxides. In response to the oxidized glutathione (GSSG) produced by these reactions, erythrocytes increase PPP metabolism to provide the NADPH necessary for the regeneration of GSH by the flavin-dependent glutathione-reductase (GR) reaction. The selective oxidation of a renewable thiol helps limit irreversible damage to erythrocyte proteins and lipids that would otherwise occur. Selenium is an essential cofactor for GPx, being incorporated into the enzyme as it is formed. Consequently, selenium deficiency can result in GPx deficiency, which may result in increased sensitivity of erythrocytes to injury by certain oxidants, as has been reported in cattle.[14]

Catalase is a heme-containing enzyme that also destroys H_2O_2 by conversion to H_2O and O_2. Recent in vitro studies suggests that catalase is of greater importance than GPx in the defense of human erythrocytes against H_2O_2-generating reactions.[12]

Except for dogs, mammalian erythrocytes generally have high catalase activities.[1] Catalase is linked metabolically to the PPP because NADPH is tightly bound to catalase.[12] The binding of NADPH prevents and reverses the accumulation of an inactive form of catalase that is generated when catalase is exposed to H_2O_2.

Vitamin E (α-tocopherol) is a lipid-soluble vitamin that acts as a free-radical scavenger within the membrane. Vitamin E deficiency increases the susceptibility of erythrocytes to peroxidative hemolysis.[15] GSH and ascorbic acid have been shown to be involved in regeneration of oxidized vitamin E.[15]

METHEMOGLOBIN FORMATION AND REDUCTION

Methemoglobin differs from hemoglobin in that the iron moiety of heme groups has been oxidized to the ferric (+3) state, which can no longer bind oxygen. Approximately 3% of hemoglobin within erythrocytes is oxidized to methemoglobin each day in normal animals[1]; however, methemoglobin usually accounts for less than 1% of total hemoglobin, because it is constantly reduced back to hemoglobin by a NADH-dependent methemoglobin reductase (cytochrome-b_5-reductase) enzyme reaction present within erythrocytes. Methemoglobin forms at much higher levels in the presence of oxidative compounds. An inherited deficiency in this enzyme results in persistent methemoglobinemia in dogs and cats that have minimal or no clinical signs.[16]

Methylene blue (MB) is used to treat toxic methemoglobinemia because it causes methemoglobin to be reduced faster than occurs by the slow NADH-dependent methemoglobin reductase reaction. MB is reduced to leukomethylene blue (LMB) by NADPH-dependent diaphorase activity (Fig. 21.1), and LMB reacts spontaneously with methemoglobin, reducing it to hemoglobin and regenerating MB.[1]

REFERENCES

1. **Harvey JW**. The erythrocyte: physiology, metabolism and biochemical disorders. In: Kaneko JJ, Harvey JW, Bruss ML, eds. Clinical biochemistry of domestic animals. 5th ed. San Diego: Academic Press, 1997;157–203.
2. **Inaba M, Yawata A, Koshino I, et al.** Defective anion transport and marked spherocytosis with membrane instability caused by hereditary total deficiency of red cell band 3 in cattle due to a nonsense mutation. J Clin Invest 1996;97:1804–1817.
3. **Ellory JC, Tucker EM**. Cation transport in red blood cells. In: Agar NS, Board PG, eds. Red blood cells of domestic mammals. Amsterdam: Elsevier, 1983;291–314.
4. **Fujise H, Higa K, Nakayama T, et al.** Incidence of dogs possessing red blood cells with high K in Japan and East Asia. J Vet Med Sci 1997;59:495–497.
5. **Fujise H, Hishiyama N, Ochiai H**. Heredity of red blood cells with high K and low glutathione (HK/LG) and high K and high glutathione (HK/HG) in a family of Japanese Shiba dogs. Exp Anim 1997;46:41–46.
6. **Baldwin SA**. Mammalian passive glucose transporters: members of an ubiquitous family of active and passive transport proteins. Biochim Biophys Acta 1993;1154:17–49.
7. **Young JD**. Erythrocyte amino acid and nucleoside transport. In: Agar NS, Board PG, eds. Red blood cells of domestic mammals. Amsterdam: Elsevier, 1983;271–290.
8. **Kim HD**. Postnatal changes in energy metabolism of mammalian red blood cells. In: Agar NS, Board PG, eds. Red blood cells of domestic mammals. Amsterdam: Elsevier, 1983;339–355.
9. **Young JD, Paterson AR, Henderson JF**. Nucleoside transport and metabolism in erythrocytes from the Yucatan miniature pig. Evidence that inosine functions as an in vivo energy substrate. Biochim Biophys Acta 1985;842:214–224.
10. **Harvey JW**. Congenital erythrocyte enzyme deficiencies. Vet Clin North Am Small Anim Pract 1996;26:1003–1011.
11. **Eda S, Kikugawa K, Beppu M**. Oxidatively damaged erythrocytes are recognized by membrane proteins of macrophages. Free Radic Res 1997;27:23–30.
12. **Gaetani GF, Ferraris AM, Rolfo M, et al.** Predominant role of catalase in the disposal of hydrogen peroxide within human erythrocytes. Blood 1996;87:1595–1599.
13. **Stockham SL, Harvey JW, Kinden DA**. Equine glucose-6-phosphate dehydrogenase deficiency. Vet Pathol 1994;31:518–527.
14. **Morris JG, Cripe WS, Chapman HL, et al.** Selenium deficiency in cattle associated with Heinz bodies and anemia. Science 1984;223:491–493.
15. **Wang JM, Huang CJ, Chow CK**. Red cell vitamin E and oxidative damage: a dual role of reducing agents. Free Radic Res 1996;24:291–298.
16. **Harvey JW**. Methemoglobinemia and Heinz-body hemolytic anemia. In: Bonagura JD, ed. Kirk's current veterinary therapy. XII. Small Animal Practice. Philadelphia: WB Saunders, 1995;443–446.

CHAPTER 22

Iron Metabolism

• GORDON A. ANDREWS and JOSEPH E. SMITH

Iron is the second most abundant metal and the fourth most common element in the earth's crust. Despite this great natural abundance, most iron in nature exists in the oxidized, insoluble, ferric (Fe^{3+}) form that is largely unavailable for most biological systems. Free iron can catalyze the formation free radicals that damage cellular membranes and DNA. Intracellular iron, therefore, is bound to or incorporated into various proteins to reduce its toxicity. Those proteins are responsible for the absorption, transport, storage, and biological activity of iron. Any study of iron metabolism involves a study of the physiologic compounds associated with it.

IRON COMPARTMENTS

Iron exists in the following compartments: hemoglobin, storage, myoglobin, labile iron, tissue iron, and transport. The compartments are defined by anatomic distribution, chemical characteristics, and function.[1]

Hemoglobin

Most iron in animals is located in erythrocytes as hemoglobin iron. Each hemoglobin molecule contains four atoms of iron and is 0.34% iron by weight. Each milliliter of erythrocytes contains 1.1 mg of iron, so the exact amount of iron depends on the animal's packed cell volume and blood volume. If the packed cell volume is constant and blood volume increases linearly with body weight, the total absolute amount of iron in hemoglobin is normally related to body weight.[2]

Storage

Iron is stored in various tissues as either a soluble, mobile fraction (ferritin) or as insoluble, aggregated deposits (hemosiderin). Storage iron concentration is the major factor affecting the relative distribution of iron between ferritin and hemosiderin in mammals. At low storage levels, more iron is stored as ferritin than as hemosiderin.[3] As the amount of iron increases, the hemosiderin proportion increases. Both hemosiderin and ferritin iron are available to the body. The liver and spleen usually have the highest storage iron concentrations, followed by the kidney, heart, skeletal muscles, and brain.[4]

Ferritin

Ferritin consists of protein (apoferritin) and iron.[5] Apoferritin is composed of 24 monomers of at least two subunit types, designated H and L. The H subunit is predominant in heart ferritin and is larger (21,000 Da) than the L subunit. The L subunit occurs in the liver and spleen and has a molecular weight of 19,000 Da. Other tissues have ferritins made up of various ratios of H and L subunits. The H:L ratio is species and tissue specific and varies from 1:9 in a horse's spleen to 8.5:1 in a horse's heart.

Each subunit is shaped like a short rod and interacts with other subunits to form a hollow sphere.[6] Pores through which iron enters or leaves the interior cavity of the ferritin molecule are formed in the exterior surface between apoferritin monomers.[7] The mineral core of ferritin is hydrated ferric oxide with some phosphate. Iron passes through the pores in the apoferritin coat as the ferrous ion. Once inside the shell, it must be oxidized to the ferric form, hydrolyzed, and polymerized to the ferric oxyhydroxide polymer. Iron can exit ferritin by reversing the process. The physiologic compounds involved in reducing the iron back to the ferrous form have not been determined.[5]

Hemosiderin

Although structurally hemosiderin seems similar to ferritin, it has a higher iron-to-protein ratio. It may be formed from soluble cytosol ferritin by lysosomal action.[8] Hemosiderin is insoluble in water and remains in tissues processed for histologic examination. It appears in unstained sections as clumps or granules of golden refractile pigment and stains readily with the Prussian blue reaction.

Myoglobin

Similar to one subunit of hemoglobin, myoglobin is found mostly in muscle. It serves as a reservoir for oxygen and can temporarily provide oxygen during anaerobic conditions. Each myoglobin molecule contains one atom of iron (0.34% iron by weight). The quantity of myoglobin in muscle tissue is species related and depends on muscular activity. The muscle myoglobin content of race horses (7.4 mg/kg) is much higher than that of man (1.2 mg/g).[9] This iron pool varies between species, because the amount of myoglobin varies among muscles within a species and among species.

Labile Iron Pool

The concept of the labile iron pool is derived from ferrokinetic studies. When radioiron disappearance curves are analyzed with a multicompartment model, an iron pool is found that is in dynamic equilibrium with the plasma iron pool.[10] Iron disappears from the plasma into this pool, but can reflux back to the plasma. Although the exact physical nature of the pool is unknown, it may be an intermediate between the plasma, storage, and hemoglobin pools.

Tissue Iron Compartment

Although the amount of iron in this compartment is small, it is extremely important. Almost half of the enzymes of the tricarboxylic acid cycle either contain iron or require it as a cofactor. The iron compounds can be classified into four categories[11]: (1) Heme-containing compounds are structurally similar to hemoglobin and include myoglobin, catalase, peroxidase, and cytochromes. Cytochromes a, b, and c are located in the mitochondria and are important in oxidative phosphorylation. Other cytochromes (such as cytochrome P-450) are located in the endoplasmic reticulum and function in the oxidative degradation of endogenous compounds and drugs. (2) Nonheme iron-containing enzymes form another large group that includes iron in nonheme such as iron sulphur compounds and metalloflavoproteins. This group includes xanthine oxidase, cytochrome c reductase, succinate dehydrogenase, and nicotinamide adenine dinucleotide dehydrogenase, which contains more iron in mitochondria than in cytochromes. (3) Enzymes requiring iron or heme as a cofactor include aconitase and tryptophan pyrrolase. (4) Enzymes containing iron in an unknown form include ribonucleotide reductase and a-glycerophosphate.

Transport Compartment

Iron is transported between some compartments by plasma transferrin. Transferrin is a single polypeptide chain glycoprotein of approximately 700 amino acids (molecular weight: ~80,000 Da). It contains two branched oligosaccharide chains that are attached to asparagine residues.[5] It has a dilobal structure; the N- and C-terminal halves form separate globular lobes connected by a short ~x-helix. Each half carries one iron-binding site that requires concomitant binding of one carbonate or bicarbonate ion with each atom of iron.

Iron as a ferric ion is bound tightly at neutral pH, but is dissociated when the pH is less than 5.5.

In domestic animals, plasma transferrin type is a polymorphic trait and can be used for parental exclusion. The genetically related, electrophoretic variability resides in both the polypeptide chain and the oligosaccharide side chains.[12,13]

The transfer of iron from transferrin to cells requires internalization of the iron-laden transferrin molecule. Ferrotransferrin binds to the transferrin receptor at neutral pH. The receptor-ferrotransferrin complex collects in specialized sites on the plasma membrane called coated pits. These pits are coated on the inner surface with a fibrous protein, clathrin. The coated-pit region of the membrane then can invaginate to form a vesicle, with the cell's outer plasma membrane and receptor-ferrotransferrin complex as the inner surface and the clathrin coat as the outer surface. The vesicles are converted into structures with the acronym CURL (compartment of uncoupling of receptor and ligand). An enzyme in the endostomal membrane exploits the energy stored in adenosine triphosphate to pump protons into the CURL lumen and, thus, lower the internal pH. At the lower pH, transferrin's affinity for iron is decreased, and the iron is released. Iron-free apotransferrin remains bound to its receptor and is transported back to the cell surface. When the coated vesicle reaches the surface, iron-free apotransferrin is released from the receptor because the affinity between the two is low at neutral pH. The iron-free apotransferrin can enter the blood plasma to bind more iron, and the receptor can be used to bind more ferrotransferrin. The free iron must escape from the CURL, cross the mitochondrial membrane, and be incorporated into heme. The exact mechanism for free-iron movement remains unknown.[14,15]

The amount of iron delivered to immature erythrocytes depends on the plasma iron concentration, percent iron saturation, and the number of membrane receptors.[16] When the percentage of transferrin containing iron is low, most transferrin is monoferric; as the percentage increases, the diferric form increases. The amount of iron delivered increases in two ways because (1) the payload of the diferric molecules is twice that of monoferric transferrin and (2) diferric transferrin has a higher affinity for the membrane receptor than monoferric transferrin and, thus, is preferentially bound to available receptors.[16] The receptor number probably increases when erythropoiesis is increased. The Belgrade rat is unable to release iron within the CURL and have an anemia resembling iron deficiency, despite being hyperferremic.[17]

Copper plays an important role in transporting iron across membranes.[18] Most of the circulating copper in plasma is attached to the serum glycoprotein, ceruloplasmin. Ceruloplasmin has ferroxidase activity and may be needed to deliver iron into the circulation. When pigs are copper deficient, they have hypoceruloplasminemia and signs of a functional iron deficiency. Iron accumulates in the liver, the macrophage-phagocyte system, and the enterocytes. Presumably, this iron deficiency results from the inability to mobilize the iron from these sites.[19] In humans, a genetic defect in the ceruloplasmin gene causes aceruloplasminemia and systemic hemosiderosis.[20] Plasma iron in laying hens is high (greater than 500 μ/dL), and approximately two thirds of it is bound to a specific phosphoprotein, phosvitin. It is responsible for transporting iron to ovocytes and egg yolks. The average egg contains approximately 1 mg of iron.[9]

GENETIC CONTROL OF IRON PROTEINS

The synthesis of ferritin heavy and light chains, the transferrin receptor, and the erythroid form of amino levulinate synthase (the rate-limiting enzyme in heme biosynthesis) are regulated at the posttranscriptional level by the interplay of iron-responsive elements (IREs) and cytosolic iron-binding proteins referred to as either IRE-binding proteins (IRE-BP) or iron regulatory proteins (IRP).[21–26] The IREs are stem-loop or hairpin structures located in the 3′ or 5′ untranslated regions of the messenger RNAs (mRNAs) that act as nucleic-acid-binding sites for the IRPs. Two IRPs are described, IRP1 and IRP2.[27] The binding affinity of IRPs for the IREs is reversibly regulated by the intracellular concentration of chelatable iron. When the intracellular concentration of iron is low, IRPs have a high affinity for the IREs, and when the cells are iron replete, the IRE-binding activity is lost. When IRP1 occurs in iron-replete cells, it is a cytosolic aconitase.[28] When iron is limiting, IRP1 exists in an alternative form that is devoid of a cubane Fe–S cluster and has a high affinity for IREs.[29] IRP2 is the product of a second gene, but its mRNA abundance and tissue distribution differ from those of IRP1. IRP2 does not have aconitase activity in an iron-adequate environment.[27]

The ferritin and amino levulinate synthase mRNAs have a single IRE in the 5′ end located between the 5′ cap site and the beginning of the coding region. Binding of the IRP under conditions of low intracellular iron prevents translation of the mRNA. When iron is high, the affinity of the IRP for the IRE is lost, and the mRNA is translated, increasing expression of ferritin to sequester the excess iron and expression of amino levulinate synthase.

The transferrin receptor has a cluster of five IREs located in the 3′ untranslated region of the mRNA. The cluster of IREs in the 3′ untranslated region confers iron-regulated control of mRNA stability. When iron is low, IRP binds to 3′ IRE and stabilizes the short-lived transferrin receptor mRNA by blocking its degradation by an endonuclease, thus increasing transferrin receptor expression. When iron is high, IRP does not bind the IREs, and transferrin receptor expression decreases. Thus, IRP exerts an iron-dependent, dual, and reciprocal control of ferritin concentrations and transferrin receptors.[21]

IRON ABSORPTION

Iron Requirements

Age, growth rate, availability of a dietary iron source, and the criteria of adequacy influence iron requirements for domestic animals. Definite iron requirements for most domestic species have not been determined. Most recommendations are estimates.[30–37] The intake for mature animals can be adequately met from the usual dietary sources. Because milk is low in iron and growth rates of neonatal animals are high relative to their weights, the young of most species can become iron deficient. Anemia should not be used to determine iron adequacy, because use of dietary iron for hemoglobin synthesis can take precedence over demands for other iron compounds.[38]

Dietary Iron

The amount of iron available for absorption by the intestine depends on the amount of iron in the diet and its bioavailability. Iron content of various foods and feeds can be divided into high (greater than 50 ppm), intermediate (10 to 50 ppm), and low (less than 10 ppm) levels. Those with high iron content include organ meats such as heart and liver, brewer's yeast, wheat germ, egg yolks, oysters, and certain dried beans and fruits. Those with intermediate iron content include most muscle meats, fish and fowl, most green vegetables, and most cereals. Foods low in iron include milk and milk products and most nongreen vegetables.[39]

Iron is absorbed as either heme or nonheme compounds. Heme is absorbed readily and independently of the composition of the diet. Nonheme iron is largely unavailable, and its absorption is affected by other ingredients in the diet. Tannates and phosphates inhibit, but meat and ascorbate enhance, nonheme iron absorption.[40]

Mechanisms of Absorption

Despite many investigations over several years, the exact mechanism of intestinal absorption of iron remains unknown. It must be a finely regulated mechanism, as control of total body iron occurs at the level of absorption. Iron absorption occurs predominantly in the duodenum. There is no formal mechanism for iron excretion. Because free iron is inherently unstable and can catalyze free-radical-mediated membrane damage, it is unlikely that iron crosses the intestinal cell wall in a free, soluble form. Iron probably is bound to a ligand that is involved in regulating its uptake. The most recent theory of iron absorption involves mucin and an intestinal protein designated mobilferrin.[41] According to this theory, gastric juice stabilizes dietary inorganic iron and prevents iron from being precipitated as insoluble ferric hydroxide. At acid pH, iron combines with mucins. Intestinal mucin delivers inorganic iron to intestinal absorptive cells in a form that is acceptable for absorption. In the small intestine, iron is transferred from mucin to the membrane integrins of the intestinal absorptive cells. Membrane integrins help the transfer of iron through the cell membrane for binding to mobilferrin. Mobilferrin serves as the shuttle protein within the absorptive cell. If an excess of iron occurs in the cell, ferritin synthesis is stimulated, and iron is deposited in ferritin to prevent oxidative damage to the cell from ionic iron. Transferrin receptors located on the basolateral membranes of the absorptive cell act to permit iron to enter the cell from plasma similar to cells in other organs.

Iron uptake is influenced by previous dietary exposure, the amount of storage iron within the body, and erythropoietic activity.[42] After one dose of iron is given orally, a second dose is absorbed more slowly.[43] Iron absorption increases 6- to 15-fold in dogs that have chronic blood-loss anemia and with increased erythropoiesis.[44]

The mucosal blockage of iron absorption has limited capacity, because higher doses of iron can overcome the blocking mechanism, resulting in iron toxicity.

TESTS FOR EVALUATING IRON METABOLISM

Hematology

With certain constraints, hematologic examination can be used to evaluate iron adequacy. Blood is obtained easily and hemoglobin iron represents the largest iron pool. However, iron is preferentially shunted from other iron pools to hemoglobin synthesis.[38] Thus, hemoglobin may be the last pool to show the effects of iron inadequacy.

A high concentration of hemoglobin in metarubricytes is a signal to stop cell division and to extrude the nucleus.[45] During severe iron deficiency, hemoglobin synthesis in immature erythrocytes is slowed, and nucleated erythrocytes continue to divide. Erythrocytes released into the circulation are small and show increased central pallor because of low hemoglobin content. Nucleated red cells may be released into circulation. Hematologic indices have been used to assess the biological availability of iron in diets, and to determine the iron requirements of various species, in spite of the drawbacks. If the erythrocyte number, packed cell volume, and hemoglobin are determined, three erythrocyte indices can be calculated: mean corpuscular hemoglobin, mean corpuscular volume, and mean corpuscular hemoglobin concentration. Classically, all three indices decrease in iron-deficiency anemia. However, similar changes can occur in any deficiency or disease that inhibits hemoglobin synthesis, such as pyridoxine-responsive anemia or copper deficiency.

Serum Iron

One can measure serum iron to assess the transport compartment. Conditions of sample collection are particularly important. Most evacuated containers used for routine serum collection are satisfactory. However, if zinc is to be determined, special trace element tubes are required, because most stoppers are contaminated with zinc.[46] Although plasma may be used, the anticoagulant should be tested for iron content. Samples must be handled carefully to avoid postsampling contamination. Glassware must be cleaned carefully with acid solution.

Disposable plastic containers and tubes offer an acceptable alterative and usually do not require acid cleansing.

Serum iron declines in severe iron deficiency, acute-phase inflammatory reactions, hypoproteinemia, hypothyroidism, renal disease, and chronic inflammation. It may be elevated in hemolytic anemia, refractory anemia, iron overload, and liver disease.[47] Measurement of serum iron, therefore, is unreliable as a predictor of total-body iron stores.

Serum Total Iron-Binding Capacity

Total transferrin can be measured by immunologic methods, but the technique is not used commonly. Transferrin usually is measured in terms of iron content after it has been saturated with iron. When transferrin is saturated with iron, the iron content is called the total iron-binding capacity (TIBC). Because transferrin can bind more iron than is normally present, the TIBC is greater than the serum iron, and the difference between them is the unsaturated iron-binding capacity (UIBC). Thus, serum iron can be expressed as a percentage of the TIBC and reported as the percent saturation.[48]

Serum Ferritin

Although ferritin functions as an iron storage compound and is primarily intracellular, it can be detected in serum. In humans, serum ferritin concentrations correlate with total-body iron stores. They are low in iron deficiency and high in iron overload.[49-53]

Serum ferritin is assayed in antibody-driven reactions such as radioimmunoassay and enzyme-linked immunosorbent assay. Unfortunately, the antibodies against ferritin are usually species specific[54]; that is, an antibody against human ferritin does not cross-react with horse ferritin. Thus, for each new species, ferritin must be isolated, an antibody must be made, and the assay conditions must be developed. Despite this difficulty, serum ferritin has been measured and correlates significantly with nonheme iron in the liver and spleen of horses, pigs, cows, dogs, and cats, but not in rats.[55-62] In calves, serum ferritin increases after iron therapy.[57]

Serum ferritin can be increased in several conditions that are not related to body stores of iron. It is an acute-phase protein and increases during inflammatory reactions when interleukin-1 is produced. Clinically, serum ferritin should be monitored relative to other acute-phase proteins such as haptoglobin, fibrinogen, or C-reactive protein, because it is possible for the low serum ferritin associated with iron deficiency to be elevated into the normal range by a concurrent infection.[63] Serum ferritin also can be increased during liver disease, hemolytic diseases, and some neoplastic disorders.[64] Serum ferritin increases and transferrin decreases with malnutrition in cattle.[65]

Bone Marrow Iron

Cytologic examinations of bone marrow smears stained with Prussian blue to detect iron are sometimes useful for evaluating disorders of iron metabolism.[66] Except for cats,[67] bone marrow from normal adult domestic animals exhibits stainable iron (hemosiderin) within macrophages. Little or no stainable iron is found in animals with iron deficiency.

Mitochondrial iron of immature erythrocytes occurs as amorphous aggregates called ferruginous micelles. Some nucleated erythrocytes in Prussian-blue-stained marrow slides contain one to three, small, blue granules in the cytoplasm. In iron deficiency, macrophages and developing erythrocytes do not contain stainable iron granules. On the other hand, when heme synthesis is impaired, mitochondria accumulate excess amorphous iron aggregates and a ring of large blue siderotic granules may encircle the erythrocyte nucleus.[1]

Erythrocyte Protoporphyrin

In the final step of heme synthesis, iron is inserted into protoporphyrin. When heme synthesis is limited by the availability of iron, protoporphyrin accumulates, and zinc substitutes for iron. The zinc chelate is stable and remains in the erythrocytes throughout their life spans. Erythrocyte protoporphyrin also increases in lead poisoning because ferrocheletase, the enzyme responsible for inserting iron into protoporphyrins, is inhibited by lead. In the anemia of chronic disease, protoporphyrin increases because of internal iron unavailability.

Tissue Nonheme Iron

Body iron stores can be determined directly by measurement of the iron concentrations in various organs.[3] Although it may be desirable to determine iron in each body tissue, nonheme iron usually is determined in organs containing large quantities of iron that are accessible for biopsy, that is, the liver and the spleen. Total tissue iron does not reflect stored iron because most tissues contain heme iron compounds such as hemoglobin, myoglobin, or heme enzymes. Only the nonheme iron fraction represents iron stored in ferritin or hemosiderin.

REFERENCES

1. **Fairbanks VF, Beutler E**. Iron Metabolism. In: Beutler E, Lichtman MA, Coller BS, Kipps TJ, eds. Williams hematology. 5th ed. New York, NY: McGraw-Hill, 1995;369–380.
2. **Stahl WR**. Scaling of respiratory variables in mammals. J Appl Physiol 1967;22:453–546.
3. **Torrance JD, Bothwell TH**. Tissue iron stores. Methods Hematol 1980;1:90–115.
4. **Underwood EJ**. Iron. Academic Press, New York, NY, 1977;13–55.
5. **Crichton RR, Charlotteaux-Wauters M**. Iron transport and storage. Eur J Biochem 1987;164:485–506.
6. **Harrison PM, Treffry A, Lilley TH**. Ferritin as a iron-storage protein: mechanisms of iron uptake. J Inorg Biochem 1986;27:287–293.
7. **Harrison PM**. Ferritin: an iron-storage molecule. Semin Hematol 1977;14:55–57.
8. **Richter GW**. Studies of iron overload–rat liver siderosome ferritin. Lab Invest 1984;50:26–35.
9. **Kolb E**. The metabolism of iron in farm animals under normal and pathologic conditions. Adv Vet Sci 1963;8:49–114.
10. **Pollycove M, Mortimer R**. The quantitative determination of iron kinetics and hemoglobin synthesis in human subjects. J Clin Invest 1961;40:753–853.
11. **Dallman PR, Beutler E, Finch CA**. Effects of iron deficiency exclusive of anaemia. Br J Haematol 1978;40:179–183.
12. **Stratil A, Glasnak V**. Partial characterization of horse transferrin heterogeneity with respect to the atypical, Tf C. Anim Genet 1981;12:113–212.
13. **Maeda K, McKenzie HA, Shaw DC**. Comparison of bovine serum transferrin A and D2. I. Amino acid residue differences. Anim Genet 1984;15:299–312.
14. **Dautry-Varsat A, Ciechanover A, Lodish HF**. pH and the recycling of transferrin during receptor-mediated endocytosis. Proc Natl Acad Sci U S A 1983;80:2258–2262.
15. **Dautry-Varsat A, Lodish HF**. How receptors bring proteins and particles into cells. Sci Am 1984;251:52–58.
16. **Huebers H, Sciba E, Huebers E, Finch CA**. Molecular advantage of diferric transferrin in delivering iron to reticulocytes: A comparative study. Proc Soc Exp Biol Med 1985;179:222–226.
17. **Edwards J, Huebers H, Kunzler C, Finch C**. Iron metabolism in the Belgrade rat. Blood 1986;67:623–628.
18. **Harris ED**. The iron-copper connection: the link to ceruloplasmin grows stronger. Nutr Rev 1996;53:170–173.
19. **Lee GR, Nacht S, Lukens JN, Cartwright GE**. Iron metabolism in copper-deficient swine. J Clin Invest 1968;47:2058–2069.
20. **Harris ZL, Takahashi Y, Miyajima H, Serizawa M, MacGillivray RTA, Gitlin JD**. Aceruloplasminemia: molecular characterization of this disorder of iron metabolism. Proc Natl Acad Sci U S A 1995;92:2539–2543.
21. **Klausner RD, Harford JB**. Cis-trans models for post-translational gene regulation. Science 1989;246:870–872.
22. **Leibold EA, Guo B**. Iron-dependent regulation of ferritin and transferrin receptor expression by the iron-responsive element binding protein. Annu Rev Nutr 1992;12:345–368.
23. **Rouault T, Klausner R, Favier AE, Neve J, Faure P**. Regulation of iron metabolism in eukaryotic cells. Trace elements and free radicals in oxidative diseases. 1994;28:8–11.
24. **Kuhn LC**. Iron and gene expression: molecular mechanisms regulating cellular iron homeostasis. Nutr Rev 1998;56:S11–S19.
25. **Addess KJ, Basilion JP, Klausner RD, Rouault TA, Pardi A**. Structure and dynamics of the iron responsive element RNA: implications for binding of the RNA by iron regulatory binding proteins. J Mol Biol 1997;274:72–83.
26. **Theil EC**. The iron responsive element (IRE) family of mRNA regulators. Regulation of iron transport and uptake compared in animals, plants, and microorganisms. Met Ions Biol Syst 1998;35:403–434.
27. **Samaniego F, Chin J, Iwai K, Rouault TA, Klausner RD**. Molecular characterization of a second iron-responsive element binding protein, iron regulatory protein 2. Structure, function, and post-translation regulation. JBC 1994;269:30904–30910.
28. **Beinert H, Kennedy MC**. Aconitase, two-faced protein: enzyme and iron regulatory factor. FASEB J 1993;7:1442–1449.
29. **Basilion JP, Rouault TA, Massinople M, Klausner RD, Burgess WH**. The iron-responsive element-binding protein: localization of the RNA-binding site to the aconitase active-site cleft. Proc Natl Acad Sci U S A 1994;91:574–578.
30. **NRC**. Nutrient requirements of sheep. National Academy of Sciences, Washington,DC, 1975:1.
31. **NRC**. Nutrient requirements of beef cattle. National Academy of Sciences, Washington, DC, 1976:9.
32. **NRC**. Nutrient requirements of horses. National Academy of Sciences, Washington,D.C. 1978:16.
33. **NRC**. Nutrient requirements of dairy cattle. National Academy of Sciences, Washington, DC, 1978:7.
34. **NRC**. Nutrient requirements of swine. National Academy of Sciences, Washington,DC, 1979:6.
35. **NRC**. Nutrient requirements of goats: angora, dairy and meat goats in temperate and tropical countries. National Academy Press, Washington,DC, 1981:7.
36. **NRC**. Nutrient requirements of beef cattle. National Academy Press, Washington, DC, 1984:17.
37. **NRC**. Nutrient requirements of dogs. National Academy Press, Washington, DC, 1985:18.
38. **Nathanson MH, McLaren GD**. Internal iron exchange in normal and iron-deficient dogs: relationship to iron absorption. Clin Res 1984;32:317.
39. **Finch CA**. Drugs effective in iron-deficiency and other hypochromic anemias. In: Gilman AG, Goodman LS, Gilman A, eds. The pharmacological basis of therapeutics. 6th ed. New York, NY: MacMillan Publishing, 1980;1315–1330.
40. **Finch CA, Cook JD**. Iron deficiency. Am J Clin Nutr 1984;39:471–477.
41. **Conrad ME, Umbreit JN**. Iron absorption-the mucin-mobilferrin-integrin pathway. A competitive pathway for metal absorption. Am J Hematol 1993;42:67–73.
42. **Finch CA, Huebers HA**. Iron metabolism. Metal Metab Dis 1985;4:5–10.
43. **Hahn RL**. Radioactive iron absorption by gastrointestinal tract. J Exp Med 1943;78:169–185.
44. **Weiden PL, Hackman RC, Deeg HJ, Graham TC, Thomas ED, Storb R**. Long-term survival and reversal of iron overload after marrow transplantation in dogs with congenital hemolytic anemia. Blood 1981;57:66–70.

45. **Stohlman F Jr, Howard D, Beland A**. Humoral regulation of erythropoiesis. XII. Effect of erythropoietin and iron on cell size in iron deficiency anemia. Proc Soc Exp Biol Med 1963;113:986–988.

46. **Handy RW**. Zn contamination in vacutainer tubes. Clin Chem 1979;25:197–198.

47. **Kaneko JJ**. Iron metabolism. In: Kaneko JJ, ed. Clinical biochemistry of domestic animals. 3rd ed. New York, NY: Academic Press, 1980;649–669.

48. **Henry RJ, Cannon DC, Winkelman JW**. Clinical chemistry: princples and techniques. 2nd ed. New York, NY: Harper & Row, 1974:687–695.

49. **Addison GM, Beamish MR, Hales CH, Hodgkins M, Jacobs A, Llewellin P**. An immunoradiometric assay for ferritin in the serum of normal subjects and patients with iron deficiency and iron overload. J Clin Pathol 1972;25:326–329.

50. **Jacobs A, Miller F, Worwood M, Beamish MR, Wardrop CA**. Ferritin in the serum of normal subjects and patients with iron deficiency and iron overload. BMJ 1972;4:206–208.

51. **Lipschitz DA, Cook JD, Finch CA**. A clinical evaluation of serum ferritin as an index of iron stores. N Engl J Med 1974;290:1213–1216.

52. **Siimes MA, Addiego JE Jr, Dallman PR**. Ferritin in serum: diagnosis of iron deficiency and iron overload in infants and children. Blood 1974;43:581–659.

53. **Walters GO, Miller FM, Worwood M**. Serum ferritin concentration and iron stores in normal subjects. J Clin Pathol 1973;26:770–772.

54. **Richter GW**. Serological cross-reactions of human, rat, horse ferritins. Exp Mol Pathol 1967;6:96–101.

55. **Smith JE, Moore K, Cipriano JE, Morris PG**. Serum ferritin as a measure of stored iron in horses. J Nutr 1984;114:677–681.

56. **Smith JE, Moore K, Boyington D**. Enzyme immunoassay for serum ferritin of pigs. Biochem Med 1983;29:293–297.

57. **Miyata Y, Furugouri K, Shijimaya K**. Developmental changes in serum ferritin concentration of dairy cattle. J Dairy Sci 1984;67:1256–1263.

58. **Weeks BR, Smith JE, Phillips RM**. Enzyme-linked immunosorbent assay for canine serum ferritin using monoclonal anti-canine ferritin. Am J Vet Res 1988;49:1193–1195.

59. **Andrews GA, Smith JE, Gray M, Chavey PS**. An improved ferritin assay for canine sera. Vet Clin Pathol 1992;21:57–60.

60. **Andrews GA, Chavey PS, Smith JE**. Enzyme linked immunosorbent assay to measure serum ferritin and the relationship between serum ferritin and nonheme iron stores in cats. Vet Pathol 1994;31:674–678.

61. **Hunter JE**. Variable effects of iron status on the concentration of ferritin in rat plasma, liver, and spleen. J Nutr 1978;108:497–595.

62. **Ward C, Saltman P, Ripley L, Ostrup R, Hegenauer J, Hatlen L, Christopher J**. Correlation of serum ferritin and liver ferritin in the anemic, normal, and iron-loaded rat. Am J Clin Nutr 1977;30:1054–1063.

63. **Lorier MA, Herron JL, Carrell RW**. Detecting iron deficiency by serum tests. Clin Chem 1985;31:337–338.

64. **Newlands CE, Houston DM, Vasconcelos DY**. Hyperferritinemia associated with malignant histiocytosis in a dog. J Am Vet Med Assoc 1994;205:849–851.

65. **Furugouri K**. Ferritin, iron and total iron-binding capacity of the serum from Holstein young steers in prolonged undernutrition. J Dairy Sci 1984;46:859–865.

66. **Fairbanks VF, Beutler E**. Iron metabolism. In: Williams WJ, Beutler E, Erslev AJ, Lichtman MA, eds. Hematology, 3rd ed. New York, NY: McGraw-Hill, 1983;300.

67. **Harvey JW**. Myeloproliferative disorders in dogs and cats. Vet Clin North Am Small Anim Pract 1981;11:349–381.

CHAPTER 23

Hemoglobin Synthesis and Destruction

• J. JERRY KANEKO

Metal porphyrin complexes are found widespread in nature and are associated with fundamental metabolic processes of life. The photosynthetic pigment of plants, chlorophyll, is a magnesium porphyrin. Iron–porphyrin complexes include the hemoglobins, myoglobins and heme-containing enzymes such as catalase, peroxidase and cytochromes. The porphyrin–metal–protein hemoglobin occupies a central role in the sustenance of animal life because of its unique role in the binding, transport, and delivery of oxygen to the tissues. In the tissues, oxygen fuels the oxidative metabolic reactions that generate the major portion of the chemical energy used in life processes. Hemoglobin (Hgb) is synthesized within developing red blood cells wherein its biochemical synthesis is exquisitely coordinated with the developmental stages of the red blood cell. Hgb synthesis is minimal at the rubriblast stage and progressively increases through the succeeding cell stages. At each stage, Hgb synthesis is finely tuned so that the protoporphyrin, iron, and globin moieties are brought together and assembled into the functional Hgb molecule. The mature red cell contains its full complement of Hgb and remains in the circulatory system until it has reached the end of its life span. At this time, the Hgb is degraded into its component protoporhyrin, iron, and globin, each of which is further catabolyzed or recycled.

HEMOGLOBIN SYNTHESIS

Hgb is a relatively small protein of 64,458 d. It consists of 2 α- and 2 β-polypeptide chains and the amino acid sequence of each is precisely known. Each chain contains a heme prosthetic group held firmly within a hydrophobic cleft or the heme pocket. The precise positioning of the heme group in the heme pocket permits the Hgb molecule to carry out its function of oxygen transport. The tetrameric Hgb molecule is a globoid protein measuring approximately 50 Å × 55 Å × 65 Å. It is this globular tetrameric form of the Hgb molecule that permits the cooperative interaction of oxygen binding that gives the familiar sigmoid oxygen–Hgb saturation curve. Approximately 25 pg of Hgb exists within a red cell (Mean Cell Hgb = MCH = 25 pg); this Hgb translates into a concentration of 33% within a red cell (Mean Cell Hgb Concentration = MCHC = 33%).

Synthesis of Porphyrins and Heme

Heme is a planar molecule composed of the tetrapyrrole protoporphyrin IX (PROTO IX) and a central iron molecule. The ultimate biochemical precursors of PROTO IX are the amino acid glycine and the Krebs cycle intermediate, succinyl-CoA. The iron for completion of heme biosynthesis is supplied by ferritin, the storage form of iron. Heme biosynthesis is an enzymatic process requiring both mitochondrial and cytosolic enzymes. Heme enzymes are highly structurally specific and in particular, the absolute specificity of coproporphyrinogen III oxidase (COPROgenIII-Ox) for coproporphyrinogen III (COPROgen III) assures that only protoporphyrin III (PROTO III), the specific precursor of PROTO IX, is synthesized. The sequential series of reactions leading to the synthesis of PROTO IX, heme, and Hgb is outlined in Figure 23.1.[1]

δ-Amino Levulinic Acid

The initial step in heme synthesis occurs in the mitochondria and involves the enzymatic condensation of glycine with succinyl-CoA to form δ-aminolevulinic acid (ALA). This reaction requires vitamin B_6 as pyridoxal phosphate and the pyridoxal–phosphate–glycine complex condenses with succinyl-CoA. The requirement for pyridoxine explains the pyridoxine responsive anemia of pyridoxine deficiency. This condensation reaction is catalyzed by ALA synthase (ALA-Syn), which is the rate-controlling enzyme for heme synthesis. ALA-Syn is induced by heme and is also suppressed by negative feedback inhibition by heme. Thus, the end product, heme, controls its own synthesis. ALA is now transferred into the cytosol.

Porphobilinogen

Within the cytosol, two moles of ALA are next condensed to form the precursor pyrrole, porphobilinogen

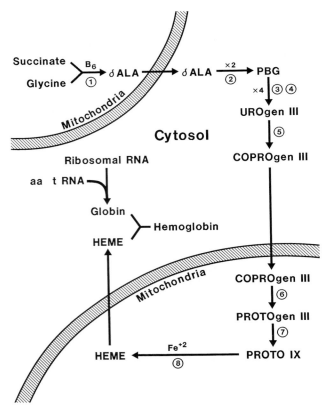

FIGURE 23.1 Pathway for protoporphyrin, heme, and hemoglobin synthesis emphasizing the partitioning of the pathway between the mitochondrial and the cytolic compartments of the cell. The circled numbers represent the following enzymes of heme synthesis: 1, ALA-Syn; 2, ALA-D; 3, UROgenI-Syn; 4, UROgenIII-Cosyn; 5, UROgen-D; 6, COPROgenIII-Ox; 7, PROTOgenIII-Ox; 8, FER-Ch. Reprinted with permission from **Kaneko JJ**. Porphyrins and the porphyrias. In: Kaneko JJ, Harvey JW, Bruss ML, eds. Clinical biochemistry of domestic animals. 5th ed. San Diego: Academic, 1997;209.

(PBG). This reaction is catalyzed by the enzyme ALA dehydrase (ALA-D), an enzyme that is strongly inhibited by lead. This accounts for the anemia of lead poisoning and a reduced-activity ALA-D is generally regarded as presumptive evidence of exposure to lead.

Uroporphyrinogen

Next, two enzymes, uroporphyrinogen I synthase (UROgenI-Syn) and uroporphrinogen III cosynthase (UROgenIII-Cosyn) act together to condense four moles of PBG into the cyclic tetrapyrrole, uroporphyrinogen III (UROgen III). UROgenI-Syn initially catalyzes the formation of a symmetric linear tetrapyrrole. In the presence of UROgenIII-Cosyn, the D ring of the tetrapyrrole is reversed or flipped and simultaneously, the pyrroles are closed into an asymmetric porphyrin ring, UROgen III. In the absence of UROgenIII-Cosyn, the symmetric linear tetrapyrrole spontaneously closes into the symmetric porphyrin, UROgen I. The hereditary absence of

UROgenIII-Cosyn is the ultimate cause of congenital erythropoietic porphyria[2] (CEP), which is characterized by the accumulation of uroporphyrin I (URO I) and coproporphyrin I (COPRO I)The resulting uroporphyrinogens contain eight carboxyl groups, four of the acetic acid and four of the propionic acid side chains.

Coproporphyrinogen

The four acetic acid side chains of the eight carboxyl-containing UROgen III are next decarboxylated into methyl groups. The result is COPROgen III, which has four methyl side chains and four propionic acid side chains. This reaction is catalyzed by the enzyme uroporphyrinogen decarboxylase (UROgen-D). The COPROgen III now moves back into the mitochondria.

Protoporphyrinogen

Within the mitochondria, COPROgenIII-Ox catalyzes the decarboxylation of the two propionic acid groups on the A and B pyrrole rings of COPROgen III to vinyl groups. The resulting product is protoporphyrinogen III (PROTOgen III) with four methyl, two vinyl, and two propionic acid side chains. The enzyme COPROgenIII-Ox is absolutely specific for COPROgen III so that only PROTOgen III and not the I form is produced. Each of the -gen forms, UROgen I or III, COPROgen I or III, and PROTOgen III, when present in excess, can be oxidized to their free forms (URO I or III, COPRO I or III, and PROTO IX), which are released into the circulation. These free porphyrins are photoreactive and in excess are the causative agents of the photosensitivity in the porphyrias.

Protoporphyrin

PROTOgen III is next oxidized at its methyl carbon bridges to form methene bridges connecting the pyrroles, which are catalyzed by PROTOgen III oxidase (PROTOgenIII-Ox). The resulting product retains its historical name, protoporphyrin IX (PROTO IX) even though it is of the type III configuration.

Iron and Heme

Iron is stored in various tissues; it is also stored in developing red cells as ferritin, an iron protein complex. The protein moiety, apoferritin consists of at least 24 monomers of either H or L subunits. Each subunit is shaped like a short rod and these rods are assembled as a hollow sphere. Apoferritin has a molecular weight of 441,000 d and can store as much as 4,500 molecules (31% iron) of iron.[3] The maximal weight of ferritin can then be approximately 800,000 d but ferritin more commonly is approximately 620,000 d with approximately 18% iron.[4] The mode of entry and exit of iron from the interior cavity of ferritin is not precisely known. Iron apparently enters as the ferrous form that is then oxidized to and stored as ferric oxide.[5] The exit of iron may be by a reversal of the process or by a proteolytic degradation of ferritin by lysosomes [6] followed by a reduction to the ferrous form. Again, the reducing mechanisms have not been determined. This ferrous iron must now enter the mitochondria where it is chelated into the PROTO IX ring catalyzed by ferrochelatase (FER-Ch), (heme synthase, heme synthetase) to form heme.[1] Iron can also be incorporated by a nonenzymic method but the enzymic iron incorporation is more than ten times that of the nonenzymic route. This heme now enters the cytoplasmic compartment where its iron is reoxidized to the ferric form, now called ferriheme, again by an unknown mechanism(s). Heme stimulates its own synthesis in developing erythroid cells and inhibits its synthesis in reticulocytes.[7]

Globin Synthesis

Synthesis of normal polypeptide globin chains, both α and β, occurs in the ribosomes and polyribosomes within the cytoplasmic compartment. There are 141 amino acid residues in the α chains, and 146 residues in the β chains of human HgbA. Each globin chain contains a cleft or heme pocket that is lined by largely nonpolar amino acid side chains that imparts a hydrophobic nature to the pocket. The nonpolar (vinyl and methyl groups) side of ferriheme is positioned in the hydrophobic pocket of each globin chain. Within the pocket, one of the two available binding sites of ferrous iron (four are bound to the N of porphyrin) is coordinately bonded to the proximal histidine moiety of the globin, at position 87 of the α chain (α87) and at position 92 of the β chain (β92). The sixth linkage site of ferrous iron is not coordinately bonded to but rather loosely bound to the distal histidine (β63 and α58). This is then followed by the formation of an α–β dimer, and two dimers combine to form the globoid Hgb tetramer. The coupling of these chains appears to be spontaneous and readily reversible.[8] This product is correctly methemoglobin because the iron is in the ferric form. Upon reduction of the iron to the ferrous form by the normal reductive processes of the red cell, fully functional Hgb results. The rate of synthesis of the globin and hemoglobin is extremely rapid, approximately 800 molecules of Hgb/s per cell.[9]

Control of Hemoglobin Synthesis

The synthesis of heme and the globin chains are finely coordinated so that there is little or no free heme or globin in the cytoplasm of developing erythroid cells. Heme apparently is the controlling factor because it governs ribosomal translation of globin chain synthesis.[10] Additionally, α- and β-chain synthesis is coordinated. Excess α chains inhibit their own synthesis while stimulating β-chain synthesis. In addition, excess β chains inhibit their own synthesis.[11]

Hemoglobin Types in Animals

During stages of gestational development and throughout adult life, synthesis of α globin chains remains con-

stant except in the earliest stages of embryonic development. Different types of non-α globin chains are synthesized and account for the different types of Hgb appearing during development and in adult life. The amino acid sequences of the α and non-α chains seems species dependent and governs the electrophoretically different types of Hgb in animals. The amino acid differences, however, do not occur in functionally active sites of the Hgb. At the embryonic stage, most animals synthesize only embryonic chains designated ε chains that constitute the embryonal Hgbs. At the fetal stage, γ chains are synthesized and two γ chains combine with two α chains to form fetal HgbF. Near mid gestation, β chains begin to be synthesized, and two β chains and two α chains combine to form adult human Hgb. Normally in humans, a small amount of δ chains are also synthesized, and two δ chains in combination with two α chains form HgbA$_2$. At birth, a mixture of adult and fetal Hgb is present. HgbF rapidly declines, but the ability to synthesize HgbF is retained and HgbF may appear in responsive anemias.

Similarly, in those animals having HgbF, such as ruminants, a mixture of HgbF and adult Hgb is present at birth. HgbF is replaced by adult Hgb in the initial month(s) after birth.[12] In animals that lack HgbF, such as cats, dogs, horses, and pigs, embryonal Hgbs are replaced by adult Hgb during the fetal period.[13,14]

No abnormal Hgbs similar to the 150 or more different abnormal Hgbs reported in humans are known to occur in any animal. These abnormal Hgbs are essentially all structural abnormalities of the globin chains with amino acid substitutions, the classic example being that of HgbS in sickle cell anemia. This is a point mutation where valine replaces glutamic acid in the β chains at position 6. Another type of abnormality occurs when there is an imbalance in the rates of synthesis of the α and the β chains as in the human thalassemias. The resulting excess of either chain leads to a precipitation of the chain and destruction of the red cell.

With the possible exception of pigs, two or more types of Hgb occur normally in several domestic animal species.[15,16] Most polymorphisms or variants of animal Hgbs are determined genetically and are usually associated with multiple amino acid substitutions.[14] Nongenetic changes in Hgb structure also contribute to Hgb variants, in particular, the glycation of Hgb as in HgbA1c.[17] A structural difference unique to cat Hgb is the presence of 8 to 10 reactive -SH groups, whereas other animals have only 2 to 4 per Hgb molecule.[18] The presence of the readily oxidizable groups is regarded as the basis for the ease of Heinz body formation in the cat.

A unique occurrence in sheep and goats is the synthesis of HgbC in response to severe anemia,[19] and this is the result of anoxia.[20] This Hgb switching from HgbA to HgbC in sheep and from HgbA and HgbB to HgbC in goats is mediated by erythropoietin (EPO).[21] Carbon dioxide decreases oxygen affinity for HgbC more than it does for normal adult Hgbs.[19,22]

HEMOGLOBIN TURNOVER

Mature red cells are unable to synthesize proteins, including those enzymes that are critical for generating the metabolic energy with which to maintain red cell proteins in a reduced and functional state. Without replenishment, these red cell enzymes lose their activity as expressed in their turnover numbers. The enzyme activities of senescent red cells near the end of their life spans will have reached a critically low level wherein their cytoskeletal, membrane, and enzyme proteins are unprotected from oxidative injury and are significantly denatured. At this point, the red cells gradually lose their deformability function. When the red cells cannot deform sufficiently to pass through the splenic capillaries, they are trapped by the splenic mononuclear phagocyte system MPS cells and their Hgb is catabolyzed. The ultimate significance of oxidative injury or of enzyme turnover in the final senescence of red cells is unknown.

When a red cell undergoes intravascular hemolysis, its Hgb is released into the circulation in the free form. Free-plasma Hgb is quickly cleared by several mechanisms, the most important of which is the binding of Hgb to haptoglobin. The Hgb–haptoglobin complex is transported to the MPS where it is taken up and catabolyzed.[23] The half-time for free-Hgb clearance is 20 to 30 m. Minor pathways for Hgb clearance are (1) oxidation to methemoglobin or ferric hemoglobin (MetHgb) that can be excreted, (2) hydrolysis of the MetHgb to release its ferriheme (ferric heme, hematin, and hemin) that is complexed to hemopexin for transport to the MPS, and (3) binding of ferriheme to albumin (Methemalbumin) for transport to the MPS. When there is excess intravascular hemolysis such that the binding capacity of plasma haptoglobin is exceeded, Hgb may be cleared via glomerular filtration. In this event, hemoglobinuria may occur, or the proximal renal tubular cells may catabolyze Hgb.[24] The catabolic functions of the cells of the MPS are primarily carried out in the spleen, with lesser activity by the MPS cells of the liver and bone marrow.

HEMOGLOBIN CATABOLISM

The major Hgb carrier form, the Hgb–haptoglobin complex, is taken up and hydrolyzed at the surface of the MPS cell to release haptoglobin, and the Hgb is transported across the cell membrane. When free Hgb is transported in the plasma to the MPS, it is also taken up at the cell surface and transported across the cell membrane. When senescent red cells are trapped by the MPS, the red cells are hemolyzed and Hgb is released. In each case, Hgb is internalized, and Hgb degradation begins by the hydrolysis of the Hgb molecule into its constituent globin and heme moieties. The globin moiety is systematically hydrolyzed by proteolytic enzymes, and its constituent amino acids are released for reuse. The catabolism of heme is of particular significance because intermediates in the pathway of its catabolism are diagnostically important in hematology and because these intermediates are toxic.

HEME CATABOLISM AND BILIRUBIN FORMATION

Approximately 80% of the heme is derived from Hgb and myoglobin with the remainder from heme enzymes, e.g., cytochromes, peroxidase, and catalase. The initial step in the catabolic pathway is the enzymatic cleavage of the heme ring at the α methene bridge to release the linear tetrapyrrole biliverdin, iron and carbon monoxide (CO). This reaction is catalyzed by microsomal heme oxygenase in the presence of cytochrome P-450, oxygen, and reduced nicotinamide adenine dinucleotide phosphate (NADPH). The release of CO is unique to heme catabolism and has been used as an index of heme catabolism and of bilirubin formation. Heme oxygenase activity is highest in the spleen, and there is some activity in the liver, bone marrow, and renal tubular cells. Iron is oxidized to the ferric form, released and transported as transferrin for storage as hemosiderin or ferritin in the liver and as ferritin in the bone marrow for subsequent reuse.[25]

Biliverdin, a green pigment, is now reduced to bilirubin, a yellow pigment, by the action of the enzyme, biliverdin reductase in the presence of NADPH. The virtual absence of biliverdin reductase in birds accounts for the green color of avian bile. Bilirubin is a nonpolar compound and to remain soluble in the aqueous plasma when it is released, it is immediately bound to albumin. This bilirubin–albumin complex is transported to the liver, and at the hepatocyte surface, albumin is released. The first step involving the hepatocyte is the uptake or transport of bilirubin across the hepatocyte membrane by a transporter system. The second step in the hepatocyte is the conjugation of bilirubin to glucuronic acid, primarily as the diglucuronide and with some monoglucuronide. This reaction is catalyzed by the enzyme glucuronyl transferase. Other carbohydrates, glucose and fructose, may also be conjugated. The bilirubin glucuronides are highly polar and are therefore soluble compounds. The third step in the hepatocyte is the transport of bilirubin glucuronide into the canaliculi and thence to the biliary system. This canalicular transport is the rate-limiting step in hepatic bilirubin metabolism.[26,27] A small amount of the glucuronides may also be transported back into the circulation so that normally, both unconjugated and conjugated bilirubins are present in the circulation.

Conjugated bilirubins now enter the intestines where they are poorly absorbed and mostly undergo bacterial reduction to the urobilinogens or stercobilinogens. Most of the urobilinogens or stercobilinogens pass into the feces. Urobilinogens that are absorbed by the intestines are transported back to the liver by means of the portal system. In the liver, urobilinogens may be extracted and reexcreted into the bile or if not extracted from the portal blood, passed into the circulatory system. This is the process generally referred to as the enterohepatic circulation of bile pigments.

The various routes of Hgb catabolism and bilirubin metabolism are diagnostically significant in hematology. Icterus is a clinically observable sign of excess hemolysis. In general, hemolytic anemias are associated with an increase in unconjugated bilirubin in plasma, whereas an increase in conjugated bilirubin is associated with cholestatic liver disease or bile duct obstruction.

REFERENCES

1. **Kaneko JJ**. Porphyrins and the porphyrias. In: Kaneko JJ, Harvey JW, Bruss ML, eds. Clinical biochemistry of domestic animals. 5th ed. San Diego: Academic Press, 1997.
2. **Levin EY, Coleman DL**. The enzymatic conversion of porphobilinogen to uroporphyrinogen catalyzed by extracts of hematopoietic mouse spleen. J Biol Chem 1967;242:4248–4253.
3. **Leibold EA, Guo B**. Iron-dependent regulation of ferritin and transferrin receptor expression by the iron-responsive element binding protein. Ann Rev Nutr 1992;12:345–368.
4. **Smith JE**. Iron metabolism and its disorders. In: Kaneko JJ, Harvey JW, Bruss ML, eds. Clinical biochemistry of domestic animals. 5th ed. San Diego: Academic Press, 1997.
5. **Crichton RR, Charlotteaux-Wauters M**. Iron transport and storage. Eur J Biochem 1987;164:485–506.
6. **Vaisman B, Fibach E, Konijin AM**. Utilization of intracellular ferritin iron for hemoglobin synthesis in developing human erythroid precursors. Blood 1997;90:831–838.
7. **Abraham NG**. Molecular regulation–biological role of heme in hematopoiesis. Blood Rev 1991;5:19–28.
8. **Harvey JW**. The erythrocyte: physiology, metabolism, and biochemical disorders. In: Kaneko JJ, Harvey JW, Bruss ML, eds. Clinical biochemistry of domestic animals. 5th ed. San Diego: Academic Press, 1997.
9. **Itano HA**. Genetic regulation of peptide synthesis in hemoglobins. J Cell Physiol 1966;67:65–76.
10. **Traugh JA**. Heme regulation of hematopoiesis. Semin Hematol 1989;26:54–62.
11. **Jandl JH**. Blood: textbook of hematology. Boston: Little Brown, 1987.
12. **Aufderheide WM, Parker, HR, Kaneko JJ**. The metabolism of 2,3-diphosphoglycerate in the developing sheep (*Ovis aries*). Comp Biochem Physiol 1980;65A:393–398.
13. **Bunn HF, Kitchen H**. Hemoglobin function in the horse: the role of 2,3-diphosphoglycerate in mogifying the oxygen affinity of maternal and fetal blood. Blood 1973;42:471–479.
14. **Kitchen H, Brett I**. Embryonic and fetal hemoglobins in animals. Ann N Y Acad Sci 1974;241:653–671.
15. **Kitchen H**. Heterogeneity of animal hemoglobins. Adv Vet Sci Comp Med 1969;13:247–330.
16. **Braend M**. Hemoglobin polymorphisms in the domestic dog. J Hered 1988;79:211–212.
17. **Kaneko JJ**. Carbohydrate metabolism and its diseases. In: Kaneko JJ, Harvey JW, Bruss ML, eds. Clinical biochemistry of domestic animals. 5th ed. San Diego: Academic Press, 1997;64–65.
18. **Mauk AG, Taketa F**. Effects of organic phosphates on oxygen equilibria and kinetics of SH reaction in feline hemoglobins. Arch Biochem Biophys 1972;150:37681.
19. **Huisman TH, Kitchen J**. Oxygen equilibria studies of the hemoglobins from normal and anemic sheep and goats. Am J Physiol 1968;215:140–146.
20. **Boyer SF, Crosby EF, Noyes AN, Kaneko JJ, Keeton K, Zinkl J**. Hemoglobin switching in non-anemic sheep. II. Response to high altitude. Johns Hopkins Med J 1968;123:92–94.
21. **Barker JE, Pierce JE, Nienhuis AW**. Hemoglobin switching in sheep: a comparison of the erythropoietin- induced switch to HbC and the fetal to adult hemoglobin switch. Blood 1980;56:488–494.
22. **Winslow RM, Swenberg M-L, Benson J, Perrella M, Benazzi L**. Gas exchange properties of goat hemoglobins A and C. J Biol Chem 1989;264:4812–4817.
23. **Jain NC**. Schalm's Veterinary Hematology. 4th ed. Philadelphia: Lea & Febiger, 1986;521.
24. **De Schepper J**. Degradation of hemoglobin to bilirubin in the kidney of the dog. Tijdschr Diergeneeskd 1974;99:699–707.
25. **Tennant BC**. Hepatic function. In: Kaneko JJ, Harvey JW, Bruss ML, eds. Clinical biochemistry of domestic animals. 5th ed. San Diego: Academic Press, 1997;329–333.
26. **Arias IM, Johnson L, Wolfson S**. Biliary excretion of injected conjugated and unconjugated bilirubin by normal and Gunn rats. Am J Physiol 1961;200:1091–1096.
27. **Jansen PLM, Chowdhury JR, Fishberg EB, Arias IM**. Enzymatic conversion of bilirubin monoglucuronide to diglucuronide by rat liver plasma membrane. J Biol Chem 1977;252:2710–2716.

Clinical and Hematologic Manifestations of Anemia

• BETSY AIRD

Anemia is the decreased ability of blood to supply tissues with adequate oxygen for proper metabolic function.[1,2] It is characterized by decreased hemoglobin (Hgb), hematocrit (HCT), or total erythrocyte count [red blood cell (RBC)] in a normally hydrated animal. Anemia is a clinical manifestation of an underlying disease process, not a diagnosis; therefore, the response to treatment of an anemia is transient unless the underlying disease process is identified.[3–6]

The cause of anemia is determined by evaluation of patient history, clinical and physical examination findings, and hematologic laboratory results. Determining the specific cause of an anemia is important to therapeutic and prognostic considerations.

CAUSES OF ANEMIA

Anemia has many causes (Table 24.1). Understanding normal bone marrow function and recognizing the systemic consequences of inadequate function is essential for characterizing the cause of an anemia and for determining the adequacy of the bone marrow response.[7] An anemia is considered regenerative if there is hematologic evidence that the bone marrow is responding appropriately to a decreased HCT. An anemia associated with an inadequate bone marrow response is termed nonregenerative.

Regenerative anemias result from excessive blood loss (hemorrhage) or RBC destruction (hemolysis). In species other than horses and ruminants, this results in increased erythropoiesis with increased numbers of young red cells (reticulocytes) present in the peripheral blood. Reticulocytes appear in the blood within 2 to 4 days of blood loss or destruction with peak production occurring within 4 to 7 days.[3] Thus erythropoiesis may appear nonregenerative early in the course of an anemia because of inadequate response time. Evaluation of regeneration is more difficult in horses because they do not reliably exhibit reticulocytosis.[8,9] Assessment of regeneration in this species is based on examination of the bone marrow or performance of serial hemograms with particular attention to the HCT, Hgb, RBC count,

and total plasma protein (TPP).[9] Nucleated RBCs and basophilic stippled RBCs are more useful indicators of erythropoiesis in ruminants.

Nonregenerative anemias are characterized by decreased or ineffective production of RBCs by the bone marrow. These may be caused by primary or, more commonly, secondary bone marrow disease. Anemias may also be relative or physiologic as well as pathologic. Physiologic anemias occur when the RBC mass is decreased as a result of normal physiologic changes such as is seen in neonates or during estrus. Relative anemias result from increased plasma volume (dilutional anemia) or sequestration of RBCs within the microcirculation (hypersplenism). These are not true anemias as the functional RBC mass is not decreased.[8] Clinical evidence of anemia is not associated with relative and physiologic anemias.[8]

CLINICAL MANIFESTATIONS

The clinical manifestations of anemia (Table 24.2) are determined in part by their specific origin and pathogenesis.[10] In general, clinical signs can be attributed to a reduction in oxygen-carrying capacity of the blood. Some of these are a direct result of tissue hypoxia, however, the majority are related to compensatory mechanisms that increase the circulating blood volume and reduce the cardiac workload.[1,3]

Clinical signs and physical examination findings suggest that the effects of anemias are varied[3–7] (Table 24.2). Severity is determined by the rapidity of onset, magnitude of decreased blood volume, and adequacy of cardiopulmonary adaptation.[10] Some animals that have severe anemia may not show clinical signs because the onset is chronic, whereas others that have mild anemia may be severely affected if the onset is acute.

COMPENSATORY MECHANISMS

Normally, in most species, approximately 1% of the senescent circulating RBCs are lost daily.[3,11] In healthy

TABLE 24.1   General Causes of Anemia

I. Blood Loss (Regenerative) (see Chapter 26)
  Coagulopathies
  Epistaxis
  Gastrointestinal hemorrhage
  Platelet disorders
  Splenic rupture
  Trauma/surgery

II. Blood Destruction/Hemolysis (Regenerative) (see Chapters 27, 29, 30)
  Fragmentation
  Immune-mediated disease (see Chapter 29)
  Infections (see Chapter 28)
  Intrinsic RBC defects
  Toxicities (see Chapters 30, 31)

III. Decreased/Ineffective Production (Nonregenerative)
  Anemia of inflammatory disease (see Chapter 35)
  Aplastic or hypoplastic anemias (see Chapters 36, 37)
  Metabolic or endocrine disease
  Neoplastic disease
  Nutritional deficiency anemias (see Chapter 32)

TABLE 24.2   Clinical and Physical Examination Findings of Anemia

General Clinical Signs of Anemia
  Pallor
  Anorexia
  Lethargy
  Weakness
  Exercise intolerance
  Dyspnea
  Collapse
  Tachypnea
  Tachycardia
  Systolic heart murmur

Clinical Signs Suggestive of Blood Loss
  Hematemesis
  Epistaxsis
  Petechiae
  Ecchymosis
  Melena
  Hematomas
  Hemarthrosis

Clinical Signs Suggestive of Hemolytic Anemia
  Icterus
  Hemoglobinemia
  Hemoglobinuria
  Splenomegaly

animals, the bone marrow effectively produces RBCs to compensate for these losses. In severe anemias, other mechanisms occur to compensate for the increased tissue hypoxia.

Decreased Oxygen Affinity

One of the earliest compensatory adjustments that occur in response to tissue hypoxia is a decrease in the affinity of Hgb for oxygen.[10] The delivery and release of oxygen to the tissues by Hgb is regulated by the RBC phosphate 2,3-diphosphoglycerate (2,3-DPG). In the presence of 2,3-DPG, Hgb can more readily release oxygen to peripheral tissues. Enhanced production of 2,3-DPG in anemic animals serves to improve tissue oxygenation and thereby diminishes the clinical signs associated with hypoxia.[10,13,14] The reason for increased synthesis of 2,3-DPG in anemia is unclear, but it probably is caused primarily by a change in the intracellular pH of red cells.[13]

Increased Tissue Perfusion

Tissue perfusion is increased by redistribution of blood from nonvital areas of the body such as the skin to organs with the greatest need for oxygen, including the heart, brain, and muscles.[14] Vasoconstriction and oxygen deprivation in the cutaneous tissue seems well tolerated by most anemic animals.

Increased Cardiac Output

Cardiac rates may increase drastically in anemic animals. The elevated heart rate increases cardiac output to keep pace with peripheral tissue oxygen demands in the face of decreased oxygen-carrying capacity. Increased cardiac output decreases the amount of oxygen that is extracted during each circulation, thereby keeping oxygen pressure high.[15] The increased output can be maintained without a measurable increase in blood pressure because vasodilation and the lower viscosity of anemic blood decrease peripheral resistance.[14,15] Tachycardia, increased jugular pulses, and systolic heart murmurs are frequent clinical signs associated with increased cardiac output. The normal myocardium tolerates a prolonged period of sustained hyperactivity; however, cardiomegaly, pulmonary congestion, ascites, and edema suggest cardiac failure.[14]

Increased Red-Cell Production

In anemia, RBC production may reach 6 to 10 times normal as a result of increased synthesis of erythropoietin by the kidney in response to hypoxia.[10] Increased erythropoietin production occurs when Hgb is decreased, when a Hgb structural problem occurs in which oxygen is not released, or at high altitudes where oxygen tension is low.[16] Clinical administration of recombinant erythropoietin is beneficial in anemias caused by systemic disease or chronic renal failure in which endogenous production of erythropoietin is low. It is not beneficial in hemolytic or blood-loss anemias in which endogenous production of erythropoietin is normal.[16]

DIAGNOSTIC TESTS

Various laboratory tests are used to further define the causes of anemia (Table 24.3). Of these, performing a

---

TABLE 24.3 Diagnostic Tests for Anemia

1. Complete Blood Count (CBC)
   a. RBC morphology
   b. Reticulocyte count
   c. RBC indices
   d. Total plasma protein (TPP)
   e. Platelet count or estimate
2. Biochemical profile
3. Urinalysis
4. Fecal examination (occult blood, parasites)
5. Bone marrow examination
6. Coagulation profile
7. Immune testing (Coombs test, antinuclear antibody test)
8. Fecal examination (occult blood, parasites)
9. Iron assays (serum iron, serum ferritin, total iron binding capacity)
10. Endocrine testing (thyroid hormone levels, adrenocorticotrophic hormone [ACTH] stimulation or dexamethasone suppression tests)
11. Body fluid examination

---

complete blood cell count (CBC) with emphasis on assessment of RBC morphology, a reticulocyte count, and a calculation of red cell indices are most important (Chapter 19).[7] Bone marrow aspiration or core biopsies are particularly useful in evaluating the cause of unexplained nonregenerative anemias in the absence of metabolic or endocrine dysfunctions (Chapter 6). Specialized tests to evaluate immune diseases include the direct Coombs test and antinuclear antibody (ANA) test (Chapter 29). Coagulation tests, occult fecal blood, fecal flotation, iron assays, and examination of body fluids are useful if hemorrhage is suspected.

Understanding the clinical and hematologic manifestations of anemia will greatly assist in identification of the cause of anemia and is useful for therapeutic and prognostic considerations.

REFERENCES

1. **Hoffbrand AV, Pettit JE, et al.** Erythropoiesis and general aspects of anaemia. In: Hoffbrand AV, Pettit JE, eds. Essential hematology. 3rd ed. Oxford: Blackwell Scientific, 1993.
2. **Jandl JH.** Blood: pathophysiology. Oxford: Blackwell Scientific, 1991;64.
3. **Jain NC.** Schalm's veterinary hematology. 4th ed. Philadelphia: Lea & Febiger, 1986;563.
4. **Jain NC.** Essentials of veterinary hematology. Philadelphia: Lea & Febiger, 1993;159.
5. **Cotter SM.** Approach to anemia. In: 20th annual waltham/OSU symposium, oncology and hematology. Vernon, CA: Waltham USA, 1996;81.
6. **Ahn AH, Cotter SM.** Approach to the anemic patient. In: Bonagura JD, ed. Kirk's current veterinary therapy. XII. Small animal practice. Philadephia: WB Saunders, 1995.
7. **Rogers KS.** Anemia. In: Ettinger SJ, ed. Textbook of veterinary internal medicine. 4th ed. Philadephia: WB Saunders, 1995;187.
8. **Tyler RD, Cowell RL.** Classification and diagnosis of anaemia. Comp Haematol Int 1996;6:1–16.
9. **Lassen ED, Swardson CJ.** Hematology and hemostasis in the horse: normal functions and common abnormalities. Vet Clin North Am Equine Pract 1995;11(3):351.
10. **Erslev AJ.** Clinical manifestations and classification of erythrocyte disorders. In: Beutler E, Lichtman MA, Coller BS, et al, eds. Williams hematology. 5th ed. New York: McGraw-Hill, 1995;441.
11. **Glassman AB.** Anemia: diagnosis and clinical considerations. In: Harmening DM, ed. Clinical hematology and fundamentals of hemostasis. 3rd ed. Philadephia: FA Davis, 1997;71.
12. **Beck WS.** Hematology. 3rd ed. Cambridge: MIT Press, 1981;91.
13. **Moore LG, Brewer GJ.** Beneficial effect of rightward hemoglobin-oxygen dissociation curve for short-term high altitude adaptation. J Lab Clin Med 1981; 98:145.
14. **Vatner SF.** Effects of hemorrhage on regional blood flow distribution in dogs and primates. J Clin Invest 1974;54:225.
15. **Sharpey-Schafer EP.** Cardiac output in severe anemia. Clin Sci 1944;5:125
16. **Erslev AJ.** Erythropoietin. N Engl J Med 1991;324:1339.

CHAPTER 25

Classification and Laboratory Evaluation of Anemia

• HAROLD TVEDTEN and DOUGLAS J. WEISS

Classification of anemia is the use of certain characteristics to place the anemia into preestablished classes or categories useful for diagnosis. Several classification systems are described and are based on laboratory evaluation of blood. The systems overlap, and classifications of one system (e.g., macrocytic hypochromic anemia) may be identifying the same change or process in erythrocytes as another classification (e.g., regenerative anemia). That is, different terms may mean the same in terms of diagnosis. Despite the classification used, the clinical diagnosis and treatment choices should be correct and appropriate.

PRESENCE AND SEVERITY OF ANEMIA

Laboratory tests commonly used to document anemia (or polycythemia) are hematocrit (HCT) or packed cell volume (PCV), total erythrocyte count (red blood cell [RBC]), and hemoglobin (Hgb) concentration. These values should be similarly lowered with reduction of erythroid mass in the sample and should reflect the severity of the anemia in the animal. If they are not similarly decreased, the erythrocyte indices (mean corpuscular volume [MCV], mean corpuscular hemoglobin concentration [MCHC]) may explain the difference. For example, in iron-deficiency anemia with severe microcytosis, the RBC may not reflect the severity of the anemia as well as the Hgb or PCV. Even normal numbers of microcytic erythrocytes do not contribute to a normal concentration of Hgb per unit volume of blood, and the smaller erythrocytes are packed into a smaller volume of the blood. There are also errors for all test procedures and these errors may be implicated as reasons for discordance among the three tests. For example, Heinz bodies may make RBCs more fragile so they lyse in the microhematocrit centrifuge, lowering the PCV; and Heinz bodies remaining in suspension after the RBCs are lysed may increase the optical density and thus Hgb. Besides the RBC indices, newer hematology analyzers graphically display cells so that abnormal erythrocytes (Fig. 25.1) and some laboratory errors may be visualized.

Severity of an anemia is often a significant factor in diagnosis. Some causes of anemia (e.g., hypothyroidism) are characteristically mild and would be excluded from consideration in a moderate to severe anemia. Severity of anemia or rapidity of decline in erythroid mass should stimulate more aggressive diagnosis and treatment, whereas mild anemia in animals that have severe inflammatory or neoplastic disorders are expected and not addressed in favor of working on the more severe problem. Table 25.1 provides some guidelines for classifying severity. Primary bone marrow disorders like chronic myelofibrosis can cause severe anemia (e.g. PCV = 8%), whereas secondary suppression of bone marrow (e.g. anemia of inflammation) is characteristically mild and PCV, Hgb and RBC values may remain within the reference range. Veterinarians tend to think in terms of PCV, so Table 25.1 uses only PCV/HCT.

CLASSIFICATION BY STRENGTH OF ERYTHROPOIESIS

Anemia not caused by bone marrow disorders should have appropriate evidence of erythropoiesis (regeneration or responsiveness). The initial and most important classification of most anemias is into regenerative and non-regenerative anemias. Regenerative anemias have good bone marrow function, so the anemia must be caused by loss of RBC from the body (external blood loss) or from lysis of the RBCs within the body (hemolytic anemia and internal blood loss). Laboratory proof of adequate regeneration may be obvious, but in other situations one must consider the severity of the anemia, the duration, the species characteristics, the treatments, and the multiple origins in classification. Poor bone marrow function causes nonregenerative anemia.

Bone marrow regeneration in species with consistent reticulocyte responses (e.g., dogs, cats, pigs, and rats) should be evaluated by the reticulocyte response. (See Chapter 19, Reticulocyte Response.) The magnitude of the absolute reticulocyte count per unit volume of blood

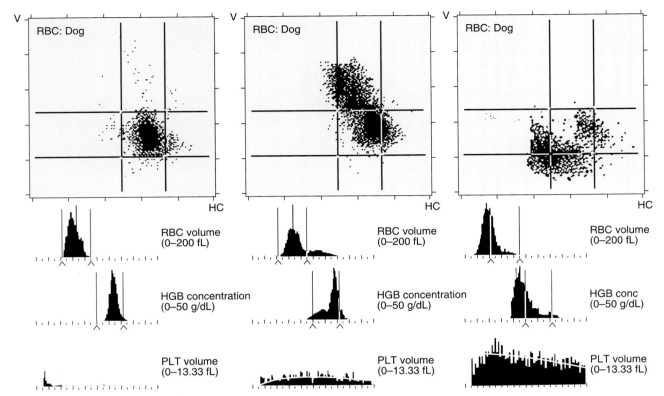

FIGURE 25.1 A composite RBC cytogram, RBC volume histogram, Hgb histogram, and platelet volume histogram from three dogs that have anemia. Graphics are part of the Bayer(Technicon) H-1 system's reports. Dog 1 had a severe normocytic normochromic anemia and an acute myeloid leukemia (HCT = 10.6%). The RBC cytogram displays each cell on the basis of volume (vertical axis) and Hgb concentration (horizontal axis). Normocytic and normochromic cells are in the center box of the 9-box cytogram. It also had a severe thrombocytopenia (9×10^9/L). Dog 2, in the middle, was hit by a car and had a moderately severe blood-loss anemia (HCT = 25%) that is regenerative. Note on the RBC cytogram a second cluster of macrocytic hypochromic cells to the upper left of normal cell cluster. These are younger erythrocytes. Reticulocytes were 10%. The normal cell cluster appears slightly to the right of the center box because the grid was not properly aligned. The RBC volume histogram demonstrates a second peak of macrocytic cells to the right of the normocytic cells. The Hgb histogram is bimodal with a small, flatter peak of hypochromic cells to the left of the normochromic cells. The histograms reflect the relative number of cells and one sees that there is at least 10% of the cells in the macrocytic or hypochromic peaks. The RBC cytogram does not allow estimation of the relative size of separate populations. The platelet histogram is smaller than normal, indicating thrombocytopenia (93×10^9/L), and extends to the right, indicating large platelets [mean platelet volume (MPV) = 6.7 fL]. The third RBC cytogram has a light cluster of normal erythrocytes on the right side of the central box, and most of the erythrocytes were microcytic and hypochromic because of iron deficiency of chronic blood loss. The RBC volume histogram has one main peak of microcytic cells to the left of the two vertical lines, indicating the normal reference range, and a small right shoulder of normocytic cells extending into the normocytic range. The Hgb histogram looks the same with hypochromic cells. The platelet histogram was large, reflecting a thrombocytosis (platelets = 707×10^9/L), and extended to the right, indicating large platelets (MCV = 6.5 fL).

reflects well bone marrow erythropoiesis and hence whether the bone marrow is responding as expected to blood loss or hemolysis (Table 25.2). The percentage of reticulocytes is a relative value affected by the severity of the anemia and the number of mature erythrocytes remaining. Absolute counts are preferred for interpretation. The corrected reticulocyte percentage and reticulocyte index are other methods of interpreting the reticulocyte response when there is a variable decrease in normal RBCs. The reticulocyte numbers are best interpreted at the time of an expected peak of reticulocytes (e.g., 4 to 7 days). Guidelines for interpreting reticulocyte numbers are useful at peak reticulocytosis but may

TABLE 25.1 Guidelines for Classification of Severity of Anemia

	Dog	Horse	Cat/Ruminant
Mild	30–37[a]	30–33	20–26
Moderate	20–29	20–29	14–19
Severe	13–19	13–19	10–13
Very Severe	<13	<13	<10

[a]Values are HCT or PCV in percent.

TABLE 25.2   Canine and Feline Reticulocyte Guidelines (Relative and Absolute)

Strength of Regeneration	Canine Reticulocytes	Feline Aggregate Reticulocytes	Feline Punctate Reticulocytes
Relative			
None	1%[a]	0–0.4%[a]	1–10%[a]
Weak	1–4	0.5–2%	10–20%
Moderate	5–20%	3–4%	20–50%
Strong	21–50%	>5%	>50%
Absolute			
None	60[b]	<15[b]	<200[b]
Weak	150	50	500
Moderate	300	100	1000
Strong	>500	>200	>1500

[a]Values are percentage of nonnucleated RBC that were reticulocytes.
Note: The percentage of canine reticulocytes or feline aggregate reticulocytes also may be used to convert the percentage of polychromatophils on a blood smear to strength of polychromasia and thus erythropoiesis.
[b]Reticulocytes $\times 10^9$/L or reticulocytes $\times 10^3$/μL.

be misleading early in an anemia (i.e., pre-regenerative) or late in an anemia when reticulocyte numbers decline (10 to 14 days). Late in an anemia the number of macrocytic hypochromic erythrocytes (Fig. 25.1) may be more reflective of the strength of regeneration than the reticulocyte number that may be declining or low.

Feline reticulocyte responses are unique in that their punctate reticulocyte with reduced RNA content has a long half-life in blood and therefore may accumulate in large numbers (>50% of nonnucleated erythroid cells). Punctate reticulocytes occur in other species but do not accumulate in numbers large enough to interfere with interpretation of a total reticulocyte count. Feline aggregate reticulocytes have responses similar to reticulocytes of other species but appear in low numbers (often less than 5%) and may not be released well unless the anemia is severe. Aggregate reticulocytes have high RNA content detectable by thiazole orange staining in flow cytometers and, on smears of blood stained with new methylene blue (or other dyes), contain large clumps or strands of RNA. Punctate reticulocytes contain only punctate granules (ribosomes) on smears and low RNA in flow cytometery. With cats, it is important that each type is interpreted separately and that laboratories indicate the type of reticulocyte identified. Note in Table 25.2 that the number of aggregate reticulocytes indicating a strongly regenerative anemia is the same number of the number of punctate reticulocytes indicating no regeneration. Duration of the regenerative response may be indicated by type of reticulocyte in abundance. A strong increase in aggregate reticulocytes along with a mild increase in punctate reticulocytes indicates an early response (3 to 6 days after the onset of anemia), whereas late in a response (9 to 20 days) there may be many punctate reticulocytes with few aggregates.

Other indicators of an appropriately active bone marrow in anemia may be less specific for erythropoiesis than reticulocytosis, but they may be useful in species

without consistent reticulocyte responses. Nucleated erythrocytes (NRBCs) are useful indicators in ruminants (e.g., cattle and llamas) to reflect regeneration. NRBC numbers are often reported as a relative ratio of NRBC:100WBC, so significant changes in WBC count can affect this ratio. Absolute numbers of NRBC/μL or /L more consistently indicate the number released into circulation. Basophilic stippling, especially in ruminants, and Howell–Jolly bodies suggest a regenerative anemia. Young erythrocytes are usually larger so macrocytosis or anisocytosis suggest active erythropoiesis and may be the only indicators in peripheral blood of horses that do not release reticulocytes into circulation. Macrocytosis and anisocytosis may be detected by the MCV (e.g., >52 fL in horses), RBC cytograms and histograms (Fig. 25.2), or blood smear evaluation. Erythroid hyperplasia on bone marrow examination demonstrates active erythropoiesis in horses.

Bone marrow evaluation is indicated in anemias for which the hemogram does not adequately provide evidence of normal bone marrow function. This most often is done in nonregenerative anemias that have had ade-

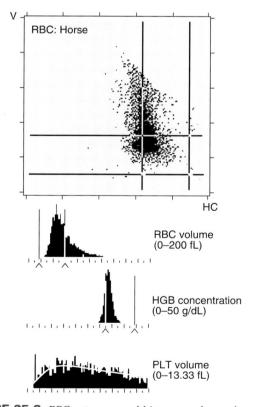

FIGURE 25.2 RBC cytogram and histograms from a horse that has severe renal hemorrhage (HCT = 16.1%) and strong regeneration reflected by macrocytosis (macrocytic normochromic). The normal erythrocytes on the RBC cytogram are below the upper horizontal line and on the RBC volume histogram the normal cells are between the two vertical lines. Based on the area of the right shoulder on the RBC volume histogram to the right of the right vertical line, one may estimate that approximately one third of the erythrocytes were macrocytic but that the MCV was only 60.6 fL.

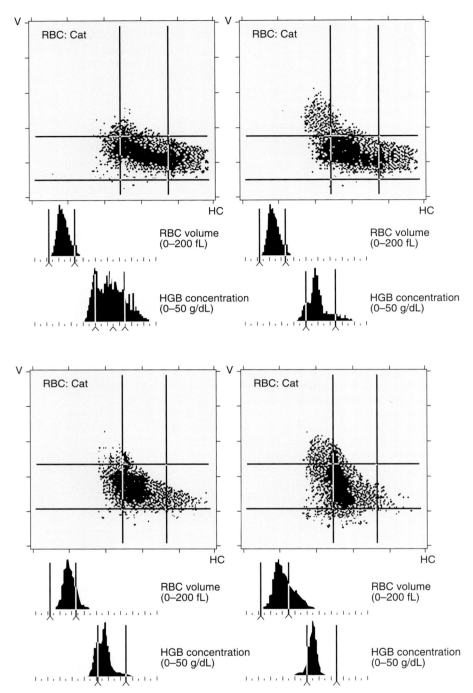

FIGURE 25.3 Composite of four sets of RBC cytograms and histograms over 1 week from a cat that had onion toxicity and Heinz-body hemolytic anemia from eating baby food with onion powder. The third set (lower left) looks the most normal and may be used for comparison. Its RBC cytogram has one dark, round cluster that is the normocytic normochromic erythrocytes. The cells should be in the center box, but the grid was not aligned well. The lightly dispersed dots extending to the right are Heinz bodies that appeared hyperchromic. Note that on the first set (upper left) this extension is dark, indicating many erythrocytes appeared hyperchromic because 84% contained Heinz bodies. The MCHC was 44 g/dL on this day. The Hgb concentration histogram was bimodal. The smaller left peak was normochromic cells (grid was offset), and the large, wider right peak are the hyperchromic-appearing cells. The final set of graphics on the lower right shows a good regenerative response with mainly macrocytic and slightly hypochromic erythrocytes extending up and to the left of the normal cells. The RBC volume histogram shows many (perhaps one fourth) of the cells were macrocytic. The Hgb histogram shows essentially no hyperchromic cells (erythrocytes with Heinz bodies dropped to 17%) and a small population of hypochromic cells. The sequence shows well the loss of hyperchromic erythrocytes with Heinz bodies and then the regenerative response with young, macrocytic cells.

TABLE 25.3   Erythrocyte Shape Changes Associated with Selected Diseases or Conditions

Spherocyte		**Eccentrocytes/Pyknocyte**	
Immune-mediated hemolytic anemias	Dog	Vitamin K treatment	Dog
Transfused blood	Dog	Onion ingestion	Dog
Blood parasite infections	Several species	Acetylphenylhydrazine	Dog
Anaplasmosis	Cattle	Hydrogen peroxide intravenously	Cattle
Hereditary spherocytosis	Goat	Glucose-6-phosphate dehydrogenase enzyme deficiency	Horse
Zinc toxicity	Dog		
Snake venom toxicity	Dog	**Hypochromasia**	
Keratocyte/shizocyte		Iron deficiency	Dog, cat, cattle, horse, pig, llama, goats, birds
DIC[a]	Dog, cat, cattle, horse	Inflammation	Birds
Congestive heart failure	Dog	Lead toxicity	Birds
Glomerulonephritis	Dog	**Macrocytosis**	
Myelofibrosis	Dog	Regenerative anemia	Many species
Hemangiosarcoma	Dog	Poodle macrocytosis	Dog
Chronic doxorubicin toxicosis	Dog	Stomatocytosis	Dog
Acanthocyte/budding Fragmentation		Feline Leukemia virus infection	Cat
DIC	Dog	Myelodysplasia	Cat
Hemangiosarcoma	Dog	Anticonvulsant (antifolate) drugs	Dog
Portosystemic shunts	Dog	Prolonged storage of blood	Many species
Chronic liver disease	Dog, cat	Hypernatremia	Cat, dog
Lymphosarcoma	Dog	**Microcytosis**	
Glomerulonephritis	Dog	Iron deficiency	Dog, cat, cow, horse, pig
Echinocyte		Hepatic protosystemic shunt	Dog
Crenation artifact	Dog, cat, cattle, horse	Hyponatremia	Dog
Lymphosarcoma	Dog	Normal breed characteristic	Dog (Akita, Shibas)
Glomerulonephritis	Dog		
Doxorubicin toxicity	Dog		
Electrolyte depletion	Horse, dog		
Heinz bodies			
Onion ingestion	Dog, cat, cow, horse, sheep		
Vitamin K (mainly K$_3$)	Dog		
Acetaminophen treatment	Cat		
Phenothiazine treatment	Horse		
Red maple leaf ingestion	Horse		
Methylene-blue treatment	Dog, cat		
Phenazopyridine treatment	Cat		
Propoylene glycol in food	Dog, cat		
Brassica spp. ingestion	Cattle		
Selenium deficiency	Cattle		
Copper toxicity	Sheep		

[a]DIC, disseminated intravascular coagulation.

quate time (e.g., 3 to 6 days) to respond. Bone marrow evaluation is best when based on cytologic evaluation of aspirated smears, histologic evaluation of a cortex to cortex section, and a complete blood count (CBC) taken on the same day. Erythroid hypoplasia, pure red cell aplasia (PRCA), myelofibrosis, aplastic pancytopenia (fatty marrow), and leukemia are the clearest conclusions obtained in nonregenerative anemia. Ineffective erythropoiesis and myelodysplasia are harder to interpret. Ineffective erythropoiesis is the appearance of adequate to increased numbers of normal-appearing erythroid cells in the marrow, and yet blood analysis

indicates no evidence of regeneration. It may result from inflammation, infections, drugs, and neoplasia. Routine morphology is often inadequate to explain poor bone marrow function. (See Chapter 6, Approaches to Evaluation of Bone Marrow.) Myelodysplasia is indicated by abnormal morphology such as megaloblastic rubricytes, dwarf megakaryocytes, binucleated cells, nuclear fragments and increased blast cells. More than 30% blast cells in the marrow's hemotopoietic cells indicates an acute leukemia. Less than 30% blast cells but increased numbers of blasts may occur in myelodysplasic syndromes and chronic leukemias.

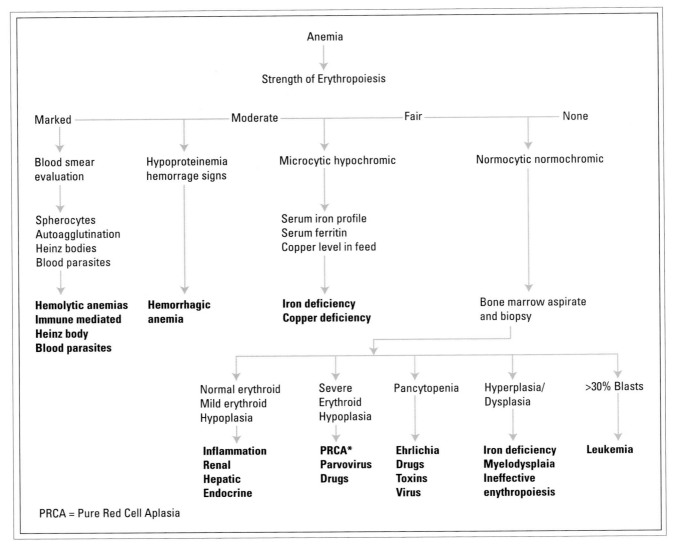

Figure 25.4. Anemia is documented and evaluated for severity. The strength of erythropoiesis (regeneration) is determined usually by reticulocyte evaluation. The significant to moderately regenerative anemias are hemolytic and hemorrhagic. Blood smear evaluation often identifies type of hemolytic anemia. Diagnoses are given in bold. Hypoproteinemia and clinical signs indicate hemorrhagic anemia. Microcytic hypochromic evidence indicates iron deficiency that varies from nonregenerative to moderately regenerative. Nonregenerative and inadequately regenerative anemias with normocytic and normochromic erythrocytes may be diagnosed by bone marrow evaluation.

CLASSIFICATION BY RED BLOOD CELL VOLUME AND HEMOGLOBIN CONCENTRATION

The RBC indices of MCV and MCHC are used for the "Morphologic Classification of Anemia." Erythrocyte volume changes are called microcytic (smaller), normocytic or macrocytic (larger). (See Chapter 33, Macrocytosis, and Chapter 34, Microcytic Anemias.) MCHC are termed hypochromic (reduced) and normochromic (normal concentration). Hyperchromic changes are usually laboratory errors (e.g., hemolysis or Heinz bodies) that imply the erythrocytes contain more Hgb per unit volume than a normal cell filled with Hgb. The three important diagnostic patterns are macrocytic hypochromic anemias (regenerative anemia with large RBCs that are not fully hemoglobinized), normocytic normochromic anemia (nonregenerative anemias with normal RBCs), and microcytic hypochromic anemias that are usually iron-deficiency anemias.

A pattern that causes confusion is macrocytic normochromic RBCs (see Chapter 33). This is the normal regenerative response of horses (Fig. 25.2). It may occur during regenerative responses of other species. In cats macrocytic normochromic RBC in the absence of polychromasia suggests feline leukemia virus (FeLV) infection or myelodysplasia. Some poodles have macrocytic RBC as an incidental finding. Swelling of RBCs is a common artifact in day-old samples. Altered erythrocytes may also swell as in stomatocytosis in dogs. In primates macrocytic normochromic RBC suggest a B-12 or folic acid deficiency or cobalt deficiency in ruminants. Macrocytosis may occur during chronic anticonvulsant therapy because some anticonvulsants antagonize folate. Folate-deficiency-induced anemia is rarely a problem in most veterinary practices. The relation between macrocytic normochromic RBCs and B-12 or folic acid deficiency has been overemphasized in veterinary medicine and has diverted attention from diagnosis of more likely causes.

Computer graphics of automated hematology systems are more sensitive in detecting changes in volume or Hgb concentration in subpopulations of erythrocytes than the MCV or MCHC (Fig. 25.1). Early in an anemia (e.g., iron deficiency) the number of microcytic hypochromic cells is often too small to affect a mean value of all erythrocytes such as MCV and MCHC. These graphic displays of each erythrocyte and populations of erythrocytes are exceptionally good tools in anemia diagnosis. In horses that lack a reticulocyte response, the cytograms and histograms may demonstrate macrocytosis (normochromic) in strongly regenerative anemias (Fig. 25.2). Cats that have macrocytic normochromic erythrocytes suggest testing for FeLV infections or myelodysplasia. Hyperchromic cells may be detected in Heinz body anemia because the Heinz bodies make the cells appear more optically dense in a laser detection system (Fig. 25.3). Canine spherocytes in immune-mediated hemolytic anemia appear normocytic and normochromic in a laser or flow cytometer system so their smaller diameter and darker color on blood smears is a three-dimensional effect of the cells not laying as flat as normal erythrocytes. The principles of morphologic classification by -cytic and -chromic are as true or truer today because instrumentation has improved sensitivity and accuracy of observations. These instruments also demonstrate when cell counts, especially platelet counts, are affected by RBC fragments or lipemia as well as other errors.

CLASSIFICATION BY BLOOD SMEAR MORPHOLOGY

Blood smear evaluation is an essential procedure in classification of anemia, especially hemolytic anemias. Many observations critical to diagnosis can only be made or are made more accurately by a person instead of an instrument. Some examples are blood parasite identification, spherocytes, autoagglutination, Heinz bodies, hypochromasia, eccentrocytes, pyknocytes, forms of erythrocyte fragmentation (Table 25.3), brown color of metHgb, clumping of platelets or leukocytes, and less-specific observations.

DIAGNOSTIC APPROACHES

The ultimate goal of diagnosis is correct classification of anemia by origin or origins in the case of multiple

---

TABLE 25.4	**Selective Causes of Hemolytic Anemias**

Immune Mediated
  Idiopathic, viral (EIA), drugs, blood parasites, neonatal iso-erythrolysis

Heinz Body
  Onions, vitamin K_3, phenothiazine, acetaminophen, phenacetin, acetanilide, phenylhydrazine-HCL, benzocaine, red maple, methylene blue, phenazopyridine, copper toxicity, selenium deficiency, *Brassica* sp. ingestion
  (Note: MetHgb caused by similar oxidative toxins and often concurrent.)

Toxic Hemolysis
  Zinc, copper, water in calves, L-sorbose

Hypophosphatemia
  Postpartiurent hemoglobinuria, refeeding syndrome, diabetes mellitus

Blood Parasites
  Anaplasma, Babesia, Haemobartonella, Eperythrozoon, Theileria, Trypanosoma, Sarcocystis, Cytauxzoon

Bacteria
  Leptospira, clostridium novyi

Hereditary RBC Enzyme Deficiencies
  Pyruvic kinase, phosphofructokinase, glucose 6-phosphate dehydrogenase

---

TABLE 25.5	**Selected Examples of Hemorrhagic Anemia**

Trauma
  Hit by car, penetrating wounds, surgical trauma

Bleeding Lesions
  Intestinal neoplasms, gastrointestinal tract ulceration, burns, infections

Parasites
  Hookworms, coccidia, haemonchus, fleas, lice

Hemostatic Disorders
  Thrombocytopenia, thrombopathy, acquired coagulopathy (e.g., Warfarin toxicity, hepatic disease), hereditary coagulopathy, von Willebrand's disease, disseminated intravascular coagulation

---

causes. The route to the final diagnosis varies with each case or situation and could begin with the cause if, for example, the cause (e.g., cat was treated with acetaminophen/paracetamol, a drug know to cause severe Heinz-body hemolytic anemia) was in the history. More typically anemia classification would begin with analysis of a typical CBC, including blood smear evaluation and in many species, reticulocyte evaluation. If the diagnosis is not obvious from the history, physical examination and CBC and then additional testing is indicated. Additional tests are chosen on the basis of the situation, the species, and the probability of different causes of anemia for a location.

A simple, algorithmic approach to selected anemias reflects the previous discussion (Fig. 25.4). One must add one's own interpretation and knowledge to any algorithm to consider additional information or factors in a given situation. After documenting the presence and severity of the anemia, determine the strength of the bone marrow's response. Hemolytic anemias are usually the most regenerative (Table 25.4). Blood smear analysis often reveals the diagnosis. Internal blood loss mimics hemolytic anemia and may be diagnosed by fluid cytology. Blood-loss anemias (Table 25.5) become less regenerative with time owing to loss of nutrients like iron and protein. Chronic, severe blood loss leads to iron-deficiency anemia that becomes progressively more nonregenerative. Nutritional iron deficiency occurs in rapidly growing animals that are still nursing milk. Microcytic hypochromic anemia is almost always iron deficiency but rarely may be copper deficiency. Anemia in canine portosystemic shunts have altered iron metabolism and a tendency toward microcytic hypochromic RBCs. Macrocytic normochromic anemia is excluded from this algorithm to de-emphasize it.

Bone marrow evaluation is indicated for normocytic, normochromic, nonregenerative anemia, especially if there is a bicytopenia or pancytopenia. Ineffective erythropoiesis, with an adequate number of normal-appearing erythroid cells in the marrow, is seen in anemia of inflammation, renal disease, hepatic disease, hypothyroidism, and hypoadrenocorticism. The primary diseases are diagnosed by other tests (e.g., clinical chemistry), and the cause of the anemia is often clinically inferred from the type of disease present (e.g., if renal failure, then anemia of renal disease). Severe decreases in only the erythroid line is called PRCA and may be caused by parvovirus in dogs. Drugs and toxins cause a wide variety of effects on the bone marrow. Some examples include estrogen; phenylbutazone sulfadiazine; cefazedone; chloramphenicol; griesofulvin; fenbendazole; quinidine; captopril; meclofenamic acid; thiacetarsamide; phenobarbital; chemotherapeutic agents: cyclophosphamide, vincristine, vinblastine, azothioprine, hydroxyurea, cytosine arabinoside, and doxorubricin. Pancytopenia is a severe deficiency of cells in all three lines, and one should test for Ehrlichia, virus of that species, and check for exposure to various drugs and toxins. Erythroid hyperplasia may occur in iron deficiency and is accompanied by a lack of hemosiderin in macrophages. Hyperplasia may also occur in ineffective erythropoiesis caused by drugs, inflammatory diseases, and viruses. Myelodysplasia should be accompanied by morphologic abnormalities in hemic cells. Blast cells exceeding 30% of hemic cells indicates an acute leukemia of one or more cell lines.

CHAPTER 26

Acute Blood Loss Anemia

• BETSY AIRD

Acute blood loss is defined as a major hemorrhage that occurs within a few minutes to several hours.[1-4] The resulting anemia is typically regenerative and has many causes (Table 26.1). Severe blood loss threatens homeostasis because it acutely decreases total blood volume and subsequently can lead to cardiovascular collapse, hypovolemic shock, and death.[1,2] Clinical manifestations of acute blood loss principally reflect the loss of blood volume rather than the loss of hemoglobin.[1] Blood volume of common domestic animals generally measures 6 to 11% of body weight or approximately 50 to 110 mL/kg.[3,4] A small amount of blood loss in relation to body weight is well tolerated, whereas a larger volume of blood loss may be fatal.[3-5] Animals that have acute blood loss of 30 to 40% exhibit hypovolemic shock, whereas, loss of 50% or more leads to death if immediate treatment is not initiated.[6] Mortality rates of young animals are often higher because their ability to respond to blood loss is less than that of adults.[7]

LABORATORY FINDINGS

Peripheral Blood

Initially, the hematocrit (HCT) is normal because red cells and plasma are lost in similar proportions. Therefore, the HCT is not an accurate indicator of severity of ongoing bleeding.[5] Splenic contraction, particularly in the horse, serves to increase the HCT and to improve oxygen transport. Within a few hours of blood loss, blood volume is rapidly restored by shifting water from the interstitial fluid compartment.[1,2] The HCT decreases approximately 12 to 24 hours after blood loss as a result of this fluid shift[5,8] and is lowest at 48 to 72 hours. A return to prehemorrhage levels occurs in approximately 2 to 4 weeks for most species but may take as long as 8 weeks in the horse.[8,9]

During acute blood loss the total protein concentration is usually decreased because of the loss of plasma proteins. This is particularly true if the blood loss is external. Internal blood loss may be more difficult to detect because plasma proteins and red blood cells are resorbed. Therefore, with blood loss that is internal, total

TABLE 26.1	Causes of Acute Blood Loss Anemia
Cause	**Primary Species Affected**
Trauma/surgery	All
Coagulation disorders	
Bracken fern poisoning	Cattle
Sweet clover hay (dicumarol) poisoning	Cattle
Warfarin poisoning	All
Thrombocytopenia	Dogs, horses
Congenital bleeding disorders	
Hemophilia A	Dogs, cats, horses
Hemophilia B	Dogs, cats
Disseminated intravascular coagulation (DIC)	All
Neoplasia/bleeding lesions	
Hemangiosarcoma	Dogs
Gastrointestinal ulcers	Dogs, cattle, swine
Parasites	
Hemonchus	Ruminants
Hookworms	Dogs
Coccidia	All

proteins may be normal or only slightly decreased, and the HCT may increase more rapidly than expected.[8] Plasma protein concentration begins to increase within 2 to 3 days and is usually normal within 5 to 7 days. A persistent decrease in plasma proteins suggest ongoing blood loss.[4]

A neutrophilic leukocytosis frequently occurs within hours after onset of acute blood loss because of a shift of neutrophils from the marginal pool and bone marrow reserve to the circulating pool.[1,2,10,11] Immature leukocytes and nucleated red blood cells may also appear in the blood, particularly in cases of severe blood loss accompanied by shock and tissue hypoxia.[1-4] Platelets may be decreased (100,000 to 200,000/ul) during active hemorrhage, thereafter, platelet numbers may increase as a result of mobilization of the splenic reserve.[4] Persistant thrombocytosis may suggest continued bleeding.[11]

Soon after acute blood loss the red blood cells appear

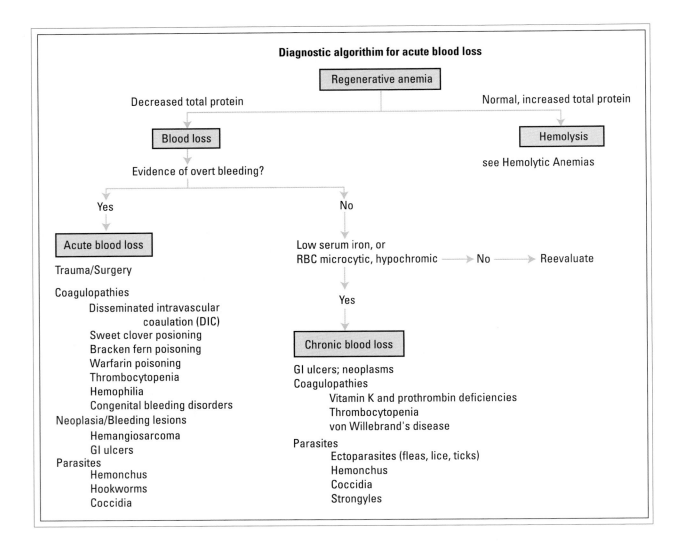

normal in size and color (i.e. normocytic, normochromic). However, as erythropoiesis intensifies in response to erythropoietin stimulation, reticulocytes are released into the peripheral blood.[4,8,11] The reticulocytes are seen as polychromatophilic macrocytes in the blood smear, and the erythrocyte indices typically show a macroctyic, hypochromic anemia. Reticulocyte counts increase approximately 2 to 3 days after acute blood loss and reach a maximum between 5 and 7 days.[3–5,11,12] The triad of anemia, hypoproteinemia, and reticulocytosis is considered a hallmark of regenerative anemia associated with acute blood loss.[4]

The reticulocyte response to acute blood loss is highly variable among species; however, the magnitude of the response is generally less than that observed in hemolytic anemias.[8] Dogs and cats exhibit the greatest degree of reticulocytosis, whereas, horses show no reticulocytosis at any magnitude of blood loss.[8,9] Therefore, a rising HCT in serial hemograms is used to indicate regeneration in horses.[9] Basophilic stippling is a characterisitic finding in ruminants and may precede macrocytosis.[3,4] The reticulocyte response of ruminants

depends on the degree of blood loss and may vary with the age of the animal.[4]

Bone Marrow

In response to tissue hypoxia, erythropoietin stimulates production of red blood cells by the bone marrow. Erythroid hyperplasia occurs as early as the second day after blood loss and is readily apparent within 5 days.[1,2] The myeloid:erythroid ratio is generally decreased. The maximum rate of red cell production is determined by the integrity of the marrow and the severity of the anemia. As long as the marrow structure is intact and iron supply to the red cell precursors is not limited, the observed increase in red cell production usually reflects the severity of the anemia.[1,2] Erythropoiesis can increase as much as six to eight times normal[4]; however, chronic renal disease, inflammation, blood transfusions, or any disorder of marrow structure can decrease the erythrocyte response.[1,2,4]

THERAPY

The first priority in the treatment of acute blood loss is to maintain adequate blood volume and prevent shock. Crystalloid and colloid solutions are commonly used and should be chosen on the basis of the inciting cause of anemia and the acid-base, electrolyte, and hydration status of the patient.[1] After plasma volume and electrolytes have been restored, red blood cell replacement can be considered. Whole-blood transfusions are necessary when hypovolemia persists or if both red cells and clotting factors are needed. However, in the normovolemic patient, packed red cells are the treatment of choice.[12] Hemoglobin substitutes may be considered for use in dogs to increase plasma hemoglobin concentrations when whole blood or packed red cells are unavailable. Therapy with Vitamin K_1 is necessary in patients that have vitamin-K-deficient coagulopathies. In general, the prognosis for anemias caused by acute blood loss is good if the inciting cause is removed and appropriate therapy is instituted.

REFERENCES

1. **Hillman RS**. Acute blood loss anemia. In: Williams WJ, Beutler E, Erslev AJ, et al, eds. Williams hematology. 4th ed. New York: McGraw-Hill, 1990;521.
2. **Hillman RS**. Acute blood loss anemia. In: Beutler E, Lichtman MA, Coller BS, et al, eds. Williams hematology. 5th ed. New York: McGraw-Hill, 1995;704.
3. **Jain NC**. Schalm's veterinary hematology. 4th ed. Philadephia: Lea & Febiger, 1986;563.
4. **Jain NC**. Essentials of veterinary hematology. Philadelphia: Lea & Febiger, 1993;159.
5. **Cotter SM**. Approach to anemia. In: 20th annual Waltham/OSU symposium, oncology and hematology. Vernon, CA: Waltham USA, 1996;81.
6. **Nelson AH**. Hypovolemic shock. Vet Clin North Am Small Anim Pract 1976;6(2):187.
7. **Willard ME, Tvedten H, Turnwald GH**. Small animal clinical diagnosis by laboratory methods. 4th ed. Philadelphia: WB Saunders, 1994;31.
8. **Tyler RD, Cowell RL**. Classification and diagnosis of anaemia. Comp Haematol Int 1996;6:1.
9. **Lassen ED, Swardson CJ**. Hematology and hemostasis in the horse: normal functions and common abnormalities. Vet Clin North Am Equine Pract 1995;11:351.
10. **Perman V, Schall WB**. Diseases of red blood cells. In: Ettinger SJ, ed. Textbook of veterinary internal medicine: diseases of the dog and cat. 2nd ed. Philadelphia: WB Saunders, 1983.
11. **Duncan JR, Prasse KW, Mahaffey EA**. Veterinary laboratory medicine. 3rd ed. Ames, IA: Iowa State University Press, 1994;3.
12. **Ahn AH, Cotter SM**. Approach to the anemic patient. In: Bonagura JD, ed. Kirk's current veterinary therapy. XII. Small animal practice. Philadephia: WB Saunders, 1995.

CHAPTER 27

Hemolytic Anemias Caused by Blood Rickettsial Agents and Protozoa

• STEPHEN D. GAUNT

Hemolytic anemia is the primary manifestation of several rickettsial and protozoal diseases in domestic animals. Erythrocytes are directly infected by the causative agents of hemobartonellosis, eperythrozoonosis, anaplasmosis, babesiosis, theileriosis, and cytauxzoonosis. In trypanosomiasis and sarcocytosis, hemolytic anemia occurs without direct infection of erythrocytes by any stage of the organism. However, infection of erythrocytes is not necessarily a pathogenic event, because the significant parasitemia in eperythrozoonosis of ruminants and llamas is not associated with hemolytic anemia.

When hemoparasites are detected on blood smears, the causal agent can be quickly identified and specific therapy instituted. Parasitemias that exceed 10^3 infected erythrocytes / μL or 0.1% infected erythrocytes are considered detectable by blood smear examination.[1,2] However, the parasitemia in rickettsial and protozoal infections is often undetected on blood smears, creating a diagnostic challenge in determining the cause of hemolytic anemia. Serologic assays are available for many of these infections, but are limited by cross reactivity between species, false-negative results during early phase of infection, and inability to differentiate carriers and acutely infected animals. The use of nucleic acid probes to detect minute quantities of an infectious agent may prove helpful in the diagnosis of acute anemias in which the parasitemia is not initially evident.[3,4]

PATHOGENESIS OF HEMOLYTIC ANEMIA

Despite the high incidence in animals of anemias associated with rickettsia and protozoa, the pathogenic mechanisms responsible for hemolysis are not fully documented. Extravascular hemolysis is the predominant cause of anemia in these infections, the result of antibody-mediated erythrocyte destruction. Antibodies, primarily gamma M immunoglobulin (IgM) and gamma G immunoglobulin (IgG), are produced to epitopes of the infectious agent, complexes of erythrocyte membrane and microbial proteins, and epitopes of the erythrocyte membrane that are exposed after infection or lysis of cell.[5–7] Antibodies, immune complexes, or complement bind to both infected and noninfected erythrocytes. Macrophages in spleen, marrow, liver, and lung phagocytize or sequester these opsonized erythrocytes. Only in babesiosis and theileriosis is intravascular hemolysis a predominant cause of erythrocyte destruction, and hemoglobinuria is often detected in those infections.

HEMATOLOGIC AND CLINICAL FINDINGS

Rickettsia and protozoa-induced hemolytic anemias are typically regenerative, with increased marrow and extramedullary erythropoiesis. The blood smear changes include polychromasia, macrocytosis, metarubricytosis, Howell-Jolly bodies, and basophilic stippling, findings similar to other regenerative anemias. However, the anemias in rickettsial and protozoal infections can specifically mimic immune-mediated hemolytic anemias. A positive Coomb's test and increased osmotic fragility of erythrocytes occur in many of the anemias caused by rickettsia and protozoa. In addition, spherocytosis, erythrophagocytosis by monocytes or macrophages, and autoagglutination may be detected on blood smears from animals infected with these agents.[8,9]

Despite evidence of active hemolysis, some rickettsial and protozoal diseases are associated with a nonregenerative anemia. The anemias in feline cytauxzoonosis, bovine trypanosomiasis, and bovine sacrocytosis are typically nonregenerative. This paradox has been attributed to the rapid onset of anemia without sufficient time for significant reticulocytosis to develop and the concurrent release of inflammatory mediators during systemic infection that specifically inhibit erythropoiesis.[10,11]

Thrombocytopenia is often associated with the hemolytic anemia caused by protozoa. Increased platelet con-

Trypanosomiasis is transmitted by saliva from blood-feeding flies, which serve as biological or mechanical vectors, depending on the species of trypanosome. The extracellular tyrpanosomes divide by binary fission in the blood of the infected animal. The parasitemia of pathogenic trypanosomes occurs intermittently, which is attributed to antigenic variation of the outer membrane glycoproteins to elude the antibody response of the host.[54] The hemolytic anemia occurs in the early stages of infection and is attributed to immune-mediated mechanisms.

Selection of drugs for treatment of trypanosomiasis depends on the species of the infective trypanosome and the infected animal. Drug resistance is a growing problem, and herd prophylaxis is often of more benefit in regions with a high incidence of infection.

Bovine Sarcocystosis

Sacrocystis cruzi causes hemolytic anemia in cattle, which are the intermediate host of this coccidian protozoa.[55] The definitive hosts for *S cruzi* are dogs and wild canids, where sexual replication occurs within intestinal epithelium. Sporocysts are excreted in feces and ingested by grazing cattle. Sporozoites invade bovine endothelial cells and undergo two or more cycles of schizogony. Merozoites are released from endothelial cells and infect mononuclear leukocytes and subsequently skeletal muscle cells where sarcocysts develop. Sarcocyts in uncooked beef are infectious for canids.

The mechanism of extravascular hemolysis in cattle that have sarcocytosis is unclear because there is no erythrocytic stage, but it is attributed to antibody-mediated removal of erythrocytes.[12,56] The anemia is nonregenerative, and its onset coincides with the second cycle of schizont formation in endothelial cells. No effective treatment is documented.

REFERENCES

1. **Gale KR, Dimmock CM, Gartside M, Leatch G**. *Anaplasma marginale*: detection of carrier cattle by PCR. Int J Parasitol 1996;26:1103–1109.
2. **Palmer GH**. Development of diagnostic reagents for anaplasmosis and babesiosis. In: Dolan TT, ed. Recent developments in the control of anaplasmosis, babesiosis, and cowdriosis. Nairobi: English Press, 1992.
3. **Gwaltney SM, Hays MP, Oberst RD**. Detection of *Eperythrozoon suis* using the polymerase chain reaction. J Vet Diagn Invest 1993;5:40–46.
4. **Torioni deEchaide S, Knowles DP, McGuire TC, Palmer GH, Suarez CE, McElwain TF**. Detection of cattle naturally infected with *Anaplasma marginale* in a region of endemicity by nested PCR and a competitive enzyme-linked immunosorbent assay using recombinant major surface protein 5. J Clin Micro 1998;36:777–782.
5. **Schmidt P, Kaspers B, Jungling A, Heinritzi K, Losch U**. Isolation of cold agglutinins in *Eperythrozoon suis*-infected pigs. Vet Immunol Immunopath 1992;31:195–201.
6. **Zulty JC, Kociba GJ**. Cold agglutinins in cats with haemobartonellosis. J Am Vet Med Assoc 1990;196:907–910.
7. **Morita T, Saeki H, Imai S, Ishii T**. Reactivity of anti-erythrocyte antibody induced by *Babesia gibsoni* infection against aged erythrocytes. Vet Parasitol 1995;58:291–299.
8. **MacWilliams PS**. Erythrocytic rickettsia and protozoa of the dog and cat. Vet Clin N Am 1987;17:1443–1461.
9. **Swenson C, Jacobs R**. Spherocytosis associated with anaplasmosis in two cows. J Am Vet Med Assoc 1986;188:1061–1064.
10. **Andrianarivo AG, Muiya P, Opollo M, Logan-Henfrey LL**. *Trypanosoma congolense*: comparative effects of a primary infection on bone marrow progenitor cells from N'Dama and Boran cattle. Exp Parasitol 1995;80:407–418.
11. **Mabbott N, Sternberg J**. Bone marrow nitric oxide production and development of anemia in *Trypanosoma brucei*-infected mice. Infect Immun 1995;63:1563–1566.
12. **Frelier PF, Lewis RM**. Hematologic and coagulation abnormalities in acute bovine sarcocystosis. Am J Vet Res 1984;45:40–48.
13. **Franks PT, Harvey JW, Shields RP, Lawman MJP**. Hematological findings in experimental feline cytauxzoonosis. J Am Anim Hosp Assoc 1988;24:395–401.
14. **Wozniak EJ, Barr BC, Thomford JW, Yamane I, McDonough SP, Moore PF, Naydan D, Robinson TW, Conrad PA**. Clinical, anatomic, and immunopathologic characterization of *Babesia gibsoni* infection in the domestic dog (*Canis familiaris*). J Parasitol 1997;83:692–699.
15. **Taboada J**. Canine babesiosis. In: Bonagura JD, ed. Kirk's current veterinary therapy: small animal practice. Philadelphia: WB Saunders, 1995.
16. **Barnwell JW, Ockenhouse CF, Knowles DM**. Monoclonal antibody OKM5 inhibits the in vitro binding of *Plasmodium falciparum*-infected erythrocytes to monocytes, endothelial, and C32 melanoma cells. J Immunol 1985;135:3494–3496.
17. **Krieg NR, Holt JG, eds**. The rickettsias and chlamydias. Bergey's manual of systematic bacteriology. Baltimore: Williams & Wilkins, 1984.
18. **Rikihisa Y, Kawahara M, Wen B, Kociba G, Fuerst P, Kawamore F, Suto C, Shibata S, Futohashi M**. Western immunoblot analysis of *Haemobartonella muris* and comparison of 16S rRNA gene sequences of *H. muris*, *H. felis*, and *Eperythrozoon suis*. J Clin Microbiol 1997:823–829.
19. **Simpson CF, Gaskin JM, Harvey JW**. Ultrastructure of erythrocytes parasitized by *Haemobartonella felis*. J Parasitol 1978;64:504–511.
20. **Jain NC, Keeton KS**. Scanning electron microscopic features of *Haemobartonella felis*. Am J Vet Res 1973;34:697–700.
21. **Zachary JF, Basgall EJ**. Erythrocyte membrane alterations associated with the attachment and replication of *Eperythrozoon suis*: a light and electron microscopic study. Vet Pathol 1985;22:164–170.
22. **Keeton KS, Jain NC**. *Eperythrozoon wenyoni*: a scanning electron microscope study. J Parasitol 1973;59(5):867–873.
23. **Harvey JW**. Haemobartonellosis. In: Greene CE, ed. Infectious diseases of the dog and cat. 2nd ed. Philadelphia: WB Saunders, 1998.
24. **Harvey JW, Gaskin JM**. Experimental feline haemobartonellosis. J Am Anim Hosp Assoc 1977;13:28–38.
25. **Loveday RK**. Porcine eperythrozoonosis In: Howard JL, ed. Current veterinary therapy. 3. Food animal practice. Philadelphia: WB Saunders, 1993
26. **Pospischil A, Hoffmann R**. *Eperythrozoon suis* in naturally infected pigs: a light and electron microscopic study. Vet Pathol 1982;19:651–657.
27. **McLaughlin BG, Evans CN, McLaughlin PS, Johnson LW, Smith AR, Zachary JF**. An Eperythrozoon-like parasite in Llamas. J Am Vet Med Assoc 1990;197:1170–1175.
28. **Reagan WJ, Garry F, Thrall MA, Colgan S, Hutchison J, Weiser MG**. The clinicopathologic, light, and scanning electron microscopic features of eperythrozoonosis in four naturally infected llamas. Vet Pathol 1990;27:426–431.
29. **Carlson GP**. Haemobartonellosis (Epyerythrozoonosis). In: Smith BP, ed. Large animal internal medicine. 2nd ed. St Louis: Mosby, 1996.
30. **Smith JA, Thrall MA, Smith JL, Salman MD, Ching SV, Collins JK**. *Eperythrozoon wenyonii* infection in dairy cattle. J Am Vet Med Assoc 1990;196:1244–1250.
31. **Stewart CG**. Ovine eperythrozoonosis. In: Howard JL, ed. Current veterinary therapy. 3. Food animal practice. Philadelphia: WB Saunders, 1993.
32. **Stoltsz WH**. Bovine anaplasmosis. In: Howard JL, ed. Current veterinary therapy. 3. Food animal practice. Philadelphia: WB Saunders, 1993.
33. **Lincoln SD**. Anaplasmosis. In: Smith BP, ed. Large animal internal medicine. 2nd ed. St Louis: Mosby, 1996.
34. **Ristic M, Watrach AM**. Studies in anaplasmosis. II. Electron microscopy of *Anaplasma marginale* in deer. Am J Vet Res 1961;22:109–115.
35. **Smith RD, Levy MG, Kuhlenschmidt MS, Adams JH, Rzechula DL, Hardt TA, Kocan KM**. Isolate of *Anaplasma marginale* not transmitted by ticks. Am J Vet Res 1986;47:127–129.
36. **French DM, McElwain TF, McGuire TC, Palmer GH**. Expression of *Anaplasma maginale* major surface protein 2 variants during persistent cyclic rickettsemia. Infect Immun 1998;66:1200–1207.
37. **Ndung'u LW, Agiurre C, Rurangirwa FR, McElwain TF, McGiure TC, Knowles DP, Palmer GH**. Detection of *Anaplasma ovis* infection in goats by major surface protein 5 competitive inhibition enzyme-linked immunosorbent assay. J Clin Microbiol 1995;33:675–679.
38. **Friedhoff KT**. Tick-borne diseases of sheep and goats caused by *Babesia*, *Theileria* or *Anaplasma* spp. Parassitologia 1997;39:99–109.
39. **Farwell GE, LeGrand EK, Cobb CC**. Clinical observations on *Babesia gibsoni* and *Babesia canis* infections in dogs. J Am Vet Med Assoc 1982;180:507–511.
40. **Breitschwerdt EB**. Babesiosis. In: Greene CE, ed. Infectious diseases of the dog and cat. 2nd ed. Philadelphia: WB Saunders, 1990.
41. **Irwin PJ, Hutchinson GW**. Clinical and pathological findings of *Babesia* infection in dogs. Austr Vet J 1992;68:204–209.
42. **DeWaal DT**. Equine piroplasmosis: a review. Br Vet J 1992;148:6–14.
43. **Bruning A**. Equine piroplasmosis an update on diagnosis, treatment and prevention. Br Vet J 1996;152:139–150.

44. **Zaugg JL**. Babesiosis. In: Smith BP, ed. Large animal internal medicine. 2nd ed. St Louis: Mosby, 1996.

45. **Holbrook AA, Johnson AJ, Madden PA**. Equine piroplasmosis: intra-erythrocytic development of *Babesia caballi* (Nuttall) and *Babesia equi* (Laveran). Am J Vet Res 1968;29:297–303.

46. **Allsopp MTEP, Cavalier-Smith T, DeWaal DT, Allsopp BA**. Phylogeny and evolution of the piroplasms. Parasitol 1994;108:147–152.

47. **DeWaal DT**. Babeisosis. In: Howard JL, ed. Current veterinary therapy. 3. Food animal practice. Philadelphia: WB Saunders, 1993.

48. **Furie WS**. Bovine Babesiosis. Comp Cont Ed 1982;4:272–277.

49. **Lawrence JA**. Theileriosis. In: Howard JL, ed. Current veterinary therapy. 3. Food animal practice. Philadelphia: WB Saunders, 1993.

50. **Hoover JP, Walker DB, Hedges JD**. Cytauxzoonosis in cats: eight cases (1985–1992). J Am Vet Med Assoc 1994;205:455–460.

51. **Kier AB**. Cytauxzonosis. In: Greene CE, ed. Infectious diseases of the dog and cat. 2nd ed. Philadelphia: WB Saunders, 1998.

52. **Garner MM, Lung NP, Citino S, Greiner EC, Harvey JW, Homer BL**. Fatal cytauxzoonosis in a captive-reared white tiger (*Panthera tigris*). Vet Pathol 1996;33:82–86.

53. **Connor RJ**. Trypanosomiasis. In: Howard JL, ed. Current veterinary therapy. 3. Food animal practice. Philadelphia: WB Saunders, 1993.

54. **Donelson JE, Hill KL, El-Sayed NM**. Multiple mechanisms of immune evasion by African trypanosomes. Mol Biochem Parasitol 1998;91:51–66.

55. **Dubey JP**. Sarcocystosis. In: Howard JL, ed. Current veterinary therapy. 3. Food animal practice. Philadelphia: WB Saunders, 1993.

56. **Mahaffey EA, George JW, Duncan JR, Prasse KW, Fayer R**. Hematologic values in calves infected with *Sarcocystis cruzi*. Vet Parasitol 1986;19:275–280.

CHAPTER 28

Anemia Associated With Bacterial and Viral Infections

• STEVEN L. STOCKHAM

Anemia is a common finding in animals that have bacterial and viral infections, but the infectious agent rarely directly causes the anemia. Most anemias associated with bacterial and viral infections are caused by the inflammatory reaction; i.e., animals develop the anemia of inflammatory disease (Chapter 35, Anemia of Inflammatory Disease). These anemias are mild to moderate and usually are not major problems for the animal. Bacterial and viral infections may cause mild to severe anemias if they result in hemorrhage (vascular damage, thrombocytopenia), erythrocyte fragmentation (vasculopathy or coagulopathy), or generalized marrow damage (marrow necrosis or replacement).

Infectious agents, their products, or the animal's specific response to the agent may cause an anemia by three major processes: (1) cause hemolysis by damaging circulating erythrocytes, (2) cause erythroid hypoplasia by damaging erythroid precursors, (3) cause general marrow hypoplasia by damaging hemopoietic or supportive stromal cells. These mechanisms are explained for each agent (Table 28.1).

YELLOW LAMB DISEASE (ENTEROTOXEMIC JAUNDICE OR YELLOWS) CAUSED BY *CLOSTRIDIUM PERFRINGENS* TYPE A (ONCE KNOWN AS *CLOSTRIDIUM WELCHII*)

Yellow lamb disease occurs in spring nursing lambs of northern California and Oregon.[1] Earlier reports describe the disorder in lambs and calves in Canada, Australia, New Zealand, and South Africa.[2] The disorder also occurs in captive Siberian ibex[3] and newborn alpacas. A *C. perfringens* infection in a horse was associated with an intravascular hemolytic anemia that was considered immune mediated.[4] Enteric disease caused by *C. perfringens* type A has been reported in chickens, wild birds, turkeys, adult horses, suckling and feeder pigs, dogs, mink, camels, ferrets, and water buffalo; but the hemolytic anemias were not described in these animals.[5]

Clinical signs in nursing lambs include depression, fever, weakness, pale mucous membranes, anemia, hemoglobinuria, and icterus. Death may occur within 6 to 12 hours of onset of illness, especially if icterus and hemoglobinuria are present.[1] Similar findings along with diarrhea were reported for calves,[2] and sudden death occurred in the ibex.[3] Anorexia, lethargy, icterus, and death in three to four days characterize less severe forms, whereas other animals may develop a persistent diarrhea and recover after several weeks.[2] Changes in the peripheral blood are consistent with a regenerative hemolytic anemia and include anisocytosis, basophilic stippling, rubricytosis, and leukocytosis.[2,6]

An α toxin, a phospholipase C, which is produced by *C. perfringens* type A, a large gram-positive bacillus, causes the erythrocyte damage. The α toxin causes hydrolysis of membrane phospholipids and thus lysis of erythrocytes, leukocytes, platelets, endothelial cells, and myocytes.[5] The α toxin's phospholipase activity was the first bacterial toxin for which the biochemical nature of its activity was established and is one of the most potent.[7]

C. perfringens type A is a part of normal intestinal flora in animals but increased growth has been associated with highly proteinaceous diets,[8] overfeeding,[9] and starchy foods.[10] After production by the bacteria, α toxin is absorbed by the intestinal mucosa and enters the blood and there damages cell membranes. Clinical findings consistent with the α toxin effects are massive intravascular hemolysis, capillary damage, inflammation, platelet aggregation, shock, cardiac effects, and death.[5,11]

Major postmortem findings include evidence of massive intravascular hemolysis, renal hemoglobin casts, destruction of capillary walls leading to intestinal mucosal necrosis, centrolobular hepatic necrosis, and serosal petechial and ecchymotic hemorrhages. In calves, abomasal hemorrhage and ulceration may be present. The small intestine is hyperemic, but rapid autolysis may obliterate the lesions; large, gram-positive bacilli may be found in the mucosa and submucosa.[12,13]

TABLE 28.1   Bacterial and Viral Infections That Cause Anemia[a]

Organism	Disease	Susceptible Mammals
Clostridium perfringens type A	Yellow lamb disease, enterotoxemic jaundice, or yellows	Lambs, calves, captive Siberian ibex, and newborn alpacas
Clostridium haemolyticum (or *C. novyi* type D)	Bacillary hemoglobinuria, red water disease, or Nevada Red Water	Cattle and sheep
Corynebacterium pseudotuberculosis	(Experimental infection)	Sheep
Leptospira interrogans serovars *pomona* and *ictohemorrhagica*	Leptospirosis	Calves, lambs, pigs, and perhaps rhinoceros
Equine infectious anemia virus	Equine infectious anemia, swamp fever, equine malarial fever, mountain fever, slow fever	Horses, ponies, donkeys, and mules
Feline leukemia virus (FeLV), FeLV-A/FeLV-C	FeLV anemia or pure red cell aplasia	Cats
Feline immunodeficiency virus (FIV)	No specific name	Cats

[a]Rickettsial bacteria not included.

One diagnoses yellow lamb disease by finding clinical and postmortem evidence and documenting the presence of the causal agent. *C. perfringens* type A is commonly recovered from intestinal tracts and environment and thus isolation from tissues of a dead animal must be interpreted with caution.[5] The number of organisms grown increases in clinical disease. Detection of α toxin in intestinal contents or blood of fresh carcasses with serum-neutralization tests in mice and guinea pigs confirms the diagnosis.[14] The α toxin gene (cpa) has been cloned and sequenced.[15–19] Polymerase chain reaction (PCR) assays have been used to detect the cpa gene of *C. perfringens* type A.[20]

BACILLARY HEMOGLOBINURIA, RED WATER DISEASE, OR NEVADA RED WATER CAUSED BY *CLOSTRIDIUM HAEMOLYTICUM* (OR *CLOSTRIDIUM NOVYI* TYPE D)

Bacillary hemoglobinuria is a highly fatal disease that occurs naturally in cattle and experimentally in sheep. It can be a seasonal disease (summer and early fall) and is associated with liver fluke migration. It is endemic in poorly drained or swampy areas of the Gulf coast states, western United States, South America, Wales, eastern Europe, and New Zealand.[8,9]

Bacillary hemoglobinuria is rarely recognized antemortem because the acute severe hemolysis causes an acute death. When seen, clinical signs include malaise, reluctance to move, arched back, bloody diarrhea, fever (40 to 41°C, 104 to 106°F but declining as death approaches), rapid and shallow breathing, and blood-tinged froth from nostrils. The classic port-wine urine, which is caused by hemoglobinuria, is uncommon.[21] If the animal survives the initial crisis and lives for a few days, icterus and evidence of increased erythropoiesis will be seen in the peripheral blood.[22]

In experimental infections, severe anemia and death is seen within 3 days of inoculation. Calves and ewes develop fever, gradual to precipitous drop in PCV values, mild to moderate leukocytosis, and increased aspartate transaminase activity[23] (from both hemoglobinemia interference and hepatocyte damage).

Erythrocyte damage is caused primarily by a β toxin, a phospholipase C or lecithinase, which splits lecithin into phosphorylcholine and diglyceride and hydrolyzes sphingomyelin. The β toxin is not related serologically to the phospholipase of other *Clostridial* sp.,[24] but the β toxin is produced by two clostridial organisms, *C. haemolyticum* and *C. novyi* type D. Other, but somewhat minor, hemolysins (lipase, proteinase, another lecithinase) have also been reported as products of *C. haemolyticum*.[25] Other nonhemolytic toxins (η and θ toxins) are also produced by the organism.

After spores are ingested, the organisms cross the intestinal mucosa and are transported to liver and other organs in macrophages. Spores may persist in Kupffer cells for a long time. Anaerobic conditions stimulate growth of organisms and production of toxins and are associated with hepatic biopsy and liver parasites—common liver fluke (*Fasciola hepatica*), lancet liver fluke (*Dicrocoelium dendriticum*), and Cysticercus cellulosae.[23,26,27] Absorption of β toxin into blood leads rapidly to intravascular hemolysis, damaged endothelial cells, icterus, hemoglobinuria, and death.[21] Death may occur within 36 to 72 hours after liver biopsy.[23]

Necropsy findings may include pale and icteric mucous membranes, petechial and ecchymotic subcutaneous hemorrhages, copious amounts of red-tinged abdominal and thoracic fluid, hemoglobinuria, renal hemoglobin casts, congested or hemorrhagic lymph nodes, extensive edema, and bloody intestinal contents. Characteristic liver lesions are foci of hepatic necrosis surrounded by a reddened reaction zone.[9] There may be thrombophlebitis in hepatic veins but not in portal veins.[23]

Diagnosis is usually made from the combination of

a sudden death and postmortem findings. Numerous gram-positive bacilli may be found in liver, spleen, blood, and abdominal fluid, but their presence must be interpreted with caution as they are normally found postmorten in these tissues. *Clostridium hemolyticum* is a common inhabitant of soils[21] and can be cultured from liver, and phospholipase C activity (β toxin) can be detected in the tissues. Extensive tests for toxins may be done but usually are not necessary if major postmortem lesions are found.

CORYNEBACTERIOSIS CAUSED BY *CORYNEBACTERIUM PSEUDOTUBERCULOSIS*

Corynebacterium pseudotuberculosis produces an exotoxin that has sphingomyelin-specific phospholipase D activity. When given intravenously in sheep, the exotoxin causes an acute, severe intravascular hemolytic anemia.[28,29] The exotoxin causes alterations in the phospholipid composition of erythrocyte membranes and leads to spherostomatocyte formation and pitting of erythrocyte membranes.[30] *C. pseudotuberculosis* causes caseous lymphadenitis in sheep and goats and other forms of abscessation. Such animals may develop an anemia, but it is probably the anemia of inflammatory disease. Natural infections with *C. pseudotuberculosis* may not cause a hemolytic anemia because infected animals produce an antitoxin against the phospholipase D during early stages of the disease.

LEPTOSPIROSIS CAUSED BY *LEPTOSPIRA INTERROGANS* SEROVARS *POMONA* AND *ICTOHEMORRHAGICA*

Leptospirae are saprophytic spirochetes that live in moist habitats throughout the world and infect humans, most domestic animals, and many wild animals.[31] However in domestic animals, the hemolytic state of leptospirosis is seen primarily in calves, lambs, and pigs.[32,33] A leptospiral infection may be a cause of acute hemolytic anemias of black rhinoceros.[34,35]

When the hemolytic state is present, the clinical signs or problems include fever, depression, anorexia, anemia, hemoglobinemia, hemoglobinuria, icterus, neutrophilia, and petechial or ecchymotic hemorrhages.[32,36–39] In experimental infections in calves, anemias were detected between the fourth and eighth day. In some calves, the precipitous drop in PCV was concurrent with the hemoglobinuria. The calves blood samples did have evidence of regeneration, including polychromasia, anisocytosis, basophilic stippling, Howell–Jolly bodies, and rubricytosis. During the anemia, two calves had increased erythrocyte fragility.[40]

Several explanations involving an immunologic response have been proposed for the hemolytic process. Experimental evidence in lambs indicates the hemolytic agent is a gamma M immunoglobulin (IgM) cold agglutinin.[41,42]

In lambs, major necropsy lesions include hemoglobinuria, icteric membranes and tissues, severe renal tubular necrosis with casts, and periacinar hepatocellular necrosis.[36,39] One confirms a hemolytic anemia caused by leptospirosis by finding leptospiral spirochetes in urine or other fluids by direct dark-field microscopic examination, cultural examinations with specific media, animal inoculation, and serologic testing. Sera from acutely ill and convalescent animals should document at least a fourfold increase in titer to either *pomona* or *ictohemorrhagica* serotypes. Either enzyme-linked immunosorbent assay (ELISA) or agglutination tests can detect IgM agglutinins within 7 to 9 days of onset of disease.[33]

EQUINE INFECTIOUS ANEMIA (SWAMP FEVER, EQUINE MALARIAL FEVER, MOUNTAIN FEVER, SLOW FEVER) CAUSED BY THE EQUINE INFECTIOUS ANEMIA VIRUS

Although more prevalent in lowland swamps, the equine infectious anemia virus (EIAV) occurs worldwide; thus the common name of swamp fever. The EIAV infection can produce clinical illness in horses, ponies, donkeys, and mules.

The EIAV in blood or other body fluids enters the horse via insect vectors or fomites and infects cells of the mononuclear-phagocytic system. The persistent replication of the virus in macrophages and the animal's response to the infection creates the disorder's clinical manifestations, which have been put into four stages[43,44] (Table 28.2).

During clinical illness, complete blood cell count (CBC) results may detect anemia, thrombocytopenia, and either a neutropenia or a neutrophilia. In the acute stage, thrombocytopenia is the most consistent hematologic abnormality and is caused by both decreased platelet survival and production.[45] Binding of either complement or immune complexes to circulating platelets causes their removal from blood by macrophages.[46] Also, it has been shown that concentrations of tumor

TABLE 28.2   Four Stages of Infection by EIAV

Stage	Clinical Signs
Acute	Acute illness may last 3–5 days, sudden fever, weakness, anemia, tachypnea, anorexia, petechial hemorrhages, thrombocytopenia, dependent edema
Subacute	Febrile episodes of several days duration occur almost monthly; see clinical signs of acute stage when febrile
Chronic	Febrile episodes at intervals of 5 months or longer; weight loss, hypergammaglobulinemia, see clinical signs of acute stage when febrile
Carrier	Asymptomatic

necrosis factor α (TNFα), transforming growth factor β (TGFβ), and interferon α (IFNα) increase before the onset of the equine infectious anemia (EIA) thrombocytopenia and that these cytokines have the ability to suppress megakaryocytes.[47]

The EIAV infection causes anemia by decreasing both erythrocyte life span and erythrocyte production.[48] During an acute stage, a horse's anemia may be accompanied by a hemoglobinemia reflecting acute intravascular hemolysis. The association of EIAV envelope glycoprotein with erythrocyte membranes activates complement that causes a coating of erythrocytes with the C3 fraction and hemolysis.[49] On the basis of studies in foals that have combined immunodeficiency, antibody binding may be necessary for the coating of erythrocytes with C3.[50] Coomb's reaction with either anticomplement or antiglobulin reagents may be positive. Morphologic changes in erythrocytes may include anisocytosis caused by macrocytosis (7 to 11 μm in diameter). Blood films contain small dense erythrocytes that could be spherocytes but definitive identification is difficult in horse blood. Sideroleukocytes can be seen, but they are uncommon. Heinz bodies have been reported to occur in the blood of EIA horses. These bodies may form because of the binding of hemoglobin to damaged erythrocyte membranes.[51]

In experimental infections, the erythrocyte life spans in four horses during the acute stage range from 28 to 87 days, and their minimum PCV values ranged from 12 to 18%. The erythrocyte life span in four horses during the subacute stage ranged from 89 to 113 days, and their minimum PCV values ranged from 29 to 37%. In the study, the mean erythrocyte life spans and PCV values for five normal horses were 136 days and 36%, respectively.[44]

The pathogenesis of the progressive nonregenerative anemia of chronic EIA is similar to the anemia of inflammatory disease; i.e., erythrocytes have decreased life span, the marrow is less responsive to erythropoietin, and changes in iron kinetics promote iron storage.[52] At least part of this process appears to be mediated by TNFα. In experimental infections, TNFα increases are associated with the onset of EIA viremia and fever. Increased TNFα is known to inhibit erythropoiesis and to stimulate macrophages.[49]

If a horse dies during the acute stage, findings may include hemorrhages in various tissues, splenomegaly, enlarged lymph nodes, subcutaneous edema, and evidence of anemia. If a horse dies during the chronic stage, findings may include the above signs plus hyperplastic marrow, enlarged liver with hemosiderin accumulation, lymphoid hyperplasia, hepatocyte necrosis, and a proliferative glomerulonephritis.

The diagnosis of EIA is confirmed by finding serologic evidence of the EIAV infection. The standard test has been an agar-gel immunodiffusion (AGID) assay (Coggins test) that detects precipitating antibody against the EIA virus' group-specific core protein, p26. A horse may produce detectable EIAV antibodies within 12 to 25 days postinoculation.[53] A competitive ELISA (CELISA) that also detects antibodies against the p26 antigen has

better analytic sensitivity but possibly lower analytic specificity. Reading the CELISA reaction is less subjective, and results are available in much less time. Immunoblot assays for antibodies against three major EIAV antigens can be used to clarify discrepancies in either AGID or CELISA results.[53] ELISA assays for the p45 antigen of EIAV have also been used.[54]

FELINE-LEUKEMIA-VIRUS-INDUCED ANEMIAS

At least half of the cats that have a feline leukemia virus (FeLV) disorder are anemic,[55] and 20 years ago, as many as 75% of anemic cats were FeLV positive.[56] The FeLV may cause an anemia either by direct or indirect methods.[56,57]

FeLV infection, by predisposing cats to other diseases, may induce the anemia of inflammatory disease. On the other hand, infecting FeLV-A-positive cats that have FeLV-C can experimentally produce the anemia of pure red cell aplasia.[58,59] The FeLV-C infection may cause pure red cell aplasia by a selective marrow depletion of blast-forming unit-erythroids[60] (BFU-Es) or by inhibition of differentiation of BFU-E to colony-forming unit-erythroids (CFU-Es).[61] FeLV infections may also lead to an aplastic anemia. Nearly 10% of FeLV-related anemias may be hemolytic anemias either because of hemobartonellosis, immune-mediated hemolysis, or other mechanisms.[62,63] Nonregenerative anemias also can be attributed to myeloproliferative, lymphoproliferative, or myelofibrosis disorders caused by the FeLV infection.

The morphologic classifications of the FeLV anemias are usually reflective of the pathologic processes that produced the anemia. An FeLV-associated anemia is usually normocytic normochromic when the FeLV infection results in a chronic inflammatory disorder, selective damage to erythroid precursors, damage to multipotential stem cells, or generalized marrow damage. If the FeLV infection leads to a hemolytic anemia, then a regenerative response may create a macrocytic normochromic or macrocytic hypochromic anemia. The major exception to this interpretative guideline is the FeLV-associated macrocytic normochromic nonregenerative anemia.[64-66] FeLV-positive cats that have macrocytic normochromic anemia typically have megablastoid rubricytes and metarubricytes in marrow samples. The process by which FeLV causes this anemia is not known, but evidence supports a dyserythropoiesis not associated with deficiencies in folate or vitamin B$_{12}$.

Clinically, it may be difficult to establish a direct relation between the FeLV infection and a cat's anemia. An ELISA or indirect fluorescent antibody (IFA) test for viral antigens typically determines the presence of the FeLV infection. A conclusion that a cat's anemia is FeLV associated is supported by findings of other hematologic abnormalities consistent with FeLV disorders and by exclusion of other causes of feline anemias.

FELINE-IMMUNODEFICIENCY-VIRUS-RELATED ANEMIAS

Cats infected with feline immunodeficiency virus (FIV) may develop various chronic debilitating disorders ranging from chronic opportunistic infections to malignant neoplasia. Anemia is found in approximately 18 to 36% of FIV-positive cats; neutropenia, lymphopenia, lymphocytosis, monocytosis, and thrombocytopenia may also be seen.[57,67-69] The presence of the FIV infection is typically determined by an ELISA, IFA, or western blot assays for antibodies against FIV.

The exact pathogenesis of the anemia in FIV-infected cats is not known. In contrast to FeLV, FIV infects megakaryocytes and marrow accessory cells but not erythroid and myeloid precursors.[70,71] The FIV-related anemia is more likely caused by the FIV-associated illness (i.e., anemia of inflammatory disease) instead of by a direct result of the FIV infection.[72]

REFERENCES

1. **McGowan B, Moulton JE, Rood SE.** Lamb losses associated with *Clostridium perfringens* type A. J Am Vet Med Assoc 1958;113:219–221.
2. **Rose AL, Edgar G.** Entero-toxaemic jaundice of sheep and cattle: a preliminary report on the aetiology of the disease. Aust Vet J 1936;12:212–220.
3. **Russel WC.** Type A enterotoxemia in captive wild goats. J Am Vet Med Assoc 1970;157:643–646.
4. **Reef VB.** *Clostridium perfringens* cellulitis and immune-mediated hemolytic anemia in a horse. J Am Vet Med Assoc 1983;182:251–254.
5. **Songer JG.** Clostridial enteric diseases of domestic animals. Clin Micro Rev 1996;9:216–234.
6. **Chamberlin WE.** The blood picture in acute cases of enzootic toxaemic jaundice in sheep. Aust Vet J 1933;9:2–9.
7. **MacFarlane MG, Knight BCJG.** The biochemistry of bacterial toxins. I. The lecithinase activity of *Cl. welchii* toxins. Biochem J 1941;35:884–902.
8. **Timoney JF, Gillespie JH, Scott FW, Barlough JE.** The Genus *Clostridium.* In: Timoney JF, Gillespie JH, Scott FW, Barlough JE, eds. Hagan and Bruner's Microbiology and infectious diseases of domestic animals. 8th ed. Ithaca: Comstock Publishing Associates, 1988;214–240.
9. **Sterne M.** Clostridial infections. Br Vet J 1981;137:443–454.
10. **Smith LDS, Williams BL.** *Clostridium perfringens.* In: Smith LDS, Williams BL, eds. The pathogenic anaerobic bacteria. 3rd ed. Springfield, IL: Charles C. Thomas, 1984;101–136.
11. **Stevens DL, Troyer BE, Merrick DT, Mitten JE, Olson RD.** Lethal effects and cardiovascular effects of purified α- and θ-toxins from *Clostridium perfringens.* J Infect Dis 1988;157:272–279.
12. **Roeder BL, Chengappa MM, Nagaraja TG, Avery TB, Kennedy GA.** Experimental induction of abdominal tympany, abomastitis, and abomasal ulceration by intraruminal inoculation of *Clostridium perfringens* type A in neonatal calves. Am J Vet Res 1988;49:201–207.
13. **Michelsen PGE.** Diseases caused by toxins of *Clostridium perfringens* (entertoxemia; yellow lamb disease; lamb dysentery; necrotic enteritis). In: Smith BP, ed. Large animal internal medicine. 2nd ed. St. Louis: Mosby, 1996; 885–890.
14. **Carter GR.** Diagnostic procedures in veterinary microbiology. Springfield, IL: Charles C. Thomas, 1984.
15. **Leslie D, Fairweather N, Pickard D, Dougan G, Kehoe M.** Phospholipase C and haemolytic activities of *Clostridium perfringens* alpha-toxin cloned in *Escherichia coli:* sequence and homology with *Bacillus cereus* phospholipase C. Mol Microbiol 1989;3:383–392.
16. **Okabe A, Inage M, Iwabuchi I, Suzuki T, Okada N, Watanabe K, Yamamoto T.** Cloning and sequencing of a phospholipase C gene of *Clostridium perfringens.* Biochem Biophys Res Commun 1989;160:33–39.
17. **Saint-Joanis B, Garnier T, Cole ST.** Gene cloning shows the alpha toxin of *Clostridium perfringens* to contain both sphingomyelinase and lecinthinase activities. Mol Gen Genet 1989;219:453–460.
18. **Titball RW, Hunter SEC, Martin KL, Morris BC, Shuttleworth AD, Rubidge T, Anderson DW, Kelly DC.** Molecular cloning and nucleotide sequence of the alpha-toxin (phospholipase C) of *Clostridium perfringens.* Infect Immun 1989;57:367–376.
19. **Tso JY, Siebel C.** Cloning and expression of the phospholipase C gene from *Clostridium perfringens* and *Clostridium bifermentans.* Infect Immun 1989; 57:468–476.
20. **Daube G, China B, Simon P, Hvala K, Mainil J.** Typing of *Clostridium*

21. **Snyder JH, Snyder SP.** Bacillary hemoglobinuria ("red water"). In: Smith BP, ed. Large animal internal medicine. 2nd ed. St. Louis: Mosby, 1996;923–925.
22. **Carlson GP.** Bacillary hemoglobinuria (Red Water). In: Smith BP, ed. Large animal internal medicine. 2nd ed. St. Louis: Mosby, 1996;1223.
23. **Olander HJ, Hughes JP, Biberstein EL.** Bacillary hemoglobinuria: induction by liver biopsy in naturally and experimentally infected animals. Pathologia Veterinaria 1966;3:421–450.
24. **Smith LDS, Williams BL.** *Clostridium haemolyticum.* In: Smith LDS, Williams BL, eds. The pathogenic anaerobic bacteria. 3rd ed. Springfield, IL: Charles C. Thomas, 1984;204–212.
25. **Lozano EA, Smith LDS.** Electrophoretic fractionation of *Clostridium hemolyticum* toxic culture fluids. Am J Vet Res 1967;28:1569–1576.
26. **Erwin BG.** Experimental induction of bacillary hemoglobinuria in cattle. Am J Vet Res 1977;38:1625–1627.
27. **Janzen ED, Orr JP, Osborne AD.** Bacillary hemoglobinuria associated with hepatic necrobacillosis in a yearling feedlot heifer. Can Vet J 1981;22:393–394.
28. **Gameel AA, Tartour G.** Haematological and plasma protein changes in sheep experimentally infected with *Corynebacterium pseudotuberculosis.* J Comp Pathol 1974;84:477–484.
29. **Hsu T, Renshaw HW, Livingston CW, Augustine JL, Zink DL, Gauer BB.** *Corynebacterium pseudotuberculosis* exotoxin: fatal hemolytic anemia induced in gnotobiotic neonatal small ruminants by parenteral administration of preparations containing exotoxin. Am J Vet Res 1985;46:1206–1211.
30. **Brogden KA, Engen RL.** Alterations in the phospholipid composition and morphology of ovine erythrocytes after intravenous inoculation of *Corynebacterium pseudotuberculosis.* Am J Vet Res 1990;51:874–877.
31. **Hartskeerl RA, Terpstra WJ.** Leptospirosis in wild animals. Vet Quarterly 1996;18(suppl 3):S149–S150.
32. **Carlson GP.** Leptospirosis. In: Smith BP, ed. Large animal internal medicine. 2nd ed. St. Louis: Mosby, 1996;1222–1223.
33. **Timoney JF, Gillespie JH, Scott FW, Barlough JE.** The Spirochetes. In: Timoney JF, Gillespie JH, Scott FW, Barlough JE, eds. Hagan and Bruner's Microbiology and infectious diseases of domestic animals. 8th ed. Ithaca: Comstock Publishing Associates, 1988;45–60.
34. **Douglass EM, Plue RE, Kord CE.** Hemolytic anemia suggestive of leptospirosis in black rhinoceros. J Am Vet Med Assoc 1980;177:921–923.
35. **Miller RE, Boever WJ.** Fatal hemolytic anemia in the black rhinoceros: case report and a survey. J Am Vet Med Assoc 1982;181:1228–1231.
36. **Smith BP, Armstrong JM.** Fatal hemolytic anemia attributed to leptospirosis in lambs. J Am Vet Med Assoc 1975;167:739–741.
37. **Nisbet DI.** *Leptospira icterohaemorrhagiae* infection in pigs. J Comp Pathol 1951;61:155–160.
38. **Hartley WJ.** Ovine leptospirosis. Aust Vet J 1952;28:169–170.
39. **Davidson JN, Hirsh DC.** Leptospirosis in lambs. J Am Vet Med Assoc 1980;176:124–125.
40. **Reinhard KR.** A clinical pathological study of experimental leptospirosis of calves. Am J Vet Res 1951;12:282–291.
41. **Decker MJ, Freeman MJ, Morter RL.** Evaluation of mechanisms of leptospiral hemolytic anemia. Am J Vet Res 1970;31:873–878.
42. **Bhasin JL, Freeman MJ, Morter RL.** Properties of a cold hemagglutinin associated with leptospiral hemolytic anemia of sheep. Infect Immun 1971;3:398–404.
43. **Ishii S.** Equine infectious anemia or swamp fever. Adv Vet Sci 1963;263–298.
44. **McGuire TC, Henson JB, Quist SE.** Viral-induced hemolysis in equine infectious anemia. Am J Vet Res 1969;30:2091–2097.
45. **Clabough DL, Gebhard D, Flaherty MT, Whetter LE, Perry ST, Coggins L, Fuller FJ.** Immune-mediated thrombocytopenia in horses infected with equine infectious anemia virus. J Virol 1991;65:6242–6251.
46. **Sellon DC.** Equine infectious anemia. Vet Clin North Am Equine Pract 1993;9:321–336.
47. **Tornquist SJ, Oaks JL, Crawford TB.** Elevation of cytokines associated with the thrombocytopenia of equine infectious anemia. J Gen Virol 1997;78:2541–2548.
48. **Cheevers WP, McGuire TC.** Equine infectious anemia virus: immunopathogenesis and persistence. Rev Infect Dis 1985;7:83–88.
49. **Costa LR, Santos IK, Issel CJ, Montelaro RC.** Tumor necrosis factor-alpha production and disease severity after immunization with enriched major core protein (p26) and/or infection with equine infectious anemia virus. Vet Immuno Immunopathol 1997;57:33–47.
50. **McGuire TC, O'Rourke KI, Perryman LE.** Immunopathogenesis of equine infectious anemia lentivirus disease. Dev Biol Stand 1990;72:31–37.
51. **McGuire TC, Henson JB, Keown GH.** Equine infectious anemia: the role of Heinz bodies in the pathogenesis of anaemia. Res Vet Sci 1970;11:354–357.
52. **McGuire TC, Henson JB, Quist SE.** Impaired bone marrow response in equine infectious anemia. Am J Vet Res 1969;30:2099–2104.
53. **Issel CJ, Cook RF.** A review of techniques for the serologic diagnosis of equine infectious anemia. J Vet Diagn Invest 1993;5:137–141.
54. **Lew AM, Thomas LM, Huntington PJ.** A comparison of ELISA, FAST-ELISA and gel diffusion tests for detecting antibody to equine infectious anaemia virus. Vet Microbiol 1993;34:1–5.

perfringens by in vitro amplification of toxin genes. J Appl Bacteriol 1994; 77:650–655.

55. **Reinacher M.** Diseases associated with spontaneous feline leukemia virus (FeLV) infection in cats. Vet Immuno Immunopathol 1989;21:85–95.
56. **Cotter SM, Hardy WD, Essex M.** Association of feline leukemia virus with lymphosarcoma and other disorders in the cat. J Am Vet Med Assoc 1975;166:449–454.
57. **Shelton GH, Linenberger ML.** Hematologic abnormalities associated with retroviral infections in the cat. Semin Vet Med Surg (Small Anim) 1995; 10:220–233.
58. **Madewell BR, Holmes PH, Onions DE.** Ferrokinetic and erythrocyte survival studies in healthy and anemic cats. Am J Vet Res 1983;44:424–427.
59. **Jarrett O, Golder MC, Toth S, Onions DE, Stewart MF.** Interaction between feline leukemia virus subgroups in the pathogenesis of erythroid hypoplasia. Int J Cancer 1984;34:283–288.
60. **Onions DE, Jarrett O, Testa N, Frassoni F, Toth S.** Selective effect of feline leukaemia virus on early erythroid precursors. Nature 1982;296:156–158.
61. **Abkowitz JL.** Retrovirus-induced feline pure red cell aplasia: pathogenesis and response to suramin. Blood 1991;77:1442–1451.
62. **Cotter SM.** Anemia associated with feline leukemia virus infection. J Am Vet Med Assoc 1979;175:1191–1194.
63. **Mackey L, Jarrett W, Jarrett O, Laird H.** Anemia associated with feline leukemia virus infection in cats. J Natl Cancer Inst 1975;54:209–217.
64. **Hirsch V, Dunn J.** Megaloblastic anemia in the cat. J Am Anim Hosp Assoc 1983;19:873–880.
65. **Weiser MG, Kociba GJ.** Erythrocyte macrocytosis in feline leukemia virus associated anemia. Vet Pathol 1983;20:687–697.
66. **Dunn JK, Hirsch VM, Searcy GP.** Serum folate and vitamin B_{12} levels in anemic cats. J Am Anim Hosp Assoc 1984;20:999–1002.
67. **Shelton GH, Linenberger ML, Grant CK, Abkowitz JL.** Hematologic manifestations of feline immunodeficiency virus infection. Blood 1990;76:1104–1109.
68. **Shelton GH, Linenberger ML, Abkowitz JL.** Hematologic abnormalities in cats seropositive for feline immunodeficiency virus. J Am Vet Med Assoc 1991;199:1353–1357.
69. **Sparkes AH, Hopper CD, Millard WG, Gruffydd-Jones TJ, Harbour DA.** Feline immunodeficiency virus infection. Clinicopathologic findings in 90 naturally occurring cases. J Vet Intern Med 1993;7:85–90.
70. **Beebe AM, Gluckstern TG, George J, Pedersen NC, Dandekar S.** Detection of feline immunodeficiency virus infection in bone marrow of cats. Vet Immuno Immunopathol 1992;35:37–49.
71. **Linenberger ML, Beebe AM, Pedersen NC, Abkowitz JL, Dandekar S.** Marrow accessory cell infection and alterations in hematopoiesis accompany severe neutropenia during experimental acute infection with feline immunodeficiency virus. Blood 1995;85:941–951.
72. **Walker C, Canfield P.** Haematological findings in cats naturally infected with feline immunodeficiency virus. Comp Haematol Intl 1996;6:77–85.

CHAPTER 29

Anemia Associated With Immune Responses

• ROBERT N. BARKER

The immune-mediated anemias, which form an important group of diseases in the domestic species, are caused by the binding of immunoproteins to red blood cells (RBC) or their precursors. The two major diseases considered here are autoimmune hemolytic anemia (AIHA), in which RBC destruction is mediated by autoantibodies, and neonatal isoerythrolysis (NI), which is caused by uptake of isologous, blood-group-specific antibodies. Anemias associated with immunoproteins that bind indirectly or nonspecifically to RBC, although not necessarily autoimmune, are described together with AIHA because many aspects of pathology are shared.

AUTOIMMUNE HEMOLYTIC ANEMIA

AIHA was one of the first conditions that was shown to have an autoimmune pathology and has been described in humans and in a wide range of domestic species. The disease is now recognized as the most frequent cause of hemolytic anemia, and the commonest manifestation of autoimmunity, in the dog.[1–14] AIHA seems less prevalent in other domestic animals but has also been described in the horse,[15–18] ox,[19,20] cat,[6,9,21] and rabbit.[22] Murine AIHA can be induced experimentally[23] and the disease develops spontaneously in the New Zealand Black mouse.[24]

Autoimmune Hemolytic Anemia Origin

The prevention and control of harmful autoimmune responses in the healthy animal appears to depend on a combination of mechanisms by which autoreactive lymphocytes are removed or rendered inherently unresponsive during their differentiation and on various forms of active immune regulation. Conditions such as AIHA result from the interaction of multiple factors that either determine susceptibility to disease or trigger autoimmune responses.[25]

In the domestic species there are few data regarding predisposing factors in autoimmune conditions, although most studies of canine AIHA have shown that certain breeds are overrepresented (Table 29.1), suggesting that there is a genetic element in determining susceptibility to the disease. Furthermore, the increased prevalence of AIHA often reported in bitches (Table 29.1) is consistent with the view that female hormones predispose to autoimmunity. The observation that ageing in humans and in animals is often associated with autoimmune phenomena may not be relevant to AIHA, because most dogs that have the disease are young adults or middle aged (Table 29.1). Although cases of canine[7,10,26] and equine[15] AIHA with concurrent neoplastic conditions have been recorded, the reason for the association is unclear. The question of whether immune dysregulation is the primary abnormality in autoimmune disease also remains unanswered. In particular, the widely held view that autoimmunity results from a defect in suppressor T lymphocytes has fallen into disrepute because of compelling evidence that these cells do not exist as a distinct subset.[27] However, T-helper lymphocytes can be classified into mutually antagonistic subsets on the basis of the cytokines that they secrete,[28] and attention is now focused on whether changes in the balance between these subpopulations can predispose toward AIHA.[29]

It is clear that, even in individuals with the appropriate predisposition to autoimmunity, environmental factors are necessary to trigger disease.[25] Infectious agents are commonly implicated, exemplified by the finding that some cases of canine AIHA are associated with infectious disease or a recent history of vaccination.[2,7,14] The mechanisms by which infectious agents may provoke autoimmunity are diverse and include cross-reactivity between the micro-organisms and the host tissues, direct infection of immune cells, deviation of the balance between T-helper subsets, and activation of autoreactive lymphocytes by exposure to inflammatory cytokines or previously hidden self-epitopes.[29]

Induction of Immune-Mediated Hemolysis by Drugs

Particular drugs can provoke immune-mediated hemolysis in susceptible individuals, but the pathology is rarely autoimmune. Indeed, the antihypertensive agent

TABLE 29.1	Breed and Sex Predisposition and Age Range in Canine AIHA		
Study	**Breed Predisposition**	**Sex Predisposition**	**Age Range**
Bennett, 1984[83]	Cocker Spaniel, Poodle, Whippet, Collie, Munsterlander	F	Young Adult
Bennett, et al, 1981[5]	Collie	None	7 m–10 yr Mean 3.6 yr
Day, 1989[9]	Old English Sheepdog, Poodle, Cocker Spaniel	F	1 yr–14 yr Mean 7.2 yr
Dodds, 1977[26]	Poodle, Cocker Spaniel, Irish Setter	NR	NR
Halliwell, 1978[3]	Poodle, Cocker Spaniel, German Shepherd Dog	F	9 m–9 yr Mean 4.7 yr
Jackson and Kruth, 1985[7]	None	F	1 yr–12 yr Mean 6.6 yr
Schalm, 1975[2]	None	F	1 yr–12 yr Mean 4.8 yr
Switzer and Jain, 1981[6]	None	M if younger than 1 yr F if 4 yr–7 yr	2 m–15 yr

NR—Not Recorded.

α-methyldopa used in human medicine is one of the few drugs that have been shown unequivocally to induce the production of true anti-RBC autoantibodies.[30] In contrast, most of the other drugs associated with immune-mediated hemolysis cause immunoproteins to react indirectly with RBC, and the mechanism varies according to whether the drug itself can bind strongly to the RBC membrane. Penicillin is the best-known example of the compounds that can provoke immune hemolytic anemia by the drug adsorption mechanism. For example, when high doses of penicillin are given to horses, the RBC can become coated with the drug, allowing any antipenicillin antibodies produced in susceptible animals to bind indirectly to the membrane.[31–33] Other drugs such as cephalosporins can cause immune-mediated hemolysis by an alternative mechanism, although they do not bind well to RBC. In these cases, drug-specific antibodies are produced and form immune complexes in the circulation, which can then bind to the RBC membrane and fix complement, even at low drug doses.[34] In domestic species other than the horse there have been few confirmed reports of drug-induced immune-mediated hemolytic anemia, although the disease has been recorded in dogs receiving levamisole[35] or cephalosporins.[36]

Autoimmune Hemolytic Anemia Pathogenesis

AIHA is characterized by the presence of autoantibodies reactive with autologous erythrocytes and a reduced RBC life span in vivo. The autoantibody may be classified as either warm or cold reactive.

Warm RBC autoantibodies react as well, or more strongly, at 37°C than at lower temperatures. Whether such antibodies are pathogenic depends on many factors, including their titre and their ability to interact with macrophage receptors or to fix complement.[11,37] In most cases of canine AIHA the autoantibody recognizes the glycophorins, which are heavily sialated RBC membrane glycoproteins.[38,39] The predominant site of RBC destruction is extravascular, and hemolysis is usually caused by immunoglobulin G (IgG) autoantibodies that can attach via their fragment, crystallizable (Fc) portion to specific receptors (Fc[γ]R) on cells of the mononuclear-phagocyte system (MPS) (Fig. 29.1A). Although blood monocytes and hepatic Kuppfer cells express the appropriate receptors for IgG, splenic macrophages appear to be the main effectors of RBC clearance. Some sensitized RBCs are only partially phagocytosed and are released back into the circulation as spherocytes, which have a short half-life because of their rigidity. Hemolysis may be accelerated if complement is fixed by the autoantibodies, because C_3b deposited on the RBC membrane enhances opsonization by interacting with specific macrophage receptors (Fig. 29.1B). Furthermore, sensitive detection methods have revealed that the RBC of canine AIHA cases are often coated with multiple immunoproteins, including IgG, IgM, IgA, and C_3 components, which may synergize strongly in causing extravascular hemolysis.[11,37] Although fixation of complement in AIHA usually seems not to progress past cleavage of C_3, in some cases warm IgM autoantibodies do trigger the entire cascade, resulting in membrane attack complex (MAC) formation and fulminant intravascular hemolysis (Fig. 29.1B).[37]

Cold RBC autoantibodies are those that react more strongly at 4°C than at higher temperatures, and the pathogenic effects of these antibodies depends not on their titre, but on their thermal amplitude. Cold autoagglutinins that bind RBC only below 10 to 15°C are harmless and can be demonstrated in the sera of many normal animals. In contrast, autoantibodies active at temperatures up to 30°C may be associated with cold hemagglu-

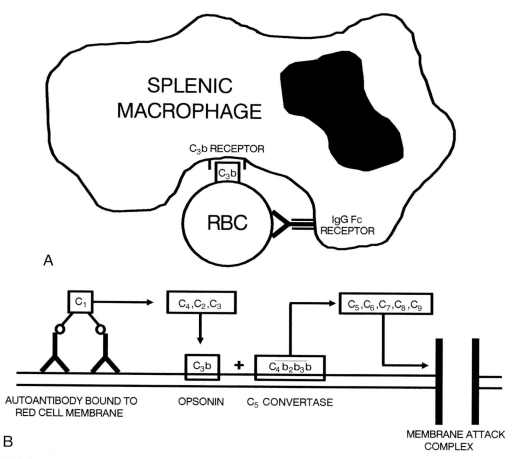

FIGURE 29.1   RBC destruction in AIHA. The predominant mechanism of RBC destruction in warm AIHA is phagocytosis by splenic macrophages bearing receptors for IgG Fc and complement components (**A**). If complement is fixed by autoantibody (**B**), phagocytosis is accelerated by the opsonin C_3b deposited on the RBC membrane. Only rarely is the entire complement cascade activated, causing MAC damage and intravascular hemolysis. Because complement fixation is triggered by two Fc portions in proximity, pentameric IgM is more efficient than monomeric IgG in activating the cascade.

tinin disease (CHAD), because temperatures in the peripheral circulation can fall below this level. The pathogenic antibody, which is usually IgM, may agglutinate RBC, blocking small blood vessels in the extremities and causing ischemic necrosis. If the complement cascade is activated and the terminal components are fixed to form MAC, there may be intravascular hemolysis (Fig. 29.1B). Cold-reactive antibodies are responsible for 8 to 24% of canine AIHA cases.[3,6,9] Another, rare, form of pathogenic cold-reactive autoantibodies are the Donath-Landsteiner (DL) hemolysins.[3] These antibodies, which are IgG, are capable of binding to RBC if the temperature is lower than 37°C and then of fixing complement when warmed again.

In some cases of AIHA, there is evidence that autoimmune reactions may be interfering with erythropoiesis, as well as causing hemolysis. Cases of canine AIHA with a persistent poor erythroid response are not unusual[37,40,41] and autoantibodies capable of suppressing erythroid cells in vitro have also been reported in pure red cell aplasia in the dog.[42]

Autoimmune Hemolytic Anemia Clinical Features

AIHA may be classified as primary, or idiopathic, in the absence of any other condition, or as secondary if there is concurrent disease. The term "secondary" does not necessarily imply a causal relation between the associated condition and the AIHA, because the presence of the two diseases may be coincidental or both may be parallel manifestations of the same underlying disorder.

In the dog, between 25 (Ref. 7) to 42% (Ref. 6) of AIHA cases have been reported to be secondary and the disease is most commonly associated with other manifestations of autoimmunity, particularly immune-mediated thrombocytopenic purpura (ITP)[6,7,9,13] or systemic lupus erythematosus.[6] AIHA has also been reported recently as part of a syndrome of multiple immunologic diseases in the Old English Sheepdog.[10] Other conditions recorded in association with canine AIHA include neoplasia[7,10] and various infectious diseases.[2,7] AIHA in the horse is also frequently associated with other diseases, including lymphoma[15] and thrombocytopenia.[15,43] In cattle, concurrent AIHA and anaplasmosis has been reported.[44] Although cats that have feline leukemia virus infection[45] or hemobartenellosis[46] have been shown to produce anti-RBC autoantibodies, often little evidence of immune-mediated hemolysis exists in these cases, and similar antibodies have been reported in many healthy controls.[45]

The clinical signs of warm AIHA in the dog range from depression and lethargy to weakness and syncope, depending on the degree of the anemia.[2,3,5–7,9] Pallor of the mucous membranes may be occasionally accompanied by icterus. In some dogs there may be splenomegaly or hepatomegaly associated with extravascular hemolysis in these organs, and there may also be lymphadenopathy or pyrexia attributable to a vigorous immune response. Dyspnea, tachycardia and a systolic heart murmur can be present in severe cases, and massive hemolysis may precipitate hemoglobinuria. However, it is important to recognize that warm AIHA is not necessarily acute in onset, with signs of fulminant hemolysis, but that the development of disease can also be insidious. Pulmonary thromboembolism has been reported in many dogs that have AIHA, but this complication is likely to have been secondary to the effects of corticosteroid treatment or to vascular injury resulting from repeated venous catheterization.[47,48]

The predominant clinical signs of canine CHAD are more likely to develop after exposure to cold temperatures and include chronic cyanosis, necrosis, and gangrene of the bodily extremities, particularly the ears, nose, and feet.[49,50] Cold RBC autoantibodies may also cause anemia of varying severity. AIHA caused by DL antibodies appears to be rare in the dog and is typified by recurrent bouts of anemia and hemoglobinuria.[3]

In horses the clinical signs of warm AIHA or immune-mediated hemolytic anemia include dullness and depression, pyrexia, icterus, and hemoglobinuria.[17] Cattle that have AIHA may be dyspneic, anorexic, depressed, and recumbent.[19,20]

Laboratory Diagnosis of Autoimmune Hemolytic Anemia

Routine hematological tests in AIHA reveal a low RBC count, packed cell volume, and blood hemoglobin concentration. The presence of spherocytes in blood smears of many species, including dogs, horses and cattle, is strongly suggestive of AIHA or immune-mediated hemolysis.[2,6,17,18,44] Indeed, a spherocyte count >50% may be diagnostic for immune-mediated anemia in the dog (D. J. Weiss, personal communication). However, it is difficult to recognize spherocytes in species that have erythrocytes smaller than those of dogs. There is also frequently a neutrophilia and a monocytosis.[2,5,6,7,13]

Most dogs that have AIHA show evidence of significant erythroid regeneration, with increased numbers of blood reticulocytes, anisocytosis, and an increased mean corpuscular volume.[3,5,7,51] However, in a minority of affected dogs,[51] perhaps as much as 35% (Ref. 51), the circulating reticulocyte count is not elevated.[2,3,5] This poor erythroid response may be caused by the normal physiologic lag of 4 to 5 days before RBC production can increase after acute hemolysis,[2] by the autoimmune reactions inhibiting RBC regeneration,[41] or by a possible underlying bone marrow disorder. AIHA must therefore be considered in the differential diagnosis of both regenerative and nonregenerative anemias.

None of the clinical signs and hematologic changes in AIHA is unique to the disease, so there is a need to identify RBC-specific autoantibodies if an unequivocal diagnosis is to be reached. In dogs, horses, and cattle the presence of autoantibody, usually of IgM class, can sometimes be revealed by autoagglutination of RBC in vitro (Fig. 29.2).[2,3,17–19] Rouleaux can be distinguished from agglutination, because they are easily dispersed by mixture of the blood sample with physiologic saline. In most cases of AIHA, however, the antibody is defined as incomplete because it does not cause autoagglutination and must be demonstrated with specific immunologic tests. The direct antiglobulin test (DAT) has been the classic tool for detecting incomplete RBC-bound autoantibodies in both veterinary[4,9,17,52] and human medicine.[34] The test can now be performed in all common domestic animals, due to the availability of a wide range of species-specific antiglobulin reagents.

In AIHA the greatest limitation of the DAT is the high proportion of false-negative results. For example, estimates of the incidence of DAT negative cases range from 14 to 32 or 42% (Refs. 4, 6, and 7, respectively) of dogs that have AIHA. Whilst the performance of the DAT can be improved by optimizing the choice of reagents and test conditions,[52,53] the technique is inherently too insensitive to detect low levels of clinically important immunoglobulins.[11,37,54] This limitation of the DAT has led to a search for more sensitive assays to detect immunoglobulins bound to RBC. One such assay, the direct enzyme-linked antiglobulin test (DELAT), uses RBCs in suspension as the solid phase of an enzyme-linked immunosorbent assay (ELISA) performed in microtitre plates and has been successfully used to detect RBC-bound immunoglobulins in DAT-negative canine AIHA and to monitor the progress of disease.[11,37,54] Furthermore, whilst sensitization with IgG alone or IgG plus C_3 are the most common DAT-positive reaction patterns in dogs that have AIHA, the DELAT has revealed that

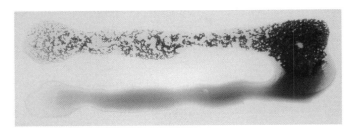

FIGURE 29.2 Slide spread with autoagglutinating blood from a dog with AIHA (top). Normal blood is shown below for comparison.

IMMUNE-MEDIATED ANEMIA

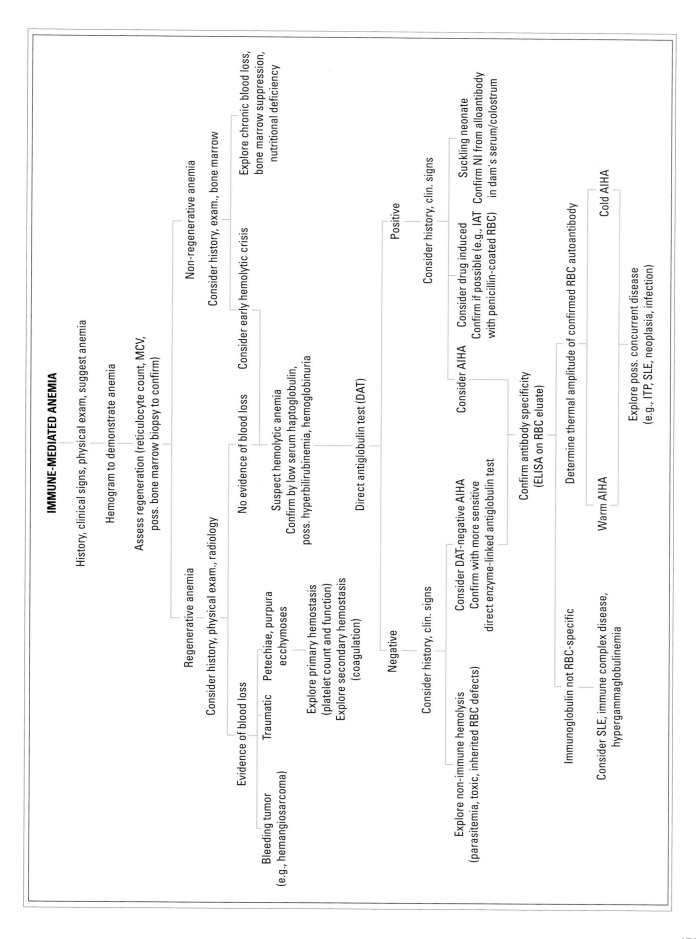

History, clinical signs, physical exam, suggest anemia

Hemogram to demonstrate anemia

Assess regeneration (reticulocyte count, MCV, poss. bone marrow biopsy to confirm)

Regenerative anemia

Non-regenerative anemia

Consider history, physical exam., radiology

Consider history, exam., bone marrow

Evidence of blood loss

No evidence of blood loss

Explore chronic blood loss, bone marrow suppression, nutritional deficiency

Traumatic

Petechiae, purpura ecchymoses

Suspect hemolytic anemia

Consider early hemolytic crisis

Bleeding tumor (e.g., hemangiosarcoma)

Explore primary hemostasis (platelet count and function)

Explore secondary hemostasis (coagulation)

Confirm by low serum haptoglobulin, poss. hyperbilirubinemia, hemoglobinuria

Direct antiglobulin test (DAT)

Negative

Positive

Consider history, clin. signs

Consider history, clin. signs

Explore non-immune hemolysis (parasitemia, toxic, inherited RBC defects)

Consider DAT-negative AIHA

Confirm with more sensitive direct enzyme-linked antiglobulin test

Consider AIHA

Consider drug induced

Suckling neonate

Confirm if possible (e.g., IAT with penicillin-coated RBC)

Confirm NI from alloantibody in dam's serum/colostrum

Confirm antibody specificity (ELISA on RBC eluate)

Immunoglobulin not RBC-specific

Determine thermal amplitude of confirmed RBC autoantibody

Consider SLE, immune complex disease, hypergammaglobulinemia

Warm AIHA

Cold AIHA

Explore poss. concurrent disease (e.g., ITP, SLE, neoplasia, infection)

the RBC of many cases are coated with IgG, IgM, IgA, and C₃.[11,37] The presence of such multiple immunoproteins bound to RBC, even at low levels, is thought to be an important factor in accelerating the rate of hemolysis.[11,37,55]

Positive DAT or DELAT reactions must also be interpreted with care, because coating of RBC with C₃ or immune complexes is common in various internal diseases in which there is no evidence of hemolysis.[3,4,11] Indeed, low levels of RBC-bound immunoprotein can be detected in as much as 78% of all dogs that have anemia,[11] and a false-positive DAT is particularly common in cats.[45] False-positive reactions may also be seen if there is cross-reactivity between the antiglobulin reagent and the RBC membrane, if immunoglobulins are nonspecifically adsorbed onto the RBC surface in hypergammaglobulinemia, or after blood transfusion.[3,9,11] Furthermore, storage of blood samples at 4°C or performance of the DAT at temperatures lower than 37°C may allow naturally occurring nonpathogenic cold autoantibodies to bind to the RBC or to fix complement.[9] One can exclude many false-positive reactions by eluting bound IgG from the RBC and testing whether it is a true autoantibody from its ability to rebind to RBC membranes specifically.[11]

No generally accepted method exists for using the DAT to demonstrate pathogenic cold autoantibodies, which dissociate from the RBC at the standard test temperature of 37°C. Some workers advocate performing a second DAT at 4°C,[3,9] although it may be difficult to distinguish between pathogenic and harmless cold antibodies unless the test is also repeated at 25 to 30°C. Others prefer to conduct the DAT only at 37°C, using C₃ alone on the RBC membrane as evidence of complement-fixing autoantibody active at lower temperatures.[1,6,52]

Under some circumstances it may be helpful to screen sera for antibodies capable of binding to RBC. For example, a modification of the indirect antiglobulin test (IAT) using penicillin-coated RBC can confirm that immune-mediated hemolysis in horses has been induced by the drug.[32] Unfortunately, in dogs that have AIHA, the IAT is almost always negative,[9,56] owing to low titres of serum autoantibody in this species[57] and to the high surface charge of canine RBC that reduces their agglutinability.[58] Although treatment of canine RBC with papain can apparently render the cells agglutinable by serum autoantibody,[56,59] the enzyme has complex effects on membranes,[58] and false-positive results are common.

Autoimmune Hemolytic Anemia Treatment

Because the underlying causes of autoantibody production in AIHA are usually unclear, conventional treatment is based on supportive care and nonspecific immunosuppression. However, in cases in which the hemolysis is possibly drug induced or secondary to another disease, attention must be paid to the primary cause of the anemia.[3,9] Animals that have pathogenic cold-reactive autoantibodies should also be protected from unnecessary exposure to low ambient temperatures.[3,49,50]

The most common treatment regime in canine warm or cold AIHA consists of high doses of short-acting glucocorticoids, such as prednisolone at 2 to 4 mg/kg per day, which are gradually tapered off over several weeks or months as the animal improves.[2,3,5–7,9,13,26] The use of glucocorticoids can prove highly effective in the dog, resulting in rapid improvements in the anemia and long-term remission of the disease in many cases.[2,3,5–7,9,13,26,37] The drugs not only downmodulate FcγR on cells of the MPS, thereby improving the survival of IgG sensitized RBC, but also rapidly suppress the production of autoantibody.[37]

In severe cases, or those which are refractory to prednisolone, the use of the cytotoxic drug cyclophosphamide is recommended (e.g., at 50 mg/M² for 4 consecutive days a week) to reduce autoantibody production.[3,6,9] Although AIHA often responds well to this treatment, cases should be monitored for the side effects of cyclophosphamide, which include bleeding into the urinary tract. Azathioprine is an alternative cytotoxic drug that can also be effective in AIHA. Transfusions should be reserved for dogs that have life-threatening anemia (e.g., packed cell volume less than 10%), because the procedure can suppress erythroid regeneration in the recipients, increase autoantibody production, or provoke a hemolytic crisis.[2,3,6,9] Splenectomy, which removes a major site of extravascular hemolysis and autoantibody synthesis, can be considered in refractory or relapsing cases[3,6,9] but may result in only temporary clinical improvement.[7]

Many novel therapies have been attempted in canine AIHA. Administration of human intravenous immunoglobulin preparations may help to stabilize some dogs that have AIHA by blocking of FcγR on cells of the MPS, but it does not improve long-term survival and repeated treatment is likely to be dangerous.[60] Danazol, a synthetic androgen with immunomodulatory properties, has been used as an adjunct to conventional treatment in too few cases to determine its efficacy.[61] Plasmapheresis[62] may be helpful in short-term stabilization, but, with the exception of cold AIHA, there is usually little unbound pathogenic autoantibody to be removed from the plasma[57] and the procedure itself can be hazardous.

The prognosis for canine AIHA treated appropriately is generally fair in the short term, with between 62% to 74% of cases recovering initially.[3,6,7] However, the response may be poor in the presence of concurrent disease,[3,6] particularly ITP,[7] or if there is intravascular hemolysis,[9] autoagglutination,[3] a weak erythroid response,[6] or severe anemia.[6] In addition, other AIHA cases may relapse despite responding to treatment initially,[3,6,7,9,37] leading to lower long-term survival rates.[7,13]

There are few reports of the efficacy of AIHA treatment in species other than the dog. Equine AIHA has been shown to respond well to dexamethasone therapy,[17,43] although cyclophosphamide and azathioprine may be necessary in refractory cases.[18] However, the success of treatment in horses that have secondary

AIHA depends on the nature of the concurrent disease.[15,17] Penicillin-induced immune-mediated anemia in horses usually resolves with supportive care after withdrawal of the drug,[31,32] but complications may arise because of the condition that originally necessitated antibiotic treatment.[31] Dexamethasone has been reported to be effective in cattle that have AIHA.[20]

NEONATAL ISOERYTHROLYSIS

Hemolytic disease of the newborn, or NI, is an important cause of anemia in horse and mule foals[63–69] and has also been described in other domestic species, including the ox,[70,71] the pig,[72,73] and the cat.[74,75] Canine NI appears to be extremely rare.[76] The pathogenesis of NI was first understood in humans,[77] and the disease has now been induced experimentally in the horse,[78] the ox,[79] the pig,[80] and the dog.[76]

Pathogenesis of Neonatal Isoerythrolysis

NI is caused by maternal alloantibodies specific for blood-group antigens entering the fetal or newborn circulation and binding to RBC. In most species except the cat, these alloantibodies are produced after sensitization of the dam with blood-group-incompatible RBC. Typically, the alloimmunization of mares[64–66,69] results from exposure to incompatible RBC from a previous fetus, caused by blood leakage through the placenta during pregnancy or at delivery when there is a danger of the circulations mixing. Alternatively, administration of products contaminated with isologous RBC, such as the anaplasmosis and babesiosis vaccines given to cattle[70,71] or a transfusion with mismatched blood may be responsible for alloimmunization. Once a dam has been sensitized against blood-group antigens, alloantibody production can persist for many years, and any further offspring bearing the target alloantigen are at risk from NI. By contrast with NI in the other domestic species, the disease reported in the cat is unique in that the pathogenic alloantibodies are naturally produced with no previous exposure of the queen to incompatible RBC.[74,75]

In all the domestic animals considered here, the alloantibodies that cause NI cannot cross the placenta but are secreted into the colostrum, ingested by the offspring, and absorbed intact into the circulation during the first hours after birth.[64–66,69,74,75,78,79] The alloantibodies, which are typically of the IgG class, bind to the neonatal RBC and can cause hemagglutination and extravascular or intravascular hemolysis. Concurrent thrombocytopenia, presumably caused by antiplatelet alloantibodies, has been reported in mule foals[69] and piglets.[72,73]

Some progress has been made in characterizing the blood group alloantigens that are important targets in NI. In one study,[64] sera from 20% of standardbred and 10% of thoroughbred mares were reactive with blood groups, including Ca, Aa, Ab, Da, Df, Ka, Ua, and Qa, with the alloantibody being secreted into the colostrum

in almost 99% of the animals. However, only alloantibodies specific for Aa and Qa appeared capable of causing NI,[64] and it has subsequently been suggested that anti-Ca alloantibodies may actually be beneficial because of preventing maternal responses against Aa.[67] Although this suggestion is not yet proved, variation in alloantibody specificity is likely to be an important factor in explaining why the frequency of NI in thoroughbreds, at approximately 1% of births, is much lower than the prevalence of maternal alloimmunity. Furthermore, 8 to 10% of mule foals suffer from NI, and this greater risk may be due to the frequent expression of a unique donkey blood group antigen that is not shared with the horse.[68,69] Canine NI can be induced experimentally by alloimmunization with the A antigen,[76] which is carried on the RBC anion channel glycoprotein.[81] The major feline blood groups A, AB, and B are similar to the human ABO system in that the polymorphisms are determined by RBC carbohydrates and that alloimmunization is unnecessary for the production of reciprocal antibodies against the antigen that is not expressed.[82] It is now clear that feline NI can be precipitated when group A or AB kittens receive naturally occurring anti-A alloantibody from group B queens.[74,75]

Clinical Features of NI

Animals that have NI are typically born healthy, and the clinical signs of NI usually do not develop until the second or third day of life, after the ingestion of alloantibody-containing colostrum.[64–66,69,74,75,78,79] The signs depend on the severity of hemolysis and range from pale mucous membranes to weakness and collapse. Icterus and hemoglobinuria can also develop, and there may be splenomegaly and hepatomegaly. If untreated, NI is often fatal, with a rapidly progressing anemia leading to respiratory distress and death within 1 week. Fulminant hemolysis in calves has been reported to trigger fatal disseminated intravascular coagulation.[70,79] Mule foals[69] and piglets[72,73] that have NI can develop concurrent anemia and thrombocytopenic purpura.

Laboratory Diagnosis of Neonatal Isoerythrolysis

Clinicians diagnose NI by use of a routine hematologic examination to demonstrate anemia in the neonate and by use of specific immunological tests to detect evidence of maternal alloimmunization.[64–66,69,74,75,78,79] In most cases the DAT (see "Laboratory Diagnosis of Autoimmune Hemolytic Anemia") on neonatal RBC is positive because of coating with maternal immunoglobulin. In addition, the production of maternal alloantibody can be confirmed by screening of the dam's plasma, serum, or colostrum for reactivity with the sire's RBC or by means of a panel of RBC bearing different blood groups.[65,66,74] High titre alloantibody from the dam's samples may directly agglutinate the RBC, and lower levels can be detected by IAT or by use of rabbit serum as a source of complement to induce hemolysis in vitro.[65] The blood-group specificity of the alloantibody from the maternal serum or colostrum may be important clinically.[64,67]

It is important to recognize that NI is not the inevitable consequence of maternal alloantibody production against fetal RBC. Several factors determine the severity of the hemolysis in the neonate, including the titre of the alloantibody in the maternal plasma and colostrum and the amount of colostrum ingested by the neonate during the critical period in which the gut can absorb immunoglobulins intact.[78,79] In addition, there is now evidence that the identity of the RBC alloantigen targeted can be important in determining the pathogenicity of alloantibody.[64,67] With the exception of the cat, naturally occurring blood-group alloantibodies do not appear to cause NI. The difficulties in identifying factors that influence hemolysis are exemplified by studies of human NI, which have not resolved the question of how to predict accurately the pathogenicity of maternal alloantibodies, although titre and IgG subclass are clearly important.[77]

Prevention and Treatment of NI

NI can be prevented in two ways: (1) by avoiding exposure to blood-group-incompatible RBC or (2) by protecting the neonate from alloantibody uptake once alloimmunization has occurred. In contrast to human NI, which can be prevented with prophylactic immunoglobulin to block maternal alloimmunization,[77] there is no specific immunologic intervention available in the domestic species.

In situations in which the risks of NI are high, such as may arise during the breeding of thoroughbred horses, it is theoretically possible to avoid pregnancy with an incompatible fetus by matching the blood types of sire and dam before mating. However, it is usually more practical to test the mare for alloantibodies during the last 2 weeks of pregnancy by screening her serum against a panel of blood-typed RBC or against the sire's RBC.[66] The sera of anaplasmosis-vaccinated cattle can also be screened for alloantibody to identify cows that are likely to produce calves that have NI.[71] If evidence of alloimmunity is detected, the offspring should not be allowed to suckle the dam for the first days of life, but given colostrum from another, alloantibody-negative female if available.[66]

When NI is diagnosed, the offspring must immediately be prevented from taking further antibodies in the dam's colostrum.[66] Supportive care of the neonate is also important, and prophylactic antibiotics should be given, particularly if no alternative source of colostrum is available. In cases in which the anemia is severe (e.g., packed cell volume less than 10%), a blood transfusion can be lifesaving, although the choice of donor is important. In the absence of a crossmatched donor that has RBCs that do not react with the maternal alloantibody, the mare's own RBCs can be considered for transfusion, provided that they have been washed extensively to remove alloantibody-containing plasma.[63] Severe NI can also be stabilized by use of glucocorticoids to reduce the rate of clearance of sensitized RBC.

REFERENCES

1. **Jain NC.** Autoimmune hemolytic anemia: a brief review. Canine Pract 1975;2:30–36.
2. **Schalm OW.** Autoimmune hemolytic anemia in the dog. Canine Pract 1975;2:37–45.
3. **Halliwell REW.** Autoimmune disease in the dog. Adv Vet Sci Comp Med 1978;22:221–263.
4. **Slappendel RJ.** The diagnostic significance of the direct antiglobulin test (DAT) in anemic dogs. Vet Immunol Immunopathol 1979;1:49–59.
5. **Bennett D, Finnett SL, Nash AS, Kirkham D.** Primary autoimmune haemolytic anaemia in the dog. Vet Rec 1981;109:150–153.
6. **Switzer JW, Jain NC.** Autoimmune hemolytic anemia in dogs and cats. Vet Clin North Am Small Anim Pract 1981;11:405–420.
7. **Jackson ML, Kruth SA.** Immune-mediated hemolytic anemia and thrombocytopenia in the dog: a retrospective study of 55 cases diagnosed from 1969 through 1983 at the Western College of Veterinary Medicine. Can Vet J 1985;26:245–250.
8. **Mills JN, Day MJ, Shaw SE, Penhale WJ.** Autoimmune haemolytic anaemia in dogs. Aust Vet J 1985;62:121–123.
9. **Day MJ.** Immune-mediated blood dyscrasias. In: University of Sydney Postgraduate Committee in Veterinary Science, Proc No 1989;118:79–104.
10. **Day MJ, Penhale WJ.** Immune-mediated disease in the Old English Sheepdog. Res Vet Sci 1992;53:87–92.
11. **Barker RN, Gruffydd-Jones TJ, Elson CJ.** Red cell bound immunoglobulins and complement measured by an enzyme-linked antiglobulin test in dogs with autoimmune haemolysis or other anaemias. Res Vet Sci 1993;54:170–178.
12. **Klag AR, Giger U, Shofer FS.** Idiopathic immune-mediated hemolytic anemia in dogs: 42 cases [1986–1990]. J Am Vet Med Assoc 1993;202:783–788.
13. **Day MJ.** Serial monitoring of clinical, haematological and immunological parameters in canine autoimmune haemolytic anaemia. J Small Anim Pract 1996;37:523–534.
14. **Duval D, Giger U.** Vaccine-associated immune-mediated hemolytic anemia in the dog. J Vet Intern Med 1996;10:290–295.
15. **Reef VB, Dyson SS, Beech J.** Lymphosarcoma and associated immune-mediated hemolytic anemia and thrombocytopenia in horses. J Am Vet Med Assoc 1984;184:313–317.
16. **Beck DJ.** A case of primary autoimmune haemolytic anaemia in a pony. Equine Vet J 1990;22:292–294.
17. **Mair TS, Taylor FGR, Hillyer MH.** Autoimmune haemolytic anaemia in eight horses. Vet Rec 1990;126:51–53.
18. **Messer NT 4th, Arnold K.** Immune-mediated hemolytic anemia in a horse. J Am Vet Med Assoc 1991;198:1415–1416.
19. **Dixon PM, Matthews AG, Brown R, Millar PM, Ritchie JSD.** Bovine autoimmune haemolytic anaemia. Vet Rec 1978;103:155–157.
20. **Fenger CK, Hoffsis GF, Kociba GJ.** Idiopathic immune-mediated hemolytic anemia in a calf. J Am Vet Med Assoc 1992;201:97–99.
21. **Schrader LA, Hurvitz AI.** Cold agglutinin disease in a cat. J Am Vet Med Assoc 1983;183:121–122.
22. **Fox RR, Meier H, Crary DD, Norberg RF, Myers DD.** Hemolytic anemia associated with thymoma in the rabbit. Genetic studies and pathological findings. Oncology 1971;25:372–382.
23. **Naysmith JD, Ortega-Pierres MG, Elson CJ.** Rat erythrocyte-induced anti-erythrocyte autoantibody production and control in normal mice. Immunol Rev 1981;55:55–87.
24. **DeHeer DH, Edgington TS.** Cellular events associated with the immunogenesis of anti-erythrocyte autoantibody responses of NZB mice. Transplant Rev 1976;31:116–155.
25. **Shoenfeld Y, Isenberg DA.** The mosaic of autoimmunity. Immunol Today 1989;10:123–126.
26. **Dodds WJ.** Autoimmune hemolytic disease and other causes of immune-mediated anemia: an overview. J Am Anim Hosp Assoc 1977;13:437–441.
27. **Möller G.** Do suppressor T cells exist? Scand J Immunol 1988;27:247–250.
28. **Mosmann TR, Coffman RL.** Heterogeneity of cytokine secretion patterns and functions of helper T-cells. Adv Immunol 1989;46:111–147.
29. **Elson CJ, Barker RN, Thompson SJ, Williams NA.** Immunologically ignorant T-cells, epitope spreading and repertoire limitation. Immunol Today 1995;16:71–76.
30. **Sokol RJ, Hewitt S, Stamps BK.** Autoimmune haemolysis: an 18-year study of 865 cases referred to a regional transfusion centre. BMJ 1981;282:2023–2027.
31. **Step DL, Blue JT, Dill SG.** Penicillin-induced hemolytic anemia and acute hepatic failure following treatment of tetanus in a horse. Cornell Vet 1991;81:13–18.
32. **McConnico RS, Roberts MC, Tompkins M.** Penicillin-induced immune-mediated hemolytic anemia in a horse. J Am Vet Med Assoc 1992;201:1402–1403.
33. **Robbins RL, Wallace SS, Brunner CJ, Gardner TR, DiFranco BJ, Spiers**

VC. Immune-mediated haemolytic disease after penicillin therapy in a horse. Equine Vet J 1993;25:462–465.

34. **Petz LD, Garratty G.** The acquired hemolytic anemias. New York: Churchill Livingstone, 1980;26–397.

35. **Atwell RB, Johnstone I, Read R, Reilly J, Wilkins B.** Haemolytic anaemia in two dogs suspected to have been induced by levamisole. Aust Vet J 1979;55:292–294.

36. **Bloom JC, Thiem PA, Sellers TS, Deldar A, Lewis HB.** Cepohalosporin-induced immune cytopenia in the dog: Demonstration of erythrocyte-, neutrophil-, and platelet-associated IgG following treatment with cefazedone. Am J Hematol 1988;28:71–78.

37. **Barker RN, Gruffydd-Jones TJ, Stokes CR, Elson CJ.** Autoimmune haemolysis in the dog: relationship between anaemia and the levels of red blood cell immunoglobulins and complement measured by an enzyme-linked antiglobulin test. Vet Immunol Immunopathol 1992:34:1–20.

38. **Barker RN, Gruffydd-Jones TJ, Stokes CR, Elson CJ.** Identification of autoantigens in canine autoimmune haemolytic anaemia. Clin Exp Immunol 1991;85:33–40.

39. **Barker RN, Elson CJ.** Red blood cell glycophorins as B and T-cell antigens in canine autoimmune haemolytic anaemia. Vet Immunol Immunopathol 1995;47:225–238.

40. **Stockham SL, Ford RB, Weiss DJ.** Canine autoimmune hemolytic disease with delayed erythroid regeneration. J Am Anim Hosp Assoc 1980;16:927–931.

41. **Jonas LD, Thrall MA, Weiser MG.** Non-regenerative form of immune-mediated hemolytic anemia in dogs. J Am Anim Hosp Assoc 1987;23:201–204.

42. **Weiss DJ.** Antibody-mediated suppression of erythropoiesis in dogs with red blood cell aplasia. Am J Vet Res 1986;47:2646–2648.

43. **Sockett DC, Traub-Dargatz J, Weiser MG.** Immune-mediated thrombocytopenia in a foal. J Am Vet Med Assoc 1987;190:308–310.

44. **Swenson C, Jacobs R.** Spherocytosis associated with anaplasmosis in two cows. J Am Vet Med Assoc 1986;188:1061–1063.

45. **Dunn JK, Searcy GP, Hirsch VM.** The diagnostic significance of a positive direct antiglobulin test in anemic cats. Can J Comp Med 1984;48:349–353.

46. **Zulty JC, Kociba GJ.** Cold agglutinins in cats with haemobartonellosis. J Am Vet Med Assoc 1990;196:907–910.

47. **Bunch SE, Metcalf MR, Crane SW, Cullen JM.** Idiopathic pleural effusion and pulmonary thromboembolism in a dog with autoimmune hemolytic anemia. J Am Vet Med Assoc 1989;195:1748–1753.

48. **Klein MK, Dow SW, Rosychuk RA.** Pulmonary thromboembolism associated with immune-mediated hemolytic anemia in dogs: ten cases. J Am Vet Med Assoc 1989;195:246–250.

49. **Slappendel RJ, Van Erp CL, Goudswaard J, Bethlehem M.** Cold hemagglutinin disease in a toy Pinscher dog. Tijdschr Diergeneeskd 1975;100:445–460.

50. **Greene CE, Kristensen F, Hoff EJ, Wiggins MD.** Cold hemagglutinin disease in a dog. J Am Vet Med Assoc 1977;170:505–510.

51. **Jones DRE, Gruffydd-Jones TJ.** The haematological consequences of immune-mediated anaemia in the dog. Comp Haematol Int 1991;1:83–90.

52. **Jones DRE, Gruffydd-Jones TJ, Stokes CR, Bourne FJ.** Investigation into factors influencing performance of the canine antiglobulin test. Res Vet Sci 1990;48:53–58.

53. **Jacobs RM, Murtaugh RJ, Crocker DB.** Use of a microtiter Coombs' test for the study of age, gender and breed distributions in immunohemolytic anemia of the dog. J Am Vet Med Assoc 1984;185:66–69.

54. **Jones DRE, Gruffydd-Jones TJ, Stokes CR, Bourne FJ.** Use of a direct enzyme-linked antiglobulin test for laboratory diagnosis of immune-mediated hemolytic anemia in dogs. Am J Vet Res 1992;53:457–465.

55. **Sokol RJ, Hewitt S, Booker DJ, Bailey A.** Erythrocyte autoantibodies, multiple immunoglobulin classes and autoimmune haemolysis. Transfusion 1990;30:714–717.

56. **Jones DRE.** Use of an enzyme indirect antiglobulin test for the diagnosis of autoimmune haemolytic anaemia in the dog. Res Vet Sci 1986;41:187–190.

57. **Barker RN, Elson CJ.** Red cell-reactive non-specific immunoglobulins and autoantibodies in the sera of normal and anaemic dogs. Vet Immunol Immunopathol 1993;39:339–354.

58. **Barker RN, Jones DRE.** Effects of papain on the agglutination of canine red cells with serum autoantibodies. Res Vet Sci 1993;55:156–161.

59. **Jones DRE, Darke PGG.** Use of papain for the detection of incomplete erythrocyte autoantibodies in autoimmune haemolytic anaemia of the dog and cat. Small Anim Pract 1975;16:273–279.

60. **Scott-Moncrieff JC, Reagan WJ.** Human intravenous immunoglobulin therapy. Semin Vet Med Surg 1997;12:178–185.

61. **Mills JN.** The use of danazol in the therapy of immune-mediated disease of dogs. Semin Vet Med Surg 1997;12:167–169.

62. **Matus RE, Schrader LA, Leifer CE, Gordon BR, Hurvitz AI.** Plasmapheresis as adjuvant therapy for autoimmune hemolytic anemia in two dogs. J Am Vet Med Assoc 1985;186:691–693.

63. **Scott AM, Jeffcott LB.** Haemolytic disease of the newborn foal. Vet Rec 1978;103:71–74.

64. **Bailey E.** Prevalence of anti-red blood cell antibodies in the serum and colostrum of mares and its relationship to neonatal erythrolysis. Am J Vet Res 1982;43:1917–1921.

65. **Becht JL, Page EH, Morter RL, Boon GD, Thacker HL.** Evaluation of a series of testing procedures to predict neonatal isoerythrolysis in the foal. Cornell Vet 1983;73:390–402.

66. **Becht JL, Semrad SD.** Hematology, blood typing and immunology of the neonatal foal. Vet Clin North Am Equine Pract 1985;1:91–116.

67. **Bailey E, Albright DG, Henney PJ.** Equine neonatal isoerythrolysis: evidence for prevention by maternal antibodies to the Ca blood group antigen. Am J Vet Res 1988;49:1218–1222.

68. **McClure JJ, Koch C, Traub-Dargatz J.** Characterization of a red blood cell antigen in donkeys and mules associated with neonatal erythrolysis. Anim Genet 1994;25:119–120.

69. **Traub-Dargatz JL, McClure JJ, Koch C, Schlipf JW Jr.** Neonatal isoerythrolysis in mule foals. J Am Vet Med Assoc 1995;206:67–70.

70. **Dowsett KF, Dimmock CK, Hill MW.** Haemolytic disease in new born calves. Aust Vet J 1978;54:65–67.

71. **Luther DG, Cox HU, Nelson WO.** Screening for neonatal isohemolytic anemia in calves. Am J Vet Res 1985;46:1078–1079.

72. **Hall SA, Rest JR, Linklater KA, McTaggart HS.** Concurrent haemolytic disease of the newborn and thrombocytopenic purpura in piglets without artificial immunisation of the dam. Vet Rec 1972;91:677–678.

73. **Linklater KA, McTaggart HS, Imlah P.** Haemolytic disease of the newborn, throbocytopenic purpura and neutropenia occurring concurrently in a litter of piglets. Br Vet J 1973;129:36–46.

74. **Cain GR, Suzuki Y.** Presumptive neonatal isoerythrolysis in cats. J Am Vet Med Assoc 1985;187:46–48.

75. **Giger U, Casal ML.** Feline colostrum—friend or foe: maternal antibodies in queens and kittens. J Reprod Fertil Suppl 1997;51:313–316.

76. **Young LE, et al.** Hemolytic disease in newborn dogs. Blood 1951;6:291.

77. **Mollison PL, Engelfriet CP, Contreras M.** The Rh blood group system. In: Blood transfusion in clinical medicine. 10th ed. Oxford: Blackwell, 1997; 151–185.

78. **Becht JL, Page EH, Morter RL, Boon GD, Thacker HL.** Experimental production of neonatal erythrolysis in the foal. Cornell Vet 1983;73:380–389.

79. **Dimmock CK, Clark IA, Hill MW.** The experimental production of haemolytic disease in newborn calves. Res Vet Sci 1976;20:244–248.

80. **Kagota K, Abe N, Tokoro K.** Production of neonatal hemolytic diseae in newborn pigs by oral administration of anti-porcine erythrocyte ovine serum. Japan J Vet Res 1982;30:94–107.

81. **Corato A, Mazza G, Hale AS, Barker RN, Day MJ.** Biochemical characterization of canine blood group antigens: immunoprecipitation of DEA 1.2, 4 and 7 and identification of a dog erythrocyte membrane antigen homologous to human Rhesus. Vet Immunol Immunopathol 1997;59:213–223.

82. **Griot-Wenk M, Pahlsson P, Chisholm-Chiat A, Spitalnik PF, Spitalnik SL, Giger U.** Biochemical characterization of the feline AB blood group system. Anim Genet 1993;24:401–407.

83. **Bennett D.** Autoimmune disease in the dog. Practice 1984;6:74–93.

CHAPTER 30

Anemias Associated With Heinz Bodies

• MICHEL DESNOYERS

R ound structures protruding from the surface of red blood cells (RBCs), with subsequent destruction of RBCs, were found by Heinz in 1890 in humans and in animals exposed to certain types of coal-tar drugs. Those structures were subsequently called Heinz bodies (HB) and can be found on the surface of RBC in several species secondary to oxidative injury to erythrocytes.

Oxygen carried by RBC is a strong oxidant because it can generate highly reactive derivatives such as the superoxide free radical (O_2-) and hydrogen peroxide (H_2O_2), and, by reacting with iron, it forms the reactive hydroxyl radical (OH). These oxidants are constantly produced and RBC have several mechanisms to prevent oxidation of hemoglobin. The enzymes superoxide dismutase (SOD), glutathione reductase (GR), glutathione peroxidase (GPx), and reduced glutathione (GSH) protect RBC against oxidative damages.[1] When these systems are overwhelmed, HB or eccentrocyte formation can occur.[1] There are two sites on RBC that are more susceptible to oxidative injury: the sulfhydryl groups on the globin chain, resulting in the formation of Heinz bodies, and heme, which when oxidized, forms methemoglobin owing to the conversion of ferrous iron to ferric iron.

Heinz bodies are denatured precipitated hemoglobin on the surface of RBC. Heinz bodies are more easily visualized with supravital stains such as new methylene blue or brilliant cresyl green and appear as dark, round protuberant bodies at the periphery of RBCs (Fig. 30.1). On Romanowsky-type stains, HBs appear also as protuberances or as clear dots on the surface of RBC, but are the same color and intensity as the rest of the RBCs (Fig. 30.2). In addition to HBs, oxidative injury to RBCs can result in the formation of eccentrocytes (Fig. 30.3). Eccentrocytes are erythrocytes that have hemoglobin concentrated on one side of the cell, leaving a pale area on the other side. Eccentrocytes are believed to be formed as a result of direct oxidative damage to the erythrocyte membrane.[2]

Anemias associated with HB or eccentrocyte formation are usually regenerative (except in the horse), with evidence of reticulocytosis and anisocytosis and with presence of nucleated RBC. This anemia may be frequently associated with a mature neutrophilia and monocytosis.[3] The hemoglobin value may be incongruously high compared with the hematocrit and RBC values. This is secondary to the presence of numerous HBs, which cause interference in the light path of the hemoglobinometer. One can circumvent this problem by centrifugating the hemolyzed blood at 8000 RPM for 20 minutes and by measuring the hemoglobin value on the supernatant.

Treatment of HB hemolysis include supportive care (fluid therapy to prevent acidosis and renal tubular damage secondary to hemoglobinuria, rest, and avoidance of stress) and, if possible, removal of the substance(s) responsible for the hemolytic crisis.[4,5] Blood transfusion and oxygen therapy should be given if warranted. Severe methemoglobinemia in dogs and cats can be treated with methylene blue (1 mg/kg given once IV).[5] However methylene blue is somewhat ineffective in horses.[4] Because Vitamin C or vitamin E are antioxidants, administration of those two substances can be useful to prevent further HB formation. The different causes of HB anemia in domestic species are the focal point of this chapter.

FELINE SPECIES

Virtually all domestic animals can develop HB, but cats are more susceptible than other species. This is because cats have eight weak sulfhydryl groups on their hemoglobin compared with two in most other species and also because of the ease of dissociation of their hemoglobin from tetramers to dimers.[6] The feline spleen, because of its nonsinusoidal nature, does not remove HB-containing RBC efficiently from the peripheral circulation. Therefore more HBs can be found in feline blood, even sometimes in nonanemic cats.[7] Because the spleen is not efficient in removing HB on the surface of RBCs, other factors are implicated in the destruction of HB-containing erythrocytes in cats. They include lipid peroxidation of the RBC membrane[7,8]; depletion of reduced GSH, which binds to the oxidized thiols in the disulfide bonds[9]; reduced membrane flexibility[10]; potassium and calcium imbalances; exposure of clustered band-3 antigens on the surface of RBCs, resulting in antibody binding[1,11]; and membrane skeletal protein cross-linking.[1] All

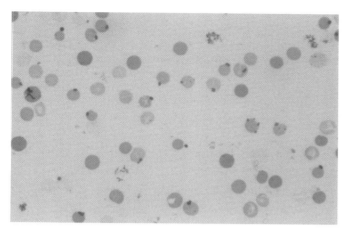

FIGURE 30.1 HBs: the HBs are dark round protuberances on the surface of erythrocytes. New methylene blue stain, 500×.

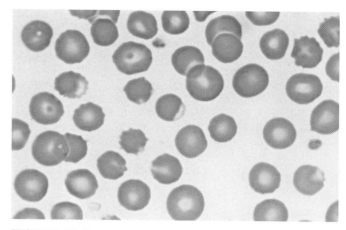

FIGURE 30.3 Eccentrocyte: the eccentrocyte is present in the center and is characterized by hemoglobin concentrated on one side of the RBC, leaving a pale area at the other extremity. Modified Wright–Giemsa stain, 1000×.

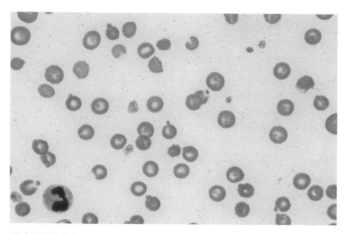

FIGURE 30.2 HBs: the HBs are protuberances on the surface of erythrocytes. Modified Wright-Giemsa stain, 500×.

these factors can result in reduced RBC life span, which may go from a normal value of 50 to 60 days to as few as 7 to 8 days.

Propylene Glycol

Propylene glycol causes HB formation in cats, but these HB are usually single and do not result in anemia.[7,12] In the past, propylene glycol was present in semimoist cat food at concentrations varying between 6 and 13%.[13] It was used as a preservative with bacteriostatic and fungistatic properties and was also a cheap source of carbohydrates. Propylene glycol is considered safe and is metabolized completely to CO_2 and H_2O, except for approximately one third that is excreted as glycol in the urine.[14] Owing to its oxidative nature, an intermediate, methylgloxal, may be responsible for the formation of HB.[14]

Kittens seem more severely affected than adults, but Bauer et al[14] found that this was secondary to the greater

intake of propylene-glycol-containing food by kittens and not their innate susceptibility to propylene glycol.

HB formation occurs within a few days and may peak after 5 to 6 weeks of consumption of the propylene-glycol-containing diet.[13,14] Although propylene glycol does not result in overt hemolysis, the RBCs from cats eating propylene-glycol-containing diets are more susceptible to oxidative injury. In a study by Weiss et al,[15] RBCs from cats eating a propylene-glycol-containing diet were more susceptible than normal RBCs to oxidative injury by acetaminophen.

Acetaminophen

Acetaminophen is a popular anti-inflammatory drug sold over-the-counter. In Europe its generic name is paracetamol.[16] It is fairly safe in humans but has been associated with serious problems of anemia and hemoglobinemia in companion animals.[16-22] The toxic effects of acetaminophen are caused by the formation of a reactive metabolite, probably N-acetyl-*p*-benzoquinoneimine, by enzymes of the microsomial cytochrome P-450 oxidase system.[17]

In cats, the toxic dosage for acetaminophen is 50 to 60 mg/kg of body weight, meaning that a single regular-strength tablet of acetaminophen can intoxicate a cat.[20] This dose is lower than that of most other species. The reason why cats are so sensitive to acetaminophen is their inability to conjugate aromatic compounds, like acetaminophen, with glucuronic acid products. Cats lack the specific glucuronyl transferases needed to conjugate the aromatic rings of several drugs.[20] This leaves a greater amount of free acetaminophen to be degraded by the cytochrome P-450 system and thus an increase in the amount of N-acetyl-*p*-benzoquinoneimine produced.[17] This, in turn, causes a depletion of the reduced

GSH stores in the RBCs with subsequent formation of methemoglobin and HBs.[23]

We had a case (Desnoyers M, Hébert P, Caouette M, DiFruscia R, unpublished data) of a cat that received two extrastrength tablets of acetaminophen (a total of 1000 mg) because it was not feeling well. On admission, the cat was cyanotic, extremely depressed, and vomiting. Blood had a chocolate brown appearance, suggesting strong methemoglobinemia. The hematocrit was within reference limits, but the majority of RBCs contained 1 or more large HBs. The methemoglobin value for this cat was 39% (reference value for our laboratory is 1%). The cat died the next day despite aggressive therapy.

Methylene Blue

Methylene blue is a dye that was used several years ago as an urinary antiseptic[24,25] and that is sometimes injected IV to visualize lymphatics, parathyroid tumors, or pancreatic islet-cell tumors.[26] This dye is usually contraindicated in cats because of its strong oxidative nature, which results in the formation of HBs.[27] However a study by Rumbeiha et al[28] showed that repeated intravenous injections of methylene blue indeed resulted in the increase of HBs on the RBC surface but did not result in clinical anemia. This finding is interesting because methylene blue is used to treat acute cases of methemoglobinemia.[5,28]

Phenazopyridine

Phenazopyridine, a urinary analgesic given orally, can result in the formation of HBs in the cat.[29] Not only phenazopyridine but also some of its metabolites are oxidants and cause RBC-membrane damage, HB formation, and hemoglobinemia.[29]

Onions

Onions were found to cause experimentally induced anemia in dogs in the 1930s,[30] but the first natural case of onion intoxication with subsequent anemia was not reported until 1974.[31] Onion intoxication is more frequent in dogs than in cats.[9,32] This is probably owing to the finicky eating nature of cats. Onions that are raw, cooked, or dehydrated can be toxic. It is also important to enquire if the cat had access to baby food because some brands contain onion powder and can result in HB formation.[33]

Propofol

Propofol (2,6-diisopropylphenol) is an intravenous anesthetic used worldwide. It is characterized by a rapid onset of action and short duration of effect.[34] A recent study that evaluated multiple 30-minute exposures of clinically healthy cats to propofol found an increase in the number of HBs after 3 days of exposure but no overt hemolysis.[34] Propofol is a phenolic compound that requires glucuronide conjugation so that it can be excreted by the kidneys. Cats have limited concentration of enzymes that catalyze glucuronide conjugation, and this may result in an increased exposure of feline RBCs to metabolites causing oxidative injury.[34]

Diabetes Mellitus

With or without concurrent ketoacidosis, diabetes mellitus is the feline disease with the greatest correlation with the presence of HB.[33,35] Cats that have ketoacidotic diabetes mellitus are frequently nonanemic, but the presence of several HBs can result in reduced RBC life span.[36] It is often important to monitor phosphorus levels in ketoacidotic cats because hypophosphatemia can precipitate a hemolytic crisis.[36]

Hyperthyroidism and Malignant Lymphoma

Hyperthyroidism is another disease that results in the formation of HBs in cats. As for diabetes mellitus, the presence of these HBs usually does not result in overt anemia. HBs are usually smaller in cats affected with hyperthyroidism than in cats that have diabetes mellitus.[35]

Malignant lymphoma can also cause HB formation. The explanation for the HB formation in this disease is not clear and varies according to the stage of clinical disease, the organs involved, therapy, and the feline leukemia virus (FeLV) status.[33,35]

CANINE SPECIES

Onions

Onion ingestion is probably the major cause of HB or eccentrocyte anemia in dogs.[3,9,19,37–40] As for cats, onions that are cooked, raw, or dehydrated can be toxic and result in a hemolytic crisis. Dogs appear to vary considerably in susceptibility to onion ingestion.[3,19,41] This means that the degree of anemia, the number and size of HBs, and the number of eccentrocytes varies from one individual to the next. After onion ingestion, HBs or eccentrocytes start to appear within 24 hours and reach a maximum number 3 days after ingestion.[3] Two compounds have been implicated as the oxidative agent responsible for the formation of either HBs or eccentrocytes. Several reports mention allyl-propyl disulfide or di-n-propyl disulfide as the culprit.[1,19,39,40] Another study found a phenolic compound with the molecular formula $C_{30}H_{18}C_{14}$ as the cause of oxidation.[42]

In addition to onions, members of the *Allium* family, such as garlic, also contain toxic components that can result in HB or eccentrocyte formation.[9]

Acetaminophen

Acetaminophen intoxication can result in HB or eccentrocyte hemolytic anemia in dogs. The toxic dosage in dogs is higher than in cats, being estimated at between 150 and 200 mg/kg of body weight.[22] Clinical signs are similar to those of cats and include weakness, tachycardia, pale mucous membranes that can be icteric or have a brownish appearance because of methemoglobinemia, facial edema, abdominal discomfort, and finally death.[18,20,22] As in cats, the toxic effects of acetaminophen are related to the formation of a toxic intermediate in the liver, N-acetyl-p-benzoquinoneimine, which is conjugated rapidly with GSH, converted to nontoxic mercapturic acid, and excreted in the urine.[18] Oxidative injury occurs when N-acetyl-p-benzoquinoneimine is formed in large quantities and depletes GSH reserves.[18] The mechanism by which N-acetyl-p-benzoquinoneimine depletes RBC GSH is not known but may represent a disruption in GSH hemostasis.[18]

Zinc

Most cases of hemolytic anemia associated with acute or subacute exposure to zinc occurred in the dog and were related to ingestion of zinc-containing foreign objects.[19,37,43–48] That the majority of cases in animals is seen in dogs may be secondary to the indiscriminate eating habits of dogs.[47] Several zinc-containing substances have been implicated but the three most common sources include skin oinments containing zinc oxide[43]; pennies minted in the United States since 1983, which contain 98% zinc per weight[45–47,49]; and metallic items such as nuts.[43,44,47,48] Other less common sources of zinc include calamine lotion, staples, nails, some fertilizers, suppositories such as Anusol, shampoos containing zinc pyrithione, and the antifungal Desenex, which contains zinc undecylenate.[45] The mechanism by which zinc induces oxidative damage to erythrocytes is still uncertain.[43,47] Proposed mechanisms include RBC enzyme inhibition, hapten-induced immune destruction of RBCs, or direct cell-membrane damage.[43] In contrast with acute and subacute zinc toxicosis, chronic zinc toxicosis results in anemia by causing interference with the absorption and use of iron and copper by RBC progenitors and by inhibition of enzymatic systems, resulting in increased erythrocyte fragility.[43,49]

Benzocaine

Benzocaine is used as a local anesthetic in both human and veterinary medicine. It is an infrequent cause of methemoglobinemia and HB anemia in dogs. To our knowledge, only three cases have been reported, all three dogs being treated by their owners with benzocaine-containing lotions or sprays (containing between 5 and 20% benzocaine) for pruritic skin condition.[50] All dogs had dark brown blood and 2 dogs had numerous HBs on their erythrocytes' surface.[50]

The rate of absorption of benzocaine depends on the amount of drug applied, the nature of the vehicle used (greatest absorption occurs with water-soluble vehicles), and nature of the surface on which it is applied. Benzocaine does not seem to be well absorbed through intact skin or the gastrointestinal tract. Therefore, absorption must occur through other routes. In all three reported cases, the dogs' skin was inflamed, resulting in greater absorption of benzocaine.[50] Moreover, the three dogs licked the skin surfaces covered with benzocaine-containing drugs causing absorption through oral mucous membranes.[50] Benzocaine metabolites responsible for the formation of methemoglobin are not known, but P-aminobenzoic acid may be responsible for the formation of Hbs.[50]

Naphtalene

Naphtalene is one of two ingredients that can be found in mothballs, the other one being paradichlorobenzene (PDB).[51] In contrast to PDB, which looks wet and oily, naphtalene looks dry. Naphtalene is more toxic than PDB and is well absorbed by the gastrointestinal tract, skin, and respiratory system.[51] Naphtalene is metabolized by the liver to α-naphtol, β-naphtol, α-naphtolquinone, and β-naphtolquinone.[51] The metabolite responsible for the hemolytic crisis and for HB anemia is α-naphtol.

Naphtalene intoxication and subsequent HB anemia is common in human medicine but rare in veterinary medicine.[51–53] To our knowledge, only one case of HB anemia after possible naphtalene ingestion has been reported in a dog.[53] The case was a 10-month-old Pekingnese dog that had clinical signs of collapse and loss of consciousness. Physical examination revealed pale and icteric mucous membranes, and blood smears revealed numerous HBs on the erythrocytes' surface. When questionned further, the owner mentioned that the dog had probably eaten naphtalene-containing moth balls.[53] The dog made an uneventful recovery after support treatment.

Vitamin K

HB anemia secondary to vitamin K administration is a rare occurrence.[54] Intravenous or intramuscular injection of vitamin K_3 (menadione) or K_1 (phytonadione) can cause oxidative damage to RBC with subsequent HB formation. It has been shown that vitamin K_3 is more toxic than vitamin K_1.[54] Vitamin K_3 reacts with hemoglobin and oxidizes oxyhemoglobin to methemoglobin with production of an intermediate, the semiquinone radical.[54] Semiquinone can combine with O_2 to produce H_2O_2 and contribute to RBC-membrane damage. Moreover, menadione can bind directly to exposed sulfhydryl groups and also to reduced GSH, depleting it.[54] This second mechanism is probably the main reason for the development of HBs. Dosage of 26 mg/kg once a day or more of menadione for several days results in HB formation.

Doses of vitamin K1 of 4 mg/kg once a day have been reported to cause HB anemia in a few dogs.[54] Because a dosage of 5 mg/kg of vitamin K_1 is recommended for anticoagulant rodenticide toxicosis, dogs on that treatment should be monitored for possible HB formation.

Phenylhydrazine

β-acetylphenylhydrazine is an oxidative drug used experimentally to induce hemolytic anemia and HB formation in dogs.[55] Hemolysis is most severe 1 week after administration of the drug. The major RBC abnormality, in addition to HB, is the presence of numerous echinocytes and, according to one study, the destruction of these echinocytes is the main reason for the hemolysis and anemia.[55]

BOVINE AND OVINE SPECIES

HB anemia does not seem to be as common in cattle and in sheep as in small animals. However, several oxidative substances can result in HB anemia in those species.

Brassica

Brassica (cabbage, kale, forage rape, etc) ingestion in cattle can result in HB anemia. Plants from the *Brassica* species are rich in S-methlylcysteine sulphoxide (SMCO).[56] Ruminal fermentation of SMCO results in the formation of dimethyl disulfide (DMDS), which is toxic to RBC. DMDS may cause HB anemia by different mechanisms[57]:

1. It may convert reduced GSH to oxidized GSH.
2. It may react with the outer sulfhydryl groups on the RBC membrane to create a mixed disulfide bond.
3. It may react with thiol groups, and this reaction may modify or even inhibit the activity of thiol enzymes, one of which is GR.[58]

All these hypothesis remain speculative and have not been tested fully in vivo.[58]

In conclusion, the effects of DMDS may be twofold: it may oxidize reduced GSH and also reduce or prevent its regeneration. This, in turn, decreases the ability of the RBC to neutralize oxidative attacks.

Plants from the *Brassica* species contain low levels of copper but high levels of sulfur, which reduce the amount of copper availability.[58] Animals on a diet rich in these plants may develop concomitant copper deficiency. This copper deficiency can lead, in turn, to hemoglobin damage by superoxide anion and to an increase in the number of HBs on the surface of erythrocytes.[59] However, there are still controversies regarding whether copper deficiency can exacerbate a *Brassica*-induced anemia.[58-60]

When fed *Brassica*-type plants, cattle develop a maximum of HBs on erythrocytes that peak at 10 days to more than 4 weeks after the beginning of feeding. The number of affected RBCs can reach as much as 80% of erythrocytes.[58] Five weeks after the beginning of feeding,

intravascular and extravascular hemolysis reduces the number of HB-containing RBCs to a minimum.[58] Destruction of erythrocytes results in a drop in the hematocrit value 1 to 4 weeks after the beginning of feeding.[60] In extreme cases, the hematocrit can fall to 30 to 50% of preanemic values.[58] The severity and rapidity at which the anemia develops is proportional to the amount of *Brassica* in the diet. A maximum level of 30% dry matter for kale and cabbage, and 40% for forage rape is recommended to avoid hemolytic crises.[58] If *Brassica* feeding is maintained, animals can still make an incomplete recovery with a slight to significant decrease in the number of HBs on the RBC surface,[60] with a return to reference values for hematocrit 9 to 10 weeks after feeding.[58] This period of recovery is, however, incomplete, and is followed by cycles of full and partial recovery if *Brassica* feeding is maintained.[58] This cycle is caused by the release of young erythrocytes in circulation that are then damaged by DMDS.[58] Total recovery is achieved when animals are completely removed from *Brassica* feeding. Erythrocyte parameters return to reference values 3 to 4 weeks after complete removal of the plants.

Onions

Cattle are more susceptible than dogs, horses, sheep, and goats to onion toxicosis.[61,62] The mechanisms by which onions cause HBs are the same as in dogs. (For a more detailed description of onion intoxication see the report by Farkas and Farkas.[31]) Onions (especially cull onions) are sometimes used as feed for sheep and cattle and can result in HB anemia.[61] However, some studies show that feeding as much as 25% dry matter chopped or crushed onions in a total mixed ration result in the appearance of HB on erythrocytes but not in the development of overt hemolysis or anemia.[61]

Deficiencies is selenium, copper, and phosphorus as well as chronic excess in copper can result in HB anemia in cattle and sheep (see Chapter 32, Nutritional Deficiency Anemias).

EQUINE SPECIES

Red Maple Leaves

Ingestion of wilted or dried leaves from red maple (*Acer rubrum*) can result in severe anemia with HB formation in horses.[63-66] Dried leaves, but not fresh ones, are toxic.[1] Clinical signs associated with this ingestion include icterus, cyanosis, pale mucous membranes, depression, and hemoglobinemia and hemoglobinuria.[64] Leaves are toxic at doses of 1.5 g/kg of body weight or more.[64] The toxin present in maple leaves causes a rapid depletion of GSH, which is caused either by overwhelming reduced GSH or by direct inhibition of the pentose phosphate pathway and GR system.[64] This toxin is not destroyed by prolonged storage or freezing.[64] HBs appear as soon as 24 hours after ingestion of maple leaves, with a peak in the number of HBs 3 days after ingestion.[64]

Wild Onions

There are few reports of onion ingestion by horses.[67] Mechanisms of action are similar to other vegetables of the Allium family (see "Onions" under "Canine Species" in this chapter).

Phenothiazine

Horses can develop HB anemia if they receive higher doses than recommended of phenothiazine.[65] Phenothiazine, an anthelmintic, is degraded in the gastrointestinal tract to phenothiazine disulfide, which is the oxidative metabolite.[65] Anemia develops usually within 1 week of exposure. There is great variation in individual susceptibility.[65]

Lymphoma

Anemia associated with lymphoma in the horse is usually immune mediated or secondary to chronic inflammation.[68] However, one case of HB anemia associated with lymphoma has been reported in a quarter horse filly.[69]

REFERENCES

1. **Harvey JW.** Erythrocyte metabolism. In: Kaneko JJ, ed. Clinical biochemistry of domestic animals. 4th ed. Toronto: Academic Press, 1989;185–224.
2. **Ham TH, Grauel JA, Dunn RF, Murphy JR, White JG, Kellermeyer RW.** Physical properties of red cells as related to effects in vivo. IV. Oxidant drugs producing abnormal intracellular concentrations of hemoglobin (eccentrocytes) with a rigid-red cell hemolytic syndrome. J Lab Clin Med 1973;82:898–910.
3. **Harvey JW, Rackear D.** Experimental onion-induced hemolytic anemia in dogs. Vet Pathol 1985;22:387–392.
4. **Warner A, Morris DD.** Hemolytic anemias. In: Robinson NE, ed. Current therapy in equine medicine. 2nd ed. Montreal: WB Saunders, 1987;295–300.
5. **Weiser MG.** Erythrocyte responses and disorders. In: Ettinger SJ, Feldman EC, eds. Textbook of veterinary internal medicine diseases of the dog and cat. 4th ed. Montreal: WB Saunders, 1989;1864–1891.
6. **Hamilton MN, Edelstein SJ.** Cat hemoglobin; pH-dependent cooperativity of oxygen binding. Science 1972;178:1104–1105.
7. **Christopher MM, White JG, Eaton JW.** Erythrocyte pathology and mechanisms of Heinz body-mediated hemolysis in cats. Vet Pathol 1990;27:299–310.
8. **Flynn TP, Allen DW, Johnson GJ, White JJ.** Oxidant damage of the lipids and proteins of the erythrocyte membranes in unstable hemoglobin disease. J Clin Invest 1983;71:1215–1223.
9. **Edwards CM, Belford CJ.** Six cases of Heinz body haemolytic anaemia induced by onion and/or garlic ingestion. Aust Vet Practit 1996;26:18–21.
10. **Reinhard WH, Sung LA, Chien S.** Quantitative relationship between Heinz body formation and red blood cell deformability. Blood 1986;68:1376–1383.
11. **Waugh SM, Williardson BM, Kannan R, Labotka RJ, Low PS.** Heinz bodies induce clustering of band 3, glycophorin, and ankyrin in sickle cell erythrocytes. J Clin Invest 1986;78:1155–1160.
12. **Hickman MA, Rogers QR, Morris JG.** Effect of diet on Heinz body formation in kittens. Am J Vet Res 1990;50:475–478.
13. **Christopher MM, Perman V, Eaton JW.** Contribution of propylene glycol-induced Heinz body formation to anemia in cats. J Am Vet Med Assoc 1989;194:1045–1056.
14. **Bauer MC, Weiss DJ, Perman V.** Hematological alterations in kittens induced by 6 and 12% dietary propylene glycol. Vet Hum Toxicol 1992;34:127–130.
15. **Weiss DJ, McClay CB, Christopher MM, Murphy M, Perman V.** Effects of propylene glycol-containing diets on acetaminophen-induced methemoglobinemia in cats. J Am Vet Med Assoc 1990;196:1816–1819.
16. **Chabre B.** Méthémoglobine, Corps de Heinz et paracétamol chez un chat. Action Vet 1991;1171:19–22.
17. **Cullison RF.** Acetaminophen toxicosis in small animals: clinical signs, mode of action, and treatment. Comp Cont Ed Pract Vet 1984;6:315–321.
18. **Hjelle JJ, Grauer GF.** Acetaminophen-induced toxicosis in dogs and cats. J Am Vet Med Assoc 1986;188:742–746.
19. **Houston DM, Myers SL.** A review of Heinz-body anemia in the dog induced by toxins. Vet Hum Toxicol 1993;35:158–161.
20. **Murphy MJ.** Toxin exposures in dogs and cats: drugs and household products. J Am Vet Med Assoc 1994;205:557–560.
21. **Rentko VT, Cotter SM.** Feline anemia: the classifications, causes, and diagnostic procedures. Vet Med 1990;6:584–604.
22. **Schlesinger DP.** Methemoglobinemia and anemia in a dog with acetaminophen toxicity. Can Vet J 1995;36:515–517.
23. **Gaunt SD, Baker DC, Green RA.** Clinicopathologic evaluation of N-acetylcysteine therapy in acetaminophen toxicosis in the cat. Am J Vet Res 1981;42:1982–1984.
24. **Schalm OW.** Methylene blue induced heinz body hemolytic anemia in a dog. Canine Pract 1978;5:20–25.
25. **Schecter RD, Schalm OW, Kaneko JJ.** Heinz body hemolytic anemia associated with the use of urinary antiseptics containing methylene blue in the cat. J Am Vet Med Assoc 1973;162:37–44.
26. **Fingeroth JM, Smeak DD.** Intravenous methylene blue infusion for intraoperative identification of parathyroid gland tumors in dogs. Part III. Clinical trials and results in three dogs. J Am Anim Hosp Assoc 1988;24:673–678.
27. **Harvey JW, Keitt AS.** Studies of the efficacy and potential hazards of methylene blue therapy in aniline-induced methemoglobinemia. Br J Haematol 1983;54:29–41.
28. **Rumbeiha WK, Oehme FW.** Methylene blue can be used to treat methemoglobinemia in cats without inducing Heinz body hemolytic anemia. Vet Hum Toxicol 1992;34:120–122.
29. **Harvey JW, Kornick HP.** Phenazopyridine toxicosis in the cat. J Am Vet Med Assoc 1976;169:327–331.
30. **Sebrell WH.** An anemia of dogs produced by feeding onions. Pub Health Rep 1930;45:1175–1177.
31. **Farkas MC, Farkas JN.** Hemolytic anemia due to ingestion of onions in a dog. J Am Anim Hosp Assoc 1974;10:65–69.
32. **Kobayashi K.** Onion poisoning in the cat. Feline Pract 1981;11:22–27.
33. **Werner LL, Christopher MM, Snipes SJ.** Spurious leukocytosis and abnormal WBC histograms associated with Heinz bodies. Vet Clin Pathol 1997;26:20.
34. **Andress JL, Day TK, Day DG.** The effects of consecutive day propofol anesthesia of feline red blood cells. Vet Surg 1995;24:277–282.
35. **Christopher MM.** Relation of endogenous Heinz bodies to disease and anemia in cats: 120 cases (1978–1987). J Am Vet Med Assoc 1989;194:1089–1095.
36. **Christopher MM.** Hematologic complications of diabetes mellitus. Vet Clin North Am Small Anim Pract 1995;25:625–637.
37. **Klag AR.** Hemolytic anemia in dogs. Comp Cont Ed Pract Vet 1992;14:1090–1098.
38. **Ogawa E, Akahori F, Kobayashi K.** In vitro studies on the breakdown of canine erythrocytes exposed to the onion extract. Jpn J Vet Sci 1985;47:719–729.
39. **Ogawa E, Shinoki T, Akahori F, Masaoka T.** Effect of onion ingestion and anti-oxidizing agents in dog erythrocytes. Jpn J Vet Sci 1986;48:685–691.
40. **Solter P, Scott R.** Onion ingestion and subsequent Heinz body anemia in a dog: a case report. J Am Anim Hosp Assoc 1987;23:544–546.
41. **Yamoto O, Maede Y.** Susceptibility to onion-induced hemolysis in dogs with hereditary high erythrocyte reduced glutathione and potassium concentration. Am J Vet Res 1992;53:134–137.
42. **Miyata D.** Isolation of a new phenolic compound from the onion (Allium cepa L. onion) and its oxidative effect on erythrocytes. Jpn J Vet Res 1990;38:65.
43. **Breitschwerdt EB, Armstrong J, Robinette CL, Dillman RC, Karl ML.** Three cases of acute zinc toxicosis in dogs. Vet Hum Toxicol 1986;28:109–117.
44. **Hornfeldt CS, Koepke TE.** A case of suspected zinc toxicity in a dog. Vet Hum Toxicol 1984;26:214.
45. **Latimer KS, Jain AV, Inglesby HB, Clarkson WD, Johnson GB.** Zinc-induced hemolytic anemia caused by ingestion of pennies by a pup. J Am Vet Med Assoc 1989;195:77–80.
46. **Luttgen PJ, Whitney MS, Wolf AM, Scruggs DW.** Heinz body hemolytic anemia associated with high zinc plasma concentration in a dog. J Am Vet Med Assoc 1990;197:1347–1350.
47. **Robinette CL.** Zinc. Vet Clin North Am Small Anim Pract 1990;20:539–544.
48. **Torrance AG, Fulton RB.** Zinc-induced hemolytic anemia in a dog. J Am Vet Med Assoc 1987;191:443–444.
49. **Meerdink GL, Reed RE, Perry D.** Zinc poisoning from the ingestion of pennies. Proc Am Assoc Vet Lab Diagn 1986;141–150.
50. **Harvey JW, Sameck JH, Burgard FJ.** Benzocaine-induced methemoglobinemia in dogs. J Am Vet Med Assoc 1979;175:1171–1175.
51. **Siegel E, Wason S.** Mothball toxicity. Pediatr Clin North Am 1986;33:369–374.
52. **Dawson JP, Thayer WW, Desforges JF.** Acute hemolytic anemia in the newborn infant due to naphtalene poisoning. Report of two cases with investigation into the mechanism of the disease. Blood 1958;13:1113–1125.
53. **Desnoyers M, Hébert P.** Heinz body anemia in a dog following possible naphtalene ingestion. Vet Clin Pathol 1995;24:124–125.

54. **Fernandez FR, Davies AP, Teachout DJ, Krake A, Christopher MM, Perman V.** Vitamin K-induced Heinz body formation in dogs. J Am Anim Hosp Assoc 1984;26:711–720.

55. **Akuzawa M, Matumoto M, Okamoto K, Nakashima F, Shinozaki M, Morizono M.** Hematological, osmotic, and scanning electron microscopic study of erythrocytes of dogs given β-acetylphenylhydrazine. Vet Pathol 1989; 26:70–74.

56. **Earl CRA, Smith RH.** Dimethyl disulphide in the blood of cattle fed on brassicas. J Sci Food Agric 1982;34:23–28.

57. **Smith RH.** Kale poisoning. Rep Rowett Inst 1974;30:112–131.

58. **Prache S.** Haemolytic anaemia in ruminants fed forage brassicas: a review. Vet Res 1994;25:497–520.

59. **Suttle NF, Jones DG.** Heinz body anemia in lambs with deficiencies of copper and selenium. Br J Nutr 1987;58:539–548.

60. **Barry TN, Reid TC, Millar KR, Sadler WA.** Nutritional evaluation of kale (Brassica oleracea) diets. 2. Copper deficiency, thyroid function, and selenium status in young cattle and sheep fed kale for prolonged periods. J Agric Sci Camb1981;96:269–282.

61. **Lincoln SD, Howell ME, Combs JJ, Hinman DD.** Hematologic effects and feeding performance in cattle fed cull domestic onions (Allium cepa). J Am Vet Med Assoc 1992;200:1090–1094.

62. **Hutchison TWS.** Onion as a cause of Heinz body anemia and death in cattle. Can Vet J 1977;18:358–360.

63. **Divers TJ, George LW, George JW.** Hemolytic anemia in horses after ingestion of red maple leaves. J Am Vet Med Assoc 1982;180:300–302.

64. **George LW, Divers TJ, Mahaffey EA, Suarez NJ.** Heinz body anemia and methemoglobinemia in ponies given red maple (Acer Rubrum L.) Leaves. Vet Pathol 1982;19:521–533.

65. **Morris DD.** Review of anemia in horses. Part II. Pathophysiologic mechanisms,specific diseases and treatment. Equine Pract 1989;11:34–46.

66. **Semrad S.** Acute hemolytic anemia from ingestion of red maple leaves. Comp Cont Ed Pract Vet 1993;15:261–267.

67. **Pierce KR, JoyceJR, England R.** Acute hemolytic anemia caused by wild onion poisoning in horses. J Am Vet Med Assoc 1972;160:323–327.

68. **Reef V, Dyson SS, Beech J.** Lymphosarcoma and associated immune mediated hemolytic anemia and thrombocytopenia in horses. J Am Vet Med Assoc 1984;184:313–317.

69. **Rollins JB, Wigton DH, Clement TH.** Heinz body anemia associated with lymphosarcoma in a horse. Equine Pract 1991;13:20–23.

CHAPTER 31

Anemias Associated With Drugs and Chemicals

• KENT A. GOSSETT

D rug- or chemical-induced anemia should be included in the differential diagnosis for all animals presenting with anemia (Table 31.1). Exposure may be accidental or intentional, and documentation of exposure may be straightforward or may require significant detective work. Anemia associated with drug administration may be related to inappropriate use or overdose, but it may also be observed in animals given recommended clinical doses. Diagnosis may be complicated by the presence of concurrent disease or the coadministration of multiple drugs associated with anemia.

CHARACTERIZATION OF THE ANEMIA

Anemia may occur as the primary clinical feature or as a secondary consequence of a more severe primary toxicity (e.g., nephrotoxicity or hepatotoxicity). All causes of anemia, including hemolysis, hemorrhage, blood loss, and decreased red blood cell production, have been associated with drug or chemical exposure. Red cells may be affected singly or in conjunction with primary or secondary effects on platelets and leukocytes.

The mechanism of toxic effect determines the type of anemia, time to onset, duration of effect, and whether persistence of the inciting agent is required for anemia to be maintained or to progress. Toxins that cause direct damage to circulating erythrocytes may cause a rapid decline in hematocrit and are generally associated with hyperbililrubinemia and bone marrow and hematologic evidence of erythrocyte regeneration. Immune-mediated hemolysis is characterized by delayed onset and the presence of the drug is generally required for erythrocyte injury to occur and for a Coomb's test to be positive. Bone marrow toxins have a delayed onset of anemia, owing in part to the long life span of circulating erythrocytes, and toxicity may persist long after the inciting agent is cleared. Certain agents have been determined or suspected to cause anemia by multiple mechanisms.

Initial characterization of the anemia should be made by standard means, including at a minimum, measurement of hematocrit or hemoglobin and review of the peripheral blood smear. Reticulocyte count and red blood cell indices may be of value if available. Bone marrow evaluation may be indicated by initial characterization. Specific tests, e.g., Coomb's test for immune-mediated hemolysis, may be required.

SELECTED DRUGS AND CHEMICALS CONFIRMED OR SUSPECTED OF INDUCING ANEMIA

Oxidants Associated With Heinz-Body Hemolytic Anemia

Exposure of red blood cells to oxidants results in production and denaturation of methemoglobin production and to coalescence of hemoglobin molecules to form Heinz bodies. The attachment of Heinz bodies to the plasma membrane increases membrane rigidity and leads to anemia by means of red blood cell lysis or premature removal from circulation. Diagnosis of oxidant-induced hemolysis can be based on identification of characteristic Heinz bodies on blood smear, new methylene blue preparation, or the presence of regenerative anemia in conjunction with documentation of exposure to an oxidant.

Methylene blue and phenazopyridine are two agents used as urinary antiseptics that have been associated with Heinz-body anemia in cats.[1,2] Cats are highly susceptible to anemia induced by acetaminophen. Dogs appear to be less susceptible to the hemolytic effects, and clinical signs are more likely to result from hepatic necrosis.[2] Phenacetin is metabolized to acetaminophen and has also been incriminated as a cause of hemolytic anemia. Phenothiazine has been associated with hemolytic anemia in horses, and occasional Heinz bodies are seen.[3] The intravenous anesthetic agent propofol may induce oxidative injury in cat red blood cells and may

TABLE 31.1 Drugs or Chemicals Confirmed or Suspected of Causing Anemia in Animals

Analgesics	**Antiparasitics**	**Chemicals/Miscellaneous**
acetaminophen—O	fenbendazole—H, D	benzene—D
phenacetin—O	levamisole—I	crude oil—O
aspirin—L		dietary
	Antiviral	onions—O
Anesthetics	azidothymidine (AZT)—D	fava beans—O
benzocaine—O		propylene glycol—O
propofol—O	**Endocrine**	plants
	estrogen—D	bracken fern—D, L
Anti-inflammatory	propylthiouracil—I, D	sweet clover—L
meclofenamic acid—D		red maple—O
naproxen—L	**Immunosuppressives**	oak—O
phenylbutazone—D	azothioprine—D	sorbose (dogs)—H
	cyclophosphamide—D	gossypol (pigs)—iron deficiency
Antibacterials		hypo-osmolality—H
cephalosporins—I, D	**Tranquilizers**	water intoxication (cattle)
chloramphenicol—D	phenothiazine—O	IV hypotonic fluids
dapsone—O		hypophosphatemia—H (hyperalimentation)
nitrofurans—O	**Urinary acidifier/antiseptics**	indole, L-tryptophan (horse)—H
penicillin—I	diphenylhydrazine—O	metals
sulfonamides—I, D	DL-methionine—O	lead—D, H
	methylene blue—O	zinc—O
Antifungals	phenazopyridine—O	copper—O, iron deficiency in pigs
amphotericin B—D		selenium—H
griseofulvin—D	**Miscellaneous drugs**	naphthalene (moth balls)—O
	benzocaine—O	pirimicarb (insecticide)—I
Antiprotozoals	gold salts—D	radiation—D
quinacrine—O	heparin (horses)—H	trichloroethylene (cattle)—D
primaquine—O	menadione (vitamin K3)—O	warfarin (dicoumarol)—L
	quinidine—D	
Antineoplastics	recombinant human erythropoietin—D	
class effect—D	vaccines (dogs)—I	

O = oxidant, Heinz-body anemia, I = immune-mediated hemolysis, H = hemolysis (other), L = blood loss, D = decreased bone marrow production.

result in Heinz-body formation if used repeatedly for several days.[4]

Ingestion of onions can result in Heinz-body anemia in dogs, cats,[5] and sheep.[6] Oxidant properties of onions are thought to be related to the presence of thiosulfate compounds.[7] Commercially available baby food is highly palatable and commonly fed to sick inappetent cats. Cats fed baby food containing 2.5% onion powder had increased Heinz-body formation, methemoglobin concentration, and decreased hematocrit.[8]

Propylene glycol was used as a preservative and source of carbohydrates in moist pet foods. Increased numbers of Heinz bodies were observed in cats fed these diets. Although anemia was rare, this finding led to removal of propylene glycol from cat food in the United States.[2,9]

Zinc toxicosis has been the subject of several published reports and is considered a common clinical disorder in dogs.[10–12] Sources of zinc are metallic hardware items, pennies, and topical formulations containing zinc oxide (e.g., Desitin and Desenex). High incidence of zinc toxicity in dogs is related to nondiscriminant eating habits. Desitin-associated hemolytic anemia has occurred after ingestion from the container or after skin application. Diagnosis is generally based on history of exposure or radiologic visualization of ingested metal objects; determination of blood zinc levels is generally unnecessary. Commonly used blood-collection tubes may con-

tain sufficient zinc to cause artifactual increases, so collection tubes specifically labeled for trace element determinations must be used.[11]

Copper accumulates in the liver of cattle, horses, swine, or chickens with high dietary copper intake. Release of copper from liver storage, often precipitated by severe stress, can result in an oxidant stress, Heinz-body formation, and acute hemolytic crisis.[13,14] Chronic copper toxicity in growing pigs can also be expressed as iron-deficiency anemia, thought to be related to impaired iron absorption.[15]

Dapsone,[16] vitamin K (menadione),[17] DL-methionine,[18] kale,[19] oak,[20] and red maple[21] leaves have or are suspected to have caused Heinz-body anemia in animals. Topical application of benzocaine induces methemoglobinemia in multiple species, however Heinz-body formation and anemia appear to be rare.[22,23]

Immune-Mediated Hemolytic Anemia

Drug-induced immune-mediated hemolytic anemia in humans is thought to occur as a result of three distinct mechanisms: (1) formation of antibodies to drug adhered to the red cell membrane (hapten), (2) binding of preformed drug-antibody complexes to the red cell membrane, or (3) induction of a true autoantibody. The first two mechanisms require a drug to be present for hemolysis to occur; the third does not.[24] Documented cases of drug-induced immune-mediated hemolytic anemia in animals are infrequent, and most probably fall into the first category (hapten). Hemolysis is a result of phagocytosis of drug-antibody-coated red cells, and laboratory findings generally include spherocytes, autoagglutination, and Coomb's positivity in the presence of drug. However, a presumptive diagnosis can be made in the absence of a positive Coomb's test, if signs of immune-mediated hemolysis resolve upon withdrawal of the drug.

Penicillin has been shown to induce immune-mediated hemolytic anemia in horses.[25–27] Cephalosporin antibiotics have been shown to cause anemia by multiple mechanisms in dogs, including immune-mediated hemolysis and bone marrow depression.[28,29] Trimethoprim-sulphamethoxazole has been suspected to cause immune-mediated hemolytic anemia in horses.[30]

Levamisole has been suspected of inducing immune-mediated hemolytic anemia in dogs that have heartworm disease.[31] Oral ingestion of the insecticide pirimicarb induced immune-mediated hemolytic anemia in dogs.[32] Propylthiouracil was associated with immune-mediated hemolytic anemia in cats treated for hyperthyroidism.[33]

Recent vaccination has been implicated as a trigger of immune-mediated hemolysis in dogs, based on a strong association between frequency of presentation of immune-mediated hemolytic anemia within 1 month of vaccination. Vaccine components stay in the blood for extended periods, making them more likely to cause an immune reaction than many other drugs.[34]

Hemolysis (Miscellaneous)

Administration of phosphate-free fluids results in decreased serum inorganic phosphate concentrations, depletion of adenosine triphosphate (ATP), increased red cell rigidity and hemolysis.[35] Excessive water ingestion in cattle (water intoxication) or intravenous administration of hypotonic fluids has resulted in hypotonic erythrocyte lysis and anemia. Heparin administration in ponies has been associated with enhanced phagocytosis of red blood cells, anemia, and hyperbilirubinemia.[36]

L-sorbose, a sugar substitute, inhibits hexokinase in canine red cells and causes severe intravascular hemolysis. Dogs that have low-potassium erythrocytes are particularly sensitive, whereas dogs that have high potassium erythrocytes and other species appear to be resistant to this effect.[37]

Selenium toxicity has been shown to cause hemolytic anemia in various animal species.[38] Lead poisoning may occur in multiple species, including dogs, cats, horses, ruminants, and pigs. Acute lead poisoning is characterized by basophilic stippling of erythrocytes and an increase in circulating nucleated erythrocytes, but anemia is uncommon. Anemia is more common in chronic lead poisoning and is considered a result of both depression of red cell production and hemolysis.[14]

L-tryptophan and indole have been shown experi-

mentally to produce intravascular hemolysis in ponies.[39,40]

Blood Loss

Nonsteroidal anti-inflammatory drugs such as naproxen have been associated with blood-loss anemia in dogs and thought to be related to gastrointestinal erosion or ulceration secondary to local irritation and inhibition of prostaglandin synthesis.[41,42] Aspirin-associated gastrointestinal irritation and platelet aggregation inhibitory activity can result in increased gastrointestinal bleeding, with hematemesis and melena in people[43] and, presumably, in animals.

Dicoumarol[44] (warfarin) and certain plants (sweet clover) interfere with vitamin-K-dependent coagulation factors, resulting in hemorrhage and blood-loss anemia. Consumption of bracken fern is associated with hemorrhagic anemia in cattle and with bone marrow aplasia and thrombocytopenia.

Bone Marrow Suppression

Bone marrow suppression is a widely recognized extension of the desired pharmacology of antineoplastic agents. Bone marrow effects are predictable, often dose limiting, generally reversible, and observed with a high incidence because these agents are dosed at or near their maximum tolerated dose.

Azidothymidine (AZT) is a dideoxynucleoside derivative reverse transcriptase inhibitor used for treatment of feline immunodeficiency virus or feline leukemia virus. Anemia develops after several weeks of treatment, and may be transient or progressive. Anemia is primarily caused by bone marrow depression, but Heinz-body formation may also be a contributing factor.[45,46] Multiple dideoxynucleoside derivatives evaluated in rats and mice resulted in a poorly regenerative anemia that was reversible with cessation of treatment.[47,48]

Ingestion of bracken fern[49] or trichloroethylene-extracted soybean feed[50] cause aplastic anemia in cattle. Benzene, a widely used industrial solvent, has been shown to induce aplastic anemia in several animal species.[51]

Aplastic anemia is observed in several species that have high endogenous or exogenous blood estrogen levels. Effects appear to be more severe in ferrets and dogs, and bone marrow panhypoplasia and pancytopenia is preceded by myeloid hyperplasia and leukocytosis. Multiple mechanisms have been incriminated for the anemia, including reduction in hemopoietic stem cell numbers, inhibition of stem cell differentiation, and decreased response to erythropoietin.[52]

The immunosuppressive agent cyclophosphamide is known to cause bone marrow suppression in dogs and cats.[53] Azothioprine, a thioguanine-derivative immunosuppressive agent, induced anemia and hypocellular bone marrow in dogs with recovery after withdrawal of the drug. Accumulation of 6-thioguanine nucleotide metabolites of azothioprine are suspected to be incorporated into bone marrow progenitor cells and cause bone marrow failure.[54]

Meclofenamic acid,[55] phenylbutazone,[55,56] quinidine,[55] and trimethoprim-sulfdiazine and fenbendazole[55,57,58] have been associated with bone marrow aplasia in dogs. Although chloramphenicol-induced bone marrow aplasia is common in humans, it appears to be infrequent in animals and has been reported to cause mild, reversible nonregenerative anemia in dogs.[59]

Recombinant human erythopoietin ([rhEPO] Epogen, Amgen Inc.) has been shown to cause increased red cell mass in cats and dogs that have renal failure[60] and in horses.[61] However, chronic therapy often results in nonregenerative anemia and bone marrow hypoplasia associated with the production of anti-rhEPO antibodies.[60,62,63] This suggests that the structure of erythropoietin is sufficiently conserved among these species and man for rhEPO to be pharmacologically active, but that the structures are sufficiently different to provoke antibody production. This drug-induced anemia appears to be reversible after the cessation of treatment with a decline in circulating anti-rhEPO antibodies.

Anemia in Toxicologic Clinical Pathology

A mild decrease in red cell mass is a common toxicity observed with high doses of many drugs and chemicals. In fact, minor nonspecific decreases in red blood cell mass are much more common than significant drug effects like those described above. Changes are often secondary to other toxicities and may be clinically similar to the anemia of inflammatory disease. Repeated withdrawal of blood for clinical pathology and toxicokinetic evaluation and suspected acclimation to the stress of repeated handling (primates) may contribute to a decrease in measured red blood cell mass over the course of toxicology studies.

Several features of toxicology studies increase the sensitivity for detection of changes in the erythron. Studies are generally well controlled, with groups of healthy, fairly homogeneous animals; concurrent controls; multiple dose groups; and controlled diet and environment. Comparison of values across treatment groups allows for detection of minor primary or secondary drug effects that, in individual animals, would not be clinically important. Samples are processed promptly and uniformly and are generally evaluated with automated instrumentation. Automated reticulocyte counts provide sufficient sensitivity and precision to identify subtle changes in erythrocyte production, prior to detection of other effects in the peripheral blood or bone marrow.

CLINICAL DIAGNOSIS OF DRUG- OR CHEMICAL-INDUCED ANEMIA

1. Other causes of anemia, e.g., infections, anemia secondary to other disorders, should be considered and ruled out.

2. Careful interrogation of the owner is needed to document exposure to drugs or chemicals known or suspected to cause anemia. Questions should include
   —Medications given
   - Prescription—e.g., chemotherapeutic, antiviral, antibiotic agents
   - Over the counter—e.g., acetaminophen, aspirin
   —Unintended access to other medications
   —Time and duration of exposure to medication
   —Exposure to household or environmental chemicals
   —Housing conditions–inside, outside, or both
   —Movement—restricted versus free roaming
   —Environmental conditions—city, suburban, rural, nearby business and industry
   —Diet—commercial versus table scraps, possible exposure to poisonous plants
3. Favorable clinical response to removal of exposure to suspected agent is critical, as many drug- or chemical-induced anemias are reversible with cessation of exposure.
4. Anemia often recurs upon rechallenge. Rechallenge is not recommended as a diagnostic tool, but it may have effectively occurred as previous multiple exposures to an inciting agent may be required before the association of the drug or chemical with the anemia can be made.
5. Measurement of blood levels of inciting agent (e.g., lead or zinc) may be helpful in confirming chemical-induced anemia. Blood levels of drugs once exposure has been confirmed is generally not required.
6. Ancillary tests may also be informative in confirming certain types of drug or chemical-induced anemia (e.g., coagulation tests for warfarin toxicity or radiology to confirm ingestion of zinc-containing objects).

REFERENCES

1. **Schechter RD, Schalm OW, Kaneko JJ.** Heinz body hemolytic anemia associated with the use of urinary antiseptics containing methylene blue in the cat. J Am Vet Med Assoc 1973;162:37–44.
2. **Harvey JW.** Methemoglobinemia and Heinz-Body Hemolytic Anemia. In: Kirk RW, ed. Kirk's Current Veterinary Therapy. XII. Small Animal Practice. 12 ed. Philadelphia: WB Saunders, 1995;443–446.
3. **Baird JD, Hutchins DR, Lepherd EE.** Phenothiazine poisoning in a thoroughbred horse. Aust Vet J 1970;46:496–499.
4. **Day TK, Andress DG, Day DG.** Effects of consecutive day propofol anesthesia on feline red blood cells. Proc Annu Meet Am College Vet Anesth 1993; 15. Abstract.
5. **Harvey JW, Rackear D.** Experimental onion-induced hemolytic anemia in dogs. Vet Pathol 1985;22:387–392.
6. **van Kampen KR, James LF, Johnson AE.** Hemolytic anemia in sheep fed wild onion (Allium validum). J Am Vet Med Assoc 1970;156:328–332.
7. **Yamato O, Hayashi M, Yamasaki M, et al.** Induction of onion-induced haemolytic anaemia in dogs with sodium n-propylthiosulphate. Vet Rec 1998;142:216–219.
8. **Robertson JE, Christopher MM, Rogers QR.** Heinz body formation in cats fed baby food containing onion powder. J Am Vet Med Assoc 1998;212:1260–1266.
9. **Christopher MM, Perman V, Eaton JW.** Contribution of propylene glycol-induced Heinz body formation to anemia in cats. J Am Vet Med Assoc 1989;194:1045–1056.
10. **Torrance AG, Fulton RB Jr.** Zinc-induced hemolytic anemia in a dog. J Am Vet Med Assoc 1987;191:443–444.
11. **Robinette CL.** Toxicology of selected pesticides, drugs, and chemicals. Zinc. Vet Clin North Am Small Anim Pract 1990;20:539–544.
12. **Latimer KS, Jain AV, Inglesby HB, et al.** Zinc-induced hemolytic anemia caused by pennies in a pup. J Am Vet Med Assoc 1989;195:77–80.
13. **Hotchkiss CE.** Diagnostic exercise: hemolytic anemia in several sheep. Lab Anim Sci 1994;44:513–516.

14. **Jain NC.** Essentials of veterinary hematology. 1st ed. 1993;198–200.
15. **Hatch RC, Blue JL, Mahaffey EA, et al.** Chronic copper toxicosis in growing swine. J Am Vet Med Assoc 1979;174:616–619.
16. **Grossman S, Budinsky R, Jollow D.** Dapsone-induced hemolytic anemia: role of glucose-6 phosphate dehydrogenase in the hemolytic response of rat erythrocytes to N-hydroxydapsone. J Pharmacol Exp Ther 1995;273:870–877.
17. **Fernandez FR, Davies AP, Teachout DJ, et al.** Vitamin K-induced Heinz-body formation in dogs. J Am Anim Hosp Assoc 1984;20:711–720.
18. **Maede Y, Hoshino T, Inaba M, et al.** Methionine toxicosis in cats. Am J Vet Res 1987;48:289–292.
19. **Greenhalgh JF, Sharman GA, Aitken JN.** Kale anaemia. I. The toxicity in various species of animal of three types of kale. Res Vet Sci. 1969;10:64–72.
20. **Garg SK, Makkar HP, Nagal KB, et al.** Oak (Quercus incana) leaf poisoning in cattle. Vet Hum Toxicol 1992;34:161–164.
21. **Stair EL, Edwards WC, Burrows GE, et al.** Suspected red maple (Acer rubrum) toxicosis with abortion in two Percheron mares. Vet Human Toxicol 1993;35:229–230.
22. **Davis JA, Greenfield RE, Brewer TG.** Benzocaine-induced methemoglobinemia attributed to topical application of the anesthetic in several laboratory animal species. Am J Vet Res 1993;54:1322–1326.
23. **Krake AC.** Cetacaine-induced methemoglobinemia in domestic cats. J Am Anim Hosp.Assoc 1985;21:527–534.
24. **Packman CH, Leddy JP.** Drug-related immune hemolytic anemia. In: Beutler E, Lichtman MA, Coller BS, Kipps TJ, eds. Williams hematology. 5th ed. New York: McGraw-Hill, 1995;691–697.
25. **Blue JT, Dinsmore RP, Anderson KL.** Immune-mediated hemolytic anemia induced by penicillin in horses. Cornell Vet 1987;77:263–276.
26. **Robbins RL, Wallace SS, Brunner CJ, et al.** Immune-mediated haemolytic disease after penicillin therapy in a horse. Equine Vet J 1993;25:462–465.
27. **McConnico RS, Roberts MC, Tompkins M.** Penicillin-induced immune-mediated hemolytic anemia in a horse. J Am Vet Med Assoc 1992;201:1402–1403.
28. **Bloom JC, Lewis HB, Sellers TS, et al.** The hematologic effects of cefonicid and cefazedone in the dog: a potential model of cephalosporin hematotoxicity in man. Toxicol Appl Pharmacol 1987;90:135–142.
29. **Bloom JC, Theim PA, Sellers TS, et al.** Cephalosporin-induced immune cytopenia in the dog: demonstration of erythrocyte-, neutrophil-, and platelet-associated IgG following treatment with cefazedone. Am J Hematol 1988;28:71–78.
30. **Thomas HL, Livesey MA.** Immune-mediated hemolytic anemia associated with trimethoprim-sulphamethoxasole administration in a horse. Can Vet J 1998;39:171–173.
31. **Atwell RB, Johnstone I, Read R, et al.** Haemolytic anaemia in two dogs suspected to have been induced by levamisole. Austr Vet J 1979;55:292–294.
32. **Jackson JA, Chart IS, Sanderson JH, et al.** Pirimicarb induced immune haemolytic anaemia in dogs. Scand J Haematol 1977;19:360–366.
33. **Peterson ME, Hurvitz AI, Leib MS, et al.** Propylthiouracil-associated hemolytic anemia, thrombocytopenia, and antinuclear antibodies in cats with hyperthyroidism. J Am Vet Med Assoc 1984;184:806–808.
34. **Duval D, Giger U.** Vaccine-associated immune-mediated hemolytic anemia in the dog. J Vet Intern Med 1996;10:290–295.
35. **Jacob HS, Yawata Y, Craddock P, et al.** Hyperalimentation hypophosphatemia: hematologic-neurologic dysfunction due to ATP depletion. Trans Assoc Am Physicians 1973;86:143–153.
36. **Engelking LH, Mariner JC.** Enhanced biliary bilirubin excretion after heparin-induced erythrocyte mass depletion. Am J Vet Res 1985;46:2175–2178.
37. **Goto I, Inaba M, Shimizu T, et al.** Mechanism of hemolysis of canine erythrocytes induced by L-sorbose. Am J Vet Res 1994;55:291–294.
38. **Halverson AW, Tsay DT, Triebwasser KC, et al.** Development of hemolytic anemia in rats fed selenite. Toxicol Appl Pharmacol 1970;17:151–159.
39. **Paradis MR, Breeze RG, Bayly WM, et al.** Acute hemolytic anemia after oral administration of L-tryptophan in ponies. Am J Vet Res 1991;52:742–747.
40. **Paradis MR, Breeze RG, Laegreid WW, et al.** Acute hemolytic anemia induced by oral administration of indole in ponies. Am J Vet Res 1991; 52:748–753.
41. **Dye TL.** Naproxen toxicosis in a puppy. Vet Hum Toxicol 1997;39:157–159.
42. **Gilmour MA, Walshaw R.** Naproxen-induced toxicosis in a dog. J Am Vet Med Assoc 1987;191:1431–1432.
43. **Hawkey CJ.** Review article: aspirin and gastrointestinal bleeding. Aliment Pharmacol Ther 1994;8:141–146.
44. **Jain NC.** Case 21 (Dog). Dicoumarol (warfarin) poisoning. In: Jain NC, ed. Schalm's Veterinary Hematology. 4th ed. Philadelphia: Lea & Febiger, 1986;1111–1112.
45. **Hart S, Nolte I.** Long-term treatment of diseased, FIV-seropositive field cats with Azidothymidine (AZT). J Vet Med Series A 1995;42:397–409.
46. **Haschek WM, Weigel RM, Scherba G, et al.** Zidovudine toxicity to cats infected with feline leukemia virus. Fundam Appl Toxicol 1990;14:764–775.
47. **Luster MI, Rosenthal GJ, Cao W, et al.** Experimental studies of the hematologic and immune system toxicity of nucleoside derivatives used against HIV infection. Int J Immunopharmacol 1991;13(Suppl 1):99–107.
48. **Thompson MB, Dunnick JK, Sutphin ME, et al.** Hematologic toxicity of AZT and ddC administered as single agents and in combination to rats and mice. Fundam Appl Toxicol 1991;17:159–176.
49. **Sippel WL.** Bracken fern poisoning. J Am Vet Med Assoc 1952;121:9–13.
50. **Pritchard WR, Rehfeld CE, Sauter JH.** Aplastic anemia of cattle associated with trichloroethylene-extracted soybean oil meal. J Am Vet Med Assoc 1952;121:1–8.
51. **Marcus WL.** Chemical of current interest–benzene. Toxicol Ind Health 1987;3:205–266.
52. **Hart JE.** Endocrine pathology of estrogens: species differences. Pharmacol Ther 1990;47:203–218.
53. **Stanton M, Legendre M.** Effects of cyclophosphamide in dogs and cats. J Am Vet Med Assoc 1986;188:1319–1322.
54. **Rinkardt NE, Kruth SA.** Azathioprine-induced bone marrow toxicity in four dogs. Can Vet J. 1996;37:612–613.
55. **Weiss DJ, Klausner JS.** Drug-associated aplastic anemia in dogs: eight cases (1984–1988). J Am Vet Med Assoc 1990;196:472–475.
56. **Watson ADJ, Wilson JT, Turner OM.** Phenylbutazone-induced blood dyscrasias suspected in three dogs. Vet Rec. 1980;107:239–241.
57. **Giger U, Werner LL, Millichamp NJ, et al.** Sulfadiazine-induced allergy in six Doberman Pinschers. J Am Anim Hosp Assoc 1985;186:479–484.
58. **Weiss DJ, Adams LG.** Aplastic anemia associated with trimethoprim-sulfadiazine and fenbendazole administration in a dog. J Am Vet Med Assoc 1985;191:1119–1120.
59. **Manyan DR, Arimuna GK, Yunis AA.** Chloramphenicol-induced suppression and bone marrow ferrochelatase activity in dogs. J Lab Clin Med 1972;79:142.
60. **Cowgill LD, James KM, Levy JK, et al.** Use of recombinant human erythropoietin for management of anemia in dogs and cats with renal failure. J Am Vet Med Assoc 1998;212:521–528.
61. **Jaussaud P, Audran M, Garaeu RL, et al.** Kinetics and haematological effects of erythropoietin in horses. Vet Res 1994;25:568–573.
62. **Piercy RJ, Swardson CJ, Hinchcliff KW.** Erythroid hypoplasia and anemia following administration of recombinant human erythropoietin to two horses. J Am Vet Med Assoc 1998;212:244–247.
63. **Woods PR, Campbell G, Cowell RL.** Nonregenerative anemia associated with administration of recombinant human erythropoietin to a thoroughbred racehorse. Equine Vet J 1997;29:326–328.

CHAPTER 32

Nutritional Deficiency Anemias

• A.D.J. WATSON and PAUL JOHN CANFIELD

Much of the literature about nutritional deficiency anemias in domestic animals is based on historical data. With few exceptions, naturally occurring deficiency anemias were often assumed to exist because of response to therapy rather than because of a demonstrated and defined nutrient deficit. Some experimental studies lacked strict controls, leaving the possibility that anemia might have resulted from interaction of several factors. In many such studies, anemia was a side issue to the main clinical and pathologic features of the deficiency state and of limited interest to researchers. Consequently, reasons for development of anemia were assumed and mechanisms remained uninvestigated. For these reasons, many older reports on nutritional anemias are inadequate.

Increasing dietary awareness over recent decades and improved feeding and management practices for pets and intensively farmed domestic species have virtually eliminated anemias resulting directly from dietary deficiency. Dietary anemia is more likely to result in these animals from mishap (for example, incorrect preparation of a batch of feed) or through interaction with other disorders, such as gastroenteropathies. However, extensively farmed animals remain vulnerable to nutrient-deficient soils and pastures but, even so, dietary supplementation can reduce deficiency states to the level of obscurity.

The focus here is on the common forms of nutritional anemia that are nonregenerative and caused by nutrient deficits. However, some nutritional abnormalities have the potential to cause hemolytic regenerative anemia with Heinz-body formation (e.g., copper intoxication, and deficiencies of copper, phosphate, and selenium) (Chapter 30, Anemias Associated with Heinz Bodies).

Table 32.1 lists the more common nutritional deficiency anemias in the major domestic species and also indicates some uncommon and rare deficiencies that may be associated with anemia.[1-7] Table 32.2 indicates nutritional and other causes of different morphologic types of nonregenerative anemia. Purported mechanisms and features of deficiency anemias are shown in Table 32.3. Because these entities are often poorly defined in veterinary patients, reference is made to the mechanisms of anemia in the corresponding human disorders where appropriate.

STARVATION

One form of nutritional anemia that probably occurs in all species, but nevertheless is not well described, is that seen in severely malnourished animals. This may be a particular problem in adverse seasons and certain geographic regions. The anemia is usually normocytic normochromic and nonregenerative, and of mild to moderate severity. It is probably attributable to combined deficiencies of protein, energy, vitamins (especially the B group), and minerals (iron, possibly copper, and cobalt). In an emaciated individual, this may be difficult to distinguish from the hypoproliferative anemia of inflammatory disease associated with underlying inflammatory, metabolic or neoplastic disorders (Chapter 35, Anemia of Inflammatory and Neoplastic Disease). Indeed, both may occur together.

IRON-DEFICIENCY ANEMIA

A wide range of disorders results in iron-deficiency anemia in people, including inadequate iron intake, iron malabsorption, chronic hemorrhage, diversion of iron to fetal or infant erythropoiesis during pregnancy or lactation, intravascular hemolysis with hemoglobinuria, and combinations of these factors.[8] By contrast, the principal cause of iron-deficiency anemia in most domestic animals is external blood loss. This is usually chronic, but depletion may occur quickly in young animals that have smaller iron reserves. The main cause is gastrointestinal hemorrhage from endoparasitism or some other process, but bloodsucking external parasites can be involved in some species. Dietary causes are rare. Signs of iron-deficiency anemia resemble those seen in any anemic disorder, but there may be additional effects owing to impaired function of various enzymes and proteins that contain iron.[8]

With bleeding, anemia is initially regenerative (macrocytic hypochromic, with reticulocytosis except in the horse), but microcytic hypochromic changes develop and reticulocytosis decreases as iron stores are depleted. Hypochromia is best seen in species that have larger erythrocytes, such as the dog; it may be unapparent in

TABLE 32.1	Specific Nutritional-Deficiency Anemias in Domesticated Animals and Man		
Species	**Major Clinical Disorders**	**Uncommon Clinical Disorders**	**Rare [and Experimental] Deficiencies[a]**
Dog	Iron deficiency[b] from chronic external blood loss caused by hookworm disease, heavy flea burden, neoplasia, hemostatic defect, overuse as blood donor	Inherited cobalamin malabsorption in giant Schnauzers[b]	Folate/cobalamin,[b] [copper, pyridoxine][1]
Cat	—	Iron deficiency[b] from heavy flea burden, gastrointestinal bleeding, dietary lack in kittens	Folate/cobalamin,[b] [pyridoxine][2]
Horse	—	Iron deficiency[b] from chronic gut bleeding, associated with strongylids[3] or other bleeding gastrointestinal lesions	Iron in foals,[b] folate[4]
Ruminants	Primary copper deficiency,[b] cobalt deficiency[b] (both occur in some regions only)	Secondary copper deficiency,[b] iron deficiency[b] from chronic intestinal parasitism, blood-sucking lice, or milk-only diets (calves, vealers)[5]	—
Pig	Dietary iron deficiency in piglets[b]	Copper-deficient diet in growing pigs[b]	Secondary iron deficiency caused by calcium carbonate (or manganese) in fattening pigs[5], [protein, lysine tryptophane, many B vitamins, vitamin E][6]
Man	Iron deficiency,[b] folate/cobalamin deficiency[b]	Deficiencies of vitamin A, vitamin C, copper[7]	Vitamin E, pyridoxine, [riboflavin][7]

[a]Anemia is often of limited importance
[b]See text for details
Data from references 1–7 with permission.

TABLE 32.2	Nutritional Deficiencies and Other Diagnostic Possibilities in Different Forms of Nonregenerative Anemia		
Type of Anemia	**Possible Nutritional Causes**	**Other Potential Causes**
Normocytic normochromic	Starvation	Chronic disease, acute blood loss (<4 days duration), primary bone marrow failure
Normocytic normochromic with some microcytes/hypochromia	Developing iron deficiency	Portosystemic shunt, anemia of chronic disease
Normocytic normochromic with some macrocytes	Folate or cobalamin deficiency, cobalt deficiency in ruminants	Dyserythropoiesis, leukemia virus in cats
Microcytic and/or hypochromic	Iron deficiency	Any nonregenerative anemia in an Akita dog, portosystemic shunt
Macrocytic	Folate or cobalamin deficiencies, cobalt deficiency in ruminant	Dyserythropoiesis, leukemia virus in cats, any nonregenerative anemia in a Poodle that had familial macrocytosis

feline blood smears.[9] Associated laboratory abnormalities include hypoproteinemia and erythrocyte fragmentation. Thrombocytosis is also common unless the cause of chronic blood loss is thrombocytopenia.

Note that transitional morphologic forms, between macrocytic regenerative anemia and the microcytic non-regenerative stage, are encountered. Furthermore, any underlying gastrointestinal disease may further alter erythrocyte morphology.

If findings suggest iron-deficiency anemia but blood loss is cryptic, urine should be tested for hemoglobin and erythrocytes. Feces should also be examined for ova

---

TABLE 32.3   Mechanisms and Hematologic Features of Nutritional-Deficiency Anemias

Type of Deficiency	Species Affected Naturally	Mechanism for Anemia	Peripheral Hematologic Features and Erythrocyte Indices	Bone Marrow Features
Starvation (attributable to combined deficiencies)	Presumed all species	Protein lack causes reduced erythropoietin, also lack of essential amino acids as precursors	Commonly normocytic normochromic if mainly protein lack	Reduced erythropoiesis
Iron	Occurs more quickly in young animals that have external blood loss, also blood loss in adults. Dietary deficiency mainly in kittens, calves and piglets on milk diets	Interference with hemoglobin synthesis, additional divisions of erythroid cells	Microcytic hypochromic, erythrocyte fragmentation, may get thrombocytosis	Ineffective erythropoiesis with asynchrony and often a shift to later rubricytes (later may get reduced erythropoiesis)
Copper	Mainly in sheep and cattle on deficient pastures. Has been reported in piglets	Impaired iron metabolism (poor absorption and inability to use intracellular iron). Molybdenum excess interferes with copper uptake	Commonly microcytic hypochromic, but may be normocytic or macrocytic in ruminants	Ineffective erythropoiesis
Pyridoxine (vitamin B_6)	Probably does not occur naturally	Interferes with the first step of heme synthesis causing iron overload	Microcytic hypochromic (with high serum iron)	Not reported
Riboflavin	Probably does not occur naturally	Not known	Either microcytic hypochromic, or normocytic normochromic in experimental deficiency	Reduced erythropoiesis
Folate/cobalamin (vitamin B_{12})	Ruminants (cobalt deficiency), dogs and cats	Impeded DNA synthesis	Commonly normocytic normochromic, but macrocytes may circulate; possibly macrocytic	Ineffective erythropoiesis with megaloblastic change in erythroid line but variable in neutrophil line
Niacin (nicotinic acid)	Probably does not occur naturally	Impedes folate synthesis in experimental deficiency in dogs	Macrocytic or normocytic	Ineffective erythropoiesis with megaloblastic erythroid changes
Vitamin C (ascorbic acid)	Only in nonhuman primates and guinea pigs	Participates in conversion of folate into active form and increases demand for iron	Either normocytic normochromic or microcytic hypochromic, depending on whether iron or folate deficient	Ineffective erythropoiesis and megaloblastic erythroid changes in monkeys
Vitamin E (α-tocopherol)	Probably does not occur naturally	Not known	Normocytic normochromic	Ineffective erythropoiesis with erythroid hyperplasia and multinucleated erythroid cells

---

of bloodsucking parasites and for occult blood. For the latter, a meat-free diet may be necessary for 3 or 4 days in carnivores, to avoid false-positive reactions.

Other laboratory findings confirming an iron-deficiency state are low values for serum iron, transferrin saturation, and ferritin concentration and bone marrow

showing erythroid hyperplasia, perhaps with late rubricyte or metarubricyte predominance,[10] and reduced stainable iron (Chapter 22, Iron Metabolism; Chapter 34, Microcytic Anemias; and Appendix Case Z).

In some species, iron deficiency can develop in young, rapidly growing individuals ingesting only milk, because milk is a poor source of iron. Subclinical iron-deficiency anemia occurs transiently in calves and kids, but is of debatable significance.[5] Veal calves, deliberately fed an iron-poor diet to produce pale meat, have the potential to develop anemia and anorexia and to grow poorly. Foals have low initial iron stores, and rapid growth could make them more susceptible than adults to iron deficiency,[11,12] although this seems not to cause problems clinically. In a small proportion of suckling kittens, however, dietary iron-deficiency anemia might be severe enough to contribute to mortality.[13] The condition is economically important in suckling piglets maintained indoors with no access to iron and causes anemia, failure to thrive, and deaths.[5]

The key step in treating iron-deficiency anemia is to identify and correct any process causing blood loss. Iron supplementation is also recommended in these cases and whenever dietary iron deficiency is suspected. Oral administration is safer and most economical, preferably given as ferrous salts and not in an enteric-coated or sustained release formulation.

COPPER-DEFICIENCY ANEMIA

Anemia can develop as part of a wider syndrome in ruminants with copper deficiency. It is more likely to occur with the severe primary form of deficiency caused by eating forage from soils where copper is deficient or unavailable; it is less common in secondary copper deficiency, where copper intake is adequate but use is impaired by high dietary molybdenum or sulfate.[14]

The anemia of copper deficiency is generally moderate in severity and microcytic hypochromic. It is attributed to impaired production of the copper-containing enzyme ceruloplasmin, which impedes use of iron (Chapter 22, Iron Metabolism; Chapter 34, Microcytic Anemias). Heinz bodies may be prominent in affected cattle, though there is no evidence of excessive hemolysis.[14] Associated clinical abnormalities include poor growth, reduced lactation, depigmentation of hair, abnormal wool fibers, diarrhea, infertility, ataxia, and osteoporosis with fractures.

Demonstration of low blood copper concentrations is useful diagnostically, but confirmation of reduced copper content in liver is preferable.[14,15] Treatment with injectable or oral copper preparations is effective.

Microcytic hypochromic anemia has occurred in growing pigs, especially whey-fed animals, and is attributed to copper deficiency and consequent maluse of iron. Signs of anemia can be accompanied by ill-thrift, limb deformities, ataxia, posterior paresis or paralysis, and cardiovascular abnormalities[16,17] Anemia and other signs respond to treatment with copper.[14]

FOLATE- AND COBALAMIN-DEFICIENCY ANEMIAS

Macrocytic normochromic, nonregenerative anemia, accompanied by neutropenia and circulating hyperseg-mented neutrophils, occurs in people who have deficiency of folate or cobalamin (vitamin B_{12}). Deficiency can be caused by poor diet or by various factors that either hinder absorption of these substances or increase the requirement for folate.[18] The resulting syndrome is dominated by signs of anemia, but neurologic abnormalities also occur with cobalamin deficiency. Hematologic abnormalities are associated with defective DNA synthesis and ineffective hemopoiesis, producing characteristic megaloblastic changes in erythroid and myeloid precursors in bone marrow.

There are few veterinary analogs of these disorders. A few cases of possible folate- or cobalamin-deficiency anemia have been reported; however, some are unconvincing, and their scantiness suggests these are not important causes of anemia in veterinary patients. However, the possible development of megaloblastic anemia during some drug treatments should be considered. Long-term treatment with anticonvulsant (phenobarbitone, phenytoin, and primidone) sometimes causes folate-deficiency anemia in people,[18] perhaps when dietary folate is marginal. Chronic therapy with phenytoin in dogs produced no evidence of folate deficiency, although suggestive hematologic changes had been seen in earlier studies.[19] Folate-deficiency anemia was suspected in one dog given primidone for 6 months; folate was not measured, but blood and bone marrow changes were suggestive and treatment response to folic acid was excellent despite continuation of phenytoin.[20]

Folate-deficiency anemia also occurs in some people given drugs that act by impairing folate metabolism, such as methotrexate, pyrimethamine, sulfasalazine, and trimethoprim. In addition, various cytotoxic agents can cause megaloblastic anemia, including azathioprine, cytarabine, 5-fluorouracil, and hydroxyurea.[18]

The absence of reports of anemias induced by therapy with these drugs in veterinary patients suggests such effects are rare or nonexistent. If anemia does occur, the blood film may not show the typical changes found in people. It has been suggested that folate and cobalamin deficiencies more likely produce normocytic normochromic anemias in dogs and cats, although there may be some circulating macrocytes and megaloblastic bone marrow changes.[21] Other data[22] generally support that view, but some uncertainty remains.

Giant Schnauzer dogs that have cobalamin malabsorption had normocytic normochromic, nonregenerative anemia, together with anisocytosis, poikilocytosis, large platelets, neutropenia, hypersegmented neutrophils, and abnormal bone marrow (giant metamyelocytes and band neutrophils and erythroid megaloblastosis). Clinical signs were inappetence, lethargy, and poor weight gain.[23] Methylmalonic aciduria and low serum cobalamin concentrations were found. The cause was an absence of intrinsic factor-cobalamin receptors in the apical brush border of ileal enterocytes, inherited as an autosomal recessive trait.[24] Affected dogs responded rapidly to vitamin B_{12}, administered parenterally but not orally. Normocytic normochromic, nonregenerative anemia also occurred in a cat that had cobalamin malabsorption, which is considered to have a hereditary origin.[25] The cat did not exhibit neutropenia or hypersegmented neutrophils. Bone marrow was not examined.

By contrast, anemia was macrocytic and nonregenerative in the dog that had a combined deficiency of folate and cobalamin; other hematologic and bone marrow changes were also compatible with megaloblastic anemia.[26] The interpretation was complicated by concurrent ehrlichiosis, but anemia lessened and folate and cobalamin concentrations normalized after treatment with doxycycline and one injection of folic acid.

Overall, evidence to date suggests that anemias caused by folate- or cobalamin-deficiency in nonhuman species are rare. Such anemias might be either normocytic or macrocytic.

COBALT DEFICIENCY IN RUMINANTS

Cobalamin-deficiency and normocytic normochromic anemia occur in ruminants grazing pastures grown on cobalt-deficient soils.[27] Sheep are more susceptible than cattle, and young animals are more vulnerable than adults. Anemia develops somewhat late in the course of the disease and, although it may be apparent clinically, the dominant signs are anorexia, wasting, pica in cattle, lacrimation in sheep, and decreased growth and productivity. Cobalt is required for rumenal bacteria to synthesize cobalamin, the absence of which causes impaired propionic acid metabolism and consequent inanition. It seems likely that malnutrition is at least partly responsible for the anemia, although macrocytosis (suggesting impaired DNA synthesis) developed in goats that have experimental cobalt-cobalamin deficiency.[28] Useful aids to diagnosis of this disorder include reduced serum cobalamin concentration, increased concentrations of methylmalonic acid in plasma and urine, and rapid response to treatment with cobalt orally or vitamin B_{12} parenterally.[27]

NUTRITIONAL DEFICIENCY ANEMIAS IN OTHER SPECIES

Laboratory animals, such as rats, rabbits, mice, guinea pigs, and nonhuman primates, now rarely suffer from anemia of this type, because of increased use of well-controlled rations. Those affected are likely to be animals kept as pets or affected by gastroenteric disease.[29] Experimentally induced and well-documented anemias have been attributed to deficiencies of protein, amino acids, pyridoxine, riboflavin, folate, vitamin E, and vitamin C. Vitamin C deficiency can occur in guinea pigs and in young monkeys fed an all-milk diet, but causes only mild anemia.[6,29]

Information about nutritional-deficiency anemias in birds is confusing, but the development of controlled diets has made the occurrence of nutritional deficiencies unlikely in production and aviary birds.[30,31] Chicks are more prone to deficiencies; macrocytic anemia can be expected with folate deficiency and microcytic anemia in copper and iron deficiencies.

No information is available on nutritional-deficiency anemias in reptiles and amphibians, but increasing interest in aquaculture and aquariums has focused some attention on fish. The available information is confusing, as naturally occurring and experimentally induced conditions are not always distinguished and the fish species involved is sometimes not stated. It appears that folate deficiency causes megaloblastic or macrocytic changes in trout and that iron deficiency induces hypochromia in sea bream and common carp.[32,33] Other deficiencies also lead to anemia, but it is likely that further refinement of fish diets will prevent their occurrence.

REFERENCES

1. **National Research Council**. Nutrient requirements in dogs. Washington: National Academy Press, 1985.
2. **National Research Council**. Nutrient requirements of cats. Washington: National Academy Press, 1986.
3. **Radostits OM, Blood DC, Gay CC**. Veterinary medicine. 8th ed. London: Ballière Tindall, 1994;1241.
4. **Jeffcott LB**. Clinical haematology of the horse. In: Archer RK, Jeffcott LB, eds. Comparative clinical haematology. Oxford: Blackwell Scientific, 1977;205.
5. **Radostits OM, Blood DC, Gay CC**. Veterinary medicine. 8th ed. London: Ballière Tindall, 1994;1398.
6. **Jain NC**. Schalm's veterinary hematology. 4th ed. Philadelphia: Lea and Febiger, 1986;655.
7. **Oski FA**. Anemia due to other nutritional deficiencies. In: Beutler E, Lichtman MA, Coller BS, Kipps TJ, eds. Williams hematology. 5th ed. New York: McGraw-Hill, 1995; 511.
8. **Fairbanks VF, Beutler E**. Iron deficiency. In: Beutler E, Lichtman MA, Coller BS, Kipps TJ, eds. Williams hematology. 5th ed. New York: McGraw-Hill, 1995;490.
9. **Fulton R, Weiser MG, Freshman JL, Gasper PW, Feltman MJ**. Electronic and morphologic characterization of erythrocytes of an adult cat with iron deficiency anemia. Vet Pathol 1988;25:521–523.
10. **Jain NC**. Schalm's veterinary hematology. 4th ed. Philadelphia: Lea and Febiger, 1986;583.
11. **Smith JE, Cipriano JE, DeBowes R, Moure K**. Iron deficiency and pseudo-iron deficiency in hospitalized horses. J Am Vet Med Assoc 1986; 188:285–287.
12. **Harvey JW, Asquith RL, Sussman WA, Kivipelto J**. Serum ferritin, serum iron, and erythrocyte values in foals. Am J Vet Res 1987;48:1348–1352.
13. **Weiser MG, Kociba GJ**. Sequential changes in erythrocyte volume distribution and microcytosis associated with iron deficiency in kittens. Vet Pathol 1983;20:1–12.
14. **Radostits OM, Blood DC, Gay CC**. In: Veterinary medicine. 8th ed. London: Baillière Tindall, 1994;1379.
15. **Maas J, Smith BP**. Copper deficiency in ruminants. In: Smith BP, ed. Large animal internal medicine. 2nd ed. St Louis: Mosby, 1996;904.
16. **Hodges RT, Fraser AJ**. Some observations on the liver copper status of pigs in the northern part of New Zealand. N Z Vet J 1983;31:96–100.
17. **National Research Council**. Nutrient requirements of swine. Washington: National Academy Press, 1988.
18. **Babior BM**. The megaloblastic anemias. In: Beutler E, Lichtmann MA, Coller BS, Kipps TJ, eds. Williams hematology. 5th ed. New York: McGraw-Hill, 1995;471.
19. **Bunch SE, Easley RJ, Cullen JM**. Hematologic values and plasma and tissue folate concentrations in dogs given phenytoin on a long-term basis. Am J Vet Res 1990;51:1865–1868.
20. **Lewis HB, Rebar AH**. Bone marrow evaluation in veterinary practice. St Louis: Ralston–Purina, 1979;46.
21. **Jain NC**. Schalm's veterinary hematology. 4th ed. Philadelphia: Lea and Febiger, 1986;658.
22. **Chanarin I, Deacon R, Lumb M, Muir M, Perry J**. Cobalamin-folate interrelations: a critical review. Blood 1985;66:479–489.
23. **Fyfe JC, Jezyk PF, Giger U, Patterson DF**. Inherited selective malabsorption of vitamin B_{12} in giant Schnauzers. J Am Anim Hosp Assoc 1989;25:533–539.
24. **Fyfe JC, Giger U, Hall CA, Jezyk PF, Klumpp SA, Levine JS, Patterson DF**. Inherited selective intestinal cobalamin malabsorption and cobalamin deficiency in dogs. Pediatr Res 1991;29:24–31.

25. **Vaden SL, Wood PA, Ledley FD, Cornwell PE, Miller RT, Page R**. Cobalamin deficiency associated with methylmalonic acidemia in a cat. J Am Vet Med Assoc 1992;200:1101–1103.
26. **Capelli J-L, Bohlay P, Barre D**. Carence en folates et vitamine B_{12} chez un chien infectè par *Ehrlichia canis*. Prat Med Chir Anim Comp 1994;29:395–402.
27. **Radostits OM, Blood DC, Gay CC**. In: Veterinary medicine. 8th ed. London: Baillière Tindall, 1994:1374.
28. **Mgongo FOK, Gombe S, Ogaa JS**. Thyroid status in cobalt and vitamin B_{12} deficiency in goats. Vet Rec 1981;109:51–53.
29. **Loeb WF, Bannerman RM, Rininger BF, Johnson AJ**. Hematologic disorders. In: Benirschke K, Garner FM, Jones TC, eds. Pathology of laboratory animals. New York: Springer-Verlag, 1978;890.
30. **Austic RE, Scott ML**. Nutritional diseases. In: Calnek BW, Barnes HJ, Beard CW, Reid WM, Yoder HW, eds. Diseases of poultry. 9th ed. Ames, IA: Iowa State University Press, 1991;45.
31. **Roudybush T**. Nutrition. In: Rosskopf WJ, Woerpel RW, eds. Diseases of cage and aviary birds. Baltimore: Williams and Wilkins, 1996;218.
32. **Ferguson HW**. Nutritional diseases. In: Fish diseases. Proceedings 106, Postgraduate Committee in Veterinary Science, University of Sydney, 1988;87.
33. **Stoskopf M**. Fish medicine. Philadelphia: WB Saunders, 1993;113.

CHAPTER 33

Macrocytosis

• GARY J. KOCIBA

An increased mean corpuscular volume (MCV) usually is an indication of an erythroid-regenerative response with the release of immature cells of increased size. In veterinary medicine, macrocytosis related to other causes is uncommon. The major differential causes of macrocytosis are presented in Table 33.1.

ERYTHROID-REGENERATIVE RESPONSES

Macrocytosis in most species indicates an erythroid-regenerative response and is accompanied by reticulocytosis. Reticulocyte size and number generally are proportional to the degree of stimulation of erythropoiesis. Macroreticulocytes are produced under conditions with intense erythropoietic stimulation and become macrocytic erythrocytes as the cells mature.[1-3] Persistent macrocytosis after reticulocytosis has been documented in rats[1], cats[4], and calves[5]. Remodeling occurs over the life span of the cells, with a gradual reduction in size to normocytic levels. In cats, macrocytic erythrocytes were detectable for at least 40 days after being produced in response to acute hemolytic anemia[4]. In the horse, which generally does not release reticulocytes into the blood, macrocytosis may provide evidence of erythroid regeneration. In horses that have hemolytic anemia, the degree of macrocytosis varies inversely with the severity of the anemia. The increase in MCV may not be drastic (0 to 15 fL), often stays within reference intervals, and is most readily detected with serial hemograms.[6] Erythroid regeneration can occur without a significant increase in MCV in some horses that have mild anemia.

GREYHOUND DOGS

Greyhounds usually have higher reference values for packed cell volume (PCV), hemoglobin concentration, MCV, and erythrocyte concentration.[7-9] The MCV of greyhounds is higher than non-greyhounds, with a mean MCV of 81.2 +/− 8.2 fL in greyhounds compared with 65.6 +/− 2.9 fL of non-greyhounds reported in one study.[8] Greyhound erythrocytes have a shorter life span (53.6 +/− 6.5 days compared with 104.3 +/−

2.2 days for non-greyhounds), which could explain the macrocytosis.[9]

MACROCYTOSIS OF POODLES

Macrocytosis is a familial condition of poodle dogs. Of 24 affected dogs, 17 (71%) in the early reports were represented by miniature or toy poodles.[10-12] The abnormality occurs in both sexes and is usually detected as an incidental finding when a hemogram is performed for an unrelated problem. The most distinctive finding is a macrocytosis with a mean MCV of 94.4 +/− 7.6 fL in data from 9 of the 24 dogs described by Schalm.[10] The dogs are not anemic and do not show evidence of reticulocytosis. The blood contains macrocytic erythrocytes along with increased nucleated erythrocytes, some of which show nuclear-cytoplasmic asynchrony. Howell–Jolly bodies are increased, may be multiple, and are of variable size with occasional cells with multiple fragments of pyknotic nuclei evident (Fig. 33.1). Megaloblastic changes are noted in erythroid precursors in the marrow, and a tendency toward hypersegmentation in neutrophils of the blood is present. The findings are reminiscent of abnormalities associated with deficiencies of vitamin B_{12} or folate; however, serum vitamin B_{12} levels, serum and erythrocyte folate levels, and transcobalamin-binding capacities are either normal or increased, and the dogs do not respond to injections of vitamin B_{12}.[10,12] The disease appears to be related to a bone marrow dyscrasia. Within the marrow, numerous abnormalities are noted in erythroid precursors. Megaloblasts with nuclear-cytoplasmic asynchrony in rubricytes and metarubricytes are common. Mitoses are increased in number and some binucleated and multinucleated erythroid cells are noted. Nuclei of the more differentiated erythroid cells show fragmentation, and unusual nuclear shapes and some incomplete nuclear divisions with frequent cells with atypical Howell–Jolly bodies are noted (Fig. 33.2).

The exact nature of the defect is unknown. The disease has been described as congenital dyserythropoieis of poodle dogs.[13] It has some similarities to the congenital dyserythropoietic anemia type I of children.[14]

HEREDITARY STOMATOCYTOSIS

Stomatocytosis has been described in Alaskan malemutes,[15,16] miniature schnauzers,[17] and Drentse-Partrijshond dogs.[18] Stomatocytes are rounded, cup-shaped cells with a slitlike indentation that is recognized as a linear area of central pallor on blood films (Fig. 33.3). Variable numbers of RBCs of affected dogs are stomatocytic with a mean of 3.7% in Alaskan malemutes and higher numbers (5 to 40%), which have been described, in the miniature schnauzers and Drenste-Partrijshonds. Stomatocytes have an increased cell volume:surface area ratio that correlates with significantly increased osmotic fragility. The diseases in the different breeds all are autosomal recessive characteristics but appear to be caused by different defects involving either cell membanes or regulation of cell volume.

The Alaskan malemutes have chondrodysplasia along with the stomatocytosis. The erythrocytes of affected Alaskan malemutes are macrocytic with MCVs in the 90- to 96-fL range. The concentration of reticulocytes is approximately twice normal, the mean corpuscular hemoglobin concentration (MCHC) is decreased, and glutathione levels are decreased to approximately 50% of normal levels in affected Alaskan malemutes. The RBC survival is shortened to less than

TABLE 33.1	Differential Causes of Macrocytosis

Erythroid-regenerative response-blood loss or hemolysis
Breed difference (greyhound dogs)
Hereditary macrocytosis of poodles
Hereditary stomatocytosis
Feline leukemia virus infection
Aplastic anemia or pure red cell aplasia
Preleukemia

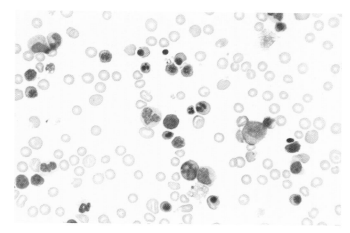

FIGURE 33.2 Erythroid precursors with atypical fragmented nuclei in bone marrow of a poodle that has macrocytosis. (Photo courtesy of Dr. Douglas Weiss, University of Minnesota, St. Paul, MN.)

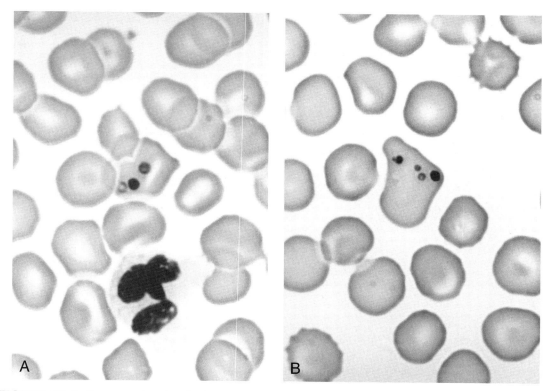

FIGURE 33.1 Two examples of multiple Howell–Jolly bodies in erythrocytes of a poodle that has macrocytosis.

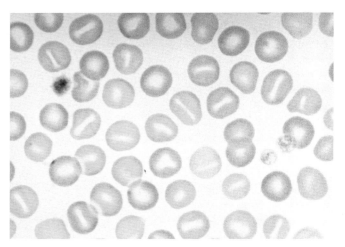

FIGURE 33.3 Stomatocytes of schnauzer-beagle mixed-breed dog. The linear zone of pallor is distinctive. (Slide courtesy of Dr. Diane Brown, Lilly Research Laboratories, Cambridge, MA.)

50% of normal in affected dogs. Cross-transfusion experiments have demonstrated short survival of erythrocytes of affected dogs in carrier littermates and normal survival of erythrocytes of carrier erythrocytes in affected dogs. Splenomegaly is associated with the defect. The stomatocytosis in Alaskan malemutes appears to be related to an increased content of monovalent cation, especially sodium, and increased cell water, reflecting either a membrane defect or a failure of a transport mechanism.[16] The effects on sodium flux with a secondary increase in water content lead to macrocytosis and decreased MCHC. A trend toward a correlation between increased sodium content and aging of the red cells of affected Alaskan malemutes was noted. This suggests that the stomatocytes develop as the aging red cells take on increased sodium and water. Heterozygous malemutes are phenotypically normal but have slightly increased MCVs and erythrocyte sodium concentrations. The erythrocytic potassium concentration is slightly increased in affected Alaskan malemutes. This appears to reflect the young age of the RBC population rather than a specific defect in the cell membrane.

In contrast to the Alaskan malemutes and Drentse-Partrijshonds, the miniature schnauzers with stomatocytosis are asymptomatic. They have macrocytosis with a high percentage of stomatocytes (5 to 40%). Although the erythrocyte life span is decreased, the erythroid-regenerative response is not intense as noted in the affected malemutes.[19]

Drentse-Partrijshond dogs that have stomatocytosis have retarded growth, diarrhea, polyuria, polydipsia, ataxia, and posterior paresis. Progressive deterioration usually leads to euthanasia while the dogs are still young. Hypertrophic gastritis resembling Menetrier's disease of human beings, progressive liver disease, polyneuropathy, and renal cysts are noted at necropsy. The MCHCs of erythrocytes of Drentse-Partrijshond dogs are normal or only slightly increased. A range of 14 to

38% of erythrocytes of Drentse-Partrijshond dogs are stomatocytic on routine blood films.[20] If the cells of Drentse-Partrijshond dogs are fixed with glutaraldehyde and examined with scanning electron microscopy, the percentage of stomatocytes is much higher with nearly all erythrocytes affected. In contrast to the erythrocytes of affected Alaskan malemutes, the erythrocytes of Drentse-Partrijshond dogs that have stomatocytosis have only a modest 6% increase in total monovalent cation content. The stomatocytosis of Drentse-Partrijshond dogs appears to be caused by a different mechanism. The erythrocytic defect in Drentse-Partrijshond dogs has been attributed to abnormal concentrations in phospholipids in the cell membranes; this defect may contribute to either membrane contraction or membrane loss.[20]

FELINE LEUKEMIA VIRUS-ASSOCIATED ANEMIA

Most cats that have anemia and feline leukemia virus (FeLV) infection have macrocytosis and increased anisocytosis.[21] Some FeLV-positive cats have normal MCV but increased anisocytosis, reflecting minor subpopulations of macrocytic erythrocytes. The macrocytosis does not correlate with reticulocytosis or other evidence of a current erythroid-regenerative response. The macrocytosis is most prominent in cats that have anemia, including both regenerative and nonregenerative anemias, but also occurs in more than 50% of nonanemic cats infected with FeLV. It has been suggested that the macrocytosis could reflect a period of intense erythroid regeneration before conversion to a hypoproliferative anemia, but the cause is unknown. In a study of cats that have experimental FeLV-induced anemia, the macrocytic changes were not as significant as noted in the naturally occurring disease, and no period of reticuolocytosis was detected over the course of the disease.[21]

PRELEUKEMIA AND APLASTIC ANEMIAS

Macrocytosis is associated with some cases of erythroid aplasia,[22] aplastic anemia,[23] or preleukemia[24] of human patients without evidence of previous erythroid regeneration. This change could reflect maximal stimulation of remaining precursors by the high levels of erythropoietin or from the emergence of abnormal clones of cells. Similar findings have been reported in erythroid aplasia of cats[21] and in myelodysplasia of dogs[25] and cats[26]. No response to vitamin B_{12} treatment has been detected.

FOLIC ACID AND VITAMIN B_{12} DEFICIENCIES

Although macrocytic anemia is associated with vitamin B_{12} deficiency in human patients, similar changes are not associated with experimental or naturally occurring vitamin B_{12} deficiency of nonhuman primates or any of the common species of domestic animals.[27-30] Vitamin B_{12} deficiency develops when ruminants are maintained on cobalt-deficient diets, but the anemia usually is normocytic and normochromic.[28] Rats and lambs that have experimental deficiencies of vitamin B_{12} develop nonregenerative anemia without macrocytosis.[27] Folic acid deficiency of monkeys, pigs, and chicks is accompanied by megaloblastic changes in the bone marrow with mild macrocytosis noted in the blood of folate-deficient pigs and chicks.[27] Megaloblastic erythroid precursors are larger than normal and have more cytoplasm relative to the size of the nucleus. Condensation of the chromatin is delayed, leading to nuclear-cytoplasmic asynchrony as the cytoplasm acquires hemoglobin. Megaloblastic changes in erythroid cells have been described in the marrow of cats depleted of folic acid but the changes are not drastic.[31] Macrocytosis in dogs that have chronic diarrhea that responded to vitamin B_{12} injections have been described in an anecdotal report.[32]

Dogs and cats on phenobarbital or primidone occasionally develop megaloblastic changes within the marrow but the changes are not accompanied by macrocytosis. In an experimental study of dogs given phenytoin on a long-term basis, neither macrocytic anemia nor megaloblastic changes were detected although erythrocyte folate content was decreased.[33]

REFERENCES

1. **Brecher G, Stohlman F**. Reticulocyte size and erythropoietic stimulation. Proc Soc Exp Biol Med 1961;107:887.
2. **Ganzoni A, Hillman R, Finch C**. Maturation of the macroreticulocyte. Br J Haematol 1969;16:119.
3. **Hillman R**. Characteristics of marrow production and reticulocyte maturation in normal man in response to anemia. J Clin Invest 1969;48:443.
4. **Weiser MG, Kociba GJ**. Persistent macrocytosis assessed by erythrocyte subpopulation analysis following erythrocyte regeneration in cats. Blood 1982;60:295–303.
5. **Schnappauf H, Stein H, Sipe C, et al**. Erythropoietic response in calves following blood loss. Am J Vet Res 1967;28:275.
6. **Radin MJ, Eubank MC, Weiser MG**. Electronic measurement of erythrocyte volume and volume heterogeneity in horses during erythrocyte regeneration associated with experimental anemias. Vet Pathol 1986;23:656–660.
7. **Porter JA, Canacay WR**. Hematologic values in mongrel and greyhound dogs being screened for research use. J Am Vet Med Assoc 1971;159:1603–1606.
8. **Sullivan PS, Evans HL, Mcdonald TP**. Platelet concentration and hemoglobin function in greyhounds. J Am Vet Med Assoc 1994;205:838–841.
9. **Novinger MS, Sullivan PS, McDonald TP**. Determination of the lifespan of erythrocytes from greyhounds, using an in vitro biotinylation technique. Am J Vet Res 1996;57:739–742.
10. **Schalm OJ**. Erythrocytic macrocytosis in miniature and toy poodles. Canine Pract 1976;3:55–57.
11. **Schalm OW**. Erythrocyte macrocytosis in miniature poodles. California Vet. 1976;30:29–33.
12. **Canfield PJ, Watson AD**. Investigations of bone marrow dyscrasia in a poodle with macrocytosis. J Comp Pathol 1989;101:269–278.
13. **Weiss DJ**. Histopathology of canine non-neoplastic bone marrow. Vet Clin Pathol 1986;15:7–11.
14. **Heimpel H**. Congenital dyserythropoietic anaemia, Type I. In: Lewis SM, Verwilghen RL, eds. Dyserythropoiesis. London, Academic Press, 1977; 55–70.
15. **Fletch SM, Pinkerton PH, Bruecker PJ**. The Alaskan malamute chondrodysplasia (dwarfism-anemia) syndrome-in review. J Am Anim Hosp Assoc 1975;11:353–361.
16. **Pinkerton PH, Fletch SM, Brueckner PJ, et al**. Hereditary stomatocytosis with hemolytic anemia in the dog. Blood 1974;44:557–567.
17. **Brown DE, Weiser MG, Thrall MA, et al**. Erythrocytic indices and volume distribution in a dog with stomatocytosis. Vet Pathol 1994;31:247–250.
18. **Slappendel RJ, van der Gaag I, Van Nes JJ, et al**. Familial stomatocytosis-hypertrophic gastritis (FSHG), a newly recognized disease in the dog (Drentse patrijshond). Vet Quart 1991;13:30–40.
19. **Giger U, Amador A, Meyers-Wallen V, et al**. Stomatocytosis in miniature schnauzers. Proceedings of Sixth Annual Veterinary Medical Formum, American College of Veterinary Internal Medicine, Washington, DC, 1988;754.
20. **Slappendel RJ, Renooij W, Debrijne JJ**. Normal cations and abnormal membrane lipids in the red blood cells of dogs with familial stomatocytosis-hypertrophic gastritis. Blood 1994;84:904–909.
21. **Weiser MG, Kociba GJ**. Erythrocyte macrocytosis in feline leukemia virus associated anemia. Vet Pathol 1983;20:687–697.
22. **Ball SE, Mcguckin CP, Jenkins G, et al**. Diamond-Blackfan anaemia in the UK: analysis of 80 cases from a 20 year cohort. Br J Haematol 1996; 94:645–653.
23. **Bessman JD, Gilmer PR Jr, Gardner FH**. Improved classification of anemias by MCV and RDW. Am J Clin Pathol 1983;80:322–326.
24. **Linman JW, Bagby GC Jr**. The preleukemic syndrome: clinical and laboratory features, natural course, and management. Blood Cells 1976;2:11.
25. **Weiss DJ, Raskin R, Zerbe C**. Myelodysplastic syndrome in two dogs. J Am Vet Med Assoc 1985;187:1038–1040.
26. **Blue JT, French TW, Kranz JS**. Non-lymphoid hematopoietic neoplasia in cats: a retrospective study of 60 cases. Cornell Vet 1988;78:21–42.
27. **Stokstad EL**. Experimental anemias in animals resulting from folic acid and vitamin B_{12} deficiencies. Vitam Horm 1968;26:443–463.
28. **Judson GJ, Gifford KE**. Haematological values in vitamin B_{12} responsive calves. Aust Vet J 1979;55:504–505.
29. **Alexander F, Davies ME**. Studies on vitamin B_{12} in the horse. Br Vet J 1969;125:169–176.
30. **Frederick GL**. Hematologic signs of vitamin B_{12} deficiency in swine. Am J Vet Res 1967;28:1447–1453.
31. **Thenen SW, Rasmussen KM**. Megaloblastic erythropoiesis and tissue depletion of folic acid in the cat. Am J Vet Res 1978;39:1205–1207.
32. **Sims MA**. Megaloblastosis in the dog. Vet Rec 1979;105:359.
33. **Bunch SE, Easley JR, Cullen JM**. Hematologic values and plasma and tissue concentrations in dogs given phenytoin on a long-term basis. Am J Vet Res 1990;51:1865–1868.

CHAPTER 34

Microcytic Anemias

• JOHN W. HARVEY

A microcytic anemia is one where the mean cell volume (MCV) is less than the reference range for the species in question. The MCV represents the average volume of a single erythrocyte in femtoliters (fL = 10^{-15} l). The MCV is determined most accurately with appropriately calibrated electronic cell counters that determine the size of individual cells and compute the MCV. It can also be determined indirectly by dividing the hematocrit (as a percentage) by the erythrocyte count (in millions of cells per microliter) and multiplying by 10. This latter method is less accurate, because two separate measurements are required. The MCV varies greatly depending on species and, in some cases, depending on a breed within a species. Some dogs from Japanese breeds (Akita and Shiba) normally have MCV values less than the reference ranges established for other breeds of dogs,[1] but these dogs are not anemic.

When hemoglobin concentration reaches a certain level in developing erythroid cells, it appears to signal the cessation of cell division. Cellular division is normal, but hemoglobin synthesis is delayed with abnormalities in heme or globin synthesis; consequently, one or more extra divisions occur during erythroid-cell development, resulting in the formation of microcytic erythrocytes. Potential causes of microcytic anemia include chronic iron deficiency, anemia of inflammatory disease, portosystemic shunts in dogs and cats, pyridoxine deficiency, copper deficiency, hereditary elliptocytosis in dogs, dyserythropoiesis, and drug or chemical toxicities.

IRON-DEFICIENCY ANEMIA

The MCV is generally normal in acute iron deficiency. If the iron-deficient state persists for weeks to months, the number of microcytic cells produced constitutes a sufficient portion of the erythrocyte population to reduce the MCV below the normal reference ranges. Chronic iron-deficiency anemia is defined as iron deficiency that results in microcytic anemia.

Causes

With the exception of young growing animals, iron deficiency in domestic animals usually results from blood loss. Chronic iron-deficiency anemia is common in adult dogs and ruminants in areas where bloodsucking parasite infestations are severe.[2,3] It appears to be rare in adult cats[4,5] and horses.[6] Chronic hemorrhage resulting in iron deficiency may also occur with intestinal neoplasms, transitional cell carcinomas, gastrointestinal ulcers, thrombocytopenia, inherited hemostatic disorders, hemorrhagic colitis, and menorrhea (primates only). Excessive removal of blood from a blood donor animal can result in an iron-deficient state.

Milk contains little iron; consequently, nursing animals can easily deplete body iron stores as they grow.[7] The potential for development of severe iron deficiency in young animals appears to be less in species that begin to eat solid food at an early age. Piglets reared in modern facilities without access to soil are especially susceptible to the development of dietary iron-deficiency anemia. The concomitant occurrence of bloodsucking parasite infestations can result in especially severe iron-deficiency anemia in nursing animals. Once the consumption of solid food begins, dietary iron deficiency usually resolves. Iron-deficiency anemia is an unavoidable consequence of feeding practices designed to produce pale meat in veal calves.

Clinical Signs and Physical Findings

Clinical signs and physical findings vary depending on the cause of the iron-deficiency anemia and the presence of other concomitant disorders. Clinical signs and physical findings that may be present include pale mucous membranes, lethargy, weakness, weight loss, diarrhea, dermatitis, hematuria, hematochezia, and melena. Asymptomatic dogs are commonly recognized serendipitously when complete blood blood cell counts (CBCs) are done as a routine screen prior to surgery and when microcytic anemia is found.

Laboratory Findings

Because erythrocyte indices are generally normal during early iron deficiency, most cases of iron deficiency go undiagnosed at this stage. As defined previously, chronic iron deficiency is characterized by the presence of microcytic anemia. Microcytic erythrocytes are produced in response to iron deficiency in nursing kittens and pups, but low MCV values may not develop postnatally because the MCV is greater than adult values at birth in these species, and some fetal macrocytes may persist during the iron-deficient nursing period. The review of erythrocyte volume histograms can reveal the presence of microcytes in iron-deficient pups and kittens that have normal MCV values.[8]

The mean cell hemoglobin concentration (MCHC) within iron-deficient erythrocytes may be low because iron is needed for normal hemoglobin synthesis. A decrease in MCV precedes a decrease in MCHC in iron-deficient animals. A low MCHC is often present in severely affected dogs and ruminants, but it is rarely present in iron-deficient horses or adult cats. The red cell distribution width (RDW) is often increased because of the presence of increased numbers of microcytes together with normocytic cells.

Erythrocytes from dogs and ruminants with iron-deficiency anemia often appear hypochromic on stained blood smears (Fig. 34.1). In species in which erythrocytes appear as discocytes, hypochromic erythrocytes have a narrow rim of lightly stained hemoglobin and a greater than normal area of central pallor. This hypochromasia results from both decreased hemoglobin concentration within cells and from the cells being thin (leptocytes). Because these microcytic leptocytes have increased diameter-to-volume ratios, they may not appear as small cells when viewed in stained blood films. Erythrocytes from members of the family Camelidae are elliptical and not biconcave. Microcytic erythrocytes from iron-

deficient llamas exhibit irregular or eccentric areas of hypochromasia within the cells.[9]

Poikilocytosis (keratocytes and schistocytes) is often present, being most pronounced in association with severe microcytosis. Poikilocytosis is common in young calves. In some cases it may result from iron deficiency, but abnormalities in protein 4.2 in the membrane and hemoglobin composition have also been suggested as causative factors.[10] Folded cells and dacrocytes are common erythrocyte shape abnormalities in iron-deficient llamas.[9]

Not only is there apparently a low incidence of this disorder in horses and adult cats, but some cases may not be recognized because hypochromasia is usually not apparent when stained blood films from iron-deficient horses and adult cats are examined. Additionally, some electronic cell counters may not count the microcytic cells present, resulting in a spuriously increased MCV. Electronic cell counters with erythrocyte histogram displays provide visual evidence that a threshold failure has occurred.[8]

Increased production and release of reticulocytes from bone marrow typically occur in response to hemorrhage in species other than the horse. Consequently, absolute reticulocytosis is often present in the early stage of iron deficiency secondary to hemorrhage (at least in the dog).[2] As iron depletion becomes more severe, there is insufficient iron for reticulocyte production, and the absolute reticulocyte count is no longer increased. Thrombocytosis is present in some cases. Plasma protein concentrations are only decreased if substantial recent or ongoing hemorrhage is present.

Serum iron concentrations are usually low in chronic iron-deficiency anemia in all species, but it can be low in other disorders as well.[7] Total iron binding capacity (TIBC) is usually normal in dogs and cats and increased in pigs, horses, and ruminants.[2,8,11] Serum ferritin concentration correlates directly with body iron stores in animals and, consequently, it is low in iron deficiency.[7] Unfortunately, this assay is not commercially available. An additional problem with ferritin is that it is an acute-phase reactant protein and serum ferritin can increase secondarily to inflammation or liver disease, resulting in an overestimate of total body iron content that might mask the presence of concomitant iron deficiency. One can confirm suspected iron deficiency by finding minimal or absent stainable iron in the bone marrow of most species. However, stainable iron is not present in the bone marrow of normal cats; consequently, a lack of stainable iron does not indicate iron deficiency in this species.

Therapy

In adult animals, the source of blood loss is eliminated, if possible, and supplemental iron is given. Iron may be given orally, as simple iron salts, parenterally, as an iron-carbohydrate complex, or as a blood transfusion if the anemia is severe.

Oral iron therapy is generally preferred in small ani-

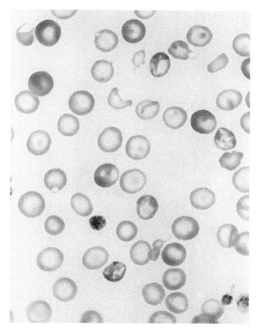

FIGURE 34.1 Hypochromasia and poikilocytosis in blood from a dog that has chronic iron deficiency. Wright–Giemsa stain.

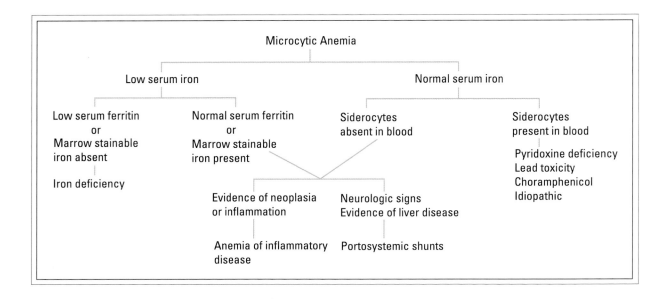

mals, because it can be given economically and safely. Ferrous salts are absorbed better than ferric salts. A total daily dosage of 15 mg ferrous sulfate (5 mg elemental iron) per kilogram of body weight divided three times a day is recommended.[2]

Several months may be required for erythrocyte parameters to return to normal, and oral iron therapy should be continued beyond the time that the hematocrit and MCV reach reference ranges to assure that iron stores are replenished. Dietary iron absorption is generally increased in iron deficiency, but it may be impaired in animals that have especially severe deficiency. In those cases, an intramuscular injection of iron dextran (10 to 20 mg/kg) should be given followed by oral iron therapy. Oral iron therapy should not be given to neonatal animals during the first week of life because of the potential danger of liver injury secondary to excess iron accumulation.[7]

Injectable iron may be given if oral iron therapy is ineffective (e.g., malabsorption), side effects occur (e.g., diarrhea), the patient is uncooperative, or the owner is unwilling to administer oral preparations. Muscle injections of iron dextran are painful, causing local irritation, and intravenous injections may cause thrombophlebitis. Both methods of administration may infrequently cause anaphylactic reactions. An intramuscular iron dextran dosage of 10 mg elemental iron per kilogram of body weight per day in divided doses has been recommended for dogs.[2] Iron deficiency in neonatal pigs is prevented by the injection of 200 mg of iron as iron dextran within the first 3 days of life and again at 10 to 14 days of age.[7]

PORTOSYSTEMIC SHUNTS

Microcytosis occurs in dogs and cats that have vascular connections between the portal and the systemic circulation. These shunts are called portosystemic shunts (PSS).

Causes

Congenital PSS are typically single vessels that fail to regress in utero. They preferentially divert portal blood around the liver. Acquired PSS are generally multiple shunts that develop secondary to portal hypertension associated with chronic primary hepatobiliary disease.[12] The cause of the microcytosis is not completely understood, but it is associated with abnormal iron metabolism, at least in dogs.

Clinical Signs and Physical Findings

Common clinical signs include encephalopathy and intermittent vomiting and diarrhea. Affected animals are generally thin and have poor hair coats. Young dogs (younger than 1 year of age) that have congenital PSS are small for their breed and age. A liver margin cannot usually be palpated because of microhepatia.[12]

Laboratory Findings

Microcytosis occurs in approximately two thirds of the dogs that have PSS. The MCV is seldom more than 7 fL less than the reference range, and the hematocrit is within or slightly less than the reference range. The MCHC is slightly decreased and the RDW is slightly increased in a majority of cases. Codocytes are commonly observed in dogs. The MCV is slightly decreased in approximately one third of the cats that have PSS. Poikilocytosis (keratocytes and elliptocytes) is common, but anemia usually is not present.[12,13]

Common clinical chemistry abnormalities in dogs include decreased serum urea, creatinine, glucose, total protein, albumin; and cholesterol and increased serum alkaline phosphatase, bile acids, and fasting plasma ammonia.[12] Serum alanine aminotransferase (ALT) and bilirubin may be slightly to moderately increased, especially in older dogs that have acquired PSS secondary to hepatobiliary disease. The urinalysis is variable, but low specific gravity and ammonium biurate crystals may be present in some cases. Similar clinical chemistry abnormalities also occur in cats that have PSS, but hypocholesterolemia and hyperbilirubinemia were not reported to occur.[13]

Approximately half of the dogs that have PSS exhibit hypoferremia with normal or slightly decreased serum TIBC. Serum ferritin and stainable iron (hemosiderin) in the liver and bone marrow are normal or high.[14–17] Although animals are not truly iron deficient, the low serum iron appears to be related to the development of microcytosis.[17]

Therapy

Congenital vascular shunts are treated by surgical ligation placement of a slow occlusion device. Hematologic values return to normal after successful treatment.

ANEMIA OF INFLAMMATORY DISEASE

A mild to moderate nonregenerative anemia often accompanies chronic inflammatory and neoplastic disorders. The anemia is generally normocytic, but may be microcytic in long-standing cases.

Origin

The cause of the anemia is multifactorial and only partially understood. Abnormalities that can contribute to the anemia include the production of inflammatory mediators that directly or indirectly inhibit erythropoiesis, decrease serum iron, shortened red blood cell (RBC) life spans, and blunted erythropoietin response to the anemia.[18]

Clinical Signs and Physical Findings

Clinical signs and physical findings vary depending on the inflammatory disorder and/or neoplasia present. Weight loss and fever are often present.

Laboratory Findings

The hematocrit is generally only slightly decreased, but it is more likely to be moderately decreased in cats. The MCV is usually in the low end of the reference range, but may occasionally be slightly less than the reference range. The MCHC and RDW are normal. The erythrocyte morphology is usually normal, except for increased rouleaux formation at times in dogs. Reticulocyte counts in blood are either low or zero. Serum iron and TIBC are normal or decreased, and serum ferritin and bone marrow stainable iron are normal or increased.[7]

Therapy

Hematologic values return to normal if the chronic disorder can be effectively treated. Examples include antibiotic therapy for infectious diseases and surgery to remove tumors.

OTHER POTENTIAL CAUSES OF MICROCYTIC ANEMIA

Pyridoxine Deficiency

Pyridoxine, vitamin B_6, is required for the first step in heme synthesis. Although natural cases of pyridoxine deficiency have not been documented in domestic animals, microcytic anemias with high serum iron values have been produced experimentally in dogs, cats, and pigs that have dietary pyridoxine deficiency.[19] Erythrocytes with iron-positive inclusions (siderocytes) may be present in blood.

TABLE 34.1 Laboratory Findings in Chronic Iron-Deficiency Anemia, Anemia of Inflammatory Disease, and Portosystemic Shunts in Dogs

Parameter	Chronic Iron Deficiency Anemia	Anemia of Inflammatory Disease	Portosystemic Shunt
Hematocrit	Sl to mk decr	Sl to mod decr	N to sl decr
MCV	Sl to mk decr	N to sl decr	N to sl decr
MCHC	N to mk decr	N	N to sl decr
RDW	Sl to mod incr	N	N to sl incr
Reticulocytes	low to incr	low	low
Serum iron	Sl to mk decrease	N to mod decr	N to mod decr
Serum TIBC	N to mod incr	N to sl decr	N to sl decr
Serum ferritin	Decr	N to incr	N
Marrow hemosiderin	Decr or absent	N to mk incr	N to sl incr

MCV = mean cell volume, MCHC = mean cell hemoglobin concentration, RDW = red cell distribution width, Reticulocytes = blood reticulocyte count, TIBC = total iron binding capacity, sl = slight, mod = moderate, mk = marked, decr = decreased, incr = increased, and N = normal.

Copper Deficiency

Prolonged copper deficiency generally results in anemia in mammals, although it was not a feature of experimental copper deficiency in the cat.[19] Erythrocyte indices are variable, with microcytic anemia being reported in some species. When present, the microcytosis may result from a functional iron deficiency because of inadequate mobilization of iron stores caused by a decreased concentration of circulating ceruloplasmin. Ceruloplasmin is the major copper-containing protein in plasma, and its ferroxidase activity appears to be important in the oxidation of ferrous iron (released from ferritin stores) to the ferric state for binding to transferrin.[19]

Toxicities

Drugs or chemicals that block heme synthesis have the potential for causing the formation of microcytic erythrocytes that may contain iron-positive inclusions.[20,21] Examples reported in animals include chloramphenicol and lead.

Dyserythropoiesis

A nonregenerative microcytic anemia with many circulating nucleated erythrocytes has been reported in three related English springer spaniels that have dyserythropoiesis, polymyopathy, and heart disease.[22] An acquired dyserythropoiesis with siderocytes and microcytosis without anemia has been reported in a dog, but the origin could not be determined.[23]

Hereditary Elliptocytosis

Persistent elliptocytosis and microcytosis have been described in a crossbred dog that lacked erythrocyte membrane band 4.1.[24] Although the animal was not anemic, the reticulocyte count was approximately twice normal in compensation for a shortened erythrocyte life span.

Thalassemia

Hereditary deficiencies in synthesis of the globin α chain (α-thalassemia) and β chain (β-thalassemia) cause microcytic hypochromic anemia in humans who have variable degrees of poikilocytosis. Both α- and β-thalassemia occur in mice, but these hereditary hemoglobinopathies have not been reported in domestic animals.[19]

DIFFERENTIAL DIAGNOSIS

Chronic iron-deficiency anemia accounts for most cases of microcytic anemia in animals. If the microcytosis is moderate to severe (e.g., MCV less than 52 fL in dogs), the anemia is nearly always the result of iron deficiency. The MCV may be slightly decreased in association with the anemia of inflammatory disease, but the MCV is at the low end of the reference range in most cases. The MCV is slightly decreased in most dogs and some cats that have portosystemic shunts and the hematocrit is within the reference range or only a slight anemia is present. Laboratory findings for the three major causes of microcytosis in dogs are compared in Table 34.1.

REFERENCES

1. **Gookin JL, Bunch SE, Rush LJ, et al.** Evaluation of microcytosis in 18 Shibas. J Am Vet Med Assoc 1998;212:1258–1259.
2. **Harvey JW, French TW, Meyer DJ.** Chronic iron deficiency anemia in dogs. J Am Anim Hosp Assoc 1982;18:946–960.
3. **Weiser G, O'Grady M.** Erythrocyte volume distribution analysis and hematologic changes in dogs with iron deficiency anemia. Vet Pathol 1983;20:230–241.
4. **French TW, Fox LE, Randolph JF, et al.** A bleeding disorder (von Willebrand's disease) in a Himalayan cat. J Am Vet Med Assoc 1987;190:437–439.
5. **Fulton R, Weiser MG, Freshman JL, et al.** Electronic and morphologic characterization of erythrocytes of an adult cat with iron deficiency anemia. Vet Pathol 1988;25:521–523.
6. **Smith JE, Cipriano JE, DeBowes R, et al.** Iron deficiency and pseudo-iron deficiency in hospitalized horses. J Am Vet Med Assoc 1986;188:285–287.
7. **Smith JE.** Iron metabolism and its disorders. In: Kaneko JJ, Harvey JW, Bruss ML, eds. Clinical biochemistry of domestic animals. 5th ed. San Diego: Academic Press, 1997;223–238.
8. **Weiser MG, Kociba GJ.** Sequential changes in erythrocyte volume distribution and microcytosis associated with iron deficiency in kittens. Vet Pathol 1983;20:1–12.
9. **Morin DE, Garry FB, Weiser MG.** Hematologic responses in llamas with experimentally-induced iron deficiency anemia. Vet Clin Pathol 1993;22:81–85.
10. **Okabe J, Tajima S, Yamato O, et al.** Hemoglobin types, erythrocyte membrane skeleton and plasma iron concentration in calves with poikilocytosis. J Vet Med Sci 1996;58:629–634.
11. **Harvey JW, Asquith RL, Sussman WA, et al.** Serum ferritin, serum iron, and erythrocyte values in foals. Am J Vet Res 1987;48:1348–1352.
12. **Center SA, Magne ML.** Historical, physical examination, and clinicopathologic features of portosystemic vascular anomalies in the dog and cat. Semin Vet Med Surg Small Anim 1990;5:83–93.
13. **Levy JK, Bunch SE, Komtebedde J.** Feline portosystemic vascular shunts. In: Bondagura JD, ed. Kirk's current veterinary therapy. XII. Small animal practice. Philadelphia: WB Saunders, 1995;743–749.
14. **Meyer DJ, Harvey JW.** Hematologic changes associated with serum and hepatic iron alterations in dogs with congenital portosystemic vascular abnormalities. J Vet Intern Med 1994;8:55–56.
15. **Laflamme DP, Mahaffey EA, Allen SW, et al.** Microcytosis and iron status in dogs with surgically induced portosystemic shunts. J Vet Intern Med 1994;8:212–216.
16. **Bunch SE, Jordan HL, Sellon RK, et al.** Characterization of iron status in young dogs with portosystemic shunt. Am J Vet Res 1995;56:853–858.
17. **Simpson KW, Meyer DJ, Boswood A, et al.** Iron status and erythrocyte volume in dogs with congenital portosystemic vascular anomalies. J Vet Intern Med 1997;11:14–19.
18. **Means RT Jr, Krantz SB.** Progress in understanding the pathogenesis of the anemia of chronic disease. Blood 1992;80:1639–1647.
19. **Harvey JW.** The erythrocyte: physiology, metabolism and biochemical disorders. In: Kaneko JJ, Harvey JW, Bruss ML, eds. Clinical biochemistry of domestic animals. 5th ed. San Diego: Academic Press, 1997;157–203.
20. **Fairbanks VF, Beutler E.** Iron deficiency. In: Beutler E, Lichtman MA, Coller BS, Kipps TJ, eds. Williams hematology. 5th ed. New York: McGraw-Hill, 1995;490–511.
21. **Beutler E.** Hereditary and acquired sideroblastic anemias. In: Beutler E, Lichtman MA, Coller BS, Kipps TJ, eds. Williams hematology. 5th ed. New York: McGraw-Hill, 1995;747–750.
22. **Holland CT, Canfield PJ, Watson ADJ, et al.** Dyserythropoiesis, polymyopathy, and cardiac disease in three related English springer spaniels. J Vet Intern Med 1991;5:151–159.
23. **Canfield PJ, Watson ADJ, Ratcliffe RCC.** Dyserythropoiesis, sideroblasts/siderocytes and hemoglobin crystallization in a dog. Vet Clin Pathol 1987;16(1):21–28.
24. **Smith JE, Moore K, Arens M, et al.** Hereditary elliptocytosis with protein band 4.1 deficiency in the dog. Blood 1983;61:373–377.

CHAPTER 35

Anemia of Inflammatory Disease

• TREVOR WANER and SHIMON HARRUS

DEFINITION

Anemia of inflammatory disease (AID) is a mild to moderate, nonregenerative, normocytic normochromic anemia, associated with inflammatory processes, chronic infections, traumatic conditions such as tissue injury and fracture, and disseminated or necrotizing neoplastic disease.[1-3] AID is a more precise name given to the previously recognized anemia of chronic disorders. The latter can be misleading as changes in hematocrit and hemoglobin concentrations can occur within 3 to 10 days.[2,4] It is the most common anemia found in small animals and probably the most common anemia encountered in veterinary medicine.[5,6] The hypoferremia resulting from AID may be considered a nonspecific antibacterial immune mechanism.[3] Iron is vital for the growth of microorganisms, and infection is discouraged by withholding of iron. This sequestration of iron is the basis of the pathogenesis of AID.

PATHOGENESIS

The pathogenesis of AID is multifactorial, mediated by cytokines secreted during inflammation.[7] AID results from decreased iron availability, a decline in erythrocyte survival, and decreased response to anemia.

Decreased Iron Availability

Decreased iron availability in AID results mostly from decreased iron reutilization. This occurs because of increased delivery of iron to macrophages and increased ferritin synthesis.[7] Apolactoferrin (iron-free lactoferrin) is an iron transport protein found in milk, certain mucosal secretions and in polymorphonuclear leukocytes.[8,9] Apolactoferrin has the capacity to bind large amounts of iron, especially at low pH as occurs in inflammatory conditions. As part of the acute-phase reaction, apolactoferrin synthesis and release is increased. Apolactoferrin synthesis and release is induced primarily by interleukin-1 (IL-1) and tumor necrosis factor α (TNFα). Activated macrophages express increased numbers of lactoferrin receptors on their surfaces, thereby permitting them to internalize lactoferrin-bound iron.[10] Within macrophages, lactoferrin-bound iron is transferred to the iron storage molecule ferritin.[11] The release of apolactoferrin by neutrophils at sites of infection leads to in situ combination with iron, thereby further reducing the availability of iron for bacterial growth. Besides its role in withholding iron, lactoferrin has been demonstrated to have an intrinsic bactericidal activity.[12] A further mechanism for decreasing iron availability is through augmented production of apoferritin by macrophages in response to inflammatory and neoplastic conditions. Consequently, a larger than normal proportion of iron enters the macrophage, effectively diverting the iron reuse from rapid-release to slow-release pathways.[13]

Intestinal epithelial cells and hepatocytes are also affected by inflammatory conditions and contribute, albeit in a minor way, to the pathogenesis of AID.[14] In AID, iron absorption from the intestinal tract is reduced owing to decreased synthesis of transferrin during the acute-phase reaction.[15-17]

Decreased Erythrocyte Survival

Erythrocyte survival is significantly, although modestly, reduced in AID. Experimental studies in cats with sterile abscesses have indicated that erythrocyte destruction seems to be a major factor in the early stage of anemia of inflammation.[4] The pathogenesis of this effect has not been definitely determined. Macrophages activated by the inflammatory process have been suggested to perform a more efficient clearing of senescent red blood cells (RBCs) and those coated with immunoglobulins. Other studies have questioned whether macrophage activation alone is sufficient to accelerate erythrocyte destruction.[19] In studies carried out in cats with experimentally induced sterile abscesses, an increased number of erythrocytes with detectable surface immunoglobulins were found. This was also associated with a significant increase in erythrophagy.[20] The results suggested that RBC surface alterations occur because of the inflammatory process and that gamma G immunoglobulin (IgG)-mediated presenescent destruction of

RBC may also be associated with the pathogenesis of anemia seen in AID. Fever *per se* has also been reported to decrease RBC survival[21]; however, not all AID patients are febrile.

Decreased Erythropoiesis

Normal bone marrow is capable of a sixfold to eightfold increase in RBC production rate and should easily compensate for a modest reduction in RBC survival. The fact that the marrow is unable to do so in AID, suggests that its impaired production capacity is of fundamental importance in the pathogenesis of AID. The defects in erythropoiesis fall into three categories: inappropriately low erythropoietin secretion, diminished marrow response to erythropoietin, and iron-limited erythropoiesis. Erythropoietin release in response to anemia is blunted in patients who have AID.[22] When stimulated by cobalt or hypoxia, erythropoiesis increases in patients who have AID, indicating that the erythropoietin secreting mechanisms retain their ability to respond to such stimuli.[23,24] However, in AID, a greater degree of hypoxia is necessary for a given level of erythropoietin secretion.

The normal inverse relation between the degree of anemia and the erythropoietin level is lost in AID.[25-27] Administration of IL-1α to mice suppressed erythropoiesis, which could be prevented by the simultaneous administration of erythropoietin.[28] IL-1α, IL-1β and TNF all inhibited hypoxia-induced erythropoietin secretion in vitro,[22] demonstrating the important role of cytokines in the pathogenesis of AID. Erythropoietin levels in cats that have experimentally induced AID were found to be slightly increased, but somewhat low for the degree of anemia that existed, suggesting that decreased erythropoietin production contributed to the decreased erythropoiesis.[4]

Treatment of AID patients with erythropoietin results in an increase in the hematocrit; however the magnitude of the shift is subnormal, suggesting decreased responsiveness of the erythroid precursors to erythropoietin.[3] This relative unresponsiveness of the bone marrow may be caused by macrophage-derived factors.[29,30] TNF has been shown to suppress erythropoiesis in laboratory animals[31] and to inhibit proliferation of primitive erythroid precursors.[32] Furthermore, a heat-stable serum factor that could not be neutralized by antibody to either γ-interferon or TNFα has been identified in human patients who have AID. This factor has been shown to render normal T cells suppressive to autologous colony-forming unit-erythroid (CFU-E).[33]

Investigations have been carried out to assess whether the decreased iron supply to the bone marrow is an adequate rationale for the erythropoietic defect seen in AID. In general, erythroid iron turnover is correlated with serum iron concentrations. Therefore, availability of iron may explain the decreased erythropoiesis in a substantial proportion of patients.[34] Similar conclusions were also made from studies in dogs.[2]

CLINICAL DESCRIPTION

AID is of little clinical significance because it is rarely severe enough to cause intrinsic clinical signs.[2] The clinical signs in patients who have AID are usually those of the underlying disease,[7] although the overall well-being of the patient is believed to be influenced by the systemic consequences of the anemia.[2]

Generally, AID in humans develops slowly over the first 1 to 2 months of illness and remains constant in degree thereafter. There is no correlation between the severity of the anemia and the duration of illness. In patients who have cancer, anemia is more severe when widespread metastases are present.[1,35]

The clinical disorder of AID has been produced experimentally in dogs, cats, rats, mice, and rabbits.[4] Cats injected with turpentine subcutaneously developed anemia within 5 to 10 days of injection.[36] In another similar study, cats developed anemia within 2 to 3 days, with an average decreased packed cell volume (PCV) of 8%.[4] Feldman et al[2] reported that a sterile abscess, produced by injection of Freund's complete adjuvant subcutaneously in dogs, was accompanied by a modest anemia.[2] RBC values began decreasing by day 5, decreased until day 11 through 13, and remained significantly decreased until day 20 postinjection.

Numerous disease states can result in AID. The major human diseases considered during evaluation of anemia that might be secondary to occult or overt inflammation are osteomyelitis, pneumonia, deep abscesses, subacute bacterial endocarditis, human immunodificiency virus infection, fungal and mycobacterial infections, systemic lupus erythematosus, rheumatoid arthritis, congestive heart failure, inflammatory bowel disease, lymphoma, sarcoma, metastatic carcinoma, and multiple myeloma.[35] The nature of the anemia associated with canine lymphoma has been investigated. It was found that anemic dogs that have lymphoma had normal values for serum iron concentrations, total iron binding capacity (TIBC), and erythropoietin levels, findings contrary to those associated with AID.[37] Renal disease is not usually considered a cause of anemia of inflammation because of its well-known association with erythropoietin deficiency.[35]

CLINICAL PATHOLOGY FINDINGS IN ANEMIA OF INFLAMMATORY DISEASE

Clinical laboratory testing is an integral element in the diagnosis of AID, and several diagnostic criteria are necessary to make a diagnosis of the condition. The more important clinical laboratory characteristics of AID are listed below.

- Mild to moderate anemia
- Normocytic normochromic erythrocyte indices
- Hypoferremia
- Decreased to normal TIBC
- Increased to normal serum ferritin

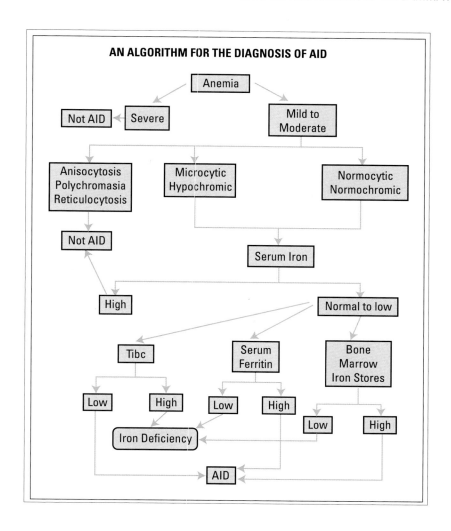

AN ALGORITHM FOR THE DIAGNOSIS OF AID

- Increased to normal bone marrow and hepatic iron stores
- Increased serum copper levels
- Increased serum zinc levels

Degree of Anemia

Mild to moderate decreases in PCV and total erythrocyte counts are typical. PCV and erythrocyte counts are usually within the lower reference range or slighlty less than it.[2] The PCV seldom drops lower than 20% in dogs and 15% in cats that have AID.[6]

Erythrocyte Indices

Anemia is consistently nonregenerative, normocytic normochromic; however mild reticulocytosis may occur. Microcytosis and hypochromia may be found occasionally, reflecting a more severe defect in iron supply.[6] It may occur in chronic AID as well as in some forms of cancer.[2]

Iron Parameters

Iron studies are the key to the diagnosis of AID. A reduction in serum iron concentration and TIBC along with increased serum ferritin concentrations are necessary for the diagnosis of AID. The level of serum ferritin correlates with tissue iron stores in humans, horses, calves, dogs, and cats and is the most reliable indicator of total-body iron stores.[38,39] Ferritin is immunologically species specific, necessitating a specific immunoassay for each species.[6]

Assessment of Bone Marrow Aspirates

The cellular pattern of the bone marrow should be nearly normal. Increases in bone marrow reticuloendothelial iron deposits are found in AID. Because of the reduced incorporation of iron into protoporphyrin, free erythrocytic protoporphyrin levels are increased.[40]

Serum Copper and Zinc Concentrations

Serum copper and zinc concentrations are modestly increased perhaps because of the increased activity of the

TABLE 35.1   Differentiation Between AID and Iron-Deficiency Anemia

Parameter	Iron Deficiency	AID
Erythrocyte indices	Microcytic hypochromic	Normocytic normochromic
Serum iron	Decreased	Decreased to normal
TIBC	High	Low to normal
Marrow iron stores	Low	Normal to increased
Ferritin	Low	Normal to increased
Platelet counts	Normal to increased	Normal

copper-zinc metalloenzyme superoxide dismutase.[41,42] There is a direct correlation between increasing superoxide dismutase activity and increasing levels of storage iron.[40]

DIAGNOSIS

A thorough clinical history and physical examination are important for diagnosis of AID, along with specific clinical laboratory tests. Elucidating the underlying pathologic condition is an essential requirement for the diagnosis and subsequent treatment of the condition. Anemia can be detected on a routine complete blood count. Erythropoietic and iron profile, as well as other biochemical findings, help in distinguishing this type of anemia from iron-deficiency anemia (Table 35.1), renal disease, drug-induced bone marrow suppression, and bone marrow myelophthisis. Differentiation of AID from iron-deficiency anemia may be difficult but should be based on the erythrocyte indices, TIBC, and values of iron stores (Table 35.1 and algorithm).

Bone marrow iron stores provide an accurate evaluation of body iron stores but has the disadvantage of being invasive. Measurement of serum ferritin concentration has the advantage of being accurate and noninvasive but is not widely available.[5]

TREATMENT

AID is not intrinsically harmful, and although it is one of the most common anemias, it is rarely severe enough to require treatment.[2] However, the primary disorder should be ascertained, and treatment efforts should focus on alleviation of the underlying disease when possible, before any specific treatment for the anemia is initiated. In human patients resolution of the anemia occurs within 3 months from alleviation of the primary disorder.[35] AID is rarely severe enough to justify blood transfusion. Iron therapy, either oral or parenteral, is of no value unless a complicating iron deficiency is present.[1,43]

Treatment of AID patients with erythropoietin results in increased hematocrit, but the response may be subnormal.[3]

REFERENCES

1. **Means RT Jr, Krantz SB**. Progress in understanding the pathogenesis of the anemia of chronic disease. Blood 1992;80:1639–1647.
2. **Feldman BF, Kaneko JJ, Farver TB**. Anemia of inflammatory disease in the dog: clinical characterization. Am J Vet Res 1981;42:1109–1113.
3. **Jurado RL**. Iron, infections and anemia of inflammation. Clin Infect Dis 1997;25:888–895.
4. **Weiss DJ, Krehbiel JD**. Studies of the pathogenesis of the anemia of inflammation: Erythrocyte survival. Am J Vet Res 1983;44:1830–1831.
5. **Stone MS, Freden GO**. Differentiation of anemia of inflammatory disease from anemia of iron deficiency. Compend Contin Educ Pract Vet 1990;12:963–966.
6. **Mahaffey EA**. Disorders of iron metabolism. In: Current Veterinary Therapy. IX. Philadelphia, WB Saunders Co, 1986;521–524.
7. **Lee GR**. The anemia of chronic disease. Semin Hematol 1983;20:61–79.
8. **Baggiolini M, deDuve C, Masson PL, Heremans JF**. Association of lactoferrin with specific granules in rabbit hetrophil leukocytes. J Exp Med 1970;131:559–570.
9. **Bennett RM, Kokocinski T**. Lactoferrin content of peripheral blood cells. Br J Haematol 1978;39:509–521.
10. **Smith RJ, Speziale SC, Bowman BJ**. Properties of interleukin-1 as a complete secretagogue for human neutrophils. Biochem Biophy Rev Commun. 1985;130:1233–1240.
11. **Richter J, Anderson T, Olson I**. Effect of tumor necrosis factor and granulocyte/macrophage colony-stimulating factor on neutrophil degranulation. J Immunol 1989;142:3199–3205.
12. **Ambroso DR, Johnston RB**. Lactoferrin enhances hydroxyl radical production by human neutrophils, neutrophil particulate fractions and an enzymatic generating system. J Clin Invest 1981;67:352–360.
13. **Konijn AM, Hershko C**. Ferritin synthesis in inflammation. I. Pathogenesis of impaired iron release. Br J Haematol 1977;37:7–16.
14. **Hershko C, Cook JD, Finch CA**. Storage of iron kinetics. VI. The effect of inflammation on iron exchange in the rat. Br J Haematol 1974;28:67–75.
15. **Haurani FI, Green D, Young K**. Iron absorption in hypoferremia. Am J Med 1965;249:537–547.
16. **Cartwright GE**. The anemia of chronic disorders. Semin Hematol 1966;3:351–357.
17. **Bresford CH, Neale RJ, Brooks OG**. Iron absorption and pyrexia. Lancet 1971;1:568–575.
18. **Leb L, Synder LM, Fortier NL, Andersen M**. Antiglobin serum mediated phagocytosis of normal, senescent and oxidized RBC: role of anti-IgM immunoglobulins in phagocytic recognition. Br J Haematol 1987;66:565–570.
19. **Singer JA, Jennings LK, Jackson CW, Dockter ME, Morrison M, Walker WS**. Erythrocyte homeostasis: antibody mediated recognition of the senescent state by macrophages. Proc Natl Acad Sci 1986;83:5498–5501.
20. **Weiss DJ, McClay CB**. Studies on the pathogenesis of the erythrocyte destruction associated with the anemia of inflammatory disease. Vet Clin Path 1988;17:90–93.
21. **Karle H**. The pathogenesis of anaemia of chronic disorders and the role of fever in erythrokinetics. Scand J Haematol 1974;13:81–86.
22. **Faquin WC, Schneinder TJ, Goldberg MA**. Effect of inflammatory cytokines on hypoxia-induced erythropoietin production. Blood 1992;79:1987–1994.
23. **Wintrobe MM, Grinstein M, Dubash JJ, et al**. The anemia of infection. VI. The influence of cobalt on the anemia associated with inflammation. Blood 1947;2:323–331.
24. **Gutnisky A, Van Dyke K**. Normal response to erythropoietin or hypoxia in rats made anemic with turpentine abscess. Proc Soc Exp Biol Med 1963;112:75–78.
25. **Ward HP, Kurnick JE, Pisarczyk MJ**. Serum levels of erythropoietin in anemias associated with chronic infection, malignancy and primary hematologic disease. J Clin Invest 1971;50:332–349.
26. **Mahmood T, Robinson WA, Vautrin R**. Granulopoietic and erythropoietic activity in patients with anemias of iron deficiency and chronic disease. Blood 1977;50:449–455.
27. **Miller CB, Jones RJ, Piantadosi S, Abeloff MD, Spivak JL**. Decreased erythropoietin response in patients with anemia of cancer. N Engl J Med 1990;322:1689–1692.
28. **Johnson CS, Chang M-J and Furmanski P**. In vivo hematopoietic effects of tumor necrosis factor-α in normal and erythroleukemic mice: characterization and therapeutic applications. Blood 1988;72:1875–1883.
29. **Roodman GD**. Mechanisms of erythroid suppression in the anemia of chronic disease. Blood Cells 1978;13:171–184.
30. **Means RT Jr, Dessypris EN, Krantz SB**. Inhibition of human erythroid colony- forming units by tumor necrosis factor requires accessory cells. J Clin Invest. 1990;86:538–541.
31. **Johnson RA, Waddelow TA, Caro J, Oliff A, Roodman GD**. Chronic expo-

sure to tumor necrosis factor in vivo preferentially inhibits erythropoiesis in nude mice. Blood 1989;74:130–138.

32. **Reissmann KR, Udupa KB**. Effect of inflammation on erythroid precursors (BFU-R and CFU-E) in bone marrow and spleen of mice. J Lab Clin Med 1978;92:22–29.
33. **Pixy JS, MacKintosh FR, Smith EA, Zanjani ED**. Anemia of inflammation: role of T lymphocyte activating factor. Pathobiology 1992;60:309–315.
34. **Douglas SW, Adamson JW**. The anemia of chronic disorders: studies of marrow regulation and iron metabolism. Blood 1975;45:55–65.
35. **Abshire TC**. The anemia of inflammation. A common cause of childhood anemia. Pediatr Clin North Am 1996;43:623–637.
36. **Mahaffey EA, Smith JE**. Depression anemia in cats. Feline Pract 1978; 8:19–22.
37. **Lucroy MD, Christopher MM, Kraegel SA, Simonson ER, Madewell BR**. Anemia associated with canine lymphoma. Comp Haematol Int 1998;3:1–6.

38. **Andrews GA, Smith JE, Chavey PS, Weeks BR**. An improved ferritin assay for canine sera. Vet Clin Path 1992;21:57–60.
39. **Andrews GA, Chavey PS, Smith JE**. Enzyme-linked immunosorbent assay to measure serum ferritin and the relationship between serum ferritin and nonheme iron stores in cats. Vet Pathol 1994;31:674–678.
40. **Feldman BF, Kaneko JJ**. The anemia of inflammatory disease in the dog. 1. Nature of the problem. Vet Res Comm 1981;4:237–252.
41. **Feldman BF, Kaneko JJ, Farver TB**. Anemia of inflammatory disease in the dog: ferrokinetics of adjuvent-induced anemia. Am J Vet Res 1981;42: 583–585.
42. **Feldman BF, Keen CL, Kaneko JJ, Farver TB**. Anemia of inflammatory disease in the dog: measurement of hepatic superoxide dismutase, hepatic nonheme iron, copper, zinc, and ceruloplasmin and serum iron, copper and zinc. Am J Vet Res 1981;42:1114–1117.
43. **Pincus T, Olsen NJ, Russell IJ, Wolfe F, Harris ER, Schnitzer TJ, Boccagno JA, Krantz SB**. Multicenter study of recombinant human erythropoietin in correction of anemia in rheumatoid arthritis. Am J Med 1990;89:161–168.

CHAPTER 36

Pure Red Cell Aplasia

• DOUGLAS J. WEISS

Pure red blood cell aplasia (PRCA) is a hematologic disorder characterized by severe nonregenerative, normocytic, normochromic, anemia associated with severe depletion of erythroid precursor cells in the bone marrow.[1-4] Granulopoiesis and thrombopoiesis are not affected, therefore, total leukocyte and platelet counts are not decreased in blood, and adequate numbers of precursors are present in bone marrow.

Both canine and feline forms of PRCA can be divided into primary and secondary types. Primary canine PRCA is caused by an immune-mediated disorder in which autoantibodies are produced that destroy erythroid precursor cells in bone marrow.[3,5] Secondary canine PRCA has been associated with canine parvovirus infection and occurs secondary to treatment with recombinant human erythropoietin.[6,7] Primary PRCA in cats is probably an immune-mediated disorder,[8] and secondary PRCA occurs in cats infected with feline leukemia virus.[9,10]

CANINE PRIMARY PURE RED BLOOD CELL APLASIA

Primary PRCA is a variant form of immune-mediated hemolytic anemia. Evidence for an immune-mediated origin includes, identifying antibodies that suppress erythropoiesis in serum of affected dogs, positive direct Coombs test in approximately half of affected dogs, spherocytes or autoagglutination in some dogs, and response to steroidal and nonsteroidal immunosuppressive therapy.[3,11,12] The clinical and hematologic features of PRCA are variable. Some cases closely resemble classical immune-mediated hemolytic anemia, but reticulocytosis is not present at the time of diagnosis.[5,11,13] The clinical history is somewhat acute and autoagglutination, spherocytes, hemoglobinuria, and positive direct Coombs test may or may not be seen. Bone marrow evaluation usually indicates erythroid maturation arrest at the rubricyte or metarubricyte stage, presumably caused by antibody-mediated destruction of late-stage precursor cells. Phagocytosis of rubricytes and metarubricytes by marrow macrophages is frequently seen. Other cases have a chronic onset, and hematocrits are

low (i.e., 6 and 13%).[3] The Coombs test may be positive in some affected dogs, but spherocytes, autoagglutination, and hemoglobinuria are not seen. The bone marrow is characterized either by complete aplasia of the erythroid series or by maturation arrest at the rubriblast or prorubricyte stage.[3]

All types of primary PRCA tend to respond to immunosuppressive therapy. Most dogs have been treated with immunosuppressive doses of prednisone (2.2 to 6.6 mg/kg/day orally). If reticulocyte count does not increase within the first 2 weeks of treatment, a nonsteroidal immunosuppressive drug, such as cyclophosphamide (2.2 mg/kg q48h orally), should be started and prednisone continued.[5,11,12] Some dogs require only short-term immunosuppressive therapy, whereas others require lifelong treatment.

CANINE SECONDARY PURE RED BLOOD CELL APLASIA

Parvovirus infection or vaccination has been incriminated as a possible cause of canine PRCA.[7] Parvovirus readily infects hemic precursor cells of dogs, cats, and humans and causes acute aplastic anemia.[7,14,15] However, hematologic recovery is usually rapid if affected animals survive the acute stage of the disease. Parvovirus infection has been incriminated as a cause of PRCA in humans.[15] Severe RBC or megakaryocytic aplasia has been reported to occur 1 day to 3 weeks after vaccination of dogs given modified live parvovirus vaccine.[7] A causal relation has been hypothesized.[7] In some dogs the aplasia was irreversible and led to death, whereas, in other cases the aplasia was reversible, and the animal recovered. The possibility that the association of parvovirus vaccination and PRCA was coincidental could not be ruled out.

Dogs consistently develop PRCA after 4 to 16 weeks of treatment with recombinant human erythropoietin.[6] All dogs recovered spontaneously 3 to 11 weeks after discontinuation of treatment. The most probable explanation of this is that the recombinant human erythropoietin induced an immune response that neutralized both the recombinant and the endogenous erythropoietin.

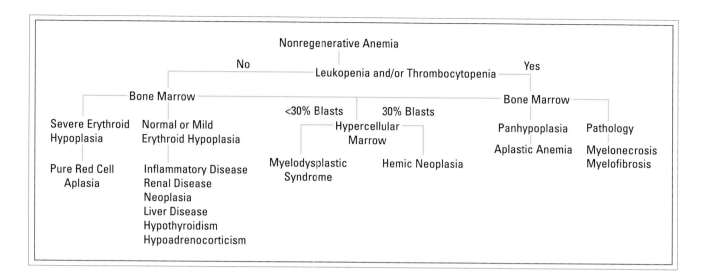

PRCA has also been reported in two horses treated with recombinant human erythropoietin.[16]

FELINE PRIMARY PURE RED BLOOD CELL APLASIA

PRCA has been reported in nine cats.[8] All cats had severe nonregenerative anemia with initial hematocrits ranging between 6 and 11%. Bone marrow aspirates were characterized by complete absence of erythroid precursor cells and an increase in small lymphocytes. All cats tested negative for feline leukemia virus and feline immunodeficiency virus and responded to immunosuppressive treatment within 3 to 4 weeks, indicating a possible immune-mediated basis for the aplasia.

FELINE SECONDARY PURE RED BLOOD CELL APLASIA

PRCA is a fairly common disease of cats infected with feline leukemia virus and has been induced by inoculation of certain strains of the virus.[9,10] PRCA developed within 3 to 5 weeks after inoculation of the Kawakami–Theilen strain of feline leukemia virus into kittens.[10]

REFERENCES

1. **Lund JE, Avolt MD**. Erythrocyte aplasia in a dog. J Am Vet Med Assoc 1972;160:1500–1503.
2. **Watson ADJ, Duff BC, Allan GS**. Erythrocyte aplasia in a dog. Aust Vet J 1975;51:94–96.
3. **Weiss DJ**. Antibody-mediated suppression of erythropoiesis in dogs with red blood cell aplasia. Am J Vet Res 1986;47:2646–2648.
4. **Glauberg A, Beaumont PR**. Acquired erythrocyte aplasia in a dog: a case report. J Am Anim Hosp Assoc 1978;14:635–637.
5. **Stockham SL, Ford RB, Weiss DJ**. Canine autoimmune hemolytic disease with a delayed erythroid regeneration. J Am Anim Hosp Assoc 1980; 16:927–931.
6. **Stokol T, Randolph J, MacLeod JN**. Pure red cell aplasia after recombinant human erythropoietin treatment in normal beagle dogs. Vet Pathol 1997;34:474.
7. **Dodds WJ**. Immune-mediated diseases of the blood. Adv Vet Sci Comp Med 1983;27:163–196.
8. **Stokol T, Blue J**. Pure red cell aplasia in nine cats (1989–1997). Vet Pathol 1997;34:475.
9. **Abkowitz JL, Holly RD, Grant CK**. Retrovirus-induced feline pure red cell aplasia. J Clin Invest 1987;80:1056–1063.
10. **Boyce JT, Hoover EA, Kociba GJ, Olsen RG**. Feline leukemia virus-induced erythroid aplasia: in vitro hemopoietic culture studies. Exp Hematol 1981;9:990–1001.
11. **Jonas LD, Thrall MA, Weiser MG**. Nonregenerative form of immune-mediated hemolytic anemia in dogs. J Am Anim Hosp Assoc 1987;23:210–204.
12. **Weiss DJ, Miller ML, Crawford MA, Johnson CA**. Primary-acquired red cell aplasia in a dog: response to glucocorticoid and cyclophosphamide therapy. J Am Anim Hosp Assoc 1984;20:951–954.
13. **Weiss DJ, Stockham SL, Willard MD, Schirmer RG**. Transient erythroid hypoplasia in the dog: report of five cases. J Am Anim Hosp Assoc 1982; 18:353–359.
14. **Boosinger TR, Rebar AH, DeNicola DB, Boon GD**. Bone marrow alterations associated with canine parvoviral enteritis. Vet Pathol 1982;19:558–561.
15. **Young N, Mortimer P**. Viruses and bone marrow failure. Blood 1984; 63:729–737.
16. **Piercy RJ, Swardson CJ, Hinchcliff KW**. Erythroid hypoplasia and anemia following administration of recombinant human erythropoietin to two horses. J Am Vet Med Assoc 1998;212:244.

CHAPTER 37

Aplastic Anemia

• DOUGLAS J. WEISS

Aplastic anemia (also termed aplastic pancytopenia) is characterized by pancytopenia in blood and panhypoplasia of bone marrow with the marrow space replaced by adipose tissue.[1,2] Excluded from this are pancytopenias associated with myelophthisic disorders, such as leukemia and myelofibrosis, myelodysplastic disorders in which the marrow is usually normocellular or hypercellular, hemophagocytic syndromes, and pure red cell aplasia in which only red blood cell (RBC) production is suppressed.

ETIOPATHOGENESIS

Regardless of the cause, aplastic anemia can be divided into acute and chronic forms.[3] Acute aplastic anemia is frequently associated with destruction of progenitor and proliferative cells in the bone marrow. Destruction of progenitor or proliferative cells results in predictable changes in the blood. Clinical signs related to leukopenia and thrombocytopenia usually develop within 2 weeks of initial marrow injury. Neutropenia develops 5 to 6 days after the marrow insult, followed by thrombocytopenia at 8 to 10 days. Because of the long RBC life span, anemia is usually mild or absent. The bone marrow has variable degrees of panhypoplasia. Multifocal areas of necrosis, degenerating hemic cells, and an increase in phagocytic macrophages may be observed. Within 10 to 14 days after the cessation of marrow injury, stem cells repopulate marrow progenitor cells, and cytopenias in the blood resolve. Dysplastic changes within erythroid, myeloid, or megakaryocytic cell lines may be observed during the recovery phase. Recovery is usually complete by 21 days. Chronic aplastic anemia results from hemopoietic stem cell injury and is characterized by neutropenia, thrombocytopenia, and moderate to severe nonregenerative anemia.[4] Marrow repopulation is uncertain and, when it occurs, may take weeks to months.

Aplastic anemia has many causes. General mechanisms that lead to decreased stem- or progenitor-cell proliferation include (1) destruction of stem or progenitor cells, (2) genetic mutations resulting in decreased proliferative capacity of stem cells, (3) hemopoietic cytokine dysregulation or stromal disorder.[5–8] Destruction of stem or progenitor cells is well established as a cause of aplastic anemia, whereas, genetic mutation and cytokine dysregulation are not. Destruction of stem or progenitor cells is frequently caused by infectious agents, drugs, and toxins (Table 37.1).

Infectious Agents

Infectious causes of aplastic anemia include parvovirus, feline leukemia virus, feline immunodeficiency virus, equine infectious anemia virus, ehrlichiosis, bacterial septicemia, and endotoxemia.[2,9] Parvovirus infection in both cats and dogs causes acute aplastic anemia perhaps as a result of virus proliferation in progenitor and proliferative cells within the marrow.[10] However, marrow injury caused by secondary endotoxemia or septicemia cannot be ruled out. The bone marrow is characterized by severe degenerative changes in hemic cells, necrosis, and increased numbers of phagocytic macrophages.[10] Hematologic recovery is usually rapid if the animal survives the acute stages of the disease. Feline leukemia virus frequently produces selective suppression of erythropoiesis (nonregenerative anemia) and thrombocytopenia, but it may cause aplastic anemia.[11,12] Equine infectious anemia virus typically causes anemia and thrombocytopenia but may cause pancytopenia. In infected foals, bone marrow is hypocellular and has an increase in intercellular homogeneous eosinophilic material.[13] Cytopenias occur in the blood of dogs and cats in both the acute and the chronic forms of ehrlichiosis.[14,15] In the acute form, bone marrow is hypercellular, suggesting that the cytopenias are the result of cell destruction in the peripheral blood. In the chronic form the marrow is hypocellular, consistent with a diagnosis of aplastic anemia.

Drug-Induced Aplasia

Dog bone marrow is highly susceptible to estrogen-induced suppression.[16,17] Estrogens, derived from endogenous as well as exogenous sources, have been incriminated in induction of aplastic anemia. Leukocyto-

| TABLE 37.1 | Reported Causes of Aplastic Anemia in Domestic Animals | | | |

Cause	Species Type of Aplasia	Number of Cases Reported	Outcome
Infectious			
Ehrlichia	D,C acute/chronic	many	reversible/irreversible
Parvovirus	D,C acute	many	reversible
Feline leukemia virus	C chronic	many	irreversible
Feline immunodefeciency virus	C chronic	many	irreversible
Equine infectious anemia virus	H chronic	few	irreversible
Drug-associated			
Estrogen	D acute/chronic	many	reversible/irreversible
Chemotherapy	D,C acute	many	reversible
Phenylbutazone	D,H acute	many	irreversible
Meclofenamic acid	D acute	one	irreversible
Trimethoprim/sulfadiazine	D,C acute	many	reversible
Quinidine	D acute	few	reversible
Thiacetarsamide	D acute	few	reversible
Griseofulvin	C acute	few	reversible
Toxins			
Brackenfern	B,S chronic	many	reversible
Trichloroethylene	B,H acute	many	irreversible
Aflatoxin B_1	P acute	few	?
Radiation	D acute	few	dose dependent
Idiopathic	D,C,H chronic	few	irreversible

D = dog, C = cat, B = bovine, H = horse, S = sheep, P = pig.

sis, thrombocytopenia, and mild but progressive anemia develop in the first 3 weeks after injection of a single large dose (1–3 mg/kg body weight) of natural or synthetic estrogens. During this period the bone marrow has normal cellularity caused by myeloid hyperplasia, but erythropoiesis and thrombocytopoiesis are depressed. Pancytopenia with associated marrow hypoplasia or aplasia develop 3 to 4 weeks after injection. Dogs begin to recover by 30 days after a single injection. In some clinical cases, severe chronic aplasia developed, particularly when multiple doses of estradiol are administered.[3] The potential reversibility of the chronic phase is uncertain. At least four reported cases, given supportive treatment only, recovered several months after initial diagnosis.[3]

Nonsteroidal anti-inflammatory drugs cause aplastic anemia in dogs and perhaps in horses.[3,18,19] Phenylbutazone-associated granulocytopenias and aplastic anemia occur sporadically, often after long-term treatment, and are not dose dependent. Phenylbutazone probably causes stem cell injury, and the prognosis for recovery is poor.

Chemotherapeutic drugs are toxic to rapidly proliferating cells, including the progenitor and proliferative cells within the marrow.[20] Because stem cells do not have a high mitotic rate, they are usually spared. Therefore, hematologic recovery usually occurs after discontinuation of the drug. Irrespective of whether aplastic anemia develops, degenerative changes, including fragmented nuclei, and dysplastic changes are seen in bone marrow

aspiration smears.[21] Drugs with high myelosuppressive potential include cyclophosphamide, cytosine arabinoside, doxorubicin, vinblastine, and hydroxyurea.[20] The associated hypoplasia or aplasia is of the acute type and is characterized by leukopenia and thrombocytopenia. Neutropenia usually develops within 5 to 7 days after initial drug administration and thrombocytopenia develops in 7 to 10 days. Neutrophil counts usually return to normal within 36 to 72 hours after treatment is discontinued.

Sulfadiazine-induced aplastic anemia has been reported in many dogs.[3,22] In Doberman pinschers, marrow dyscrasias are part of a systemic hypersensitivity reaction. Clinical signs included polyarthritis, lymphadenopathy, retinitis, glomerulonephritis, polymyositis, anemia, leukopenia, and thrombocytopenia. Clinical signs resolved after discontinuing treatment. In non-Doberman breeds of dogs and in cats, sulfadiazine induces acute aplastic anemia.[3] The hematologic dyscrasia usually resolves within 2 weeks after discontinuation of treatment.

Other drugs causally associated with aplastic anemia in the dog include cephalosporins, albendazole, captopril, phenothiazine, tranquilizers, quinidine, griseofulvin, and thiacetarsamide. Drugs associated with aplastic anemia in cats include albendazole and griseofulvin.[23] In general, the animals recovered promptly after discontinuation of the drug.[3,9] Chloramphenicol, when given in therapeutic doses, may cause mild bone marrow suppression in both dogs and cats, but the severe aplastic

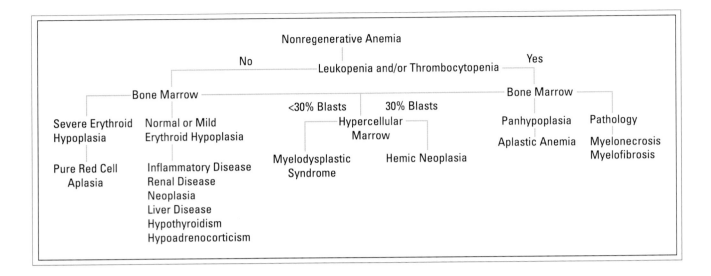

anemia reported in human patients has not been documented.[24]

Aplastic Anemia Associated With Toxins and Radiation

Toxins associated with aplastic anemia include aflatoxin B_1, brackenfern, and trichloroethylene. Aflatoxin B_1 toxicity has been reported in horses, cattle, dogs, and pigs.[25] The major lesion reported for all species is hepatocellular necrosis. Aplastic anemia has only been reported in experimental studies in pigs. Consumption of trichloroethylene-extracted soybean oil meal by cattle produces aplastic anemia.[26] Cattle grazing on brackenfern develop aplastic anemia.[27] Total-body irradiation of sufficient dosage induces aplastic anemia in all species.[28]

Idiopathic Aplastic Anemia

Less than 10 cases of idiopathic aplastic anemia have been reported in dogs, cats, horses, and cattle.[29] This paucity of reported cases suggests that idiopathic aplastic anemia similar to that which occurs in human beings does not occur in domestic animals. Idiopathic aplastic anemia accounts for 40 to 90% of all human cases of aplastic anemia. Cell-mediated cytotoxicity, marrow stromal defects, overproduction of inhibitory hemopoietic cytokines, deficiency of stem cell factor, and genetic mutation have been proposed as causes of human idiopathic aplastic anemia.[6-8,29]

DIAGNOSIS

Minimum clinical evaluation of patients who have suspected aplastic anemia includes a complete history with questions pertaining to exposure to drugs, chemicals, and infectious agents; complete blood count; blood smear evaluation; and bone marrow aspiration and core biopsy (see Algorithm). A diagnosis of aplastic anemia cannot be made without evaluation of bone marrow. Bone marrow aspiration smears permit identification of individual cells, whereas core biopsy sections are essential for evaluating marrow cellularity and architecture. Cellularity in the core biopsy is assessed by estimating the relative percentage of the marrow space occupied by hemic cells. In aplastic anemia, hemic tissue occupies 0 to 25% of the marrow space with the remainder replaced by adipose tissue. Frequently only small islands of hemic cells remain and consist mainly of lymphocytes and plasma cells. In acute toxic plastic anemia, rapid destruction of hemic cells may result in many lysed and degenerating cells, an increase in phagocytic macrophages in marrow smears, and multifocal areas of necrosis in core biopsy sections.

In acute aplastic anemia, particular attention should be given to drug or chemical exposure 2 to 3 weeks before clinical signs developed. Patients who have acute aplastic anemia present with signs referable to neutropenia (fever and infection) and thrombocytopenia (petechial hemorrhage, epistaxis, and hematuria). Anemia is usually mild but may progress over time.

In chronic aplastic anemia, animals usually present with signs referable to severe nonregenerative anemia. Although variable degrees of leukopenia and thrombocytopenia accompany the anemia, enough residual granulopoiesis and thrombopoiesis remains to prevent infection and hemorrhage and to permit development of anemia over weeks or months.

TREATMENT

Severe leukopenia (i.e., segmented neutrophils <500/μL) is associated with significantly increased susceptibility to bacterial infection.[23] Administration of broad-spectrum antibiotic drugs are essential to control infection. Severe thrombocytopenia (i.e., platelet count <5,000/μL) should be treated by administration of platelet transfusions. Severe anemia (i.e., packed cell volume [PCV] <10%) should be treated by administration of RBC transfusions. Because repeated RBC transfusion may be needed, donors of similar blood type should be used and RBC crossmatching should be done before each transfusion.

Specific treatments for aplastic anemia have not been extensively evaluated for domestic animals. An immune-mediated mechanism for aplastic anemia has not been established, therefore, there is no indication for immunosuppressive therapy. Anabolic steroid treatment is probably of no benefit. Recombinant hemopoietic growth factors have become available for clinical use in dogs. Studies of human aplastic anemia patients indicate that treatment with granulocyte-macrophage colony-stimulating factor, interleukin-3, or stem cell factor may result in increased cell counts in blood but do not appear to be curative.[8] Therefore, these factors probably stimulate existing residual hemopoiesis but do not alleviate the underlying defect in hemopoiesis. Bone marrow transplantation for aplastic anemia is limited by a lack of compatible donors. Studies of humans who have aplastic anemia suggest that transplantation is superior to immunosuppressive therapy only when human leukocyte antigen (HLA)-identical related donors are available.

PROGNOSIS

The outcome of aplastic anemia depends on the cause and whether the anemia is acute or chronic. In general, acute aplastic anemias tend to be reversible after elimination of initiating agents and if adequate supportive care is given. Nonsteroidal anti-inflammatory drugs are an exception. With present approaches to treatment of phenylbutazone-associated aplastic anemia, most affected dogs do not recover.

Chronic aplastic anemia is less amenable to treatment. Many affected animals have been euthanatized shortly after diagnosis. However, with supportive care, recovery weeks to months after initial diagnosis has been reported.[3] In the future, more extensive use of blood component therapy, recombinant hemopoietic growth factors, and bone marrow transplantation should further increase survival time and remission rates.

REFERENCES

1. Tvedten H. Erythrocyte disorders. In: Willard M, Tvedten H, Turnwald GH, eds. Small animal clinical diagnosis by laboratory method. 2nd ed. Philadelphia: WB Saunders, 1994.
2. Weiss DJ, Armstrong PJ. Nonregenerative Anemias in the Dog. Compend Contin Educ Pract Vet 1984;6: 452–460.
3. Weiss DJ, Klausner JS. Drug-associated aplastic anemia in dogs: eight cases (1984–1988). J AM Vet Med Assoc 1990;196:472–479.
4. Steinberg S. Aplastic anemia in a dog. J Am Vet Med Assoc 1970;157: 966–967.
5. Oglivie GK, Obradovich J. Use of colony-stimulating factors in human and veterinary medicine. Proc 8th Am Coll Vet Intern Med Forum. Washington, DC, 1990;917.
6. Hus HC, Tsai WH, Chen LY, Hsu ML, Ho BCHH, Lin CK. Production of hematopoietic regulatory cytokines by peripheral blood mononuclear cells in patients with aplastic anemia. Exp Hematol 1996;24:31–36.
7. Moralespolanco MR, Sanchezvalle E, Guerrerorivera S, Gutierrezalamillo L, Delgadomarquez B. Treatment results of 23 cases of severe aplastic anemia with lymphocytaphoresis. Arch Med Res 1997;28:85–90.
8. Scopes J, Daly S, Atkinson R, Ball SE, Gordonsmith EC. Aplastic anemia—evidence for dysfunctional bone marrow progenitor cells and the corrective effect of granulocyte colony-stimulating factor in vitro. Blood 1996;87:3179–3185.
9. Shelly SM. Causes of canine pancytopenia. Compend Contin Educ Pract Vet 1988;10:9–17.
10. Boosinger TR, Rebar AH, DeNicola DB, Boon GD. Bone marrow alterations associated with canine parvoviral enteritis. Vet Pathol 1982;19:558–561.
11. Dornsife RE, Gasper PW, Mullins JI, Hoover EA. In vitro erythrocytopathic activity of an aplastic anemia-inducing feline retrovirus. Exp Hematol 1989;17:138–144.
12. Dornsife RE, Gasper PW, Mullins JI, Hoover EA. Induction of aplastic anemia by intra-bone marrow inoculation of molecularly cloned feline retrovirus. 1989;13:745–755.
13. Wardrop KJ, Baszler TV, Relich E, Crawford TB. A morphometric study of bone marrow megakaryocytes in foals infected with equine infectious anemia virus. Vet Pathol 1996;33:222–227.
14. Kuehn NF, Gaunt SD. Clinical and hematologic findings in canine ehrlichiosis. J Am Vet Med Assoc 1985;186:355–358.
15. Peavy GM, Holland CJ, Dutta SK, Smith G. Moore A, Rich LJ, Lappin MR, Richter K. Suspected ehrlichial infection in five cats from a household. J Am Vet Med Assoc 1997;210:231.
16. Bowen RA, Olson PN, Behrendt MD, Wheeler SL. Efficacy and toxicity of estrogens commonly used to terminate canine pregnancy. J Am Vet Med Assoc 1985;186:783–788.
17. Sherding RG, Wilson GP, Kociba GJ. Bone marrow hypoplasia in eight dogs with sertoli cells tumors. J Am Vet Med Assoc 1981;178:497–501.
18. Berggren PC. Aplastic anemia in a horse. J Am Vet Med Assoc 1981; 179:1400–1402.
19. Lavoie JP, Morris DD, Zinkl JG, Lloyd K, Divers TJ. Pancytopenia caused by bone marrow aplasia in a horse. J Am Vet Med Assoc 1987;191:1462–1464.
20. Couto CG. Toxicity of anticancer chemotherapy. In: Campfield WW, ed. Kal Kan symposium for the treatment of small animal diseases. Vermon, CA: Kal Kan Pet Foods, 1986; 37.
21. Alleman AR, Harvey JW. The morphologic effects of vincristine sulfate on canine bone marrow cells. Vet Clin Path 1993;22:36–41.
22. Fox LE, Ford S, Alleman AR, Homer BL, Harvey JW. Aplastic anemia associated with prolonged high-dose trimethoprim-sulfadiazine administration in two dogs. Vet Clin Path 1993;22:89–92.
23. Weiss DJ. Leukocyte response to toxic injury. Toxicol Pathol 1993;21: 135–140.
24. Watson ADJ. Further observation on chlormaphenicol toxicosis in cats. Am J Vet Res 1980;41:293–294.
25. Cukrova V, Langrova E, Akao M. Effects of aflatoxin B$_1$ on myelopoiesis in vitro. Toxicology 1991;70:203–211.
26. McKinney LL, Weakley FB, Cambell RE, Eldridge AC, Cowan JC. Toxic protein from trichloroethylene-extracted soybean oil meal. J Am Oil Chem 1957;34;461–466.
27. Dalton RG. The effects of batyl alcohol on the haematology of cattle poisoned with bracken. Vet Rec 1964;76:411–416.
28. Bond VP, Cronkite EP. Effects of radiation on mannals. Annu Rev Physiol 1957;19:299–328.
28. Weiss DJ. Idiopathic aplastic anemia in the dog. Vet Clin Pathol 1985; 14:23–25.
29. Marsh JCW, Geary CG. Is aplastic anemia a pre-leukemic disorder? Br J Haematol 1991;77:447–451.

CHAPTER 38

Erythrocytosis and Polycythemia

• A.D.J. WATSON

An increase in erythrocyte [red blood cell (RBC)] count in peripheral blood is referred to as erythrocytosis; hematocrit [packed cell volume (PCV)] and hemoglobin (Hgb) concentration are usually increased similarly. Polycythemia can be used as a synonym for erythrocytosis, but it is also implied sometimes to denote erythrocytosis accompanied by leukocytosis and thrombocytosis. The term erythrocytosis is preferred here, because the focus is on erythrocyte changes.

Various disorders cause erythrocytosis in domestic animals. These can be divided into four or five groups depending on the cause (Table 38.1) and laboratory features (Table 38.2).

CLASSIFICATION OF ERYTHROCYTOSIS

Relative Erythrocytosis

In the common form of relative erythrocytosis, the total volume of RBCs in the body red cell mass is normal, but PCV, Hgb, and RBC count are increased because of dehydration and hemoconcentration. The usual causes are reduced intake or increased losses of fluid through vomiting, diarrhea, or polyuria. Erythrocytosis is accompanied by increased total plasma protein and albumen concentrations, unless protein synthesis is impaired or losses are enhanced by concurrent disease.

Relative erythrocytosis can also occur in excitable individuals as a result of catecholamine-induced splenic contraction. This redistributes RBCs by forcing stored cells into the circulation, but plasma protein concentrations and osmolality are not affected. It should be suspected when erythrocytosis is a transient finding in an otherwise normal animal or if the patient was fearful or excited at blood collection. In these instances, changes suggesting physiologic leukocytosis may also be present: namely, mature neutrophilia and lymphocytosis and possibly monocytosis or eosinophilia.

Absolute Erythrocytosis

In absolute erythrocytosis, the high RBC count is caused by a true increase in red cell mass, rather than by hemo-concentration or RBC redistribution. Absolute erythrocytosis is much less common than the relative form and can be classified as primary or secondary, depending on whether excessive erythropoietin (EPO) production is involved in its development.

Primary Erythrocytosis

In primary erythrocytosis, erythroid cells proliferate to excess in the absence of substantial concentrations of EPO in blood. This form of myeloproliferative disease is rarely diagnosed in domestic species other than the cat and the dog. It has some similarities to polycythemia vera, a better-defined entity that occurs in people, but differs in that leukocytosis, thrombocytosis, and splenomegaly are less often found in veterinary cases.

Human polycythemia vera is a hemopoietic disorder characterized by uncontrolled proliferation of erythroid, granulocytic, and megakaryocytic cells. This clonal defect arises by transformation of a single stem cell into a cell line with selective growth advantage that gradually becomes the predominant source of marrow precursors.[1] The abnormal population may proliferate in the absence of EPO or be hyperresponsive to it.

The important diagnostic features of human polycythemia vera are erythrocytosis (in almost all cases), leukocytosis (in two thirds), thrombocytosis (in one half), and splenomegaly (in three quarters). Frequently only two or three of these components, and sometimes just one (mostly erythrocytosis), are found initially. The onset is gradual and progression is slow. Other changes may evolve in later stages, namely progressive marrow fibrosis, anemia, and increasing splenomegaly. An increased incidence of lymphoid neoplasia has also been documented.[1] Some patients who have erythrocytosis alone never develop other features of polycythemia vera, even after many years.

The pathogenesis of primary erythrocytosis has not been investigated thoroughly in domestic species, but probably involves proliferation of an erythroid clone in an EPO-independent or EPO-hyperresponsive fashion, as was demonstrated in one cat.[2] The disorder is rare and should be diagnosed only after careful exclusion of alternative possibilities, especially the nonhypoxemic form of secondary erythrocytosis.

TABLE 38.1	Classification of Erythrocytosis
Type	**Cause**
Relative	Dehydration and hemoconcentration
	Splenic contraction
Absolute	
Primary	Myeloproliferative disorder
Secondary	
Appropriate	Right-to-left cardiovascular shunting
	Pulmonary disease
	High altitude
	Hemoglobin with high oxygen affinity
Inappropriate	Other tumor
	Renal tumor or other nephropathy
Atypical	Mixed or unknown

TABLE 38.2	Expected Features in Erythrocytosis	
Type	**Arterial P_{O_2}**	**Serum Erythropoietin Concentration**
Relative	Normal	Normal
Primary	Normal or slightly low	Low or normal
Secondary	—	—
Appropriate	Low[a]	High
Inappropriate	Normal	High
Atypical	Normal	High

[a]Normal in hemoglobinopathy with high oxygen affinity.

Secondary Erythrocytosis

In secondary erythrocytosis, there is also an increased red cell mass, but the mechanism involves increased EPO production. This may occur appropriately in response to tissue hypoxia or inappropriately when EPO production is independent of tissue oxygenation.

Appropriate Secondary Erythrocytosis Secondary erythrocytosis associated with hypoxemia (reduced arterial P_{O_2}) can be seen in patients who have congenital cardiovascular disorders in which right-to-left shunting of blood bypasses the lungs. These occur infrequently and are accompanied by dyspnea, cyanosis, heart murmur, and poor growth. Secondary erythrocytosis can also develop appropriately when chronic, severe pulmonary disease causes substantial ventilation-perfusion mismatch or seriously hinders gas diffusion. Typical signs of pneumonopathy, especially dyspnea, should be evident in such cases. Living at high altitude induces several physiologic responses to hypoxemia, including erythrocytosis. Although species sensitivities to altitude effects vary,[3] erythrocytosis seems unlikely to occur at altitudes less than 1800 m (6000 ft) above sea level.

Appropriate secondary erythrocytosis can also develop when tissue hypoxia occurs in the absence of hy-

poxemia: for example, a circulating stable variant of Hgb that binds oxygen more readily than normal may be less able to release it to tissues.[4] These inherited hemoglobinopathies are rare in people and have not been described in domestic animals. Similarly, impaired tissue oxygenation can lead to secondary erythrocytosis despite normal arterial P_{O_2} when there is prolonged carboxyhemoglobinemia (carbon monoxide poisoning) or in some forms of methemoglobinemia.

Inappropriate Secondary Erythrocytosis This form of erythrocytosis is characterized by increased EPO secretion without general tissue hypoxia. Mechanisms identified in people involve release of EPO from the kidneys, in response to structural or functional renal abnormalities, or from tumors in other sites.[5] Some renal lesions (tumors, cysts, and hydronephrosis) may cause EPO overproduction through pressure-induced hypoxia in adjacent renal parenchyma. Nonrenal tumors associated with erythrocytosis include uterine myoma, cerebellar hemangioma, hepatoma, and some endocrine tumors.[5]

Atypical Erythrocytosis

Some human patients have erythrocytosis and increased EPO concentration in the absence of any disorder known to increase EPO production, whereas others have both an increased EPO concentration and an autonomous erythroid clone. Such cases are difficult to classify satisfactorily.[5]

EFFECTS OF ERYTHROCYTOSIS

In most patients who have erythrocytosis, abnormal signs and findings are directly attributable to an underlying disease (for example, gastroenteropathy, cardiopulmonary disease, renal tumor) rather than to erythrocytosis per se; erythrocytosis here is generally not severe and consequent signs are absent or mild. However, even a mild but sustained increase in erythrocyte production, as occurs with severe hypoxemia, primary erythrocytosis, or inappropriate secondary erythrocytosis, may increase blood volume and viscosity sufficiently to affect the patient adversely. Affected people report headaches, dizziness, tinnitus, and feelings of fullness of face and neck; these may be caused by increased viscosity and vascular dilation.[6] Alertness is also impaired.[7]

An obvious manifestation of erythrocytosis is deep red to purplish-red mucous membranes and skin. There may be slight cyanosis because blood flow is sluggish, allowing excessive deoxygenation of blood. The slow blood flow and capillary distention also promote hemorrhages and thrombosis.

Optimum oxygen transport probably occurs in most species at PCV values corresponding to normal reference ranges.[6] Higher PCVs increase blood viscosity, slowing blood flow and decreasing oxygen transport. This effect is blunted somewhat by improved cardiac output caused by hypervolemia, so that optimum oxygen transport occurs at higher PCV values in hypervolemia than under normovolemic conditions.[6] However, beyond a certain point the increased viscosity further reduces tissue perfusion and clinical effects can be expected.

Many of the abnormalities observed in domestic animals that have moderate to severe erythrocytosis can be accounted for by these processes. Polydipsia and polyuria are not reported in affected people but are seen in some veterinary patients; studies in two dogs that have erythrocytosis suggest these effects might be caused by impaired vasopressin release.[8]

ERYTHROCYTOSIS IN DOMESTIC ANIMALS

Relative Erythrocytosis

Relative erythrocytosis from dehydration and hemoconcentration is common. The clinical signs and findings reflect the underlying disease, and erythrocytosis, usually mild or moderate, is an indicator of hemoconcentration rather than of concern in itself. Significant erythrocytosis (PCV >0.60 l/l) occurs rarely and may be associated with additional adverse effects.

Splenic contraction as a cause of relative erythrocytosis is likely to occur only in excitable individuals of some species, such as dogs and horses.[9] It is mild, transient, and clinically unimportant.

Appropriate Secondary Erythrocytosis

Congenital cardiac diseases with right-to-left shunting of blood, hypoxemia, and secondary erythrocytosis occur in all species. Although not common in large domestic animals, they are recognized with some frequency in the dog and are also encountered in the cat. The most frequent causes in small animals are tetralogy of Fallot and forms of Eisenmenger's syndrome. Erythrocytosis secondary to congestive heart failure or chronic pneumonopathy is uncommon in any species and is usually mild when it occurs. With cardiovascular or cardiopulmonary disease the predominant clinical signs are likely to be dyspnea, reduced exercise tolerance, and failure to thrive; cyanosis may be present as well. Concurrent arterial hypoxemia is an important diagnostic finding.

Hemoglobinopathies causing erythrocytosis are rare in all domestic species. Erythrocytosis, presumably inherited, has been observed in some dogs that have methemoglobin reductase deficiency and in a cat[10]; it has also been observed in cats that have suspected carbon monoxide poisoning.[11] However, inherited hemoglobinopathies with increased oxygen affinity causing tissue hypoxia have not been reported in the veterinary literature.

Primary Erythrocytosis and Inappropriate Secondary Erythrocytosis

It is convenient to consider primary erythrocytosis (PE) and inappropriate secondary erythrocytosis (ISE) together because they can be similar clinically and because distinguishing between them is sometimes difficult even after thorough investigation. Both are rare in all species, with most cases reported in cats and in dogs and few cases reported in other animals.

Cats

PE is the more common diagnosis in the cat. ISE has been identified rarely in this species.[2,12–15]

Cats that have PE are usually older animals (median age reported 6 or 7 years). A male:female ratio of 2:1 is evident amongst 41 reported cases. Common clinical signs include neurologic disturbances (seizures, blindness, ataxia, abnormal behavior, and apparent mental depression) and occasionally lethargy, anorexia, polyuria or polydipsia, and vomiting. Hyperemia of mucous membranes is the main abnormal physical finding, and approximately 20% have splenomegaly. Initial PCV values reported were 0.56 to 0.84 l/l, and usually ≥0.70 l/l (in 12 of 14 cases). Leukocytosis or thrombocytosis was rarely observed: stress leukocyte changes occurred in some cats and panleukocytosis in one.[2] Concurrent hypoglucosemia in some patients could be an in vitro artifact associated with high cell counts.

Serum EPO concentration in cats that have PE is generally within reference limits (62% of 39 cases) or low (31%); three other cats that have features compatible with PE had high EPO concentrations, although the value was subnormal on retesting in one of them.[12,13,15] Serum EPO concentrations in four cats that have renal tumors and ISE were within reference limits in three and low in one; two other cats that have nonneoplastic renal disease and ISE had high EPO values.[12,15]

Dogs

PE also appears more common than ISE in the dog. Reported cases of PE outnumber ISE cases by approximately 2:1.[16–32]

Approximately 40 dogs are recorded as having PE, but some reports are incomplete and earlier cases preceded the development of radioimmunoassays that made measurement of EPO more accessible. Furthermore, some dogs had renal lesions that might have been the cause or a consequence of erythrocytosis, or which might have been an incidental finding.[9,23,24]

PE occurs in dogs at any age (median around 7 years) and affects more females than males (ratio 2:1). Clinical signs vary, but include lethargy, inappetence, diverse neurologic signs (seizures, collapse, posterior ataxia, and disorientation), hemorrhages, and polyuria or polydipsia. The main physical abnormality is reddening of skin and mucous membranes. Splenomegaly is rare. Hematologic abnormalities in most cases are confined to erythrocytosis; leukocytosis occurs in a minority, and thrombocytosis is rare. Microcytic RBCs sometimes circulate, possibly reflecting relative iron deficiency. Bone marrow aspirates may appear normal or hypercellular, sometimes with erythroid hyperplasia.

Of 16 dogs potentially having ISE,[8,12,21,25–32] 13 had renal tumors (7 carcinoma, 3 lymphosarcoma, 3 other) and 1 had nasal fibrosarcoma. In two cases the diagnosis seems questionable: cryptococcal nephritis in one[28] may have caused erythrocytosis or been coincidental to PE (EPO was not measured), and pulmonary metastases from renal carcinoma in another[32] could have induced hypoxemic erythrocytosis (arterial P_{O_2} was not determined). No sex predisposition is apparent within the ISE group. Clinical signs in dogs that have ISE resemble those in PE but often with additional features caused by the underlying disease, namely anorexia, weight loss, and an intra-abdominal mass. Erythrocytosis is the main hematologic finding, but leukocyte changes sometimes reflect stress, inflammation, or necrosis associated with the causative lesion.

Serum EPO concentration was within or less than reference limits in 14 of 15 dogs that have PE. It was increased in 7 of 8 dogs (normal in 1) that have ISE.[12,21–23,26–28,30]

Horses

There are few reports of absolute erythrocytosis without hypoxemia in horses: PE was the likely diagnosis in three and ISE in two.[33–37] In the latter, the underlying lesions were hepatocellular carcinoma with metastatic spread in one, and a disseminated carcinoma in the other.

Cattle

ISE has not been recorded in cattle. PE was described in one Hereford steer and a group of inbred Jersey calves.[38,39] PE in Jerseys did not behave like a clonal bone marrow disorder: PCV values were normal at birth, decreased during the first month, then increased until 6 or 7 months of age when most calves died. In survivors, erythrocytosis gradually abated over the next 12 months. It was suggested that erythrocytosis resulted from transient overcorrection of normal neonatal anemia. A simple autosomal recessive mode of inheritance was proposed.

Other Animals

ISE without identifiable cause was diagnosed in a llama.[40] ISE associated with glomerulonephropathy has been reported in a brown lemur.[41]

Atypical Erythrocytosis

A few cases classified above as PE or ISE (in two cats, one dog, and one llama) might be regarded as atypical erythrocytosis, because available data are interpretable either as PE with unexpectedly high EPO concentration or as ISE without identifiable underlying cause.[12,15,40] These cases were not investigated to exclude tissue hypoxia caused by a hemoglobin variant with high oxygen affinity. Investigation of similar cases should include hemoglobin electrophoresis and determination of hemoglobin P_{50} (the oxygen tension at which hemoglobin is 50% saturated).

DIAGNOSIS

The investigative path in erythrocytosis depends on the case and availability of resources (see Algorithm). The following is suggested as a logical sequence:

- Verify that erythrocytosis is a repeatable finding: exclude laboratory error.
- Evaluate for relative erythrocytosis. Consider possibility of excitement and splenic contraction. Evaluate for underlying disease causing increased fluid losses or reduced intake. Check for dehydration and hemoconcentration by looking for suggestive physical and laboratory test abnormalities. Intravenous fluid therapy should reduce PCV rapidly in dehydration but will not change PCV much in absolute erythrocytosis, unless combined with phlebotomy.
- Assess color of mucous membranes. Mucosal color in severe erythrocytosis is generally deep red to purplish red. Sluggish local flow may cause slight cyanosis, but overt cyanosis suggests hypoxemia from severe pulmonary disease, or blood bypassing the lungs. Methemoglobinemia may produce brownish-blue discoloration and carbon monoxide a cherry-red color.
- Examine further for cardiopulmonary disease, using thoracic palpation, auscultation and radiography, and ultrasonic examination if indicated. Arterial blood gas analysis is important: hypoxemia (P_{O_2} <80 mm Hg, O_2 saturation <92%) makes appropriate secondary erythrocytosis likely, although mild hypoxemia can occur with other forms of erythrocytosis too.
- Investigate for possible renal lesions, if not hypoxemic. Renal ultrasonography, with optional guided biopsy, is helpful but intravenous urography may also assist. Glomerulonephropathy can be the cause or a consequence of erythrocytosis and warrants further investigation.
- Look for neoplasia elsewhere if renal lesions are absent or of questionable significance. Abdominal ultrasonography is indicated, with thorough physical examination and thoracic radiographs if not already done.
- Sample serum for EPO determination. This may help further distinguish PE from secondary and atypical forms.
- Consider other procedures if data are equivocal. If further differentiation between relative and absolute forms is required, measure total red cell mass with radioisotope-labeled autologous RBCs. Bone marrow

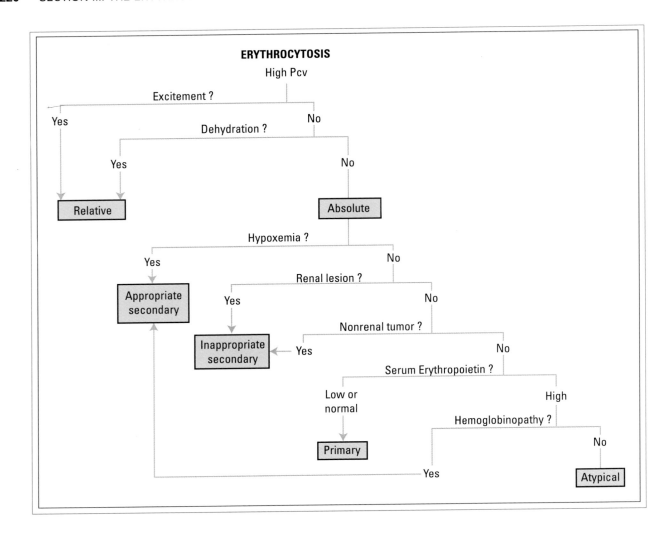

ERYTHROCYTOSIS

High Pcv

Excitement ?

Yes   No

Dehydration ?

Yes   No

Relative   Absolute

Hypoxemia ?

Yes   No

Renal lesion ?

Appropriate secondary

Yes   No

Inappropriate secondary ← Yes   Nonrenal tumor ?

No

Serum Erythropoietin ?

Low or normal   High

Hemoglobinopathy ?

Primary   No

Yes   Atypical

hemopoietic cell culture could be done to examine for EPO-independent or EPO-hyperresponsive erythroid progenitors. In patients that have apparent ISE but no identifiable cause or that have apparent PE but increased EPO, an abnormal Hgb with high oxygen affinity might be present; determine P_{50} of hemoglobin, and perform hemoglobin electrophoresis. Other investigative procedures may be available through specialized laboratories. Bone marrow evaluation is not generally diagnostically useful.

TREATMENT

Where appropriate, dehydration and underlying diseases should be identified and treated. If secondary erythrocytosis is an appropriate response to tissue hypoxia, treatment to reduce erythrocytosis may be unwise. However, if PCV is high and consequent signs are severe, one can consider removal of blood and replacement by an equivalent volume of intravenous fluids so that blood viscosity is reduced and tissue perfusion improved. This is best done in small amounts (5 mL/

kg) repeated as necessary, with careful assessment of the response.

For animals that have ISE, surgery may be possible to remove the causal lesion (renal mass or other tumor). Presurgical reduction in PCV by phlebotomy could be advantageous and can be done more vigorously: removal of 20 mL/kg of blood with PCV 0.70 l/l and replacement by 20 mL/kg of intravenous fluid should reduce PCV to approximately 0.55 l/l in a dog or 0.50 l/l in a cat.

There are several treatment options in PE. Provided the patient, owner, and veterinarian are willing, repeated phlebotomy can be used successfully.[24] The goal is to maintain PCV at a high normal value. Long-term iron supplements may be advisable to avoid iron deficiency. Surprisingly, one dog treated only with three phlebotomies in the first week remained alive, with PCV in the reference range, 18 months later.[22] Alternatively, hydroxyurea or radioactive phosphorus (^{32}P) can be administered alone or with an initial phlebotomy or repeated phlebotomies. In dogs, hydroxyurea can be given orally at 30 mg/kg once daily for 7 to 10 days, after which dose and frequency are adjusted according to hematologic response.[42] A suggested regimen for cats is 125 mg every second day for 2 weeks, then 250 mg twice weekly for 2 weeks, followed by 500 mg once weekly.[13] The interval is increased to 10 or 14 days once the target PCV (0.40 to 0.45 l/l) is reached. Regular hematologic monitoring is required and hydroxyurea treatment suspended if neutropenia, thrombocytopenia or anemia occur. Methemoglobinemia and hemolytic anemia are other potential complications of therapy in cats.[13] Treatment with ^{32}P may be available in some institutions and has given excellent long-term control after a single intravenous dose in some cases.[18]

REFERENCES

1. **Beutler E.** Polycythemia vera. In: Beutler E, Lichtman MA, Coller BS, Kipps TJ, eds. Williams hematology. 5th ed. New York: McGraw-Hill, 1995:324.
2. **Khanna C, Bienzle D.** Polycythemia vera in a cat: bone marrow culture in erythropoietin-deficient medium. J Am Anim Hosp Assoc 1994;30:45–49.
3. **Radostits OM, Blood DC, Gay CC.** Veterinary medicine. 8th ed. Baillière Tindall: London, 1994:1457.
4. **Benz EJ.** Hemoglobinopathies with altered solubility or oxygen affinity. In: Bennet JC, Plum P, eds. Cecil textbook of medicine. 20th ed. Philadelphia: Saunders, 1996:873.
5. **Erslev AJ.** Secondary polycythemia (erythrocytosis). In: Beutler E, Lichtman MA, Coller BS, Kipps TJ, eds. Williams hematology. 5th ed. New York: McGraw-Hill, 1995:714.
6. **Erslev AJ.** Clinical manifestations and classification of erythrocyte disorders. In: Beutler E, Lichtman MA, Coller BS, Kipps TJ, eds. Williams hematology. 5th ed. New York: McGraw-Hill, 1995:441.
7. **Willison JR, Thomas DJ, du Boulay GH, Marshall J, Paul EA, Pearson TC, Russell RW, Symon L, Wetherley-Mein G.** Effect of high haematocrit on alertness. Lancet 1980;1(8173):846–848.
8. **van Vonderen IK, Meyer HP, Kraus JS, Kooistra HS.** Polyuria and polydipsia and disturbed vasopressin release in 2 dogs with secondary polycythemia. J Vet Intern Med 1997;11:300–303.
9. **Jain NC.** Schalm's veterinary hematology. 4th ed. Philadelphia: Lea and Febiger, 1985:563.
10. **Harvey JW, Dahl M, High ME.** Methemoglobin reductase deficiency in a cat. J Am Vet Med Assoc 1994;205:1290–1291.
11. **Hopkins J.** Suspected carbon monoxide poisoning in cats. Vet Rec 1995; 136:204.
12. **Cook SM, Lothrop CD.** Serum erythropoietin concentrations measured by radioimmunoassay in normal, polycythemic, and anemic dogs and cats. J Vet Intern Med 1994;8:18–25.
13. **Watson ADJ, Moore AS, Helfand SC.** Primary erythrocytosis in the cat: treatment with hydroxyurea. J Small Anim Pract 1994;35:320–325.
14. **Evans LM, Caylor KB.** Polycythemia vera in a cat and management with hydroxyurea. J Am Anim Hosp Assoc 1995;31:434–438.
15. **Hasler AH, Giger U.** Serum erythropoietin values in polycythemic cats. J Am Anim Hosp Assoc 1996;32:294–301.
16. **Watson ADJ, Yates JA.** Primary polycythaemia in a dog. Aust Vet J 1984; 61:61–63.
17. **Holden AR.** Polycythaemia vera in a dog. Vet Rec 1987;120:473–475.
18. **Smith M, Turrel JM.** Radiophosphorus (^{32}P) treatment of bone marrow disorders in dogs: 11 cases (1970–1987). J Am Vet Med Assoc 1989;194: 98–102.
19. **Page RL, Stiff ME, McEntee MC, Walter LG.** Transient glomerulonephropathy associated with primary erythrocytosis in a dog. J Am Vet med Assoc 1990;196:620–622.
20. **Wysoke JM, van Heerden J.** Polycythaemia vera in a dog. J S Afr Vet Assoc 1990;61:182–183.
21. **Giger U.** Serum erythropoietin concentrations in polycythemic and anemic dogs. 9th American College of Veterinary Internal Medicine Forum Proceedings, New Orleans, LA, 1991;143–145.
22. **Codner EC.** Transient erythrocytosis (polycythaemia vera) in a dog. Comp Hematol Int 1992;2:111–113.
23. **Quesnel AD, Kruth SA.** Polycythemia vera and glomerulonephritis in a dog. Can Vet J 1992;33:671–672.
24. **Meyer HP, Slappendel RJ, Greydanus-van der Putten SWM.** Polycythaemia vera in a dog treated by repeated phlebotomies. Vet Q 1993;15:108–111.
25. **Scott RC, Patnaik AK.** Renal carcinoma with secondary polycythemia in the dog. J Am Anim Hosp Assoc 1972;8:275–283.
26. **Peterson ME, Zanjani ED.** Inappropriate erythropoietin production from a renal carcinoma in a dog with polycythemia. J Am Vet Med Assoc 1981;179:995–996.
27. **Nelson RW, Hager D, Zanjani ED.** Renal lymphosarcoma with inappropriate erythropoietin production in a dog. J Am Vet Med Assoc 1983;182:1396–1397.
28. **Waters DJ, Preuter JC.** Secondary polycythemia associated with renal disease in the dog: two case reports and review of the literature. J Am Anim Hosp Assoc 1988;24:109–114.
29. **Gorse MJ.** Polycythemia associated with renal fibrosarcoma in a dog. J Am Vet Med Assoc 1988;192:793–794.
30. **Couto CG, Boudrieau RJ, Zanjani ED.** Tumor-associated erythrocytosis in a dog with nasal fibrosarcoma. J Vet Intern Med 1989;3:183–185.
31. **Gentile A, Guglielmini C, Cipone M.** Eritrocitosi secondaria ad emangiopericitoma renale in un cane. Veterinaria (Cremona) 1994;8:29–33.
32. **Crow SE, Allen DP, Murphy CJ, Culbertson R.** Concurrent renal adenocarcinoma and polycythemia in a dog. J Am Anim Hosp Assoc 1995;31:29–33.
33. **Beech J, Bloom JC, Hodge TG.** Erythrocytosis in a horse. J Am Vet Med Assoc 1984;184:986–989.
34. **Steiger R, Feige K.** Fallbericht: polyglobie bei einem pferd. Schweiz Arch Tierheilkd 1995;137:306–311.
35. **McFarlane D, Sellon DC, Parker B.** Primary erythrocytosis in a 2-year-old Arabian gelding. J Vet Intern Med 1998;12:384–388.
36. **Roby KAW, Beech J, Bloom JC, Black M.** Hepatocellular carcinoma associated with erythrocytosis and hypoglycemia in a yearling filly. J Am Vet Med Assoc 1990;196:465–467.
37. **Cook G, Divers TJ, Rowland PH.** Hypercalcemia and erythrocytosis in a mare associated with a metastatic carcinoma. Equine Vet J 1995;25:316–318.
38. **Fowler ME, Cornelius CE, Baker NF.** Clinical and erythrokinetic studies on a case of bovine polycythemia vera. Cornell Vet 1964;54:153–160.
39. **Tennant B, Harrold D, Reina-Guerra M, Laben RC.** Arterial pH, PO_2 and PCO_2 of calves with familial bovine polycythemia. Cornell Vet 1969;59:594–604.
40. **Gentz EJ, Pearson EG, Lassen ED, Snyder SP, Sharpnack E.** Polycythemia in a llama. J Am Vet Med Assoc 1994;204:1490–1492.
41. **Fox LE, Heard DJ, Garner MM.** Glomerulonephritis-associated secondary polycythemia in a brown lemur (*Petterus fulvus*). J Zoo Wildl Med 1994; 25:585–589.
42. **Couto CG.** Erythrocytosis. In: Nelson RW, Couto CG, eds. Small animal internal medicine. 2nd ed. St Louis: Mosby, 1998;1174.

SECTION IV
Leukocytes–Lymphocytes
Erik Teske

CHAPTER 39

Structure and Function of the Hemopoietic System

• VICTOR EDWIN VALLI and ROBERT MANUEL JACOBS

HISTORICAL PERSPECTIVE

In framing the context for the fifth edition of Schalm's Veterinary Hematology, it is appropriate to recognize the seminal contributions of our predecessors in veterinary hematology, including Dr. Oscar Schalm, as well the workers of the previous centuries who have provided us with the foundation for our current understanding of the hemopoietic system. Those who have an interest in the origins of hematology will appreciate the book Hematology, The Blossoming of a Science: A Story of Inspiration and Effort, by Maxwell M. Wintrobe, Lea & Febiger, Philadelphia, 1985. In contrast to the study of gross anatomy of which there was a wealth of knowledge and understanding by the Middle Ages, the study of blood, a fluid tissue that had the property to become solid on injury to its containing vascular structure, required the development of the microscope for detailed studies to begin. The first complete account of red blood cells was made by Antoni van Leeuwenhoek (1632–1723) of Delft, a city hall custodian whose hobby was grinding lenses.[1] The development of the microscope lead to the description of capillaries as a conduit of blood from the arteries to the veins by Marcello Malpighi (1628–1694), who, as professor of anatomy successively at Bologna, Pisa, and Messina, also described the red cells but mistook them for fat globules. Knowledge came slowly in an era that, since antiquity, illness was felt to be punishment for sins. Harvey's discovery of the circulation of the blood, in itself a cornerstone of understanding, gave greater impetus to the understanding of the body as a whole and to integration of the organ systems and then to an understanding of blood itself. Thomas Hodgkin (1798–1866) described diffuse glandular disease associated with splenomegaly in a paper entitled, "On some morbid appearances of the absorbant glands and spleen" in 1832, although the work was largely ignored for nearly 30 years.[2] Rudolf Virchow (1821–1902) introduced the concept of cellular pathology and is generally credited as the father of modern pathology. The first descriptions of leukemia were published concurrently by Virchow and John Hughes Bennett (1822–1875) of Edinburgh at a time when the distinction between inflammatory and neoplastic diseases of the spleen and nodes were not distinguished. Virchow felt that leukemia, a condition of white blood was a primary autonomous disease of spleen and lymphatic glands, whereas Bennett attributed the increase in cells to an accumulation of pus cells in the blood.[3] At this time, the lymphadenopathy, splenomegaly, and intermittent fever associated with malaria were well known, but neither the malarial parasites or the tubercle bacillus had been identified. As yet, the origin of the blood leukocytes was not understood and Virchow, for one, thought that the pus cells observed in inflammatory exudates arose from within various connective tissues and were not related to the leukocytes in the blood. William Addison (1802–1881), a British practitioner, described the white cells in blood and also concluded that they were identical with the cells seen in pus.[4] Subsequently, Julius Cohnheim (1839–1884) and Friederich von Recklinghausen (1833–1910), both students of Virchow, were able to convince him of the correctness of Addison's observations.

At this time iron-deficiency anemia was not recognized as such, but the green sickness or chlorosis of young women was recognized and associated with pallor of cheeks and mucus membranes and palpitation of the heart with minimal exertion. This disease was common in the seventeenth century and was a favorite subject of the painters of that period. Thomas Sydenham (1624–1689), a graduate of Oxford and considered the father of English medicine, recognized the value of iron filings, or chalybeate, for the treatment of chlorosis. Remarkably, it was not until 1832 when Pierre Blaud popularized the use of pills containing ferrous sulphate and potassium carbonate that the treatment of iron-deficiency anemia was routinely and specifically treated. In 1872 Antoine Biermer (1827–1892) of Zurich described 15 cases of anemia under the description progressive pernicious anemia, which, judged by his descriptions, were likely megaloblastic anemia.[5] About the same time, changes in the color of the urine, intermittent albuminuria and chromaturia, was reported in what was likely paroxysmal cold hemoglobinuria. Later, march hemoglobinuria in military personnel was described in Germany. Other forms of hemolytic anemia that were not characterized by hemoglobinuria remained undescribed.

Furthermore, hemophilia had been recognized already in Roman times. The Babylonian Talmud notes the decision of a Rabbi to not circumcise a son of a woman who had three previous sons that bled to death after that rite.[6]

The concept of the bone marrow as the seed bed of the blood was stoutly opposed when suggested in 1868 by Ernst Neumann (1823–1918), professor at Konigsberg in East Prussia.[7] Similar observations were published by Giulio Bizzozero (1849–1901), a 21-year-old graduate of Pavia at the time his work was published.[8] Bone marrow had been considered, since the time of Hippocrates and Galen, to be nutrient to the bone. This latter concept was supported by the eighteenth century anatomists who were impressed by the extensive vascularity of bone marrow. Part of the reluctance to accept the marrow as the source of blood-cell production seems caused by the difficulty in accepting the production of anucleated red cells from the highly cellular structure of bone marrow.

In 1908, the Nobel Prize for Medicine was shared by Ilya Metchnikoff (1845–1916) and Paul Ehrlich (1854–1915). Metchnikoff received the award for his recognition of phagocytosis and Ehrlich for the introduction of aniline dyes for the staining of blood cells. Ehrlich's methods of fixing and staining blood cells for microscopic examination subsequently added to by Romanowsky, Giemsa, and Wright, led him to be recognized as the founder of modern hematology. Besides his many other contributions, Ehrlich is known for bringing the laboratory to the bedside, an approach that persists well into the current century. Metchnikoff's work stimulated many other studies, including the suggestion of a system of cells throughout the body with the capability of removing foreign material described as the reticuloendothelial system by Ludwig Aschoff (1866–1942).[9] Despite the use of the term reticuloendothelial in this text, the system has become more correctly known as the mononuclear-phagocytic system since neither endothelium nor cells elaborating reticulin fibers are involved in the phagocytic process.[10] Deriving from the above, the term "reticulum cell" describing a cell with a vesicular nucleus that did not produce reticulin fibers and referred to a large lymphocyte thankfully, is no longer in use.

The Howell–Jolly bodies, familiar to veterinarians, derived their description from Justin Jolly (1870–1953) of Paris, who described the process by which mammalian rubricytes loose their nuclei and by W. H. Howell (1860–1945) while working at Ann Arbor and later at Johns Hopkins.

In 1901, Karl Landsteiner (1868–1943) working at the Institute of Pathologic Anatomy at the University of Vienna reported on the reactions between red cells and sera of 22 of his laboratory associates. His research laid the foundations for the ABO blood group system[11] and transfusion medicine.

The discovery of the platelet is credited to Max Schultze (1825–1874) of Freiburg and to William Osler (1849–1919). Osler who studied medicine first at Toronto and then at McGill, taught students of both human and veterinary medicine and is known as the first American hematologist. Osler, first a student of microscopy before studying medicine, subsequently brought microscopy to the clinic and demonstrated the power of bedside examinations. Osler subsequently moved from Montreal to Philadelphia and then to Baltimore where, with Halsted and Welch, he was involved in the origins of the Johns Hopkins Hospital. For years, students at the Ontario Veterinary College who were winners of the Schofield Prize in pathology received the two-volume text by Harvey Cushing entitled, *The Life of Sir William Osler* (Oxford Press, 1940), a most inspirational and treasured award.

The understanding of myeloid leukemias was advanced by the proposal by Giovanni DiGuglielmo (1886–1961) that malignancies of primitive myeloid tissue would occur along morphological and functional lines of the erythroid, myeloid, and megakaryocytic systems. DiGuglielmo further proposed that these malignancies would not only occur singly, but in various combinations. Two of these syndromes which initially bore his name have become more familiarly known as erythroleukemia, a mixed tumor of both myeloid and erythroid systems, and erythremic myelosis, a tumor of the erythroid system that occurs in both acute and chronic forms. Subsequent hematologists like Artur Pappenheim (1870–1916) published a beautifully illustrated text describing blood-cell production and destruction. Hal Downey (1877–1959) of the University of Minnesota edited a four-volume *Handbook of Hematology* in 1938 that was an encyclopedic compendium on the hemopoietic system. Downey contributed to the concept of the hemopoietic stem cell system as a theory that was subsequently identified in functional and mathematic terms in the spleen colony assay of mice, developed at Princess Margaret Hospital in Toronto by Till and McCulloch.[12]

HEMOPOIETIC SYSTEM CELLS AND ORGANS

The hemopoietic system consists of the cascade of cells produced by the bone marrow as well as their specialized conducting and supporting systems consisting of vascular endothelium and the connective tissue cells supporting the sinuses of the lymph nodes and spleen. Other highly specialized supporting structures of the hemopoietic system include the epithelial cells of the thymus, which sheath the blood vessels and form the saccular structures of the thymic cortex by which developing T cells gain their recognition of normal self-antigens. The cells themselves consist of the full range of differentiated products of pluripotential stem cells, including monocyte-macrophage and granulocytic cells of the neutrophil, eosinophil, and basophil series as well as the precursors of peripheral red blood cells and platelets and the thymic and the bone-marrow-dependent arms of the lymphoid system responsible for cellular and humoral immunity, respectively.

The vascular endothelium of the hemopoietic system includes the apparently regionally undifferentiated cells lining the lymphatics as well as the regionally differentiated endothelial cells of the blood vascular system. The latter includes high endothelial venules of the lymph node paracortex that bear specific receptors permitting the adhesion of lymphocytes in transit and their transmural migration to exit the blood and enter the node paracortex. These specialized hemopoietic cells and their conducting and supporting structures are uniquely packed in a series of organs of either separate design like the thymus, lymph nodes, and spleen or are incorporated into other organs such as the marrow core of the skeletal system, the phagocytic cells of the liver, and the mucosal-associated lymphoid tissue contained within the lining structures of the respiratory and enteric systems. The integration of these cells and organs to the blood vascular system of the body constitutes a remarkably well-integrated series of systems.

The blood cells circulate in an isotonic solution of plasma containing electrolytes and proteins, including the clotting factors produced by the liver. The red cells carry oxygen to all areas of the body, whereas the platelets maintain endothelial integrity and react with the clotting proteins to contain injury to the vascular system. Foreign material, including infectious agents, are targeted by the cellular and humoral arms of the lymphoid system and the phagocytic cells. Containment of invading organisms involving solid tissues are accomplished by filtration of lymph through the regional lymph nodes, whereas invasion of the blood is prevented by filtration of the entire volume of the blood through the sinus filtering system of the spleen at least once each day. The system is maintained in homeostasis by constant sensing of antigenic stimuli on the surface area of the body, primarily in the respiratory and enteric systems and to a lesser extent through the skin.

HEMOPOIETIC AND IMMUNE SYSTEMS PHYLOGENY AND ONTOGENY

Phylogeny

The development of intercellular recognition systems is present in single-celled organisms, such as protozoa, which may be capable of phagocytosis but do not attack members of the same species. Specific antibody defenses associated with T- and B-lymphocyte differentiation are not found in invertebrates. However, many multicellular organisms, such as sponges, are able to demonstrate fusion between identical types and rejection of unrelated species. Circulating cellular defenses appear first in echinoderms (star fish) and annelids such as earthworms and form leukocytes in their coelomic cavity. These cells seem to combine some functions of both lymphocytes and granulocytes and act defensively. Defensive humoral factors are produced by earthworms; hemolysins, and hemagglutinins occur in star fish and shell fish, but they are not antibodies and act in a generic rather than in an antigen-specific sense. Cells resembling T and B lymphocytes are present in teleost fishes but are not clearly defined in the agnatha, which include cyclostomes, hag fish, lampreys, and eels. The thymus first appears in cartilaginous fish such as sharks and rays,

which have blood granulocytes and lymphocytes and are capable of cell-mediated immunity. Bony fishes add the beginnings of bone marrow as well as the previous capabilities, whereas amphibians, reptiles, birds, and mammals have thymus and bone marrow. Reptiles have weak, slow-reacting cell-mediated defenses, and birds lack lymph glands but have the specialized cloacal bursa of Fabricius. Thus, in the evolution from primitive fishes to mammals, the full range of immune cells, organs, and functions have appeared and are developed to a greater or lesser extent of activity.[13]

Ontogeny

Ontogeny refers to the development of the hemopoietic system within an individual of a given species. Much of our knowledge of hemopoietic development comes from the study of nonmammalian species, particularly the chick embryo for the first evidence of hemopoiesis in the yolk sac. In contrast to the avian species in which yolk-sac structures persist throughout embryogenesis, in mammals, the yolk sac is a transitory structure; however, in both phyla, the yolk sac forms blood islands that contain the primordeal blood cells. Hemopoiesis is first observed in yolk sac mesoderm, but it appears that inductive stimuli probably arise from the other cell layers. The fact that the blood islands, which are a site of the development of embryonic pluripotential stem cells, develop at a distance from the embryo has been suggested to indicate a unique role for the yolk sac in separating these primitive cells from the array of growth factors present within the embryo and that might trigger their early differentiation rather than cell proliferation. The hemopoietic potential appears to be determined at an early stage in preprimitive streak blastoderm. Through a series of foldings and migrations, the predetermined cells of the epiblast form the middle germ layer that is arranged in a horseshoe-shaped configuration around the developing primitive streak of the embryo. The mesangial differentiation within the erythropoietic areas of the blastoderm differentiate into two cellular streams, forming a flattened network of spindle-shaped cells that form the walls and conduits of the blood islands while the central cells roundup and detach from their peripheral surroundings and develop the cytoplasmic basophilia and primitive-appearing nuclei of hemopoietic stem cells. The movement of these precursor cells to the rudimentary organs of the developing embryo constitutes a stream of cells that seeds the primordeal hemopoietic organs in both birds and mammals.

In all species, primary lymphoid development first begins in the thymus. The development of subsequent tissues is then similar for birds and mammals, with the exception that in mammals hemopoiesis begins at an early stage in the liver, whereas in the bird during embryogenesis, hemopoiesis continues in the blood islands of the yolk sac. The production of primitive blood cells can be detected by 2 days of egg incubation in the chicken and by 1 week in the mouse, 2 weeks in the pig, and 3 to 4 weeks in humans. Early on, the liver becomes intensely hemopoietic in mammals, with production beginning at 11 days of gestation in the mouse, 30 days in the lamb and pig, and 42 days in humans.

The embryonic pharyngeal pouch formation begins at 2 days of embryonic development in the chick, 8 days in the mouse, 17 days in the lamb and pig, and 30 to 35 days in humans. The third and fourth pharyngeal pouches have developed and are beginning their migration to form the thymic epithelial anlagen by 6 to 7 days of embryogenesis in the chicken, 10 days in the mouse, 30 days in the lamb, 31 days in the pig, and 40 days in humans. Colonization of the rudimentary thymus by large lymphocytes begins shortly thereafter in all species.

Concurrent with development of the epithelial- and connective-tissue structure of the thymus, the splenic rudiment appears at day 8 in the chicken and day 13 in the mouse and at comparable periods later in other mammals. Splenic erythropoiesis begins 3 days later in both the chick and the mouse embryo, and splenic lymphopoiesis begins a week later in the chick embryo and slightly earlier in the mouse. Marrow hemopoiesis occurs concurrently with that in the spleen and depends on the formation of the marrow cavity with growth and remodeling of embryonic bones. The lymph nodes develop as outpouchings of endothelial ducts with supporting connective tissues and develop concurrently with the spleen becoming active sites of lymphoid production in the mouse embryo at 18 days, 45 days in the lamb, 52 days in the pig, and 70 to 100 days in humans. Birds do not develop lymph nodes, but the bursa of Fabricius begins formation as early as 4 to 5 days of incubation, with attainment of normal architecture by day 11 of embryonic development and becomes colonized by lymphocytes by day 14 of incubation. The earliest stages of hemopoiesis are largely of erythroid cells, with the full range of cellular production present by hatching of birds and midgestation of mammals. Lymphopoiesis does not occur in the yolk sac but rather through differentiation of cells migrating from the yolk-sac blood islands. In the mouse, the blood islands are connected by a capillary network by day 9 of gestation. A day later, with initiation of cardiac contraction, free communication between the blood islands of the yolk sac and the primordeal hemopoietic organs of the embryo occurs. Careful extirpation of the blood islands before development of communicating sinusoids results in a complete absence of blood cells within the embryonic circulation. Embryonic and fetal hemoglobin synthesis is chiefly or exclusively of the fetal type, and in human fetuses, comprises 85% of total hemoglobin at birth.

In early postnatal development, hemopoiesis becomes rapidly centered in bone marrow with a few foci of hemopoiesis remaining in the liver of pigs at birth and continuing in the spleen of mice throughout life. Unusual demands for hemopoiesis result in production returning to extramedullary sites. Throughout postnatal life, streams of primitive and uncommitted lymphocytes leave the bone marrow and undergo development in the thymic cortex into T cells and in the enteric mucosa into B cells. More recently, it has been demonstrated that the intestinal lymphoid tissue is a site for peripheral maturation of T cells analogous to that occurring in the thymus gland.[14] In general, mammals are not born with well-developed germinal centers unless there has been fetal infection and induction of terminal development of the B- and T-lymphocyte systems.[15]

FUNCTIONAL ANATOMY OF THE HEMOPOIETIC SYSTEM

Bone Marrow

In birds and mammals, a close relation between bone and hemopoiesis is a constant finding. As noted above, fetal hemopoiesis is largely erythroid. The full expression of all cell lines in maturity is largely confined to bone marrow. The relation between hemopoiesis and bone is sufficiently interdependent that in maturity, intramedullary blood production is predominately within 200 micrometers of bone. This intimate relation is the result of the pattern of blood flow in which capillaries of cortical bone derived from periosteal vessels arborize on the endosteal surface, forming a second capillary system that flows centripetally to drain into the central venous sinus of the bone marrow. Thus a bone–bone marrow portal capillary system exists, which suggests that blood that has traversed bone forms a preferential microenvironment for hemopoiesis. Remarkably, this relation is constant and responsible for the seeding of hemopoietic stem cells into ectopic or metaplastic bone.

In the neonate, bone marrow is solidly cellular, as remodeling of the cartilaginous framework for bones forms the initial marrow cavity. The marrow remains solidly hemopoietic in early postnatal life as the increase in body size and red cell mass requires highly accelerated red cell production. With the onset of maturity, bone marrow recedes to cancellous areas in the ends of long bones as well as the vertebrae and the flat bones, including ribs and calvarium. As hemopoiesis declines on a regional basis, the space is occupied by fat cells. Even in hemopoietic areas, the fat may occupy 50% of marrow volume under conditions of homeostasis. Conversion from red or hemopoietic to yellow or fatty marrow varies regionally with species. In humans and dogs, the iliac crest remains hemopoietic throughout life, but in cattle, the sternum or vertebral processes are the only reliable sites for bone marrow biopsy after 1 to 2 months of age.

Hemopoiesis is extravascular and occurs in solid tissue spaces between the marrow sinuses. The wall of the bone marrow sinus is trilaminar with the endothelium overlying a discontinuous basement membrane supported by the processes of reticular cells forming a fine supporting network that arborizes in marrow from the surface of bone and the adventitia of small arteries. The endothelial cells are without tight junctions, permitting specialized cells from the marrow to egress both between and through the endothelial membranes. Within the hemopoietic areas, there is an organization of trilineage production such that the nonmotile cells of the erythroid and megakaryocytic system are next to the endothelial surfaces, whereas granulopoiesis tends to occur more deeply within the marrow cords (Figs. 39.1 and 39.2).

The redness of bone marrow observed on gross examination is caused by blood within these thin-walled vascular sinuses. The walls of these sinuses are highly plastic, and the diameter of the sinuses may vary with the degree of marrow activity. Thus, the bone marrow may

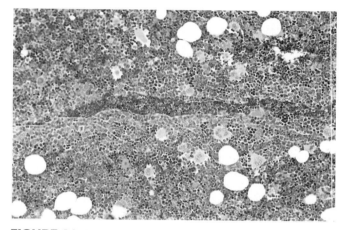

FIGURE 39.1 Central femoral bone marrow from a normal rat. The bone marrow is 70 to 90% hemopoietic in the normal young adult, and decreases to fairly equal portions of hemopoietic and fat cells with age. The marrow sinusoids drain centripetally into the central venous sinus for delivery to the peripheral circulation. The darker cells in the marrow represent islands of erythropoiesis, and the lighter staining areas on either side of the central vein are largely occupied by myeloid precursors and their progeny. H&E × 160.

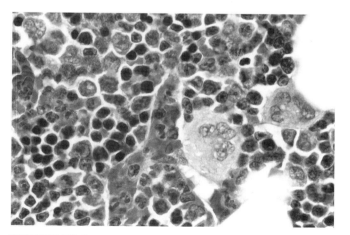

FIGURE 39.2 Details of Figure 39.1. A thin-walled capillary (center) is closely aligned with developing erythroid cells and megakaryocytes with the more motile myeloid cells tending to be further from the capillary wall. H&E × 800.

become solid and pale when there is hemopoietic hyperplasia and may even become infarcted in leukemias. In contrast, because the marrow is a closed cavity, sudden increases in demand for marrow cells, such as occurs in hemorrhagic anemia, acute infection or stem cell injury, result in contraction of the hemopoietic cords with corresponding dilation of the venous sinuses creating the appearance of a reddened marrow that may be erroneously described grossly as hyperactive. This distinction is important because in conditions of marrow failure, such as might occur at the acute stage of infection with feline panleukopenia or equine infectious anemia viruses, the marrow may appear grossly red, but this should not be interpreted as evidence of increased hemopoietic activity. When there is increased demand for hemopoiesis that persists for several weeks or months, the conversion of fat to red marrow occurs first in subendosteal areas that may form a cuff of hemopoietic marrow around the fatty central cavity of long bones. The process of conversion is slow; mature animals that have red marrow in the central cavity of long bones can be considered to have had increased demands for hemopoiesis for several months.

The cells of bone marrow consist of proliferative and maturation compartments of the myeloid (including monocytic), erythroid, and megakaryocytic systems as well as a small number of lymphocytes that are usually 5% or less of nucleated cells in normal animals.[10] Lymphoid germinal centers may occur in bone marrow but not in normal animals and can be considered indicative of prolonged immune stimulation. In addition to the specialized cells of the bone marrow, there are both myelinated and nonmyelinated nerve fibers that appear both to be sensory and to innervate blood vessels. Sensory capability of the bone marrow is immediately evident on aspiration of marrow from a nonanesthetized animal.

Thymus

In both architectural and cellular components, the thymus differs significantly from bone marrow. Although the bone marrow is cytologically diverse, containing a small population of pluripotential stem cells, plus proliferative and maturation phases of the erythroid myeloid and megakaryocytic cell lines, the marrow as a tissue is homogeneous. Thus, in the absence of neoplasia, red marrow anywhere in the body can be expected to have a similar proportion of its constituent cells. In contrast, the thymus is cytologically simple but unique in containing both lymphocytes and epithelial cells, but unlike marrow, it is architecturally complex in having a lobular structure differentiated into cortical and medullary areas (Figs. 39.3 and 39.4). The epithelial cells of the thymus are derived from the third and fourth pharyngeal pouches, which migrate in two streams to form paired lobes of the thymus within the anterior mediastinum. This migration occurs early in embryologic development and is followed by seeding of the thymus with progenitor cells from the blood islands of the yolk sac.

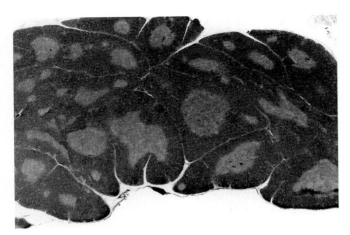

FIGURE 39.3 Thymus from a young adult male rat. The organ is composed of closely faceted lobules with a sharp distinction between the darker cortex and the lighter medullary areas of each lobule. H&E × 16.

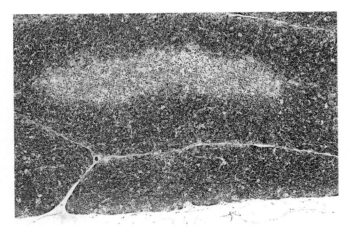

FIGURE 39.4 In mammals, the medulla and cortex are sharply delineated in young healthy animals, with the width of the cortices and medulla approximately equal to one-third the width of the lobe. H&E × 80.

The first stream of epithelial migration forms the isolated reticular epithelial cells of the cortex and the medulla of the adult thymic lobule. The second epithelial migration forms the thymic duct epithelium and later the Hassall's corpuscles of the thymic medulla. The early reticular epithelial migration forms loose cuffs around small vessels that persist in adult life and become obvious in conditions of lymphoid atrophy. Also, in early development, the second or ductular component of epithelium forms the branching system that communicates between the lobules of a single thymic lobe. These embryologic relations are important owing to the mimicry of embryologic events in thymic lesions of adult life. Thus, a thymic lesion with loss of corticomedullary distinction that might be medullary hyperplasia or thymoma can be differentiated by the presence of the reticular cuffs

around the vessels of a thymoma. These epithelial cuffs of thymic vessels form a barrier to bloodborne antigens and, because the thymus lacks afferent lymphatics, the prolymphocytes of marrow receive their immunologic training solely from the reticular epithelial cells. The medullary epithelium produces trophic hormones that assist lymphocytic colonization and are the source of cysts lined by ciliated epithelium that commonly develop in adult life but are seldom of clinical significance. An additional cellular component to the supporting connective tissue, vascular structures, lymphocytes, and epithelium of the thymus are known as the myoid cells because of their cross striations. They surround the Hassell's corpuscles (Fig. 39.5) and are important in the immunopathogenesis of myasthenia gravis.[16] In most species, the thymus reaches its maximal development about the time of puberty and then slowly decreases in size throughout adult life. An unusual antigenic stimulation during adolescent life may result in benign thymic hyperplasia to a remarkable degree, which in the calf, may result in a chain of thymic lobules that extend from the rami of the mandibles to the base of the heart.

At the physiologic level, the postnatal thymic cortex receives a continuous stream of uncommitted lymphocytes of bone marrow origin that undergo immunologic selection for tolerance to self-antigens. Uncommitted lymphocytes contact the reticular epithelial cells that form thin-walled pouches or caveolae in cortical tissue. Paradoxically, the thymic cortical lymphocytes have small densely stained nuclei without nucleoli, yet this is a region of intense cellular proliferation in which the majority of the progeny die and are removed by tingible body macrophages (Fig. 39.6). These latter cells become more prominent in conditions resulting in cortical lympholysis such as viral infection, irradiation, or corticosteroid therapy. In the normal state, the vesicular nuclei of the cortical macrophages resembles that of the

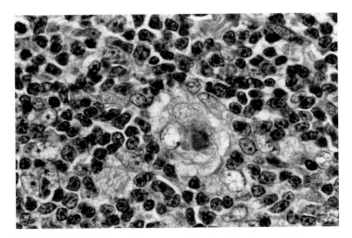

FIGURE 39.5 Hassall's corpuscle in the thymic medullary area consisting of concentric laminations of squamous epithelial cells. The surrounding lymphocytes are characteristically a mixture of small and medium cells with moderately abundant cytoplasm separating the nuclei and giving the medulla a less dense appearance on histological examination. H&E × 800.

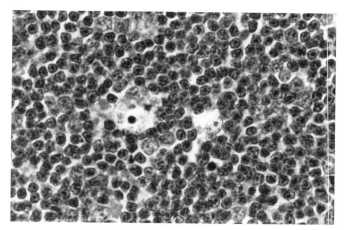

FIGURE 39.6 Thymic cortex composed of densely packed
small lymphocytes. A macrophage in the center has a larger, more
vesicular nucleus, and the cytoplasm contains several pyknotic
structures (tingible bodies) representing nuclei of apoptotic cortical
thymocytes. The larger vesicular nuclei above, below, and to the
right of the macrophage likely represent epithelial cells involved in
the self-recognition selection process of developing T lymphocytes.
H&E × 800.

reticular epithelial cells and may not be identifiable with
routine stains unless cytoplasmic nuclear debris is present. Marrow-derived lymphocytes entering the thymic
cortex have the cell surface molecules for selective homing to thymic cortical vascular endothelium, but they
lack helper, suppressor, or killer-cell functions. In gaining these characteristics on migration through the thymic cortex, thymocytes also acquire homing receptors
shortly before release by which most of the progeny
enter the paracortex of lymph nodes through the high
endothelial venules.

Medullary lymphocytes are larger than the cortical
cells with a larger and more lightly staining nucleus.
This greater cytoplasmic volume prevents tight packing
of nuclei giving the medullary area a less dense appearance on histologic examination (Fig. 39.5). Physiologic
development continues in the lymphocytes entering the
medullary areas, resulting in progeny with preferential
homing of cells to the intestinal mucosa and Peyer's
patches.

In young animals, particularly in rabbits, heterophils
are common in the lobular connective tissue of the thymus. Eosinophils may occasionally be found in the thymic connective tissues of other species, and mast cells
are present in the thymic capsules in most species and
are particularly frequent in the rat. Thymic hyperplasia
is accomplished largely through an increase in the number of lobules rather than increased lobule size, whereas
thymic atrophy results in a blurring of the corticomedullary distinction. Thymic function does not necessarily
vary in proportion to thymic size, and in the adult, a
small thymic remnant may be responsible for a persistent autoimmune disease. B lymphocytes are seldom a
normal component of the thymus, and the presence of
actual germinal centers within the thymus are consid-

ered a hallmark of autoimmune disease. Recent work
suggests that terminal maturation of T lymphocytes may
occur in the intestinal tract as well as in the thymus.[14]
It would not be surprising if similar activity was found
in both the lung and the skin, which would provide a
more comprehensive explanation for aberrant lymphoid
reactions in both benign and malignant states.

Spleen

The spleen is essentially an organ that filters blood
through a sinusoidal system. It has additional functions
in lymphopoiesis, antibody production, and hemopoiesis under conditions of increased demand for blood cells.
The latter is accomplished by colonization of sinusoids
with pluripotential stem cells. Species with the genetic
potential for athletic activity such as humans, dogs, cats,
and horses have spleens with a somewhat contractile
muscular capsule supported by internal and equally
contractile fibromuscular trabeculae. In contrast, species
that tend to group aggregations, such as ruminants for
protection against their more agile predators, tend to
have spleens whose capsules are largely connective tissue with less capability for contraction. In addition to
cellular components and antibodies, the spleen may also
produce some clotting factors, but the major hazard
to life after splenectomy appears to be bacteremia and
septicemia. The spleen forms early in embryonic life and
is a site of active erythropoiesis during the fetal period.
The spleen is both architecturally and cytologically complex. It not only contains a wide variety of cells that
may vary in proportion in reactive and disease states,
but it also has a diverse regional anatomy based on a
complex vascular system that has the added feature of
altering internal anatomy with changes in overall size
and volume.

The spleen is like the thymus in having efferent but
no afferent lymphatics. Thus, all antigen enters the
spleen through the blood vascular system. Both the major arterial supply and the venous outflow enter through
the hilus of the spleen and arborize together throughout
its length. This arborization is fairly random in mammals, but in reptiles there is a system somewhat analogous to the bone marrow with a major central venous
sinus. At the level of small- and medium-sized arterioles,
the vessels are sheathed in a cuff of small thymic-derived
lymphocytes known as the periarteriolar lymphoid
sheaths. Small branches from these central arteries give
rise to germinal centers that are foci of B-cell proliferation. Surrounding the dense cuff of small lymphocytes
constituting the periarteriolar lymphoid sheath is a more
loosely aggregated area of small lymphocytes constituting the mantle layer that is a mixture of T and B lymphocytes (Figs. 39.7 and 39.8). This layer of mantle cells also
surrounds the germinal centers that arise adjacent to the
central arterioles, and in these areas, a third layer of
lymphocytes, known as the marginal zone, with less
definite boundaries also of mixed phenotype occurs.
Whereas the cells of the periarteriolar sheath and germinal center are composed of resident cells with movement

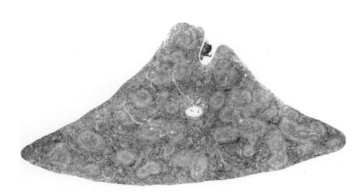

FIGURE 39.7 Cross section of spleen from a young adult male rat. At the architectural level of histologic examination, the spleen is occupied by multiple but dispersed round darker areas representing lymphoid nodules with the intervening lighter areas consisting of blood sinuses and extramedullary hemopoiesis. The lymphoid or white pulp areas can be seen to consist of central areas of darker tissue consisting of the periarteriolar lymphoid sheaths surrounded by the lighter mantle and marginal zone areas. H&E × 10.

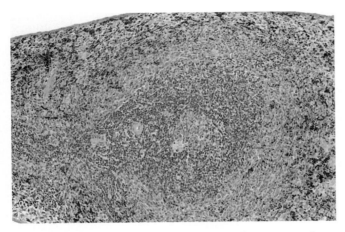

FIGURE 39.8 Details of Figure 39.7. Unlike larger mammals, rats tend not to have well-formed splenic germinal centers. In the center, a lighter zone constitutes the center of an ill-defined germinal center eccentric to and abutting a small muscular arteriole on the lower left margin. This center is surrounded by a cuff of darker mantle lymphocytes which, itself, has an outer envelope of lighter-staining marginal zone cells that interface with the surrounding splenic red pulp. H&E × 125.

largely through senescence and replenishment, the cells of the mantle layer tend to be in low-level interchange with the cells in the surrounding vascular sinuses, and cells in the marginal zone are in constant interchange with their environment and are most representative of leukocytes within the peripheral circulation. The small branches of the central arteriole may terminate in germinal centers or pass through mantle and

marginal zones to terminate in a penicillary array of small branches that feed directly into the sinusoids. The penicillary vessels are ensheathed by a few plump reticular cells forming a contractile ellipsoid that under neural and hormonal control adjust the level of blood entering venous sinuses.

The venous sinuses of the spleen constitute the expansile regions of the organ and thus may vary greatly in their content of blood in species with a high level of smooth muscle in the splenic capsule. The walls of the splenic sinusoids are unique in consisting of elongated endothelial cells arranged like the staves of a barrel, which are without tight junctions to their neighbors but are maintained in alignment by a discontinuous encirclement of fine reticular fibers. The lumen of these sinuses communicates directly to the exiting vein of the spleen, whereas the exterior of these veins is in contact with the filtering area of spleen consisting of macrophages suspended in a loose reticular supporting framework. It is estimated that under normal circumstances 97% of the arteriolar blood entering the spleen exits directly via the penicillary vessels into a major sinus and then quickly reenters the central circulation. The remaining 3% passes into the filtering extrasinusoidal area to regain the peripheral circulation by passing between the walls of the sinus endothelial cells. Immature and normal red cells and leukocytes readily achieve this transit back into the circulation, whereas aged red cells, those containing Howell–Jolly bodies, senescent leukocytes, and foreign material are phagocytosed by the macrophages of the red pulp areas (Fig. 39.9). By this process, the entire blood volume passes through the filtering system of the spleen once each day. In a muscular spleen in the contracted state, all of the blood would pass directly from the arteriole to the venous system in a closed circulation permitting maximal use of blood cells in the systemic circulation. In contrast, any influence that tends to cause the splenic capsule to dilate, such as anesthesia, portal hypertension caused by hepatic fibrosis or sig-

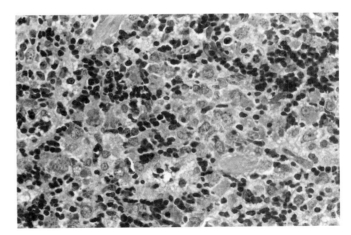

FIGURE 39.9 Splenic sinus area demonstrating the interposition of large hemosiderin-bearing macrophages and thin-walled capillaries facilitating the filtering system of the spleen. H&E × 500.

nificant increase in extrasinusoidal macrophages, or extramedullary hemopoiesis, results in a greater proportion of blood passing through the filtering system. Because of the slow flow of blood through the red pulp, there is in these areas lower glucose, cholesterol, and pH than in the central circulation. Collectively, these biochemical changes can contribute to a premature aging of red cells and result in increased destruction. Thus, an enlarged spleen of any cause is a distinct hazard to red cell life span. The same implications apply for blood platelets, whereas the granulocytes are less affected by these conditions because they are normally replaced at the rate of 3 to 4 times per day.[18]

Various changes occur in the spleen in response to systemic states. Acute toxic diseases result in lysis of lymphocytes in the germinal centers and replacement by residual proteinaceous debris referred to as follicular hyalinosis. Diagnosticians are aided by the fact that nuclear debris after acute lympholysis is cleared within 24 hours, but the hyalin debris may remain for weeks or months. In systemic amyloidosis, the germinal centers may become sites of amyloid deposition, whereas atrophic changes caused by starvation, aging, cancer, or chemotherapy may result in atrophy that affects one or both of the thymic-dependent arteriolar sheaths or bone-marrow-dependent germinal center systems. In chronic hemolytic anemias, there is an expected significant increase in hemosiderin-bearing macrophages in sinus areas. Iron deposition may occur normally in the connective tissue of the spleen, particularly in aged dogs.

Lymph Nodes

Histogenetically, lymph nodes form at the confluence of an afferent lymphatic sprig with a dilated sheath of vascular serosa. The blood vessels covered by the serosal sheath then produce a fine arborization of vessels within this area of dilation, thus forming an architectural framework for lymphocytic colonization. The vascular distribution to lymph nodes is highly organized with the arteriolar and the venous branches arborizing through the medullary cords to form microcirculatory units that become the functional basis for germinal center formation. Specialized high endothelial venules form in the paracortical areas between, and never within, the germinal centers and present specific adhesion molecules by which transmural lymphocyte traffic from blood to node paracortex is regulated.[19] The normal development of lymph nodes depends on cells and antigens entering through the afferent lymphatics that drain into the peripheral capsule of the node.

Nonactivated lymphocytes apparently circulate randomly in the blood and vascular systems; however, once these cells are involved in antigen recognition in the node cortex, their further migration becomes altered. Activated B cells migrate preferentially to mucosa-associated lymphoid tissues, whereas T cells preferentially migrate to peripheral lymph nodes.[20] This selectivity is achieved through recirculating lymphocytes selectively binding to the endothelium of high endothe-

lial venules while passing within vessels lined by other types of endothelium. Lymphocyte binding to endothelium is generally followed by migration into the associated tissues. The interaction between lymphocyte and high endothelium seems to codepend on endothelial height related to the intensity of lymphocyte passage. On the other hand, antigenic stimulation of a lymph node results in an increase in prominence and number of high endothelial or postcapillary venules, and macrophage depletion abrogates this effect.[21] Blockage of the afferent lymphatic results in lymphoid atrophy of varying degrees and in flattening of the endothelium of postcapillary venules.[22]

This system of organ-specific lymphocyte homing receptors functions in neoplastic as well as in inflammatory conditions with the spread of malignant lymphocytes limited by their ability to migrate into various tissues. Malignant lymphocytes tend to mimic their benign counterparts such that B-cell neoplasms have binding behavior similar to that of reactive B cells and bind to endothelial venules in various sites. Thus, the spread of lymphoma to lymphoid structures is not a function of the tumor cells' ability to enter the peripheral blood, but rather it is an indication that the cells have successfully bound to site-specific endothelial venules.[23] Remarkably, migration of lymphocytes through the postcapillary venule endothelium is largely transcellular rather than via the intracellular spaces.[24]

The afferent lymphatics, the peripheral capsule, and the subcapsular sinus are the delivery systems whereby lymph, blood cells, and antigens are delivered to the interior of the lymph node (Fig. 39.10). The peripheral capsule is thin and taut in conditions in which there has been rapid enlargement of a lymph node of benign or malignant causes. On the other hand, lymph node atrophy results in the histologic appearance of a capsule that is thickened and wavy, with the peripheral sinus

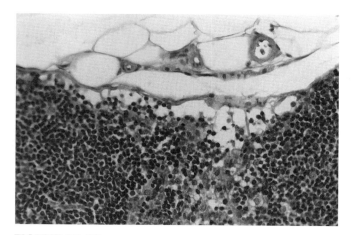

FIGURE 39.10 Mesenteric lymph node from a normal male rat. Outer cortex with an afferent lymphatic leading into the peripheral sinus beneath the node capsule. The sinus is moderately open and contains a few cells in transit, whereas to the left and right, the sinus is compressed by developing germinal centers. H&E × 300.

widened. Chronic stimulation of the node results in sclerosis of the capsule with significant thickening and with the formation of fibrous raphe that penetrates the cortex of the node and may terminate in a dense collagenous network within the node medulla. Remarkably, in cattle and likely in other species, the lymph node capsule is contractile and under neural control, thus assisting lymph flow.[25] Benign lymphoid hyperplasia may compress the peripheral capsule but never destroys it, whereas in lymphoma the peripheral sinus tends to be only focally invaded in indolent small cell lymphomas and tends to be diffusely infiltrated in aggressive high-grade lymphoma. Colonization of the node capsule by lymphocytes is not a criterion of malignancy and neither is colonization of perinodal tissues. Benign diseases characterized by persistent and high-level antigenemia, such as equine infectious anemia and bovine trypanosomiasis, are both characterized by lymphoid colonization of the lymph node capsule and perinodal structures.

The lymphoid cortex and germinal centers form the first order of filtering system through channels extending from the inner lining of the peripheral sinus to the microcirculatory units in the node cortex. A fully developed germinal center is a highly organized structure consisting of a progression of cell types in a proliferative gradient that provides the germinal center cut in proper orientation with an easily recognized polarity (Fig. 39.11). This polarity is always oriented to the source of antigen regardless of tissue in which the germinal center is located, be it tonsil, Peyer's patch, or lymph node cortex.[26] The polarity gradient of the germinal center consists of a cuff of small lymphocytes at the superficial pole that is just beneath the inner lining of the peripheral sinus in a normally stimulated lymph node. Antigen sorting and processing occurs through a focusing process with the dendritic reticular cells in the

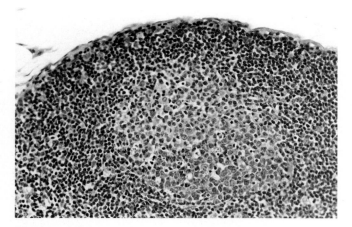

FIGURE 39.11 Node cortex with germinal center having a polarity aimed at antigens being delivered from the peripheral sinus into the superficial pole of small lymphocytes. In the middle of the reaction, there are a mixture of small and large lymphocytes with macrophages removing apoptotic lymphocyte nuclei. Near the bottom of the picture, the deep-pole area consists of large lymphocytes selected for immunoglobulin production against a single antigen. H&E × 250.

middle of the germinal center that is characterized by a high level of tingible body macrophages. The deep pole of the germinal center is characterized by closely packed large lymphocytes, numerous mitoses, and a lot of variation in chromatin and nuclear outline. This entire progression of cells is surrounded by a mantle layer of small lymphocytes. Thus the architecture of the germinal center may be likened to an egg that if sectioned through its long axis presents a progression of apical albumin and yolk and a deep cuff of albumin, whereas, in contrast, if the egg was cut across at its maximum width, the structure would largely be yolk with a fairly thin and uniform rim of albumin. For this reason, in follicular hyperplasias, the germinal centers beneath the node capsule are usually sectioned in a plane that allows their antigen orientation to be recognized, but those in medullary areas are oriented in various planes such that all levels of the proliferative progression of cells are viewed. This point is worth emphasizing because it is essential to recognize polarity of germinal centers to distinguish benign and atypical follicular hyperplasias from follicular lymphomas. Follicular lymphomas whether of small cleaved cells, mixed-cell type, or large cells, have a mantle of small lymphocytes as in benign lymphoid proliferations, but the mantle cuff may be thinned and discontinuous. Further distinction between true follicular lesions, whether benign or malignant, and pseudofollicular lesions is that the postcapillary venules are always between the follicular or nodular proliferations and are never within them.

The dendritic reticulum cells are apparently bone marrow derived. Langerhans's cells from the skin may migrate to nodes and form dendritic antigen-focusing cells.[27–29] Phenotypic characteristics of dendritic cells vary with anatomic site.[30–32] Ultrastructurally, the dendritic cells are characterized by cytoplasmic tendrils that are joined by tight junctions. In conditions of lymphoid depletion, the dendritic cells become exposed in germinal centers as the eosinophilic background of large pale cells. In highly toxigenic reactions, there may be an amorphous accumulation of protein within the germinal centers of node and spleen termed "follicular hyalinosis," which was noted to be the characteristic lesion in fatal cases of human diphtheria. It is suspected that the dendritic cells themselves may be the cell of origin for certain types of tumors that have a sarcomatous appearance.[33–35] Degenerative changes in lymph nodes may result in mineralization of the germinal centers that may be penetrated by thick-walled vessels, resulting in a lesion known as lymphoid hyperplasia of the hyaline-vascular type. This disease is rare in humans and animals and is seen most often in aged sheep and goats.

One of the more difficult decisions in examining lymph nodes is the distinction between florid hyperplasia and lymphoma. The syndrome of transformation of germinal centers to malignant disease is described in humans,[36,37] and it seems that in animals, chronic lymphoid proliferation of any cause can be a serious risk factor for lymphoma. Examples of this type of association in animals includes infection with feline leukemia virus (FeLV) and bovine leukemia virus (BLV) and immunoproliferative small intestinal disease (IPSID) of idiopathic cause. A type of nodular or follicular lymphoma in which the malignant cells are derived from the corona of small cells surrounding the germinal center occurs in both humans and animals and is known as mantle-cell lymphoma. Morphologically, the disease is characterized by coalescing proliferations of lymphocytes surrounding fading germinal centers.[38,39]

In the paracortex of lymph nodes, there are nodular structures distinct from germinal centers, which are particularly common in the mesenteric nodes of mature rats. These deep cortical units form as a result of antigenic stimulation, with cellular input from a distinct afferent lymphatic radical (Fig. 39.12). They form semicircular or oval structures beneath the germinal centers of the outer cortex and are most easily seen in lymph nodes in which there is some degree of paracortical atrophy, making the nodules more apparent. Central areas of these nodules are somewhat mottled in appearance owing to varying proportions of large and small lymphocytes with some macrophages and postcapillary venules (Fig. 39.13). The edges of the nodules gradually meld with the surrounding medullary cords and sinuses and are apparently the areas where cells exiting these nodules enter the efferent lymph channels. The main significance of the deep cortical nodules is to recognize that they are normal structures and not to confuse them with malignant lymphoid proliferation.[19,40]

The medullary cords and medullary sinuses may best be considered together since they form an interwoven matrix that may wax and wane in unison or at the expense of each other (Fig. 39.14). A medullary unit consists of a radical of vascular structures from the deep pole of the node hilus consisting of an artery, vein, and lymphatics surrounded by a variable amount of connective tissue and invested with a thin single-cell-thick endothelial covering. These vascular structures form the

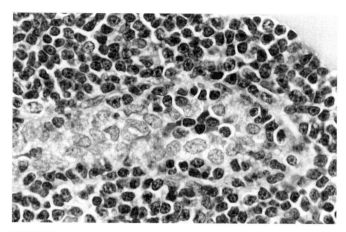

FIGURE 39.13 Node paracortex with a high endothelial postcapillary venule in the center. Several lymphocytes within the wall of the venule can be seen to be in transluminal transit exiting the blood to enter the node cortex. A thin-walled lymphatic is present in the upper right, with the lumen containing lymph but no red cells. H&E × 800.

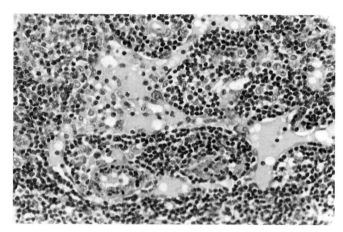

FIGURE 39.14 Lymph-node medulla with cords and sinuses. The cords are densely cellular and surrounded by a thin endothelial membrane with the sinuses containing a few fixed macrophages and cells in transit in a background of lymph. H&E × 300.

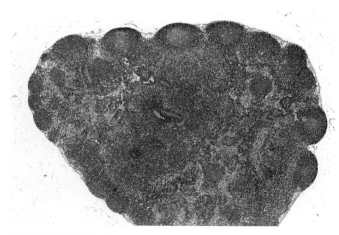

FIGURE 39.12 Cross section of rat mesenteric lymph node. The periphery of the node is occupied by germinal centers with lighter central areas occupying the top and right side of the node. The medullary cords and sinuses lie along the right side of the node and abut a large uniformly dense oval deep cortical unit that lies obliquely across the cut surface of the node. H&E × 30.

center of many of the medullary sinuses as they are seen in a cross-sectional profile. The sinus area constitutes the space between the endothelial wall of the vascular structures and the similar endothelial wall of the medullary cords. The medullary sinuses may extend up to the inner surface of the subcapsular sinus in nodes in which there is severe paracortical and follicular atrophy. Such a circumstance occurs in the mesenteric nodes of cattle dying of the acute form of Bovine Virus Diarrhea with massive B-cell lysis in which the sinuses tend to be filled with macrophages, thus forming sinus histiocytosis.

The cellularity of the medullary sinuses varies widely depending on the cellular economy of the animal. In diseases characterized by chronic immune stimulation, there is usually a high level of sinus macrophages that are apparently suspended in a syncytial network somewhat similar to the sinus areas of the spleen. In nodes, draining areas of chronic dermatitis, the macrophages of the superficial cortex, and those of the medullary sinuses frequently contain abundant normal-appearing melanin granules. Similarly, nodes draining areas of hemorrhage have numerous hemosiderin-bearing macrophages in medullary areas. The transit of red cells from areas of hemorrhage to the node medulla is surprisingly rapid and may occur during excisional biopsy of lymph nodes if there is an opportunity for hemorrhage into the afferent lymph to reach the peripheral sinus. The process of erythrocyte intracellular degradation is remarkably rapid and has been shown to be approximately 6 hours,[41] thus any amount of erythrophagocytosis by medullary macrophages must be looked on as a recent event.

The medullary sinuses may become involved in septic processes but usually not until there are also foci of neutrophilic or granulomatous reactions in the outer cortex. Foci of metastatic carcinoma appear in the medullary sinuses but usually not until they are much more evident in the peripheral sinus. Infiltration of lymph nodes draining a mast cell tumor occurs with isolated tumor cells suspended in the meshwork of the medullary sinuses, while individual cells or small clusters of tumor cells will be more obvious in the peripheral sinus. In leukemias and lymphomas, when there is impending marrow failure, the medullary sinuses may be empty and compressed both as a result of medullary cord expansion and phthisis of the marrow precursors by the tumor cells.

The medullary cords contain the recirculating lymphocytes composed of small or medium lymphocytes or plasma cells. Evidence for the persistence plasma cells is seen by their accumulation in medullary cords of nodes where the germinal centers have become atrophic through steroid or antineoplastic treatment. The fine reticular network of the medullary cords forms a fertile microenvironment for bone marrow stem cells in situations in which there is significant marrow hyperplasia or marrow phthisis with displacement of pluripotent stem cells. In lymphoproliferative diseases with extra medullary hemopoiesis in the medullary cords, it is likely that the disease has invaded marrow or is primarily a leukemia. In myeloid leukemias, the malignant cells also colonize the medullary cords, and under these circumstances, there may be both tumor and benign extramedullary hemopoiesis coexisting, and with progression there may be extrusion of the benign cells that then colonize the medullary sinuses.

LYMPHOID SYSTEMS OF BODY SURFACES

In the context referred to herein, body surfaces include the skin as well as the lining of the upper and the lower respiratory and enteric systems. The hemopoietic organs of the body are often referred to as primary, referring to the bone marrow and the thymus and, to a lesser extent, the spleen and the lymph nodes. Secondary lymphoid organs constitute the focal and diffuse lymphoid populations of skin, lung, and enteric systems. In the bird, it is clear that the stream of cells from the bone marrow gain their orientation to T-cell function in the thymus and B-cell function in the bursa of Fabricius. This segmentation of central and peripheral training grounds lead to the feeling that in mammals the Peyer's patches and diffuse lymphoid areas of the intestinal lamina propria may constitute a mammalian counterpart to the avian bursa. As information is gained, it appears that these distinctions are not as clear-cut and that the gut may function as training ground for both B and T lymphocytes. It is likely that the same situation occurs in the lymphoid tissue of the lung and, to a lesser extent, in the skin.[42] Such a process would make it easier to understand the array of immune-mediated diseases that may affect each of these three body surface areas in a fairly selective manner. What has become clear on body surface areas is that intraepithelial lymphocytes in all three of these locations are not primarily cells on the way to being lost to the exterior but rather cells in training, which after their specific sensitization in surface areas return to deeper lymphoid structures to perform a specific function in differentiation and proliferation.

In the skin, keratinocytes constitute 85% of the epidermis, with the remaining cells constituting melanocytes, Langerhans' cells, Merkel cells, and dendritic cells of uncertain type (Figs. 39.15 and 39.16). In humans and in cattle, the Langerhans' cells contain a typical rod-shaped cytoplasmic organelle visible only on ultrastructural examination with a unipolar bulb. The Langerhans' cells are products of the mononuclear-phagocytic system and constitute the major antigen-presenting cell of the epidermis.[43] The presence of the specific cytoplasmic organelle, known as a Birbeck granule, permitted identification of Langerhans' cells in the paracortex of lymph nodes draining skin. It is assumed that these cells gain a form of antigenic training in the epidermis and dermis

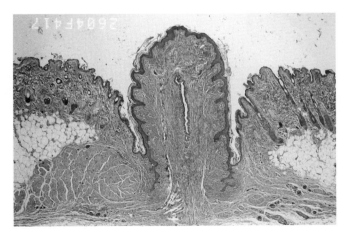

FIGURE 39.15 Abdominal skin with nipple from a normal female rat. Normal architecture of all structures without focal accumulation of inflammatory or immune cells. H&E × 10.

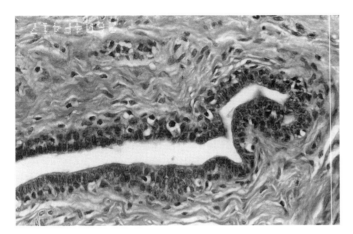

FIGURE 39.16 Details of Figure 39.15, showing the nipple duct lining with a moderate number of intraepithelial lymphocytes appearing as small dark nuclei within a clear vacuole. H&E × 300.

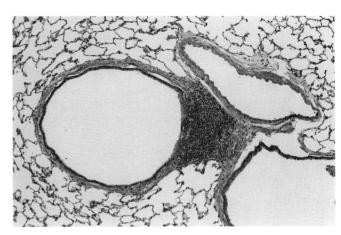

FIGURE 39.17 Lung from a normal male rat with an eccentric area of peribronchiolar lymphoid proliferation lying beneath normal and intact respiratory epithelium. H&E × 80.

and then migrate to the local lymph nodes and appear to be the index cell involved in contact sensitization of the skin. Both T and B cells are present in the skin, and there, their function is largely unknown. A fairly consistent proportion of cutaneous lymphocytes are suppressor T cells that may be resident in situ to dampen cutaneous immune sensitization.

The mucosal-associated lymphoid tissue of the respiratory and enteric systems is in common in the tonsils and pharyngeal areas, which in humans, is collectively known as Waldeyer's ring. In the respiratory system, the epithelium of the nasal mucosa as well as the larynx, trachea, and bronchi are infiltrated to a variable degree with lymphocytes and to a lesser extent neutrophils and macrophages. Mucosal infiltration is also more prominent above areas of submucosal lymphoid proliferation such as occurs in the tonsil and in bronchiolar-associated lymphoid tissues. In general, the level of reactivity in these areas is related to the level of antigenic stimulation. Lymphoid proliferation in the tonsil is usually characterized by prominent germinal center formation, whereas in the lower lung, in conditions of health, the lymphoid tissue may be minimal and restricted to diffuse accumulations of cells between the bronchial epithelium and the supporting smooth muscle and cartilaginous plates (Fig. 39.17).[44] The effect of air quality, in terms of freedom from dust particles and airborne infectious agents, is immediately apparent in the histology of laboratory animals. Those animals maintained in facilities in which the air is well filtered have minimal bronchiolar-associated lymph node tissue and few intraepithelial lymphocytes. In contrast, animals maintained in less pristine circumstances characteristically have diffuse lymphoid proliferation in the proximal trachea and laryngeal areas with heavy and mixed cellular infiltration of the surface epithelium. In the lower lung, the lymphoid proliferation, which may contain germinal centers but is usually diffuse, may be of sufficient volume to partially occlude airways. As in other areas, the lymph nodes draining the lung at the base of the heart and in the caudal medias-

tinum bear the evidence of past environmental experiences, including contact with smoke and other inhaled particulate matter.

The gut-associated lymphoid tissue forms a fairly continuous chain from the oral cavity to the anus, although there are generally few lymphocytes in the epithelium and mucosa of the esophagus. Lymphoid proliferation with germinal center formation is somewhat common beneath the gastric epithelium where lymphomas are fairly common in both humans and animals. In recent years, with discovery of the association between Helicobacter and human gastric ulceration, it has become apparent that most of the lymphoid tissue present in these cases is antigen dependent and rapidly recedes with long-term antibiotic therapy. Even more remarkably, cases of human gastric lymphoma, in at least early stages of development, seem antigen-dependent and may regress with antibiotic treatment alone. The organized areas of lymphoid tissue in the lower small intestine, including the Peyer's patches, are estimated to equal the thymus gland in young animals (Fig. 39.18). The epithelium overlying the intestinal germinal centers is generally devoid of goblet cells and villi and glandular crypts are absent (Fig. 39.19). In these areas, the epithelium contains specialized cells with complex folding of the surface epithelium known as M cells. M cells enfold lymphocytes within their membranes and function as antigen trephocytic cells able to metabolize particulate antigen and instruct the associated lymphocytes to specific immune reaction.[45,46] Much of the immunoglobulin produced in these areas is of the gamma A immunoglobulin (IgA) type with luminal and mucosal concentrations higher than that in the blood, demonstrating local production. Humans and animals are frequently affected with a destructive sensitization of lymphoid tissue in the small intestine, resulting in the florid proliferation of lymphoid cells in the lamina propria of the intestine known as lymphocytic-plasmacytic enteritis. When persistent, this lesion may become malignant, and full-blown intestinal lymphoma is seen. Malignancy in this

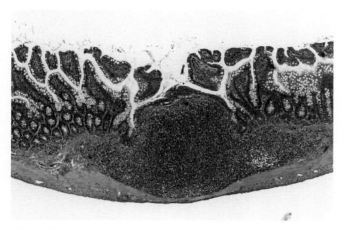

FIGURE 39.18 Small intestine of normal male rat. A focal submucosal proliferation of lymphocytes in a dome area characterized by absent villi and modified epithelium to assist antigen recognition and sorting. H&E × 50.

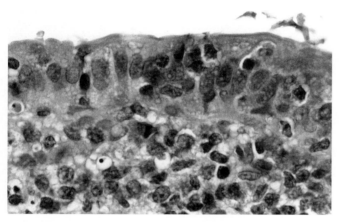

FIGURE 39.19 Details of Figure 39.18 at the mucosal surface. The epithelium is modified to contain M cells that have a deeply folded cellular membranes that enclose intraepithelial lymphocytes. The M cells are capable of uptake and of processing antigen from the intestinal lumen and providing immune instruction to maturing lymphocytes. An M cell to the left of the center is surrounded by a somewhat clear area of cytoplasm with the intraepithelial lymphocytes appearing as small dark nuclei approximately half the size of the epithelial nuclei. H&E × 800.

area is characterized by a lymphoepithelial lesion in which the tumor cells are observed invading and destroying mucosal glands. Remarkably, the mucosal-associated lymphoid tumors seem highly targeted to the mucosal system, and surgical excision of focal lymphoid tumor in the intestinal tract may result in prolonged remission.

HEMOPOIETIC SYSTEM AS AN ORGAN RESPONSIVE TO PHYSIOLOGIC CHALLENGES

In conditions of homeostasis, the central or primary and peripheral or secondary organs of the hemopoietic and immune systems are maintained by the normal turnover of cells in the peripheral circulation and in the various hemopoietic and lymphopoietic organs. The system is facilitated by a low level of circulation of hemopoietic stem cells that are capable of seeding peripheral tissues as required and on a complex interaction of trophic hormones called interleukins, which titer the level of production to the level of need in various body sites. It is apparent that all animals, including humans, live in a fairly constant but low level of inflammatory response that maintains normal functions and freedom from infectious agents. Evidence for this interpretation is present in the hematology of germ-free animals in which the numbers of circulating granulocytes are reduced to low levels, and peripheral blood lymphocytes are reduced to a proportionately lesser degree with a proportionate increase in erythroid precursors in marrow that supports a normal level of circulating red cells. In a similar fashion, humans and animals with congenital immune deficiencies have a characteristic loss of B- or T-dependent areas in peripheral lymphoid tissues or of both systems in combined immunodeficiency. At the other end of the spectrum, chronic benign stimulation of both the hemopoietic and the lymphopoietic systems may, over a period of months or years, result in conversion to a malignant process. In the bone marrow, this is seen in various myeloid dysplasias usually associated with peripheral cytopenias and in lymphoid tissues by chronic follicular hyperplasias. It is apparent in viewing lymphoproliferative lesions in various tissue areas that lymphomas of the skin, gut, and lymphoid tissues are frequently observed in a background of chronic benign hyperplastic reaction that may have persisted for a matter of months or years.

Taken as a total functional organ system, immune and hemopoietic systems are remarkable for their diversity of responsiveness and for the wealth of information that is available through careful examination and interpretation of reactions in these systems as defined in the succeeding pages of this volume.

REFERENCES

1. **Haden RL.** The origin of the microscope, Ann Med Hist, Ser 1939;3(1):30–44.
2. **Kass AM.** Dr. Thomas Hodgkin's friendship with Sir Moses Montefiore. N Engl J Med 1984;310:401–404.
3. **Seufert W, Seufert WD.** The recognition of leukemia as a systemic disease. J Hist Med 1982;37:34–50.
4. **Craddock CG.** Defenses of the body. In: Wintrobe MM, ed. Blood pure and eloquent. New York: McGraw Hill, 1980;13:420.
5. **Castle WB.** The conquest of pernicious anemia. In: Wintrobe MM, ed. Blood pure and eloquent. New York: McGraw Hill, 1980;10:283–317.
6. **Ratnoff OD.** Why do people bleed? In: Wintrobe MM, ed. Blood pure and eloquent. New York: McGraw Hill, 1980;18:625.
7. **Neumann E.** Eüeber die Bedeutung des Knochenmarkes für die Butbildung. Zentralbl Med Weissensch 1868;6:689.
8. **Bizzozero G.** Sulla funzion hematopoetica del midollo delle ossa. Zentralbl Med Weissensch 1868;6:885.
9. **Talbot JH.** Biographical history of medicine. New York: Grune and Stratton, 1970;916.
10. **Van Furth R, Cohn ZA, Hirsch JG, Humphrey JH, Spector WG, Langevoort NL.** The mononuclear phagocyte system: a new classification of macrophages, monocytes, and their precursor cells. Bull Wld Hlth Org 1972;46:845–852.
11. **Diamond LK.** The story of our blood groups. In: Wintrobe MM, ed. Blood pure and eloquent. New York: McGraw Hill, 1980;20:691.
12. **Till JE, McCulloch AE.** A direct measurement of the radiation sensitivity of normal mouse bone marrow cells. Radiation Research 1961;14:213–222.

13. **Sell S.** Immunology, immunopathology and immunity. 4th ed. New York: Elsevier, 1987;9–13.
14. **Lefrançois L, Puddington L.** Extrathymic intestinal T-cell development: virtual reality? Immunology Today 1995;16:16–21.
15. **Metcalf D, Moore MAS.** Hematopoietic cells. In: Embryonic aspects of haemopoiesis. New York: Elsevier, 1971;4:172–266.
16. **Valli VE, Villeneuve DC, Reed B, Barsoum N, Smith Gl.** Evaluation of blood and bone marrow, rat. In: Jones TC et al., eds. Hematopoietic system. Monographs on pathology of laboratory animals. Berlin: Springer-Verlag, 1990;9–26.
17. **Shier KJ.** The thymus according to Schambacher: medullary ducts and reticular epithelium of the thymus and thymomas. Cancer 1981;48:1183–1199.
18. **Schmidt EE, McDonald IC, and Groom AC.** Circulatory pathways in the sinusal spleen of the dog. A study by scanning electron microscopy of microcorrosion casts. J Morphol 1983;178:1111–1123.
19. **Belisle C, Sainte-Marie G, Peng F-S.** Tridimensional study of the deep cortex of the rat lymph node. Am J Pathol 1982;107:70–78.
20. **Duijvestijn A, Hamann A.** Mechanisms and regulation of lymphocyte migration. Immunol Today 1989;10:23–28.
21. **Mebius RE, Bauer J, Twisk AJT, Breve J, Kraal G.** The functional activity of high endothelial venules: a role for the subcapsular sinus macrophages in the lymph node. Immunobiol 1991;182:277–291.
22. **Hoshi J, Kamiya K, Aijima H, Yoshida K, Endo E.** Histological observations on rat popliteal lymph nodes after blockage of their afferent lymphatics. Arch Histo Jap 1985;48:135–148.
23. **Stauder R, Hamader S, Fasching B, Kemmler G, Thaler J, Huber H.** Adhesion to high endothelial venules: a model for dissemination mechanisms in non-Hodgkins' lymphoma. Blood 1993;82:262–267.
24. **Farr AG, De Bruyn PPH.** The mode of lymphocyte migration through postcapillary venule endothelium in lymph node. Am J Anat 1975;143:59–92.
25. **Hughes GA, Allen JM.** Neural modulation of bovine mesenteric lymph node contraction. Exp Physiol 1993;78:663–674.
26. **Millikin PD.** Anatomy of germinal centers in human lymphoid tissue. Arch Path 1966;82:499–505.
27. **Cumberbatch M, Gould SJ, Peters SW, Kimber I.** MHC class II expression by Langerhans' cells and lymph node dendritic cells: possible evidence for maturation of Langerhans' cells following contact sensitization. Immunol 1991;74:414–419.
28. **Fossum S.** Lymph-borne dendritic leucocytes do not recirculate, but enter the lymph node paracortex to become interdigitating cells. Scand J Immunol 1988;27:97–105.
29. **Shamoto M., Shinzato M, Hosokawa S, Kaneko C, Hakuno T, Nomoto K.** Langerhans cells in the lymph node: mirror section and immunoelectron microscopic studies. Virchows Archiv B Cell Pathol 1992;61:337–341.
30. **Petrasch S, Perez-Alvarez C, Schmitz J, Kosco M, Brittinger G.** Antigenic phenotyping of human follicular dendritic cells isolated from nonmalignant and malignant lymphatic tissue. Eur J Immunol 1990;20:1013–1018.
31. **Tew JG, Thorbecke G, Steinman RM.** Dendritic cells in the immune response: characteristics and recommended nomenclature (a report from the reticuloendothelial society committee on nomenclature). J Reticulo Soc 1982;31:371–380.
32. **Van Der Valk P, van der Loo EM, Jansen J, Daha MR, Meijer CJLM.** Analysis of lymphoid and dendritic cells in human lymph node, tonsil and spleen. A study using monoclonal and heterologous antibodies. Cell Pathol 1984;45:169–185.
33. **Monda L, Warnke R, Rosai J.** A primary lymph node malignancy with features suggestive of dendritic reticulum cell differentiation. A report of 4 cases. Am J Pathol 1986;122:562–572.
34. **Rabkin MS, Kjeldsberg CR, Hammond ME, Wittwer CT, Nathwani B.** Clinical, ultrastructural immunohistochemical and DNA content analysis of lymphomas having features of interdigitating reticulum cells. Cancer 1988;61:1594–1601.
35. **Van Der Valk P, Ruiter DJ, Den Ottolander GJ, Te Velde J, Spaander PJ, Meijer CJLM.** Dendritic reticulum cell sarcoma? Four cases of a lymphoma probably derived from dendritic reticulum cells of the follicular compartment. Histopathology 1982;6:269–287.
36. **Ferry JA, Zukerberg LR, Harris NL.** Florid progressive transformation of germinal centers. A syndrome affecting young men, without early progression to nodular lymphocyte predominance Hodgkin's disease. Am J Surg Pathol 1992;16:252–258.
37. **Schnitzer B.** Reactive lymphadenopathies. In: Knowles DN, ed. Neoplastic hematopathology. Baltimore: Williams & Wilkins, 1992;14:427–457.
38. **Koopman G, Pals ST.** Cellular interactions in the germinal center: role of adhesion receptors and significance for the pathogenesis of AIDS and malignant lymphoma. Immunol Rev 1992;126:21–45.
39. **Poppema S, Kaleta J, Hugh J, Visser L.** Neoplastic changes involving follicles: morphological, immunophenotypic and genetic diversity of lymphoproliferations derived from germinal center and mantle zone. Immunol Rev 1992;126:164–178.
40. **Van Rooijen N.** The "in situ" immune response in lymph nodes: a review. Anat Rec 1987; 218:359–364.
41. **Sasaki K.** Three-dimensional analysis of erythrophagosomes in rat mesenteric lymph node macrophages. Am J Anat 1990;188:373–380.
42. **Walsh LJ, Lavker RM, Murphy GF.** Biology of disease. Determinants of immune cell trafficking in the skin. Lab Invest 1990;63:592–600.
43. **Streilein JW, Bergstresser PR.** Langerhans cells: antigen presenting cells of the epidermis. Immunobiol 1984;168:285–300.
44. **Semenzato G, Bortolin M, Facco M, Tassinari C, Sancetta R, Agostini C.** Lung lymphocytes: origin, biological functions, and laboratory techniques for their study in immune-mediated pulmonary disorders. Crit Rev Clin Lab Sci 1996;33:423–455.
45. **Fujimura Y, Hosobe M, Kihara T.** Ultrastructural study of M cells from colonic lymphoid nodules obtained by colonoscopic biopsy. Dig Dis Sci 1992;37:1089–1098.
46. **Parsons KR, Bland AP, Hall GA.** Follicle associated epithelium of the gut associated lymphoid tissue of cattle. Vet Pathol 1991;28:22–29.

CHAPTER 40

Biology of Lymphocytes and Plasma Cells

• MICHAEL J. DAY

The lymphoid cells are the key components of the adaptive immune system. Several lymphoid subsets are now defined (Table 40.1), and these cells regulate the production of antibodies (humoral immunity) and are responsible for cell-mediated immune effects such as cytotoxicity or delayed-type hypersensitivity. Animals that have genetic inability to produce normal lymphoid cells (severe combined immunodeficiency) are profoundly immunodeficient and readily succumb to infectious disease.[1]

Lymphocyte subsets may be defined:

- phenotypically, by the expression of particular surface molecules
- anatomically, by their developmental pathways and distribution within lymphoid tissue
- functionally, by their end effects in an immune response that relates to expression of particular membrane molecules and the release of specific profiles of soluble factors (cytokines).

Lymphocyte biology is best defined in humans and experimental rodents, but most features are highly conserved and have parallels in veterinary species.

T LYMPHOCYTES

Definition and Development

T lymphocytes are defined by the expression of a T-cell receptor (TCR) that confers a unique antigen specificity to the cell. The TCR complex comprises a central two-chain transmembrane portion involved in antigen recognition that is associated with a series of minor components (collectively called CD3 and comprising CD3γ, CD3δ, CD3ε, and ζ chain) that act as signal transducers after recognition of specific antigen (Fig. 40.1). The majority of T cells use α and β chains in forming the central portion of the TCR complex, and a second group of T cells have $\gamma\delta$ TCRs. The diverse specificity of TCRs is achieved by the variable genetic combination of an array of gene segments that encode portions of the TCR chains. The total repertoire of TCRs in the body is sufficient to allow an animal potential recognition of any possible antigen that it may encounter. Most mature T cells also express one of two mutually exclusive surface molecules, CD4 or CD8 that define nonoverlapping T-cell subsets; however double-negative (CD4$^-$CD8$^-$) or double-positive (CD4$^+$CD8$^+$) T cells are found at certain stages of development.

All lymphoid cells, including T lymphocytes, arise from the common bone marrow stem cell. Immature T-cell precursors are then exported from the marrow to undergo development and maturation within the thymus.[2] Intrathymic development of T cells is complex and involves a series of interactions between the developing thymocytes and populations of antigen-presenting cells (APCs) such as thymic epithelial cells or dendritic cells. These tests of developing thymocytes determine whether the cells express a functional TCR capable of antigen recognition (positive selection) or a TCR that may recognize self-antigens and induce autoimmunity (negative selection); T cells that fail either test undergo apoptosis (programmed cell death or cell suicide) within the thymus, and the remnants of the cell are phagocytosed by macrophages (Fig. 40.2).

Mature CD4$^+$ or CD8$^+$ T cells leave the thymus and seed the peripheral lymphoid tissue, particularly the lymph node paracortex, splenic periarteriolar lymphoid sheath, or perifollicular regions of mucosa-associated lymphoid tissue (Fig. 40.3). However, lymphocytes do not remain static within these locations. There is continual and massive recirculation of lymphoid cells throughout the body, via the pathway depicted in Figure 40.4. Such recirculation is necessary to optimize the chance of contact with specific antigen and to orchestrate and regulate an immune response in the appropriate area of the body. Lymphocyte recirculation and vascular egress of these cells is carefully regulated by a complex network of adhesion molecules expressed by the recirculating lymphocytes (and other leukocytes) and modified vascular endothelium [high endothelial venules (HEV)] found normally in some lymphoid tissues or induced at sites of inflammation.[3]

Lymphocytes are considered functionally naive until they encounter the antigen that they are programmed to recognize via their specific TCR; after participation in an immune response, a population of memory lym-

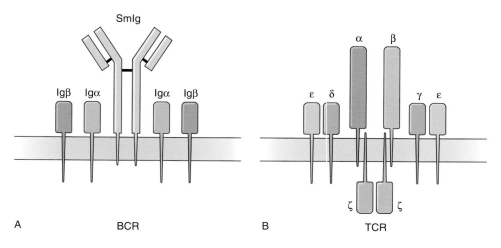

FIGURE 40.1 Diagrammatic representation of the B-cell receptor (BCR) and T-cell receptor (TCR). Antigen recognition is mediated by the SmIg of the BCR or the $\alpha\beta$ chains (alternative $\gamma\delta$ chains not shown) of the TCR. The signal transduction molecules of the BCR are collectively known as CD79 and those of the TCR as CD3.

TABLE 40.1   Lymphocyte Subsets

Cell Type	Function
B lymphocyte	plasma cell precursor
Plasma cell	immunoglobulin secretion
T lymphocytes	
$\alpha\beta$ TCR$^+$ CD4$^+$	immunoregulatory
Th1	cell-mediated immunity, limited help for antibody production (type 1 immune response)
Th2	antibody production, particularly IgE, IgG subclass, IgA (type 2 immune response)
Th3	oral tolerance
Tr1	suppression of Th1 cells
$\alpha\beta$TCR$^+$ CD8$^+$	cytotoxic (type 1 and type 2 populations are defined)
$\gamma\delta$TCR$^+$	antibacterial (type 1 and type 2 populations are defined)
NK cells	cytotoxicity, antibody-dependent cell-mediated cytotoxicity (ADCC)

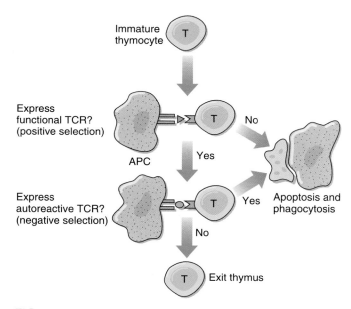

FIGURE 40.2 Intrathymic development of T lymphocytes. Developing thymocytes must express a T-cell receptor able to interact productively with MHC and peptide, but they must not recognize self-antigens and be capable of inducing an autoimmune response. Only T cells that satisfy these requirements are permitted to leave the thymus and enter the peripheral recirculation pathway.

phocytes persists for generation of the more effective anamnestic (memory) immune response.

T-Lymphocyte Activation

T lymphocytes have specialized requirements for activation. Intact antigen is generally unable to stimulate T cells and must first be processed and presented by populations of APCs.[4] Naive T cells are most effectively activated when antigen is presented to them by dendritic cells, but macrophages and B lymphocytes can also present antigen, and in some circumstances a wide variety of other cells (e.g., endothelia, epithelia, and fibroblasts) can be induced to present antigen (nonprofessional APC). There are two broad pathways of antigen presentation. Most exogenous antigens (the majority of anti-

gens such as infectious agents or allergens) are taken up by the APC (phagocytosis or macropinocytosis) and placed within a cytoplasmic compartment where they are enzymatically degraded to small peptide fragments that associate with Class II molecules of the major histocompatibility complex (MHC). The combination of antigenic peptide with MHC is then expressed on the surface of the APC in a manner that can be recognized by the TCR. Endogenous antigens (derived from the cell cytoplasm such as viral, tumor, or self-molecules) undergo an alternative process involving degradation within a cytoplasmic proteasome and transport into the endoplasmic reticulum (mediated by transporter proteins),

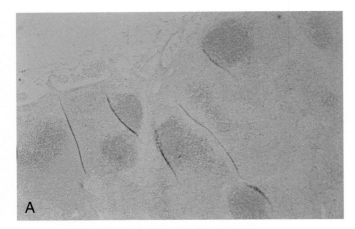

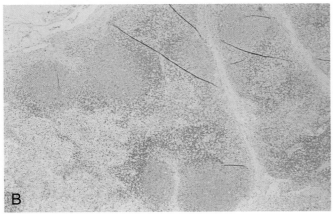

FIGURE 40.3 Sections of canine lymph node stained immunohistochemically for expression (**A**) of CD79 and (**B**) of CD3. The two antibodies clearly delineate cortical aggregates (**A**) of B lymphocytes and (**B**) the surrounding paracortical T cells.

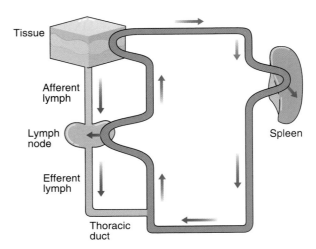

FIGURE 40.4 Pathways of lymphocyte recirculation. Lymphoid cells from the tissues drain to regional lymph nodes via the afferent lymph and exit the lymph node through efferent lymph, subsequently entering the blood circulation via the thoracic duct. Lymphocytes circulate within the bloodstream and may leave the vasculature to enter lymphoid tissue or other body tissues where there is expression of appropriate adhesion molecules by the local vascular endothelium.

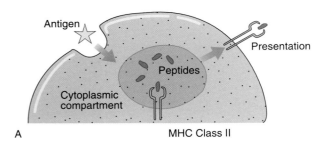

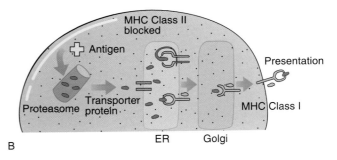

FIGURE 40.5 Processing and presentation (**A**) of exogenous antigen and (**B**) of endogenous antigen. Exogenous antigen is degraded within a cytoplasmic compartment in which there is association between peptide fragments of antigen and Class II molecules of the MHC. Endogenously derived antigen is degraded within the cytoplasmic proteasome and transported to the endoplasmic reticulum where peptide fragments become associated with MHC Class I molecules. In each case, the processed antigen is presented on the surface of the antigen-presenting cell by MHC for T-cell recognition.

where they associate with Class I MHC molecules. After transfer to the Golgi apparatus, the combination of antigenic peptide-MHC is similarly expressed on the surface of the APC (Fig. 40.5). Endogenous peptides may also be presented by MHC Class II molecules.

T-cell activation requires the delivery of intracytoplasmic signals after

- recognition of antigenic peptide and MHC residues by the TCR
- cognate interaction of the APC and T cell by an array of other surface molecules (e.g., B7 and CD28). In one such interaction, the CD4 molecule binds to MHC Class II and CD8 to MHC Class I. This renders the CD4⁺ T cells susceptible to stimulation only when antigen is presented by Class II, and CD8⁺ T cells to activation only after recognition of peptide in the context of Class I.
- release of costimulatory cytokines by the APC that bind cytokine receptors on the T cell.

After activation, the T cell undergoes blast transformation and cytokine secretion [e.g., interleukin-2 (IL-2)] and the process of clonal proliferation and differentiation, whereby large numbers of T cells with identical antigen-MHC specificity are generated to participate as effector cells in the immune response. Such T-cell activation generally occurs within the secondary lymphoid tissue, and activated T lymphocytes enter the recirculation pathway to arrive at the site of antigen exposure or at other lymphoid tissues.

T-Lymphocyte Functions

The result of T-cell activation is orchestration of some component of an antigen-specific immune response. T cells may be regulatory, providing either positive (helper) or negative (suppressor) signals to other leukocytes, or be cytotoxic in function.

Function of CD4⁺ T Lymphocytes

T lymphocytes bearing the CD4 molecule regulate the function of various leukocytes or cross regulate the function of each other. The recognition of CD4⁺ T-cell subsets has fundamentally reshaped study of the immune response in recent years. First recognized were two subsets of $\alpha\beta$TCR⁺CD4⁺ T cells, known as Th1 (T helper) and Th2.[5,6] Although phenotypically indistinguishable, these subpopulations have distinct function conferred upon them by the secretion of two nonoverlapping cytokine profiles (Fig. 40.6). Th1 cells selectively secrete the cytokines IL-2 and interferon gamma (IFNγ) and enhance the cytotoxic effects of CD8⁺ and natural killer (NK) cells, the killing of intracytoplasmic pathogens (e.g., *Leishmania, Mycobacterium*) by macrophages, and the selective production of antibody of a specific immunoglob-

ulin G subclass (IgG2a in mice).[7] Th2 cells selectively secrete IL-4, -5, -6, -9, -10, and -13 and provide help for B-cell and plasma cell development and for secretion of immunoglobulin E (IgE), immunoglobulin A (IgA), and another subclass of IgG (IgG1 in mice). The two subsets are mutually exclusive in function as the cytokines produced by each are antagonistic of the other population. For example, IFNγ downregulates the function of Th2 cells, whereas IL-4, -10, and -13 are suppressive of Th1 function. In practice, this exclusivity is not absolute, as elements of Th1 and Th2 immunology are involved in many immune responses, although some examples of distinctly polarized responses exist (e.g., Th1 requirement for resolution of intracellular infections or Th2 requirement for expression of type I hypersensitivity disease). Th1 and Th2 cells may follow selective recirculation pathways to different tissue sites as they may express particular adhesion molecules[8] and be chemotactically attracted by specific molecules (chemokines) for which they bear receptors.[9]

Th1 and Th2 subsets are proposed to be related through a common Th0 precursor that secretes elements of both cytokine profiles. In any particular immune response, the response can be driven toward either type 1 (Th1) or type 2 (Th2) function by a range of factors including:

- antigen type, dose, and route of delivery
- nature of the APC presenting the antigen
- local cytokine and hormonal environment in the lymphoid tissue generating the response. For example, the presence of high concentrations of endogenous corticosteroid or IL-4 may preferentially activate a Th2 response, whereas IL-12 drives forward a Th1 response.

Two further CD4⁺ T-cell subsets have recently been proposed. A Th3 cell, producing transforming growth factor beta (TGFβ) has been suggested to mediate the phenomenon of oral tolerance (failure to respond to systemic administration of antigen after previous feeding of the antigen),[10] and a population that selectively secretes IL-10 [T regulatory 1 (Tr1) cells] may underlie the suppression of particular Th1-driven inflammatory or autoimmune responses.[11]

Function of CD8⁺ T Lymphocytes

The major function of CD8⁺ T cells is mediation of cytotoxicity, and such cells are positively influenced by the effects of the Th1-regulatory population. However, it has also been recognized that CD8⁺ T cells are capable of producing type 2 cytokines (e.g., IL-4), and subsets of type 1 and type 2 CD8⁺ T cells are proposed.[12] The cytotoxic effect of lymphoid cells follows a similar sequence of events (Fig. 40.7) that are initiated after recognition of the target cell (e.g., virally infected, neoplastic, or incompatible graft cell) by cytotoxic cells.[13] In the case of CD8⁺ T cells, recognition involves TCR interaction with endogenous peptide presented by MHC Class I. A range of other surface molecular interactions between

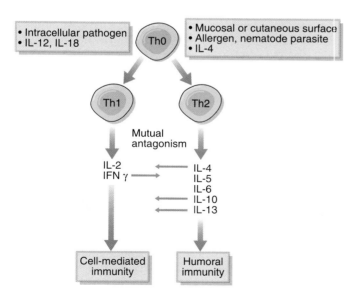

FIGURE 40.6 Two subsets of CD4⁺ T lymphocytes (Th1 and Th2) produce nonoverlapping cytokine profiles, mediate different immune functions, and are mutually antagonistic. The subsets have a common precursor (Th0) and several factors determine which of the subsets predominate in any particular immune response.

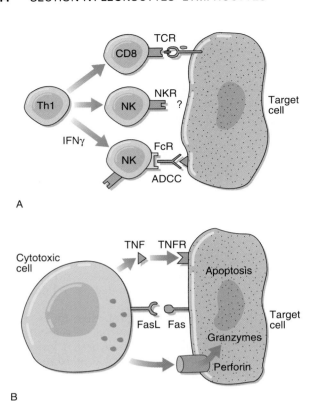

A

B

FIGURE 40.7 (**A**) Cytotoxic destruction of a target cell may be mediated by CD8+ T lymphocytes or NK cells. These populations are positively influenced by Th1 CD4+ T lymphocytes. (**B**) Cytotoxic process involves induction of target-cell apoptosis by the interactions of Fas–Fas Ligand and TNF–TNF receptor, membrane pore formation and osmotic imbalance, and cytoplasmic damage caused by granzymes released from the cytotoxic cell.

the two cells are also required. After recognition, the cytotoxic effects may be mediated by

■ induction of target-cell apoptosis triggered by intracellular signals delivered after molecular interactions such as between Fas (on the target cell) and Fas-ligand (on the cytotoxic cell) or cytotoxic cell-derived tumor necrosis factor (TNF) binding TNF receptor on the target cell.

■ osmotic and enzymatic effects produced by the release of substances from the cytotoxic cell that form membrane channels in the target cell (perforins), allowing osmotic imbalance or the delivery of toxic substances (granzymes) to the target-cell cytoplasm.

Cytotoxic cells may then disengage from the killed target cell and subsequently attack further targets.

Function of Natural Killer Cells

The NK cell is observed microscopically as a circulating large granular lymphocyte and is defined by the presence of a poorly characterized NK receptor that mediates the cytotoxic interaction with the target cell (Fig. 40.7). The cytotoxic function of an NK cell can be inhibited

by the interaction of a second class of receptor [killer inhibitory receptors (KIR)], which recognizes MHC Class I molecules on the target cell.[14] The NK cell may also recognize the target cell by interaction of the membrane (Fc) immunoglobulin receptor and antibody bound to the target cell in the process of antibody-dependent cell-mediated cytotoxicity (ADCC; Fig. 40.7).

Function of $\gamma\delta$ T Lymphocytes

In most species, T cells expressing the $\gamma\delta$ TCR with a CD3 complex are primarily located in the skin and mucosal sites of the body; however, in ruminants, a significant proportion of blood T cells may be of this phenotype.[15] $\gamma\delta$ T cells are poorly characterized but are known to develop in the thymus early in ontogeny. The $\gamma\delta$ TCR has limited heterogeneity and may largely recognize conserved microbial (especially bacterial) molecules and thus have a role in the early immune response to such agents. The receptor may recognize antigen directly or in association with particular forms of MHC Class I molecules. Functional subsets of $\gamma\delta$ T cells able to produce either IFNγ or IL-4 have been proposed and may be important in creating a cytokine milieu for subsequent development of the CD4+ $\alpha\beta$+-cell response.[16]

B LYMPHOCYTES AND PLASMA CELLS

B lymphocytes are defined by the expression of surface membrane immunoglobulin (SmIg) with a transmembrane domain that is associated with the signal transducing molecules immunoglobulin α (Igα) and immunoglobulin β (Igβ) (CD79). The complex is collectively referred to as the B-cell receptor (BCR; Fig. 40.1). Each B cell expresses a unique BCR of single specificity, and this diversity in the B-cell repertoire is achieved by genetic combination of BCR gene segments in a similar fashion to formation of the TCR. A range of other surface molecules (e.g., Fc and complement receptors) are expressed by B cells.

B cells are derived from the bone marrow stem cell and are thought to undergo their development and maturation within the fetal liver and bone marrow of mammals. In some species, evidence suggests that the intestinal tract may be an alternative site of B-cell development. The stages of B-cell development are less well understood than for the T lymphocyte, but the principle of cellular interactions with marrow stroma, with deletion of nonfunctional or autoreactive B cells by apoptosis, is likely similar. B-cell development relies on direct contact with stromal cells that also provide appropriate growth factors (e.g., IL-7). Developing B cells first express cytoplasmic immunoglobulin μ heavy chain, and after development to the naive stage, express antigen-specific SmIg of both the IgM and IgD classes. B lymphocytes are exported from the marrow to particular anatomic locations (lymphoid follicles of

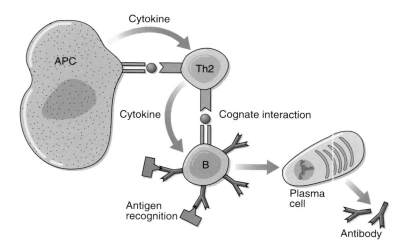

FIGURE 40.8 Activation of B lymphocytes requires recognition of antigen by surface membrane immunoglobulin and a range of interactions with the helper Th2 lymphocyte. These latter include direct interaction of membrane molecules and binding of T-cell-derived cytokines by specific receptors. B-cell differentiation involves transformation to a plasma cell that secretes immunoglobulin.

the lymph node cortex, splenic white pulp, or mucosal lamina propria) (Fig. 40.3) and recirculate around the body in the manner described for T cells.

B-cell activation occurs in lymphoid tissue and requires a similar array of signals to those described for the T lymphocyte. The SmIg of the BCR recognizes antigenic epitopes directly, without the need for antigen processing or presentation by APC. The epitope may be larger and have conformational or planar shape, although peptides may also be recognized. B cells require costimulatory signals delivered by $CD4^+$ helper T lymphocytes (Th2 or Th1). These take the form of cognate interactions between surface membrane molecules on the two cells (including TCR recognition of antigenic peptide presented on MHC Class II by the B cell) and the cytokines derived from the T cell that bind receptors on the B cell (Fig. 40.8). Some antigens (thymus-independent antigens) can directly activate B cells in the absence of T-cell help.

After activation, the B lymphocyte undergoes transformation to a lymphoblast (that may secrete IgM) and clonal proliferation and differentiation as described for the T cell. As part of the differentiation process, the B cell undergoes the immunoglobulin class switch, involving DNA rearrangement with substitution of the μ and δ genes by one of the other constant region genes to produce SmIg of the IgG, IgA, or IgE class. This process may be cytokine directed.

The initial contact of antigen-specific B and Th2 cells with APC (dendritic cells) and antigen occurs in the T-cell zones of lymphoid tissue (e.g., lymph node paracortex) after egress of the T and B cells from the HEV. Next, there is B cell proliferation and activated B and T cells migrate from this primary focus to the B-cell area (primary follicle) to form a germinal center within the follicle.[17] These activated B cells (centroblasts) accumulate within the dark zone of the germinal center of this secondary follicle and then migrate to the edge of the germinal center (light zone) where as centrocytes they reencounter antigen on follicular dendritic cells. The mantle zone of this secondary follicle is composed of

inactive B cells that are not specific for the antigen driving the immune response. Most of the centrocytes have BCRs that recognize antigen with low affinity, and this interaction causes them to undergo apoptosis. However, those centrocytes with appropriate receptors undergo further interactions with Th cells and leave the germinal centers to differentiate into plasma cells (that secrete immunoglobulin but do not have SmIg) or into the population of memory B cells that mediate the secondary immune response on reencounter with antigen. Plasma cells migrate as precursor plasmablasts and are largely located in lymph node medullary cords, splenic red pulp, bone marrow, and the mucosal lamina propria. They have a limited life span (weeks) at these sites. Memory T and B lymphocytes are long lived cells that may be periodically restimulated by depots of antigen that persists, associated with dendritic cells in lymphoid tissue, or is reintroduced to the body by vaccination or exposure to micro-organisms bearing cross-reactive epitopes.[18,19]

REFERENCES

1. **Shin EK, Perryman LE, Meek K.** A kinase-negative mutation of DNA-PK$_{CS}$ in equine SCID results in defective coding and signal joint formation. J Immunol 1997;158:3565–3569.
2. **Ardavin C.** Thymic dendritic cells. Immunology Today 1997;18:350–361.
3. **Springer TA.** Adhesion receptors of the immune system. Nature 1990; 346:425–434.
4. **Banchereau J, Steinman RM.** Dendritic cells and the control of immunity. Nature 1998;392:245–251.
5. **Romagnani S.** The Th1/Th2 paradigm. Immunology Today 1997;18: 263–266.
6. **Abbas AK, Murphy KM, Sher A.** Functional diversity of helper T lymphocytes. Nature 1996;383:787–793.
7. **Powrie F, Correa-Oliveira R, Mauze S, Coffman RL.** Regulatory interactions between CD45RB^high and CD45RB^low CD4$^+$ T cells are important for the balance between protective and pathogenic cell-mediated immunity. J Exp Med 1994;179:589–600.
8. **Austrup F, Vestweber D, Borges E, Lohning M, Brauer R, Herz U, Renz H, Hallmann R, Scheffold A, Radbruch A, Hamann A.** P- and E-selectin mediate recruitment of T-helper-1 but not T-helper-2 cells into inflamed tissues. Nature 1997;385:81–83.
9. **Bonecchi R, Bianchi G, Bordignon PP, D'Ambrosio D, Lang R, Borsatti A, Sozzani S, Allavena P, Gray PA, Mantovani A, Sinigaglia F.** Differential expression of chemokine receptors and chemotactic responsiveness of type 1 T helper cells (Th1s) and Th2s. J Exp Med 1998;187:129–134.

10. **Weiner HL.** Oral tolerance: immune mechanisms and treatment of autoimmune diseases. Immunology Today 1997;18:335–343.
11. **Groux H, O'Garra A, Bigler M, Rouleau M, Antonenko S, de Vries JE, Roncarolo MG.** A CD4⁺ T-cell subset inhibits antigen-specific T-cell responses and prevents colitis. Nature 1997;389:737–741.
12. **Erard F, Le Gros G.** Th2-like CD8 T cells: their role in protection against infectious diseases. Parasitology Today 1994;10:313–315.
13. **Chouaib S, Asselin-Paturel C, Mami-Chouaib F, Caignard A, Blay JY.** The host-tumor immune conflict: from immunosuppression to resistance and destruction. Immunology Today 1997;18:493–497.
14. **Mingari MC, Moretta A, Moretta L.** Regulation of KIR expression in human T cells: a safety mechanism that may impair protective T-cell responses. Immunology Today 1998;19:153–157.
15. **Hein WR, Dudler L.** TCR⁺ cells are prominent in normal bovine skin and express a diverse repertoire of antigen receptors. Immunology 1997;91:58–64.
16. **Ferrick DA, Schrenzel MD, Mulvania T, Hsieh B, Ferlin WG, Lepper H.** Differential production of interferon-γ and interleukin-4 in response to Th1- and Th2-stimulating pathogens by γδ T cells in vivo. Nature 1995;373:255–257.
17. **Lindhout E, Koopman G, Pals ST, de Groot C.** Triple check for antigen specificity of B cells during germinal centre reactions. Immunology Today 1997;18:573–577.
18. **Bell EB, Sparshott SM, Bunce C.** CD4⁺ T-cell memory, CD45R subsets and the persistence of antigen-a unifying concept. Immunology Today 1998;19:60–64.
19. **Gray D, Matzinger P.** T cell memory is short-lived in the absence of antigen. J Exp Med 1991;174:969–974.

CHAPTER 41

Lymphocytes: Differentiation Molecules in Diagnosis and Prognosis

• PETER F. MOORE and WILLIAM VERNAU

LYMPHOCYTE DEVELOPMENT

Thymus

The thymus is the central lymphoid organ in which T lymphocytes are educated and selected for self-major-histocompatibility-complex (MHC) restriction and self-tolerance. T-cells originate from committed lymphoid stem cells in bone marrow. T-cell precursors (CD7+) that express terminal deoxyribonucleotidyl transferase (TdT) migrate to the thymus and are recognizable in the outer cortex. These thymic immigrants undergo an orderly differentiation process as they pass through the thymic cortex and medulla. During this process thymocytes rearrange T-cell antigen receptor genes (TCR; A, B, G, and D) by a process of somatic recombination that requires the activity of the recombinase genes (RAG-1 and RAG-2). The rearrangement process brings variable (V), diversity (D) and joining (J) gene segments together. The multiple combinatorial possibilities for the joining of the different gene segments, coupled with the addition of nontemplate encoded (N) nucleotides between V, D, and J segments (that is, V-N-D-N-J) by TdT, result in the generation of a large repertoire of T-cell specificities within two recognized lineages: $\alpha\beta$ and $\gamma\delta$ T-cells. TCR-$\alpha\beta$+CD4+CD8+ cortical thymocytes interact with MHC molecules, which are expressed by cortical epithelial cells, bone-marrow-derived macrophages and dendritic cells (antigen-presenting cells or [APC]), and undergo selection processes that shape the T-cell repertoire toward self-MHC restriction and self-tolerance by processes of positive and negative selection, respectively. Thymocytes that do not pass the applied selection criteria usually die by the process of *apoptosis* (programmed cell death).[1]

Surviving TCR$\alpha\beta$+ thymocytes mature and join one of two sublineages: either TCR $\alpha\beta$ +CD4+ cells that leave the thymus and become peripheral T-helper or inducer cells that are restricted to interact with antigen presented in the context of self-MHC Class II on the surface of APC or TCR$\alpha\beta$+CD8+ cells that leave the thymus and become T-cytotoxic cells that interact with antigen presented in the context of MHC Class I on the cell surface of almost any cell in the body.[1] Adaptive immune responses are the province of $\alpha\beta$ T-cells, which comprise the dominant population in blood and peripheral lymphoid tissues.

Extrathymic T-cell populations differ significantly in swine with respect to the expression pattern of CD4 and CD8. Two further T-cell populations exist. Double negative CD4−CD8− T-cells, which constitute the TCR-$\gamma\delta$+ T-cells in blood, and double positive CD4+CD8+$\alpha\beta$ T-cells. The ratio of these 2 populations varies with age: juveniles have a high proportion of CD4−CD8− T-cells and few CD4+CD8+ T-cells; in adults the ratio is reversed.[2] Cattle and sheep also have a high prevalence of CD4−CD8−$\gamma\delta$ T-cells in juveniles, but lack the prevalent CD4+CD8+$\alpha\beta$ T-cell populations, which seem unique to swine.[2]

In humans, mice and dogs TCR$\gamma\delta$+ T-cells occur as CD4−CD8− or CD8+ cells, which form a minor T-cell lineage in blood. They are most numerous within gut epithelia and the splenic red pulp in humans and also in the splenic red pulp in dogs (McDonough SP and Moore PF, submitted). The functions of $\gamma\delta$ T-cells are still uncertain, but it is known that they have a role in the control of certain types of infectious disease (especially intracellular pathogens). They are among the earliest cells to respond to invading pathogens and perhaps shape the responses that follow.[3]

Bone Marrow

Bone marrow is the major central lymphoid organ in mammalian B-cell development. B- and T-lymphocyte precursors develop in bone marrow from committed lymphoid stem cells that are derived from the pluripotent stem cell responsible for all myeloid and lymphoid lineages. B-cell development in bone marrow in primates and mice follows a well-defined series of stages resulting in the production of mature virgin B-lymphocytes. In the process, B-cells rearrange multiple V, J, and D immunoglobulin (Ig) gene segments, initially their heavy chain Ig genes (V_HDJ), and later either kappa or lambda light chain Ig genes (V_LJ only).[1] This process of somatic recombination was first described for Ig genes and resembles the description of the process already outlined for T-cells. A further property of Ig genes is the propensity to undergo V region somatic mutation particularly during secondary antibody responses in germinal centers of follicles in peripheral lymphoid organs.[1] In addition, secondary V-(D)-J rearrangement has also been described in germinal centers of mice through reactivation of recombinase genes, which were previously thought active only in central lymphoid organs.[4] By these mechanisms, antibodies of high affinity are produced in secondary lymphoid responses (affinity maturation).

Stages in B-cell development are not recognizable morphologically in bone marrow in contrast to myeloid lineages. Instead, maturation of B cells has been best characterized by the acquisition of more- or less-specific cell membrane markers of B-cell differentiation in an orderly sequence (CD79a, CD79b, CD45, CD45R, CD19, CD20, CD21, and CD22). Logically, surface IgM and IgD expression can only occur after the stage of somatic Ig gene recombination. In primates and mice, B-cells expressing both surface IgM (sIgM) and IgD (sIgD) are mature virgin B-cells of the conventional B-2 lineage that leave bone marrow and populate peripheral lymphoid organs.[1] IgD has only been found in primates and rodents so far. B-2 B-cells are continuously generated throughout life in the bone marrow. In contrast, B-1 B-cells are dominant B-cells in the fetus and neonate; they are characterized by predominant expression of sIgM, not sIgD, and by expression of CD5 in some species (humans, mice, and ruminants).[1,5] CD5 expression by B-1 B-cells has not been adequately evaluated in dogs, cats, horses, and swine. B-1 B-cells form a self-renewing population, which does not seem to be continuously generated from bone marrow throughout life. B-1 B-cells are sparse in peripheral lymphoid organs (lymph nodes and spleen), but predominate in peritoneal and pleural cavities where they respond with broad specificity to polysaccharide antigens of bacteria.[1] In chickens and rabbits, B-cells in all peripheral locations are of the B-1 lineage.[5] B-1 B-cells are expanded in B-cell chronic lymphocytic leukemia (B-CLL) of humans[6] and in the lymphocytosis or leukemia induced by Bovine Leukemia Virus (BLV) in cattle.[7]

Bursa of Fabricius

The Bursa of Fabricius is the central lymphoid organ responsible for the generation of Ig receptor diversity in B-lymphocyte development in birds. It is a saccular, lymphoepithelial structure attached to the cloaca. The bursa undergoes age-related involution, and it can undergo premature involution with resulting immunodeficiency in specific viral infections that affect it. B-cells arise in bone marrow in birds. A single V_H segment and a single V_L segment rearranges (the same ones in all individuals). These invariant B-cells traffic to the Bursa, where they interact with a self-ligand present on bursal epithelium, via their unique sIg receptor. They proliferate and exchange small stretches of their other V_H and V_L gene segments (V_H and V_L pseudogenes) with the single rearranged V_H gene segments, which is a process of gene conversion (templated mutation) that creates antigen-receptor diversity. The essential function of the bursa is not to generate B-cells, but rather to generate Ig-receptor diversity in B-cells.[1]

Terminal Ileal Peyer's

The terminal ileal Peyer's patch also behaves as a central lymphoid organ in B-cell development in ruminants. In ruminants the terminal ileal Peyer's patch is approximately 1 to 2 m long and undergoes age-related involution, much as occurs in the bursa of birds. The randomly distributed, more proximal, discontinuous Peyer's patches do not undergo age-related involution and presumably function as peripheral lymphoid organs. The antibody repertoire of horses, cattle, sheep, and swine develops from a small number of V_H and V_L genes. Ruminants and swine appear to use gene conversion (templated mutation) or somatic mutation (untemplated mutation) to diversify the Ig repertoire. These events occur in the terminal ileal Peyer's patch. Data on generation of Ig receptor diversity are unavailable for horses, dogs, and cats.[5]

Regulation of Ig Light Chain Expression

Regulation of Ig light chain expression differs significantly between species. The ratio of expressed κ and λ light chains varies significantly between species. Dogs, cats, horses, cattle, and sheep express almost exclusively λ light chains.[5,8] Also, chickens lack a κ locus and express λ light chains exclusively.[5] Mice and rabbits express almost exclusively κ light chains.[5] Humans and swine have a similar $\kappa:\lambda$ chain ratio of approximately 1:1.5.[5,8] Consequently, the sensitivity of examining light chain restriction as an indicator of clonal B-cell expansion is significantly reduced in species that have heavily skewed light chain expression patterns normally.

IMMUNOPHENOTYPING

Lessons from the Human Experience

The usefulness of immunophenotypic assessment of lymphoproliferative disease has been firmly established in humans. Immunophenotypic assessment significantly impacts diagnosis, prognosis, and therapy.[6,9] This is because the diagnosis and precise classification of hematopoietic malignancies, both leukemias and lymphomas, by morphologic criteria alone is limited.[9] The basic premise of immunophenotyping is that leukemias and lymphomas are the neoplastic counterparts of subpopulations of normal lymphoid and myeloid cells.[10] In general terms, they tend to maintain a constellation of antigen expression similar to their normal counterparts that reflects both their lineage and their stage of maturation arrest and clonal expansion. This paradigm has not only proved useful in the diagnosis and classification of hemopoietic neoplasia but also has assisted in the determination of normal hematopoietic ontogeny. For many reasons, immunophenotyping in humans has achieved a much greater level of complexity, sophistication, and importance than currently exists in veterinary medicine. Nevertheless, the same principles apply, and as this discipline develops in veterinary medicine, it is clear that similar useful information can be derived from immunophenotypic studies in animals (see below). There are a multitude of both surface and cytoplasmic antigens or markers that are used in these studies. These antigens are usually assigned cluster of differentiation (CD) numbers. This nomenclature greatly assists in the use and comparison of a vast array of antibodies that have been developed to detect the presence and level of expression of these antigens. Methods of detection include flow cytometric assessment of both surface and cytoplasmic antigens in fluid samples[11] and immunochemistry of tissue-sections, smears, and cytospin preparations.

Immunophenotyping is one of the primary diagnostic modalities for assessment of acute leukemias in humans. It is helpful in differentiating acute myeloid leukemia (AML) from acute lymphoblastic leukemia (ALL) and determining the various subtypes of both AML and ALL.[6,9,10] These subtypes have significantly differing prognoses and therapies. It is also helpful in characterizing, and hence determining, the prognosis of the inevitable acute or blastic stage of chronic myelogenous leukemia in humans. More recently, precise enumeration and immunophenotypic characterization of blast-cell populations in bone marrow has been achieved by flow cytometric techniques that use a combination of CD45 staining and side-scatter characteristics to isolate these populations.[12] This is especially helpful when there are significant numbers of residual normal cells admixed with the tumor cells. Flow cytometry has also assumed an important role in the detection of minimal residual disease (MRD) in humans. In general terms, flow cytometry is far more sensitive than routine morphologic assessment in the detection of MRD. Reported sensitivities of detection are in the range of from 0.01 to 1.0%, depending on the phenotype of the neoplastic cells.[6,9] These studies generally use multiparameter staining to detect tumor-specific antigen combinations. Immunophenotyping is also one of the primary diagnostic modalities (along with routine morphology and complete blood count [CBC]) for the assessment of chronic B-, T-, and natural-killer (NK)-cell lymphoproliferative diseases.[6,9,10] In humans, the chronic lymphoproliferative disorders (CLPD) are characterized by a malignant proliferation of mature, small, lymphoid cells.[9] Each of the CLPD have typical cytologic features. However, because of overlap of these features, morphology alone is not always sufficient for consistent separation of the various entities, which differ significantly in prognosis and therapy. Included in this group are B-CLL, prolymphocytic leukemia, T-cell CLL (T-CLL), hairy-cell leukemia, the leukemic phase of B-cell lymphoma, large granular lymphocytoses (LGL), and Sezary syndrome among others.

Immunophenotyping is a crucial adjunct in the diagnostic workup of lymphoma in humans. It is considered essential for a precise, reproducible, and clinically relevant classification of lymphoma.[9] Techniques include routine immunohistochemistry of tissue sections, flow cytometric evaluation of appropriately processed tissue biopsies and aspirates of lymph nodes and other tissues and flow cytometric evaluation of blood and bone marrow.

Diagnostically Important CD Molecules in Leukocytic Disorders in Animals

The nomenclature and complexity pertaining to the biology of leukocyte surface molecules is intimidating. There are currently 166 CDs assigned in the human immune system, as well as many other defined molecules that have not yet been assigned to clusters of differentiation.[13,14] Comprehensive reports of recent leukocyte antigen workshops have been published for ruminants,[15] swine,[16] and horses.[17] A single workshop was convened to identify canine leukocyte antigens,[18] and none has been conducted for cats. Despite the large number of CD molecules identified, not all are useful in immunodiagnostics. The following glossary consists of the CD and related molecules of most importance in veterinary immunodiagnostics for which monoclonal antibodies (mAb) are available. Many more specificities exist for some domestic species, but in no case do they approach the comprehensive array of CD molecules identified in mice and humans. In most instances, these CD molecules are detectable only in unfixed cells, which can include unfixed air-dried cytologic preparations, anticoagulated blood or bone marrow, and fresh tissue that has been carefully snap frozen and sectioned. In some instances, antibodies that detect epitopes resistant to the deleterious effects of formalin fixation have been developed; these are valuable reagents for the study of archived tissue in paraffin blocks and routinely processed pathologic material.[19]

CD1

There are 5 CD1 genes (A–E); the protein products of these genes are CD1a–e. The classical CD1 molecules consist of CD1a, CD1b, and CD1c, which are differentially expressed on leukocyte populations. CD1 molecules are distantly related to MHC Class I molecules; they present peptide, lipid, and glycolipid antigens to T-cells.[14] CD1-specific mAbs are available in dogs, cats, cattle, sheep, and swine. CD1 molecules are expressed by cortical thymocytes but not by mature T-cells. CD1 molecules are the best markers of dendritic APC, although subpopulations of B-cells and monocytes express CD1c. The majority of histiocytic proliferative disorders in dogs involve dendritic APC and are best defined by expression of CD1 molecules, lack of expression of lineage-specific lymphoid markers (CD3 and CD79a), and coexpression of molecules of functional importance to dendritic APC such as CD11c and MHC II.[19] CD1 molecules are also frequently expressed in canine B-CLL.[20]

T-Cell Antigen-Receptor Complex

The TCR/CD3 complex is expressed only on the surface of mature T-cells (and thymocytes). CD5 and CD4 or CD8 associate with TCR/CD3 in the majority of $\alpha\beta$ T-cells to form a coreceptor complex. There are two types of TCR: $\alpha\beta$ and $\gamma\delta$; each is associated with the CD3 complex (five polypeptides: CD3γ, CD3δ, CD3ε, CD3ζ, and CD3η) (Fig. 41.1), which is the signal transduction portion of the receptor complex in both TCR types.[14] In dogs, mAbs are available for both lineages[19] and only for TCR$\gamma\delta$ in cattle, sheep, and swine.[15,16] The biology of T-cells differs significantly between species. In ruminants, the coordinate expression of the WC1 molecule, a member of the scavenger receptor cysteine-rich family that includes CD5, defines a major $\gamma\delta$ T-cell subset that lacks expression of CD2. The distribution and frequency of WC1−CD2+$\gamma\delta$ T-cells in ruminants closely match that of $\gamma\delta$ T-cells in dogs and humans. Conversely, WC1+CD2−$\gamma\delta$ T-cells of ruminants form a unique subset that is especially prevalent in peripheral blood of young calves and can account for as much as 60 to 80% of the lymphocytes in blood of neonates.[21] Analogous, but more complexly organized, populations of $\gamma\delta$ T-cells occur in swine.[2,22]

Evaluation of CD3 expression is possible in formalin-fixed tissue with either a mAb (CD3-12, Serotec, Oxford, UK) or a rabbit polyclonal antibody(#A452, Dako, Carpinteria, CA) specific for a highly conserved peptide sequence from the cytoplasmic domain of CD3ε from diverse species (dogs, cats, horses, cattle, swine, rabbits, chickens, humans, mice, etc.). CD3ε expression is largely limited to mature T-cells, although activated human NK cells can express CD3ε in their cytoplasm. Demonstration of CD3ε expression is one of the most useful immunophenotypic analyses currently performed and is used for the diagnosis of T-cell lymphoma and T-cell leukemia. CD3 expression, with rare exceptions, confirms the presence of T-cells in a lesion, although it does not distinguish $\alpha\beta$ and $\gamma\delta$ T-cells. Usually, mAbs specific for the extracellular domains of CD3 are species specific and do not react in formalin-fixed tissue, although they are the reagents of choice for identification of T-cell lymphoproliferative processes by surface staining of leukocytes derived from blood or bone marrow with flow cytometry. In dogs, horses, cattle, and swine mAbs specific for extracellular domains of CD3 are available. Further dissection of the T-cells comprising a lesion relies on the availability of mAbs specific for TCR.

CD4

The CD4 molecule functions as a TCR-associated coreceptor for MHC Class II in T-helper cells. The known ligands for CD4 include MHC II and interleukin (IL) −16. CD4 expression is not limited to T-cells. Monocytes, macrophages, and dendritic APC either express or can upregulate CD4 in some instances. Canine neutrophils constitutively express CD4 and in this respect differ from neutrophils of other species.[23] Dendritic APC, which comprise a major cell population in the lesions of reactive Langerhans cell histiocytosis (cutaneous and systemic histiocytosis) in dogs, consistently express CD4 and Thy-1 (CD90). In this respect they differ from neoplastic dendritic APC present in histiocytoma, histiocytic sarcoma, and malignant histiocytosis, which do not consistently express these molecules.[19]

CD5

CD5 is expressed on mature T-cells, thymocytes, and the B-1 subset of B cells. CD5 is associated with the TCR and B-cell antigen receptor (BCR). CD5 modulates signaling through the antigen-specific receptor complexes. In peripheral mature T-cells CD5 acts as a costimulatory signal receptor. CD5-specific mAbs have been identified for dogs, cats, horses, cattle, sheep, and swine. CD5 is a marker of the B-1 subset of B cells that are expanded in B-CLL of humans[6] and in the lymphocytosis or leukemia of cattle induced by BLV.[7] CD5 is not expressed in B-CLL in dogs.[20]

CD8

The CD8 molecule functions as a TCR-associated coreceptor for MHC Class I in T-cytotoxic cells. T-cells that use TCR$\alpha\beta$ usually express CD8$\alpha\beta$ heterodimers; although a subset can express CD8$\alpha\alpha$ homodimers. Subsets of NK cells and $\gamma\delta$ T-cells may also express CD8$\alpha\alpha$ homodimers. CD8α expression is required for the expression of CD8β.[14]

T-Cell Lymphoproliferative Disease

Case studies in canine lymphoma have revealed an adverse prognostic correlation with presence of a T-cell phenotype despite the overall predominance of B-cell lymphoma.[24–26] Lymphoma-associated hypercalcemia

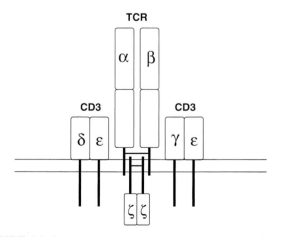

FIGURE 41.1 Components of the TCR complex: TCRβ/CD3; TCR/CD3 complex is similarly arranged. Adapted from **Janeway C, Travers P**. Immunobiology: the immune system in health and disease. New York: Garland Publishing, 1997.

was exclusively correlated with CD4+ T-cell phenotype in one large study,[26] although we have observed hypercalcemia in canine B-cell lymphomas and also in canine histiocytic diseases, albeit rarely.

Investigation of cutaneous epitheliotropic T-cell lymphoma (mycosis fungoides [MF]) in dogs revealed that in the majority of instances neoplastic T-cells expressed CD8 rather than CD4 as in human MF.[27] Loss of CD5 expression in neoplastic T cells in human MF is a marker of clinical disease progression.[28] Studies in canine MF did not demonstrate a clear correlation of clinical disease stage and CD5 expression.[19] Furthermore, almost 70% of canine MF cases involved proliferation of $\gamma\delta$ T-cells instead of $\alpha\beta$ T-cells, which are the most common T-cell lineage in human MF.[19,27] Interestingly, the Pagetoid form of canine MF, which is characterized initially by intraepidermal T-cell infiltration without dermal involvement, is exclusively a $\gamma\delta$ T-cell disease[19]

Canine chronic lymphocytic leukemia (CLL) differs significantly from human CLL; the latter is largely a B-cell proliferative disease. T-CLL, however, is the most common form of CLL in dogs (approximately 70% of CLL). B-CLL only accounts for approximately 30% of canine CLL.[20] The large granular lymphocyte (LGL) form of T-CLL is most prevalent (approximately 55% of CLL) (Fig. 41.2). Canine T-CLL is predominantly a CD8+ T-cell proliferative disease. In LGL T-CLL, the novel leukointegrin $\alpha D\beta2$ (CD11d/CD18) is expressed by LGL in more than 90% of cases (McDonough SP and Moore PF, submitted) (Figs. 41.3 and 41.4). Early splenomegaly and late bone marrow infiltration characterize this disease, which often follows an indolent clinical course with minimal therapeutic intervention. Interestingly, CD11d expression is somewhat constrained in tissue; the splenic red pulp is the dominant site of CD11d expression in the hematopoietic system in both dogs and cats.[29] Expression of CD11d in feline LGL leukemia is much less prevalent, indeed in many instances this disease is associated with intestinal lymphoma, likely of T-

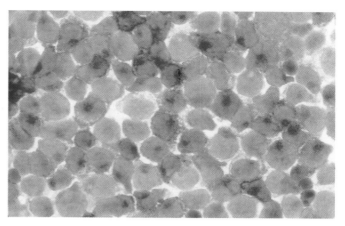

FIGURE 41.3 Immunocytochemical stain of a cytospin preparation of canine LGLs stained with mAbS to $\alpha D\beta2$ (CD11d). Note the diffuse and paranuclear dot staining.

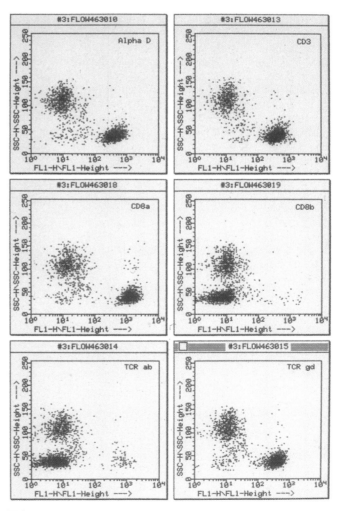

FIGURE 41.4 Flow-cytometry dot plots of a typical case of canine LGL CLL. Fluorescence intensity is depicted on the x axis. The LGLs in this case are CD3+, TCR$\gamma\delta^+$, $\alpha D\beta2^+$ (CD11d+), and CD8+.

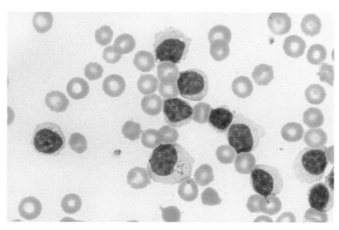

FIGURE 41.2 Photomicrograph of a typical canine LGL CLL illustrating variable cytoplasmic azurophilic granulation.

cell origin.[30] Expression of integrins and other molecules normally expressed in the intestinal mucosa, for example αEβ7, has been associated with feline LGL leukemia or lymphoma under these circumstances (Roccabianca P and Moore PF, unpublished). It is important to recognize that feline LGL leukemia or lymphoma is a rapidly progressive disease with a poor prognosis; a significant difference from canine LGL CLL.

B-Cell Antigen-Receptor Complex

The BCR consists of sIg complexed with two invariant molecules that function as signal transduction molecules (CD79a, CD79b). Other components, which form the BCR coreceptor complex, include CD19, CD81, and two complement receptors (CR): CD21 (C3dg receptor or CR2) and CD35 (CR1) (Fig. 41.5). B-cell detection mAbs include HM57 (Dako), which is specific for a cytoplasmic peptide sequence of CD79a that is well conserved in diverse species (humans and mice) and is detectable in formalin-fixed tissue sections.[31] HM57 also has good reactivity with B cells in dogs, cats, horses, cattle, and swine, although CD79a sequence is unavailable in these species. For the extracellular domains of CD79a and CD79b, specific mAbs have not been described for domestic animal species. CD79a (mb-1) is expressed throughout all stages of B-cell development and persists into the plasma cell stage (despite absent or diminished sIg on plasma cells). CD79a is a useful marker for establishing the diagnosis of B-cell lymphoma and leukemia, because it is present in the BCR of all B-cells regardless of the isotype of the sIg receptor. Background associated with Ig stains in tissues is also less of an issue. CD79a is also useful in the diagnosis of canine cutaneous plasmacytoma (approximately 80% have focal to diffuse expression).[32]

CD21 is expressed on mature B-cells and follicular dendritic cells of the germinal center. CD21-specific mAbs are available in dogs, cats, cattle, sheep, and swine. CD19 is also an important B-cell lineage associated molecule in humans. However, monoclonal antibodies specific for CD19 have not been described in domestic animal species. Detection of CD21 is useful in the diagnosis of canine B-cell lymphoma[25] and B-CLL, which is a leukemia of mature B cells in dogs.[20] Detection of Ig components of the BCR was reported in an immunophenotypic study of bovine enzootic lymphoma associated with BLV infection. Expression of MHC II, IgG heavy chain, and lambda light chain was found consistently.[33] Also, BLV-induced lymphocytosis or leukemia is a B-1 B-cell expansion in which B cells express both sIg and CD5.[7]

CD11 and CD18

The β2 integrins (CD11/CD18) are the major leukocyte adhesion molecule family. The absence of β2 integrins owing to mutations in CD18 results in leukocyte adhesion deficiency syndrome (LAD-I) described in humans, Irish Setters, and Holstein cattle.[34-36] Afflicted individuals are unable to mount effective inflammatory reactions; they die from sepsis within a few months after birth. Most leukocytes express one or more members of this family. CD18 is the β2 subunit that pairs with one of four α subunits to form a heterodimer. Expression of β2 is required for surface expression of the α subunits. Staining for CD18 indicates the presence of the β2 subunit, but it does not indicate which of the four integrin molecules is present. The four α subunits are CD11a (all leukocytes), CD11b (granulocytes, monocytes, and some macrophages), CD11c (granulocytes, monocytes, and dendritic APCs), and CD11d(αDβ2) (LGLs and macrophages and T-cells in splenic red pulp).[29,37,38] Macrophages and granulocytes express approximately tenfold

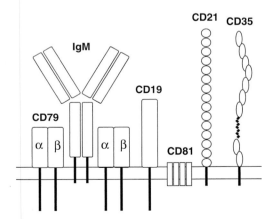

FIGURE 41.5 Components of the BCR and coreceptor complex. Adapted from **Janeway C, Travers P**. Immunobiology: The immune system in health and disease. New York: Garland Publishing, 1997 and **Barclay A, Brown M, Law S, McKnight A, Tomlinson M, van der Merwe P**. The leukocyte antigen facts book. 2nd ed. London: Academic Press, 1997.

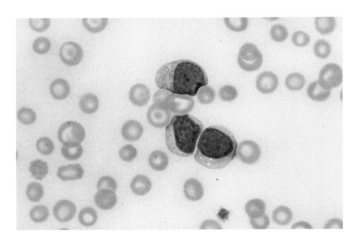

FIGURE 41.6 Photomicrograph of a case of canine lymphoid leukemia (white blood cell [WBC] = 70,700/μL) that was originally classified as CLL. However, the presence of significant pancytopenia was considered unusual for CLL (see Fig. 41.7).

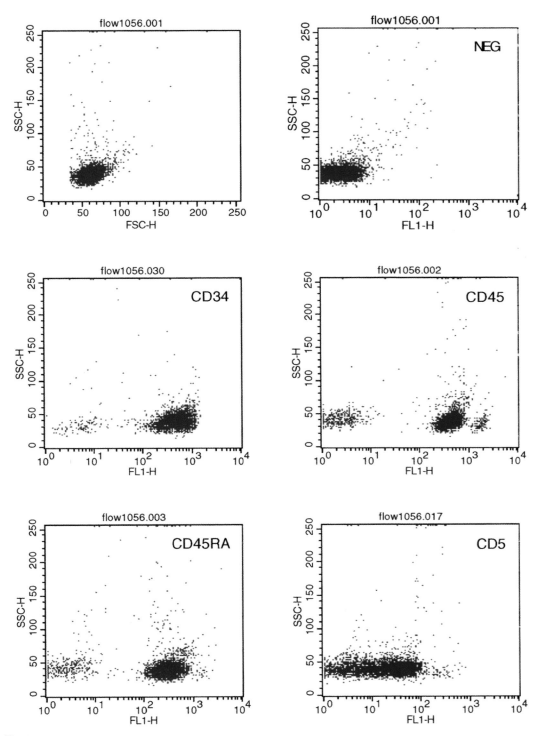

FIGURE 41.7 Flow-cytometry dot plots of the case described in Figure 41.6. The cells strongly express CD34, a hematopoietic stem-cell marker (see panel middle left). This resulted in reclassification of the case to ALL.

more CD18 than do lymphocytes.[38] CD11- and CD18-specific mAbs have been described in dogs, cats, horses, cattle, sheep, and swine. Canine and feline CD18 and canine CD11d are detectable with species-specific mAbs in formalin-fixed tissue sections. In the absence of CD3 or CD79a expression, abundant CD18 expression by large mononuclear cells is preliminary evidence of macrophage or dendritic APC differentiation. Frozen sections or unfixed cytologic smears stained for CD1 and CD11c molecules would provide definitive confirmation.[19]

CD34

The heavily glycosylated surface glycoprotein, CD34, is expressed on early lymphohematopoietic stem and progenitor cells, small-vessel endothelial cells, embryonic fibroblasts and bone marrow stromal cells.[39] CD34-specific mAbs have been described in humans, mice, and dogs.[39,40] CD34+ bone marrow cells comprise approximately 1 to 2% of marrow mononuclear cells but contain precursors for all lymphohematopoietic lineages as evidenced by the ability of CD34+ bone marrow cells to reconstitute hematopoiesis in primates, mice, and dogs after bone marrow radioablation.[39] Ligands for CD34 include L-selectin (CD62-L) and E-selectin (CD62-E); hence CD34 may play a role in leukocyte endothelial interactions.[14,39] CD34 expression has proved useful in diagnosis of acute, immature cell leukemias of both myeloid and lymphoid types in humans.[39] CD34 is not expressed in CLL, lymphoma, or myeloma, which are malignancies of more mature cells.[39] Similarly, mAbs specific for canine CD34 have proved useful in the differentiation of acute lymphoid leukemia from lymphoma with leukemic involvement or chronic lymphocytic leukemia (Figs. 41.6 and 41.7). A high proportion of acute myeloid and acute lymphoid leukemias express CD34 in dogs.[20]

CD45

The leukocyte common antigen family is the former nomenclature for CD45. CD45 is a membrane-bound tyrosine phosphatase that is critically important in antigen-receptor-mediated T- and B-cell activation and perhaps in receptor-mediated activation of other leukocytes.[13] One or more CD45 isoforms are expressed on all cells of hematopoietic origin, except erythrocytes. Alternate messenger RNA (mRNA) splicing generates eight possible isoforms from three alternatively spliced exons (A, B, and C). The isoforms are expressed differentially on leukocytes as revealed by mAbs specific for sequences derived from the spliced exons: CD45RA, CD45RB, and CD45RC. The CD45R0 epitope is formed by the junction of the constantly expressed exons at the potential point of insertion of alternatively spliced exons, which, in this instance, are missing.[14] The mAbs that detect epitopes in the constantly expressed exons detect all isoforms of CD45 (Fig. 41.8). B-cells express a high molecular-weight isoform of CD45 containing all of the spliced exons. Naive CD4+ T-cells express CD45

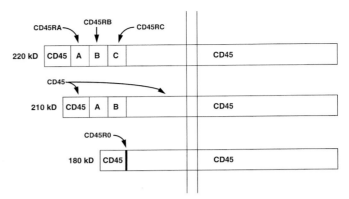

FIGURE 41.8 Illustration of three of eight possible CD45 isoforms generated by alternative splicing of exons A, B, and C. The 220 kD form is prevalent in B-cells and naive T-cells. The 180 kD form is prevalent in memory T-cells.

molecules containing one or two alternate exons. Memory CD4+ T-cells predominantly express CD45R0 (i.e., no spliced exons). Monoclonal antibodies specific for one or more isoforms of CD45 have been described in dogs, cats, cattle, sheep, and swine. Canine CD45RA is detectable with mAbs in formalin-fixed tissue sections.[19] CD45RA is expressed by all B-cells and by 100% of B-cell lymphomas involving lymph nodes.[25] Peripheral T-cell lymphomas usually occur in memory T cells in older individuals. Memory cells switch from expressing CD45RA to CD45R0. Memory cells preferentially traffic to cutaneous and mucosal sites, and T-cell lymphomas (CD3ε+) in these sites usually do not express CD45RA.[19,27,28] Canine transmissible venereal tumor cells express canine CD45 and CD45RA, but no other leukocyte differentiation antigens that indicate a lineage commitment. This unusual pattern is useful for diagnosis in frozen sections, and even in formalin-fixed tissue sections (Moore PF, unpublished).

Caveats and Limitations

The same major caveats apply to use of immunophenotyping in all species. Correlating the clinical outcome with specific antigens rather than the total phenotype is probably not useful. Additionally, the optimal use of immunophenotypic data in patient care should include integration of all historical, clinical, morphologic, and other (i.e., cytochemical and cytogenetic) information.

Current limitations include definitive confirmation of lineage in acute leukemia and identification of NK cells in lymphoproliferative disease. The development of mAbs specific for CD13, CD33, and myeloperoxidase in companion animal species would illuminate the myeloid disorders. The availability of mAbs specific for CD7, CD10, and CD19 would be useful adjuncts to typing of acute lymphoblastic leukemia, as would mAbs for TdT. There are no lineage-specific markers for NK cells. Detection of NK-associated killer-inhibitory receptors (KIR) and lack of surface CD3 would permit definitive identification of NK cells and their distinction from NK-like T-cells.

Unequivocal confirmation of neoplasia is rarely possible solely by the use of immunophenotyping. Careful assessment of clinical and morphologic criteria are critical. Molecular techniques developed for analysis of human lymphoproliferative disease hold promise for the demonstration of clonal lymphocyte populations expected in lymphoma and leukemia in animals. These techniques rely on amplification by polymerase chain reaction (PCR) of the V–D–J splice junctions of TCR or BCR in lymphocytes. The heterogeneity of N nucleotide addition between these junctions provides a sensitive and specific target for the demonstration of unique (clonal) or diverse (polyclonal) lymphocyte populations in a lymphoproliferative disease. This technology has been developed for the dog[20] and is under development for the cat in our laboratory.

REFERENCES

1. **Janeway C, Travers P**. Immunobiology: The immune system in health and disease. New York: Garland Publishing, 1997.
2. **Saalmuller A**. Antigen-specific immune response of porcine T lymphocytes to various pathogens. Rev Sci Tech 1998;17:71–83.
3. **Ferrick DA, Schrenzel MD, Mulvania T, Hsieh B, Ferlin WG, Lepper H**. Differential production of interferon-gamma and interleukin-4 in response to Th1- and Th2-stimulating pathogens by gamma delta T cells in vivo. Nature 1995;373:255–257.
4. **Han S, Zheng B, Takahashi Y, Kelsoe G**. Distinctive characteristics of germinal center B cells. Semin Immunol 1997;9:255–260.
5. **Butler JE**. Immunoglobulin diversity, B-cell and antibody repertoire development in large farm animals. Rev Sci Tech 1998; 17:43-70.
6. **Jennings CD, Foon KA**. Recent advances in flow cytometry: application to the diagnosis of hematologic malignancy. Blood 1997;90:2863–2892.
7. **Meirom R, Brenner J, Trainin Z**. BLV-infected lymphocytes exhibit two patterns of expression as determined by Ig and CD5 markers. Vet Immunol Immunopathol 1993;36:179–186.
8. **Arun SS, Breuer W, Hermanns W**. Immunohistochemical examination of light-chain expression (lambda / kappa ratio) in canine, feline, equine, bovine and porcine plasma cells. Zentralbl Veterinarmed A 1996;43:573–576.
9. **Davis BH, Foucar K, Szczarkowski W, Ball E, Witzig T, Foon KA, Wells D, Kotylo P, Johnson R, Hanson C, Bessman D**. U.S.-Canadian consensus recommendations on the immunophenotypic analysis of hematologic neoplasia by flow cytometry: medical indications. Cytometry 1997;30:249–263.
10. **Freedman AS**. Cell surface antigens in leukemias and lymphomas. Cancer Invest 1996;14:252–276.
11. **Knapp W, Strobl H, Majdic O**. Flow cytometric analysis of cell-surface and intracellular antigens in leukemia diagnosis. Cytometry 1994;18:187–198.
12. **Borowitz MJ, Guenther KL, Shults KE, Stelzer GT**. Immunophenotyping of acute leukemia by flow cytometric analysis. Use of CD45 and right-angle light scatter to gate on leukemic blasts in three-color analysis. Am J Clin Pathol 1993;100:534–540.
13. **Shaw S, Katz K, Turni L**. Protein reviews on the web. http://www.ncbi.nlm.nih.gov/prow/. National Center for Biotechnology Information, 1998.
14. **Barclay A, Brown M, Law S, McKnight A, Tomlinson M, van der Merwe P**. The leukocyte antigen facts book. 2nd ed. London: Academic Press, 1997.
15. **Naessens J, Howard CJ, Hopkins J**. Nomenclature and characterization of leukocyte differentiation antigens in ruminants. Immunol Today 1997;18:365–368.
16. **Saalmuller A**. Characterization of swine leukocyte differentiation antigens. Immunol Today 1996;17:352–354.
17. **Lunn DP, Holmes MA, Antczak DF, Agerwal N, Baker J, Bendali-Ahcene S, Blanchard-Channell M, Byrne KM, Cannizzo K, Davis W, Hamilton MJ, Hannant D, Kondo T, Kydd JH, Monier MC, Moore PF, O'Neil T, Schram BR, Sheoran A, Stott JL, Sugiura T, Vagnoni KE**. Report of the

second equine Leucocyte Antigen Workshop, Squaw Valley, California, July 1995 [In Process Citation]. Vet Immunol Immunopathol 1998;62:101–143.
18. **Cobbold S, Metcalfe S**. Monoclonal antibodies that define canine homologues of human CD antigens: summary of the First International Canine Leukocyte Antigen Workshop (CLAW). Tissue Antigens 1994;43:137–154.
19. **Moore P, Affolter V, Olivry T, Schrenzel M**. The use of immunological reagents in defining the pathogenesis of canine skin diseases involving proliferation of leukocytes. In: Kwotchka K, Willemse T, von Tscharner C, eds. Advances in veterinary dermatology. Vol 3. Oxford: Butterworth Heinmann, 1998;77–94.
20. **Vernau W, Moore PF**. An immunophenotypic study of canine leukemias and preliminary assessment of clonality by polymerase chain reaction. Vet Immunol Immunopathol 1999;69:145–164.
21. **Davis WC, Brown WC, Hamilton MJ, Wyatt CR, Orden JA, Khalid AM, Naessens J**. Analysis of monoclonal antibodies specific for the gamma delta TCR. Vet Immunol Immunopathol 1996;52:275–283.
22. **Davis WC, Zuckermann FA, Hamilton MJ, Barbosa JI, Saalmuller A, Binns RM, Licence ST**: Analysis of monoclonal antibodies that recognize gamma delta T / null cells. Vet Immunol Immunopathol 1998;60:305–316.
23. **Moore PF, Rossitto PV, Danilenko DM, Wielenga JJ, Raff RF, Severns E**. Monoclonal antibodies specific for canine CD4 and CD8 define functional T-lymphocyte subsets and high-density expression of CD4 by canine neutrophils. Tissue Antigens 1992;40:75–85.
24. **Teske E, van Heerde P, Rutteman GR, Kurzman ID, Moore PF, MacEwen EG**. Prognostic factors for treatment of malignant lymphoma in dogs. J Am Vet Med Assoc 1994;205:1722–1728.
25. **Teske E, Wisman P, Moore PF, van Heerde P**. Histologic classification and immunophenotyping of canine non-Hodgkin's lymphomas: unexpected high frequency of T cell lymphomas with B cell morphology. Exp Hematol 1994;22:1179–1187.
26. **Ruslander DA, Gebhard DH, Tompkins MB, Grindem CB, Page RL**. Immunophenotypic characterization of canine lymphoproliferative disorders. In Vivo 1997;11:169–172.
27. **Moore PF, Olivry T, Naydan D**. Canine cutaneous epitheliotropic lymphoma (mycosis fungoides) is a proliferative disorder of CD8+ T cells. Am J Pathol 1994;144:421–429.
28. **Knowles DM**. Immunophenotypic and antigen receptor gene rearrangement analysis in T cell neoplasia. Am J Pathol 1989;134:761–785.
29. **Danilenko DM, Rossitto PV, Van der Vieren M, Le Trong H, McDonough SP, Affolter VK, Moore PF**. A novel canine leukointegrin, alpha d beta 2, is expressed by specific macrophage subpopulations in tissue and a minor CD8+ lymphocyte subpopulation in peripheral blood. J Immunol 1995;155:35–44.
30. **Darbes J, Majzoub M, Breuer W, Hermanns W**. Large granular lymphocyte leukemia / lymphoma in six cats. Vet Pathol 1998;35:323–460.
31. **Jones M, Cordell JL, Beyers AD, Tse AG, Mason DY**. Detection of T and B cells in many animal species using cross-reactive anti-peptide antibodies. J Immunol 1993;150:5429–5435.
32. **Schrenzel M, Naydan D, Moore P**. Leukocyte antigen expression in cutaneous plasmacytomas in dogs. Vet Dermatol 1998;9:33–41.
33. **Vernau W, Jacobs RM, Valli VE, Heeney JL**. The immunophenotypic characterization of bovine lymphomas. Vet Pathol 1997;34:222–225.
34. **Anderson DC, Springer TA**. Leukocyte adhesion deficiency: an inherited defect in the Mac-1, LFA-1, and p150,95 glycoproteins. Annu Rev Med 1987;38:175–194.
35. **Kehrli ME Jr, Ackermann MR, Shuster DE, van der Maaten MJ, Schmalstieg FC, Anderson DC, Hughes BJ**. Bovine leukocyte adhesion deficiency. Beta 2 integrin deficiency in young Holstein cattle. Am J Pathol 1992;140:1489–1492.
36. **Giger U, Boxer LA, Simpson PJ, Lucchesi BR, Todd RFd**. Deficiency of leukocyte surface glycoproteins Mo1, LFA-1, and Leu M5 in a dog that has recurrent bacterial infections: an animal model. Blood 1987;69:1622–1630.
37. **Moore PF, Rossitto PV, Danilenko DM**. Canine leukocyte integrins: characterization of a CD18 homologue. Tissue Antigens 1990;36:211–220.
38. **Danilenko DM, Moore PF, Rossitto PV**. Canine leukocyte cell adhesion molecules (LeuCAMs): characterization of the CD11/CD18 family. Tissue Antigens 1992;40:13–21.
39. **Krause DS, Fackler MJ, Civin CI, May WS**. CD34: structure, biology, and clinical utility. Blood 1996;87:1–13.
40. **McSweeney PA, Rouleau KA, Wallace PM, Bruno B, Andrews RG, Krizanac-Bengez L, Sandmaier BM, Storb R, Wayner E, Nash RA**. Characterization of monoclonal antibodies that recognize canine CD34. Blood 1998; 91:1977–1986.

CHAPTER 42

Cytokines and the Immune Response to Infection

• MARY B. TOMPKINS and WAYNE A.F. TOMPKINS

The immune system can be categorized into two distinct but interlocking components: the innate, or nonspecific response, and the acquired, or specific response. The innate immune system, consisting of neutrophils, macrophages (MPs) and natural killer (NK) cells, is the first line of defense against an invading pathogen and is characterized by immediacy in its response, lack of antigen specificity, and failure to develop immunologic memory. If a pathogen gets past the cells of the innate system, it induces an inflammatory response and activates the acquired immune system.

The acquired immune response is characterized by antigen specificity and the development of memory, and unlike the innate response, requires uptake and processing of antigens by antigen-presenting cells (APCs). The APC presents antigen to specific CD4+ T helper (Th) cells and, in the presence of the appropriate cytokine microenvironment, antibody- and cell-mediated immunity develops. It is now believed that antibody- and cell-mediated immune responses are under the direction of two distinct CD4+ helper cell subsets: Th1 cells, which secrete interleukin-2 (IL-2) and interferon-gamma (IFNγ, and Th2 cells, which secrete IL-4, IL-5, IL-6, IL-10, and transforming growth factor beta (TGFβ). The initial antigen-APC-Th cell interactions that result in high levels of the IL-12 and IFNγ, but little IL-4, leads to the preferential expansion of the Th1 CD4+ subset and a Th1 immune response, including activation of MPs, cytotoxic CD8+ cells, and NK cells. Numerous studies have established that a Th1 immune response is necessary for resistance to intracellular parasites, bacteria, and viruses. In contrast, antigen-APC-CD4+ interactions that lead to IL-4 production initiate Th2-dependent gamma G immunoglobulin (IgG[1]) and gamma E immunoglobulin (IgE) humoral immune responses that are a characteristic of immunity to extracellular bacteria, helminth parasites, and environmental allergens. Although, it is tempting to polarize protective immune responses to infectious agents as either Th1 or Th2, exceptions to this paradigm are numerous, and it is impor-

tant to keep in mind that in many cases, a combination of Th1 and Th 2 cytokines may be required for successful immunity. In addition, there are numerous examples, in particular the immunodeficiency-inducing lentiviruses, which do not adhere to the Th1-Th2 subset paradigm. Evidence suggests that these lentiviruses concurrently induce some Th1 and Th2 cytokines, whereas other Th1 and Th2 cytokines are depressed.

INNATE IMMUNE RESPONSE

One of the most important cells involved in innate resistance is the MP. Although resting MPs can ingest microorganisms, they do not effectively destroy organisms unless activated by IFNγ and other cytokines. MP activation is biphasic in that IFNγ produced by NK cells is an early step in the innate response, whereas a second, delayed MP activation occurs as a result of the specific immune response depends on IFNγ production by Th1-type CD4+ cells. This second level of activation is necessary for complete elimination of intracellular pathogens.

Several studies in which various intracellular pathogens such as *Listeria*, *Toxoplasma*, and *Mycobacterium* have demonstrated that, in addition to IFNγ, tumor necrosis factor alpha (TNFα) and IL-2 are also important in the early innate response.[1-3] However, MP activation and IL-12 production actually depend on autocrine priming by MP-produced IFNγ and TNFα. Sibley et al.[4] demonstrated that IFNγ-primed macrophages would not express enhanced antitoxoplasma activity unless they received an additional signal from TNFα. The initial interaction of the MP and pathogen induces synthesis of small amounts of IFNγ and TNFα that act in an autocrine manner to activate MP, as well as to stimulate the production of IL-12 by the MP. This MP-derived IL-12, in collaboration with TNFα, stimulates the NK cell to make high levels of IFNγ. The IFNγ, in a paracrine feedback loop, increases the IL-12 production by the MP as well as enhances the MPs microbicidal capability. In addition to activating microbicidal MPs, TNFα, IFNγ, and IL-12 are necessary cytokines for driving the Th1 immune response.

Th1 IMMUNE RESPONSE

While it is not fully understood what signals a naive T cell to differentiate into a Th1 or Th2 cell, data suggest that it is the cytokine microenvironment at the time of antigen presentation. In the case of the Th1 response, it is the IL-12 and IFNγ generated during the innate response that determines the differentiation from a naive Th0 cell into a Th1 cell. The importance of these two cytokines is demonstrated by the fact that if the production of IL-12 is blocked, high levels of IFNγ do not appear, and the IL-4-dependent Th2 default pathway dominates instead.[5] Recent evidence suggests that naive or precursor T cells (Tp) stimulated with the APC-peptide complex, presented by MHC Class II molecules, initially produce IL-2 and develop into Th0 cells that are capable of producing a number of cytokines, including IL-2, IFNγ, IL-4, IL-5, IL-6 and IL-10, and of differentiating into either Th1 or Th2 subsets.[6] In the presence of IL-12 and IFNγ, the CD4+ Th0 cell becomes a Th1 type cell and begins to secrete IL-2 and IFNγ. It is now clear that, at least in the mouse, IFNγ upregulates the IL-12 receptor β2 chain (IL-12Rβ2), leading to the formation of the high affinity IL-12 β1/β2 receptors on Th0 and Th1 cells and increased responsiveness to IL-12[5]. The interaction of the T cell with antigen presented by APC also stimulates the T cell to express high affinity receptors for IL-2, the T cell growth factor.

A number of other studies have provided evidence that IFNγ is not the only mediator of the IL-12 driven Th1 protective immune response. As discussed above, TNFα, in collaboration with IL-12 and IFNγ, is a critical molecule in the activation of microbial macrophages against numerous intracellular microorganisms. It is now becoming evident that TNFα is also an important cytokine in bridging the innate and Th1 acquired immune responses. Knockout mice lacking the p55 TNFα receptor fail to make IL-12 in response to infection, suggesting that TNFα also plays an important role in priming for an acquired T cell immune response.[2] Macrophages from gene deletion mutant mice lacking either the IFNγ or TNFα (p55) receptor failed to produce IL-12 in vitro after mycobacterial infection,[2] suggesting that IL-12 production is dependent on priming by both IFNγ and TNFα. These observations further emphasize the importance of IFNγ and TNFα not only for macrophage priming for IL-12 production, but for driving the Th1 immune response. These three cytokines, in collaboration with IL-2, stimulate T cell proliferation and production of a Th1 response.

EFFECTOR ARM OF THE Th1 IMMUNE RESPONSE

The antigen-specific effector cell of a Th1 response is the CD8+ T cell. CD8+ T cells recognize antigen presented by MHC Class I molecules and therefore, the APC must also present antigen in Class I molecules. The APC, when presenting antigen, not only secretes IFNγ and IL-12, it also secretes IFNα, which is an important stimulatory signal for CD8+ cell activation. In the presence of IFNα (from the APC) and IL-2 (from the stimulated CD4+ cells), CD8+ cells begin to undergo clonal expansion. This generation phase of the immune response, the activation and clonal expansion of T cells (both CD4+ and CD8+), occurs in the lymph nodes that drain the sites of infection or, in the case of a blood borne pathogen, in the spleen. Either APCs capture antigen at the site of infection and migrated to the local node or they trap antigen carried by lymph to the local node. Once the activated T cells have undergone clonal expansion, they leave the nodes and migrate (via the blood) to the site of infection, where the effector phase of the response occurs. Activated T cells express tissue-selective molecules (integrins) on their surface that allow them to enter the infection site through the recognition and binding to adhesion molecules that have been expressed on the surface of endothelial cells as a result of the inflammatory cytokines (IL-1, IL-6, and TNFα) and chemokines (IL-8, macrophage inflammatory protein [MIP] 1α, MIP1β, and RANTES).

The CD4+ cells secrete many cytokines that function to recruit and activate CD8+ cells, NK cells, and MPs, including IFNγ, TNFα, and IL-2. CD8+ cells function as cytotoxic T cells (CTL), recognizing and killing virus-infected cells in an antigen-specific manner. They are probably the most important defense mechanism against viruses and other intracellular pathogens that infect cells other than MPs. A population of CD8+ cells exist that secrete IFNγ, which has both antiviral and MP-activating activity. The most important defense mechanism against intracellular pathogens that infect MPs is the activated MP. However, as noted in the discussion on innate resistance, for complete success at eliminating the pathogen, the MP must receive a final activation signal consisting of IFNγ secreted by the T cells. Activation of the MP results in enhanced viricidal and bactericidal activity and IFN production. Remember that although this final activation of MPs occurs as a result of the antigen-specific immune response, the activated MP is nonspecific in its activity.

As the effector cells begin to eliminate the infected cells and inactivate the pathogen, the stimulus for maintaining production of the cytokines described above declines. It has also been shown that IL-12 produced by the MP acts in an autocrine feedback loop to stimulate the production of IL-10 by these cells. IL-10, traditionally thought of as a Th2 cytokine that suppresses Th1 responses, is a potent anti-inflammatory cytokine necessary for controlling the level of inflammation. This IL-10 production is probably necessary to turn off the immune and inflammatory response as the infection is controlled. For example, gene knockout mice deficient in IL-10 die from T. gondii infection caused by an uncontrolled inflammation despite their ability to mount a strong Th1 response.[7] IL-10 exerts much of its immunosuppressive effects by inhibiting synthesis of inflammatory cytokines such as TNFα, IL-1β, IL-6, and IFNγ by activated MP.

Th2 IMMUNE RESPONSE

Just as the Th1 cytokine-cell-mediated immunity (CMI) paradigm developed from the observations that expression of Th1 cytokines was necessary for resistance to intracellular pathogens, the dogma that Th2 cytokines protected against extracellular parasites evolved from the observation that resistance to pathogens such as helminthic parasites depended on, in many cases, a humoral immune response regulated by the Th2 cytokines IL-4, IL-5, IL-6, and IL-9. Although it is well established that differentiation of Th0 cells into Th1 cells is largely triggered by IL-12 derived from the APC, the factors that promote the Th2 pathway are less understood. However, CD4+ cells activated in vitro in the presence of IL-4 differentiate into Th2 cytokine secreting cells[8] and IL-4$^{-/-}$ knockout mice do not develop Th2 cytokines.[9] The source of the IL-4 is unclear, but some evidence suggests an early cytokine milieu, including IL-5 and IL-9 generated by non-T cells at the early stage of infection, may be responsible for a rapid T-cell differentiation to IL-4-producing Th0 and Th2 cells.[10]

Although the early cytokines initiating a Th2 immune response remain illusive, the cytokines responsible for driving the Th2 proliferation and regulating immunoglobulin (Ig) isotype switching are well defined. Th2 cells are effective B-cell activators and are associated with elevated levels of IL-4, IL-5, IL-6, IL-9, IL-10, and TGF-β. To undergo clonal expansion, form germinal centers, and differentiate into plasma cells, B cells must first interact with Th2 cells, thus a T-cell-dependent antibody response cannot occur until after Th2 cells have been generated. B cells bind and internalize antigen, with their Ig receptors; process the antigen; and present it in Class II molecules on their surface. The Th2 cell can then recognize the antigen and interact with the B cell. The B-cell-Th2-cell interaction stimulates the T cell to secrete IL-4, which drives the B-cell clonal expansion. As the B cells begin to divide, three additional cytokines, IL-5, IL-6, and, TGF-β contribute to further cell proliferation and differentiation into plasma cells.

Although early antibody production is predominantly gamma M Ig (IgM), T-dependent antibody responses are characterized by isotype switch to IgG, gamma A immunoglobulin (IgA), or IgE, and the resulting isotype depends on the cytokine environment. IL-4 directs class switching to IgG1 and IgE, whereas IL-5 promotes IgA-producing plasma cells. TGF-β, which is also a product of Th2 cells, induces switching to IgG2b and IgA. Although Th1 cells are poor stimulators of antibody response, they do promote the production of IgG2a through secretion of IFNγ.

Th1–Th2 PARADIGM AND DISEASE

Whether a Th1 or Th2 response occurs after infection can have drastic consequences, not all of which are beneficial. For example, humans infected with *M. leprae* can follow one of two clinical courses, depending on whether a Th1 or a Th2 response occurs. A Th1 response, characterized by high levels of IL-12, IL-2, IFNγ, and TNFα production, results in tuberculoid leprosy, with few organisms found in MP, slowly progressing disease, and patient survival. However, if a Th2 response develops, characterized by high levels of IL-4, IL-5, and IL-10, lepromatous leprosy develops in which organisms grow abundantly in MPs, major tissue destruction occurs, and patient survival is poor.[11]

What determines the early dominance of Th1 or Th2 cytokines is not known. However, recent studies in the mouse suggest that early commitment to the Th2 pathway may represent a default mechanism stemming from deficiencies in IFNγ necessary for maintaining expression of the high affinity IL-12Rβ1/β2 on Th1 cells and responsiveness to IL-12. Szabo et al.[5] demonstrated that when IL-4 was neutralized by antibodies, T-cell antigen receptor (TCR) activation alone is sufficient for inducing IL-2Rβ2-chain expression and commitment to the Th1 phenotype. However, when even low levels of IL-4 are present, expression of the IL-12Rβ2 chain is inhibited. Inhibition of IL-2Rβ2 chain expression leads to loss of IL-12 signaling and subsequent stabilization of the Th2 response. These authors also observed that exogenous IFNγ overrides the IL-4-induced inhibition of IL-12-Rβ2-chain expression, suggesting that the balance between IL-4 and IFNγ during the early stages of APC-Th0 interaction may determine IL-12 responsiveness and commitment of cells to the Th1 or Th2 pathway. These findings are directly relevant to the understanding how different pathogens may induce different immune responses. The fact that IL-4 appears to inhibit expression of the IL-12β2 subunit imposes an early requirement for IFNγ for a Th1 immune response. In the case of pathogens that induce limited amounts of IFNγ, IL-4 may inhibit IL-12Rβ2 expression and severely curtail a Th1 response in favor of a Th2 response. In contrast, intracellular pathogens that produce high levels of MP- or NK-derived IFNγ early would override the IL-4 default pathway and promote a protective Th1 immune response.

Despite Th1 cytokines being important features of the cell-mediated immune response and resistance to intracellular pathogens, the distinction between Th1 and Th2 responses as polarized cytokine profiles is not always evident. For example, both Th1 and Th2 cells in the human produce IL-10,[12] a cytokine made only by mouse Th2 cells and thought to promote a Th2 response by suppression of a Th1 cytokines. The interspecies functional dichotomy of the Th1–Th2 paradigm is further emphasized by the finding that in the human, IFNα but not IFNγ, upregulates the IL-12 Rβ2 chain on T cells,[13] whereas the reverse is true in the mouse.[5] The concept of an exclusive Th1 or Th2 response as defined by a specific cytokine pattern is also confounded by various infectious agents that induce mixed cytokine profiles. Human immunodeficiency virus (HIV) immunopathogenesis has long been dominated by the paradigm of a virus-induced Th1 to Th2 cytokine shift,[14] yet T cells from infected patients constitutively and concurrently synthesized high levels of the type 2 cytokine

IL-10, as well as IFNγ and TNFα, the prototypical Th1 cytokines.[15]

Levy et al.[16] also recently presented strong evidence against a strict Th1–Th2 paradigm in the feline acquired immunodeficiency syndrome (AIDS) model. In contrast to the predicted Th1 to Th2 shift, based on increased susceptibility to facultative intracellular pathogens, these authors reported an increase in Th1 cytokines, IFNγ and TNFα, as well as the Th2 cytokine IL-10 in cats infected with feline immunodeficiency virus (FIV), Bucci et al.[17] demonstrated that this unusual cytokine profile (high IFNγ and high IL-10) was accompanied by a strong CD8+ antiviral response that correlated with a significant decrease in cell-associated and plasma viremia. Preliminary studies indicate that the CD8+ antiviral cells may be the source of the elevated levels of IL-10 and IFNγ found in HIV-infected and FIV-infected subjects. Thus, protective immunity in these cases may be mediated by CD8+ cells with a chimeric Th1 or Th2 (IFNγ or IL-10) cytokine profile.

Studies with the intracellular parasite *T. gondii* further demonstrate that it is not possible to generalize about the benefit-to-risk ratio of a Th1 or a Th2 cytokine response in an infection. Although numerous studies have clearly demonstrated that IFNγ is essential for resistance to *T. gondii*, the presence of Th1 cells is not necessary, as administration of IL-12 to severe combined immunodeficiency (SCID) mice induces high levels of IFNγ from NK cells and confers protection against *T. gondii* in the absence of Th1 cells.[3] Further confounding the Th1–Th2 paradigm is the observation that mice deficient in IL-10, a Th2 anti-inflammatory cytokine, die from *T. gondii* infection caused by an unrestrained inflammatory response, despite their ability to mount a vigorous Th1 response.[7] In contrast, conventional mice administered high levels of IL-10 and infected with *T. cruzi* succumb to the infection, presumably because of IL-10-induced suppression of the MP microbicidal response.[18] These observations show that negative regulation signals, such as IL-10, may be as important as positive signals in the overall response to infection. Thus, while it is evident that Th1 cytokines are critical components for controlling most intracellular pathogens, a Th1 cytokine response is not by itself inherently protective, and strong Th1 and Th2 cytokine responses are not mutually exclusive.

CONCLUSIONS

It is evident from the above discussion that a complex network of cells that is orchestrated by multiple cytokines and their specific receptors regulates the immune response to an antigen. Regulation of this intricate system is balanced by positive and negative transduction signals that are in turn regulated by the differentiation state of cells, specific receptor expression, and the cytokine microenvironment. In a physiologic setting, these cytokine-receptor interactions produce an ordered sequence of immune response, inflammation, and resolution of the lesion. In a nonphysiologic setting, they may lead to serious immunopathologic conditions.

REFERENCES

1. **Dunn PL, North RJ.** Early gamma interferon production by natural killer cells is important in defense against murine listeriosis. Infect Immun 1991;59:2892.
2. **Flesch IE, Hess JH, Huang S, Aguet M, Rothe J, Bluethmann H, Kaufmann SH.** Early interleukin 12 production by macrophages in response to mycobacterial infection depends on interferon gamma and tumor necrosis factor alpha. J Exp Med 1995;181:1615.
3. **Gazzinelli RT, Hieny S, Wynn TA, Wolf S, Sher A.** Interleukin 12 is required for the T-lymphocyte-independent induction of interferon gamma by an intracellular parasite and induces resistance in T-cell-deficient hosts. Proc Natl Acad Sci U S A 1993;90:6115.
4. **Sibley LD, Adams LB, Fukutomi Y, Krahenbuhl JL.** Tumor necrosis factor-alpha triggers antitoxoplasmal activity of IFN-gamma primed macrophages. J Immunol 147:2340.
5. **Szabo S, Dighe A, Gubler U, Murphy K.** Regulation of the interleukin (IL)-12R beta 2 subunit expression in developing T helper 1 (Th1) and Th2 cells. J Exp Med 1997;185:817.
6. **Mosmann T, Coffman R.** TH1 and TH2 cells: different patterns of lymphokine secretion lead to different functional properties. Annu Rev Immunol 1989;7:145.
7. **Gazzinelli R, Wysocki M, Hieny S, Scharton KT, Cheever A, Kuhn R, Muller W, Trinchieri G, Sher A.** In the absence of endogenous IL-10, mice acutely infected with Toxoplasma gondii succumb to a lethal immune response dependent on CD4+ T cells and accompanied by overproduction of IL-12, IFN-gamma and TNF-alpha. J Immunol 1996;157:798.
8. **Parronchi P, De Carli M. Manetti R, Simonelli C, Sampognaro S, Piccinni M-P, Macchia D, Maggi E, Del Prete G, Romagnani S.** IL-4 and IFN (alpha and gamma) exert opposite regulatory effects on the development of cytolytic potential by Th1 or Th2 human T cell clones. J Immunol 1992;149:2977.
9. **Noben-Trauth N, Kropf P, Muller I.** Susceptibility to Leishmania major infection in interleukin-4-deficient mice. Science 1996;271:987.
10. **Svetic A, Madden K, Zhou X, Lu P, Katona I, Finkelman F, Urban JJ, Gause W.** A primary intestinal helminthic infection rapidly induces a gut-associated elevation of Th2-associated cytokines and IL-3. J Immunol 1993;150:3434.
11. **Yamamura M, Uyemura K, Deans R, Weinberg K, Rea T, Bloom B, Modlin R.** Defining protective responses to pathogens: cytokine profiles in leprosy lesions [published erratum appears in Science 1992;255(5040):12]. Science 1991;254:277.
12. **Del Prete G, De Carli M, Almerigogna F, Giudizi M, Biagiotti R, Romagnani S.** Human IL-10 is produced by both type 1 helper (Th1) and type 2 helper (Th2) T cell clones and inhibits their antigen-specific proliferation and cytokine production. J Immunol 1993;150:353.
13. **Rogge L, Barberis ML, Biffi M, Passini N, Presky D, Gubler U, Sinigaglia F.** Selective expression of an interleukin-12 receptor component by human T helper 1 cells. J Exp Med 1997;185:825.
14. **Clerici M, Shearer GM.** A TH1 to TH2 switch is a critical step in the etiology of HIV infection. Immunol Today 1993;14:107.
15. **Graziosi C, Gantt K, Vaccarezza M, Demarest J, Daucher M, Saag M, Shaw G, Quinn T, Cohen O, Welbon C, Pantaleo G, Fauci A.** Kinetics of cytokine expression during primary human immunodeficiency virus type 1 infection. Proc Natl Acad Sci U S A 1996;93:4386.
16. **Levy J, Ritchey J, Rottman J, Davidson M, Liang Y-H, Jordan H, Tompkins W, Tompkins M.** Elevated IL10:IL12 ratio in FIV-Infected cats predicts loss of type 1 immunity to T. gondii. J Infect Dis 1998;178:503.
17. **Bucci J, English R, Jordan H, Childers T, Tompkins M, Tompkins W.** Mucosally transmitted feline immunodeficiency virus induces a CD8+ antiviral response that correlates with the reduction of cell-associated virus. J Infect Dis 1998;177:18.
18. **Reed S, Brownell C, Russo D, Silva J, Grabstein K, Morrissey P.** IL-10 mediates susceptibility to Trypanosoma cruzi infection. J Immunol 1994;153:3135.

CHAPTER 43

Immunodeficiency Disease

• PETER J. FELSBURG

Immunodeficiency diseases, which are characterized clinically by an increased susceptibility to infection, are a diverse group of diseases that result from abnormalities in one or more components of the immune system. Immunodeficiency diseases can be broadly divided into two main categories: primary or genetic immunodeficiencies and secondary or acquired immunodeficiencies. Primary immunodeficiencies are diseases in which the animal is born with a genetic defect involving its immune system and any clinical disease observed in these animals is a direct consequence of the hereditary defect. Secondary immunodeficiencies are diseases in which the animal is born with an intact immune system, but as a result of some underlying disease process, their immune system becomes transiently or permanently impaired. This chapter is majorly devoted to the primary immunodeficiencies that have been documented in domestic animals.

Animals that have immunodeficiencies generally suffer from recurrent or chronic infections. Some of the more common conditions associated with immunodeficiency diseases are respiratory infections, otitis, dermatitis and pyoderma, diarrhea, growth retardation, adverse reactions to modified-live vaccines, and infection with usually nonpathogenic organisms (opportunistic infections). Although the possibility of an immunodeficiency should be considered in any animal that has too many infections, immunodeficiency diseases are fairly uncommon, so it is important to consider other conditions that may lead to infection. Most of these conditions can be determined after a careful history and physical examination and can be confirmed by appropriate laboratory tests. When there is no apparent explanation for the recurrent infections, a primary immunodeficiency should be considered. Because the primary immunodeficiency diseases are genetic, the majority of affected patients are neonates or young animals.

DIAGNOSIS OF IMMUNODEFICIENCIES

The severity of the defect and which part of the immune system is affected influence the type of infection involved and the clinical signs. Defects in the B-cell (hu-moral immune) system usually increase susceptibility to bacterial infections. Animals with T-cell (cell-mediated immune) deficiencies usually have an increased susceptibility to intracellular microorganisms such as fungal, protozoal, and viral infections. Note that since a humoral immune response highly depends on the T-cell system, certain T-cell deficiencies may also present as humoral immune deficiencies even though the B cell itself may be normal. Disorders of the phagocytic system are usually associated with superficial skin infections or systemic infections with pyogenic microorganisms. Complement deficiencies are usually associated with recurrent infections with pyogenic microorganisms.

Although the clinical history and findings may be highly suggestive of an immunodeficiency, the diagnosis must be established by appropriate clinical immunologic testing. Many tests of immune function are available, however. The clinical immunologic tests below are commonly used to determine the competence of the various components of the immune system. These basic tests are becoming more available to the veterinary practitioner. Once an immunodeficiency has been established, other more sophisticated tests can be performed to localize the defect more narrowly.

- B-Cell System:
    —Quantitation of serum immunoglobulin A (IgA), immunoglobulin G (IgG), and immunoglobulin M (IgM)
    —Phenotypic evaluation of B cells
- T-cell System:
    —Lymphocyte transformation test
    —Phenotypic evaluation of T cells
- Phagocytic System:
    —Bactericidal assay
- Complement System:
    —Quantitation of serum C3

The most practical test for evaluating the B-cell (humoral immune) system is to quantitate the serum concentrations of IgG, IgM, and IgA. Since the only published normal values for the dog and cat are from normal adult animals, it is extremely important not to overemphasize the significance of low immunoglobulin concentrations in young animals. Serum immunoglobulin concentrations are greatly influenced by age. For example, in the dog, IgM concentrations reach normal adult values within several months; however, IgG concentrations do not reach normal adult values until the dog is approximately 10 to 12 months of age and IgA concentrations until the dog is approximately 15 to 18 months of age. It is imperative to compare the immunoglobulin concentrations of young animals with age-matched normal animals. If the immunoglobulin concentrations are less than 95% confidence limits for age-matched normal animals, a diagnosis of a deficiency in one or more of the immunoglobulin classes (antibody deficiency) may be made.

The lymphocyte transformation (blastogenesis) test is the simplest and most widely accepted in vitro test to evaluate the competence of the T-cell system. This test evaluates the ability of T cells to proliferate after stimulation. Animals with T-cell deficiencies have an absent or a significantly reduced response to stimulation. If an abnormal lymphocyte transformation response is found in an animal, it is important to test the animal on at least two occasions to eliminate the possibility of a transient T-cell suppression from a concurrent viral infection.

Since the main function of the phagocytic (neutrophil) system is to phagocytize and eliminate microorganisms from the body, neutrophil function is most commonly evaluated by bactericidal assays. This in vitro test measures the ability of neutrophils to kill bacteria. Neutrophils from normal animals will be more than 95% of the bacteria in this assay. It is important to test a normal animal at the same time as the patient to control for test variables.

Several tests of the complement system exist. However, since the only documented complement deficiency is a C3 deficiency, quantitation of serum C3 concentrations is sufficient.

CANINE PRIMARY IMMUNODEFICIENCIES

X-Linked Severe Combined Immunodeficiency

Severe combined immunodeficiency (SCID) is the most serious of all the primary immunodeficiencies. SCID describes a heterogeneous group of disorders that have the common feature of severely deficient humoral (B cell) and cell-mediated (T cell) immune responses resulting in an increased susceptibility to a wide spectrum of microbial agents with untreated patients rarely surviving past infancy.

A form of X-linked SCID (XSCID) has been documented in the dog.[1,2] Problems with infections in the neonatal period are rare owing to the presence of maternal antibody. Recurrent or chronic infections begin to appear between 4 and 8 weeks of age with clinical signs that include pyoderma, otitis, diarrhea, and respiratory infections. These infections, usually of bacterial origin, are nonresponsive to antibiotic therapy. A universal finding in affected dogs is a failure to thrive (stunted growth). On physical examination, there is an absence of

any palpable lymph nodes and tonsils are not noticeable. Affected puppies usually die before 3 to 4 months of age either from overwhelming bacterial infections or viral infections. Several affected puppies vaccinated with a modified-live distemper vaccine died 2 to 3 weeks later of distemper induced by the vaccine.

XSCID is caused by mutations in the common gamma chain (γc) gene that encodes for an essential component of the receptors for interleukin (IL) -2, IL-4, IL-7, IL-9, and IL-15. The shared usuage of the γc by receptors of cytokines essential for normal B- and T-cell development and function explains the profound immunologic abnormalities and clinical severity of this disease.

In XSCID, only males are affected, whereas females may be carriers in the disease. In the dog, approximately half of the males in a litter from a carrier female are affected, and half of the females are potential carriers. Note that carrier females show no clinical or immunologic abnormalities. When a male is diagnosed and the mutation determined, a polymerase-chain-reaction-based DNA test can be developed to detect female carriers of the disease within that family or line of dogs.

Lymphocyte counts are usually low, averaging $1000/mm^3$, but can be within normal range. Affected dogs have normal or elevated proportions of peripheral B cells and low to near normal proportions of nonfunctional peripheral T cells. Laboratory findings include normal serum concentrations of IgM but low to absent serum IgG and IgA. IgG may be normal during the first few weeks owing to maternal antibody. The patient's T cells fail to proliferate after mitogenic or antigenic stimulation in the lymphocyte transformation (blastogenesis) test. Flow-cytometric analysis of activated lymphocytes demonstrates the absence of functional IL-2 receptors. The typical postmortem findings are a small thymus characterized by thymic dysplasia and a lack of lymph nodes, tonsils, and Peyer's patches.

The only successful means of treating XSCID is bone marrow transplantation. Although normal immune function can be successfully reconstituted in XSCID dogs after bone marrow transplantation, currently, in veterinary medicine, this is not a practical treatment.

Selective IgA Deficiency

Selective IgA deficiency (IgAd) represents a heterogeneous group of diseases consisting of three major types: severe IgAd as defined by undetectable IgA measured by radial immunodiffusion, partial IgAd as defined by detectable IgA but less than two standard deviations of the mean value for age-matched normal dogs, and transient IgAd as defined by undetectable or low IgA with subsequent development of normal IgA concentrations. All three forms of IgAd have been documented in the dog.[3-5] There does not appear to be a difference in the clinical manifestations between dogs that have severe IgAd and dogs that have partial IgAd. It has been suggested that IgAd alone in human patients who have severe IgAd is sufficient to cause clinical disease, whereas in parital IgAd patients, a concomitant IgG subclass deficiency predisposes to disease. IgG subclasses have not been examined in canine IgAd.

The most common clinical problems in dogs that have IgAd include recurrent infections, usually upper respiratory infections caused by *Bordetella bronchiseptica* and canine parainfluenza virus, otitis, staphylococcal dermatitis, diarrhea, and atopic dermatitis. The infections associated with IgAd are usually not severe or life threatening. Several dogs have experienced convulsive episodes. Older dogs may develop autoantibodies and, possibly, autoimmune disease. There appears to be a high incidence of IgAd in Shar-peis that may be a reflection of their predisposition to upper respiratory infections and atopic disease.

The only abnormal laboratory finding is an absence or a significantly low concentration of serum IgA compared with values of age-matched normal dogs. There is a possibility that some young dogs diagnosed as IgAd may have a transient IgAd and that as they become adults, will outgrow their tendency for recurrent infections.

Treatment of IgAd is mainly symptomatic. Immune globulin, if available, is contraindicated because IgAd patients have been reported to make anti-IgA antibodies that may lead to an anaphylactic reaction when treated with immune globulin.

Immunodeficiency Syndrome in Shar-pei Dogs

Immunodeficiency syndrome in Shar-pei dogs is a recently described late-onset immunodeficiency that seems similar to common variable immunodeficiency in humans.[6] The mean age at clinical onset in affected dogs is 3 years of age. Intermittent fever and recurrent infection of the skin, respiratory system, and gastrointestinal system, including ulcerative colitis, characterize the disease. Several of the reported cases died of intestinal adenocarcinoma and lymphoma. Although the immunologic defect is unknown, both B- and T-cell abnormalities are observed in affected dogs.

Laboratory findings include low serum concentrations of one or more of the serum immunoglobulins (IgG, IgM, and IgA). In approximately half of the patients, the in vitro proliferative response of the lymphocytes to mitogenic stimulation is depressed.

Leukocyte Adhesion Deficiency

For phagocytes to perform their major function of ingesting and killing microorganisms, they must be able to adhere to and migrate across the vascular endothelium and to phagocytosize and kill the micoorganism. In addition, the effector function of cytotoxic T cells and natural killer (NK) cells requires adherence to the target cell. Many of these functions are regulated by glycoproteins of the integrin family that are found on the surface of leukocytes, including CD11a, CD11b, CD11c and their common β chain component, CD18. Leukocyte adherence deficiency (LAD) is caused by a deficiency of the common β subunit that results in the dysfunction of all three integrins and is characterized by defective phagocytic function and suppressed cell-mediated immunity. LAD in humans can have an X-linked as well as an autosomal recessive mode of inheritance.

An autosomal recessive form of LAD has been reported in Irish Setters in the United States and Europe.[7-9] Clinical signs begin at a few weeks of age and primarily consist of recurrent pyogenic infections, including pyoderma, pododermatitis, gingivitis, pneumonia, thrombophlebitis, and osteomyelitis. Poor wound healing is a common feature. Infection sites usually exhibit a localized cellulitis with minimal pus formation.

Laboratory findings include a persistent significant leukocytosis (possibly >200,000/mm³) with most of the cells being mature, hypersegmented neutrophils. Flowcytometric analysis of leukocytes with monoclonal antibodies show a lack of CD11b or CD18. Neutrophil function tests are uniformly abnormal. Lymphocytes from affected dogs also have a significantly suppressed blastogenic response after mitogenic stimulation.

Canine Cyclic Hemopoiesis

Neutropenia is the most common disorder of the polymorphonuclear phagocytic system in man and results in increased susceptibility to severe bacterial infections and a poor response to antibiotic treatment. Cyclic hematopoiesis is characterized by a periodic production and maturation defect of hemopoietic cells in the bone marrow and can either be acquired or hereditary.

A hereditary form of cyclic hemopoiesis that has an autosomal recessive mode of inheritance has been documented in collies.[10,11] Affected collies have hypopigmentation and their coat appears silvery gray or light tan, thus the term gray-collie syndrome. Unlike cyclic neutropenia in humans, the disease in the dog is characterized by cyclic fluctuation of not only peripheral blood neutrophils but also of all cellular blood elements, including platelets. The blood cell elements cycle at 10 to 14 day intervals, lasting for 2 to 4 days. The clinical signs are cyclic and are present only during the periods of severe neutropenia (<1000/mm³). Affected dogs suffer from severe, recurrent bacterial infections primarily involving the respiratory and gastrointestinal tracts. Epistaxis or profuse hemorrhage may be present owing to the associated thrombocytopenia. Affected dogs rarely survive past 3 years of age.

The reason for the recurrent infections was originally thought to be caused by the lack of sufficient numbers of functional neutrophils during the periods of neutropenia. It is now evident that metabolic abnormalities, including a myeloperoxidase deficiency and a defect in iodination, result in the impaired ability of neutrophils from affected animals to kill bacteria. No other immunologic abnormalities have been documented in this disorder.

The laboratory diagnosis is based on the demonstration of a cyclic neutropenia as well as an abnormal bactericidal assay. Treatment of this condition is primarily supportive antibiotic therapy to control infections. Although lithium carbonate has been shown effective in controlling the cycling of the neutrophils and platelets, it is only effective at high and toxic doses. Once treatment is stopped, the cycling of cells and clinical signs reappear.

C3 Deficiency

C3 is a component of the complement system that is important in the opsonization of bacteria. A C3 deficiency, with an autosomal recessive mode of inheritance, has been reported in the Brittany spaniel.[12] Dogs that are homozygous for the trait have no detectable C3, whereas dogs that are heterozygous have C3 concentrations that are approximately 50% of normal. Clinical signs are only observed in dogs that are homozygous for the C3 deficiency and are related to an increased susceptibility to bacterial infections, including septicemia primarily involving gram-negative organisms and clostridia. The C3 deficient dog is also susceptible to type I membranoproliferative glomerulonephritis. The major laboratory finding is the absence of serum C3.

Miscellaneous Neutrophil Deficiencies

A neutrophil oxidative metabolic defect has been independently described by two groups in a total of 64 related Weimaraner dogs.[13,14] The clinical signs included recurrent episodes of fever, vomiting, diarrhea, pneumonia, pyoderma, lymphadenopathy, and osteomyelitis. Neurologic signs consisting of disorientation, ataxia, head pressing, and seizures were observed in some of the dogs. The only abnormal immunologic finding appears to be the inability of the neutrophils to kill bacteria because of their metabolic defect.

A defect in the bacterial killing capacity of neutrophils has also been reported in eight related Doberman pinschers that had a history of recurrent respiratory infections since birth.[15] These dogs had normal neutrophil counts, and laboratory tests of the B- and T-cell systems were normal.

Transient Hypogammaglobulinemia of Infancy

Transient hypogammaglobulinemia of infancy is a self-limiting immunoglobulin deficiency resulting from an abnormally delayed onset of IgG and IgA production by the neonate or young puppy.[16] Affected puppies are clinically normal during the time they possess maternal antibody. However, when the maternal antibody disappears they have an increased susceptibility to infection, primarily chronic or recurrent bacterial infections of the respiratory tract. Spontaneous recovery occurs between 5 to 7 months of age when the animal's own humoral immune system begins to produce sufficient immuno-

globulin. It may be necessary to treat the animal symptomatically during the period of hypogammaglobulinemia.

The only significant laboratory finding is significantly reduced concentrations of serum immunoglobulins after the disappearance of maternal antibody, at approximately 2 months of age, that persists until their own humoral immune system becomes operational, usually between 5 and 7 months of age. Monitoring of immunoglobulin concentrations in puppies diagnosed as immunoglobulin deficient is essential for determining whether the deficiency is a permanent or a transient defect.

FELINE PRIMARY IMMUNODEFICIENCIES

Hypotrichosis With Thymic Aplasia (Nude Kittens)

Birman cats have been diagnosed with an autosomal recessive disease that appears to be the homologue of that found in the nude mouse.[17] The disease is characterized by the lack of hair growth and thymic development and a severe immunodeficiency. Kittens are born with no hair and fail to thrive, resulting in death within a few days. Necropsy findings include the lack of a thymus and the presence of severely aplastic lymph nodes, if the latter are detected at all.

Chediak–Higashi Syndrome

Characterized by the presence of abnormally large, eosinophilic granules in neutrophils, basophils, and eosinophils, Chediak–Higashi Syndrome is an autosomal recessive genetic disease of humans and other species, including blue-smoke Persian cats.[18] Enlarged melanin granules are observed in the skin and hair shaft of affected animals.

Affected cats show an increased susceptibility to infection, particularly to neonatal septicemia and viral respiratory infections. Sudden death caused by an increased bleeding tendency may occur. The tendency for increased bleeding is thought to be caused by abnormal platelet function and can result in major bleeding problems after even minor surgery and hematoma formation after venipuncture. The abnormal melanin granules cause abnormally light coat colors in affected blue-smoke Persian cats. Affected cats may also have light-colored irises, reduced fundic pigmentation, photophobia, and increased incidence of congenital cataracts.

Neutrophils from affected cats exhibit impaired chemotaxis and a defect in intracellular killing of bacteria. Treatment is symptomatic.

EQUINE PRIMARY IMMUNODEFICIENCIES

Severe Combined Immunodeficiency

SCID in the horse is characterized by impaired humoral and cell-mediated immune responses caused by an absence of both B and T lymphocytes.[19,20] It primarily occurs in Arabian and part Arabian horses, although it has been reported in other breeds, and has an autosomal mode of inheritance. It has been estimated that 25% of the Arabian horses are carriers of the disease and that 2 to to 3% of the Arabian foals in the United States are born with SCID.

Affected foals appear normal at birth, but develop infections within the first 2 months of life and rarely survive past 5 months of age. Foals that have this disease are susceptible to various infections, including bacterial, fungal, parasitic, and viral infections. A common clinical finding is bronchopneumonia, often caused by adenovirus or *Pneumocystis carinii*. Another common clinical finding is diarrhea caused by *Cryptosporidia*. Both *Pneumocystis* and *Cryptosporidia* are considered opportunistic infections that are only seen in immune-compromised hosts.

The primary immunologic defect appears to be the inability of the lymphoid stem cell to differentiate into mature B and T lymphocytes. Recent reports have shown that the defect in Arabian foals is caused by defective variable (V), diversity (D), and joining (J) genes, V-D-J recombination, which is necessary for the differentiation and maturation of B and T lymphocytes.[21,22]

Laboratory findings of SCID include an absolute lymphopenia (usually $<1000/mm^3$); absence of B and T lymphocytes, the few lymphocytes present are probably NK cells; and low to absent serum IgA, IgG, and IgM. Antemortem diagnosis is usually based on the presence of the absolute lymphopenia ($<1000/mm^3$) and absence of IgM 3 weeks after birth (by this time any maternal IgM obtained through the colostrum should have been depleted).

Selective IgM Deficiency

Traits that characterize selective IgM deficiency are reduced or absent serum IgM with normal or elevated serum concentrations of other immunoglobulin classes.[23,24] Although it occurs in different breeds of horses, it is most common in Arabians and quarter horses. The mode of inheritance is unknown. Three forms of the disease have been described. The most common form occurs in foals that develop severe pneumonia, arthritis, enteritis, and possibly septicemia. The bacterial infections are frequently caused by *Klebsiella* sp. Most of these foals die before 10 months of age. The second form also occurs in foals, but these foals may respond temporarily to antibiotic therapy resulting in recurrent infections and poor development. These foals usually die between 1 to 2 years of age. The third form occurs in horses between 2 to 5 years of age. These horses do not necessarily have recurrent infections but have chronic weight loss and depression. Approximately half of these horsesdevelop lymphosarcoma.

The only significant laboratory abnormality is an absent or low serum IgM and is the basis for the diagnosis of this disease. Other than supportive care and antibiotic therapy, there is no effective treatment for selective IgM deficiency.

Agammaglobulinemia

Agammaglobulinemia is a rare immunodeficiency that has been reported in thoroughbreds and standardbreds.[25,26] It has only been reported in males, suggesting an X-linked mode of inheritance with many similarities to X-linked agammaglobulinemia in humans. Affected horses suffer from recurrent bacterial infections such as pneumonia, enteritis, laminitis, and arthritis. Clinical signs begin between 2 and 6 months of age with most affected horses dying before 2 years of age from generalized infections.

The two major laboratory findings are the lack of peripheral B lymphocytes and low or absent serum IgA, IgG, and IgM. Specific antibody responses are also severely depressed.

Treatment is symptomatic, including antibiotic therapy. Although administration of plasma may temporily control infections, the long-term prognosis is poor.

BOVINE PRIMARY IMMUNODEFICIENCIES

Leukocyte Adhesion Deficiency

Bovine leukocyte adhesion deficiency is an autosomal recessive disease that was first described in Holstein cattle in 1984.[27] The clinical and laboratory findings are similar to those described previously for canine LAD. At birth, affected calves appear normal, but clinical signs develop within the first few weeks of life and are usually fatal before the calf is 1 year of age. Bovine LAD is characterized by recurrent or chronic bacterial infections. Typical clinical findings include fever, stomatitis, gingivitis, bronchopneumonia, diarrhea, vasculitis, dermatitis, and peripheral lymphadenopathy. The lack of pus formation is a common feature. Hematologic findings include a mature neutrophilia ($>40,000/mm^3$), lymphocytosis, and monocytosis. Leukocytes lack surface expression of the CD11b or CD18 complex.[28]

Bovine LAD has been reported to be caused by a single point mutation in the gene-encoding bovine CD18.[29] It has been shown that all cattle with the mutant allele, D128G, are related to one bull. In the United States, it has been estimated that the carrier fequency is 15% among bulls and 6% among cows, which results in approximately 16,000 Holstein calves born each year with LAD. Because the mutation is known, diagnostic tests are available to detect heterozygous carriers as well as homozygous (affected) calves.

REFERENCES

1. **Felsburg PJ, Somberg RL, Hartnett BJ, Henthorn PS, Carding SR.** (1998a). Canine X-linked severe combined immunodeficiency. A model for investigating the requirement for the common gamma chain (gc) in human lymphocyte development and function. Immunol Res 1998;17: 63–73.
2. **Felsburg PJ, Hartnett BJ, Henthorn PS, Moore PF, Krakowka S, Och HD.**

Canine X-linked severe combined immunodeficiency. Vet Immunol Immunopathol 1999;69:127–135.

3. **Felsburg PJ, Glickman LT, Jezyk PF.** Selective IgA deficiency in the dog. Clin Immunol Immunopathol 1985;36: 297–305.
4. **Felsburg PJ, HogenEsch H, Shofer F, Kirkpatrick CE, Glickman LT.** Clinical, epidemiologic and immunologic characteristics of canine selective IgA deficiency. Adv Exp Med Biol 1987;216B:1461–1470.
5. **Moroff SD, Hurvitz AI, Peterson ME, Saunders L, Noone K.** IgA deficiency in Shar-pei dogs. Vet Immunol Immunopathol 1986;13:181–188.
6. **Rivas AL, Tintle L, Argentieri D, Kimball ES, Goodman MG, Anderson DW, Capetola RJ, Quimby FW.** A primary immunodeficiency syndrome in Shar-Pei dogs. Clin Immunol Immunopathol 1995;74:243–251.
7. **Renshaw HW, Davis WC.** Canine granulocytopathy syndrome: an inherited disorder of leucocyte function. Am J Pathol 1979;95:731–745.
8. **Giger U, Boxer LA, Simpson PJ, Lucchesi BR, Todd RF.** Deficiency of leukocyte surface glycoprotein Mo1, LFA-1, and Leu M5 in a dog with recurrent bacterial infections: an animal model. Blood 1987;69: 1622–1630.
9. **Trowald-Wigh G, Hakansson L, Johannisson A, Norrgren L, Segerstad CH.** Leucocyte adhesion protein deficiency in Irish setter dogs. Vet Immunol Immunopathol 1992;32:261–280.
10. **Lund JE, Padgett GA, Ott RL.** Cyclic neutropenia in grey collie dogs. Blood 1967;29:452–461.
11. **Dale DC, Alling DW, Wolff SM.** Cylcic hematopoiesis: the mechanism of cyclic neutropenia in grey collie dogs. J Clin Invest 1972;51:2197–2204.
12. **Blum JR, Cork LC, Morris JM, Olsen JL, Winkelstein JA.** The clinical manifestations of a genetically determined deficiency in the third component of complement in the dog. Clin Immunol Immunopathol 1985;24:304–315.
13. **Studdert VP, Phillips WA, Studdert MJ, Hosking CS.** Recurrent and persistent infections in related Weimaraner dogs. Aust Vet J 1984;61:261–263.
14. **Couto CG, Krakowka S, Johnson G, Ciekot P, Hill R, Lafrado L, Kociba G.** In vitro immunologic features of Weimaraner dogs with neutrophil abnormalities and recurrent infections. Vet Immunol Immunopathol 1989;23:103–112.
15. **Breitschwerdt EB, Brown TT, DeBuyssher EV, Anderson BR, Thrall DE, Hager E, Ananaba G, Degen MA, Ward MD.** Rhinitis, pneumonia and defective neutrophil function in the Doberman pinscher. Am J Vet Res 1987;48:1054–1062.
16. **Felsburg PJ.** Overview of the immune system and immunodeficiency disease. Vet Clin North Am Small Anim Pract 1994;24:629–653.
17. **Casal ML, Strauman U, Sigg C, Arnold S, Rusch P.** Congenital hypotrichosis with thymic aplasia in nine Birman kittens. J Am Anim Hosp Assoc 1994;30: 600–602.
18. **Kramer JW, Davis WC, Prieur DJ.** The Chediak–Higashi syndrome of cats. Lab Invest 1977;36:554–562.
19. **McGuire TC, Poppie MJ, Banks KL.** Combined (B- and T-lymphocyte) immunodeficiency: A fatal genetic disease in Arabian foals. J Am Vet Med Assoc 1974;164:70–75.
20. **McGuire TC, Banks KL, Poppie MJ.** Combined immunodeficiency in horses. Characterization of the lymphocyte defect. Clin Immunol Immunopathol 1975;3:555–566.
21. **Wiler R, Leber R, Moore BB, VanDyk LF, Perryman LE, Meek K.** Equine severe combined immunodeficiency: a defect in V(D)J recombination and DNA-dependent protein kinase activity. Proc Nat Acad Sci U S A 1985;92:11485–11489.
22. **Shin EK, Perryman LE, Meek K.** A Kinase-negative mutation of DNA-PK$_{cs}$ in equine SCID results in defective coding and signal joint formation. J Immunol 1997;158:3565–3569.
23. **Perryman LE, McGuire TC, Hilbert BJ.** Selective immunoglobulin M deficiency in foals. J Am Vet Med Assoc 1977;170: 212–215.
24. **Weldon AD, Zhang C, Antxzak DF, Rebhun WC.** Selective IgM deficiency and abnormal B cell response in foals. J Am Vet Med Assoc 1992;201:1396–1398.
25. **Banks KL, Mc Guire TC, Jerrells TR.** Absence of B-lymphocytes in horses with primary agammaglobulinemia. Clin Immunol Immunopathol 1976;5: 282–290.
26. **Deem DA, Traver DS, Thacker HL.** Agammaglobulinemia in the horse. J Am Vet Med Assoc 1979;175:469–472.
27. **Muller KE, Bernadinia WE, Kalsbeek HC, Hoek A, Tutten VPMG, Wentink GH.** Bovine leukocyte adherence deficiency–clinical course and laboratory findings in eight affected animals. Vet Quarterly 1994;16:27–33.
28. **Kehrli ME, Schmalstiey FC, Anderson DC, Van Der Maaten MJ, Hughes BJ, Ackermann MR, Wilhelmsen CL, Brown GB, Stevens MG, Whetstone CA.** Molecular definition of the bovine granulocytopathy syndrome: identification of deficiency of the Mac-1 (CD11b/CD18) complex. Am J Vet Res 1990;51:1826–1836.
29. **Shuster DE, Kehrli ME, Ackermann MR, Gilbert RO.** Identification and prevalence of a genetic defect that causes leukocyte adhesion deficiency in Holstein cattle. Proc Nat Acad Sci U S A 1992;89:9225–9229.

CHAPTER 44

Benign Lymphadenopathy

• C. GUILLERMO COUTO and RANCE M. GAMBLIN

The lymph nodes constitute a major component of the mononuclear phagocytic and immunologic systems. Because of their dynamic state, they constantly reshape and change in size in response to various stimuli. Most tissue changes within these structures result in lymph-node enlargement. This enlargement oftentimes represents the only abnormality on physical examination in an otherwise healthy patient and alerts the clinician to an ongoing disease process.

LYMPH NODE ANATOMY

The microscopic architecture of the lymph node is beyond the scope of this chapter. However, lymph-node architecture is reviewed in-depth elsewhere in this text as well as in other sources.[1,2]

From the clinical standpoint, it is important to become familiar with the characteristics of palpable lymph nodes in normal dogs and cats so that subtle changes can be easily detected. Palpable lymph nodes in small animals include the mandibular, prescapular (or superficial cervical), axillary, superficial inguinal, and popliteal. Other lymph nodes become palpable only when enlarged; these include the facial, retropharyngeal, and iliac (or sublumbar) nodes.[1]

LYMPHADENOPATHY

Definitions

In the context of this chapter, the term lymphadenopathy refers to lymph node enlargement, although lymph node atrophy, for example, should also be considered a lymphadenopathy. Solitary or isolated lymphadenopathy refers to enlargement of a single lymph node. Regional lymphadenopathy describes the enlargement of more than one lymph node draining a specific anatomic area; these nodes are usually interconnected. Generalized lymphadenopathy refers to multicentric lymph node enlargement affecting more than one anatomic area. Lymphadenopathies can also be classified as superficial or deep, according to their anatomic location.

Pathogenesis

Lymph nodes are in a dynamic state that results in constant reshaping. Lymph node enlargement usually occurs as a consequence of either proliferation of normal cells within the node or infiltration with normal or abnormal cells. When normal cells proliferate within a node, the term reactive lymphadenopathy is used. Proliferation of normal lymphoid or mononuclear phagocytic cells occurs in response to various stimuli, mainly infectious and immunologic, although occasionally the clinician encounters a dog or cat with reactive lymphadenopathy in which a causal agent cannot be identified (i.e., idiopathic reactive lymphadenopathy). When polymorphonuclear leukocytes or inflammatory macrophages predominate in the lymph node infiltrate, the term lymphadenitis is used; this process is usually secondary to infectious agents. If neutrophils predominate, the lymphadenitis is considered suppurative; if macrophages are the predominant cell, then the inflammation is granulomatous; if macrophages and neutrophils occur, the term pyogranulomatous lymphadenitis is preferred.[1] Infectious diseases associated with lymphadenopathy in dogs and cats and their typical cellular infiltrate on lymph node cytology are listed in Table 44.1.

Infiltrative lymphadenopathies result from displacement of normal lymph node tissue by neoplastic or inflammatory cells. Inflammatory lymphadenopathies are classified by the predominant cell type as described above. Neoplasms involving the lymph nodes can be either primary hemopoietic malignancies or secondary (metastatic) neoplasms. Neoplastic causes of lymphadenopathy are discussed elsewhere in this text. Table 44.1 provides a classification scheme for lymphadenopathy in dogs and cats.

TABLE 44.1	Classification of Lymphadenopathy in Dogs and Cats		

Type	Species	Type	Species
Proliferative Lymphadenopathies		*Viral* (cellular infiltrate varies with agent)	
Infectious		Infectious canine hepatitis	D
Bacterial (neutrophilic/suppurative)[a]		Canine herpesvirus	D
Streptococci	C, D	Canine viral enteritides	D
Corynebacterium	C	Feline retroviruses	C
Brucella	D	Feline infectious peritonitis	C
Mycobacteria	C, D	*Noninfectious*	
Actinomyces sp.	C, D	Postvaccinal	C, D
Nocardia sp.	C, D	Immune-mediated disorders	
Localized bacterial infection	C, D	Systemic lupus erythematosus	D
Yersinia pestis	C	Rheumatoid arthritis	D
Francisella tularensis	C, D	Immune-mediated polyarthritides	C, D
Rickettsial (plasmacytic)		Localized inflammation	C, D
Ehrlichiosis	D, C	Aluminosilicate	D
Rocky Mountain spotted fever	D	Idiopathic	C, D
Salmon poisoning	D	*Infiltrative Lymphadenopathies*	
Fungal (granulomatous/pyogranulomatous)		*Neoplastic*	
Histoplasmosis	C, D	*Primary Hemopoietic Neoplasms*	
Blastomycosis	C,D	Lymphomas	C, D
Cryptococcosis	C, D	Malignant histiocytosis	D
Coccidioidomycoss	C, D	Leukemias	C, D
Aspergillosis	C, D	Multiple myeloma	C, D
Sporotrichosis	C, D	Systemic mast cell disease	C, D
Phaeohyphomycosis	C, D	*Metastatic Neoplasms*	
Phycomycosis	C, D	Carcinomas	C, D
Algal (granulomatous/pyogranulomatous)	C, D	Sarcomas	C, D
Protothecosis	C, D	Mast cell tumors	C, D
Parasitic (cellular infiltrate varies with agent		Malignant melanomas	D
Demodicosis	C, D	*Nonneoplastic*	
Trypanosomiasis	D	Mast cell infiltration (nonneoplastic	C, D
Leishmaniasis	D	Eosinophilic granuloma complex	C, D?
Hepatozoonosis	D	Lysosomal storage diseases	D, C?
Babesiosis	D		
Toxoplasmosis	C, D		

[a]Typical cellular infiltrates on cytology are listed in parenthesis.
C: cats; D: dogs

Evaluation of the Patient With Lymphadenopathy

Thorough evaluation of the patient that has lymphadenopathy is essential for establishing an accurate diagnosis. Several reviews of this subject are available,[1,3] but a brief summary of proper patient evaluation is included below.

Historical and Physical Examination Findings

Several important clues of diagnostic value can be deduced from the history. A detailed travel history should be obtained in dogs presented for evaluation of generalized lymphadenopathy, since certain diseases have a definite geographic distribution (e.g., ehrlichiosis in the southwestern or southeastern United States). Other dis-

eases associated with lymphadenopathy have a seasonal distribution (e.g., Rocky Mountain spotted fever [RMSF] in the spring and summer). A vaccination history should also be obtained, because generalized reactive lymphadenopathy shortly after vaccination is fairly common.

The presence or absence of systemic clinical signs is also helpful in guiding the clinician to a specific diagnosis in dogs or cats that have generalized lymphadenopathy, because severe systemic signs are more common in association with certain diseases, such as systemic mycoses, Salmon poisoning, RMSF, leishmaniasis, and acute leukemias. In contrast, systemic signs are usually absent or are mild in dogs and cats that have lymphoma or chronic leukemia.

The distribution of the lymphadenopathy is also of diagnostic relevance. When evaluating a patient that has solitary or regional lymphadenopathy, the clinician should focus attention on the area drained by the lymph node or nodes, since with almost certainty that is where the primary lesion will be found. In our experience, most dogs and cats that have superficial solitary or regional lymphadenopathy have localized inflammatory (or infectious) processes or metastatic neoplasia, whereas most patients that have deep (i.e., intraabdominal or intrathoracic) solitary or regional lymphadenopathy have metastatic neoplasia or systemic infectious diseases (e.g., systemic mycoses). In contrast, most dogs and cats that have generalized lymphadenopathy have systemic fungal or rickettsial infections, idiopathic lymph node hyperplasia, or hemopoietic neoplasia.

The palpable characteristics of the nodes are also important. In most dogs and cats that have lymphadenopathy, regardless of whether it is solitary, regional, or generalized, the lymph nodes are firmer than usual, irregular, and painless; have normal temperature to the touch (i.e., cold lymphadenopathies); and do not adhere to the surrounding tissues. The main exception to this rule occurs in patients that have lymphadenitis in which the nodes may be softer, tender (i.e., painful lymphadenopathy), warmer than normal, and adhere to surrounding structures (i.e.. fixed lymphadenopathy).

From the clinical standpoint, the size of the affected lymph nodes is also important. In our experience, marked lymphadenopathy (i.e., lymph node size five to ten times normal) occurs almost exclusively with lymphadenitis (e.g., lymph node abscessation and tuberculosis) and with lymphomas. Occasionally, metastatic lymph nodes enlarge to this degree. Dogs that have Salmon poisoning may also present with significant generalized lymphadenopathy preceded by (or in conjunction with) bloody diarrhea.[4,5] Cats that have idiopathic reactive lymphadenopathy usually have significant generalized lymph node enlargement.[6-8] Mild lymph node enlargement (i.e., two to four times normal size) occurs mostly in association with various reactive lymphadenopathies and lymphadenitidies (e.g., ehrlichiosis, RMSF, systemic mycoses) and in leukemias.[9-12]

As noted, a thorough examination of the area or areas draining the enlarged lymph node or nodes should always be performed, paying particular attention to the skin, subcutis, and musculoskeletal structures. In patients that have generalized lymphadenopathy, it is important to evaluate other hemolymphatic organs, including the spleen, liver, and bone marrow.

Hematology and Serum Biochemistry

Obtaining a complete blood count (CBC) and a serum biochemical profile are of importance, particularly during evaluation of patients that have generalized lymphadenopathy. Changes in the CBC may suggest a systemic inflammatory process (e.g., leukocytosis caused by neutrophilia, left shift, and monocytosis in a dog that has histoplasmosis or blastomycosis) or a diagnosis of hemopoietic neoplasia (e.g., presence of circulating blasts or of significant lymphocytosis suggestive of chronic lymphocytic leukemia). Occasionally, the causal agent may be identified by examination of a blood or buffy coat smear (i.e., histoplasmosis, trypanosomiasis, babesiosis, or ehrlichiosis).

Anemia in patients that have lymphadenopathy may be caused by several mechanisms. Briefly, anemia of chronic disease can be seen in inflammatory, infectious, or neoplastic disorders; hemolytic anemia is usually present in patients that have hemoparasitic lymphadenopathies or histiocytic malignancies; severe nonregenerative anemia may be observed in dogs that have chronic ehrlichiosis or immune-mediated disorders, in cats that have retroviral infections, and in dogs and cats that have primary bone marrow neoplasms (i.e., leukemias). Intraabdominal lymphadenopathy in a dog that has iron deficiency anemia suggests the presence of a gastrointestinal neoplasm.[13,14]

Thrombocytopenia is a common finding in patients that have ehrlichiosis, RMSF, sepsis, lymphoma, leukemias, multiple myeloma, systemic mastocytosis, malignant histiocytosis, retroviral infections, and some immune-mediated disorders.[9-12,15-18] Pancytopenia is common in dogs that have chronic ehrlichiosis, malignant histiocytosis, and systemic immune-mediated disorders; in dogs and cats that have leukemia; and in cats that have retroviral disorders.[9-12,18,19]

Two major serum biochemical abnormalities are of diagnostic value in dogs and cats that have lymphadenopathy: hypercalcemia and hyperglobulinemia. Hypercalcemia is a paraneoplastic syndrome that occurs in approximately 10 to 20% of dogs that have lymphoma[15] and multiple myeloma[16]; it has also been documented in dogs that have blastomycosis.[20] Hypercalcemia is extremely rare in cats; neoplasms associated with hypercalcemia in this species include lymphoma, squamous cell carcinoma, fibrosarcoma, myeloma, and parathyroid tumors.[21-26] (JP Paola, AS Hammer, DJ Chew, unpublished observations, 1992) Monoclonal hyperglobulinemia may occur in dogs and cats that have multiple myeloma,[21,26] in dogs that have chronic lymphocytic leukemia[11] (CLL) and occasionally in dogs that have lymphoma,[15] ehrlichiosis,[27] and leishmaniasis (A Font, personal communication, 1989). Polyclonal hyperglobulinemia commonly occurs in dogs and cats that have systemic mycoses, in cats that have feline infectious peritonitis (FIP), and in dogs that have ehrlichiosis or lymphoma.[9,15,21,27,28]

Imaging

Radiographic abnormalities in dogs that have lymphadenopathy vary with the primary disorder. Generally, plain radiographs are beneficial in patients that have deep regional lymphadenopathy involving the thoracic and the abdominal cavities. Ultrasonography is a noninvasive procedure that provides great benefit in evaluating intra-abdominal lymphadenopathy. With this technique, lymph nodes can be accurately imaged and measured so that therapeutic progress can be monitored.[29] Moreover, ultrasound-guided aspirates or biopsies can be performed in these patients with minimal complications.[30]

Bone Marrow Findings

Evaluation of bone marrow aspirates or core biopsies may be beneficial in patients that have generalized lymphadenopathy caused by hemopoietic neoplasia or systemic infectious diseases (e.g., histoplasmosis, ehrlichiosis, leishmaniasis).

Lymph Node Aspirate

Cytologic evaluation of lymph node aspirates provides the clinician with a wealth of information and is often the definitive diagnostic procedure in most patients that have lymphadenopathy. Superficial lymph nodes can be aspirated with minimal difficulty; the successful aspiration of intrathoracic or intra-abdominal lymph nodes requires some expertise. For a fine needle aspirate of a superficial node to be obtained, the area does not need to be surgically prepared. Aspiration of intrathoracic and intra-abdominal structures requires surgical preparation of the area and adequate restraint of the patient; in addition, ultrasonographic imaging may be beneficial in obtaining the desired specimen. The technique for fine-needle aspiration (FNA) of lymph nodes is reviewed elsewhere.[1]

Several reviews of cytologic evaluation of lymphoid tissues have appeared in the veterinary literature.[31,32] Briefly, normal lymph nodes are composed primarily of small lymphocytes (80 to 90% of all cells); a low number of macrophages, medium or large lymphocytes, plasma cells, and mast cells can also be found. Reactive lymph nodes are characterized by variable numbers of lymphoid cells in different stages of development (i.e., small, medium, and large lymphocytes; immunoblasts; and plasma cells). As discussed above, the cytologic features of lymphadenitis vary with the causal agent and the type of reaction elicited (i.e., neutrophils in suppurative inflammation; macrophages in granulomatous reactions; an admixture of both in pyogranulomatous reactions). Causal agents can usually be identified in cytologic specimens obtained from affected nodes.[21,32] Metastatic neoplasms have different cytologic features, depending on the degree of involvement and the cell type. Primary lymphoid neoplasms (lymphomas) are characterized by a monomorphic population of lymphoid cells, which are usually immature (lymphoblasts).

Lymph Node Biopsy

When cytologic examination of an enlarged lymph node fails to provide a definitive diagnosis, excision of the affected node for histopathologic examination is indicated. In this regard, it is preferable to excise the whole node, since core or needle biopsies are difficult to interpret because the lymph node architecture is not preserved. Care should be exerted in handling the node during surgical manipulation, since trauma may induce considerable artifact and preclude interpretation of the specimen. The popliteal lymph nodes are easily accessible and are the ones usually excised in dogs and cats that have generalized lymphadenopathy.[21]

Once a node is excised, it should be halved lengthwise; impression smears should be made for cytology; and the node should be fixed in 10% buffered formalin, at a rate of one part of tissue to nine parts of fixative.

The specimen is then ready to be referred to a laboratory for evaluation. Unfixed tissue can also be submitted in a sterile container for bacterial or fungal culture.[21]

Selected Disorders Associated With Benign Lymphadenopathy in Dogs and Cats

As mentioned above, various infectious and noninfectious diseases are commonly associated with lymphadenopathy in small animals. In-depth discussion of all causes of lymphadenopathy is beyond the scope of this chapter, but Table 44.1 outlines the most common origins. The reader is referred to specific references regarding each condition or infectious agent. A discussion of a few unusual conditions causing lymphadenopathy follows.

Bacterial Lymphadenitis

Two syndromes presumptively associated with pyogenic bacterial infections and lymphadenitis, contagious streptococcal lymphadenitis of cats and puppy strangles, have been described in small animals.[21] Also, localized streptococcal and staphylococcal infections may result in solitary or regional lymphadenopathy in these species.

Contagious streptococcal lymphadenitis was described in several kittens in a cat colony.[21] The kittens developed diarrhea and fever at 4 weeks of age, followed by cervical lymphadenopathy 2 weeks later. The lymph nodes in these cats were significantly enlarged and developed draining purulent lesions. An adult, unrelated cat housed with these kittens also developed similar signs and lesions, and the disease could be transmitted orally by administration of lymph-node material from the affected cats.[21] All the cats were negative for circulating feline leukemia virus (FeLV) p27 antigen. Lancefield group G beta-hemolytic streptococci were isolated from the abscessed lymph nodes and from heart blood in one of the kittens that died of septicemia. Most cats responded to treatment with penicillin.

Puppy strangles is a disorder associated with cutaneous cellulitis of the head and neck and cervical lymphadenopathy in 4- to 12-week-old dogs.[21] Pups usually present with fever, deep facial pyoderma, and cervical lymphadenopathy; more than one pup in the litter are commonly affected. FNA of affected lymph nodes reveals purulent lymphadenitis; staphylococcal or streptococcal organisms may be cultured. However, because of the lack of response to antibiotic therapy in a high proportion of cases, the absence of bacteria in most cultures obtained from affected areas, and the subsequent response to immunosuppressive doses of corticosteroids, a hypersensitivity reaction to staphylococcal antigens is suspected.

Idiopathic Lymphadenopathies

Three recent reports describe syndromes of idiopathic lymphadenopathy in cats.[6–8] In one report, 14 cats that had generalized lymphadenopathy and that ranged in ages from 5 months to 2 years were evaluated.[6] The term distinctive peripheral lymph-node hyperplasia (DPLH) was chosen by the authors for this condition. Eight cats were clinically normal on initial physical examination, except for the presence of lymphadenopathy; clinical signs in the other six cats included fever (five cats), lethargy (three cats), anorexia (three cats), pallor, hematuria, eczema, vomiting, and mastitis (one cat each).[6] Of the 14 cats for which CBCs were available, 9 had anemia; 1 cat had neutrophilia and lymphocytosis; and 3 cats had neutropenia. Six of nine cats evaluated for FeLV antigens in peripheral blood were positive.

Therapy in affected cats included antibiotics, corticosteroids, and fluids. In six cats the lymphadenopathy resolved within 2 weeks to 4 months; one of these cats subsequently developed intrathoracic lymphoma and died; one additional cat had recurrence of the lymphadenopathy over 5 years and was euthanized; three cats had persistent lymphadenopathy and were also euthanized within a month of the initial diagnosis; four cats were lost to follow up.[6] Histologic changes in the affected nodes included distortion of the architecture; proliferation of histiocytes, lymphocytes, plasma cells, and immunoblasts in the paracortical regions; and numerous prominent postcapillary venules.[6] These changes were similar to the ones observed in 7 cats that have experimental FeLV infection.[6] Based on these changes and on the fact that six of the nine cats evaluated were FeLV positive, the authors postulated that this syndrome is secondary to retroviral infection.

Mooney et al[7] recently described six young cats that have significant generalized lymphadenopathy resembling lymphoma. The cats ranged in age from 1 to 4 years, and three of them were Main Coon cats. Most peripheral nodes were 2 to 3 cm in diameter and firm. Four cats had leukocytosis and one had leukopenia. One of the cats was anemic, and atypical lymphocytes were visualized in the blood smear. Five cats evaluated for FeLV viremia were negative. Serum protein electrophoresis in five cats revealed the presence of polyclonal gammopathies; one cat was hypercalcemic. Histologic features were suggestive of lymphoma and included loss of normal lymph node architecture, presence of a uniform population of lymphoid cells in the paracortical areas, capsular and perinodal infiltration, and presence of large follicular structures without germinal centers. However, other features were not compatible with malignancy, including abundant vascularity; lymphoid follicles with active germinal centers; and mixed population of lymphoid cells, plasma cells, histiocytes, and granulocytes in the sinuses.[7] One of the cats was euthanized on presentation; the remaining five cats were not treated. Resolution of the lymphadenopathy was seen in all cats within 5 to 120 days; all cats were alive 12 to 84 months after initial diagnosis.[7]

The clinical and pathologic features in cats that have idiopathic reactive lymphadenopathy are similar to those observed in cats naturally or experimentally infected with feline immunodeficiency virus (FIV).[33,34] It is unlikely that all cats that have idiopathic reactive

lymphadenopathy are infected with FIV; more likely, FIV represents one of the agents that can induce such changes in the lymph nodes of domestic cats. Indeed, a recent report found few differences between FIV-infected cats and seronegative cats with regards to lymph-node pathology.[35]

A clinical syndrome characterized by solitary cervical or inguinal lymphadenopathy in cats ranging in ages from 3 to 14 years and referred to as plexiform vascularization of lymph nodes was recently described.[8] The lesions were unilateral in seven of nine cases studied. Most cats were asymptomatic, and the FeLV status was not reported. Surgical removal of the affected nodes resulted in uneventful recovery in most cats; however, postoperative edema occurred in two of the cats. Histologically, the nodes showed replacement of the interfollicular pulp by a plexiform proliferation of small capillary-sized vascular channels and lymphoid atrophy. The pathogenesis of this syndrome has not yet been elucidated.[8]

REFERENCES

1. **Couto CG, Hammer AS.** Diseases of the lymph nodes and spleen. In: Ettinger SJ, Feldman EC, eds. Textbook of veterinary internal medicine. 4th ed. Philadelphia: WB Saunders, 1995.
2. **Rogers KS, Barton CL, Landis M.** Canine and feline lymph nodes. Part I. Anatomy and function. Comp Cont Ed 1993;15:397–409.
3. **Rogers KS, Barton CL, Landis M.** Canine and feline lymph nodes. Part II. Diagnostic evaluation of lymphadenopathy. Comp Cont Ed 1993;15:1493–1503.
4. **Gorham JR, Foreyt WJ.** Salmon poisoning disease. In: Greene CE, ed. Clinical microbiology and infectious diseases of the dog and cat. Philadelphia: WB Saunders, 1984.
5. **Hibler SC, Hoskins JD, Greene CE.** Rickettsial infections in dogs. Part III. Salmon disease complex and hemobartonellosis. Comp Cont Ed 1986;8:251.
6. **Moore FM, Emerson WE, Cotter SM, et al.** Distinctive peripheral lymph node hyperplasia of young cats. Vet Pathol 1986;23:386.
7. **Mooney SC, Patnaik AK, Hayes AA, et al.** Generalized lymphadenopathy resembling lymphoma in cats: six cases (1972–1976). J Am Vet Med Assoc 1987;190:897.
8. **Lucke YM, Davies JD, Wood CM, et al.** Plexiform vascularization of lymph nodes: An unusual but distinctive lymphadenopathy in cats. J Comp Path 1987;97:109.
9. **Hibler SC, Hoskins JD, Greene CE.** Rickettsial infections in dogs. Part I. Rocky Mountain spotted fever and coxiella infections. Comp Cont Ed 1985;7:856.
10. **Hibler SC, Hoskins JD, Greene CE.** Rickettsial infections in dogs. Part II. Ehrlichiosis and infectious cyclic thrombocytopenia. Comp Cont Ed 1986;8:106.
11. **Leifer CE, Matus RE.** Chronic lymphocytic leukemia in the dog: 22 cases (1974-1984). J Am Vet Med Assoc 1986;189:214.
12. **Couto CG.** Clinicopathologic aspects of acute leukemia in the dog. J Am Vet Med Assoc 1985;186:681.
13. **Couto CG, Rutgers HC, Sherding RG, Rojko J.** Gastrointestinal lymphoma in 20 dogs. A retrospective study. J Vet Intern Med 1989;3:73.
14. **Birchard SJ, Couto CG, Johnson S.** Nonlymphoid intestinal neoplasia in 32 dogs and 14 cats. J Am Anim Hosp Assoc 1986;22:533.
15. **Couto CG.** Canine lymphomas: Something old, something new. Comp Cont Ed 1985;7:291.
16. **Matus RE, Leifer CE, MacEwen EG, et al.** Prognostic factors for multiple myeloma in the dog. J Am Vet Med Assoc 1986;188:1288.
17. **O'Keefe DA, Couto CG, Burke-Schwartz C, et al.** Systemic mastocytosis in 16 dogs. J Vet Int Med 1987;1:75.
18. **Wellman ML, Davenport DJ, Morton D, et al.** Malignant histiocytosis in 4 dogs. J Am Vet Med Assoc 1985;187:919.
19. **Cotter SM.** Feline viral neoplasia. In: Greene CE, ed. Clinical microbiology and infectious diseases of the dog and cat. Philadelphia: WB Saunders, 1984.
20. **Dow SW, Legendre AM, Stiff M, et al.** Hypercalcemia associated with blastomycosis in dogs. J Am Vet Med Assoc 1986;188:706.
21. **Couto CG.** Diseases of the lymph nodes and the spleen. In: Ettinger SJ, ed. Textbook of veterinary internal medicine. 3rd ed. Philadelphia: WB Saunders, 1989.
22. **Dust A, Norris AM, Valli VEO.** Cutaneous lymphosarcoma with IgG monoclonal gammopathy, serum hyperviscosity, and hypercalcemia in a cat. Can Vet J 1982;23:235.

23. **Engelman RW, Tyler RD, Good RA, et al.** Hypercalcemia in cats with feline leukemia virus-associated leukemia-lymphoma. Cancer 1985;56:777.
24. **Klausner JS, Bell FW, Hayden DW, et al.** Hypercalcemia in two cats with squamous cell carcinomas. J Am Vet Med Assoc 1990;196:103.
25. **McMillan F.** Hypercalcemia associated with lymphoid neoplasia in two cats. Feline Pract 1985;15:31.
26. **Zenoble RD, Rowland GN.** Hypercalcemia and proliferative myelosclerotic bone reactions associated with feline leukemia virus infection in a cat. J Am Vet Med Assoc 1979;175:591.
27. **Breitschwerdt EB, Woody BJ, Zerbe CA, et al.** Monoclonal gammopathy associated with naturally occurring canine ehrlichiosis. J Vet Intern Med 1987;1:2.
28. **Pedersen NC.** Feline coronavirus infections. In: Greene CE, ed. Clinical microbiology and infectious diseases of the dog and cat. Philadelphia: WB Saunders, 1984.
29. **Nyland TG, Kantrowitz BM.** Ultrasound in diagnosis and staging of abdominal neoplasia. In: Gorman NT, ed. Oncology. Churchill Livingstone, 1986.
30. **Smith S.** Ultrasound-guided biopsy. Vet Clin North Am 1985;15:1249.
31. **Mills JN.** Diagnoses from lymph node fine-aspiration cytology. Austr Vet Practit 1984;14:14.
32. **Thrall MA.** Cytology of lymphoid tissues. Comp Cont Ed 1987;9:104.
33. **Brown PJ, Hopper CD, Harbour DA.** Pathological features of lymphoid tissues in cats with natural feline immunodeficiency virus infection. J Comp Pathol 1991;104:345.
34. **Callanan JJ, Thompson H, Toth SR, et al.** Clinical and pathological findings in feline immunodeficiency virus experimental infection. Vet Immunol Immunopathol 1992;35:3.
35. **Rideout BA, Lowenstine LJ, Hutson CA, Moore PF, Pedersen NC.** Characterization of morphologic changes and lymphocyte subset distribution in lymph nodes from cats with naturally acquired feline immunodeficiency virus infection. Vet Pathol 1992;29:391.

CHAPTER 45

Disorders of the Spleen

• JOHN L. ROBERTSON and SHELLEY J. NEWMAN

The spleen can be a site of primary disease, or it can be affected by disease elsewhere, especially in circulating erythrocytes and leukocytes. This chapter provides a brief overview of splenic disorders.[1]

ANATOMY

The spleen is a discrete organ located adjacent to the stomach, and attached to the omentum, in most higher vertebrates (birds and mammals). It varies considerably in size and shape, depending on species. However, in most mammals, the spleen is oblong, is reddish blue or mahogany colored, has a smooth surface, and is covered by a somewhat tenacious capsule. The spleen of sheep and goats is more triangular. In birds, the spleen is more rounded. Measurements of size are imprecise, given the considerable variation caused by physiologic conditions (see Physiology). The spleen is approximately 0.1% of the body weight of herbivorous animals and 0.2% of the body weight of omnivores and carnivores (pigs and dogs).[1]

Blood is supplied to the spleen in mammals by the splenic artery, a branch of the celiac artery. Blood is drained by the splenic vein into the portal vein. The spleen is richly invested with lymphatic channels and nerves.

Microscopically, the spleen is formed from several structural components. A distensible capsule of fibrous connective tissue covers the spleen. Bands of fibrous connective tissue extend from the capsule into the parenchyma. Smooth muscle, also present in these anastomosing bands, facilitates splenic contraction (see Physiology). Beneath the capsule and interspersed between fibromuscular bands, the parenchyma is segregated into erythrocyte-rich regions (the red pulp) and lymphoreticular regions (the white pulp).

Branches of the splenic artery divide into arterioles, which then shunt blood to either red or white pulp. Within the canine spleen (for example), much of the circulation passes into sinusoidal channels lined with various immunocytes and endothelial and phagocytic cells (splenic macrophages). In other species, such as cats, open-ended venous channels and perforated endo-thelial channels form much of the intrasplenic circulation.[2] A portion of the arterial circulation divides into penicilliary or sheathed arterioles that terminate within the white pulp. These vessels are surrounded by a collar of T lymphocytes and are adjacent to germinal centers formed from a core of B lymphocytes and a mantle of surrounding T lymphocytes.[3]

During fetal development, the red pulp is a site of significant extramedullary hemopoiesis. Clusters of erythrocytes and precursors in stages of maturation may be found scattered throughout the red pulp. When there is significant physiologic demand creating hypoxia, extramedullary hemopoiesis also occurs in the spleen of adult animals. This is especially common in rodents.

PHYSIOLOGY

The spleen performs five primary physiologic functions. These are phagocytosis, hemopoiesis, lymphocyto-poiesis or maturation, hemoglobin processing, and storage and release of blood cells, especially erythrocytes.

Fixed macrophages (also referred to as reticuloendo-thelial [RE] cells) and circulating monocytes within splenic sinusoids phagocytose particulate matter from within the circulation. The primary targets of splenic phagocytosis are damaged erythrocytes, circulating foreign particular debris such as infectious microorganisms, circulating degraded cellular material, and macromolecules. Studies of splenic phagocytic activity indicate it is labile. When overwhelmed with particulate debris, the phagocytic system becomes hypofunctional (RE blockade).[4] Conversely, the continual presentation of particulate matter may induce a state of phagocytic hyperfunction, commonly manifested by splenomegaly (see Algorithm).

In response to physiologic demand, the spleen becomes a site of significant erythropoiesis, leukopoiesis, and lymphocytopoiesis. Damaged erythrocytes are removed from the circulation by RE cells (fixed macrophages) throughout the body, but primarily by RE cells in the spleen. The degradation of hemoglobin within the spleen allows cells to remove and to retain iron in the form of ferritin and hemosiderin. The spleen is an

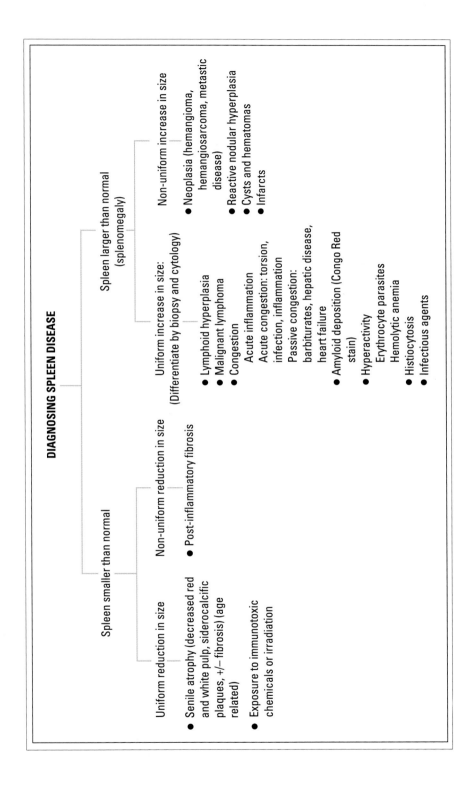

DIAGNOSING SPLEEN DISEASE

Spleen smaller than normal

Uniform reduction in size
- Senile atrophy (decreased red and white pulp, siderocalcific plaques, +/– fibrosis) (age related)
- Exposure to immunotoxic chemicals or irradiation

Non-uniform reduction in size
- Post-inflammatory fibrosis

Spleen larger than normal (splenomegaly)

Uniform increase in size:
(Differentiate by biopsy and cytology)
- Lymphoid hyperplasia
- Malignant lymphoma
- Congestion
  Acute inflammation
  Acute congestion: torsion, infection, inflammation
  Passive congestion: barbiturates, hepatic disease, heart failure
- Amyloid deposition (Congo Red stain)
- Hyperactivity
  Erythrocyte parasites
  Hemolytic anemia
- Histiocytosis
- Infectious agents

Non-uniform increase in size
- Neoplasia (hemangioma, hemangiosarcoma, metastic disease)
- Reactive nodular hyperplasia
- Cysts and hematomas
- Infarcts

important site of iron storage for later use in hemoglobin synthesis.

Splenic stores of erythrocytes and leukocytes are an important source of these cells during periods of unusual physiologic demand. The spleen may contract to one half to one quarter of normal size after, e.g. hemorrhage, releasing cells into the circulation. Such contraction is mediated by circulating pressors and also by direct nerve action on splenic smooth muscle. The ability of the spleen to act as a reservoir for cells and fluid is variable, depending on species. However, it is an important mechanism for preservation of homeostasis and for circulation of blood volume.

SPLENIC DISORDERS

Many disease processes affect the spleen directly or indirectly. These are considered in a fairly classical manner–by means of a disease process or a pathologic mechanism. A diagnostic algorithm, based on gross morphology, is included on the previous page.

Developmental Defects

Diffuse or focal enlargement of the spleen may occur when there is reactive hyperplasia of white pulp lymphoid elements. The stimulus for hyperplasia may be known in some instances, such as chronic antigenic stimulation (e.g., with osteomyelitis or bacterial endocarditis). In other cases, the cause of enlargement is often not known. It is common to find foci of nodular hyperplasia in dog and cat spleens at necropsy.

Small, vascularized splenic fragments (accessory splenic nodules) are incidental findings at necropsy. These are attached to the omentum, with a separate blood supply from the main body of the spleen. Small accessory splenic nodules (a few millimeters in diameter) may be found scattered widely in the omentum. Occasionally, larger fragments, roughly the size of one half of the spleen, are found. It has long been presumed that traumatic rupture of the spleen is the source of accessory spleens. This has been demonstrated in animals sustaining blunt abdominal trauma. However, the presence of splenic fragments in nontraumatized animals suggests formation de novo during embryogenesis. During laparotomy these accessory splenic nodules should not be mistaken for tumor metastases.

Circulatory Disturbances

Changes in splenic morphology and function may accompany alterations in splenic circulation. Active congestion of the spleen, with pooling of red cells and leukocytes in the splenic red pulp may occur during episodes of generalized inflammation, infection, or toxemia, such as clostridial endotoxemia in calves.[5] There is also active splenic congestion during episodes of gastric or splenic torsion.

Splenic torsion, a cause of acute congestion, is seen primarily in dogs and pigs. In dogs, the majority of cases are found in association with gastric dilation and torsion in deep-chested, large-breed dogs. Torsion of the spleen on its vascular pedicle without gastric displacement is considered uncommon.[6] After torsion, the spleen enlarges, as arterial blood fills sinusoids that cannot drain because of venous impairment. Thrombosis of splenic veins has been reported as a consequence of partial or complete torsion and venous occlusion. Stagnation and breakdown of blood and splenic tissue may result in the release of pigments in the circulation.[5]

Occlusion of venous drainage of the spleen produces passive splenic congestion and varying degrees of splenomegaly. Hepatic disease, with increased portal pressure, induces splenic congestion. Right-sided congestive heart failure produces venous stasis in the liver and secondary venous stasis in the spleen. In cattle, constrictive pericarditis, secondary to traumatic reticulitis, also produces venous back pressure and splenic congestion. In addition, the growth of occlusive intra-abdominal masses, such as neoplasms, adhesions, and abscesses, alters venous return from the spleen, producing passive congestion.

The administration of intravenous barbiturates also causes passive splenic congestion and splenomegaly in several species. Barbiturates relax smooth muscle tone, allowing for pooling of blood in splenic sinusoids. This should be accounted for during evaluation of an enlarged spleen in an animal anaesthetized with a barbiturate.

Interruption of the arterial blood supply to the spleen causes splenic infarction. Thromboemboli from vegetations in the left heart or in the cranial mesenteric artery of horses and other species produce infarcts. Splenic torsion may occlude arterial and venous circulation, leading to infarction. Splenic infarction has also been seen in cases of immune-mediated hemolytic anemia, purpura hemorrhagica, consumptive coagulopathies, and hypercoagulable states, and it has been associated with disseminated necrosis of abdominal viscera (pancreatic necrosis).[5]

Traumatic Lesions

Blunt abdominal trauma may rupture the splenic capsule. This can lead to loss of parenchyma, acute and severe hemorrhage, and death. In horses especially, rupture of the spleen is seen after splenic infarction, although this may also occur in other species.[7] When splenomegaly is present, splenic rupture is fairly common, as the connective tissue of the capsule is significantly distended and attenuated.[5]

Splenectomy is indicated when there is severe trauma compromising organ viability and also when physiologic actions of the spleen are deleterious to health. Splenectomy is also used when persistent infection of the splenic parenchyma acts to propagate serious bloodborne or systemic disease.

Immune and Inflammatory Disorders

Infectious organisms may affect the spleen, stimulating an acute inflammatory response (acute splenitis). In fact, it is common to see acute splenic inflammation in both septicemia or with focal infection or inflammation as pathogens and necrotic debris are filtered in the spleen and phagocytized by RE cells.

During episodes of immune-mediated hemolytic anemia, antibody-coated erythrocytes are removed from the circulation by splenic macrophages. Hemolytic anemia may also result from infection of erythrocytes by protozoan and rickettsial parasites, from exposure to oxidative toxins (onions, zinc, propylene glycol, phenothiazines, or copper), or from erythrocyte metabolic deficiencies.[8] Pigments derived from the breakdown of hemoglobin and iron accumulate in the spleen. Splenomegaly is a common finding in hemolytic anemia as intact and damaged erythrocytes fill splenic sinusoids.

Primary splenic amyloidosis is rare. However, amyloid fibrils deposit around splenic arterioles or in the walls of sinusoids in cases of systemic amyloidosis. Deposits may be difficult to appreciate without special stains, such as Congo Red. As with other tissues in which amyloid is present, deposits may displace normal splenic cells and interfere with cell nutrition, leading to organ enlargement and dysfunction.[5]

Thrombocytopenia has been associated with several types of splenic infections,[9,10] splenic infarction,[11] and commonly with hemangiosarcoma.[12] Splenic enlargement, decreased or stagnant circulation, ischemia, necrosis, and the presence of abnormal or transformed endothelium are all factors that favor sequestration of thrombocytes within the spleen.

Several pathogens may cause primary splenic infections or may produce splenic lesions as a result of systemic disease. The latter situation is more common. The most frequent pathologic consequences of infection of the spleen include splenomegaly, multifocal necrosis of white or red pulp, lymphoid depletion, hemorrhage, congestion or vasculitis, or thrombosis.

The causative agents may be grouped in the following categories: bacteria, viruses, fungi, and protozoa. A few of the more important agents that produce splenic disease are reviewed here.

Bacterial Pathogens

Anthrax, a disease produced by *Bacillus anthracis,* is an example of a primary splenic infection. The classic lesion of anthrax is splenic enlargement and softening. When infected, the splenic parenchyma is dark red and has a currant jelly consistency when cut. Histologic examination shows congested sinusoidal areas and hypocellular, widely separated lymphoid follicles. Bacilli may be found on impression smears. The disease is most commonly recognized in cattle, but wild ruminants, elephants, and less commonly pigs, horses, and dogs have been affected.[13–15]

Various other bacterial agents affect the spleen as a part of the systemic illness that they cause. Several of the more common examples include *Salmonella, Erysipelas, Yersinia, Francisella,* and *Streptococcus.*

Salmonella sp. are notorious for producing intestinal disease, but splenic lesions often occur secondary to the presence of markedly increased numbers of splenic macrophages that contain this intracellular organisms. Typically, these organisms and their metabolic byproducts produce splenic enlargement, capsular petechiation, parenchymal congestion and, less often, miliary foci of necrosis or reactive granulomatous nodules.[16] Degenerate organisms can be seen commonly within macrophages and neutrophils and occasionally in extracellular locations.

Yersinia is a gastrointestinal pathogen that may infect the spleen when septicemia is present. Splenomegaly is common. Multifocal areas of parenchymal necrosis, with central bacterial colonies surrounded by a rim of fragmented leukocytes and macrophages, may be present. Lymphoid and histiocytic hyperplasia is also commonly noted. *Y. pseudotuberculosis* is primarily a pathogen of ruminants, but lesions have been documented in farmed cervids,[17] nonhuman primates,[18] and chinchillas.[19]

Infection with *F. tularensis* produces various nondiagnostic gross lesions.[20] Histologically, there is discrete focal splenic necrosis, composed of centrally located neutrophil foci rimmed by macrophages and reactive fibroblasts. The disease has been reported recently in cats.[20]

Brucella sp. cause specific lesions in the spleen because of the presence of this intracellular organism within RE cells. Brucellosis is most commonly a disease of domesticated ruminants, but splenic lesions have been documented in cetaceans, seals, otters,[21] and fish.[22] Typical lesions include activated lymphoid elements, granuloma formation,[23] and necrotizing splenitis.[24] In experimental infections in mice, lesions included decreased white pulp area, increased macrophage numbers, expanded marginal zones,[25] focal granulomas, increased mature neutrophils, depletion of periarteriolar sheaths lymphoid tissue, and extramedullary hemopoiesis.[26]

E. rhusiopathiae infection may cause active splenic hyperemia in pigs.

Goat kids and calves also develop acute splenic hyperemia when infected with *S. pneumoniae.* Infection with this pathogen produces a fulminating septicemia with mucous membrane petechiation and significant splenomegaly. Streptococcosis in nonmammalian species such as aquarium fish (zebra danios) produces splenic acellularity and necrosis but no granulomatous lesions.[27]

Hemophilus septicemia in lambs produces similar splenic lesions to those pathogens already described.

Viral Pathogens

Several viruses cause characteristic splenic pathology in several domestic species. Some of the most important viral diseases are reviewed here.

Although an exotic disease to the North American continent, African swine fever virus is a good example of a splenic viral pathogen. This virus attacks mononuclear cells causing friability, necrosis, and acute splenic infarction, which is a pathognomonic lesion for this infection. The infarcts appear grossly as single or multiple dark red pyramidal foci, usually along the peripheral margin of the capsule. Splenic follicular changes such as swelling, hyalinization of vessel walls, and occlusion of vascular lumens are the underlying causes of infarction in many cases. A recent study of lesions showed that splenic cords macrophages first increased in number and then clustered around muscle cells. After the development of this initial lesion, macrophages disappeared and then erythrocytes and fibrin flooded the areas formerly filled with macrophages.[28]

Equine infectious anemia lentivirus is another primary splenic pathogen. After infection, horses develop turgid splenomegaly, capsular hemorrhages, swollen but indistinct lymphoid follicles (white pulp). Histologic changes include congestion, enlarged but hypocellular follicles, sinusoidal stromal-cell proliferation, hemosiderosis, and macrophage and plasma cell proliferation.

Herpesvirus infections produce splenic pathology in various exotic species, particularly including nonhuman primates,[29] catfish,[30] goldfish,[31] pigeons,[32] parrots,[33] budgerigars,[34] snowy owls,[35] hedgehogs,[36] raccoons,[37] and rabbits[38] as well as the more traditional species, including cows,[39] horses,[40] pigs,[41] and dogs.[42] The lesions produced by these include splenomegaly with multifocal necrosis, hemorrhage, and, less consistently, vasculitis and perivascular accumulations of splenic monocytes and cells with intranuclear viral inclusion bodies.

Fungal Pathogens

Fungal organisms are the least common of the overall groups of agents to induce splenic pathology. The most common splenic fungal infection occurs in the horse and is caused by *Histoplasma capsulatum*.[43,44] Recently, fungal splenic disease was reported in a badger.[45] Splenic lesions include splenic enlargement, white intraparenchymal nodules that are abscesses formed by macrophages containing the intracellular organism, and areas of lymphoid atrophy.

Protozoa and Rickettsial Pathogens

Protozoal and rickettsial infections of blood cells invariably induce splenic hyperactivity and splenomegaly. The mechanism by which these organisms produce lesions is similar. Infected, damaged, or antibody-coated erythrocytes are removed from the circulation by the action of splenic macrophages. Additionally, the chronic antigenic stimulation produced by some infection induces splenic lymphoid hyperplasia. Several organisms, such as *Cytauxzooan* and *Plasmodium,* have proliferative exoerythrocytic cycles within endothelium or splenic RE cells, which damage splenic cells and disrupt vasculature.[46] The most important infectious protozoans include *Plasmodium, Babesia, Trypanosoma,* and *Cytauxzooan.* Pathogenic rickettsial organisms of importance are *Anaplasma, Eperythrozooan,* and *Hemobartonella.* Several species of *Plasmodium* cause avian malaria, characterized

by significant morbidity and mortality (as much as 80%) in domesticated and wild birds. Details of the life cycles of these agents and information on pathogenesis are found elsewhere.[46,47]

Toxic and Physical Agents Producing Splenic Disease

As noted above, the administration of intravenous barbiturates relaxes splenic smooth muscle and leads to both congestion and relative ischemia. Several immunosuppressive drugs also have a direct effect on splenic lymphoid tissue. Corticoids and chemotherapeutic agents such as azathioprine suppress lymphoid activity and produce lymphoid hypocellularity. It is likely that many more immunotoxic agents (e.g., pesticides, estrogen analogues, and aromatic hydrocarbons) that produce functional or morphologic lymphoid suppression in the spleen will be identified in the future. The effects of ionizing irradiation on splenic lymphoid tissue is similar to that of corticoids and chemotherapeutic agents.

Degenerative Disorders

Senile atrophy of the spleen occurs primarily in dogs and horses in association with starvation or wasting. In some species (dogs, cats, and pigs), chronic passive splenic congestion, leading to ischemia and fibrosis results in atrophy of the spleen. Deposits of calcium and hemosiderin (siderocalcific plaques) may be present in abundance on the capsule of atrophic spleens.

Hemosiderosis of the spleen is a consequence of excessive red cell breakdown. A normal activity of the healthy spleen is to remove, to sequester, and then to transport iron derived from hemoglobin for synthesis of new hemoglobin and erythrocytes. However, when there is a significant increase in red cell degradation (hemolysis), normal metabolic processes may be overwhelmed and hemosiderin accumulates. Any disease that alters splenic metabolism also results in hemosiderin accumulation. In affected spleens, pigment is present within macrophages and in connective tissue.

Metabolic storage diseases may affect splenic cells as well as other target cells within the body. In particular, splenic macrophages may accumulate material (lipofuscin) when they are unable to metabolize these substances effectively.

Neoplastic Disease

In the dog, splenic neoplasms are considered a major cause of splenomegaly, although splenic hematoma and reactive hyperplasia are the most frequent causes of splenomegaly.[48] Hemangiosarcoma is the most frequent tumor of the spleen; the instances of its occurrence are as much as all other splenic tumors combined. Hemopoietic tumors (e.g., malignant lymphoma and malignant histiocytosis) and hemangiomas are other important tumors of the spleen in the dog. In the cat, primary and metastatic neoplasia account for one third of all splenic lesions. In this species, however, the frequency of occurrence is different from the dog, with mast cell tumors being the most frequent and hemangiosarcomas a less frequent tumor type.[49]

Malignant histiocytosis is a disease primarily affecting purebred or crossbred Bernese Mountain dogs, although other breeds like Rottweilers, golden retrievers, and flat-coated retrievers may also be afflicted.[50] A few cases of malignant histiocytosis in the cat have been published.[51] In the Bernese mountain dog, malignant histiocytosis has been proved to be inherited by means of a polygenic mode of inheritance. The disease is characterized by the aggregation of atypical histiocytes in various organs, including the spleen, liver, and lymph nodes.[52] Hematologic abnormalities, including a nonregenerative anemia, thrombocytopenia, and leukocytosis, are present in affected dogs, and organ dysfunction may be related to the presence of infiltrating histiocytes. Discernible splenomegaly is seen in approximately 50% of dogs. The rapidly progressive character of the disease in most cases necessitates euthanasia. There have only been less than a dozen cases on symptomatic treatment and chemotherapy in this disease. No treatment has been successful.

In both the alimentary and the multicentric form of malignant lymphoma in dogs, cats, and cattle, the spleen may become involved in the disease process and become enlarged owing to infiltration with neoplastic lymphoblasts and lymphocytes. Single involvement of the spleen in malignant lymphoma is uncommon.[53] The splenic form of lymphosarcoma in horses may produce dramatic splenomegaly and leukemia.[7] Malignant lymphoma is discussed further in Section IX.

Splenic hemangiomas and hemangiosarcomas occur more commonly in dogs, prevalence 0.3 to 2%,[54,55] than in any other species. Especially prone to develop these tumors are middle- and older-aged large-breed dogs, with German Shepherd dogs having an unusually high incidence.[56] These tumors typically appear as large, solitary friable nodules that penetrate the capsule and that bleed easily and uncontrollably. Multiple nodules have also been seen. In dogs that have hemangiosarcoma, regenerative anemia and thrombocytopenia are common because of bleeding within and from the tumor. Some dogs die from hemorrhage after rupture of splenic hemangiosarcomas. At the time when many of these tumors are diagnosed cytologically or with biopsy, they have metastasized to liver and lung.

Although surgical resection of hemangiosarcoma has been the mainstay of treatment in dogs, survival times have been short. In dogs that have splenic hemangiosarcoma, reported median survival times after surgery alone are between 19 and 65 days.[54,56,57] Clinical staging may have some prognostic value. In one study, dogs with splenic hemangiosarcoma and hemoperitoneum had a median survival of 17 days. In contrast, the median survival of dogs with hemangiosarcoma, splenectomized before developing hemoperitoneum, was 121 days.[54] However, two other studies could not confirm

this observation.[56,57] Chemotherapy with doxorubicin (30 mg/m² every other 3 weeks) and cyclophosphamide (50 to 75 mg/m² during 3 days, every other 3 weeks) as an adjuvant therapy to surgery in dogs that have splenic hemangiosarcoma has been reported to prolong median survival to 180 days.[58,59]

Metastatic disease may also occur in the spleen, but it is not common. In dogs and horses that have myelogenous leukemia, the spleen may be significantly enlarged owing to the filling of splenic sinusoids with neoplastic cells.[60]

REFERENCES

1. **Getty R.** Sisson and Grossman's anatomy of the domestic animals. 5th ed. Philadelphia: WB Saunders, 1975.
2. **Dial SM.** The hematopoietic system, lymph nodes, and spleen. In: Goldston RT, Hoskins JD, eds. Geriatrics and gerontology of the dog and cat. Philadelphia: WB Saunders, 1995.
3. **Sell S.** Immunology and immunopathology. San Diego: Academic Press, 1987.
4. **Breazile JE.** Blood. In: Breazile JT, Beames CG, Cardielhac PT, Newcomer WS, eds. Textbook of veterinary physiology. Philadelphia: Lea & Febiger, 1971.
5. **Jubb KVF, Kennedy PC, Palmer N.** Pathology of domestic animals. 4th ed. San Diego: Academic Press, 1993.
6. **Stead AC, Frankland AL, Borthwick R.** Splenic torsion in dogs. J Small Anim Pract 1983;24:549–554.
7. **Rooney JR, Robertson JL.** Equine pathology. Ames, IA: Iowa State University Press, 1996.
8. **Searcy GP.** Hematopoietic system. In: Carlton WW, McGavin MD, eds. Thomson's special veterinary pathology. 2nd ed. St. Louis, MO: Mosby, 1995.
9. **Farrar ET, Washabau RJ, Saunders HM.** Hepatic abscesses in dogs: 14 cases. J Am Vet Med Assoc 1996;208:243–247.
10. **Clinkenbeard KD, Tyler RD, Cowell RL.** Thrombocytopenia associated with disseminated histoplasmosis in dogs. Comp Cont Educ Pract Vet 1989; 11:301–304.
11. **Ellison GW, King RR, Calderwood-Mays M.** Medical and surgical management of multiple organ infarctions secondary to bacterial endocarditis in a dog. J Am Vet Med Assoc 1988;193:1289–1291.
12. **Kessler M, Maurus Y, Kostlin R.** Clinical manifestations of splenic hemangiosarcoma in 52 dogs. Tierarztl Prax 1997;25:651–656.
13. **Mustafa AH.** Isolation of anthrax bacillus from an elephant in Bangladesh. Vet Rec 1984;114:590.
14. **Lodh C, Chakrabarti A, Choudhury MN, Biswas S, Majumber BK.** Histopathological lesion of Anthrax bacilli [Bacillus anthracis] infected zoo deer. Environment and Ecology 1992;10:462–463.
15. **McGee ED, Fritz DL, Ezzel JW, Newcomb HC, Brown RJ, Jaax NK.** Anthrax in a dog. Vet Pathol 1994;31:471–473.
16. **Mastroeni P, Skepper JN, Hormaeche CE.** Effect of anti-tumor necrosis factor alpha antibodies on histopathology of primary Salmonella infections. Infect Immunol 1995;63:3674–3682.
17. **Sanford SE.** Outbreaks of yersiniosis caused by Yersinia pseudotuberculosis in farmed cervids. J Vet Diagn Invest 1995;7:78–81.
18. **Skavlen PA, Stills HF, Steffan EK, Middleton CC.** Naturally occurring Yersinia enterocolitis septicemia in patas monkeys (Erythrocebus patas). Lab Anim Sci 1985;35:488–490.
19. **Vasil'-ova Z.** Yersinia infection is a serious disease of chinchillas in Slovakia. Slovensky Veterinary Casopis 1994;19:129–130.
20. **Baldwin CJ, Panciera RJ, Morton RJ, Cowell AK, Waurzyniak BJ.** Acute tularemia in three domestic cats. J Am Vet Med Assoc 1991;199:1602–1605.
21. **Foster G, Jahans KL, Reid RJ, Ross HM.** Isolation of Brucella species from cetaceans, seals and an otter. Vet Rec 1996;24:583–586.
22. **Salem SF, Mohsen A.** Brucellosis in fish. Vet Med 1997;42:5–7.
23. **Doghiem RE, El-Giabaly SM, Nafady AA, Mousa AA, Hamoda MA, Montaser AM.** Morphological and immunopathological studies on sheep and goats infected with brucellosis. Proceedings of the third Scientific Congress Egyptian Society for Cattle Diseases. Vol 2. Assiut-Egypt, December 3–5, 1995;243–265.
24. **Abdel-Hafeez MM, Ab del-Kadder HA, Bastawros AF, El Ballal SS, Hamdy MER.** Bacteriological and pathological studies on Brucella melitensis infection in a dairy farm. Proceedings of the Third Scientific Congress Egyptian Society for Cattle Diseases. Vol 2. Assiut-Egypt, December 3–5, 1995;266–274.
25. **Palmer MV, Cheville NF, Tatum FM.** Morphometric and histopathologic analysis of lymphoid depletion in murine spleens following infection with Brucella abortus strains 2308 or RB51 or an htrA deletion mutant. Vet Pathol 1996;138:583–586.
26. **Enright FM, Araya LN, Elkzer PH, Rowe GE, Winter AJ.** Comparative

histopathology in BALB/c mice infected with virulent strains of Brucella abortus. Vet Immunol Immunopathol 1990;26:171–82.

27. **Ferguson HW, Morales JA, Ostland VE.** Streptococcosis in aquarium fish. Dis Acquatic Organisms 1994;19:1–6.

28. **Carrasco L, Bautista MJ, Gomez-Villamondos JC, Mulas JM, de la Lara FCM, Wilkinson PJ, Sierra MA.** Development of microscopic lesions in splenic cords of pigs infected with African swine fever virus. Vet Res 1997;28:93–99.

29. **Carlson CS, O'Sullivan MG, Jayo MJ, Anderson DK, Harber ES, Jerome WG, Bullock BC, Heberling RL.** Fatal disseminated cercopithecine herpesvirus 1 (Herpes B) infection in cynomologus monkeys (Macaca fascicularis). Vet Pathol 1997;34:405–414.

30. **Alborali L, Bovo G, Lavazza A, Cappellaro H, Guadagnini PF.** Isolation of an herpesvirus in breeding catfish (Ictalurus mela). Bull Eur Assoc Fish Pathol 1996;16:134–137.

31. **Jung SJ, Miyazaki T.** Herpesviral haematopoietic necrosis of goldfish, Carassius auratus (L.). J Fish Dis 1995;18:211–220.

32. **Allam IH, Aly HAE, Hamoda MS, Tawfik A, Shaker MHM, Hafez MAM, Orabi F, Ayoub NNK.** An outbreak in pigeons associated with a herpes virus encephalomyelitis. Egyptian J Comp Pathol Clin Pathol 1991; 4:173–186.

33. **Widen F, Roken BO, Gavier-Widen D.** Pacheco's parrot disease diagnosed in parrots for the first time in Sweden. Svensk-Veterinartidning 1992;44:255–258.

34. **Ramis A, Tarres F, Fondevila D, Ferrer L.** Immunocytochemical study of the pathogenesis of Pacheco's parrot disease in budgerigars. Vet Microbiol 1996;52:49–61.

35. **Gough RE, Drury SEN, Higgins RJ, Harcourt-Brown NH.** Isolation of a herpes virus from a snowy owl (Nyctea scandiaca). Vet Rec 1995;136:541–542.

36. **Widen F, Gavier-Widen D, Nikiila T, Morner T.** Fatal herpesvirus infection in a hedgehog (Erinaceus europaeus). Vet Rec 1996;139:237–239.

37. **Hamir AN, Moser G, Kao M, Raju N, Rupprecht CE.** Herpesvirus-like infection in a raccoon (Procyon lotor). J Wildl Dis 1995;31:420–423.

38. **Onderka DK, Papp-Vid G, Perry AW.** Fatal herpesvirus infection in commercial rabbits. Can Vet J 1992;33:539–543.

39. **Lopez OJ, Galeota JA, Osorio FA.** Bovine herpesvirus type-4 (BHV-4) persistently infects cells of the marginal zone of spleen in cattle. Microb Pathog 1996;21:47–58.

40. **Dunn KA, Smith KC, Blunden AS, Wood JLN, Jagger DW.** EHV-1 infection in twin equine fetuses. Vet Rec 1993;133:580.

41. **Nauwynck HF, Pensaret MB.** Abortion induced by cell associated pseudorabies virus in vaccinated sows. Am J Vet Res 1992;53:489–493.

42. **Seo IB, Lim CH.** Study on the pathogenesis of canine herpesvirus infection. II. Immunohistochemical observation. Korean J Vet Res 1994;34:583.

43. **Johnston PF, Reams R, Jakovljevic S, Andrews DA, Heath SE, DeNicola D.** Disseminated histoplasmosis in a horse. Can Vet J 1995;36:707–709.

44. **Herve V, Gall-Campodonico-P-le, Blanc F, Improvisi L, Dupont B, Mathiot C, Gall-F-le.** Histoplasmosis due to Histoplasma farciminosum in an African horse. J Mycol Med 1994;4:54.

45. **Jensen HE, Bioch B, Henriksen P, Dietz HH, Schonheyder H, Kaufman L.** Disseminated histoplasmosis in a badger (Meles meles) in Denmark. PMIS—Acta Pathologica Microbiologica et Immunolgica Scandinavica 1992;100:586–592.

46. **Soulsby EJL.** Helminths, arthropods and protozoa of domesticated animals. London: Balliére, Tindall, and Cassell, 1968.

47. **Hoskins JD.** Canine haemobartonellosis, canine hepatozoonosis, and feline cytauxzoonosis. Vet Clin N Am–Small 1991;21:129–140.

48. **Spangler WL, Culbertson MR.** Prevalence, type, and importance of splenic diseases in dogs: 1,480 cases (1985–1989). J Am Vet Med Assoc 1992;200:829–834.

49. **Spangler WL, Culbertson MR.** Prevalence and type of splenic diseases in cats: 455 cases (1985–1991). J Am Vet Med Assoc 1992;201:773–776.

50. **Schaiken LC, Evans SM, Goldschmidt MH.** Radiographic findings in canine malignant histiocytosis. Vet Radiol 1991;32:237–242.

51. **Gafner F, Bestetti GE.** Feline malignant histiocytosis and the lysozyme immunoenzyme technique. Schweiz Arch Tierheilkd 1988;130:349–356.

52. **Kohn B, Arnold P, Kaser-Hotz B, Hauser B, Fluckiger M, Suter PF.** Malignant histiocytosis of the dog: 26 cases. Kleintierpraxis 1993;38:409–424.

53. **Teske E.** Canine malignant lymphoma: a review and comparison with human non-Hodgkin's lymphoma. Vet Quart 1994;16:209–219.

54. **Prymak C, McKee LJ, Goldschmidt MH, Glickman LT.** Epidemiologic, clinic, pathologic, and prognostic characteristics of splenic hemangiosarcoma and splenic hematoma in dogs: 217 cases (1985). J Am Vet Med Assoc 1988;193:706–712.

55. **Priester WA, McKay FW.** The occurrence of tumors in domestic animals. NCI Monograph 54, NIH Publ no 80–2046. NCI Monograph. Bethesda, MD, 1980;167.

56. **Johnson KA, Powers BE, Withrow SJ, Sheetz MJ, Curtis CR, Wrigley RH.** Splenomegaly in dogs. Predictors of neoplasia and survival after splenectomy. J Vet Intern Med 1989;3:160–166.

57. **Brown NO, Patnaik AK, MacEwen EG.** Canine hemangiosarcoma: retrospective analysis of 104 cases. J Am Vet Med Assoc 1985;186:56–58.

58. **Sorenmo KU, Jeglum KA, Helfland SC.** Chemotherapy of canine hemangiosarcoma with doxorubicin and cyclophosphamide. J Vet Intern Med 1993;7:370–376.

59. **Hammer AS, Couto CG, Filppi J, Getzy D, Shank K.** Efficacy and toxicity of VAC chemotherapy (vincristine, doxorubicin, and cyclophosphamide) in dogs with hemangiosarcoma. J Vet Intern Med 1991;5:160–166.

60. **Buechner-Maxwell V, Zhang C, Robertson JL, Jain NC, Antczak D, Feldman BF, Murray MJ.** Intravascular leukostasis and systemic aspergillosis in a horse with subacute subleukemic myelomonocytic leukemia. J Vet Intern Med 1994;8:258–263.

SECTION V
Leukocytes–Nonlymphoid Leukocytes
Kenneth S. Latimer

CHAPTER 46

Neutrophils

• GRAHAM S. SMITH

Neutrophilic leukocytes are a critical component of the host defense system, forming the first line of cellular defense against invading organisms. Neutrophils normally are released from bone marrow as mature cells, which, after a brief period in circulation, transmigrate through the vascular endothelium into tissues. Their primary function is ingestion and killing of bacteria; however, they also can damage or destroy fungi, yeasts, algae, parasites, and viruses.[1-5] In addition, neutrophils may induce antibody-dependent cellular cytotoxicity (ADCC) to destroy infected or transformed cells.[3,4] To perform its functions, neutrophils employ mediators that promote inflammation and eliminate invading microorganisms. In the event that the acute insult cannot be resolved, neutrophils subsequently may contribute to host tissue damage, by production or release of these same mediators in certain subacute and chronic inflammatory states.[6,7] Mounting evidence indicates that neutrophils are not only end-stage effectors of the inflammatory response, but also may secrete or induce production of cytokines that modulate the immune response.[8] Recent major advances have been made in understanding the complex interactions leading to neutrophil recruitment at sites of infection and inflammation. These finely balanced processes involve an array of soluble mediators and cell–cell adhesion molecules expressed by both vascular endothelium and circulating neutrophils.[9] The molecular understanding of these and other events integral to neutrophil kinetics and function has provided potential targets for the therapy of inflammation.[6] An overview of aspects of neutrophil production, kinetics, function, and response to various physiologic and disease states follows and is based on current knowledge in animals and humans. More species-specific descriptions of these features of neutrophils are provided in other chapters of this book.

MORPHOLOGY

Neutrophils in the blood are relatively large cells (approximately 10 to 15 μm in diameter).[10] They contain a large, multilobed nucleus (hence their other name, polymorphonuclear leukocyte), cytoplasm containing two or three types of granules (primary, secondary, and tertiary), centrally located Golgi apparatus, little endoplasmic reticulum, and few mitochondria. A narrow rim of cytoplasm around the periphery of the cell is generally free of organelles and inclusions (glycogen, lipid, etc.) but contains cytoskeletal proteins consisting of microtubules and microfilaments.[11-14] Light microscopic, ultrastructural, and morphometric characterization of neutrophils from various animal species have been reviewed.[11,15,16]

Species differences in neutrophil morphology can be seen at the light microscopic level. Nuclear segmentation varies with species. Only a slight indentation separates nuclear lobes in mature neutrophils from dogs and cats. Mature equine neutrophils may have a distinctly multilobulated nucleus or sharp jagged nuclear margins with less distinct lobulation. A nuclear appendage or extra chromatin lobe, resembling a drumstick and known as the Barr body, is present in varying numbers of neutrophils of the female of various species. These appendages contain an inactivated X chromosome. Ultrastructurally, the mature nucleus is primarily composed of heterochromatin and rarely contains a nucleolus.[11,15,16] Barr bodies may occasionally be observed in males that have chromosomal mosaicism (Kleinfelter's syndrome, XXY syndrome; e.g., male calico cats).

The neutrophil cytoplasm contains numerous granules, typically neutral in their affinity for the acidic and basic dyes used with Romanowsky stains. Granule staining intensity varies with species, and in some species (e.g., rats and dogs) staining can be so light that granules are difficult to discern. In contrast, nonhuman primates have readily identifiable, prominent granules with such stains.[15,17] Neutrophils of the chicken and laboratory animals such as guinea pigs and rabbits have pink-red staining granules. Such cells are called heterophils.[15] Two types of neutrophil granules can be differentiated based on peroxidase activity. Peroxidase-positive granules are also known as azurophil or primary granules, while peroxidase-negative granules are specific or secondary granules. Primary and secondary granules are pleomorphic within and between species. Bovine neutrophils have a larger cell granule volume than neutrophils of other domestic animals.[11] Rabbit heterophils have unique, large, irregularly shaped, eosinophilic granules.[17]

Neutrophil granule contents and structure in animals have been reviewed.[11,15,16] There appear to be more than two major granule populations in the rat,[10,18] guinea pig,[18,19] rabbit,[20] cow,[21,22] sheep,[23] goat,[23] horse,[24] dog,[25] and cat[26,27] as well as in humans.[28] Primary and secondary granules contain microbicidal factors and digestive enzymes that function in conjunction with membrane-bound and cytoplasmic enzymes in killing and digesting phagocytosed microbes. Granule contents are described in several references.[11,15,29,30,31] Some typical contents of primary and secondary granules are listed in Table 46.1. The third granule type in cattle contains bactenecins, lactoferrin, and cationic proteins, but lacks peroxidase activity, lysosomal hydrolases, and metalloproteinases.[21,32,33] Tertiary granules in humans are peroxidase-negative, contain gelatinase, and, in contrast to specific granules, lack lactoferrin.[31]

Interspecies variation in granule morphometry, cytochemical reactivity, and granule contents are reviewed by Bertram.[11] Neutrophil defensins have been cited as present in rabbits, guinea pigs, hamsters, rats, and cattle but seem lacking in the mouse, pig, and horse.[30] The microbicidal peptides, cathelicidins, have been found in neutrophils of cattle, pigs, rabbits, and mice.[30] The antibacterial and antiviral protein inhibitors, equinins, are present in horse neutrophil granules.[34] Myeloperoxidase (MPO) and lysozyme granule activities are reduced in cattle and sheep compared with other animals evaluated.[11] Chicken heterophils have been reported to lack MPO activity,[35] and consequently have been used as a model to study MPO deficiency in humans. However, a recent report indicates that chicken heterophils do contain slight MPO activity.[36]

Neutrophils in animals and humans have been shown to be heterogeneous based on differences in protein synthesis, receptor expression, oxidative metabolism, cytochemical staining, or function. Whether the heterogeneity reflects true neutrophil subpopulations that originate from distinct stem cells or represents maturational differences within a common cell line is not known. Also,

the pathophysiologic significance of the heterogeneity is unknown.[11,16,37]

GRANULOPOIESIS, MYELOID DIFFERENTIATION, AND GRANULOKINETICS

A continuous turnover and resupply of neutrophils to tissues is critical to prevent infection. Under normal physiologic conditions, a stable equilibrium exists between bone marrow neutrophil production and peripheral tissue use. The hemopoietic stem cell has the potential for self-renewal or lineage-specific differentiation.[38] Mature neutrophils are produced in bone marrow, under the influence of cytokines, from stem cells after a process involving proliferation, commitment to differentiation along the granulocytic lineage, and terminal maturation before release into the circulation.[39]

Erythrocytes, granulocytes, monocytes, and megakaryocytes are related through a pluripotential stem cell. Neutrophils and monocytes originate from the subsequent bipotential progenitor cell, colony-forming unit-granulocyte macrophage (CFU-GM), in the bone marrow. Myeloid differentiation is regulated primarily by transcriptional regulatory proteins; dysfunction of such regulators may be involved in most disorders of neutrophil maturation.[38]

Several populations of cells support and maintain hemopoiesis. These include monocytes, natural killer (NK) cells, T lymphocytes, and the fixed stromal elements such as endothelial cells and fibroblasts. These cells deliver hemopoietic growth factors. The stromal cells and associated extracellular matrix also provide an adhesive environment that optimizes cell–cell and cell–matrix interactions.[40] The function, cellular sources, and colony targets for myelopoietic growth factors recently have been reviewed.[41] Several hemopoietic growth factors, including stem-cell factor (SCF), granulocyte-colony-stimulating factor (G-CSF), granulocyte-macrophage-colony-stimulating factor (GM-CSF), interleukin-3 (IL-3), and interleukin-6 (IL-6), are positive regulators of granulopoiesis that act at different stages of cell development (Figure 46.1).[42,43,44] Most of the positive regulatory cytokines support the proliferation of early myeloid progenitor cells and have a limited influence on differentiation and maturation. The earliest hemopoietic progenitors, in G_0 arrest, are triggered to proliferate by early-acting cytokines such as SCF and IL-6. The proliferation of primitive progenitors with multilineage potential is promoted by intermediate factors such as IL-3, which is not lineage specific. GM-CSF and G-CSF are the principal cytokines invloved in neutrophil differentiation, although more broadly acting cytokines (SCF, IL-3, and IL-6) act synergistically.[38] G-CSF is lineage specific and is the major growth factor responsible for regulating granulopoiesis and promotes the survival, proliferation, functional activation, and maturation of neutrophils. These biologic activities of G-CSF are mediated by distinct functional subdomains in its cognate G-CSF receptor (G-CSFR), with subsequent signal trans-

---

TABLE 46.1   Some Contents of Primary and Secondary Granules of Neutrophils

Primary Granules	Secondary Granules
Microbicidal elements	*Microbicidal elements*
Myeloperoxidase	Lactoferrin
Lysozyme	Lysozyme
Defensins	Cathelicidins
Bactericidal permeability-inducing protein (BPI)	
Enzymes	*Enzymes*
Acid hydrolases	Alkaline phosphatase
Neutral proteases	Collagenase
Elastase	Apolactoferrin
	C5a splitting enzyme

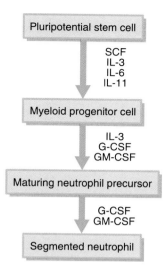

FIGURE 46.1 Influence of cytokines on myeloid proliferation and neutrophil differentiation.

duction. G-CSFR numbers on granulocyte progenitor cells increase with neutrophilic differentiation, with mature human neutrophils displaying approximately 200 to 1000 receptors per cell. The molecular characterization and biological role of G-CSF, as well as the role of mutations in this receptor in the pathogenesis of disorders of granulopoiesis, has recently been described.[45] The application of in vitro models of hemopoiesis and of cytokine technology have been reviewed.[46,47]

During myeloid differentiation, the pluripotent stem cell passes through several well-defined morphologic stages within the bone marrow by proliferation and subsequent maturation through the myeloblast, promyelocyte, myelocyte, metamyelocyte, band, and segmenter stages of development. The light microscopic and ultrastuctural appearance of these cells have been characterized.[15,16] Changes associated with granulopoiesis include progressive nuclear lobulation or segmentation and acquisition of stage-specific granules. Developing neutrophils in marrow can be differentiated from eosinophils and basophils as early as the promyelocyte stage, based on granule structure.[15] Myeloid lineage immunophenotypic differentiation has not been as fully characterized as for lymphocytes.[48]

The earliest recognizable granulocyte precursor is the myeloblast, typified by a round nucleus, finely stippled chromatin, one or more nucleoli, and moderately basophilic cytoplasm. Subtypes I and II are recognized in veterinary medicine. The type I myeloblast has an agranular cytoplasm, whereas the type II myeloblast has a few, small azurophilic cytoplasmic granules.[15,16,41]

The promyelocyte stage has similar nuclear features but is characterized by numerous dispersed azurophilic (primary or nonspecific) granules (approximately 0.4 μm in diameter) that persist in decreasing numbers in later phases of neutrophil maturation. The cytoplasm is lightly basophilic and more abundant with more granules than the type II myeloblast. As the promyelocyte

undergoes the transition to myelocyte, it acquires secondary (specific) granules. The appearance of these relatively smaller (approximately 0.3 μm in diameter) secondary granules indicates a commitment to development along the neutrophil lineage. Formation of primary granules is generally stated to cease with the appearance of the secondary granules,[15,16,41] although evidence in the cat indicates that peroxidase-positive granules also are formed in late (nondividing) neutrophils.[27] Stage-specific transcription factors govern the successive expression of genes for granule proteins, and the protein composition of the granules varies with the timing of their appearance during development.[31,38] The myelocyte varies in size as it may divide twice. Its nucleus is round to slightly indented and lacks a nucleolus.

The metamyelocyte has an indented, kidney-bean-shaped nucleus, or it is wide and elongated with fat ends. It varies in size and has similar cytoplasmic features to the myelocyte.

The band neutrophil approximates the size and has similar features to the mature multilobulated neutrophil but is distinguished by a slender, nonsegmented nucleus with a smooth contour and parallel-appearing sides. The nuclear chromatin pattern usually is less condensed than that of segmented neutrophils. The cytoplasm is clear and contains pale granules as per the segmented neutrophil.[15,16]

Bone marrow neutrophils may be divided into two compartments. The proliferation (mitotic) compartment normally contains approximately 10 to 30% of marrow neutrophils that are capable of cell division (i.e., myeloblasts, promyelocytes, and myelocytes). Each myeloblast undergoes 4 to 5 divisions producing 16 to 32 cells. Approximately 65 to 90% of marrow neutrophils are metamyelocytes, bands, and segmenters constituting the maturation and storage compartment.[49] These are functionally mature nonreplicating cells.[50,51] Transit time in each of proliferative and storage compartments is approximately 2 to 3 days in both dogs[52] and cats.[53] Thus, the transit time from bone marrow myeloblast to blood segmenter takes approximately 6 days in dogs and cats.[50,51] Autoradiographic study in normal calves demonstrated that neutrophils were present in the blood approximately 7 days after marrow precursors were labeled.[54] The transit time from bone marrow to blood has been reported to take as many as 14 days in humans.[40] Transit time can be shortened by early release of immature neutrophils into circulation to meet significant tissue demand. The release of cells from marrow into blood is age ordered with most mature cells (i.e., segmenters and bands) being released first.[50] In the dog, the marrow reserve contains approximately a 5-day supply of cells at a normal rate of depletion. Similar reserves have been demonstrated in the rabbit, mouse, and guinea pig.[55] If tissue demand for neutrophils intensifies, the bone marrow storage pool of mature segmenter cells becomes depleted; progressively less mature forms appear in the circulation constituting a left shift.[51] Species differences in neutrophil response to acute infections appear to depend on the rapidity with which compensatory myeloid proliferation occurs.[56]

Hemopoiesis (including granulopoiesis) in healthy adults of most domestic animal species is largely confined to bone marrow, but infrequently occurs in extramedullary sites when bone marrow production is insufficient for several reasons (e.g., myelofibrosis). In contrast, extramedullary hemopoiesis, particularly in the spleen, occurs commonly in rats and mice.[57,58]

Neutrophils in peripheral blood are distributed in one of two interchanging pools known as the marginal neutrophil pool (MNP) and circulating neutrophil pool (CNP). Neutrophils in peripheral blood may move more slowly than red blood cells and plasma in postcapillary venules because of adhesion molecules on neutrophils and endothelial cells. Neutrophils moving with red blood cells and plasma within vessels represent the CNP and are sampled by venipuncture to yield the white blood cell (WBC) count. Neutrophils that intermittently adhere to the vascular endothelium, MNP, are not included in routine WBC counts. Together, the CNP and MNP neutrophils constitute the total blood neutrophil pool. Blood granulokinetic data for many animal species is summarized by Jain[15,16] The number of granulocytes in the MNP approximates those in the CNP in the horse[59] and dog,[52] whereas, in the cat, the MNP is approximately threefold the size of the CNP.[60] In health, neutrophils move randomly and in a unidirectional manner from blood to tissues, with an average blood transit time of approximately 10 hours. Neutrophil circulating half-life is generally approximately 5.5 to 7.6 hours in dogs[52] and cats[60] and 10.5 hours in horses.[59] Neutrophils marginate and emigrate into tissues in a random (non-age-ordered) manner where they survive for 1 to 4 days.[40] Subsequently, they are phagocytosed by tissue macrophages or are lost from the body by transmucosal migration. Once recruited to sites of inflammation and having exerted their activity, neutrophils die by programmed cell death or apoptosis. Apoptosis induces the recognition and phagocytosis of senescent neutrophils by macrophages, thus permitting the demise and removal of intact neutrophils at tissue sites while avoiding the release of potentially toxic intracellular contents.[29,61] As neutrophils progress through apoptosis, functional activity declines, with loss of CD16 (Fcγ type III receptor) and CD43 expression, as well as loss of the ability to degranulate, mount a respiratory burst, or undergo shape changes in response to stimuli. The process of neutrophil apoptosis can be delayed by certain proinflammatory compounds (e.g., lipopolysaccharide [LPS]), by various cytokines (e.g., G-CSF, GM-CSF, IL-2, interferon-γ (IFN-γ), by tumor necrosis factor α (TNFα), and by anti-inflammatory glucocorticoids.[29,62,63]

The circulating neutrophil count reflects a balance of the following factors: rate of marrow release, distribution between marginal and circulating pools, and rate of egress from blood into tissues. Tissue sequestration also may influence circulating neutrophil counts.[15,51] Counts are maintained within fairly broad ranges according to species Table 46.2.[17,50] Circulating neutrophil counts may be low in healthy laboratory rodents. Diurnal variation in leukocyte and neutrophil counts has been reported in domestic species. The highest neutro-

TABLE 46.2 Peripheral Blood Segmented Neutrophil Counts for Various Animal Species

Species	Reference Interval ($\times 10^3/\mu$L)
Dog[a]	2.9–12.0
Cat[a]	2.5–12.5
Cow[a]	0.6–4.0
Horse[a]	2.9–8.5
Rat[b]	0.1–3.0
Mouse[b]	0.3–2.5
Hamster[b]	0.5–3.5
Guinea Pig[b]	0.5–4.5
Rabbit[b]	1.0–6.0
Ferret[b]	2.0–11.0
Monkey[b]	0.5–9.0

[a]Duncan JR, Prasse KW, Mahaffey EA. Leukocytes. In: Veterinary laboratory medicine: clinical pathology. Ames, IA: Iowa State University Press, 1994;37–62.
[b]Hall RL. Clinical pathology of laboratory animals. In: Gad S, Chengelis C, eds. Animal models of toxicology, Marcel Dekker, 1992;765–811.

phil numbers are noted in late afternoon in healthy dogs, which is similar to the pattern reported in humans, cattle, and pigs. The diurnal changes in dogs are mild and not of sufficient magnitude to confound clinical interpretation.[64]

Increased neutrophil production and delivery to the circulation in response to inflammation may be effected by one or more of the following mechanisms which may occur simultaneously:

1. Multiple signals, including endotoxin, IFN-α, and IL-3, stimulate the secretion of cytokines which, in turn, stimulate differentiation and proliferation of stem cells. Approximately 3 to 5 days are required for influencing the number of blood neutrophils.[40,50]
2. Increased effective granulopoiesis (decreased myelocyte attrition or additional divisons within the proliferation pool) may result in increased peripheral blood neutrophil counts in 2 to 3 days.[50]
3. The early neutrophilia (within 2 days) that follows the initial tissue demand is a result of G-CSF, IL-1, or TNF-mediated increased release of maturing cells from the bone marrow storage pool.[50,61] G-CSF blood levels increase drastically during the inflammatory response, and thereafter return to low basal levels.

The suggestion of feedback regulation of neutropil production when circulating neutrophil levels are high has been proposed. Suggested mechanisms include neutrophil receptor-mediated endocytosis and degradation of G-CSF.[40]

Inhibitor regulatory molecules tend to suppress primitive progenitors while favoring growth of mature progenitors. Examples are IL-8, IFN-inducible protein-10, macrophage inflammatory protein-1α, and macrophage chemotactic and activating factor.[41]

INTERPRETATION OF NEUTROPHIL RESPONSES

Peripheral Blood

Leukocyte and neutrophil peripheral blood counts may change substantially in altered physiologic and disease states. Absolute cell numbers, rather than relative percentages, should be used in interpreting leukocyte responses. Multiple leukograms performed over time may be required to determine the response pattern. Examples of causes of neutrophilia and neutropenia in animals are summarized in several articles and texts.[50,51,65]

Neutrophilia

Increased peripheral blood neutrophil counts or neutrophilia, may reflect physiologic-, pathologic-, or xenobiotic-induced states. Physiologic neutrophilia occurs most commonly in young animals in response to fear, excitement, or strenuous exercise. This physiologic change is actually a pseudoneutrophilia mediated by epinephrine, resulting in a mobilization of MNP with cell redistribution into the CNP; the total blood neutrophil pool remains unchanged. The hematologic result is a mild, transient, short-lived (10 to 20 minute) neutrophilia (as much as twofold the normal) that may be accompanied by lymphocytosis, particularly in cats and nonhuman primates. Numbers of other peripheral blood leukocytes remain within the reference interval.[17,51]

Corticosteroid-induced mild to moderate neutrophilia results in approximately twofold to threefold increase in neutrophil counts, according to species. WBC counts as much as $40 \times 10^3/\mu L$ in dogs–less in other species–may occur after either endogenous corticosteroid release caused by acute disease or stress (e.g., pain or pyrexia) or after therapeutic corticosteroid administration. In dogs, peak response occurs approximately 6 to 8 hours after a single oral dose of prednisolone, with return to baseline values at 12 to 24 hours after a single dose. The neutrophilia is mainly caused by increased bone marrow release of neutrophils, but it also reflects decreased migration of neutrophils from circulation into tissues as well as decreased adherence of neutrophils with a consequent shift of cells from the MNP to the CNP. The neutrophilia is typically without a left shift and accompanied by lymphopenia, eosinopenia, and monocytosis.[51,66]

Inflammation occurs in response to mediators related to infectious agents or to products of tissue injury or necrosis. Cytokines and growth factors are major mediators that are involved in the proliferation, maturation, bone marrow release into blood, and tissue migration of neutrophils. The number of neutrophils in blood during purulent tissue inflammation reflects the balance between the rate of tissue emigration or use and bone marrow release of cells. Therefore, nearly any WBC count from low to high can occur, depending on this balance. In the dog, neutrophil counts over $30 \times 10^3/\mu L$ are common, and counts greater than 50 to 100 $\times$ $10^3/\mu L$ may be achieved. WBC counts exceeding 30 $\times$

$10^3/\mu L$ are less frequent in other species in response to inflammation. Localized purulent diseases such as pyometra, empyema, or abscessation stimulate greater neutrophilic responses than generalized infections or septicemias. Sustained neutrophilia results when the rate of marrow neutrophil release to blood exceeds emigration from blood to tissues. Both total blood and circulating neutrophil pools are increased. Neutrophilia with a left shift is the classic response to inflammation. When the demand for neutrophils depletes the storage pool of segmenters, bands and potentially earlier forms are released. Left shifts can extend to early precursors in circulation, and, if associated with extreme leukocytosis, this results in a leukemoid reaction. A degenerative left shift describes a normal or decreased neutrophil count with more immature than mature neutrophils. However, mild or long-standing inflammation may not produce a left shift because production is balanced with usage. Toxic changes may be present in segmenters and neutrophil precursors according to the degree of systemic toxicity or severity of the disease process. The neutrophilia of inflammation commonly is accompanied by lymphopenia and eosinopenia, reflecting endogenous steroid release. Monocytosis is an inconsistent finding, and may reflect a response to endogenous steroids or effects of mediators of inflammation.[16,50,51] Inflammatory lesions in the rat and mouse cause a neutrophilic leukocytosis, often accompanied by a lymphocytosis. Chronic lesions (e.g., cage sores, ulcerated tumors) in older rats and mice commonly are associated with WBC counts greater than $50 \times 10^3/\mu L$.[17]

Increased bone marrow release of neutrophils may be associated with hemorrhage, resulting in a mild, mature neutrophilia. The neutrophilia, lymphopenia, and monocytosis that are common in hemolytic anemias can be attributed to the effects of both hemolysis and endogenous corticosteroids. Phagocytic hemolysis is characterized by neutrophilia and monocytosis. A left shift may occur, particularly when the hemolysis is immune mediated. WBC counts in the dog frequently approach $50 \times 10^3/\mu L$.[50,51]

Myeloproliferative disorders are interrelated dysplastic and neoplastic conditions that originate from a clonal transformation of nonlymphoid stem cells and their progeny. These disorders may result in increased numbers of neutrophils, abnormal neutrophil maturation (or other cell lines derived from the common pluripotential stem cell), or cytopenia (including neutropenia) in bone marrow and blood. Classification of these disorders in veterinary medicine, based on morphologic and cytochemical characteristics, was established by the Animal Leukemia Study Group of the American Society for Veterinary Clinical Pathology.[41,67] Major categories of myeloproliferative disorders in dogs and cats are myelodysplastic syndrome (preleukemia), acute and chronic myeloid leukemias, and acute undifferentiated leukemia. These are further classified according to the cell line of differentiation and degree of cellular maturity (e.g., myeloblastic, promyelocytic, myelomonocytic, and undifferentiated forms of acute myeloid leukemia). Granulocytic leukemia is described in rats and mice, but spontaneous occurrence is rare.[68,69,70] Myeloproliferative disorders occur less commonly than lymphoproliferative disorders.[50]

Neutropenia

An absolute neutrophil count that is less than the reference range for the species, gender, and age is referred to as neutropenia. Neutropenia may be a reflection of decreased marrow production and release of neutrophils, increased tissue demands in excess of marrow production capacity, or a shift in neutrophils from the CNP to the MNP.

Examples of causes of neutropenia caused by decreased marrow granulopoiesis include radiation, drugs and chemicals (e.g., estrogens in dogs and ferrets, nonsteroidal anti-inflammatory drugs [NSAIDS], sulfonamides, antithyroid drugs, phenothiazines, anticonvulsants, benzene, aflatoxin), certain viral infections (e.g., canine and feline parvovirus, feline leukemia virus, feline immunodeficiency virus), other infectious agents (e.g., *Ehrlichia canis*), myelophthisis originating from several causes, and cyclic stem-cell proliferation.[40,51,71–74] Because the marrow has a large reserve capacity, only widespread and severe marrow damage to neutrophil precursors results in neutropenia.

Although some agents, particularly chemotherapeutic cytotoxic agents, cause predictable toxicity of rapidly proliferating marrow precursors,[75,76] many agents produce idiosyncratic marrow damage (e.g., chloramphenicol, phenylbutazone, cephalosporin antibiotics).[73] Drugs or other agents that produce neutropenia may effect the pluripotential stem cell, committed multilineage or lineage restricted progenitors, differentiated cells, or marrow microenvironment cells, including endothelium and connective tissue stromal cells. The onset of neutropenia and time to recovery of blood neutrophil counts depends on the target-cell population and time of activity of the agent during the cell cycle.[73] With acute destruction of the proliferative pool, neutropenia develops within 5 to 7 days, and recovery usually occurs within 36 to 72 hours of discontinuing drug exposure. The onset of peripheral blood hematotoxicity is variable after stem-cell injury, and damage is often permanent. Pluripotential stem-cell destruction results in suppression of all hemic cell lines and is termed aplastic anemia (pancytopenia). In acute aplastic anemia, marrow suppression of stem cells is severe, resulting in clinical signs referable to neutropenia and thrombocytopenia which usually occur within the first 2 to 3 weeks of drug treatment. However, anemia is not usually present, reflecting the longer circulating half-life of erythrocytes. In chronic aplastic anemia, hemopoiesis, although reduced, is still adequate to maintain neutrophil and platelet levels that prevent sepsis and hemorrhage. The bone marrow is significantly hypoplastic in acute and chronic aplastic anemia. Drug-related immune-mediated neutropenia may occur acutely or months or years after treatment and is frequently non-dose-dependent and idiosyncratic. With aplastic anemia and immune-mediated hematotoxicity, recovery after discontinuation of drug

treatment is variable. Mutagenic drugs or toxins can induce various hemopoietic disorders, including aplastic anemia, myelodysplasia, and leukemia. Drug-induced suppression of granulopoiesis is reviewed succinctly by Weiss.[73] In vitro screening of potential myelotoxicity has application in the development of new therapeutic candidates.[77]

Mechanisms and time course associated with development of neutropenias because of various infections in dogs and cats are reviewed by Latimer and Rakich.[51] The etiopathogenesis of the neutropenia may be multifaceted. For example, canine parvovirus causes destruction of mitotically active tissue such as cells of the neutrophil marrow proliferative pool. Thus, neutropenia is most severe approximately 5 to 8 days after viral infection and may be accompanied by a left shift. Other mechanisms may contribute to the development of neutropenia in canine parvovirus such as depletion of marrow neutrophil stores by excessive tissue demand, a shift from circulating to marginal pools caused by secondary endotoxemia, and ineffective granulopoiesis.

Canine cyclic hemopoiesis is an hereditary stem-cell disease of gray-collie dogs that is transmitted in an autosomal recessive manner. Leukocyte, reticulocyte, and platelet counts fluctuate in a cyclic pattern approximately every 11.5 days. Neutropenia lasts 2 to 4 days after which a rebound neutrophilia may occur.[78] Cyclic hemopoiesis also has been reported in other dog breeds,[51] in feline leukemia virus infection in cats,[79] as well as in association with cyclophosphamide administration in dogs,[80] and has been experimentally induced in mice.[81]

In neutropenias of severe inflammation, the rate of emigration of neutrophils into tissues exceeds the rate of supply from the bone marrow, despite increased marrow production and release. The inflammation may result from various causes, including primary or secondary bacterial or fungal infections, endotoxemia, tissue necrosis, and immune-mediated disorders. Left shifts and toxic changes are common, and marrow granulocytic hyperplasia is generally present.[51]

Immune-mediated mechanisms with reduced intravascular survival of leukocytes can lead to neutropenia. Although evidence for spontaneous immune-mediated neutropenia in animals is presumptive, steroid-responsive neutropenias in animals have been observed.[82] Confirmation of immune-mediated neutropenia requires the demonstration of antineutrophil antibodies.[83] Animals treated with heterologous growth factors may develop anemia caused by the development of neutralizing antibodies that inhibit the function of endogenous growth factors.[84] Neonatal alloimmune neutropenia occurs in humans when maternal neutrophil-specific antibodies cross the placenta and mediate the destruction of the infant's neutrophils. Recurrent otitis media, pneumonia, meningitis, and sepsis may result. Antineutrophil antibodies are demonstrable in 80 to 100% of patients.[85,86]

Severe congenital neutropenia occurs in several syndromes in humans, including congenital agranulocytosis, Shwachman–Diamond syndrome, myelokathexis,

Chédiak–Higashi syndrome, inborn errors of metabolism, and immunologic disorders. Idiopathic neutropenia occurs in individuals without evidence for congenital, neoplastic, inflammatory or immunologic causes for neutropenia.[74,85] The etiopathogenesis underlying disorders such as congenital agranulocytois, cyclic neutropenia, and idiopathic neutropenia is unknown. Hypotheses considered include the defective production of G-CSF or the defective response of neutrophil precursors to G-CSF or other hemopoietic growth factors.[74]

A pattern of infections are associated with neutropenias. Oropharyngeal lesions (ulcers, gingivitis, or pharyngitis), respiratory, and skin infections are common. The most common causes of infection are staphylococci and streptococci present on body surfaces. Pneumonia caused by gram-negative or anaerobic bacteria, deep-tissue abscesses (e.g., caused by *Clostridium* sp.), and bacteremia occur less frequently but are life threatening.[74]

Bone Marrow

Accurate interpretation of hematologic responses generally involves integration of peripheral blood data with bone marrow findings as well as findings in other organ systems. Marrow responses may reflect local or systemic manifestations of inflammation, necrosis, toxic insult, or pharmacologic response. A brief description of anticipated marrow granulocyte findings in concert with peripheral neutrophil changes in disease follows. Marrow response in various disease states is covered more fully elsewhere in this book.

Whenever significant inflammation occurs at any site in the body, expansion of the marrow granulocytic pool and granulocytic hyperplasia results. The features of the response vary with the type, duration, and severity of inflammation. The earliest change is depletion of the storage pool of mature granulocytes, usually correlating with a mature neutrophilia. If immature neutrophils (bands and possibly earlier stages) appear in peripheral blood in response to ongoing severe inflammation, then increased numbers of immature granulocytes will be present in marrow. Under these circumstances, the myeloid maturation index (sum of myeloid maturation phase cells divided by the sum of the myeloid proliferative cell phase) will be decreased. If the myeloid response is adequate, then expansion of more mature neutrophils will follow and the neutrophil storage pool will be replenished over several days. In chronic inflammation, all marrow neutrophil compartments are expanded, marrow is hypercellular, and the myeloid-to-erythroid ratio is high.[49,87]

Marrow granulocytic hypoplasia and neutropenia may occur alone or in combination with hypoplasia of red cell and platelet precursors. Causes of decreased marrow granulopoiesis are described in the Neutropenia section of this chapter.

Granulocytic hyperplasia or hypoplasia with associated changes in peripheral blood neutrophil counts are anticipated findings in preclinical toxicology studies when the test material is a cytokine or growth factor.[87,88] Qualitative abnormalities in bone marrow are a reflection of local response to injury and may take the form of maturation abnormalities (dysplasia), toxicity, necrosis, reactivity, or myelofibrosis. Nuclear maturation defects result in nuclear or cytoplasmic asynchrony and megaloblastosis that is most readily seen in red cell precursors but also may be apparent in neutrophil precursors. Among the causes are agents such as methotrexate and its analogues that inhibit the action of folic acid, which is essential for nuclear maturation and cell division. Systemic toxicity may result in morphologic changes in circulating neutrophils (see Morphologic Abnormalities) that also are present in marrow precursors. These changes are most easily recognized in metamyelocytes, bands, and segmenters, reflecting maturation abnormalities. Neutrophil nuclear changes of toxicity are less common than cytoplasmic changes but may appear as hypersegmentation, hyposegmentation, giant neutrophils with more than one nucleus, and nuclear vacuolation. Donut-shaped cells are normal forms of rodent metamyelocytes but are indicators of granulocytic toxicity in dogs and primates.[49,87]

ROLE OF NEUTROPHILS IN HOST DEFENSE

Neutrophils are attracted to sites of inflammation or infection by directed migration or chemotaxis along gradients of mediators or chemoattractants. Many of these chemoattractants (e.g., N-formylated peptides [N-FMLP], the fifth component of complement [C5a], leukotriene B4 [LTB4], IL-8, Rantes, etc.) bind to heptahelical G-protein coupled-cell surface receptors on the neutrophil. As a result of the chemoattractant receptor activation, neutrophils are stimulated to rearrange their cytoskeleton, adhere to and detach from vascular endothelium, transmigrate across the endothelium into tissues, phagocytose microorganisms, secrete granule contents containing degradative enzymes and antimicrobial agents, and activate nicotinamide adenine dinucleotide phosphate (NADPH) oxidase to generate toxic metabolites of oxygen (Fig. 46.2).[89,90]

CHEMOTAXIS AND MIGRATION INTO TISSUES

Binding of a chemoattractant to its neutrophil receptor results in the activation of the associated G protein with subsequent activation of protein kinase (PKC) and Ca^{2+}-dependent and Ca^{2+}-independent pathways through signal transduction. Activated low-molecular-weight guanosine triphosphatases (GTPases) of the Ras superfamily regulate pathways leading to cytoskeletal assembly (actin polymerization or depolymerization) and motility. A comprehensive description of the potential pathways involved in leukocyte activation after chemoattractant signaling is provided by Bokoch.[89]

FIGURE 46.2 Neutrophil chemotaxis and function in response to infection.
Abbreviations: PSGL-1, P-selectin glycoprotein ligand-1; LFA-1, leukocyte function antigen-1; ICAM-1, intercellular adhesion molecule-1; ICAM-2, intercellular adhesion molecule-2; MAC-1, CD11b/CD18; PECAM, platelet-endothelia cell-adhesion molecule; IAP, integrin-associated protein.

Neutrophil

Key Molecules

A. Normal flow in post capillary venule

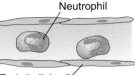

Endothelial cell

B. Rolling

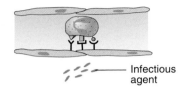

Infectious agent

C. Integrin activation and adherence

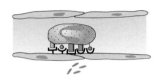

D. Transendothelial migration and migration through extra cellular matrix

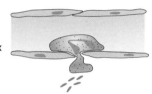

E. Phagocytosis and microbicidal activity

Invagination, opsonization and engulfment

Phagosome formation, and activation of microbicidal systems

Intracellular degranulation and microbial killing

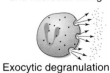

Exocytic degranulation

▽ L-Selectin
Y L-Selectin receptor
▯ PSGL-1
⊤ P-selectin
• E-selectin receptor
Y E-selectin

▯ LFA-1
⊔ ICAM-2
◦ Mac-1
∪ ICAM-1

PECAM
IAP

Oxygen-dependent killing:

O_2^- $^1O_2$
H_2O_2 HOCl
OH

Oxygen-independent killing:

defensins
lysozyme
hydrolases
neutral and acid proteases
lactoferrin

Chemotactic inflammatory stimuli lead to accumulation of neutrophils along the endothelia of postcapillary venules, followed by extravasation through the endothelium into tissue. An array of soluble mediators and cell–cell adhesion molecules expressed by vascular endothelium and by neutrophils themselves mediate the process. Based on structural homology four superfamilies of cell–cell adhesion molecules have been identified: integrins, immunoglobulin (Ig)-like proteins, selectins, and the mucin-like selectin ligands.[9]

Integrins are heterodimeric proteins consisting of noncovalently associated α and β subunits. Different α and β subunits combine to form unique molecules. Leukocytes constitutively express three integrins that share a common β_2 subunit (CD18) and distinct α subunits: leukocyte function-associated antigen-1 (LFA-1) (CD11a/CD18), Mac-1 (CD11b/CD18), and glycoprotein (gp) 150,95 (CD11c/CD18). LFA-1 is constitutively expressed on the cell surface, and several agonists including chemoattractants increase its avidity for relevant ligands. Leukocytes contain storage pools of Mac-1 that are translocated to the cell surface upon cellular stimulation. The integrin, $\alpha_4\beta_1$ (very late activation 4 [VLA-4]), is expressed on lymphocytes, monocytes, and eosinophils but not on neutrophils.[91]

Ig-like proteins serve as counterreceptors for integrins. Intercellular adhesion molecule-1 (ICAM-1) is constitutively expressed by endothelial cells, and its synthesis is upregulated severalfold by agonists such as IL-1 and TNF produced by resident macrophages, and bacterial endotoxins such as LPS. ICAM-1 interacts with both LFA-1 and Mac-1 on leukocytes. ICAM-2 is a noninducible molecule, expressed by endothelial cells and platelets, that binds to LFA-1. VCAM-1, the ligand for VLA-4, is expressed by cytokine and LPS-stimulated endothelial cells. The cellular ligand for gp150,95 has not been well characterized.

Selectins are calcium-dependent, carbohydrate-binding (lectin) integral membrane proteins. Three selectins have been identified. L-selectin is expressed constitutively by neutrophils as well as other leukocytes and is important in transendothelial migration. L-selectin is shed from the plasma membrane through proteolytic cleavage during the process of neutrophil activation. P-selectin is expressed in α granules and Weibel–Palade body membranes of resting platelets and unstimulated endothelial cells and is translocated to the external membrane after stimulation with mediators of inflammation such as thrombin, platelet-activating factor (PAF), histamine, or cytokines (TNF; IL-1). P-selectin on endothelium or platelets interacts with P-selectin glycoprotein ligand-1 (PSGL-1) on neutrophils. E-selectin is synthesized by cytokine or LPS-stimulated endothelial cells. E-selectin may be less important in initial interactions between neutrophils and endothelium than P- and L-selectin.

Mucins are heavily glycosylated proteins rich in serine and threonine. PSGL-1 is the best characterized member of this family and is constitutively expressed on monocytes, neutrophils, and certain lymphocyte subsets.[6,9,29]

Cell-adhesion molecules and their repective ligands are depicted in Figure 46.1 and are reviewed by Elangbam et al.[91] Leukocyte accumulation in tissues occurs through a series of processes and phases. A multi-step model characterizes transendothelial migration (Fig. 46.2).[6]

Rolling

Early events enhance expression of adhesion molecules on endothelial cells overlying the inflammatory focus. At sites of vascular damage and platelet deposition, leukocytes decelerate their transit along the vascular endothelium, a process known as rolling. P-selectin on endothelium and L-selectin on neutrophils act sequentially in the initial margination or rolling process, which is enhanced by blood flow conditions. Bonds between neutrophils and endothelium are made and broken rapidly. In the presence of shear stress, this leads to neutrophil rolling and spreading along the endothelial monolayer. Selectins appear to be responsible for the initial rolling.[6,9,92]

Integrin Activation

The second step in neutrophil transmigration is integrin activation. Leukocyte integrins can exist in two states with respect to adhesion. In circulating unactivated cells, integrins are of low avidity and do not mediate adhesion, even if ligand is expressed on endothelium. On activation, the integrin avidity for ligand is increased significantly. Leukocyte integrins, activated by various chemoattractants to undergo conformational change, bind to Ig-like proteins such as ICAM-1, whose synthesis by vascular endothelium is upregulated during the inflammatory process. In turn, the adhesion of neutrophils is downregulated by nitric oxide (NO) generated by endothelial cells in response to cytokines or LPS.[29] In the absence of β_2 integrins, neutrophils cannot migrate to most extravascular sites of infection.[6,9] Canine, bovine, and human leukocyte adhesion deficiency (LAD-1) results from mutations in the gene encoding CD18, the β_2 leukocyte integrin subunit. LAD-1 is characterized by recurrent infections and delayed wound healing. Neutrophilia is associated with incongruent decreased neutrophilic infiltration into inflamed tissue. Decreased neutrophil adherence, chemotaxis, and phagocytosis have been described.[93–97]

Adherence

Binding of neutrophils with increased integrin avidity to endothelium expressing ligand leads to the arrest of the rolling neutrophils, with close and stable cell–cell adhesion. This is the third step in neutrophil transmigration.

Endothelial Transmigration

The fourth step in extravasation is the actual endothelial transmigration. PAF and IL-8 play a role in guiding neutrophils across the endothelial monolayer wherein transmigration appears to occur at interendothelial junctions. Two molecules found at these junctions, as well as expressed on neutrophils that are involved in the process are platelet-endothelial cell-adhesion molecule (PECAM; CD31) and integrin-associated protein (IAP; CD47). Neutrophil adhesion triggers disruption of endothelial tight junctions, thus permitting neutrophil migration. Limited digestion of both the vascular basement membrane and the tissue matrix by serine proteases such as cathepsin G, elastase, and proteinase 3 expressed on the cell surface of migrating cells occurs. Migration is directed by gradients of chemotaxins generated locally. A series of chemokines belonging to the CXC supergene family are important to neutrophil migration through the extravascular space because of their resistance to inactivation by hydrolytic enzymes and oxidants. Extravasated neutrophils may favor secondary waves of cell recruitment caused by their ability to produce IL-8, PAF, and leukotrine B_4 (LTB$_4$).[6,29]

Migration Through Extracellular Matrix

Having migrated through the endothelial barrier, the extravasated neutrophil migrates through extracellular matrix (ECM) to the site of inflammation or infection. This involves expression of several neutrophil integrins that bind a large number of ECM proteins. Integrins released from interaction with ECM move through the cell to be reexpressed on the surface and reactivated to begin the adhesion–detachment cycle again.[6]

PHAGOCYTOSIS

Once neutrophils have reached an inflammatory focus, the offending organism must be internalized by phagocytosis. Phagocytosis is a process used by neutrophils and mononuclear phagocytes to ingest and clear large particles (0.5 μm), including infectious agents, senescent cells, and cellular debris. The process is facilitated by opsonization, which increases the rate of cell recognition of target material and of attachment to that material. The opsonins involved are Igs and complement, primarily through the third component of complement.[97,98] Opsonic receptors, including fragment, crystallizable (Fc) receptors and complement receptors, and additional receptors such as the fibronectin receptor are involved in phagocytosis. The importance of opsonization is highlighted in the report on Irish Setters that had defective integrin expression. Neutrophils from these dogs could not or had impaired ability to ingest particles opsonized with C3b or immunoglobulin G (IgG) and could not overcome infections.[99]

Particle internalization is initiated by the interaction of specific receptors on the surface of the phagocyte with ligands on the surface of the particle. Ligation of phagocytic receptors leads to localized actin polymerization at the site of particle ingestion, pseudopod extension, and particle internalization with phagosome formation. Actin is shed from the phagosome after internalization, and the phagosome matures by a series of fusion and fission events involved in the endocytic pathway. The next phase of phagosome maturation is mediated by a microtubule-based system. Maturation of phagosomes provides an environment that generally leads to the sterilization of infectious agents. However, many pathogens have evolved, each using a unique mechanism, to evade killing within the phagosomes. For example, *Listeria monocytogenes* escapes from the vacuole, whereas *Mycobacterium tuberculosis* modifies the maturation of the phagosome.[100] *Hemophilus somnus* may evade killing by inducing apoptosis in bovine neutrophils.[101]

ANTIMICROBICIDAL ACTIVITY

At the same time that phagocytosis is occurring, the cells begin to mobilize for the killing or disposal of internalized microorganisms. Neutrophils possess oxygen-dependent and oxygen-independent systems that are contained in the granules and act in concert with membrane and cytoplasmic enzymes.

Oxidative mechanisms represent the most potent means for neutrophil killing of microorganisms. Neutrophils produce various oxidizing agents by reducing molecular oxygen (O_2) in a process referred to as the respiratory burst. The burst is accompanied by increases in superoxide anion (O_2^-) and hydrogen peroxide (H_2O_2) production, and glucose oxidation via the hexose monophosphate shunt (HMPS). The basis of the respiratory burst is the activation of a membrane-bound flavoprotein oxidase, NADPH oxidase, which facilitates the formation of superoxide (O_2^-) by means of the reaction: $2O_2 + NADPH \rightarrow 2O_2^- + NADP$. NADPH oxidase is stored in the resting cell associated with the membrane as well as free within the cytosol. The rapid assembly of NADPH oxidase is associated with membrane depolarization and changes in intracellular cyclic adenosine monophosphate (cAMP) concentration and is mediated through activation of diaglycerol and PKC. The oxygen radical produced in the reaction is the precursor for a series of microbicidal oxidants. Dismutation of O_2^- to H_2O_2 occurs spontaneously or is catalyzed by superoxide dismutase. Increased availability of NADP increases HMPS activity. Other reactive oxygen derivatives include the hydroxyl radical (OH), singlet oxygen ($^1O_2$), and hypochlorous acid (HOCl). The oxygen free radicals produced are unstable compounds that rapidly interact with the lipid of cell membranes. HOCl is formed by a reaction combining myeloperoxidase with H_2O_2 to form an enzyme–substrate complex that oxidizes halides to form toxic products.[11,12,97]

Oxygen-independent killing mechanisms may function in the presence or absence of oxygen. Effectors include cationic proteins and enzymes such as defensins, lysozyme, hydrolases, neutral and acid proteases, and lactoferrin.[11] Species differences in antimicrobial systems are present. For example, normal bovine, monkey, sheep, and goat neutrophils have little or no lysozyme activity, whereas rabbit heterophils are rich in cationic proteins but have low concentrations of other antimicrobial enzymes.[11]

INTEGRATION OF MOLECULAR ASPECTS OF NEUTROPHIL ACTIVATION, RECRUITMENT, AND FUNCTION

Neutrophils circulate in blood as resting cells, endowed with a low number of surface proteins or glycoproteins acting as adhesion molecules or receptors. Neutrophils exist in one of three states: quiescent, primed, or activated.[102] Receptors on the cell surface function cooperatively in the activation process, and neutrophils possess at least three different classes of receptors: the G-protein-linked seven-transmembrane-domain receptors, such as those for N-FMLP, PAF, C5a, substance P, and IL-8; the single-transmembrane-domain receptors that require immoblilzation or cross-linking rather than occupancy for activation, such as the integrins and Fc receptors; and the single-transmembrane-domain receptors for growth-regulating cytokines such as TNFα and GM-CSF.[102] Whether the signal for leukocyte activation comes from a chemotaxin, a leukotriene, a complement fragment, or ECM, β_2 integrins have an important role in many functions of the activated cell.[6] Activation results in both phenotypic and functional changes. Similarities exist between the activation signals and the mechanisms effecting adhesion, chemotaxis, phagocytosis, and microbicidal activity. These processes appear to be regulated by messengers such as low-molecular-weight GTPases of the RAS superfamily, and by cAMP generation and catabolism.[29,89,102]

IMMUNOREGULATORY ROLE

Recent evidence indicates that neutrophils may have an active role in the immune system. GM-CSF and IFN-γ induce the expression of human leukocyte antigen DR (HLA-DR) on the surface of neutrophils. Cellular HLA-DR expression relates to the cell's ability to present antigens to helper T cells. Also, neutrophils can synthesize and release immunoregulatory cytokines, including IL-1, IL-6, IL-8, TNFα, GM-CSF, and transforming growth factor (TGF-β). A list of proinflammatory and anti-inflammatory cytokines produced by neutrophils, inducing stimuli, and potential roles of these cytokines is provided by Fujishima.[13] Thus, neutrophils are not only terminal effector cells but also are immunoregulatory cells capable of communicating with other inflammatory cells.[13,29]

NEUTROPHIL PATHOPHYSIOLOGY

Defects in neutrophils may be quantitative or qualitative, both potentially leading to increased susceptibility to infection. Such defects may be acquired or inherited.[103] Quantitative defects (neutropenia) already have been described.

Morphologic Abnormalities

Changes in neutrophil morphology can be important in interpreting changes in the leukon as well as for identifying underlying etiopathogenesis of disease. In general, changes in neutrophil morphology may reflect aging changes, toxic changes, degenerative changes, changes or inclusions indicating infectious diseases, and changes representing underlying myeloproliferative or genetic disorders. Morphologic changes may be associated with functional alterations.[51]

Aging changes, such as nuclear hypersegmentation or pyknosis, occur as a normal physiologic process. However, neutrophils usually exit peripheral blood before aging changes are discernable. Thus, when aging changes are recognized in peripheral blood smears, conditions that extend neutrophil transit time should be considered (e.g., excessive plasma concentrations of glucocorticoids).[65]

Toxic changes develop in neutrophils during their development in bone marrow under the influence of severe inflammation from bacterial infection or, occasionally, in instances of drug toxicity. Toxic changes present in peripheral blood neutrophils are most commonly noted as cytoplasmic changes. Cytoplasmic basophilia results from RNA and ribosomes remaining in the cytoplasm after maturation. Cytoplasmic vacuolation presents as small- to medium-sized clear vacuoles (the cytoplasm of normal mature neutrophils is devoid of vacuoles). The cause of the vacuoles is uncertain but may reflect autodigestion. Toxic granulation represents intensely stained primary granules resulting from retention of acid mucopolysaccharides. Döhle bodies are gray inclusions in the cytoplasm of mature neutrophils, representing retention and aggregation of rough endoplasmic reticulum. Döhle bodies and other toxic changes are seen more frequently in cats than in dogs or other species. Nuclear toxic changes include polyploidy, hyposegmentation, and nuclear ring forms. Giant neutrophils may reflect a further manifestation of toxicity.[51,65,104] Döhle bodies, cytoplasmic vacuolation, and toxic granulation are expected findings after G-CSF administration and do not necessarily indicate sepsis in that situation.[105]

Degenerative changes such as karyolysis occur in neutrophils only after they have exited peripheral blood.[50]

Examples of infectious agents that have been identified in circulating neutrophils and other leukocytes include *Histoplasma capsulatum*, *Hepatozoon canis*, and rickettsial morulae in dogs infected with *Ehrlichia canis* and *Ehrlichia equi*. Canine distemper inclusions are round to irregularly shaped magenta inclusions present in leukocytes or erythrocytes.[51]

Several hereditary diseases or syndromes in animals present with characteristic neutrophil morphologic abnormalities (reviewed by Latimer and Rakich[51]) including the Pelger–Huët anomaly of rabbits, dogs, and cats; the Birman cat neutrophil granulation anomaly; Chédiak–Higashi syndrome in several species; and lysosmal storage diseases such as mucopolysaccharidosis type VI and type VII in cats and dogs.

Myeloproliferative disorders involving granulocytes may present as well differentiated granulocytic or myelomonocytic leukemia or as poorly differentiated forms exhibiting atypical or blastic cellular features.[41,50]

Functional Alterations

Neutrophil function testing is described fully in another chapter, and therefore receives only a brief overview here. Major bacterial infections are most commonly associated with neutropenia or an abnormality of Igs or complement. Occasionally, repeated infections cannot be attributed to these causes. In such cases, an abnormality in neutrophil function should be considered. Abnormalities in function may involve disorders of adhesion, chemotaxis, phagocytosis, degranulation, respiratory burst activity, bacterial killing, and associated events (e.g., aggregation or chemiluminescence) singly or in combination. A logical approach to screening for defects in neutrophil function is to use a battery of tests that evaluate each major step in neutrophil activity and a tiered approach to testing has been recommended.[106] However, defects of neutrophil function are rare, and animals that have persistent and recurring infections should be evaluated carefully for underlying disease before primary neutrophil function testing is pursued. There are important species differences that must be considered in evaluating neutrophil function. For example, N-FMLP derived from bacteria, is a common chemotactic stimulus used for in vitro evaluation of human neutrophils. However, neutrophils from dogs, cats, cattle, and pigs lack receptors for N-FMLP.[107]

Impaired neutrophil functions have been identified in a number of disease states in animals. Neutrophil function may be altered in individuals that have genetic defects, inadequate nutrition, or after exposure to infectious agents, xenobiotics, or toxins.[4,51,97,106]

Chédiak-Higashi syndrome is a rare autosomal recessive disorder of animals and humans with typical features that include partial oculocutaneous albinism and the presence of giant lysosomal granules in neutrophils and other blood cells.[51,93,96] Affected Persian cats did not have increased occurrence of infection despite defective neutrophil chemotaxis, but were predisposed to bleeding.[51] Hereditary deficiencies of integrin molecules have been identified in cattle, dogs, and humans (described as Leukocyte Adhesion Defect or LAD).[93–97]

Chronic granulomatous disease (CGD) in humans is an X-linked autosomal recessive disorder characterized by recurrent life-threatening infections with catalase positive bacteria and fungi, reflecting a defect in any of four genes encoding subunits of the superoxide generating phagocyte NADPH oxidase.[93,96] A canine counterpart for the human disease was reported previously in Irish

Setters[108]; however, this defect may have resulted from an adhesion molecule defect that failed to stimulate NADPH oxidase.[97] Defective killing mechanisms have been identified in related Doberman pinschers.[109] This may be an animal counterpart for CGD; however, a receptor deficiency has not been excluded.[97]

Other inherited neutrophil function disorders in humans include neutrophil glucose-6-phosphate dehydrogenase (G6PD) deficiency, myeloperoxidase deficiency, congenital absence of specific granules, juvenile periodontitis, and hyperimmunoglobulinemia E syndrome.[93,96]

Several agents have been found to augment particular neutrophil functions. These include some antimicrobials, G-CSF, GM-CSF, IFN-γ, IL-5, ascorbic acid, and levamisole.[4,61,93,103,110,111] The effect of G-CSF on neutrophil function has been explored in a number of nonneutropenic infectious disease animal models, including neonatal sepsis, pneumonia, burn wound infection, intra-abdominal sepsis, and intramuscular infection.[61] Increased neutrophil function has been reported as a secondary phenomenon in noninfectious diseases with active inflammation.[93]

Bone marrow transplantation has been used successfully to achieve permanent cure of disorders such as LAD-1 and CGD, where marrow progenitors or stem cells are the appropriate target.[96] Only a small number of patients that have congenital or acquired severe chronic neutropenia have been treated by bone marrow transplantation.[74] Allogenic bone marrow transplantation corrected the neutrophil migration defect and platelet storage pool deficiency in Chédiak–Higashi cats but had no effect on lysosme distribution in liver and kidney cells.[112]

Use of recombinant hemopoietic growth factors has potential in the therapy of neutropenias of varying causes; however, the development of neutralizing antibodies has largely precluded the use of recombinant human G-CSF (rhG-CSF) in veterinary patients.[105] The initial increase in leukocyte counts after daily administration of rhG-CSF in dogs that had cyclic hemopoiesis was followed by a decline after 23 days of therapy, coincident with development of neutralizing antibodies.[113] Reports are cited by Henry et al[105] indicating that rhG-CSF may alleviate myelosuppression associated with chemotherapy-induced neutropenia in dogs and cats. Injection of rhG-CSF in cows induced a threefold to fivefold increase in peripheral blood mature neutrophils.[114] In human medicine, severe chronic neutropenia is a global descriptive term for several disorders of varied origins in which neutrophil concentrations are consistently or recurrently at less than 0.5×10^6 cells/μL. Despite this heterogeneity of origin, administration of rhG-CSF results in an increase in neutrophil counts in most patients. The neutrophilia after G-CSF administration is due to release of maturing cells from bone marrow as well as stimulation of proliferation of precursors through the myelocyte stage of development. Administration of GM-CSF or G-CSF has resulted in stimulation of neutrophil counts after chemotherapy or radiotherapy in animal preclinical and human clinical studies. Administration of these factors may be associated with alterations in neutrophil function.[40,74,85,115]

The therapeutic use of exogenously administered bactericidal permeability-inducing protein (BPI) has been evaluated in patients with bacterial infections.[30] BPI is a constituent of neutrophil primary granules that has bactericidal and endotoxin-neutralizing properties.

ROLE OF NEUTROPHILS IN TISSUE INJURY

In various noninfectious diseases characterized by extravascular recruitment of neutrophils, these leukocytes play a crucial role in tissue injury that ultimately may lead to irreversible destruction of normal tissue architecture with consequent organ dysfunction. Tissue injury has been attributed mainly to effects of extracellular release of granule content (neutrophils contain more than 40 hydrolytic enzymes and toxic molecules) and oxygen radicals with resultant proteolytic and oxidative toxicity (Fig. 46.3). Hypochlorous acid, generated by the MPO catalyzed transformation of H_2O_2, is the most toxic oxidant generated during neutrophilic inflammation. It exerts several unwanted effects, two of which are particularly harmful. First, hypochlorous acid depletes adenosine triphosphate (ATP) in tissue cells with consequent dysfunction and necrosis. Secondly, it inactivates $\alpha1$-antitrypsin, which is an inhibitor of neutrophil elastase, thus favoring the uncontrolled proteolytic activity of elastase. Neutrophils also contain metalloproteinases, including collagenase, gelatinase, and stromelysin that can digest collagen, gelatin, and proteogylcan, respectively.[29] Also, neutrophils can produce or induce both proinflammatory and anti-inflammatory cytokines, thereby contributing to tissue injury in some circumstances.[103] Neutrophil-mediated tissue injury may play an important role in numerous disease states in animals, including inflammatory dermatoses in dogs[116] and pneumonic pasteurellosis in cattle.[117,118] IL-8 appears to have a major role in neutrophil recruitment into lesions of pneumonic pasteurellosis.[117] Neutrophil-mediated tissue injury is implicated in numerous disease states in humans, including acute respiratory distress and multiple organ dysfunction syndromes,[13] systemic vasculitis,[119] ischemia-reperfusion injury,[120] ulcerative colitis,[121] liver injury,[7] cardiopulmonary bypass, dermatologic disorders, and other conditions.[103]

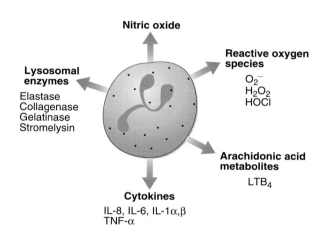

FIGURE 46.3 Examples of neutrophil-derived cytotoxic substances.

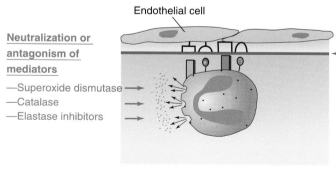

FIGURE 46.4 Potential therapeutic approaches for pharmacologic modulation of neutrophil-mediated tissue injury.

Neutralization or antagonism of mediators

—Superoxide dismutase
—Catalase
—Elastase inhibitors

Anti-adhesion therapy

—Monoclonal antibodies (anti-CAM)
—Adhesion-inhibiting peptides (based on sequences of P-selectins, E-selectins, ICAM-1)
—Antisense oligonucleotides (inhibit expression of E-selectins, ICAM-1, neutrophil integrins)

Inhibition/Modulation of neutrophil activation

—Decreased generation of chemotaxins (corticosteroids)
—Limit upregulation of surface expression of integrins (NSAIDS)
—Decreased local generation of proinflammatory cytokines such as IL-1, IL-8, TNF (NSAIDS)
—Interference with signal transduction/post-receptor signals (PDE-IV inhibitors)

In humans, antineutrophil cytoplasmic antibodies (ANCA) are implicated in the pathogenesis of clinically diverse diseases. ANCA are diagnostic markers for some forms of inflammatory vascular injury associated with autoimmune diseases that include primary systemic vasculidites, systemic lupus erythematosus, rheumatoid arthritis, and collagen vascular disease.[122,123]

Pharmacologic Modulation of Neutrophil-Mediated Tissue Injury

Although the best therapeutic approach to tissue injury in neutrophilic inflammation is origin driven, the knowledge of the mechanisms and pathways underlying inflammation and neutrophil activation provide opportunities to develop physiopathologic therapeutic strategies to prevent or to reduce tissue injuries associated with neutrophil influx. Three major targets for pharmacologic intervention can be considered (Fig. 46.4). The first two approaches either modulate receptor binding on neutrophils or endothelium or modulate signal transduction.[13] A third approach to limiting tissue injury in neutrophilic inflammation is inactivation of neutrophil-derived oxidants or proteases and neutralization or blockade of already activated protease.[13,29]

Although various molecules can inhibit neutrophil function in vitro or in vivo, their use is not necessarily applicable in vivo, as neutrophils share many receptors, signal transduction pathways, and mediators with other cells. Thus, nonspecific inhibition would interfere with function of other cell types. Also, complete inhibition of neutrophil function or neutrophil depletion is disadvantageous in view of the indispensable role of neutrophils in host defense.

REFERENCES

1. **Diamond RD, Krzesicki R, Epstein B, Wellington J.** Damage to hyphal forms of fungi by human leukocytes in vitro. A possible host defense mechanism in aspergillosis and mucormycosis. Am J Pathol 1978; 91:313–328.
2. **Rouse BT, Babiuk LA, Henson PM.** Neutrophils in antiviral immunity: inhibition of virus replication by a mediator produced by bovine neutrophils. J Infect Dis 1980;141:223–232.
3. **Babiuk LA, van Drunen Littel-van den Hurk S, Tikoo SK.** Immunology of bovine herpesvirus 1 infection. Vet Microbiol 1996;53:31–42.
4. **Smith GS, Lumsden JH.** Review of neutrophil adherence, chemotaxis, phagocytosis and killing. Vet Immunol Immunopathol 1983;4:177–236.
5. **Williams MR, Bunch KJ.** Variation among cows in the ability of their blood polymorphonuclear leukocytes to kill *Escherichia coli* and *Staphylococcus aureus*. Res Vet Sci 1981;30:298–302.
6. **Brown E.** Neutrophil adhesion and the therapy of inflammation. Semin Hematol 1997;34:319–326.
7. **Jaeschke H, Smith CW, Clemens MG, Ganey PE, Roth RA.** Contemporary issues in toxicology. Mechanisms of inflammatory liver injury: adhesion molecules and cytotoxicity of neutrophils. Toxicol Appl Pharmacol 1996; 139:213–226.
8. **Cassatella MA.** The production of cytokines by polymorphonuclear neutrophils. Immunol Today 1995;16:21–26.
9. **Celi A, Lorenzet R, Furie B, Furie BC.** Platelet-leukocyte-endothelial cell interaction on the blood vessel wall. Semin Hematol 1997;34:327–335.
10. **Calamai EG, Spitznagel JK.** Characterization of rat polymorphonuclear leukocyte subcellular granules. Lab Invest 1982;46:597–604.
11. **Bertram TA.** Neutrophil leukocyte structure and function in domestic animals. Adv Vet Sci Comp Med 1985;30:91–129.
12. **Henderson LM, Chappell JB.** Review. NADPH oxidase of neutrophils. Biochem Biophys Acta 1996;1273:87–107.
13. **Fujishima S, Aikawa N.** Neutrophil-mediated tissue injury and its modulation. Intensive Care Med 1995;21:277–285.
14. **Klebanoff SJ, Clark RA.** Structure. In: The neutrophil. Function and clinical disorders. Amsterdam: Elsevier/North Holland Biomedical Press, 1978; 5–72.
15. **Jain NC.** The neutrophils. In: Schalm's veterinary hematology. Philadelphia: Lea & Feibiger, 1986;676–730.
16. **Jain NC.** The neutrophils. In: Comparative hematology of common domestic animals. Essentials of veterinary hematology. Philadelphia: Lea & Febiger, 1993;222–246.
17. **Hall RL.** Clinical pathology of laboratory animals. In: Gad S, Chengelis C, eds. Animal models of toxicology. Marcel Dekker, 1992;765–811.
18. **Brederoo P, van der Meulen J.** Granule formation in guinea pig and rat heterophil promyelocytes. Cell Biol Int 1981;5:468.
19. **Brederoo P, Daems WT.** A new type of primary granule in guinea pig heterophil granulocytes. Cell Biol Int 1977;1:363–368.
20. **Spicer SS, Hardin JH.** Ultrastructure, cytochemistry and function of neutrophil leukocyte granules: a review. Lab Invest 1969;20:488–497.
21. **Gennaro R, Dewald B, Horisberger U, Gubler HU, Baggiolini M.** A novel type of cytoplasmic granule in bovine neutrophils. J Cell Biol 1983;96:1651–1661.
22. **Gennaro R, Dolzani L, Romeo D.** Potency of bactericidal proteins purified from the large granules of bovine neutrophils. Infect Immun 1983; 40:684–690.
23. **Baggiolini M, Horisberger U, Gennaro R, Dewald B.** Identification of three types of granules in neutrophils of ruminants. Ultrastructure of circulating and maturing cells. Lab Invest 1985;52:151–158.
24. **Bertram TA, Coignoul FL.** Morphometry of equine neutrophils isolated at different temperatures. Vet Pathol 1982;19:534–543.
25. **O'Donnell RT, Andersen BR.** Characterization of canine neutrophil granules. Infect Immun 1982;38:351–359.
26. **Fittschen C, Parmley RT, Austin RL.** Ultrastructural cytochemistry of complex carbohydrates in developing feline neutrophils. Am J Anat 1988;181:149–162.
27. **Fittschen C, Parmley RT, Bishop SP, Williams JC.** Morphometry of feline neutrophil granule genesis. Am J Anat 1988;181:195–202.
28. **Borregaard N, Lollike K, Kjeldsen L.** Human neutrophil granules and secretory vesicles. Eur J Haematol 1993;51:187–198.
29. **Dallgeri F, Ottonello L.** Tissue injury in neutrophilic inflammation. Inflamm Res 1997;46:382–391.
30. **Ganz T, Weiss J.** Antimicrobial peptides of phagocytes and epithelia. Semin Hematol 1997;34:343–354.
31. **Gullberg U, Andersson E, Garwicz D, Lindmark A, Olsson I.** Review article. Biosynthesis, processing and sorting of neutrophil proteins: insight into neutrophil granule development. Eur J Haematol 1997;58:137–153.
32. **Selsted ME, Novotny MJ, Morris WL, Tong YQ, Smith W, Cullor JS.** Indolicidin, a novel bactericidal tridecapeptide amide from neutrophils. J Biol Chem 1992;267:4292–4295.
33. **Zanetti M, Litteri L, Gennaro R, Horstmann H, Romeo D.** Bactenecins, defense polypeptides of bovine neutrophils, are generated from precursor molecules stored in large granules. J Cell Biol 1990;111:1363–1371.
34. **Pellegrini A, Kalkinc M, Hermann M, Grunig B, Winder C, Von Fellenberg R.** Equinins in equine neutrophils: quantification in tracheobronchial secretions as an aid in the diagnosis of chronic pulmonary disease. Vet J 1998;155:257–262.
35. **Brune K, Leffell MS, Spitznagel JK.** Microbicidal activity of peroxidaseless chicken heterophile leukocytes. Infect Immun 1972;5:283–287.
36. **Lam KM.** Myeloperoxidase activity in chicken heterophils and adherent cells. Vet Immunol Immunopathol 1997;57:327–335.
37. **Gallin JI.** Human neutrophil heterogeneity exists, but is it meaningful? Blood 1984;63:977–983.
38. **Sigurdsson F, Khanna-Gupta A, Lawson N, Berliner N.** Control of late neutrophil-specific gene expression: insights into regulation of myeloid differentiation. Semin Hematol 1997;34:303–310.
39. **Ogawa M.** Differentiation and proliferation of hematopoietic stem cells. Blood 1993;81:2844–2853.
40. **Kim SK, Demetri GD.** Chemotherapy and neutropenia. Hematol Oncol Clin North Am 1996;10:377–395.
41. **Raskin RE.** Myelopoiesis and myeloproliferative disorders. Vet Clin North Am Small Anim Pract 1996;26:1023–1042.
42. **Metcalf D.** The molecular control of cell division, differentiation, commitment and maturation in hematopoietic cells. Nature 1989;339:27–30.
43. **Metcalf D.** Control of granulocytes and macrophages: molecular, cellular and clinical aspects. Science 1991;254:529–533.
44. **Murphy PM.** Neutrophil receptors for interleukin-8 and related CXC chemokines. Semin Hematol 1997;34:311–318.
45. **Avalos BR.** Molecular analysis of the granulocyte colony-stimulating factor receptor. Blood 1996;88:761–777.
46. **Deldar A, Stevens CE.** Development and application of in vitro models of hematopoiesis to drug development. Toxicol Pathol 1993;21:231–240.
47. **House RV.** Cytokine technology in basic and applied research on the hematopoietic system. Toxicol Pathol 1993;21:251–257.
48. **Grindem CB.** Blood cell markers. Vet Clin North Am Small Anim Pract 1996;26:1043–1064.

49. **Grindem CB.** Bone marrow biopsy and evaluation, Vet Clin North Am Small Anim Pract 1989;19:669–696.
50. **Duncan JR, Prasse KW, Mahaffey EA.** Leukocytes. In: Veterinary laboratory medicine: clinical pathology. Ames, IA: Iowa State University Press, 1994;37–62.
51. **Latimer KS, Rakich PM.** Clinical interpretation of leukocyte responses. Vet Clin North Am Small Anim Pract 1989;19:637–668.
52. **Deubeleiss KA, Dancey JT, Harker LA, Finch CA.** Neutrophil kinetics in the dog. J Clin Invest 1975;55:833–839.
53. **Prasse KW, Seagrave RC, Kaeberle ML, Ramsey FK.** A model of granulopoiesis in cats. Lab Invest 1973;28:292–299.
54. **Valli VEO, Hulland TJ, McSherry BJ, Robinson GA, Gilman JPW.** The kinetics of hematopoiesis in the calf. I. An autoradiographical study of myelopoiesis in normal, anemic, and endotoxin treated calves. Res Vet Sci 1971;12:535–550.
55. **Boggs DR.** The kinetics of neutrophil leukocytes in health and disease. Semin Hematol 1967;4:359–386.
56. **Valli VE, McSherry BJ, Robinson GA, Willoughby RA.** Leukopheresis in calves and dogs by extracorporeal circulation of blood through siliconized glass wool. Res Vet Sci 1969;10:267–270.
57. **Seifert MF, Marks SC Jr.** The regulation of hemopoiesis in the spleen. Exp 1985;41:192–199.
58. **Valli VE, Villeneuve DC, Reed B, Barsoum N, Smith G.** Evaluation of blood and bone marrow, rat. In: Jones TC, Ward JM, Mohr U, Hunt RD eds. Hemopoietic system. Berlin Heidelberg: Springer-Verlag, 1990;9–26.
59. **Carakostas MC, Moore WE, Smith JE.** Intravascular neutrophil granulocyte kinetics in horses. Am J Vet Res 1981;42:623–625.
60. **Prasse KW, Kaeberle ML, Ramsey FK.** Blood neutrophilic granulocyte kinetics in cats. Am J Vet Res 1973;34:1021–1025.
61. **Dale DC, Liles WC, Summer WR, Nelson S.** Review: granulocyte colony-stimulating factor-role and relationships in infectious disease. J Infect Dis 1995;75:1061–1075.
62. **Liles WC, Klebanoff SJ.** Regulation of apoptosis in neutrophils-fas track to death. J Immunol 1995;155:3289–3291.
63. **Sendo F, Tsuchida H, Takeda Y, Gon S, Takei H, Kato T, Hachiya O, Watanabe H.** Regulation of neutrophil apoptosis—its biological significance in inflammation and the immune response. Hum Cell 1996;9:215–222.
64. **Lilliehook I.** Diurnal variation of canine blood leukocyte counts. Vet Clin Pathol 1997;26:113–117.
65. **Tyler RD, Cowell RL, Clinkenbeard KD, MacAllister CG.** Hematologic values in horses and interpretation of hematologic data. Vet Clinics North Am Equine Pract 1987;3:461–484.
66. **Wong CW, Smith SE, Thong TH, Opdebeeck JR, Thornton JR.** Effects of exercise stress on various immune functions. Am J Vet Res 1992;53:1414–1417.
67. **Jain NC.** Classification of myeloproliferative disorders in cats using criteria proposed by the Animal Leukemia Study Group: A retrospective study of 181 cases (1969–1992). Comp Hematol Int 1993;3:125–134.
68. **Frith CH, Ward JM, Chandra M.** The morphology, immunohistochemistry, and incidence of hematopoietic neoplasms in mice and rats. Toxicol Pathol 1993;21:206–208.
69. **Gal F, Sugar J, Csuka O.** Granulocytic leukemia, rat. In: Jones TC, Ward JM, Mohr RD, Hunt RD, eds. Hemopoietic system. Berlin Heidelberg: Springer-Verlag, 1990;39–45.
70. **Seki M, Inoue T.** Granulocytic leukemia, mouse. In: Jones TC, Ward JM, Mohr U, Hunt RD eds. Hemopoietic system. Berlin Heidelberg: Springer-Verlag, 1990;46–50.
71. **Reagen WJ.** A review of myelofibrosis in dogs. Toxicol Pathol 1993;21:164–169.
72. **Shelly SM.** Causes of canine pancytopenia. Compend Contin Educ Pract Vet 1988;10:9–16.
73. **Weiss DJ.** Leukocyte response to toxic injury. Toxicol Pathol 1993;21:135–140.
74. **Welte K, Boxer LA.** Severe chronic neutropenia: pathophysiology and therapy. Semin Hematol 1997;34:267–278.
75. **Hahn KA, Rohrbach BW, Legendre AM, Frazier DL, Nolan ML.** Hematologic changes associated with weekly low-dose cisplatin administration in dogs. Vet Clin Pathol 1997;26:29–31.
76. **Reynolds JA, Davies MH, Perigard CJ, Dufrain RJ, Mezza LE, Hirth RS.** The hematologic toxicity of the anticancer agent taxol. Toxicol Pathol 1992;20:635.
77. **Parchment RE, Huang M, Erickson-Miller CL.** Roles for in vitro myelotoxicity tests in preclinical drug development and clinical trial planning. Toxicol Pathol 1993;21:241–250.
78. **Campbell KL.** Canine cyclic hematopoiesis. Compend Contin Educ Pract Vet 1985;7:57–62.
79. **Swenson CL, Kociba GJ, O'Keefe DA, Crisp MS, Jacobs RM, Rojko JL.** Cyclic hematopoiesis associated with feline leukemia virus infection in two cats. J Am Vet Med Assoc 1987;191:93–96.
80. **Morely A, Stohlman F.** Cyclophosphamide-induced cyclical neutropenia. N Engl J Med 1970;282:643–646.
81. **Jones JB, Lange RD.** Cyclic hematopoiesis: animal models. Immunol Hematol Res Mono 1983;1:33–42.
82. **Willard MD.** Corticosteroid-responsive leukopenia and neutropenia associated with FeLV infection in 2 cats. Mod Vet Pract 1985;66:719–722.
83. **Chickering WR, Prasse KW.** Immune mediated neutropenia in man and animals: a review. Vet Clin Pathol 1981;10:6–16.
84. **Reagen WJ, Murphy D, Battaglino M, Bonney P, Boone TC.** Antibodies to canine granulocyte colony-stimulating factor induce persistent neutropenia. Vet Pathol 1995;32:374–378.
85. **Sievers EL, Dale DC.** Non-malignant neutropenia. Blood Rev 1996;10:95–100.
86. **Winkelstein A, Kiss JE.** Immunohematologic disorders. JAMA 1997;278:1982–1992.
87. **Rebar AH.** General responses of the bone marrow to injury. Toxicol Pathol 1993;21:118–129.
88. **Anderson TA.** Cytokine-induced changes in the leukon. Toxicol Pathol 1993;21:147–157.
89. **Bokoch GM.** Chemoattractant signaling and leukocyte activation. Blood 1995;86:1649–1660.
90. **Zwahlen RD, Spreng D, Wyder-Walther M.** In vitro and in vivo activity of human interleukin-8 in dogs. Vet Pathol 1994;31:61–66.
91. **Elangbam CS, Qualls CW, Dahlgren RR.** Cell adhesion molecules-update. Vet Pathol 1997;34:61–73.
92. **Dore M, Simon SI, Hughes BJ, Entman ML, Smith CW.** P-selectin and CD18- mediated recruitment of canine neutrophils under conditions of shear stress. Vet Pathol 1995;32:258–268.
93. **Bogomolski-Yahalom V, Matzner Y.** Disorders of neutrophil function. Blood Rev 1995;9:183–190.
94. **Gerardi AS.** Bovine leukocyte adhesion deficiency: a review of a modern disease and its implications. Res Vet Sci 1996;61:183–186.
95. **Gerardi AS.** Bovine leukocyte deficiency: a brief overview of a modern disease and its implications. Acta Vet Hung 1996; 44:1–8.
96. **Malech HL, Nauseef WM.** Primary inherited defects in neutrophil function: etiology and treatment. Semin Hematol 1997;34:279–290.
97. **Stickle JE.** The neutrophil. Function, disorders, and testing. Vet Clin North Am Small Anim Pract 1996;26:1013–1021.
98. **Sengelov H.** Complement receptors in neutrophils. Crit Rev Immunol 1995;15:107–131.
99. **Trowald-Wigh G, Hakansson L, Johannisson A, Norrgren L, af Sergerstad CH.** Leukocyte adhesion protein deficiency in Irish Setter dogs. Vet Immunol Immunopathol 1992;32:261–280.
100. **Allen LA, Aderem A.** Mechanisms of phagocytosis. Curr Opin Immunol 1996;8:36–40.
101. **Yang YF, Sylte MJ, Czuprynski CJ.** Apoptosis: a possible tactic of *Haemophilus somnus* for evasion of killing by bovine neutrophils? Microb Pathog 1998;24:351–359.
102. **Hallett MB, Lloyds D.** Neutrophil priming: the cellular signals that say 'amber' but not 'green'. Immunol Today 1995;16:264–268.
103. **Matzner Y.** Acquired neutrophil dysfunction and diseases with an inflammatory component. Semin Hematol 1997;34:291–302.
104. **Gossett KA, MacWilliams PS.** Ultrastructure of canine toxic neutrophils. Am J Vet Res 1982;43:1634–1637.
105. **Henry CJ, Buss MS, Lothrop CD.** Veterinary uses of recombinant human granulocyte colony-stimulating factor. Part I. Oncology. Compend Contin Educ Pract Vet 1998;20:728–733.
106. **Roth JA.** Evaluation of the influence of potential toxins on neutrophil function. Toxicol Pathol 1993;21:141–146.
107. **Styrt B.** Species variation in neutrophil biochemistry and function. J Leukocyte Biol 1989;46:63–74.
108. **Renshaw HW, Chatburn C, Bryan GM, Bartsch RC, Davis WC.** Canine granulocytopathy syndrome: neutrophil dysfunction in a dog with recurrent infections. J Am Vet Med 1975;166:443–447.
109. **Breitschwerdt EB, Brown TT, De Buysscher EV, Andersen BR, Thrall DE, Hager E, Ananaba G, Degan MA, Ward MDW.** Rhinitis, pneumonia, and defective neutrophil function in the Doberman pinscher. Am J Vet Res 1987;48:1054–1062.
110. **Roth JA, Kaeberle ML.** Effect of levamisole on lymphocyte blastogenesis and neutrophil function in dexamethasone-treated cattle. Am J Vet Res 1984;45:1781–1784.
111. **Roth JA, Kaeberle ML.** In vivo effect of ascorbic acid on neutrophil function in healthy and dexamethasone-treated cattle. Am J Vet Res 1985;46:2434–2436.
112. **Colgan SP, Hull-Thrall MA, Gasper PW, Gould DH, Rose BJ, Fulton R, Blanquaert AM, Bruyninckx, WJ.** Restoration of neutrophil and platelet function in feline Chediak-Higashi syndrome by bone marrow transplantation. Bone Marrow Transplant 1991;7:365–374.
113. **Lothrop CD, Warren DJ, Souza LM, Jones JB, Moore MAS.** Correction of canine cyclic hematopoiesis with recombinant human granulocyte colony-stimulating factor. Blood 1988;72:1324–1328.
114. **Cullor JS, Fairley N, Smith WL, Wood SL, Dellinger JD, Inokuma MS, Souza LM.** Hemogram changes in lactating dairy cows given human recombinant granulocyte colony stimulating factor (r-MethuG-CSF). Vet Pathol 1990;27:311–316.

115. **Hoglund M, Hakansson L, Venge P.** Effects of in vivo administration of G-CSF on neutrophil functions in healthy volunteers. Eur J Haematol 1997;58:195–202.

116. **Krogsgaard Thomsen M.** Review paper. The role of neutrophil activating mediators in canine health and disease with special reference to the role of leukotrienes in inflammatory dermatoses. J Vet Pharmacol Ther 1991;14:113–133.

117. **Caswell JL, Middleton DM, Sorden SD, Gordon JR.** Expression of the neutrophil chemoattractant interleukin-8 in the lesions of bovine pneumonic pasteurellosis. Vet Pathol 1998;35:124–131.

118. **Slocombe RF, Malark J, Ingersoll R, Derksen FJ, Robinson NE.** Importance of neutrophils in the pathogenesis of acute pneumonic pasteurellosis in calves. Am J Vet Res 1985;46:2253–2258.

119. **Nowack R, Flores-Suarez LP, van der Woude FJ.** New developments in pathogenesis of systemic vasculitis. Curr Opin Rheumatol 1998;10:3–11.

120. **Thiagarajan RR, Winn RK, Harlan JM.** The role of leukocyte and endothelial adhesion molecules in ischemia-reperfusion injury. Thromb Haemost 1997;78:310–314.

121. **Grisham MB, Granger DN.** Neutrophil-mediated mucosal injury. Role of reactive oxygen metabolites. Dig Dis Sci 1988;33:6S–15S.

122. **Schultz DR, Tozman EC.** Antineutrophil cytoplasmic autoantibodies: major autoantigens, pathophysiology, and disease associations. Semin Arthritis Rheum 1995;25:143–159.

123. **Schnabel A, Hauschild S, Gross WL.** Anti-neutrophil cytoplasmic antibodies in generalised autoimmune disease. Int Arch Allergy Immunol 1996;109:201–206.

CHAPTER 47

Eosinophils

• KAREN M. YOUNG

The course granular cell described by Jones in 1846 was named the eosinophil by Ehrlich, based on its affinity for anionic dyes, such as eosin.[1] This eye-catching cell has been an enigma, because it can both enhance and dampen inflammatory reactions. Serving roles as defender against helminthic parasites, pacifist in basophil- or mast cell-mediated inflammation, and dangerous enemy of host tissues, the eosinophil challenges us to make sense of these contradictory roles and, importantly, to understand its function in a given situation so that intervention is approached rationally and effectively. This chapter emphasizes structure–function relations to explicate the eosinophil's varying roles in many complex processes; variations among species undoubtedly exist, and known distinctions are highlighted. For more detailed information, the reader is referred to several comprehensive reviews.[2–10]

REGULATION, PRODUCTION, RELEASE

Eosinophils develop in bone marrow and to a lesser extent in the thymus, the spleen, and the lymph nodes in some laboratory species.[11] They are derived from a distinct progenitor cell, the colony-forming unit-eosinophil (CFU-EO), under the tutelage of several T-cell-derived cytokines, interleukin (IL)-3, granulocyte-macrophage-colony-stimulating factor (GM-CSF), and IL-5.[12,13] Of these, IL-5 is most selective for eosinophils; it promotes differentiation, proliferation, maturation, and functional aspects of eosinophils and, in addition, prolongs their survival at inflammatory sites by preventing apoptosis.[14,15] This 40 to 55 kD glycoprotein mediates the eosinophilia found in helminthic infections, hypereosinophilic syndrome, and human eosinophilia-myalgia syndrome.[16] Coordinated expression of IL-3, GM-CSF, and IL-5 is suggested by the clustering of their genes on the long arm of chromosome 5 in people, the production of all three cytokines by a subset of T-helper cells (TH$_2$ clones), and the structural similarity of their receptors (type 1 hemopoietin cytokine receptor family).[10] Although the α subunit is unique to each cytokine, they share a β chain that confers high affinity to the receptor and is required for signal transduction.

Eosinophils become recognizable morphologically with the appearance of specific, or secondary, granules at the progranulocyte stage. Myelocytes have numerous immature specific granules, as well as an extensive Golgi complex and abundant rough endoplasmic reticulum (RER). Granules continue to mature in the band and segmented forms, whereas the nucleus undergoes its characteristic shape changes, resulting in nuclear segmentation. Eosinophils can also be identified cytochemically. Eosinophil peroxidase (EPO) can be found in progranulocytes and myelocytes in the RER, perinuclear cisterna, Golgi cisternae and smooth vesicles, and specific granules (Fig. 47.1). Thereafter, EPO is located solely in specific granules.[17,18]

Eosinophils differentiate and mature in bone marrow over a period of 2 to 6 days, depending on the species. They comprise less than 10% of marrow nucleated cells, and the marrow:peripheral blood eosinophils ratio varies from 300:1 in guinea pigs to 3.4:1 in people. Generation and emergence times are shortened in animals that have *Trichinella* infections. In rats, eosinophils travel to the spleen to complete maturation. In healthy individuals, the half-life of eosinophils in circulation varies from <1 hour in the dog to as long as 18 hours in people, and migration into tissues occurs randomly.[4,10] Under pathologic conditions, it is possible for eosinophils to reenter circulation.[19]

TISSUE DISTRIBUTION AND METABOLISM

Eosinophils are tissue-dwelling cells, residing in the loose connective tissue of organs that serve as entry points for foreign substances, predominantly the skin and the respiratory and the gastrointestinal tracts. The location and number of eosinophils vary with species, stage of estrous cycle, diet, and histamine content of the tissue. Estimates of the ratio of blood to tissue eosinophils range from 1:100 in people to 1:300 in guinea pigs. The life span of eosinophils in tissues is approximately 6 days in healthy people and is increased under the influence of cytokines. Anaerobic glycolysis provides the major source of energy.[4,6,8]

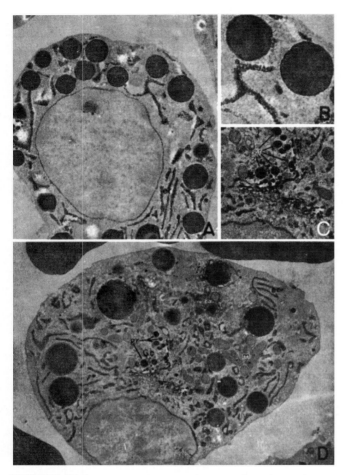

those of ruminants are small; feline granules are rod-shaped and numerous; and the canine eosinophil contains round granules that vary in size and number within and among cells, with extensive vacuolation characterizing the cytoplasm of the eosinophils of Greyhound dogs.

At the ultrastructural level, eosinophils contain four types of granules: specific granules, primary granules, small dense granules, and microgranules. In addition, lipid bodies, mitochondria, free ribosomes, sparse RER, coated vesicles, a small Golgi, and glycogen particles and aggregates are present.[17-18] Specific or secondary granules comprise the majority of the granule population in eosinophils (Fig. 47.2b) and are characterized by

FIGURE 47.1 Eosinophil progranulocyte and myelocyte from canine bone marrow stained for EPO. (**A**) A progranulocyte contains dense, homogeneous granules and cisternae of rough endoplasmic reticulum (er), highlighted in (**B**). The myelocyte shown in (**D**) contains condensing granules of varying morphology, an active Golgi complex (Gc) producing granules (gr), profiles of rough endoplasmic reticulum, and numerous mitochondria (m). (**C**) is an enlargement of the Golgi area from the cell in (**D**). EPO activity is characterized by the electron-dense material in the perinuclear cisterna, rough endoplasmic reticulum, Golgi complex, and the specific granules. A, ×10,080; B, ×18,900; C, ×14,280; D, ×10,080. (Reprinted from *Schalm's Veterinary Hematology*, 4th edition, p. 732)

STRUCTURE AND MORPHOLOGY

Eosinophils are slightly larger than neutrophils and have a nucleus that may be less segmented, but it is nevertheless polymorphic. Specific granules housing potent cytotoxic proteins constitute the most striking structural feature. At the light microscopic level, these granules stain red orange with acidic dyes in Romanowsky stains and aquamarine with Luxol fast blue, highlighting the intensely basic nature of the granule (Fig. 47.2a). The shape, size, and number of granules vary drastically among species: For example, the granules of the equine eosinophil are round, large, and numerous;

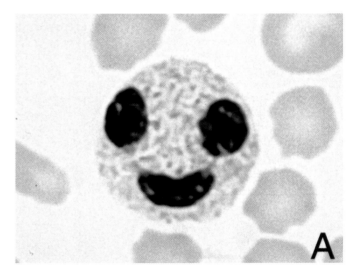

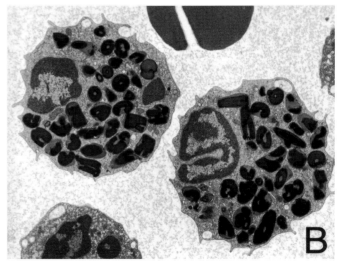

FIGURE 47.2 Feline eosinophils in peripheral blood. (**A**) Rod-shaped specific granules fill the cytoplasm and stain red orange with Romanowsky stains. ×1000. (Photomicrograph courtesy of Dr. Charles K. Henrikson.) (**B**) Transmission electron micrograph of two eosinophils containing numerous heterogeneous bicompartmental granules. ×4500 (Micrograph by Dr. Richard L. Meadows)

a bicompartmental structure in many species, including humans, rhesus monkeys, cats, goats, rabbits, opossum, guinea pigs, rats, and mice.[4,8,17] The granule has a distinctive electron-dense core, or crystalloid, that exhibits both longitudinal and cross-sectional periodicity and is surrounded by a more lucent matrix. Cores vary in density, size, and shape among species, and there is especially wide variation in cats (Fig. 47.3 and Fig. 47.4). In dogs, approximately 10% of the granules display distinct cores.[20] Equine eosinophil granules, previously reported to be homogeneous (Fig. 47.5), also contain dense cores that lack crystalline patterns, are often located eccentrically, and are surrounded by a less dense matrix.[21] Homogeneous granules are found in the eosinophils from cattle, mink, and gorillas.[4,8]

The constituents of specific granules have been well defined in some species, including guinea pigs and humans, and comprise a group of highly toxic proteins.[18,22] Features of the four major proteins are described in Table 47.1. Major basic protein (MBP) comprises >50% of the granule protein content and is located in the core or crystalloid. Its precursor is acidic, possibly protecting the eosinophil from the cytotoxicity of the arginine-rich basic protein during transport and storage. Deposits of MBP can be found in tissues at sites of eosinophilic inflammation. The other proteins are found in the matrix. EPO is distinct from and more potent than myeloperoxidase, but its antibacterial role is controversial.[17] This enzyme has been reported to be absent from feline eosinophils, but better detection methods are being used to refute this assertion. EPO deficiency in people has no known consequences. Eosinophil cationic protein (ECP) constitutes ~30% of the protein found in granules and damages membranes by a colloid osmotic process, causing formation of transmembrane non-ion-selective pores. Eosinophil-derived neurotoxin (EDN) damages myelinated nerve fibers, but has no cytotoxic actions on parasites or mammalian cells. Other constituents of granules include catalase, peroxisomal lipid B oxidation enzymes (enoyl-CoA hydratase, 3-ketoacyl-CoA thiolase), flavoprotein (acyl-CoA oxidase), β-glucuronidase, cathepsin D, serine:pyruvate aminotransferase, and zinc.[4,18] Acid phosphatase and arylsulfatase activities may be unmasked in the matrix when eosinophils are activated.[18] Recently, four basic proteins were isolated from equine eosinophils but could not be correlated definitively to the human proteins, although one is likely the analogue of human MBP.[23]

Crystalloid-free, membrane-bound primary granules are most numerous in the progranulocyte, but they can be found in all stages of eosinophils in some species. Their lysophospholipase activity resides in the Charcot–Leyden crystal protein (CLCP), comprising 7 to 10% of total eosinophil protein.[18,24] CLCP is a 13-kD protein in reduced form and may also be located in the plasma membrane. It polymerizes to form hexagonal crystals deposited in tissues at sites of eosinophilic inflammation, even when intact eosinophils are no longer visible. Lysophospholipase diminishes inflammation by impeding generation of arachidonic acid metabolites. CLCP is also found in basophils that may take up CLCP, as well

as EPO, from eosinophils and store these products in their granules. A third type of granule, the small dense granule, contains acid phosphatase, arylsulfatase, and perhaps ECP, catalase, and peroxidase.

Finally, microgranules, better termed vesiculotubular structures (VTS), are unique to eosinophils and are markers of this lineage.[18] VTS have a double membrane and are round, C-shaped, or elongated (Fig. 47.3). They transport proteins from their site of synthesis within the cell to the specific granule, thereby protecting the cell from the toxic effects of these potent proteins. In addition to playing a role in granule formation, VTS probably contribute to degranulation by delivering proteins from the granule to the tissue or target, leaving an empty granule behind. This process can be selective, e.g., EPO can be transported out of the granule leaving the other proteins behind.[6]

Lipid bodies are spherical stores of arachidonic acid, chiefly in esterified forms, used in the generation of lipid mediators such as leukotrienes and prostaglandins (Figs. 47.3D and 47.4).[18] Eosinophils also synthesize cytokines, proteoglycans, vitamin B-binding proteins, and numerous enzymes, including collagenase, histaminase, phospholipase D, and nonspecific esterases. The plasma membrane contains nicotinamide adenine dinucleotide phosphate (NADPH) oxidase to generate an oxidative burst and alkaline phosphatase in some species (cattle, horses, dogs, and cats).[4] Eosinophils lack the bactericidal agents lysozyme, lactoferrin, and phagocytin.[25]

SURFACE MOLECULES

The surface of eosinophils, as visualized by scanning electron microscopy, has short blunt processes and sparse microvilli (Fig. 47.5). This innocuous appearance belies a surface teeming with communication devices, mostly in the form of receptors (Table 47.2).[6,10] These surface molecules are essential for effective eosinophil function in the surrounding environment. Cytokine primers attach to eosinophils to deliver a wake-up call, rousing them to respond to other stimuli. Adhesion receptors link eosinophils with endothelial cells or extracellular matrix components, allowing them to leave circulation and directing their movement in tissues and extracellular spaces. Chemotactic factors are inflammatory calling cards and bind to receptors on eosinophils to ensure their presence at the inflammatory site. Many factors, including lipid mediators, immunoglobulins, and complement components, act through receptors to activate eosinophils to perform their effector functions and to connect them with their targets, be they parasites in need of killing, mast cells in need of discipline, or immune complexes in need of removal.[4,6]

STRUCTURE–FUNCTION RELATIONS IN EOSINOPHILIC INFLAMMATION

Hauling a veritable arsenal of preformed toxins, eosinophils enter the field of battle, communicating by means

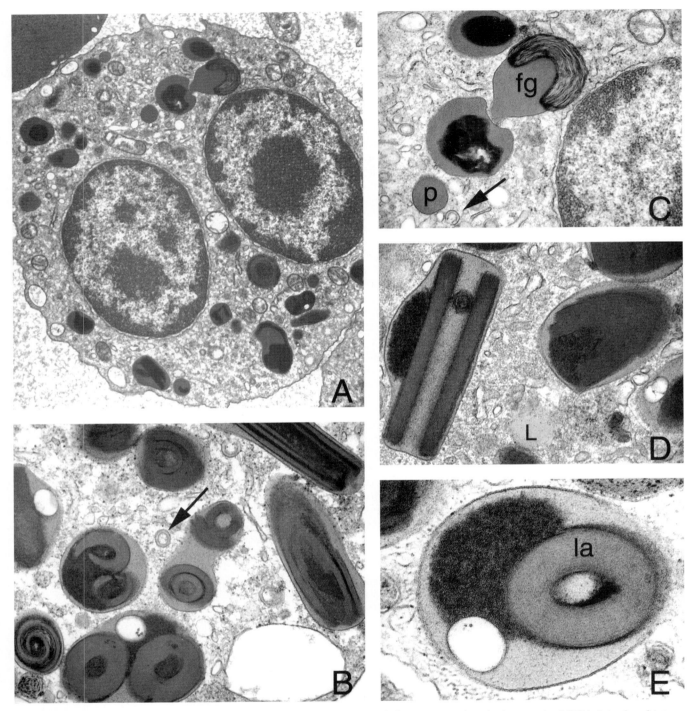

FIGURE 47.3 Transmission electron micrographs of feline eosinophils with forming granules. As the putative MBP is introduced into the granule, it appears as disorganized aggregates of electron-dense material, sometimes in swirls or wavy patterns, that eventually coalesce into a more organized core structure. The mature granules are elongated in longitudinal section, and the electron-dense cores may be hollow in cross section, multiple within a single granule, and peripherally rather than centrally located within the granule. (**A**) Developing eosinophil with forming granules exhibiting wide variation in morphology. ×18,000. (**B**) Multiple electron-dense cores are surrounded by a more lucent matrix in these forming granules. The arrow indicates a round VTS. ×40,000. (**C**) Enlargement of the granules in (**A**). The core of the forming granule (fg) exhibits a wavy pattern that progresses to a lamellar pattern. A primary granule (p) and C-shaped, round, and elongate VTS (arrow) are also evident. ×40,000. (**D**) Possible incorporation of electron-dense clouds of core material into the adjacent rod-shaped cores. A lipid body (L) is present. ×40,000. (**E**) Cross-sectional view of a hollow core, with its lamellar pattern (la), surrounded by an electron-dense cloud of core material. The vacuole may be a VTS participating in granule formation. ×65,000. (Micrographs by Dr. Richard L. Meadows.)

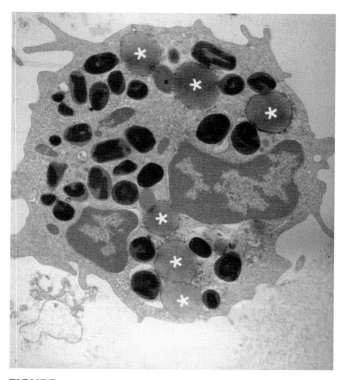

FIGURE 47.4 Transmission electron micrograph of an activated eosinophil from a transtracheal wash performed on a cat that has allergic bronchitis. Lipid bodies (astericks) are increased. ×9100.

of surface molecules to ascertain when and where to go, what interactions to explore, and which weapons to use. The following sequence of events describes the path leading the circulating eosinophil to participate in inflammatory processes:[7]

1. To migrate into tissues from circulation, the eosinophil must engage in close contact with endothelium. Quiescent eosinophils express L-selectin, which is downregulated in activated eosinophils.[26] This lectin receptor binds reversibly and with weak affinity to carbohydrate ligands on the surface of postcapillary venule endothelium, permitting the eosinophil to slow its fast-paced travel and roll along the vessel wall.[6,7,27]

2. During this slow cruising, the eosinophil meets a priming stimulus, released from perivascular immune cells, endothelial cells, and the local inflammatory site. Priming, or preactivation, prepares the cell to react to stimuli that have little or no effect on the naive cell. Eosinophil primers include the cytokines IL-3, GM-CSF, and IL-5, whose generation occurs through immunologic events, namely, antigen-driven stimulation of B cells and a subset of T lymphocytes (TH$_2$ clones).[28] Another cytokine elaborated is IL-4, which mediates ε isotype switching and brisk production of immunoglobulin E (IgE).[29] IL-5 initiates signal transduction in eosinophils, not by changes in intracellular calcium concentrations or activation of protein kinase C, but probably through the Janus

family of kinases/signal transducers and activators of transcription (JAK/STAT) pathway resulting in expression of genes for surface receptors, structural and secreted proteins, and transcription factors.[28,30,31] Priming leads to adhesion, chemotaxis, degranulation, release of lipid mediators, and oxidative burst.

3. The primed eosinophil expresses both β1 (very late activation [VLA]-4) and β2 (Mac-1 and leukocyte function-associated antigen [LFA]-1) integrins that mediate secure adhesion to the endothelial ligands vascular cell-adhesion molecule (VCAM)-1, induced by IL-4 and IL-13, and intercellular-adhesion molecule (ICAM)-1, induced by IL-1 and tumor necrosis factor α (TNFα), respectively.[16,27,32,33] Although the latter pathway is also used by neutrophils, the VLA-4/VCAM-1 pathway is selective for eosinophils and basophils.[27] Adhesion further primes the eosinophil to respond to chemoattractants and lipid mediators.

4. Recruited by various chemotactic factors, the primed eosinophil flattens against the endothelium and migrates between cells into the interstitial space.[34]

5. The eosinophil approaches its final destination, guided by interactions with adhesion molecules in the extracellular matrix, e.g., fibronectin, laminin, and fibrinogen, and a concentration gradient of chemoattractants, including C5a, N-formyl-methionyl peptides, leukotrienes, platelet-activating factor (PAF), hydroxyeicosatetraenoic acids (HETEs), hydroxyheptadecatrienoic acids (HHTs), monocyte chemotactic peptide-3 (MCP-3), macrophage inflammatory protein-1α (MIP-1α), eosinophil chemotactic factor of anaphylaxis (ECF-A), histamine, parasite-derived factors, and chemokines like RANTES (regulated upon activation in normal T cells expressed and secreted).[6,7,34] Many of these factors also recruit neutrophils, monocytes, and other inflammatory cells; eotaxin, a chemokine acting synergistically with IL-5, is more selective for eosinophils.[35,36]

6. As the eosinophil travels to its final destination, it is being activated by cytokines, lipid mediators, chemoattractants, and immunoglobulins to release granule proteins, lipid mediators, and oxygen radicals.

7. Eosinophil survival is enhanced through exposure to inflammatory cytokines, such as IL-5, which can prevent apoptosis and reprime or reactivate listless eosinophils to their proinflammatory state.[3,7,15]

The events described above mediate the participation of many types of cells in inflammatory processes, hence the common phenomenon of mixed inflammation. The predominance of eosinophils in certain disorders, such as parasitic disease and asthma, is likely mediated by several eosinophil-selective processes, including adhesion pathways (VLA-4/VCAM-1), primers (IL-5), chemoattractants (eotaxin), and prolongation of survival (IL-5). Finally, a major consequence of chronic eosinophilic inflammation is tissue damage. The injury to airway epithelium and other cells mediated by MBP seems reversible, but myocardial fibrosis, perhaps induced by granule proteins or transforming growth

TABLE 47.1   Four Preformed Proteins Released from Eosinophil Specific Granules[22]

	Location	Characteristics	Actions
Major basic protein (MBP)	Specific granule core; Also found in basophils	Cationic protein, 14 kD, pI 10.9, 117 amino acid single polypeptide rich in arginine. Premolecule (207 aa) has a pI of 6.2 owing to a 90 aa acidic portion thought to protect cell from toxic effects of MBP during transport.	Cytotoxic to parasites, protozoa, bacteria, normal mammalian epithelial cells, murine tumor cells; induces release of histamine from basophils, mast cells; neutralizes heparin; activates platelets, basophils, mast cells, neutrophils; induces bronchospasm; no enzymatic activity.
Eosinophil peroxidase (EPO)	Specific granule matrix	Heavy (58 kD) and light (14 kD) subunits; pI 10.8; genetically and biochemically distinct from myeloperoxidase.	In presence of H_2O_2 and halide, generates oxygen radicals toxic to helminths, bacteria, mycoplasma, fungi, protozoa, viruses, tumor cells. In absence of H_2O_2 acts as cationic toxin; toxic to host respiratory epithelium; induces release of granules, histamine from mast cells; inactivates leukotrienes.
Eosinophil cationic protein (ECP)	Specific granule matrix	Cationic protein, 18–21 kD, pI 10.8, 133 aa. Secreted and stored forms differ. Ribonuclease gene superfamily; 66% sequence homology with EDN.	Toxic to helminths, protozoa, bacteria, tracheal epithelium; neurotoxic; neutralizes heparin.
Eosinophil-derived neurotoxin (EDN; protein X, EPX)	Specific granule matrix	Cationic protein, 18–19 kD, pI 8.9, 134 aa. Ribonuclease gene superfamily; 66% sequence homology with ECP.	Toxic to myelinated nerve fibers; significant ribonuclease activity.

Abbreviations: aa, amino acid; EPX, eosinophil protein x.

factors (TGFs), is permanent in hypereosinophilic syndrome.[2,7,16,37]

EFFECTOR FUNCTIONS

What objective the eosinophil ultimately pursues is determined by the concentration and mixture of activators that greet the conscript along its path. Both preformed and newly synthesized mediators play important roles as the eosinophil executes its charge.[3]

Defense Against Helminthic Parasites

Although eosinophils are capable of phagocytosis, their preferred victims are too large for this approach; therefore, they secrete mediators directly onto the target, rather than modeling the strategy of neutrophils and macrophages that engulf material and secrete toxic mediators into intracellular lysosomes. Helminthic parasites are assailed by eosinophils, working in concert with T cell-derived perforins that bind to larvae opsonized with immunoglobulin G (IgG), IgE, or complement; flatten against the integument; release a barrage of basic toxins and hydrolytic enzymes directly onto the target; and migrate under the damaged larval skin.[6,8,38–40] The

oxidative burst in eosinophils may contribute to antihelminthic action, however, the cytotoxic effect of MBP to schistosomula of *Schistosoma mansoni* occurs independent of oxygen metabolites.[7] Parasite cytotoxicity is enhanced by IL-5. A cautionary note is in order regarding the role of eosinophils as essential effector cells in helminthic cytotoxicity. Parasitized mice in which eosinophil and IgE responses were ablated by administering anti-IL-5 antibody had no changes in parasite burden or resistance to infection compared with mice that had intact eosinophil responses.[41,42] After all these years, the beneficial role of eosinophils in control of parasite infection remains to be fully understood, whereas pathologic changes in the host may be a consequence of the antihelminthic function.

Modulation of Inflammation

Eosinophils impart an immunosuppressive function to immediate hypersensitivity reactions by removing immune complexes and granular debris released from mast cells, inactivating mediators released by basophils and mast cells and inhibiting their degranulation, and preventing the generation of active metabolites.[5,7] Spe-

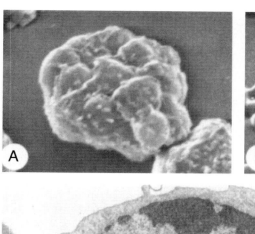
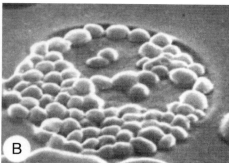
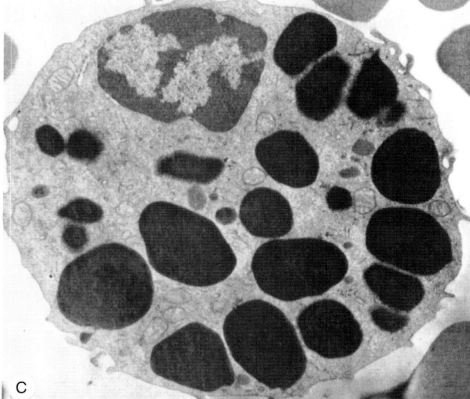

FIGURE 47.5 Equine esoinophils. (**A**) Scanning electron micrograph showing granule contours and surface. ×4400. (**B**) Scanning electron micrograph showing distinctly dispersed granules in a cell with a collapsed nucleus and cell membrane. ×3000. (**C**) Transmission electron micrograph of an eosinophil with specific granules that are large, round, and homogeneous. Bicompartmental granules, not shown here, have now been demonstrated in equine eosinophils (see reference 21). ×10,000. (Reprinted from *Schalm's Veterinary Hematology,* 4th ed, p. 735).

cifically, eosinophils phagocytose immune complexes, peroxidize mast cell granule debris, and release histaminase to neutralize histamine, phospholipase B to inactivate mast cell PAF, MBP to inactivate mast cell heparin, plasminogen to reduce local thrombin activity, arylsulfatase B and hypochlorous acid to inactivate leukotrienes (slow-reacting substance of anaphylaxis), prostaglandin E_1 (PGE_1) and PGE_2 to inhibit degranulation of basophils and mast cells, and lysophospholipase to prevent generation of arachidonic acid metabolites. The importance of the modulatory effects of eosinophils in mast cell-mediated inflammation has been questioned, and it may be that this role is confined to homeostatic conditions.[8,9]

Effector Cells in Asthma and Allergic Disease

Eosinophils are now thought to be the major effectors of tissue damage in late-phase allergic diseases, such as asthma.[43,44] Eosinophils are recruited into the lung, and other tissues, where they promote damage and dysfunction through elaboration of proinflammatory mediators, such as leukotriene C_4, PAF, and eicosanoids, and release of granule proteins. MBP in particular is toxic to airway epithelium and causes bronchial hyperreactivity.[8,22] Recruitment is associated with allergen-induced release by CD4+ lymphocytes of IL-5 and GM-CSF, cytokines that also enhance effector function and prolong

TABLE 47.2   Surface Molecules of Human Eosinophils[6,10,27]

Cytokine/Chemokine Receptors	Adhesion Molecules
IL-3[a], GM-CSF, IL-5[a], and IL-16 (CD4) TNFα RANTES[a]	β1 integrins[a] (induced): VLA-4 and VLA-6 β2 integrins (induced): LFA-1 and Mac-1 Immunoglobulin superfamily: ICAM-1 Selectins; P-selectin, L-selectin (downregulated)
Complement Protein Receptors	**Receptors for Lipid Mediators**
C1q, C3a, C3b/4b (CR1), iC3b (CR3), C3d, and C5a (fewer than neutrophils; expression of some increased after stimulation by chemotactic factors)	PGE, LTB$_4$, PAF (upregulated)
Receptors for Immunoglobulin	**Other**
IgG (FcγRII, Cdw32; FcγRI and FcγRIII may be induced) IgE[a] (FcεRII)?? IgA (FcαR)	HLA-DR, CD4, CD69, IL-2R (induced or upregulated) Corticosteroids, histamine, fMLP

[a]Expressed on eosinophils, but not neutrophils.
Abbreviations: CD, cluster of differentiation; Fc, fragment, crystallizable; HLA-DR, human leukocyte antigen-DR; fMLP, formylmethionylleucylphenylalanine.
See text for role of surface molecules in eosinophil functions.

survival of eosinophils, preventing the termination of eosinophilic inflammation. Selectivity for eosinophil recruitment may be mediated by IL-2, IL-16, and the synergistic activities of IL-5 and eotaxin. In an amplification loop, eosinophils themselves may recruit CD4+ cells into tissues by releasing IL-16. Priming cytokines, CD4+ T cells, and primed eosinophils are found in both the peripheral blood and the airways of patients who have asthma and allergic pulmonary disorders. IgE-mediated mast cell degranulation, induced upon reexposure to allergens and parasite antigens, also plays a role in eosinophil recruitment in hypersensitivity disorders.[6]

Phagocytosis

Eosinophils have the capacity to phagocytose immune complexes, antibody-coated erythrocytes, mast cell granules, inert particles, yeast, and bacteria, including mycoplasma organisms. They are decidedly less efficient at killing bacteria than neutrophils despite having higher levels of peroxidase activity, oxidative responses, and H$_2$O$_2$ production.[4,5,25,45] Eosinophils lack several bactericidal substances (see Structure and Morphology, above) and have a lower density of complement receptors than neutrophils.

Antitumor Effect

Eosinophil-mediated tumor cytotoxicity is recognized, but the mechanisms are unclear. In vitro studies demonstrate the capacity of eosinophil-derived proteins to kill tumor cells.[46] In some neoplasms, local infiltration by eosinophils in the absence of peripheral eosinophilia improves prognosis.[47]

Other

Eosinophils participate in T cell-mediated immunity through recognition and presentation of antigen, perhaps related to their location at surfaces in contact with the outside environment; their capacity to respond to particulate antigens, e.g., inhaled, ingested, or granuloma-encapsulated antigens; and their expression of Fc is standard (doesn't require explanation) receptors for IgG, IgE, and immunoglobulin A (IgA).[44] Eosinophils may contribute to wound healing, or sclerosis, by secretion of TGF, procoagulation through activation of factor XII by ECP, and fibrinolysis by activation of plasminogen.[10,48–50]

MECHANISMS OF EOSINOPHIL EFFECTOR FUNCTION

Eosinophil degranulation occurs through several mechanisms, including piecemeal degranulation, exocytosis, and cell necrosis.[18] Piecemeal degranulation is a noncytotoxic mechanism in which VTS transport some or all of the granule constituents from the granule to the exterior of the cell, leaving behind an empty granule membrane. Triggered by binding of immunoglobulin or complement, this process can be selective. For example, IgE induces release of EPO, IgA binding can cause release of ECP and EPO, whereas IgG binding results in release of ECP and EDN.[6,8,51] Equine eosinophils degranulate through a complex process of compound exocytosis and cumulative fusion in which multiple granules fuse with one another after fusion by one granule with the plasma membrane, resulting in a degranulation sac and focal release of granule proteins, targeting the cytotoxicity to the intended victim and away from host cells.[52]

Release of Lipid Mediators

Eosinophils not only respond to PAF, they produce and secrete it on activation. PAF enhances many eosinophil activities: adherence to endothelium, chemotaxis, binding of IgE, production and release of oxygen radicals, release of granule proteins and subsequent decrease in cell density, and synthesis of prostanoids.[53] Other lipid mediators released by eosinophils include leukotrienes (LTB$_4$ and LTC$_4$), thromboxane A$_2$, and prostaglandins, i.e., PGD$_2$, PGE, PGF$_1$, and PGF$_{2\alpha}$.[6,7,54] With the exception of PGE, which may downregulate eosinophil effector functions, lipid mediators contribute to host dysfunction, such as bronchial hyperreactivity.[7,55]

Cytokine Release

Eosinophils exhibit paracrine regulation of other inflammatory cells, endothelial cells, and fibroblasts through release of IL-1, TNFα, TNFβ, IL4, IL-6, IL-8, and RANTES. Autocrine control results from elaboration of IL-3, IL-5, and GM-CSF by eosinophils.[16,44]

SIGNS OF ACTIVATION

Activation results in various changes in morphology, cell surface characteristics, and functional activities.[6,16,18] Although these changes generally are acquired by eosinophils subsequent to exiting circulation, they are found in circulating eosinophils from patients who have allergic disease and hypereosinophilic syndrome. Activated human eosinophils are typically hypodense, house fewer specific granules, and have increased numbers of lipid bodies and VTS. Similar changes are seen in feline eosinophils (Fig. 47.4). In a canine model of asthma, two populations of eosinophils are found in bronchoalveolar lavage fluid: one with a typical morphology with respect to nuclear segmentation and another with an atypical appearance of a globule leukocyte. Ultrastructurally, the latter cell contains many microgranules or VTS, suggestive of the eosinophil lineage.[56] Lipid bodies serve as a repository of arachidonate-containing lipids for oxidative metabolism and synthesis of lipid mediators, and VTS are increased to deliver granule products to the tissues, resulting in a decrease in the specific granule content. Other changes noted in human eosinophils are increases in primary granules containing CLCP, small dense granules, and other vesicles and tubules. Functionally, cytotoxicity to parasites and mammalian cells is increased; there is enhanced generation of reactive oxygen species; and enzymes, such as acid phosphatase, are activated.

SIMILARITY WITH BASOPHILS

Eosinophils and basophils share many features.[3,9,18] IL-3, GM-CSF, and IL-5 are trophic and priming factors for both lineages, with IL-5 having a dominant effect on eosinophils, whereas basophils respond preferentially to IL-3. They share many surface receptors, including the β1 and β2 integrins, generate LTC_4, and contain MBP and CLCP, although there is evidence that basophils may acquire these proteins from the site of eosinophilic inflammation.[7,18]

MECHANISMS OF EOSINOPHILIA AND EOSINOPENIA

Factors influencing the number of eosinophils in circulation include diurnal variation related to cortisol levels, age, exercise, and exposure to environmental stimuli.[4,57] Eosinophils are enumerated in several ways. The least accurate is the differential leukocyte count performed on a stained blood film, but this method is useful in most situations. Eosinophil counting chambers also can be used, but automated methods that stain peroxidase provide the most accurate counts. Eosinophil peroxidase is not detected by this method in all animal species, especially cats. The reference range for eosinophils varies among species and geographic regions. Eosinophilia is not always present in the face of eosinophilic inflammation in tissues where eosinophil survival is increased.

Eosinophilia

The pathway to eosinophilia common to most causes of eosinophilic inflammation is the elaboration of eosinophilopoietic factors, principally IL-5, by sensitized T cells. T cell dependence has been demonstrated in multiple ways, and the central role of IL-5 is shown by the abrogation of eosinophilia after administration of anti-IL-5 antibodies.[41,42] Lymphocytes are likely the chief source of IL-5, whereas IL-5 derived from mast cells and eosinophils probably plays a local role in priming eosinophils, enhancing their function, and prolonging their survival.

What sensitizes T cells varies with the disease process. Parasite antigens induce production of IgG and IgE as well as activation of complement. What makes an antigen allergenic in diseases such as atopy, drug allergy, and asthma is unclear. In the syndrome of pulmonary infiltrates with eosinophilia (PIE), hypersensitivity may be initiated by heartworm infection, migration of larval parasites, exogenous proteins, and antigens associated with chronic infections. Chronic eosinophilia is associated with inflammatory disorders of mast cell-rich organs, namely skin, lungs, gastrointestinal tract, and uterus, in which mast cell degranulation provokes eosinophils. Some neoplasms, such as lymphoma, mast cell tumor, and solid tumors, are associated with eosinophilia caused by tumor cell elaboration of IL-5 and other cytokines.[58] Eosinophilic leukemia is a rare disease, and the diagnosis depends on ruling out other causes and measuring serum IgE levels. In hypereosinophilic syndrome (HES), characterized by persistent eosinophilia of unknown origin, increased survival of eosinophils in circulation, tissue infiltrates, and organ dysfunction, a proposed mechanism of eosinophilia is clonal expansion of T cells generating eosinophilopoietic factors.[37] Increased levels of IL-5 in these patients may override the apoptotic effects of corticosteroids, resulting in steroid resistance. Novel therapeutic approaches to eosinophilic inflammation are being investigated and include anti-IL-5 antibody, receptor antagonists, inhibitors of eosinophil chemotaxis and IgE synthesis, and corticosteroids that act more specifically to affect adhesion and production of proinflammatory cytokines.[7,16]

Eosinopenia

Detection of low numbers of eosinophils, especially on a routine differential leukocyte count, has limited significance, and some healthy animals have no eosinophils detected in a complete blood count. However, there are several known associations with eosinopenia,[4,57] although the underlying mechanisms are unclear. For example:

1. Corticosteroids effect eosinopenia, perhaps by neutralization of circulating histamine and inhibition of mast cell degranulation. The lympholytic effect of steroids may attract eosinophils into lymphoid tissues after release of cytokines; alternatively, production of cytokines promoting growth and function of eosinophils may be diminished. Finally, steroids induce apoptosis of eosinophils.[15]
2. Catecholamines induce eosinopenia through a β-adrenergic effect, as the effect is eliminated by β-blockers.
3. In acute inflammation or infection, eosinopenia may result, in part, from release of corticosteroids and catecholamines.

REFERENCES

1. **Hirsch JG, Hirsch BI.** Paul Ehrlich and the discovery of the eosinophil. In: Mahmoud AAF, Austen KF, eds. The eosinophil in health and disease. New York: Grune and Stratton, 1980;3–24.
2. **Gleich GJ, Adolphson CR, Leiferman KM.** The biology of the eosinophil leukocyte. Annu Rev Med 1993;44:85–101.
3. **Hirai K, Miyamasu M, Takaishi T, Morita Y.** Regulation of the function of eosinophils and basophils. Crit Rev Immunol 1997;17:325–352.
4. **Jain NC.** The eosinophils. In: Jain NC, ed. Schalm's veterinary hematology. 4th ed. Philadelphia: Lea & Febiger, 1986;731–755.
5. **Jandl JH.** Granulocytes. In: Blood. Textbook of hematology. 2nd ed. Boston: Little, Brown and Co, 1996;618–622.
6. **Kroegel C, Virchow JC Jr, Luttman W, Walker C, Warner JA.** Pulmonary immune cells in health and disease: the eosinophil leucocyte (Part I). Eur Respir J 1994;7:519–543.
7. **Kroegel C, Warner JA, Virchow JC Jr, Matthys H.** Pulmonary immune cells in health and disease: the eosinophil leucocyte (Part II). Eur Respir J 1994;7:743–760.
8. **McEwen BJ.** Eosinophils: A review. Vet Res Commun 1992;16:11–44.
9. **Shurin SB.** Eosinophil and basophil structure and function. In: Hoffman R, Benz EJ Jr, Shattil SJ, Furie B, Cohen HJ, Silberstein LE, eds. Hematology. Basic principles and practice. 2nd ed. New York: Churchill Livingstone, 1995;762–768.
10. **Wardlaw AJ, Kay AB.** Eosinophils: production, biochemistry, and function. In: Beutler E, Lichtman MA, Coller BS, Kipps T, eds. Williams hematology. 5th ed. New York: McGraw-Hill, 1995;798–805.
11. **Hudson G.** Quantitative study of the eosinophil granulocytes. Semin Hematol 1968;5:166–186.
12. **Quesenberry PJ.** Hemopoietic stem cells, progenitor cells, and cytokines. In: Beutler E, Lichtman MA, Coller BS, Kipps T, eds. Williams hematology. 5th ed. New York: McGraw-Hill, 1995;211–228.
13. **Young KM, Moriello KA, Peickert H.** Characterization of eosinophil progenitor cells in feline bone marrow. Am J Vet Res 1997;58:348–353.
14. **Clutterbuck EJ, Hirst EM, Sanderson CJ.** Human interleukin-5 (IL-5) regulates the production of eosinophils in human bone marrow cultures: comparison and interaction with IL-1, IL-3, IL-6, and GMCSF. Blood 1989;73:1504–1512.
15. **Yamaguchi T, Suda T, Ohta S, Tominaga K, Miura Y, Kasahara T.** Analysis of the survival of mature human eosinophils: interleukin-5 prevents apoptosis in mature human eosinophils. Blood 1991;78:2542–2547.
16. **Boyce JA.** The pathobiology of eosinophilic inflammation. Allergy Asthma Proc 1997;18:293–300.
17. **Bainton DF.** Morphology of neutrophils, eosinophils, and basophils. In: Beutler E, Lichtman MA, Coller BS, Kipps T, eds. Williams hematology. 5th ed. New York: McGraw-Hill, 1995;753–765.
18. **Dvorak AM, Ackerman SJ, Weller PF.** Subcellular morphology and biochemistry of eosinophils. In: Harris JR, ed. Blood cell biochemistry. Vol 2. New York: Plenum Press, 1991;237–344.
19. **Dale DC, Hubert RT, Fauci AS.** Eosinophil kinetics in the hypereosinophilic syndrome. J Lab Clin Med 1976;87:487–495.
20. **Hung KS.** Electron microscopic observations on eosinophil leukocyte granules in dog blood. Anat Rec 1972;174:165–173.
21. **Stockert JC, Trigosos CI, Tato A, Ferrer JM.** Electron microscopical morphology of cytoplasmic granules from horse eosinophil leucocytes. Z Naturforsch 1993;48:669–671.
22. **Gleich GJ, Adolphson CR, Leiferman KM.** Eosinophils. In: Gallin JI, Goldstein IM, Snyderman R, eds. Inflammation: basic principles and clinical correlates. 2nd ed. New York: Raven, 1992;663–700.
23. **Piller K, Portmann P.** Isolation and characterization of four basic proteins from horse eosinophilic granules. Biochem Biophys Res Commun 1993;192:373–380.
24. **Dvorak AM, Letourneau L, Login GR, Weller PF, Ackerman SJ.** Ultrastructural localization of the Charcot-Leyden crystal protein (lysophospholipase) to a distinct crystalloid-free granule population in mature human eosinophils. Blood 1988;72:150–158.
25. **DeChatelet LR, Migler RA, Shirley PS, Muss HB, Szejda, Bass DA.** Comparison of intracellular bactericidal activities of human neutrophils and eosinophils. Blood 1978;52:609–617.
26. **Mengelers HJ, Maikoe T, Hooibrank B, Kuypers TW, Kreukniet J, Lammers JW, Koenderman L.** Down modulation of L-selectin expression on eosinophils recovered from bronchoalveolar lavage fluid after allergen provocation. Clin Exp Allergy 1993;23:196–204.
27. **Bochner BS, Schleimer RP.** The role of adhesion molecules in human eosinophil and basophil recruitment. J Allergy Clin Immunol 1994;94:427–438.
28. **Koenderman L, van der Bruggen T, Schweizer RC, Warringa RAJ, Coffer P, Caldenhoven E, Lammers J-WJ, Raaijmakers JAM.** Eosinophil priming by cytokines: from cellular signal to in vivo modulation. Eur Respir J 1996;9(suppl 22):119S–125S.
29. **Gauchat JF, Roncarolo MG, Yssel H, Spits H, de Vries JE.** Human B-cell clones can be induced to proliferate and switch to IgE and IgG4 synthesis by IL-4 and a signal provided by activated CD4+ T-cell clones. J Exp Med 1991;173:747–750.
30. **Ihle JN, Witthuhn BA, Quelle FW, Yamamoto K, Thierfelder WE, Kreider B, Silvennoinen O.** Signaling by the cytokine receptor superfamily: JAKs and STATs. Trends Biochem Sci 1994;19:222–227.
31. **van der Bruggen T, Caldenhoven E, Kanters D, Coffer P, Raaijmakers JA, Lammers JW, Koenderman L.** Interleukin-5 signaling in human eosinophils involves JAK2 tyrosine kinase and Stat1 alpha. Blood 1995;85:1442–1448.
32. **Schleimer RP, Sterbinsky SA, Kaiser J, Bickel CA, Klunk DA, Tomioka K, Newman W, Luscinskas FW, Gimbrone MA Jr, McIntyre BW.** IL-4 induces adherence of human eosinophils and basophils but not neutrophils to endothelium. Association with expression of VCAM-1. J Immunol 1992;148:1086–1092.
33. **Bochner BS, Klunk DA, Sterbinski SA, Coffman RL, Schleimer RP.** IL-13 selectively induces vascular adhesion molecule-1 expression in human endothelial cells. J Immunol 1995;154:799–803.
34. **Knol EF, Roos D.** Mechanisms regulating eosinophil extravasation in asthma. Eur Respir J 1996;9(suppl 22):136S–140S.
35. **Jose PJ, Griffiths-Johnson DA, Collins PD, Walsh DT, Moqbel R, Totty NF, Truong O, Hsuan JJ, Williams TJ.** Eotaxin: a potent eosinophil chemoattractant cytokine detected in a guinea pig model of allergic airways inflammation. J Exp Med 1994;179:881–887.
36. **Collins PD, Marleau S, Griffiths-Johnson DA, Jose PJ, Williams TJ.** Cooperation between interleukin-5 and the chemokine eotaxin to induce eosinophil accumulation in vivo. J Exp Med 1995;182:1169–1174.
37. **Weller PF, Bubley GJ.** The idiopathic hypereosinophilic syndrome. Blood 1994;83:2759–2779.
38. **Butterworth AE, Wassom DL, Gleich GJ, Loegering DA, David JR.** Damage to schistosomula of Schistosoma mansoni induced directly by eosinophil major basic protein. J Immunol 1979;122:221–229.
39. **Caulfield JP, Lenzi HL, Elsas P, Dessein AJ.** Ultrastructure of the attack of eosinophils stimulated by blood mononuclear cell products on schistosomula of Schistosoma mansoni. Am J Pathol 1985;120:380–390.
40. **McLaren DJ, Mackenzie CD, Ramahlo-Pinto FJ.** Ultrastructural observations on the in vitro interaction between rat eosinophils and some parasitic helminths (Schistosoma mansoni, Trichinella spiralis and Nippostrongylus brasiliensis). Clin Exp Immunol 1977;30:105–118.
41. **Herndon FJ, Kayes SG.** Depletion of eosinophils by anti-IL-5 monoclonal antibody treatment of mice infected with Trichinella spiralis does not alter parasite burden or immunologic resistance to reinfection. J Immunol 1992;149:3642–3647.
42. **Sher A, Coffman RL, Hieny S, Cheever AW.** Ablation of eosinophil and IgE responses with anti-IL-5 or IL-4 antibodies fails to affect immunity against Schistosoma mansoni in the mouse. J Immunol 1990;145:3911–3916.
43. **Corrigan CJ, Kay AB.** T-cell/eosinophil interactions in the induction of asthma. Eur Respir J 1996;9(suppl 2):72S–78S.
44. **Weller PF, Lim K, Wan H-C, Dvorak AM, Wong DTW, Cruikshank WW, Kornfeld H, Center DM.** Role of the eosinophil in allergic reactions. Eur Respir J 1996;9(suppl 2):109S–115S.
45. **Bujak JS, Root RK.** The role of peroxidase in the bactericidal activity of human blood eosinophils. Blood 1974;43:727–736.
46. **Jong EC, Klebanoff SJ.** Eosinophil-mediated mammalian tumor cell cytotoxicity: Role of the peroxidase system. J Immunol 1980;124:1949–1953.
47. **Lowe D, Jorizzo J, Hutt MSR.** Tumour-associated eosinophilia: a review. J Clin Pathol 1981;34:1343–1348.
48. **Capron M, Tomassini, Torpier G, Kusnierz JP, MacDonald S, Capron A.** Selectivity of mediators released by eosinophils. Int Arch Allergy Appl Immunol 1989;88:54–58.

49. **Venge P, Dahl R, Hallgren R.** Enhancement of factor XII dependent reactions by eosinophil cationic protein. Thromb Res 1979;14:641–649.
50. **Dahl R, Venge P.** Enhancement of urokinase-induced plasminogen activation by the cationic protein of human eosinophil granulocytes. Thromb Res 1979;14:599–608.
51. **Khalife J, Capron M, Cesbron JY, Tai PC, Taelman H, Prin L, Capron A.** Role of specific IgE antibodies in peroxidase (EPO) release from human eosinophils. J Immunol 1986;137:1659–1664.
52. **Scepek S, Lindau M.** Focal exocytosis by eosinophils-compound exocytosis and cumulative fusion. EMBO J 1993;12:1811–1817.
53. **Zimmerman GA, Prescott SM, McIntyre TM.** Platelet-activating factor. A fluid phase and cell-associated mediator of inflammation. In: Gallin JI, Goldstein IM, Snyderman R, eds. Inflammation: basic principles and clinical correlates. 2nd ed. New York: Raven, 1992;149–176.
54. **Sun FF, Crittenden NJ, Czuk CI, Taylor BM, Stout BK, Johnson HG.** Biochemical and functional differences between eosinophils from animal species and man. J Leukoc Biol 1991;50:140–150.
55. **Giembycz MA, Kroegel C, Barnes PJ.** Platelet activating factor stimulates cyclo-oxygenase activity in guinea pig eosinophils. Concerted biosynthesis of thromboxane A2 and E-series prostaglandins. J Immunol 1990;144:3489–3497.
56. **Baldwin F, Becker AB.** Bronchoalveolar eosinophilic cells in a canine model of asthma: Two distinctive populations. Vet Pathol 1993;30:97–103.
57. **Wardlaw AJ, Kay AB.** Eosinopenia and eosinophilia. In: Beutler E, Lichtman MA, Coller BS, Kipps T, eds. Williams hematology. 5th ed. New York: McGraw-Hill, 1995; 844–852.
58. **Fermand JP, Mitjavila MT, Le Couedic JP, Tsapsi A, Berger R, Modigliani R, Seligmann M, Brouet JC, Vainchenker W.** Role of granulocyte-macrophage colony-stimulating factor, interleukin-3, and interleukin-5 in the eosinophilia associated with T cell lymphoma. Br J Haematol 1993;83:359–364.

CHAPTER 48

Basophils and Mast Cells

• MICHAEL A. SCOTT and STEVEN L. STOCKHAM

B asophils and mast cells were first described by Paul Ehrlich in the late nineteenth century. As the only mammalian cells known to synthesize histamine and have high-affinity receptors for IgE, they frequently have been described and discussed jointly as sister cells.[1] However, they have many distinct differences and here are discussed independently.

Much of the body of knowledge relating to basophils and mast cells stems from studies of human, mouse, and guinea pig cells; much less has been derived from studies of our common domestic species. The available information has been synthesized and expressed in several valuable review articles.[1-13] Although the existing information serves as an important interpretive aid and as a guide for directing future clinical and laboratory investigations, caution should be exercised in extrapolating information from one species to another.

BASOPHILS

Production and Distribution

The collective evidence supports the conclusion that basophils, like eosinophils and neutrophils, are terminally differentiated granulocytes. They originate from CD34+ cells in the bone marrow[14,15] where they can be recognized by routine hematologic stains after developing into basophilic myelocytes. They normally complete their maturation through metamyelocytes, bands and mature basophils within the bone marrow before being released into the blood.[16] The process of maturation and release normally requires at least 2.5 days.[17] The circulating half-life of basophils is approximately 6 hours, but in vitro survival studies suggest that they may survive for as long as 2 weeks once they reach the tissues.[6,18,19] Basophils retain their granulocytic appearance in the tissues but are generally unidentifiable by histologic evaluation of routinely fixed and routinely stained sections.

The growth and differentiation of basophils from progenitor cells seems controlled primarily by interleukin (IL)-3, but granulocyte-macrophage-colony-stimulating

factor (GM-CSF) and IL-5 also contribute to the process.[5,14] Lymphocytes continue to influence the functions of mature basophils by means of persisting cell receptors for these cytokines.

Functions

Pure basophil deficiency has not yet been identified, but the occurrence of IgE-mediated anaphylaxis in genetically mast cell deficient mice is strong indirect evidence that basophils can play a primary role in type I hypersensitivity responses.[20] Extensive anatomic and functional evidence from other studies also exists to support a major role for basophils in allergic conditions, including hives or urticaria, allergic rhinitis, allergic conjunctivitis, asthma, allergic gastroenteritis, and anaphylaxis caused by drug reactions or insect stings.[2,21] Mast cells are considered the primary mediators of the initial clinical signs of allergic responses. The subsequent recruitment of basophils and other leukocytes then leads to the late-phase reaction, hours to days later, with recurrence of clinical signs and continued pathologic effects.[2,4,22] Basophils play a similar role in the resistance to parasitic infections, but their relative importance appears to vary with the parasite, the host species, and the site of infection.[4,23,24] Basophil infiltration and degranulation frequently have been associated with tick bites, and in some cases with resistance to and rejection of ticks.[23,25-30] Heartworms in dogs and cats also may induce a basophil response, both in the tissues and in the blood.[31-33] The degree to which these basophil responses are protective and the specific mechanism of protection they offer are unclear.

Basophils may have other influential roles as well. They may antagonize or promote hemostasis by means of the anticoagulant actions of secreted heparin and the procoagulant effects of kallikrein generated by secreted proteases. They may promote lipolysis by means of the activation of lipoprotein lipase by secreted heparin. There is also mounting evidence that basophils are involved in delayed hypersensitivity reactions in the human skin and lung, in host defense against bacterial and viral infections, in some chronic and fibrotic disorders affecting several organs, and possibly in tumor cytotoxicity.[1] However, the precise function of basophils in these responses is unknown. The phagocytic potential of basophils is small.[34]

Effectors of Basophil Responses

The functional responses of basophils are driven primarily by cytokines, immunoglobulins, and complement proteins that each bind to their respective, specific, membrane receptors (Table 48.1).[35,36] IL-3 appears to be the major cytokine effector of basophil function, promoting basophilia and upregulating essentially all basophil responses.[2,37] Other cytokines either induce mediator release or augment release stimulated by other agonists.[6,38] Several chemokines (chemotactic cytokines, Table 48.1) can also induce or potentiate some or all basophil release functions in addition to directing basophils to inflammatory sites.[39–44] As with mast cells, antigen-induced activation is mediated by high-affinity Fc (fragment, crystallizable) receptors for IgE (FcεRI). In sensitized individuals, the Fc ends of specific IgE molecules are bound to FcεRI with their antigen-binding sites directed outward. Cell activation occurs with re-exposure to reactive allergens that bind and cross-link their specifically reactive surface-bound IgE molecules.[4] Immunologically nonspecific activation can occur with binding of the anaphylatoxin C5a. Other basophil agonists that may be nonimmunologic triggers of anaphylactoid reactions include neutrophil lysosomal proteins, insect venoms, radiocontrast solutions, cold, trauma, calcium ionophores, narcotics, muscle relaxants, bacterial lipopolysaccharide, and some viruses or viral products.[1,4,6,14] Pharmacologic inhibitors of basophil function include corticosteroids,[6,45–47] cyclosporine A,[6,48] and theophylline.[6,49]

Adhesion and Emigration

For basophils to reach sites of inflammation, they must attach to endothelial cells by specific adhesion molecules and emigrate from the bloodstream in response to chemotactic agents (Table 48.1).[39–42,50,51] Basophil selectins tether the cells loosely to their carbohydrate counterligands on endothelial cells until firm adhesion is effected by integrins and members of the immunoglobulin superfamily.[14,21] Adhesion is enhanced by basophil activation and by induction of endothelial cell-adhesion molecules by means of IL-1, tumor necrosis factor α (TNFα), or endotoxin. Transendothelial migration and movement through the extracellular matrix also are mediated largely by integrins and members of the immunoglobulin adhesion molecule superfamily.[6]

Basophil Products and Their Effects

With sufficient activation, basophils discharge their preformed granular stores of primary mediators and synthesize secondary mediators de novo. The secretion of preformed granules may be rapid and explosive as occurs with anaphylaxis, or, as is seen with contact allergies, it may be a slower, piecemeal release.[52] Once ex-

tracellular, the granules may lyse slowly over several days and contribute to delayed allergic effects. There is evidence that at least some basophils can then regranulate while maintaining their mature nuclear structure.[53,54]

The primary substances stored in basophil granules include biogenic amines, enzymes, proteoglycans, and major basic protein (Table 48.1).[4,55,56] Biogenic amines, principally histamine, contribute to local increases in vascular permeability, smooth muscle contraction, glandular secretion, and bronchoconstriction. Stored enzymes lead to the generation of kinins and activated components of complement. The function of proteoglycans is largely unknown, but they may contribute to the packaging and storage of granular contents like histamine,[4] and they appear to be responsible for the characteristic staining of most basophil granules. Heparin may inhibit coagulation via antithrombin III and promote lipolysis by activating lipoprotein lipase. Major basic protein, which is more abundant in eosinophils, has parasiticidal activities.[56]

The secondary products that are synthesized de novo by activated basophils include lipid-derived mediators and protein cytokines (Table 48.1).[1,57,58] Leukotriene (LT) C$_4$ is the major product of arachidonic acid metabolism, and it contributes to clinical signs by increasing vascular permeability and stimulating smooth muscle contractions.[1,59] Cytokines modulate the activity of other cells and therefore the immune response.[1,4,37] IL-4, the major cytokine synthesized by basophils, recruits eosinophils and helps drive immunoglobulin class switching and IgE production.[4,37,45,58,60,61] It is also important in selective tissue infiltration by basophils, eosinophils, and lymphocytes.[37,62]

Interactions With Eosinophils

Basophils and eosinophils frequently participate together in inflammatory reactions with each probably having both protective and pathologic functions. In the late-phase response of allergic processes in the nose, skin, and lungs, basophil influx has been documented to occur slightly after eosinophil influx.[22] This occurrence may partially be the result of increased basophil response secondary to IL-1, IL-3, IL-5, and GM-CSF released by eosinophils. Eosinophil-derived major basic protein and platelet-acitivating factor (PAF) can stimulate basophil degranulation, and PAF can induce basophil LTC$_4$ production that is augmented by the presence of neutrophils.[22]

Differentiation From Mast Cells

Despite similarities in appearance and function, basophils and mast cells have many distinct differences (Table 48.1). They function independently[3,63] and are immunophenotypically distinct from each other and from other hemopoietic cells.[4,14,55] In rare cases, patients that

TABLE 48.1   **Major Features of Basophils and Mast Cells (Species Variations Exist)**[2,4,6,8,9,11,14,39,96,127–129]

Features	Basophils	Mast Cells
Pluripotential stem cell	CD34+ (differentiation to CFU-Ba)	CD34+
Site of differentiation	Bone marrow	Extramedullary tissue (a few in marrow)
Nucleus	Long, variably segmented	Round to oval
Circulation in blood	Present at low concentrations	Rarely recognized
Life span in tissue	Days, possibly weeks	Weeks to months
Mitotic potential	Not reported	Present
Major mediator of differentiation and proliferation	IL-3	SCF
Agonists		
Cytokines	IL-1, IL-2, IL-3, IL-4, IL-5, IL-8, CD40 ligand, GM-CSF, IFNγ, IGF-I, IGF-II, TGF-β, NGF, and chemokines	IL-3, IL-4, IL-9, IL-10, NGF, GM-CSF, SCF, and endothelins
Chemotaxins	IL-3, GM-CSF, IL-5, IL-8, PAF, C5a, and chemokines	—
Chemokines	MCP-1, MCP-2, MCP-3, RANTES, MIP-1α, FIC, CTAP III, eotaxin, eotaxin-2	IL-8, CTAP-III, MCP-1, MIP-1α, RANTES
Complement proteins	C1, C3, C4, and C5a	C3a and C5a
Immunoglobulin receptors on cells	FcεRI and FcγRII	FcεRI and FcγRIII
Major cell products		
Stored in cytoplasmic granules		
Biogenic amines	Histamine, adenosine, serotonin (rats and mice)	Histamine, serotonin (rats and mice)
Enzymes	Neutral proteases with bradykinin-generating activity, elastase, β-glucoronidase, and cathepsin G-like enzyme	α-tryptase, β-tryptase, chymase (M$_{TC}$), carboxypeptidase (M$_{TC}$), cathepsin G (M$_{TC}$), acid hydrolases, phospholipase A$_2$, aminopeptidase, and hexosaminodase
Proteoglycans	Chondroitin sulfate, heparin, and dermatan sulfate	Heparin, chrondroitin sulfate
Other	Major basic protein	—
Mediators synthesized *de novo*		
Arachidonic acid products	LTC$_4$	PgD$_2$, LTC$_4$, LTB$_4$, LTD$_4$, LTE$_4$, TxB$_2$, and PGE$_2$
Cytokines	IL-4, IL-8, IL-13, TNF-α, and MIP-1α	SCF, TNF-α, IL-1, IL-1α, IL-1β, IL-3, IL-4, IL-5, IL-6, IL-8, IL-10, IL-13, IL-16, GM-CSF, MCP-1, MIP-1α, MIP-1β, bFGF, RANTES, endothelin, and lympholactin
Other	PAF	PAF
Metachromatic staining with basic dyes	At acid but not neutral pH	At acid and neutral pH
Cytochemical staining		
Chloracetate activity	Usually negative (except cats)	Positive
Tryptase activity	Negative	Positive

bFGF (basic fibroblast growth factor), CD34+ (stem cell with CD34 antigen), CFU-Ba (colony-forming unit, basophil), CTAP-III (connective tissue-activating protein III), FIC (fibroblast-induced cytokine), FcεRI (plasma membrane receptors that bind with high affinity the Fc portion of IgE), FcγRII (plasma membrane receptors that bind the Fc portion of IgG), GM-CSF (granulocyte-macrophage colony-stimulating factor), IFNγ (interferon-γ), IGF (Insulin Growth Factor), IL (interleukin), LTB$_4$ (leukotriene B$_4$), LTC$_4$ (leukotriene C$_4$), LTD$_4$ (leukotriene D$_4$), LTE$_4$ (leukotriene E$_4$), MCP (monocyte chemotactic protein), MIP (macrophage inflammatory protein), NGF (nerve growth factor), PAF (platelet-activating factor), PGD$_2$ (prostaglandin D$_2$), PGE$_2$ (prostaglandin E$_2$), RANTES (regulated on activation, normal T-cell expressed and secreted), SCF (stem cell factor), TNF (tumor necrosis factor), TGF-β (transforming growth factor-β), TxB$_2$ (thromboxane B$_2$)

have defects in basophilopoiesis or function have had no concurrent mast cell problems.[64,65]

Laboratory Evaluation of Basophils

Appearance

On blood smears, normal mammalian basophils generally appear larger than neutrophils, having a diameter similar to that of well-spread monocytes and eosinophils. They contain round to oval, variably sized, cytoplasmic granules that generally stain metachromatically with basic dyes (e.g., Alcian blue, toluidine blue) at low pH.[4,66,67] Staining is termed metachromatic when objects take on a color that is different from that of any of the dyes or combinations of the dyes in the stain. In most species, the cytoplasmic granules are conspicuous and often mask the nucleus (Fig. 48.1). With routine hematologic stains, the granules are dark purple, similar in color to the darkest parts of the nucleus, though often somewhat redder. In contrast, canine basophils often have fewer of these purplish, sometimes smudged, granules scattered unevenly across a basophilic (gray-blue) cytoplasm (Fig. 48.2). When the granules are inconspicuous, canine basophils may be misidentified as monocytes or neutrophils. Feline basophils have numerous round to oval granules that densely pack the cytoplasm to the extent that individual granules may not be discerned, especially if the cell is not spread flat (Figs. 48.3 and 48.4A). With routine Romanowsky stains, these granules are pale and appear gray or lavender with a slight pinkish or orangish tint. Because of the pale staining and dense packaging of these granules, feline basophils also may be mistaken for monocytes or neutrophils. Misidentification of these cells occurs frequently in human clinical pathology laboratories because of their unique appearance.

Basophil granules may be abnormal in form or number in myeloproliferative and myelodysplastic disorders, and they may be unapparent after degranulation. They may be enlarged and atypical in animals that have Chédiak–Higashi syndrome (Fig. 48.4B).[68] Enlarged purplish granules were reported in basophil-like cells of a cat that has mucopolysaccharidosis,[69] and circulating feline basophils may contain darkly stained granules as is seen in their developing basophilic myelocytes within the bone marrow.[70]

In most mammalian species, basophil nuclei are mildly lobulated with fairly condensed chromatin, but they often are obscured by the dark cytoplasmic granules. The nuclei of canine and feline basophils are generally long and ribbon shaped, appearing twisted or folded with less segmentation than mature neutrophils and with few nuclear filaments. The nuclei often extend to the margins of the cells, and the chromatin is less clumped than that of mature neutrophils. Nuclear shape and smaller cell size are features that help to differentiate basophils from circulating or contaminating mast cells. In birds, however, basophil nuclei are usually nonlobulated and eccentrically placed.[13,71–73] Basophil nuclei also

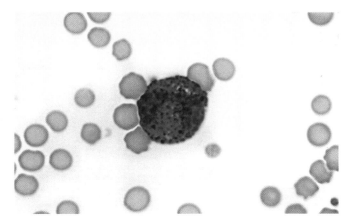

FIGURE 48.1 Equine basophil: the cytoplasmic granules stain similarly to those of mast cells (48.6), but the barely visible bilobed nucleus defines the cell as a basophil. (Hematek Stain, Ames; 1650×)

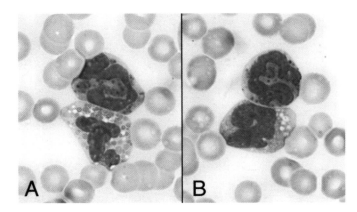

FIGURE 48.2 Canine basophils are similar in size to monocytes and eosinophils, but their long, ribbon-like nuclei and scattered purplish granules define them as basophils. **A.** Basophil (top) and eosinophil (bottom); **B.** Basophil (top) and monocyte (bottom). (Hematek Stain, Ames; 1650×)

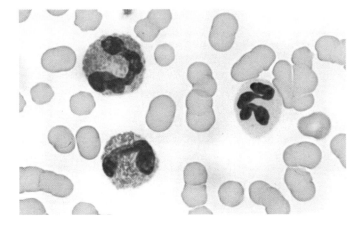

FIGURE 48.3 Feline granulocytes: the basophil (top left) and eosinophil (bottom left) are larger than the neutrophil (right). The basophil has the longest nucleus and densely packed, oval, gray to lavender, cytoplasmic granules. The eosinophil's granules are short, eosinophilic rods. (Hematek Stain, Ames; 1650×)

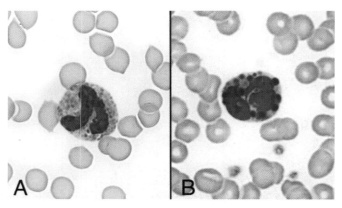

FIGURE 48.4 Normal and abnormal feline basophils: **A.** The round to oval cytoplasmic granules of normal feline basophils are densely packed and pale staining (Hematek Stain, Ames; 1650×); **B.** Basophil granules are sometimes abnormally large and dark in cats that have Chédiak–Higashi syndrome. (Hematek Stain, Ames; 1650×)

may be round in mammals that have Pelger–Huët anomaly.[74]

Basophil Counts

Automated methods for counting basophils vary considerably among manufacturers,[75] and their accuracy for detecting basophils from our common domestic species is largely unknown. The Technicon H1, however, has failed to detect basophils in cats and dogs that have significant basophilias,[76,77] and it has indicated the presence of basophilias in cats and horses when basophilias were not detected by blood smear inspection.[76]

Because basophils account for much less than 2% of the leukocytes in most species,[78–83] 100-cell manual differential counts are imprecise. If just 1 of the 100 counted cells was a basophil, and the white blood cell concentration was 40,000/μL, there would be an apparent basophilia (400 basophils/μL). If the differential count was done in a different area of the smear where no basophils were counted, the basophil concentration would appear normal (0 basophils/μL). For precise counts, one must count thousands of cells or use direct counting methods with a hemacytometer and a basophil stain.[84,85]

Basophilia

Only substantial or persistent mild increases in basophil concentrations greater than 200 to 300 cells/μL should be considered abnormal in domestic mammals. Abnormal mild increases may be present at lower concentrations, but they are undetectable by routine methods. Rabbits may have mildly to significantly higher concentrations of basophils,[70,86,87] and in some nonmammalian species such as turtles and tortoises, basophils can amount to 30 to 60% of the leukocyte population.[88,89]

The cause of basophilia in a particular patient may be unapparent, even after careful diagnostic evaluation. Primary consideration should be given to immediate or delayed allergic diseases and parasitism. Causes of localized or systemic allergic responses include drugs, foods, inhalants, insect stings or bites, and flea bites. Parasites that can lead to basophil recruitment and the accumulation of tissue basophils include ectoparasites such as fleas[66] and ticks,[23,25–30] gastrointestinal parasites such as nematodes,[90] vascular parasites such as *Dirofilaria immitis* and *Dipetalonema reconditum*,[31,32] and other parasites within various tissues. Detectable basophilias may accompany tissue infiltration.[32,33]

When allergic and parasitic diseases cannot be detected in patients that have basophilia, other inflammatory or neoplastic conditions should be considered.[91] They may be the result of primary neoplasia or occur as a secondary response to other neoplastic processes. Primary basophilic leukemia is rare, but it has been reported in dogs and cats,[92–95] and it may be associated with clinical signs related to hyperhistaminemia.[96] Differentiation from other leukemias such as mast cell leukemia can be difficult; however, cytochemical stains may help, and immunophenotyping should be useful when available. Basophilia is a recognized feature of other human leukemias and myeloproliferative diseases such as polycythemia vera, idiopathic myelofibrosis, and thrombocythemia[96]; it may similarly occur with these conditions in other species. Basophilias may also occur with mast cell neoplasia, with or without mastocytemia,[97,98] and in dogs that have lymphomatoid granulomatosis.[99] The potential for basophilia to occur secondary to other forms of cancer also exists.[96]

Hyperlipidemia has frequently been mentioned as a cause of basophilia, but there is no good evidence that clinical basophilias occur with hyperlipidemia. A significant correlation between basophil and triglyceride concentrations was reported in a small group of normolipemic people; however, the increases in basophil concentration would not be detectable by routine methods, and there was no significant correlation in hyperlipemic patients.[100]

Basopenia

Because basophils often are absent from 100-cell differential counts, basopenias cannot be detected with routine complete blood cell counts (CBCs). However, with more sensitive enumeration techniques, one can detect depression of basophil concentrations with some inflammatory conditions, anaphylaxis, and corticosteroid administration. Adrenocorticotropic hormone (ACTH) and corticosteroids cause rapid reductions in basophil and eosinophil concentrations, though basophils may not be depressed as completely as eosinophils.[70,101–103] When basophilias occur without eosinophilias, one should consider the possibility that endogenous or exogenous corticosteroid influences have depressed eosinophil concentrations to a greater extent than basophil concentrations.[70] In birds, the stress of climatic or nutritional changes may actually cause a basophilia.[13]

Basophil Function

Assays for basophil histamine release have been developed to assess hypersensitivity states in several species, including horses[104,105] and sheep.[106] Functional studies with human basophils have shown that the basophils of as much as 20% of human donors are nonresponsive to IgE-mediated stimulation.[35] The significance of this observation is unknown, but similar variability may occur in other species.

MAST CELLS

Mast cells have long been recognized as a tissue cell with critical roles in type I hypersensitivity reactions. Within the past decade, mast cells have been established as a tissue leukocyte with key roles not only in allergic responses but also in other inflammatory reactions. Most of what we know about mast cells comes from studies in rodents and man, and knowing major facts and processes increases the understanding of clinical mast cell disorders in domestic mammals. An extensive review of mast cell production and function is beyond the scope of this chapter but is available in the published literature.[8–12] Major features of mast cells are listed in Table 48.1.

Production and Function

In people, mast cells originate from a CD34+ pluripotential hemopoietic stem cell that differentiates into a distinct and separate lineage from monocyte or macrophage and from granulocytic precursors.[8,107,108] Mast cell differentiation is promoted by a mast cell hemopoietin called stem cell factor (SCF; also called kit ligand [KL], c-*kit* ligand, Steel factor, or mast cell growth factor) that is produced by fibroblasts, endothelial cells, epithelial cells, and other culture cell lines.[109] Other factors such as IL-3, IL-4, IL-9, IL-10, and nerve growth factor (NGF) augment murine mast cell proliferation. GM-CSF, interferon-γ (IFN-γ) and tumor growth factor-β (TGF-β) inhibit mast cell proliferation.

The committed mast cell precursors move from marrow to blood to tissues as nongranulated mononuclear cells. In mice, the precursor mononuclear cell may be as rare as 90 per million peripheral mononuclear cells.[110] As they establish residence in tissues, mast cell subset differentiation and cell growth are promoted by ILs (IL-3, IL-4, IL-9, and IL-10).

Mast cells contain or produce various substances that promote inflammatory reactions, and release of these substances can be stimulated by various mediators (Table 48.1). Also, mast cells interact with other leukocytes to promote or to modulate inflammatory responses. Mast cell functions include: promoting hypersensitivity reactions characterized by vasodilation, increased vascular permeability, bronchoconstriction, mucus secretion, and nerve stimulation; modulating immune responses by means of stimulating T cells; defending a host against tissue parasites; and promoting acute and chronic inflammatory responses by stimulating leukocyte migration, endothelial-leukocyte adhesion, angiogenesis, fibrin deposition, fibroblast proliferation, and fibrosis.[9]

In people, most mast cells in intestinal and respiratory mucosal tissues belong to a mast cell subset that contains tryptase and is designated as MC_T. Mast cells of MC_T phenotype have primary roles in host defense, are more common in allergic and parasitic reactions, and are decreased in acquired immunodeficiency syndrome (AIDS) and chronic immunodeficiency diseases.[11] Another mast cell subset is located predominately in intestinal submucosa and tissues adjacent to microvascular and neural tissues. This second subset contains both tryptase and chymase and is designated as the MC_{TC} subset. Mast cells of MC_{TC} phenotype are more involved in angiogenesis and tissue repair and thus are more involved with fibrotic disease; they are not decreased in AIDS and chronic immunodeficiency diseases.[11] There may be a third subset that contains chymase but not tryptase. There are comparable but different mast cell subsets in rats and mice that are designated as mucosaltype mast cells (MMC) and connective tissue-type mast cells (CTMC).

Laboratory Evaluation of Patients

Mast cells are normal residents of many tissues, including bone marrow and lymph nodes. In healthy dogs, 11 of 46 fine-needle lymph node aspirates had 1 to 16 mast cells per slide; 2 of 51 bone marrow aspirates had 1 mast cell per slide; and 0 of 53 blood buffy coat preparations had mast cells.[111] Occasional mast cells are found in various nonneoplastic lymph node and bone marrow samples of clinically ill animals. Differentiated mast cells do circulate in the blood of healthy Golden hamsters[112] but are not recognized in blood of healthy domestic mammals.

A Romanowsky stain, such as a Wright's stain, is an ideal stain for mast cells. If a stain provides differential staining of blood cells, then it should work well for mast cell identification. The major exceptions to this rule are the manual quick stains such as Diff-Quik or Quik-Dip. With these manual stains, mast cell granules may stain poorly or not at all (Fig. 48.5). Lack of staining may be associated with dissolution of mast cell granules by these largely aqueous stains if fixation is inadequate.

In a Romanowsky-stained preparation, mast cells are round cells with round to oval, usually central nuclei and have variable quantities of cytoplasm that contain varying shades of red to purple, variably sized granules. If not packed with granules, cytoplasms can be clear, pale pink, or blue. Nuclear chromatin patterns range from coarsely granular to finely stippled, depending on cell maturity. Mast cell nuclei may stain pale blue, especially when numerous, highly granulated mast cells are present in the sample. This may result from the

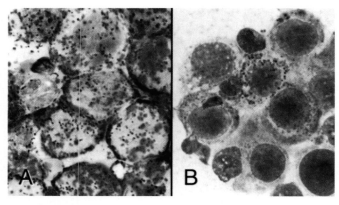

FIGURE 48.5 Mast cell neoplasia in a canine lymph node aspirate; fields A & B from same sample but with different stains. **A.** Mast cell granules are pink to reddish purple, but nuclei of mast cells are poorly stained. (Wright-Giemsa Stain, Fisher Diagnostics; 1650×); **B.** Some mast cells contain darkly stained granules, whereas granules in other cells are poorly stained; mast cell nuclei stained intensely. (Quik-Dip, Mercedes Medical, Inc. 1650×)

high affinity of mast cell granules for the stain, with subsequent understaining of nuclear DNA. Prominent nucleoli are not a common finding but may be seen in mast cell neoplasia.

Because of their unique staining, mast cells can be detected microscopically in stained preparations with scanning objectives but their identity should be confirmed with higher magnifications (400 to 1000×). In some species, highly granulated basophils can be confused with mast cells at lower magnifications. Because of their size, mast cells tend to accumulate in the feathered edges of blood films. Examination of blood buffy coat preparations increases the chances of finding blood mast cells.

Conditions Associated With Mastocytemia (Mastocythemia) or Marrow Mastocytosis

An increased number of mast cells in tissues (mastocytosis) or blood (mastocytemia or mastocythemia) may represent either a reactive or neoplastic state (Chapter 110, Systemic Mastocytosis and Mast-Cell Leukemia). In fact, there is evidence that benign forms of systemic mastocytosis in people may represent a hyperplastic response to SCF overproduction,[113] but other studies have shown the monoclonality of neoplasia.[114] Several forms of mastocytosis reflecting tissue distribution and clinical manifestations are recognized in people and different classification schemes are described.[115–117] Other than the atypical mast cells of mast cell leukemia, mastocytemia is not an expected feature of human mastocytosis disorders. Poorly differentiated mast cells have been found in the blood of a person who has had aggressive systemic mastocytosis.[118]

Mastocytemia occurs in cats that have systemic mastocytosis, and the mast cells can be erythrophagocytic

(Fig. 48.6C).[119] Cats that have mastocytemia in systemic mastocytosis have survived from 7 to 34 months after splenectomy.[120–123]

In dogs, cutaneous mastocytoma is the most common mast cell disorder, and the neoplasia may spread to lymph nodes, spleen, liver, bone marrow, blood, and other tissues.[98] When few mast cells are present in potential metastatic sites, it is difficult or impossible to determine if the mastocytosis represents metastatic neoplasia, mast cell hyperplasia, or a nonpathologic state.

For many years, finding mast cells in a dog's blood was considered highly suggestive of mast cell neoplasia or representative of contamination of sample with cutaneous mast cells. However, canine mastocytemia may be seen in various disorders other than mast cell neoplasia (Table 48.2). In nonneoplastic states, mast cell granularity can vary from significant granulation to almost an

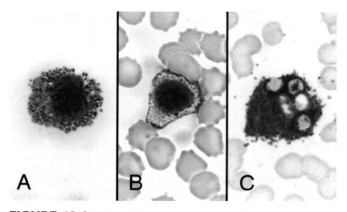

FIGURE 48.6 Mast cells from mastocytemic disorders: **A.** Highly granulated mast cell in the blood of a dog that has an inflammatory disease; nucleus covered with granules (Wright–Giemsa Stain, Fisher Diagnostics; 1650×); **B.** Poorly granulated mast cell in the blood of a dog that has parvovirus enteritis; cell conforms to space available (Hematek Stain, Ames; 1650×); **C.** Highly granulated, erythrophagocytic mast cell in the bone marrow of a cat that has systemic mastocytosis; erythrophagocytic mast cells were also present in peripheral blood. (Hematek Stain, Ames; 1650×)

TABLE 48.2	**Nonneoplastic Disorders Reported to be Associated With Mastocytemia in Dogs[124–126]**

Inflammatory Disorders
  Enteritis, probably parvovirus
  Fibrinous pericarditis and pleuritis
  Bacterial peritonitis
  Aspiration pneumonia
  Acute pancreatic necrosis
  Immune-mediated hemolytic anemias
  Renal failure associated with acute inflammation
  Inflammatory skin diseases (flea-bite hypersensitivity, atopy, sarcoptic mange, food allergy; some with secondary pyoderma)
Hemorrhage secondary to hemophilia
Gastric torsion

absence of granulation; the more poorly granulated mast cells tend to conform to the space available to them (Figs. 48.6A and 48.6B). In one study involving 19 mastocytemic dogs, all but one had acute inflammatory leukograms, including toxic change of neutrophils.[124] In another study, inflammatory leukograms also were reported to be common in the mastocytemic dogs.[125] CBC results were not detailed in a report describing the association of mastocytemia and inflammatory skin disease.[126] Considering that proliferation and differentiation of mast cell precursors are affected by inflammatory cytokines, one could speculate that finding an inflammatory mastocytemia may represent a form of mast cell hyperplasia and the movement of mast cells from bone marrow to inflamed tissues. On the other hand, mastocytemia might represent tissue mast cells that gained entrance into blood through lymph or other means because of the inflammatory reaction.

A search for mast cells in blood, bone marrow, and lymph nodes is frequently a part of the clinical staging of mast cell neoplasia in dogs. In such cases, mast cells can be found in the routine blood film (especially in the feathered edge) and in buffy coat examinations. However, the finding of mast cells in such clinical investigations should be interpreted with caution.

Extensive involvement or obliteration of marrow or lymph node by mast cells would confirm the spread of mast cell neoplasia, but finding occasional to rare mast cells in lymph node or marrow samples may represent metastasis. A leukocytosis caused by a mastocytemia is considered diagnostic of mast cell neoplasia or mast cell leukemia. Unless there is extensive blood involvement, the number of mast cells seen in the blood samples cannot be used to distinguish nonmalignant from malignant mastocytemia. More than a thousand mast cells per buffy coat preparation were described in nonneoplastic disorders of dogs.[125] Neoplastic and nonneoplastic mast cells often do not have unique morphologic features and thus the observed mast cells may or may not be neoplastic. Lastly, finding mastocytemia in dogs that have mast cell neoplasia might suggest a poorer prognosis, but data to substantiate such a conclusion have not been reported.

REFERENCES

1. **Marone G, Casolaro V, Patella V, Florio G, Triggiani M.** Molecular and cellular biology of mast cells and basophils. Int Arch Allergy Immunol 1997;114:207–217.
2. **Knol EF, Mul FJ, Lie WJ, Verhoeven AJ, Roos D.** The role of basophils in allergic disease. Eur Respir J Suppl 1996;22:126S–131S.
3. **Charlesworth EN.** The role of basophils and mast cells in acute and late reactions in the skin. Allergy 1997;52(suppl 34):31–43.
4. **Costa JJ, Weller PF, Galli SJ.** The cells of the allergic response: mast cells, basophils, and eosinophils. JAMA 1997;278:1815–1822.
5. **Enerbäck L.** The differentiation and maturation of inflammatory cells involved in the allergic response: mast cells and basophils. Allergy 1997;52:4–10.
6. **Hirai K, Miyamasu M, Takaishi T, Morita Y.** Regulation of the function of eosinophils and basophils. Crit Rev Immunol 1997;17:325–352.
7. **Alam R, Grant JA.** The chemokines and the histamine-releasing factors: modulation of function of basophils, mast cells and eosinophils. Chem Immunol 1995;61:148–160.
8. **Metcalfe DD, Baram D, Mekori YA.** Mast cells. Physiol Rev 1997;77:1033–1079.
9. **McNeil HP.** The mast cell and inflammation. Aust N Z J Med 1996;26:216–225.
10. **Abraham SN, Malaviya R.** Mast cells in infection and immunity. Infect Immun 1997;65:3501–3508.
11. **Church MK, Levi-Schaffer F.** The human mast cell. J Allergy Clin Immunol 1997;99:155–160.
12. **Welle M.** Development, significance, and heterogeneity of mast cells with particular regard to the mast cell-specific proteases chymase and tryptase. J Leukoc Biol 1997;61:233–245.
13. **Maxwell MH, Robertson GW.** The avian basophilic leukocyte: a review. World's Poultry Sci J 1995;51:307–325.
14. **Valent P.** Immunophenotypic characterization of human basophils and mast cells. Chem Immunol 1995;61:34–48.
15. **Kirshenbaum AS, Goff JP, Kessler SW, Mican JM, Zsebo KM, Metcalfe DD.** Effect of IL-3 and stem cell factor on the appearance of human basophils and mast cells from CD34+ pluripotent progenitor cells. J Immunol 1992;148:772–777.
16. **Dvorak AM, Monahan RA.** Guinea pig bone marrow basophilopoiesis. J Exp Pathol 1985;2:13–24.
17. **Murakami I, Ogawa M, Amo H, Ota K.** Studies of kinetics of human leukocytes in vivo with ³H-thymidine autoradiography. II. eosinophils and basophils. Acta Haematol Jpn 1969;32:384–390.
18. **Osgood EE.** Culture of human marrow; length of life of the neutrophils, eosinophils and basophils of normal blood as determined by comparative cultures of blood and sternal marrow from healthy persons. JAMA 1937;109:933–937.
19. **Yamaguchi M, Hirai K, Morita Y, Takaishi T, Ohta K, Suzuki S, Motoyoshi K, Kawanami O, Ito K.** Hemopoietic growth factors regulate the survival of human basophils in vitro. Int Arch Allergy Immunol 1992;97:322–329.
20. **Ha T, Reed ND.** Systemic anaphylaxis in mast cell-deficient mice of W/W^v and Sl/Sl^d genotypes. Expl Cell Biol 1987;55:63–68.
21. **Bochner BS, Sterbinsky SA, Knol EF, Katz BJ, Lichtenstein LM, MacGlashan DW Jr, Schleimer RP.** Function and expression of adhesion molecules on human basophils. J Allergy Clin Immunol 1994;94:1157–1162.
22. **Thomas LL.** Basophil and eosinophil interactions in health and disease. Chem Immunol 1995;61:186–207.
23. **Gill HS.** Kinetics of mast cell, basophil and eosinophil populations at *Hyalomma anatolicum anatolicum* feeding sites on cattle and the acquistion of resistance. Parasitology 1986;93:305–315.
24. **Neitz AWH, Gothe R, Pawlas S, Groeneveld HT.** Investigations into lymphocyte transformation and histamine release by basophils in sheep repeatly infested with *Rhipicephalus evertsi evertsi* ticks. Exp Appl Acarol 1993;17:551–559.
25. **Allen JR.** Immunology of interactions between ticks and laboratory animals. Exp Appl Acarol 1989;7:5–13.
26. **Brown SJ, Galli SJ, Gleich GJ, Askenase PW.** Ablation of immunity to *Amblyomma americanum* by anti-basophil serum: cooperation between basophils and eosinophils in expression of immunity to ectoparasites (ticks) in guinea pigs. J Immunol 1982;129:790–796.
27. **Brown SJ, Askenase PW.** Rejection of ticks from guinea pigs by anti-hapten- antibody-mediated degranulation of basophils at cutaneous basophil hypersensitivity sites: role of mediators other than histamine. J Immunol 1985;134:1160–1165.
28. **Brown SJ, Barker RW, Askenase PW.** Bovine resistance to *Amblyomma americanum* ticks: an acquired immune response characterized by cutaneous basophil infiltrates. Vet Parasitol 1984;16:147–165.
29. **Brown SJ, Bagnall BG, Askenase PW.** *Ixodes holocyclus*: kinetics of cutaneous basophil responses in naive, and actively and passively sensitized guinea pigs. Exp Parasitol 1984;57:40–47.
30. **Gill HS, Walker AR.** Differential cellular responses at *Hyalomma anatolicum anatolicum* feeding sites on susceptible and tick-resistant rabbits. Parasitology 1985;91:591–607.
31. **Rawlings CA, Prestwood AK, Beck BB.** Eosinophilia and basophilia in *Dirofilaria immitis* and *Dipetalonema reconditum* infections. J Am Anim Hosp Assoc 1980;16:699–704.
32. **Calvert CA, Rawlings CA.** Diagnosis and management of canine heartworm disease. In: Kirk RW, ed. Current veterinary therapy VIII. Philadelphia: WB Saunders, 1983;348–359.
33. **Atkins CE, DeFrancesco TC, Miller MW, Meurs KM, Keene B.** Prevalence of heartworm infection in cats with signs of cardiorespiratory abnormalities. J Am Vet Med Assoc 1998;212:517–520.
34. **Dvorak AM, Dvorak HF.** The basophil: its morphology, biochemistry, motility, release reactions, recovery, and role in the inflammatory responses of IgE-mediated and cell-mediated origin. Arch Pathol Lab Med 1979;103:551–557.
35. **MacGlashan D Jr.** Signal transduction: mechanisms in basophils. J Allergy Clin Immunol 1994;94:1146–1151.
36. **Hamawy MM, Mergenhagen SE, Siraganian RP.** Protein tyrosine phosphorylation as a mechanism of signalling in mast cells and basophils. Cell Signal 1995;7:535–544.
37. **Schroeder JT, Kagey-Sobotka A, MacGlashan DW, Lichtenstein LM.** The interaction of cytokines with human basophils and mast cells. Int Arch Allergy Immunol 1995;107:79–81.
38. **Bischoff SC, De Weck AL, Dahinden CA.** Interleukin 3 and granulocyte/

macrophage-colony-stimulating factor render human basophils responsive to low concentrations of complement component C3a. Proc Natl Acad Sci U S A 1990;87:6813–6817.

39. **Wardlaw AJ, Walsh GM, Symon FA.** Mechanisms of eosinophil and basophil migration. Allergy 1994;49:797–807.

40. **Weber M, Uguccioni M, Ochensberger B, Baggiolini M, Clark-Lewis I, Dahinden CA.** Monocyte chemotactic protein MCP-2 activates human basophil and eosinophil leukocytes similar to MCP-3. J Immunol 1995; 154:4166–4172.

41. **Alam R, Forsythe P, Stafford S, Heinrich J, Bravo R, Proost P, Van Damme J.** Monocyte chemotactic protein-2, monocyte chemotactic protein-3, and fibroblast-induced cytokine: three new chemokines induce chemotaxis and activation of basophils. J Immunol 1994;153:3155–3159.

42. **Kuna P, Reddigari SR, Rucinski D, Schall TJ, Kaplan AP.** Chemokines of the α, β-subclass inhibit human basophils' responsiveness to monocyte chemotactic and activating factor/monocyte chemoattractant protein-1. J Allergy Clin Immunol 1995;95:574–586.

43. **Forssmann U, Uguccioni M, Loetscher P, Dahinden CA, Langen H, Thelen M, Baggiolini M.** Eotaxin-2, a novel CC chemokine that is selective for the chemokine receptor CCR3, and acts like eotaxin on human eosinophil and basophil leukocytes. J Exp Med 1997;185:2171–2176.

44. **Yamada H, Hirai K, Miyamasu M, Iikura M, Misaki Y, Shoji S, Takaishi T, Kasahara T, Morita Y, Ito K.** Eotaxin is a potent chemotaxin for human basophils. Biochem Biophys Res Commun 1997;231:365–368.

45. **Schroeder JT, MacGlashan DW Jr.** New concepts: the basophil. J Allergy Clin Immunol 1997;99:429–433.

46. **Schleimer RP, Lichtenstein LM, Gillespie E.** Inhibition of basophil histamine release by anti-inflammatory steroids. Nature 1981;292:454–455.

47. **Schleimer RP, MacGlashan D Jr, Gillespie E, Lichtenstein LM.** Inhibition of basophil histamine release by anti-inflammatory steroids: II. Studies on the mechanism of action. J Immunol 1982;129:1632–1636.

48. **Cirillo R, Triggiani M, Siri L, Ciccarelli A, Pettit GR, Condorelli M, Marone G.** Cyclosporin A rapidly inhibits mediator release from human basophils presumably by interacting with cyclophilin. J Immunol 1990; 144:3891–3897.

49. **Toll JBC, Andersson RGG.** Effects of enprofylline and theophylline on purified human basophils. Allergy 1984;39:515–520.

50. **Tanimoto Y, Takahashi K, Kimura I.** Effects of cytokines on human basophil chemotaxis. Clin Exp Allergy 1992;22:1020–1025.

51. **Yamaguchi M, Hirai K, Shoji S, Takaishi T, Ohta K, Morita Y, Suzuki S, Ito K.** Haemopoietic growth factors induce human basophil migration in vitro. Clin Exp Allergy 1992;22:379–384.

52. **Dvorak AM.** Ultrastructural analysis of human mast cells and basophils. Chem Immunol 1995;61:1–33.

53. **Dvorak AM.** Ultrastructural localization of histamine in human basophils and mast cells; changes associated with anaphylactic degranulation and recovery demonstrated with a diamine oxidase-gold probe. Allergy 1997; 52:14–24.

54. **Dvorak AM, Galli SJ, Morgan E, Galli AS, Hammond ME, Dvorak HF.** Anaphylactic degranulation of guinea pig basophilic leukocytes: II. evidence for regranulation of mature basophils during recovery from degranulation in vitro. Lab Invest 1982;46:461–475.

55. **Schwartz LB, Kepley C.** Development of markers for human basophils and mast cells. J Allergy Clin Immunol 1994;94:1231–1240.

56. **Ackerman SJ, Kephart GM, Habermann TM, Greipp PR, Gleich GJ.** Localization of eosinophil granule major basic protein in human basophils. J Exp Med 1983;158:946–961.

57. **Brunner T, De Weck AL, Dahinden CA.** Platelet-activating factor induces mediator release by human basophils primed with IL-3, granulocyte-macrophage colony-stimulating factor, or IL-5. J Immunol 1991;147:237–242.

58. **Li H, Sim TC, Alam R.** IL-13 released by and localized in human basophils. J Immunol 1996;156:4833–4838.

59. **MacGlashan D Jr, Hubbard WC.** IL-3 alters free arachidonic acid generation in C5a-stimulated human basophils. J Immunol 1993;151:6358–6369.

60. **MacGlashan D Jr, White JM, Huang S, Ono SJ, Schroeder JT, Lichtenstein LM.** Secretion of IL-4 from human basophils: the relationship between IL-4 mRNA and protein in resting and stimulated basophils. J Immunol 1994;152:3006–3016.

61. **Spiegelberg HL.** The role of interleukin-4 in IgE and IgG subclass formation. Springer Semin Immunopathol 1990;12:365–383.

62. **Schleimer RP, Sterbinsky SA, Kaiser J, Bickel CA, Klunk DA, Tomioka K, Newman W, Luscinskas FW, Gimbrone MA Jr, McIntyre BW, Bochner BS.** IL-4 induces adherence of human eosinophils and basophils but not neutrophils to endothelium: association with expression of VCAM-1. J Immunol 1992;148:1086–1092.

63. **Casolaro V, Spadaro G, Marone G.** Human basophil releasability: VI. changes in basophil releasability in patients with allergic rhinitis or bronchial asthma. Am Rev Respir Dis 1990;142:1108–1111.

64. **Juhlin L, Michaelsson G.** A new syndrome characterized by absence of eosinophils and basophils. Lancet 1977;1:1233–1235.

65. **Galli SJ, Colvin RB, Orenstein NS, Dvorak AM, Dvorak HF.** Patients without basophils. Lancet 1977;2:409 (letter).

66. **Halliwell REW, Schemmer KR.** The role of basophils in the immunopatho-

67. **Vogt RF Jr, Hynes NA, Dannenberg AM Jr, Castracane S, Weiss L.** Improved techniques using giemsa stained glycol methacrylate tissue sections to quantitate basophils and other leukocytes in inflammatory skin lesions. Stain Technol 1983;58:193–205.

68. **Davis WC, Spicer SS, Greene WB, Padgett GA.** Ultrastructure of cells in bone marrow and peripheral blood on normal mink and mink with the homologue of the Chediak-Higashi trait of humans: II. cytoplasmic granules in eosinophils, basophils, mononuclear cells and platelets. Am J Pathol 1971;411–432.

69. **Cowell KR, Jezyk PF, Haskins ME, Patterson DF.** Mucopolysaccharidosis in a cat. J Am Vet Med Assoc 1976;169:334–339.

70. **Jain NC.** The basophil and the mast cell. In: Jain NC, ed. Schalm's veterinary hematology. 4th ed. Philadelphia: Lea & Febiger, 1986;756–767.

71. **Maxwell MH.** Comparison of heterophil and basophil ultrastructure in six species of domestic birds. J Anat 1973;115:187–202.

72. **Zinsmeister VAP.** Light microscopic study of granulocytes of Pygoscelid penguins (Pygoscelis adeliae) of Antarctica. Am J Vet Res 1988;49:1402–1406.

73. **Campbell TW.** Avian hematology and cytology. 2nd ed. Ames, IA: Iowa State University Press, 1995.

74. **Latimer KS.** Leukocytes in health and disease. In: Ettinger SJ, Feldman EC, eds. Textbook of veterinary internal medicine: diseases of the dog and cat. 4th ed. Philadelphia: WB Saunders Company, 1995;1892–1929.

75. **Groner W, Simson E.** Description of modern systems. In: Groner W, Simson E, eds. Practical guide to modern hematology analyzers. Chichester, PA: John Wiley & Sons, 1995;51–93.

76. **Tvedten H, Korcal D.** Automated differential leukocyte count in horses, cattle, and cats using the Technicon H-1E hematology system. Vet Clin Path 1996;25:14–22.

77. **Tvedten H, Haines C.** Canine automated differential leukocyte count: study using a hematology analyzer system. Vet Clin Path 1994;23:90–96.

78. **Hoover JP, Baldwin CA.** Changes in physiologic and clinicopathologic values in domestic ferrets from 12 to 47 weeks of age. Companion Anim Pract 1988;2:40–44.

79. **Zinkl JG, Mae D, Merida PG, Farver TB, Humble JA.** Reference ranges and the influence of age and sex on hematologic and serum biochemical values in donkeys (Equus asinus). Am J Vet Res 1990;51:408–413.

80. **Miller LD, Thoen CO, Throlson KJ, Himes EM, Morgan RL.** Serum biochemical and hematologic values of normal and Mycobacterium bovis-infected American bison. J Vet Diagn Invest 1989;1:219–222.

81. **Hawkey CM, Hart MG.** Haematological reference values for adult pumas, lions, tigers, leopards, jaguars and cheetahs. Res Vet Sci 1986;41:268–269.

82. **Clevenger AB, Marsh WL, Peery TM.** Clinical laboratory studies of the gorilla, chimpanzee, and orangutan. Am J Clin Pathol 1971;55:479–488.

83. **Fowler ME, Zinkl JG.** Reference ranges for hematologic and serum biochemical values in llamas (Lama glama). Am J Vet Res 1989;50:2049–2053.

84. **Moore JE III, James GW III.** A simple direct method for absolute basophil leucocyte count. Proc Soc Exp Biol Med 1953;82:601–603.

85. **Mettler L, Shirwani D.** Direct basophil count for timing ovulation. Fertil Steril 1974;25:718–723.

86. **Jain NC.** Normal values in blood of laboratory, fur-bearing, and miscellaneous zoo, domestic, and wild animals. In: Jain NC, ed. Schalm's veterinary hematology. 4th ed. Philadelphia: Lea & Febiger, 1986;274–349.

87. **Schermer S.** The Rabbit. In: Schermer S, ed. The blood morphology of laboratory animals. 3rd ed. Philadelphia: FA Davis Company, 1967;5–24.

88. **Alleman AR, Jacobson ER, Raskin RE.** Morphologic and cytochemical characteristics of blood cells from the desert tortoise (Gopherus agassizii). Am J Vet Res 1992;53:1645–1651.

89. **Sypek JP, Borysenko M, Findlay SR.** Anti-immunoglobin induced histamine release from naturally abundant basophils in the snapping turtle, Chelydra serpentina. Dev Comp Immunol 1984;8:359–366.

90. **Cross DA, Klesius PH, Hanrahan LA, Hayens TB.** Dermal cellular responses of helminth-free and Ostertagia ostertagi-infected calves to intradermal injections of soluble extracts from O. ostertagi L3 Larvae. Vet Parasitol 1987;23:257–264.

91. **Athreya BH, Moser G, Raghavan TES.** Increased circulating basophils in juvenile rheumatoid arthritis. Am J Dis Child 1975;129:935–937.

92. **Alroy J.** Basophilic leukemia in a dog. Vet Pathol 1972;9:90–95.

93. **MacEwen EG, Drazner FH, McClelland AJ, Wilkins RJ.** Treatment of basophilic leukemia in a dog. J Am Vet Med Assoc 1975;166:376–380.

94. **Mahaffey EA, Brown TP, Duncan JR, Latimer KS, Brown SA.** Basophilic leukaemia in a dog. J Comp Pathol 1987;97:393–399.

95. **Latimer KS, Meyer DJ.** Leukocytes in health and disease. In: Ettinger SJ, ed. Textbook of veterinary internal medicine: diseases of the dog and cat. 3rd ed. Philadelphia: WB Saunders Company, 1989;2181–2224.

96. **Lichtman MA.** Basophilopenia, basophilia, and mastocytosis. In: Beutler E, Lichtman MA, Coller BS, Kipps TJ, eds. Williams hematology. 5th ed. New York: McGraw-Hill, 1995;852–858.

97. **Davies AP, Hayden DW, Klausner JS, Perman V.** Noncutaneous systemic mastocytosis and mast cell leukemia in a dog: case report and literature review. J Am Anim Hosp Assoc 1981;17:361–368.

98. **O'Keefe DA, Couto CG, Burke-Schwartz C, Jacobs RM.** Systemic mastocytosis in 16 dogs. J Vet Intern Med 1987;1:75–80.
99. **Postorino NC, Wheeler SL, Park RD, Powers BE, Withrow SJ.** A syndrome resembling lymphomatoid granulomatosis in the dog. J Vet Intern Med 1989;3:15–19.
100. **Braunsteiner H, Sailer S, Sandhofer F.** The relationship between level of triglycerides in plasma and number of basophils in blood. Metabolism 1965;14:1071–1075.
101. **Dunsky EH, Zweiman B, Fischler E, Levy DA.** Early effects of corticosteroids on basophils, leukocyte histamine, and tissue histamine. J Allergy Clin Immunol 1979;63:426–432.
102. **Saavedra-Delgado AMP, Mathews KP, Pan PM, Kay DR, Muilenberg ML.** Dose-response studies of the suppression of whole blood histamine and basophil counts by prednisone. J Allergy Clin Immunol 1980;66:464–471.
103. **Boseila AA.** Hormonal influence on blood and tissue basophilic granulocytes. Ann N Y Acad Sci 1963;103:394–408.
104. **Magro AM, Rudofsky UH, Schrader WP, Prendergast J.** Characterisation of IgE-mediated histamine release from equine basophils in vitro. Equine Vet J 1988;20:352–356.
105. **Dirscherl P, Grabner A, Buschmann H.** Responsiveness of basophil granulocytes of horses suffering from chronic obstructive pulmonary disease to various allergens. Vet Immuno Immunopathol 1993;38:217–227.
106. **Pfeffer A, Phegan MD, Bany J.** Detection of homocytotropic antibody in lambs infested with the louse, *Bovicola ovis*, using a basophil histamine-release assay. Vet Immuno Immunopathol 1997;57:315–325.
107. **Fodinger M, Fritsch G, Winkler K, et al.** Origin of human mast cells: development from transplanted hematopoietic stem cells after allogeneic bone marrow transplantation. Blood 1994;84:2954–2959.
108. **Agis H, Willheim M, Sperr WR, et al.** Monocytes do not make mast cells when cultured in the presence of SCF: characterization of the circulating mast cell progenitor as a c-kit⁺, CD34⁺, Ly⁻, CD14⁻, CD17⁻, colony-forming unit. J Immunol 1993;151:4221–4227.
109. **Denburg JA.** Differentiation of human basophils and mast cells. Chem Immunol 1995;61:49–71.
110. **Rottem M, Hull G, Metcalfe DD.** Demonstration of differential effects of cytokines on mast cells derived from murine bone marrow and peripheral blood mononuclear cells. Exp Hematol 1994;22:1147–1155.
111. **Bookbinder PF, Butt MT, Harvey HJ.** Determination of the number of mast cells in lymph node, bone marrow, and buffy coat cytologic specimens from dogs. J Am Vet Med Assoc 1992;200:1648–1650.
112. **Desai RG.** Hematology and microcirculation. In: Hoffman RA, Robinson RF, Magalhaes H, eds. The golden hamster; its biology and use in medical research. Ames, IA: Iowa State University Press, 1968:187.
113. **Longley JB Jr, Morganroth GS, Tyrrell L, Ding TG, Anderson DM, Williams DE, Halaban R.** Altered metabolism of mast cell growth factor (*c-kit* ligand) in cutaneous mastocytosis. N Engl J Med 1993;328:1302–1307.
114. **Kröber SM, Horny H-P, Ruck P, Kämmerer U, Geiselhart A, Handgretinger R, Griesser H, Menke DM, Kaiserling E.** Mastocytosis: reactive or neoplastic? J Clin Pathol 1997;50:525–527.
115. **Golkar L, Bernhard JD.** Mastocytosis. Lancet 1997;349:1379–1385.
116. **Gruchalla RS.** Southwestern Internal Medicine Conference: mastocytosis: developments during the past decade. Am J Med Sci 1995;309:328–338.
117. **Schneider I, Schwartz RA.** Mast cell disease. Cutis 1997;59:63–66.
118. **Castells MC, Friend DS, Bunnell CA, Hu X, Kraus M, Osteen RT, Austen, KF.** The presence of membrane-bound stem cell factor on highly immature nonmetachromatic mast cells in the peripheral blood of a patient with aggressive systemic mastocytosis. J Allergy Clin Immunol 1996;98:831–840.
119. **Madewell BR, Gunn C, Gribble DH.** Mast cell phagocytosis of red blood cells in a cat. Vet Pathol 1983;20:638–640.
120. **Weller RE.** Systemic mastocytosis and mastocytemia in a cat. Mod Vet Pract 1978;59:41–43.
121. **Confer AW, Langloss JM.** Long-term survival of two cats with mastocytosis. J Am Vet Med Assoc 1978;172:160–161.
122. **Guerre R, Millet P, Groulade P.** Systemic mastocytosis in a cat: remission after splenectomy. J Small Anim Pract 1979;20:769–772.
123. **Liska WD, MacEwen EG, Zaki FA, Garvey M.** Feline systemic mastocytosis: a review and results of splenectomy in seven cases. J Am Anim Hosp Assoc 1979;15:589–597.
124. **Stockham SL, Basel DL, Schmidt DA.** Mastocytemia in dogs with acute inflammatory diseases. Vet Clin Path 1986;15:16–21.
125. **McManus PM.** Frequency and severity of mastocytemia in dogs with and without mast cell tumors: 120 cases. J Am Vet Med Assoc 1999;215:355–357.
126. **Cayatte SM, McManus PM, Miller WH Jr, Scott DW.** Identification of mast cells in buffy coat preparations from dogs with inflammatory skin diseases. J Am Vet Med Assoc 1995;206:325–326.
127. **Galli SJ, Dvorak AM.** Production, biochemistry, and function of basophils and mast cells. In: Beutler E, Lichtman MA, Coller BS, Kipps TJ, eds. Williams hematology. 5th ed. New York: McGraw-Hill, 1995;805–810.
128. **Ehrenreich H, Burd PR, Rottem M, Hültner L, Hylton JB, Garfield M, Coligan JE, Metcalfe DD, Fauci AS.** Endothelins belong to the assortment of mast cell-derived and mast cell-bound cytokines. New Biol 1992;4:147–156.
129. **Yamamura H, Nabe T, Kohno S, Ohata K.** Endothelin-1, one of the most potent histamine releasers in mouse peritoneal mast cells. Eur J Pharmacol 1994;265:9–15.

CHAPTER 49

Monocytes and Macrophages

• DOROTHEE BIENZLE

Monocytes and tissue macrophages comprise the mononuclear phagocytic system (MPS). Members of this system are present in virtually all tissues and serosal cavities, such as the Kupffer cells in the liver, alveolar and interstitial macrophages in the lung, type A synoviocytes in joint fluid, and microglia in the brain. The cells function in the phagocytosis and digestion of cellular debris, microorganisms, and particulate matter; secretion of cytokines and chemical mediators of inflammation; presentation of antigen to lymphocytes to initiate immune responses; and exertion of cytotoxicity against tumor or foreign cells. Although monocytes are a fairly inconspicuous component of the leukogram, they are the precursors of macrophages, which are essential for life. Monocytes circulate only transiently in the peripheral blood, exit the vasculature either randomly or at specific sites of inflammation, and differentiate into long-lived macrophages under the influence of specific tissue factors. Monocytes normally do not reenter the circulation.

PRODUCTION AND DISTRIBUTION

Monocytes are produced in the bone marrow and descend from pluripotent hemopoietic stem cells in common with all other blood cells. A bipotential cell, the colony-forming unit-granulocyte macrophage (CFU-GM), is the common precursor cell for mature granulocytes and monocytes (Fig. 49.1). Differentiation of CFU-GM into monoblasts, promonocytes, and monocytes is influenced by specific growth factors that induce transcription factors uniquely expressed in this particular cell lineage.[1,2] The cytokines promoting monocyte development and function are interleukin-3 (IL-3), granulocyte-macrophage colony stimulating factor (GM-CSF), and macrophage stimulating factor (M-CSF) (Fig. 49.1).[3] Canine and bovine GM-CSFs have been produced as recombinant proteins and act analogously to their human counterpart.[4,5] Administration produces a dose-dependent neutrophilia and monocytosis that abate rapidly with discontinuation of the growth factor. Thrombocytopenia caused by increased platelet destruction occurred in dogs at doses inducing significant monocytosis. This consumptive thrombocytopenia has been attributed to excessive phagocytic activation of macrophages.[6]

Monoblasts are morphologically indistinct and are defined functionally as a transition stage between CFU-GM and promonocytes. Promonocytes have features in common with mature monocytes such as cytoplasmic vacuolation, and irregular cell membranes. Neither promonocytes nor monocytes are stored in the bone marrow; therefore, these cells are observed infrequently in bone marrow preparations from healthy animals. An exception are mice who have been reported to store two to three times more monocytes in the bone marrow than in the blood.[7] Human blood monocytes appear 13 to 26 hours after the last cell division,[8] and studies in cattle indicate a similar release rate.[9] Thus, under homeostatic conditions, monocytes are released from the bone marrow approximately 6 days after initiation of stem cell division. A bone marrow storage pool comparable to that for granulocytes does not exist.

Once in the peripheral blood, the circulating half-life of human monocytes is approximately 70 hours,[8] the circulating half-life of mouse monocytes is 18 hours,[10] and that of bovine monocytes 20 to 23 hours.[9] Studies of the circulating half-life are influenced by the experimental technique: removal of leukocytes for in vitro labeling manipulations generally result in shorter half-lives than those methods relying on direct in vivo administration of a label. The values cited above are based on either in vivo or bone marrow precursor labeling of monocytes and thus should provide a close estimate of the actual circulating half-life. In humans, monocytes are unequally distributed between circulating and marginal cell pools in a 1:3.5 ratio.[11] Rabbits also have a large pool of monocytes transiently trapped in the pulmonary vasculature[8]; and approximately 60% of blood monocytes of mice are marginated.[7] As a result, certain stimuli, such as infectious agents, may result in a monocytosis owing to redistribution of intravascular monocytes. Whether a similar phenomenon exists in other domesticated animals is unresolved; however, the monocytosis observed after glucocorticoid administration in dogs suggests that a marginal pool exists in this species. In inflammatory conditions, the circulating half-life of monocytes in the blood is shortened with increased numbers entering the bone marrow and leaving the circulation.

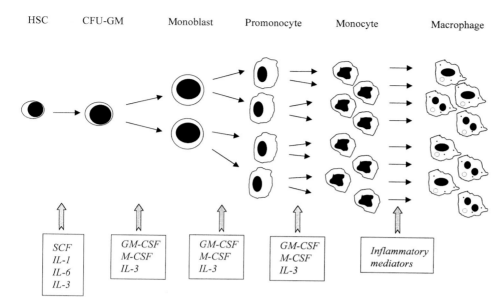

FIGURE 49.1 Hemopoietic stem cells (HSC) gives rise to CFU-GM. These cells differentiate to both monocytic and granulocytic precursors. Mature monocytes are released from the bone marrow approximately 3 days later. Monocytes differentiate to tissue or serosal cavity macrophages in response to inflammatory mediators and cytokines.

Monocytes exit from the circulation in an apparent random manner in the absence of inflammatory stimuli. However, in response to inflammation, monocytes accumulate specifically at the site of the lesion, though in lesser numbers than neutrophils. Although tissue macrophages are capable of cell division, less than 5% of the resident macrophage population arise de novo.[11] Most macrophages in inflammatory sites have been recruited from the blood. In human recipients of marrow transplants, autologous macrophage populations are replaced over approximately 100 days with donor-derived cells.[8] In contrast, studies in mice indicate that replacement of tissue macrophages in the absence of inflammation occurs gradually, suggesting that the natural life span of macrophages may exceed 1 year.[10] Thus, the exact life span of macrophages in tissues is unknown, but it appears that resident macrophages are long lived, whereas monocytes or macrophages responding to inflammatory stimuli are short lived. Multinucleated giant cells are observed at sites of chronic inflammation, and arise from fusion of resident macrophages.[3]

MORPHOLOGY AND CYTOCHEMISTRY

In stained blood smears, because of their propensity to adhere and to spread on glass surfaces, monocytes appear larger than neutrophils. Flow-cytometric evaluation of animal leukoytes indicates that fresh monocytes are actually of similar size or slightly smaller than neutrophils but are larger than lymphocytes. Monocytes have irregular cytoplasmic boundaries and may appear round to angular in blood films. The cytoplasm is abundant and typically has a gray-blue, ground glass appearance with Romanowsky stains (Fig. 49.2). Cytoplasmic vacuoles, consistently mentioned as an identifying feature of monocytes, are primarily an artifact of sample handling in most blood specimens but may be associated

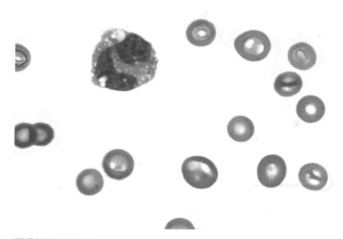

FIGURE 49.2 Mature canine monocyte in the peripheral blood (Wright's stain). Monocytes have irregular nuclei with loose and evenly distributed chromatin. The cytoplasm is abundant and stains pale blue; a few vacuoles may be evident. Monocytes appear larger than neutrophils in blood smears.

with increased phagocytic activity in some diseases.[11] Monocytes also may have fine pink to azurophilic granules (lysosomes) in the cytoplasm. The nucleus is highly pleiomorphic and may be horseshoe-shaped, butterfly-shaped, folded, or ovoid. The nuclear margins are distinct, and the chromatin pattern is reticular or lacy. Cytoplasmic margins may have small projections or pseudopodia. Canine monocytes may have a more granular cytoplasm and nuclei resembling those of immature neutrophils. Such changes are especially noticeable in stained blood smears from dogs that have a leukocytosis accompanying immune hemolytic anemia. However, the gray-blue color of the cytoplasm and the dispersed chromatin pattern should allow distinction of monocytes from immature neutrophils that have paler cytoplasmic staining and clumped chromatin. Promonocytes are infrequently observed in the bone marrow unless the animal has profound neutropenia, monocytic leukemia, or myelomonocytic leukemia. Promonocytes are larger than monocytes and are characterized by a higher nuclear-to-cytoplasmic ratio, a large irregular nucleus (Fig. 49.3), and an occasional nucleolus.[7] Cytoplasmic features are similar to mature monocytes. Monoblasts are indistinguishable from myeloblasts by light microscopy.

The cytochemical characteristics of monocytes and macrophages are summarized in Table 49.1. Although species differences are apparent and the enzymatic properties of monocytic granule contents in animals differ slightly from those in humans, monocytes generally are devoid of staining or stain weakly for peroxidase, arylsulfatase, β-glucoronidase, and acid phosphatase.[7]

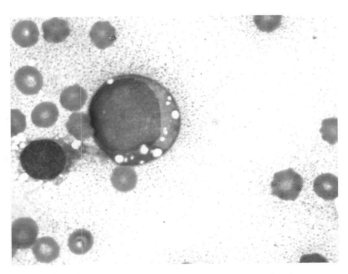

FIGURE 49.3 Promonocyte in the bone marrow of a dog (Wright's stain). Promonocytes are infrequently observed in normal bone marrow and have a higher nuclear-to-cytoplasmic ratio than mature monocytes. The chromatin is more darkly staining, and one or more nucleoli are apparent. There is a perinuclear clear area that corresponds to the Golgi apparatus.

However, they characteristically have diffuse cytoplasmic staining for nonspecific esterase (α-naphthyl acetate esterase) activity. Nonspecific esterase activity is absent in neutrophil granules of dogs, cats, cows, and sheep, and only faintly present in horses and goats.[7] Esterase activity in monocytes is inhibited by sodium fluoride treatment, allowing differentiation from esterase activity in immature granulocytic cells and T lymphocytes. Macrophages are heterogenous regarding the enzymatic content of their granules. Resident and early exudate macrophages are reported to have peroxidase-positive nuclear envelopes, whereas those in inflammatory lesions are peroxidase negative.[7] With cellular activation the hydrolytic enzyme content of macrophage lysosomes increases. More pronounced staining for esterase and β-glucuronidase activity may be observed.

ULTRASTRUCTURE

Monocytes and macrophages have a distinct appearance on electron microscopy. The monocyte surface is extensively ruffled, correlating with the cell's motility and phagocytic ability. The cytoplasm contains vacuoles, small heterogenous granules, numerous mitochondria, a variable quantity of ribosomes, and few profiles of endoplasmic reticulum. Small nucleoli may be observed in the nucleus. Macrophages have similar membrane features; however, the cytoplasmic characteristics reflect the degree of differentiation and phagocytic activity of the cell. Lysomes are numerous, and identified as electron-dense, membrane-bound vesicles that may be fusing with phagosomes to form secondary lysosomes called phagolysosomes. Digested material may be apparent within phagolysosomes. In macrophages the Golgi apparatus is well developed and situated adjacent to the nucleus. The nucleus often contains prominent nucleoli.

CELL RECEPTORS AND CYTOKINE PRODUCTION

In human and mouse studies macrophage surface receptors have been extensively characterized. In many cases, the existence of analogous molecules in domestic ani-

TABLE 49-1	Cytochemical Properties of Monocytes in Domestic Animals[a]						
Cytochemical Marker	**Dog**	**Cat**	**Horse**	**Cow**	**Sheep**	**Goat**	**Human**
Acid phosphatase	±[b]	±	±	±	±	±	++[c]
Alkaline phosphatase	−	−	−	−	−	−	−
Chloroacetate esterase	−	−	+[d]	±	±	±	±
Glycogen	±	−	±	±	±	±	±
Nonspecific esterase	++	++	+	+	+	+	++
Peroxidase	±	−	±	−	−	−	+
Sudan black B	±	±	±	±	−	±	−

[a]Adapted from references 7, 40 and 41.
[b]Occasional cells stain positive.
[c]Strongly positive staining.
[d]Most cells stain positive.

mals has been confirmed.[12,13] Receptors for the crystalliz-able fragment region (FcR) of immunoglobulins (Ig) are essential for binding of antigen–antibody complexes or antibody-coated particles and thus are expressed at high density on mononuclear phagocytes. Binding of comple-ment components, through receptors for different frag-ments of C3 and for C5a and C1q, allows macrophages to recognize organisms opsonized with complement on their surface. The iC3b receptor (CR3) is a member of the β_2 integrin family, which mediates cell-to-cell adhesion. Thus, in addition to binding complement, the receptors function in promoting the interaction of macrophages with other cells of the immune system. Another major receptor expressed on macrophages is CD14, which in-teracts with lipopolysaccharide (LPS) on gram-negative bacteria. By a different mechanism, the CD14 molecule also may mediate phagocytosis of apoptotic cells.[14] Bind-ing of LPS induces macrophages to elaborate inflamma-tory cytokines such as tumor necrosis factor (TNF) and interleukin (IL)-1. In contrast, the clearance of apoptotic cells is disassociated from inflammatory cytokine pro-duction. Macrophages are major antigen-presenting cells (APC) and accordingly express high levels of major histocompatibility complex (MHC) I and II antigens. In addition, macrophages possess receptors for hundreds of different molecules, including cytokines, hormones, lipoproteins, small peptide sequences, arachidonic acid metabolites, coagulants and anticoagulants, lectins, and catecholamines. The presence of receptors varies ac-cording to the tissue-specific function of the phagocyte. Expression of such a broad range of receptors highlights the central role macrophages play in immunity, in-flammation, hemostasis, and hormonal physiology.

BIOCHEMISTRY AND FUNCTION

Mononuclear phagocytes derive their metabolic energy largely from glycolysis, except for alveolar macrophages in which oxidative phosphorylation contributes to the generation of adenosine triphosphate (ATP). Monocytes and nonfixed macrophages are motile, moving toward chemotactic signals through the use of contractile cellu-lar proteins such as actin and myosin. Substances that can induce mononuclear phagocyte chemotaxis include N-formylated bacterial peptides, complement compo-nents (C3a and C5a), leukotriene B$_4$, collagen and elastin fragments, thrombin, platelet factor 4 and platelet-derived growth factor (PDGF), and chemokines such as macrophage inflammatory proteins (MIP)-1α, MIP-1β, and RANTES (regulated upon activation, normal T ex-pressed and secreted).[15,16] Other factors, like macrophage migration inhibitory factor (MIF), produced by T lym-phocytes and eosinophils, arrest macrophage migration and are strong stimuli for cytokine production, thus acting in a proinflammatory manner.[15]

Phagocytes that are motile are not necessarily acti-vated. Macrophage activation refers to enhanced cyto-toxic properties or an enhanced ability to restrict the replication of intracellular organisms. Hence increased production of reactive oxygen metabolites and proteo-

lytic enzymes, as well as upregulation of MHC Class II expression, characterize the activated state. Macro-phages become activated in response to cytokines, in particular by interferon (IFN) γ secreted by lymphocytes or nonhemopoietic cells . Therefore, chemokines may recruit macrophages to a site of inflammation, but ap-propriate stimulation by IFNγ and other cytokines is required for activating macrophages. Once a primed macrophage binds a particle coated with Ig, cytotoxic molecules such as TNFα and proteases are secreted, and lysis of the target results from antibody-dependent cellular cytotoxicity (ADCC). Recognition of neoplastic or allogeneic cells may induce macrophages to release cytostatic compounds including nitric oxide, prosta-glandins, and cytokines. Complement-marked micro-bial organisms engulfed by macrophages are seques-tered in cytoplasmic phagosomes that subsequently fuse with lysosomes. The phagolysosomes becomes acidi-fied, resulting in activation of the proteolytic enzymes and oxidative compounds contained within lysosomes. In this environment most microbial organisms are killed; however, some have developed mechanisms to inhibit vacuolar acidification or phagolysosomal fusion. Organ-isms characterized by their ability to survive in macro-phages are *Mycobacterium* sp., *Leishmania* sp., *Listeria monocytogenes,* and *Cryptococcus neoformans.* Thus, effec-tive macrophage function depends on the highly coordi-nated and complex interactions of chemotactic factors, activating cytokines, costimulatory signals from sur-rounding cells, and generation of effector molecules.

MONOCYTOPENIA AND MONOCYTE DYSFUNCTION

A decreased monocyte count is rarely appreciated in domestic animals, and no specific significance is associ-ated with monocytopenia. Lack of monocyte production accompanies the complete hemopoietic failure of aplas-tic anemia and the leukopenia observed in many myelo-proliferative diseases. However, monocytopenia is of lesser importance compared with life-threatening neu-tropenia. Recovery of monocyte numbers precedes the reappearance of neutrophils in the blood. This is espe-cially noticeable in panleukopenia secondary to parvovi-ral infections, estrogen toxicity, or chemotherapy. In these circumstances, a monocytopenia followed by re-covering monocyte counts or a monocytosis heralds the return of neutrophil production. As discussed pre-viously, monocytes are produced in 3 days, whereas neutrophils are produced in 6 days from a common bipotential precursor cell (e.g., CFU-GM). Although there are few specific disease conditions associated with monocytopenia in animals, monitoring the monocyte count may be beneficial in evaluating leukopenic and neutropenic states.[11]

Animal lentiviruses, analogous to the human immu-nodeficiency virus (HIV), infect monocytes and macro-phages. Although the immunodeficiency syndrome re-sulting from feline immunodeficiency virus (FIV) and HIV infection is attributed to the loss of function and numbers of CD4+ lymphocytes, monocytes and macrophages are susceptible to infection as well.[17,18] In fact, infection of monocytes is characteristic of early HIV infection and is considered by most researchers an obligate stage of the viral life cycle.[19] The temporal and pathogenic association of FIV infection of monocytes with disease progression remains to be determined; however, the neurologic syndrome of FIV infection is attributed to infection of monocyte-derived cells in the central nervous system.[20] Furthermore, peritoneal macrophages from FIV-infected cats produced less IL-1 than those of uninfected cats even in the early stage of infection.[21]

In other animal lentiviral infections, an immunodeficient stage that correlates with predominant viral tropism for macrophages and lack of lymphopenia is not observed. Although various cells are susceptible to infection by sheep lentiviruses (Maedi–Visna virus), only macrophages are permissive for viral replication.[22] Tissue-specific infection of macrophages correlates with the lymphoproliferative and inflammatory lesions observed in naturally infected animals that have pneumonia, mastitis, polyarthritis or synovitis, encephalomyelitis, and vasculitis.[22] Infection of goats with the caprine arthritis encephalitis virus is characterized by similar lesions. Viral infection alters the expression of cytokines by infected macrophages, a phenomenon well described in HIV disease.[23] Monocytes in the peripheral blood are susceptible to infection by the equine infectious anemia virus; however, viral expression correlates with differentiation of monocytes to macrophages.[24] Little effect on monocyte function has been observed in experimental infections of cattle with the bovine immunodeficiency virus (BIV), but this may reflect the general lack of disease induced by the virus or the low levels of infection achieved.[25] Thus, macrophages are the main target of pathogenic infections by animal lentiviruses. The lesions produced are generally attributed to altered cytokine secretion and altered function of the phagocytes in inflammation.

Several other viruses infect macrophages and probably contribute to the manifestations of disease. However, less is known about the functional aspects of infection. Many herpesviruses infect macrophages, producing recurrent inflammatory lesions that may well result from aberrant cytokine production. Macrophage infection with the feline leukemia virus (FeLV) subgroup C may induce erythroid aplasia in cats, which has been shown to be associated with increased production of TNFα by macrophages.[26] Thus, it is likely that our limited ability to detect subtle changes in macrophage function, especially in inaccessible tissues, precludes detailed analysis of the results of infection. The changes that occur in virally infected macrophages are rarely life threatening, whereas widespread impairment of macrophage function is incompatible with life. In congenital and acquired lysosomal storage disorders specific steps of the degradative pathway in macrophages are defective. As a result, intermediate breakdown products of complex molecules (such as mucopolysaccharides) accumulate,

leading to loss of functional macrophages, tissue and organ dysfunction, and eventual death of the patient.

BENIGN AND MALIGNANT PROLIFERATION

Benign elevations in blood monocyte numbers are generally of modest magnitude and may reflect a variety of pathophysiological conditions. Situations requiring increased macrophage numbers are usually met by increased bone marrow production of monocytes and their recruitment from the blood. The complete blood cell count may not reflect the increased transit of monocytes through the vascular compartment. In this respect, monocytes are distinctly different from neutrophils for which increased tissue demand generally is accompanied by neutrophilia. A reactive monocytosis characteristically results from excess corticosteroids in dogs and has been reported in inflammatory diseases such as pancreatitis and abcessation in dogs and in disorders involving tissue necrosis or malignancies.[11,27] Bacterial endocarditis in humans[28] and in animals[11,27] has been linked to a reactive monocytosis (Fig. 49.4). Furthermore, chronic mycobacterial or ehrlichial infections also may present with a monocytosis.

Neoplastic proliferations involving monocytes or their precursors are rare, but have been reported in all domestic animals species. Leukemias of monocytic cells usually present as an acute illness in a compromised host with severe cytopenias. Myelomonocytic leukemia (type M4) involves the uncontrolled proliferation of granulocytic and monocytic cells.[29] In these cases, the bipotential precursor cell shared by neutrophils and monocytes undergoes neoplastic transformation. Mono-

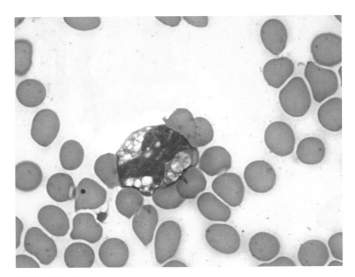

FIGURE 49.4 Reactive monocytosis in a dog that has bacteremia (Wright's stain). Monocytes comprise 22% of the leukocyte count. The cytoplasm of all monocytes was highly vacuolated and the nuclei convoluted.

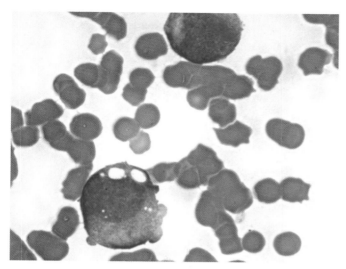

FIGURE 49.5 Monocytic leukemia in a horse (type M5a), buffy coat smear (Wright's stain). Monoblasts in the peripheral blood are characterized by round to oval nuclei with open chromatin patterns and large, prominent nucleoli. The cytoplasm is vacuolated and stains pale blue.

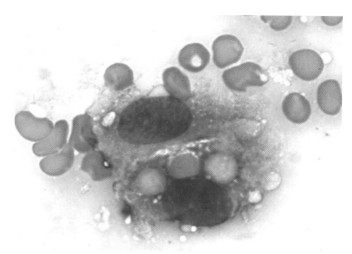

FIGURE 49.7 Malignant histiocytosis in a Golden Retriever, buffy coat smear (Wright's stain). Many of the cells are large, occasionally binucleate, and have oval to round nuclei with prominent nucleoli. The cytoplasm is profoundly vacuolated, and phagocytosed red cells, neutrophils, or cellular debris were evident in most cells. Cells with a similar morphology were present in lymph nodes, spleen, and pleural fluid.

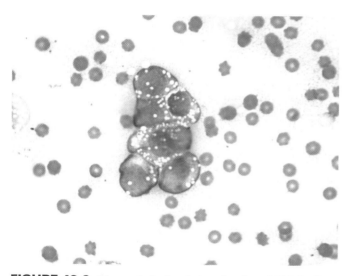

FIGURE 49.6 Monocytic leukemia in a dog (type M5a), buffy coat smear (Wright's stain). The monoblasts have a similar appearance to those in Figure 49.5 and react positively for nonspecific esterase content.

cytic leukemias, of types M5a or M5b are characterized by a predominance of monoblasts or monocytes, respectively (Figs. 49.5 and 49.6).[11,28,30]

Proliferative disorders of macrophages are well characterized in companion animals, and frequently appear analogous to those diseases described in humans.[31,32] The hemophagocytic syndrome consists of an exaggerated histiocytic inflammatory response to systemic infectious or metabolic disorders.[31] In humans, the disorder frequently presents as a severe illness in viral infections;

spontaneous recovery is common. In animals this disorder has been associated with bicytopenia and erythrophagocytosis by macrophages in the bone marrow.[33] The syndrome has been reported in four dogs and in one cat.[33] Two of the dogs were diagnosed with myeloproliferative disease and all five animals either died or were euthanized owing to clinical deterioration.[33] These findings suggest that the hemophagocytic syndrome is more severe in animals than in humans or that the histiocytic reaction is an epiphenomenon of a different and more severe disease.

Malignant histiocytosis is a neoplastic condition with a high prevalence in Bernese Mountain dogs.[34] It has also been reported in many other large-breed dogs[35] and in cats.[36,37] Proliferating masses of pleiomorphic macrophages have been observed in the lungs, lymph nodes, liver, nervous system, and bone marrow. The neoplastic macrophages frequently phagocytose red cells, leukocytes, and thrombocytes. Therefore, cytopenias are common and often severe. Nonspecific esterase reactivity and expression of immunoreactive lysozyme are diagnostic features of the neoplastic cell population.[35,37] Malignant macrophages occasionally may be observed on blood smears (Figs. 49.7 and 49.8). Malignant histiocytosis is an aggressive neoplastic disease. Treatment has largely been unsuccessful.

Systemic histiocytosis is a proliferative disorder of histiocytes most commonly observed in Bernese Mountain dogs. This disease may manifest with nodular cutaneous masses.[38] The mucosae and skin of the face and head are affected most frequently. Immunoreactivity studies indicate that the proliferating cells are likely of dermal Langerhans cell origin.[39] This breed-associated

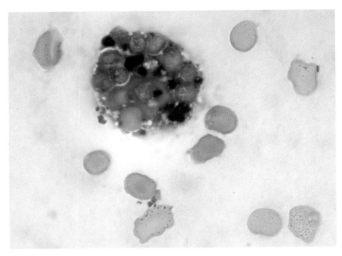

FIGURE 49.8 Malignant histiocytosis in a Golden Retriever, buffy coat smear, α-naphthyl acetate esterase reactivity. This sample is from the same dog as in Figure 49.7. All the large vacuolated cells are reactive with a substrate for nonspecific esterase, confirming a diagnosis of malignant histiocytosis.

disorder has a more prevalent and benign counterpart, the cutaneous histiocytoma. This benign tumor occurs most commonly in young dogs and consists of localized accumulations of dermal Langerhans cells. Cutaneous histiocytomas regress spontaneously coincident with infiltration by CD8[+] T lymphocytes.[39]

In summary, monocytes are inconspicuous elements of the peripheral blood that give rise to tissue macrophages. Few disorders other than leukemia are associated with pathognomonic changes in blood monocyte numbers; however, abnormal monocyte counts and morphology may reflect neutrophil kinetics or various infectious states. Macrophages are essential in inflammatory reactions, immune responses, and metabolic processes. Lack or dysfunction of tissue phagocytes as well as neoplastic proliferation of these cells results in severe clinical disease or death.

REFERENCES

1. **Hamilton JA.** Colony stimulating factors, cytokines and monocyte-macrophages—some controversies. Immunol Today 1998;14:18–24.
2. **Valledor AF, Borràs FE, Cullell-Young, Celada A.** Transcription factors that regulate monocyte/macrophage differentiation. J Leukoc Biol 1998; 63:405–417.
3. **Metcalf D.** Control of granulocytes and macrophages: molecular, cellular and clinical aspects. Science 1991;254:529–533.
4. **Nash RA, Schuening F, Appelbaum F, Hammond WP, Boone T, Morris CF, Slichter S, Storb R.** Molecular cloning and in vivo evaluation of canine granulocyte-macrophage colony-stimulating factor. Blood 1991;78:930–937.
5. **Tao W, Dougherty R, Johnston P, Pickett W.** Recombinant bovine GM-CSF primes superoxide production but not degranulation induced by recombinant bovine interleukin1 beta in bovine neutrophils. J Leukoc Biol 1993; 53:679–684.
6. **Nash RA, Burstein SA, Storb R, Yang W, Abrams K, Appelbaum FR, Boon T, Deeg HJ, Durack LD, Schuening FG, McDonough S, Moore P, Nelp WB, Slichter S.** Thrombocytopenia in dogs induced by granulocyte-macrophage colony-stimulating factor: increased destruction of circulating platelets. Blood 1995;86:1765–1775.
7. **Jain NC.** Schalm's veterinary hematology. 4th ed. Philadelphia: Lea & Febiger, 1986;768–789.
8. **Ganz T, Lehrer RI.** Production, distribution, and fate of monocytes and macrophages. In: Beutler E, Lichtman MA, Coler BS, Kipps TJ, eds. Williams hematology. 5th ed. New York: McGraw-Hill, 1995;875–878.
9. **Allzzi SA, Maxie MG, Valli VE, Wilkie BN, Johnson JA.** The kinetics of mononuclear phagocytes in normal calves given Corynebacterium parvum. Can J Comp Med 1982;46:138–145.
10. **van Furth R, Diesselhoff-den Dulk MMC, Sluiter W, van Dissel JT.** Production and migration of monocytes and kinetics of macrophages. In: van Furth R, ed. Mononuclear phagocytes: Characteristics, physiology and function. Dordrecht: Kluwer Academic Publishers, 1985;201–210.
11. **Latimer KS.** Leukocytes in health and disease. In: Ettinger SJ, Feldman EC, eds. Textbook of veterinary internal medicine. Diseases of the dog and cat, Vol 2. 4th ed. Philadelphia: WB Saunders Co, 1995;1982–1992.
12. **Lucas DL, Bowles CA, Robinson DM.** Characterization of canine monocytes in vitro: increased receptor activity for Fc, C3, and heterologous erythrocytes. Transplantation 1980;29:133–139.
13. **Birmingham JR, Jeska EL.** The isolation, long-term cultivation and characterization of bovine peripheral blood monocytes. Immunology 1980;41: 807–814.
14. **Devitt A, Moffatt OD, Raykundalia C, Capra JD, Simmons DL, Gregory CD.** Human CD14 mediates recognition and phagocytosis of apoptotic cells. Nature 1998;392:505–509.
15. **Lehrer RI, Ganz T.** Biochemistry and function of monocytes and macrophages. In: Beutler E, Lichtman MA, Coler BS, Kipps TJ, eds. Williams hematology. 5th ed. New York: McGraw-Hill, 1995;869–873.
16. **Donnelly SC, Bucala R.** Macrophage migration inhibitory factor: a regulator of glucocorticoid activity with a critical role in inflammatory disease. Mol Med Today 1997;3:502–507.
17. **van't Wout AB, Kootstra NA, MulderKampinga GA, et al.** Macrophagetropic variants initiate human immunodeficiency virus type 1 infection after sexual, parenteral, and vertical transmission. J Clin Invest 1994; 94:2060–2067.
18. **Willett BJ, Flynn JN, Hosie MJ.** FIV infection of the domestic cat: an animal model for AIDS. Immunol Today 1997;18:182–189.
19. **Granelli-Piperno A, Delgado E, Finkel V, et al.** Immature dendritic cells selectively replicate macrophagetropic (M-tropic) human immunodeficiency virus type 1, while mature cells efficiently transmit both M- and T-tropic virus to T cells. J Virol 1998;72:2733–2737.
20. **Dow S, Poss M, Hoover E.** Feline immunodeficiency virus: a neurotropic lentivirus. J Acquir Immune Defic Syndr Hum Retrovirol 1990;3:658–668.
21. **Lin DS, Bowman DD.** Macrophage functions in cats experimentally infected with feline immunodeficiency virus and Toxoplasma gondii. Vet Immunol Immunopathol 1992;33:69–78.
22. **Brodie SJ, Pearson LD, Zink MC, Bickle HM, Anderson BC, Marcom KA, DeMartini JC.** Ovine lentivirus expression and disease. Am J Pathol 1995;146:250–263.
23. **Lechner F, Machado J, Bertoni G, Seow HF, Dobellaere DAE, Peterhans E.** Caprine arthritis encephalitis virus dysregulates the expression of cytokines in macrophages. J Virol 1997;71:7488–7497.
24. **Maury W.** Monocyte maturation controls expression of equine infectious anemia virus. J Virol 1994;68:6270–6279.
25. **Rovid AH, Carpenter S, Roth JA.** Monocyte function in cattle experimentally infected with bovine immunodeficiency virus-like virus. Vet Immunol Immunopathol 1995;45:31–43.
26. **Khan KN, Kociba GJ, Wellman ML.** Macrophage tropism of feline leukemia virus (FeLV) of subgroup-C and increased production of tumor necrosis factor-alpha by FeLV-infected macrophages. Blood 1993;15:2585–2590.
27. **Duncan JR, Prasse KW, Mahaffey EA.** Leukocytes. In: Duncan JR, Prasse KW, Mahaffey EA. Veterinary laboratory medicine. 3rd ed. Ames: Iowa State University Press, 1994;37–62.
28. **Lichtman MA.** Monocytosis and monocytopenia. In: Beutler E, Lichtman MA, Coler BS, Kipps TJ, eds. Williams hematology. 5th ed. New York: McGraw-Hill, 1995;881–883.
29. **Jain NC, Blue JT, Grindem CB, Harvey JW, Kociba GJ, Krehbiel JD, Latimer KS, Raskin RE, Thrall MA, Zinkl JG.** Proposed criteria for classification of acute myeloid leukemia in dogs and cats. Vet Clin Pathol 1991; 20:63–82.
30. **Bienzle D, Hughson SL, Vernau W.** Acute myelogenous leukemia in a horse. Can Vet J 1993;34:36–40.
31. **Moschella SL.** An update of the benign proliferative monocyte-macrophage and dendritic cell disorders. J Dermatol 1996;23:805–815.
32. **Schmidt D.** Monocyte-macrophage system and malignancies. Med Pediatr Oncol 1994;23:444–451.
33. **Watlon RM, Modiano JF, Thrall MA, Wheeler SL.** Bone marrow cytological findings in 4 dogs and a cat with hemophagocytic syndrome. J Vet Intern Med 1996;10:7–14.
34. **Moore PF, Rosin A.** Malignant histiocytosis of Bernese Mountain dogs. Vet Pathol 1986;23:1–10.
35. **Brown DE, Thrall MA, Getzy DM, Weiser MG, Ogilvie GK.** Cytology of canine malignant histiocytosis. Vet Clin Pathol 1994;23:118–122.
36. **Court EA, Earnest-Koons KA, Bar SC, Gould WJ.** Malignant histiocytosis in a cat. J Am Vet Med Assoc 1993;203:1300–1302.
37. **Walton RM, Brown DE, Burkhard MJ, Donnelly KB, Frank AA, Obert**

LA, Withrow SJ, Thrall MA. Malignant histiocytosis in a domestic cat: cytomorphologic and immunohistochemical features. Vet Clin Pathol 1997; 26:56–60.

38. **Moore PF.** Systemic histiocytosis of Bernese Mountain dogs. Vet Pathol 1984;21:554–563.

39. **Moore PF, Schrenzel MD, Affolter VK, Olivry T, Naydan D.** Canine cutaneous histiocytoma is an epidermotropic Langerhans cell histiocytosis that expresses CD1 and specific β2-integrin molecules. Am J Pathol 1996; 148:1699–1708.

40. **Douglas SD, Ho WZ.** Morphology of monocytes and macrophages. In: Beutler E, Lichtman MA, Coler BS, Kipps TJ, eds. Williams hematology. 5th ed. New York: McGraw-Hill, 1995;861–868.

41. **Grindem CB, Stevens JB, Perman V.** Cytochemical reactions in cells from leukemic dogs. Vet Pathol 1986;23:103–109.

CHAPTER 50

Ultrastructural Features of Leukocytes

• W.L. STEFFENS III

The light microscope generally is used for the identification and classifcation of leukocytes in Romanowsky-stained blood and bone marrow specimens. Under optimal conditions, the light microscope is capable of resolving features as small as 0.2 μm, which gives it a useful upper magnification of approximately 1000× (the resolution of the human eye is approximately 200 μm). Because the light microscope uses full-spectrum white light as an illumination source, specific chromatic stains, such as traditional and rapid (Diff-Quik) modifications of Romanowsky (Wright, Giemsa, and Leishman) stains, can be used to identify morphologic features of leukocytes. These features include larger organelles such as primary and secondary (specific) granules, the nucleus, and nucleoli.

Occasionally, the need arises to resolve cellular features beyond that of the light microscope, in which case the electron microscope becomes the instrument of choice. Most modern electron microscopes have a routine resolution of 1 nm and a useful magnification range as high as 300,000×. Thus imaging to the macromolecular or supramolecular level is possible. Ultrastructural examination of leukocytes may be of benefit in the identification of virions and viral inclusions, lysosomal storage products, and early granule development. Specific diagnosis of leukemias, which may appear undifferentiated by light microscopy, is sometimes possible by routine electron microscopy or with ultrastructural immunocytochemistry or immunoelectron microscopy.

Although the transmission electron microscope can easily resolve detail that cannot be imaged by the light microscope, it uses a beam of electrons rather than full-spectrum white light for illumination. The result is a monochrome image, produced by electrons interacting with a phosphor screen. Thus an inability exists to differentiate leukocyte types and features based on specific chromatic staining (e.g., eosinophilic versus basophilic granules). Identification of leukocytes in electron microscopic images of blood, bone marrow, biopsy, and necropsy materials is based entirely on morphologic information such as type and distribution of nuclear chromatin; presence or absence of specific granules or inclusions; and the type, amount, and distribution of cellular organelles.

CONSIDERATIONS IN SPECIMEN COLLECTION AND PROCESSING

Particular care must be taken when collecting cells and tissues for electron microscopy. Rapid deterioration of many ultrastructural features commences immediately after either the removal of cells and tissues from the living animal or the death of the individual. These ultrastructural changes can and often do lead to misinterpretation of data; therefore it is essential that samples be processed rapidly and optimally as possible. The mechanisms behind processing artifacts are many and diverse, with the most significant being related to autolysis, anoxia, and altered fluid balance. These effects on living cells are minimized by fixation. The benefits of fixation include (1) inactivation of endogenous enzymes to prevent autolysis; (2) inactivation of respiratory pathway components to minimize the morphologic outcomes of anoxia, including autolysis; (3) inactivation of membrane transport proteins under isotonic conditions to prevent volume changes of cells and organelles; and (4) stabilization of structural components, such as proteins, to minimize their loss during the subsequent processing steps, including specimen dehydration, embedding, and staining.

PRECAUTIONS IN INTERPRETATION

Poor fixation results not only in difficulty of cell identification and interpretation of findings, but also can mimic some important pathologic changes, leading to an erroneous diagnosis. For example, cell and tissue anoxia may cause condensation and margination of chromatin that resembles apoptosis, and focal autolysis with a loss of cellular integrity may be misinterpreted as tissue necrosis. Also, fixation under extremely hypotonic conditions or excessive perfusion pressures results in massive fluid uptake by cells and tissues, which can be misinterpreted as edema. Cells and tissues vary in their resistance to fixation artifacts; however, leukocytes and other blood cellular components are sensitive to these effects. Leukocyte ultrastructural morphology may be grossly abnormal to unrecognizable.

These artifacts may largely be avoided by use of a fixation protocol that is appropriate for the cells or tissues being processed and by minimization of the elapsed time (seconds to a few minutes) between blood or tissue collection (antemortem or immediately postmortem) and immersion into the fixative. In some cases however, samples may be acquired at necropsy several hours postmortem or may be received in a fixative (such as 10% formalin) that is not specifically designed for electron microscopy. In such instances, sample handling and fixation artifacts will be present and likely will be extensive. Therefore the electron microscopic images should be interpreted cautiously. Numerous detailed references exist describing optimal collection and processing of animal cells and tissues for electron microscopy.[1–7]

Another significant problem in interpreting electron photomicrographs lies in the geometry of the electron micrograph image itself. Cells processed for transmission electron microscopy typically are sectioned to an optimal thickness of 50 to 65 nm, compared with the 3 to 6 μm routinely required for histopathology sections observed by light microscopy. Thus a typical cell can be sectioned for electron microscopy approximately tenfold more times than similar cells sectioned for light microscopy. Consequently, a spherical cell always appears smaller than actual size in thin sections unless it has been sectioned precisely through its equatorial plane. Therefore, cell size determinations are meaningless unless a large number of similar cells are observed and measured and the data subjected to statistical analysis. The accepted size ranges (diameters) of the various leukocytes generally are based on light microscopic measurements of leukocytes in Wright-stained smears. Because cell size is somewhat meaningless in electron micrographs, it is only mentioned here for comparative purposes. Organelle distribution also may be uneven, and the plane of section may pass through an area that is not representative of the entire cell. This is particularly true in the case of cells with acentric nuclei, which may be missed entirely in the thin section plane or may be obliquely sectioned, resulting in atypical chromatin distribution. Additionally, irregularly shaped cells, such as macrophages, almost never appear in a profile that is truly representative of their actual shape. Thus, when attempting to identify leukocytes in electron micrographs, it is extremely important to remember that any morphologic anomalies observed could be a result of misorientation. When more precise information regarding organelle number and distribution or cell size, shape, or volume are needed, appropriate computer planar morphometric methods may be employed. Such methods are described for application in hematology.[8]

SAMPLE TYPES FOR ULTRASTRUCTURAL IMAGING OF LEUKOCYTES

Leukocytes may be imaged in virtually any animal specimen that can be adequately processed for electron microscopy, including whole blood, buffy coats, bone marrow, biopsy and necropsy tissues, lavage fluids, enrichments from columns or gradients, and cell culture. Because of the low frequency of leukocytes in whole blood under normal conditions and the small sample size observable by means of electron microscopy, buffy coats and enriched preparations are most productive for examination of a given leukocyte type. However, the techniques used to prepare leukocyte enrichments often leads to handling artifacts. These artifacts may not be readily observable by means of light microscopy but may cause obvious ultrastructural changes that could mimic cellular pathology. In particular, granulocytes may appear to be degranulating, and surface decorations such as microvilli may be lost or reduced in length and number.

The ultrastructural features of most mature circulating or tissue leukocytes have been well documented for the past 3 decades in the literature, histology texts, and ultrastructural atlases. Only recently, however, have some of the early bone-marrow-derived lines been convincingly differentiated and described[9–12] as a consequence of greatly improved cellular enrichment, labeling, and culture techniques. In most cases, each leukocyte type has distinguishing ultrastructural features for specific identification. However, cell identification based on ultrastructure alone is not always as readily and confidently accomplished as is identification of similar cells in appropriately stained smears. A general familiarity with biological ultrastructure is likely the greatest asset that one can have for competent identification of leukocytes by means of electron microscopy.

NEUTROPHILS

Neutrophilic and heterophilic polymorphonuclear neutrophil leukocytes (PMNs) have been studied ultrastructurally for many species, including humans,[13] dogs,[14–16] cats,[17–20] horses,[21–23] cows,[24,25] goats,[24] sheep,[24,26–28] pigs,[29] birds,[30,31] guinea pigs,[32] rats,[33,34] and frogs.[35] These frequently encountered leukocytes comprise approximately 50 to 80% of the total leukocyte volume, depending on the health of the animal. Ultrastructurally, PMNs must be distinguished from basophils and eosinophils, which lack crystalline structures within their granules. In buffy coat preparations from blood, PMNs appear as rounded cells, decorated with a few short microvilli (Fig. 50.1). In tissues, they tend to localize near the vessel walls, particularly in the postcapillary and muscular venules. Microvilli probably play a significant role in the adhesion of the PMNs to vascular endothelium against the force of blood flow.[36] As PMNs become phagocytic during migration from the circulatory system into the extravascular space, they become elongated and acquire long pseudopodia with cytoplasm that is temporarily devoid of organelles and is referred to as hyaloplasm. The extravascular morphology of PMNs is consistent with their motile, phagocytic role.

The nucleus of immature PMNs may appear poorly lobed, whereas the nucleus of a mature PMN has a typical multilobed appearance, contributing to the term

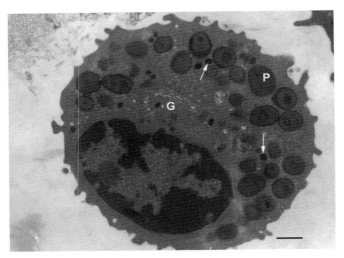

FIGURE 50.1 Immature heterophil from chicken buffy coat. Golgi (G), Primary granule (P), Secondary granules (arrows). Bar, 1 μm.

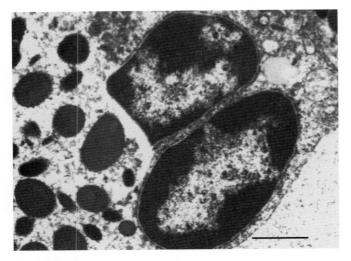

FIGURE 50.2 PMN nucleus. Bar, 1 μm.

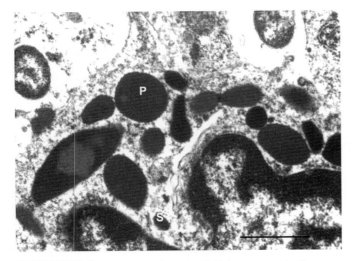

FIGURE 50.3 PMN granule types. P, Primary granule. S, Specific granule. Bar, 1 μm.

polymorph for neutrophil and heterophil granulocytes. Nuclear lobes are pronounced and may be connected by only a thin strand of nucleoplasm. The nucleus is heavily heterochromatic (Fig. 50.2), with strands of euchromatin occupying the center. However a progressive increase in euchromatinization has been described in the case of certain active infections.[37] A nucleolus is often absent or poorly defined if present. There are noticeably fewer profiles of nuclear pores evident than in basophils and eosinophils.

Except for the population of PMN granules, the cytoplasm is poorly endowed with organelles, the greater bulk being occupied by glycogen particles. Mitochondria are scarce, thin, and elongated. Golgi and other endomembranes are rudimentary when visible in immature PMNs. The granules are membrane-bound structures and consist of two distinct populations, the primary (azurophilic) granules and the secondary (specific) granules (Fig. 50.3). The larger primary granules (average 0.5 μm) represent lysosomes and may be stained for peroxidase and several acid hydrolases concerned with antimicrobial and digestive functions. With suitable fixation, they tend to be less densely stained than the secondary granules and may contain electron lucent areas. Their shape is variable, ranging from rounded to football-shaped, depending on the species. Frequently, both granule appearances occur simultaneously. The secondary granules are more numerous and approximately half the size of the primary granules. They lack specific lysosomal enzymes but can be stained for alkaline phosphatase. Small membrane vesicles lacking any visible contents often are observed and considered degranulated secondary granules.

The degranulation of PMNs is observed frequently, particularly when inflammation or active infection are present. Considerable ultrastructural change is noted in these toxic neutrophils, and these changes are well documented in several species. The earliest changes in toxic PMNs include a progressive increase in cell diameter and vacuolization owing to edema (Fig. 50.4), a decrease in nuclear heterochromatin, nuclear blebbing, and dissolution of the granule matrix. Degranulation is intracellular and occurs similar to the process in eosinophils. If material has been phagocytized, the primary granules may be seen to fuse with phagocytic vacuoles to form tertiary lysosomes. Degranulation in the presence of a significant stimulus such as a pathogen or toxin is usually irreversible, with the neutrophil degenerating in the process.

MONOCYTES

Monocytes are the largest of the circulating leukocytes in health, averaging 15 μm in diameter. They develop in the bone marrow, continue maturation in the circulatory system, and subsequently migrate across the postcapillary venules to become macrophages. In circulation, monocytes are round to oval in profile (Fig. 50.5) but become pleomorphic as they migrate through the connective tissue as macrophages.

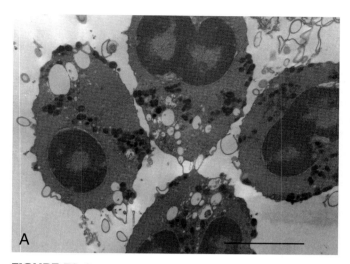
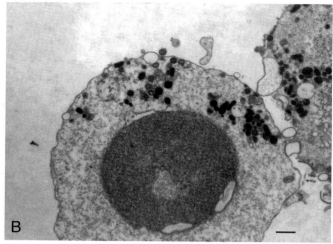

FIGURE 50.4 **A.** Toxic heterophil showing early degranulation. Bar, 10 μm. **B.** Toxic heterophil showing late degranulation. Bar, 1 μm.

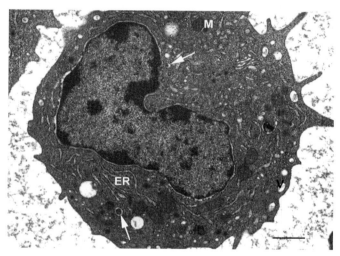

FIGURE 50.5 Avian monocyte from buffy coat. Endoplasmic reticulum (ER), Submembrane Vacuolation (V), Mitochondrion (M), azurophilic granules (arrows). Bar, 2 μm.

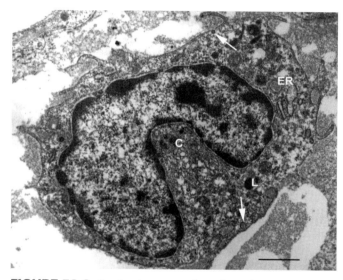

FIGURE 50.6 Porcine free macrophage from skin. Endoplasmic reticulum (ER), Centriole (C), Primary lysosome (L), Clathrin-coated pits (arrows). Bar, 2 μm.

The monocyte cytoplasm contains fewer free ribosomes than most other leukocytes and thus stains less intensely in both light and electron microscopic preparations. The cell surface contains a few irregular short microvilli and the cytoplasm below the plasma membrane is often vacuolated. The nucleus is generally kidney- to horseshoe-shaped and lies acentrically within the cell. There is an abundance of small, round mitochondria and short profiles of rough endoplasmic reticulum. The Golgi apparatus is usually well developed and prominent. Centrioles also are encountered frequently. The azurophilic granules constitute a variable population of small, membrane-bound vesicles. These granules are produced by the Golgi and are lysosomal in nature, containing peroxidase and hydrolytic enzymes. Degran-

ulation is intracellular and generally occurs only after differentiation into a macrophage.

Macrophages are phagocytic to secretory cells derived from monocytes. They share some common features with monocytes during differentiation. As fixed or wandering cells, macrophages are encountered in every organ where there is richly vascularized connective tissue. They frequently are found among leukocytes that have left circulation. Fixed macrophages may have a diversity of shapes ranging from flat and spindle-shaped to angular, whereas free macrophages tend to be rounded in profile (Fig. 50.6). Free and actively phagocytic macrophages often possess a surface adorned with extended processes such as pseudopodia and microvilli. A single short flagellum or cilium may occasionally be present. The nucleus is oval to highly elongated with numerous indentations, several nucleoli, and an abundance of marginated heterochromatin. There is considerable cytoplasm that in some species (mouse or rat) contains a large amount of rough endoplasmic reticulum. The Golgi is prominent, producing numerous smooth vesicles. Mitochondria are oval and generally few in number. Clathrin-coated pits (pinocytotic invaginations) at the plasma membrane surface and cytoplasmic coated vesicles also are common. These structures indicate that macrophages actively accumulate molecules from the extracellular environment. Vacuoles, lysosomes, and ingested material are often in evidence, attesting to the phagocytic nature of these cells.

LYMPHOCYTES

In recent years, considerable information has surfaced regarding the role and function of lymphocytes in immunity. Although this new information has considerably restructured our knowledge of immunity and disease processes, it has done little to change the accepted view of lymphocyte ultrastructure. The two immunologically and functionally distinct populations of lymphocytes, the thymic-derived T lymphocytes and the bone-marrow-derived B lymphocytes are not sufficiently distinct ultrastructurally to allow a reliable differentiation by microscopy alone without the aid of specifically localizing special surface markers or antigens. A single notable exception is the antigen-stimulated B lymphocyte that has begun plasma-cell transformation and has acquired some of the distinctive ultrastructural features that define the plasma cell.

Although lymphocytes are classified as agranular leukocytes, some of them have a few small azurophilic granules that are most evident when imaged by electron microscopy. The function of these granules is poorly understood. All lymphocytes are nearly spherical in shape but differ drastically in size, depending on the tissue or organ in which they reside. Traditionally, lymphocytes are morphologically classified as small, medium, or large lymphocytes (lymphoblast). Actually, the size range for lymphocytes is a continuum, varying from approximately 6 to 18 μm. The small, intermediate, and large size classification is conveniently applied to relate lymphocyte morphology to other factors such as location and immunologic state. The principal structural difference between these three types of lymphocytes relates to the amount of cytoplasm relative to the nucleus (nuclear : cytoplasmic [N : C] ratio).

Small lymphocytes (average diameter of 6 μm) are the most numerous, being found in blood, lymphatic circulation, and in the coronal zone of lymph nodes. The cell profile is normally round or nearly round with a few short surface microvilli. The nucleus is round, often with shallow indentations, and averages 5 μm in diameter, giving the small lymphocyte a high N : C ratio

(Fig. 50.7). Nucleoli usually are absent. The heterochromatin is extensive and highly marginated at the nuclear envelope and scattered throughout the nucleoplasm. The cartwheel arrangement of heterochromatin usually associated with plasma cells is frequently observed in this lymphocyte (Fig. 50.7). The cytoplasm often appears as a thin band surrounding the nucleus and is dominated by free ribosomes. Other organelles, including mitochondria, Golgi, and endoplasmic reticulum are not well represented. Approximately 10% of the small lymphocytes in mammals reportedly contain a few azurophilic granules that are membrane bound, often stain darkly, and measure approximately 0.25 to 0.5 μm.

Medium-sized lymphocytes, which constitute approximately 10% of the total lymphocyte population, average 8 to 9 μm in diameter or are slightly larger. The nucleus is slightly indented with a thin layer of marginated heterochromatin and a considerable amount of euchromatin. One or two nucleoli are normally evident. Generally, there are more free ribosomes than in small lymphocytes but fewer polyribosomes than are seen in large lymphocytes. The Golgi is usually present but small. The number of other organelles, such as mitochondria and endoplasmic reticulum, is variable but is now related to the direction of lymphocyte differentiation. If differentiation to a plasma cell is underway, there is a considerable increase in the rough endoplasmic reticulum, and the nucleus remains spherical and becomes acentrically located within the cytoplasm.

Large lymphocytes (lymphoblasts) are found in the germinal centers of lymphatic nodules in Peyer's patches, lymph nodes, and spleen and are not normally found in circulation. These cells average 14 μm or more in diameter and are round to ovoid with an occasional microvillus. The nucleus is round with more numerous and deeper indentations than seen in the small lymphocytes. The nucleus is highly euchromatic, with the heterochromatin entirely marginated in a thin band along the nuclear membrane. A large, coarsely granular nucle-

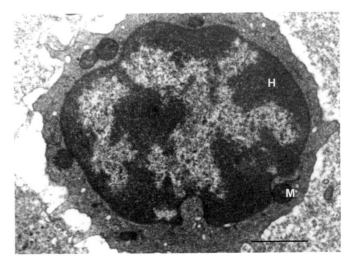

FIGURE 50.7 Porcine lymphocyte from spleen. Mitochondrion (M), Heterochromatin in cartwheel arrangement (H). Bar, 1 μm.

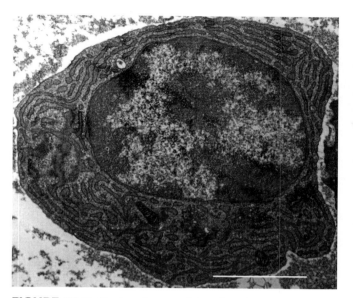

FIGURE 50.8 Porcine plasma cell from lymph node. Bar, 3 μm.

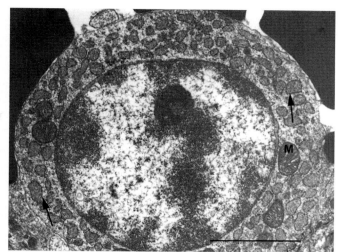

FIGURE 50.9 Porcine plasma cell with Russell's Bodies. Mitochondrion (M), Russell's bodies (arrows). Bar, 3 μm.

olus, connected at one end to the chromatin on the nuclear envelope, is characteristic for this cell. The N:C ratio is smaller for the large lymphocyte than for the small lymphocyte, resulting in a cytoplasmic band approximately 2 to 3 μm in width around the nucleus. The cytoplasm is predominated by free ribosomes, polyribosomes, and a few short profiles of rough endoplasmic reticulum; round mitochondria also may be evident. As a rule, the Golgi apparatus is lacking.

Plasma cells, resulting from the antigenic stimulation and subsequent blast transformation, mitosis, differentiation, and maturation of B-lymphocytes, are ultrastructurally distinctive cells. They commonly are encountered in antigen-stimulated lymph nodes and other active lymphoid tissues such as the spleen and bone marrow. Plasma cells appear rounded with cytoplasm predominated by rough endoplasmic reticulum, which usually contains a darkly staining granular material (Fig. 50.8). Mitochondria are more numerous than in unstimulated lymphocytes and are usually elongated. The nucleus contains patchy areas of heterochromatin that may be attached at the nuclear envelope producing a characteristic cartwheel pattern. Actively secreting plasma cells often contain profiles of grossly hypertrophied vesicles derived from the endoplasmic reticulum. These vesicles, termed Russell bodies, contain a granular to flocculent material that represents newly synthesized immunoglobulin molecules (Fig. 50.9).

EOSINOPHILS

Eosinophils are the second most frequent granulocyte in blood except in some avian and reptilian species. Because of their distinctive granule features, eosinophils tend to be more easily identified than other granulocytes in ultrastructural preparations. In recent years, eosino-

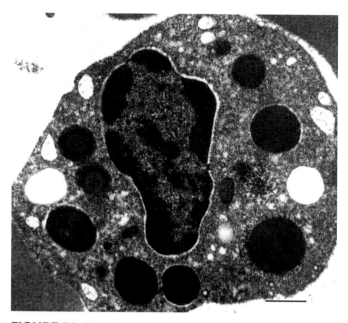

FIGURE 50.10 Canine eosinophil from buffy coat. Bar, 1 μm.

phils have become one of the most studied of the granulocytes both ultrastructurally and biochemically. Several good reviews and detailed studies have been published.[38-42] In tissues, they commonly occur in the lamina propria of the intestinal tract and the respiratory system. They are fragile cells and are easily ruptured during handling and processing for electron microscopy. Eosinophils are larger than basophils and neutrophils, averaging 10 to 15 μm in diameter. The cell shape may be rounded to slightly irregular and the membrane decorated with short, poorly defined microvilli. The nucleus is bilobed and similar morphologically to the basophil nucleus (Fig. 50.10); however, nuclear pleomorphism is described in response to certain infections making positive cellular identification possible only by granule ultrastructure.[43] Nucleoli, although not always evident in smears, are usually obvious in electron micrographs. The cytoplasm contains larger and more clearly defined mitochondria and Golgi than do basophils or neutrophils. Ribosomes, glycogen particles, and profiles of rough and smooth endoplasmic reticulum usually are evident.

Eosinophils are most easily delineated from other granulocytes by the presence and morphology of the granules. The granules are heterogeneous, particularly between species, and their true complexity has only begun to become evident in recent times. Two novel fluorescent staining procedures for the specific elucidation of eosinophil granules recently have been developed.[44,45] As seen with electron microscopy, the granules are normally rounded, measuring approximately 1 μm or greater, and often contain components that are intensely osmiophilic (Fig. 50.11). The membrane bounding the granules is often not easily visible owing to poor stainability. The granule contents may stain differentially, depending on the species, and include a lighter staining, amorphous, finely granular matrix and one to several densely stained regions that often appear as an angular or bar-shaped crystalloid structure. In some species, the crystalloid inclusion may be infrequent or lacking, and considerable intraspecies heterogeneity may occur (Fig. 50.11).[44] The eosinophil granules are produced by the Golgi complex and are known to have lysosomal function; they may be stained specifically for peroxidase activity and several hydrolytic enzymes. Other proteins, including Charcot–Leyden crystal protein,[46] urokinase,[47] and major basic protein,[48] have been localized ultrastructurally in specific eosinophil granules, suggesting that the granules may be composed of several subtypes.

Processes that lead to eosinophil activation, migration, adhesion, and ultimately degranulation have been well documented only in recent years. These processes have not been documented ultrastructurally in many species. Several types and degrees of eosinophil degranulation are described. In addition to intracellular degranulation, as in neutrophils with the granules fusing with phagocytic vacuoles to form darkly stained tertiary lysosomes, there may be classical degranulation by exocytosis[49] as well as explosive degranulation, resulting in cellular lysis (Fig. 50.12) and the release of eosinophil granules into the surrounding tissues.[50-52]

BASOPHILS

Basophils are the rarest of the PMNs in most species except some birds and reptiles. Basophils constitute approximately 0.5% of the total leukocytes in peripheral blood. They are the least likely leukocyte to be encountered except in enriched preparations or tissue infiltrates. Developmental stages are observable in bone marrow preparations; however, specific cytochemical markers are required for distinguishing them from resi-

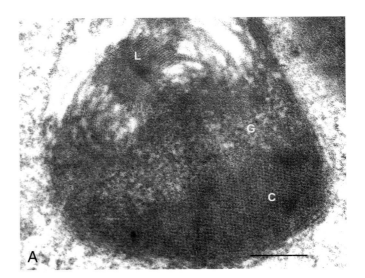

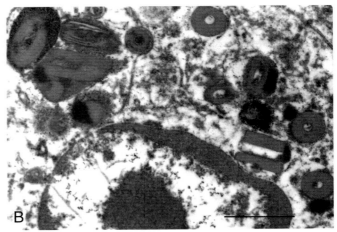

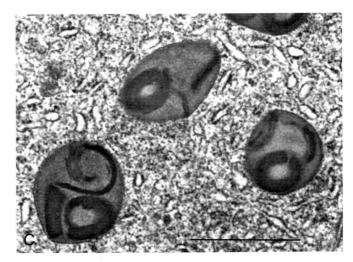

FIGURE 50.11 Eosinophil granules. **A.** Canine. Lamellar component (L), Granular component (G), Crystalloid component (C). Bar, 250 nm. **B.** Feline. Bar, 2 μm. **C.** Equine. Bar, 2 μm.

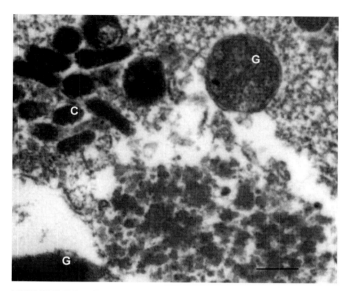

FIGURE 50.12 Eosinophil explosive degranulation in a feline cornea. Eosinophil granules (G) and the crystalloid cores (C) of granules are dispersed within the corneal stroma. Bar, 1 μm.

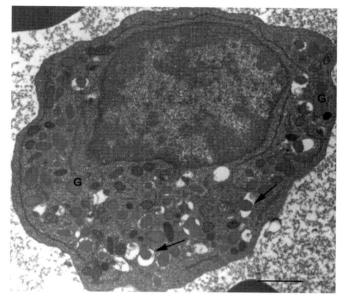

FIGURE 50.13 Porcine basophil from bone marrow. Intact granules (G) and dissolving granules (arrows). Bar, 1 μm.

dent mast cells and other myelocytes.[10,12] Basophils may be somewhat difficult to distinguish ultrastructurally from other granulocytes, unless they occur in large numbers. They frequently are observed singly in normal tissues but may be numerous as infiltrates in pathologic tissues. Because of their low frequency in blood, basophils are seen infrequently in sections of whole blood, capillaries, and other vessels. In processed buffy coats, basophils may be scattered among other granulocytes. Their specific identification may be difficult if specimen collection and fixation are not optimal. This is caused in part by the water solubility of basophil granules, which can lead to considerable change in their ultrastructure. If the fixed sample has been allowed to remain in an aqueous state for an extended period, the basophil granules frequently lose considerable electron density. Affected basophils subsequently may resemble degranulating neutrophils or eosinophils. A good review of basophil cell biology is found in the study by Dvorak.[12]

In general, basophils appear round and measure approximately 8 to 10 μm in diameter. A well-defined and sometimes darkly stained plasma membrane decorated with numerous surface folds and microvilli usually is observed (Fig. 50.13).[53] In well-preserved mature basophils, the cytoplasm contains few electron-lucent areas. The cytoplasm primarily is occupied by the characteristic basophil granules, as well as numerous ribosomes, polyribosomes, and glycogen granules. Glycogen, when present, often appears transparent, particularly if heavy metal stains are incorporated before embedment. In this instance, glycogen is partially extracted, resulting in a negative image. Other organelles such as mitochondria, endoplasmic reticulum, and a well-developed central Golgi usually are present, although these organelles tend to regress as the cell matures. Cytoskeletal elements are evident and include microtubules, actin, and inter-

mediate filaments,[54] which are thought to have a regulatory role during degranulation.[55]

The single nucleus is multilobed or kidney shaped, which in sectional profile may appear as two to three nuclear segments. The nuclear segments are irregularly shaped and contain a considerable amount of heterochromatin, which tends to marginate heavily around the inner nuclear envelope. Euchromatin also is present and tends to be heavily granular. Nucleoli, when present, are irregularly shaped and are usually confined to only one nuclear segment.

Although the basophil granule is the key to that cell's identification in Wright-stained smears, ultrastructural aspects of the granules may not provide many useful aids to differentiate the basophil from other granulocytes. Although basophil granules tend to be homogeneous, their structure in electron microscopic preparations may be variable owing to their water solubility. A vacuolated appearance or an electron-lucent area surrounding some granules is a commonly observed feature, reflecting the water solubility of some granule components (Fig. 50.14). Considerable species variation exists in the number, size, and ultrastructure of basophil granules. The granules originate in the Golgi complex, and have a similar ontogeny to lysosomes, although they are not lysosomal in function. Specific staining reveals that they contain histamine (or serotonin in rodents) and heparin. Morphologically, basophil granules average 1 μm in diameter and are membrane-bound round, oval, or slightly angular structures that appear homogeneous at lower magnifications. When examined at higher magnifications, the matrix may consist of fine granules measuring approximately 15 nm in diameter,[56] of fibrils, or of lamellae.[57–59] The matrix appearance varies with the animal species, with internal structure being

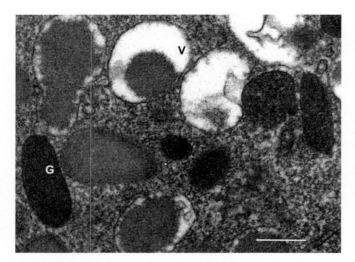

FIGURE 50.14 Porcine basophil granules. Intact granule (G). Vacuolated granule (V) in process of dissolution. Bar, 0.5 μm.

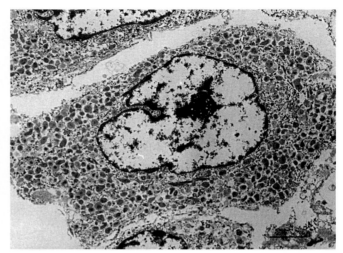

FIGURE 50.15 Chicken tissue mast cell from skin. Bar, 2 μm.

irregularly arranged in immature granules and becoming more regular and aligned in mature particles, producing a banded pattern. Small basophil granules frequently are observed in the process of coalescing into larger ones.

Degranulation of basophils is sometimes observed and is well documented ultrastructurally.[60–63] Although the basophils may appear to be lysed, the process is actually a prolonged extensive exocytosis, where the granule membrane fuses with the basophil membrane forming a pore (or in some species, multiple pores) through which the granule contents are expelled to the extracellular environment. During the degranulation process, new granules are continually being formed by the Golgi and rapidly mature. Unlike neutrophils, however, the basophil usually recovers once stimulus is stopped, and it regenerates granules and returns to resting or normal state.

The relation between tissue mast cells and basophils has been a topic of debate for several decades. Only recently have convincing answers begun to emerge.[11] Mast cells commonly are encountered within tissues close to blood vessels. They are also abundant in connective tissues and in the parenchyma of many organs. Mast cells average 12 to 15 μm in diameter and have a profile that may be round, irregular, or stellate (Fig. 50.15). The cell surface is generally smooth with a few short microvilli. Although there is ample cytoplasm, few ribosomes are present and a poorly developed rough endoplasmic reticulum exists in short profiles. Mitochondria tend to be scarce and are generally rounded. The major part of the cytoplasm is occupied by secretory granules that may be so numerous that the nucleus is obscured (as is the case in light microscopic preparations). When visualized, the nucleus is round, often centrally located, and has a considerable amount of marginated heterochromatin.

The greater part of the mast-cell cytoplasm is occupied by the secretory granules. These structures measure

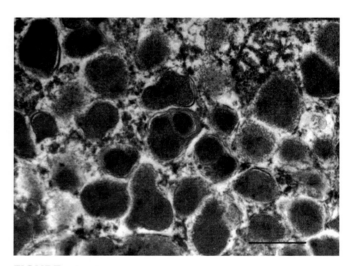

FIGURE 50.16 Chicken mast-cell granules. Bar, 1 μm.

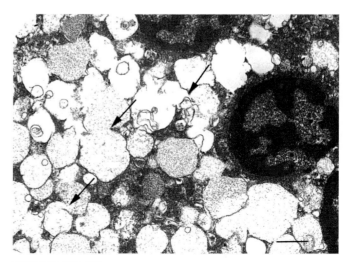

FIGURE 50.17 Degranulating mast cell from feline skin. Coalescing granules (arrows). Bar, 0.5 μm.

approximately 1 μm in diameter. They are bounded by a membrane that is often difficult to preserve and that appears lacking (Fig. 50.16). The granule membrane encloses a finely granular matrix, which often contain membranous structures resembling scrolls. The granular contents are known to include heparin and biogenic amines, including serotonin and histamine. Degranulation of mast cells results from numerous stimuli and contributes to the inflammatory process. The degranulation process is similar to that described for basophils and involves fusion of the granule membrane with the cell membrane and externalization of their contents through exocytosis. At the onset of degranulation, the granules increase in size and decrease in stainability (Fig. 50.17), a reaction possibly caused by the solubilization of their contents before release.[64] As is the case with basophils, mast cells that have degranulated under a strong stimulus may appear to be lysed owing to massive granule exocytosis; however, granule regeneration and recovery is reported to occur.

REFERENCES

1. **Postek MT, Howard KS, Johnson AH, McMichael K.** Scanning electron microscopy—a students handbook. Burlington, Vt: Ladd Research Industries, 1979.
2. **Hayat MA.** Fixation for electron microscopy. New York: Academic Press, 1981.
3. **Hayat MA.** Basic techniques for transmission electron microscopy. Orlando: Academic Press, 1986.
4. **Dawes CJ.** Introduction to biological electron microscopy: theory and techniques. Burlington, VT: Ladd Research Industries, 1988.
5. **Crang R FE, Klomparens KL.** Artifacts in biological electron microscopy. New York: Plenum Press, 1988.
6. **Bozzola JJ, Russell LD.** Electron microscopy: principles and techniques for biologists. Boston: Jones and Bartlett, 1992.
7. **Dykstra MJ.** Biological electron microscopy. New York: Plenum Press, 1992.
8. **Sokol RJ Hudson G, Wales J, James NT.** Morphometry of human blood leukocyte ultrastructure: its potential value in haematology. Haematologia (Budap) 1988;21(3):129–139.
9. **Anosa VO.** Ultrastructure of developing and mature caprine leukocytes. Anat Histol Embryol 1993;22:328–341.
10. **Okada M, Nawa Y, Hori Y, Kitamura T, Arizono N.** Development of basophils in Mongolian gerbils: formation of basophilic cell clusters in the bone marrow after *Nippostrongylus brasiliensis* infection. Lab Invest 1997;76:89–97.
11. **Dvorak AM.** New aspects of mast cell biology. Int Arch Allergy Immunol 1997;114:1–9.
12. **Dvorak AM.** Cell biology of the basophil. Int Rev Cytol 1998;180:87–236.
13. **Saito N, Takemori N, Hirai K, Onodera R.** An ultrastructural study of primary granule subtypes in human neutrophils. Hum Cell 1995;8:25–34.
14. **O'Donnell RT, Anderson BR.** Characterization of canine neutrophil granules. Infect Immun 1982;38:351–359.
15. **Shively JN, Feldt C., Davis D.** Fine structure of formed elements in canine blood. Am J Vet Res 1969;30:893–905.
16. **Sonoda M, Kobayashi K.** Neutrophils of canine peripheral blood in electron microscopy. Jpn J Vet Res 1970;18:37.
17. **Canfield PJ.** An ultrastructural study of granulocytic development of feline bone marrow. Anat Histol Embryol 1984;13:97–107.
18. **Grindem CB.** Ultrastructural morphology of leukemic cells in the cat. Vet Pathol 1985;22:147–155.
19. **Sonoda M, Kobayashi K.** Feline neutrophils in electron microscopy. Jpn J Vet Res 1970;18:63–65.
20. **Ward JW, Wright JF, Wharran GH.** Ultrastructure of granulocytes in the peripheral blood of the cat. J Ultrastruct Res 1972;39:389–396.
21. **Bertram TA, Coignoul FL.** Morphometry of equine neutrophils isolated at different temperatures. Vet Pathol 1982;19:534–543.
22. **Coignoul FL, Bertram TA, Roth JA, Cheville NF.** Functional and ultrastructural evaluation of neutrophils from foals and lactating and nonlactating mares. Am J Vet Res 1984;45:898–902.
23. **Sonoda M, Kobayashi K.** Electron microscopic observations on the blood of the horse. I. Neutrophils in the peripheral blood of the clinically healthy horse. Jpn J Vet Res 1966;14:71–78.
24. **Baggiolini M, Horisberger U, Gennaro R, Dewald B.** Identification of three types of granules in neutrophils of ruminants; ultrastructures of circulating and maturing cells. Lab Invest 1985;52:151–158.
25. **Gennaro R, Dewald B, Horisberger U, Gubler HU, Baggiolini M.** A novel type of cytoplasmic granule in bovine neutrophils. J Cell Biol 1983; 96:1651–1661.
26. **Rudolph R, Schnabl W.** Fine structure of blood leukocytes and electron-optical demonstration of peroxidase and acid phosphatase in sheep granulocytes. Zentralbl Veterinarmed A 1981;28A:282–295.
27. **Yamada Y.** The leukocytes of ovine peripheral blood in electron microscopy. Jpn J Vet Res 1970;18:99–106.
28. **Yamada Y, Sonoda M.** Neutrophils of ovine peripheral blood in electron microscopy. Jpn J Vet Res 1970;18:83–89.
29. **Nafstad HJ, Nafstad I.** An electron microscopic study of normal blood and bone marrow in pigs. Vet Pathol 1968;5:451–470.
30. **Maxwell MH.** Comparison of heterophil and basophil ultrastructure in six species of domestic birds. J Anat 1973;115:187–202.
31. **Robertson GW, Maxwell MH.** Fine structure of secondary granule inclusions in fowl heterophils after ruthenium tetroxide fixation. Res Vet Sci 1991;50:121–122.
32. **Brederdoo P, Daems WT.** The ultrastructure of guinea pig heterophil granulocytes and the heterogeneity of the granules. Cell Tissue Res 1978; 194:183–205.
33. **Brederoo P, van der Meulen J.** Development of the granule population in heterophil granulocytes from rat bone marrow. Cell Tissue Res 1983; 228:433–449.
34. **Tang XM, Clermont Y.** Granule formation and polarity of the golgi apparatus in neutrophil granulocytes of the rat. Anat Rec 1989;223:128–138.
35. **Frank G.** Granulopoiesis in tadpoles of *Rana esculenta*. Ultrastructural observations on the morphology and development of heterophil and basophil granules. J Anat 1989;163:107–116.
36. **Shao JY, Ting-Beall HP, Hochmuth RM.** Static and dynamic lengths of neutrophil microvilli. Proc Natl Acad Sci U S A 1998;95:6797–6802.
37. **Avdeeva MG, Evglevskii AA, Moisova DL, Shubich MG.** Leukocyte chromatin anisotropy in patients with leptospirosis. Klin Lab Diagn 1997; 11:36–39.
38. **McEwen BJ.** Eosinophils: a review. Vet Res Commun 1992;16:11–144.
39. **Kishimoto T.** Advance of the examination of eosinophil: methodology and clinical significance—morphological examination—electron microscopic examination by immuno-SEM. Nippon Rinsho 1993;51:696–699.
40. **Jones DG.** The eosinophil. J Comp Pathol 1993;108:317–335.
41. **Dvorak AM, Ishizaka T.** Human eosinophils in vitro. An ultrastructural morphology primer. Histol Histopathol 1994;9:339–374.
42. **Weller PF.** Eosinophils: structure and function. Curr Opin Immunol 1994; 6:85–90.
43. **Bardenstein DS, Lass JH, Kazura JW, Pearlman E.** Pleomorphism of stromal eosinophils in murine experimental onchocercal keratitis. Ocul Immunol Inflamm 1997;5:157–163.
44. **Stockert JC, Trigoso CI.** Fluorescence of eosinophil leukocyte granules induced by the fluorogenic reagent 2-methoxy-2, 4-diphenyl-3 (2H)-furanone. Blood Cells 1993;19:423–430.
45. **Trigoso CI, Stockert JC.** Fluorescence of the natural dye saffron: selective reaction with eosinophil leucocyte granules. Histochem Cell Biol 1995; 104:75–77.
46. **Calafat J, Janssen H, Knol EF, Weller PF, Egesten A.** Ultrastructural localization of Charcot-Leyden crystal protein in human eosinophils and basophils. Eur J Haematol 1997;58:56–66.
47. **Mabilat-Pragnon C, Janin A, Michel L, Thomaidis A, Legrand Y, Soria C, Lu H.** Urokinase localization and activity in isolated eosinophils. Thromb Res 1997;88:373–379.
48. **Dvorak AM, Furitsu T, Estrella P, Letourneau L, Ishizaka T, Ackerman SJ.** Ultrastructural localization of major basic protein in the human eosinophil lineage in vitro. J Histochem Cytochem 1994;42:1443–1451.
49. **Weiler CR, Kita H, Hukee M, Gleich GJ.** Eosinophil viability during immunoglobulin-induced degranulation. J Leukoc Biol 1996;60:493–501.
50. **Cheng JF, Ott NL, Peterson EA, George TJ, Hukee MJ, Gleich GJ, Leiferman KM.** Dermal eosinophils in atopic dermatidis undergo cytolytic degeneration. J Allergy Clin Immunol 1997;99:683–692.
51. **Persson CG, Erjefalt JS.** Ultimate activation of eosinophils in vivo: lysis and release of clusters of free eosinophil granules (Cfegs). Thorax 1997; 52:569–574.
52. **Persson CG, Erjefalt JS.** Eosinophil lysis and free granules: an in vivo paradigm for cell activation and drug development. Trends Pharmacol Sci 1997;18:117–123.
53. **Galli SJ, Dvorak AM, Hammond ME, Morgan E, Galli AS, Dvorak HF.** Guinea pig basophil morphology in vitro. I. Ultrastructure of uropod-bearing (motile) basophils and modulation of motile structures by serum and substrate effects. J Immunol 1981;126:1066–1074.
54. **Hastie R, Chir B.** Study of the ultrastructure of human basophil leukocytes. Clin Lab Invest 1974;31:223–231.
55. **Grant JA, Dupree E, Thueson DO.** Complement-mediated release of histamine from human basophils. III. Possible regulatory role of microtubules and microfilaments. J Allergy Clin Immunol 1977;60:306–311.

56. **Yamada Y, Sonoda M.** Basophils of ovine peripheral blood in electron microscopy. Jpn J Vet Sci 1972;34:29–32.

57. **Terry RW, Bainton DF, Farquhar MG.** Formation and structure of specific granules in basophilic leukocytes of the guinea pig. Lab Invest 1969;21: 65–76.

58. **Wetzel BK.** The fine structure and cytochemistry of developing granulocytes with special reference to the rabbit. In: Gordon AS, ed. Regulation of hematopoiesis. Vol. 2. New York: Appleton-Century-Crofts, 1970.

59. **Wetzel BK.** The comparative fine structure of normal and diseased mammalian granulocytes. In: Gordon AS, ed. Regulation of hematopoiesis. Vol. 2. New York: Appleton-Century-Crofts, 1970.

60. **Dvorak AM, Osage JE, Dvorak HF, Galli SF.** Surface membrane alterations in guinea pig basophils undergoing anaphylactic degranulation: a scanning electron microscope study. Lab Invest 1981;45:58–66.

61. **Dvorak AM, Galli SJ, Morgan E, Galli AS, Hammond ME, Dvorak HF.** Anaphylactic degranulation of guinea pig basophilic leukocytes. I. Fusion of granular membranes and cytoplasmic vesicles: formation and resolution of degranulation sacs. Lab Invest 1981;44:174–191.

62. **Dvorak AM, Galli SJ, Morgan E, Galli AS, Hammond ME, Dvorak HF.** Anaphylactic degranulation of guinea pig basophilic leukocytes. II. Evidence for regranulation of mature basophils during recovery from degranulation in vitro. Lab Invest 1982;46:461–475.

63. **Dvorak AM, Galli SJ, Schulman ES, Lichtenstein LM, Dvorak HF.** Basophil and mast cell degranulation: ultrastructural analysis of mechanisms of mediator release. Fed Proc 1983;42:2510–2515.

64. **Caulfield JP, Lewis RA, Hein A, Austen KF.** Secretion of dissociated human pulmonary mast cells: evidence for solubilization granule contents before discharge. J Cell Biol 1980;85:299–312.

CHAPTER 51

Cytochemistry of Normal Leukocytes

• ROSE E. RASKIN and AMY VALENCIANO

GENERAL PRINCIPLES OF CYTOCHEMISTRY

Cytochemistry is the use of special stains in the microscopic examination of cellular constituents such as lipids, carbohydrates, and enzymes.[1] These stains may distinguish normal cell types and identify the lineage of poorly differentiated blast cells (see Section X). Cytochemistry is ideal as a diagnostic technique because it involves minimal cost and is readily performed at many veterinary colleges. This technique may be used with hemolymphatic tissues (blood, bone marrow, lymph nodes, spleen, and thymus) or with liver. These specimens may include fresh imprints or aspirates, frozen tissues,[2] or plastic-embedded tissues.[3] In contrast, paraffin-embedded tissues may not be stained for nonspecific esterase (NSE) activity because the enzyme is unstable during tissue processing. In addition to light microscopic preparations, cytochemical staining also has been applied to electron microscopic specimens.[4]

To insure proper sample handling, the clinician should contact the laboratory performing the cytochemical staining before submitting materials. Multiple unfixed slides usually are preferred so a panel of stains can be performed. During cytochemical staining, appropriate control slides are used as positive and negative stain markers to assure quality control for the procedure(s). Although cytochemistry is applicable to the cells of various species, it is noteworthy that incubation times, staining patterns, and the presence of substrates may differ, even among the various avian, reptile, and fish species.

CYTOCHEMISTRY OF HEMATOPOIETIC CELLS

A summary of reactions for selected cytochemical stains in several animal species is provided in Table 51.1.

NEUTROPHILS/HETEROPHILS

Primary or azurophilic lysosomal granules contain the enzyme myeloperoxidase. Peroxidase (PER) activity is readily demonstrated from the promyelocyte stage through mature segmenters (Fig. 51.1). In electron microscopic preparations, PER activity also may be visualized in the nuclear membrane, rough endoplasmic reticulum, and Golgi apparatus of myeloblasts.[5] PER reactivity generally is absent in heterophils of rabbits, certain birds, and reptiles.[6-8] Neutrophils with eosinophilic prominence, such as those of the manatee, possess myeloperoxidase and stain intensely.[6]

Secondary or specific granules contain lipids, which stain positively with Sudan black B (SBB) (Fig. 51.2). SBB staining is found to a lesser extent within primary granules. Because both primary and secondary granules stain with SBB, all stages of neutrophil maturation are detected.

Primary and secondary neutrophilic granules also contain chloroacetate esterase (CAE) activity (Fig. 51.3). The cytochemical stain technique detects enzymatic activity, producing moderate to strong reactions in all maturation stages of neutrophils (Fig. 51.4).

Leukocyte alkaline phosphatase (LAP) is found predominantly in the secondary granules of most species, including humans, horses, rabbits, and ruminants (Fig. 51.5). However, this enzyme is absent in more mature neutrophils of dogs and cats. Equine and caprine neutrophils stained for NSE activity may show variable reactivity; neutrophils from most other species are cytochemically unreactive.[5,9] Acid phosphatase (ACP) activity is present in the primary granules of neutrophils. Enzymatic activity is higher in immature neutrophils than in bands or segmenters. Stain reactivity, however, is of modest intensity.

EOSINOPHILS

The PER that is present in eosinophils differs both structurally and biochemically from that found in neutrophils and megakaryocytes. This enzyme is present in the matrix of large eosinophilic granules, but not within the crystalloid core (Fig. 51.1). Unlike eosinophils of most species, feline eosinophils do not stain with either PER or SBB techniques. However, within birds and reptiles, PER and SBB reactivity may be observed in avian and reptilian eosinophils.[7,10,11] In general, eosinophils do not stain with CAE technique; however, reactivity has been

TABLE 51.1 Summary of Selected Cytochemical Staining Reactions for Normal Blood Cells in Various Animal Species

Species/Cell Type	PER	SBB	CAE	LAP	PAS	NSE	NSE/Fluoride	ACP	ACP/T	βG
Bovine										
Neutrophil	pos	pos	pos	pos	pos	neg	neg	pos/neg	—	—
Eosinophil	pos	pos	neg	pos	pos/neg	pos/neg	—	pos/neg	—	—
Basophil	neg	pos/neg	pos/neg	pos/neg	pos/neg	neg	neg	neg	neg	—
Monocyte	neg	pos/neg	pos/neg	neg	pos/neg	pos/neg	pos/neg	pos/neg	—	—
Lymphocyte	neg	neg	neg	neg	pos/neg	pos/neg	pos	pos/neg	neg	—
Cat										
Neutrophil	pos	pos	pos	neg	pos	neg	neg	pos/neg	neg	neg
Eosinophil	neg	neg	neg	pos	pos/neg	neg	neg	pos	pos	neg
Basophil	neg	neg	pos	pos/neg	pos/neg	neg	neg	pos	neg	
Monocyte	pos/neg	pos/neg	neg	neg	pos/neg	pos/neg	neg	pos/neg	neg	pos
Lymphocyte	neg	neg	neg	neg	neg	pos/neg	pos/neg	pos/neg	neg	pos/neg
Platelet/Megakaryocyte	neg	neg	pos/neg	neg	pos/neg	pos/neg	neg	pos/neg	neg	pos/neg
Dog										
Neutrophil	pos	pos	pos	neg	pos	neg	neg	pos/neg	neg	—
Eosinophil	pos	pos	neg	pos/neg	pos/neg	neg	neg	pos	pos	—
Basophil	neg	neg	pos	pos/neg	pos/neg	neg	neg	pos-neg	pos	—
Monocyte	pos/neg	pos/neg	neg	neg	pos/neg	pos/neg	neg	pos	neg	—
Lymphocyte	neg	neg	neg	pos/neg	pos/neg	pos/neg	pos	pos/neg	neg	—
Platelet/Megakaryocyte	neg	neg	pos/neg	neg	pos	pos	pos/neg	pos	neg	—
Horse										
Neutrophil	pos	pos	pos	pos	pos	pos/neg	—	pos/neg	—	—
Eosinophil	pos	pos	neg	pos/neg	pos/neg	pos/neg	—	pos/neg	—	—
Basophil	neg	neg	pos/neg	neg	pos	neg	—	neg	—	—
Monocyte	pos/neg	pos/neg	pos/neg	neg	pos/neg	pos/neg	—	pos/neg	—	—
Lymphocyte	neg	neg	neg	neg	pos/neg	pos/neg	—	pos/neg	—	—
Platelet/Megakaryocyte	neg	neg	—	neg	—	—	—	pos	—	—
Chicken										
Heterophil	neg	neg	neg	neg	pos/neg	neg	—	neg	—	—
Eosinophil	pos	pos	neg	neg	neg	neg	—	pos	—	—
Monocyte	pos/neg	pos/neg	—	neg	pos/neg	pos	—	pos	—	—
Lymphocyte	neg	neg	—	neg	neg	pos/neg	—	pos/neg	—	—
Thrombocyte	—	—	—	—	pos	—	—	—	—	—
Yellow Rat Snake										
Heterophil	neg	neg	pos	neg	pos	pos	—	neg	—	—
Basophil	—	—	neg	neg	—	neg	—	neg	—	—
Azurophil	pos	pos	pos	neg	pos	pos	—	pos	—	—
Lymphocyte	neg	neg	neg	neg	pos/neg	neg	—	pos	—	—
Thrombocyte	neg	neg	neg	neg	pos	neg	—	pos	—	—
Alligator										
Heterophil	neg	—	neg	pos	pos	pos	—	pos	—	—
Eosinophil	pos	—	neg	pos	pos	neg	—	neg	—	—
Basophil	neg	—	neg	neg	pos	neg	—	pos	—	—
Monocyte	neg	—	pos/neg	neg	pos	neg	—	neg	—	—
Lymphocyte	neg	—	pos	pos	pos	pos	—	pos	—	—
Thrombocyte	neg	—	neg	neg	pos	neg	—	neg	—	—
Green Sea Turtle										
Heterophil	neg	neg	neg	—	pos	pos	—	neg	—	—
Eosinophil	neg	neg	pos	—	pos/neg	neg	—	neg	—	—
Basophil	—	—	—	—	—	—	—	—	—	—
Monocyte	neg	neg	neg	—	pos	pos/neg	—	pos	—	—
Lymphocyte	neg	neg	neg	—	neg	neg	—	neg	—	—
Thrombocyte	neg	neg	neg	—	pos	pos	—	neg	—	—
Channel Catfish										
Neutrophil	pos	pos	neg	neg	pos	neg	—	pos	—	pos/neg
Basophil	neg	neg	neg	neg	pos	neg	—	neg	—	neg
Monocyte	neg	neg	neg	neg	neg	pos/neg	—	pos	—	neg
Lymphocyte	neg	pos/neg	neg	neg	neg	neg	—	pos/neg	—	neg
Thrombocyte	neg	neg	neg	neg	pos/neg	neg	—	neg	—	neg

PER, peroxidase; SBB, Sudan black B; CAE, chloroacetate esterase; LAP, leukocyte alkaline phosphatase; PAS, periodic acid-Schiff; NSE, nonspecific esterase; ACP, acid phosphatase; ACP/T, acid phosphatase with tartrate; βG, β glucuronidase; neg, no reaction; pos, easily detectable; pos/neg, weak or occasional reactivity; — = undetermined.

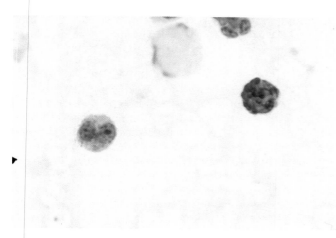

FIGURE 51.1 PER reaction in canine blood showing strong reaction in an eosinophil and moderate reaction in a segmented neutrophil. 500× original magnification.

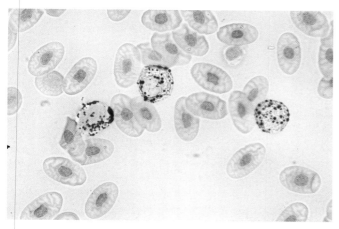

FIGURE 51.2 SBB reaction in two heterophils and one azurophil from boa snake blood. 250× original magnification.

moderately positive reaction in canine and feline basophils, whereas bovine and equine basophils are weakly positive for enzyme reactivity. Basophils of the dog, cat, horse, and cow are negative for NSE activity. ACP activity occasionally may be observed in canine and feline basophils; enzymatic activity is tartrate resistant.[12,13] Alcian blue stains positively for mucosubstances in basophil granules of many species.[16] Omega-exonuclease (OEN) activity is present in basophils and mast cells of dogs and cats (Fig. 51.10), but it is absent in both equine and bovine basophils.[16,17] Toluidine blue (TB) staining may be metachromatic (purple) for basophil granules of domestic animals under acidic conditions, but this characteristic is not observed at neutral pH.[18] TB staining also has been demonstrated in basophils from the alligator and desert tortoise.[7,11]

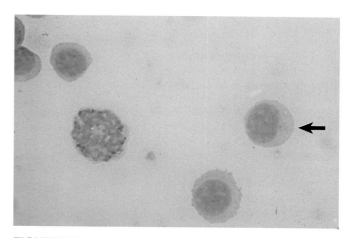

FIGURE 51.3 Canine blood stained with chloroacetate esterase showing strong positive reaction in a neutrophil and focal reaction in a lymphocyte. 500× original magnification.

observed in green turtle eosinophils.[8] NSE activity is absent in canine and feline eosinophils, but occasionally may be observed in equine and ruminant eosinophils.[5] Eosinophils, especially those of the cat, stain strongly for ACP activity in the intergranular areas. Enzymatic activity is present in both canine and feline eosinophils and is tartrate resistant.[12,13] LAP activity is found intracellularly between the specific granules of eosinophils. The strongest reactivity occurs within the eosinophils of the horse. Specific eosinophil stains, such as Luna[14] and Luxol fast blue,[15] also have been helpful in cell identification.

BASOPHILS

Basophils are negative for SBB and PER reactivity. Feline basophils may demonstrate occasional positive reactions for LAP activity.[5] The CAE technique produces a

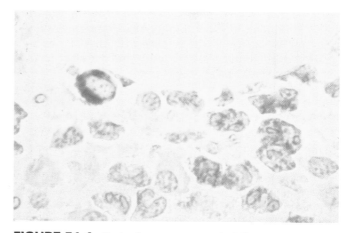

FIGURE 51.4 Canine bone marrow with diffuse positive chloroacetate reaction in granulocytic precursors. Plastic-embedded section. 500× original magnification.

MONOCYTES

Monocytes of some species show diffuse, weakly positive reactivity for PER and SBB.[19] PER activity may be more evident when copper nitrate is used to intensify the enzymatic reaction within the lysosomes. Generally, monocytes do not contain CAE activity; however, trace positive reactivity may be observed in bovine, equine, ovine, and caprine monocytes.[5] NSEs are present in cells of monocytic origin, resulting in diffuse, finely granular reactivity that is most intense within macrophages.[20,21] NSE reactivity is inhibited with sodium fluoride because of the presence of the enzymes on the plasma membrane.[22–24] ACP reactivity is present in a diffuse manner, similar to that observed for the NSEs. ACP reactivity is of moderate intensity in monocytes and increases with maturity into macrophages.

LYMPHOCYTES

Traditionally, lymphocytes lack reactivity to many of the cytochemical techniques used to identify granulocytic and monocytic cells. PER activity is absent, although rare cases in human medicine exhibit PER expression as detected by molecular studies.[25] Rare cases of human lymphocytes with lipid-filled vacuoles also stain positively. LAP activity may be observed in a B-cell subtype associated with the mantle zone of lymph nodes in dogs.[2] Stain reactiivity is discerned in a fine, diffusely granular pattern involving the plasma membrane. CAE reactivity is rare in lymphocytes (Fig. 51.3), but slight staining has been reported in bovine and equine lymphocytes.[5] Occasional punctate staining has been associated with non-T-cell large granular lymphocytes in people.[26] NSE activity results in a focally discrete staining reaction within the intracellular organelles of lymphocytes from humans, dogs, cats, cattle, horses, sheep, and chickens. This focal staining has been associated with lymphocytes of a T-cell origin.[2,12,13,24,26–31] Cells consistent with canine natural killer (NK) cell activity have weak, focal staining with the NSE and periodic acid-Schiff (PAS) techniques.[32] Weak PAS staining has been demonstrated in lymphocytes from cattle, dogs, horses, and sheep.[5] Positive reactivity for ACP has been observed in canine NK cells with and without tartrate incubation (Fig. 51.7).[32]

PLATELETS AND MEGAKARYOCYTES

Platelets contain a specific PER that is only apparent in ultrastructural preparations (not in light microscopic specimens). This specific PER is present within the endoplasmic reticulum and nuclear membrane of megakaryocytes and within the tubular system of the platelets. Slight CAE reactivity in canine and feline megakaryocytes has been reported, similar to that observed in human cells.[12,13] PAS staining is often apparent within platelets and megakaryocytes of many animal species,

including thrombocytes of birds and reptiles (Fig. 51.6).[11,33] Positive reactivity to LAP- or SBB-staining techniques has not been demonstrated within platelets. Megakaryocytes and platelets exhibit reactivity for NSEs; these reactions are mildly to totally inhibited with sodium fluoride.[34] Both megakaryocytes and platelets are strongly reactive for ACP activity. Synacril black AN, a textile dye,[35] selectively stains acid mucopolysaccharides found in the megakaryocytic cytoplasm (Fig. 51.11); metachromatic staining is observed. Acetylcholinesterase reactivity is another marker that primarily identifies megakaryocytes and platelets of dogs, cats, and rats.[36]

ERYTHROID CELLS

Reactivity of erythroid cells to routine cytochemical stains is observed infrequently. Exceptions include a diffuse blush of positive reactivity caused by endogenous PER activity. Similar observations occur with SBB cytochemistry. ACP, beta glucuronidase, PAS (Fig. 51.6), and naphthyl butyrate esterase techniques may result in diffuse granular staining of various stages of erythroid precursors.[12,13,37]

MAST CELLS

Canine and feline mast cells exhibit variable reactivity with the CAE, PAS, alcian blue, toluidine blue, and OEN cytochemical techniques (similar to basophils from these species).[17] Mast cells, like basophils, are negative for PER and SBB reactivity. LAP activity is not present in canine and feline mast cells, whereas ACP reactivity results only in weak staining. NSE reactivity may have variable intensity in mast cells from some species like the pig, dog, and cat.

CYTOCHEMICAL STAIN METHODS

A summary of cytochemical stain techniques and their application is provided in Table 51.2. These are the methods used by the primary author. Other methods and kits may be used for a similar result.

MYELOPEROXIDASE

This cytochemical technique is used as a marker for myeloid cells, particularly neutrophils, eosinophils, and monocytes (Fig. 51.1). The PER enzymes are sensitive to tissue processing. Therefore, enzymatic reactivity is demonstrable only in fresh tissues and not in paraffin-embedded tissues. PER reactivity diminishes over time, especially in samples older than 2 weeks of age. PER reactivity may be less intense if smears are over three days old.[38] The most sensitive method to detect PER activity involves benzidine compounds that are potentially carcinogenic.[39] Copper salts enhance the benzidine

TABLE 51.2 Summary of Cytochemical Staining Techniques for Selected Procedures

Cytochemical Reaction	Fixative	Substrate	Coupler Dye	Counterstain	Reaction	Reference/Kit
Myeloperoxidase	Formalin-acetone	Diaminobenzidine tetra-hydrochloride	—	Hematoxylin	Red orange to brown black	Ref 39 Sigma #391-A
	Formalin-acetone	3-amino-9-ethylcarbazole	—	Hematoxylin	Fine red granules	Ref 40
Sudan black B	Formaldehyde fumes	Sudan black B	—	Giemsa	Black granules	Ref 41 Sigma #380-B
Chloroacetate esterase	Formalin-acetone	Naphthol AS-D chloro-acetate	Fast Corinth V salt	Hematoxylin	Fine red granules	Ref 42 Sigma #90-C2
Leukocyte alkaline phosphatase	Methanol-formalin	Naphthol AS-BI phosphate	Fast red-violet LB or fast blue RR salts	Hematoxylin	Red or blue-black granules	Ref 5 or Ref 44 Sigma #85L
Periodic acid-Schiff	Formalin	Schiff reagent	—	Alcian blue or hematoxylin	Magenta	Ref 46
Alpha naphthyl acetate esterase with sodium fluoride inhibition	Formalin-acetone	Alpha naphthyl acetate	Hexazotized para-rosaniline or fast blue RR salt	Hematoxylin	Red or blue-black diffuse granules or focal reaction	Ref 20 Sigma #90-A1 (monocytes)
Alpha naphthyl butyrate esterase	Formalin-acetone	Alpha naphthyl butyrate	Hexzotized para-rosaniline	Hematoxylin	Fine red granules or focal reaction	Ref 5 Sigma #181-B (lymphocytes) Sigma #180-B (lymphocytes)
Acid phosphatase with tartrate solution	Formalin-acetone	Naphthol AS-BI phosphate	Hexazotized para-rosaniline	Hematoxylin	Fine red granules or focal reaction	Ref 3 Sigma #181A
β-glucuronidase	Citrate-acetone-formaldehyde	Naphthol AS-BI beta-D-glucuronic acid	Hexazotized para-rosaniline	Methylene blue	Red focal re-action	Ref 49 Sigma #181-C

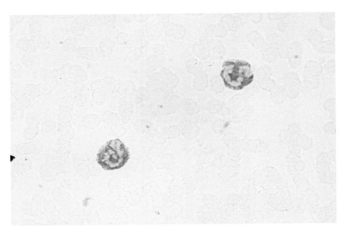

FIGURE 51.5 Equine blood with positive leukocyte alkaline phosphatase in two neutrophils. 250× original magnification.

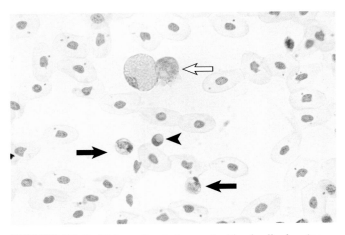

FIGURE 51.6 PAS reaction in boa snake blood cells showing strong reaction in thrombocytes (closed arrows), moderate reaction in an azurophil (open arrow), trace reaction in a heterophil, and punctate reaction in erythrocytes. Note lymphocyte with inclusion body (arrowhead). 250× original magnification.

fail to stain. The sudanophilic material within cells is stable to heat and storage.

CHLOROACETATE ESTERASE

Referred to as specific esterase, the CAE reaction is likely produced by a group of enzymes. This reaction is considered more specific for neutrophils (Fig. 51.3) than PER or SBB reactivity, although the CAE technique is less sensitive. CAE reactivity is strongest from the promyelocyte to the segmented stage; weaker reactivity is observed in myeloblasts (Fig. 51.4). The CAE reaction also is specific for mast cells. Enzymatic reactivity in the CAE procedure probably involves chymotrypsin and elastase. These enzymes are capable of hydrolyzing esters linked to the substrate naphthol AS-D chloroacetate that, when liberated, complex with a stable diazonium salt to produce an insoluble, colored product at the site of enzyme activity.[42] This esterase group can be distinguished biochemically from NSEs on the basis of isoenzyme separation in gel electrophoresis.[43] The specific esterase group is resistant to sodium fluoride inhibition. The CAE cytochemical reaction is stable and may be used in paraffin-embedded tissues.

LEUKOCYTE ALKALINE PHOSPHATASE

Enzymes with LAP activity hydrolyze naphthol AS-BI phosphate at an alkaline pH, releasing naphthol to complex with a diazonium salt, forming an insoluble, colored product near the site of enzyme activity.[44] This group of enzymes is present in granulocytes (Fig. 51.5), osteoblasts, histiocytes, vascular endothelial cells, and a subset of lymphocytes.[43] In human neutrophils, LAP activity is present in a subset of granules associated with

reaction, producing a gray-black product rather than an orange-brown chromagen. An acceptable alternative substrate to diaminobenzidine tetrahydrochloride is 3-amino-9-carbazole.[40]

SUDAN BLACK B

Lipids (including phospholipids, neutral fats, and sterols) within neutrophils, eosinophils, azurophils, and occasional monocytes are identified (Fig. 51.2) by a gray-black reaction using SBB dye.[41] This staining technique is as sensitive as the PER reaction. The mechanism of cellular staining may involve an enzymatic reaction because eosinophils from patients that have eosinophil-PER deficiency do not stain after SBB application. The same may be true in cats because their eosinophils also

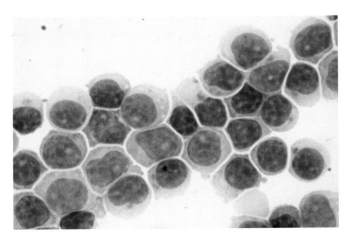

FIGURE 51.7 Focal stain reaction with ACP in canine lymphocytes having NK-cell activity. 250× original magnification.

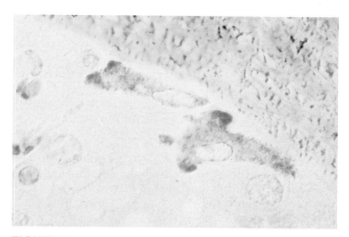

FIGURE 51.8 Bovine bone marrow with diffuse positive ACP reaction in reticuloendothelial cells. Plastic-embedded section. 500× original magnification.

the plasma membrane. The LAP reactivity of neutrophils varies with the species. In people, metamyelocyte and earlier stages are devoid of reactivity, whereas more mature cells (such as segmenters) stain more intensely. LAP reactivity is normal to increased in leukocytosis or leukemoid reaction, but it is decreased in neoplastic neutrophils (e.g, chronic myelogenous leukemia). LAP reactivity, similar to that in people, occurs in rabbits, rats, guinea pigs, horses, cattle, sheep, goats, and monkeys.[5] In dogs and cats, the late stages of neutrophils are devoid of LAP activity whereas enzymatic activity is present in myeloblast and promyelocyte stages. The LAP technique, therefore, has been helpful in identifying myelogenous leukemia. LAP activity is absent in human eosinophils. In contrast, LAP activity is strong in the equine eosinophils, moderate in bovine eosinophils, and mild in canine and feline eosinophils. In each instance, enzymatic activity is observed in the cytoplasm between the specific granules. A subset of B lymphocytes, present in the mantle zone of lymph nodes, exhibits cellular membrane staining with LAP technique in people, dogs, rats, and mice.[2,45] LAP reactivity, though present in a wide variety of cells and tissues, also is helpful for the identification of hemolymphatic cells from mammalian and certain reptilian species.

PERIODIC ACID-SCHIFF

In the PAS technique, periodic acid oxidizes carbohydrates to form aldehydes that react with Schiff's reagent to produce a dye product.[46] The bright red or magenta reaction product is focal, diffuse, or granular. Depending on the species, PAS positivity may be found within a wide variety of cells, including neutrophils, heterophils, eosinophils, basophils, monocytes, azurophils, lymphocytes, platelets, thrombocytes, and erythrocytes (Fig. 51.6). The materials stained include glycoproteins, mucoproteins, glycolipids, and high-mo-

lecular-weight carbohydrates. In blood cells, glycogen usually is the substance demonstrated; if the sample is predigested with diastase, glycogen staining is eliminated.

NONSPECIFIC ESTERASES AND SODIUM FLUORIDE INHIBITION

NSEs are a group of enzymes capable of hydrolyzing esters to liberate naphthol products that bind with a coupler dye. These esterases demonstrate a wide range of substrate specificity and stain pH environment for various blood cells; therefore, they are termed nonspecific. Many of the esterases, as determined by polyacrylamide gel electrophoresis, are cell specific. Monocytes, granulocytes, and a subset of lymphocytes exhibit unique patterns of reactivity. A red-to-pink, diffusely granular pattern is seen in monocytes, histiocytes stain more intensely, and a single focal or punctate reaction product is seen in T lymphocytes. The NSE activity in monocytes is inhibited by the addition of sodium fluoride to the incubation medium, whereas T lymphocytes are resistant. Differentiated histiocytes or macrophages have weakened or abolished reactivity in the presence of sufficient sodium fluoride. Sensitivity to sodium fluoride inhibition also has been observed in megakaryocytes, platelets, and plasma cells.[24,34] The difference in inhibition relates to the location of the enzyme in these cells. For example, the NSEs alpha naphthyl acetate esterase (αNAE) and alpha naphthyl butyrate esterase (αNBE) have been identified mostly on the plasma membrane of monocytes but only within intracellular organelles of lymphocytes.[22,23,26] The intracellular location of the enzyme appears to be protective. The activity of these enzymes is unstable, being sensitive to heat, fixatives, and storage. Fresh blood smears or tissue imprints are preferred to paraffin-embedded tissues that may not demonstrate the reaction.

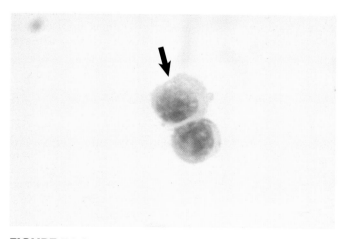

FIGURE 51.9 Faint punctate stain reaction (arrow) with βG in canine lymphocytes. 500× original magnification.

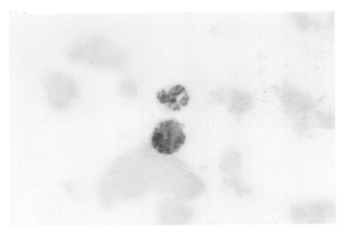

FIGURE 51.10 Positive stain reaction with OEN in a feline basophil. Blood. 250× original magnification.

Alpha Naphthyl Acetate Esterase

Cell specificity for αNAE activity may be demonstrated by altering the pH of the medium, temperature, and length of incubation.[1,23,47] Monocytes are best stained in an acidic medium, whereas both granulocytes and monocytes may show enzymatic activity when the same substrate is used in a neutral medium. Lymphocytes are best demonstrated only with acid conditions and prolonged incubation. Compared with αNBE, αNAE is more sensitive and less specific in identifying monocytes, macrophages, and T lymphocytes. Therefore, sodium fluoride inhibition is necessary to differentiate the cell types. T lymphocytes have been identified by a focal staining pattern in humans, dogs, and chickens.[27,30,31] The stain reaction may be weak in megakaryocytes, platelets, and plasma cells, all of which are sodium fluoride sensitive.[34]

Alpha Naphthyl Butyrate Esterase

Similar to the αNAE technique, differential staining of cells requires changing the pH of the incubation medium.[23] Sodium fluoride inhibition often is not used with αNBE owing to its greater specificity for monocytes compared with αNAE.

ACID PHOSPHATE WITH TARTRATE

ACPs are a group of enzymes that hydrolyze phosphate esters in an acidic environment. There are erythrocyte and leukocyte isoenzymes that are specific for different cells. Many cell types react in the ACP cytochemical technique, including lymphocytes, monocytes, histiocytes, granulocytes (particularly eosinophils), platelets, megakaryocytes, plasma cells, and erythroid precursors.[3,12] The reaction product gives a diffuse pattern in monocytes, with histiocytes staining more intensely. A single focal or punctate reaction product in the Golgi area occurs in T lymphocytes.[30] Canine lymphocytes with NK-cell activity also react in the ACP technique with focal staining (Fig. 51.7).[48] Approximately one third of canine NK cells stained positively, and a small percentage remained positive with tartrate incubation.[32] Tartrate resistance was found in eosinophils and basophils from normal dogs and cats.[12,13] Tartrate resistance is most helpful in human medicine for recognition of hairy-cell leukemia, a condition not recognized in veterinary medicine.[1] All ACPs are sensitive to tissue processing and heat. Therefore, the ACP technique is recommended only for fresh cytologic or plastic-embedded materials (Fig. 51.8) and not for paraffin-embedded tissues.

β-GLUCURONIDASE

A hydrolytic enzyme with a pattern of reactivity similar to that of the esterases is β-glucuronidase (βG). βG hydrolyzes the substrate to produce liberated naphthol compounds which subsequently bind to a colored dye. Enzymatic activity is demonstrable in blood lymphocytes, monocytes, and granulocytes (Fig. 51.9). Both monocytes and neutrophils display weak, diffuse, cytoplasmic reactivity, whereas T lymphocytes produce a focal or distinct granular reaction.[49] In feline specimens, βG activity appears in monocytes, granulocytes, lymphocytes, and platelets; the strongest reactivity is observed in monocytes.[37] Weakly positive reactivity has been observed in neutrophils of channel catfish.[50] For human blood, the βG staining procedure appears to have little advantage over the NSEs in detecting T lymphocytes.[49]

MISCELLANEOUS STAINS

Toluidine Blue

This common histologic stain is helpful for the evaluation of basophil and mast cell populations from many

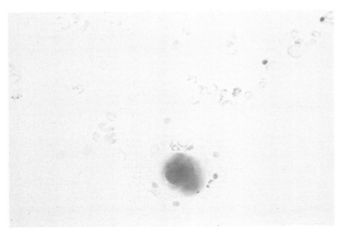

FIGURE 51.11 Feline megakaryocyte with magenta reaction stained with Synacril black AN (Megacolor). Bone marrow. 100× original magnification.

species.[17,20] Toluidine blue is a basic dye that reacts with the acid mucopolysaccharides to form metachromatic complexes that appear red purple. Basophils stain readily in acidic toluidine blue but not in neutral toluidine blue.[18]

Omega-Exonuclease

OEN is an enzymatic staining technique for basophils or mast cells and their precursors in several species, particularly humans, dogs, cats (Fig. 51.10), and primates such as the Rhesus monkey and the gibbon. Enzymatic activity is not found in normal basophils of the horse, cow, goat, pig, or alpaca.[17] This enzyme is an alkaline phosphodiesterase found within the cytoplasm and not in the specific granules. Therefore, it is said that OEN activity is more helpful than toluidine blue in identifying poorly differentiated or degranulated cells. Positive OEN reactivity produces diffuse, red-brown, granular, cytoplasmic deposits.

Synacril Black AN

Synacril black AN application results in selective metachromatic staining of acid mucopolysaccharides found in the megakaryocytic cytoplasm.[35] This substance is a textile dye available commercially as Megacolor from Cytocolor, Inc. After fixation with formaldehyde-acetic acid-ethanol solution, specimens are pretreated with ribonuclease to remove ribonucleic acid. The dye stains the cytoplasm of mature and immature megakaryocytes with a red-violet to violet reaction product (Fig. 51.11). All other cells are pale yellow to yellow brown except for eosinophils whose granules appear pink. In one report, normal equine megakaryocytes along with normal and neoplastic canine megakaryocytes from paraffin-embedded samples stained with a magenta reaction with this dye.[51]

Acetylcholinesterase

Acetylcholinesterase is another enzymatic marker that specifically identifies mature megakaryocytes and platelets from dogs, cats, and rats.[36,52] In addition, acetylcholinesterase also is found within human and murine erythroid precursors.[53] Specimens for cytochemical staining are incubated in a medium containing acetylthiocholine iodide as substrate. The subsequent reaction product is brown.

SUMMARY

Cytochemical staining is inexpensive and provides a convenient manner to identify the chemical constituents of blood cells. These staining procedures are particularly useful in categorizing unknown cell types from a wide variety of animal species, including birds, reptiles, amphibians, fish, and invertebrates.

REFERENCES

1. **Li C-Y, Yam LT.** Cytochemistry and immunochemistry in hematologic diagnoses. Hematol Oncol Clin North Am 1994;8:665–681.
2. **Raskin RE, Nipper MN.** Cytochemical staining characteristics of lymph nodes from normal and lymphoma-affected dogs. Vet Clin Pathol 1992; 21:62–67.
3. **Beckstead JH, et al.** Enzyme histochemistry and immunohistochemistry on biopsy specimens of pathologic human bone marrow. Blood 1981;57:1088–1098.
4. **Kadota K, et al.** Ultrastructure of swine myelogenous leukaemic cells, with particular reference to intracytoplasmic granules. J Comp Pathol 1987; 97:401–406.
5. **Jain NC.** Cytochemistry of normal and leukemic leukocytes. In: Jain NC, ed. Philadelphia: Lea & Febiger, 1986;909–939.
6. **Kiehl AR, Schiller CA.** A study of manatee leukocytes using peroxidase stain. Vet Clin Pathol 1994;23:50–53.
7. **Alleman AR, et al.** Morphologic and cytochemical characteristics of blood cells from the desert tortoise (Gopherus agassizii). Am J Vet Res 1992; 53:1645–1651.
8. **Work TM, et al.** Morphologic and cytochemical characteristics of blood cells from Hawaiian green turtles. Am J Vet Res 1998;59:1252–1257.
9. **Tschudi P, et al.** Cytochemical staining of equine blood and bone marrow cells. Equine Vet J 1977;9:205–207.
10. **Andreasen CB, Latimer KS.** Cytochemical staining characteristics of chicken heterophils and eosinophils. Vet Clin Pathol 1990;19:2:51–54.
11. **Mateo MR, et al.** Morphologic, cytochemical, and functional studies of peripheral blood cells of young healthy American alligators (Alligator mississippiensis). Am J Vet Res 1984;45:1046–1053.
12. **Facklam NR, Kociba GJ.** Cytochemical characterization of leukemic cells from 20 dogs. Vet Pathol 1985;22:363–369.
13. **Facklam NR, Kociba GJ.** Cytochemical characterization of feline leukemic cells. Vet Pathol 1986;23:155–161.
14. **Luna LG.** Luna's method for erythrocytes and eosinophil granules. In: Luna LG, ed. New York: McGraw-Hill, 1968;111–112.
15. **Young KM, et al.** Characterization of eosinophil progenitor cells in feline bone marrow. Am J Vet Res 1997;58:348–353.
16. **Raskin RE, MacKay M.** Cytochemical staining characteristics of basophils and mast cells Vet Pathol 1994;31:580–580.
17. **Jain NC, Kono CS.** Omega-exonuclease activity in basophils of certain animal species. Comp Haematol Int 1991;1:166–168.
18. **Jain NC.** The basophils and mast cells. In: Jain NC, ed. Philadelphia: Lea & Febiger, 1993;258–265.
19. **Al-Izzi SA, et al.** Morphology and cytochemistry of bovine bone marrow mononuclear phagocytes. Can J Comp Med 1982;46:130–132.
20. **Yam LT, et al.** Cytochemical identification of monocytes and granulocytes. Am J Pathol 1971;55:283–290.
21. **Inoue M, et al.** Ultrastructural cytochemical characterization of alpha-naphthyl acetate esterase in chicken monocytic cell lines. J Vet Med Sci 1991; 53:415–418.
22. **Drexler HG, et al.** Lineage-specific monocytic esterase, a distinct marker for leukemias of monocytic origin: cytochemical, isoenzymatic and biochemical features. Leuk Lymphoma 1991;4:295–312.
23. **Bozdech MJ, Bainton DF.** Identification of α-naphthyl butyrate esterase as a plasma membrane ectoenzyme of monocytes and as a discrete intracellular membrane-bounded organelle in lymphocytes. J Exp Med 1981;153:182–195.
24. **Dulac RW, Yang TJ.** Differential sodium fluoride sensitivity of alpha-naphthyl acetate esterase in human, bovine, canine, and murine monocytes and lymphocytes. Exp Hematol 1991;19:59–62.
25. **Hu Z-B, et al.** Myeloperoxidase: expression and modulation in a large panel of human leukemia-lymphoma cell lines. Blood 1993;82:1599–1607.
26. **Heumann D, et al.** Human large granular lymphocytes contain an esterase activity usually considered as specific for the myeloid series. Eur J Immunol 1983;13:254–258.
27. **Wulff JC, et al.** Nonspecific acid esterase activity as a marker for canine T lymphocytes. Exp Hematol 1981;9:865–870.
28. **Raich PC, et al.** Cytochemical reactions in bovine and ovine lymphosarcoma. Vet Pathol 1983;20:322–329.
29. **Wellman ML, et al.** Lymphoma involving large granular lymphocytes in cats: 11 cases (1982–1991). J Am Vet Med Assoc 1992;201:1265–1269.
30. **Yang K, et al.** Acid phosphatase and alpha-naphthyl acetate esterase in neoplastic and non-neoplastic lymphocytes. A statistical analysis. Am J Clin Pathol 1982;78:141–149.
31. **Odend'hal S, Player EC.** Histochemical localization of T-cells in tissue section. Avian Dis 1979;24:886–895.
32. **Knapp DW, et al.** Ultrastructure and cytochemical staining characteristics of canine natural killer cells. Anat Rec 1995;243:509–515.
33. **Swayne DE, et al.** Cytochemical properties of chicken blood cells resembling both thrombocytes and lymphocytes. Vet Clin Pathol 1986;15:17–24.
34. **Grindem CB, et al.** Cytochemical reactions in cells from leukemic dogs. Vet Pathol 1986;23:103–109.
35. **Kass L.** Synacril black AN. A new stain for normal and abnormal human megakaryocytes. Am J Clin Pathol 1986;86:506–510.

36. **Joshi BC, Jain NC.** Experimental immunologic thrombocytopenia in dogs: a study of thrombocytopenia and megakaryocytopoiesis. Res Vet Sci 1977; 22:11–17.
37. **Tsujimoto H, et al.** A cytochemical study on feline blood cells. Jpn J Vet Sci 1983;45:373–382.
38. **Grindem CB, et al.** Cytochemical reactions in cells from leukemic cats. Vet Clin Pathol 1985;14:6–12.
39. **Kaplow LS.** Simplified myeloperoxidase stain using benzidine dihydrochloride. Blood 1965;26:215–219.
40. **Jain NC, et al.** A comparison of cytochemical techniques to demonstrate peroxidase activity in canine leukocytes. Vet Clin Pathol 1989;17:87–89.
41. **Sheehan HL, Storey GW.** An improved method of staining leukocyte granules with Sudan black B. J Pathol Bacteriol 1947;59:336–337.
42. **Moloney WC, et al.** Esterase activity in leukocytes demonstrated by the use of naphthol AS-D chloroacetate substrate. J Histochem Cytochem 1960; 8:200–207.
43. **Elghetany MT, et al.** The use of cytochemical procedures in the diagnosis and management of acute and chronic myeloid leukemia. Clin Lab Med 1990;10:707–720.
44. **Ackerman GA.** Substituted naphthol AS phosphate derivatives for the localization of leukocyte alkaline phosphatase activity. Lab Invest 1962;11: 563–567.
45. **Nanba K, et al.** Alkaline phosphatase-positive malignant lymphoma. A subtype of B-cell lymphomas. Am J Clin Pathol 1977;68:535–542.
46. **Luna LG.** McManus' method for glycogen (PAS). In: Luna LG, ed. New York: McGraw-Hill, 196;158–160.
47. **Osbaldison GW, et al.** Cytochemical determination of esterases in peripheral blood leukocytes. Am J Vet Res 1978;39:683–685.
48. **Raskin RE.** Natural killer cell activity in canine lymphoid malignancies. PhD Dissertation, Michigan State University,1987.
49. **Machin GA, et al.** Cytochemically demonstrable β-glucuronidase activity in normal and neoplastic human lymphoid cells. Blood 1980;56:1111–1119.
50. **Zinkl JG, et al.** Morphology and cytochemistry of leukocytes and thrombocytes of six species of fish. Comp Haematol Int 1991;1:187–195.
51. **Lester GD, et al.** Malignant histiocytosis in an Arabian filly. Equine Vet J 1993;25:471–473.
52. **Jackson CW.** Cholinesterase as a possible marker for early cells of the megakaryocytic series. Blood 1973;42:413–421.
53. **Koekebakker M, Barr RD.** Acetylcholinesterase in the human erythron. I. Cytochemistry. Am J Hematol 1988;28:252–259.

Bone marrow

| Proliferation pool | Storage pool | Blood | Tissue |

Healthy

1a. Decreased Production

1b. Ineffective Production

2. Overwhelming Demand by the Tissues

3. Shift From Circulating to Marginal Pool

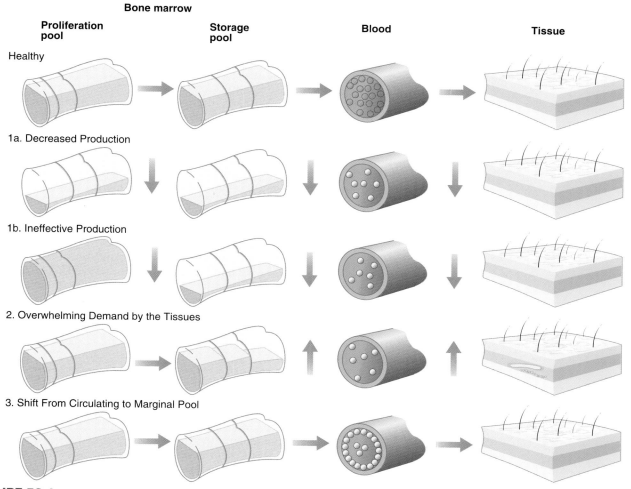

FIGURE 53.1 Mechanisms of neutropenia. The arrows represent the numbers of cells supplied by marrow compartments to the blood and the tissues in the various conditions compared to a healthy patient. Normal numbers are represented by an arrow pointing left to right, increased numbers are represented by an upward pointing arrow, and decreased numbers are represented by a downward pointing arrow. Each condition is further represented by the amount of marrow in the cavity and the distribution and number of cells in the blood. Modified from an illustration by Terry Lawrence.

sue demand are generally acute or peracute infections caused by gram-negative bacteria. These conditions most often involve large surface areas, such as the peritoneum after bowel rupture. Horses and cattle appear more susceptible to this type of neutropenia.

3. Neutropenia Caused by a Shift From the Circulating Neutrophil Pool to the Marginal Neutrophil Pool

Neutropenia because of neutrophil margination is a transient condition found in the initial minutes to hours of an endotoxemia[10–15] or anaphylactic shock.[16,17] These conditions cause the neutrophils in the circulating neutrophil pool to enter the marginal neutrophil pool (Fig. 53.1-3). During anaphylactic shock, an immune-mediated hypersensitivity reaction causes many tissue mast cells to degranulate, releasing large quantities of histamine. Endotoxemia is caused by the release of a

toxin from the cell wall of certain gram-negative bacteria. These substances cause neutrophils to marginate from the circulating pool, thereby reducing the number reported on the leukogram. Initially, neutropenia from bacterial endotoxemia often is caused by a combination of sequestration caused by the endotoxin and subsequently by an excessive tissue demand because of the chemotactic response to the bacteria.

CONGENITAL DISEASES WITH ASSOCIATED NEUTROPENIA

Cyclic neutropenia (cyclic hemopoiesis) of gray collies is the best documented of the congenital abnormalities resulting in neutropenia in domestic animals.[18–26] This syndrome is characterized by cyclic fluctuations in peripheral blood neutrophils, monocytes, lymphocytes, eosinophils, platelets, and reticulocytes. The specific pathophysiologic mechanism has not been determined, but a defect in a granulocytic colony-stimulating factor postreceptor signal transduction is hypothesized.[19] A similar problem was reported in a colony of gray collie crossbred research dogs.[27] Animals that have cyclic neutropenia are prone to infections and secondary amyloidosis. Functional abnormalities have been demonstrated in neutrophils from affected collies.

Chédiak–Higashi Syndrome (CHS) is a hereditary abnormality characterized by abnormal fusion of granules, resulting in altered granule size and shape visible by light microscopy. This defect occurs in humans, mink, cats, cattle, and has been reported in a killer whale.[25] Neutropenia occasionally is observed in cats that have CHS.[28] The mechanism of the neutropenia has not been determined in these cases, although an effect at the marrow level, mediated through either destruction of intramedullary neutrophils or aberrations in regulation of myelopoiesis relating to dysfunction of natural-killer-cell activity, has been proposed as the cause.

Neutropenia and neutrophil hypersegmentation associated with nonregenerative anemia occurs in giant schnauzers.[29] Affected dogs were inappetent, lethargic, and cachectic. Methylmalonic aciduria and low serum B_{12} concentration indicated that vitamin B_{12} deficiency resulted from selective malabsorption of vitamin B_{12}. Parenteral administration of vitamin B_{12} resulted in normalization of the laboratory abnormalities and resolution of the clinical signs. An autosomal recessive mode of inheritance is hypothesized as the cause of this congenital abnormality.

A familial syndrome of myeloid and megakaryocytic hypoplasia occurs in standardbred horses.[30] The neutropenia is cyclic in some horses and is accompanied by thrombocytopenia. The bone marrow of affected animals is severely depleted of myeloid precursors and megakaryocytes. Bone marrow cultures suggested a defect in the marrow microenvironment, a dysfunction or lack of marrow growth factors, or a lack of pluripotential stem cells. Three of eight horses of one report died from fatal hemorrhage, likely resulting from or complicated by thrombocytopenia.

Myelofibrosis was reported in 11 of 16 related pygmy goats.[31] Affected animals were lethargic, had pale mucous membranes, and failed to gain weight normally. Anemia and neutropenia resulted in the death of 6- to 12-week-old goats. The number of circulating red blood cells, platelets, and neutrophils declined progressively from birth. Numerous nucleated red blood cells were noted in blood smears at 7 days of age, but the number declined as the animals aged. Well-differentiated fibrocytes and abundant collagen replaced the active bone marrow. Focal megakaryocyte hyperplasia in association with areas of marrow fibrotic regions as well as areas of megakaryocyte necrosis and emperipolesis of hemopoietic cells in megakaryocytes was found in the bone marrow. This syndrome of myelofibrosis is believed to be a hereditary disorder in pygmy goats. There are some similarities to disorders of megakaryocytopoiesis in humans.

Persistent neutropenia with marrow myeloid hyperplasia was diagnosed in related Border collie puppies.[32]

These pups had periodic fever and osteomyelitis, which were attributed to infectious processes relating to persistent leukopenia. The pathogenesis of the neutropenia was not established, but an inability of neutrophils to migrate from the marrow into the peripheral circulation was suspected. An autosomal recessive mode of inheritance was hypothesized.

In humans, there are multiple congenital syndromes associated with neutropenia.[9,24,33,34] In addition to cyclic neutropenia described above, neutropenia has been associated with abnormalities of lymphoid cells and with congenital cutaneous and skeletal abnormalities. With the exception of cyclic neutropenia, comparable syndromes are not reported in domestic animals.

The authors have documented rare cases of apparently benign, transitory neutropenia in young dogs. The affected puppies either were clinically normal or had minimal depression. Random neutrophils counts assessed over a 6- to 9-month period revealed peripheral blood neutrophil counts of less than 2000 cells/μl. Bone marrow aspirates revealed myeloid hyperplasia with normal maturation. Other hematologic parameters were normal. The neutropenia resolved without specific treatment.

ACQUIRED CAUSES OF NEUTROPENIA

Neutropenia commonly occurs during the course of infectious disease. Viral infections commonly cause neutropenia in many different species of animals. Such viral infections include feline leukemia virus, feline immunodeficiency virus, and parvoviral infections in cats; herpes, adenoviral, and influenza viral infections in horses; bovine viral diarrhea in cattle; and parvoviral infections in dogs.[35–42] Cyclic neutropenia associated with cyclic oscillation of varying hemopoietic cells, including eosinophils, lymphocytes, platelets and reticulocytes, has been associated with feline leukemia virus infection.[43–45] Resolution of the cyclic hemopoiesis occurred with prednisone treatment, whereas spontaneous recovery was noted in one cat. Myelosuppression and myelodysplasia can result from feline leukemia virus infection. Affected animals may have various cytopenias, including neutropenia associated with abnormal myeloid precursors in the marrow and decreased number of postmitotic granulocytes. Rarely, feline leukemia virus results in diffuse myelofibrosis with accompanying pancytopenia.[46] Chronic, persistent leukopenia and neutropenia has been reported in a cat that had feline immunodeficiency virus infection.[47] Bone marrow aspirates from this cat were unremarkable, and the pathogenesis of the neutropenia was not established.

Gram-negative bacterial infections frequently cause neutropenia.[10,48] The neutrophils are shunted from the circulating and bone marrow pools into the marginal pool. This effect is believed to be mediated through endotoxin. Horses and cattle may be more prone to the neutropenic manifestation of endotoxemia because of the small leukocyte reserve.

Horses and dogs infected with ehrlichiae may be neutropenic.[25] The mechanism of the neutropenia varies. In *Ehrlichia canis* infection in dogs, diffuse bone marrow suppression results in thrombocytopenia, anemia, and leukopenia. Granulocytic ehrlichiosis may be associated with mild neutropenia in dogs and in horses, although the mechanism of the neutropenia has not been investigated. Recurrent neutropenia and thrombocytopenia was documented in a 3-year-old Pomeranian dog in which irregular cycles of neutropenia and thrombocytopenia were associated with episodes of anorexia and depression for an 8- to 12-month interval.[49] Although *E. canis* titers were negative, peripheral blood monocytes contained ehrlichial-type inclusions. Treatment with tetracycline resolved the clinical signs. *Ehrlichia phagocytophila*, a neutrophilic ehrlichial agent documented in ruminants in Europe, causes neutrophil dysfunction and neutropenia.[50–52] Animals infected with *E. phagocytophila* are prone to infections with other bacteria.

Fungal infections may also result in various cytopenias. Disseminated histoplasmosis has been associated with anemia, neutropenia, and thrombocytopenia in dogs and cats.[53,54]

Various drugs and toxins may cause neutropenia.[46,55–59] Chemotherapeutic agents routinely cause neutropenia through the effects of the drugs on bone marrow precursors. The peripheral blood neutrophil count is used to monitor the effects of these drugs in the course of chemotherapy. Cyclophosphamide also can induce cyclic neutropenia in some dogs dosed at 1.5 to 3.7 mg/kg administered orally.[60] Oscillations in the neutrophil counts have a periodicity of 11 to 17 days in these dogs.

Chronic exposure to endogenous (estrus in ferrets) or exogenous estrogens results in pancytopenia from bone marrow hypoplasia.[61] The mechanism of estrogen-induced bone marrow suppression is believed to be caused by the induction of myelopoiesis inhibitory substances from the thymus.[62,63] Other drugs that have been periodically associated with neutropenia through effects on bone marrow precursor cells include griseofulvin, trimethoprim or sulfadiazine, cephalosporins, phenobarbitol, chloramphenical, and phenylbutazone.[25,64–66] Bracken fern poisoning causes leukopenia and thrombocytopenia from diffuse bone marrow hypoplasia.[67] Mycotoxins are also incriminated as causes of neutropenia in horses and cattle.[68] Herd outbreaks of thrombocytopenia and granulocytopenia in cattle were attributed to mycotoxicosis.[69–71] Irradiation causes depletion of bone marrow stem cells and resultant pancytopenia. This effect is used in the preparation of animals for bone marrow transplantation for the treatment of lysosomal storage diseases.

Bone marrow necrosis is rarely documented in animals.[72] Neutropenia is commonly manifested in cases of suspected or documented marrow necrosis. Hematologic malignancies may progress to myelophthisis or marrow fibrosis with pancytopenia. Myelofibrosis also can accompany some congenital disorders and may occur in the course of viral disease (such as with feline leukemia virus).[25] In some instances, the cause of myelofibrosis cannot be determined. Myelofibrosis is accompanied by anemia, leukopenia, and neutropenia.

Immune-mediated cytopenia, especially immune-mediated hemolytic anemia and thrombocyotopenia, are seen commonly in domestic animals, especially in dogs.[25,46] Immune-mediated neutropenia is documented in humans by demonstration of antineutrophil antibodies in affected patients.[34,73,74] Techniques have been developed to detect neutrophil-associated antibodies in cats and in horses, but few cases of immune-mediated neutropenia have been documented.[73,75–79] Immune mechanisms were hypothesized as a cause of thrombocytopenia and neutropenia in a litter of newborn piglets and in leukopenia of newborn foals.[73] In humans, there are no specific clinical characteristics of immune-mediated neutropenia. Neutropenia is accompanied by marrow myeloid hyperplasia in most cases, with the exception being cases in which antibody is directed against myeloid precursor cells.[34,74] Other immune-mediated disease syndromes, such as immune-mediated thrombocytopenia, rheumatoid arthritis, and lupus erythematosus, may accompany the neutropenia. Drugs, infectious agents, and neoplasms may stimulate immune responses that trigger immune-mediated neutropenia.[73]

In cats, persistent neutropenia and bone marrow myeloid hyperplasia are relatively common, stimulating assessment of a series of these patients for the presence of antineutrophil antibody. Antibody was not detected, and the pathogenesis of this syndrome remains unidentified.[76]

Experimentally, a form of immune-mediated neutropenia has been induced in dogs by the administration of recombinant human granulocyte colony-stimulating factor.[80] The neutropenia is antibody mediated, but the precise mechanism for neutropenia has not been elicited.

In humans, a syndrome of chronic idiopathic neutropenia (CIN) has been reported in which persistent neutropenia occurs concurrent with decreased or ineffective myelopoiesis.[9,81] There is variable susceptibility to infectious disease and spontaneous remissions have been reported. Persistent neutropenia with decreased marrow myelopoiesis was reported in a 4-year-old, domestic, female, spayed, short hair cat.[82] The case had similarities to human CIN, but unlike some CIN in certain human patients, the cat showed no response to cortisone therapy.

Neutropenia and leukopenia have been associated with iron deficiency in baby pigs[83,84] and with taurine deficiency in cats.[85] In the pigs, iron supplementation resolved the neutropenia.

REFERENCES

1. **Carakostas MC, Moore WE, Smith JE**, Intravascular neutrophilic granulocyte kinetics in horses. Am J Vet Res 1981;42:623–625.
2. **Carakostas MC, Moore WE, Smith JE.** Procedure for granulokinetic studies in the horse with chromium-51. Am J Vet Res 1981;42:620–622.
3. **Deubelbeiss KA, Dancey JT, Harker LA, Finch CA.** Neutrophil kinetics in the dog. J Clin Invest 1975;55:833–839.
4. **Mary JY.** Normal human granulopoiesis revisited. I. Blood data. Biomed Pharmacother 1984;38:33–43.
5. **Mary JY.** Normal human granulopoiesis revisited. II. Bone marrow data. Biomed Pharmacother 1985;39:66–77.
6. **Walker RI, Willemze R.** Neurophil kinetics and the regulation of granulopoiesis. Rev Infect Dis 1980;2:282–292.

7. **Cronkite EP, Burlington H, Chanana AD, Joel DD.** Regulation of granulopoiesis. Prog Clin Biol Res 1985;184:129–144.

8. **Duncan R, Prasse K, Mahaffey E.** Leukocytes. Veterinary laboratory medicine: clinical pathology. 3rd ed. Ames, IA: Iowa State University Press, 1994;37–62.

9. **Dale D.** Neutropenia. In: Beutler E, Lichtman M, Coller B, Kipps T, eds. Williams hematology. 5th ed. New York: McGraw-Hill, 1995;815–824.

10. **Cybulsky MI, Cybulsky IJ, Movat HZ.** Neutropenic responses to intradermal injections of Escherichia coli. Effects on the kinetics of polymorphonuclear leukocyte emigration. Am J Pathol 1986;124:1–9.

11. **Miert Av, Duin CTMv, Wensing T, Van Miert A, Van Duin CTM.** Fever and acute phase response induced in dwarf goats by endotoxin and bovine and human recombinant tumour necrosis factor alpha. J Vet Pharmacol Thera 1992;15:332–342.

12. **Ward DS, Fessler JF, Bottoms GD, Turek J.** Equine endotoxemia: cardiovascular, eicosanoid, hematologic, blood chemical, and plasma enzyme alterations. Am J Vet Res 1987;48:1150–1156.

13. **Jain NC, Paape MJ, Berning L, Salgar SK, Worku M.** Functional competence and monoclonal antibody reactivity of neutrophils from cows injected with Escherichia coli endotoxin. Comp Haematol Int 1991;1:10–20.

14. **Jain NC, Lasmanis J.** Leucocytic changes in cows given intravenous injections of Escherichia coli endotoxin. Res Vet Sci 1978;24:386–387.

15. **Weld JM, Kamenling SG, Combie JD, et al.** The effect of naloxone on endotoxic and hemorrhagic shock in horses. Res Commun Chem Pathol Pharmacol 1984;44:227–238.

16. **Wassef NM, Johnson SH, Graeber GM, et al.** Anaphylactoid reactions mediated by autoantibodies to cholesterol in miniature pigs. J Immunol 1989;143:2990–2995.

17. **Wells PW, Eyre P, Lumsden JH.** Hematological and pathological changes in acute systemic anaphylaxis in calves: effects of pharmacological agents. Can J Comp Med 1973;119–129.

18. **Allen WM, Pocock PI, Dalton PM, Richards HE, Aitken MM.** Cyclic neutropenia in collies. Vet Rec 1996;138:371–372.

19. **Avalos BR, Broudy VC, Ceselski SK, Druker BJ, Griffin JD, Hammond EP.** Abnormal response to granulocyte colony-stimulating factor (G-SCF) in canine cyclic hematopoiesis is not caused by altered G-CSF receptor expression. Blood 1994;84:789–794.

20. **Chusid MJ, Bujak JS, Dale DC.** Defective polymorphonuclear leukocyte metabolism and function in canine cyclic neutropenia. Blood 1975;46:921–930.

21. **Dale DC, Alling DW, Wolff SM.** Cyclic hematopoiesis: the mechanism of cyclic neutropenia in grey collie dogs. J Clin Invest 1972;51:2197–2204.

22. **Dale DC, Ward SB, Kimball HR, Wolff SM.** Studies of neutrophil production and turnover in grey collie dogs with cyclic neutropenia. J Clin Invest 1972;51:2190–2196.

23. **DiGiacomo RF, Hammond WP, Kunz LL, Cox PA.** Clinical and pathologic features of cyclic hematopoiesis in Grey Collie dogs. Am J Pathol 1983;111:224–233.

24. **Lange RD, Jones JB.** Cyclic neutropenia. Review of clinical manifestations and management. Am J Pediatr Hematol Oncol 1981;3:363–367.

25. **Meyer DJ, Harvey JW.** Evaluation of leukocytic disorders. In: Meyer DJ, Harvey JW, eds. Veterinary laboratory medicine. 2nd ed. Philadelphia: WB Saunders, 1998;98–99.

26. **Yang TJ, Jones ES, Lange RD.** Serum colony-stimulating activity of dog with cyclic neutropenia. Blood 1974;41–48.

27. **Jones JB, Lange RD, Jones ES.** Cyclic hematopoiesis in a colony of dogs. J Am Vet Med Assoc 1975;365–367.

28. **Prieur DJ, Collier LL.** Neutropenia in cats with the Chediak-Higashi syndrome. Can J Vet Res 1987;51:407–408.

29. **Fyfe JC, Jezyk PF, Giger U, Patterson DF.** Inherited selective malabsorption of vitamin B_{12} in Giant Schnauzers. J Am Anim Hosp Assoc 1989;25:533–539.

30. **Kohn CW, Swardson C, Provost P, Gilbert RO, Couto CG.** Myeloid and megakaryocytic hypoplasia in related standardbreds. J Vet Intern Med 1995;9:315–323.

31. **Cain GR, East N, Moore PF.** Myelofibrosis in young pygmy goats. Comp Haematol Int 1994;4:167–172.

32. **Allan FJ, Thompson KG, Jones BR, Burbidge HM, McKinley RL.** Neutropenia with a probable hereditary basis in Border Colliers. N Z Vet J 1996;44:67–72.

33. **Baehner RL, Miller DR.** Disorders of granulopoiesis. In: Miller DR, Baehner RL, eds. Blood diseases of infancy and childhood. 7th ed. St. Louis, MO: Mosby, 1995;562–576.

34. **Curnutte JT.** Disorders of granulocytes function and granulopoiesis. In: Nathan DG, Oski RA, eds. Hematology of infancy and childhood. 4th ed. Philadelphia: WB Saunders, 1993;939–950.

35. **Coignoul FL, Bertram TA, Cheville NF.** Pathogenicity of equine herpesvirus 1 subtype 2 for foals and adult pony mares. Vet Microbiol 1984;9:533–542.

36. **Hardy WD Jr.** Immunopathology induced by the feline leukemia virus. Springer Semin Immunopathol 1982;5:75–106.

37. **Allen BV, Frank CJ.** Haematological changes in 2 ponies before and during an infection with equine influenza. Equine Vet J 1982;14:171–172.

38. **Linenberger ML, Beebe AM, Pedersen NC, Abkowitz JL, Dandekar S.** Marrow accessory cell infection and alterations in hematopoiesis accompany severe neutropenia during experimental acute infection with feline immunodeficiency virus. Blood 1995;85:941–951.

39. **Mandell CP, Sparger EE, Pedersen NC, Jain NC.** Long-term haematological changes in cats experimentally infected with feline immunodeficiency virus (FIV). Comp Haematol Int 1992;2:8–17.

40. **McChesney AE, England JJ.** Adenoviral infection in foals. J Am Vet Med Assoc 1975;166:83–85.

41. **Parrish CR.** Pathogenesis of feline panleukopenia virus and canine parvovirus. Baillieres Clin Haematol 1995;8:57–71.

42. **Shelton GH, Linenberger ML, Abkowitz JL.** Hematologic abnormalities in cats seropositive for feline immunodeficiency virus. J Am Vet Med Assoc 1991;199:1353–1357.

43. **Gabbert NH.** Cyclic neutropenia in a feline leukemia-positive cat: a case report. J Am Anim Hosp Assoc 1984;20:343–347.

44. **Lester SJ, Searcy GP.** Hematologic abnormalities preceding apparent recovery from feline leukemia virus infection. J Am Vet Med Assoc 1981;178:471–474.

45. **Swenson CL, Kociba GJ, O'Keefe DA, Crisp MS, Jacobs RM, Rojko JL.** Cyclic hematopoiesis associated with feline leukemia virus infection in two cats. J Am Vet Med Assoc 1987;191:93–96.

46. **Latimer KS.** Leukocytes in Health and Disease. In: Ettinger SJ, Feldman EC, eds. Textbook of Veterinary Internal Medicine. 4 ed. Philadelphia: WB Saunders, Co., 1994;1892–1929.

47. **Shelton GH, Abkowitz JL, Linenberger ML, Russell RG, Grant CK.** Chronic leukopenia associated with feline immunodeficiency virus infection in cats. J Am Vet Med Assoc 1989;194:253–255.

48. **Dorn CR, Coffman JR, Schmidt DA, Garner HE, Addison JB, McCune EL.** Neutropenia and salmonellosis in hospitalized horses. J Am Vet Med Assoc 1975;65–67.

49. **Alexander JW, Jones JB, Michel RL.** Recurrent neutropenia in a Pomeranian: a case report. J Am Anim Hosp Assoc 1981;17:841–844.

50. **Woldehiwet Z.** The effects of tick-borne fever on some functions of polymorphonuclear cells of sheep. J Comparative Pathology. 1987;97:481–485.

51. **Larsen HJS, Overnes G, Waldeland H, Johansen GM.** Immunosuppression in sheep experimentally infected with Ehrlichia phagocytophila. Res Vet Sci 1994;56:216–224.

52. **Madigan JE.** Veterinary infections with granulocytotropic ehrlichiae, Ehrlichia phagocytophila and Ehrlichia equi. In: Smith BP, ed. Large animal internal medicine: diseases of horses, cattle, sheep, and goats. 2nd ed. St. Louis: Mosby 1996;1244–1245.

53. **Clinkenbeard KD, Cowell RL, Tyler RD.** Disseminated histoplasmosis in cats: 12 cases (1981–1986). J Am Vet Med Assoc 1987;190:1445–1448.

54. **Clinkenbeard KD, Cowell RL, Tyler RD.** Disseminated histoplasmosis in dogs: 12 cases (1981–1986). J Am Vet Med Assoc 1988;193:1443–1447.

55. **Beale KM, Altman D, Clemmons RR, Bolon B.** System toxicosis associated with azathioprine administration in domestic cats. Am J Vet Res 1997;53:1236–1240.

56. **Hammer AS, Couto CG, Filppi J, Getzy D, Shank K.** Efficacy and toxicity of VAC chemotherapy (vincristine, doxorubicin, and cyclophosphamide) in dogs with hemangiosarcoma. J Vet Int Med 1991;5:160–166.

57. **Hauck ML, Price GS, Ogilvie GK, et al.** Phase I evaluation of mitoxantrone alone and combined with whole body hyperthermia in dogs with lymphoma. Int J Hyperthermia 1996;12:309–320.

58. **Henry CJ, Brewer WG Jr, Stutler SA.** Early-onset leukopenia and severe thrombocytopenia following doxorubicin chemotherapy for tonsillar squamous cell carcinoma in a dog. Cornell Vet 1993;83:163–168.

59. **O'Keefe DA, Schaeffer DJ.** Hematologic toxicosis associated with doxorubicin administration in cats. J Vet Int Med 1992;6:276–282.

60. **Morley A, Stohlman F Jr.** Cyclophosphamide-induced cyclical neutropenia. An animal model of a human periodic disease. N Engl J Med 1970;282:643–646.

61. **Gaunt SD, Pierce KR.** Effects of estradiol on hematopoietic and marrow adherent cells of dogs. Am J Vet Res 1986;47:906–909.

62. **Farris GM, Benjamin SA.** Inhibition of myelopoiesis by serum from dogs exposed to estrogen. Am J Vet Res 1993;54:1374–1379.

63. **Farris GM, Benjamin SA.** Inhibition of myelopoiesis by conditioned medium from cultured canine thymic cells exposed to extrogen. Am J Vet Res 1993;54:1366–1373.

64. **Jacobs G, Calvert C, Kaufman A.** Neutropenia and thrombocytopenia in three dogs treated with anticonvulsants. J Am Vet Med Assoc 1998;212:681–684.

65. **MacKay RJ, French TW, Nguyen HT, Mayhew IG.** Effects of large doses of phanylbutazone administration to horses. Am J Vet Res 1983;44:774–780.

66. **Shelton GH, Grant CK, Linenberger ML, Abkowitz JL.** Severe neutropenia associated with griseofulvin therapy in cats with feline immunodeficiency virus infection. J Vet Int Med 1990;4:317–319.

67. **Galey FD.** Disorders caused by toxicants in large animal internal medicine. In: Smith BP, ed. Large animal internal medicine: diseases of horses, cattle, sheep, and goats. 2nd ed. St. Louis, MD:Mosby, 1996;1883.

68. **Wilkins PA, Vaala WE, Zivotofaky D, Twitchell ED.** A herd outbreak of equine leukoencephalomalacia. Cornell Vet 1994;84:53–59.

69. **Jeffers M, Lenghaus C.** Granulocytopaenia and thrombocytopaenia in dairy cattle—a suspected mycotoxicosis. Aust Vet J 1986;63:262–264.

70. **Nicholls TJ, Shiel MJ, Westbury HA, Walker DM.** Granulocytopaenia and thrombocytopaenia in cattle. Aust Vet J 1985;62:67–68.
71. **Sheldon IM.** A field-case of granulocytopenic disease of calves. Vet Rec 1994;135:408.
72. **Weiss DJ, Armstrong PJ, Reimann K.** Bone marrow necrosis in the dog. J Am Vet Med Assoc 1985;187:54–59.
73. **Chickering WP, Prasse KW.** Immune mediated neutropenia in man and animals: a review. Vet Clin Pathol 1981;10:6–16.
74. **Lichtman MA.** Classification and clinical manifestations of neutrophil disorders. In: Williams WJ, ed. Hematology. New York: McGraw-Hill 1990;802–806.
75. **Chickering WR. Brown J, Prasse KW, Dawe DL.** Effects of heterologous antineutrophil antibody in the cat. Am J Vet Res 1985;46:1815–1819.
76. **Chickering WR, Prasse KW, Dawe DL.** Development and clinical application of methods for detection of antineutrophil antibody in serum of the cat. Am J Vet Res 1985;46:1809–1814.
77. **Jain NC, Vegad JL, Kono CS.** Methods for detection of immune-mediated neutropenia in horses, using antineutrophil serum of rabbit origin. Am J Vet Res 1990;51:1026–1031.
78. **Jain NC, Vegad JL, Dhawedkar RG, Kono CS, Kabbur MB.** Ultrastructural and biochemical observations on antineutrophil antibody- and complement-induced immuno-injury to equine neutrophils. J Comp Pathol 1991;104:389–402.
79. **Jain NC, Stott JL, Vegad JL, Dhawedkar RG.** Detection of anti-equine neutrophil antibody by use of flow cytometry. Am J Vet Res 1991;52:1883–1890.
80. **Hammond WP, Csiba E, Canin A, et al.** Chronic neutropenia. A new canine model induced by human granulocyte colony-stimulating factor. J Clin Invest 1991;87:704–710.
81. **Kyle RA, Linman JW.** Chronic idiopathic neutropenia. A newly recognized entity? N Engl J Med 1968;279:1015–1019.
82. **Swenson CL, Kociba GJ, Arnold P.** Chronic idiopathic neutropenia in a cat. J Vet Int Med 1988;2:100–102.
83. **Gainer JH, Guarnieri J, Das NK.** Neutropenia in iron deficient baby pigs. Abstract of papers presented at the 65th Annual Meeting of the Conference of Research Workers in Animal Disease, Chicago, IL. 1984;314.
84. **Gainer JH, Guarnieri J.** Effects of poly I:C in porcine iron deficient neutropenia. Cornell Vet 1985;75:454–465.
85. **Schuller-Levis G, Mehta PD, Rudelli R, Sturman J.** Immunologic consequences of taurine deficiency in cats. J Leukoc Biol 1990;47:321–331.

CHAPTER 54

Neutrophil Functional Abnormalities

• CLAIRE B. ANDREASEN and JAMES A. ROTH

Neutrophils are phagocytic leukocytes that are an essential component of host defense against many bacterial, viral, and fungal infections. The analogous cells in avians, reptiles, and several mammalian species are termed heterophils because of the different staining qualities of the granules. Mammalian neutrophils and neutrophil function are discussed in this chapter. Any factor that interferes with neutrophil production or suppresses neutrophil function rapidly makes the animal more susceptible to infectious diseases.[1]

Neutrophil function may be decreased in individuals that have genetic defects, inadequate nutrition, or in individuals exposed to infectious agents, pharmaceuticals, or various toxins. Defects in neutrophil function may range from mild to severe. Mild defects in neutrophil function, such as that induced by cortisol,[2] leave animals with a moderately increased susceptibility to an infectious challenge. Severe defects in neutrophil function, as in patients that have leukocyte adhesion deficiency (LAD), are life threatening owing to increased susceptibility to infection with pathogens or opportunistic microorganisms.[1] An evaluation of neutrophil function is indicated when there is evidence of increased susceptibility to infection, the presence of chronic recurrent infections, or a poor response to the treatment of infectious diseases. The physiology of neutrophil function recently has been reviewed,[1] and several references describe methods for evaluation of neutrophil function.[3–6]

Neutrophils undergo a complex series of events in their role to control bacterial, viral, and fungal infections. These events include adherence to endothelial cells; exit from postcapillary venules by means of diapedesis; directed migration in response to chemotactic factors; adherence to and ingestion of particles; generation of oxygen radicals, hydrogen peroxide, aldehydes, and hypochlorous acid; release of enzymes from lysosomes; and cytotoxic destruction of antibody-coated and foreign cells. These events are regulated by a series of intracellular signaling mechanisms.

When a thorough evaluation of neutrophil function is conducted, each of these events should be evaluated. There is no single assay that can adequately screen for all defects in neutrophil function. Even to evaluate a single function, such as bacterial killing, various assays are needed because the neutrophil has redundant bactericidal mechanisms that are important for killing different bacteria. The lack of a bactericidal defect in neutrophils for one species of bacteria may be incorrectly interpreted as meaning there is no defect in neutrophil function.

A logical approach to screening for defects in neutrophil function is to use a battery of assays that evaluate each major step in neutrophil activity. Assays that are useful in screening for defects in neutrophil function are listed in Table 54.1. Considerations during testing are

1. to use a sufficiently large number of animals to satisfy the requirements for statistical evaluation.
2. to use a second tier of assays to characterize the molecular basis for a defect in neutrophil function detected with this battery of assays.
3. to assay neutrophils from normal animals and from patients in parallel on the same days; this is important because neutrophil function tests often have significant day-to-day variability.
4. to perform neutrophil function assays soon after blood collection; this is essential because neutrophils have a short life span.
5. to transport, store, and handle the normal control neutrophils (if necessary to transport blood long distances or to hold it overnight) in the same manner as those from the test subject.

NEUTROPHIL TESTING

Neutrophils (and heterophils) from various species behave similarly in the inflammatory response and the control of infectious diseases, but species differences do exist. The basic assays listed in Table 54.1 generally work in the various species in which they have been attempted. However, modifications of assays and neutrophil isolation techniques often are required for each individual species.[6–8] There may be wide variation between species reference intervals for various neutrophil function assays. Reference interval values for neutrophil

TABLE 54.1   Summary of Tests Used to Evaluate Neutrophil Function and Principle Behind Each of the Tests

Neutrophil Function Evaluated	Neutrophil Function Test	Principle of the Test
Adherence	Flow cytometry to quantitate surface expression of L-selectin and/or β_2 integrins[9]	L-selectin mediates rolling adhesion to endothelial cells; β_2 integrins mediate tight adhesion to endothelial cells
	Adherence to plastic, glass, fiber columns, or endothelial cell monolayers[5,90]	Thought to correlate with adherence to endothelium
Migration/chemotaxis	Boyden Chambers[91]	Neutrophils migrate through a porous filter either randomly or toward a chemotactic factor on the other side of the membrane
	Migration under agarose[10]	Neutrophils migrate under agar in a petri plate either randomly or toward a gradient of chemotactic factors placed in an adjacent well in the agar
Ingestion	Microscopic observation of ingestion of particles[92]	Particle ingestion is directly observed
	Ingestion of radiolabeled *S. aureus*[4]	Extracellular *S. aureus* is removed with lysostaphin; uptake of radioactivity is quantitated
	Flow cytometric quantitation of ingestion of fluorescent particles[93,94]	Flow cytometer quantitates particle ingestion by individual cells
	Ingestion of live bacteria[95]	Perform colony counts to quantitate bacteria removed from the supernatant or released from lysed neutrophils
Oxidative metabolism	Cytochrome C reduction or nitroblue tetrazolium reduction[96]	Cytochrome C and nitroblue tetrazolium are reduced by superoxide anion causing a change in color and light absorption.
	Chemiluminescence[4,97]	The oxidative burst of metabolism generates photons of light that can be detected with a photomultiplier tube
	Spectrofluorometric measurement of kinetics of oxidant production[98]	H_2O_2 oxidizes p-hydroxy phenylacetate to a fluorescent product
Degranulation	Myeloperoxidase (MPO) release[99]	MPO released from primary granules with H_2O_2 oxidizes 3, 3'; 5,5' tetramethylbenzidine resulting in a color change
	Microscopic observation of loss of granules[100]	Direct observation by electron microscopy and morphometry
	Spectrofluorometric measurement of elastase release[101]	Elastase released from primary granules acts on a substrate to release a fluorescent product
MPO–H_2O_2–halide antibacterial system	Iodination[102]	MPO released from primary granules catalyzes a reaction involving H_2O_2 generated during the oxidative burst resulting in binding of ^{125}I to protein
Bacterial killing	Bactericidal activity[92]	Perform colony counts to quantitate bacteria remaining alive
	Tetrazolium dye reduction[103]	Bacteria that are not killed reduce tetrazolium dye during metabolism
	Acridine orange[104]	Live bacteria in the phagosome fluoresce green, and dead bacteria fluoresce red after incubation in acridine orange
	Radioassay for ^3H-thymidine incorporation[92]	Live bacteria incorporates ^3H thymidine into DNA during growth
Cytotoxicity	^{51}Chromium release[15]	Live target cells retain ^{51}Cr intracellulary, dead cells release ^{51}Cr

function must be established for each species, for each laboratory, and even for each day that the assays are run within a particular laboratory.

Adherence

To control infection, neutrophils emigrate from the bloodstream into the tissues; therefore, they must be able to adhere to endothelial cells. On their surface, normal neutrophils have the adhesion molecule L-selectin that loosely adheres them to endothelial cells, resulting in margination or in rolling adhesion of neutrophils to endothelial cells. If an inflammatory signal is received by endothelial cells and neutrophils, then the neutrophil upregulates expression of beta 2 (β2) integrin adhesion molecules that mediate tight adhesion of neutrophils to endothelial cells. The tightly adherent neutrophil then leaves the bloodstream by diapedesis and enters the tissues. The surface expression of L-selectin and β2 integrins can be quantitated with specific monoclonal antibodies and flow cytometry.[9] There also are several in vitro assays in which neutrophil adherence to plastic, glass, fiber columns, or endothelial-cell monolayers are used as a correlate of neutrophil adherence to endothelial cells in vivo (Table 54.1).

Chemotaxis and Migration

After neutrophils arrive in the tissues, they must migrate to the site of infection. This requires functional microtubules and microfilaments for extension of pseudopodia and forward flow of cytoplasm. Chemotactic factors generated at the site of infection form a gradient that the neutrophil is capable of following. In the absence of chemotactic factors, neutrophils move in an undirected or random fashion. Neutrophil random migration and chemotaxis can be evaluated with Boyden chambers in which the neutrophils migrate through porous filters or with an under agarose technique in which neutrophils placed in petri plate agar wells migrate under the agarose.[10] Chemotactic factors (chemoattractants) can be placed on the opposite side of the membrane in the Boyden chambers or in an adjacent well in the under-agarose technique.

Phagocytosis

After neutrophils arrive at the site of infection they must be capable of ingesting (phagocytosing) infectious agents to kill them efficiently. Neutrophils are capable of phagocytosing particles that are more hydrophobic than their own membrane. To ingest hydrophilic particles efficiently, these particles must be opsonized with either an appropriate class of antibody or with the C3b component of complement. There are several methods listed in Table 54.1 for evaluating neutrophil phagocytosis. For the phagocytic assays, it is important to differentiate surface adherence from true internalization of the particles in a cytoplasmic phagosome.

Bacterial Killing

After the neutrophil ingests the infectious agent, there are two steps that are important for efficient killing of the agent. These steps include the oxidative burst of metabolism and release of lysosomal (granule) contents into the phagosome. The oxidative burst of metabolism is rapidly initiated on contact of the neutrophil with an appropriately opsonized particle. This activates a multicomponent nicotinamide adenine dinucleotide phosphate (NADPH) oxidase enzyme in the membrane of the neutrophil. This enzyme converts oxygen into a superoxide anion (O_{2-}) that spontaneously dismutates to form hydrogen peroxide (H_2O_2). The O_{2-} and H_2O_2 react together to form hydroxyl radicals (OH^-). These are all potent unstable molecules that are capable of directly damaging bacterial organisms and result in the generation of aldehydes. In the presence of myeloperoxidase (MPO), they also cause the generation of hypochlorous acid ($HOCl^-$). All of these components are capable of damaging or destroying infectious agents, as well as host tissues. Several assays have been used to evaluate the burst of neutrophil oxidative metabolism (Table 54.1).

The nonoxidative mechanisms of bacterial killing involve various enzymes and granule cationic proteins and peptides. Defensins, described in several species, are cationic peptides stored in lysosomes that insert into microbial target-cell membranes to increase cell permeability and to act as opsonins to increase phagocytosis.[11] Release of neutrophil lysosomal contents can be quantitated by measurement of the presence or activity of granule contents in cell supernatants when the cells are treated with cytochalasin B and stimulated to induce degranulation to the cell exterior. MPO and elastase are some of the more commonly measured granule contents. Degranulation also can be evaluated with an electron microscope to observe for the loss of neutrophil intracytoplasmic lysosomal granules.

The most potent oxidative killing mechanism that neutrophils have apparently is the myeloperoxidase–hydrogen peroxide–halide (MPO–H_2O_2–halide) antibacterial system. By allowing neutrophils to ingest opsonized particles in the presence of Na[125]I, it is possible to directly measure the activity of the MPO–H_2O_2–halide system. This iodination reaction depends on degranulation and the burst of oxidative metabolism. Avian heterophils do not stain for[12] or have a demonstrable chemical reaction for MPO[13] and have minimal oxidant production compared with mammals.[8] It has been thought that avian heterophils primarily use oxygen-independent killing, but recently the demonstration of a heterophil DNA sequence with homology to human MPO has renewed investigations into oxygen-dependent bactericidal pathways.[14]

Bactericidal assays are typically performed by incubating neutrophils in the presence of bacteria that have been opsonized with antibody or complement for various time periods. The decrease in bacterial numbers from the supernatant can be quantitated, as well as the numbers of viable bacteria released from neutrophils after neutrophil lysis. This gives an indication of the proportion of bacteria that have been removed and killed by phagocytosis. When performing bactericidal assays using colony counts, it is important to avoid agglutinating the bacteria during the opsonization process. Agglutination reduces the number of colony-forming units observed, because a clump of agglutinated bacteria is only capable of forming one confluent colony. If a defect in bactericidal activity is observed, further tests are needed to determine the nature of the defect. Bactericidal assays (Table 54.1), which depend on metabolic activity of surviving bacteria, do not have the same susceptibility to artifact induced by agglutination. If bactericidal activity seems normal, it is possible there are serious defects in neutrophil function, but the bacteria involved in the assay are easily killed by additional functional mechanisms.

Cytotoxicity

Neutrophils are capable of attacking and killing target cells that are coated with antibody. This is called antibody-dependent cell-mediated cytotoxicity (ADCC) and is thought to be an important mechanism for killing certain virus-infected cells. Neutrophils attach to the antibody coating the target cell through fragment, crystallizable (Fc) receptors in the neutrophil membrane. The subsequent generation of oxygen radicals and release of granule contents contribute to the destruction of the target cell. This can be evaluated by prelabeling target cells with ^{51}Cr. The ^{51}Cr is retained in the cytoplasm of live cells but is released into the supernatant once a cell dies.[15] In some species, neutrophils can lyse target cells without antibody, and this is evaluated by antibody-independent cell-mediated cytotoxicity (AICC) assays.[16]

NEUTROPHIL FUNCTION DEFECTS

Emphasis in this section is primarily on the qualitative defects in neutrophil function or the findings of normal neutrophil function in animals in which the analogous syndrome in human beings produces neutrophil dysfunction. To date, chronic granulomatous disease or MPO deficiency seen in human beings has not been documented in animals. Because neutrophil kinetics are covered in Chapter 46, quantitative neutrophil defects primarily will be discussed when neutrophil function also has been examined (Table 54.2).

Age-Related Neutrophil Function

In general, neutrophil function is thought to increase during the first weeks to months of life. There are many studies, especially in large animals, that have variable results for individual function tests but tend to support the assumption that neutrophils from neonates have functional deficits when compared with adult animals.

Young and aged beagles were found to have comparable capacity to generate a respiratory burst.[17] Age-

| TABLE 54.2 | Overview of the Classification of Neutrophil Qualitative Disorders |

Qualitative Disorders of Neutrophils

A. Defective adhesion of neutrophils
1. Bovine leukocyte adhesion deficiency[38,41]
2. Canine leukocyte adhesion deficiency (canine granulocytopathy syndrome)[42–44]

B. Defective chemotaxis/migration
1. Feline leukemia virus[82]
2. Failure of immune production of cytotaxins[5]
3. Inhibitory factors from cells or bacteria[5]
4. Canine pyoderma (variable results)[75,76]

C. Defective phagocytosis
1. Canine leukocyte adhesion deficiency (canine granulocytopathy syndrome)[42–44]
2. Bovine leukocyte adhesion deficiency[38,41]
3. Failure of opsonization or generation of complement[5,70]

D. Defective microbial killing/respiratory burst
1. Feline leukemia virus[83]
2. Canine leukocyte adhesion deficiency (canine granulocytopathy syndrome)[42–44]
3. Bovine leukocyte adhesion deficiency[38,41]
4. Cyclic neutropenia of Gray-Collie dogs[27,31,34]

E. Multiple or mixed functional disorders
1. Nutritional[48–50]
2. Drugs[64,65]
3. Infectious[72–74,80,82]

F. Abnormal structure of the nucleus or an organelle
1. Pelger–Huët anomaly—Majority of heterozygous dogs have no functional defects[35,36]
2. Chédiak–Higashi syndrome—Species variable functional defects[26,28]
3. Birman cat neutrophil granulation anomaly—No functional defects[45]

related differences were not found for random or directed neutrophil migration, but a gender difference was observed with possible progesterone suppression of chemotaxis.[18] It was thought that these differences were too subtle to have a clinical effect.

In calves, neutrophils from neonates produce less superoxide anion in response to phorbol myristate acetate (PMA) than neutrophils from either fetal calves (210 to 220 days gestation) or adult cattle.[19] Neutrophils from neonatal calves also have decreased Fc receptor expression, decreased capping of concanavalin A (Con A) binding sites, and decreased MPO content compared with neutrophils from adult cattle.[20] Deficits in superoxide anion generation, iodination, ADCC, chemotaxis, random migration, and MPO content were found in calves as old as 4 months of age compared with adult cattle.[21,22]

Foal neutrophil function is influenced by age with decreased killing capacity and increased phagocytic capacity until 113 days of age, after which a reversal in this trend occurred.[23] The values for foal neutrophil phagocytosis and bacterial killing were similar to adult horses. Neonatal foals varied in their neutrophil killing of *Rhodoccocus equi* but had similar bactericidal function compared with young and adult horses.[24]

Hereditary or Genetic Neutrophil Abnormalities

Chédiak–Higashi Syndrome Described in human beings, Chédiak–Higashi syndrome is inherited as an autosomal recessive trait with an analogous syndrome in mink; Arctic foxes; Persian cats; Hereford, Japanese black,[25] and Brangus cattle; beige mice; and a killer whale.[26,27] These species have abnormal lysosomal granule formation and degranulation, and in mink, mice, cattle, cats, and human beings abnormal microtubule formation that can result in a decreased chemotactic responsiveness has been reported.[26,28] Abnormal giant granules appear to occur after fusion of lysosomes in neutrophils, eosinophils, renal tubular cells, epithelial cells, and Kupffer cells of humans, mink, cats, and cattle (Fig. 54.1). Pink to magenta staining characteristics of the granules are similar in all species. Neutrophil lysosomal calcium transport and bacterial killing are defective in human beings and mice.[26,29] In some cattle breeds[25,27] and mice,[26] an increased susceptibility to bacterial infections caused by impaired neutrophil function has been demonstrated. Initially, neutrophil dysfunction was not detected in cats,[26] but recent studies have documented neutrophil defects, including chemotaxis, for which improvement occurred after treatment with recombinant canine granulocyte colony-stimulating factor.[28] In most species, there is an increased tendency to bleed because of platelet granule defects[25] and partial oculocutaneous albinism caused by abnormal melanin distribution.[26] The beige mouse and the Aleutian mink exemplify the hair coat pigment dilution seen in the syndrome. Diagnosis is based on pigment dilution, presence of giant granules, hemorrhagic tendencies, and possible increased susceptibility to infections.

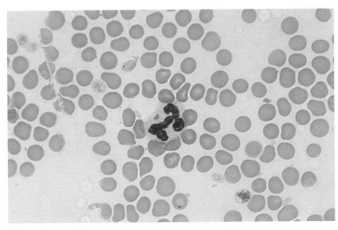

FIGURE 54.1 Giant lysosomes in the neutrophil cytoplasm of a cat that has Chédiak–Higashi.

Cyclic Hemopoiesis in Gray Collies (Gray-Collie Syndrome, Canine Cyclic Neutropenia) Cyclic hematopoiesis is an inherited autosomal recessive immunodeficiency characterized by a profound cyclic neutropenia, overwhelming recurrent bacterial infections, bleeding, and coat color dilution.[30] The molecular basis is a cyclic bone marrow maturation defect at the level of the pluripotential hemopoietic stem cells.[27,31,32] It is suggested that there is a defect in the granulocyte-colony-stimulating factor (G-CSF) signal-transduction pathway.[33] Arrest of neutrophil maturation occurs at regular cycles of 11 to 14 day intervals, and the peripheral neutropenia lasts 3 to 4 days and is followed by a neutrophilia. All other hemopoietic cells, including lymphocytes, are cyclic with the same intervals but occur at different times compared with the neutropenic phase. Hemopoietic growth factors (e.g., erythropoietin) and other hormones (e.g., cortisol) also have been demonstrated to have a cyclic pattern.[31] Affected puppies often die at birth or during the first week, and rarely live longer than 1 year. Surviving dogs may be stunted and weak and, during periods of neutropenia, may develop serious recurrent bacterial infections characterized by fever, septicemia, pneumonia, and gastroenteritis. They also develop amyloidosis in many tissues, including kidney and liver, resulting in renal disease and coagulopathies.[27] All affected dogs have a diluted coat color. Diagnosis is based on clinical signs and repeated serial complete blood counts over a minimum 3- to 6-week period. Increased susceptibility to bacterial infections is caused by the neutropenia and defective bactericidal activity because the affected neutrophils have decreased MPO activity.[34] Bone marrow transplantation at an early age eliminates the cyclic hemopoiesis and effects a clinical cure. In one study, administration of human recombinant G-CSF (rhG-CSF) temporarily eliminated the cyclic hemopoiesis until the dogs were assumed to have produced neutralizing antibodies.[31] Canine G-CSF also has been used for long-term therapy.[32]

Pelger–Huët Anomaly An inherited condition of human beings, rabbits, dogs, and cats, Pelger-Huët anomaly is characterized by failure of granulocytes to lobulate from the band form to the segmented form (Fig. 54.2).[27] Because megakaryocytes also are hyposegmented, this suggests a stem-cell defect.[27] Inheritance appears to be by means of autosomal dominance in most species. Heterozygote dogs do not exhibit clinical signs, and this anomaly is usually an incidental laboratory finding. The granulocytes, particularly the neutrophils, are hyposegmented, and the chromatin is condensed; the complete blood count shows an apparent pseudo left shift with a normal total leukocyte count. Recognition of this syndrome is important to prevent an incorrect association with diseases that do produce a left shift. Affected dog breeds include Australian shepherds; Australian blue heelers; Basenjis, border collies; cocker spaniels; black and tan, bluetick, and redbone coonhounds; German shepherds; English-American (Walker) foxhounds; Samoyeds; and mongrels.[27] Initial investiga-

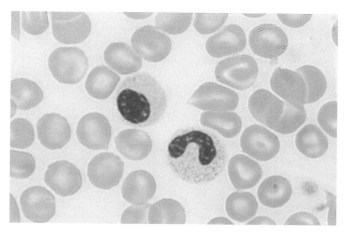

FIGURE 54.2 Band and myelocyte neutrophils from a border collie that has Pelger–Huët anomaly. (Dr. K. S. Latimer, University of Georgia, Athens, Georgia.)

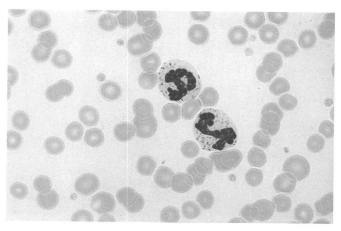

FIGURE 54.3 Birman cat neutrophil granulation anomaly with azurophilic cytoplasmic granules. (Dr. K. S. Latimer, University of Georgia, Athens, Georgia.)

tions indicate decreased neutrophil chemotaxis in affected foxhounds,[35] but subsequent studies did not support this finding in other breeds.[36] Leukocyte function, examined in affected dogs, indicated no significant difference in neutrophil adherence, random movement, chemotaxis, phagocytosis, and bacterial killing.[36] Additionally, lymphocyte blastogenesis was not decreased. The homozygous state, described in rabbits and in one kitten,[37] is usually lethal and associated with skeletal deformities and increased susceptibility to infection. The term pseudo-Pelger-Huët anomaly refers to acquired hyposegmentation of granulocytes secondary to chronic infections, viral diseases, drug therapy, and neoplasia.

Bovine Leukocyte Adhesion Deficiency

An autosomal recessive disorder that occurs in Holstein cattle that have the homozygous genotype resulting in premature death is called bovine leukocyte adhesion deficiency (BLAD).[38] The leukocytes lack or have partial absence of adhesion glycoproteins (β integrins) that are essential for normal leukocyte to endothelial adherence and emigration. The genetic defect can be traced to a common sire and is identified as a single amino acid substitution in a 26 amino acid sequence of the common β subunit found in all 3 members of the leukocyte integrin family.[39] The disease is characterized by recurrent bacterial infections, persistent neutrophilia (often exceeding 100,000 neutrophils/μL), increased lymphocytes, and death usually between 2 weeks and 8 months of age. Calves often are stunted and have recurrent pneumonia, ulcerative stomatitis, enteritis, and periodontitis.[40] Tissue examination reveals the existence of few neutrophils except within vessel lumens, because they persist in circulation and are unable to enter the tissues. Neutrophil functional defects include decreased adherence, phagocytosis, bacterial killing, superoxide generation, chemiluminescence activity, and MPO-catalyzed iodination.[41] Testing is available to detect carrier animals.

Canine Leukocyte Adhesion Deficiency (Canine Granulocytopathy Syndrome)

A defect in neutrophil function was identified in an Irish setter that had recurrent bacterial infections and a persistent leukocytosis. Defects in bactericidal activity, reduced glucose oxidation by the hexose monophosphate shunt, and an increased capacity to reduce nitroblue tetrazolium dye were documented.[42] This syndrome was probably similar to an additional Irish Setter in which CD11/CD18 antibodies failed to detect expression of leukocyte Mo1, leukocyte function-associated antigen-1 (LFA-1), and Leu M5 glycoproteins, indicating a deficiency of the common β integrin subunit. This dog had defects in neutrophil chemotaxis, induced aggregation, and phagocytosis of opsonized particles.[43] A litter of Irish Setter puppies with the same defect had decreased adherence, phagocytosis, and a defective respiratory burst, but normal random migration and chemotactic responses.[44]

Birman Cat Neutrophil Granulation Anomaly

Inherited as an autosomal recessive trait in some Birman cats, Birman cat neutrophil granulation anomaly is an abnormality of neutrophil granules, characterized by fine, azurophilic (nonmetachromatic) granules similar to progranulocyte granules in the bone marrow myeloid precursors (Fig. 54.3).[45] Neutrophil ultrastructure, cytochemistry, phagocytosis, oxidative metabolism, and bactericidal activity were reported to be within normal limits.[45] These cats are not predisposed to clinical disease. The neutrophil granulation has to be differentiated from toxic granulation and mucopolysaccharidosis types VI and VII.

Primary Ciliary Dyskinesia

A defective microtubular system in the respiratory cilia is the defining characteristic of primary ciliary dyskinesia. Some affected dogs had increased neutrophil function caused by breed differences or concurrent bacterial infections. Decreased function was not found in dogs that have congenital ciliary dyskinesia, indicating that the neutrophils do not have the microtubular defect.[46,47]

Nutritional Influences on Neutrophil Function

Many nutritional studies of neutrophil function have involved large-animal species. Nutritional deficiencies also have been shown to be associated with increased incidence of infectious diseases and decreased neutrophil function in ruminants. Nutritional deficiencies that have been shown to decrease neutrophil function in ruminants include deficiencies in copper,[48] cobalt,[49] selenium,[50] molybdenum, thiamine, and sulfur.[48]

Hormonal, Endocrinal, and Pharmaceutical Influences on Neutrophil Function

Glucocorticoids   Because of downregulation of neutrophil adherence molecules, glucocorticoids are reported to decrease neutrophil egress from vessels.[9] In human beings, glucocorticoids result in impaired locomotion, chemotaxis, ingestion, degranulation, and aggregation.[51] Results in animal studies have been mixed, probably owing to species differences; dosage, duration, and type of glucocorticoid administered; study criteria; if endogenous cortisol was evaluated; or the type of stressors imposed. Stress-induced cortisol during pig blood sampling did not affect neutrophil phagocytosis,[52] and swine neutrophils have been shown to be resistant to glucocorticoid suppression.[53] Elevated cortisol levels are known to suppress neutrophil function in cattle.[2,54] Dexamethasone is capable of strongly suppressing neutrophil function, as well as other aspects of immune function, in ruminants.[9,54] The alteration of neutrophil function is mediated by at least 2 mechanisms. Dexamethasone treatment of cattle inhibits the production of lipoxygenase products of arachidonic acid metabolism in neutrophils and is responsible for a decrease in neutrophil-oxidative metabolism and iodination activity.[55] Suppression of neutrophil ADCC activity and the enhancement of random migration observed after dexamethasone treatment in cattle apparently is mediated through glucocorticoid effects on monocytes that subsequently release factors altering neutrophil function.[56] In horses, random migration, bacterial phagocytosis, and bacterial killing were influenced, but not impaired, after one dose of hydrocortisone sodium succinate.[57]

Progesterone and Estrogen   Administration of pharmacologic dosages of progesterone to bovine steers has been shown to inhibit neutrophil iodination and enhance neutrophil random migration.[58] This correlates with alterations of neutrophil function during the normal estrous cycle in cows. When progesterone is high during the estrous cycle, neutrophil-oxidative metabolism, iodination, and ADCC are depressed, whereas random migration is enhanced.[59] Bacterial killing by neutro-

phils is unchanged in ovariectomized mares given estradiol or progesterone.[60] Bovine neutrophil function is suppressed during the periparturient period and this may be related to fluctuations in hormone concentrations.[61] This may be partially responsible for the increased incidence of mastitis during this time period.

Diabetes Mellitus   Neutrophil adherence, random migration, and chemotaxis were found to be comparable in control dogs and in subject dogs with well-controlled diabetes.[62,63] Neutrophil adherence was significantly decreased in subject dogs with poorly controlled diabetes.[63]

Drugs and Toxins   Certain antibiotics, including tetracycline, gentamicin, and particularly chloramphenicol, also have been shown to inhibit bovine neutrophil function.[64,65] Numerous drugs and toxins have an affect on neutrophil kinetics by means of bone marrow suppression. These affects often lead to pancytopenias and a quantitative neutrophil depression. Examples would include estrogen, chemotherapy drugs, phenylbutazone, anticonvulsants, cephalosporins, chloramphenicol, and bracken fern, to name a few.[27]

Humoral Immune Dysfunction

Immune-Mediated Neutropenia   A presumptive diagnosis of primary immune-mediated neutropenia (autoantibody neutropenia) may be made when a profound neutropenia exists with no associated diseases to explain the neutropenia and other hemopoietic elements are unaffected. Autoantibodies also may produce qualitative defects in neutrophil function, including defects similar to LAD and decreased bacterial phagocytosis.[66] Confirmation of the diagnosis requires demonstration of antineutrophil antibodies in the serum or on the neutrophil surface by leukoagglutination or immunofluorescent techniques.[27,67] Secondary immune-mediated neutropenia may occur in association with other immune diseases such as systemic lupus erythematosus, immune-mediated thrombocytopenias or anemias, lymphoma, rheumatoid arthritis, or drug therapy, as occurs in human beings.[68] Several reports have discussed the detection of antineutrophil antibodies in domestic species.[67,69] Detection of autoimmune neutropenia has been reviewed in human beings and these techniques may find future application in veterinary medicine.[66,68]

Immune Humoral Dysfunction   Failure to generate complement components[70] or antibodies for opsonization are humoral abnormalities associated with neutrophil dysfunction, especially phagocytosis. Failure to generate chemoattractants or cytotaxins impair neutrophil migration.[5]

Infectious Diseases

Bacteria and Endotoxin   Bacterial infections may increase or decrease neutrophil function, depending on bacterial virulence factors and which cytokines or bacterial products are produced.[71] Various recurrent bacterial infections or chronic bacterial diseases have been attributed to underlying granulocyte defects.[72–74] Neutrophil function in canine staphylococcal pyoderma has been examined, because neutrophil defects have been documented in human beings that have this syndrome. Neutrophil chemotactic defects have been documented in dogs that have bacterial pyodermas.[75] Additional studies of canine pyodermas failed to find differences in chemotaxis, phagocytosis, and bacterial killing between affected and healthy dogs.[76] The variable results may be because of the multiple factors that underlie the pyodermas and the sampling times (active versus quiescent infections). Virulence factors from bacterial pathogens also have been shown to interfere directly with neutrophil function. For example, *Pasteurella haemolytica* has a leukotoxin that is cytotoxic for bovine neutrophils as well as other leukocytes.[77] Also, capsular material and lipopolysaccharide from *P. haemolytica* have been shown to impair bovine neutrophil function.[78,79]

Viral Diseases In humans and in animals, viral diseases can induce depression of neutrophil function.[80] Feline leukemia virus is known to have various effects on hematologic cells. Cyclic neutropenia (from 8 to 16 days), in combination with other peripheral blood cells, has been observed in 3 cats.[81] Neutrophils from clinically affected viremic cats had significantly lower chemotactic responses than did cells from subclinical viremic cats.[82] Feline leukemia positive cats also have a decreased chemiluminescent response compared with healthy age-matched control cats.[83]

Some viral diseases in cattle produce decreased neutrophil functions. Cattle that are persistently infected with bovine viral diarrhea (BVD) virus after in utero infection have decreased random migration, *Staphylococcus aureus* ingestion, superoxide anion generation, iodination, AICC, and cytoplasmic calcium flux in response to stimuli.[84] Nonpersistent infection with BVD virus and exposure to modified-live BVD vaccines also suppress neutrophil function.[85] Infection of cattle with parainfluenza 3 virus results in decreased oxidative metabolism and iodination activity in neutrophils.[86] Infection with bovine herpes virus 1 results in reduced neutrophil random migration but enhanced neutrophil *S. aureus* ingestion.[86] Infection with bovine immunodeficiency-like virus ([BIV], a bovine lentivirus) is associated with a significant decrease in neutrophil ADCC and iodination activities but, as yet, has not been associated with increased susceptibility to infectious disease.[87]

Parasitic Diseases Infection with coccidia has been shown to suppress neutrophil function in cattle and to be associated with increased susceptibility to bacterial pneumonia. Both subclinical and clinical infections with *Eimeria* sp. were found to be associated with decreased neutrophil-oxidative metabolism and iodination activity.[88] In a dog infected with *Prototheca zopfii*, patient serum resulted in inhibition of chemotaxis.[89]

REFERENCES

1. **Naussef WM, Clark RA.** Granulocytic phagocytes. In: Mandell GL, Dolin R, Bennett JE, eds. Principles and practice of infectious diseases. 5th ed. New York: Churchill Livingstone, 2000;89–111.
2. **Roth JA, Kaeberle ML, Hsu WH.** Effects of ACTH administration on bovine polymorphonuclear leukocyte function and lymphocyte blastogenesis. Am J Vet Res 1982;43:412–416.
3. **Metcalf JA, Gallin JI, Nauseef WM, et al.** Laboratory manual of neutrophil function. New York: Raven Press, 1986.
4. **Roth JA, Kaeberle ML.** Evaluation of bovine polymorphonuclear leukocyte function. Vet Immunol Immunopathol 1981;2:157–174.
5. **Smith GS, Lumsden JH.** Review of neutrophil adherence, chemotaxis, phagocytosis and killing. Vet Immunol Immunopathol 1983;4:177–236.
6. **Barta O.** Veterinary clinical immunology laboratory. 2. Blacksburg, VA: BAR-LAB 1993; B2-1–B3-29.
7. **Styrt B.** Species variation in neutrophil biochemistry and function. J Leukoc Biol 1989;46:63–74.
8. **Brooks RL, Bounous DI, Andreasen CB.** Functional comparison of avian heterophils with human and canine neutrophils. Comp Haematol Int 1996;6:153–159.
9. **Burton JL, Kehrli M, Kapil S, Horst RL.** Regulation of L-selection and CD18 on bovine neutrophils by glucocorticoids: effects of cortisol and dexamethasone. J Leukoc Biol 1995;57:317–325.
10. **Nelson RD, Quie PG, Simmons RL.** Chemotaxis under agarose: a new and simple method for measuring chemotaxis and spontaneous migration of human polymorphonuclear leukocytes and monocytes. J Immunol 1975;115:1650–1656.
11. **Evans EW, Harmon BG.** A review of antimicrobial peptides: defensins and related cationic peptides. Vet Clin Pathol 1995;24:109–116.
12. **Andreasen CB, Latimer KS.** Cytochemical staining characteristics of chicken heterophils and eosinophils. Vet Clin Pathol 1990;19:51–54.
13. **Brune K, Spitznagel JK.** Peroxidaseless chicken leukocytes: isolation and characterization of antibacterial granules. J Infect Dis 1973;127:84–94.
14. **Lam KM.** Myeloperoxidase activity in chicken heterophils and adherent cells. Vet Immunol Immunopathol 1997;57:327–335.
15. **Wardley RC, Babiuk LA, Rouse BT.** Polymorph-mediated antibody-dependent cytotoxicity–modulation of activity by drugs and immune interferon. Can J Microbiol 1976;22:1222–1228.
16. **Lukacs K, Roth JA, Kaeberle ML.** Activation of neutrophils by antigen-induced lymphokine with emphasis on antibody-independent cytotoxicity. J Leukoc Biol 1985;38:557–572.
17. **Johnson DD, Renshaw HW, Warner DH, Browder EJ, Williams JD.** Characteristics of the phagocytically induced respiratory burst in leukocytes from young adult and aged beagle dogs. Gerontology 1984;30:167–177.
18. **Krogsgarrd-Thomsen M, Strom H.** Biological variation in random and leukotriene B4-directed migration of canine neutrophils. Vet Immunol Immunopathol 1989;21:219–224.
19. **Clifford CB, Slauson DO, Neilsen NR, Suyemoto MM, Zwahlen RD, Schlafer DH.** Ontogeny of inflammatory cell responsiveness: superoxide anion generation by phorbol ester-stimulated fetal, neonatal, and adult bovine neutrophils. Inflammation 1989;13:221–231.
20. **Zwahlen RD, Wyder-Walther M, Roth DR.** Fc receptor expression, concanavalin A capping, and enzyme content of bovine neonatal neutrophils: A comparative study with adult cattle. J Leukoc Biol 1992;51:264–269.
21. **Hauser MA, Koob MD, Roth JA.** Variation of neutrophil function with age in calves. Am J Vet Res 1986;47:152–153.
22. **Lee CC, Roth JA.** Differences in neutrophil function in young and mature cattle and their response to IFN-gamma. Comp Haematol Int 1992; 2:140–147.
23. **Wichtel MG, Anderson KL, Johnson TV, Nathan U, Smith L.** Influence of age on neutrophil function in foals. Equine Vet J 1991;23:466–469.
24. **Martens JG, Martens RJ, Renshaw HW.** *Rhodococcus (Corynebacterium) equi*: Bactericidal capacity of neutrophils from neonatal and adult horses. Am J Vet Res 1988;49:295–299.
25. **Ogawa H, Tu CH, Kagamizono H, Soki K, Inoue Y, Akatsuka H, Nagata S, Wada T, Ikeya M, Makimura S, et al.** Clinical, morphologic, and biochemical characteristics of Chediak-Higashi syndrome in fifty-six Japanese black cattle. Am J Vet Res 1997;58:1221–1226.
26. **Styrt B.** Species variation in neutrophil biochemistry and function. J Leukoc Biol 1989;46:63–74.
27. **Latimer KS.** Leukocytes in health and disease. Ettinger SJ, Feldman EC, eds. Textbook of veterinary internal medicine, diseases of the dog and cat. 4th ed. Philadelphia: WB Saunders, 1995;1897–1921.
28. **Colgan SP, Gasper PW, Thrall MA, Boone TC, Blancquaert AM, Bruyninckx WJ.** Neutrophil function in normal and Chediak-Higashi syndrome in cats following administration of recombinant canine granulocyte colony-stimulating factor. Exp Hematol 1992;20:1229–1234.
29. **Styrt B, Pollack CR, Klempner MS.** An abnormal calcium uptake pump in Chediak-Higashi neutrophil lysosomes. J Leukoc Biol 1988;44:130–135.
30. **Cheville NF, Cutlip RC, Moon HW.** Microscopic pathology of the grey collie syndrome. Vet Pathol 1970;7:225–245.
31. **Lothrop CD, Warren DJ, Souza LM, Jones JB, Moore MA.** Correction of

canine cyclic hematopoiesis with recombinant human granulocyte colony-stimulating factor. Blood 1988;72:1324–1328.

32. **Dale DC, Rodger E, Cebon J, Ramesh N, Hammond WP, Zsebo KM.** Long-term treatment of canine cyclic hematopoiesis with recombinant canine stem cell factor. Blood 1995;85:74–79.

33. **Avalos BR, Broudy VC, Ceselski SK, Druker BJ, Griffin JD, Hammond WP.** Abnormal response to granulocyte colony-stimulating factor (G-CSF) in canine cyclic hematopoiesis is not caused by altered G-CSF receptor expression. Blood 1994;84:789–794.

34. **Pratt HL, Carroll RC, McClendon S, Smathers EC, Souza LM, Lothrop CD.** Effects of recombinant granulocyte colony-stimulating factor treatment on hematopoietic cycles and cellular defects associated with canine cyclic hematopoiesis. Exp Hematol 1990;18:1199–1203.

35. **Bowles CA, Alsaker RD, Wolfe TL.** Studies of Pelger-Huët anomaly in foxhounds. J Pathol 1979;96:237–247.

36. **Latimer KS, Kircher IM, Lindl PA, Dawe DL, Brown J.** Leukocyte function in Pelger-Huët anomaly of dogs. J Leukoc Biol 1989;45:301–310.

37. **Latimer KS, Rowland GN, Mahaffey MB.** Homozygous Pelger-Huët anomaly and chondrodysplasia in a stillborn kitten. Vet Pathol 1988;25:325–328.

38. **Kehrli ME, Shuster DE, Ackermann MR.** Leukocyte adhesion deficiency among Holstein cattle. Cornell Vet 1992;82:103–109.

39. **Shuster DE, Bosworth BT, Kehrli ME Jr.** Sequence of the bovine CD18-encoding cDNA: comparison with the human and murine glycoproteins. Gene 1992;114:267–271.

40. **Gilbert RO, Rebhun WC, Kim CA, Kehrli ME Jr., Shuster DE, Ackermann MR.** Clinical manifestations of leukocyte adhesion deficiency in cattle: 14 cases (1977–1991). J Am Vet Med Assoc 1993;202:445–449.

41. **Kehrli ME Jr, Schmalstieg FC, Anderson DC, Van der Maaten MJ, Hughes BJ, Ackermann MR, Wilhelmsen CL, Brown GB, Stevens MG, Whetstone CA.** Molecular definition of the bovine granulocytopathy syndrome: Identification of deficiency of the Mac-1 (CD11b/CD18) glycoprotein. Am J Vet Res 1990;51:1826–1836.

42. **Renshaw HW, Davis WC, Renshaw SJ.** Canine granulocytopathy syndrome: defective bactericidal capacity of neutrophils from a dog with recurrent infections. Clin Immunol Immunopathol 1977;8:385–395.

43. **Giger U, Boxer LA, Simpson PJ, Lucchesi BR, Todd RF III.** Deficiency of leukocyte surface glycoproteins Mo 1, LFA-1, and Leu M5 in a dog with recurrent bacterial infections: An animal model. Blood 1987;69:1622–1630.

44. **Trowald-Wigh G, Hakansson L, Johannisson A, Norrgren L, Hard af Segerstad C.** Leucocyte adhesion protein deficiency in Irish setter dogs. Vet Immunol Immunopathol 1992;32:261–280.

45. **Hirsh VM, Cunningham TA.** Hereditary anomaly of neutrophil granulation in Birman cats. Am J Vet Res 1984;45:2170–2174.

46. **Maddux JM, Edwards DF, Barnhill MA, Sanders WL.** Neutrophil function in dogs with congenital ciliary dyskinesia. Vet Pathol 1991;28:347–353.

47. **Morrison WB, Frank DE, Roth JA, Wilsman NJ.** Assessment of neutrophil function in dogs with primary ciliary dyskinesia. J Am Vet Med Assoc 1987;191:425–430.

48. **Olkowski AA, Gooneratne SR, Christensen DA.** Effects of diets of high sulphur content and varied concentrations of copper, molybdenum and thiamine on in vitro phagocytic and candidacidal activity of neutrophils in sheep. Res Vet Sci 1990;48:82–86.

49. **MacPherson A, Gray D, Mitchell GB, Taylor CN.** Ostertagia infection and neutrophil function in cobalt-deficient and cobalt-supplemented cattle. Br Vet J 1987;143:348–353.

50. **Aziz E, Klesius PH.** Effect of selenium deficiency on caprine polymorphonuclear leukocyte production of leukotriene B₄ and its neutrophil chemotactic activity. Am J Vet Res 1986;47:426–428.

51. **Boxer LA.** Neutrophil disorders: Qualitative abnormalities of neutrophils. In: Williams WJ, Beutler E, Erslev AJ, Lichtman MA, eds. Hematology. 4th ed. New York: McGraw-Hill, 1990;821–901.

52. **Magnusson U, Wattrang E, Tsuma V, Fossum C.** Effects of stress resulting from short-term restraint on in vitro functional capacity of leukocytes obtained from pigs. Am J Vet Res 1998;59:421–425.

53. **Fleming KP, Goff BL, Frank DE, Roth JA.** Pigs are relatively resistant to dexamethasone induced immunosuppression. Comp Haematol Int 1994;4:218–225.

54. **Roth JA, Kaeberle ML.** Effects of glucocorticoids on the bovine immune system. J Am Vet Med Assoc 1982;180:894–901.

55. **Webb DS, Roth JA.** Relationship of glucocorticoid suppression of arachidonic acid metabolism to alteration of neutrophil function. J Leukoc Biol 1987;41:156–164.

56. **Frank DE, Roth JA.** Factors secreted by untreated and hydrocortisone-treated monocytes that modulate neutrophil function. J Leukoc Biol 1986;40:693–707.

57. **Morris DD, Strzemienski PJ, Gaulin G, Spencer P.** The effects of corticosteroid administrations on the migration, phagocytosis and bactericidal capacity of equine neutrophils. Cornell Vet 1988;78:243–252.

58. **Roth JA, Kaeberle ML, Hsu WH.** Effect of estradiol and progesterone on lymphocyte and neutrophil functions in steers. Infect Immun 1982;35:997–1002.

59. **Roth JA, Kaeberle ML, Appell LH, Nachreiner RF.** Association of increased estradiol and progesterone blood values with altered bovine polymorphonuclear leukocyte function. Am J Vet Res 1983;44:247–253.

60. **Strzemienski PJ, Dyer RM, Kenny RM.** Effect of estradiol and progesterone on antistaphylococcal activity of neutrophils from ovariectomized mares. Am J Vet Res 1987;48:1638–1641.

61. **Kehrli ME Jr., Nonnecke BJ, Roth JA.** Alterations in bovine neutrophil function during the periparturient period. Am J Vet Res 1989;50:207–214.

62. **Stickle JE, Tvedten HW, Schall WD, Smith CW.** Adherence of neutrophils from dogs with diabetes mellitus. Am J Vet Res 1986;47:541–543.

63. **Latimer KS, Mahaffey EA.** Neutrophil adherence and movement in poorly and well-controlled diabetic dogs. Am J Vet Res 1984;45:1498–1500.

64. **Paape MJ, Miller RH, Ziv G.** Effects of florfenicol, chloramphenicol, and thiamphenicol on phagocytosis, chemiluminescence, and morphology of bovine polymorphonuclear neutrophil leukocytes. J Dairy Sci 1990;73:1734–1744.

65. **Paape MJ, Nickerson SC, Ziv G.** In vivo effects of chloramphenicol, tetracycline, and gentamicin on bovine neutrophil function and morphologic features. Am J Vet Res 1990;51:1055–1061.

66. **Shastri KA, Logue GL.** Autoimmune neutropenia. Blood 1993;81:1984–1995.

67. **Chickering WR, Prasse KW, Dawe DL.** Development and clinical application of methods for detection of antineutrophil antibody in serum of the cat. Am J Vet Res 1985;46:1809–1814.

68. **Bux J, Mueller-Eckhardt C.** Autoimmune neutropenia. Semin Hematol 1992;29:45–53.

69. **Jain NC, Vegad JL, Kono CS.** Method for detection of immune-mediated neutropenia in horses, using anti-neutrophil serum of rabbit origin. Am J Vet Res 1990;51:1026–1031.

70. **Winkelstein JA, Cork LC, Griffin DE, Griffin JW, Adams RJ, Price DL.** Genetically determined deficiency of the third component of complement in the dog. Science 1981;212:1169–1170.

71. **Roth JA.** Enhancement of nonspecific resistance to bacterial infection by biologic response modifiers. In: Roth JA, ed. Virulence mechanisms of bacterial pathogens. Washington, DC: American Society for Microbiology, 1988;329–342.

72. **Breitschwerdt EB, Brown TT, DeBuysscher EV, Anderson BR, Thrall DE, Hager E, Ananaba G, Degen MA, Ward MD.** Rhinitis, pneumonia, and defective neutrophil function in the Doberman Pinscher. Am J Vet Res 1987;48:1054–1062.

73. **Couto CG, Krakowka S, Johnson G, Ciekot TP, Hill R, Lafrado L, Kociba G.** In vitro immunologic features of Weimaraner dogs with neutrophil abnormalities and recurrent infections. Vet Immunol Immunopathol 1989;23:103–112.

74. **Andreasen JR, Andreasen CB, Anwer M, Sonn AE.** Heterophil chemotaxis in chickens with natural Staphylococcal infections. Avian Dis 1993;37:284–289.

75. **Latimer KS, Prasse KW, Mahaffey EA, Dawe DL, Lorenz MD, Duncan JR.** Neutrophil movement in selected canine skin diseases. Am J Vet Res 1983;44:601–605.

76. **Chammas PPC, Hagiwara MK.** Evaluation of neutrophilic function (chemotaxis, phagocytosis and microbicidal activity) in healthy dogs and in dogs suffering from recurrent deep pyoderma. Vet Immunol Immunopathol 1998;64:123–131.

77. **O'Brien JK, Duffus WP.** Pasteurella haemolytica cytotoxin: relative susceptibility of bovine leucocytes. Vet Microbiol 1987;13:321–334.

78. **Czuprynski CJ, Noel EJ, Adlam C.** Modulation of bovine neutrophil antibacterial activities by Pasteurella haemolytica A1 purified capsular polysaccharide. Microb Pathog 1989;6:133–141.

79. **Paulsen DB, Confer AW, Clinkenbeard KD, Mosier DA.** Pasteurella haemolytica lipopolysaccharide-induced arachidonic acid release from and neutrophil adherence to bovine pulmonary artery endothelial cells. Am J Vet Res 1990;51:1635–1639.

80. **Abramson JS, Mills EL.** Depression of neutrophil function induced by viruses and its role in secondary microbial infections. Rev Infect Dis 1988;10:326–341.

81. **Swenson CL, Kociba GJ, Arnold P.** Chronic idiopathic neutropenia in a cat. J Vet Intern Med 1988;2:100–102.

82. **Kiehl AR, Fettman MJ, Quachenbush SL, Hoover EA.** Effects of feline leukemia virus infection on neutrophil chemotaxis in vitro. Am J Vet Res 1987;48:76–80.

83. **Lewis MG, Duska GO, Stiff MI, Lafrado LJ, Olsen RG.** Polymorphonuclear leukocyte dysfunction associated with feline leukaemia virus infection. J Gen Virol 1986;67:2113–2118.

84. **Brown GB, Bolin SR, Frank DE, Roth JA.** Defective function of leukocytes from cattle persistently infected with bovine viral diarrhea virus, and the influence of recombinant cytokines. Am J Vet Res 1991;52:381–387.

85. **Roth JA, Kaeberle ML.** Suppression of neutrophil and lymphocyte function induced by a vaccinal strain of bovine viral diarrhea virus with and without the concurrent administration of ACTH. Am J Vet Res 1983;44:2366–2372.

86. **Briggs RE, Kehrli M, Frank GH.** Effects of infection with parainfluenza-3 virus and infectious bovine rhinotracheitis virus on neutrophil functions in calves. Am J Vet Res 1988;49:682–686.

87. **Fleming K, vander Maaten M, Whetstone C, Carpenter S, Frank D, Roth**

J. The effect of bovine immunodeficiency-like virus on immune function in experimentally-infected cattle. Vet Immunol Immunopathol 1993; 36:91–105.

88. **Roth JA, Jarvinen JA, Frank DE, Fox JE.** Alteration of neutrophil function associated with coccidiosis in cattle: Influence of decoquinate and dexamethasone. Am J Vet Res 1989;50:1250–1253.

89. **Rakich PM, Latimer KS.** Altered immune function in a dog with disseminated protothecosis. J Am Vet Med Assoc 1984;185:681–683.

90. **MacGregor RR.** Granulocyte adherence. In: Glynn LE, Houck JC, Weissmann G, eds. Handbook of inflammation 2. The cell biology of inflammation. New York: Elsevier North-Holland Biomedical Press, 1980;267–298.

91. **Zigmond SH.** A model for understanding millipore filter assay systems. In: Gallin JI, Quie PG, eds. Leukocyte chemotaxis: methods, physiology and clinical implication. New York: Raven Press, 1978;87–95.

92. **Babior BM, Cohen HJ.** Measurement of neutrophil function: phagocytosis, degranulation, the respiratory burst and bacterial killing. In: Cline MF, ed. Leukocyte function. New York: Churchill Livingstone, 1981;1–38.

93. **Andreasen CB, Latimer KS, Harmon BG, Glisson JR, Golden JM, Brown J.** Heterophil function in healthy chickens and in chickens with experimentally induced Staphylococcal tenosynovitis. Vet Pathol 1991;28:419–427.

94. **Stewart CC, Lehnert BE, Steinkamp JA.** *In vitro* and *in vivo* measurement of phagocytosis by flow cytometry. Methods Enzymol 1986;132:183–193.

95. **VanFurth R, VanZwet TL, Leijh PCJ.** In vitro determination of phagocytosis and intracellular killing by polymorphonuclear and mononuclear phagocytes. In: Weir DM, ed. Handbook of experimental immunology. 3rd ed. Oxford: Alden Press, 1978;32.1–32.19.

96. **Baehner RL, Nathan DG.** Quantitative nitroblue tetrazolium test in chronic granulomatous disease. N Engl J Med 1968;278:971–976.

97. **Allen RC, Stjernholm RL, Steel RH.** Evidence for the generation of an electronic excitation state(s) in human polymorphonuclear leukocytes and its participation in bactericidal activity. Biochem Biophys Res Commun 1972;47:679–684.

98. **Hyslop PA, Sklar LA.** A quantitative fluorometric assay for the determination of oxidant production by polymorphonuclear leukocytes: its use in the simultaneous fluorometric assay of cellular activation processes. Anal Biochem 1984;141:280–286.

99. **Quade MJ, Roth JA.** A rapid, direct assay to measure degranulation of bovine neutrophil primary granules. Vet Immunol Immunopathol 1997;58:239–248.

100. **Bertram TA, Canning PC, Roth JA.** Preferential inhibition of primary granule release from bovine neutrophils by a *Brucella abortus* extract. Infect Immun 1986;52:285–292.

101. **Sklar LA, McNeil VM, Jesaitis AJ, Painter RG, Cochrane CG.** A continuous spectroscopic analysis of the kinetics of elastase secretion by neutrophils. The dependence of secretion upon receptor occupancy. J Biol Chem 1982;257:5471–5475.

102. **Klebanoff SJ, Clark RA.** Iodination by human polymorphonuclear leukocytes: a re-evaluation. J Lab Clin Med 1977;89:675–686.

103. **Stevens MG, Kehrli ME Jr, Canning PC.** A colorimetric assay for quantitating bovine neutrophil bactericidal activity. Vet Immunol Immunopathol 1991;28:45–56.

104. **Goren MB, Mor N.** Recent developments in studies on phagosome-lysosome fusion in cultured macrophages. In: Roth JA, ed. Virulence mechanisms of bacterial pathogens. Washington, DC: American Society for Microbiology, 1988;184–199.

CHAPTER 55

Interpretation of Canine Leukocyte Responses

• A. ERIC SCHULTZE

The complete blood count is an essential screening test used to evaluate the hematologic status of dogs. It provides quantitative and qualitative assessment of the erythron, leukon, and thrombon. The total leukocyte count, relative and absolute differential leukocyte counts, and the assessment of leukocyte morphology are collectively referred to as the leukogram. Evaluation of the leukogram provides valuable information regarding pathologic and physiologic leukocyte responses to various stimuli, severity of disease, response to treatment, and prognosis.[1-5]

Accurate interpretation of leukograms is based on calculated absolute differential leukocyte counts (percent leukocyte type × total leukocyte count) rather than on the relative differential counts. This absolute count better reflects the total number of each cell type within the overall leukocyte population. These calculated absolute counts are then compared with predetermined reference intervals.[3] The numbers of several types of leukocytes may change simultaneously, and the pattern of response is important during consideration of a list of differential diagnoses. Serial leukograms and bone marrow analyses performed over several days to weeks may be necessary to accurately assess specific response patterns in certain conditions.

The total leukocyte count in healthy dogs varies from 5,000 to 14,100 cells/μL blood.[3] Leukocytes recognized in the blood of dogs include neutrophils, eosinophils, basophils, monocytes, and lymphocytes. The neutrophil is the most commonly encountered leukocyte in the blood of healthy dogs. Lymphocytes occur often but are less numerous than neutrophils. Monocytes and eosinophils are seen less frequently, whereas basophils are rare.

Total leukocyte counts are highest in puppies, and the counts gradually decrease with increasing age throughout life. Alterations in the total leukocyte count primarily are caused by changes in the numbers of lymphocytes and neutrophils. Both cell types decrease in number with advancing age. Eosinophils also decrease in number but have minimal effect on the total leukocyte count. Monocytes tend to increase slightly in number with advancing age.[3,4]

Diurnal variation in the total leukocyte count and absolute numbers of neutrophils, lymphocytes, and eosinophils can be detected in conditioned dogs kept under controlled light, feeding, and activity. The total leukocyte and absolute neutrophil counts increase with time, reaching maximum values in the late afternoon (7 PM). Lymphocyte counts are highest in late evening (11 PM) and lowest in the early morning (7 AM). Eosinophil counts reach a zenith in late evening (11 PM) with the nadir at midday (12 PM). Although statistically different, diurnal variation has minimal effect on cell counts. Therefore, these daily cellular fluctuations would be unlikely to cause problems in interpretation of clinical data from patients in which comparison is made to standard reference intervals.[6]

CLASSICAL CANINE LEUKOGRAM PATTERNS

Historically, dogs have been kept as companions for many years, and they are often presented for veterinary care. In addition, dogs are frequently used as research subjects. Therefore, much is known regarding the hematology of this particular species. Several leukogram patterns that are seen frequently in dogs are described below and the mechanisms of alteration in cellular distribution are explained briefly.

Physiologic Leukocytosis

Dogs that experience fear, excitement, or engage in brief periods of strenuous exercise may develop physiologic leukocytosis. This reaction is more common in puppies and is seldom seen in the adult dog. The leukogram is characterized by mild, mature neutrophilia and lymphocytosis. The monocyte and eosinophil counts may remain within the reference intervals or increase slightly. The magnitude of lymphocytosis may exceed that of the neutrophilia. Physiologic leukocytosis is a transient alteration in the leukogram that occurs within minutes of the stimulus and usually resolves within 30 minutes.

The mechanism of neutrophilia involves an epinephrine-mediated demargination of neutrophils from the marginal pool into the circulating pool, where they can be quantitated by the leukocyte count. Because the total number of neutrophils in the blood (sum of the marginal and circulating pools) does not change, this reaction is often termed psuedoneutrophilia. The lymphocytosis is believed to be caused by epinephrine-mediated blockade of lymphocytes entering lymphoid tissues or by mobilization of lymphocytes from the thoracic duct.[1-4]

Corticosteroid-Induced Leukocytosis

Endogenous release of glucocorticoids because of severe stress or hyperadrenocorticism (Cushing's syndrome), and administration of exogenous glucocorticoids or adrenocorticotropic hormone (ACTH) may cause corticosteroid-induced leukocytosis in the dog. Total leukocyte counts usually range from 15,000 to 25,000/μL blood, but may occasionally reach 40,000/μL blood. The leukogram is characterized by mature neutrophilia, lymphopenia, monocytosis, and eosinopenia. Rarely, a mild left shift may occur if the bone marrow storage pool is depleted at the time of stimulation by corticosteroids. The leukogram alterations occur within 4 to 8 hours after a single administration of glucocorticoids and usually resolve within 24 hours. Leukograms from dogs given long-term corticosteroid therapy (>10 days) may require 2 to 3 days to return to baseline values after treatment ceases. The neutrophilia usually resolves prior to lymphopenia. The mature neutrophilia is the result of several factors, including: decreased emigration of neutrophils from blood into tissues, increased release of mature neutrophils from the bone marrow, and decreased margination of neutrophils within the vasculature. The lymphopenia is attributed to redistribution of circulating lymphocytes. Long-term use of corticosteroids may cause lympholysis. The monocytosis may be the result of mobilization of marginated cells within the blood vasculature, similar to the mechanism of neutrophilia. Eosinopenia occurs because of inhibition of eosinophil release from the bone marrow and sequestration of eosinophils within tissues.[1-5]

Inflammatory Leukocytosis

The leukogram is an excellent method to monitor inflammation in the dog. Infections caused by bacteria, rickettsia, viruses, fungi, and parasites may cause alterations in the leukogram. Immune-mediated diseases, tissue necrosis, and neoplasia may elicit inflammatory reactions. Because neutrophils respond within hours to various chemotactic stimuli during inflammation, the time of phlebotomy relative to initial inflammatory stimulus is extremely important in interpretation of the leukogram.

Peracute Inflammation

Sudden onset of an overwhelming infection or other inflammatory reactions may cause leukopenia characterized primarily by neutropenia. Transient neutropenia may be detected within 1 to 3 hours after exposure to endotoxin. Overwhelming sepsis caused by infection of the lungs, thorax, uterus, or peritoneum by gram-negative bacteria may cause similar responses. The neutropenia, which persists for 2 to 3 hours, is caused by endotoxin-mediated neutrophil margination within the vasculature, shortened neutrophil half-life, and increased cell emigration into tissues.[1-4]

Acute Inflammation

Within 6 to 8 hours after an initial inflammatory stimulus, the bone marrow compensates by accelerated release of neutrophils, which results in neutrophilia. The acute inflammatory leukogram in the dog is characterized by leukocytosis. Total leukocyte counts usually range from 20,000 to 30,000/μL blood and are characterized by neutrophilia with a left shift (>450 bands or other neutrophil precursors/μL blood). The neutrophilia and left shift occur because the production and early release of neutrophils by the bone marrow exceed the tissue demand for phagocytes. The left shift is usually orderly in that the number of bands > metamyelocytes > myelocytes. Toxic change may be observed in the neutrophils. Concurrent lymphopenia and eosinopenia are typical owing to release of endogenous corticosteroids. Monocytosis is an inconsistent observation but may be present, particularly if a stress response is superimposed on the inflammatory leukogram.[1-5]

Chronic Inflammation

Established inflammation of days to weeks duration may result in characteristic alterations in the bone marrow, including expansion of the proliferation pool and maturation and storage pool of neutrophils to meet tissue demand for these cells. The leukogram is characterized by leukocytosis with neutrophilia; a left shift may be mild or absent.[1,5,7] Alterations in the numbers of other leukocytes may be variable.

Leukemoid Reactions and Extreme Neutrophilia

Leukemoid reactions in the dog are uncommon. The term leukemoid refers to leukograms that resemble granulocytic leukemia in cell numbers and differential cell counts but are caused by benign processes. Typical leukemoid reactions are characterized by significant neutrophilic leukocytosis ranging from 50,000 to 100,000 cells/μL blood with a concurrent, orderly left shift that may extend to myelocytes or promyelocytes.[7] Toxic change in neutrophils may or may not be present. Rarely, leukemoid reactions involve significant lymphocytosis or eosinophilia.[5,8] The common causes of leukemoid reactions are listed in Table 55.1.[1-5,7-16] Pyometra and peritonitis are frequent causes of this reaction.[1,5] Dogs that have immune-mediated hemolytic anemia,[1] CD11-CD18 neutrophil protein adhesion deficiency (canine granulocytopathy syndrome),[9,10] and *Hepatozoon canis* infection[11] develop leukemoid reactions. Neutrophilic leu-

TABLE 55.1	Causes of Leukemoid Reactions and Extreme Neutrophilia in Dogs[1–5,7–16]
Infections/infectious agents:	Chronic active peritonitis, *H. canis* infection, internal abscesses, pyometra, salmon disease (lymphoid and monocytoid reaction?)
Neoplasia:	Metastatic fibrosarcoma, pulmonary adenocarcinoma, rectal adenomatous polyp, renal tubular carcinoma, renal tubular adenocarcinoma
Immune mediated:	Immune-mediated hemolytic anemia
Other:	Canine granulocytopathy syndrome (leukocyte glycoprotein CD11/CD18 deficiency), extreme eosinophilia from nonneoplastic causes (eosinophilic reaction)

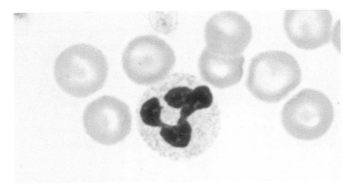

FIGURE 55.1 Normal canine neutrophil with distinct nuclear lobulation, Wright's stain.

kemoid reactions have been reported in dogs that have paraneoplastic syndromes secondary to renal tubular carcinoma,[12,13] metastatic fibrosarcoma,[14] metastatic pulmonary adenocarcinoma,[15] and rectal adenomatous polyp.[16] Terminology may vary slightly among clinical pathologists when leukemoid reactions of extreme degree or of varied cell types are described. Leukograms characterized by neutrophilic leukocytosis (>100,000/μL blood) with a left shift and no evidence of hemopoietic neoplasia are sometimes referred to as extreme neutrophilic leukocytoses.[1] The term leukoerythroblastic response is used to describe a typical leukemoid reaction that is accompanied by normoblastemia.[7] Differentiation of benign leukemoid reactions from chronic myelogenous leukemia can be challenging and often requires serial complete blood counts and bone marrow examinations. The diagnosis of chronic myelogenous leukemia is made by exclusion of causes of inflammation, presence of a disorderly left shift, or observation of abnormal granulocyte morphology in blood or bone marrow smears.

NEUTROPHILIA AND NEUTROPENIA

Canine neutrophils have two to five nuclear lobes that are separated by constrictions. The nuclear outline is slightly irregular, and the chromatin is tightly condensed. The cytoplasm is moderate in amount and is filled with a myriad of granules that appear faintly pink in Romanowsky-stained blood films (Fig. 55.1). Neutrophils are the most numerous leukocyte in the blood of dogs, and they function as the primary line of defense against microorganisms. In addition, neutrophils destroy transformed cells, modulate acute inflammatory reactions, and control granulopoiesis.[17,18] The half-life of circulating blood neutrophils is approximately 7.4

hours. After emigration into the tissues, they live an additional 24 to 48 hours and then are phagocytized by the mononuclear phagocyte system or are sloughed from mucosal surfaces.[17,19] The number of neutrophils within the blood of dogs depends on several factors, including rate of release from the bone marrow, shifting of neutrophils between the marginal pool and the circulating pool in the blood, and the emigration rate of neutrophils from blood into tissues.[2]

Neutrophilia, defined as >12,000 neutrophils/μL blood, is a common observation in canine blood films.[3] Causes of neutrophilia in dogs are listed in Table 55.2.[1–5,10,17–60] The more common causes of neutrophilia in dogs include physiologic leukocytosis, corticosteroid-induced leukocytosis, and inflammation. Additional causes of neutrophilia in dogs include hemolysis, hemorrhage, genetic defects in leukocyte adhesion molecules, and immune-mediated diseases. Several benign and malignant neoplastic conditions cause paraneoplastic syndromes that may result in neutrophilia. Thrombosis, infarction, burns, and uremia also may cause neutrophilia.[1–4]

Inflammation is the most common cause of neutrophilia. The intensity of the underlying disease process has a direct effect on the magnitude of the total neutrophil response.[1,4] Localized purulent lesions, like abscesses, induce greater neutrophilia than do more generalized diseases such as septicemia. Neutrophilia with a left shift is the hallmark of acute inflammatory reactions. The degree of the left shift is considered a direct indication of the severity of disease.[1,4] Left shifts of great magnitude may occur in dogs that have pleuritis, peritonitis, pyoderma, or pyometra. The early release of immature neutrophils from the bone marrow is related to the increased tissue demand of purulent inflammation associated with necrosis, fungi, foreign bodies, or pyogenic bacteria. In some diseases, inflammation is too mild to induce a left shift. A degenerative left shift, which occurs when the number of immature neutrophils is greater than that of mature neutrophils, is a poor prognostic sign. The total number of blood neutrophils may be decreased or normal. Degenerative left shifts occur when tissue demand depletes the bone marrow storage pool and exceeds the capability of the bone marrow to produce neutrophils.[1-3]

Insignificant or extremely mild left shifts may occur in seborrheic dermatitits, catarrhal enteritis, and hemorrhagic cystitis, conditions in which tissue demand for neutrophils is minimal.[1,4] In general, the magnitude of the left shift in inflammatory leukograms decreases as the bone marrow compensates and produces more neutrophils to fill the postmitotic or maturation and storage pool.

Neutropenia, defined as <2,900 neutrophils/μL blood, occurs less frequently than neutrophilia in dogs. Because neutrophils are the primary line of defense against microorgansims, prolonged neutropenia results in increased risk of infection. The more severe the degree of neutropenia, the greater the risk of infection. Three common mechanisms of neutropenia include decreased production of neutrophils in the bone marrow, cellular shifting from the circulating to the marginal pool, and increased tissue emigration in excess of bone marrow release of neutrophils (Table 55.2).[1,4]

Decreased production of neutrophils occurs in dogs treated with total-body ionizing irradiation, certain chemotherapeutic agents, and estrogen toxicosis. These conditions kill hemopoietic stem cells or inhibit their replication. Significant neutropenia results from a single treatment of 12 Gray in dogs that have total-body irradiation. Bone marrow transplant or infusion of hemopoietic stem cells is necessary to repopulate the bone marrow and prevent death.[1] Predictable neutropenia occurs in dogs treated with the chemotherapeutic agents, including azathioprine, cyclophosphamide, daunomycin, dimethyl myleran, doxorubicin, 6-thioguanine, cisplatin, carboplatin, and mitoxantrone.[1,4,20] The onset of

neutropenia occurs within several days and recovery may require as long as 20 to 40 days.[1] Male dogs that have Sertoli cell tumors and those treated with estrogen for perianal gland tumors may develop estrogen toxicosis. Female dogs given diethylstilbestrol or estradiol cyclopentylpropionate for urinary incontinence, infertility, or mismating may also develop neutropenia within 72 hours. Pancytopenia may develop. Recovery is prolonged and may require 3 months.[1,21]

Idiosyncratic drug reactions may cause neutropenia and pancytopenia in dogs. Phenylbutazone and cephalosporin antibiotics are reported to cause severe neutropenia that resolves within 1 week of cessation of treatment. Administration of trimethoprim-sulfadiazine or thiacetarsamide and ingestion of commerically available skin cream (Noxema, Noxema Chemical Company of Canada) has caused neutropenia and pancytopenia in dogs.[1,22-24]

The neutropenia and leukopenia of canine parvoviral enteritis can be attributed to several mechanisms. The virus is cytotoxic for hemopoietic stem cells. Endotoxemia and gastrointestinal necrosis cause depletion of the maturation and storage pools of neutrophils within the bone marrow. Endotoxemia may cause increased margination of neutrophils within the vasculature. Finally, increased ineffective neutrophil production occurs, evidenced by leukophagocytosis within bone marrow aspirates.[1,25,26]

Decreased production of neutrophils occurs in <30% of dogs that have chronic ehrlichiosis[27-31] and in some giant schnauzer dogs that have inherited malabsorption of vitamin B_{12}.[32,33] Because of decreased hemopoietic space, bone marrow necrosis, myelofibrosis, and osteopetrosis result in neutropenia in dogs.[1,34-36] Infre-

---

TABLE 55.2   Causes of Neutrophilia and Neutropenia in the Dog[1-5,10,17-60]

Neutrophilia	**Neutropenia**
Chemical and drug toxicity (estrogen [acute phase only], recombinant granulocyte-CSF)	Decreased production of neutrophils in the bone marrow
Corticosteroid-induced leukocytosis	Bone marrow necrosis
Genetic adhesion molecule (CD11-CD18) deficiency (canine granulocytopathy syndrome)	Cyclic hematopoiesis gray collies (congenital), cyclophosphamide administration
Hemolysis	Drug administration
Hemorrhage	Predictable (estrogen toxicity [late], chemotherapeutic agents) idiosyncratic (cephalosporins, phenylbutazone, thiacetarsamide, Noxema ingestion)
Immune-mediated diseases	Inherited malabsorption of vitamin B_{12} in giant schnauzers
Hemolytic anemia, systemic lupus erythematosus, polymyositis, polyserositis, rheumatoid arthritis, systemic necrotizing vasculitis	Myelofibrosis and osteopetrosis
Infections	Myeloproliferative and lymphoproliferative diseases (several types of leukemia and lymphosarcoma)
Bacteria (many species), viruses—canine distemper virus, fungi (many organisms), parasites (many species), rickettsia (Rocky Mountain spotted fever)	Radiation
Inflammatory leukocytosis (acute, chronic, or leukemoid responses)	Cellular shifting from the circulating to the marginal pool
Leukemia (several types, acute or chronic)	Anaphylaxis
Necrosis (thrombosis, infarction, burns)	Endotoxemia
Physiologic leukocytosis	Increased tissue emigration in excess of bone marrow release
Tissue neoplasia/paraneoplastic syndromes (several benign and malignant tumors)	Infection
Toxemia (endotoxemia, uremia)	Bacteria (many), Rickettsia (ehrlichiosis), viruses (parvoviral enteritis, canine distemper virus), parasites (*B. canis*)
	Immune-mediated disease (suspected but not proven in dogs)

quently, disseminated granulomatous disease secondary to histoplasmosis[37] and myelophthisis secondary to proliferation of neoplastic cells within the marrow causes neutropenia in dogs.[38,61] Myelophthisis has been associated with various leukemias and metastatic neoplasia in the bone marrow.

Cyclic hemopoiesis is an autosomal recessive disease of gray-collie dogs. It is characterized by regular fluctuations in leukocytes, reticulocytes, and platelets that occur at 10- to 12-day intervals. This stem-cell defect results in profound cyclic neutropenia. Untreated the disease is fatal within 3 years. Repeated endotoxin injections and administration of lithium carbonate control the neutropenia.[1,62] Long-term control of the disease requires bone marrow transplantation. Recently, similar cyclic hemopoietic disease has been reported in cocker spaniels and Pomeranian dogs.[1] Administration of cyclophosphamide also results in cyclic neutropenia.[1]

A second mechanism of neutropenia is cellular shifting from the circulating to marginal pool. Rapid margination of neutrophils occurs with anaphylaxis and endotoxemia in dogs.[1,3]

The third major mechanism of neutropenia is increased tissue emigration in excess of bone marrow release of neutrophils. Rapid use of neutrophils occurs with localized infections by pyogenic bacteria. Intense, acute, purulent infection of the lungs, uterus, gastrointestinal tract, or body cavities may cause moderate to significant neutropenia.[1,3]

Morphologic Alterations in Neutrophils

Nuclear Alterations in Neutrophils

Asynchronous Nuclear Maturation An indication of dysplasia, asynchronous nuclear maturation is characterized by a lobulated nucleus with an immature chromatin pattern. The neutrophil may appear slightly swollen and may have some degree of toxic change. Nuclear lobes may be enlarged or coiled in unusual configurations, and the chromatin may appear dispersed. This uncommon nuclear alteration occurs in dogs that have significant resurgent neutrophilia, myeloid leukemia, and myelodysplastic or preleukemic syndromes.[3]

Nuclear Hypersegmentation Neutrophils with >5 nuclear lobes are seldom observed in the blood of dogs (Fig. 55.2). These hypersegmented neutrophils are associated with prolonged transit times in the vasculature and occur secondary to severe stress (endogenous corticosteroid release), hyperadrenocorticism, and exogenous corticosteroid administration. Few normal to slightly larger, hypersegmented neutrophils are reported in toy and miniature poodles that have congenital erythrocytic macrocytosis. Giant hypersegmented neutrophils have been observed in myelodysplastic syndromes and in granulocytic leukemia.[1,3,4]

Nuclear Hyposegmentation Hyposegmentation of the neutrophil nucleus may occur in the left shift

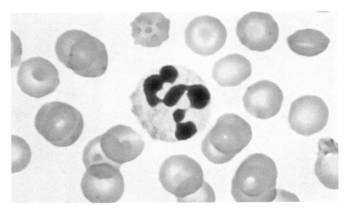

FIGURE 55.2 Hypersegmented neutrophil from a dog that has hyperadrenocorticism, Wright's stain.

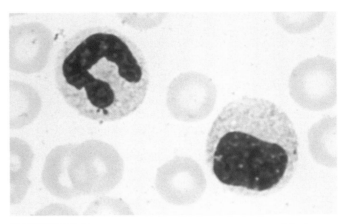

FIGURE 55.3 Late-band and metamyelocyte neutrophils from a dog that has inflammation, Wright's stain.

of inflammation or infection, Pelger–Huët anomaly, or pseudo-Pelger–Huët anomaly (Fig. 55.3). The key to differentiation between neutrophil immaturity and Pelger–Huët anomaly is assessment of the maturity of nuclear chromatin and observation of other immature neutrophilic cells in the blood smear that might support a left shift. The chromatin in bands and metamyelocytes is progressively less condensed than that of neutrophils in Pelger–Huët anomaly in which there is a failure of the nucleus to segment.[3,5]

Pelger–Huët Anomaly Reported in several breeds of dogs, Pelger–Huët anomaly is a benign condition. (Fig. 55.4). This hereditary disorder of granulocyte development is presumed transmitted as an autosomal dominant trait and is characterized by granulocytes and monocytes with hyposegmented nuclei and mature chromatin patterns. The nucleus of neutrophils, eosinophils, and basophils typically has a band or peanut-shaped nucleus with tightly condensed chromatin. Most dogs that have Pelger–Huët anomaly are heterozygous for the condition, and the neutrophils have normal function. Therefore, there is no predisposition for infection.[1,63–65]

Cytoplasmic Alterations/Inclusions in Neutrophils

Ethylenediamine-Tetra-Acetic-Acid-Induced Artifact The change to an ethylenediamine-tetra-acetic-acid (EDTA) -induced artifact may occur in canine neutrophils when there is a prolonged delay in smear preparation.[66] When whole blood is collected in EDTA and allowed to incubate at room temperature, neutrophils develop a few, clear vacuoles within the cytoplasm and an irregular distribution of cytoplasmic granules. Cell membranes appear irregular, and mild pyknosis may occur. Cytoplasmic basophilia and foamy vacuolation are not observed in EDTA-induced artifactual change.

Toxic Change A set of disease-induced morphologic alterations in neutrophils, including cytoplasmic vacuolation, cytoplasmic basophilia, Döhle bodies, or prominently stained primary granules (toxic granulation) is referred to as a toxic change (Fig. 55.5).[3,5] These cytoplasmic lesions may be seen in cases of intense, localized or systemic infection[67–69]; sterile inflammation[70]; and drug toxicity.[1,4] Observation of toxic change warrants a guarded prognosis, because these frequently encountered, cytoplasmic alterations indicate compromised production and function of neutrophils.

Cytoplasmic vacuolation occurs in neutrophils when bone marrow production of these cells is disrupted, resulting in loss of granule and membrane integrity. Persistent ribosomes impart the cytoplasm with its characteristic basophilia. Döhle bodies are angular, blue-to-gray, cytoplasmic inclusions that stain with variable intensity and measure approximately 0.5 to 2.0 μm in diameter. They represent lamellar aggregates of retained rough endoplasmic reticulum. Increased permeability of primary granule membranes to Romanowsky stains results in toxic granulation, a change seldom seen in canine neutrophils.[71,72] Resolution of toxic change in neutrophils after appropriate treatment of the underlying disease is a favorable prognostic indicator in the dog.

Infectious Agents Bacterial rods and cocci may be detected infrequently within the cytoplasm of neutrophils and other blood phagocytes during septicemic crises.[73] The bacteria may stain positively or negatively in Romanowsky-stained blood films and buffy coat preparations (Fig. 55.6). Although clinical signs and leukograms may provide supportive evidence for bacteremia, the diagnosis is best confirmed by blood culture.

Canine distemper virus inclusion bodies may be observed infrequently in neutrophils from dogs that have naturally occurring viral disease or postvaccination (Fig. 55.7). The intracytoplasmic inclusions are round to irregularly shaped, homogenous, magenta to gray-blue structures that may occur in blood cells, including erythrocytes and several types of leukocytes.[1,4,74]

Hepatozoon canis and *Hepatozoon americanum* gametocytes may be detected in the cytoplasm of neutrophils or monocytes. Parsitemia varies from high to low levels. It may be necessary to examine several blood films, capillary blood smears, or buffy coat preparations to identify gametocytes (Fig. 55.8). The oval gametocytes measure 5×10 μm and are unstained to ice-blue within the cytoplasm of monocytes and neutrophils in Romanowsky-stained blood smears. Infection often is associated with neutrophilic leukocytosis.[11,75,76]

Histoplasma capsulatum is a yeast-like fungus that may be observed within neutrophils, monocytes, and eosinophils in Romanowsky-stained blood films and buffy coats from dogs that have disseminated disease (Fig. 55.9). The organisms are round, 2 to 4 μm in diameter, and have thin walls. They have a small round, purple nucleus, and may occur singly or in clusters within the cytoplasm.[37,77]

Leishmania donovani amastigotes have rarely been identified in neutrophils from dogs that have disseminated leishmaniasis.[78,79] Leukocytosis with neutrophilic left shift is common. The amistogotes are small, round to oval organisms and occur 1 to 2 organisms per neutro-

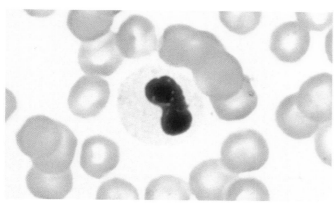

FIGURE 55.4 Neutrophil with Pelger–Hüet anomaly. Notice coarse mature chromatin pattern, Wright's stain.

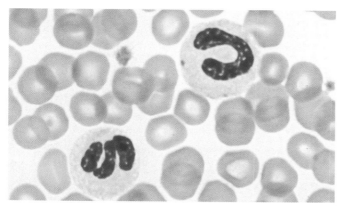

FIGURE 55.5 Canine segmented (left bottom) and band (right top) neutrophils with toxic change, including cytoplasmic basophilia and Döhle bodies, Wright's stain.

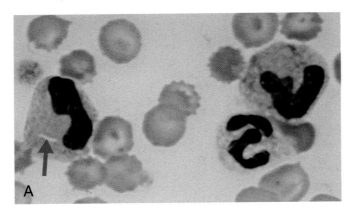

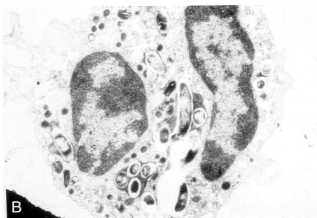

FIGURE 55.6 **A**. Neutrophil with negatively stained intracellular bacillus (arrow) in blood smear from a dog that has mycobacteriosis, Wright's stain. **B**. Transmission electron micrograph of a neutrophil from the same dog that has several bacilli. (Courtesy of Dr. Harold W. Tvedten, Michigan State University, East Lansing, MI).

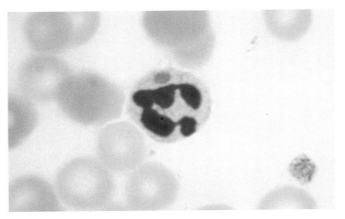

FIGURE 55.7 Magenta-colored canine distemper virus inclusion in a neutrophil, Wright's stain.

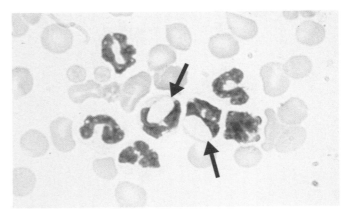

FIGURE 55.8 Two segmented neutrophils with intracytoplasmic, clear to ice-blue *H. canis* gametocytes, Wright's stain. (Courtesy of Dr. Robert Green, Texas A&M University, College Station, TX).

phil. They have an oval nucleus, basophilic ventral kinetoplast, and light blue cytoplasm. Amastiogotes have been identified in approximately 3% of circulating neutrophils.

Rickettsia morulae are rarely observed in the cytoplasm of neutrophils and other granulocytes in blood and buffy coats from some dogs infected with *Ehrlichia ewingii* and *Ehrlichia equi*.[27–29,80,81] *Ehrlichia canis* morulae may be observed infrequently within monocytes. The morulae vary from magenta to blue gray in color and resemble a mulberry (Fig. 55.10). The identity of the specific agent is established by polymerase chain reaction or by determination of acute and convalescent serum antibody titers.

Miscellaneous Inclusions *Hemosiderin* granules have been observed within the cytoplasm of occasional neutrophils and monocytes from three dogs that have immune-mediated hemolytic anemia after transfusion therapy. The brown granules, which were positive for iron with Prussian blue staining, measured 1 to 4 μm in diameter (Fig. 55.11). Multiple granules were observed

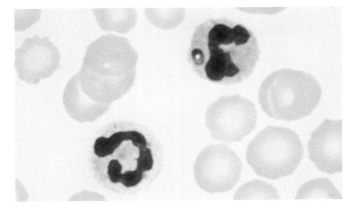

FIGURE 55.9 Segmented neutrophil with intracytoplasmic *H. capsulatum*, Wright's stain.

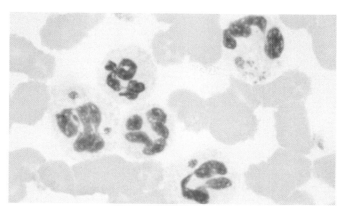

FIGURE 55.10 Three neutrophils containing morulae of *E. ewingii*, Wright's stain. (Courtesy of Dr. Steven L. Stockham, University of Missouri, Columbia, MO).

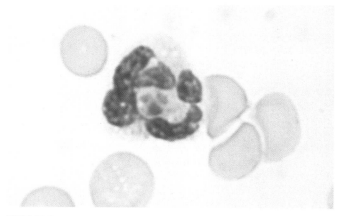

FIGURE 55.11 Segmented neutrophil with *hemosiderin* crystal from a dog that has immune-mediated hemolytic anemia, Wright's stain. (Courtesy of Dr. Stephen Gaunt, Louisiana State University, Baton Rouge, LA).

within some cells. The mechanism of their occurrence within neutrophils was uncertain.[82]

Mucopolysaccharidosisis type VI (arylsulfatase B deficiency) and type VII (β-glucuronidase deficiency) are lysosomal storage diseases that have been reported rarely in the dog. Neutrophils and lymphocytes from affected dogs may have large, pink-to-purple staining inclusions (Alder–Reilly bodies) within the cytoplasm in routine Romanowsky-stained blood films (Fig. 55.12). The inclusions in mucopolysaccharidosis type VII may stain metachromatically with 1% toluidine blue dye. The granules represent intermediate products that accumulate within cells caused by the arylsulfatase B (type VI) or β-glucuronidase deficiency (type VII). Disease inheritance is by means of an autosomal recessive pattern.[83,84]

EOSINOPHILIA AND EOSINOPENIA

In Romanowsky-stained blood films, canine eosinophils have a bilobed or trilobed nucleus with condensed chro-

matin and abundant cytoplasm that contains round, red-orange granules (Fig. 55.13). The granules may vary considerably in number and size. In some dogs, eosinophils appear degranulated or vacuolated. The primary functions of eosinophils are to destroy parasites (primarily helminths) and to modulate hypersensitivity reactions.[4,85,86] Alternatively, they also may promote inflammation. Although eosinophils are capable of phagocytosis, they are not effective in protection from most bacterial infections.[3,4]

Eosinophilia, defined as >1300 eosinophils/μL blood, is a common occurrence in the dog.[3] The causes of eosinophilia are listed in Table 55.3.[1–5,16,81,85–112] By far the most common cause of eosinophilia in the dog is parasitism. Both endoparasites and ectoparasites may cause eosinophilia. However, this alteration occurs more often and is of greater magnitude with endoparasites that migrate within the tissues and have prolonged host-tissue contact. Sensitized T lymphocytes initiate and maintain the eosinophilia by means of production of

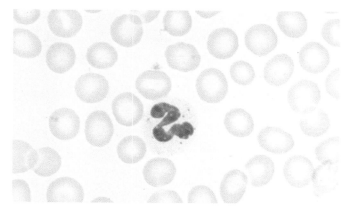

FIGURE 55.12 Segmented neutrophil with Alder–Reilly bodies from a dog that has mucopolysaccharidosis type VII, Wright's stain. (Courtesy of Dr. Mary Anna Thrall, Colorado State University, Ft. Collins, CO and Dr. Mark Haskins, University of Pennsylvania, Philadelphia, PA).

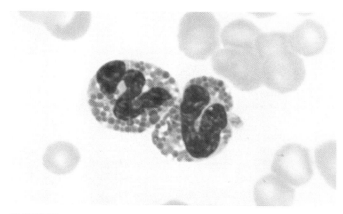

FIGURE 55.13 Two normal canine eosinophils, Wright's stain.

TABLE 55.3   Causes of Eosinophilia and Eosinopenia in Dogs[1–5,16,57,85–112]

Eosinophilia
Drug administration
  Recombinant interleukin-2 administration, tetracycline
Hypoadrenocorticism
Hypersensitivity reactions (alimentary, genitourinary, respiratory systems, skin and special senses may be affected)
  Oral granuloma
  Ulcerative/eosinophilic gastroenteritis
  Gastrointestinal eosinophilic granuloma
  Pyometra
  Myositis
  Panosteitis
  Pulmonary infiltrates with eosinophilia
  Canine eosinophilic granuloma
  Sterile eosinophilic pustulosis
Fungi/Yeastlike fungi
  Aspergillus fumigatus, Cryptococcus neoformans, Pythium insidiosum
Parasites
  Nematodes
    Ancylostoma sp.*, Angiostrongylus vasorum, Ascarids, Dipetalonema reconditum, Dirofilaria immitis, Oslerus (Filaroides) osleri, Filaroides hirthi, Physaloptera* sp.*, Spirocerca lupi, Trichinella spiralis, Trichuris vulpis*
  Trematodes
    Heterobilharzia americana, Pargonimus kellicotti, Alaria sp.
  Arthropods
    Dermatobia hominis, Fleas, Ticks, *Sarcoptes scabiei var canis*, Pentastomes
  Protozoa
    Babesia canis, Hepatozoon canis, Pneumocystis carinii
Neoplasia
  Idiopathic hypereosinophilic syndrome, myeloid leukemia, paraneoplastic syndromes (fibrosarcoma, lymphomatoid granulomatosis, mammary carcinoma, disseminated mastocytosis, rectal polyp, thymoma)

Eosinopenia
Corticosteroids
  Endogenous
    Hyperadrenocorticism
    Stress
  Exogenous
    Corticosteroid treatment
Acute infection/inflammation

interleukin 5. Subsequent exposure to the same parasite elicits a quicker and more drastic eosinophilia.[1,3,4,87]

Inflammation or local hypersensitivity reactions in the alimentary, respiratory, and genitourinary systems and in skin that are mediated by mast cell degranulation cause eosinophilia. In some dogs, localized tissue eosinophilia may occur in the presence of normal blood eosinophil counts. The stimulus for eosinophil accumulation at the sites of inflammation may be mediated by products of mast cell or basophil degranulation, deposition of immune complexes within tissues, cytokines and vasoactive amines, or complement-derived chemotactic factors.[4,88,89]

Eosinophilia may occur as a paraneoplastic syndrome in some dogs.[90,91] Although many malignant and few benign neoplasms have been reported to cause eosinophilia, disseminated mast cell neoplasia most commonly causes this alteration in the dog.[92] The mechanism of eosinophilia is unknown. However, T-lymphocyte-derived cytokine mediators, such as interleukins 2 and 5, are probably involved.[1] Idiopathic hypereosinophilic syndrome occurs rarely in dogs and is characterized by persistent eosinophilia with extensive tissue infiltration and organ dysfunction of unknown cause.[93] It may be difficult to differentiate hypereosinophilic syndrome from eosinophilic leukemia. Rarely, eosinophilia is reported after administration of certain drugs in the dog. Eosinophilia has been associated with tetracycline and recombinant interleukin-2 administration.[94,95]

Eosinophil counts in healthy dogs range from 0 to 1300 eosinophils/μL blood.[3] Because many normal dogs may routinely have eosinophil counts of 0/μL, true eosinopenia is difficult to document and is of limited clinical significance. Determination of absolute eosinophil counts with a hemocytometer and eosin-based diluent is recommended to confirm suspected cases of eosinopenia and may be valuable in monitoring responses to o,p'-DDD (mitotane) treatment in dogs that have hyperadrenocorticism.[4]

Eosinopenia may occur in dogs that have emotional or physical stress owing to release of adrenocorticosteroids.[5,96] The mechanism of the decrease in eosinophil numbers is uncertain but is believed caused by intravascular lysis, decreased release from bone marrow, sequestration in organs such as spleen and liver, and increased tissue migration.[5] It is hypothesized that corticosteroids inhibit histamine release, neutralize circulating histamine, and initiate release of cytokines that mediate these alterations in eosinophil distribution. Eosinopenia from a single dose of corticosteroids occurs within 1 to 6 hours and counts return to normal within 12 to 24 hours.[2]

Eosinopenia may occur in dogs that have hyperadrenocorticism (Cushing's syndrome).[97] Administration of ACTH or exogenous corticosteroids also may cause eosinopenia in dogs.[1,98,99] The dose and duration of corticosteroid administration affects eosinophil kinetics. Long-term use of high-dose corticosteroids depresses eosinophil production by the bone marrow.[1]

Eosinopenia occurs in some acute infections and inflammatory reactions. Although the mechanism of eosinopenia is unknown, it is hypothesized because of the effect of corticosteroid release.[5] Other investigators suggest that sequestration, degranulation, or eosinophil destruction within inflammatory lesions may account for the eosinopenia. Decreased release of eosinophils from the bone marrow also may occur.[100]

BASOPHILIA AND BASOPENIA

Basophils are seen infrequently in blood films submitted for hematologic evaluation. These unique cells, which are slightly larger than segmented neutrophils, usually account for <2% of the differential leukocyte count or an absolute count of 0 to 140 basophils/μL.[3] Basophils have a poorly lobulated nucleus that has been described as a twisted ribbon (Fig. 55.14). The blue-gray cytoplasm contains widely scattered, round, metachromatic granules that vary greatly in size and number.[1,5]

Basophil granules contain preformed mediators, including histamine and heparin. When stimulated, these cells synthesize platelet-activating factor; thromboxane A_2; and leukotrienes C_4, D_4, and E_4.[5] Basophils are intricately involved in host defense by means of gamma-E-immunoglobulin (IgE)-mediated inflammatory reactions.[113] They participate in several important physiologic processes, including initiation of plasma lipolysis,[114] stimulation and inhibition of hemostasis[115,116] and rejection of certain parasites such as ticks.[117] They also may be involved in cytotoxicity of neoplastic cells during immune surveillance.[118–120]

Basophilia, defined as a prolonged increase in circulating numbers of basophils (>140 basophils/μL blood), is a rare event. Because numbers of circulating basophils are low in health, the routine differential cell count is a rather insensitive measure of basophil numbers. Only sustained increases in basophil numbers of >3 to 6% of the differential cell count can be detected on routine blood smears.[1]

The most frequently reported causes of basophilia in dogs are listed in Table 55.4.[1–5,75,89,92,111,113–130] Usually, basophilia accompanies eosinophilia but can occur independently. The most common cause of basophilia in the dog is infection with the canine heartworm, *Dirofilaria immitis*.[1,121–123] Basophilia also is reported owing to infection with several other parasites and infectious agents.[53,124] In addition, basophilia is associated with various hypersensitivity or inflammatory conditions,[89,125] several neoplastic diseases,[92,111,126–129] and as an infrequent consequence of the administration of certain drugs.[1] Although it has been suggested that basophilia is a result of lipemia associated with chronic liver disease, nephrotic syndrome, and endocrine disturbances, including diabetes mellitus and hyperadrenocorticism,[4] these assertions have not been confirmed in many cases. Significant basophilia caused by basophilic leukemia is rare.[130]

Basophil counts in healthy dogs range from 0 to 140

TABLE 55.4	Causes of Basophilia in Dogs[1–5,75,89,92,111,113–130]

Drug administration
  Heparin, penicillin

Hypersensitivity and/or inflammatory lesions
  Allergic respiratory disease, cutaneous eosinophilic granuloma, eosinophilic gastroenteritis, experimental *Candida crusei* and *Candida albicans* administration, osteomyelitis, pulmonary eosinophilic granuloma, pulmonary infiltrates with eosinophilia

Neoplasia
  Basophilic leukemia, disseminated mast cell neoplasia, essential thrombocythemia, lymphomatoid granulomatosis, thymoma

Parasitic diseases
  Ancylostoma and *Uncinaria* sp., *Dirofilaria immitis, Dipetalonema reconditum, Hepatozoon canis*

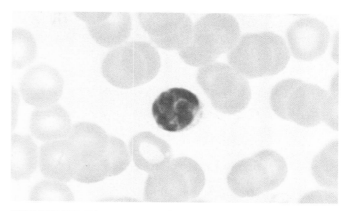

FIGURE 55.15   Normal canine lymphocyte, Wright's stain.

basophils/μL.[3] Because many normal dogs may routinely have basophil counts of 0/μL, basopenia is difficult to document with currently available methods and is considered clinically insignificant at this time.

LYMPHOCYTOSIS AND LYMPHOPENIA

Canine lymphocytes are small, round mononuclear cells. They have a round to oval nucleus with aggregated chromatin and indistinct nucleoli. The blue cytoplasm is scant and may contain few azurophilic granules (Fig. 55.15). In healthy dogs, the lymphocyte is the second most commonly encountered leukocyte. B lymphocytes function in humoral immunity, and the T lymphocytes are components of cell-mediated immunity. B and T lymphocytes appear similar by light microscopic examination of Romanowsky-stained blood films. However, the majority of lymphocytes in the blood are T lymphocytes.[3] In general, B cells are short-lived (days to weeks) compared with T cells (months to years). Lymphocytes are unique among leukocytes in their ability to recirculate and undergo mitosis.[4,5]

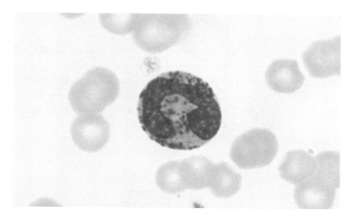

FIGURE 55.14   Normal canine basophil, Wright's stain.

Lymphocytosis, defined as >2900 lymphocytes/ μL blood, is an uncommon occurrence in the dog. The causes of lymphocytosis are listed in Table 55.5.[1–5,7,25,28,109,131–157] Physiologic leukocytosis may cause a transient lymphocytosis. Although the complete mechanism of lymphocytosis in physiologic leukocytosis is unknown, epinephrine is a likely mediator of this alteration. Current hypotheses suggest that epinephrine-mediated release of lymphocytes from the thoracic duct or inhibition of lymphocyte recirculation by means of alterations of surface receptors on endothelial cells and lymphocytes may account for the lymphocytosis.[1] Physiologic lymphocytosis does not occur frequently in the adult dog and is more common in puppies. This form of lymphocytosis can be avoided if animals are not overly excited at time of venipuncture. Examination of a second sample of blood, collected at a later time from the calmed or tranquilized dog, can be used to distinguish transient lymphocytosis of physiologic leukocytosis from lymphocytosis of pathologic origin.[1]

Persistent antigenic stimulation of chronic infection or inflammatory reactions may cause lymphocytosis in dogs. Chronic canine ehrlichiosis[28,131] and Rocky Mountain spotted fever are diseases that result in proliferation of lymphocytes and expansion of the blood lymphocyte pool. Trypanosomiasis,[132–134] leishmaniasis,[135] and brucellosis[136] also may cause lymphocytosis by a similar mechanism.

Lymphoid neoplasia may cause lymphocytosis.[137] Lymphosarcoma, acute or chronic lymphocytic leukemia, and thymoma have been associated with lymphocytosis.[138] The highest lymphocyte counts usually are associated with chronic lymphocytic leukemia.[139] Lymphosarcoma, a neoplastic proliferation of lymphocytes within tissue, may also produce lymphocytosis in approximately 10% of dogs that have this disease.[140]

Hypoadrenocorticism (Addison's disease) has been reported to cause lymphocytosis in 11 to 20% of affected dogs.[109,141] The lack of lymphopenia in a severely stressed dog would provide supportive evidence for glucocorticoid deficiency.[109]

Lymphopenia, defined as <400 lymphocytes/μL blood, is a common occurrence in dogs and may result from several different mechanisms.[3] Causes of lymphopenia are listed in Table 55.5. Physical stresses such as extremes in temperature or pain, that result in excess corticosteroid release causes lymphopenia of transient and predictable nature. Exogenous administration of corticosteroids or ACTH and hyperadrenocorticism also causes lymphopenia. The common mechanism of lymphopenia after corticosteroid exposure is redistribution of lymphocytes to bone marrow or body compartments.[1,4] The lympholysis and depletion of lymphoid tissues that occurs when dogs receive high doses of corticosteroids for prolonged periods also may contribute to lymphopenia.[142,143]

Acute infections may cause lymphopenia by means of stress-induced corticosteroid release and redistribution of lymphocytes.[1,4] Specific antigens may cause lymphocytes to become trapped in lymphoid tissues. Lymphopenia may occur when lymphocytes are recruited to antigenically stimulated lymph nodes and then emigrate into tissues.[1] Inflamed lymph nodes may occlude efferent lymph flow, thus preventing lymphocyte recirculation and compounding lymphopenia.[144] Certain viruses, particularly canine distemper virus and canine parvovirus, cause lymphocyte destruction, atrophy of lymphoid tissues, and depletion of lymphocyte subpopulations.[1,5,25]

Some cases of protein-losing enteropathy, lymphangiectasia, ulcerative enteritis, and granulomatous enteritis in dogs may cause lymphopenia by means of loss of lymphocyte-rich fluid into the intestinal lumen.[145] Chylothorax and chyloperitoneum may result in lymphopenia caused by sequestration of lymphocyte-rich fluids in body cavities.[146] Repeated centesis and removal of chyle from body cavities may exacerbate lymphopenia. Occlusion of the flow of lymph caused by disseminated granulomatous inflamation or neoplasia also can result in lymphopenia.

Rarely lymphopenia may be the result of congenital lymphocyte deficiency.[147] Basset hounds that have combined immunodeficiency may have lymphopenia and recurrent infections such as mycobacteriosis.[148]

TABLE 55.5 **Causes of Lymphocytosis and Lymphopenia in Dogs**[1–5,7,25,28,109,131–157]

Lymphocytosis
Chronic antigenic stimulation
  Aspergillosis, Actinomyces, Babesia canis, Blastomycosis, Brucellosis, Ehrlichiosis, Encephalitozoonosis, Leishmaniasis, Pneumocystis pneumonia, Rocky Mountain spotted fever, Trypanosoma cruzi gambiense
Hypoadrenocorticism
Lymphoid neoplasia
  lymphocytic leukemia (acute or chronic), lymphosarcoma, thymoma
Physiologic leukocytosis
  (not common in the dog)

Lymphopenia
Acute systemic bacterial infections
  Septicemia, endotoxemia
Corticosteroids
  Stress-induced leukocytosis (pain, extremes in body temperature), hyperadrenocorticism (Cushing's syndrome), exogenous corticosteroid therapy or ACTH administration
Disruption of lymph node architecture
  Generalized granulomatous disease, multicentric lymphosarcoma
Immunodeficiency syndromes
  Combined T- and B-cell deficiency of basset hounds
Immunosuppressive drugs
Loss of lymphocyte rich fluids
  Protein-losing enteropathy (lymphangiectasia), ulcerative enteritis, granulomatous enteritis, chylothorax, chyloperitoneum
Malignant neoplasia
  Lymphosarcoma, lymphocytic leukemia
Radiation
Viral infections (acute stages usually)
  Canine distemper, infectious canine hepatitis, coronavirus enteritis, canine parvovirus?

Morphologic Alterations in Lymphocytes

Reactive lymphocytes (immunocytes and transformed lymphocytes) are antigentically stimulated lymphoid cells that are occasionally seen in the blood of dogs (Fig. 55.16). These lymphoid cells are likely T cells but also may be B cells. They are slightly larger than normal small lymphocytes and have deeply basophilic cytoplasm. The nucleus contains aggregated chromatin and may have a scalloped margin. Nucleoli usually are indistinct. The cytoplasm may have a perinuclear Golgi zone and may contain a few vacuoles.[1,3]

Plasma cells are rare in the blood of dogs and are usually observed in bone marrow or lymph-node aspirates (Fig. 55.17). They are large B-lymphoid cells with intensely basophilic cytoplasm and a prominent, pale-staining, perinuclear Golgi zone. The nucleus is usually eccentrically located and has condensed chromatin.[1,3]

Granular lymphocytes or natural killer cells are null lymphoid cells that are seen infrequently in blood

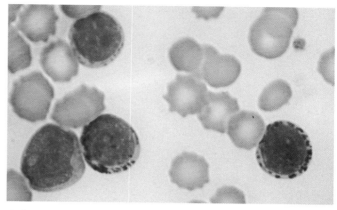

FIGURE 55.18 Large granular lymphocytes in a canine blood smear, Wright's stain. (Courtesy of Dr. Maxey L. Wellman, The Ohio State University, Columbus, OH).

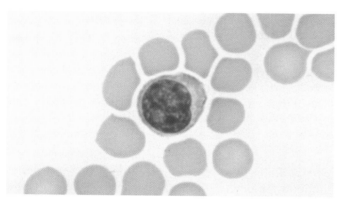

FIGURE 55.16 Reactive lymphocyte (immunocyte and transformed lymphocyte) in a canine blood smear, Wright's stain.

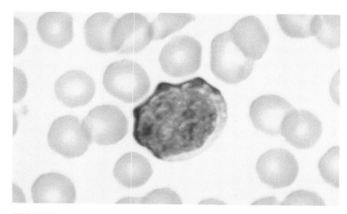

FIGURE 55.19 Lymphoblast in blood smear of a dog that has lymphosarcoma, Wright's stain. Notice the prominent nucleoli. (Courtesy of Dr. Rose Raskin, University of Florida, Gainesville, FL).

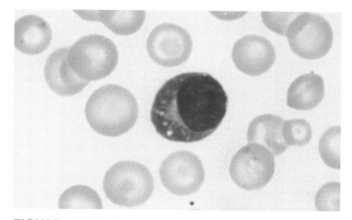

FIGURE 55.17 Plasma cell in canine blood smear, Wright's stain. (Courtesy of Dr. Steven L. Stockham, Columbia, MO).

smears (Fig. 55.18). They have few distinct azurophilic granules that tend to cluster at the nuclear margin or indentation.[1,149]

Lymphoblasts are large lymphoid cells that are observed frequently in disseminated lymphosarcoma and lymphoblastic leukemia (Fig. 55.19). Lymphoblasts have a large nucleus with vesicular chromatin and prominent nucleoli. The cytoplasm is abundant and has a deep blue hue.[1,3]

MONOCYTOSIS AND MONOCYTOPENIA

Canine monocytes are large cells with pleomorphic (round, oval, bilobed, or multilobed) nuclei and fine lacy

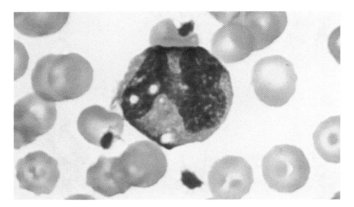

FIGURE 55.20 Normal canine monocyte, Wright's stain. Notice the large cell size, irregularly shaped nucleus, and cytoplasmic vacuoles.

TABLE 55.6	Causes of Monocytosis in Dogs[1-5,40,53,54,76,110,136,150,158-167]

Inflammatory lesions (acute or chronic)
  Bacteremia/septicemia, bacterial endocarditis, immune-mediated injury (hemolytic anemia), necrosis/suppuration (tissue or body cavities), osteomyelitis, pyogranulomatous disease

Miscellaneous causes
  Corticosteroid-induced leukocytosis, hemorrhage/hemolysis, rebound neutropenia/cyclic hematopoiesis, recombinant G-CSF administration, trauma

Neoplasia
  Benign tumors (rectal polyp), malignant tumors (chondrosarcoma, hemangiosarcoma, lymphosarcoma), malignant histiocytosis, monocytic leukemia, myelomonocytic leukemia

Parasitic diseases
  Hepatozoon canis infection, *Pneumocystis carinii* pneumonia, *Trypanosoma brucei* infection, *Angiostrongylus vasorum* infection

nuclear chromatin patterns (Fig. 55.20). Monocytes have large amounts of blue-gray cytoplasm that may contain numerous small vacuoles and few pink-to-azurophilic granules (lysosomes). Amoeboid or short hairlike processes (pseudopodia) may bulge from the cytoplasmic membrane.[3] The functions of monocytes are numerous and diverse and include phagocytosis and killing of infectious agents (certain bacteria, rickettsia, chlamydia, fungi, protozoa, and viruses), phagocytosis and digestion of foreign matter and effete cells, production of cytokines and colony-stimulating factors required for hemopoiesis, secretion of inflammatory mediators, tissue remodeling, immune recognition, and surveillance of virus-infected and tumor cells. In addition, monocytes are the source for many types of tissue macrophages.[1,3]

Monocytes occur in low numbers in the blood of healthy dogs. Monocytosis, defined by numbers that exceed 1400 monocytes/μL blood, may occur because of various reasons and may be associated with acute or chronic diseases.[3] In general, monocytosis occurs with neutrophilia, but rarely it may occur as a single alteration in a leukogram.[1,3] Causes of monocytosis in dogs are listed in Table 55.6.[1-5,40,53,76,110,136,150,158-167] Monocytosis is a fairly common leukogram alteration that often is associated with necrosis, suppuration, malignant neoplasia,[158-160] pyogranulomatous lesions, internal hemorrhage, hemolysis, trauma,[1] and immune-mediated diseases. It is an inconsistent finding in the leukogram of dogs responding to corticosteroids. It may be observed in the leukograms of dogs that have bacterial endocarditis or bacteremia. Monocytosis is seen often in cases of rebound from neutropenia such as in cyclic hemopoiesis of gray-collie dogs.[64,161] Significant, persistent monocytosis, with counts >50,000/μL blood, may be detected in monocytic or myelomonocytic leukemia. Abnormal monocyte morphology and numerous blast cells may be detected in the blood or bone marrow during these neoplastic diseases.

Reference intervals for monocyte counts in the blood from healthy dogs are fairly large. Therefore, it is difficult to document true, repeatable monocytopenia. Thus,

this alteration is of little clinical significance at this time. However, monocytopenia may be detected in some cases of acute pancytopenia that may be the result of several causes.[1]

Leukemia

The definition of leukemia is the neoplastic proliferation of hemopoietic cells originating in the bone marrow. Leukemias are classified by cell type and differentiation, time course of disease process (acute or chronic), and presence or absence of neoplastic cells in circulation. Myeloproliferative disorders reported in the dog include granulocytic (neutrophilic or myeloid) leukemia, myelomonocytic leukemia, monocytic leukemia, basophilic leukemia, mast cell leukemia, erythremic myelosis, polycythemia vera, megakaryocytic leukemia, and essential thrombocythemia. Lymphoproliferative diseases reported in the dog include lymphocytic leukemia and plasma cell leukemia. Diagnosis of these disorders is facilitated by examination of Romanowsky-stained blood films and bone marrow aspirate biopsies. Histologic examination of bone marrow core biopsies may be required in some cases. Use of immunohistochemistry greatly aides diagnosis in poorly differentiated cell types.[1-4] The diagnosis, classification, and clinical behavior of the various leukemias are reported in Sections IX and X.

REFERENCES

1. **Latimer KS.** Leukocytes in health and disease. In: Ettinger SJ, Feldman EC, eds. Textbook of veterinary internal medicine. Diseases of the dog and cat. 4th ed. Philadelphia: WB Saunders, 1995;1892–1946.
2. **Latimer KS, Rakich PM.** Clinical interpretation of leukocyte responses. Vet Clin North Am Small Anim Pract 1989;19:637–668.
3. **Duncan RJ, Prasse KW, Mahaffey EA.** Veterinary laboratory medicine; clinical pathology. 3rd ed. Ames, IA: Iowa State University Press, 1994;37–62.
4. **Jain NC.** Schalm's veterinary hematology. 4th ed. Philadelphia: Lea & Febiger, 1986.

5. **Jain NC.** Essentials of veterinary hematology. Philadelphia: Lea & Febiger, 1993.

6. **Lilliehöök I.** Diurnal variation of canine blood leukocyte counts. Vet Clin Pathol 1997;26:113–117.

7. **Meyer DJ, Coles EH, Rich LJ.** Veterinary laboratory medicine: interpretation and diagnosis. Philadelphia: WB Saunders, 1992.

8. **Jensen AL, Nielson OL.** Eosinophilic leukemoid reaction in a dog. J Small Anim Pract 1992;33:337–340.

9. **Giger U, Boxer LA, Simpson PJ, Lucchesi BR, Todd RF III.** Deficiency of leukocyte surface glycoproteins Mol, LFA-1, and Leu M5 in a dog with recurrent bacterial infections: an animal model. Blood 1987;69:1622–1630.

10. **Trowald-Wigh G, Hakansson L, Johannisson A, Norrgren L, Hard-af-Segerstad C.** Leukocyte adhesion protein deficiency in Irish setter dogs. Vet Immunol Immunopathol 1992;32:261–280.

11. **Gaunt PS, Gaunt SD, Craig TM.** Extreme neutrophilic leukocytosis in a dog with hepatozoonosis. J Am Vet Med Assoc 1983;182:409–410.

12. **Lappin MR, Latimer KS.** Hematuria and extreme neutrophilic leukocytosis in a dog with renal tubular carcinoma. J Am Vet Med Assoc 1988;192:1289–1292.

13. **Madewell BR, Wilson DW, Hornof WJ, Gregory CR.** Leukemoid blood response and bone infarcts in a dog with renal tubular adenocarcinoma. J Am Vet Med Assoc 1990;197:1623–1625.

14. **Chinn DR, Myers RK, Matthews JA.** Neutrophilic leukocytosis associated with metastatic fibrosarcoma in a dog. J Am Vet Med Assoc 1985;186:806–809.

15. **Tomlinson MJ, Jennings PB, Wendt JB, Meriwether WA, Crumrine MH.** Adenocarcinoma of the lung with secondary pericardial effusion and leukemoid response in a dog. J Am Vet Med Assoc 1973;63:257–258.

16. **Thompson JP, Christopher MM, Ellison GW, Homer BL, Buchanan BA.** Paraneoplastic leukocytosis associated with a rectal adenomatous polyp in a dog. J Am Vet Med Assoc 1992;201:737–738.

17. **Wade BH, Mandell GL.** Polymorphonuclear phagocytes: Dedicated professional phagocytes. Am J Med 1983;74:686–693.

18. **Wright DG.** The neutrophil as a secretory organ of host defense. In: Gallin JA, Fauci AS, eds. Advances in host defense mechanisms, vol 1. New York: Raven Press, 1982;75–110.

19. **Raab SO, Athens JW, Haab OP, Boggs DR, Ashenbrucker H, Cartwright GE, Wintrobe MM.** Granulokinetics in normal dogs. Am J Physiol 1964;206:83–88.

20. **Frimberger AE, Cotter SM.** Principles of chemotherapy. In: Hahn KA, Richardson RC, eds. Cancer chemotherapy, a veterinary handbook. Philadelphia: Williams and Wilkins, 1995;47–62.

21. **Gaunt SD, Pierce KR.** Effects of estradiol on hematopoietic and marrow adherent cells of dogs. Am J Vet Res 1986;47:906–909.

22. **Badame FG, van Slyke W, Hayes MA.** Reversible phenylbutazone-induced pancytopenia in a dog. Can J Vet 1984;25:269–270.

23. **Giger U, Werner LL, Millichamp NJ, Gorman NT.** Sulfadiazine-induced allergy in six Doberman Pinschers. J Am Vet Med Assoc 1985;186:479–484.

24. **Weiss DJ, Adams LG.** Aplastic anemia associated with trimethoprim-sulfadiazine and fenbendazole administration in a dog. J Am Vet Med Assoc 1987;191:1119–1120.

25. **Young N, Mortimer P.** Viruses and bone marrow failure. Blood 1984;63:729–737.

26. **Pollock RVH.** The parvoviruses. Part II. Canine parvovirus. Comp Contin Educ Pract Vet 1984;6:653–664.

27. **Stockham SL, Schmidt DA, Tyler JW.** Canine granulocytic ehrlichiosis in dogs from Central Missouri: A possible cause of polyarthritis. Vet Med Rev 1985;6:2–5.

28. **Stockham SL, Tyler JW, Schmidt DA, Curtis KS.** Experimental transmission of granulocytic ehrlichial organisms in dogs. Vet Clin Pathol 1990;19:99–104.

29. **Stockham SL, Schmidt DA, Curtis KS, Schauf BG, Tyler JW, Simpson ST.** Evaluation of granulocytic ehrlichiosis in dogs of Missouri including serologic status to *Ehrlichia canis*, *Ehrlichia equi* and *Borrelia burgdorferi*. Am J Vet Res 1992;53:63–68.

30. **Codner EC, Farris-Smith LL.** Characterization of the subclinical phase of ehrlichiosis in dogs. J Am Vet Med Assoc 1986;189:47–50.

31. **Cowell RL, Tyler RD, Clinkenbeard KD, Meinkoth JH.** Ehrlichiosis and polyarthritis in three dogs. J Am Vet Med Assoc 1988;192:1093–1095.

32. **Fyfe JC, Jezyk PF, Giger U, Patterson DF.** Inherited selective malabsorption of vitamin B$_{12}$ in Giant Schnauzers. J Am Anim Hosp Assoc 1989;25:533–539.

33. **Fyfe JC, Giger U, Hall CA, Jezyk PF, Klumpp SA, Levine JS, Patterson DF.** Inherited selective intestinal cobalamin malabsorption and cobalamin deficiency in dogs. Pediatr Res 1991;29:24–31.

34. **Weiss DJ, Armstrong PJ.** Secondary myelofibrosis in three dogs. J Am Vet Med Assoc 1985;187:423–425.

35. **Hoenig M.** Six dogs with features compatible with myelonecrosis and myelofibrosis. J Am Anim Hosp Assoc 1989;25:335–339.

36. **Hoff B, Lumsden JL, Valli VEO, Kruth SA.** Myelofibrosis: review of clinical and pathological features in fourteen dogs. Can Vet J 1991;32:357–361.

37. **Clinkenbeard KD, Cowell RL, Tyler RD.** Disseminated histoplasmosis in dogs: 12 cases (1981–1986). J Am Vet Med Assoc 1988;193:1443–1447.

38. **Couto CG, Kallet AJ.** Preleukemic syndrome in a dog. J Am Vet Med Assoc 1984;184:1389–1392.

39. **Albassam MA, Houston BJ, Greaves P, Barsoum N.** Polyarteritis in a Beagle. J Am Vet Med Assoc 1989;194:1595–1597.

40. **Allen WM, Pocock PI, Dalton PM, Richards HE, Aitken MM.** Cyclic neutropenia in collies. Vet Rec 1996;138:371–372.

41. **Axthelm MK, Krakowka S.** Canine distemper virus-induced thrombocytopenia. Am J Vet Res 1987;48:1269–1275.

42. **Calvert CA.** Salmonella infections in hospitalized dogs: epizootiology, diagnosis and prognosis. J Am Anim Hosp Assoc 1985;21:499–503.

43. **Dale DC, Graw RC Jr.** Transplantation of allogeneic bone marrow in canine cyclic neutropenia. Science 1974;183:83–84.

44. **Deldar A, Lewis H, Bloom J, Weiss L.** Cephalosporin-induced changes in the ultrastructure of canine bone marrow. Vet Pathol 1988;25:211–218.

45. **Donnolly D.** Canine granulocytopathy syndrome in Irish setters. J Small Anim Pract 1997;38:591.

46. **Hammer AS, Couto CG, Filppi J, Getzy D, Shank K.** Efficacy and toxicity of VAC chemotherapy (vincristine, doxorubicin, and cyclophosphamide) in dogs with hemagiosarcoma J Vet Intern Med 1991;5:160–166.

47. **Harris CK, Beck ER, Gasper PW.** Bone marrow transplantation in the dog. Comp Contin Educ Pract Vet 1986;8:337–344.

48. **Liefer CE, Matus RE, Patnaik AK, MacEwen EG.** Chronic myelogenous leukemia in the dog. J Am Vet Med Assoc 1983;183:686–689.

49. **Lund JE, Padgett GA.** Animal models of human disease: canine cyclic neutropenia. Comp Pathol Bull 1973;5:2,4.

50. **Macartney L, McCandlish IAP, Thompson H, Cornwell HJC.** Canine parvovirus enteritis 1: clinical, haematological and pathological features of experimental infection. Vet Rec 1984;115:201–210.

51. **Maddison JE, Hoff B, Johnson RP.** Steroid responsive neutropenia in a dog. J Am Anim Hosp Assoc 1983;19:881–886.

52. **Messick J, Carothers M, Wellman M.** Identification and characterization of megakaryoblasts in acute megakaryoblastic leukemia in a dog. Vet Pathol 1990;27:212–214.

53. **Mishu L, Callahan G, Allebban Z, Maddux JM, Boone TC, Souza LM, Lothrop CD.** Effects of recombinant canine granulocyte colony-stimulating factor on white blood cell production in clinically normal and neutropenic dogs. J Am Vet Med Assoc 1992;200:1957–1964.

54. **Renshaw HW, Chatburn C, Bryan GM, Bartsch RC, Davis WC.** Canine granulocytopathy syndrome: neutrophil dysfunction with recurrent infections. J Am Vet Med Assoc 1975;166:443–447.

55. **Scott-Moncrieff JCR, Snyder PW, Glickman LT, Davis EL, Felsburg PJ.** Systemic necrotizing vasculitis in nine young Beagles. J Am Vet Med Assoc 1992;201:1553–1558.

56. **Van Vechten M, Helfand SC, Jeglum KA.** Treatment of relapsed canine lymphoma with doxorubicin and dacarbazine. J Vet Intern Med 1990;4:187–191.

57. **Vercammen F, de Deken R , Maes I, de Deken R.** Haematological and biochemical profile in experimental canine babesiosis (Babesia canis). Vlaams Diergeneeskundig Tijdschrift 1997;66:174–178.

58. **Weiden PL, Robinett B, Graham TC, Adamson J, Storb R.** Canine cyclic neutropenia: a stem cell defect. J Clin Invest 1974;53:950–953.

59. **Weiss DJ, Armstrong PJ, Reimann K.** Bone marrow necrosis in the dog. J Am Vet Med Assoc 1985;187:54–59.

60. **Weiss DJ, Raskin R, Zerbe C.** Myelodysplastic syndrome in two dogs. J Am Vet Med Assoc 1985;187:1038–1040.

61. **Shull RM, DeNovo RC, McCraken MD.** Megakaryoblastic leukemia in a dog. Vet Pathol 1986;23:533–536.

62. **Campbell KL.** Canine cyclic hematopoiesis. Comp Contin Educ Pract Vet 1985;7:57–60.

63. **Bertram TA.** Neutrophilic leukocyte structure and function in domestic animals. Adv Vet Sci Comp Med 1985;30:91–129.

64. **Latimer KS, Duncan JR, Kircher IM.** Nuclear segmentation, ultrastructure and cytochemistry of blood cells from dogs with Pelger-Huët anomaly. J Comp Pathol 1987;97:61–72.

65. **Latimer KS, Kircher IM, Lindl PA, Dawe DL, Brown J.** Leukocyte function in Pelger-Huët anomaly of dogs. J Leukoc Biol 1989;45:301–310.

66. **Gossett KA, Carakostas MC.** Effect of EDTA on morphology of neutrophils of healthy dogs and dogs with inflammation. Vet Clin Pathol 1984;13:22–25.

67. **Barsanti JA, Finco DR.** Evaluation of techniques for diagnosis of canine prostatic diseases. J Am Vet Med Assoc 1984;185:198–200.

68. **Hirsh CD, Jang SS, Biberstein DL.** Blood culture of the canine patient. J Am Vet Med Assoc 1984;184:175–178.

69. **Salisbury KS, Lantz GC, Nelson RW, Kazacos EA.** Pancreatic abscess in dogs: six cases (1978–1986). J Am Vet Med Assoc 1988;193:1104–1108.

70. **Gossett KA, MacWilliams PS, Enright FM, Cleghorn B.** *In vitro* function of canine neutrophils during experimental inflammatory disease. Vet Immunol Immunopathol 1983;5:151–159.

71. **Gossett KA, MacWilliams PS.** Ultrastructure of canine toxic neutrophils. Am J Vet Res 1982;43:1624–1637.

72. **Gossett KA, MacWilliams PS, Cleghorn B.** Sequential morphological and

quantitative changes in blood and bone marrow neutrophils in dogs with acute inflammation. Can J Comp Med 1985;49:291–297.

73. **Tvedten HW, Walker RD, DiPinto NM.** Mycobacterium bacteremia in a dog: diagnosis of septicemia by microscopical evaluation of blood. J Am Anim Hosp Assoc 1990;26:359–363.

74. **McLaughlin BG, Adams PS, Cornell WD, Elkins AD.** Canine distemper viral inclusions in blood cells of four vaccinated dogs. Can Vet J 1985; 26:368–372.

75. **Baker JL, Craig TM, Barton CCL, Scott DW.** Hepatozoon canis infection in dog with oral pyogranulomas and neurological disease. Cornell Vet 1988;78:179–180.

76. **Makimura S, Kinjo H.** Cytochemical identification of canine circulating leukocytes parasitized with the gametocyte of Hepatozoon canis. J Vet Med Sci 1991;53:963–965.

77. **van Steenhouse JL, DeNovo RC.** Atypical *Histoplasma capsulatum* infection in a dog. J Am Vet Med Assoc 1986;188:527–528.

78. **Domina F, Catarsini O.** Unusual report of Leishmania in circulating cells. Atti della Societa Italiana delle Scienze Veterinarie 1984;37:359–361.

79. **Schalm OW.** Uncommon hematologic disorders: spirochetosis, trypanosomiasis, leishmaniasis, Pelger-Huët anomaly. Can Pract 1979;6:46–49.

80. **Troy GC, Forrester SD.** Canine ehrlichiosis. In: Infectious diseases of the dog and cat. Philadelphia: WB Saunders, 1990; 404–418.

81. **Goldman EE, Breitschwerdt EB, Grindem CB, Hegarty BC, Walls JJ, Dumler JS.** Granulocytic ehrlichiosis in dogs from North Carolina and Virginia. J Vet Intern Med 1998;12:61–70.

82. **Gaunt SD, Baker DC.** Hemosiderin in leukocytes of dogs with immune-mediated hemolytic anemia. Vet Clin Pathol 1986;15:8–10.

83. **Haskins ME, Desnick RJ, DiFerrante N, Jezyk PF, Patterson DF.** Beta-glucuronidase deficiency in a dog: a model of human mucopolysaccharidosis VII. Pediatr Res 1984;18:980–984.

84. **Neer TM, Dial SM, Pechman R, Wang P, Oliver JL, Giger U.** Clinical vignette. Mucopolysaccharidosis VI in a miniature pinscher. J Vet Intern Med 1995;9:429–433.

85. **Butterworth AE, David JR.** Eosinophil function. N Engl J Med 1981; 304:154–156.

86. **Beeson PB.** Cancer and eosinophilia. N Engl J Med 1983;309:792–793.

87. **Sanderson CJ.** Interleukin-5, eosinophils, and disease. Blood 1992;79:3101–3109.

88. **Tavassoli M.** Eosinophil, eosinophilia and eosinophilic disorders. Crit Rev Clin Lab Sci 1981;16:35–83.

89. **Corcoran BM, Thoday KL, Henfrey JI, Simpson JW, Burnie AG, Mooney CT.** Pulmonary infiltration of eosinophils in 14 dogs. J Small Anim Pract 1991;32:494–502.

90. **Couto CG.** Tumor-associated eosinophilia in a dog. J Am Vet Med Assoc 1984;184:837.

91. **Losco PE.** Local and peripheral eosinophilia in a dog with anaplastic mammary carcinoma. Vet Pathol 1986;23:536–538.

92. **O'Keefe DA, Couto CG, Burke-Schwartz C, Jacobs RM.** Systemic mastocytosis in 16 dogs. J Vet Intern Med 1987;1:75–80.

93. **Ballmer Rusca E, Hauser B.** Case report: persistent eosinophilia in a dog. Hypereosinophilic syndrome? Kleintierpraxis 1993;38:137–138.

94. **Cain GR, Kawakami T, Taylor N, Champlin R.** Effects of administration of recombinant human interleukin-2 in dogs Comp Haematol Int 1992;2:201–207.

95. **Domina F, Giudice E, Britti D.** Tetracycline-induced eosinophilia in the dog. J Vet Pharmacol Ther 1997;20(suppl1):259–260.

96. **Millis DL, Hauptman JG, Richter M.** Preoperative and postoperative hemostatic profiles of dogs undergoing ovariohysterectomy. Cornell Vet 1992;82:465–470.

97. **Ling GV, Stabenfeldt GH, Comer KM, Gribble DH, Schechter RD.** Canine hyperadrenocorticism: pretreatment clinical and laboratory evaluation of 117 cases. J Am Vet Med Assoc 1979;174:1211–1215.

98. **Osbaldiston GW, Greve T.** Estimating adrenal cortical function in dogs with ACTH. Cornell Vet 1978;68:308–316.

99. **Dillon AR, Spano JS, Powers RD.** Prednisolone induced hematologic, biochemical, and histologic changes in the dog. J Am Anim Hosp Assoc 1980;16:831–837.

100. **Lee GR, Bithell TC, Foerster J, Athens JW, Leukens JN, Kushner J,** eds. Wintrobe's clinical hematology. 9th ed. Philadelphia: Lea & Febiger, 1993.

101. **Arlian LG, Morgan MS, Rapp CM, Vyszenski Moher DL.** Some effects of sarcoptic mange on dogs. J Pathol 1995;81:698–702.

102. **Bourdeau P, Klap DF, Mialot M.** Dermatobia hominis myiasis. Case report in a dog. Recueil de Medecine Veterinaire 1988;164:901–906.

103. **Brocklebank J.** Canine Cryptococcus neoformans. Can Vet J 1997;38:724.

104. **Guelfi JF.** Symptoms and diagnosis of cardiopulmonary strongylosis in the dog. Animal de Compagnie 1976;11:49–56.

105. **Jones GW, Neal C, Turner GRJ.** Angiostrongylus vasorum infection in dogs in Cornwall. Vet Rec 1980;106:83.

106. **Lowry S.** Challenging cases in internal medicine: what's your diagnosis? [Addison's disease]. Vet Med 1993;88:716–723.

107. **Moon M.** Pulmonary infiltrates with eosinophilia. J Small Anim Pract 1992;33:19–23.

108. **Patton CS, Hake R, Newton J, Toal RL.** Esophagitis due to Phythium insidiosum infection in two dogs. J Vet Intern Med 1996;10:139–142.

109. **Rakich PM, Lorenz MD.** Clinical signs and laboratory abnormalities in 23 dogs with spontaneous hypoadrenocorticism. J Am Anim Hosp Assoc 1984;20:647–649.

110. **Ramsey IK, Foster A, McKay J, Herrtage ME.** Pneumocystis carinii pneumonia in two Cavalier King Charles spaniels. Vet Rec 1997;140:372–373.

111. **Simpson RM, Waters DJ, Gebhard DH, Casey HW.** Massive thymoma with medullar differentiation in a dog. Vet Pathol 1992;29:416–419.

112. **Torgerson PR, McCarthy G, Donnelly WJC.** Filaroides hirthi verminous pneumonia in a West Highland white terrier bred in Ireland. J Small Anim Pract 1997;38:217–219.

113. **Halliwell REW, Schemmer KR.** The role of basophils in the immunopathogenesis of hypersensitivity to fleas (*Ctenocephalides felis*) in dogs. Vet Immuno Immunopathol 1987;15:203–213.

114. **Jasper DE, Jain NC.** Postprandial lipemia in dogs. Calif Vet 1964;18:27.

115. **Dvorak AM, Dvorak HF.** The basophil: its morphology, biochemistry, motility, release reactions, recovery, and role in the inflammatory responses of IgE-mediated and cell-mediated origin. Arch Pathol Lab Med 1979; 103:551–557.

116. **Newball HH, Meier HL, Lichtenstein LM.** Basophil mediators and their release, with emphasis on BK-A. J Invest Dermatol 1980;74:344–348.

117. **Brown SJ, Askenase PW.** Immune rejection of ectoparasites (ticks) by T-cell and IgG$_1$ antibody recruitment of basophils and eosinophils. Fed Proc 1983;42:1744–1749.

118. **Anthony HM.** Blood basophils in lung cancer. Br J Cancer 1982;45:209–216.

119. **May ME, Waddell CC.** Basophils in peripheral blood and bone marrow: a retrospective review. Am J Med 1984;76:509–511.

120. **Huntley JF.** Mast cells and basophils: a review of their heterogeneity and function. J Comp Pathol 1992;107:349–372.

121. **Matic SE, Herrtage ME.** Diagnosis and treatment of occult dirofilariasis in an imported dog. J Small Anim Pract 1987;28:183–196.

122. **Rawlings CA, Prestood AK, Beck BB.** Eosinophilia and basophilia in Dirofilaria immitis and Dipetalonema reconditum infections. J Am Anim Hosp Assoc 1980;16:699–704.

123. **Rawlings CA.** Clinical laboratory evaluations of seven heartworm infected Beagles: during disease development and following treatment. Cornell Vet 1982;72:49–56.

124. **Begovic S, Kadic M, Tafro A.** Experimental basophilia in dogs, sheep and rabbits. Veterinaria 1972;21:447–458.

125. **Varsheny AC, Singh H.** Haematological alterations in osteomyelitis in dogs. Indian J Vet Med 1993;13:19–20.

126. **Pollack MJ, Flanders JA, Johnson RC.** Disseminated malignant mastocytoma in a dog. J Am Anim Hosp Assoc 1991;27:435–440.

127. **Postorino NC, Wheeler SL, Park RD, Powers BE, Withrow SJ.** A syndrome resembling lymphomatoid granulomatosis in the dog. J Vet Intern Med 1989;3:15–19.

128. **Hopper PE, Mandell CP, Turrel JM, Jain NC, Tablin F, Zinkl JG.** Probable essential thrombocythemia in a dog. J Vet Intern Med 1989;3:79–85.

129. **Calvert CA, Mahaffey MB, Lappin MR, Farrell RL.** Pulmonary and disseminated eosinophilic granulomatosis in dogs. J Am Anim Hosp Assoc 1988;24:311–320.

130. **Mears EA, Raskin RE, Legendre AM.** Basophilic leukemia in a dog. J Vet Intern Med 1997;11:92–94.

131. **Breitschwerdt EB, Woody BJ, Zerbe CA, De Buysscher EV, Barta O.** Monoclonal gammopathy associated with naturally occurring canine ehrlichiosis. J Vet Intern Med 1987;1:2–9.

132. **Barr SC, Gossett KA, Klei TR.** Clinical, clinicopathologic, and parasitologic observations of trypanosomiasis in dogs infected with North American Trypanosoma cruzi isolates. Am J Vet Res 1991;52:954–960.

133. **Schoning B.** The dogs as reservoir host of Trypanosoma (Trypanozoon) brucei gambiense: a comparative study on the susceptibility of European and West African dogs to T. gambiense and T. brucei and on the course of infection. J Nr 1990;1481:113.

134. **Weiser MG, Thrall MA, Fulton R, Beck ER, Wise LA, van Steenhouse JL.** Granular lymphocytosis and hyperproteinemia in dogs with chronic ehrlichiosis. J Am Anim Hosp Assoc 1991;27:84–88.

135. **Groulade P.** Canine leishmaniasis. Clinical haematology and biology of leishmaniasis. Animal de Compagnie 1977;12:121–128.

136. **Villalba EJ, Garrido A, Molina JM, Poveda JB, Portero JM.** Haemogram in canine brucellosis. Medicina Veterinaria 1990;9:99–100, 102–104.

137. **Raskin RE, Krehbiel JD.** Prevalence of leukemic blood and bone marrow in dogs with multicentric lymphoma. J Am Vet Med Assoc 1989;194:1427–1429.

138. **Matus RE, Leifer CE, MacEwen EG.** Acute lymphoblastic leukemia in the dog: a review of 30 cases. J Am Vet Med Assoc 1983;183:859–862.

139. **Leifer CE, Matus RE.** Chronic lymphocytic leukemia in the dog: 22 cases (1974–1984) J Am Vet Med Assoc 1986;189:214–217.

140. **Madewell BR.** Hematological and bone marrow cytological abnormalities in 75 dogs with malignant lymphoma. J Am Anim Hosp Assoc 1986; 22:235–240.

141. **Willard MD, Schall WD, McCaw DE, Nachreiner RF.** Canine hypoadreno-

corticism: report of 37 cases and review 39 previously reported cases. J Am Vet Med Assoc 1982;180:59–62.

142. **Jasper DE, Jain NC.** The influence of adrenocorticotropic hormone and prednisolone upon marrow and circulating leukocytes in the dog. Am J Vet Res 1965;26:844–850.

143. **Schuyler MR, Gerblich A, Urda G.** Prednisolone and T-cell subpopulations. Arch Intern Med 1984;144:973–975.

144. **Hopkins J, McConnell I.** Immunological aspects of lymphocyte recirculation. Vet Immunol Immunopathol 1984;6:3–33.

145. **Meschter CL, Rakich PM, Tyler DE.** Intestinal lymphangiectasia with lipogranulomatous lymphangitis in a dog. J Am Vet Med Assoc 1987; 190:427–430.

146. **Fossum TW, Birchard SJ, Jacobs RM.** Chylothorax in 34 dogs. J Am Vet Med Assoc 1986;188:1315–1318.

147. **Felsburg PJ, Jezyk PF, Haskins ME.** A canine model for variable combined immunodeficiency Clin Res 1982;30:347A

148. **Carpenter JL, Myers AM, Conner MW, Schelling SH, Kennedy FA, Reimann KA.** Tuberculosis in five Basset Hounds. J Am Vet Med Assoc 1988;192:1563–1568.

149. **Kay NE.** Natural killer cells. Crit Rev Clin Lab Sci 1986;22:343–359.

150. **Canfield PJ, Church DB, Malik R.** Pneumocystis pneumonia in a dog. Aust Vet Pract 1993;23:150–154.

151. **Hennet P.** What is your diagnosis? [aspergillosis of the nasal cavities in a Siberian Husky dog]. Point Veterinaire 1994;25:805–809.

152. **Kagiwara MK, Holzchuh MP, Hagiwara MK.** Experimental infection of dogs with Babesia canis. I. Evaluation of leukocyte changes during the evolution of the disease. Arquivo Brasilerio de Medicina Veterinaria e Zootecnia 1987;39:745–755.

153. **Kelly WD.** The thymus and lymphoid morphogenesis in the dog. Fed Proc 1963;22:600.

154. **Krakowka S, Higgins RJ, Koestner A.** Canine distemper virus: review of structural and function modulations in lymphoid tissues. Am J Vet Res 1980;41:284–292.

155. **McElhaney LM, Jones MP.** Challenging cases in internal medicine: what's your diagnosis? [Actinomyces infection]. Vet Med 1993;88:1032–1038.

156. **Szabo JR.** Observations on the pathogenesis of canine encephalitozoonosis. Dissertation Abstracts International-B 1985;46:1126.

157. **Szabo JR, Shadduck JA.** Experimental encepalitozoonosis in neonatal dogs. Vet Pathol 1987;24:99–108.

158. **LaRock RG, Ginn PI, Burrows CF, Newell SM, Henson KL.** Primary mesenchymal chondrosarcoma in the pericardium of a dog. J Vet Diagn Invest 1997;9:410–413.

159. **Hoskins JD, Davis CK.** Compendium challenge. [haemangiosarcoma in the heart base and aorta in a Poodle]. Comp Cont Educ Pract Vet 1994;16:895–900.

160. **McCaw DL, Turk MAM, Schmidt DA, Da-Silva-Curiel JMA.** Multiple mucocutaneous lymphosarcoma in a dog. Can Vet J 1988;29:1001–1002.

161. **Pfeil R.** Long-term haematological studies on dogs with spontaneous parvovirus infection. Kleinteirpraxis 1984;29:413–422.

162. **Cobb MA, Fisher MA.** Angiostrongylus vasorum: transmission in south east England. Vet Rec 1990;126:529.

163. **Dunn JK, Dennis R, Houston JEF.** Successful treatment of two cases of metaphyseal osteomyelitis in the dog. J Small Anim Pract 1992;33:85–89.

164. **Koch J, Jensen AL, Monrad J.** Angiostrongylus vasorum infection in a Scottish terrier associated with gastric dilation. J Small Anim Pract 1992; 33:239–241.

165. **Kohn B, Arnold P, Kaser-Holtz B, Hauser B, Fluckiger M, Suter PF.** Malignant histiocytosis of the dog: 26 cases (1989–1992). Kleintierpraxis 1993;38:409–424.

166. **Luttgen PJ, Whitney MS, Wolf AM, Scruggs DW.** Heinz body hemolytic anemia associated with high plasma zinc concentration in a dog. J Am Vet Med Assoc 1990;197:1347–1350.

167. **Nwosu CO, Ikeme MM.** Parsitaemia and clinical manifestations in Trypansoma brucei infected dogs. Revue d'Elevage et de Medecine Veterinaire des Pays Tropicaux 1992;45:273–277.

CHAPTER 56

Interpretation of Feline Leukocyte Responses

• RICK L. COWELL and LILLI S. DECKER

The complete blood cell count (CBC) is a vital component of the minimum laboratory database used in the evaluation of feline illnesses. The CBC provides quantitative and qualitative information regarding the status of red cells (hemogram), platelets (thrombogram), and leukocytes (leukogram). The leukogram includes a total white blood cell (WBC) or leukocyte count with absolute and relative quantification of leukocyte cell types and comments on leukocyte morphology. Leukocytes include both granulocytes (neutrophils, eosinophils, and basophils) and mononuclear cells (monocytes and lymphocytes). Assessment of the WBC count, leukocyte morphology, and some general patterns of differential cell counts may aid in the diagnosis or identification of specific pathologic or physiologic processes. Although some general rules regarding leukogram interpretation may be applied to all species, some unique characteristics must be considered and recognized during evaluation of the feline leukogram.

The leukocyte or WBC count, is a quantification of all the types of leukocytes present in 1 μL of circulating blood. The WBC count may be done by manual (e.g., Unopette system and hemocytometer) or automated techniques. Both methods enumerate all nucleated cells in the blood, including nucleated red blood cells (nRBCs) such as rubricytes and metarubricytes. The distinction between the leukocytes and nRBCs is made on the stained blood smear. In a typical leukocyte differential count, 100 consecutive leukocytes are classified by subtype. At the same time, any nRBCs observed are quantitated separately and reported as the number of nRBCs per 100 WBCs. Correction of the leukocyte count for the presence of nRBCs should be performed when >5 nRBCs are encountered per 100 WBCs. The formula for correction of the leukocyte count is

$$\text{Corrected WBC count} = \frac{\text{Initial WBC count}/\mu\text{L} \times 100}{100 + \text{nRBC}/100 \text{ WBCs}}$$

Differential cell counts may be reported as relative percentages (%) of the leukocyte population or as absolute values (cells per microliter of blood). Calculated absolute values (percent cell type × total WBC per microliter of blood) are best for interpretation, as they reflect total numbers of individual cell types comprising the total WBC count. In normal cats, the total leukocyte population is composed primarily of mature neutrophils and lesser numbers of lymphocytes. Monocytes, eosinophils, and basophils usually do not contribute significantly to the total WBC count.

LEUKOCYTE MORPHOLOGIC ARTIFACTS

Peripheral blood samples that are collected in ethylenediamine tetra-acetic acid (EDTA) anticoagulant and allowed to sit for several hours before a blood smear is made tend to develop artifactual leukocyte nuclear hypersegmentation, pyknosis, or cytoplasmic vacuolation. Once these changes occur, the cells cannot be identified; the interpretive value of leukocyte morphology is lost (Fig. 56.1). Artifactual cytoplasmic vacuolation also may be confused for toxic change of neutrophils. When nucleated cells rupture or are stripped of their cytoplasm during blood smear preparation, the nuclear chromatin spreads out and stains eosinophilic. These eosinophilic masses are referred to as basket cells. Attempts should not be made to identify or to classify basket cells. When more than 10% of the leukocytes are pyknotic or basket cells, the leukocyte differential count is invalid.

NONPATHOLOGIC LEUKOCYTE RESPONSES

Various physiologic and pharmacologic processes can cause changes in the total leukocyte count. Because neutrophils are the predominant blood leukocyte in the cat,

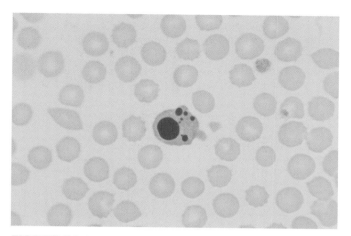

FIGURE 56.1 Wright-stained blood smear from a cat. Improper sample handling has resulted in altered leukocyte morphology. A leukocyte shows pyknosis, karyorrhexis, and karyolysis. Courtesy of Oklahoma State University, College of Veterinary Medicine teaching files.

alterations in the WBC count often parallel alterations in the absolute neutrophil count. Nonpathologic leukogram changes are primarily the result of influences over neutrophil kinetics and subsequent shifts in neutrophil populations. Granulopoiesis is directed by cytokines primarily secreted from macrophages within the bone marrow. Maturation of neutrophils occurs in approximately 3.5 to 6 days.[1] Three distinct pools of neutrophils exist. The first pool is the bone marrow neutrophil pool (BMNP) of developing and mature neutrophils. Neutrophils are released from the bone marrow in an age-ordered fashion. Once they have entered systemic circulation, they are distributed between one of two remaining pools, the marginated neutrophil pool (MNP) or the circulating neutrophil pool (CNP). Marginated neutrophils adhere to endothelial venules and capillaries primarily in the spleen, lungs, and splanchnic vessels, whereas neutrophils of the CNP remain free in the vasculature. Only circulating neutrophils are collected during venipuncture sampling. In the cat,[2] the MNP:CNP ratio is approximately 3:1. Blood neutrophils remain in a dynamic equilibrium, and many processes may cause a redistribution of neutrophils between these blood neutrophil pools. Shifts are dynamic and may occur rapidly, drastically altering circulating neutrophil numbers as reflected by the total WBC and neutrophil counts. Two distinct patterns of nonpathologic leukograms have been identified.

Physiologic Leukocytosis

In physiologic leukocytosis, the leukogram is characterized by a mild to moderate leukocytosis. Mild, mature neutrophilia and lymphocytosis exist. The lymphocytosis is often of greater magnitude than the neutrophilia[1,2] and is thought to be caused by a redistribution of lymphocytes between the blood, lymphatics, and lymphoid organs. The neutrophilia reflects the redistribution of neutrophils from the MNP to the CNP secondary to the effects of epinephrine. This leukogram pattern generally is seen in young, healthy cats that become excited or frightened by environmental stresses (e.g., fear, excitement, restraint, venipuncture). Leukogram changes are immediate but transient, lasting approximately 20 to 30 minutes. The short duration of the physiologic leukocytosis and lymphocytosis helps to distinguish this physiologic state from other pathologic processes that can cause a persistent lymphocytosis (e.g., lymphoma and lymphocytic leukemia). Young cats typically have a higher number of circulating lymphocytes than older cats, and an epinephrine-associated lymphocytosis rarely may exceed 20,000 lymphocytes/μL of blood.[2]

Stress (Glucocorticoid-Associated) Leukogram

Elevations in endogenous or exogenous glucocorticoids tend to cause a mild to moderate leukocytosis characterized by a mature neutrophilia, lymphopenia, and eosinopenia. Monocytosis generally is not observed in cats, and an eosinopenia is difficult to demonstrate in any species. Glucocorticoids induce neutrophilia primarily by enhancing the release of mature neutrophils from the bone marrow into the blood. Secondarily, glucocorticoids promote the shift of marginated neutrophils into the CNP and the decrease in egress of circulating neutrophils into tissue. The normal blood transit time of circulating neutrophils is approximately 10 to 12 hours, but the blood transit time may be prolonged slightly secondary to glucocorticoid administration. Finally, chronic glucocorticoid influence stimulates granulopoiesis. The lymphopenia occurs owing to sequestration of circulating lymphocytes; lysis of immature or uncommitted lymphocytes occurs only with high dosages of corticosteroids given over prolonged periods. Glucocorticoids also exert a neutralizing effect on histamine, a major chemoattractant for eosinophils.[3] The eosinopenia occurs owing to a sequestration of eosinophils in the microcirculation, but delayed release from the bone marrow may also play a role. The corticosteroid response is delayed. It may be seen in approximately 4 hours and peaks 6 to 8 hours poststress or after administration of corticosteroids. Neutrophil values return to reference intervals within 24 hours after a single 5-mg dose of prednisolone and within 48 to 96 hours after cessation of prolonged corticosteroid therapy.[1]

PATHOLOGIC LEUKOCYTE RESPONSES

Because neutrophils are the predominant leukocyte in the cat, alterations in the total WBC count often parallel alterations in neutrophil numbers. Many factors, including physiologic, pharmacologic, and pathologic processes can cause changes in the absolute neutrophil count in blood.

Inflammatory Leukogram

In a normal animal, homeostasis is maintained between production and loss of neutrophils. Neutrophil use or destruction, bone marrow production, and tissue sequestration all can be affected by various disease processes. With an increased tissue demand for neutrophils, the bone marrow responds by increasing the release of mature neutrophils into circulation. In the cat, a significant, mature neutrophilic leukocytosis indicates inflammation. With established inflammation, a sustained neutrophilia indicates that bone marrow release of mature neutrophils exceeds neutrophil emigration into tissues. Bone marrow evaluation usually reveals granulocytic hyperplasia. These findings reflect the bone marrow's ability to produce enough mature neutrophils to combat the inciting agent and also suggest that the inflammatory process has probably been present for several days. The demand for neutrophils depends on the chronicity and severity of the disease process.

Inflammatory Leukogram With a Left Shift

When the demand for neutrophils exceeds bone marrow reserve capacity, the storage pool of mature neutrophils may be exhausted. Immature neutrophils are then released into the systemic circulation. An increase in the number of band cells (or immature neutrophils) into the blood is referred to as a left shift. A clinically significant left shift is the hallmark of an inflammatory leukogram. In the cat, a left shift is considered clinically significant when immature neutrophils exceed 500 to 1000 bands/μL with a normal or elevated total WBC count.[4] A left shift may be categorized as either regenerative or degenerative, which may be useful clinically as a prognostic indicator of disease severity. A regenerative left shift is defined as a neutrophilic leukocytosis in which the number of immature neutrophils does not exceed the number of segmented neutrophils. A regenerative left shift indicates that the bone marrow is meeting the body's need for neutrophils. In contrast, a degenerative left shift is present when the number of immature neutrophils exceeds the number of segmented neutrophils.[3] A degenerative left shift indicates that the bone marrow cannot meet the tissue demands for neutrophils, indicating a severe disease process with a guarded to poor prognosis. Degenerative left shifts can occur in conditions such as septicemia, endotoxemia, and severe inflammation of large-surface areas (peritonitis, pleuritis, pneumonia, gastroenteritis, placentitis). Commonly, a left shift is limited to band neutrophils, but with chronicity or severity of disease, metamyelocytes, myelocytes, and promyelocytes (progranulocytes) may appear in the blood. These immature stages are more likely to be associated with a degenerative left shift. Giant neutrophils or metamyelocytes are more common in the cat than in any other species and may be seen after recovery from severe neutropenia. Toxic neutrophils often are seen with inflammatory responses and are discussed later. Occasionally, an inflammatory process may induce an extreme neutrophilia (>50,000 cells/μL) with an associated left shift that may include band, metamyelocyte, myelocyte, and promyelocyte stages. This is a leukemoid response that may be difficult to distinguish from granulocytic (neutrophilic) or myelomonocytic leukemia. These forms of leukemia, which also can cause extremely high neutrophil counts, often have a left shift to myeloblasts.

NEUTROPHIL RESPONSES

Neutrophilia

As previously stated, blood neutrophil counts may be increased by physiologic (epinephrine and glucocorticoid) or pathologic mechanisms. Inflammation is the most common cause of a pathologic neutrophilia. Inflammation may stem from infectious or noninfectious origins. Infectious disease processes include bacterial, viral, fungal, and parasitic infections that may be localized or generalized (systemic). Examples of localized infections include pyothorax, pyometra, peritonitis, pleuritis, and abscesses.[1] The magnitude of the neutrophilia and the presence or absence of a left shift depends on the severity and duration of disease, as well as the competency of the bone marrow to produce and release neutrophils as needed. With prolonged duration, localized inflammatory processes may result in some of the most intense neutrophilic leukocytoses. These cases are often associated with a left shift and toxic change of neutrophils. A neutrophilia with a declining left shift may indicate either a decreased tissue demand, which may reflect diminishing severity of the infectious process, or an accelerated production of neutrophils from the bone marrow. Occasionally, the inflammatory nidus is obscure. In such cases, exudative loss of neutrophils into large-surface areas should be considered. Such sites of loss include the skin, gastrointestinal tract, genitourinary tract, respiratory tract, and joints. Surgical removal of the inciting cause (e.g., abscess) often results in a transient increase in neutrophil numbers secondary to granulocytic hyperplasia in the bone marrow. Medical treatment involving the administration of glucocorticoids may induce a transient glucocorticoid (stress) leukogram. Generalized or systemic infectious processes also may cause a neutrophilia, but the magnitude of the neutrophilia is generally less severe than localized infectious processes. Some specific examples would include feline viral rhinotracheitis and feline infectious peritonitis. Infrequently, these diseases may present with neutropenia, but this finding is less common. Various noninfectious causes of tissue cell necrosis may induce mild to moderate neutrophilia. Any process that leads to tissue necrosis may result in an inflammatory response. As expected, the magnitude of the neutrophilia and the presence of a left shift depends on the disease process severity and chronicity. A few examples include soft-tissue trauma, immune-mediated diseases (e.g., hemolytic anemia), hemorrhage, and nonleukemic neoplasia that results in tissue necrosis secondary to loss of perfusion (outgrow their blood supply).

Neutropenia

Neutropenia (<2500 neutrophils/μL) can result from several causes and various mechanisms.[2] General mechanisms of neutropenia include increased tissue use or destruction in which neutrophil egress or loss exceeds bone marrow production, decreased bone marrow production or release of neutrophils, and redistribution or sequestration of neutrophils. A single cause (e.g., endotoxemia) may act by several different mechanisms to produce neutropenia.

Increased Use or Destruction

When tissue demand for neutrophils exceeds replacement by the bone marrow, neutropenia occurs. Massive emigration of neutrophils into tissue is often caused by acute inflammatory processes. Acute or peracute bacterial infection of highly vascular organs is probably the most common cause of increased tissue use of neutrophils in cats. With time, inflammatory responses secondary to bacterial infections generally progress to a neutrophilic leukocytosis, assuming there is adequate bone marrow response. Endotoxemia, often associated with bacterial infections, induces a neutropenia by several mechanisms. Neutrophil circulation time is decreased, whereas egress into tissues is enhanced. Endotoxemia also activates complement and production of complement fragment C5a may induce intravascular neutrophil aggregation (leukoagglutination) and subsequent neutrophil consumption. Immune-mediated neutropenia has been experimentally induced in cats. Excessively high body temperature (e.g., heatstroke) may result in the destruction of neutrophils and neutrophil precursors in the bone marrow.

Deficient Production

Decreased bone marrow production of neutrophils can be secondary to various causes. Basic mechanisms include hemopoietic stem-cell death, seen with certain infectious agents (e.g., feline immunodeficiency virus [FIV], feline leukemia virus [FeLV], or feline parvovirus) and some drugs (e.g., chloramphenicol), as well as myelophthisic diseases (e.g., neoplasia and marrow fibrosis) with subsequent loss of hemopoietic space. Although bone marrow suppression usually involves all hemopoietic elements (pancytopenia), the earliest change in the blood picture is often a neutropenia.

Approximately 50% of cats that have FeLV-related illness present with a neutropenia and are often leukopenic.[1,2,4] Three FeLV-associated leukogram patterns have been described. A mild neutropenia with normal marrow hemopoiesis is the most common form. A moderate to severe neutropenia, with concurrent marrow granulocytic hypoplasia is referred to as a panleukopenia-like syndrome, although gastrointestinal signs

are not associated with this form of FeLV infection. Presentation with a severe, persistent neutropenia and concurrent bone marrow granulocytic hyperplasia has been referred to as hemopoietic dysplasia, preleukemia, or subleukemic granulocytic leukemia. Mechanisms of neutropenia include virally induced stem-cell destruction and retarded maturation and bone marrow release of neutrophils. Cyclic hemopoiesis, characterized by a neutropenia with cycle lengths ranging from 8 to 16 days, has been documented in FeLV-positive cats.[5] Neutropenia also may be seen in cats infected with FIV, an immunosuppressive retrovirus.

Administration of chemotherapeutic drugs and chloramphenicol can induce neutropenia in cats by suppression of bone marrow granulopoiesis. Toxic changes, notably Döhle bodies and cytoplasmic vacuolation, may be present in blood neutrophils. Chloramphenicol toxicity may be seen with high dosages or with chronic administration of lower dosages.[6] Drug-induced myelosuppression is reversible; the neutropenia generally resolves within 7 days after cessation of drug administration.

Neutropenia may be seen with many myelophthisic diseases, including leukemias, certain granulomatous inflammatory conditions (i.e., disseminated histoplasmosis), metastatic neoplasms, myelofibrosis (proliferation of bone marrow stromal cells), and osteopetrosis (bone deposition). Often, myelophthisic diseases affect other hemopoietic cell lines, resulting in a panleukopenia (nonregenerative anemia, thrombocytopenia, and leukopenia). Examination of a bone marrow aspirate and core biopsy may provide a definitive diagnosis when myelophthisic disease is suspected.

Redistribution and Sequestration

Pathologic processes may cause sequestration or shifts in neutrophil populations. Early endotoxemia enhances margination of circulating neutrophils, and a rapid, drastic neutropenia may ensue after initial endotoxin exposure. This effect is transient, and is often followed by a neutrophilia in 1 to 3 hours.[1] Sequestration of neutrophils may be seen posttransfusion or with processes such as hypersplenism.

Neutrophil Morphology

Alterations in neutrophil morphology, when present, may assist in identifying pathologic processes. Toxic changes occur in neutrophils during maturation in the bone marrow and mainly affect the myelocytic and metamyelocytic stages of development. These maturational defects are caused by toxic substances that may be associated with strong inflammatory conditions such as severe bacterial infections, septicemias, acute inflammatory conditions, and extensive burns. Toxic change may be seen in both mature and immature neutrophils and generally is associated with a left shift. Toxic changes should not be confused with degenerative changes. Degenerative neutrophils are formed in the tissues as a result of endotoxin, causing the neutrophils to undergo hydropic degeneration. Degenerative neutrophils appear swollen, and their chromatin stains more eosinophilic and is less tightly clumped. Toxic changes can be observed on Romanowsky-stained blood smears. Although both nuclear and cytoplasmic toxic changes occur, the cytoplasmic changes are more reliable and occur more frequently. Although all cell types are exposed to the same insult, toxic change is evaluated only in neutrophils in the stained blood smear. Mechanical stresses during slide preparation can induce artifactual changes in cell morphology at the feathered edge of the smear. The type of toxic change always should be indicated and semiquantitated as either 1+ to 4+, or as slight, mild, moderate, or severe. Toxic changes include diffuse cytoplasmic basophilia, cytoplasmic vacuolation, Döhle bodies, and toxic granulation, with the latter change being infrequent to rare. Diffuse cytoplasmic basophilia occurs when polyribosomes are retained in the cytoplasm. Cytoplasmic vacuolation may occur secondary to systemic toxemia, or it might occur artifactually. Cytoplasmic vacuolation generally occurs in association with diffuse basophilia. Döhle bodies are intracytoplasmic clumps of endoplasmic reticulum that typically stain a light blue with most Romanowsky-type stains (Fig. 56.2). Döhle bodies occur commonly in cat neutrophils. Regardless of the number of neutrophils containing Döhle bodies, their presence should never be interpreted as meaning anything more than a mild toxic change. Toxic granulation occurs when primary granules within neutrophils retain sufficient amounts of mucopolysaccharide so that these granules stain red purple. Diffuse cytoplasmic basophilia, cytoplasmic vacuolation, and toxic granulation are graded as slight (1+) to severe (4+), depending on the number of neutrophils affected and the degree of toxic change.

Pelger–Huët anomaly is an inherited or acquired (pseudoPelger–Huët) defect in granulocyte nuclear segmentation.[7,8,9] In Pelger–Huët anomaly, hyposegmented nuclei characteristically have a mature chromatin pattern in contrast to nuclear hyposegmentation of infection where band cells have finely granular chromatin. The lack of toxic change in the face of a significant to degenerative left shift is also a hint to consider Pelger–Huët anomaly in the differential diagnosis. Pelger–Huët neutrophils function (phagocytize and kill bacteria) normally. Cats that have this anomaly are not predisposed to infection.

Hypersegmented neutrophils contain ≥ 5 distinct nuclear lobes. Hypersegmentation may occur as an in vivo aging change caused by prolonged blood transit time. More commonly, neutrophilic hypersegmentation, as well as pyknosis, represent an in vitro artifactual aging change that may be seen on smears of EDTA-anticoagulated blood that has been allowed to sit for several hours.

Mucopolysaccharidosis is caused by inborn errors of mucopolysaccharide (glycosaminoglycan) metabolism[10,11] and has been reported in cats.[10,12] Circulating neutrophils contain a few to many coarse, reddish-purple, intracytoplasmic granules on Romanowsky-stained blood smears. Basophils granules often are enlarged and metachromatic (Fig. 56.3A, B).

Chédiak–Higashi syndrome occurs in Persian cats.[13,14] Circulating neutrophils and lymphocytes contain single to multiple, pink to reddish, intracytoplasmic granules (Fig. 56.4). Eosinophil granules also may be enlarged.

Cytoplasmic vacuolation of neutrophils may be observed with high doses of chloramphenicol or phenylbutazone. Also, cholesteryl ester storage disease is associated with subtle cytoplasmic vacuolation of neutrophils, lymphocytes, and monocytes on fresh blood smears.[15]

A neutrophil granulation anomaly has been identified in Birman cats. The anomaly is characterized by the presence of azurophilic cytoplasmic granules that resemble toxic granulation.[16] The anomaly is inherited as an autosomal recessive trait and is innocuous.

Histoplasma capsulatum organisms are observed occasionally in blood and buffy coat leukocytes made from cats with disseminated histoplasmosis. These organisms are identified by their small size and round shape. They are 2 to 4 μm in diameter with a darkly staining, eccentrically located nucleus and a thin clear cell wall that resembles a halo.

Monocytes

Monocytes are the largest of the leukocytes in the blood of healthy cats. These cells have a variably shaped nucleus (e.g., round, oval, lobated, indented, or twisted) with a lacy chromatin pattern. The cytoplasm may be vacuolated. Cytoplasmic vacuolation also may be a feature of cholesteryl ester storage disease of Siamese cats.[15] The bone marrow does not contain a storage pool of monocytes. Thus, the bone marrow transit time is short, approximating 1 to 2.5 days. After monocytes enter the blood, they exit the vasculature randomly. The blood transit half-life of monocytes is 8.4 hours, and these cells do not recirculate.

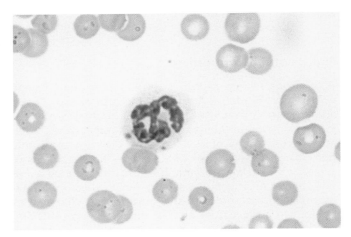

FIGURE 56.2 Wright-stained blood smear from a cat. A neutrophil contains Döhle bodies. Courtesy of Oklahoma State University, College of Veterinary Medicine teaching files.

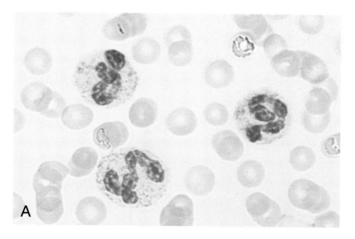

FIGURE 56.3 Wright-stained blood smear from a cat that has mucopolysaccharidosis type VI. **A**. Three neutrophils contain granular, purple, intracytoplasmic inclusions. **B**. A neutrophil with intracytoplasmic inclusions and a basophil with dark blue-black granules. Courtesy of Oklahoma State University, College of Veterinary Medicine teaching files.

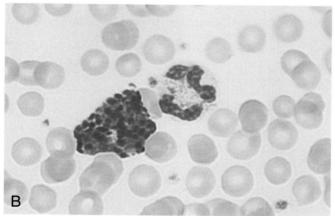

FIGURE 56.4 Wright-stained blood smear from a cat that has Chédiak–Higashi syndrome. **A**. The neutrophils have large, pink lysosomes in their cytoplasms. **B**. The basophils have large, round, lavender granules. Courtesy of Oklahoma State University, College of Veterinary Medicine teaching files.

MONOCYTOSIS

In the cat, an absolute monocyte count of >850 cells/μL is considered a monocytosis.[1,2] Monocytosis is a non-specific finding that has been reported to occur in approximately 11% of the leukograms of hospitalized cats.[1] Monocytosis is not a characteristic feature of the stress leukogram in cats as it is in dogs. Monocytosis occurs in many conditions, including both acute and chronic conditions, associated with inflammation, tissue destruction, and neutrophilia. Some of the reported causes of a monocytosis include trauma-related injuries, suppuration, necrosis, pyogranulomatous inflammation, hemolysis, hemorrhage, malignancy, and immune-mediated disorders.

MONOCYTOPENIA

Persistent monocytopenia is clinically unimportant in cats and seldom documented, because the low end of the reference range is zero cells/μL of blood. With severe leukopenia, the clinical focus is on neutropenia and prevention of sepsis; little attention is given to any coexisting monocytopenia.

LYMPHOCYTES

Lymphocytes are the second most common leukocyte in the blood of healthy cats. Most blood lymphocytes are small-sized, long-lived, T lymphocytes that are capable of recirculation. In health, they are fairly uniform in size and in morphologic appearance. Small lymphocytes have a round, slightly indented nucleus with a coarse chromatin pattern. Nucleoli are not visible. Lymphocytes have scant pale to light blue cytoplasm and are smaller than neutrophils. Antigenically stimulated lymphocytes (e.g., reactive lymphocytes, immunocytes) are larger and have more abundant, dark blue cytoplasm. Rarely, immune-stimulated lymphocytes may exhibit plasmacytoid differentiation. Such cells have a round, eccentric nucleus with coarse nuclear chromatin; abundant dark blue cytoplasm; and a pale-staining Golgi zone located between the nucleus and the largest volume of cytoplasm. Also, large granular lymphocytes, which are natural killer cells and in the null cell group, may be observed. These cells are identified by distinctive azurophilic granules, usually in the vicinity of the nuclear indentation. In contrast, lymphoblasts (immature lymphocytes) are large lymphocytes (equal to or larger than neutrophils) with finely stippled nuclear chromatin and multiple, prominent nucleoli. Lymphocyte vacuolation has been associated with cholesteryl ester storage disease of Siamese cats and mannosidosis of Persian cats.[15,17]

Lymphocytes are evaluated by both their morphology and their absolute number. Peripheral blood lymphocyte numbers are influenced by physiologic states, disease, and drug administration, causing changes in lymphocyte production, distribution, margination, recirculation, sequestration, destruction, or loss.

LYMPHOCYTOSIS

Lymphocytosis (>7000 lymphocytes/μL) is generally secondary to epinephrine-mediated physiologic responses, hypoadrenocorticism, chronic antigenic stimulation (e.g., FeLV), or lymphoid neoplasia. Young animals also have higher absolute lymphocyte counts than middle-aged or old cats.[2] Young, healthy cats (especially those <1 year of age) are especially prone to lymphocytosis secondary to excitement or fear (physiologic leukocytosis). With physiologic leukocytosis, the absolute lymphocyte count is usually less than 20,000 cells/μL but has been reported to exceed 36,000 cells/μL.[1] Physiologic lymphocytosis is thought to be caused by epinephrine and is short lived. If another blood sample can be collected from the cat after it has been allowed to calm down, the absolute lymphocyte count should be within the reference interval, allowing differentiation from a pathologic cause of lymphocytosis. Also, lymphocytosis is present in 20% of cats that have glucocorticoid deficiency (hypoadrenocorticism).[1]

Chronic antigenic stimulation causes lymphocyte proliferation and may result in lymphocytosis. An example of chronic antigenic stimulation is the lymphocytosis seen with FeLV-associated peripheral lymph-node hyperplasia. Lymphocytosis also may be seen a few days postvaccination. Reactive lymphocytes (immunocytes) are a more common finding with antigenic stimulation than is lymphocytosis. Reactive lymphocytes, when present, must be differentiated from atypical (immature) lymphocytes that would suggest lymphoid neoplasia.

LYMPHOPENIA

Lymphopenia is recognized by an absolute lymphocyte count of less than 1500 to 2500 lymphocytes/μL of blood.[1,2] The younger the cat, the higher the lymphocyte count that can be classified as a lymphopenia (i.e., a lymphopenia in young cats is less than 2500 lymphocytes/μL, whereas that in old cats is less than 1500 lymphocytes/μL). The most common cause of lymphopenia is corticosteroid-induced redistribution of lymphocytes. Some other causes include viral infections (e.g., panleukopenia, FeLV, and FIV), septicemia or endotoxemia, lymphocyte-rich thoracic effusions (chylothorax from thoracic duct rupture, cardiovascular disease, nonexfoliating neoplasia, lymphosarcoma, or thymoma), and gastrointestinal disease (e.g., ulcerative enteritis, granulomatous enteritis, lymphosarcoma, and other neoplasias).

EOSINOPHILS

Feline eosinophils contain numerous, rod-shaped, bright red-orange granules. These granules are secondary granules that develop in the myelocyte stage, making this the first recognizable stage of eosinophil development in the bone marrow. Like neutrophils, the bone marrow has a storage pool of eosinophils. Eosinophils have many functions, including the destruction of parasites, the modulation of hypersensitivity reactions, and a proinflammatory function.

EOSINOPHILIA

The absolute number of eosinophils that constitutes an eosinophilia varies with different geographic areas, but it generally represents absolute eosinophil counts in excess of 750 to 1500 eosinophils/μL. Some causes of eosinophilia include hypersensitivity or inflammatory lesions (e.g., ulcerative gastroenteritis, food allergy, flea allergy dermatitis, atopy, eosinophilic keratitis, or feline eosinophilic granuloma complex), parasites (endoparasites and ectoparasites), idiopathic hypereosinophilic syndrome, FELV-associated eosinophilia, tumor-associated eosinophilia, and miscellaneous conditions (e.g., hyperthyroidism and hypoadrenocorticism).[1,2,18,19]

EOSINOPENIA

Eosinopenia is sometimes difficult to recognize clinically because the lower end of the reference interval for feline eosinophil counts is 0 cells/μL. Eosinopenia usually is associated with exogenous administration or stress-related endogenous release of glucocorticoids. Acute infections are associated with an eosinopenia, but this is likely glucocorticoid induced.

BASOPHILS

Basophils are the least numerous of the blood leukocytes in healthy cats, accounting for less than 2% of the leukocyte differential count.[1] Cat basophils are large cells (approximately the size of a monocyte) with a lobated nu-

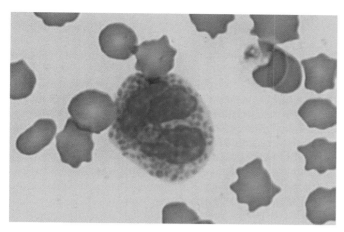

FIGURE 56.5 Wright-stained blood smear from a cat. A feline basophil contains numerous, small, round, lavender, intracytoplasmic granules. Courtesy of Oklahoma State University, College of Veterinary Medicine teaching files.

cleus, and many, small, rounded, cytoplasmic granules that stain pale lavender (Fig. 56.5). Cat basophils often are misclassified as toxic neutrophils by technicians unfamiliar with feline blood. Occasionally, some basophils are present with a few typical dark purple granules. Basophil granules from cats that have mucopolysaccharidosis stain blue black. Enlarged granules are seen with Chédiak–Higashi syndrome.

BASOPHILIA

A basophilia is recognized by an increased absolute basophil count (>200 basophils/μL) and generally occurs with a concomitant eosinophilia. Some causes of basophilia in cats are allergic respiratory conditions, heartworm disease, eosinophilic granuloma complex, basophilic leukemia, myeloid leukemia, and polycythemia vera.[1,2,18]

BASOPENIA

Because basophils are rarely observed in blood smears of cats, basopenia is not a recognized clinical problem.

LEUKEMIAS (MYELOPROLIFERATIVE AND LYMPHOPROLIFERATIVE DISORDERS)

Leukemias and myeloproliferative disorders (MPD) originate in the bone marrow. Most of the MPDs and leukemias in cats are FeLV-associated and some also have been associated with FIV infection. MPDs include neoplastic proliferation of granulocytes, monocytes, erythrocytes, and megakaryocytes. The acute MPD disorders include acute undifferentiated leukemia (AUL) and the acute myeloid leukemias (French-American

British [FAB] classification M1–M7).[20] Chronic MPD categories include chronic myeloid leukemias, polycythemia vera, idiopathic myelofibrosis, myeloid metaplasia, and essential thrombocythemia.[20] The other leukemias are lymphoproliferative leukemias, including acute lymphoblastic leukemia and chronic lymphocytic leukemia. Leukemias are encountered less frequently than lymphoma, which is the most common lymphoproliferative neoplasm in the cat.[20] Cats that have leukemia generally have vague and variable clinical signs, including anorexia, weight loss, and lethargy. Clinical findings often include organomegaly, anemia, fever, emaciation, and petechiae.[1] Some leukemias are discussed briefly below. Their classification, diagnosis, and clinical behavior are described in more detail in Sections IX and X.

Leukemia usually is associated with a high total WBC count, but it occasionally may present with a normal WBC count or leukopenia. If the neoplastic cell line exhibits cellular differentiation, the type of leukemia often can be identified by examination of Wright-stained blood and bone marrow smears. However, many blast cells appear similar morphologically.[21] Therefore, cytochemical staining may be needed to identify the neoplastic cell line.[21] When atypical cells that cannot be identified are seen in peripheral blood smears, the slides should be referred to a veterinary clinical pathologist or hematologist for evaluation if leukemia is suspected.

Granulocytic, myelomonocytic, and monocytic leukemias all occur in cats. If adequate cellular differentiation is not present, cytochemical staining may be needed to differentiate these leukemias. Granulocytic leukemia must be differentiated from a leukemoid response or extreme neutrophilic leukocytosis secondary to an inflammatory focus (e.g., infection and tumor with a necrotic center).

Eosinophilic leukemia is rare and may be impossible to differentiate from idiopathic hypereosinophilic syndrome. Basophilic leukemia also is rare and should not be confused with mast cell neoplasia. In cats, mast cell neoplasia usually is associated with splenic enlargement or gastrointestinal neoplasms with circulating mast cells. Mast cells can readily be differentiated from feline basophils. Mast cells appear as large round cells with a round to oval nucleus and abundant small, round red-purple granules that may partially obscure the nucleus (Fig. 56.6). Cat basophils have a segmented nucleus and numerous small, rounded, lavender-staining granules.

Erythremic myelosis and erythroleukemia are common in cats, but polycythemia vera is infrequently observed. Erythremic myelosis generally is recognized by the presence of severe nonregenerative anemia (lack of reticulocytosis) in the presence of numerous nRBCs and a few to many rubriblasts in the circulation (Fig. 56.7). Nuclear to cytoplasmic asynchrony and megaloblastic change are common findings. Erythremic myelosis may evolve into erythroleukemia, which is the neoplastic proliferation of both erythrocytes and granulocytes. Polycythemia vera is the neoplastic proliferation of mature erythrocytes. Cats that have polycythemia vera have high packed-cell volume, hemoglobin concentra-

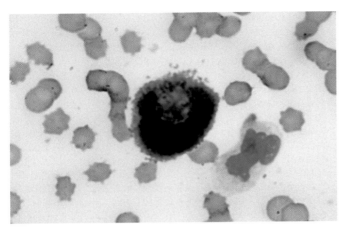

FIGURE 56.6 Wright-stained blood smear from a cat that has mast cell leukemia. Mast cells have a round to oval nucleus and numerous small, red-purple granules. Courtesy of Oklahoma State University, College of Veterinary Medicine teaching files.

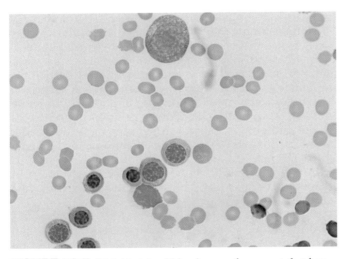

FIGURE 56.7 Wright-stained blood smear from a cat that has erythremic myelosis. A rubriblast and several rubricytes and metarubricytes are shown. Courtesy of Oklahoma State University, College of Veterinary Medicine teaching files.

tion, and erythrocyte count caused by the increased red cell mass. The PaO_2 is within the reference interval, whereas the erythropoietin concentration is variable. The diagnostic workup of polycythemic cats should eliminate causes of relative polycythemia (dehydration and splenic contraction) and secondary polycythemia.

Megakaryocytic leukemia and essential thrombocythemia are rare in cats and may be FeLV-test positive or negative. They are classically associated with a significant thrombocytosis, and megakaryoblasts may be found in the stained blood smear.

Lymphocytic leukemia is fairly common in cats. Acute lymphoblastic leukemia is characterized by the presence of circulating lymphoblasts, whereas chronic lymphocytic leukemia is characterized by many small, well-differentiated lymphocytes. Chronic lymphocytic leukemia must be differentiated from a physiologic lymphocytosis, which is a transient response.

REFERENCES

1. **Latimer KS.** Leukocytes in health and disease. In: Ettinger SJ, Feldman EC, eds. Textbook of veterinary internal medicine. Philadelphia: WB Saunders, 1995.
2. **Hall RL.** Interpreting the leukogram. In: August JR, ed. Consultations in feline internal medicine. 2nd ed. Philadelphia: WB Saunders, 1994.
3. **Jain NC.** Essentials of veterinary hematology. Philadelphia: Lea & Febiger, 1993:303.
4. **Prasse KW.** Clinical, hematological and postmortem findings in feline leukovirus infected cats: a retrospective study of 95 naturally occurring cases. In: Proceedings of the 31st Annual Meeting of the American College of Veterinary Pathology, New Orleans, 1980.
5. **Swenson CL, Kociba GJ, O'Keefe DA, et al.** Cyclic hematopoiesis associated with feline leukemia virus infections in two cats. J Am Vet Med Assoc 1987;191:93–96.
6. **Watson ADJ, Middleton DJ.** Chloramphenicol toxicosis in cats. Am J Vet Res 1978;39:1199.
7. **Weber SE, Feldman BF, Evans DA.** Pelger-Huët anomaly of the granulocytic leukocytes in two feline littermates. Feline Pract 1981;11:44–47.
8. **Latimer KS, Rakich PM, Thompson DF.** Pelger-Huët anomaly in cats. Vet Pathol 1985;22:370–374.
9. **Latimer KS, Rakich PM.** Clinical interpretation of leukocyte responses. Vet Clin North Am Small Anim Pract 1989;19:637–668.
10. **Haskins ME, Aguirre GD, Jezyk PF, et al.** The pathology of the feline model of mucopolysaccharidosis VI. Am J Pathol 1980;101:657–674.
11. **Glew RH, Basu A, Prence EM, et al.** Biology of disease: Lysosomal storage diseases. Lab Invest 1985;53:250–269.
12. **Gitzelmann R, Bosshard NU, Superti-Furga A, Spycher MA, Briner J, Wiesmann U, Lutz H, Litschi B.** Feline mucopolysaccharidosis VII due to β-glucuronidase deficiency. Vet Pathol 1994;31:435–443.
13. **Kramer JW, Davis WC, Prieur DJ.** An inherited disorder of Persian cats with intracytoplasmic inclusions in neutrophils. J Am Vet Med Assoc 1975;166:1103–1104.
14. **Kramer JW, Davis WC, Prieur DJ.** The Chediak-Higashi syndrome of cats. Lab Invest 1977;36:554–562.
15. **Thrall MA, Mitchell T, Lappin M, et al.** Cholesteryl ester storage disease in two cats. In: Proceedings of the 42nd Annual Meeting of the American College of Veterinary Pathologists, Orlando, FL, 1991.
16. **Hirsch VM, Cunningham TA.** Hereditary anomaly of neutrophil granulation in Birman cats. Am J Vet Res 1984;45:2170.
17. **Maenhout T, et al.** Mannosidosis in a litter of Persian cats. Vet Rec 1988;122:351.
18. **Center SA, Randolph JF.** Eosinophilia. In: August JR, ed. Consultations in feline internal medicine. Philadelphia: WB Saunders, 1991.
19. **Center SA, Randolph JF, Erb HN, et al.** Eosinophilia in the cat: a retrospective study of 312 cases (1975 to 1986). J Am Anim Hosp Assoc 1990;26:349–358.
20. **Grindem CB.** Classification of myeloproliferative diseases. In: August JR, ed. Consultation in feline internal medicine. 3rd ed. Philadelphia: WB Saunders, 1997.
21. **Jain NC, Blue JT, Grindem CB, et al.** Proposed criteria for classification of acute myeloid leukemia in dogs and cats. Vet Clin Pathol 1991;20:63–82.

CHAPTER 57

Leukocyte Responses in Ruminants

• JUDITH A. TAYLOR

Leukocyte responses in ruminants often differ from those observed in other species. Seldom are the hematologic changes specific for a particular disorder, but rather support trends or are suggestive of diagnostic considerations such as septicemia or endotoxemia. Acute bacterial sepsis often is characterized by neutropenia rather than neutrophilia, and there is less tendency for ruminants to develop a significant neutrophilia.[1] Total white cell counts of 20 to 30 × 10^3/μL are significant in cattle compared with counts of 50 to 100 × 10^3/μL under similar conditions in the dog.[2] Increased concentrations of acute-phase reactant proteins, such as fibrinogen and haptoglobin, may be more sensitive indicators of acute or chronic inflammation in ruminants than changes in total leukocyte counts.[1,3,4] Often altered leukocyte differential counts with normal total leukocyte counts characterize the inflammatory response. The normally low neutrophil-to-lymphocyte ratio (0.5 in the cow) compared with other species (3.5 in the dog, 1.8 in the cat) may predispose the ruminant to delays in granulopoietic response because of a slower rate of acceleration of myelopoiesis. Thus, there is an inability to mount a rapid, significant leukocytosis.[5-7] This lack of response has been attributed by some authors to a lower bone marrow granulocyte reserve in cattle. However, Valli[8] found that bone marrow reserves were similar in the dog and cow and that the rate of recovery of bone marrow granulocyte reserves was the factor most responsible for the observed species differences in leukocyte responses. Dog bone marrow reserves recovered quicker (2 to 3 days) than calves (6 days) during granulocyte demand. Studies of myelopoiesis, with labeled bone marrow cells showed that the mean production time of peripheral blood granulocytes was 7.01 days, with a 5-hour circulating life span of the segmented neutrophil in normal calves.[6]

Toxic leukocyte changes often accompany ruminant hematologic responses to acute inflammation or sepsis (Figs. 57.1 and 57.2). Cytoplasmic basophilia is often more striking in these species because of the eosinophilic cytoplasm characteristic of neutrophils in health. Cytoplasmic vacuolation or foaminess, azurophilic granules, Döhle bodies, or nuclear dysmaturation resemble changes induced in other species under similar disease conditions.

ENVIRONMENTAL EFFECTS ON THE LEUKOGRAM

Hematologic examination of colostrum-fed (CF) and colostrum-deprived (CD) calves during the first 48 hours postdelivery revealed significantly higher leukocyte counts in CF calves owing to a transient mature neutrophilia. Neutrophil counts ranged from 10 to 15.5 × 10^3 cells/L in CF calves compared with 6 to 10 × 10^3 cells/μL in CD calves. The high neutrophil-to-lymphocyte ratio observed at birth reversed in both groups during the 48- to 72-hour sampling period.[9] Veal calves have been reported to have lower leukocyte counts than healthy calves (5.5 to 6.5 × 10^3 cells/μL compared with 8.87 × 10^3/μL, respectively).[10]

Seasonal variations in bovine leukocyte counts have been reported with highest counts observed in summer.[11] Dietary influences on the hemogram in cattle also have been studied. Leukocytosis and monocytosis were reported in cows fed grass silage compared with cows fed green forage.[12]

The effects of cold stress have been examined in cattle[13] and sheep.[14] Hematologic values did not differ significantly between hypothermic calves and noncold-stressed calves, although a linear trend of lowered total leukocyte counts with neutropenia was observed in cooled animals when compared with baseline values. A significant eosinopenia was noted during cold exposure of shorn mature wethers.

PHYSIOLOGIC INFLUENCES ON THE LEUKOGRAM

Effects of Age

Neonatal calves had the highest leukocyte counts at birth (5.7 to 20.5 × 10^3/μL).[15] Total leukocyte counts declined within the first few days of life and stabilized by 3 days of age (4.9 to 13.3 × 10^3/μL). Neutrophils declined from birth over the first 5 days, ranging from 4.2 to 14.8 × 10^3/μL (day 1) to 0.9 to 6.0 × 10^3/μL (day 6). Lymphocytes increased from a range of 0.9 to 4.6 × 10^3/μL to 2.8 to 7.2 × 10^3/μL by 6 days of age. The neutrophil-to-lymphocyte ratio was 2.8 at birth and re-

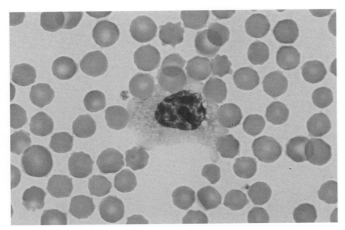

FIGURE 57.1 Peripheral blood, cow, *E. coli* mastitis. Hematologic findings included a leukocytosis (15 × 10³/μL) with a significant degenerative left shift (neutrophils: 0.45 × 10³/μL; bands: 1.2 × 10³/μL; metamyelocytes and younger: 6.45 × 10³/μL). Toxic changes (cytoplasmic basophilia and Döhle bodies) were noted in most cells of the neutrophil series. A neutrophil myelocyte demonstrates basophilic cytoplasm. 500×.

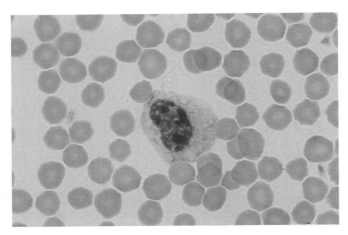

FIGURE 57.2 Same case as in Figure 57.1. A neutrophil metamyelocyte with cytoplasmic basophilia and vacuolation supporting the significant left shift and leukocyte toxicity in this hemogram. 500×.

versed during the first 5 days to 0.5, which is closer to the ratio observed in older calves and adults. Monocytes are present in low numbers (mean 3%) at birth but increase during the first week; this increase is followed by a decline in numbers during the second and third weeks of life. Band neutrophils are present in low numbers but are somewhat variable among calves. Examination of bone marrow of calves at birth reveals a significantly lower myeloid-to-erythroid ratio than in adults, likely reflecting a commitment to erythropoiesis and suggesting that the neutrophil response occurs just before or during parturition.

Hematologic findings in the neonatal lamb indicated that the total leukocyte count doubled by 12 hours postbirth, and declined over the next 12 to 14 hours. The leukocyte count peaked at approximately 3 months of age. Examination of sheep bone marrow indicated vast differences in myeloid-to-erythroid (M:E) ratios between investigations; however, the ratio ranged from 0.59 to 1.1 with a high proportion of eosinophils (18.5 to 25.4%).[16] The reference interval for adult sheep leukocytes has been reported at 4 to 12×10³/μL, with a mean of 8×10³cells/μL.[17]

Leukocyte changes in the goat occur with advancing age as the leukocyte count rises from birth to peak at approximately the third or fourth month. Adult values are gradually attained and resemble those at birth.[17] Mbassa[18] studied leukocyte profiles in Dwarf and Landrace kids from birth to 12 months of age and found that the reference intervals depended on age, breed, environment, and individual variations (Table 57.1). This same study found that lymphocyte and neutrophil counts were low at birth and increased to maximal values by 6 to 12 months of age. Bands, eosinophils, basophils, and monocytes are low in number in all ages. The early increase in the leukocyte count is caused by increases in lymphocytes. Neutrophils composed 55% of the differential count in the first 2 weeks of life, 23% by 3 months of age, and 49% at 2 years of age.[19] Lymphocytes were found to comprise 41% of the differential count at birth, 73% at 3 months of age, and fell to 42% of the total count at 2 years of age. The total leukocyte counts during the first 2 weeks after birth, at 3 months, and 2 years of age were 7.5, 18.0, and 8×10³/μL, respectively.[19] Bone marrow studies showed a mean M:E ratio of 0.69 in goats that have fewer eosinophils than in sheep (4.3% of total nucleated marrow cells).[20]

Excitement and Stress

Epinephrine-induced physiologic leukocytosis in cattle is characterized by a neutrophilic leukocytosis with increases in lymphocytes and monocytes with a mild eosinopenia. Exogenous or endogenous corticosteroid-induced leukocyte changes include a mature neutrophilia, lymphopenia, eosinopenia, and monocytosis.[21] The observed changes in both these conditions are similar to those observed in other species, albeit to a lesser degree in cattle. Similar corticosteroid responses have been observed in goats[22] and sheep.[23]

Parturition

Changes in the leukocyte count of periparturient cows and in calves have been reported.[24,25] Studies have indicated gradually increasing leukocyte counts in the dam as parturition approached, peaking at approximately 13 × 10³/μL by 9 hours postcalving, with a return to normal values at 3 days postpartum. Calves had the highest leukocyte counts at 9 hours postdelivery (mean, 11.0 × 10³ leukocytes/μL and 5.5 × 10³ neutrophils/μL), which then decreased to reference intervals by 6 days of age. Parturition in sheep was associated with

TABLE 57.1   Comparison of Mean Reference Intervals of Caprine Leukocyte Counts × 10³/μL According to Age by Different Authors[18]

Age (days)	WBC	Lymphocytes	Neutrophils	Bands	Eosinophils	Monocytes	Basophils
0–7	8.1	3.04	4.88	0.01	0.06	0.16	—
0–30	12.3	8.12	3.74	0.01	0.16	0.30	—
30–60	12.2	10.84	—	—	—	—	—
0–30	15.8	9.55	6.52	—	0.16	0.24	0
0–30	9–14	0.5–8.2	3.3–5.8	0.2–0.6	0–0.14	0.02–0.22	—
0–30	6.7	3.70	2.50	—	0.15	0.29	—
0–30	12.3	9.23	2.71	0.16	0.02	—	—
0–7	7.10	2.60	3.90	0.27	0.28	0.64	0.23
0–7	7.00	4.10	2.30	0.70	0.50	0.80	0.30
7–30	8.00	4.40	4.10	0.31	0.53	0.36	0.16
7–30	8.30	5.20	2.60	0.20	0.40	1.80	0.60

Data from Mbassa GK, Poulsen JSD. Leukocyte profile in growing Dwarf and Landrace kids. J Am Vet Med Assoc 1991;38:389–397 with permission.

significant neutrophilia, lymphopenia, and mild eosinopenia that normalized by day 14 postpartum.[23]

Plasma glucocorticoid concentration has been reported to increase fourfold in cows at parturition.[26] In calves, glucocorticoid levels also are high at birth, decreasing rapidly within 6 hours postdelivery, and reaching a plateau by 48 hours after birth.[27] Burton et al[28] reported that in vivo administration of glucocorticoids to Holstein cows induced significant downregulation of CD62L and CD18 expression on blood neutrophils. The expression of CD62L on neutrophils in cows and calves is diminished at parturition.[24] Because CD62L mediates endothelial adhesion of neutrophils, the initial step in transendothelial migration, decreased expression contributes to reduced neutrophil margination and impaired neutrophil surveillance of tissues and may be a factor in increased disease incidence in the periparturient period.[24,29]

Leukocyte counts in ewes indicated that the percentage of neutrophils rose during gestation to 60% of the total leukocyte count and then declined to 45% by day 14 of lactation.[30] Band neutrophils were present at birth (0.8%) and decreased to 0.4% by 2 weeks into lactation. Lymphopenia and eosinopenia have been reported at parturition and have returned to baseline by 2 weeks postpartum.[23]

The activity of acyloxyacyl hydrolase in bovine neutrophils decreased to approximately 20% less than prepartum activity between 10 and 26 days postpartum.[31] This enzyme hydrolyzes a specific linkage of fatty acyl chains within the lipid A portion of endotoxin, resulting in decreased toxicity of lipopolysaccharide (LPS). Reduced enzyme activity may contribute to an increased susceptibility of dairy cows to coliform mastitis during early lactation.

Experimentally induced hypocalcemia and the development of milk fever did not significantly influence the hematology of postpartum cows.[32] Cows that have retained placenta develop leukopenia, left shift (to metamyelocytes), and monocytosis between 2 and 5 days postpartum with decreased bone marrow granulocyte reserves.[2]

LEUKOCYTE RESPONSES IN INFECTIOUS AND INFLAMMATORY DISEASE

Bacterial Diseases

Endocarditis

In a review of 31 cases of bovine endocarditis in adult cows, neutrophilia was a typical hematologic finding in early disease.[33] Leukocytosis (>12 × 10³/μL) was found in 45% (14 of 31) of affected cattle, and neutrophilia (>4 × 10³/μL) was found in 77% (24 of 31) of the hemograms. *Corynebacterium pyogenes* was the most frequently isolated organism.

Small-Intestinal Volvulus

Medical records of 35 cattle that had small-intestinal volvulus revealed a trend for affected cows to have a leukocytosis (mean leukocyte count of 15.1 × 10³/μL) with a mild left shift.[34] This may have been caused by inflammation resulting from intestinal necrosis or concurrent disease that was identified in 39% of the cases.[12]

Meningitis

In a retrospective study of 32 neonatal calves that had meningitis, *Escherichia coli* was the organism most frequently isolated (11 of 16; 69%).[35] Hematologic investigation revealed a leukocytosis and left shift in 12 of 16 (75%) of calves. The significant leukocytosis (mean leukocyte count 30.0 $\times$ $10^3/\mu L$, range 13.0 to 50.0 $\times$ $10^3/\mu L$) was thought to indicate the severity of the systemic disease secondary to sepsis.

Endotoxin

Calves challenged with endotoxin show dose-dependent hematologic changes.[5,37] At low doses, endotoxin administration causes a leukocytosis, whereas higher doses produce a characteristic biphasic response. High doses of endotoxin caused a profound decrease in the leukocyte count with leukopenia noted as early as 5 minutes postinfusion, with a neutropenia, lymphopenia, and increase in the number of metarubricytes.[36,37] Mean leukocyte counts dropped from 11.6 to 4.9 $\times$ $10^3/\mu L$, and neutrophils decreased from 6.9 to 1.4 $\times$ $10^3/\mu L$ at 2 hours postendotoxin administration.[36] Surviving calves showed a leukopenia followed by a rebound neutrophilia. Endotoxin-mediated changes are caused by enhanced margination and sequestration of the neutrophils, especially in the lung, whereas lymphopenia has been attributed to endogenous hypercortisolemia and redistribution.

Cows given intramammary inoculations of *E. coli* endotoxin showed characteristic leukogram changes of neutropenic leukopenia, left shift (to the myelocyte stage) and subsequent leukocytosis. These peripheral blood observations were accompanied by depletion of bone marrow reserves followed by increased granulopoietic activity in the bone marrow.[38] Within 4 to 6 hours of inoculation, the neutrophil count dropped from 4.6 $\times$ $10^3/\mu L$ to 0.6 $\times$ $10^3/\mu L$ as a result of endotoxin-mediated neutrophil margination, complement activation and cytolysis, and diapedesis into the mammary gland. A degenerative left shift was noted with a band neutrophil count of 2.45 $\times$ $10^3/\mu L$ with myelocytes, supporting intense mobilization of cells from the bone marrow reserve pool. Upon recovery within the following 24 to 72 hours, the neutrophil count decreased a second time, possibly because of intravascular distribution of cells to restore the neutrophil marginal pool, and then increased to baseline values or greater by day 6 or 7 owing to continuous marrow release and replenishment of marrow granulocyte reserves. In another study, leukopenia was noted 4 hours after injection of endotoxin, and 16 hours after intramammary infection of *E. coli* in mature lactating cows.[39]

Mastitis

Bovine mastitis has been used as a model for investigation of neutrophil kinetics in response to tissue injury. Concurrent evaluation of bone marrow, peripheral blood, and milk leukocytes has allowed the examination of the responses of all three compartments to acute and chronic infections.

Hemograms from a normal cow and four cows that had mastitis showed normal total leukocyte counts of 5.8 $\times$ $10^3/\mu L$ and 6.4 to 9.5 $\times$ $10^3/\mu L$, with 31% and 36.5 to 41.5% neutrophils, respectively. The bone mar-

row M:E ratio was <1.0 in normal cows and generally >1.0 in mastitic cows.[40]

Pasteurella Haemolytica

Neutrophils play an important role in the pathogenesis of pneumonic pasteurellosis and constitute the primary leukocytic response after the initial macrophage-mediated defenses. Pasteurella-haemolytica-induced changes in neutrophil morphology indicative of irreversible cell injury and compatible with the mechanism of action of pore-forming cytolysins have been demonstrated in vitro[41,42] and in vivo.[43] Significant leukopenia, primarily caused by neutropenia, has been reported as a result of *Pasteurella* sp. infection, possibly because of substantial pulmonary sequestration of leukocytes.[44,45]

Salmonellosis

CF calves experimentally inoculated with *Salmonella typhimurium* demonstrated variable hematologic profiles.[46] There was a tendency for the total leukocyte and neutrophil counts to be within or less than reference intervals during the first 48 to 72 hours, followed by a return to normal at approximately 5 days postinoculation. Leukocyte counts varied between 2.5 and 27.6 $\times$ $10^3/\mu L$ with neutrophil counts between 0.2 and 23.6 $\times$ $10^3/\mu L$. Left shifts with 12% bands were observed in the hemograms of some calves. Neutropenia was observed to be more variable in calves in this study than in other species infected with *Salmonella* sp., but this may have been caused by variability in the inoculum dosages and age of calves at the time of infection. Injection of *S. typhimurium* endotoxin into calves induced profound leukopenia (1.1 $\times$ $10^3/\mu L$ compared with 9.1 $\times$ $10^3/\mu L$ preinjection), mainly by increased adherence of leukocytes with a shift to the marginating pool.[47] Experimental salmonellosis in goats induced neutrophilia with pyrexia and diarrhea.[48]

Corynebacterium Pseudotuberculosis Infection

Sheep experimentally infected with *C. pseudotuberculosis* isolated from a prescapular lymph node from a naturally infected animal developed increases in their leukocyte counts (18 to 20 $\times$ $10^3/\mu L$) with a reversal of the neutrophil-to-lymphocyte ratio on the second day postinfection (PI).[49] A monocytosis also has been reported in association with caseous lymphadenitis in a previous study.[50]

Viral Diseases

Bovine Viral Diarrhea Virus Infection

Of the hematologic changes produced by bovine viral diarrhea virus (BVDV) infection, leukopenia and thrombocytopenia are most frequently reported.[51,52,53] Carlsson and colleagues[52] reported that heifers experimentally infected with a cytopathic strain of BVDV developed a leukopenia 5 days postinoculation. Leukopenia was detected 1 week postexposure in a naturally infected heifer. When a noncytopathic field strain was used in naturally infected calves, BVDV caused a significant decrease in the total leukocyte count and lymphopenia 4 days PI.[54] Calves demonstrated significant leukopenia, neutropenia, left shift to metamyelocytes, toxic changes, and lymphopenia 7 to 8 days postexperimental infection with a noncytopathic virus (Fig. 57.3) (Table 57.2).[53] (D. Wood, personal communication, 1998). BVDV infection of bone marrow myeloid cells and megakaryocytes has been demonstrated.[55,56] Experimental BVDV infection of lambs resulted in leukopenia with lymphopenia and provided support that BVDV infection in lambs modulates the ability of lymphocytes to respond to lectins or antigenic stimulation.[57] The pathogenesis of the hematologic changes in BVDV infection is currently poorly understood.

Bovine Leukemia Virus Infection

Cattle, sheep, and goats may be infected with a transforming retrovirus known as bovine leukemia virus (BLV). BLV infection may result in leukocytosis in cattle because of a benign lymphoproliferative response in 30 to 70% of infected cows.[58] This polyclonal B-cell expansion is referred to as persistent lymphocytosis (PL). Only 0.1 to 10% of BLV-infected cows develop lymphocytic leukemia.[1] Experimental infection of sheep results in either PL caused by proliferation of CD5+ B cells or, in some cases, lymphoid neoplasia.[59,60] Reports of lymphomagenesis in experimentally infected goats are rare.[61,62] Eosinophilia has also been reported in cows serologically positive for BLV that had concurrent eosinophil infiltration into peripheral lymph nodes, suggesting a possible role of eosinophils in the regulation of immune responses to BLV.[63]

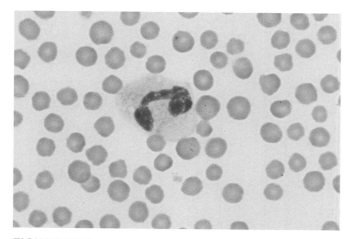

FIGURE 57.3 Peripheral blood, BVD. Yearling calf on day 8 PI with noncytopathic BVD virus had inappetance, watery diarrhea, pyrexia, and depression. Hematologic findings included leukopenia $(3.2 \times 10^3/\mu L)$ and neutropenia $(0.5 \times 10^3/\mu L)$. Platelet numbers were adequate at the time of sampling. A mature neutrophil with basophilic cytoplasm and Döhle bodies illustrates toxic changes. $500\times$

Bovine Herpesvirus and Bovine Immunodeficiency Virus

During a study of field outbreaks of bovine herpes virus (BHV-4), severe leukopenia was observed to last several weeks in infected animals.[64] Experimental infection of calves that have bovine immunodeficiency-like virus resulted in higher numbers of circulating lymphocytes.[65] A possible link between bovine immunodeficiency virus (BIV) infection and bovine paraplegic syndrome, which is characterized by leukocytosis, lymphopenia, and monocytopenia, has been suggested.[66] Sheep experimentally inoculated with BIV had significantly increased numbers of neutrophils and eosinophils at 3 months and 6 to 8 months postinoculation, respectively.[67]

Bovine Ephemeral Fever

In a study of a natural outbreak[68] and experimental infection[69] with bovine ephemeral fever, all affected cows showed similar hematologic changes of neutrophilia and lymphopenia. In the natural outbreak, cattle showed varying degrees of leukocytosis (mean of $14 \times 10^3/\mu L$) with an absolute neutrophilia (mean of $8 \times 10^3/\mu L$) and a mild left shift (30% bands). The peak of neutrophilia and left shift coincided with the peak rise in temperature, after which the leukogram normalized within 24 to 48 hours.

Blue Tongue Virus

Experimental intravenous infection with blue tongue virus (BTV), an orbivirus, was accompanied by a profound neutropenia in inoculated calves; infected sheep developed a transient leukopenia on days 7 to 8 PI (BTV-infected sheep white blood cells [WBCs] ranged from 3.0 to $3.5 \times 10^9/\mu L$).[70,71]

Caprine Arthritis-Encephalitis Virus

In a 10-year study of 60 goats that had caprine arthritis-encephalitis (CAE), a persistent retroviral disease, affected animals had occasional mild anemia and moderate monocytosis in otherwise unremarkable hemograms.[72] A 52-goat herd affected with CAE had leukocyte counts ranging from 8.2 to $19.8 \times 10^3/\mu L$; these ranges were not significantly different from normal reported values of $13.3 \pm 2.7 \times 10^3/\mu L$.[73]

Maedi-Visna Virus

Sheep flocks in Italy affected with maedi-visna virus were investigated. Infected animals were anemic and leukopenic (mean leukocyte count of 3.0 to $4.5 \times 10^3/\mu L$) with an inversion of the neutrophil-to-lymphocyte ratio (neutrophils were 60% or more of differential). Progression of the disease was inevitably fatal.[74] A review of ovine progressive pneumonia stated a persistent leukocytosis is associated with clinical disease, although data was not shown.[75]

TABLE 57.2   Analysis of Terminal (Premortem) Blood and Bone Marrow (Postmortem) From BVDV-infected Calves

Parameter	Calf No. 1	Calf No. 3	Calf No. 6	Calf No. 7	Calf No. 2290	Calf No. 6395	Reference Values†
Total leukocyte count ($\times10^3/\mu$L)	1.9	4.5	4.4	1.40	2.20	2.2	7.67–13.8
Segmented neutrophils ($\times10^3/\mu$L)	0.114	1.035	0.440	0.098	0.286	0.308	1.451–4.203
Band neutrophils ($\times10^3/\mu$L)	0.019	0.495	0.440	0.070	0.176	0.198	0–0.80
Metamyelocyte neutrophils ($\times10^3/\mu$L)	—	—	—	—	—	—	—
Eosinophils ($\times10^3/\mu$L)	—	—	—	—	—	—	0–0.448
Lymphocytes ($\times10^3/\mu$L)	1.710	2.880	2.904	1.190	1.694	1.672	4.682–9.040
Monocytes ($\times10^3/\mu$L)	0.057	0.090	0.616	0.042	0.022	0.022	0.524–1.064
Toxic change	1+	1+	1+	1+	1+	1+	—
Platelets ($\times10^3/\mu$L)	<100‡	20	167	103	121	<10	192–892
Erythrocyte count ($\times10^6/\mu$L)	9.10	10.25	6.85	6.30	8.73	8.25	8.50–10.5
Hemoglobin (g/dL)	9.2	10.1	7.5	6.9	9.0	8.7	9.7–12.7
Hematocrit (%)	29.9	31.6	22.5	20.6	28.0	26.6	32.0–40.0
Mean corpuscular volume (fL)	32.9	30.8	32.8	32.7	32.1	32.3	34.6–41.0
Mean corpuscular hemoglobin (pg)	10.1	9.9	10.9	11.0	10.3	10.5	10.2–13.4
Mean corpuscular hemoglobin Concentration (g/dL)	30.8	32.0	33.3	33.5	32.1	32.7	28.4–34.0
Plasma proteins (g/dL)	5.6	4.8	4.6	4.5	4.8	4.5	5.6–6.8
Fibrinogen (mg/dL)	600	300	500	600	400	400	0–280
Protein:Fibrinogen ratio	8:1	15:1	8:1	7:1	11:1	10:1	>15:1
Bone marrow	hypoplasia	hypoplasia necrosis	hypoplasia	ND†	hypoplasia necrosis	hypoplasia	—
Day of euthanasia	12	10	11	10	10	10	—

†ND = not done.
‡Aged blood sample (2 days old) precluded automated platelet count; platelet count estimated from blood smear.
§Not applicable due to platelet clumping.
Reference values for 3–16 wk old calves from: Jain NC. Comparative hematology of common domestic animals. In: Essential of veterinary hematology. Philadelphia, Lea & Febiger: 1993;36.
Adapted from Ellis JA, West KH, Cortese VS, Myers SL, Carman S, Martin KM, Haines DM. Lesions and distribution of viral antigen following an experimental infection of young seronegative calves with virulent bovine virus diarrhea virus-type II. Can J Vet Res 1998;62(3):161–169 with permission.

Parasitic Diseases

Eosinophils are potent proinflammatory cells that play an integral role in the body's defense mechanisms, in particular against ectoparasites and endoparasites and allergic responses. They also may be involved in host-tissue damage. Calves severely infested with *Psoroptes ovis* developed neutropenia, lymphopenia, and variable eosinophilia.[76,77] Examination of bone marrow revealed myeloid hyperplasia with reduced bone marrow granulocyte reserves and decreased eosinophils in infected calves, leading to the conclusion that the neutropenia was not caused by mite-induced bone marrow suppression but rather by poorly compensated efflux of neutrophils into the epidermis.[78,77] A neutropenia with mild basophilia developed in calves that had acquired immunity to experimental infection with *Amblyomma americanum* ticks, suggesting a role for basophils in the immune response to ticks in this species.[79] In natural infections of Hereford steers that had Gulf Coast ticks (*Amblyomma maculatum* var Koch), lymphopenia, neutrophilia, and basophilia were reported.[80]

Experimental and natural parasitic diseases in sheep are inconsistently associated with eosinophilia.[17] Total leukocyte counts are often unaffected, although there may be a shift in the differential toward an increase in neutrophils at the expense of lymphocytes.[81] In a study of hemopoiesis in nematode-infected sheep, observed hematologic changes during experimental infection with *Telodorsagia circumcincta* included a decrease in neutrophils, a biphasic eosinophil response that peaked between 5 and 10 days PI and again at 16 to 21 days PI, and insignificant changes in the lymphocytes or monocytes.[82] High eosinophil counts correlated with low fecal egg counts in nematode-resistant-infected sheep.[83] The degree of eosinophilia has been correlated with the expression of resistance in sheep to nematodes, and together with fecal egg counts has been suggested to be an indication of host responsiveness to infection rather than an indicator of helminthiasis.[84,85] Experimental *Dic-*

tyocaulus filaria infection of sheep and goats resulted in higher percentages of eosinophils in inoculated animals when compared with control subjects, and the eosinophil response was higher in sheep than goats (17 to 58% and 9% eosinophils, respectively).[86]

Experimental *Schistosoma bovis* infection of goats resulted in eosinophilia during periods of high fecal egg excretion,[87,88] although other studies did not concur with these findings.[89] Monrad et al[88] reported mild eosinophilias of 1.9 and 2.4 × 10³/μL at 4 to 6 and 18 to 22 weeks PI, respectively.[88] Eosinophilia was apparent in experimental infections of *Elaphostrongylus rangiferi* in goats,[90,91] and in natural infections with *Fasciola hepatica*.[92] Heavy infestation of lambs and kids that had *Ctenocephalides felis felis* resulted in severe anemia and eosinophilia (eosinophil percentages ranged from 16.3 to 26.2%; absolute leukocyte counts not shown) associated with an exudative dermatitis.[93]

Trypanosoma congolense infection in goats was associated with leukocytosis (neutropenia and lymphocytosis) in more resistant breeds such as the West African Dwarf and leukopenia (neutrophilia and lymphopenia) in susceptible breeds such as the Red Sokoto.[94]

Miscellaneous Infectious Diseases

Hematologic changes were similar among calves experimentally infected with heartwater (*Cowdria ruminantium*); infected animals developed variable mild leukocytosis (13.2 to 16.1 × 10³/μL) with transient neutropenia (0.46 to 0.53 × 10³/μL) and lymphocytosis (12.0 to 13.2 × 10³/μL).[91] Goats that were infected experimentally with a Nigerian isolate of *C. ruminantium* developed anemia and significant leukopenia with lymphopenia and neutropenia.[96]

Experimental intravenous inoculation of goats, sheep, and calves with a strain of *Mycoplasma mycoides* subsp. *mycoides* isolated from a goat that had polyarthritis induced a neutropenic leukopenia with thrombocytopenia and disseminated intravascular coagulation in the inoculated goats (Figs. 57.4 and 57.5).[97] Preinoculation average leukocyte count was 10.6 ± 2.9 × 10³/μL, and after infection the average leukocyte count decreased to 4.3 ± 2.1 × 10³/μL with a significant decrease in the number of neutrophils. Inoculated calves and sheep showed no significant hematologic changes.

Calves inoculated with *Mycoplasma bovis* intra-articularly developed arthritis, pneumonia, and neutrophilia.[98] The mean leukocyte count rose from 8.5 to 19.0 × 10³/μL, and mean neutrophil counts rose from 3.5 to 12.0 × 10³/μL by 7 weeks PI.

A reported herd outbreak of *Mycoplasma putrefaciens* resulted in mastitis and arthritis that required destruction of nearly 700 goats. Hematologic changes during the investigation detailed unremarkable changes in the leukograms of the adults and mild to severe leukocytosis in the kids (12.4 to 24.0 × 10³/μL).[99]

In goats, neutrophilic leukocytosis was reported in experimental challenges with *Aspergillus fumigatus*,[100] and a novel spotted fever group *Rickettsia*.[101] The former

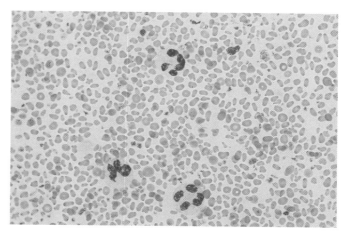

FIGURE 57.4 Peripheral blood, 4-week-old Alpine goat that has weakness, fibrinous bronchopneumonia, polyarthritis, and myocarditis. *M. mycoides*, subsp *mycoides* was isolated. An obvious neutrophil-to-lymphocyte shift is evident in the field of view. The hemogram revealed a normal leukocyte count (8.9 × 10³/μL) with 5.2 × 10³/μL segmented neutrophils, 0.1 × 10³/μL bands, and 3.4 × 10³/μL lymphocytes. 200×.

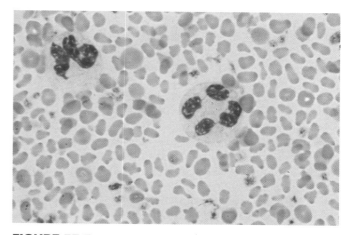

FIGURE 57.5 Higher magnification of mature neutrophils predominating the blood picture in caprine mycoplasma infection. 500×.

study showed leukocytes increasing only slightly from 9.0 × 10³/μL (± 0.79) to 11.2 × 10³/μL (± 1.22) on day 6 postinoculation with neutrophils peaking at approximately 60% of the differential count on day 3 postinoculation. *A. fumigatus* also has been reported as a cause of mastitis and lymphadenitis in dairy sheep, but hematologic findings were not reported.[102]

GENETIC DISORDERS

Bovine Leukocyte Adhesion Deficiency

Bovine leukocyte adhesion deficiency (BLAD), formerly known as bovine granulocytopathy) is an autosomal recessive lethal condition of Holstein cattle, resulting in impaired leukocyte expression of the beta-2 integrin glycoproteins Mac-1 (CD11b/CD18), LFA-1, and p150, 95.[103] Affected animals have defective neutrophil adhesion and diapedesis and are susceptible to various chronic and recurrent infections because of impaired chemotaxis and phagocytosis.[104,105] Gingivitis, periodontitis, pneumonia, diarrhea, stunted growth, impaired wound healing, and chronic dermatitis frequently are reported in affected calves.[106] Hematologic findings in cattle that have BLAD range from mild to severe mature neutrophilia. A left shift was inconsistent and depended on disease stage.[106] Leukocyte counts of $14.0 \times 10^3/\mu L$ at birth and increasing to $100 \times 10^3/\mu L$ with greater than 85% neutrophils were reported in a Holstein calf that died at 48 days of age.[107,108] In another study of 4 affected Holstein calves, the mean number of total leukocytes from affected calves ranged from 48.1 to $188 \times 10^3/\mu L$, with mean neutrophil counts of 35.3 to $163.1 \times 10^3/\mu L$.[105] Left shifts without toxic changes were reported with mean band counts of 4.6 to $20.3 \times 10^3/\mu L$. Bone marrow observations included striking myeloid hyperplasia with prominent extramedullary myelopoiesis.[109] M:E ratios of 9:1 have been seen in such cases.[104] Characteristic findings on postmortem include various necrotizing lesions with prominent intravascular leukocytosis and a lack of tissue neutrophil infiltration, consistent with the underlying physiologic defect.[109]

Immunomodulatory and Hormone Therapy

The potential use of cytokines as immunomodulators has stimulated interest in the effects of various recombinant growth factors on hemopoietic progenitors and on the hemogram. Use of cytokines as immunotherapeutics in the dairy cow to prevent immunosuppression and infectious diseases during the periparturient period has been of particular interest.

Recombinant bovine granulocyte-colony-stimulating factor (rboG-CSF) given to periparturient cows produced a striking prepartum and postpartum leukocytosis (35.6 and $53.5 \times 10^3/\mu L$, respectively), with a mature neutrophilia (24.0 and $38.1 \times 10^3/\mu L$) and monocytosis (7.6 and $9.8 \times 10^3/\mu L$) prepartum and postpartum.[110] The rboG-CSF also was shown to enhance neutrophil adhesiveness, bacterial ingestion, and cytotoxicity. In studies of limited numbers of cows given intramammary bacterial challenge after pretreatment with granulocyte-colony-stimulating factor (G-CSF), the rate of new infections, as well as the duration and severity of infection were reduced in cytokine-treated cattle.[111]

Cattle treated with a natural recombinant bovine G-CSF or a recombinant synthetic analogue of bovine G-CSF demonstrated a large increase in the bone marrow M:E ratio, with the maximum ratio of 6.71 achieved on day 14 of treatment with the synthetic analogue.[111] M:E increases were characterized by an increase in both the mitotic and the maturation pools of neutrophils.

A neutrophilia with an initial left shift (bands, meta-myelocytes, and myelocytes) was reported within 2 days of treating lactating dairy cows with recombinant human G-CSF (rhG-CSF).[112,113] By the last treatment on day 15, maximum neutrophil counts observed ranged from 22.5 to $45.6 \times 10^3/\mu L$. Lymphocytes and monocytes did not vary significantly from baseline values. Discontinuation of treatment resulted in a steady and rapid decline in neutrophil counts over the subsequent 3 days.

Cows treated with rhG-CSF responded with a leukocytosis of $30.2 \times 10^3/\mu L$ compared with the mean leukocyte count in control subjects of $8.7 \times 10^3/\mu L$. Intramammary challenge with *Staphylococcus aureus* of a small number of rhG-CSF-treated cows resulted in a reduction in the incidence of intramammary infections compared with untreated control cows.[114]

In an additional study involving intramammary bacterial challenge of rhG-CSF-treated cows during which *Klebsiella pneumonia* was used, reduced duration of bacterial recovery and shortened duration of clinical symptoms were reported.[111] These findings were attributed to the potential of rhG-CSF to enhance the marginating pool of neutrophils and somatic cell counts, leading to intensification of the local response to bacterial infection.

Dwarf goats injected with recombinant bovine tumor necrosis factor alpha (rBo-TNF alpha) or *E. coli* endotoxin (LPS) developed similar hematologic findings, namely, lymphopenia and neutropenia followed by neutrophilia. However with rBo-TNF alpha, leukopenia was longer lasting and was followed by less of a neutrophilia and a more persistent lymphopenia compared with LPS injection.[115] Similar acute-phase responses were noted in goats treated with human interferon-alpha 2a or poly I: poly C (an interferon inducer).[116]

Neutrophilia has been observed in adult Jersey cattle treated with Interleukin-1-β (IL-1-β). The neutrophilia reportedly declined within a few days of cessation of treatment.[111] Calves treated with recombinant bovine IL-1-β with bovine herpes virus-1 vaccine had higher leukocyte counts, primarily owing to a mature neutrophilia and monocytosis.[117]

In vitro eosinophil-potentiating activity (EPA) was demonstated during exposure of sheep bone marrow eosinophils to recombinant ovine granulocyte-macrophage colony-stimulating factor and recombinant ovine IL-3. Recombinant mouse IL-5 and recombinant human IL-5 showed similar effects in the same assay. EPA was measured by use of microassays for eosinophil peroxidase and arylsulfatase.[118]

The total leukocyte counts of cows treated with exogenous bovine somatotropin tended to increase primarily because of a higher segmented neutrophil count. The presence of band neutrophils, basophils, monocytes, and eosinophils in the blood remained unaffected.[119]

Neoplasia

Significant leukocytosis with severe anemia, thrombocytopenia, and atypical or poorly differentiated cells are characteristic hemogram findings in ruminants with hemopoietic neoplasia. Myelomonocytic, monocytic, and lymphocytic leukemias have been reported.[120,121,122] In a calf that has acute myelomonocytic leukemia, the leukocyte count exceeded $100 \times 10^3/\mu L$ and was predominated by atypical blast cells.[120] In calves that had acute lymphocytic leukemia, there was a notable decrease in the number of B-cells and a significant unresponsiveness to mitogenic stimulation (Figs. 57.6 and 57.7). Similar findings have been reported for a cow that had persistent lymphocytosis that underwent transformation to leukemia.[122]

Leukopenia was reported in a 4-year-old Nubian goat that had systemic mastocytosis.[123] Total white cell counts were as low as $2.8 \times 10^3/\mu L$ and were accompanied by a severe macrocytic hypochromic anemia (packed cell volume [PCV], 12%; hemoglobin, 4.0 g/dL).

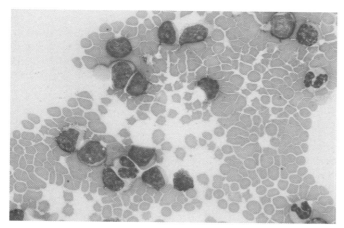

FIGURE 57.6 Peripheral blood, sporadic bovine leukosis in a 3-month-old calf with a history of lethargy and peripheral lymphadenopathy. Hemogram revealed a leukocytosis (31.6 × 10³/μL) with an absolute lymphocytosis (18.5 × 10³/μL). The calf was anemic (hematocrit [HCT]: 0.18%; hemoglobin [Hgb]: 6.9 g/dL), and thrombocytopenic (149 × 10³/μL). 200×

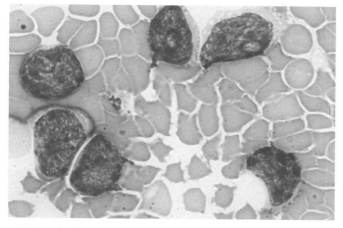

FIGURE 57.7 Same case as in Figure 57.6. Examination of the blood smear revealed a monomorphic population of large lymphocytes, some with nucleoli and nucleolar rings, and frequent lytic cells. 500×

Toxic and Nutritional Causes of Leukocyte Alterations

Blue-Green Alga

Intraruminal inoculation of sheep with *Microcystis aeruginosa* resulted in a mild neutrophilia (mean leukocyte count of 8.8 to $11.3 \times 10^3/\mu L$, with a 50% increase in neutrophils over baseline) and a significant left shift (reported as a 40-fold increase in the mean number of immature neutrophils) in lethally dosed animals.[124] Experimental infections of two sheep with *Nodularia spumigena* mimicked the findings of naturally infected sheep that had the same alga. Leukopenia (<2.0 and 4.5×10^3 leukocytes/μL) were reported before death in experimentally dosed animals, and bone marrow smears were not supportive of myeloid hypoplasia.[125] Both studies attributed the leukocyte changes to peripheral consumption secondary to massive hepatic necrosis that was identified at postmortem.

Botulism Type-D

A dairy herd suffered mortality in 64% of their lactating cows suspected to be caused by type-D botulism.[126] Hemograms of affected cows revealed variable leukocytosis (12.5 to $20.9 \times 10^3/\mu L$) with neutrophilia, lymphopenia, and eosinopenia.

Bracken Fern

Leukopenia has been reported in cattle that developed bracken fern poisoning with leukocyte counts reported as low as $0.7 \times 10^3/\mu L$.[127,128] Yearling cattle fed a bracken diet during experiments developed severe leukopenia ($<2.0 \times 10^3$ leukocytes/μL) prior to the development of clinical symptoms.[127] In one animal that died as a result of the poisoning, hematologic findings indicated a severe neutropenia ($0 \times 10^3/\mu L$) terminally. Marrow examination revealed significant myeloid and megakaryocytic hypoplasia with early sparing of the erythroid series. These hematologic findings were confirmed in field outbreaks of bracken fern toxicity. Although the selective eating habits and reported tolerance to bracken fern in sheep render them less likely to be involved in poisonings, reports of bracken fern toxicity have been associated with leukopenia and thrombocytopenia in this species.[17,129]

Copper Deficiency

Copper deficiency has been associated with an increased incidence of microbial infections in domestic animals,[130] stimulating interest in the identification of hematologic alterations that may arise as a direct result of this nutritional disorder, and possibly predispose to enhanced disease incidence. Experimental studies inducing copper deficiency in molybdenum- and sulfate-supplemented calves demonstrated increases in peripheral blood monocytes as the only significant hematologic alteration. Monocytes increased from 0.5 to 1.2 × 10³/μL in treated calves, and this change was accompanied by alterations in B-lymphocyte subpopulations, impaired phagocytosis of sheep red blood cells, and decreased neutrophil nitroblue tetrazolium (NBT) reduction.[131] Another study of experimentally induced molybdenum-induced copper deficiency in 12 angus × hereford heifers identified neutrophilia without alterations in chemotaxis or adhesion molecule expression.[132]

Ethylene Glycol Toxicosis

Ethylene glycol toxicity was induced experimentally in calves and cows, which subsequently developed neutrophilia consistently throughout the study.[133] Absolute numbers of neutrophils increased 2- to 20-fold greater than baseline values 24 hours postadministration. Lymphocyte numbers remained unchanged or increased slightly. Experimental testing was prompted by a clinical case in a calf. Toxicosis had not been previously reported in this species.

Fluorosis

In calves born to fluoride-intoxicated cows, osteopenia and atrophy of bone marrow cells with serous atrophy of bone marrow fat were reported with signs of congenital fluorosis. Hematologic findings were not reported.[134] Excessive dietary fluoride has been associated with eosinophilia.[135,136] In the latter study, mean eosinophil percentages ranged from 5.0 ± 1.5 to 11.5 ± 2.0 with normal total leukocyte counts.

Furazolidone Toxicity

Granulocytopenic disease in calves is characterized by pyrexia, hypersalivation, nasal discharge, oral and intestinal necrotic lesions, and neutropenic leukopenia with myeloid hypoplasia in the bone marrow. It is associated with chronic ingestion of furazolidone, and caused by the inhibition of several enzymes required for the aerobic oxidation of glucose and other carbohydrate substrates.[137]

Monensin Toxicity

Calves experimentally dosed with 40 mg/kg of mycelial monensin developed leukocytosis with signs of anorexia, lethargy, and diarrhea.[138] A mean leukocyte count of $16 \times 10^3/\mu L$ with neutrophilia (mean $7 \times 10^3/\mu L$) and a mild left shift ($0.23 \times 10^3/\mu L$) were reported. A significant decline in baseline lymphocyte counts also was noted. Toxicosis also has been reported in sheep,[139,140] although changes in total leukocyte counts were not observed in this species.[139]

Mycotoxins

Sheep and calves poisoned with trichothecenes (T-2 toxin) developed lymphopenia and leukopenia, with decreased lymphocyte function and altered immune responses.[141,142] Diacetoxyscirpenol (DAS) is a mycotoxin produced by some strains of *Fusarium* sp., and acute hematologic changes of intoxication have been reported.[143] Although cattle were the most resistent of the species tested, a significant left shift to the myelocyte stage with signs of toxicity (Döhle bodies), metarubricytes, immature lymphocytes, and evidence of bone marrow necrosis were reported. Stachybotryotoxicosis has been reported in cattle and sheep and is characterized by progressive and severe leukopenia and thrombocytopenia with focal bone marrow necrosis and significant myeloid hypoplasia. Field cases in sheep had leukocyte counts reported as low as $2.3 \times 10^3/\mu L$.[144]

Plant Toxicity

Ingestion of the green leaves of *Ipomoea carnea*, a tropical plant of the family Convolvulacae, has caused the death of goats in the Sudan. These goats were observed to have hematologic changes, including anemia and decreased leukocyte counts, possibly caused by bone marrow depression.[145] Experimental and field cases of acute toxicity with prickly paddy melon (*Cucumis myriocarpus*) in calves have been associated with neutrophilia, a left shift, and toxic changes of neutrophils on day 2 postingestion.[146]

Uranyl Nitrate

Experimental injection of uranyl nitrate into goats resulted in acute nephrotoxicity, systemic shock, and death. Hematologic findings in treated animals included neutrophilic leukocytosis with left shift, eosinopenia, and monocytopenia.[147] By 24 hours, mean leukocyte counts of $16.6 \times 10^3/\mu L$ with bands and segmented neutrophils comprising 60% of the differential count were reported.

Leukopenia

Leukopenia in the ruminant is often caused by lymphopenia, or lymphopenia with concurrent neutropenia. This develops because the lymphocyte is the predominant cell in the differential count, as evidenced by the normally low neutrophil-to-lymphocyte ratio found in ruminants. Leukopenia is a common hematologic response to a wide array of pathologic conditions.

In a retrospective study of 4287 bovine hemograms (3639 cows), Andresen[12] reported the highest incidence of leukopenia ($<5.0 \times 10^3/\mu L$) in cows that had diseases of the digestive system (Fig 57.8), mammary gland, and reproductive tract. Neutropenia was present in 47.5% of all leukopenias. Low leukocyte counts were observed more frequently within the first month postpartum and more often in the winter months. The recovery rate among leukopenic cows compared with hematologically normal cows was 61.0% and 82.9%, respectively.

There have been sporadic reports of pancytopenia in cattle compared with other species.[148,149] Underlying causes such as bone marrow necrosis, hematologic neoplasia, idiosyncratic drug reactions, exposure to toxins, and unknown causes are suspected or demonstrated in

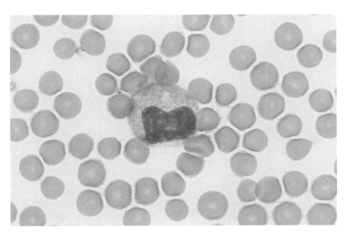

FIGURE 57.8 Peripheral blood, cow, left displaced abomasum and septic arthritis. Hematologic findings included leukopenia ($2.4 \times 10^3/\mu$L) with a degenerative left shift (21% segmented neutrophils, 24% bands) and significant toxicity (cytoplasmic basophilia, vacuolation, and Döhle bodies). A toxic metamyelocyte is pictured here. 500×

such cases. Profound leukopenia, neutropenia, and toxic changes of neutrophils, found in association with nonregenerative anemia, thrombocytopenia, and bone marrow hypocellularity, are the hallmark findings. Fatal aplastic anemia has been reported in cattle fed trichloroethylene-extracted feed that produced renal and bone marrow injury.[150] The toxic substance was identified as S-(1,2-dichlorovinyl)-L-cysteine (DCVC).

Neutropenia has been experimentally induced in calves,[151] sheep,[152] and goats[153] by injection of hydroxyurea in the former two and either nitrogen mustard or hydroxyurea in the latter to investigate the role of neutrophils in the pathogenesis of various inflammatory diseases. Profoundly decreased neutrophil counts (as low as $0.032 \times 10^3/\mu$L) were obtained.[154] Partial to complete selective myeloid destruction was observed in the bone marrow.[151] Severe anemia and neutropenia with moderate leukopenia occurred in 11 of 16 pygmy goats that had widespread myelofibrosis.[155] Mean neutrophil counts of 0.164 to $0.195 \times 10^3/\mu$L and 0.966 to $2.146 \times 10^3/\mu$L were reported in affected and normal kids, respectively. Although the cause of the marrow fibrosis was undetermined, breeding practices implicated an inherited disorder.

REFERENCES

1. **Weiss DJ, Perman V.** Assessment of the hematopoietic system in ruminants. Vet Clin North Am Food Anim Pract 1992;8(2):411–428.
2. **Jain NC.** Comparative hematology of common domestic animals. In: essentials of veterinary hematology. Philadelphia: Lea & Febiger, 1993.
3. **Godson DL, Campos M, Attah-Poku SK, Redmond MJ, Cordeiro DM, Sethi MS, Harland RJ, Babiuk LA.** Serum Haptoglobin as an indicator of the acute phase response in bovine respiratory disease. Vet Immunol Immunopath 1996;51:277–292.
4. **Skinner JG, Brown RAL, Roberts L.** Bovine haptoglobin response in clinically defined field conditions. Vet Rec 1991;128:147–149.
5. **Lumsden JH, Valli VEO, McSherry BJ, Willoughby RA.** The Piromen test as an assay of bone marrow granulocyte reserves in the calf. I. Studies on bone marrow and peripheral blood leukocytes. Can J Comp Med 1974;38:56–64.
6. **Valli VEO, Hulland TJ, McSherry BJ, Robinson GA, Gilman JPW.** The kinetics of haematopoiesis in the calf. I. An autoradiographical study of myelopoiesis in normal, anaemic and endotoxin treated calves. Res Vet Sci 1971;12:535–550.
7. **Valli VEO.** The hematopoietic system. In: Jubb KVF, Kennedy PC, Palmer N, eds. Pathology of domestic animals. 4th ed. San Diego: Academic Press, 1993.
8. **Valli VEO.** M.Sc. thesis. University of Guelph, 1966.
9. **Clover CK, Zarkower A.** immunologic responses in colostrum-fed and colostrum-deprived calves. Am J Vet Res 1980;41(7):1002–1007.
10. **Doxey DL.** Haematology of the ox. In: Archer RK, Jeffcott LB, eds. Comparative clinical hematology. London: Blackwell Scientific Publications, 1977.
11. **Abt DA, Ipsen J, Hare WCD, Marshak RR, Sahl J.** Circadian and seasonal variations in the hemogram of mature dairy cattle. Cornell Vet 1966; 56:479–520.
12. **Andresen HA.** Evaluation of leukopenia in cattle. J Am Vet Med Assoc 1970;156(7):858–867.
13. **Olson DP, South PJ, Hendrix K.** Hematologic values in hypothermic and rewarmed young calves. Am J Vet Res 1983;44(4):572–576.
14. **Alexander G, Bell AW, Hales JRS.** The effect of cold exposure on the plasma levels of glucose, lactate, free fatty acids and glycerol and on the blood gas and acid-base status in young lambs. Biol Neonate 1972;20:9–21.
15. **Tennant B, Harrold D, Reina-Guerra M, Kendrick JW, Laben RC.** Hematology of the neonatal calf. I. Erythrocyte and leukocyte values of normal calves. Cornell Vet 1974;64:516–532.
16. **Winter H.** The myelogram of normal sheep. J Comp Pathol Ther 1964; 74:205–209.
17. **Greenwood B.** haematology of the sheep and goat. In: Archer RK, Jeffcott LB, eds. Comparative clinical hematology. London: Blackwell Scientific Publications, 1977.
18. **Mbassa GK, Poulsen JSD.** Leukocyte profile in growing dwarf and landrace kids. J Am Vet Med Assoc 1991;38:389–397.
19. **Holman HH, Dew SM.** The blood picture of the goat. IV. Changes in coagulation times, platelet counts and leucocyte numbers associated with age. Res Vet Sci 1965;6:510–521.
20. **Winquist G.** Morphology of the blood and the haematopoietic organs in cattle under normal and some experimental conditions. Acta Anat 1954; 22(suppl 21–1):1–159.
21. **Jacobs RM, Horney B, Beiner L.** Cutaneous response to PHA-M and hematologic changes in corticosteroid treated cows. Can J Comp Med 1981;45:384–387.
22. **van Miert AS, van Duin CT, Wensing T.** The effects of ACTH, prednisolone and Escheria coli endotoxin on some clinical haematological and blood biochemical parameters in dwarf goats. Vet Q 1986;8(3):195–203.
23. **Anosa VO, Ogbogu DA.** The effect of parturition on the blood picture of sheep. Res Vet Sci 1979;26(3):380–382.
24. **Lee EK, Kehrli ME Jr.** Expression of adhesion molecules on neutrophils of periparturient cows and neonatal calves. Am J Vet Res 1998;59(1):37–43.
25. **Kehrli ME Jr, Nonnecke BJ, Roth JA.** Alterations in bovine neutrophil function during the periparturient period. Am J Vet Res 1989;50:207–214.
26. **Goff JP, Kehrli ME Jr, Horst RL.** Periparturient hypocalcemia in cows: prevention using intramuscular parathyroid hormone. J Dairy Sci 1989; 72:1182–1187.
27. **Hoyer C, Grunert E, Jochle W.** Plasma glucocorticoid concentrations in calves as an indicator of stress during parturition. Am J Vet Res 1990; 51:1882–1884.
28. **Burton JL, Kehrli ME Jr, Horst RL.** Regulation of L-selectin and CD18 on bovine neutrophils by glucocorticoids: effects of cortisol and dexamethasone. J Leukoc Biol 1995;57:317–325.
29. **Kehrli ME Jr, Goff JP.** Periparturient hypocalcemia in cows: effects on peripheral blood neutrophil and lymphocyte function. J Dairy Sci 1989; 72:1188–1196.
30. **Ullrey DE, Miller ER, Long CH, Vincet BH.** Sheep hematology from birth to maturity 1. Erythrocyte population, size, and hemoglobin concentration. J Anim Sci 1965;24:134–140.
31. **Dosgne H, Capuco AV, Paape MJ, Roets E, Burvenich C, Fenwick B.** Reduction of acyloxyacyl hydrolase activity in circulating neutrophils from cows after parturition. J Dairy Sci 1998;81(3):672–677.
32. **Kehrli ME Jr, Jesse JR, Goff JP Harp JA Thurston JR.** Effects of preventing periparturient hypocalcemia in cows by parathyroid hormone administration on hematology, conglutinin, immunoglobulin, and shedding of Staphylococcus aureus in milk. J Dairy Sci 1990;73:2103–2111.
33. **Power HT, Rebhun WC.** Bacterial endocarditis in adult dairy cattle. J Am Vet Med Assoc 1983;182(8):806–808.
34. **Anderson DE, Constable PD, St Jean G, Hull BL.** Small-intestinal volvulus in cattle: 35 cases (1967–1992). J Am Vet Med Assoc 1993;203(8):1178–1183.
35. **Green SL, Smith LL.** Meningitis is neonatal calves: 32 cases (1983–1990). J Am Vet Med Assoc 1992;201(1):125–128.
36. **Constable PD, Schmall LM, Muir WW, Hoffsis GF.** Respiratory, renal, hematologic, and serum biochemical effects of hypertonic saline solution in endotoxemic calves. Am J Vet Res 1991;52(7):990–998.

37. **Tennant B, Harrold D, Reina-Guerra M.** Hematology of the neonatal calf. II. Response associated with acute enteric infections, gram-negative septicemia, and experimental endotoxemia. Cornell Vet 1975;65(4):457–475.
38. **Jain NC, Schalm OW, Lasmanis J.** Neutrophil kinetics in endotoxin-induced mastitis. Am J Vet Res 1978;39(10):1662–1667.
39. **Griel LC, Zarkower A, Eberhart RJ.** Clinical and clinico-pathological effects of escherichia coli endotoxin in mature cattle. Can J Comp Med 1975;39:1–6.
40. **Schalm OW, Lasmanis J.** Cytologic features of bone marrow in normal and mastitic cows. Am J Vet Res 1976;37(4):359–363.
41. **Clinkenbeard KD, Mosier DA, Confer AW.** Effects of *Pasteurella haemolytica* leukotoxin on isolated bovine neutrophils. Toxicon 1989;27:797–804.
42. **Clinkenbeard KD, Mosier DA, Confer AW.** Transmembrane pore size and role of cell swelling in cytotoxicity caused by *Pasteurella haemolytica* leukotoxin. Infect Immun 1989;57:420–425.
43. **Clarke CR, Confer AW, Mosier DA.** In vivo effect of Pasteurella haemolytica infection on bovine neutrophil morphology. Am J Vet Res 1998; 59(5):588–592.
44. **Linden A, Desmecht D, Amory H, Daube G, Lecomte S, Lekeux P.** Pulmonary ventilation, mechanics, gas exchange and haemodynamics in calves following intratracheal inoculation of *Pasteurella haemolytica*. J Am Vet Med Assoc 1995;42:531–544.
45. **Slocombe RF, Derksen FJ, Robinson NE, Trapp A, Gupta A, Newman JP.** Interactions of cold stress and Pasteurella haemolytica in the pathogenesis of pneumonic pasteurellosis in calves: method of induction and hematologic and pathologic changes. Am J Vet Res 1984;45:1757–1763.
46. **Smith BP, Habasha F, Reina-Guerra M, Hardy AJ.** Bovine salmonellosis: experimental production and characterization of the disease in calves, using oral challenge with *Salmonella typhimurium*. Am J Vet Res 1979;40(11):1510–1513.
47. **Luthman J, Kindahl H, Jacobsson SO.** The influence of flunixin on the response to Salmonella typhimurium endotoxin in calves. Acta Vet Scand 1989;30(3):295–300.
48. **Otesile EB, Ahmed G, Adetosoye AI.** Experimental infection of Red Sokoto goats with Salmonella typhimurium. Rev Elev Med Vet Pays Trop 1990;43(1):49–53.
49. **Gameel AA, Tartour G.** Haematological and plasma protein changes in sheep experimentally infected with *Corynebacterium pseudotuberculosis*. J Comp Path 1974;84:477–484.
50. **Nadim MA, Mahmoud AH, Soliman MK.** The significance of the blood picture in the diagnosis and prognosis of caseous lymphadenitis in sheep. Zentralbl Veterinarmed A 1966;13:715–718.
51. **Bolin SR, Ridpath JF.** Assessment of protection from systemic infection or disease afforded by low to intermediate titers of passively acquired neutralizing antibody against bovine viral diarrhea virus in calves. Am J Vet Res 1995;56(6):754–759.
52. **Carlsson U, Fredriksson G, Alenius S, Kindahl H.** Bovine virus diarrhoea virus, a cause of early pregnancy failure in the cow. Zentralb Veterinarmed A 1989; 36: 15–23.
53. **Ellis JA, West KH, Cortese VS, Myers SL, Carman S, Martin KM, Haines DM.** Lesions and distribution of viral antigen following an experimental infection of young seronegative calves with virulent bovine virus diarrhea virus-type II. Can J Vet Res 1998;62(3):161–169.
54. **Traven M, Alenius S, Fossum C, Larsson B.** Primary bovine viral diarrhoea virus infection in calves following direct contact with a persistently viraemic calf. Zentralb Veterinarmed B 1991;38:453–462.
55. **Marshall DJ, Moxley RA, Kelling CL.** Distribution of virus and viral antigen in specific pathogen-free calves following inoculation with noncytopathic bovine viral diarrhea virus. Vet Pathol 1996;33:311–328.
56. **Spagnuolo M, Kennedy S, Foster JC, Moffett DA, Adair BM.** Bovine viral diarrhoea virus infection in bone marrow of experimentally infected calves. J Comp Pathol 1997;116:97–100.
57. **Lamontagne L, Lafortune P, Fournel M.** Modulation of the cellular immune responses to T cell-dependent and T cell-independent antigens in lambs with induced bovine viral diarrhea virus infection. Am J Vet Res 1989;50(9):1604–1608.
58. **Burny A, Bruck C, Cleuter Y, Couez D, Deschamps J, Gregoire D, Ghysdael J, Kettmann R, Mammerickx M, Marbaix G, Portetelle D.** Bovine leukaemia virus and enzootic bovine leukosis. Onderstepoort J Vet Res 1985;52:133–144.
59. **Chevallier N, Berthelemy M, Le Rhun D, Laine V, Levy D, Schwartz-Cornil I.** Bovine leukemia virus-induced lymphocytosis and increased cell survival mainly involve the CD11b: B-lymphocyte subset in sheep. J Virol 1998;72(5):4413–4420.
60. **Birkebak TA, Palmer GH, Davis WC, Knowles DP, McElwain TF.** Association of GP51 expression and persistent CD5+ B-lymphocyte expansion with lymphomagenesis in bovine leukemia virus infected sheep. Leukemia 1994;8(11):1890–1899.
61. **Olson C, Kettmann R, Burny A, Kaja R.** Goat lymphosarcoma from bovine leukemia virus. J Natl Cancer Inst 1981;67:671–675.
62. **Kettmann R, Mammerickx M, Portetelle D, Gregoire D, Burny A.** Experimental infection of sheep and goat with bovine leukemia virus: localization of proviral information on the target cells. Leuk Res 1984;8(6):937–944.
63. **Levkut M, Levkutova M, Konrad V, Polacek M.** Eosinophils in lymph nodes of cows infected by bovine leukaemia virus. Acta Vet Hung 1995;43(1):145–151.
64. **Van Opdenbosch E, Wellemans G, Ooms La, Degryse AD.** BHV4 (bovine herpes virus 4) related disorders in Belgian cattle: a study of two problem herds. Vet Res Commun 1988;12(4–5):347–353.
65. **Carpenter S, Miller LD, Alexandersen S, Whetstone CA, VanDerMaaten MJ, Viuff B, Wannemuehler Y, Miller JM, Roth JA.** Characterization of early pathogenic effects after experimental infection of calves with bovine immunodeficiency-like virus. J Virol 1992;66(2):1074–1083.
66. **Walder R, Kalvatchev Z, Tobin GJ, Barrios MN, Garzaro DJ, Gonda MA.** Possible role of bovine immunodeficiency virus in bovine paraplegic syndrome: evidence from immunochemical, virological and seroprevalence studies. Res Virol 1995;146(5):313–323.
67. **Jacobs RM, Smith HE, Whetstone CA, Suarez DL, Jefferson B, Valli VE.** Haematological and lymphocyte subset analyses in sheep inoculated with bovine immunodeficiency-like virus. Vet Res Commun 1994;18(6):471–482.
68. **Uren MF, Murphy GM.** Studies on the pathogenesis of bovine ephemeral fever in sentinel cattle. II Haematological and biochemical data. Vet Microbiol 1985;10:505–515.
69. **Uren MF, St George TD, Zakrezewski H.** The effect of anti-inflammatory agents on the clinical expression of bovine ephemeral fever. Vet Microbiol 1989;19(2):99–111.
70. **Ellis JA, Luedke AJ, Davis WC, Wechsler SJ, Mecham JO, Pratt DL, Elliot JD.** T lymphocyte subset alterations following bluetongue virus infection in sheep and cattle. Vet Immunol Immunopath 1990;24(1):49–67.
71. **MacLachlan NJ, Thompson J.** Bluetongue virus-induced interferon in cattle. Am J Vet Res 1985;46(6):1238–1241.
72. **Crawford TB, Adams DS.** Caprine arthritis-encephalitis: clinical features and presence of antibody in selected goat populations. J Am Vet Med Assoc 1981;178(7):713–719.
73. **Woodard JC, Gaskin JM, Poulos PW, MadKay RJ, Burridge MJ.** Caprine arthritis-encephalitis: clinicopathologic study. Am J Vet Res 1982; 43(12):2085–2096.
74. **Caporale VP, Foglini A, Lelli R, Mantovani A, Nannini D, Simoni P.** Preliminary observations on the presence of visna-maedi in Italy. Vet Res Commun 1983;6(1):31–35.
75. **Bulgin MS.** Ovine progressive pneumonia, caprine arthritis-encephalitis, and related lentiviral diseases of sheep and goats. Vet Clin North Am Food Anim Pract 1990;6(3):691–704.
76. **Stromberg PC, Fisher WF, Guillot FS, Pruett JH, Price RE, Green RA.** Systemic pathologic responses in experimental Psoroptes ovis infestation of Hereford calves. Am J Vet Res 1986;47(6):1326–1331.
77. **Stromberg PC, Guillot FS.** Pathogenesis of psoroptic scabies in Hereford heifer calves. Am J Vet Res 1989;50(4):594–601.
78. **Stromberg PC, Guillot FS.** Bone marrow response in cattle with chronic dermatitis caused by Psoroptes ovis. Vet Pathol 1987;24(5):365–370.
79. **Brown SJ, Barker RW, Askenase PW.** Bovine resistance to Amblyomma americanum ticks: an acquired immune response characterized by cutaneous basophil infiltrates. Vet Parasitol 1984;16(1–2):147–165.
80. **Williams RE, Hair JA, McNew RW.** Effects of Gulf Coast ticks on blood composition and weights of pastured Hereford steers. J Parasitol 1978; 64(2):336–342.
81. **Gallagher CH.** Studies on trichostrongylosis of sheep: plasma volume, haemoglobin concentration, and blood cell count. Aust J Agric Res 1963;14:349–363.
82. **Haig DM, Stevenson LM, Thomson J, Percival A, Smith WD.** Haemopoietic cell responses in the blood and bone marrow of sheep infected with the abomasal nematode *Telodorsagia circumcincta*. J Comp Pathol 1995; 112:151–164.
83. **Hohenhaus MA, Josey MJ, Dobson C, Outteridge PM.** The eosinophil leucocyte, a phenotypic marker of resistance to nematode parasites, is associated with calm behaviour in sheep. Immunol Cell Biol 1998; 76(2):153–158.
84. **Buddle BM, Jowett G, Green RS, Douch PG, Risdon PL.** Association of blood eosinophilia with the expression of resistance in Romney lambs to nematodes. Int J Parasitol 1992;22(7):955–960.
85. **Dawkins HJ, Windon RG, Eagleson GK.** Eosinophil responses in sheep selected for high and low responsiveness to Trichostrongylus colubriformis. Int J Parasitol 1989;19(2):199–205.
86. **Wilson GI.** The strength and duration of immunity to Dictyocaulus filaria infection in sheep and goats. Res Vet Sci 1970;11(1):7–17.
87. **Monrad J, Christensen NO, Nansen P.** Acquired resistance in goats following a single primary Schistosoma bovis infection. Acta Trop 1990; 48(1):69–77.
88. **Monrad J, Christensen NO, Nansen P, Johansen MV, Lindberg R.** Acquired resistance against Schistosoma bovis after single or repeated low-level primary infections in goats. Res Vet Sci 1995;58(1):42–45.
89. **Kassuku A, Christensen NO, Nansen P, Monrad J.** Clinical pathology of Schistosoma bovis infection in goats. Res Vet Sci 1986;40(1):44–47.
90. **Handeland K, Skorping A.** The early migration of Elaphostrongylus rangiferi in goats. Zentralbl Veterinarmed B 1992;39(4):263–272.

91. **Handeland K, Skorping A.** Experimental cerebrospinal elaphostrongylosis (Elaphostrongylus rangiferi) in goats. I. Clinical observations. Zentralb Veterinarmed B 1993;40(2):141–147.

92. **Leathers CW, Foreyt WJ, Fetcher A, Foreyt KM.** Clinical fascioliasis in domestic goats in Montana. J Am Vet Med Assoc 1982;180(12):1451–1454.

93. **Yeruham I, Rosen S, Perl S.** An apparent flea-allergy dermatitis in kids and lambs. Zentralbl Veterinarmed A 1997;44(7):391–397.

94. **Adah MI, Otesile EB, Joshua RA.** Susceptibility of Nigerian West African Dwarf and Red Sokoto goats to a strain of Trypanosoma congolense. Vet Parasitol 1993;47(3–4):177–188.

95. **Van Amstel SR, Reyers F, Guthrie AJ, Oberem PT, Bertschinger H.** The clinical pathology of Heartwater. I. Haematology and blood chemistry. Onderstepoort J Vet Res 1988;55:37–45.

96. **Illemobade AA, Blotkamp C.** Clinico-pathological study of heartwater in goats. Tropenmed Parasitol 1978;29(1):71–76.

97. **Rosendal S.** Experimental infection of goats, sheep and calves with the large colony type of Mycoplasma mycoides subsp. mycoides. Vet Pathol 1981;18(1):71–81.

98. **Ryan MJ, Wyand DS, Hill DL, Tourtellotte ME, Yang TJ.** Morphologic changes following intraarticular inoculation of Mycoplasma bovis in calves. Vet Pathol 1983;20(4):472–487.

99. **DaMassa AJ, Brooks DL, Holmber CA, Moe AI.** Caprine mycoplasmosis: an outbreak of mastitis and arthritis requiring destruction of 700 goats. Vet Rec 1987;120:409–413.

100. **Mandal PC, Gupta PP.** Experimental aspergillosis in goats: clinical, haematological and mycological studies. Zentralbl Veterinarmed B 1993; 40(4):283–286.

101. **Kelly PJ, Mason PR, Rhode C, Dziva F, Matthewman L.** Transient infections of goats with a novel spotted fever group rickettsia from Zimbabwe. Res Vet Sci 1991;51(3):268–271.

102. **Perez V, Corpa JM, Garcia Marin JF, Aduriz JJ, Jensen HE.** Mammary and systemic aspergillosis in dairy sheep. Vet Pathol 1998;35:235–240.

103. **Ackermann MR, Kehrli ME Jr, Morfitt DC.** Ventral dermatitis and vasculitis in a calf with bovine leukocyte adhesion deficiency. J Am Vet Med Assoc 1993;202(3):413–415.

104. **Gerardi AS.** Bovine leucocyte adhesion deficiency: a review of a modern disease and its implications. Res Vet Sci 1996;6(3)183–186.

105. **Nagahata H, Kehrli ME, Murata H, Okada H, Noda H, Kociba GJ.** Neutrophil function and pathologic findings in Holstein calves with leukocyte adhesion deficiency. Am J Vet Res 1994;55(1):40–48.

106. **Muller KE, Bernadina WE, Kalsbeek HC, Hoek A, Rutten VP, Wentink GH.** Bovine leukocyte adhesion deficiency-clinical course and laboratory findings in eight affected animals. Vet Q 1994;16(2):65–71.

107. **Kehrli ME Jr, Schmalstieg FC, Anderson DC, Van der Maaten MJ, Hughes BJ, Ackermann MR, Wilhelmsen CL, Brown GB, Stevens MG, Whetstone CA.** Molecular definition of the bovine granulocytopathy syndrome: identification of deficiency of the Mac-1 (CD11b/CD18) glycoprotein. Am J Vet Res 1990;51(11):1826–1836.

108. **Kehrli ME, Shuster DE, Ackermann MR.** Leukocyte adhesion deficiency among Holstein cattle. Cornell Vet 1992;82(2):103–109.

109. **van Garderen E, Muller KE, Wentink GH, van den Ingh TS.** Post-mortem findings in calves suffering from bovine leukocyte adhesion deficiency (BLAD). Vet Q 1994;16(1):24–26.

110. **Kehrli ME, Jesse JR, Goff P, Stevens MG, Boone TC.** Effects of granulocyte colony-stimulating factor administration to periparturient cows on neutrophils and bacterial shedding. J Dairy Sci 1991;74:2448–2458.

111. **Kehrli ME, Cullor JS, Nickerson SC.** Immunobiology of hematopoietic colony- stimulating factors: potential application to disease prevention in the bovine. J Dairy Sci 1991;74:4399–4412.

112. **Cullor JS, Fairley N, Smith WL, Wood SL, Dellinger JD, Inokuma M, Souza LM.** Hemogram changes in lactating dairy cows given human recombinant granulocyte colony-stimulating factor (r-MethuG-CSF). Vet Pathol 1990;27:311.

113. **Cullor JS, Smith W, Fairley N, Wood SL, Dellinger JD, Souza L.** Effects of human recombinant granulocyte colony stimulating factor (HR-GCSF) on the hemogram of lactating dairy cattle. Vet Clin Pathol 1990;19:9–12.

114. **Nickerson SC, Owens WE, Watts JL.** Effects of recombinant granulocyte colony- stimulating factor on Staphylococcus aureus mastitis in lactating dairy cows. J Dairy Sci 1989;72:3286.

115. **van Miert AS, van Duin CT, Wensing T.** Fever and acute phase response induced in dwarf goats by endotoxin and bovine and human recombinant tumor necrosis factor alpha. J Vet Pharmacol Ther 1992;15(4):332–342.

116. **Koot M, van Duin CT, Wensing T, van Miert AS.** Comparative observations of fever and associated clinical, haematological and blood biochemical changes after parenteral administration of poly I: poly C, interferon-alpha 2a and Escherichia coli endotoxin in goats. Vet Q 1989;11(1):41–50.

117. **Reddy DN, Reddy PG, Minocha HC, Fenwick BW, Baker PE, Davis WC, Blecha F.** Adjuvanticity of recombinant bovine interleukin-1 beta: influence on immunity, infection and latency in a bovine herpesvirus-1 infection. Lymphokine Res 1990;9(3):295–307.

118. **Stevenson LM, Jones DG.** Cross-reactivity amongst recombinant haematopoietic cytokines from different species for sheep bone-marrow eosinophils. J Comp Pathol 1994;111(1):99–106.

119. **Eppard PJ, White TC, Sorbet RH, Weiser MG, Cole WJ, Hartnell GF, Hintz RL, Lanza GM, Vincini JL, Collier RJ.** Effect of exogenous somatotropin on hematological variables of lactating cows and their offspring. J Dairy Sci 1997;80:1582–1591.

120. **Woods Pr, Gossett RE, Jain NC, Smith R III, Rappaport ES, Kasari TR.** Acute myelomonocytic leukemia in a calf. J Am Vet Med Assoc 1993; 11(1):1579–1582.

121. **Mackay LJ, Jarrett WFH, Wiseman A.** Monocytic leukemia in a cow. Res Vet Sci 1972;13:287–289.

122. **Muscoplat CC, Johnson DW, Pomeroy KA, Olson JM, Larson VL, Stevens JB, Sorensen DK.** Lymphocyte subpopulations and immunodeficiency in calves with acute lymphocytic leukemia. Am J Vet Res 1974;35(12):1571–1573.

123. **Khan KN, Sagartz JE, Koenig G, Tanaka K.** Systemic mastocytosis in a goat. Vet Pathol 1995;32(6):719–721.

124. **Jackson AR, McInnes A, Falconer IR, Runnegar MT.** Clinical and pathological changes in sheep experimentally poisoned by the blue-green alga Microcystis aeruginosa. Vet Pathol 1984;21(1):102–113.

125. **Main DC, Berry PH, Peet RL, Robertson JP.** Sheep mortalities associated with the blue-green alga Nodularia spumigena. Aust Vet J 1977;53:578–581.

126. **Abbitt B, Murphy MJ, Ray AC, Reagor JC, Eugster AK, Gayle LG, Whitford HW, Sutherland RJ, Fiske RA, Pusok J.** Catastrophic death losses in a dairy herd attributed to type D botulism. J Am Vet Med Assoc 1984; 185(7):798–801.

127. **Evans WC, Evans ETR, Hughes LE.** Studies on bracken poisoning in cattle-part I-III. Br Vet J 1954;110:295–306,365–380,426–444.

128. **Schofield FW.** Agranulocytosis associated with leukopenia in bracken poisoning in cattle. Rep Ont Vet Coll 1947;127.

129. **Moon FE, McKeand JM.** Observations on the vitamin C status and hematology of bracken-fed ruminants. Br Vet J 1953;109:321.

130. **Suttle NF, Jones DG.** Copper and disease resistance in sheep: a rare natural confirmation of interaction between a specific nutrient and infection. Proc Nutr Soc 1986;45:317–325.

131. **Cerone SI, Sansinanea AS, Streitenberger SA, Carcia MC, Auza NJ.** The effect of copper deficiency on the peripheral blood cells of cattle. Vet Res Commun 1998;22:47–57.

132. **Arthington JD, Spell AR, Corah LR, Blecha F.** Effect of molybdenum-induced copper deficiency on in vivo and in vitro measures of neutrophil chemotaxis both before and following an inflammatory stressor. J Anim Sci 1996;74(11):2759–2764.

133. **Crowell WA, Whitlock RH, Stout RC, Tyler DE.** Ethylene glycol toxicosis in cattle. Cornell Vet 1979;69(3):272–279.

134. **Maylin GA, Eckerlin RH, Krook L.** Fluoride intoxication in dairy calves. Cornell Vet 1987;77:84–98.

135. **Hoogstratten B, Leone NC, Shupe JL, Greenwood DA, Lieberman J.** Effects of fluorides on the hematopoietic system, liver and thyroid gland in cattle. JAMA 1965;192:26.

136. **Hillman D, Bolenbaugh DL, Convey EM.** Hypothyroidism and anemia related to fluoride in dairy cattle. J Dairy Sci 1979;62:416–423.

137. **Sheldon IM.** A field case of granulocytopenic disease of calves. Vet Rec 1994;135:408.

138. **Van Vleet JF, Amstutz HE, Weirich WE, Rebar AH, Ferrans VJ.** Clinical, clinicopathologic, and pathologic alterations in acute monensin toxicosis in cattle. Am J Vet Res 1983;44(11):2133–2144.

139. **Anderson TD, Van Alstine WG, Ficken MD, Miskimins DW, Carson TL, Osweiler GD.** Acute monensin toxicosis in sheep: light and electron microscopic changes. Am J Vet Res1984;45(6):1142–1147.

140. **Donev B, Stoianov K, Dzhurov A, Dilov P.** [Acute and subchronic monensin toxicity for lambs] [Bulgarian]. Vet Med Nauki 1980;17(1):17–25.

141. **Friend SCE, Hancock DS, Schiefer HB, Babiuk LA.** Experimental T-2 toxicosis in sheep. Can J Comp Med 1983;47:291–297.

142. **Sharma RP.** Immunotoxicity of mycotoxins. J Dairy Sci 1993;76:892–897.

143. **Coppock RW, Hoffmann WE, Gelberg HB, Bass D, Buck WB.** Hematologic changes induced by intravenous administration of diacetoxyscirpenol in pigs, dogs, and calves. Am J Vet Res 1989;50(3):411–415.

144. **Schneider DJ, Marasas WFO, Dale Kuys JC, Kriek NPJ, Van Schalkwyk GC.** A field outbreak of suspected Stachybotryotoxicosis in sheep. J S Afr Vet Assoc 1979;50(2):73–81.

145. **Tartour G, Adam SEI, Obeid HM, Idriss OF.** Development of anaemia in goats fed with Ipomoea carnea. Br Vet J 1974;130:271–279.

146. **McKenzie RA, Newman RD, Rayner AC, Dunster PJ.** Prickly paddy melon (Cucumis myriocarpus) poisoning of cattle. Aust Vet J 1988; 65:167–170.

147. **Dash PK, Joshi HC.** Clinico-biochemical studies on acute toxic nephropathy in goats due to uranyl nitrate. Vet Hum Toxicol 1989;31(1):5–9.

148. **Ammann VJ, Fecteau G, Helie P, Desnoyer M, Hebert P, Babkine M.** Pancytopenia associated with bone marrow aplasia in a holstein heifer. Can Vet J 1996;37:493–495.

149. **Strafuss AC, Sautter JH.** Clinical and general pathologic finding of aplastic anemia associated with S-(chlorovinyl)-L-cysteine in calves. Am J Vet Res 1967;28:25–37.

150. **Weiss DJ, Miller DC.** Bone marrow necrosis associated with pancytopenia in a cow. Vet Pathol 1985;22:90–92.

151. **Lock EA, Sani Y, Moore RB, Finkelstein MB, Anders MW, Seawright AA.** Bone marrow and renal injury associated with haloalkene cysteine conjugates in calves. Arch Toxicol 1996;70(10):607–619.

152. **Slocombe RF, Malark J, Ingersoll R, Derksen FJ, Robinson NE.** Neutrophil depletion of calves with hydroxyurea: methods and clinical and pathologic effects. Am J Vet Res 1986;47(10):2313–2317.

153. **Heflin AC, Brigham KL.** Prevention by granulocyte depletion of increased vascular permeability of sheep lung following endotoxemia. J Clin Invest 1981;68:1253–1260.

154. **Winn R, Maunder R, Chie E, Harlan J.** Neutrophil depletion does not prevent lung edema after endotoxin infusion in goats. J Appl Physiol 1987;62(1):116–121.

155. **Cain GR, East N, Moore PF.** Myelofibrosis in young pygmy goats. Comp Haematol Int 1994;4:167–172.

CHAPTER 58

Clinical Interpretation of Equine Leukograms

• ELIZABETH G. WELLES

Leukocyte production, blood transit, and tissue use are dynamic processes; therefore, a single blood sample taken for a complete blood count (CBC) is analogous to one frame of a movie or video. Often a specific disease diagnosis is not made, but general information about the disease process, severity, and prognosis can be obtained. Serial leukograms may be helpful in assessing the response to therapy, detecting a change in health status, or documenting the presence of disease.

The leukogram is that portion of the CBC concerning white blood cells (WBCs) or leukocytes. Most leukocytes (neutrophils, monocytes, eosinophils, and basophils) obtained from peripheral blood are in transit from the bone marrow (where they are produced) to the tissues (where they function and die). Lymphocytes are exceptions. Most of the lymphocytes in circulation are long-lived, recirculating cells that spend time in one of the secondary lymphoid organs, periodically enter the peripheral blood, circulate for minutes to hours, and then return to lymphoid organs.

To interpret leukogram data, there must be an appreciation of the production, kinetics, and fate of the various leukocytes, because each cell type is kinetically and functionally independent. However, patterns of combined cellular alterations are observed with specific clinical interpretations.

Leukocyte function, production, and kinetics in horses are similar to those described in other species. Kinetics of equine neutrophils have been studied, and it has been determined that they circulate in the blood for approximately 10.5 hours[1] and that they are equally distributed in two pools designated the circulating and the marginated neutrophil pools.[2]

General Considerations in Equine Leukogram Interpretation

Samples for CBC in horses should be handled with similar care as in other species. Refrigerated equine samples maintain morphologic integrity fairly well for approximately 24 hours.[3] If samples are processed after refrigeration of 48 hours or more, leukocytes may be severely smudged or unidentifiable in the stained blood smear.

If the WBC count is increased, 14,000 to 20,000 leukocytes/μL is considered moderate leukocytosis, 20,000 to 30,000 leukocytes/μL is considered significant leukocytosis, and >30,000 leukocytes/μL is considered extreme leukocytosis.[3] Significant leukocytosis in horses is apparent at lower cell counts than in dogs and cats.

Leukopenia is a significant finding and usually results from neutropenia because neutrophils are the predominant circulating leukocytes in healthy horses. Diseases that cause leukopenia (neutropenia) are generally acute and severe. Neutropenia places the patient at increased risk for secondary bacterial infection.

Reference intervals determined by most laboratories are fairly wide because values from horses of different breeds, ages, and sexes are included. Reference intervals for a specific breed of horse may have a much tighter interval. Differences between sexes are insignificant, but some age-related differences are important (Table 58.1).

Cell Morphology

The expected appearance of equine leukocytes in Romanowsky-stained (Wright, Giemsa, Wright-Giemsa, Diff-Quik, Leukostat, etc) blood smears has been described.[4] Lymphocytes, basophils, and monocytes appear similar to those in other species. Segmented neutrophils have nearly colorless cytoplasm with a jagged, ribbon-shaped nucleus rather than smooth-edged lobules typical of canine neutrophils (Fig. 58.1). Band neutrophils often are slightly larger and have nearly parallel nuclear margins. The cytoplasm is colorless to pale blue. Toxic neutrophils may be enlarged. Toxic changes primarily affect the neutrophil cytoplasm and are caused by exposure to endotoxin or other cellular toxins while neutrophils are developing in the bone marrow. Toxic changes of the cytoplasm include increased basophilia (increased staining of RNA), vacuolation (from burst

TABLE 58.1	**Leukocyte Reference Intervals Established for the Clinical Pathology Laboratory, Auburn University**
Cell Type	Reference Interval (cells/μL)
WBC count	6,000–12,000
Segmented neutrophils	3,000–6,000
Band neutrophils	0–100
Lymphocytes	1,500–5,000
Monocytes	0–600
Eosinophils	0–800
Basophils	rare

Data from Duncan JR, Prasse KW, Mahaffey EA. Veterinary laboratory medicine, clinical pathology. 3rd ed. Ames, IA: Iowa State University Press. 1994; 37–62 and Latimer KS. In: Colaha PT, Mayhew IG, Merritt AM, Moore JN, eds. Equine medicine and surgery. 4th ed. Goleta, CA: American Veterinary Publications, 1991; 1762–1764, with permission.

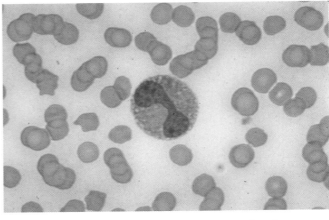

FIGURE 58.2 Toxic neutrophil band with cytoplasmic basophilia and vacuolation.

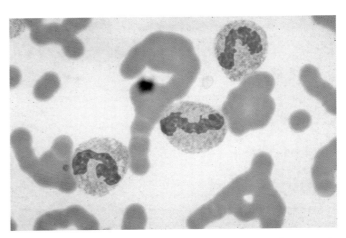

FIGURE 58.3 Segmented and band neutrophils displaying toxic granulation.

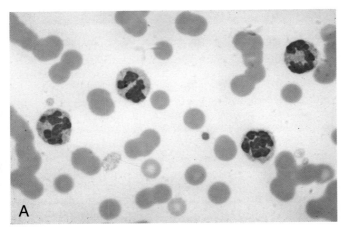

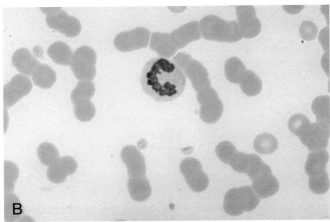

FIGURE 58.1 **A**. Four segmented neutrophils are present that have distinct lobulation. **B**. A single mature neutrophil is present that shows jagged nuclear margins instead of nuclear lobulation.

granules), Döhle bodies (lamellar stacks of rough [granular] endoplasmic reticulum [RER] that appear blue gray), and toxic granulation (primary granules with increased permeability to stains) appear purple (Figs. 58.2 and 58.3). Horses that have *Ehrlichia equi* infection[5] may have neutrophils that contain morulae or mulberrylike inclusions in the cytoplasm (Fig. 58.4). In contrast, inclusions have not been observed in leukocytes from horses infected with *Ehrlichia risticii* (monocytic ehrlichiosis, Potomac horse fever, ehrlichial colitis).[6] Eosinophils are larger than neutrophils and have a lobulated nucleus with less condensed chromatin than neutrophils. Described as raspberrylike, eosinophils contain multiple, large, fairly uniformly sized, round, bright, red-orange granules (Fig. 58.5).

Age-Related Leukogram Changes

At birth, healthy foals have more neutrophils (2.5 times more) than lymphocytes, variable numbers of mono-

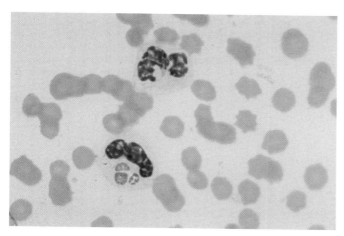

FIGURE 58.4 Morula of *E. equi* in cytoplasm of neutrophil (bottom).

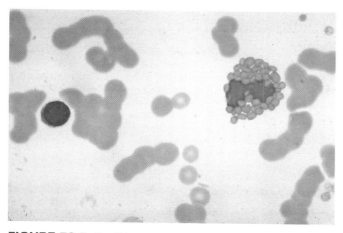

FIGURE 58.5 Small lymphocyte (left) and eosinophil (right).

cytes, and an absence of eosinophils.[3] Absolute neutrophil counts often exceed the reference interval for adult horses for several months, whereas lymphocyte counts are slightly less than the reference interval. By 3 to 4 months of age, these leukocyte values reach adult reference intervals. Eosinophils gradually increase in number over several months, probably in response to intestinal parasite exposure and burden. Premature foals have significantly lower neutrophil counts than term foals for the first several hours of life.[7] Premature foals that survive may have nearly equal neutrophil and lymphocyte counts at birth, with the neutrophil proportion rapidly increasing within the first 18 hours of life. In contrast, the neutrophil-to-lymphocyte ratio does not increase significantly in nonsurviving premature foals. However, these findings may not be evident before 35 hours after birth.

RECOGNITION OF LEUKOGRAM RESPONSE PATTERNS

Although leukocyte types are kinetically independent and respond differently to various stimuli, they collectively demonstrate certain distinct response patterns.

Leukograms Characterized by Leukocytosis

Physiologic Leukocytosis

Physiologic leukocytosis[8] is a transient (20 to 30 minutes) but moderate increase in total leukocyte count, often reaching 12,000 to 25,000 cells/μL. Typically, a modest mature neutrophilia exists in the absence of a left shift or toxic change. Lymphocytosis (6,000 to 14,000 lymphocytes/μL) often is observed[1] and may be proportionately greater than the neutrophil count. In frightful, painful, or exciting conditions or after vigorous exercise or activity, catecholamines increase cardiac output, hydrostatic blood pressure, and muscular activity. Neutrophils subsequently are swept from the marginated pool into the circulating pool, transiently increasing the numbers of cells quantitated by the WBC count. The causes of lymphocytosis are not as well documented; however, muscular activity may force cells in lymphatics into circulation, whereas catecholamines may alter receptors on postcapillary venular endothelial cells and lymphocytes, blocking normal lymphocyte recirculating patterns.[1] Horses have a marginated pool of neutrophils at least as large as the circulating pool; therefore, total cell counts may double with excitement. Physiologic leukocytosis is observed somewhat commonly in horses because they are easily excited, especially young hotblooded horses and most horses that are minimally handled.

Stress and Corticosteroid Effects

Stress and corticosteroid leukograms are characterized by a moderate neutrophilia, usually no left shift, lymphopenia, eosinopenia, and variable monocyte counts.[1,9,10] This response is mediated by glucocorticoids of either endogenous or exogenous origin. Neutrophilia is caused predominately by early release of neutrophils from the bone marrow storage pool and to a lesser extent by decreased margination and emigration from the blood, causing neutrophils to circulate longer. Sometimes hypersegmented neutrophils are observed on the blood smear. These cells have five or more nuclear lobes and represent older cells that have remained within the vasculature longer than normally expected. Lymphopenia is caused by temporary sequestration of cells in lymphoid tissues, whereas eosinopenia is caused by temporary sequestration of cells in the bone marrow. Lymphocytes and eosinophils generally are not killed at the concentrations of glucocorticoids obtained physiologically or achieved through most therapeutic uses of corticosteroids in horses. This response pattern may be seen in horses secondary to endogenous corticosteroid release in acute and severe diseases, pituitary adenoma, or after administration of exogenous corticosteroids.

Inflammation-Infection-Associated Effects

Inflammatory changes in the leukogram have variable appearances, depending on the severity and duration of the inciting agent, lesion, or condition.[1,11] The hallmark of inflammation is a left shift, which is the presence of immature neutrophils in circulation. Typically, these are band neutrophils, but less mature precursors also may be present. A significant left shift is present if there are >300 bands/μL, and the total WBC is within or greater than the reference interval.[1] In the presence of neutropenia (leukopenia), a significant left shift exists if bands comprise at least 10% of the neutrophil population. The extent of the left shift can be used as a prognostic indicator. If the number of immature neutrophils exceeds the number of mature segmented neutrophils, a degenerative left shift exists, and a guarded prognosis is issued. The presence of toxic changes in neutrophils along with neutropenia and a degenerative left shift indicate a poor prognosis. Immature neutrophils and neutrophils demonstrating toxic changes have decreased functional ability[12] compared with mature neutrophils. Therefore, toxic bands or metamyelocytes may have significantly decreased functional capabilities compared with mature segmented neutrophils.

Toxic changes are graded on a subjective scale from +1 to +4 in most laboratories; the greater the number, the more severe the toxic change. If the source of the toxin is removed, the cytologic alterations resolve within 12 to 24 hours. The decrease or disappearance of toxic changes in neutrophils and an increasing neutrophil count are favorable prognostic signs.[4]

Leukograms indicative of acute inflammation usually have a significant left shift with or without toxic changes in the neutrophils. Established or chronic inflammation may be more difficult to recognize. Typically, leukocytosis is accompanied by mature neutrophilia because increased granulopoiesis over sufficient time (at least a week or more) has replenished the bone marrow storage pool such that only mature neutrophils are released into circulation. Additional information may be helpful for leukogram interpretation, including physical examination, history, previous leukogram data, and plasma protein-to-fibrinogen ratio. Fibrinogen is produced in large quantities by hepatocytes as an acute-phase reactant protein. Comparison of fibrinogen to plasma protein values allows adjustment for alterations that are present because of dehydration and hemoconcentration. A plasma protein-to-fibrinogen ratio of <10 is indicative of inflammation.[1] This ratio has usefulness in diagnosis of acute inflammation, especially in the absence of a left shift.

Eosinophilia

Eosinophilia is uncommon in horses and may be subtle when present. It usually is related to parasite or allergen exposure[13]; however, some horses that have heavy intestinal parasite burdens have normal to low eosinophil counts.[3] This may be related to the stress of disease (endogenous corticosteroid release). Horses may have significant tissue infiltration by eosinophils without a concurrent eosinophilia because of the short blood transit time and long life span of eosinophils within tissues.[14] Cutaneous eosinophilic granulomas, either idiopathic

or associated with parasite infection, may be accompanied by eosinophilia. Hypereosinophilic syndromes involving the gastrointestinal tract and pancreas or multiple organs have been reported intermittently in horses.[15] Cases of lymphoid leukemia or lymphosarcoma[16] in horses have been reported with a concurrent hypereosinophilic syndrome. Such observations are similar to paraneoplastic syndromes in human patients in whom production of interleukin (IL)-5 by neoplastic T lymphocytes causes selective differentiation and activation of eosinophils.

Lymphocytosis

Lymphocytosis is a component of physiologic leukocytosis. Infrequently, lymphocytosis may be observed after antigenic exposure or with lymphoid neoplasia.

Leukemias

Hematopoietic neoplasia that originates in the bone marrow is called leukemia. Leukemias are rare in horses, but lymphocytic,[4] granulocytic,[17] monocytic,[18] eosinophilic,[19] and myelomonocytic[20] leukemias have been reported. Lymphocytic leukemia is the most common presentation of leukemia in horses, followed by myelomonocytic leukemia. Total and differential leukocyte counts of the affected cell line(s) can be less than, within, or, in most cases, greater than reference intervals. Abnormal or immature cells (blast cells) are often observed in stained blood smears. A preponderance of these cells is apparent in Romanowsky-stained bone marrow smears and aspirates or biopsies of other tissues and organs. Lymphoid leukemia has been reported as a primary disorder[21]; however, a leukemic blood picture also may be apparent with lymphosarcoma.[22,23] The leukocyte and lymphocyte counts may be within the reference interval, but abnormal cells (30 to 50%) may be observed on the stained blood smear.[24] Chronic lymphocytic leukemia has been diagnosed in two aged horses, one was a T-cell variant and the other was a B-cell variant with a monoclonal gammopathy (gamma G immunoglobulin [IgG]) and light-chain proteinuria.[25]

Leukograms Characterized by Cytopenias

Lymphopenia

Lymphopenia is a predictable component of the stress-corticosteroid-associated leukogram pattern. In addition, lymphopenia may be observed with acute, severe inflammatory disorders and infections. In such conditions, endogenous corticosteroid release may be facilitated. Furthermore, antigen-induced sequestration and trapping of cells in lymphoid tissues and organs occurs in response to infectious agents. In horses, lymphopenia is rarely caused by loss of lymphocyte-rich lymph into the thorax. Chylothorax has rarely been diagnosed (J. Schumacher, 1997, personal communication) in horses, but it has not been associated with lymphopenia. Combined immunodeficiency in Arabian and Arabian-cross

TABLE 58.2	Serial Inflammatory Leukogram Findings and Their Interpretation	
Leukogram Finding	Favorable Prognostic Sign	Unfavorable Prognostic Sign

Neutropenia	Increase in absolute neutrophil count	Continued neutropenia
		  Development of greater left shift
		  Development of toxic changes

Degenerative left shift	Increase in segmented neutrophils Decrease or lack of band neutrophils	Continued degenerative left shift
Toxic changes	Resolution of toxic changes	Continued toxic changes
Concurrent lymphopenia	Increase in absolute lymphocyte count	Continued lymphopenia

foals is characterized by severe lymphopenia (<1000/ μL) and lack of gamma M immunoglobulin (IgM) production.[26,27] A deficiency of both T and B cells exists. Hypoplasia of lymph nodes may be apparent in biopsy specimens. Alternatively, the presence of hypoplasia in other lymphoid tissues and organs can be documented more extensively during postmortem examination.

Monocytopenia and Basopenia

Monocytopenia, if present, is not clinically significant. Eosinopenia may be part of the stress and corticosteroid leukogram. Basopenia is not clinically significant, if recognized at all.

Neutropenia

Neutropenia has significant clinical significance because it predisposes the patient to infection. Three major mechanisms result in neutropenia. First, lack or ineffective production of neutrophils may occur rarely. A group of eight related young standardbred horses that had significant neutropenia and intermittent thrombocytopenia have been reported.[28] Bone marrow cultures from these horses revealed that myeloid precursor cells were present and capable of responding to growth factors. Therefore, the investigators concluded that the cytopenias were caused by a familial bone marrow microenvironmental or a growth factor defect. Seven of the eight horses either died or were euthanized. Defective neutrophil production also has been associated with myelophthisis with crowding of the marrow space by neoplastic cells (e.g., lymphosarcoma).[29] Second, neutrophils may be rapidly redistributed from the circulating to the marginated pool after endotoxin exposure.[30] This causes an upregulation of cell adhesion molecules[31] on both neutrophils and endothelial cells. As neutrophils enter the marginated cell pool, they cannot be quantitated by the WBC count. If endotoxin exposure is terminated, a rebound neutrophilia occurs within 24 hours. However, if exposure is continued, then the mechanism of neutropenia is likely redistribution and increased peripheral usage of cells. Third, increased peripheral usage or reduced survival of neutrophils may occur. This is the most common cause of neutropenia. Tissue demand for neutrophils exceeds the bone marrow's capacity to supply them. The transit time from bone marrow release to migration into tissues is usually shortened. Once in

the tissues, the neutrophils encounter a hostile environment, resulting in a shortened life span. Horses have approximately a 5-day supply of mature neutrophils in the bone marrow storage compartment in health,[1] but this reserve can be rapidly depleted by demands of acute, severe infectious disease. Continued neutropenia with a left shift and toxic changes over several days in the face of appropriate therapy warrants a poor to grave prognosis.

Leukograms observed in foals or adult horses that have suspected septicemia or endotoxemia can have a variable appearance and must be interpreted in conjunction with other information collected from the patient. A moderate to significant leukopenia with left shift and toxic change are leukogram findings highly consistent with septicemia or endotoxemia and are observed in most cases.[32,33] Even with adequate passive transfer, most neonatal foals that have severe disease have leukopenia, neutropenia, and significant left shift with toxic changes in the neutrophils within 24 hours after admission to the hospital.[34]

Benefit of Serial Leukograms

Performance and interpretation of leukograms for 2 or more days are valuable in determining the response to therapy, clinical prognosis, or confirmation of a diagnosis.[1,4,32] Favorable and unfavorable prognostic signs related to data derived from serial leukograms are presented in Table 58.2.

REFERENCES

1. **Carakostas MC, Moore WE, Smith JE.** Intravascular neutrophilic granulocyte kinetics in horses. Am J Vet Res 1981;42:623–625.
2. **Duncan JR, Prasse KW, Mahaffey EA.** Veterinary laboratory medicine, clinical pathology. 3rd ed. Ames, IA: Iowa State University Press, 1994;37–62.
3. **Jain NC,** ed. Schalm's veterinary hematology. 4th ed. Philadelphia: Lea & Febiger, 1986;140–177.
4. **Latimer KS.** In: Colaha PT, Mayhew IG, Merritt AM, Moore JN, eds. Equine medicine and surgery. 4th ed. Goleta, CA: American Veterinary Publications, 1991;1762–1764.
5. **Madigan JE, Gribble D.** Equine ehrlichiosis in northern California: 49 cases (1968–1981). J Am Vet Med Assoc 1987;190:445–448.
6. **Ziemer EL, Whitlock RH, Palmer JE, Spencer PA.** Clinical and hematologic variables in ponies with experimentally induced equine ehrlichial colitis (Potomac horse fever). Am J Vet Res 1987;48:63–67.
7. **Chavatte P, Brown G, Ousey JC, Silver M, Cottrill C, Fowden AL, McGladdery AJ, Rossdale PD.** Studies of bone marrow and leucocyte counts in peripheral blood of fetal and newborn foals. J Reprod Fertil Suppl 1991;44:603–608.
8. **Schalm OW, Hughes JP.** Some observations on physiologic leukocytosis in the cat and horse. Calif Vet 1964;18:23–25.
9. **Carakostas MC, Moore WE, Smith JE, Johnson D.** Effects of etiocholanolone

and prednisolone on intravascular granulocyte kinetics in horses. Am J Vet Res 1981;42:626–628.

10. **Osbaldiston GW, Johnson JH**. Effect of ACTH and selected glucorticoids on circulating blood cells in horses. J Am Vet Med Assoc 1972;161:53–56.

11. **Schalm OW**. Leukocyte responses to disease in various domestic animals. J Am Vet Med Assoc 1962;140:557–589.

12. **Silva ID, Jain NC, George LW**. Phagocytic and nitroblue tetrazolium reductive properties of mature and immature neutrophils and eosinophils from blood and bone marrow of cows. Am J Vet Res 1989;50:778–781.

13. **McCraw BM, Slocombe JO**. Strongylus equinus: development and pathological effects in the equine host. Can J Comp Med 1985; 49:372–383.

14. **Pass DA, Bolton JR**. Chronic eosinophilic gastroenteritis in the horse. Vet Pathol 1982;19:486–496.

15. **Latimer KS, Bounous DI, Collatos C, Carmichael KP, Howerth EW**. Extreme eosinophilia with disseminated eosinophilic granulomatous disease in a horse. Vet Clin Pathol 1996;25:23–26.

16. **LaPerle KM, Piercy RJ, Long JF, Blomme EA**. Multisystemic, eosinophilic, epitheliotropic disease with intestinal lymphosarcoma in a horse. Vet Pathol 1998;35:144–146.

17. **Search GP, Orr JP**. Chronic granulocytic leukemia in a horse. Can Vet J 1981;22:148–151.

18. **Burkhardt E, v Saldern F, Huskamp B**. Monocytic leukemia in a horse. Vet Pathol 1984;21:394–398.

19. **Morris DD, Bloom JC, Roby KAW, Woods K, Tablin F**. Eosinophilic myeloproliferative disorder in a horse. J Am Vet Med Assoc 1984;185:993–996.

20. **Mori T, Ishida T, Washizu T, Yamagami T, Umeda M, Sugiyama M, Motoyoshi S**. Acute myelomonocytic leukemia in a horse. Vet Pathol 1991;28:344–346.

21. **Bernard WV, Sweeny CR, Morris F**. Primary lymphocytic leukemia in a horse. Equine Pract 1988;10;(10):24–30.

22. **Madewell BR, Carlson GP, MacLachlan NJ, Feldman BF**. Lymphosarcoma with leukemia in a horse. AM J Vet Res 1982;43:807–812.

23. **Platt H**. Alimentary lymphomas in the horse. J Comp Pathol 1987;97:1–10.

24. **Van Den Hoven R, Franken P**. Clinical aspects of lymphosarcoma in the horse. Equine Vet J 1983;15:49–53.

25. **Dascanio JJ, Zhang CH, Antczak DF, Blue JT, Simmons TR**. Differentiation of chronic lymphocytic leukemia in the horse. A report of two cases. J Vet Intern Med 1992;6:225–229.

26. **Riggs MW**. Evaluation of foals for immune deficiency disorders. Vet Clin North Am 1987;3:515–528.

27. **Lew AM, Hosking CS. Studdert MJ**. Immunologic aspects of combined immunodeficiency disease in Arabian Foals. Am J Vet Res 1980;41:1161–1166.

28. **Kohn CW, Swardson C, Provost P, Gilbert RO, Couto CG**. Myeloid and megakaryocytic hypoplasia in related standardbreds. J Vet Intern Med 1995;9:315–323.

29. **Morris DD**. Diseases of the hemolymphatic system In: Colahan PT, Mayhew IG, Merritt AM, Moore JN, eds. Equine medicine and surgery. Goleta, CA: American Veterinary Publishers, 1991;1573–1857.

30. **Ewert KM, Fessler JF, Templeton CB, Bottoms GD, Latshaw HS, Johnson MA**. Endotoxin-induced hematologic and blood chemical changes in ponies: effects of flunixin meglumine, dexamethasone, and prednisolone. Am J Vet Res 1985;46:24–30.

31. **Yong K, Khwaja A**. Leucocyte cellular adhesion molecules. Blood Rev 1990;4:211–225.

32. **Knottenbelt DC**. Rhodococcus equi infection in foals: a report of an outbreak on a thoroughbred stud in Zimbabwe. Vet Rec 1993;132:79–85.

33. **Moore JN, Morris DD**. Endotoxemia and septicemia in horses: experimental and clinical correlates. J Am Vet Med Assoc 1992;200:1903–1914.

34. **East LM, Savage CJ, Traub-Dargatz JL, Dickinson CE, Ellis RP**. Enterocolitis associated with Clostridium perfringens infection in neonatal foals: 54 cases (1988–1997). J Am Vet Med Assoc 1998;212:1751–1756.

CHAPTER 59

Interpretation of Porcine Leukocyte Responses

• ELLEN W. EVANS

The literature regarding leukocytes in pigs has primarily addressed leukograms of normal pigs of different breeds, ages, and stages of life. Little has been published concerning porcine leukograms during disease states. This chapter is a review of the existing literature that addresses normal porcine leukocyte counts and differentials at various ages and physiologic states of pigs, as well as influences of stressful situations and a few disease states.

General reference intervals for pigs are presented in Table 59.1. The development of reference intervals for pigs poses some challenges. Overall differences in breeds, including miniature and standard swine, are minor,[1] but considerable variation exists between normal individuals and for a given individual on different days or at different time points.[2-7] Pigs are notoriously excitable and unused to handling[8] and can develop physiologic leukocytosis or stress leukograms readily. Age, sex, season, circadian rhythm, physiologic state, environmental conditions, social interactions, and feeding impose significant influences on the swine leukogram (Table 59.2).[2,3,9-14] For these reasons, reference ranges in field conditions tend to be wide, and values seen in disease states often overlap with those seen in normal animals, complicating interpretation.[2,9,15,16] Researchers are well advised to include control animals in all studies and to keep environmental conditions and sampling times, particularly in relation to feeding, uniform. They also are encouraged to develop reference intervals specific to their subjects' age groups, sex, and husbandry. Samples should be obtained with minimal restraint, and animals sampled should be accustomed to handling.

BLOOD AND BONE MARROW COLLECTION

Limitations of blood collection procedures are discussed by Friendship and Henry.[7] Sites that have been recommended for single samples include the jugular, ear, and cephalic veins, tail vessels, orbital sinus, heart, and ante-rior vena cava[8,14,17]; good descriptions of various venipuncture and restraint techniques are provided by Straw and Meuten.[8] Repeated sampling can be accomplished with a catheter placed in one of several sites.[14]

Bone marrow can be obtained from the medial or lateral tibial tuberosity of piglets or small pigs, and from the sternum of older or larger pigs. Another recommended site is the wing of the ilium.[17] Myeloid-to-erythroid (M:E) ratios vary from 1.0 to 3.0, and lymphocytes make up 4.2 to 30% of cells counted, with plasma cells representing fewer than 0.8% of cells in normal porcine marrow.[9] As in other species, marrow cellularity is highest and fat is lowest in the newborn, with the proportions of cellularity and fat cells reversing as the pig ages.[17]

The morphology of porcine white blood cells (WBC) is similar to that of other species. Therefore, identification of cell types should be straightforward to the experienced hematologist. Note that a wide range of lymphocyte sizes (5 to 18 μm in diameter) is seen in normal pigs,[6,9,18] but the majority are small (5 to 7 μm in diameter) or medium.[9,18]

INFLUENCE OF AGE

WBCs are first seen, in some individuals, at 35 to 40 days postconception, after which time the WBC count gradually increases. By day 45, most fetuses have both lymphocytes and myeloid cells in peripheral blood.[19] Average WBC counts increased from approximately 1400/μL at 51 days to approximately 4200 to 6000/μL at term in one study.[20] Brooks and Davis[21] found WBC counts of 4100 to 5500/μL 16 days before birth, with the number increasing to 9000/μL at birth. Other researchers also found higher term WBC counts in the range 8,000 to 26,000/μL,[4,19,22-24] than did Waddill and colleagues.[20] Clearly, considerable variability occurs in newborn WBC counts.[24,25]

During most of the gestational period, which averages 114 days,[26] the leukocytes of the fetus are predominantly lymphocytes. Between gestation days 110 and 112, Upcott et al[19] found a drastic reversal of the neutrophil-to-lymphocyte (N:L) ratio so that neutrophils predominated at birth, although Brooks and Davis[21] did not see a reversal in the ratio even at 6 days after birth. Most studies have demonstrated that the typical percentage of neutrophils at birth is approximately 60 to 85%.[18–20,25] Immature neutrophils may be seen in large numbers at birth and during the weeks immediately after birth.[19] Unlike lymphocytes, granulocytes are considered fully functional at birth.[27]

Shortly after birth, peripheral blood neutrophils begin to decrease, and, to a lesser extent, lymphocytes increase, resulting in a decrease in WBC count and a shift in the percentages of neutrophils and lymphocytes. As a result, lymphocytes predominate by the age of 1 to 2 weeks and essentially remain the predominant cell type in health.[3,4,9,24,25,28] There is great variability in the time at which the shift in N:L ratio occurs.[28]

Eosinophil numbers are lowest at birth and begin to increase as early as day 2 of life or as late as week 4 after birth.[13,18,29,30] In general, eosinophils contribute little to the total WBC count in normal pigs, regardless of age.[4] Monocyte numbers fluctuate and researchers are not in agreement as to when numbers are highest and lowest in healthy growing piglets, but generally numbers contribute little (<10%) to the total WBC count. Basophil numbers remain low at all ages.[9,18,19]

For the first 2 weeks after birth, the WBC count decreases; at 2 to 3 weeks of age, the WBC count begins to increase, largely because of increases in the number of lymphocytes.[27,29,31] As the number of lymphocytes increases, the proportion of functionally mature lymphocytes also increases, so that by 3 to 4 weeks of age, lymphocyte maturity, subset proportions, and function are similar to those of adults.[27]

At the age of 2 to 7 months, average total WBC counts have increased to a range of 13,300 to 22,000/μL.[4,18,30,32] WBC counts are higher in 8- to 16-week-old pigs than in older pigs.[4] Although monocyte and eosinophil counts are higher at points during this age range than at younger ages,[30] the major influence on the WBC count is still the lymphocyte count. Within the time period of 9 to 15 weeks of age, one or two peaks occur in lymphocyte counts,[4,18,31] and higher lymphocyte counts have been

TABLE 59.1	Reference Intervals for Cross-bred Pigs (Predominantly Gilts and Sows) Ranging in Age From 6-weeks-old to Mature Adults ($n = 114$).

Parameter	Interval
WBC $\times$ 10^3/μL	6.0–32.5
Neutrophilic segmenters $\times$ 10^3/μL	1.2–25.7
Neutrophilic bands 10^3/μL	0
Lymphocytes $\times$ 10^3/μL	1.0–22.8
Monocytes $\times$ 10^3/μL	0–3.9
Eosinophils $\times$ 10^3/μL	0–5.2
Basophils $\times$ 10^3/μL	0

Intervals were established by range test (66). Courtesy of Dr. Frances M. Moore, Marshfield Laboratories, Veterinary Division, Marshfield, WI.

TABLE 59.2	Influence of Age and Husbandry on the Leukograms of Young Duroc-Jersey Pigs.*

Age (days)	Value	WBC ($\times$10^3/μL)	Differential Leukocyte Count					
			Neutrophil %	Band %	Lymphocyte %	Monocyte %	Eosinophil %	Basophil %
1	Min.	7.6	64.5	1.0	16.0	0.5	0	0
	Max.	15.3	75.5	7.0	31.0	7.5	2.0	1.0
	Av.	11.5	71	3.6	20	4.7	0.9	0.2
3	Min.	6.3	38.0	1.0	23.5	6.0	0	0
	Max.	13.4	61.5	5.5	54.0	9.5	1.5	0
	Av.	9.4	51	3.3	37.6	6.8	0.8	0
6	Min.	7.4	33.0	1.0	32.5	2.0	0	0
	Max.	10.5	60.5	3.3	55	10.5	1.0	0
	Av.	8.2	45.4	2	45.3	4.9	0.3	0
10	Min.	5.6	8.0	0	36.5	1.0	0	0
	Max.	19.1	51.0	2.0	82.0	10.0	0.5	0.5
	Av.	10.9	27	1	64	7	0.1	0.05
20	Min.	6.2	13.5	0	55.0	2.0	0	0
	Max.	10.5	39.5	3.5	82.0	7.0	2.0	0.5
	Av.	7.7	25.7	1.4	66.8	4.3	0.8	0.05
36	Min.	12.7	28.0	0	40.0	3.0	3.5	0
	Max.	20.9	43.0	5.0	68.0	10.5	14.0	1.5
	Av.	16.3	33	1.8	52	6	7	0.5

*Modified from Jain's *Essentials of Veterinary Hematology*.
Ranges and means for a single litter of five males and four females; pigs kept on concrete until 10 days of age and then placed on soil.[1]

observed at 12 weeks than at 24 weeks.[33,34] McTaggart[31] reported a mean peak height of approximately 16,000 lymphocytes/μL and individual peak counts that approached 30,000/μL. Caution is advised in interpreting WBC and lymphocyte counts during the peak period, because this normal increase in lymphocyte counts may be mistaken for the lymphocytosis that occurs in lymphosarcoma of young pigs. There should be a difference in morphology; in the normal young pig, only occasional lymphoblasts are seen, but with lymphosarcoma, poorly differentiated lymphocytes are encountered frequently in peripheral blood.[31]

By 8 to 9 months of age, WBC counts are lower than at 8 to 16 weeks.[4] The average mean WBC counts show little age dependency after maturity is reached at 10 months,[35] with average counts ranging from 11,000 to 16,000 cells/μL in pigs older than 1 year of age.[4,18,35]

Summary of Age-Related Effects

In general, the developing pig fetus has myeloid cells and lymphocytes by the day 45 after conception. The predominant cell type in peripheral blood during fetal development is the lymphocyte, but near the end of gestation a reversal occurs so that most piglets are born with a predominantly neutrophilic leukogram. WBC counts are high at birth, decrease over 2 weeks, and then begin to increase at 2 to 3 weeks of age. By week 2 of life, a N:L reversal occurs, resulting in a predominantly lymphocytic leukogram that essentially remains throughout life. The WBC count increases for most pigs between the ages of 8 and 16 weeks, primarily because of an increase in lymphocytes; but by 8 to 9 months of age the WBC counts are similar to those of adults. Fluctuations in the proportions of neutrophils and lymphocytes occur at various stages of life.

INFLUENCE OF PHYSIOLOGIC STATE

Feeding

At variable times after feeding, from immediately to 5 hours later, pig WBC counts increase dramatically.[2,4,5,36,37] The increased WBC count is caused by approximately a 12 to 50% increase in mature neutrophil numbers and percentages in peripheral blood, and typically the N:L ratio increases.[3,9] Lymphocytes may increase, may decrease, or may be unchanged,[3,4,36] but generally remain the predominant leukocyte.[4] By 12 hours, the leukogram should be similar to the prefeeding leukogram.[3]

Estrus, Gestation, Parturition, and Lactation

At days 14 and 19 of estrus, the time of luteolysis, sows have significantly higher WBC counts than on day 2. By day 21, values are less than day 2 values.[38]

During most of gestation, the sow's WBC count remains essentially the same; however, mean lymphocyte and eosinophil numbers increase, and neutrophil and monocyte numbers decrease, compared with estrus.[39] Then, during the last trimester and particularly at parturition, increases in neutrophil numbers, with or without nonsegmented neutrophils, and decreases in lymphocytes, with or without eosinopenia, occur.[3,39-43] The shift of N:L ratio can occur from as early as 3 weeks prepartum[39] to as late as after farrowing has begun, but usually occurs 6 to 30 hours prepartum.[40] The normal sow's nongestational ratio of neutrophils and lymphocytes is restored within 1 to 8 days postpartum,[40] and mild eosinophilia may be seen at 48 to 72 hours after parturition.[43] The increases in neutrophils and decreases in lymphocytes or eosinophils are typical of a stress leukogram mediated by increased plasma corticosteroid concentrations. Increased plasma cortisol concentrations have been demonstrated around parturition in sows.[43] During lactation, a physiologic leukocytosis, caused by lymphocytosis with or without neutrophilia, may occur.[9,37,42]

INFLUENCES OF SEX, BREED, AND HUSBANDRY

Differences Owing to Sex

In general, because of higher neutrophil counts, male swine have higher WBC counts than do female swine.[12,35,44] One researcher found that neonatal males have higher WBC counts than neonatal females,[20] whereas in another study the mean WBC count of males and females was equal until maturity, at which time boars averaged 2000 cells/μL higher than gilts.[35] In the latter study, eosinophil counts spiked in females (female mean of 13,500 cells/μL versus male mean of 306 cells/μL) at the age of 3 months, corresponding with the beginning of puberty. After that time, the mean eosinophil count in females was only slightly higher than that of males. At intervals from 6 to 36 months, male eosinophil counts generally remained in the 300s to the low 600s/μL, whereas female eosinophil counts were in the 500s and 600s/μL.[35]

Differences Owing to Breed

In the few studies that have been undertaken to address differences in leukograms between different breeds, only minor differences have been seen. Although the ranges of individual values overlapped, German Country Pigs (Landschweine) had consistently lower WBC counts (by 3000 to 4000 cells/μL) than Hanford miniature pigs at 2 to 6 months of age.[32] Purebred Yorkshire pigs had higher WBC counts (mean of approximately 6000 cells/μL) than did cross-bred pigs (mean of approximately 4000 cells/μL) at birth,[20] and Landrace and Poland Chinas had higher WBC counts than Durocs and Hampshires.[20] Morgan et al[45] compared Duroc and Hampshire piglets and found that WBC counts were similar, but relative numbers of neutrophils and lymphocytes varied.

Miniature pig leukograms have been found to be similar to domestic pigs in cell numbers and subset proportions, influences of husbandry, age, sex, and disease.[13,34,35,46]

Differences Owing to Husbandry

Not surprisingly, germ-free, microbiologically defined, and specific pathogen-free miniature piglets of three different breeds had fewer leukocytes and a lower percentage of neutrophils and monocytes than did their conventional counterparts.[13,34,46] White blood counts for germ-free Minnesota mini piglets stayed the same from birth to the age of 8 weeks, whereas conventional piglets of the same breed doubled their WBC counts during the same period.[46]

Large White pigs in Nigeria had lower WBC counts and higher eosinophil counts when raised under substandard local husbandry conditions than did pigs raised under improved husbandry, in concrete pens that were cleaned daily.[30] These differences corresponded to differences in incidence of husbandry-related diseases such as dermatitis, ectoparasites, and gastrointestinal parasites.[30] Conversely, in a German study, pigs kept in balance pens had 25% fewer leukocytes than pigs kept in typical farm conditions.[5] Typical local farm conditions, however, may have been different between Nigeria and Germany.

PHYSIOLOGIC LEUKOCYTOSIS

As in other species, experimental epinephrine administration or endogenous epinephrine release because of restraint, excitement, weaning, or sudden change in environment or diet, typically causes a transient, mild increase in WBC count, usually characterized by a mature neutrophilia or lymphocytosis.[36,47] In pigs, neutrophilia is typical, but there may or may not be an accompanying lymphocytosis.[16,12] Increased eosinophils and monocytes are seen occasionally.[16]

To reduce restraint and handling effects, research pigs that are frequently bled should be accustomed to handling and ideally should be catheterized for optimal sample collection.[36]

INFLUENCE OF STRESS

Circumstances that stimulate a stress response in pigs include shipping, exercise, handling, changes in body or ambient temperature, pain, surgery, trauma, and parturition.[3,6,15,16,39,48–50] Leukograms in response to stress (corticosteroid mediated) in pigs are similar to stress leukograms in other species in that lymphocytes and eosinophils typically decrease and neutrophils increase in number and percentage,[15,16,50,51] often resulting in a reversal of the N:L ratio. Indeed, in one study of pigs, the increase in neutrophil counts caused by shipping correlated with increases in plasma cortisol concentra-

tion.[50] However, because of the wide reference intervals in normal pigs, stress leukograms may go unappreciated in individual pigs.[15,16] Unlike dogs, pigs do not typically have a monocytosis as part of their stress leukogram.

The changes seen in porcine leukograms because of stressful conditions can be reproduced with administration of exogenous corticosteroids or adrenal corticotrophic hormone (ACTH) within as little as 2 to 6 hours,[3,12,29,48,52,53] although some studies with ACTH or corticosteroids have not been able to reproduce the phenomenon[54] or have only reproduced the lymphocyte changes.[53]

Eosinophils deserve special mention, because their measurement has historically been used as a crude assessment of adrenal function. They usually decrease [12,29] under the influence of corticosteroids, and their numbers have been shown to be negatively proportional to 17-hydroxycorticosteroid levels.[29] Adrenalectomy results in an increase in eosinophils. However, one study found an increase in eosinophils with ACTH administration,[48] and eosinophilia owing to other causes may mask a stress-induced eosinopenia.

Peak effects with corticosteroid or ACTH administration occur at variable times and may be different for different leukocyte types.[48] There may also be drastic fluctuations over time.[48]

Stress-susceptible pigs have lower WBC and lymphocyte counts prestress than do stress-resistant pigs. However, by 60 or 120 minutes poststress, WBC and neutrophil counts are higher and lymphocyte and eosinophil counts are lower for stress-susceptible pigs than for stress-resistant pigs, suggesting a greater production and more rapid use of corticosteroids by stress-susceptible pigs.[51]

INFLUENCE OF DISEASE

Responses of leukocytes to disease have not been well documented for pigs. For this reason and because porcine leukocyte reference intervals are broad, interpretation of leukograms in evaluating disease states is limited. Measurement of plasma fibrinogen may be a more useful tool in diagnosing inflammation.

In general, the leukocyte behavior of swine is similar to that of other species. Typical leukocyte responses seen in a limited number of disease states are discussed in this section. Bacterial infections cause inflammatory responses of increased WBC with a neutrophilia, typically with a left shift, and lymphocytes decrease, likely owing to a stress component. Acute infections resulting in intense tissue demand for neutrophils or bacterial endotoxin may produce a leukopenia and neutropenia. Degenerative left shifts are common in porcine WBC counts of less than 10,000 cells/μL.[26] Viral infections typically cause a decrease in WBC counts, largely owing to lymphopenia, and parasitic infections may or may not present with an eosinophilia depending on the degree of tissue invasion or hypersensitivity.

Bacterial Infections

Endotoxin injection causes a significant decrease in circulating granulocytes within 30 minutes in pigs. The major cause of this decrease is sequestration of neutrophils within the lungs.[55]

Shortly after parturition, leukopenia, caused by neutropenia or lymphopenia, caused by *Escherichia coli, Klebsiella pneumoniae,* or *Proteus* sp. occurs in sow agalactia or mastitis. [56,57] The neutropenia is likely bacterial endotoxin-induced, and lymphopenia is likely a stress response. Endotoxin has been shown to stimulate cortisol secretion in pigs.[57]

Acute salmonellosis or erysipelas infection usually is accompanied by a leukocytosis.[9] Eosinophilia (>2,000 eosinophils/μL) has occurred in septicemia caused by *Erysipelothrix rhusiopathiae.*[26]

Viral Diseases

Acute hog cholera (HC) is generally accompanied by a leukopenia, caused by neutropenia and eosinopenia, by days 2 to 6, which correlates with increased body temperature. Leukopenia may be intermittent until death.[58,59] Secondary pneumonia or the presence of parasites may mask the neutropenia (granulocytopenia) usually seen with HC virus.[9] In chronic HC, leukopenia may not occur for 10 days after infection,[58] but it is then a consistent finding until the terminal phase, when leukocytosis may occur.[59] Leukopenia may be the only sign of subclinical HC produced by strains of low virulence.[59] Vaccination for HC also may decrease the WBC count, with a return to normal within 9 to 14 days.[58]

Decreases in WBC count have been associated with several other viral diseases of pigs. Bovine viral diarrhea (BVD) virus in pigs,[60] swine influenza,[61] or porcine parvovirus[62] may present with leukopenia. Transmissible gastroenteritis virus in pigs may produce a moderate leukopenia in the acute phase, followed by leukocytosis in convalescence.[63]

In most cases, African swine fever causes a decrease in WBC (approximately 50%) owing to lymphopenia. An increase of immature neutrophils in peripheral blood is generally seen.[64]

Parasites

Pigs may develop eosinophilia within 6 to 10 days after infection with *Ascaris* sp. ova. The magnitude of response is greater with higher dosage levels or multiple exposures. Peak levels, at days 10 to 15, correlate with periods of ecdysis.[65] Other researchers have found that ascarid infection can increase peripheral blood eosinophils to approximately 24% of WBC, with the peak at 16 to 20 days postinfection and a return to normal in 4 to 6 weeks.[4]

Neoplasia

Hereditary lymphosarcoma of young pigs usually is accompanied by lymphocytosis ($\geq$80% of a WBC count that may be normal or may approximate 30,000 cells/μL). This neoplastic lymphocytosis usually can be distinguished from the normal young pig lymphocytosis by the presence of significant numbers of lymphoblasts and poorly differentiated lymphocytes and by the presence of clinical signs suggestive of lymphosarcoma.[31]

REFERENCES

1. **Jain NC.** Essentials of veterinary hematology. Philadelphia:Lea and Febiger, 1993:19–53.
2. **Cole CG.** Leucocyte counts on the blood of normal, cholera-infected and recently immunized pigs. J Am Vet Med Assoc 1932;81:392–401.
3. **Pond WG, Houpt KA.** The biology of the pig. Ithaca, NY: Cornell University Press, 1978.
4. **Luke D.** The differential leucocyte count in the normal pig. J Comp Pathol 1953;63:346–354.
5. **Slesingr L.** Hämatologische Ergebnisse bei gesunden Schweinen, die in Bilanzkäfigen gehalten wurden. Berliner und Münchener tierärztliche Wochenschrift 1967;80:291–293.
6. **Palmer CC.** Morphology of normal pigs' blood. J Agr Res 1917;9:131–140.
7. **Friendship RM, Henry SC.** Cardiovascular system, hematology, and clinical chemistry. In: Leman AD, Straw BE, Mengeling WL, D'Allaire S, Taylor DJ, eds. Diseases of swine. 7th ed. Ames, IA: Iowa State University Press, 1992.
8. **Straw BE, Meuten DJ.** Physical examination.In: Leman AD, Straw BE, Mengeling WL, D'Allaire S, Taylor DJ, eds. Diseases of swine. 7th ed. Ames,IA: Iowa State University Press, 1992.
9. **Calhoun ML, Brown EM.** Hematology and hematopoietic organs. In: Dunne HW, Leman AD, eds. Diseases of swine. 4th ed. Ames, IA: Iowa State University Press, 1975.
10. **Gabris J.** Differences between the sexes and during summer and winter in the blood picture of unweaned piglets. Folia Vet 1973;17:303–312.
11. **Tumbleson ME, Badger TM, Baker PC, Hutcheson DP.** Systematic oscillations of serum biochemical and hematologic parameters in Sinclair (S-1) miniature swine. J Anim Sci 1972;35:48–50.
12. **Romack FE, Lasley JF, Day BN.** A study of the circulating leucocytes in swine. Mo Ag Exp Sta Res Bull 1962;804.
13. **Gregor VG.** Hämatologische und biochemische Untersuchungen am Miniaturschwein Mini-Lewe I. Mitteilung: Blutbild und Serumproteine. Z. Versuchstierk 1979;21:92–106.
14. **Schmidt DA, Tumbleson ME.** Swine hematology. In: Tumbleson ME, ed. Swine in biomedical research, vol. 2. New York: Plenum Press, 1986.
15. **Duncan JR, Prasse KW.** Veterinary laboratory medicine. 2nd ed. Ames, IA: Iowa State University Press, 1986;31–60.
16. **Kidd R.** Interpreting the leukogram: noninfectious factors that affect leukocyte production. Vet Med 1991;86:472–479.
17. **Kohler H.** Knochenmark und Blutbild des Ferkels 1. Mitteilung: das gesunde Ferkel. Vet Med 1956;3:359–395.
18. **Fraser AC.** A study of the blood of pigs. Br Vet J 1938;94:3–21.
19. **Upcott DH, Hebert CN, Robins M.** Erythrocyte and leukocyte parameters in fetal and neonatal piglets. Res Vet Sci 1973;15:8–12.
20. **Waddill DG, Ullrey DE, Miller ER, Sprague JI, Alexander EA, Hoefer JA.** Blood cell populations and serum protein concentrations in the fetal pig. J Anim Sci 1962;21:583–587.
21. **Brooks CC, Davis JW.** Changes in hematology of the perinatal pig. J Anim Sci 1969;28:517–522.
22. **Gabris J.** Changes in the relationship between leucocytes, neutrophil and lymphocyte counts in the blood of pig fetuses and unweaned piglets. Vet Med 1974;19:591–601.
23. **Tumbleson ME, Kalish PR.** Serum biochemical and hematological parameters in crossbred swine from birth through eight weeks of age. Can J Comp Med 1972;36:202–208.
24. **Lie H.** Thrombocytes, leucocytes and packed red cell volume in piglets during the first two weeks of life. Acta Vet Scand 1968;9:105–111.
25. **Mount LE, Ingram DL.** The pig as a laboratory animal. London: Academic Press, 1971;73.
26. **Jain NC.** Schalm's veterinary hematology. 4th ed. Philadelphia: Lea and Febiger, 1986:240–255.
27. **Schwager J, Schulze J.** Maturation of the mitogen responsiveness, and IL2 and IL6 production by neonatal swine leukocytes. Vet Immunol Immunopathol 1997;57:105–119.
28. **Gardiner MR, Sippel WL, McCormick WC.** The blood picture in newborn pigs. Am J Vet Res 1953;14:68–71.
29. **Dvorak M.** Eosinophil levels in the blood of piglets with normal and retarded development. Docum Vet Brno 1968;7:199–206.
30. **Saror DI, Santiago F.** Haematological parameters of large white pigs in Nigeria. Bull Anim Health Prod Africa 1981;29:129–133.
31. **McTaggart HS.** Lymphocytosis in normal young pigs. Br Vet J 1975;131:574–579.
32. **Kircher GH.** Beitrag zur Bestimmung hämatologischer und biochemischer Normprofile des Hanford Miniaturschweines und des Deutschen Land-

schweines in Abhängigkeit vom Lebensalter [Dissertation]. Munich: Fachbereich Tiermedizin der Ludwig-Maximilians-Universität, 1976.

33. **Grimoldi RJ, Marquez AG.** Hemograma en el cerdo Landrace. Rev Med Vet Argentina 1976;57:232–239.

34. **Bollen PJA, Ellegaard L.** Developments in breeding Göttingen minipigs. In: Tumbleson ME, Schook LB, eds. Advances in swine in biomedical research, vol. 1. New York: Plenum Press, 1996.

35. **Burks MF, Tumbleson ME, Hicklin KW, Hutcheson DP, Middleton CC.** Age and sex related changes of hematologic parameters in Sinclair (S-1) miniature swine. Growth 1977;41:51–62.

36. **Bickhardt VK, Wirtz A.** Der Einfluss von Anbindestress und Fütterung auf Blutmesswerte des Schweines. Deutsche Tierärztliche Wochenschrift 1978;85:457–496.

37. **Duncan JR, Prasse KW, Mahaffey EM.** Veterinary laboratory medicine. 3rd ed. Ames, IA: Iowa State University Press, 1994:37–62.

38. **Tewes H, Steinbach J, Smidt D.** Investigations on the blood composition of sows during the reproductive cycle. I. Blood changes during the oestrous cycle. Zuchthyg 1977;12:117–124.

39. **Tewes H, Steinbach J, Smidt D.** Investigations on the blood composition of sows during the reproductive cycle. II. Blood changes during pregnancy. Zuchthyg 1979;14:111–116.

40. **Luke D.** The reaction of the white blood cells at parturition in the sow. Br Vet J 1953;109:241–244.

41. **Gabris J.** Relationship between the numbers of leucocytes, neutrophils, granulocytes, and lymphocytes in sows before and during parturition and during lactation. Folia Vet 1975;19:151–161.

42. **Tumbleson ME, Burks MF, Spate MP, Hutcheson DP, Middleton CC.** Serum biochemical and hematological parameters of Sinclair (S-1) miniature sows during gestation and lactation. Can J Comp Med 1970;34:312–319.

43. **Nachreiner RF, Ginther OJ.** Gestational and periparturient periods of sows: serum chemical, hematologic, and clinical changes during the periparturient period. Am J Vet Res 1972;33:2233–2238.

44. **Crookshank HR, Smalley HE, Steel E.** Hematological parameters of American-Essex swine [Abstract]. J Anim Sci 1975;40:190.

45. **Morgan RM, Goertel J, Schipper IA.** Comparative hemograms of Hampshire and Duroc piglets. Southwestern Vet 1966;1:35–41.

46. **Mandel I, TravniFek J.** Haematology of conventional and germfree miniature Minnesota piglets I. Blood picture. Z Versuchstierk 1982;24:299–307.

47. **McClellan RO, Vogt GS, Ragan HA.** Age-related changes in hematological and serum biochemical parameters in miniature swine. In: Bustad LK, McClellan RO, Burns MP, eds. Swine in biomedical research. Seattle, WA: Frayn Printing, 1966.

48. **Luke D.** The effect of adrenocorticotrophic hormone and adrenal cortical extract on the differential white cell count in the pig. Br Vet J 1953;109:434–436.

49. **Wronska J.** Changes in the leukocyte picture, protein levels and total choles-

terol in fat swine under preslaughter conditions. Med Weterynaryjna 1982;38:230–232.

50. **McGlone JJ, Salak JL, Lumpkin EA, Nicholson RI, Gibson M, Norman RL.** Shipping stress and social status effects on pigs performance, plasma cortisol, natural killer cell activity, and leukocyte numbers. J Anim Sci 1993;71:888–896.

51. **Ellersieck MR, Veum TL, Durham TL, McVickers WR, McWilliams SN, Lasley JF.** Response of stress-susceptible and stress-resistant Hampshire pigs to electrical stress II. effects on blood cells and blood minerals. J Anim Sci 1979;48:453–458.

52. **Mutsumi M.** Influence of adrenocorticotropic hormone upon the circulating leukocyte count of peripheral blood in pigs [Abstract]. Nat Inst Anim Hlth Quarterly 1974;14:104.

53. **Salak-Johnson JL, McGlone JJ, Norman RL.** In vivo glucocorticoid effects on porcine natural killer cell activity and circulating leukocytes. J Anim Sci 1996;74:584–592.

54. **Blecha F.** Effects of in vivo ACTH on leukocyte numbers and din vivo and in vitro cellular immunity in pigs [Abstract]. J Anim Sci 1984;59(suppl 1):189.

55. **Olson NC.** Porcine endotoxemia: chemical mediators and therapeutic interventions. In: Tumbleson ME, Schook LB, eds. Advances in swine in biomedical research, vol. 1. New York: Plenum Press, 1996.

56. **Ross RF, Zimmerman BS, Wagner WC, Cox DF.** A field study of coliform mastitis in sows. J Am Vet Med Assoc 1975;167:231–235.

57. **Lofstedt J, Roth JA, Ross RF, Wagner WC.** Depression of polymorphonuclear leukocyte function associated with experimentally induced *Escherichia coli* mastitis in sows. Am J Vet Res 1983;44:1224–1228.

58. **Dunne HW.** Hog cholera. In: Dunne HW, Leman AD, eds. Diseases of swine. 4th ed. Ames, IA: Iowa State University press, 1975.

59. **Van Oirschot JT.** Hog cholera. In: Leman AD, Straw BE, Mengeling WL, D'Allaire S, Taylor DJ, eds. Diseases of swine. 7th ed. Ames, IA: Iowa State University Press, 1992.

60. **Vannier P, Leforban Y.** Bovine viral diarrhea and border disease. In: Leman AD, Straw BE, Mengeling WL, D'Allaire S, Taylor DJ, eds. Diseases of swine. 7th ed. Ames, IA: Iowa State University Press, 1992.

61. **Easterday BC.** Swine Influenza. In: Dunne HW, Leman AD, eds. Diseases of swine. 4th ed. Ames, IA: Iowa State University Press, 1975.

62. **Mengeling WL.** Porcine parvovirus. In: Leman AD, Straw BE, Mengeling WL, D'Allaire S, Taylor DJ, eds. Diseases of swine. 7th ed. Ames, IA: Iowa State University Press, 1992.

63. **Bohl EH.** Transmissible gastroenteritis. In: Dunne HW, Leman AD, eds. Diseases of swine. 4th ed. Ames, IA: Iowa State University Press, 1975.

64. **Maurer FD.** African swine fever. In: Dunne HW, Leman AD, eds. Diseases of swine. 4th ed. Ames, IA: Iowa State University press, 1975.

65. **Moncol DJ, Batte EG.** Peripheral blood eosinophilia in porcine ascariasis. Cornell Vet 1967;57:96–107.

66. **Solberg HE.** Establishment and use of reference values. In: Burtis CA, Ashwood ER, eds. Tietz fundamentals of clinical chemistry. 4th ed. Philadelphia: WB Saunders, 1996.

CHAPTER 60

Determination and Interpretation of the Avian Leukogram

• KENNETH S. LATIMER and DOROTHEE BIENZLE

Complete blood cell (CBC) counts are performed routinely in mammals to detect changes in the health status. Leukocyte responses are particularly useful because blood leukocyte numbers and morphology are fairly stable in health but may change drastically in disease. Although leukocyte responses are seldom pathognomonic for a specific disease, they can provide clinical information to establish a differential diagnosis, to monitor a patient's response to treatment, or to suggest a clinical prognosis.[1] Changes in leukocyte homeostasis are detected by performing a white blood cell (WBC) or leukocyte count, which is part of the CBC count. The component parts of this process include determination of the total and differential WBC counts, calculation of the absolute numbers of various leukocyte types per microliter of blood, and morphologic examination of leukocytes on the stained blood smear. This information constitutes the leukogram.[1]

Mammalian hematology has advanced rapidly over the past three decades owing to the introduction of semi-automated or automated technology (which may provide total leukocyte counts and complete or 2- to 3-part differential counts). In addition, reference intervals have been developed for various mammalian species to identify abnormal laboratory test results. Furthermore, numerous experimental studies have been done to clarify leukocyte responses. Finally, substantial published literature exists detailing clinical hematologic responses to disease.[2,3] In contrast, avian hematology is still in its infancy. Descriptive accounts of avian blood-cell morphology[4–6] and techniques of performing avian leukocyte counts[5,7–10] have been published. However, the progress of avian hematology has been inhibited by lack of automated technology, lack of appropriate reference intervals for all major avian species, and lack of carefully controlled experimental studies to interpret avian leukocyte responses. Presented in this chapter is a brief overview of avian leukocytes with respect to quantitation of leukocyte data, establishment of reference intervals, and interpretation of leukocyte responses in health and disease. Much of the research to date has been done in domestic poultry, which provides a model for avian leukocyte development and function.[11] Although generalizations can be drawn concerning avian leukocyte production, morphology, function, and response in health and disease, differences are sometimes apparent among and between species of birds. Avian hematology will advance rapidly as our understanding of leukocyte responses increases.

LEUKOCYTE COUNT

In avian hematology, only the red blood cell count can be determined routinely by automated methods (electronic particle counter).[9] Therefore, three manual approaches are used to determine or estimate the leukocyte count. These include (1) the direct leukocyte count with a hemacytometer and Natt and Herrick's solution, (2) the indirect leukocyte count with a hemacytometer and eosinophil Unopette® in conjunction with the stained blood smear, and (3) the estimated leukocyte count with the stained blood smear. Specific technical procedures for these counting methods may be found in the literature.[5,10,12–14]

The avian leukocyte count is determined directly with a Neubauer-ruled hemacytometer, pipettes, and methyl violet 2B diluent.[7] The advantages of this technique are that all leukocytes are visualized and enumerated. The disadvantages are that this leukocyte counting technique is labor intensive, care must be taken to differentiate thrombocytes from small lymphocytes, and leukocytes may distort if analysis of the diluted specimen is delayed.[11,15] This method works well for an in-house laboratory but may cause difficulty in samples that are mailed to a diagnostic laboratory. In the latter instance, prolonged exposure to ethylenediamine tetra-acetic acid (EDTA) anticoagulant may cause erythrolysis and viscosity changes of hematologic specimens from crowned cranes, crows, jays, brush turkeys, hornbills, magpies, and some ratites.[9,16,17] In addition, leukocyte morphology may be altered upon prolonged exposure to EDTA.[2]

Specimens collected in heparin eventually clot, and heparin also interferes with Romanowsky staining of blood smears.

The leukocyte count can be quantitated indirectly with the eosinophil Unopette #5877 system. In this technique, which was described originally in 1931,[18] heterophils and eosinophils are selectively stained by phloxine dye and counted in the hemacytometer.[8,12] Based on the leukocyte differential count of the stained blood smear, the combined heterophil and eosinophil hemacytometer count is mathematically corrected to account for basophils and mononuclear cells (lymphocytes and monocytes) that were not counted. Thus, the total leukocyte count per microliter of blood has been determined indirectly. Advantages of this system are that heterophils and eosinophils are directly identified and counted in the hemacytometer. There also is no confusion between lymphocytes and thrombocytes because they are not counted with the hemacytometer. However, several disadvantages of the eosinophil Unopette method are apparent. Hemacytometer counts are labor intensive. A greater potential for mathematical errors exists because both the hemacytometer-derived count and indirect total leukocyte count must be calculated. Ultimately, the indirect leukocyte count depends on leukocyte distribution on the stained blood smear; leukocytes may not be randomly distributed in a poorly prepared smear. Finally, anticoagulated blood samples mailed to a diagnostic laboratory may be labile as mentioned above.

One can estimate leukocyte counts from the stained blood smear by multiplying the average number of leukocytes per field of view by a given factor (the factor is usually 1500 or 2000 for the 40 to 45× high-dry or 50× oil-immersion microscope objectives, respectively).[2] Advantages of this technique include the stability of the preparation (air-dried blood smear) submitted to the diagnostic laboratory and the labor-efficient process of leukocyte count estimation. The major disadvantage is that the leukocyte count is estimated instead of quantitated. Thus, estimated leukocyte counts may not be reproducible, poor smear technique may influence the estimate because of cell lysis or maldistribution, and too much emphasis may be placed on the data in a clinical setting.[19] In summary, an estimated leukocyte count is no substitute for a properly performed quantitative leukocyte count, although the former technique may have some benefit in an emergency situation in which time is critical.

Quantitative leukocyte counts with hemacytometers are superior to estimated leukocyte counts. Studies have shown the coefficient of variation to be 12.7% for hemacytometer-derived leukocyte counts (eosinophil Unopette method) as opposed to 28% for estimated leukocyte counts from the stained blood smear.[20] However, the latter technique may be useful to indicate hematologic trends for which the lability or volume of the blood specimen would otherwise preclude hematologic study. Ultimately, the future of avian hematology depends on the development of semiautomated or automated techniques to determine avian leukocyte counts in a rapid, accurate, economical, and labor-efficient manner.

STAINED BLOOD SMEAR

The stained blood smear is used to perform the leukocyte differential count and morphologic examination of leukocytes. Although considerable discussion has revolved around the best method to produce acceptable avian blood smears, both the wedge technique (with two glass slides) and coverslip technique (with two square glass coverslips) can be used. The major factors in producing high-quality smears are manual dexterity and practice.

It is generally assumed that leukocytes are randomly distributed in the blood smear, which may not be the case. Hematologic studies have shown that leukocytes are more randomly distributed in coverslip smears than in wedge smears where large cells, such as monocytes, may be carried to the lateral margins and feathered edge of the smear.[2] Furthermore, this problem is magnified with poor smear technique, such as moving the spreader slide too slowly, which carries almost all leukocytes to the margins of the smear. Depending on the type of smear and the method of examination (e.g., the battlement method where the lateral margins of a wedge smear are included in the WBC differential count), leukocyte differential counts may vary somewhat.

Leukocyte differential counts still vary even if the same general area of the smear is reexamined (two leukocyte differential counts from the same stained blood smear are rarely identical). Therefore, the accuracy of the leukocyte differential count can only be increased by counting more cells. To increase the accuracy of the differential count significantly, one must perform a 400-cell as opposed to 100-cell leukocyte differential count.[3] The trade-off is increased expense through increased labor costs.

In summary, the importance of producing high-quality avian blood smears cannot be over emphasized. The smear quality directly influences the accuracy of the differential and estimated leukocyte counts. Also, smears that are made at the time of blood specimen collection reflect the morphologic changes in leukocytes at that point. If smears are made from the blood specimen at a later time, artifacts include increased numbers of smudge cells, distortion of leukocytes and thrombocytes, vacuolation of monocytes, swelling of lymphocytes, and changes in leukocyte tinctorial properties.[2,11] Specific stain-induced artifacts in leukocytes are discussed below.

LEUKOCYTE DIFFERENTIAL COUNT

One performs a leukocyte differential count by classifying 100 consecutive leukocytes as segmented or band heterophils, lymphocytes, monocytes, eosinophils, or basophils (in certain disease states, the leukocyte differential count may be modified to include juvenile heterophils or blast cells). When performing avian leukocyte counts, one must remember that leukocyte morphology may vary between species. Examples include the ap-

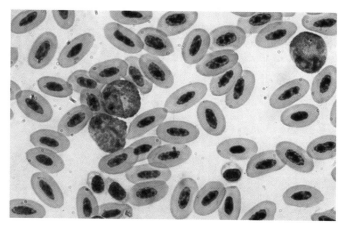

FIGURE 60.1 Blood smear from an African grey parrot. A left shift is indicated by the presence of immature heterophils (band, metamyelocyte, and myelocyte). All of these cells display mild toxic change (cytoplasmic basophilia).

tion than mammalian neutrophils.[11] Furthermore, heterophil granules tend to obscure nuclear morphology in Romanowsky-stained blood smears. With these preparations, only severe left shifts can be easily identified (Fig. 60.1). Promyelocytes, which contain both basophilic and eosinophilic granules,[23] indicate an intense left shift[11,24] (Fig. 60.5). Subtle left shifts can be accurately quantitated by examination of hematoxylin-stained blood smears in which the nucleus is stained but the granules remain unstained.[11] This technique allows determination of a nuclear lobulation score, a sensitive indicator of a left shift. However, this technique is more labor intensive.

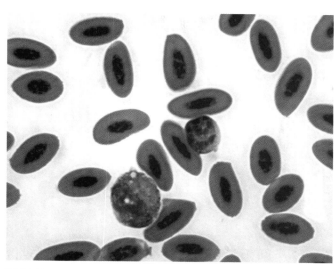

FIGURE 60.3 Blood smear from a great horned owl. A monocyte (lower left) and lymphocyte (upper right) are present.

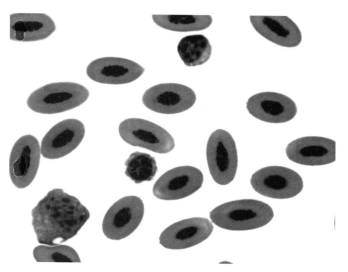

FIGURE 60.2 Blood smear from a great horned owl. A monocyte (lower left), thrombocyte (center), and lymphocyte (top) are present.

pearance of granule morphology and cytoplasmic coloration of raptor eosinophils[6] and the shape of heterophil granules in certain species of birds.[9] With currently accepted criteria of leukocyte identification, performance of the leukocyte differential count in healthy and sick birds may be challenging and requires practice. Problems may be encountered in identifying left shifts in the heterophil population[11] (Fig. 60.1) and in distinguishing some small lymphocytes from thrombocytes[21] (Fig. 60.2), monocytes from large lymphocytes[22] (Fig. 60.3), reactive lymphocytes from rubricytes,[5] heterophils from eosinophils[5,9] (Fig. 60.4), and extremely toxic promyelocytes (mesomyelocytes) from basophils[13] (Fig. 60.5).

Detection of left shifts in avian blood is more difficult because avian heterophils exhibit less nuclear segmenta-

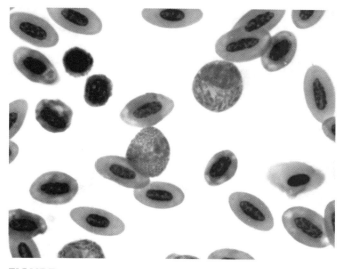

FIGURE 60.4 Blood smear from a red-tailed hawk. The myelocytic heterophil (top right) has needle-shaped, dull red granules, whereas the eosinophil (left) has round, bright, red-orange granules.

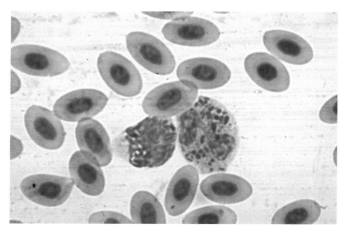

FIGURE 60.5 Blood smear from a chicken. Segmented heterophil and toxic heterophil promyelocyte. Note purple and red granules in the promyelocyte.

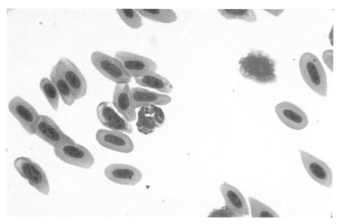

FIGURE 60.6 Blood smear from an Amazon parrot that has septicemia. Note the phagocytosed cocci within a heterophil.

CHANGES IN LEUKOCYTE MORPHOLOGY

Changes in leukocyte morphology are important observations that allow assessment of the severity of the disease process. Occasionally, morphologic changes in leukocytes may provided a definitive medical diagnosis.

Toxic Changes

Variable degrees of degranulation, cytoplasmic basophilia, cytoplasmic vacuolation, and cellular swelling constitute toxic changes in avian heterophils[25] (Figs. 60.1 and 60.5). Ultrastructurally, cellular swelling and cytoplasmic vacuolation are the result of intracellular edema. Degranulation is a sequel to dissolution of the granule matrix. Cytoplasmic basophilia is explained by the persistence of ribosomes. In Romanowsky-stained avian blood smears, cytoplasmic basophilia is the last manifestation of toxic change to disappear with convalescence.

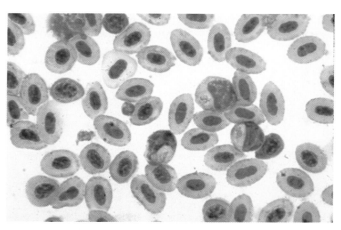

FIGURE 60.7 Blood smear form a Bali mynah that has disseminated atoxoplasmosis. Note round to oval intracytoplasmic organisms within the mononuclear cells.

Infectious Disease

Inclusions in avian leukocytes are seen infrequently but may provide a definitive diagnosis when observed. Examples include phagocytosed bacteria within heterophils of septicemic birds (Fig. 60.6), *Atoxoplasma* sp. organisms in the cytoplasm of monocytes (Fig. 60.7), *Leukocytozoon* sp. organisms within the cytoplasm of leukocytes or erythrocytes (Fig. 60.8), and elementary bodies of *Chlamydia psittaci* in the cytoplasm of various leukocytes (Fig. 60.9).

After exposure to antigens and stimulation of the immune system, scattered lymphocytes may appear reactive (a prelude to blast transformation or plasmacytoid differentiation) and have dark blue granular cytoplasm. Such cells are classified as lymphocytes on the leukocyte differential count, but they are designated as immunocytes or reactive lymphocytes morphologically. In

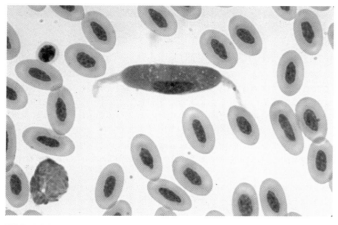

FIGURE 60.8 Blood smear from a great horned owl. *Leukocytozoon* sp. gametocyte is present within a leukocyte. The affected cell is enlarged, elongated, and has pointed cell margins.

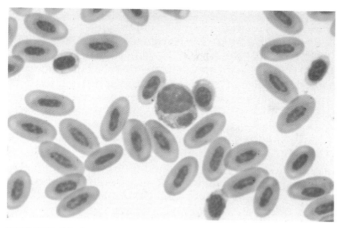

FIGURE 60.9 Blood smear from parrot that has chlamydiosis. Intracytoplasmic elementary bodies of *C. psittaci* are present in a monocyte. Blood smear courtesy of Dr. Michele Menard, Veterinary Cytopathology, Gresham, OR.

lymphoid neoplasia, the majority of lymphocytes may appear immature or reactive.

The clinician also should be familiar with stain-induced changes in cellular morphology. Stain-induced artifacts such as degranulation and intensified cytoplasmic coloration of heterophils in Diff-Quik-stained preparations should not be mistaken for toxic changes.[11] Also, partial heterophil degranulation, especially with aqueous-based stains coupled with short fixation times, may leave a round granule core, causing affected cells to resemble eosinophils.[11,26,27] Cytochemical staining has the potential to reliably distinguish heterophils from eosinophils for which cellular identification is uncertain.[28]

As avian hematology progresses, laboratories should undertake a coordinated effort to modernize avian leukocyte nomenclature (mesomyelocyte versus promyelocyte), uniformly evaluate morphologic changes in blood cells, and consistently report semiquantitative hematologic data.[29] Standardized guidelines will facilitate comparison of hematologic data between laboratories.

REFERENCE INTERVALS

Reference intervals are used to identify laboratory test results or values that discriminate between health and disease. These intervals were previously known as normal intervals; however, a normal state was difficult, if not impossible, to define. Therefore, the ambiguous term normal interval was replaced by the term reference interval.

Establishment of meaningful reference intervals requires data collection from an adequate number of individuals constituting a precisely defined population. The population must be defined precisely because test values may be influenced by species of bird, age, sex, health and reproductive status, diet, and climate or environ-

ment (age-related changes in the leukogram are of special importance and are covered below). In addition, the method of specimen collection and analytical technique may influence test results. Usually, a minimum of 40 to 60 individuals should be sampled unless significant variation in test values is observed. In such cases, 120 individuals should be sampled. Once test values are determined, the data are statistically manipulated to reduce all-encompassing reference ranges into more narrow reference intervals. With these intervals, laboratory test values suggestive of health or disease may be distinguished more reliably.

Reference intervals for various species of companion and exotic birds have been published in journals and textbooks. Several of these publications are especially noteworthy based on the large numbers of individuals sampled, a defined reference population, and attention to age-related changes in hematologic data.[30-38] However, those reference intervals based on quantitative leukocyte counts[31-33,37] provide superior data to those reference intervals based on estimated leukocyte counts.[30,35,36] Sometimes, avian clinicians are presented with ill patients that are rare exotic birds or juvenile birds of common species for which extensive reference intervals do not exist. In such cases, analysis of control blood samples from clinically healthy birds of the same species, age, sex, and environment may allow identification of abnormal hematologic trends.[20,39-49]

HEMOPOIESIS WITH EMPHASIS ON LEUKOCYTE PRODUCTION

Primitive cells in the yolk sac initiate blood-cell development during the first few days of embryonic incubation. By 10 to 15 days of incubation, hemopoietic activity peaks in the yolk sac and is widespread in other tissues, including bone marrow, liver, kidney, spleen, thymus, bursa of Fabricius, aorta, heart, pharynx, cranial nerves, spinal ganglia, subcutaneous tissues, and muscles.[50,51] Although the bone marrow is the major site of hemopoietic activity posthatching, foci of hemopoiesis also may be observed commonly in the liver, spleen, and kidney of companion birds. In mammals, much of the extramedullary hemopoiesis observed specifically involves erythropoiesis and is largely limited to the liver and spleen. In birds, extramedullary hemopoiesis is widespread and involves granulopoiesis, wherein the majority of the cells contain eosinophilic granules and nuclei in various stages of lobulation. Granulopoiesis is especially prominent in the liver, kidney, and spleen, but it may involve the heart and subdural spaces. Granulopoiesis, especially in the spleen, bursa, and thymus, involves production of heterophils.[50]

In mammals, marrow hemopoietic activity (production of erythrocytes, leukocytes, and megakaryocytes) is extravascular. In birds, granulopoiesis occurs in the extravascular spaces, whereas erythropoiesis and thrombopoiesis occur within the bone marrow vascular sinuses. Sites of hemopoiesis in birds involve non-pneumatized long bones and the axial skeleton. A practical example is the acquisition of bone marrow aspirates from the tibia because the humerus and femur frequently are pneumatized. During early life, hemopoiesis is distributed throughout the skeleton, except for the skull.[52]

Lymphocyte production, however, occurs in primary (thymus, bursa of Fabricius) and secondary (spleen; gut-associated lymphoid tissue, including cecal tonsils; bronchial-associated lymphoid tissues; paraocular tissues, including conjunctival-associated lymphoid tissue; paranasal sinuses, and miscellaneous lymphoid follicles along lymphatic vessels) extramedullary tissues. Lymphocytes are present in the thymus and bursa of the embryo by 10 to 14 days of incubation. As lymphopoiesis progresses, the secondary lymphoid tissues produce the majority of the lymphocytes, whereas the primary lymphoid tissues (thymus and bursa) involute with sexual maturity.

Comparative studies of blood-cell development indicate that all blood-cell components are derived from pluripotential stem cells that are present in the bone marrow and blood. Stem cells are an absolute requirement for blood-cell production because differentiated blood cells, with the exception of lymphocytes and some macrophages, are incapable of mitosis. Stem cells can repopulate the bone marrow, and hemopoiesis may resume after severe bone marrow damage (e.g., viral infections), but the proliferative capacity of stem cells appears to decrease with age.

Comparative studies, primarily in mammalian cell systems, have partially elucidated the regulation of hematopoiesis by interleukins.[2] The ability of interleukins to function across species lines suggests a similar role in avian hemopoiesis. Although knowledge of comparable avian cytokines exists, colony-stimulating factor and interleukin activities have not been demonstrated.[53] Extramedullary hemopoiesis (especially granulopoiesis) in the adult bird may resume in conjunction with severe body requirements for leukocytes, with certain forms of liver disease, and in localized (e.g., myelolipoma) or generalized (e.g., myeloblastosis) neoplasia.

LEUKOCYTE FUNCTION AND RESPONSE IN HEALTH AND DISEASE

Interpretation of avian leukograms should be based on absolute leukocyte values per microliter of blood. This results in fewer erroneous interpretations than reliance on relative percentages alone.[1,2] Although diurnal rhythms of leukocyte counts have been demonstrated occasionally in birds (e.g., chickens),[54–58] these fluctuations have little effect on leukogram interpretations in a clinical setting.

Review of the published avian literature, particularly concerning clinical hematology of companion birds, has revealed numerous instances of incorrect interpretation of avian leukocyte responses. The following discussion is offered to correct these deficiencies.

Few scientifically controlled studies have been per-formed to evaluate avian leukocyte responses.[11] Therefore, interpretation of avian leukograms has relied on extrapolations from the veterinary literature and individual clinical experience. Although hematologic studies of patients with spontaneous disease have increased our knowledge of avian hematology, precise interpretation of avian leukocyte responses is obscured by numerous variables and incomplete patient data concerning sample collection, method of analysis, restraint, drug administration, etc. The following discussion is intended to provide basic guidelines for leukogram interpretation. It is hoped that these guidelines will be refined as our knowledge of avian leukocyte responses increases.

HETEROPHIL OR LYMPHOCYTE PREDOMINANCE IN THE BLOOD IN STATES OF RELATIVE HEALTH

Birds are similar to rodents in that the primary circulating leukocyte in some species is the heterophil, whereas in other species the lymphocyte predominates. Examples of birds that have a predominance of heterophils include greater sulfur-crested cockatoos, herring gulls, hyacinth macaws, rainbow lorikeets, yellow-crowned Amazon parrots, African grey parrots, and pigeons.[16,39,40,42,44,49] Examples of birds that have a predominance of lymphocytes include budgerigars, canaries, cockatiels, finches, Rose-ringed parakeets, and many species of Amazon parrots.[14,16,30,37]

Hematologic studies of some species of adult birds, such as flamingos [34,48] and white-naped cranes,[41,59] are contradictory in that either heterophils or lymphocytes have been identified as the major circulating leukocyte in health. Possible explanations of these divergent observations should include stress of capture, handling, caging, social interactions, and environmental conditions. These variables, singly or in combination, could induce heterophilia or lymphopenia, resulting in aberrant reference intervals.[40,44,60–63]

Hematologic study of neonatal and juvenile birds indicates that heterophilic leukocytosis may be observed with some frequency.[31–33,46] The presumed mechanism for this observation is stress. Furthermore, some birds that have a predominance of lymphocytes in the adult leukogram often have a predominance of heterophils during the posthatch and juvenile periods.[46] Transition to the normal adult leukogram eventually occurs with age (generally 8 to 12 weeks of age), a similar process typically occurs in young ruminants by weaning age. Total leukocyte counts frequently are elevated posthatch (a stressful period of neonatal life) and decrease with age.

From the discussion and examples given above, one can readily appreciate the need for reference intervals so that avian leukograms from birds of various species and ages are interpreted correctly. In the case of expensive or rare birds, an annual physical examination and CBC count provides individual reference data to detect subtle changes in individual health status. This procedure is expensive, but it has proved to be highly effective in human health care.

LEUKOCYTOSIS AND LEUKOPENIA

Leukocytosis

Leukocytosis, an elevated total leukocyte count, is commonly the result of physiologic processes, infection, or inflammation. Physiologic leukocytosis is precipitated by excitement, fear, forced flight, and excessive muscular activity. Increases in heterophils or lymphocytes may account for the leukocytosis. If the mechanism in birds mimics that of mammals, leukocytosis could be related to epinephrine release or muscular exertion, both of which cause increased cardiac output, increased blood pressure, and an outpouring or washout of leukocytes from the microvasculature into the mainstream of circulation.[2] Physiologic lymphocytosis, presumably an epinephrine-mediated effect interfering with lymphocyte homing and recirculation, is understood incompletely in mammals and has not been studied to any extent in birds.

In inflammatory and infectious conditions of birds, heterophilia often is observed and the degree of heterophilia may be more pronounced than comparable neutrophilia in mammals. Examples include acute chlamydiosis, mycobacteriosis, and disseminated mycosis where the total leukocyte count may exceed 100,000 cells/μL of blood.[64] In the case of birds that have a predominance of lymphocytes such as chickens, a heterophil-lymphocyte reversal that is reminiscent of an adult bovine leukocyte response may be observed.[11] In some infectious conditions of birds, a lymphocytosis may be noted. An example is chronic chlamydiosis wherein the immune system has been stimulated as observed by plasmacytosis, most notable in sections of liver and spleen.[65] The mechanism of lymphocytosis is nonspecific immune system stimulation.

Leukopenia

Leukopenia in birds that have a predominance of heterophils usually is the result of heteropenia. In birds that have a predominance of lymphocytes, leukopenia often is synonymous with lymphopenia. Causes of leukopenia vary, depending on whether heterophils, lymphocytes, or both cell lines are affected. Specific causes of heteropenia and lymphopenia, including those mechanisms resulting in leukopenia, are discussed in detail below.

HETEROPHIL RESPONSES

Heterophils generally are considered the avian equivalent of the mammalian neutrophil. Heterophils, in conjunction with humoral immunity, provide one of the body's first lines of defense against infection. However, avian heterophils and mammalian neutrophils differ both morphologically and biochemically. Morphologically, avian heterophils are identified by the presence of large, dull red, often needle-shaped granules (see Fig. 60.4). The presence of these eosin-staining granules has given rise to the term heterophil (*heteros* from the Greek meaning different), as opposed to the mammalian neutrophil whose granules are generally neutral in Romanowsky-stained blood smears. In some disease conditions, heterophil morphology may be altered. A left shift exists when excess band heterophils are present in the blood. Because avian heterophils are less segmented in health compared with mammalian neutrophils, identification of left shifts is more challenging in avian species.[11,25,26] Toxic changes of heterophils include cytoplasmic basophilia, cytoplasmic vacuolation, variable degranulation, and cellular swelling (see Figs. 60.1 & 60.5). Toxic degranulation must be distinguished from stain-induced degranulation. Toxic degranulation is the result of severe inflammation or infection and is associated with cytoplasmic basophilia. Stain-induced degranulation results from partial or complete granule dissolution when heterophils on the blood smear are exposed to aqueous-based stains (such as Diff-Quik stain) with a short fixation time.[11,25,26]

Biochemically, avian heterophils lack myeloperoxidase, an enzyme that is largely responsible for the efficient oxidative bactericidal activity of mammalian neutrophils.[28,66–68] A measurable oxidative burst has been observed for avian heterophils, but it is insignificant in bacterial killing. Avian heterophils accomplish effective nonoxidative bacterial killing by myeloperoxidase-independent methods with granule-derived proteins.[67,68] These substances include lysozyme, acid phosphatase, cathepsin, and β-glucuronidase (hydrolase) activities, and cationic proteins.[69,70] The cationic proteins include β-defensins (e.g., gallinacins, chicken heterophil antimicrobial peptides, and turkey heterophil antimicrobial peptides), which are natural antibiotics. In addition to bacteria (*Staphylococcus albus*, *Serratia marcescens*, *Escherichia coli*, *Pasteurella multocida*), avian heterophils also have been shown to kill yeast (*Candida albicans*).[66]

Recent studies indicate that avian heterophil function (adherence, chemotaxis, phagocytosis, and bacterial killing) is fairly efficient[71–74] in host defense against bacteria in conjunction with the humoral immune system. Mammalian neutrophil functions are well characterized and include killing or inactivation of bacteria, fungi, yeast, algae, parasites, and viruses. In addition, neutrophils can kill infected and transformed cells, amplify and modulate acute inflammatory reactions, enhance immunocompetent cell function, and regulate granulopoiesis.[2] Avian heterophil functions are less well understood and will provide an area for future research.

Heterophil responses in clinical practice are typically divided into heterophilia or heteropenia (Table 60.1). Mechanisms for these changes in the leukogram are discussed below. Heterophilia may result from physiologic responses, corticosteroid administration or endogenous corticosterone release, and inflammation and/or infection.

TABLE 60.1	**Causes of Heterophilia and Heteropenia in Birds**

Heterophilia
  Physiologic response
  Infection
    Bacteria
    Viruses
    Fungi
    Parasites
  Tissue destruction or necrosis
    Thrombosis and infarction
    Inflammation
  Drug administration
    Corticosteroids
    Estrogen
  Miscellaneous
    Acute, severe stress
    Foreign bodies
    Hemorrhage or hemolytic disease

Heteropenia
  Infection
    Overwhelming bacterial infection
    Viral-induced hemopoietic cell destruction
  Drug administration
    Predictable
      Cyclophosphamide
      Progesterone
    Idiosyncratic
      Piperacillin or doxycycline
  Neoplasia
    Leukemia
    Metastatic disease (disseminated lymphosarcoma)
  Radiation exposure

Physiologic Heterophilia

One can observe physiologic heterophilia after excitement, fear, or short-term strenuous exercise (the fright or flight response). The heterophilia occurs rapidly but is transient. The presumed mechanism, based on studies in other species, is an epinephrine- or exercise-mediated increase in microvascular blood flow that shifts heterophils into the mainstream of circulation. Concurrent lymphocytosis also may be observed (and may overshadow the heterophilia), especially in those species that have higher lymphocyte counts in health. Because of the frequent occurrence of physiologic heterophilia (leukocytosis), it may be wise to obtain hematologic specimens before the patient is unduly perturbed. Physiologic responses are frequently confused with stress leukograms where lymphopenia is expected.[76]

Corticosteroid-Associated Heterophilia

Corticosteroid-induced heterophilia is observed sporadically in diseased or severely stressed birds and is the result of corticosterone release from the adrenal cortex. An example of developing heterophilia in response to forced confinement has been reported in captive herring gulls.[44] Corticosteroid-induced heterophilia is observed more frequently with exogenous corticosteroid administration[77,78] or injection of adrenocorticotropic hormone (ACTH), which stimulates endogenous corticosterone release.[61] The phenomenon is dosage and route dependent, wherein higher corticosteroid dosages produce greater heterophilia and more rapid heterophilia occurs with injection of the drug as opposed to oral medication. In mammals, this response also depends on the type of corticosteroid, dosage, and route of administration.[1] Developing or concurrent lymphopenia separates this response from physiologic leukocytosis. In mammals, neutrophilia primarily is the result of facilitated release of neutrophils from the bone marrow and minor redistribution of neutrophils from the marginal to circulating neutrophil pools. A similar mechanism probably occurs in birds.

Inflammation- or Infection-Induced Heterophilia

Heterophilia is frequently observed in conjunction with tissue damage induced by inflammation or bacterial infection (including chlamydiosis).[11,24,34,40–43,64,73,79,82] Occasionally, the source of tissue damage provoking heterophilia may be obscure. Examples include hemorrhage or oxidative injury and subsequent destruction of erythrocytes.[83,84] Experimental studies have shown that significant heterophilia can occur within 6 hours of induced inflammation and that cell counts peak fourfold greater than baseline values by 12 hours postinflammation.[11] As bone marrow reserves of segmented heterophils are depleted, a left shift accompanied by toxic changes of heterophils may appear within 24 hours. The presence of progranulocytes (cells with round nuclei and a mixture of purple and red cytoplasmic granules) indicates an intense shift.[11,24,34,64] As the bone marrow responds to tissue demands for heterophils, the leukocytosis and heterophilia intensify. A return toward baseline values with disappearance of the left shift and toxic change indicates convalescence. As a final note, birds often exhibit a drastic heterophilic leukocytosis in comparison with neutrophilia in mammals.[11,73,79] In companion birds, total leukocyte counts may exceed 100,000 cells/μL in chronic chlamydiosis and mycobacteriosis, especially in grey cheek parakeets and macaws.[14,76]

Heteropenia

The three most common mechanisms for production of neutropenia in mammals include deficient neutrophil production in the bone marrow, a shift in neutrophils from the circulating to marginal cell pool (where they cannot be quantitated by the WBC count), and emigration of neutrophils from the blood into the tissues at a rate that exceeds neutrophil replacement into the blood from the bone marrow.[1,2] Similar mechanisms undoubtedly exist in birds but have not received detailed study. However, anecdotal reports in the literature and personal observations tend to support these mechanisms.

Any instance of heteropenia indicates a guarded prognosis until favorable resolution of the condition can be ascertained by additional hematologic study.

Deficient Heterophil Production

Deficient heterophil production can be the result of hemopoietic stem cell death from infectious agents, drugs, or ionizing radiation and myelophthisis-associated loss of hemopoietic space.

Leukopenia and heteropenia have been reported in pet birds that have presumed viral infections (herpesvirus, polyomavirus, and psittacine reovirus); however, such reports largely represent undocumented clinical or laboratory impressions.[14,76,85] One hematologic study of Quaker Parrots that had experimental Pacheco's disease failed to document heteropenia.[86] Drug-induced myelosuppression may be predictable, as observed in cyclophosphamide-treated chickens and turkeys,[87,88] or may be an idiosyncratic adverse drug reaction, as observed in a budgerigar after antibiotic (piperacillin or doxycycline) treatment.[89] Toxic change of heterophils and vacuolation of hemopoietic precursor cells may be observed with drug toxicity.

Myelophthisis-associated loss of hemopoietic space is observed infrequently in clinical practice. In our experience, this cause of heteropenia has been associated with disseminated lymphoid neoplasia wherein proliferating neoplastic lymphocytes replace normal hemopoietic cells.

Heterophil Shifts From the Circulating to Marginal Pool

In mammals, early endotoxemia or gram-negative sepsis results in a shift of neutrophils from the circulating to marginal cell pools where they cannot be quantitated by the leukocyte count. The neutropenia is transient (1 to 3 hours duration) and is followed by a rebound leukocytosis if the patient survives.[2] This mechanism may occur in birds but is not well documented.

Severe Tissue Demands for Heterophils

Overwhelming tissue demand for heterophils at a rate that exceeds cell replacement in the blood from the bone marrow also produces heteropenia. Examples include acute severe peritonitis[34] and necrotizing enteritis. Heteropenia may be accompanied by a degenerative left shift and toxic change of heterophils.

LYMPHOCYTE RESPONSES

As mentioned previously, lymphocytes may be the major circulating leukocyte in the blood of some avian species (see Figs. 60.2 & 60.3). Characterization of the blood lymphocyte population in mammals indicates that the majority of these cells are small, mature, long-lived, T-lymphocyte memory cells.[2] This probably is the case in avian species. For example, chicken peripheral blood lymphocytes have shown to be approximately 14% B lymphocytes and 72% T lymphocytes by direct and indirect immunofluoresence, respectively.[90] The remaining blood lymphocytes (approximately 14%) are probably null cells.

Lymphocytosis

Physiologic lymphocytosis represents a transient phenomenon in birds after excitement, fright, or struggling during venipuncture (Table 60.2). Lymphocytosis may overshadow any heterophilia. This response may be especially noticable in healthy birds that have high circulating lymphocyte counts.[76,78]

Lymphocytosis secondary to antigenic stimulation may be observed commonly in birds that have chronic infectious (bacterial, viral, fungal, or parasitic) or inflammatory diseases wherein the blood lymphocyte pool is expanded because of persistent antigen exposure, most notably in chronic bacterial or viral diseases.[11,12,34,40–42,79,82,91] Occasionally, the lymphocytosis may be extreme as in a crane that had granulomatous disease and an absolute lymphocyte count of 45,900 cells/μL.[41]

Lymphoid neoplasia such as lymphosarcoma with a leukemic blood picture[92,93] (Fig. 60.10) or lymphoid leukemia (Fig. 60.11) may be associated with lymphocytosis. In our experience, lymphoid leukemias produce more drastic or extreme elevations in the absolute lymphocyte count (as much as 200,000 lymphocytes/μL).

Lymphopenia

Lymphopenia is commonly the result of severe stress-induced endogenous corticosterone release or exogenous corticosteroid administration (Table 60.2). Corticosteroid administration produces a rapid, predictable, transient redistribution of mammalian T lymphocytes

---

TABLE 60.2	Causes of Lymphocytosis and Lymphopenia

Lymphocytosis
  Physiologic response
  Antigenic stimulation
    Chronic viral infection
    Chronic bacterial infection
    Chronic fungal infection
    Parasitic diseases
  Lymphoid neoplasia
    Lymphosarcoma
    Lymphocytic leukemia

Lymphopenia
  Acute systemic infection
  Corticosteroid-induced
    Exogenous corticosteroid administration
    Endogenous corticosterone release (acute, severe stress)
  Immunosuppressive drugs, radiation

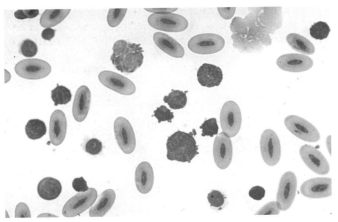

FIGURE 60.10 Blood smear from an emu that has disseminated lymphoma. Immature, neoplastic lymphocytes within the blood smear have dark blue cytoplasm with broad pseudopodia.

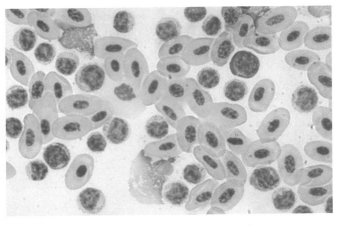

FIGURE 60.11 Blood smear from a cockatoo that has lymphocytic leukemia. The leukocytes are predominately mature, well-differentiated lymphocytes.

to the bone marrow or other tissue compartments, resulting in lymphopenia.[1] Studies in chickens have documented a rapidly developing but transient lymphopenia after corticosteroid administration. The magnitude and duration of the lymphopenia depends on the type of drug preparation (long- versus short-acting corticosteroids), dosage (the higher the dosage the more severe the lymphopenia), and route of administration (more rapid lymphopenia with parenteral as opposed to oral drug dosing).[61,77,78]

Stress-associated lymphopenia is more variable and often difficult to document hematologically in an apparently clinically stressed bird. Heterophilia and concurrent lymphopenia are the hallmarks of a stress leukogram and may be observed in diseased[34,40,42,81] or severely stressed birds, such as those subjected to forced molting through severe feed restriction.[94]

Lymphopenia of acute infection may have a complex origin, involving one or more mechanisms. These mechanisms include endogenous corticosterone release with temporary lymphocyte redistribution, temporary trapping of recirculating lymphocytes within lymphoid tissues to promote antigen contact, and direct destruction of lymphoid tissue, especially during viral infection.[1]

Last, drug-induced lymphopenia (other than corticosteroids) may be observed infrequently after drug administration or ingestion of toxicants. Examples include cyclophosphamide administration in chickens and turkeys[87,88] and crude oil ingestion by gulls.[84]

MONOCYTE RESPONSES

The monocyte-macrophage system is composed of stem cells, monoblasts, and promonocytes in the bone marrow; monocytes in the bone marrow and blood; and macrophages within various tissues of the body. Blood monocytes can be envisioned as somewhat immature cells that constitute a replacement pool for tissue macrophages. Diverse functions of the monocyte-macrophage system (best characterized in mammalian cell systems) include: defense against infectious agents (bacteria, fungi, protozoa, and viruses), phagocytic removal of damaged or aged cells, elimination of virus-infected and tumor cells, and remodeling of tissues during growth and healing. Macrophages secrete a diverse array of proteins, including components and regulators of the complement, kinin, and hemostasis or fibrinolysis cascades and interleukins that are involved in granulopoiesis, stimulation of T lymphocytes, and production of fever.[2] Studies in turkeys indicate that phagocytic uptake of blood particulate material occurs predominantly by macrophages in the liver, spleen, and bone marrow.[95]

Monocytes are produced in the bone marrow and released into the blood at an early age compared with heterophils. A bone marrow storage pool of monocytes apparently does not exist as these cells are rare in most Romanowsky-stained bone marrow aspirates except from some heteropenic birds (with compensatory monocytosis). Once released into the blood, monocytes circulate for a short time and emigrate from the blood vessels into the tissues (see Figs. 60.3 and 60.12). Those monocytes that mature into tissue macrophages may have an extended life span ranging from days to months.[2]

Tissue demands for macrophages are met primarily by recruiting monocytes from the blood and increasing monocyte production in the bone marrow.[2,96] Macrophages can undergo limited mitosis in situ, but such activity generally accounts for less than 5% of the total macrophage population.[2]

Monocytes are generally the largest circulating leukocyte in avian blood in health and typically account for 1 to 3% of the circulating leukocyte population. These cells have round to oval nuclei, slightly condensed chromatin, gray cytoplasm, and occasional pseudopodia. Cytoplasmic vacuolation also may be observed, but is more common if the blood stands for a while before smears are made. Difficulty may be encountered in distinguishing monocytes from large lymphocytes in some birds. In such cases, cytochemistry can be used for definitive cell identification if necessary.[97] Intracytoplasmic inclusions are rare, but may be diagnostic of disease when present (e.g., atoxoplasma gametocytes and chlamydial elementary bodies; Figs. 60.7 and 60.9).

Monocytosis

Monocytosis often is associated with chronic diseases such as granulomatous lesions,[14,64,98] nonspecific tissue necrosis, bacterial infections, including mycobacteriosis[14,15,40,42,64,82,98] and chlamydiosis,[14,98] deep mycosis such as aspergillosis,[64] parasitism,[12] and zinc deficient diets[99] (Table 60.3). A frequent misconception among avian clinicians, however, is that monocytosis is only seen in chronic diseases and, when present, is indicative of granulomatous inflammation.[14,76,98,100] In fact, monocytosis may be observed in both acute and chronic diseases. Experimental studies in chickens have shown that significant monocytosis can be observed in the blood within 12 hours of induced inflammation or bacterial airsacculitis, with peak monocyte counts occurring within 24 to 48 hours.[11,101] These hematologic findings corroborate earlier observations in experimentally induced bacterial infection of chicken wing webs.[96] Studies of induced infection of wing webs demonstrated that tissue exudation peaked at 12 hours postinfection. These exudates were monocyte-macrophage rich as a result of cell recruitment from the blood. Furthermore, monocyte-macrophages participated in phagocytosis of bacteria in conjunction with heterophils.[96] Perhaps the misconception that monocytosis is a feature of chronic disease is related to many birds being presented for diagnosis and laboratory testing late in the course of disease or after protracted illness. Avian clinicians should remember that both acute and chronic illnesses should be considered in an avian patient that has monocytosis.[11]

Monocytopenia

Monocytopenia is clinically unimportant and difficult to document because of the wide range in avian monocyte counts. In instances of pancytopenia, such as viral-induced (e.g., chicken anemia agent) hemopoietic cell damage, heteropenia deserves more clinical attention because of the possibility of secondary infections.[102]

BASOPHIL RESPONSES

Avian basophils are recognized by their round to oval nucleus and prominent, round, purple granules in Romanowsky-stained blood smears (Fig. 60.12). In healthy birds, basophils usually are more numerous in the blood than are eosinophils. This observation has been made in many avian species, including chickens; pheasants[4]; macaws[20,33]; various species of cockatoos[32]; African grey,[40] Amazon,[35] and eclectus parrots[31]; finches; canaries; lovebirds; budgerigars; parakeets[30,36]; and gulls.[103]

Functions ascribed to mammalian basophils include participation in immune-mediated reactions such as anaphylaxis and cutaneous hypersensitivity; both prevention (heparin release) and promotion (basophil kallikrein-like activity) of hemostasis; involvement in plasma lipolysis (heparin activates lipoprotein lipase); rejection of parasites, especially ticks; and possible tumor cytotoxicity.[2] In addition, a proinflammatory role for these cells has been suggested in joint, intestinal, pulmonary, coronary, and myocardial diseases.[104]

Functions of avian basophils apparently are similar, but investigations of cell function are sparse or anecdotal. The involvement of avian basophils in acute inflammation is well documented. In chickens, basophilic infiltration of tissues has been observed with early (1.5 to 3 hours) inflammation of skin,[96,105–109] wattle,[110] skeletal muscle,[111] and mesentery.[112] Involvement of basophils has also been demonstrated in avian cutaneous hypersensitivity and systemic anaphylaxis.[113] Clinical and experimental evidence also suggests that avian basophils are involved in the host response to internal and external parasites, including schistosomes,[114] soft-bodied ticks,[115] and air sac mites.[116] Evidence also exists for basophil-associated tumor cytotoxicity wherein intense baso-

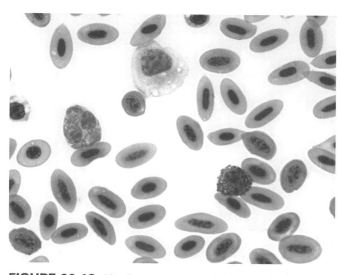

FIGURE 60.12 Blood smear from a red-tailed hawk. A heterophil, monocyte, and basophil are present.

TABLE 60.3   Causes of Monocytosis in Birds

Granulomatous inflammation

Acute inflammation

Bacterial infection
  Mycobacteriosis
  Chlamydiosis (chronic)

Fungal infection
  Aspergillosis

Parasitism

Zinc-deficient diets

philic infiltrates have been observed in experimentally induced Rous sarcomas in chicken wing webs.[117] In contrast to mammalian basophils, avian basophils also are actively phagocytic.[118]

Basophilia

Generally, only sustained overt basophilia can be detected by routine hematologic methods wherein basophils constitute at least 3 to 6% of the leukocyte differential count. Although absolute basophil counts with a hemacytometer and toluidine blue diluent have been performed in birds,[113,117] reports of blood basophil responses in disease are sporadic. Causes of basophilia in birds are listed in Table 60.4.

Basophilia is reported to occur with respiratory diseases and severe tissue damage in pet birds.[116] This finding is partially corroborated by a trend toward development of basophilia in chickens that have experimentally induced salmonellosis wherein basophil counts tended to increase within the first week of bacterial infection.[79] Blood basophilia, however, may be sporadic in avian inflammation.[11] Although the mechanism of basophilia is unknown, it may be related to the proinflammatory response observed in human beings.[104]

Blood basophilia also has been observed in internal and external parasitism. Examples include experimental infection of chickens that have the intravascular marine schistosome *Austrobilharzia variglandis*,[114] experimental cutaneous infestation of pigeons with soft-bodied ticks,[115] and natural infestation of canaries and finches with air sac mites.[116] Basophilia may occur alone or in conjunction with eosinophilia (air-sac mite infestations).

Basophilia also has been observed in chickens[119,120] and ducks after significant feed restriction and is presumed to be a harbinger of severe stress.[120] Apparently birds differ from mammals in that basophilia occurs in stress and that blood basophil counts apparently are unaffected by corticosteroid administration.[120]

Last, basophilia has been reported in chickens presumably in response to mycotoxin-contaminated feed.[121,122] The mechanism for basophilia was not given, but may be related to stress.

Basopenia

Basopenia cannot be detected reliably without performing absolute basophil counts.[107,117] The presence of basopenia in other species is of limited clinical importance in routine health care, as may be the case in avian patients.

EOSINOPHIL RESPONSES

Avian eosinophils are recognized by their round, often red-orange granules, and light blue cytoplasm in Romanowsky-stained blood smears. However, raptor eosinophil granules may occasionally be rod shaped, and granule tinctorial properties may vary slightly between species.[6] Eosinophils generally are the least frequently encountered leukocyte in avian blood smears, with the exception of raptors in which these cells may account for 15% of the leukocyte differential count.[6] In some species of birds, such as Amazon parrots, a leukocyte with round, colorless to light blue granules may be observed in the stained blood smear.[5] Obviously, the granules are not eosinophilic, which technically precludes cell identification as an eosinophil. However, the common practice is to identify such cells as eosinophils because typical eosinophils with red-orange granules have not been observed. Ultimate identification of this unusual leukocyte will require both ultrastructural and cytochemical study.

Eosinophil functions include modulation of hypersensitivity reactions, killing of certain parasites, and a proinflammatory function.[2] In mammals, eosinophil production in the bone marrow has been shown to be regulated by interleukin-3 and interleukin-5 production by T lymphocytes. These cells generally have a tendency to localize in subepithelial sites such as skin, respiratory tract, gastrointestinal tract, and genitourinary tract. Because of the presence of estrogen receptors, eosinophil counts in females may fluctuate with the reproductive cycle. Clinically, a paradox exists in that significant eosinophil infiltration may occur in tissues in the absence of blood eosinophilia.

In mammals, T lymphocytes play an important role in the production and maintenance of sustained eosinophilia. This lymphocyte–eosinophil interaction is analogous to the generation of an immune response in that a delayed onset of eosinophilia occurs at the first exposure to an antigen. The second exposure to the same antigen produces a more drastic and rapid eosinophilia, an antigen-specific memory response.[2]

TABLE 60.4   Causes of Basophilia in Birds

Tissue damage or perturbation
  Acute inflammation
    Skin, wattle, muscle, mesentery
  Severe nonspecific tissue damage
  Bacterial infection
  Respiratory disease
  Systemic anaphylaxis

Stress
  Feed restriction
  Starvation
  Forced molting

Parasitism
  Shistosomes
  Ticks
  Air sac mites

Miscellaneous
  Ingestion of mytoxin-contaminated feed

TABLE 60.5	Causes of Eosinophilia and Eosinopenia in Birds

Eosinophilia
  Facial edema
  Parasitism
  Exposure to foreign antigens
    Horse serum
    Bovine serum albumin

Eosinopenia
  Severe stress
  Corticosteroid administration

Eosinophilia

Avian species are similar to horses in that eosinophilia is observed infrequently in species other than raptors although parasitism is observed commonly[123] (Table 60.5). Eosinophilia has been observed in chickens that have facial edema[124]; chickens experimentally infected with schistosomes[114] or naturally infected with *Trichostrongylus tenuis*[125]; and in quails, chickens, and ducks injected intraperitoneally with horse serum or bovine serum albumin.[126–129] The magnitude of the eosinophilia may range from 6 to 56% of the leukocyte differential count in both experimental and natural disease. Furthermore, lymphocyte–eosinophil interaction has been demonstrated indirectly. This is apparent in that more drastic secondary eosinophilic responses have been observed in chickens and ducks after repeated antigen administration.[126] Irradiation has been shown to depress development of eosinophilia in chickens, whereas thymectomy had little effect.[129] The reason for this apparent paradoxical observation is that total-body irradiation affects all lymphocytes. Thymectomy in chickens is difficult because multiple lobules of thymic tissue extend along the neck to the thoracic inlet. In addition, T lymphocytes may be found in a localized area of the bursa of Fabricius as well as within secondary lymphoid tissues such as spleen.[97]

Eosinopenia

Eosinopenia is best defined by clinical experience in routine hematology. Because eosinophils are infrequently encountered in avian blood except for raptors, absolute eosinophil counts are necessary for a quantitative study of avian eosinopenia. A problem is readily apparent in that it may be difficult to distinguish eosinophils from heterophils in absolute counts (e.g., eosinophil Unopette) unless cytochemistry can be adapted.[28]

In mammals, eosinopenia is observed after corticosteroid or ACTH administration. Single-dose administration results in sequestration of eosinophils in the microvasculature (the cells are not destroyed), with a return to baseline values in 12 to 24 hours. Short-term corticosteroid administration (1.5 to 12 days) results in delayed eosinophil release from the bone marrow. Prolonged high-dose corticosteroid treatment causes decreased eosinophil production. Therefore, eosinopenia associated with corticosteroid therapy may be a combination of vascular sequestration, impaired bone marrow release of eosinophils, and ultimately, arrest of eosinophil production.[2] Eosinopenia of acute infection has been attributed to endogenous corticosteroid release, but this hypothesis has not been supported by determination of blood steroid levels. The precise mechanism of eosinopenia remains unknown, but cell margination within blood vessels or emigration into the tissues is postulated.[2]

Eosinophil responses in sick birds are seldom mentioned, although indication of eosinopenia sometimes is apparent.[24] Injection of long-acting ACTH in immature chickens has shown a suggestion of slight eosinopenia, but routine hematologic methods lacked the sensitivity needed for adequate quantitation of the cellular response.[61] In summary, clarification of avian eosinophil responses in blood (especially eosinopenia) relies on evaluation of absolute cell counts. In addition, the importance of avian eosinophil responses within the tissues will only be clarified by immunohistochemical staining to distinguish eosinophils from heterophils reliably.[28,128]

REMARKS ON PROGNOSIS AND HEMATOLOGIC TRENDS

Heterophil:Lymphocyte Ratios

Introduced as an indicator of stress in chickens, the heterophil:lymphocyte (H:L) ratio has been calculated on the basis of both absolute heterophil and lymphocyte counts or upon relative percentages of these leukocytes from the stained blood smear.[62,63] It was felt that the H:L ratio was less variable than either the absolute or relative percentage of these two types of leukocytes in the blood. When interpreting H:L ratios, one must remember that the ratio may increase with absolute heterophilia when the lymphocyte count is within the reference interval or with absolute lymphopenia when heterophil counts are within the reference interval. The true stress response, which is observed after corticosteroid administration, is absolute heterophilia in conjunction with developing lymphopenia.[77,78] In an experiment on feed restriction, ducks showed no change in H:L ratios; however, H:L ratios were increased in chickens and turkeys.[120] In this study, it was felt that developing basophilia in chickens, turkeys, and ducks was a more uniform hematologic change denoting severe stress. In our opinion, H:L ratios currently represent another mathematical manipulation of limited clinical value in assessing stress in birds (until more definitive scientific data can be collected and evaluated).

Guarded Prognosis

A guarded prognosis is indicated with heteropenia of any cause, especially if a left shift and toxic changes of heterophils are observed. If a left shift in the heterophil series intensifies or becomes degenerative (where band heterophils and younger forms outnumber segmented heterophils), a guarded prognosis is indicated. Extreme leukocytosis also has a guarded prognosis until chlamydiosis, mycobacteriosis, deep mycosis, and leukemia are excluded.

Favorable Hematologic Trends

Hematologic trends in birds that are suggestive of recovery include resolution of extreme leukocytosis, leukopenia, heteropenia, left shift, toxic changes of heterophils, and lymphopenia.

REFERENCES

1. **Latimer KS, Rakich PM.** Clinical interpretation of leukocyte responses. Vet Clin North Am Small Anim Pract 1989;19:637–668.
2. **Latimer KS.** Leukocytes in health and disease. In: Ettinger SJ, Feldman EC, ed. Textbook of veterinary internal medicine. Diseases of the dog and cat, vol 2. 3rd ed . Philadelphia: WB Saunders, 1995;1892–1929.
3. **Lee GR, Bithell TC, Foerster J, Athens JW, Lukens JN,** eds. Wintrobe's clinical hematology, 9th ed. Philadelphia: Lea & Febiger, 1993.
4. **Lucas AM, Jamroz C.** Atlas of avian hematology. USDA Agricultural Monograph 25. Washington, DC: US Government Printing Office, 1961.
5. **Campbell TW:** Avian hematology. 2nd ed. Ames, IA: Iowa State University Press, 1995.
6. **Lind PJ, Wolff PL, Petrini KR, Keyler CW, Olson DE, Redig PT.** Morphology of the eosinophil in raptors. J Assoc Avian Vet 1990;4:33–38.
7. **Natt MP, Herrick CA.** A new blood diluent for counting the erythrocytes and leukocytes of the chicken. Poult Sci 1952;31:735–738.
8. **Campbell TW, Dein FJ.** Avian hematology: The basics. Vet Clin North Am Small Anim Pract 1984;14:223–248.
9. **Dein FJ.** Laboratory manual of avian hematology. East Northport: Association of Avian Veterinarians, 1984.
10. **Zinkl JG.** Avian hematology. In: Jain NC, ed. Schalm's veterinary hematology. 4th ed. Philadelphia: Lea & Febiger, 1986;256–273.
11. **Latimer KS, Tang K-N, Goodwin MA, Steffens WL, Brown J.** Leukocyte changes associated with acute inflammation in chickens. Avian Dis 1988;32:760–772.
12. **Ferris M, Bacha WJ.** A new method for the identification and enumeration of chicken heterophils and eosinophils. Avian Dis 1984;28:179–182.
13. **Lane R.** Basic techniques in pet avian clinical pathology. Vet Clin North Am Small Anim Pract 1991;21:1157–1179.
14. **Fudge AM.** Avian hematology identification and interpretation. Proc Annu Conf Assoc Avian Vet, Seattle, WA, 1989;284–292.
15. **Gross WB.** Differential and total avian blood cell counts by the hemacytometer method. Avian Exotic Pract 1984;1:31–36.
16. **Dein FJ.** Hematology. In: Harrison GJ, Harrison LR eds: Clinical avian medicine and surgery. Philadelphia: WB Saunders, 1986;174–191.
17. **Robertson GW, Maxwell MH.** Importance of optimal mixtures of EDTA anticoagulant: blood for the preparation of well-stained avian blood cells. Br Poult Sci 1993;34:615–617.
18. **Wiseman BK.** An improved direct method for obtaining the total white cell count in avian blood. Proc Soc Exp Biol Med 1931;28:1030–1033.
19. **Latimer KS.** Response to avian hematology letters. J Assoc Avian Vet 1991;5:121–124.
20. **Russo EA, McEntee L, Applegate L, Baker JS.** Comparison of two methods for determination of white blood cell counts in macaws. J Am Vet Med Assoc 1986;189:1013–1016.
21. **Swayne DE, Johnson GS.** Cytochemical properties of chicken blood cells resembling both thrombocytes and lymphocytes. Vet Clin Pathol 1986;15:17–24.
22. **Sturkie PD, Griminger P.** Blood: Physical characteristics, formed elements, hemoglobin, and coagulation. In: Sturkie PD, ed. Avian physiology. 3rd ed. New York: Springer-Verlag, 1976;65–70.
23. **Hamre CJ.** Origin and differentiation of heterophil, eosinophil and basophil leucocytes of chickens. Anat Rec 1952;112:339–340.
24. **Hawkey CM, Pugsley SL, Knight JA.** Abnormal heterophils in a king shag with aspergillosis. Vet Rec 1984;114:322–324.
25. **Latimer KS, Steffens WL, Goodwin M.** Ultrastructural changes in avian toxic heterophils. Proc 46th Annu Meet Electron Microscopic Society of America, San Francisco, California, 1988;360–361.
26. **Natt MP, Herrick CA.** Variations in the shape of the rod-like granules of the chicken heterophil leucocyte and its possible significance. Poult Sci 1954;33:828–830.
27. **Robertson GW, Maxwell MH.** Modified staining techniques for avian blood cells. Br Poult Sci 1990;31:881–886.
28. **Andreasen CB, Latimer KS.** Cytochemical staining characteristics of chicken heterophils and eosinophils. Vet Clin Pathol 1990;19:51–54.
29. **Weiss DJ.** Uniform evaluation and semiquantitative reporting of hematologic data in veterinary laboratories. Vet Clin Pathol 1984;13:27–31.
30. **Woerpel RW, Rosskopf WJ.** Clinical experience with avian diagnostics. Vet Clin North Am Small Anim Pract 1984;14:249–286.
31. **Clubb SL, Schubot RM, Joyner K, Zinkl JG, Wolf S, Escobar J, Clubb KJ, Kabbur MB.** Hematologic and serum biochemical reference intervals in juvenile eclectus parrots (Eclectus roratus). J Assoc Avian Vet 1990;4:218–225.
32. **Clubb SL, Schubot RM, Joyner K, Zinkl JG, Wolf S, Escobar J, Kabbur MB.** Hematologic and serum biochemical reference intervals in juvenile cockatoos. J Assoc Avian Vet 1991;5:16–26.
33. **Clubb SL, Schubot RM, Joyner K, Zinkl JG, Wolf S, Escobar J, Kabbur MB.** Hematologic and serum biochemical reference intervals in juvenile macaws (Ara sp.). J Assoc Avian Vet 1991;5:154–162.
34. **Hawkey C, Hart MG, Samour HJ, Knight JA, Hutton RE.** Haematological findings in healthy and sick captive rosy flamingos (Phoenicopterus ruber ruber). Avian Pathol 1984;13:163–172.
35. **Rosskopf WJ, Woerpel RW, Rosskopf G, Van De Water D.** Hematologic and blood chemistry values for Amazon parrots (Amazona spp.). Avian Exotic Pract 1984;1:30–33.
36. **Rosskopf WJ, Woerpel RW, Rosskopf G, Van De Water D.** Hematologic and blood chemistry values for the budgerigar. Calif Vet 1982;36:11–13.
37. **Tell LA, Citino SB.** Hematologic and serum chemistry reference intervals for Cuban amazon parrots (Amazona leucocephala leucocephala). J Zoo Wildl Med 1992;23:62–64.
38. **Ritchie BW, Harrison GJ, Harrison LR,** eds. Avian medicine: principles and application. Lake Worth: Wingers Publishing, 1994.
39. **Calle PP, Stewart CA.** Heamtologic and serum chemistry values of captive hyacinth macaws (Anodorhynchus hyacinthinus). J Zoo Anim Med 1987;18:98–99.
40. **Hawkey CM, Hart MG, Knight JA, Samour JH, Jones DM.** Haematological findings in healthy and sick African grey parrots (Psittacus erithacus). Vet Rec 1982;111:580–582.
41. **Hawkey C, Samour JH, Ashton DG, Hart MG, Cindery RN, Ffinch JM, Jones DM.** Normal and clinical haematology of captive cranes (Gruiformes). Avian Pathol 1983;12:73–84.
42. **Hawkey CM, Hart MG, Samour HJ.** Normal and clinical haematology of greater and lesser flamingos (Phoenicopterus roseus and Phoeniconaias minor). Avian Pathol 1985;14:537–541.
43. **Hawkey C, Samour HJ, Henderson GM, Hart MG.** Haematological findings in captive gentoo penguins (Pygoscelis papua) with bumblefoot. Avian Pathol 1985;14:251–256.
44. **Hoffman AM, Leighton FA.** Hemograms and microscopic lesions of herring gulls during captivity. J Am Vet Med Assoc 1985;187:1125–1128.
45. **Lane R.** Abnormal findings in avian hematology. Proc First Int Conf Zool Avian Med, Oahu, Hawaii, 1987;287–289.
46. **Lane RA, Rosskopf WJ, Allen KA.** Avian pediatric hematology: Preliminary studies of the transition from the neonatal hemogram to the adult hemogram in selected psittacine species: African greys, Amazons & macaws. Proc Annu Conf Assoc Avian Vet, Houston, Texas, 1988;231–238.
47. **Palomeque J, Pintó, Viscor G.** Hematologic and blood chemistry values of the Masai ostrich (Struthio camelus). J Wildlife Dis 1991;27:34–40.
48. **Peinado VI, Polo FJ, Viscor G, Palomeque J.** Haematology and blood chemistry values for several flamingo species. Avian Pathol 1992;21:55–64.
49. **Peinado VI, Polo FJ, Celdrán JF, Viscor G, Palomeque J.** Hematology and plasma chemistry in endangered pigeons. J Zoo Wildlife Med 1992;23:56–71.
50. **Maxwell MH.** Granulocyte differentiation in the lymphoid organs of chick embryos after antigenic and mitogenic stimulation. Dev Comp Immunol 1985;9:93–106.
51. **Riddell C.** Avian histopathology. 1st ed. Kennett Square, PA: American Association of Avian Pathologists, 1987.
52. **Schepelmann K.** Erythropoietic bone marrow in the pigeon: development of its distribution and volume during growth and pneumatization of bones. J Morphol 1990;203:21–34.
53. **Klasing KC.** Avian leukocytic cytokines. Poult Sci 1994;73:1035–1043.
54. **Kondo Y, Cahyaningsih U, Abe A, Tanabe A.** Presence of the diurnal rhythms of monocyte count and macrophage activities in chicks. Poult Sci 1992;71:296–301.
55. **Cahyaningsih U, Kondo Y, Abe A, Tanabe A.** The diurnal rhythms in lymphocyte counts and antibody formation in chicks. Jpn Poult Sci 1990;27:29–37.
56. **Cahyaningsih U, Kondo Y, Abe A, Tanabe A.** Presence of the diurnal rhythms of granulocyte counts and heterophil activities in chicks. Jpn Poult Sci 1990;27:281–290.
57. **Glick B.** Leukocyte count variation in young chicks during an 18 hour period. J Appl Physiol 1960;15:965.
58. **Maxwell MH.** Leucocyte diurnal rhythms in normal and pinealectomized juvenile female fowls. Res Vet Sci 1981;31:113–115.
59. **Cook RA, Moretti RA, Duffelmeyer JA.** Hematology of the white naped

crane (*Grus vipio*). Proc 1st Int Conf Zool Avian Med, Oahu, Hawaii, 1987;417–418.

60. **Burton R, Guion CW.** The differential leucocyte blood count: its precision and individuality in the chicken. Poult Sci 1968;47:1945–1949.

61. **Davison TF, Flack IH.** Changes in the peripheral blood leucocyte populations following an injection of corticotrophin in the immature chicken. Res Vet Sci 1981;30:79–82.

62. **Gross WB, Siegel HS.** Evaluation of the heterophil/lymphocyte ratio as a measure of stress in chickens. Avian Dis 1983;27:972–979.

63. **Gross WB, Siegel PB.** Effects of initial and second periods of fasting on heterophil/lymphocyte ratios and body weight. Avian Dis 1986; 30:345–346.

64. **Bienzle D, Pare JA, Smith DA.** Leukocyte changes in diseased non-domestic birds. Vet Clin Pathol 1997;26:76–84.

65. **Graham DL.** Histopathologic lesions associated with chlamydiosis in psittacine birds. J Am Vet Med Assoc 1989;195:1571–1573.

66. **Brune K, Leffell MS, Spitznagel JK.** Microbicidal activity of peroxidaseless chicken heterophile leukocytes. Infect Immun 1972;5:283–287.

67. **Brune K, Spitznagel JK.** Peroxidaseless chicken leukocytes: isolation and characterization of antibacterial granules. J Infect Dis 1973;127:84–94.

68. **Rausch P, Moore TG.** Granule enzymes of polymorphonuclear neutrophils: a phylogenetic comparison. Blood 1975;46:913–919.

69. **Harmon BG.** Avian heterophils in inflammation and disease resistance. Poult Sci 1998;77:972–977.

70. **Evans EW, Beach GG, Wunderlich J, Harmon BG.** Isolation of antimicrobial peptides from avian heterophils. J Leukocyte Biol 1994;56:661–665.

71. **Evans EW, Beach FG, Moore KM, Jackwood MW, Glisson JR, Harmon BG.** Antimicrobial activity of chicken and turkey heterophil peptides CHP1, CHP2, THP1, and THP3. Vet Microbiol 1995;47:295–303.

72. **Andreasen CB, Latimer KS, Steffens WL.** Evaluation of chicken heterophil adherence. Avian Dis 1990;34:639–642.

73. **Andreasen CB, Latimer KS, Harmon BG, Golden JM, Brown J.** Heterophil function in healthy chickens and in chickens with experimentally induced staphylococcal tenosynovitis. Vet Pathol 1991;28:419–427.

74. **Andreasen JR, Andreasen CB, Anwar M, Sonn AE.** Heterophil chemotaxis in chickens with natural staphylococcal infections. Avian Dis 1993; 37:284–289.

75. **Latimer KS, Harmon BG, Glisson JR, Kircher IM, Brown J.** Turkey heterophil chemotaxis to Pasteurella multocida (serotype 3,4)-generated chemotactic factors. Avian Dis 1990;34:137–140.

76. **Rosskopf WJ, Woerpel RW.** Pet avian hematology trends. Proc Annu Conf Assoc Avian Vet, Chicago, Illinois, 1991;98–111.

77. **Gross WB, Siegel PB, DuBose RT.** Some effects of feeding corticosterone to chickens. Poult Sci 1980;59:516–522.

78. **Davison TF, Rpwell JG, Rea J.** Effects of dietary corticosterone on peripheral blood lymphocyte and granulocyte populations in immature domestic fowl. Res Vet Sci 1983;34:236–239.

79. **Allan D, Duffus WPH.** The immunopathology in fowls (*Gallus domesticus*) of acute and subacute *Salmonella gallinarum* infection. Res Vet Sci 1971;12:140–151.

80. **Bounous DI, Schaeffer DO, Roy A.** Coagulase-negative *Staphylococcus* sp septicemia in a lovebird. J Am Vet Med Assoc 1989;195:1120–1122.

81. **Ficken MD, Barnes HJ.** Effect of cyclophosphamide on selected hematologic parameters of the turkey. Avian Dis 1988;32:812–817.

82. **Henderson GM, Gulland FMD, Hawkey CM.** Haematological findings in budgerigars with megabacterium and trichomonas infections associated with 'going light.' Vet Rec 1988;123:492–494.

83. **Maxwell MH.** Production of body anaemia in the domestic fowl after ingestion of dimethyl disulfide: a haematological and ultrastructural study. Res Vet Sci 1981;30:233–238.

84. **Leighton FA.** Clinical, gross, and histological findings in Herring gulls and Atlantic puffins that ingested Prudhoe Bay crude oil. Vet Pathol 1986;23:254–263.

85. **Rosskopf WJ, Woerpel RW, Howard EB, Holshuh HJ.** Chronic endocrine disorder associated with inclusion body hepatitis in a sulfur-crested cockatoo. J Am Vet Med Assoc 1981;179:1273–1276.

86. **Godwin JS, Jacobson ER, Gaskin JM.** Effects of Pacheco's parrot disease virus on hematologic and blood chemistry values of Quaker parrots (*Myopsitta monachus*). J Zoo Anim Med 1982;13:127–132.

87. **Ficken MD, Barnes HJ.** Effect of cyclophosphamide on selected hematologic parameters of the turkey. Avian Dis 1988;32:812–817.

88. **Fulton RM, Reed WM, Thacker HL, DeNicola DB.** Cyclophosphamide (Cytoxan)- induced hematologic alterations in specific-pathogen-free chickens. Avian Dis 1996;40:1–12.

89. **Rosskopf WJ, Woerpel RW.** Avian diagnosis: laboratory interpretations and case reports, part 3. Companion Anim Pract 1989;19:41–48.

90. **Nowak JS, Kai O, Peck R, Franklin RM.** The effects of cyclosporin A on the chicken immune system. Eur J Immunol 1982;12:867–876.

91. **Sijtsma SR, Rambout JHWM, Kiepurski A, West CE, van der Zijpp AJ.** Changes in lymphoid organs and blood lymphocytes induced by vitamin A deficiency and Newcastle disease virus infection in chickens. Dev Comp Immunol 1991;15:349–356.

92. **Newell SM, McMillan MC, Moore FM.** Diagnosis and treatment of lymphocytic leukemia and malignant lymphoma in a Pekin duck (*Anas platyrhynchos domesticus*). J Assoc Avian Vet 1991;5:83–86.

93. **Gregory CR, Latimer KS, Mahaffey EA, Doker T.** Lymphoma and leukemic blood picture in an emu (*Dromaius novaehollandiae*). Vet Clin Pathol 1996;25:136–139.

94. **Holt PS.** Effects of induced moulting on immune responses of hens. Br Poult Sci 1992;33:165–175.

95. **McEntee MF, Ficken MD.** Blood clearance of radiolabeled gold colloid by the turkey mononuclear phagocytic system. Avian Dis 1990;34:393–397.

96. **Carlson HC, Allen JR.** The acute inflammatory reaction in chicken skin: blood cellular response. Avian Dis 1969;14:817–833.

97. **Odend'hal S, Player EC.** Histochemical localization of T-cells in tissue sections. Avian Dis 1980;24:886–895.

98. **Campbell TW, Coles EH.** Avian clinical pathology. In: Coles EH, ed. Veterinary clinical pathology. 4th ed. Philadelphia: WB Saunders, 1986;279–301.

99. **Wight PAL, Dewar WA, MacKenzie GM.** Monocytosis in experimental zinc deficiency of domestic birds. Avian Pathol 1980;9:61–66.

100. **Rosskopf WJ, Woerpel RW.** Avian diagnosis: laboratory interpretations and case reports, part 1. Companion Anim Pract 1988;2:24–28.

101. **Gross WB:** Blood cultures, blood counts and temperature records in an experimentally produced "air sac disease" and uncomplicated *Escherichia coli* infection of chickens. Poult Sci 1961;41:691–700.

102. **McNulty MS.** Chicken anemia agent: a review. Avian Pathol 1991;20:187–203.

103. **Averbeck C.** Haematology and blood chemistry of healthy and clinically abnormal Great Black-backed Gulls (*Larus marinus*) and Herring Gulls (*Larus argentatus*). Avian Pathol 1992;21:215–223.

104. **Marone G, Casolaro V, Cirillo R, Stellato C, Genovese A.** Pathophysiology of human basophils and mast cells in allergic disorders. Clin Immunol Immunopathol 1989;50:S24–S40.

105. **Awadhiya RP, Vegad JL, Kolte GN.** A microscopic study of increased vascular permeability and leucocyte emigration in thermal injury in the chicken skin. Avian Pathol 1981;10:313–320.

106. **Awadhiya RP, Vegad JL, Kolte GN.** Microscopic study of increased permeability and leucocyte emigration in the chicken wing web. Res Vet Sci 1981;31:231–235.

107. **Chand N, Carlson HC, Eyre P.** Passive cutaneous anaphylaxis in domestic fowl. Int Arch Allergy Immunol 1975;51:508–517.

108. **Nair MK:.** The early inflammatory reaction in the fowl. A light microscopical, ultrastructural and autoradiographic study. Acta Vet Scand Suppl 1973;42:1–13.

109. **Stadecker MJ, Lukic M, Dvorak A, Leskowitz S.** The cutaneous basophil response to phytohemagglutinin in chickens. J Immunol 1977;118:1564–1568.

110. **McCorkle F, Olah I, Glick B.** The morphology of the phytohemagglutinin-induced cell response in the chicken's wattle. Poult Sci 1980;59:616–623.

111. **Carlson HC.** The acute inflammatory reaction in chicken breast muscle. Avian Dis 1972;16:553–558.

112. **Awadhiya RP, Vegad JL, Kolte GN.** Studies on acute inflammation in the chicken using mesentery as a test system. Res Vet Sci 1980;29:172–180.

113. **Chand N, Eyre P.** Rapid method for basophil count in domestic fowl. Avian Dis 1978;22:639–645.

114. **Ferris M, Bacha WJ.** Response of leukocytes in chickens infected with the avian schistosome *Austrobilharzia variglandis* (Trematoda). Avian Dis 1986;30:683–686.

115. **Dusbabek F, Skarkovaspakova V, Vitovec J, Sterba J.** Cutaneous and blood leucocyte response of pigeons to larval *Argas polonicus* feeding. Polia Parasitologica 1988;35:259–268.

116. **Woerpel RW, Rosskopf WJ, Monahan-Brennan M.** Clinical pathology and laboratory diagnostic tools. In: Burr EW, ed. Companion bird medicine. Ames, IA: Iowa State University Press, 1987;180–196.

117. **Burton AL, Higginbotham RD.** Response to blood basophils to Rous sarcoma virus infection in chicks and its significance. J Reticulo-Endothelial Society 1966;3:314–326.

118. **Dhodapkar BS, Vegad JL, Kolte GN.** Demonstration of the phagocytic activity of chicken basophils in the reversed Arthus reaction using colloidal carbon. Res Vet Sci 1982;33:377–379.

119. **Maxwell MH, Robertson GW, Spence S, McCorquodale CC.** Comparison of haematological values in restricted- and *ad libitum*-fed domestic fowls: White blood cells and thrombocytes. Br Poult Sci 1990;31:399–405.

120. **Maxwell MH, Hocking PM, Robertson GW.** Differential leucocyte responses to various degrees of food restriction in broilers, turkeys, and ducks. Br Poult Sci 1992;33:177–187.

121. **Nordio C, Rosi F.** Possible significance of the increase of basophils in blood differential count of farm animals. Atti Societa Italiana Scienze Veterinarie 1979;32:254.

122. **Rosi F, Nordio C.** Observations on the increase of basophils in leucocyte differential count of farm animals. La Clinica Veterinaria 1979;102:353–371.

123. **Latimer KS.** Diseases affecting leukocytes. In: Colahan PT, et al, eds. Equine medicine and surgery, vol 2. 4th ed. Goleta, CA: American Veterinary Publications, 1991;1809–1815.

124. **Maxwell MH, Siller WG, MacKenzie GM.** Eosinophilia associated with facial oedema in fowls. Vet Rec 1979;105:232–233.

125. **Maxwell MH, Burns RB.** Blood eosinophilia in adult bantams naturally infected with *Trichostrongylus tenuis*. Res Vet Sci 1985;39:122–123.

126. **Maxwell MH, Burns RB.** Experimental eosinophilia in domestic fowls and ducks following horse serum stimulation. Vet Res Commun 1982;5:369–376.

127. **Maxwell MH.** Ultrastructural and cytochemical studies in normal Japanese quail (*Coturnix coturnix japonica*) eosinophils and in those from birds with experimentally induced eosinophilia. Res Vet Sci 1986;41:149–161.

128. **Maxwell MH.** Fine structural and cytochemical studies of eosinophils from fowls and ducks with eosinophilia. Res Vet Sci 1986;41:135–148.

129. **Maxwell MH, Burns RB.** Experimental stimulation of eosinophil production in the domestic fowl (*Gallus gallus domesticus*). Res Vet Sci 1986;41:114–123.

CHAPTER 61

Fish Leukocyte Responses

• EDWARD J. NOGA

The leukocyte response is one of the most useful clinical tools in veterinary medicine and is a cornerstone of baseline health analysis. Although the leukocyte (white blood cell [WBC]) count also can be used as a clinical tool in aquatic medicine, the clinician must be aware of impediments that may limit its reliable interpretation.[1] The most important biological factor limiting accurate WBC analysis is the tremendous variation in types, numbers, and appearance of leukocytes in different fish species. Also, fish are highly affected by their environment and normal differences in water quality, especially temperature, also can affect the leukogram. Iatrogenic changes in the leukogram are a serious concern in terms of evaluation. Acute stress can cause a significant change in the WBC count.[2] These changes can be extremely rapid. For example, cold shock induces leukopenia within 3 minutes in mummichog minnows.[3] Stress often affects osmoregulation. The resulting hemoconcentration or hemodilution may alter leukocyte concentrations. Thus, samples from fish that have been collected at the clinic, rather than being sampled directly on site, should be interpreted cautiously.

The considerable variation in reported leukocyte values from healthy fish, even within a species, is also partly caused by differences in methodology as well as in investigator interpretation of cell types. All cells in peripheral blood of fish (including erythrocytes and thrombocytes, the platelet analog) are nucleated, preventing the use of automated cell counting. Even many peer-reviewed, experimental studies of leukocyte responses have used somewhat inaccurate measurements of total cell counts such as buffy coat thickness (leukocrit) or estimated cell counts from stained blood smears. This is caused in large part by the problem of differentiating various leukocyte types in stained cell suspensions with a hemacytometer,[4] which is needed to obtain an accurate count.

Improper sample handling can cause problems in cell identification. For example, prolonged blood storage before preparing smears causes thrombocytes to round up, making them difficult to distinguish from lymphocytes. Prolonged storage also may lead to other artifacts, such as cytoplasmic vacuolation or apparent pseudopodia.[4] Immature leukocytes and erythrocytes are common in peripheral blood,[4] adding to the confusion in cell identification. Although species-specific lymphocyte and granulocyte markers (antibodies) have been developed for a small number of fish species (e.g., trout, catfish, carp), they are not commercially available. There are no universal markers for specific fish leukocyte types that could allow their definitive differentiation. Special cytochemical stains for various cell types can be used. However, this is not routinely feasible in a clinical practice. There also is considerable variability in the cytochemical staining properties of different cell types among fish species.

FISH LEUKOCYTES TYPES

Fish possess the same major types of peripheral blood leukocytes as observed in higher vertebrates, namely, lymphocytes, monocytes, and granulocytes.[4] These leukocytes often possess the same morphology and physiologic functions of analagous cell types in mammals. However, as mentioned previously, there is significant variability in the morphology of fish leukocytes from one species to another. For commercially important aquaculture species, such as salmonids (salmon, trout), channel catfish, or cyprinids (carp, koi, goldfish), the cell types are fairly well defined. In contrast, the overwhelming majority of fish species (over 40,000 described to date) are not well studied, and most have never been studied. Thus, confident use of the leukogram in clinical diagnosis may require the establishment of baseline data from healthy individuals to allow any rational interpretations. Because of the considerable leukocyte variation in different environments, it is also advisable to have data on individuals from the specific site (e.g., farm) being examined. This may be justified in the case of large commercial aquaculture operations or for experimental research protocols, but it is not feasible for a single, sporadic case seen in practice.

Another limitation is that in many cases, description of cell types is solely based on morphologic criteria (e.g., staining reaction with Romanowsky-type stain). The similar appearance of totally unrelated cell types (e.g., lymphocytes and thrombocytes; monocytes and granulocytes) makes leukocyte identification a serious problem for the microscopist. It is important to realize that cell function should be the primary characteristic of importance in identifying blood cell types, whereas morphology is simply a useful tool for making these distinctions between cells with different functions. Resolution of this problem will probably never be complete until the stem cells responsible for each cell lineage in fish are defined.

MONONUCLEAR CELLS

Lymphocytes

Lymphocytes are responsible for typical B- and T-cell-mediated specific immune responses in fish, including antibody production and specific cell-mediated immunity. Fish lymphocytes have specialized properties like those in lymphocytes of higher vertebrates, including responsiveness to cytokines and mitogens. Lymphocytes usually are the most abundant leukocytes in peripheral blood and are the most sensitive leukocyte to stress.

Fish lymphocytes resemble those of birds and mammals. They are typically round with a high nuclear-to-cytoplasmic ratio. The scant, homogeneous, blue cytoplasm surrounds a dark purple nucleus with coarsely clumped chromatin. Red cytoplasmic granules may be seen occasionally. Lymphocytes vary in size from one third to nearly equal in size to erythrocytes. Larger lymphocytes tend to have a larger proportion of cytoplasm.

Monocytes

Monocytes often are present in the peripheral blood of fish. They are avid phagocytes and are influenced by cytokines. They probably also participate in many specific immune responses. Mononuclear phagocytes are common in chronic inflammation (e.g., mycobacteriosis, bacterial kidney disease), but their relation to changes in the leukogram is less well defined. Monocytes are usually less abundant than lymphocytes or granulocytes. They are large cells with blue gray to blue cytoplasm that usually occupies at least half the cell volume. The variably shaped nucleus may be round to oval and often is indented. Unlike lymphocytes, the chromatin is not coarsely clumped but is rather granular.

GRANULOCYTES

Neutrophils

The neutrophil (also referred to as the heterophil) is the most common fish granulocyte and has been identified in most fish species that have been examined.[5] The primary role of the neutrophil in the mammalian immune response is phagocytosis and destruction of foreign agents. Neutrophil phagocytosis has been demonstrated in many fish species. Neutrophils are often the first cells to respond within the first 24 hours of an acute insult.[6]

The fish neutrophil is typically round to oval with an eccentric nucleus. In some species, the nucleus may be lobated, but this is not a consistent finding. More typically, the nucleus is round to oval with an indentation. The chromatin is coarsely clumped and stains dark purple. The cytoplasm is typically pale gray and has granules that stain variably (gray to blue to red), depending on cell maturity. As many as four subtypes of neutrophils have been described for some fish species, making the literature even more confusing.[5]

Eosinophils and Basophils

So-called eosinophilic granular cells are normally resident in various tissues of many fish and may accumulate in certain inflammatory processes, especially in response to parasite infections.[5] However, true circulating eosinophils or basophils have only been observed in a small number of species. The most characteristic feature of the eosinophil is rod-shaped or spherical granules. Basophils are even rarer than eosinophils.

Thrombocytes

Thrombocytes are not true leukocytes. However, they must be differentiated from leukocytes to obtain an accurate WBC count. In addition, some disease processes in fish have been associated with abnormal thrombocyte numbers. Thrombocytes are pleiomorphic and may be round, oblong, fusiform, or dumbbell shaped. The method of blood smear preparation has a large influence on morphology. For example, thrombocytes in freshly prepared smears often appear different from those in older samples. Being the platelet analog, they clump in poorly prepared smears or sometimes in stressed fish. The nucleus has dark purple, densely clumped chromatin. The cytoplasm is colorless to light blue.

FISH LEUKOCYTE RESPONSE CHARACTERISTICS

General Response to Stress

Change in leukocyte numbers is a sensitive indicator of stress in fish.[2] Although the response to environmental insults varies with the type and severity of the stress, it often leads to a leukopenia associated with lymphopenia and sometimes neutrophilia, which is similar to the classic leukocytic response to stress in mammals. Leukopenia has been associated with stress imposed by several

TABLE 61.1 Leukocyte Responses of Fish to Various Noninfectious and Infectious Diseases: Management/Environment

Species	Stressor	Total Leukocytes	Lymphocytes	Monocytes	Granulocytes	Thrombocytes	Other	References
Mummichog	Cold shock	decr						(3)
Channel catfish	Transport	decr	decr		incr			(7)
Channel catfish	Temperature	nc	nc	nc	nc			(8)
Channel catfish	Season	nc	nc	nc	nc			(8)
Striped bass	Season (fall-winter)	incr						(9)
Hybrid striped bass	High temperature	nc	decr					(10)
Snakehead	Starvation	decr						(11)
Dab	Restraint		decr			decr	inc "phagocytes"	(12)
Atlantic salmon/sea trout	Smoltification	incr	incr					(13)
Chinook salmon	Handling	incr	incr					(14)
Brown trout	Handling	decr	decr		nc	nc		(15)
Rainbow trout	Surgery	decr						(16)
Rainbow trout/coho salmon	Crowding + high temperature	decr						(17)
Rainbow trout	Chronic crowding		decr		nc	decr		(18)
Spiny dogfish shark	Confinement	decr						(19)

incr = increase; decr = decrease; nc = no change.
Data from references 3, 7–19 with permission.

TABLE 61.2 Leukocyte Responses of Fish to Various Noninfectious and Infectious Diseases: Toxins

Species	Toxin	Total Leukocytes	Lymphocytes	Monocytes	Granulocytes	Thrombocytes	Other	References
Spiny dogfish shark	Copper	decr						(20)
Spiny dogfish shark	Zinc	incr						(19)
Rosy barb	Cadmium		incr	incr	decr	decr	"basophilia"	(21)
American eel	Cadmium	incr						(22)
Rainbow trout	Pulp mill effluent	decr						(17)
Rainbow trout	Benzo-(a)-pyrene	nc			nc	nc		(23)
Rainbow trout	ozone	decr						(24)

incr = increase; decr = decrease; nc = no change.
Data from references 17, 19–24 with permission.

TABLE 61.3 Leukocyte Responses of Fish to Various Noninfectious and Infectious Diseases: Viral Infections

Species	Disease	Total Leukocytes	Lymphocytes	Monocytes	Granulocytes	Thrombocytes	Other	References
Salmonids	Infectious hematopoetic necrosis (IHN)	decr						(25)
Salmonids	Viral hemorrhagic septicemia (VHS)	decr						(25)
Carp	Spring viremia of carp (SVC)	decr						(25)

incr = increase; decr = decrease; nc = no change.
Data from Wolf K. The viruses and viral diseases of fish. Ithaca, NY: Cornell University Press, 1988, with permission.

TABLE 61.4 Leukocyte Responses of Fish to Various Noninfectious and Infectious Diseases: Bacterial Infections

Species	Disease	Total Leukocytes	Lymphocytes	Monocytes	Granulocytes	Thrombocytes	Other	References
Goldfish	*Aeromonas hydrophila*		decr	incr	incr			(26)
Channel catfish	*Aeromonas/Flexibacter*		decr		incr			(8)
Salmonids	Furunculosis (*Aeromonas salmonicida*)	decr						(27)
Salmonids	Enteric redmouth (*Yersinia ruckeri*)	decr	decr	incr	incr	decr		(28)
Channel catfish	Enteric septicemia (*Edwardsiella ictaluri*)	decr						(29)
Rainbow trout/Atlantic salmon/coho salmon	Bacterial kidney disease	incr		incr	incr	incr		(30–32)
Salmonids	*Piscirickettsia salmonis*			incr	incr			(33, 34)

incr = increase; decr = decrease; nc = no change
Data from references 8, 26–34 with permission

TABLE 61.5 Leukocyte Responses of Fish to Various Noninfectious and Infectious Diseases: Fungal/Parasitic Infections

Species	Disease	Total Leukocytes	Lymphocytes	Monocytes	Granulocytes	Thrombocytes	Other	References
Brown trout	Water mold		decr		decr			(35)
Atlantic salmon	Water mold (*Saprolegnia*) and sea louse (*Salmincola*)	incr						(36)
Carp	Ich	nc	decr		incr		basophilia	(37)
Channel catfish	Ich		decr		incr			(8)
Rainbow trout	Proliferative kidney disease	nc						(38)
Rainbow trout	*Cryptobia*	nc			incr	nc		(39)
Stinging catfish	Digenean worm	incr			incr		incr granuloblasts	(40)

incr = increase; decr = decrease; nc = no change
Data from references 8, 35–40 with permission.

factors, including high temperature, temperature shock, crowding, transport, confinement, and some toxins (Tables 61.1 to 61.5).[3,7–40] Even brief stresses (less than 1 minute of handling) may cause a transient lymphopenia.[2]

Response to Infectious Disease

One must be cautious in making broad generalizations about leukocyte responses to various infectious diseases of fish, because studies have been sporadic and in some cases contradictory. However, a fairly consistent leukocyte response is seen to certain rhabdoviral infections, such as infectious hemopoietic necrosis, spring viremia of carp, and viral hemorrhagic septicemia, which cause severe leukopenia caused by damage of the hemopoietic organs.[8] Leukopenia also has been associated with many gram-negative bacterial infections, including *Aeromonas, Yersinia,* and *Edwardsiella* spp. (Table 61.2). Both lymphopenia and neutrophilia have been reported in some of these infections. Leukocytic responses to parasites are variable. Eosinophilia has not been reported as a feature of parasitosis, although eosinophillike cells are often seen in inflammatory responses to metazoan parasites.[5]

SUMMARY

Complete blood counts are most useful in assessing the health of fish species in which the leukogram has been well characterized and for which blood samples are fresh and collected without iatrogenic stress. It is also advisable that a good history of the normal baseline blood values for the affected population (e.g., fish farm or natural water body) be available, which will allow the clinician to compare values to what is normal for that population. Although the WBC count also can be used in less ideal situations (especially if there are profound deviations from the normal state), it must be interpreted more cautiously because of increased technical and biological variables.

REFERENCES

 1. **Klontz GW.** Fish hematology. In: Stolen JS, Fletcher TC, Rowley AF, Zelikoff JT, Kaattari SL, Smith SA, eds. Techniques in fish immunology-3. Fair Haven: SOS Publications, 1994;121–131.
 2. **Barton BA, Iwama GK.** Physiological changes in fish from stress in aquaculture with emphasis on the response and effects of corticosteroids. Ann Rev Fish Dis 1991;1:3–26.
 3. **Pickford GE, Srivastava AK, Slicher AM, Pang PKT.** The stress response in the abundance of circulating leukocytes in the killifish, *Fundulus heteroclitus.* J Exp Zool 1971;177:89–96.
 4. **Rowley AF, Hunt TC, Page M, Mainwaring G.** Fish. In: Rowley AF, Ratcliffe NA, eds. Vertebrate blood cells. Cambridge: Cambridge University Press, 1988;19–127.
 5. **Ainsworth AJ.** Fish granulocytes: Morphology, distribution and function. Ann Rev Fish Dis 1992;2:123–148.
 6. **Suzuki Y, Iida T.** Fish granulocytes in the process of inflammation. Ann Rev Fish Dis 1992; 2:149–160.
 7. **Ellsaesser C, Clem LW.** Hematological and immunological changes in channel catfish stressed by handling and transport. J Fish Biol 1986;28:511–521.
 8. **Ellsaesser CF, Miller NW, Cuchens MA, Lobb CJ, Clem LW.** Analysis of channel catfish peripheral blood leucocytes by brightfield microscopy and flow cytometry. Trans Am Fish Soc 1985;114:279–285.
 9. **Lochmiller RL, Weichman JD, Zale AV.** Hematological assessment of temperature and oxygen stress in a reservoir population of striped bass (*Morone saxatilis*). Comp Biochem Physiol 1989;93A:535–541.
10. **Carlson RE, Baker EP, Fuller RE.** Immunological assessment of hybrid striped bass at three culture temperatures. Fish Shellfish Immunol 1995;5:359–373.
11. **Raizada MN, Singh CP.** Effect of starvation on the blood of *Ophiocephalus punctatus* (Bloch). Experientia 1981;37:1206–1207.
12. **Pulsford AL, Lemaire-Gony S, Tomlinson M, Collingwood N, Glynn PJ.** Effects of acute stress on the immune system of the dab, *Limanda limanda.* Comp Biochem Physiol 1994;109C:129–139.
13. **Muona M, Soivio A.** Changes in plasma lysozyme and blood leucocyte levels of hatchery-reared Atlantic salmon (*Salmo salar* L.) and sea trout (*Salmo trutta* L.) during parr-smolt transformation. Aquacult 1992;106:75–87.
14. **Salonius K, Iwama GK.** Effects of early rearing environment on stress response, immune function, and disease resistance in juvenile coho (*Oncorhynchus kisutch*) and chinook salmon (*O. tshawytscha*). Can J Fish Aquatic Sci 1992;50:759–766.
15. **Pickering AD, Pottinger TG, Christie P.** Recovery of the brown trout, *Salmo trutta* L., from acute handling stress: A time-course study. J Fish Biol 1982;20:229–244.
16. **Bry C, Zohar Y.** Dorsal aorta catheterization in rainbow trout *Salmo gairdneri* 2. Glucocorticoid levels, hematological data and resumption of feeding for 5 days after surgery. Reprod Nutr Dev 1980;20:1825–1834.
17. **McLeay DJ, Gordon MR.** Leucocrit: A simple hematological technique for measuring acute stress in salmonid fish including stressful concentrations of pulpmill effluent. J Fish Res Bd Can 1977;34:2164–2175.
18. **Pickering AD, Pottinger TG.** Crowding causes prolonged leucopenia in salmonid fish, despite interrenal acclimation. J Fish Biol 1987;30:701–712.
19. **Torres P, Tort L, Planas J, Flos R.** Effects of confinement stress and additional zinc treatment on some blood parameters in the dogfish *Scyliorhinus canicula.* Comp Biochem Physiol 1986;83C:89–92.
20. **Tort L, Torres P, Flos R.** Effects on dogfish haematology and liver composition after acute copper exposure. Comp Biochem Physiol 1987;87C:349–353.
21. **Gill TS, Pant JC.** Erythrocytic and leukocytic responses to cadmium poisoning in a freshwater fish, *Puntius conchionus* (Ham). Environ Res 1985;36:327–337.
22. **Gill TS, Epple A.** Stress-related changes in the hematological profile of the American eel (*Anguilla rostrata*). Ecotoxicol Environ Saf 1993;25:227–235.
23. **Walczak BZ, Blunt BR, Hodson PV.** Phagocytic function of monocytes and hematological changes in rainbow trout injected intraperitoneally with benzo-a-pyrene B-A-P and benzo-a-anthrcene B-A-A. J Fish Biol 1987;31 (suppl A):251–253.
24. **Wedemeyer GA, Nelson NC, Yasutake WT.** Physiological and biochemical aspects of ozone toxicity to rainbow trout (*Salmo gairdneri*). J Fish Res Bd Can 1979;36:605–614.
25. **Wolf K.** The viruses and viral diseases of fish. Ithaca, NY: Cornell University Press, 1988.
26. **Brenden RA, Huizinga HW.** Pathophysiology of experimental *Aeromonas hydrophila* infection in goldfish, *Carassius auratus* (L.). J Fish Dis 1986;9:163–167.
27. **Munro ALS, Hastings TS.** Furunculosis. In: Inglis V, Roberts RJ, Bromage NA, eds. Bacterial diseases of fish. New York: John Wiley and Sons, 1993;122–142.
28. **Lehmann J, Sturenberg F-J, Mock D.** The changes in haemogram of rainbow trout (*Salmo gairdneri* Richardson) to an artifical and natural challenge with *Yersinia ruckeri.* J Appl Ichthyol 1987;3:174–183.
29. **Areechon N, Plumb JA.** Pathogenesis of *Edwardsiella ictaluri* in channel catfish, *Ictalurus punctatus.* J World Maricult Soc 1983;14:249–260.
30. **Bruno DW, Munro ALS.** Hematological assessment of rainbow trout *Salmo gairdneri* and Atlantic salmon *Salmo salar* infected with *Renibacterium salmoninarum.* J Fish Dis 1986;9:195–204.
31. **Iwama GK, Greer GL, Randall DJ.** Changes in selected hematological parameters in juvenile chinook salmon subjected to a bacterial challenge and a toxicant. J Fish Biol 1986;28:563–572.
32. **Suzumoto BK, Schreck CB, McIntyre JD.** Relative resistances of 3 transferrin genotypes of coho salmon *Oncorhynchus kisutch* and ther hematological responses to bacterial kidney disease. J Fish Res Bd Can 1977;34:1–8.
33. **Branson EJ, Diaz-Munoz DN.** Description of a new disease condition occurring farmed coho salmon, *Oncorhynchus kisutch* (Walbaum) in South America. J Fish Dis 1991;14:147–156
34. **Cvitanich JD, Garate NO, Smith CE.** The isolation of a rickettsia-like organism causing disease and mortality in Chilean salmonids and its confirmation by Koch's postulates. J.Fish Dis 1991;14:121–145.
35. **Alvarez F, Razquin B, Villena A, Lopez Fierro P, Zapata A.** Alterations in peripheral lymphoid organs and differential leukocyte counts in *Saprolegnia-*

infected brown trout, *Salmo trutta fario*. Vet Immunol Immunopathol 1988;18:181–193.

36. **Johnson C, Gray RW, McLennan A, Paterson A.** Effects of photoperiod, temperature and diet on the reconditioning response, blood chemistry and gonad maturation of Atlantic salmon kelts *Salmo salar* held in freshwater. Can J Fish Aquatic Sci 1987;44:702–711.

37. **Hines RS, Spira DT.** Ichthyophthiriasis in mirror carp II. Leukocyte response. J Fish Biol 1973;5:527–534.

38. **Hoffman R, Lommel R.** Hematological studies in proliferative kidney disease of rainbow trout *Salmo gairdneri*. J Fish Dis 1984;7:323–326.

39. **Lowe-Jinde L.** Hematological changes in *Cryptobia* infection in rainbow trout *Salmo gairdneri*. Can J Zool 1986;64:1352–1355.

40. **Murad A, Mustafa S.** Blood parameters of catfish, *Heteropneustes fossilis* (Bloch), parasitized by metacercariae of *Diplostomulum* sp. J Fish Dis 1988;11:365–368.

SECTION VI

Hemostasis: Platelets—
Platelet Structure and Function

Fern Tablin

CHAPTER 62

Megakaryocytes

• ROBERT M. LEVEN

MEGAKARYOCYTOPOIESIS

Megakaryocyte Progenitors

Clinicians first analyzed megakaryocyte (MK) progenitors by taking advantage of the fact that in some species (cat, dog, rat, and mouse) acetylcholine esterase is a specific marker of the megakaryocytic lineage.[1] Small acetylcholine positive cells were identified as late MK progenitors.[2] The enzyme activity is found in the Golgi apparatus of immature cells and membrane that gives rise to the platelet-dense tubular system in more mature MKs.[2]

Like other hemopoietic cells, MKs arise by the commitment of multipotential progenitor cells. MKs develop from CD34+ myeloid cells that are resident in hemopoietic tissue and circulate in the blood.[3] Different subpopulations of CD34+ cells represent MK progenitors at different levels of maturation. CD34+/CD38− cells may contain more primitive progenitors,[4] whereas CD34+/CD38+ cells contain more mature, short-term MK progenitors.[5] Two percent of CD34+ cells also express specific MK markers. As MK progenitors mature, they acquire MK-specific markers, such as glycoprotein (GP)IIb-IIIa and GPIb, but lose CD34+ expression.[6] The development of CD34+ cells into MKs in vitro requires stimulation by growth factors. Interleukin (IL) -3, IL-6, IL-11, stem cell factor (SCF), Flt-3 ligand, and thrombopoietin (TPO) have been used in various combinations to stimulate the development of MKs from CD34+ cells.[7-10]

MK colonies grown in culture were first described by Metcalf et al[11] and can develop from a multipotent progenitor as part of a mixed colony of granulocytic, erythroid, macrophage, and MKs (colony-forming unit-granulocyte, erythroid, monocyte, megakaryocyte [CFU-GEMM]) or as a pure MK colony.[12] Pure colonies may arise from the CFU-MK or the more primitive burst-forming unit-MK (BFU-MK). The precise relationship of MK colony-forming cells and CD34+ cells committed to megakaryocytopoiesis is not clear. Quantitation of multipotent progenitor-cell commitment to the megakaryocytic lineage can be determined from changes in the number of CFU-MK or BFU-MK. In vivo, the number of CFU-MK and the ploidy (DNA content) of CFU-

MK-derived MKs increases in response to thrombocytopenia.[13] Therefore, recruitment of more progenitors into the MK lineage is part of the response to thrombocytopenia. In vitro, the addition of several growth factors, including IL-3, IL-6, IL-11, and TPO increases the number of CFU-MK that develop from marrow cells and the size and maturation of MKs in colonies.

Megakaryocyte Morphology

Once MK progenitors are recognizable in a marrow smear, a series of well-defined cytoplasmic changes have already occurred. MKs are classified into three stages with the following characteristics observed in Wright–Giemsa stained marrow smears (Fig. 62.1). **Stage I** is a cell of 15 to 50 μm in diameter. The nucleus can be circular, oval, or an indented kidney shape. The cytoplasm is a relatively regular rim of approximately 5 μm, which shows intense basophilia as the result of abundant ribosomes.(Fig. 62.1A) **Stage II** is slightly larger than Stage I, as much as approximately 75 μm. Nuclear morphology is similar to Stage I, although there may be increased lobulation. The cytoplasm, of greater volume than the Stage I cell, is polychromatophilic, and azurophilic granules also may be observed (Fig 62.1B). **Stage III** is the completely mature MK, with a diameter of as much as 150 μm. The nucleus is lobulated with thin bands of chromatin connecting lobules. The cytoplasm is variable in volume; however, on the average, it is larger than Stage II, and staining is completely eosinophilic with numerous azurophilic granules (Fig. 62.1C). The regulation of MK size is complex. Average MK size increases as maturation progresses, but size is also proportional to ploidy. Despite this relation between size and ploidy, it has been demonstrated that size can be regulated independent of ploidy or cytoplasmic maturation.[14]

By observation of tritiated thymidine incorporation into rat MKs in vivo, Ebbe and Stohlman[15] showed that DNA synthesis, and consequently the development of polyploidy is almost complete before progenitors become recognizable as MKs. Only a small percent of Stage I MKs are capable of DNA synthesis, most have reached their final ploidy level. Normally, the ploidy distribution

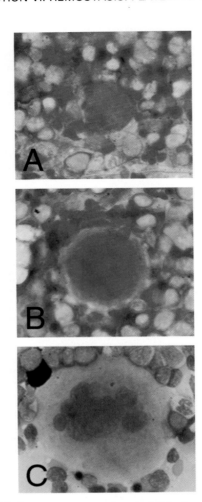

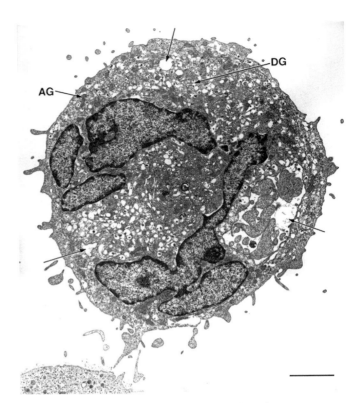

FIGURE 62.2 Demonstrates the organization of a mature guinea pig MK. Dense granules (DG) and alpha granules (AG) are distributed throughout the cytoplasm. In the perinuclear zone there is an extensive Golgi system (G). DMS (→) is present throughout the cell, and areas of dilated DMS represent sites of DMS fusion and eventual process formation. Photograph donated by Dr. Fern Tablin.

FIGURE 62.1 **A**. Stage I MK. Note the bilobed nucleus with basophilic cytoplasm, evidence of the abundant rough endoplasmic reticulum and prominent ribosomes. **B**. Stage II MK. The cell volume has increased and a peripheral zone devoid of organelles except ribosomes is present. A multilobulated nucleus is present. **C**. Stage III MK. This large, polyploid cell has abundant eosinophilic cytoplasm, which, by electron microscopy, contains an extensive demarcation membrane system along with α and dense granules.

is approximately log normal with a peak at 16N and most mature MKs having from 8N to as many as 32N, although values of as much as 128N may occur, especially in cattle.[16] Consequently, it was found that cytoplasmic maturation occurs after the development of polyploidy is complete, and occurs in MKs of all ploidy classes above 4N. This study also demonstrated that the three stages of megakaryocytopoiesis are chronologically sequential stages of maturation and that there is independent regulation of ploidy and cytoplasmic maturation.

Mature Megakaryocytes

MKs comprise approximately 0.1 to 0.5% of nucleated marrow cells. Both mature and immature MKs are located adjacent to vascular sinuses in the marrow.[17] The cytoplasm of the mature MK is typically divided into three zones (Fig. 62.2): a peripheral organelle poor zone, an intermediate zone, and a perinuclear zone. The peripheral zone, inconsistent in size and form, is characterized by a lack of membrane-bound organelles, but it contains many microfilaments and some glycogen particles. Rarely, the connection of the demarcation membrane system with the plasma membrane is observed in the peripheral zone. This zone may be entirely absent in MKs that appear to be near platelet formation or may form pseudopods that can be mistaken for platelet formation. The intermediate zone, which is the majority of the cytoplasm, is dominated by the demarcation membrane system (DMS).[18] The structural and immunochemical similarities of the DMS and platelet plasma membrane support the hypothesis that the DMS is the precursor pool for the platelet plasma membrane.[19,20] In addition to the DMS, a separate membrane system that becomes the dense tubular system of platelets develops during the cytoplasmic maturation of MKs. The intermediate zone also contains lysosomes, ribosomes, mitochondria, microtubules and microfilaments, and developing granules.[21] The perinuclear zone mostly contains the Golgi apparatus, of which there may be several, rough endoplasmic reticulum and free ribosomes.

The primary secretory granule of platelets, the α-granule, appears to develop from a multivesicular body precursor[22] and contains all of the proteins found in platelet α-granules. These proteins are probably of dual origin, of intrinsic synthesis in the MK, and of endocytosis of extracellular proteins. In addition to secretory proteins, the intrinsic membrane proteins, platelet glycoproteins Ib and IX, CD63, αIIbβ3, αvβ3, and p-selectin are also found in MK α-granules.[23,24] MKs also contain precursors to dense granules[25] that are capable of serotonin accumulation (Fig. 62.2).

Most platelet membrane glycoproteins are present on the plasma membrane of MKs.[26] In addition, the integrins α2β1, α4β1, α5β1, α6β1, αIIbβ3, αvβ3, and αvβ5 have all been observed on the MK surface. The adhesive functions of these ligands have not been well characterized in MKs to the extent that they have been in platelets. It is known that bovine MKs can adhere to fibronectin, collagen, and vitronectin. Adhesion to fibronectin and collagen is by means of β1 integrin.[27] Adhesion to vitronectin is through the αvβ3 integrin. The αIIbβ3 integrin can be activated by adenosine diphosphate (ADP) or thrombin as in platelets, allowing for increased MK adhesion and spreading on a broad range of substrates. Analogous to platelet activation, MK activation by platelet agonists is associated with secretion of granules and the alteration of the MK cytoskeleton.

Mature MKs have an extensive microfilament and microtubule network. Other than a layer of subcortical microfilaments in the peripheral zone, there is no obvious spatial organization of these cytoskeletal structures. The microfilaments have associated myosin, α-actinin, and actin-binding protein and can organize into stress fiberlike structures after stimulation with platelet activators. Numerous microtubules are seen throughout the intermediate zone cytoplasm of MKs, often in association with the DMS. The formation of microtubule coils, the hallmark of the microtubule arrays in platelets, has been seen in spread- and pseudopod-forming MKs in culture. The formation of these coils may be part of the more extensive microtubule reorganization that occurs during platelet formation as described below.

Mechanism of Platelet Formation

The culminating event of megakaryocytopoiesis is platelet formation. Though the regulation of platelet production is well understood, the mechanism by which platelets are formed still remains unclear. There is little doubt that the DMS plays an important role in platelet formation, however, the exact mechanism of action remains to be completely elucidated. The prevailing data suggests that the DMS provides additional membrane for the extension of pseudopodia during platelet formation.[28] In vivo, pseudopodia have been observed crossing the bone marrow sinus endothelium and waving free in the vascular spaces (Fig. 62.3). In vitro, pseudopodia production is associated with fragmentation in culture. MK pseudopodia, both in vivo and in vitro form periodic beaded constrictions, which have been observed to

separate spontaneously into smaller chains and individual platelet-size fragments with the internal organelle organization of platelets. These fragments also are reactive to platelet agonists. Pseudopodia formation requires reorganization of both microtubules and microfilaments. Though it is not certain how pseudopodia separate into individual platelets, cytoplasmic vesicles appear to fuse with the plasma membrane at constriction sites that may lead to separation of individual platelets.[29,30]

Humoral Regulation of Megakaryocytopoiesis

Studies on the humoral regulation of megakaryocytopoiesis have been largely based on the supposition that a single molecule regulates platelet production. The action of this molecule would have to account for the

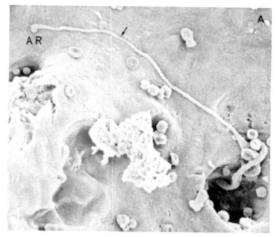
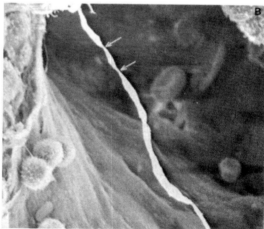

FIGURE 62.3 Scanning electron photomicrographs of canine bone marrow depicting long slender extensions of proplatelets within sinusoidal lumen. Platelets may be shed by grafmentation of a proplatelet at the apical region (AR) or areas of intermittent constrictions (arrows). **A**, × 721; **B**, × 2,540. (Photograph donated by Dr. Prem Handagama.)

various aspects of megakaryocytopoiesis that had been demonstrated to be targets of regulation, including lineage specificity, changes in response to the circulating platelet mass in MK progenitor number; mature MK number, size, and ploidy; maturation rate; and platelet number and size. Recently, the availability of recombinant growth factors has allowed investigators to more clearly define the role of these molecules in vivo. Though no one factor has been shown to have strict lineage specificity in its' effects, by cloning thrombopoietin, a relative understanding of the humoral regulation of megakaryocytopoiesis and the clinical use of these factors in the treatment of thrombocytopenia is now possible.

SCF acts synergistically with IL-3 or granulocyte-macrophage colony-stimulating factor (GM-CSF) in stimulation of CFU-MK growth and also may effect polyploidization and cytoplasmic maturation.[31] In vivo, SCF appears to play an important role in megakaryocytopoiesis. Mutant mice lacking this factor (Sl/Sld) or its receptor (W/Wv) both have abnormal megakaryocytopoiesis.[32] IL-3 is another cytokine with broad biological effects, including stimulation of megakaryocytopoiesis. In vitro, IL-3 alone can stimulate some CFU-MK growth, which is increased when IL-3 is used in combination with other factors such as IL-6, IL-11, TPO, or GM-CSF. A hybrid IL-3/GM-CSF molecule (PIXY321) also stimulates CFU-MK growth.

A group of cytokines, including IL-6, IL-11, leukemia inhibitory factor (LIF), ciliary neurotrophic factor (CNTF), cardiotrophin-1 and Oncostatin-m have overlapping effects owing to the closely related cell surface receptors that share a common signal transduction molecule (GP130). In vitro, IL-6 potentiates IL-3 stimulated CFU-MK growth, increased MK size, ploidy, and pseudopod formation.[33] In vivo administration of IL-6 leads to increased platelet counts in both normal and thrombocytopenic animals.[33] Clinical use for treatment of thrombocytopenia has not been pursued because of drug-related toxicity. LIF augments IL-3-stimulated CFU-MK growth. In vivo, LIF increases the number of MK progenitors, mature MKs, and platelet counts.[34] In nonhuman primates, splenomegaly and loss of subcutaneous fat are observed after LIF treatment.[34] IL-11 also increases the number and size of MK colonies and their ploidy when cells are grown in the presence of IL-3. In vivo, IL-11 increases bone marrow MK progenitor numbers, MK size and ploidy, and circulating platelet counts in rodents, dogs, nonhuman primates and humans.[35] Minimal drug related toxicity has led to the introduction of IL-11 as the first cytokine for effective clinical treatment of thrombocytopenia.

The isolation and cloning of TPO[36] was an event long anticipated in the field of megakaryocytopoiesis. Experiments with the purified and cloned TPO established that it demonstrates all properties predicted for the primary regulator of this lineage, except for strict lineage specificity. In vitro, TPO increases MK size and ploidy and CFU-MK growth, as well as MK pseudopod formation and release of functional platelets.[37] In vivo, TPO administration in normal animals causes an increase in circulating platelet levels, the number of CFU-MK, and the size and ploidy of MKs.[38] Knockout mice that do not express TPO or do not express c-mpl (the TPO receptor) both have an 85 to 90% decrease in platelet count,[39] however, other myeloid progenitor cells also are decreased in these knockout mice. An important characteristic of a physiologic regulator of megakaryocytopoiesis demonstrated by TPO is the inverse relation between circulating TPO and platelet levels.

REFERENCES

1. **Tranum-Jensen J, Behnke O.** Acetylcholinesterase in the platelet-megakaryocyte system. II. Structural localization in megakaryocytes of the rat, mouse and cat. Eur J Cell Biol 1981;24:281–286.
2. **Young KM, Weiss L.** Megakaryocytopoiesis: incorporation of tritiated thymidine by small acetylcholinesterase-positive cells in murine bone marrow during antibody-induced thrombocytopenia. Blood 1987;69:290–295.
3. **Zucker-Franklin D, Yang JS, Grusky G.** Characterization of glycoprotein IIb/IIIa positive cells in human umbilical cord blood: their potential usefulness as megakaryocyte progenitors. Blood 1992;79:347–355.
4. **Schipper LF, Brand A, Reniers NC, Melief CJ, Willemze R, Fibbe WE.** Effects of thrombopoietin on the proliferation and differentiation of primitive and mature haemopoietic progenitor cells in cord blood. Br J Haematol 1998;101:425–435.
5. **Nichol JL, Hornkolh MM, Choi ES, Hokom MM, Ponting I, Schuening FW, Hunt P.** Enrichment and characterization of peripheral blood-derived megakaryocyte progenitors that mature in short-term liquid culture. Stem Cells 1994;12:494–505.
6. **Debili N, Issaad C, Masse JM, Guichard J, Katz A, Breton-Gorius J, Vainchenker W.** Expression of CD34 and platelet glycoproteins during human megakaryocytic differentiation. Blood 1995;86:2516–2525.
7. **Debili N, Masse JM, Katz A, Guichard J, Breton-Gorius J, Vainchenker W.** Effects of the recombinant hematopoietic growth factors interleukin-3, interleukin-6, stem cell factor, and leukemia inhibitory factor on the megakaryocytic differentiation of CD34+ cells. Blood 1993;82:84–95.
8. **Kaushansky K, Lok S, Holly RD, Broudy VC, Lin N, Bailey MC, Forstrom JW, Buddle MM, Oort PJ, Hagen FS, Roth GJ, Papayannopoulou T, Foster DC.** Promotion of megakaryocyte progenitor expansion and differentiation by the c-MPL ligand thrombopoietin. Nature 1994;369:568–571.
9. **Zeigler FC, de Sauvage F, Widmer HR, Keller GA, Donahue C, Schreiber RD, Malloy B, Hass P, Eaton D, Matthews W.** In vitro megakaryocytopoietic and thrombopoietic activity of c-mpl ligand (TPO) on purified murine hematopoietic stem cells. Blood 1994;84:4045–4052.
10. **Ku H, Yonemura Y, Kaushansky K, Ogawa M.** Thrombopoietin, the ligand for the Mpl receptor, synergizes with steel factor and other early acting cytokines in supporting proliferation of primitive hematopoietic progenitors of mice. Blood 1996;87:4544–4551.
11. **Metcalf D, MacDonald HR, Odartchenko N, Sordat B.** Growth of mouse megakaryocyte colonies in vitro. Proc Natl Acad Sci U S A 1975;72:1744–1748.
12. **Gewirtz AM.** Human megakaryocytopoiesis. Semin Hematol 1986;23:27–42.
13. **Levin J, Levin FC, Penington DG, Metcalf D.** Measurement of ploidy distribution in megakaryocyte colonies obtained from culture: with studies of the effects of thrombopoietin. Blood 1981;57:287–297.
14. **Ebbe S, Yee T, Carpenter D, Phalen E.** Megakaryocytes increase in size within ploidy groups in response to the stimulus of thrombocytopenia. Exp Hematol 1988;16:55–61.
15. **Ebbe S, Stohlman F Jr.** Megakaryocytopoiesis in the rat. Blood 1965; 26:20–35.
16. **Topp K.S, Tablin F, Levin J.** Culture of isolated bovine megakaryocytes on reconstituted basement membrane matrix leads to proplatelet process formation. Blood 1990;76:912–924.
17. **Lichtman MA, Chamberlain JK, Simon W, Santillo PA.** Parasinusoidal location of megacaryocytes in marrow: A determinant of platelet release. Am J Hematol 1978;4:303–312.
18. **MacPherson GG.** Origin and development of the demarcation system in megakaryocytes of rat bone marrow. J Ultrastruc Res 1972;40:167–177.
19. **Bentfeld-Barker ME, Bainton DF.** Ultrastructure of rat megakaryocytes after prolonged thrombocytopenia. J Ultrastruc Res 1977; 61:201–214.
20. **Zucker-Franklin D, Peterssen S.** Thrombocytopoiesis-analysis by membrane tracer and freeze-fracture studies on fresh human and cultured mouse megakaryocytes. J Cell Biol 1984;99:390–402.
21. **Menard M, Meyers KM, Prieur DJ.** Primary and secondary lysosomes in megakaryocytes and platelets from cattle with the Chediak-Higashi syndrome. Thromb Haemost 1990;64:156–160.
22. **Heijnen HF, Debili N, Vainchencker W, Breton-Gorius J, Geuze HJ, Sixma**

JJ. Multivesicular bodies are an intermediate stage in the formation of platelet alpha-granules. Blood 1998;91:2313–2325.

23. **Poujol C, Nurden AT, Nurden P.** Ultrastructural analysis of the distribution of the vitronectin receptor (alpha v beta 3) in human platelets and megakaryocytes reveals an intracellular pool and labeling of the alpha-granule membrane. Br J Haematol 1997;96:823–835.

24. **Berger G, Masse JM, Cramer EM.** Alpha-granule membrane mirrors the platelet plasma membrane and contains the glycoproteins Ib, IX and V. Blood 1996;87:1385–1395.

25. **Menard M, Myers KM.** Storage pool deficiency in cattle with the Chediak-Higashi syndrome results from an absence of dense granule precursors in their megakaryocytes. Blood 1988;72:1726–1734.

26. **van Pampus EC, Denkers IA, van Geel BJ, Huijgens PC, Zevenbergen A, Ossenkoppele GJ, Langenhuijsen MM.** Expression of adhesion antigens of human bone marrow megakaryocytes, circulating megakaryocytes and blood platelets. Eur J Haematol 1992;49:122–127.

27. **Topp KS, Tablin F.** Bovine megakaryocyte integrins: their association with extracellular matrix in vivo. Comp Haematol Int 1991;1:135–144.

28. **Radley JM, Haler CJ.** The demarcation membrane system of the megakaryocyte: a misnomer? Blood 1982;60:213–219.

29. **Tablin F, Castro M, Leven RM.** Blood platelet formation in vitro. The role of the cytoskeleton in megakaryocyte fragmentation. J Cell Sci 1990;97:59–70.

30. **Choi ES, Nichol JL, Hokom MM, Hornkohl AC, Hunt P.** Platelets generated in vitro from proplatelet-displaying human megakaryocytes are functional. Blood 1995;85:402–413.

31. **Avraham H, Vannier E, Cowley S, Jiang S, Chi S, Dinarell CA, Zsebo KM, Groopman JE.** Effects of the stem cell factor, c-kit ligand, on human megakaryocytic cells. Blood 1992;79:365–371.

32. **Ebbe S, Phalen E, Stohlman F Jr.** Abnormalities of megakaryocytes in Sl-Sld mice. Blood 1973;42:857–871.

33. **Ishibashi T, Kimura H, Shikama Y, Uchida T, Shigeo K, Hirano T, Kishimoto T, Takatsuki F, Akiyama Y.** Interleukin 6 is a potent thrombopoietic factor in vivo in mice. Blood 1989;74:1241–1244.

34. **Akiyama Y, Kajimura N, Matsuzaki J, Kikuchi Y, Imai N, Tanigawa M, Yamaguchi K.** In vivo effect of recombinant human leukemia inhibitory factor in primates. Jpn J Cancer Res 1997;88:578–583.

35. **Weich NS, Wang A, Fitzgerald M, Neben TY, Donaldson D, Giannotti J, Yetz-Aldape J, Leven RM, Turner KJ.** Recombinant human interleukin-11 directly promotes megakaryocytopoiesis in vitro. Blood 1997;90:3893–3902.

36. **Eaton D.** The purification and cloning of human thrombopoietin. In: Kuter DJ, Hunt P, Sheridan W, Zucker-Franklin D, eds. Thrombopoiesis and thrombopoietins. Totowa, NJ: Humana Press, 1997;135–142.

37. **Choi E.** Regulation of proplatelet and platelet formation in vitro. In: Kuter DJ, Hunt P, Sheridan W, Zucker-Franklin D, eds. Thrombopoiesis and thrombopoietins. : Humana Press, 1997;271–284.

38. **Harker LA, Toombs CF, Stead RB.** In vivo-dose response effects of mpl ligands on platelet production and function. In: Kuter DJ, Hunt P, Sheridan W, Zucker-Franklin D, eds. Thrombopoiesis and Thrombopoietins. : Humana Press, 1997;301–320.

39. **de Sauvage FJ, Moore MW.** Genetic manipulation of mpl ligand and thrombopoietin in vivo. In: Kuter DJ, Hunt P, Sheridan W, Zucker-Franklin D, eds. Thrombopoiesis and thrombopoietins. Totowa, NJ: Humana Press, 1997;349–358.

CHAPTER 63

Platelet Structure and Function

• FERN TABLIN

Platelets travel through the circulation as discoid anucleate cytoplasmic fragments. Resting platelets, when observed by scanning electron microscopy or differential intereference light microscopy, have no filopodia or microspikes typical of leukocytes, but instead appear to have a smooth surface with random indentations that represent the membranous invaginations known as the open canalicular system (OCS).

Platelets are small, 5 to 7 μm long, and often less than 3 μm wide. Occasionally, in the horse and guinea pig, larger more lentiform platelets, as long as 20 μm and termed proplatelets, can be observed in the circulation. These are thought to represent partially fragmented platelet processes from parent megakaryocytes.

For such a small cytoplasmic fragment, the platelet contains an extensive and complicated array of transmembrane proteins that participate in activation, adhesion, and coagulation, as well as numerous organelles and an extensive network of cytoskeletal filaments.

MEMBRANE DOMAIN

The platelet membrane domain can be divided into the most exterior region (the glycocalyx) and the plasma membrane and its invaginated OCS. The glycocalyx is reported to be 15 to 20 nm thick and can be labeled with various electron-dense tracer molecules that bind glycosylated molecules. Many of these molecules (including but not limited to lanathum, horseradish peroxidase, cationized ferritin, and ruthenium red) have been used to stain the extracellular domain of the plasma membrane as well as to define the continuity of the OCS with the plasma membrane.[1] The OCS, also termed the surface-connected canalicular system is present in humans, rats, mice, guinea pigs, rabbits, dogs, cats, primates, and horses but is virtually absent from bovine platelets.[2]

Biochemically, much of the glycocalyx is composed of the extracellular domains of glycoproteins, some of which are members of the integrin superfamily, the leucine-rich glycoprotein family, the immunoglobulin superfamily, and the selectins.

INTEGRINS

Integrins are an extensive and highly dispersed gene family that mediate a large number of cellular interactions. Platelet integrins are necessary for aggregation and adhesive spreading of platelets during hemostasis. Integrins consist of an α subunit noncovalently bound to a β subunit. Both subunits have extracellular domains that bind divalent cation (in particular Ca2+) necessary for ligand binding. The N-terminus and the majority of the subunits are extracellular, and a single-pass membrane unit is connected to a short C-terminus cytoplasmic tail[3] (Fig. 63.1). This tail is associated with a wide variety of signaling molecules as well as with the cell's cytoskeleton. Although specific actin-associated proteins link the integrin β-cytoplasmic domains with the internal platelet cytoskeleton, it is the complex signaling by means of G proteins, tyrosine kinases, and phosphoinositides and their association with integrins that ultimately controls platelet function.

More than seven β subunits have been identified; however, only two β subunits, β1 and β3 have thus far been demonstrated to be present on platelets. The platelet β1 family is associated with at least three different α subunits, and these heterodimeric glycoprotein receptors on platelets can bind collagen (α2β1), fibronectin (α5β1), and laminin (α6β1).[3] These receptors are ubiquitous throughout eukaryotic cell systems. The platelet β3 family includes glycoprotein (GP) IIb-IIIa (αIIbβ3a) and αvβ3, the vitronectin receptor. GPIIb-IIIa is the most abundant integrin on both platelets and megakaryocytes and is unique to the megakaryocyte lineage. In addition to being present on the surface of platelets, additional pools of this integrin are present on the membranes of the OCS, as well as in α and dense granules. GP IIb-IIIa has a high affinity for the soluble adhesive ligand fibrinogen and can also bind to von Willebrand factor (vWF), fibronectin, and vitronectin. There are relatively few copies of αvβ3 on platelets, however, this integrin is abundant on the membranes of progenitor megakaryocytes and has been postulated to play an important role in platelet formation.

Integrin signaling is the information that is sent back and forth between the integrin cytoplasmic domains and

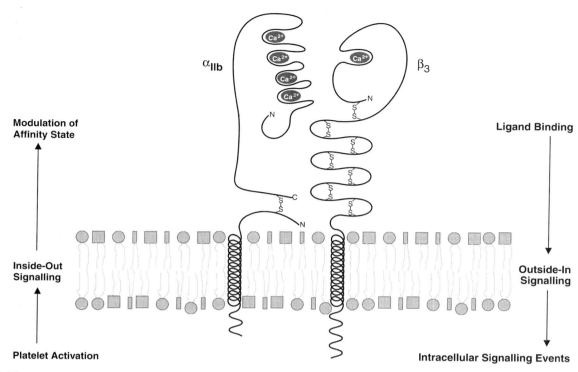

α_{IIb}

β_3

Modulation of
Affinity State

Ligand Binding

Inside-Out
Signalling

Outside-In
Signalling

Platelet Activation

Intracellular Signalling Events

FIGURE 63.1 Typical platelet integrin. GPIIb/IIIa. A diagram of the abundant platelet integrin GPIIb/IIIa ($\alpha IIb\beta3a$) demonstrates the extensive extracellular domain. Note the four calcium binding sites on the α subunit; divalent cations are required for integrin interaction with ligand and modulate the correct folding of the heterodimer to bind its ligand. Both the α and the β subunits each have two distinct binding sites for fibrinogen. The beta cytoplasmic tail is associated with the actin cytoskeleton.

the N-terminal globular heads.[4] Platelet GPIIb-IIIa has been the best studied of these molecules, and its signaling is described herein. A distinction can be made between inside-out and outside-in signaling. Inside-out signaling occurs when an agonist (such as thrombin or adenosine diphosphate [ADP]) binds to its plasma membrane receptor that then leads to a change in the integrin receptor from a low avidity/affinity complex to a high avidity/affinity complex. A change in affinity of the integrin receptor results in a conformation change such that greater ligand binding occurs, whereas a change in avidity suggests a functional change in affinity of the receptor for multivalent ligands as occurs with integrin clustering.[4] During the conformational change of GPIIb-IIIa a ligand-induced binding site (LIBS) for fibrinogen is exposed. These studies also demonstrated significant interspecies variation in this site and suggested that unlike human, monkey, dog, and rabbit platelets, pig platelets may undergo a variable form of conformation change during activation.[5]

Outside-in signaling occurs when an integrin has bound its multivalent ligand, oligermized (clustered), and in conjunction with signals from other plasma membrane G-protein-linked receptors, sets off a series of downstream signals. Many of these signals are regulated by tyrosine kinases that ultimately result in calcium release from the dense tubular system (DTS), actin polymerization, shape change, granule secretion, the flip flop of anionic phospholipids from the inner to the outer

leaflet of the membrane, formation of large platelet aggregates, and ultimately in clot retraction.[6]

LEUCINE-RICH GLYCOPROTEIN FAMILY

In platelets, this family primarily involves glycoprotein (GP) Ib-IX-V complex all of which have a large leucine-rich domain. This complex is a sialoglycoprotein and as such contributes to the net negative charge on the platelet surface. GPIb consists of two disulfide-linked subunits GPIbα and GPIbβ that are tightly complexed to GP IX and GP V[7] (Fig. 63.2). The N-terminal globular domain of GPIbα has seven tandem, leucine-rich repeats as well as a highly glycosylated macroglycopepetide mucin core. This globular domain contains the site of vWF and thrombin binding. Its single transmembrane sequence is linked to a short cytoplasmic tail that is associated with the actin cytoskeleton by its binding to actin-binding protein (ABP).[7] GPIbβ has a single leucine-rich repeat and is associated with GPIbα through a disulfide linkage located adjacent to the extracellular domain of the lipid bilayer. It has a single transmembrane sequence, and its cytoplasmic domain contains a site for protein kinase A phosphorylation that appears to play a role in cytoskeletal rearrangement in response to agonist stimulation.[8] GPIX, as does GPIbβ, has a single leucine-rich domain and a single transmembrane sequence. However, it has a short cytoplasmic tail that may be

FIGURE 63.2 GPIb-IX-V Complex. GPIb has both an α and a β subunit associated through a disulfide linkage. GPIbα has seven leucine-rich repeats and a highly glycosylated mucin core. The globular head domains of all of these glycoproteins contain leucine-rich repeats. GPIb α and β are associated with GP IX in a 1:1 complex. The complex is associated with the platelet cytoskeleton by binding of the cytoplasmic tail of GPIbα to actin-binding protein.

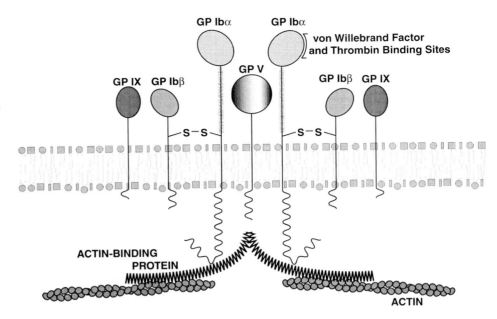

anchored to the plasma membrane by covalent modifications of myristoylation or palmitoylation.[7,8] GPIX is associated with GPIb in a 1:1 complex. GPV has 15 leucine-rich repeats, and similar to GPIX, has a short cytoplasmic tail. It is thought to bridge adjacent GPIb-IX complexes through its interaction with GPIbα.[7,8]

Previous studies have shown GPIb to be present in virtually all species except cats.[9] However, recent research from our laboratory has shown that both components of GPIb are indeed present on the platelets of domestic cats (Fig. 63.3). The primary function of the GPIb-IX-V complex is early in hemostasis, serving to adhere platelets to the initial site of vascular damage. The complex does not bind to soluble vWF, but binds only to immobilized vWF, which is proposed to expose an otherwise cryptic binding site for GPIb-IX-V.[7] vWF also binds to GPIb-IX-V complex under high shear; such binding has been suggested to alter the conformation of either vWF or the GPIb complex although the exact mechanism by which this occurs is unknown. It has been suggested that the interaction of GPIb-IX-V with the subendothelium is similar to that of selectins that mediate leukocyte rolling.

In addition to its ability to bind vWF, thrombin binds within the N-terminal domain of GPIbα. Although the agonist action of thrombin on platelets is primarily through its binding to the 7-transmembrane spanning domain thrombin receptors,[7] the binding of thrombin by GPIb-IX-V has been shown to enhance platelet response to low concentrations of thrombin.[7,8]

Downstream events of GPIb-IX-V binding to vWF are increases in cytoplasmic Ca^{2+} and activation of protein kinases, as well as association of activated phosphatidyl-inositol-3-kinase and src with the cytoskeleton.[8] Subsequent events include activation of phospholipase A_2 and the synthesis of arachidonic acid and thromboxane A_2—

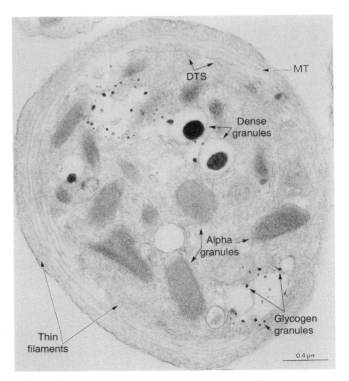

FIGURE 63.3 Bovine platelet. A transmission electron micrograph of a resting bovine platelet clearly demonstrates its granule components; α, dense, and glycogen granules are present as are the membranes of the DTS. The cytoskeleton is composed of thin filaments (F-actin) and the circumferential microtubule (MT) coil, both of which contribute to the discoid shape of the resting cell.

the mechanisms of which are covered in the next several chapters.

ADDITIONAL PLATELET RECEPTORS

The most notable of these receptors is the thrombin receptor. This G-protein-coupled receptor is characterized by a single polypeptide with seven transmembrane-spanning domains. Receptor activation is due to a unique mechanism in which α-thrombin (the serine protease found in plasma) cleaves its receptor, creating a new N-terminus that serves as its own tethered ligand.[10] Downstream signaling from the thrombin receptor is characterized by tyrosine kinase phosphorylation and subsequent activation of GP IIb-IIIa.[10,11] Additional receptors on the platelet surface, including P-selectin (platelet activation-dependent granule–external membrane [PADGEM] or granule membrane protein-140 [GMP-140]), an α granule membrane protein (and a member of the selectin superfamily) that is expressed on the platelet surface subsequent to α granule secretion. Platelet-endothelial cell adhesion molecule (PECAM)-1, a member of the immunoglobulin superfamily is also present subsequent to α granule secretion. CD 36 (GP IV) a receptor for thrombospondin, is present as well. The ADP receptor, although cloned and expressed in cell lines, has yet to be definitely identified on the platelet plasma membrane.

CYTOSKELETON

Many of the platelet transmembrane receptors are intimately associated with a unique membrane skeleton composed of short actin filaments linked to receptors by actin-associated proteins, including α-actinin, talin, vinculin, spectrin. This arrangement facilitates the clustering of receptors necessary for signal transduction, evagination of the OCS and platelet activation.

Actin filaments are the essential contractile element of the platelet. Filament organization–the dynamic rearrangements from G (monomeric) to F (filamentous) actin–is regulated by a group of actin sequestering, capping, severing, nucleating, and binding proteins. Together with these proteins along with changes in the intracellular calcium concentration and in association with platelet myosin, actin filaments regulate shape change, extension of pseudopodia, platelet spreading and adhesion, platelet aggregation, secretion, and clot retraction.[12]

Additional major cytoskeletal elements include microtubules and intermediate filaments. In resting platelets microtubules assume a unique array in the form of a coil. The microtubule coil helps to maintain the discoid arrangement of the resting platelet as a result of its palmitoylation and association with the plasma membrane.[13] Upon activation, microtubules reorganize into linear arrays, and in activated bovine platelets, lacking an OCS, the linear microtubule array is essential for granule translocation and secretion.[14]

Intermediate filaments composed of vimentin have been shown to be present in bovine and human platelets and are presumably present in other species as well. These short nondynamic filaments make up the backbone of the discoid cell and may participate in the stabilization of other cytoskeletal elements during activation.

Overall, the cytoskeleton forms a dense submembranous zone; internal to this area is the central portion of the platelet, consisting of α and dense granules, mitochondria, and the membrane complexes of the dense tubular system (DTS) and the OCS (Fig. 63.3).

ORGANELLES

Three major membrane-bound granule populations are present in platelets. Lysosomes, membrane-bound reservoirs of hydrolases, can either degrade endocytic material or can fuse with the membranes of the OCS and release their contents into the extracellular milieu. The expression of lysosomal membrane components during activation, in particular, CD63 (GP 53), can be used in flow cytometry as a marker of platelet activation. The α granules are the largest granule population and contain coagulation factors (albumin, factor V, and fibrinogen), platelet-specific proteins (β-thromboglobulin and platelet factor 4), growth factors (platelet-derived growth factor [PDGF], β-transforming growth factor [TGF-β], epidermal growth factor [EGF], and endothelial cell growth factor [ECGF]) and glycoproteins.[15] In addition both thrombospondin and fibronectin can be found within the α granule contents. GPIb, GPIIb-IIIa, and the α granule specific protein P-selectin are among the α granule membrane proteins. Antibodies to P-selectin are often used to detect platelet activation by flow cytometry.

Dense granules are storage sites for the nucleotides adenosine triphosphate (ATP), guanosine triphosphate (GTP), ADP, and guanosine diphosphate (GDP), as well as for Ca^{2+} and Mg^{2+}. In addition serotonin and its precursor 5'hydroxytryptamine are dense granule components. Of all the species studied, pig platelet dense granules release the most Mg^{2+}; however, there is significant species variability between relase of Ca^{2+}, Mg^{2+}, ATP, and ADP.[16] Similar to α granules and lysosomes, the membranes of dense granules contain the major platelet glycoproteins, GPIIb-IIIa and GPIb.

The DTS of platelets is derived from the endoplasmic reticulum of the parent megakaryocyte and serves as the reservoir for calcium. A calcium-activated adenosine triphosphatase (ATPase) is one mechanism for release and uptake of cytosolic calcium.

Glycogen granules are found free in the cytoplasm of the platelet. They are especially numerous in bovine platelets, but are generally present in all species. Glycogen is the primary source of energy metabolism of resting platelets, and its breakdown is controlled by the enzyme systems amylo-1, 6-glucosidase and glycogen phosphorylase. Platelets also are capable of active uptake of glucose that can be metabolized in two major directions: degraded through glycolysis or metabolized through the hexose monophosphate shunt.[17]

PHYSIOLOGIC RESPONSES OF PLATELETS

Platelet responses to either agonists in vivo or in vitro are characterized by a series of events, including platelet shape change, secretion, aggregation and clot retraction.

Platelet shape change is characterized by a morphologic transformation of resting discoid platelets into spiny spherical cells with numerous filopodia. This is accompanied by activation of small G proteins and actin polymerization, a rise in cytosolic calcium, and some eversion of the OCS. Shape change occurs in response to most agonists as well as in response to chilling and is reversible in some but not all cases.

Granule secretion occurs subsequent to ligand binding and receptor activation. In the case of either the GPIIb-IIIa or GPIb receptor pathways, the ligand is bound and a resulting set of signaling cascades proceed before actual secretion. These pathways are well characterized and have been reviewed in depth elsewhere.[5,18] Subsequent to ligand binding and signaling there is a rise in intracellular calcium, resulting in actin polymerization. Contraction of the actin-myosin cytoskeleton and its association with integral membrane proteins is required for granule secretion. This contractile shell results in the centralization of α, dense, and lysosomal granules that ultimately fuse with the invaginated membranes of the OCS and release their contents into the extracellular milieu. This pattern is similar in all species except the bovine, which lacks an OCS. In bovine platelets, granule secretion occurs by movement of granules via microtubules to the plasma membrane and their subsequent fusion and release of contents. Release of granular contents stimulates platelet aggregation, as many of the granular contents (such as ADP, thrombospondin, and fibrinogen) are themselves platelet agonists.

REFERENCES

1. **White JG.** Anatomy and structural organization of the platelet. In: Colman RW, Hirsh J, Marder VJ, Salzman EW, eds. Hemostasis and thrombosis, basic principles and clinical practice. 3rd ed. Philadelphia: JB Lippincott Company, 1994;397–507.
2. **White JG.** The secretory pathway of bovine platelets. Blood 1987;69:878–885.
3. **Ginsberg MH, Du X, O'Toole TE, Loftus JC.** Platelet integrins. Throm Haemost 1995;74:352–359.
4. **Shattil SJ, Kashiwagi H, Pampori N.** Integrin signaling: the platelet paradigm Blood 1998;91:2645–2657.
5. **Jennings LK, White MM, Mandrell TD.** Interspecies comparison of platelet aggregation, LIBS expression and clot retraction: observed differences in GP IIb-IIIa functional activity. Thromb Haemost 1995;74:1551–1556.
6. **Fox JEB.** Platelet activation: new aspects. Haemostasis 1996;26(suppl 4):102–131.
7. **Lopez JA, Dong JF.** Structure and function of the glycoprotein Ib-IX-V complex. Curr Opin Hematol 1997;4:323–329.
8. **Andrews RK, Lopez JA, Berndt MC.** Molecular mechanisms of platelet adhesion and activation. Int J Biochem Cell Biol 1997;29:91–105.
9. **Nurden AT.** A different organization of bound carbohydrate within cat platelets membranes. Thromb Haemost 1977;37:358–360.
10. **Brass LF, Molino M.** Protease-activated G protein-coupled receptors on human platelets and endothelial cells. Thromb Haemost 1997 78:234–241.
11. **Denning PM, Brendt MC.** The thrombin receptor Clin Exp Pharmcol Physiol 1994;21:349–358.
12. **Hartwig JH.** Mechanisms of actin rearrangements mediating platelet activation. J Cell Biol 1992;118:1421–1442.
13. **Caron JM.** Posttranslational modification of tubulin by palmitoylation: I. In vivo and cell-free studies. Mol Biol Cell 1997;8:621–636.
14. **Tablin F, Castro MD.** Bovine platelets contain a 280kDa microtubule-associated protein antigenically related to brain MAP2. Eur J Cell Biol 1991;56:415–421.
15. **Corash L, Costa JL, Shafer B, Donlon JA, Murphy D.** Heterogeneity of human whole blood platelet subpopulations: III. Density-dependent differences in subcellular constituents. Blood 1984;64:185–193.
16. **Meyers KM, Holman H, Seachord CL.** Comparative study of platelet dense granule constituents. Am J Physiol 1982;243:R454–R461.
17. **Holmsen H.** Platelet secretion and energy metabolism. In: Colman RW, Hirsh J, Marder VJ, Salzman EW, eds. Hemostasis and thrombosis, basic principles and clinical practice. 3rd ed. Philadelphia: JB Lippincort Company, 1994;524–545.
18. **Shattil SJ, Ginsberg MH, Brugge JS.** Adhesive signaling in platelets. Curr Opin Cell Biol 1994;6:695–704.

CHAPTER 64

Platelet Lipids and Prostaglandins

• PATRICIA A. GENTRY and KWASI NYARKO

In platelets, as in other cells, membrane phospholipids play an essential role in homeostasis by providing a barrier between the cell and its external environment and by serving as a source of intracellular messenger molecules and active metabolites that modulate intracellular and intercellular responses after platelet stimulation. Much of the knowledge of platelet lipid biochemistry has been derived from studies with human platelets, in part because of clinical interest in the association between platelet membrane levels of n-3 polyunsaturated fatty acids and cardiovascular disease. However, studies on lipid composition and metabolism from various species suggest that differences between platelets from people and domestic and laboratory animals are quantitative rather than qualitative. For example, the turnover of membrane phospholipids in activated human and bovine platelets is similar despite their ultrastructural differences.[1]

PLATELET MEMBRANE PHOSPHOLIPIDS

Platelet membranes, like those of other cells, are composed of a phospholipid bilayer containing transmembrane and peripheral proteins that function as membrane receptors. Phospholipids (phosphoglycerides) are functionally the most important group of membrane lipids, and they also constitute the largest component, (e.g., in pig and human platelets they comprise 63% and 57% of the total lipid content, respectively).[2] Phospholipids are esters, characterized by having two fatty acyl groups and phosphoric acid esterified to a glycerol or sphingosine backbone. The fatty acid portion of the molecule is lipophilic, whereas the dipolar anionic portions are hydrophilic. These properties allow the phospholipid molecules to form two opposing rows within the membrane with the polar portion projecting inward. Individual phospholipids are asymmetrically distributed within the membrane in the typical manner found in other mammalian cell types. In unstimulated platelets the negatively charged phospholipids (or aminophospholipids), such as phosphatidylserine (PS) and phosphatidyl enthanolamine (PE), are found predominantly in the inner leaflet, whereas neutral phospholipids, like

phosphatidylcholine (PC) and sphingosine (SP) are distributed in the outer leaflet.[3] These four compounds comprise the major portion of the lipid content in platelet membranes, and their relative distribution appears similar in nonruminant and ruminant platelets with $PC \geq PE > SP > PS$. Other lipids present within the membrane include, phosphatidyl inositol (PI), lysolecithin, and various neutral lipids. The differences in free fatty acid (FFA) composition in membrane phospholipids may contribute to the different membrane stabilities observed in ex vivo studies of platelets from different species.

When platelets are activated, three major alterations in membrane phospholipids occur: (i) PI turnover is enhanced with the formation of the intracellular signal transducers, inositol triphosphate (IP_3), and 1,2-diacylglycerol (DAG); (ii) arachidonic acid (AA) is liberated from PC, and to a lesser extent from PE, to be metabolized to various biologically active compounds; and (iii) PS is translocated from the inner membrane to the platelet surface where it functions as an essential cofactor in protein–protein interactions that regulate the rate of thrombin generation.[3–5] However, before these reactions can proceed the circulating, quiescent platelet must be prompted into action by one, or more, of several soluble activators, e.g., thrombin, adenosine diphosphate (ADP), or platelet-activating factor (PAF), or by components of the extracellular matrix, e.g., collagen, which interact with their specific receptor(s) on the platelet membrane.

Platelet Membrane Activation

All the specific platelet agonist receptors currently identified are members of the large family of transmembrane guanosine triphosphate binding proteins, or G proteins. These G-protein receptors are characterized by an external ligand-binding domain, seven hydrophobic regions spanning the membrane, and a hydrophilic cytoplasmic domain that serves as an effector. Thrombin receptors are distinguished by the need for thrombin to first cleave the amino terminal of the exodomain of the G-coupled receptor. This proteolytic cleavage unmasks a tethered peptide ligand that then, by binding intramolecularly to the body of the receptor, activates it and induces transmembrane signaling.[6] As occurs in other cells, depending on the agonist and the type of G-protein complex activated, an array of stimulatory or inhibitory intracellular reactions are triggered by agonist–receptor binding. The key intracellular messenger systems that modulate platelet responses are listed in Tables 64.1 and 64.2. Because of the rapidity of the intracellular response to agonist–receptor interactions and because of the synergy between secondary messenger compounds, it is not possible to organize the various effector systems into a temporal sequence. Among mammalian platelets the elevation of intracellular free calcium levels and the initiation of phosphoinositol hydrolysis through activation of endogenous phospholipase C (PLC) appear to be universal.

The elevation of free cytosolic calcium, as a result of receptor mediated influx of extracellular calcium and the secondary release of calcium from the dense tubular system and in some species the dense granules, is one of the critical biochemical events in platelet activation and occurs after stimulation with all types of platelet activators.[5] Calcium is directly involved in regulating phospholipid metabolism through the calcium-dependent enzymes PLC and phospholipase A_2 (PLA$_2$). At the same time calcium initiates protein phosphorylation reactions (Table 64.1). For example, protein kinase C (PKC) is activated, which increases platelet adhesion and fibrinogen binding through a conformation change in the glycoprotein (GP) IIb/IIIa receptor on the platelet membrane. The elevation in free calcium also results in the lowering of intracellular cyclic adenosine monophosphate (cAMP) levels through activation of cAMP phosphodiesterase, which indirectly enhances platelet aggregation (Tables 64.1 and 64.2). These various reactions exert a positive feedback effect on platelet reactivity. A consistent observation among mammalian platelets is the suppression of platelet aggregation by drugs, such as verapamil and diltiazem, which function as calcium channel blockers.

TABLE 64.1   Intracellular Signal Transduction Systems That Enhance Platelet Activation and Aggregation

Effector	Actions
↑ Intracellular Calcium	Activation of phospholipase C (PLC) and phospholipase A_2 (PLA$_2$) Activation of myokinase light chain kinase ⇒ granule secretion Activation of phosphodiesterase ⇒ ⇓ cAMP
PLC	Hydrolysis of PI to IP$_3$ and DAG
IP$_3$	Activation of Ca^{2+}-dependent transporting ATPase ⇒ Ca^{2+} release from dense tubular system and dense granules
DAG	Activation of protein kinase C ⇒ GPIIb/IIIa conformational change ⇒ increased adhesion
PLA$_2$	Hydrolysis of phosphatidylcholine ⇒ release of AA and PAF precursor, lyso-PAF

TABLE 64.2   Intracellular Signal Transducer Systems That Suppress Platelet Reactivity

Effector	Actions
Prostaglandin I$_2$	⇓ PLC binding to membranes ⇒ inhibition of PI hydrolysis Activation of adenyl cyclase ⇒ ⇑ intracellular cAMP
cAMP	⇓ PLC binding to membranes ⇒ inhibition of PI hydrolysis ⇓ thrombin binding
Nitric oxide	Inhibition of phospholipase C activity ⇑ intracellular cGMP ⇒ ⇓ intracellular free Ca^{2+} levels

PHOSPHOINOSITOL METABOLISM

PI constitutes only approximately 5% of the total platelet phospholipids, which is high relative to total protein in comparison with other cell types.[2,7] In unstimulated platelets PI exists in equilibrium with its phosphorylated derivatives, inositol-1-phosphate (PIP) and phosphatidyl 4,5 biophosphate (PIP$_2$). After activation by collagen, thrombin, ADP, or PAF, PIP$_2$ undergoes diesteric cleavage by PLC to yield lipophilic DAG and hydrophilic IP$_3$. Because of the synergistic action of these two signal transducers, they initiate all aspects of the basic platelet response, including shape change and conformation change of receptors to a high avidity binding state, aggregation, and secretion of granular contents (Table 64.1). IP$_3$ mobilizes calcium from the dense tubular and open canalicular systems through activation of a calcium transporting adenosine triphosphatase (ATPase). DAG activates PKC, which then can phosphorylate pleckstrin, a 47 kDa protein that, in turn, mediates a change in the GPIIb/IIIa receptor from a low affinity or avidity to a high affinity or avidity that results in greater strength of ligand binding. The continued functioning of the IP$_3$–DAG system depends on the continued agonist–receptor-mediated activation of PLC because both IP$_3$ and DAG exist transiently within the cell. IP$_3$ is dephosphorylated to inositol, which can be reincorporated into PI within the platelet membrane, whereas DAG undergoes deacylation to either monoglyceride or phosphatidic acid (PA). The PA is used for the resynthesis of platelet PI. The recycling of PI intermediates seems a consistent phenomenon in mammalian platelets. For instance, in vitro studies have shown that when [1-^{14}CAA] is incorporated into human, rabbit, or bovine platelet phospholipids and the distribution of radiolabel examined after either thrombin or PAF stimulation, the reduc-

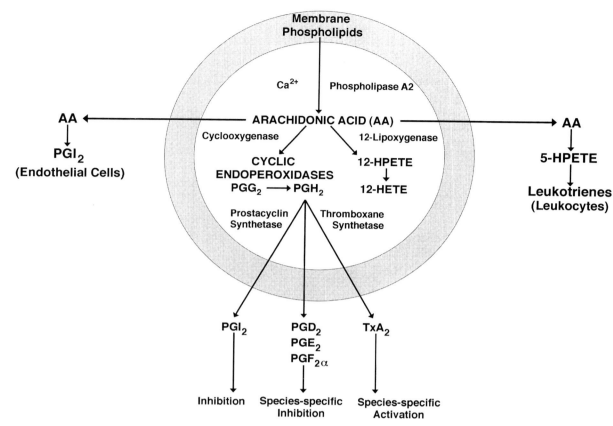

FIGURE 64.1 Eicosanoid biosynthesis from AA released from membrane phospholipids, PC and PE. Platelet stimulation is followed by the activation of phospholipases (PLA$_2$); AA is transformed into unstable intermediates by distinct oxygenases. PGH$_2$ is further metabolized by specific enzymes, with TxA$_2$ being the major metabolite in activated platelets. The lipophilic AA may also be released to be used by other platelets, by endothelial cells for the production of PGI$_2$, and by leukocytes for LT formation.

tion in PI and the concomitant increase in PA and FFA labeling is similar in each species.[1]

ARACHIDONIC ACID METABOLISM

The main metabolic end products of AA metabolism in mammalian platelets are shown in Figure 64.1. AA (a C20:4n-6 FFA) is important for both structural and functional integrity of cell membranes, and it is the precursor for all oxygenated derivatives, including prostaglandins (PGs), thromboxanes (Txs), leukotrienes (LTs) and hydroxyeicostetranoic acids (HETEs), which are collectively termed eicosanoids. Although the level of platelet AA varies between species, in all types of platelets, it is the major FFA in platelet membranes and granules.[8] AA exists in esterified form with phospholipids, and before it can be metabolised it must be released into the cytosolic medium. This is achieved through the calcium-dependent action of the acyl hydrolase, PLA$_2$, which cleaves the sn-2 acyl bond of PC or PE to release AA and lysophospholipids. In general, AA metabolites are characterized as being lipid soluble, labile products that can function as intracellular or extracellular messengers. In platelets two enzymes are involved in AA metabolism, cyclooxygenase (COX), which is also known as prostaglandin H synthetase (PGHS), and a 12-lipoxygenase. Only the constitutively expressed form of COX, COX-1, is present in platelets, whereas a second cytokine-inducible form, COX-2, is found in many nucleated cell types, including endothelial cells.[9] Both forms of COX possess two catalytic activities. AA is first oxidized and cyclyzed to form PGG$_2$, which then undergoes peroxidation to PGH$_2$ (Fig. 64.1). Both of these cyclic endoperoxides are chemically unstable and are rapidly metabolized to (i) TxA$_2$ by Tx synthetase, (ii) prostacyclin (PGI$_2$) by PGI synthetase or, (iii) PGD$_2$, PGE$_2$, and PGF$_2$ by isomerases that have yet to be fully characterized. In platelets, TxA$_2$ is the major metabolite, although the amount of TxA$_2$ produced depends on both the type of agonist and platelet. Because of the labile nature of TxA$_2$, the stable metabolite TxB$_2$ is used to evaluate the extent of AA metabolism by Tx synthetase in stimulated platelets. Collagen- or thrombin-stimulated platelets produce more TxB$_2$ than the same platelets stimulated with ADP or PAF. Likewise, human, horse, and cat platelets produce approximately tenfold more TxB$_2$ after thrombin stimulation than cow, pig, sheep, and mink platelets. The amount of TxB$_2$ produced by canine platelets is breed dependent, and in rats it is strain dependent. The ability of AA and TxA$_2$ to act as platelet agonists and induce platelet aggregation also varies between species. Human, horse, rabbit, and guinea pig platelets, as well as platelets from some breeds of dogs respond well to these metabolites and to the endoperoxide analog, U46619. In contrast, bovine, rat, and elephant platelets are fairly insensitive, especially to TxA$_2$ and U46619.[5] These variable responses may be related to TxA$_2$-receptor populations on the platelet membrane. A TxA$_2$-receptor antagonist, vapipost, inhibits collagen-, AA-, or U46619-stimulated platelets from various species with the sensitivity of human $\geq$ guinea pig > rat > rabbit platelets. It is likely that the different sensitivity to AA and TxA$_2$ between species is not a unique platelet response. For example, at least under in vitro conditions, bovine neutrophils and corneal epithelial cells, like bovine platelets, are nonresponsive to exogenous AA.

The variations between species observed for the in vitro aggregation responses to AA and its metabolites are most likely irrelevant for the in vivo aggregation response. Within the circulation, platelets are simultaneously exposed to various agonists that trigger the multiple, interrelated signaling mechanisms. However, the dependence on AA metabolism to generate platelet reactive intermediates is clinically relevant because drugs, especially nonsteroidal anti-inflammatory drugs (NSAIDs) such as aspirin and indomethacin, that function through inhibition of specific enzymes involved in AA metabolism are ineffective in reducing platelet reactivity in those species where platelet aggregation can proceed at physiologically relevant rates through AA-independent pathways.[5]

At least in some species, AA released from activated platelets may be more important as a substrate for other cells than for platelet function. For example, although PGI$_2$ (prostacyclin) is a minor metabolite in platelets, it is a major AA metabolite in endothelial cells because of the higher levels of PGI synthetase in these cells compared with platelets (Fig. 64.1, Table 64.2). PGI$_2$ appears to be a universal inhibitor of platelet aggregation, being effective in platelets from species that are both sensitive and insensitive to TxA$_2$. It is a more potent inhibitor of ADP-induced aggregation in human, dog, rat, sheep, and horse platelets than PGD$_2$, PGE$_2$ or PGF$_{2\alpha}$. Likewise, leukocytes contain different lipoxygenase enzymes than are present in platelets, and this permits more extensive LT formation from AA.[9]

PLATELET-ACTIVATING FACTOR

Although the first biological role identified for PAF was that of a platelet agonist, it is a phospholipid that has a critical role in inflammatory responses and is produced by many cell types. In platelets, as in other cells, PAF is derived from the intermediate lyso-PAF that is released from PC by the action of PLA$_2$. The sensitivity of platelets from different species to PAF stimulation varies. Whether PAF stimulates aggregation by a TxA$_2$-dependent or TxA$_2$-independent mechanism also varies between species. Platelets from most species, including

people, cows, sheep, horses, pigs, dogs, cats, elephants, and guinea pigs, are activated by PAF with various degrees of sensitivity, whereas platelets from mice, hamsters, and rats are unresponsive to PAF.[5] The fact that inflammatory mediators frequently induce platelet activation in a PAF-dependent fashion has clinical implications for some species. For example, because bovine platelets aggregate to PAF through AA- and TxA$_2$-independent pathways, anti-inflammatory drugs that serve as COX and lipoxygenase inhibitors do not prevent the aggregatory and procoagulant responses in stimulated platelets in cattle.[5] However, PAF antagonists, such as WEB 2086, which is not a PAF analog but a diazepine compound, can ameliorate the platelet activation response in cattle, as occurs in other species.

PLATELET LIPIDS AND PROCOAGULANT ACTIVITY

The lipid asymmetry within the platelet membrane is similar to that in other cells with the same three distinct activities involved in regulating the intramembrane phospholipid distribution. An adenosine triphosphate (ATP)-dependent aminotranslocase transports PS and PE, but not PC, from the outer to the inner membrane leaflet in nonactivated platelets, whereas a less specific and slower-acting ATP-requiring enzyme, termed floppase, transports PC and some PS, from the inner to the outer membrane.[3] The maintenance of membrane asymmetry in the unstimulated platelet depends on both a source of ATP and on the maintenance of physiologic (low) intracellular calcium concentrations. When the concentration of intracellular calcium rises after platelet activation, the activity of the translocase and floppase enzymes is inhibited, and phospholipids can move rapidly back and forth between the two membranes. Specific membrane proteins, referred to as lipid scramblase activity, are involved in this non-ATP-dependent mechanism. The anionic phospholipids, particularly PS, that congregate on the surface of activated platelets are essential in promoting the membrane-binding and membrane-enhancing catalytic activity of two key enzyme complexes involved in thrombin generation. This membrane PS-related function is referred to as platelet procoagulant activity (PCA).

During platelet activation, in addition to PS expression, two high affinity binding sites become available for the plasma proteins, factors (fs) VIIIa and Va, which are involved in the formation of the tenase and prothrombinase complexes, respectively (Fig. 64.2). These enzyme complexes interact sequentially to rapidly form the serine proteases, fXa and thrombin, on the surface of the activated platelet. In the first reaction, activated fIX (fIXa), a serine protease, combines with PS, fVIIIa, and calcium on the platelet surface to form the highly reactive tenase complex that activates fX. The second reaction involves the formation of the prothrombinase complex, which consists of fXa, PS, fVa and calcium, which converts prothrombin to thrombin. The importance of these reactions in maintaining normal hemosta-

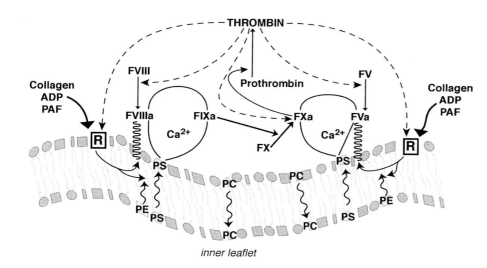

inner leaflet

FIGURE 64.2 Schematic diagram of the interaction of plasma proteins with the negatively charged PS, also known as PCA, expressed on the surface of the activated platelet that promotes thrombin generation. The interaction of agonists with their specific platelet surface receptor (R) induces expression of binding sites for both fVIIIa and fVa on the platelet surface, facilitating the formation of the tenase (fVIIIa-PS-Ca-fIXa) and prothrombinase (fVa-PS-Ca-fXa) complexes, respectively. The dotted lines represent the positive feedback reactions of thrombin.

sis is illustrated by the clinical bleeding tendency observed in people who have the inherited disease Scott syndrome.[3] In these patients the calcium-induced scramblase activation mechanism is defective; this causes a deficiency of surface PS in activated platelets, resulting in the loss of platelet procoagulant activity. Platelet activation and aggregation are normal in Scott syndrome patients, but only a low number of fVa and fVIIIa binding sites are expressed on the surface of their activated platelets.

The generation of PCA through the surface expression of PS occurs after platelet aggregates have begun to form at a site of vascular damage. Platelet PCA is not involved in the initial events at a site of vascular damage that trigger the first few molecules of thrombin formation, but it is essential to sustain thrombin generation, and subsequent fibrin formation, at a physiologically viable rate. By themselves, strong agonists like thrombin and collagen cause the membrane translocation of PS, but weaker agonists, such as ADP and PAF, only do so in combination with another agonist.[5] Platelet procoagulant activity can also be generated by the complement membrane attack complex C5b-9, which has the additional effect of recruiting leukocytes through binding of platelet-exposed PS to the leukocyte L-selectin. This provides one mechanism that links platelet activation and aggregation with the inflammatory response.

LIPID-MODULATED INHIBITORY ACTIVITIES

Several regulatory mechanisms function to suppress platelet reactivity and ensure that, once initiated, platelet activation and aggregation do not proceed unchecked. One of the most important ways in which both platelet inhibition is locally promoted within the vasculature and the antithrombotic property of endothelial cells is maintained, is the generation of PGI_2 in endothelial cells.[10,11] The formation of PGI_2 is rapidly but transiently stimulated, as much as at least 100-fold over basal levels, in endothelial cells by platelet agonists, by inflammatory mediators such as histamine and bradykinin and, by AA and other soluble mediators, such as ADP, released from activated platelets. Hence, activated platelets can initiate negative feedback for their inhibition (Table 64.2).

In addition to acting as a vasodilator, PGI_2 functions as an inhibitor of platelet adhesion and aggregation through its interaction with a specific membrane receptor coupled to a stimulatory G protein that, in turn, activates membrane-bound adenylate cyclase.[10,11] It is likely that all the prostacyclin-induced platelet responses are mediated through elevation of intracellular cAMP and the subsequent activation of a cAMP-protein kinase (PKA). PKA stimulates the phosphorylation of a low-molecular-weight guanosine triphosphate (GTP)-binding protein, rap 1B, which causes it to dissociate from the membrane and to inhibit PLC membrane binding (Table 64.2). The net effect of this response is to suppress PI hydrolysis and to reduce intracellular levels of IP_3 and DAG (Table 64.2). In addition to the effects on phospholipid metabolism, a rise in cAMP levels can reduce platelet reactivity by inhibiting agonist surface binding through a reduction of GPIIb/IIIa expression and by reducing the magnitude and duration of the elevation of cytosolic free calcium after platelet activation.

Activated endothelial cells can also suppress platelet reactivity by increasing the rate of nitric oxide (NO) production. It has been shown that unlike PGI_2, NO is endogenously synthesized by human endothelial cells at a sufficiently high basal rate to influence vascular tone continually and to inhibit platelet reactivity (Table 64.2). NO appears to be an even better inhibitor of the human platelet adhesion response than PGI_2.[10,11] The NO-induced downregulation of platelet activation results from an increase in intracellular cyclic guanosine monophosphate (cGMP) levels. This, in turn, induces the activation of cGMP-dependent protein kinases that cause intracellular free calcium levels to decrease. Although the inhibitory mechanism of this cGMP pathway is not yet fully understood, it has been shown that the cGMP-dependent protein kinase shares a common substrate, a 46/50 protein known as VASP, with the cAMP-dependent PKA and that the phosphorylation of this protein correlates well with the extent of human platelet inhibition responses.[11] It has yet to be determined whether the NO pathway has an important role in modulating the reactivity of platelets from domestic and companion animals.

REFERENCES

1. **Grandoni KM, Gentry PA, Holub BJ, Yagen B.** Trichothecene mycotoxins inhibit phosphoinositide hydrolysis in bovine platelets stimulated with platelet activating factor. Toxicology 1992;72:51–60.
2. **Schick PK.** Megakaryocyte and platelet lipids. In: Colman RW, Hirsh J, Marder VJ, Salzman EW, eds. Hemostasis and thrombosis: basic principles and clinical practice. 3rd ed. Philadelphia: JB Lippincort Company, 1994;574.
3. **Zwaal RFA, Schroit AJ.** Pathophysiologic implications of membrane phospholipid asymmetry in blood cells. Blood 1997;89:1121–1132.
4. **Barritt GJ.** The plasma-membrane receptors and GTP-binding proteins. In: Barritt GJ, ed. Communication within animal cells. New York: Oxford University Press, 1992;53.
5. **Hawiger J, Brass LF, Salzman EW.** Signal transduction and intracellular regulatory processes in platelets. In: Colman RW, Hirsh J, Marder VJ, Salzman EW, eds. Hemostasis and thrombosis: basic principles and clinical practice. 3rd ed. Philadelphia: JB Lippincott Company, 1994:603.
6. **Coughlin SR.** How thrombin 'talks' to cells. Molecular mechanisms and roles in vivo. Arterioscler Thromb Vasc Biol 1998;18:514–518.
7. **Marcus AJ.** Molecular eicosanoids and other metabolic interactions of platelets and other cells. In: Colman RW, Hirsh J, Marder VJ, Salzman EW, eds. Hemostasis and thrombosis: basic principles and clinical practice. 3rd edition. Philadelphia: JB Lippincott Company, 1994:590.
8. **Hwang DH.** Species variation in platelet aggregation. In: Longenecker GL, ed. The platelets: physiology and pharmacology. New York: Academic Press, 1985:289.
9. **Maclouf J, Folco G, Patrono C.** Eicosanoids and iso-eicosanoids: constitutive, inducible and transcellular biosynthesis in vascular disease. Thromb Haemost 1998;79:691–705.
10. **Gentry PA.** The mammalian blood platelets: its role in haemostasis, inflammation and tissue repair. J Comp Pathol 1992;107:243–270.
11. **de Groot PG, Sixma JJ.** Regulation of platelet-rich thrombus formation by the endothelium. In: van Hinsbergh VWM, ed. Vascular control of hemostasis. Amsterdam: Harwood Academic Publishers, 1996:127.

CHAPTER 65

Platelet Biology

• PATRICIA A. GENTRY

Blood platelets are the first line of host defense when blood vessels are damaged. They function to minimize blood loss by adhering to the subendothelium, aggregating, recruiting additional platelets to the area, and facilitating the localized formation of thrombin and fibrin in a microenvironment that ensures rapid thrombus formation. In addition to their critical function in hemostasis, platelets also play an essential role in inflammation and wound healing through direct cell–cell interactions and the release of soluble mediators from activated platelets that modulate the activity of other blood cells and the vascular endothelium. The majority of literature reports describe in vitro studies with human platelets, in part because of the rapidity with which platelet mediated intracellular and intercellular reactions occur in vivo, and also owing to the accessibility of blood platelets for experimentation. Although it is well documented that biochemical differences exits among platelets from different species,[1] it is clear that the overall platelet biological response to vascular trauma, inflammation, and participation in tissue repair are fundamentally similar in all mammals.

PLATELET ADHESION REACTIONS

Circulating platelets do not normally interact with intact vascular endothelium, with each other, or with other blood cells, but they adhere rapidly to thrombotic surfaces that develop after perturbations of the vascular endothelium.[2] The initial adhesion of single platelets to a surface (Fig. 65.1A) triggers a cascade of reactions leading to recruitment and adhesion of additional platelets (Fig. 65.1B) followed by the platelet coadhesion that constitutes aggregation (Fig. 65.1C). The initial adhesion phase involves two concurrent events: the adhesion of unstimulated platelets and their transition to an activated state. When trauma to the vasculature is sufficiently extensive to expose collagen fibers in the subendothelium, they serve as a potent agonist for platelet activation. Under less traumatic conditions von Willebrand factor (vWF), synthesized and secreted by endothelial cells, and fibrinogen, which can absorb to and infiltrate the vessel wall, are the major protein determinants of platelet adhesion. Initially, platelets adhere as a single layer, and their membranes undergo conforma-

tional changes causing activation of glycoprotein (GP) IIb/IIIa (CD41/CD61) receptors that have the dual role of supporting platelet adhesion to both fibrinogen and vWF. When blood flow occurs at low shear rates, the interaction between fibrinogen and the GPIIb/IIIa receptors is sufficient to facilitate the congregation and aggregation of platelets. However, at high shear rates, platelets are more readily activated and adhere more efficiently through interactions between vWF and GPIb/IX/V (CD42b+CD42c/CD42a/CD42d) platelet receptor complexes.[3] These supplementary adhesion sites ensure that the adherent platelets are not dislodged by turbulent flow around sites of vascular damage. This sequence of reactions appears similar for all species and involves the loss of the unstimulated platelet discoid shape (shape change) and the formation of long filopodia. The specific mechanisms that induce the second phase of adhesion, which involves platelet–platelet interactions and secretion of granular contents, are variable among mammalian species. For example, in species whose platelets possess an open canalicular system (OCS), such as humans, pigs, and rabbits, aggregate formation proceeds through (i) the spreading of the adherent platelets, which is associated with the development of cytoplasmic-filled pseudopods, (ii) the centripetal movement of α-granules and dense bodies that precedes their fusion with the OCS and, (iii) the dilation and vagination of the OCS to the external cell surface. These events not only provide a route for the secretion of granular contents but also expose additional platelet surface receptors derived from the α-granule membranes. Platelet spreading and pseudopod formation appears less extensive in species, e.g., bovine and Asian elephant, lacking an OCS. Further, in these platelets, as platelets coadhere their granules migrate to the periphery of the cell where they fuse with the external plasma membrane before releasing their contents.[1]

PLATELET BIOCHEMISTRY

Platelet Aggregation

The recruitment of circulating platelets and their incorporation into the developing platelet plug is facilitated by agonists, including adenosine diphosphate (ADP),

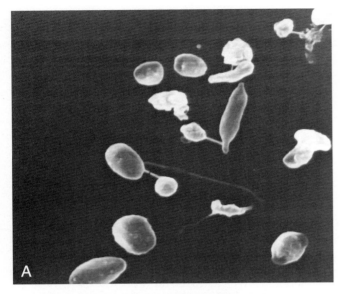

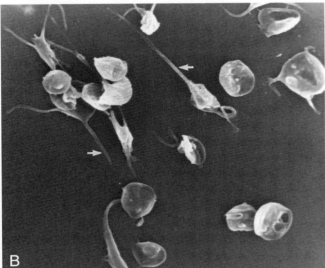

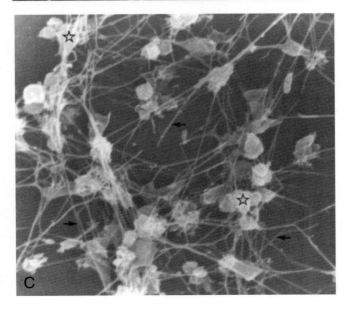

serotonin, and epinephrine, released from dense storage granules and the release of newly synthesized reactive molecules, such as platelet-activating factor (PAF) and thromboxane (Tx) A_2 from activated platelets (Fig. 65.2). Collectively these agonists function to accelerate the development of an irreversible platelet aggregate by recruiting additional platelets and inducing their activation and cohesion to the already adherent platelets.

Endogenous Agonists

Mammalian platelet aggregation is generally investigated in vitro by observation of the rate and extent of aggregate formation after the addition of an agonist to stirred suspensions of platelet-rich plasma or washed platelets. With the exception of thrombin and collagen, which consistently induce rapid irreversible aggregation in all mammalian platelets, a wide variation in response to other agonists is observed between species. This variation in sensitivity to a single agonist is related to several factors, including (i) whether the platelet has an OCS, (ii) the type and number of agonist receptors, and (iii) the ability of the platelet to synthesize and respond to TxA_2. For example, in OCS-containing platelets, the biochemical response to ADP is the extravasation of the OCS, resulting in an increased number of GPIIb/IIIa-fibrinogen bindings sites and the secretion of dense granule contents, including additional ADP, thus producing a higher local concentration that augments the initial stimulus.[4] Hence, in this type of platelet, irreversible aggregation is the typical response to even low doses of exogenous agonists. In contrast, low doses of these agonists generally induce only reversible aggregation in platelets that lack an OCS, although irreversible aggregation does occur with pharmacologic doses. Morphologic analysis of both bovine and elephant platelets undergoing a reversible aggregation response, as a result of stimulation with low, physiologic doses of ADP or PAF, reveal only limited intracellular granular movement with the majority of platelets displaying an intact granule complement. This indicates that there is limited release of dense granular contents to supplement the initial stimulus, and hence, irreversible aggregation is not induced. Unlike mammalian platelets, which consistently show some degree of response to ADP, nucleated

FIGURE 65.1 Scanning electron micrographs of washed bovine platelets adhering to a negatively charged surface (**A**) with no agonist stimulation, (**B**) with mild agonist stimulation by ADP, and (**C**) in the presence of thrombin. In the unstimulated sample (**A**) a majority of the adherent platelets have the characteristic discoid shape. When ADP is added to the platelet suspension (**B**) some platelets assume a crescent shape and exhibit the formation of filiform processes (arrows), and a few platelet–platelet interactions (stars) are visible. Platelets treated with thrombin (**C**) show increased adhesion and spreading, filiform process extensions (arrows), and evidence of aggregate formation (stars). (7,000 × magnification, 1.4-cm scale bar = 2 μm)

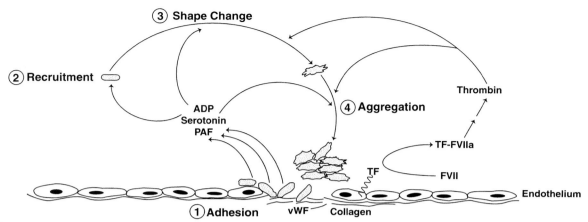

FIGURE 65.2 Diagrammatic representation of initial stages of the hemostatic process. (1) Damage to endothelial cells initiates platelet adhesion to collagen fibers and to the cell surface, resulting in release of ADP, serotonin, and PAF that collectively (2) recruit additional platelets to the site, (3) activate them so that they undergo shape change with the generation of surface binding sites that facilitate (4) the platelet–platelet cohesion reactions that constitute aggregation. The process is accelerated by actions of the potent agonist, thrombin, which is generated at the site of vascular damage on endothelial cells through the action of the TF-fVII pathway.

thrombocytes from birds and reptiles are insensitive to this agonist.[1]

The addition of either serotonin or epinephrine to mammalian platelet suspensions induces either no reaction or a weak aggregation response. Serotonin only induces the initial shape change reaction in rat, guinea pig, and dog platelets that is extended to a weak aggregation response in human, rabbit, cat, pig, sheep, cow, and horse platelets.[5] Only human, primate, feline, and canine platelets appear responsive to epinephrine. However, when all types of platelets are exposed to either serotonin or epinephrine in conjunction with another agonist, a synergistic strong aggregation response is consistently observed.[3] Because circulating levels of serotonin and epinephrine can become elevated in response to various physiologic events unrelated to vascular damage, the relative insensitivity of mammalian platelets to these agonists may serve as a protective mechanism to ensure that inappropriate platelet aggregation that could cause thrombotic disease does not occur.

Unlike human platelets that are less responsive to PAF than ADP, bovine, elephant, equine, and ovine platelets respond to nanomolar concentrations of PAF but only to micromolar concentrations of ADP.[1] Primate, canine, guinea pig, and rabbit platelets also aggregate after exposure to PAF, whereas mouse and rat platelets are insensitive to this agonist. Conversely, human platelets are more sensitive to TxA$_2$ stimulation than are platelets from domestic animals. For instance, both arachidonic acid (AA) and TxA$_2$ are potent agonists for human, guinea pig, and rabbit platelets but are weak agonists for equine platelets and fail to induce a response in bovine, elephant, rat, mink, and miniature pig platelets.[1,5] AA can also act as a strong agonist in some breeds of dogs and some inbred strains of mice but not in other breeds and strains.

Although the different platelet sensitivities and responses to an agonist in vitro are useful in elucidating the underlying intracellular biochemical mechanism involved in platelet function, it is likely that they have limited relevance to the in vivo situation. Within the circulation, platelets are simultaneously exposed to multiple agonists released from activated platelets (Fig. 65.2) and to additional agonists released from blood cells that become trapped within the developing thrombus. For example, erythrocytes release ADP, and PAF is generated by activated white cells, resulting in high local agonist concentrations.

Thrombin

In addition to initiating platelet adhesion, activated endothelial cells express on their surface the transmembrane protein tissue factor (TF). TF interacts with circulating factor VII (fVII) to form a proteolytic active complex, TF-fVIIa, that triggers a sequence of biochemical reactions that culminates in thrombin formation (see Fig. 65.2). Thrombin is a universal platelet agonist that initiates the entire cascade of events that constitute the basic platelet reaction: shape change, aggregation, secretion of granular contents, and synthesis of reactive compounds. Thrombin, through selective proteolytic cleavages causes the conversion of soluble fibrinogen to insoluble fibrin polymers. Although the fibrinogen content of platelet α-granules is low relative to the circulating plasma levels, local secretion can provide additional substrate molecules for thrombin.[6] The combined actions of thrombin in exposing binding sites on activated platelets and on fibrin formation result in a significant enhancement in the rate and extent of development of the fibrinogen or fibrin bridges between activated platelets. These stabilize the aggregates and accelerate thrombus formation because of potent procoagulant activity generated in this microenvironment.[2,3]

Energy Metabolism

Like all cells, platelets depend on adequate intracellular levels of adenosine triphosphate (ATP) to maintain cellular integrity in the unstimulated state and to support adhesion and aggregation reactions. In nonactivated platelets much of the available ATP is consumed to maintain osmotic equilibrium, to regulate cyclic adenosine monophosphate (cAMP) levels, and to maintain intramembrane phospholipid conformations.[4] Intracellular glycogen stores and glucose are the major energy sources for ATP production. Although circulating platelets are able to take up glucose from the circulation through membrane glucose transporters, glycogen granules are derived from megakaryocytes rather than from de novo synthesis. Both glycogen and glucose are metabolized to ATP and pyruvic acid by glycolysis. Because platelets contain few mitochondria, pyruvic acid is reduced to lactic acid, which diffuses out of the cell. These reactions explain the need to supplement platelet concentrates with both an energy source and a buffering capacity to retain platelet viability during storage. In activated platelets, glycogen phosphorolysis is stimulated by the immediate increase in cytosolic calcium. ATP generated by glycolysis appears more important than mitochondrial-derived ATP for sustaining platelet aggregation. The hexose monophosphate shunt pathway is functional within platelets, but the contribution of this pathway to maintaining glycolytic intermediates is poorly understood, as are the roles of fatty acids and amino acids in ATP production.[4]

MAINTENANCE OF VASCULAR INTEGRITY

The maintenance of integrity and patency of blood vessels requires that (i) thrombus formation be locally contained at sites of vascular damage, (ii) the thrombus be protected from premature degradation, and (iii) the thrombus be dissolved after vascular repair has occurred. Platelets participate directly or indirectly in each of these events.

Platelets and Hemostasis

Unstimulated platelets have little procoagulant activity because of the virtual absence of phosphatidyl serine (PS), formerly referred to as platelet factor 3 (PF3), on their outer surface.[1] As described in Chapter 63, Platelet Structure, Membrane Proteins, Cytoskeleton, Granules, and Secretory Pathways, when platelets are activated, PS is translocated to the outer membrane where it is readily available to function as an essential cofactor in the key proteolytic reactions, tenase and prothrombinase, involved in thrombin formation. The localized generation of thrombin further accelerates thrombus formation by (i) converting soluble fibrinogen to insoluble fibrin that forms the impermeable meshwork around the platelet aggregates, (ii) attracting and activating additional platelets to the area, and (iii) positive feedback

activation of procoagulant proteins, including fV, fIX, fVIII, and fX, which sustains a high local concentration of thrombin. Because they lack TF, platelets are unable to initiate thrombin formation, but they are essential for sustaining local thrombin generation at a site of vascular injury.

Regulation of Thrombus Formation

The two basic physiologic events that function to limit the size of thrombi are (a) the local release of inhibitory components from activated endothelial cells and (b) the suppression of thrombin generation on the surface of activated platelets (Fig. 65.3). At least three thromboregulatory substances are released when endothelial cells are activated.[7] Prostacyclin (PGI_2) is a major product of eicosanoid metabolism that acts as an inhibitor of mammalian platelets by elevating intracellular cAMP levels that suppress platelet reactivity. Vascular endothelial cells can synthesize endothelium-dependent relaxing factor/nitric oxide (EDRF/NO) that, in human platelets at least, functions to raise intracellular cyclic guanosine monophosphate (cGMP) levels which, like elevated cAMP, blocks agonist-induced aggregation. The third mechanism of suppression of platelet activation involves ectoadenosine diphosphatase (ecto-ADPase) activity in activated endothelial cells that metabolizes adenosine diphosphate (ADP) released from platelets to AMP and adenosine (Fig. 65.3).

The primary mechanism that limits the rate of thrombin formation on the platelet surface is proteolytic cleavage of fVIIIa and fVa to their respective inactive forms, FVIIIi and fVi by activated protein C (APC) (Fig. 65.3). Because fVIIIa and fVa are protein cofactors that regulate the rate of formation of the proteolytic complexes tenase and prothrombinase, their inactivation results in suppression of thrombin generation. APC formation is initiated by the thrombin-induced expression of thrombomodulin on endothelial cell membranes. Thrombin then binds to thrombomodulin, producing a highly reactive complex that converts plasma protein C to APC. The formation of APC is one of the few negative feedback actions of thrombin. The inhibitory action of APC is enhanced though its interaction with a plasma cofactor, Protein S, and PS exposed on the activated platelet surface. The effect of APC formation on the platelet surface in proximity to procoagulant complexes effectively blocks both fXa and thrombin generation.[1] A second platelet-mediated inhibitory mechanism involves tissue factor pathway inhibitor (TFPI), a potent inhibitor of prothrombin activation via the TF-fVIIa-fXa pathway.[8] The portion of TFPI that circulates in association with platelet membranes is released after platelet activation. Hence, platelet-associated TFPI can suppress TF-initiated coagulation in the microenvironment of platelet aggregates.

Control of Thrombolysis

Platelet-rich thrombi are fairly resistant to fibrinolysis. Before a clot can be dissolved, plasmin must be gen-

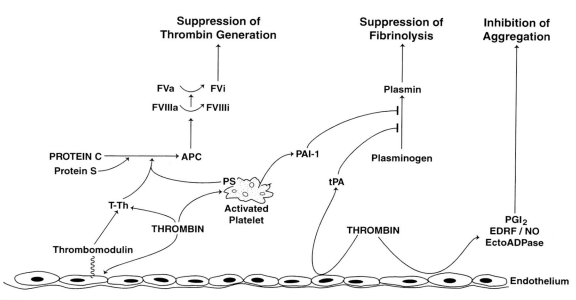

FIGURE 65.3 Diagrammatic representation of major platelet-mediated pathways that limit thrombus formation. In response to thrombin, vascular endothelial cells synthesize PGI$_2$, EDRF/NO, and ecto-ADPase that all can inhibit platelet function. Thrombin combines with thrombomodulin expressed on thrombin-activated endothelial surfaces and coverts protein C (PC) to its inhibitory form, APC, in a reaction requiring platelet surface PS. APC suppresses thrombin generation by converting the activated cofactors, fVIII and fV to inactive forms, fVIIIi and fVi, respectively. The fibrin strands that form around the platelet aggregates in the thrombus are protected from premature destruction by the inhibition of plasmin formation by PAI-1 released from activated platelets. Without PAI-1, tPA released from the thrombin-activated endothelial cells can initiate the fibrinolytic process.

erated by proteolytic cleavage of the plasminogen molecules that became embedded within the fibrin meshwork during thrombus formation. The tissue plasminogen activator (tPA) required to catalyze this reaction is released from thrombin-stimulated endothelial cells. Several proteolytic inhibitors are secreted by activated platelets, including plasminogen activator inhibitor (PAI-1). PAI-1 promotes clot stabilization at sites of hemostatic plug formation by serving as an inhibitor of both APC and tPA (Fig. 65.3). This platelet-derived PAI-1 ensures that thrombin generation, and hence fibrin formation, is sustained and that fibrinolysis is not initiated until the thrombus is consolidated and wound healing is well advanced. The physiologic significance of other inhibitors, including α_1-protease inhibitor, α_2 macroglobulin, C1 inhibitor, α_2 antiplasmin, and protease nexin 1, in regulating proteolytic activity in the microenvironment of a blood clot or during inflammation has yet to be established.[9]

PLATELETS AND INFLAMMATION

Interaction with Neutrophils

Mounting evidence exists from clinical studies in both people and animals that platelets play an essential role in inflammation through the release of vasoactive compounds, such as serotonin and PAF, the production of cytokines, e.g., interleukin (IL)-I, and the interaction of platelets with polymorphonuclear leukocytes (PMNs).

The ability of platelets and their release products to modulate PMN function is well established, but both stimulatory and inhibitory platelet effects have been reported.[6,10] It is probable that this apparent dicotomy reflects the parallel role of platelets in hemostasis and in inflammation: early platelet response reactions, e.g., exposure of P-selectin binding sites and release of nucleotides and PAF function to activate neutrophils, whereas secondary secretory products, e.g., β-thromboglobulin, released in the later stages of aggregation, exert an inhibitory effect.

Like platelets, PMNs, at low to moderate shear rates, can adhere to fibrin in an integrin-independent manner. At higher shear rates, P-selectin and GPIIb/IIIa binding sites presented on the surface of activated platelets are needed to tether PMNs and colocalize them within a thrombus. Platelet–PMN adhesion requires activated platelets but not prior PMN activation and, as occurs during platelet aggregation, results in enhanced reactivity of both cell types. Platelet–PMN interactions increase PMN production of reactive oxygen species through the release of platelet purine nucleotides. The somewhat low levels of PAF synthesized by activated platelets are sufficient to stimulate PAF production by PMNs that, along with platelet-generated AA metabolites, stimulate PMNs to release their granular contents and produce superoxide anions that function in combination to enhance the inflammatory response. At least with human platelets, this type of cross talk between platelets and PMNs also occurs through the action of cathepsin G, an agonist with a potency and biochemical action that

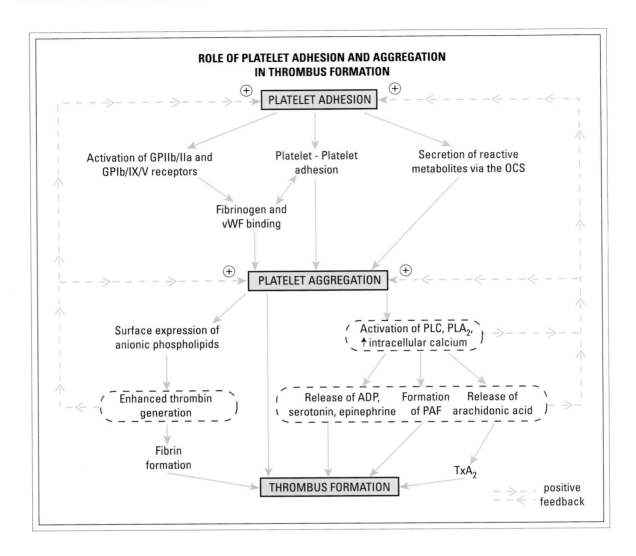

resembles thrombin that is released from activated neutrophils. In turn, a neutrophil-activating peptide (NAP-2) can be generated by cathepsin G from platelet α-granule precursor proteins that are resistant to proteolysis by thrombin or plasmin.[10] Platelets can also alleviate the extent of tissue damage by inhibiting the formation of reactive oxygen metabolites in activated neutrophils.[6]

Platelets as Inflammatory Cells

Circulating platelets can be directly activated by several inflammatory agents, including bacteria, viruses, and antibody-antigen complexes.[1,11] The biochemical consequences of such stimulations are similar to that of the endothelial cell-mediated hemostatic response. Hence, platelet activation is an early event of inflammation, and platelet release products contribute to the inflammatory response through the recruitment of additional cells and through the release of proteases, e.g., collagenase and elastase, and acid hydrolases from storage sites in lysosomes. The lysosomal secretory process differs from that of the α granules and dense granules. Not only are higher concentrations of agonist required, but release proceeds more slowly and is rarely complete. In platelets, as in other cells, the primary physiologic role of lysosomal enzymes is to degrade materials that have been endocytosed. Phagocytic and bactericidal activities toward material that has been internalized through the OCS system have been demonstrated for both rabbit and human platelets.[1] The fact that a greater number of lysosomes are found in bovine platelets (without an OCS) compared with human and rat platelets (that have an OCS) suggests that lysosomal enzymes have an important intracellular function in all types of platelets. Further, the thrombospondin that is released from activated platelets can mediate bacterial adherence at sites of platelet aggregates.[1]

PLATELETS AND TISSUE REPAIR

Platelets contain several potent mitogens, including platelet-derived growth factor (PDGF), epidermal

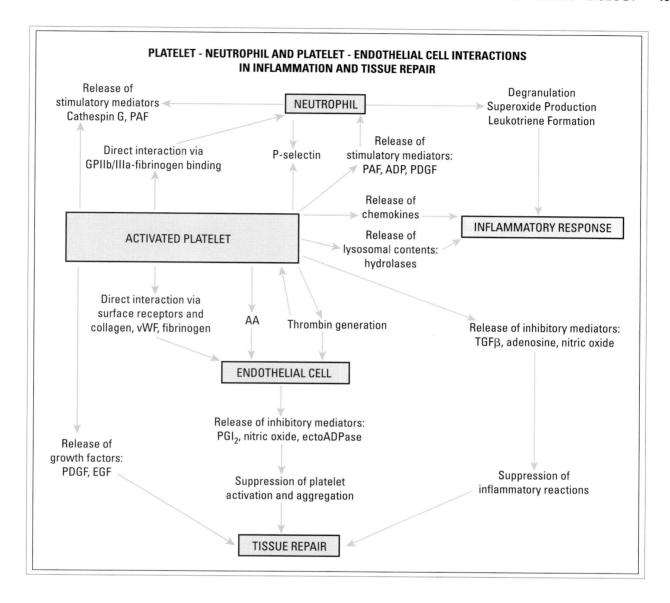

**PLATELET - NEUTROPHIL AND PLATELET - ENDOTHELIAL CELL INTERACTIONS
IN INFLAMMATION AND TISSUE REPAIR**

growth factor (EGF) and β-transforming growth factor (TGFβ). Megakaryocytes are the source of the PDGF, which is sequestered in α granules at a concentration several thousand times greater than the circulating plasma concentration.[9] When released from aggregating platelets, PDGF promotes wound healing by stimulating mitogenesis of smooth muscle cells and fibroblasts. PDGF is also important in inflammatory reactions associated with fibroproliferative responses because it is chemotactic for both monocytes and neutrophils. The localized release of PDGF from activated platelets is associated with the development of disorders associated with excessive cell growth, such as atherosclerosis and tumor production.[1,11] Unlike PDGF and EGF, which both promote wound fibroblast proliferation, TGF-β inhibits proliferation of many cell types, including endothelial cells. However, because it can also selectively increase production of integrins, decrease the synthesis of proteases that degrade extracellular matrix proteins, and in-

crease formation of several protease inhibitors, TGF-β, released at wound sites can function to modulate the extent of proteolysis of the vasculature and thus indirectly promote tissue repair.

REFERENCES

1. **Gentry PA.** The mammalian blood platelet: its role in haemostasis, inflammation and tissue repair. J Comp Pathol 1992;107:243–270.
2. **Ruggeri ZM.** New insights into the mechanisms of platelet adhesion and aggregation. Semin Hematol 1994;31:229–239.
3. **Colman RW, Cook JJ, Niewiarowski S.** Mechanisms of platelet aggregation. In: Colman RW, Hirsh J, Marder VJ, Salzman EW, eds. Hemostasis and thrombosis: basic principles and clinical practice. 3rd ed. Philadelphia: JB Lippincott Company, 1994:508.
4. **Holmsen H.** Platelet secretion and energy metabolism. In: Colman RW, Hirsh J, Marder VJ, Salzman EW, eds. Hemostasis and thrombosis: basic principles and clinical practice. 3rd ed. Philadelphia: JB Lippincott Company, 1994:524.
5. **Meyers KM.** Species differences. In: Holmsen H, ed. Platelet responses and metabolism, vol. 1. Boca Raton, FL: CRC Press, 1986:209.

6. **Allegrezza-Giuliettis A, Serretti R, Beccerica E, Muti S, Ferretti G, Cervini C.** Platelet release products modulate some aspects of polymorphonuclear leukocyte activation. J Cell Biochem 1991;47:242–250.
7. **Marcus AJ, Safier LB.** Thromboregulation: multicellular modulation of platelet reactivity in hemostasis and thrombosis. FASEB J 1993;7:516–522.
8. **Broze GJ.** The role of tissue factor pathway inhibitor in a revised coagulation cascade. Semin Hemost 1992;29:159–169.
9. **Niewiarowski S, Holt JC, Cook JJ.** Biochemistry and physiology of secreted platelet proteins. In: Colman RW, Hirsh J, Marder VJ, Salzman EW, eds. Hemostasis and thrombosis: basic principles and clinical practice. 3rd ed. Philadelphia: JB Lippincott Company, 1994:546.
10. **Flad HD, Harter L, Petersen F, Ehlert JE, Ludwig A, Bock L, Brandt E.** Regulation of neutrophils activation by proteolytic processing of platelet derived α- chemokines. Adv Exp Med Biol 1997;421:223–230.
11. **Boudreaux MK.** Platelets and coagulation. Vet Clin North Am Small Anim Pract 1996;26:1065–1087.

SECTION VII

Hemostasis: Platelets—Clinical Platelet Disorders

Annemarie T. Kristensen

CHAPTER 66

Platelet Production Defects

• DOUGLAS J. WEISS

Thrombocytopenia is a frequent clinical problem in dogs and cats and occurs in other domestic species.[1] At present, there is no noninvasive test that consistently differentiates thrombocytopenia caused by platelet destruction or consumption from thrombocytopenia caused by decreased platelet production. Thrombopoiesis has classically been assessed by bone marrow examination. However, the invasive nature of the procedure and the difficulty in accurately quantifying the number of megakaryocytes in bone marrow limits the usefulness of this procedure. The presence of large platelets (i.e., shift platelets) in blood smears has been associated with increased platelet production.[1,2] Large platelets were reported in blood smears from 50% of dogs that have immune-mediated thrombocytopenia but in less than 25% of dogs that have neoplasia and inflammatory diseases.[1] However, an increase in mean platelet volume has not correlated with increased platelet production. Increased mean platelet volume was detected in only 3 of 17 dogs that have disseminated intravascular coagulopathy, whereas, 3 of 9 dogs that have a primary bone marrow disorder had increased mean platelet volume.[3] Immature platelets have been identified in human beings and dogs by detecting increased ribonucleic acid content.[4] This technique is similar to the technique used for enumeration of reticulocytes.[5] One can identify immature (i.e., reticulated) platelets by staining with the fluorescent nucleic acid dye thiazole orange and quantifying platelet fluorescence intensity by use of flow cytometry.[6] In one study, 36 of 45 thrombocytopenic dogs had increased reticulated platelets compared with values for the healthy nonthrombocytopenic dogs.[4,5] Most dogs that have increased reticulated platelets had disease conditions in which the thrombocytopenia was attributed to destruction or consumption of platelets, whereas, those that did not have increased reticulated platelet had conditions associated with decreased thrombopoiesis. Therefore, determination of reticulated platelet numbers may be useful in differentiating platelet destruction or consumption from decreased production.

The percentage of cases of thrombocytopenia that result from decreased production versus those that result from destruction or consumption has not been determined, however, it seems probable that the majority of cases result from destruction or consumption. Thrombocytopenia caused by decreased production can be divided into disorders associated with pure megakaryocyte hypoplasia, marrow panhypoplasia, and dysthrombopoiesis (Table 66.1).

AMEGAKARYOCYTIC IMMUNE-MEDIATED THROMBOCYTOPENIA

Amegakaryocytic immune-mediated thrombocytopenia is a rare form of immune-mediated thrombocytopenia in which the putative autoantibody destroys megakaryocytes. Megakaryocytes are decreased or absent in marrow aspirates or core biopsy specimens. At least 3 bone marrow aspiration smears should be examined before megakaryocyte hypoplasia is diagnosed. Amegakaryocytic immune-mediated thrombocytopenia has been reported in a dog and a cat.[7,8] Both cases had severe thrombocytopenia and no megakaryocytes were observed in bone marrow aspiration smears. The cat had an associated immune-mediated hemolytic anemia. The dog recovered after treatment with steroidal and nonsteroidal immunosuppressive drugs and antibiotics, but the cat failed to respond to immunosuppressive therapy and was euthanatized. Anecdotal reports indicate that amegakaryocytic immune-mediated thrombocytopenia responds poorly to immunosuppressive or other therapies.

INFECTIOUS CAUSES OF DECREASED PLATELET PRODUCTION

Infectious causes of pure megakaryocytic hypoplasia include ehrlichiosis, feline leukemia virus infection, feline immunodeficiency virus infection, equine infectious anemia virus infection, African swine fever virus infection, and bovine virus diarrhea virus infection (Table 66.1). Thrombocytopenia is frequently associated with leukopenia or nonregenerative anemia but may occur as a pure thrombocytopenia. Thrombocytopenia is the most frequent hematologic abnormality occurring in canine ehrlichiosis. In acute ehrlichiosis, thrombocytopenia probably results from immune-mediated destruc-

TABLE 66.1	Reported Causes of Megakaryocyte Hypoplasia in Domestic Animals	
Pure Megakaryocytic Hypoplasia		
Immune-mediated		Dog, Cat
Infectious		
Ehrlichia		Dog, Cat
Feline leukemia virus		Cat
Feline immunodeficiency virus		Cat
Equine infectious anemia virus		Horse
African Swine fever virus		Pig
Bovine virus diarrhea virus		Cow
Vaccination		Dog, Cat, Pig
Panhypoplasia		
Infectious		
Ehrlichia		Dog, Cat
Parvovirus		Dog, Cat
Feline leukemia virus		Cat
Feline immunodeficiency virus		Cat
Equine infectious anemia virus		Horse
Bovine virus diarrhea virus		Cow
Drug-associated		
Estrogen		Dog
Chemotherapy		Dog, Cat
Phenylbutazone		Dog, Horse
Meclofenamic acid		Dog
Sulfadiazine		Dog, Cat
Cefazedone		Dog
Quinidine		Dog
Thiacetarsamide		Dog
Griseofulvin		Cat
Methimazole		Cat
Toxins		
Brackenfern		Cow, Sheep
Trichloroethylene		Cow, Horse
Aflatoxin B_1		Pig
Radiation		Dog
Dysthrombopoiesis		
Myelodysplastic syndrome		Dog, Cat
Megakaryoblastic leukemia		Dog

tion of platelets in the circulation, but in chronic ehrlichiosis, thrombocytopenia probably results from decreased production.[9] The mechanism responsible for thrombocytopenia associated with viral infections is poorly understood. Feline leukemia and immunodeficiency viruses, African swine fever virus, and bovine virus diarrhea virus directly invade bone marrow and may destroy megakaryocytes and other hemopoietic cells.[10–12] African swine fever virus infects megakaryocytes and induced severe thrombocytopenia by day 7 after infection. Degenerative changes in megakaryocytes, including swelling and vacuolization, were observed by day 2 postinfection, and megakaryocytes appeared necrotic at day 4 post infection.[10] Of 5 thrombocytopenic cattle infected with bovine virus diarrhea virus, no megakaryocytes were observed in bone marrow aspiration smears from 2 and megakaryocytes were normal to increased in 3.[11] Viruses can also infect marrow stromal cells, resulting in decreased production of hemopoietic cytokines or production of he-

mopoietic suppresser substances.[13] Feline leukemia virus and equine infectious anemia virus may suppress hemopoiesis by increasing production of tumor necrosis factor.[14]

VACCINATION-INDUCED THROMBOCYTOPENIA

After administration of modified-live measles, distemper, and parvovirus vaccinations, vaccination-induced thrombocytopenia has been reported in dogs; it has been reported in cats after feline panleukopenia virus vaccination; and in pigs after hog cholera vaccination.[15,16] Mild to moderate thrombocytopenia usually begins 3 to 5 days after vaccination. Clinical bleeding tendencies have not been observed and treatment is unnecessary. The mechanism responsible for the thrombocytopenia is unknown and bone marrow studies have not been done.

DRUG-INDUCED SUPPRESSION OF THROMBOPOIESIS

Rarely, drug-induced suppression of thrombopoiesis selectively suppresses megakaryocytes. In acute drug toxicity, neutropenia usually develops at approximately day 5, and thrombocytopenia develops between days 8 and 10.[17] Because of the long red blood cell (RBC) life span, animals are usually not anemic. Drugs frequently associated with suppression of hemopoiesis include chemotherapeutic agents, sulfadiazine, estrogen compounds, and nonsteroidal anti-inflammatory drugs.[17,18]

TOXIN-INDUCED SUPPRESSION OF THROMBOPOIESIS

Toxins that induce thrombocytopenia include aflatoxin B_1, brackenfern, and trichloroethylene.[19–21] All of these compounds produce suppression of all marrow cell lines and result in aplastic anemia.

DYSTHROMBOPOIESIS

Dysthrombopoiesis is defined as disordered production of platelets and has been associated with myelodysplastic syndromes and megakaryoblastic leukemia. Myelodysplastic disorders are characterized by cytopenias in the blood and hypercellular bone marrow with dysplastic changes in one or more cell lines.[22–24] Features of dysthrombopoiesis include macrothrombocytes with increased granulation in blood and megakaryocytes characterized by immaturity, increased nuclear-to-cytoplasmic ratio, asynchronous nuclear-to-cytoplasmic maturation, dispersed nuclei, or anisokaryosis.[23] The cause of dysthrombopoiesis is poorly understood. In cats, feline leukemia virus infection is the major cause of dysthrombopoiesis. In dogs, inherited and acquired genetic mutation, treatment with chemotherapeutic drugs and cephalosporins, and vitamin B_{12} and folic acid deficiencies have been identified as causes of myelodysplasia.[23,24]

Megakaryoblastic leukemia is a rare form of leukemia in dogs. Both spontaneously occurring and radiation-induced forms have been described.[25,26] Large bizarre platelets are usually seen in blood, and megakaryoblasts may be present. Increased numbers of immature and atypical megakaryocytes are seen in bone marrow.

TREATMENT OF PLATELET PRODUCTION DEFECTS

Definitive guidelines for treatment of platelet production disorders in animals have not been described. General approaches to treatment include administration of platelet-rich plasma transfusions, immunosuppressive therapy, removal of causative agents, and stimulation of residual thrombopoiesis. Platelet transfusions are indicated for animals that have signs of clinical bleeding or those that have severe thrombocytopenia (i.e., $<2,000/\mu L$). The indications and techniques for platelet transfusion have been described.[27] Steroidal or nonsteroidal immunosuppressive therapy is indicated in cases of immune-mediated thrombocytopenia (Chapter 68, Immune-Mediated Thrombocytopenia). Removal of causative agents includes specific treatment for causative infectious agents, discontinuation of potentially causative drugs, and elimination of exposure to potential toxins. Recently, thrombopoietin has been characterized and a recombinant human product is available for therapeutic use.[28] Thrombopoietin is the primary regulator of megakaryocyte and platelet production. Thrombopoietin appears to stimulate proliferation of primitive hemopoietic stem cells as well as megakaryocytic precursor cells. Presumably, platelet production defects other than those caused by decreased thrombopoietin production, should have high levels of thrombopoietin in the blood. It remains to be determined if administration of exogenous thrombopoietin will be beneficial.

CONCLUSION

Decreased platelet production is most frequently associated with generalized suppression of hemopoiesis (i.e., aplastic anemia). Pure megakaryocyte hypoplasia and dysthrombopoiesis are rare causes of decreased production. Differentiation of the various causes of decreased platelet production is based on careful evaluation of blood and bone marrow and evaluation of exposure to infectious agents, drugs, and toxins.

REFERENCES

1. **Grindem CB, Breitschwerdt EB, Corbett WT, Jans HE.** Epidemiologic survey of thrombocytopenia in dogs: a report on 987 cases. Vet Clin Pathol 1991;20:38–43.
2. **Jain NC.** Essentials of veterinary hematology. Philadelphia: Lea & Febiger, 1993.
3. **Northern J, Tvedten HW.** Diagnosis of microthrombosis and immunemediated thrombocytopenia in dogs with thrombocytopenia: 68 cases (1987–1989). J Am Vet Med Assoc 1992;200:368–372.
4. **Weiss DJ, Townsend E.** Evaluation of reticulated platelets in dogs. Comp Haematol Int 1998;8:166–170.
5. **Corberand JX.** Reticulocyte analysis using flow cytometry. Hematol Cell Ther 1996;38:487–494.
6. **Kienast J, Schmitz G.** Flow cytometric analysis of thiazole orange uptake by platelets: a diagnostic aid in the evaluation of thrombocytopenic disorders. Blood 1990;75:116–121.
7. **Murtaugh RJ, Jacobs RM.** Suspected immune-mediated megakaryocytic hypoplasia. J Am Vet Med Assoc 1985;186:1313–1315.
8. **Gaschen FP, Smith Meyer B, Harvey JW.** Amegakaryocytic thrombocytopenia and immune-mediated haemolytic anemia in a cat. Comp Haematol Int 1992;2:175–178.
9. **Waner T, Harris S, Weiss DJ.** Detection of serum antiplatelet antibodies in experimental acute canine ehrlichiosis. Vet Immunol Immunopath 1995;48:177–182.
10. **Calderon NL, Paasch LH, Bouda J.** Haematological and histological bone marrow findings in experimental classical swine fever. Acta Vet Brno 1997;66:171.
11. **Rebhun WC, French TW, Perdrizet JA, Dubovi EJ, Dill SG, Karcher LF.** Thrombocytopenia associated with acute bovine virus diarrhea infection in cattle. J Vet Intern Med 1989;3:42–46.
12. **Shelton GH, Linenberger ML.** Hematologic abnormalities associated with retroviral infections in the cat. Semin Vet Med Surg 1995;10:220–233.
13. **Linenberger ML, Dow SW, Abkowitz JL.** Feline leukemia virus infection downmodulates the production of growth-inhibitory activity by marrow stromal cells. Exp Hematol 1995;23:1069–1079.
14. **Tornquist SJ, Oaks JL, Crawford TB.** The role of TNF-α and TGF-β in suppression of megakaryocytopoiesis in equine infectious anemia. Vet Pathol 1996;33:576.
15. **Dodds WJ.** Immune-mediated diseases of the blood. Adv Vet Sci Comp Med 1983;27:163–196.
16. **Stokol T, Parry BW.** The effects of modified-live vaccination on the platelet count and von Willebrand factor antigen. Vet Pathol 1995;32:549.
17. **Weiss DJ, Klausner JS.** Drug-associated aplastic anemia in dogs: eight cases (1984–1988). J Am Vet Med Assoc 1990;196:472.
18. **Handagama P, Feldman BF.** Thrombocytopenia and drugs. Vet Clin North Am 1988;18:51–65.
19. **Cukrova V, Langrova E, Akao M.** Effects of aflatoxin B_1 on myelopoiesis in vitro. Toxicology 1991;70:203–211.
20. **McKinney LL, Weakley FB, Cambell RE, Eldridge AC, Cowan JC.** Toxic protein from trichloroethylene-extracted soybean oil meal. J Am Oil Chem 1957;34:461–466.
21. **Dalton RG.** The effects of batyl alcohol on the haematology of cattle poisoned with bracken. Vet Rec 1964;76:411–416.
22. **Raskin RE, Krehbiel JD.** Myelodysplastic changes in a cat with myelomonocytic leukemia. J Am Vet Med Assoc 1985;187:171–174.
23. **Weiss DJ, Raskin R.** Myelodysplastic syndrome in the dog. J Am Vet Med Assoc 1985;187:1038–1041.
24. **Couto CG, Kallet AJ.** Preleukemia syndrome in a dog. J Am Vet Med Assoc 1984;184:1389–1392.
25. **Shull RM, DeNovo RC, McCraken MD.** Megakaryoblastic leukemia in a dog. Vet Pathol 1986;23:533–536.
26. **Cain B, Kawakami TC, Jain NC.** Radiation-induced megakaryoblastic leukemia in a dog. Vet Pathol 1985;22:641.
27. **Cotter SM.** Transfusion of platelets. Adv Vet Sci Comp Med 1991;36:209–210.
28. **Ramsfjell V, Borge OJ, Jacobsen SEW.** Thrombopoietin directly and potently stimulates multilineage growth and progenitor cells expansion from primitive (CD34 (+) CD38 (−)) human bone marrow progenitor cells—distinct and key interactions with the ligands for C-kit and FLT3, and inhibitory effects of TGF-beta and TNF-alpha. J Immunol 1997;158:5169–5177.

CHAPTER 67

Drug-Induced Thrombocytopenias

• KURT L. ZIMMERMAN

T hrombocytopenia is one of the most commonly recognized hematologic disorders seen in veterinary medicine. It is essential for the clinician to understand the common pathogeneses and origins involved in the development of thrombocytopenias. In this chapter, thrombocytopenias arising as a result of drug administration is the focus. Drug-induced thrombocytopenias (DITs) are caused by several different mechanisms: decreased platelet production; increased platelet consumption; platelet sequestration; and excessive platelet loss.[1] Some of these mechanisms are shared with other disease processes leading to thrombocytopenias. The incidence of DIT in animals is not known, but several reports exist documenting the problem.[2,3]

CLINICAL PRESENTATION

Clinical symptoms of DIT are similar to those observed in other types of thrombocytopenias. Hemorrhage is not likely unless the platelet count is less than 25,000–50,000/μL.[4,5] If symptoms consistent with hemorrhage caused by thrombocytopenia are present, petechiation and ecchymosis, a platelet count and buccal bleeding time are indicated.

A thorough patient history exploring exposure to any medication is always indicated in any case in which a low platelet count is encountered. It is important to remember that not only are prescription medications capable of inducing a thrombocytopenia but that many of the over-the-counter medications have also been incriminated.[6] In an examination of the United States Pharmacopia Drug Information Volume I text, "Drug Information for the Health Care Professional", listing over 11,000 different prescription and over-the-counter drugs, there are 812 references to the risk of thrombocytopenia as a potential complication associated with therapy.[7]

PATHOGENESIS OF DRUG-INDUCED THROMBOCYTOPENIAS

Drug-Induced Marrow-Mediated Thrombocytopenia

Suppression

Bone marrow suppression caused by drug administration may be directly caused by the cytotoxic effect on the bone marrow progenitor cells as observed with most chemotherapeutic medications used in veterinary medicine (Table 67.1) or may be caused by an idiosyncratic reaction. Marrow cells are predisposed to such damage because of their high mitotic rate.[8] Because the life span of the platelet varies from 3 to 10 days, depending on the species, and the granulocytic cell line has a much shorter life span in the peripheral circulation, abnormalities are typically first observed in the white blood cell indexes.[9] Table 67.1 contains a list of myelosuppressive chemotherapeutic agents capable of inducing thrombocytopenia. These agents tend to exert their effect in a dose-related response, and therefore the resulting thrombocytopenia tends to be predictable and more easily controlled.

Other directly cytotoxic agents may have a more unpredictable manifestation of their toxic side effects. Chloramphenicol has been associated with both regenerative and nonregenerative aplastic anemias in both the dog and the cat.[10] The regenerative aplastic anemia tends to follow a dose-related directly cytotoxic linear relation directed at the mitochondria, whereas the nonregenerative aplastic anemia manifestation is idiopathic. This latter presentation is believed to involve bacterial metabolites of the drug, which are formed in the gut and reabsorbed. These metabolites then undergo further metabolic transformation in the bone marrow with in situ production of toxic intermediates, which then have a direct cytotoxic effect on the marrow cells.[11]

The administration of estrogen derivatives has also been noted to produce marrow suppression resulting

TABLE 67.1	Drugs Known to Cause Thrombocytopenia by Bone Marrow Suppression[17]	

Antibiotics
  Chloramphenicol
  Streptomycin
 	
Antimicrobial Agents
  Isoniazid
  Sulfonamides
  Quinacrine
  Organic arsenicals
 	
Anticonvulsants
  Methylhydantoin
  Trimethadione
  Paramethadione
 	
Anti-inflammatory Agents
  Colchicine
  Phenylbutazone
  Gold salts
  Indomethacin
	Chemotherapeutic[8]
	  5-Fluorouracil
	  6-Mercaptopurine
	  Actinomycin D
	  Carboplatin[18–20]
	  Cisplatin
	  Cyclophosphamide
	  Cystine Arabinoside
	  Doxorubicin
	  Hydroxyurea
	  Melphalan
	  Methotrexate
	  Mitomycin C
	  Mitoxantrone
	  Vinblastine
	  Vincristine
		Antiviral
		  Ribavirin[21]
		
		Miscellaneous
		  Estrogens
		  Prednisolone
		  Interferon[15]
		  Thiacetarsamide[22]
		  Griseofulvin[22]
		
		Diuretics
		  Thiazide derivatives
		  Acetazolamide

Data from references 8, 15, 17–22 with permission.

in thrombocytopenia. The canine patient seems much more susceptible to estrogen-induced marrow suppression than other species.[12] Within the canine population, much individual variability as to the susceptibility to the toxic effect seems to exist. This has made it difficult to predict the precise dosages, which may elicit the reaction, all this suggesting a genetic predisposition to the syndrome.[13] Marrow suppression because of estrogen therapy initially produces a thrombocytopenia, a progressive nonregenerative anemia, and an initial increased neutrophil granulopoiesis and leukocytosis followed by a pancytopenia.[1]

Interferon administration may induce apoptosis of marrow stem cells in man and mice, leading to inhibition of hemopoiesis by means of the destruction of stem cells and more mature progenitor cells.[14,15]

Bone marrow aspiration and biopsies from the affected animals contain decreased numbers of megakaryocytes. In the normal canine patient, aspirates contain 1 to 3 megakaryocytes per low-power field.[16] This can be a useful parameter in distinguishing the underlying cause for the thrombocytopenia because drug-induced immune-mediated mechanisms often elicit increased numbers of megakaryocytes.[17] However, in human patients who have immune-mediated thrombocytopenia, 30% of the cases are associated with a decrease in megakaryocytes.[4] Many isolated case reports of marrow suppression by various classes of drugs exist. Table 67.1 contains a listing of some of the more commonly reported agents in these classes.[8,15,18–22]

Immune-Mediated

Drug-induced immune-mediated destruction of platelets has been observed in humans and dogs.[23] Although the immunologic mechanisms are similar peripherally and at the marrow level, an increase in megakaryocytes

is present with the former and a decrease with the latter.[4] In veterinary medicine only a few suspected cases of DIT caused by pure immune-mediated bone marrow destruction of megakaryocytes have been reported. Megakaryocytes are more commonly damaged concurrently while one of the peripherally mediated immune mechanisms, which are discussed later, is at work.

Drug-Induced Peripherally Mediated Thrombocytopenia

Once platelets have been released into the peripheral circulation, they are vulnerable to being prematurely removed from circulation by one of two categories of mechanism: immune-mediated and nonimmune-mediated.

Drug-Induced Immune-Mediated

The most common underlying mechanism documented in drug-induced peripheral thrombocytopenias in dogs, cats, and horses is immune-mediated. This drug induced immune-mediated destruction can be further classified as being due to either a primary or a secondary mechanism.

Primary Primary drug-induced immune-mediated thrombocytopenia is rare. Compounds included in the primary category are those few drugs capable of inducing an immune-mediated thrombocytopenia independent of the continued presence of the eliciting drug. These compounds seem to provoke an immune response directed at an unadulterated antigen on the platelet's surface membrane. Methyldopa and levodopa are two such compounds capable of inducing a true autoimmune response directed against platelets and red blood cells than can persist for months after discontinuation of therapy.[5] Gold therapy may also seem to fall within this group because clinical manifestation of an immune-mediated thrombocytopenia in dogs and humans may become evident months after the discontinuation of therapy.[17] Likely though, the immune reaction induced by gold therapy is of the secondary type in which the drug itself plays a role as a hapten interacting with the platelet membrane and immunoglobulin. This is possible because of the prolonged half-life (months) of gold compounds in the body.

Secondary Novel Exposure The more common manifestation of a drug-induced immune-mediated thrombocytopenia is secondary in which the concurrent presence of the drug is required for the manifestation of the immune-mediated destruction. Within this secondary category, the agents can be further subdivided into two subclasses based on the exposure history to the drug (first time exposure versus repeat exposure).

In the first subclass, novel, a few drugs have been recognized to elicit immune-mediated thrombocytopenias without previous sensitization of the patient to the medication or without the long-term use of the drug. Two commonly used medications fall into this category: heparin and quinine.

Heparin has been recognized as inducing thrombocytopenia in humans and horses after its administration. In people approximately 10% of the patients treated with unfractionated heparin develop platelet counts less than 150,000/μL. This seems to be mediated by preformed platelet-activating antibodies directed not at heparin itself but at the complex formed between heparin and platelet factor 4 found in the α granules of the platelet.[24,25]

Quinine, an antimalarial drug, is another medication that appears capable producing a thrombocytopenia in humans by reacting with specific glycoprotein (GP) molecules on the platelet's surface membrane, specifically GP1b and GPIX.[26] Evidence suggests that it is the hypervariable region of a drug-dependent antibody that binds to a second domain-specific region of the target platelet while binding to the attached quinine that then leads to platelet activation.[27]

Secondary Previous Exposure In the second subclass, previous, the drug-induced immune-mediated thrombocytopenia occurs at least a week or more after the initiation of a drug or at least 3 days after its subsequent reintroduction to the animal and has been seen in dogs, cats, and horses.[5,17] It is in this final category, where most of the encountered drug offenders lie and unfortunately, this is where most of the confusion over the precise immunologic bases of the resulting platelet destruction also resides.

Regardless of the exact underlying mechanism, the affected platelets are ultimately destroyed by the interaction of the FC portion of the immunoglobulin and attached platelet with macrophages in the spleen and liver.[5] The immunoglobulins (Igs) involved may be of the gamma G Ig (IgG) or the gamma M Ig (IgM) class

but are frequently of the IgG type in dogs.[5] The modes of interaction between the platelet and immunoglobulins can be varied and hard to predict. Generally, one of five interactions can occur:

1. The drug in question binds with a plasma protein that then forms a complex with the Ig directed against this drug-protein unit. The entire complex then is absorbed onto the platelet's surface.
2. The drug-protein complex binds directly to the platelet's surface and the Ig then binds to the protein-drug complex attached to the platelet's surface.
3. The drug in question binds directly to the platelet's membrane and the Ig then discreetly binds to the attached drug.
4. The same mechanism as in number 3, except the Ig attaches to a combination of the attached drug and a platelet surface antigen.
5. The drug attaches to the platelet, and doing so induces the expression of new surface antigens to which the Ig attaches.[17,27]

As this category accounts for the majority of the reported occurrences of drug-induced immune-mediated thrombocytopenias, no attempt is made here to present the reader with an all-inclusive list of the offending compounds.[28] However, mention of the most common culprits can be made, and Table 67.2 is provided as a general listing of compounds that have provoked such thrombocytopenias in canine, feline, equine, and bovine patients. In one study of human cases of drug-induced thrombocytopenias over a 23-year period, sulfamethoxazole and trimethoprim were the most commonly reported single drugs, and nonsteroid anti-inflammatory drugs were the most frequently reported category of drugs involved.[28] Cases involving trimethoprim have been reported in the veterinary literature involving dogs.[29–31] However, it is important to realize that such reactions can occur with virtually any medication (Table 67.2).[22,32–35]

Nonimmune Mechanisms

Medications may cause direct agglutination, sequestration, and loss or may induce platelet consumption by means of the normal platelet activation and coagulation pathways.

Iron supplementation, in the form of both injectable iron dextran and oral supplementation has been incriminated in thrombocytopenia in a horse.[36] The mechanism suggested consumption of platelets because of disseminated intravascular coagulation. Iron toxicity leads to interference with thrombin function and its production, and the suppression of other components of the intrinsic coagulation pathway.[36] Prolongation of both the activated partial thromboplastin time (APTT) and the prothrombin time (PT) would be expected in such cases.

Although anticoagulation rodenticides are not employed as common therapeutic agents, patients are inadvertently exposed to them frequently. Thrombocytopenias induced by hemorrhage are typically mild in the canine patient that has counts typically reported as less

TABLE 67.2   Drugs Associated with Increased Platelet Destruction[6]

Antibiotics	Anti-inflammatory Agents	Hormones
Cephalosporins	Acetaminophen	Estrogens
Sulfonamides	Aspirin	
Trimethoprim	Phenylbutazone	Miscellaneous
Penicillins	Gold salts	Protamine sulfate
Novobiocin		Heparin
Oxytetracycline	Cardiovascular Drugs	Phenobarbital
Streptomycin	Digitoxin	Diazepam
Erythromycin	Digoxin	Para-aminosalicylic acid
Methicillin	Nitroglycerin	Desipramine
Rifamycin	Methyldopa	Chlorpheniramine
Rifampicin[32]	Levodopa	Lidocaine
	Hydralazine	Methimazole[35]
Antimicrobial Agents		Propylthiouracil[22]
Dinitrophenol	Diuretics	DL-Methionine[22]
Quinine	Thiazide derivatives	
Organic arsenicals	Furosemide[33]	
Dapsone		
	Vaccine	
Helminthicide	Modified live canine	
Fenbendazole[22]	distemper virus[34]	

Data from references 6, 22, 32–35 with permission.

than 150,000.[37] However, there have been reported cases in which the count has reached as low as 20,000 platelets/μL of blood before transfusion and hemodilution and may be owing to peripheral consumption of platelets or the direct suppression of the bone marrow.[37] For this reason the clinician must consider anticoagulation rodenticides as a possibility in cases in which a mild to moderated thrombocytopenia is present; there is clinical evidence of some form of hemorrhage (often no petechiation); and in which the APTT, and PT values are increased along with normal fibrin degradation products (FDPs) levels.

Ristocetin, an antibiotic, has been documented as causing the direct agglutination of platelets in humans, dogs, cattle, camelidae, and mice.[17] The mechanism of the agglutination is related to the interaction between von Willebrand's cofactor, the antibiotic, and GPIb on the platelet's surface.[38–43] The agglutination reaction is irreversible, and its intensity is correlated with the concentration of von Willebrand's factor present, making it a useful research and diagnostic tool in the study of von Willebrand's disease.

DIAGNOSIS

Because the underlying mechanism involved in the production of any one particular drug-induced thrombocytopenic episode is often unknown, a clinical approach is often employed in the identification of the adverse drug reaction. Feldman and others have suggested the use of the following four criteria in the identification of compounds suspected of inducing a thrombocytopenia:

1. The thrombocytopenia develops after a lag that coincides with the minimum time needed to produce a primary immune response.

2. Rapid recovery is observed in the platelet numbers after the drug is discontinued.
3. There is immediate reoccurrence of the thrombocytopenia after reexposure to the drug.
4. There are normal or increased numbers of megakaryocytes in the bone marrow.[17]

Assessment as to the adequacy of thrombopoiesis in the bone marrow can be of great help in determining the cause of an observed thrombocytopenia. Generally, in patients in which a thrombocytopenia is associated with a drug-induced immune-mediated mechanism, there is hyperplasia of megakaryocytes with a maturation shift to the left visible in a bone marrow aspirate from the patient.[4] The presence of a low number of platelets in the patient's peripheral blood sample should not preclude the clinician from proceeding with a marrow biopsy or aspirate if it is needed as part of the diagnostic workup. Clinical experience has shown that the risk of hemorrhage is minimal in such individuals.

It has been demonstrated that one can predict a normal or a proliferation of the number of megakaryocytes present in the bone marrow by analyzing the mean platelet volume of the circulating platelets in the patient's blood. Platelet volumes greater than 12.00 μm^3 were associated with a normal to a hyperplastic bone marrow megakaryocyte production level, and the measurement had a predictive positive value of 96%.[44] Unfortunately, in another study, it was demonstrated that a microthrombocytosis was identified in 17 of 31 dogs experiencing an immune-mediated thrombocytopenia.[45] In animals that have lower mean platelet volume values, the possibility of megakaryocytic hyperplasia or normoplasia could not be ruled out; therefore it is necessary to obtain a marrow sample so that megakaryocyte numbers can be evaluated. In patients experiencing thrombocytopenias caused by marrow suppression from a drug,

TABLE 67.3   Diagnostic Database[16]

Complete History	Physical Examination	Clinical Pathology	Antiplatelet Antibody
Recent vaccinations, drugs, illness, travel to regions endemic with Ehrlichia, Rickettsia, Histoplasma, or dirofilaria	Distribution of hemorrhage: Cutaneous: Inspection of pinnae, pressure points, and ventral abdomen Mucosal: Examination of oral, nasal, and urogenital mucosa Ocular: Ophthalmic examination	Direct blood smear: Rapidly estimate platelet and megathrombocyte numbers and detects erythrocyte and leukocyte involvement	Antiplatelet antibody measured if suitable test readily available Treatment not delayed pending results.
		Complete hemogram	
		Serum biochemical profile	
	Exploration for concurrent disease: Including abdominal palpation for neoplasia or splenomegaly	Urinalysis	
		Coagulation profile with FDP[a]	
		Bone marrow aspiration and biopsy	

[a] Test added to original list by current author.

the resulting marrow aspirate is typically depicted by a hypocellular sample with the exception of early estrogen toxicity and its associated granulocytic hyperplasia.[1]

Various tests have been used to identify antiplatelet antibodies thought to be drug induced. There are two tests routinely employed for this purpose: the platelet factor 3 (PF3) test and the megakaryocyte direct immunofluorescence (MDIF) test. In the PF3 test, a sample of the patient's serum is collected and incubated in the presence of the suspected offending drug. If the patient's serum contains Ig that interact with the drug and the homologous platelets, the homologous platelets will release an increased amount of PF3 that increases the rate of clot formation compared with a control sample.[46] This test has sensitivity that is highly variable, ranging from 28 to 80%.[5] Several variations of this test have been presented in the literature.[44] For the other test, MDIF, to be performed, adequate numbers of megakaryocytes in the marrow must be present. A positive test occurs with the addition of a species-specific fluorescein-linked Ig reacting with the test patient's megakaryocytes coated with the drug-induced Ig and the drug in question.[16] Variations of different immunologic tests have been developed to detect platelet-associated antibodies. Both radio immuno assays, and direct and indirect enzyme-linked immunosorbent assay (ELISA) tests have been developed with the direct method detecting platelet-bound IgG and the indirect, detecting serum platelet-bindable immunoglobulins. It has been reported that the direct test has a greater sensitivity of 94% compared with 34% with the indirect version.[5] Flow-cytometric assays have also been successfully employed in the identification of platelet-associated antibodies.[47] However, these later immunologic tests have limited availability. Along with the aforementioned diagnostic tests, a minimal database for a patient experiencing a thrombocytopenia has been included in Table 67.3.

TREATMENT

The cornerstone of treatment in any case in which an episode of DIT is suspected is the immediate discontinuation of all of the medications that the patient may be receiving.[17] Most cases of drug-induced immune-mediated thrombocytopenia resolve within 2 weeks of the discontinuation of the offending drug, and often no further intervention is required.[5]

In cases in which the thrombocytopenia is endangering the life of the patient, transfusions with platelet–rich plasma (10 mL/kg) or whole blood (20 mL/kg) may be warranted.[16] The quantities of blood needed to maintain adequate platelet levels may not be practical, particularly if thrombocyte numbers do not stay elevated by 5,000 to 10,000 for at least 2 hours posttransfusion.[5,16] Glucocorticoids are often administered in such cases both orally (prednisone at 2 to 4 mg/kg/day) and intravenously (dexamethasone at 0.2 mg/kg as single dose). In cases in which there is evidence of persistence of immune-mediated destruction of platelets or a poor response to the above therapy is seen, more potent immunosuppressive agents may be considered. Azathioprine (2 mg/kg orally once daily with a gradual tapering of the dosage) or cyclophosphamide (50 mg/m² orally the first 4 days of the week for a maximum of 4 to 5 months) may be added to the therapy.[16] In patients suffering from thrombocytopenia caused by marrow suppression, the use of anabolic steroids, lithium, and hemopoietic growth factors may be worth considering.[48]

REFERENCES

1. **Jain NC.** The platelet. In: Mundorff GH, ed. Essentials of veterinary hematology. Philadelphia: Lee & Febiger, 1993;125–131.
2. **Grindem CB, Breitschwerdt EB, Corbett WT, et al.** Epidemiologic survey of thrombocytopenia in dogs: a report on 987 cases. Vet Clin Pathol 1991;20:38–43.
3. **Jordan HL, Grindem CB, Breitschwerdt EB.** Diseases associated with feline

thrombocytopenia: a retrospective review of 41 cases. Vet Clin Pathol 1991;20;22.
4. **Mackin A.** Canine immune-mediated thrombocytopenia–part I. Compend Cont Educ Pract Vet 1995;17:515–535.
5. **Lewis DC, Meyers KM.** Canine idiopathic thrombocytopenic purpura. J Vet Intern Med 1996;10:207–218.
6. **Feldman BF.** Disorders of platelets. In: Robert DVM, Kirk W, eds. Current veterinary therapy. X. Small animal practice. Philadelphia: WB Saunders, 1989;387–493.
7. **USPC.** Drug Information for the Heath Care Professional, vol. 1 and vol. 2. 3rd ed. Englewood, CO: Dyma Test Corporation, 1998.
8. **Hammer AS.** Prevention and treatment of chemotherapy complications. In: Robert DVM, Kirk W, eds. Current veterinary therapy. XI. Small animal practice. Philadelphia: WB Saunders, 1992;387–493.
9. **Jain NC.** Schalm's veterinary hematology. 4th ed. Philadelphia: Lea & Febiger, 1986.
10. **Jain NC.** Schalm's veterinary hematology. 4th ed. Philadelphia: Lea & Febiger, 1986.
11. **Yunis AA.** Chloramphenicol toxicity: 25 years of research. Am J Med 1989;87:44N–48N.
12. **Jain NC.** Schalm's veterinary hematology. 4th ed. Philadelphia: Lea & Febiger, 1986.
13. **Castellan E, Burgat Sacaze V, Petit C, et al.** Iatrogenic toxicity of oestrogens in the dog. Rev Med Vet 1993;144:285–289.
14. **McCune JS, Liles D, Lindley C.** Precipitous fall in platelet count with anagrelide: case report and critique of dosing recommendations. Pharmacother 1997;17:822–826.
15. **Selleri C, Maciejewski JP, Sato T, et al.** Interferon-gamma constitutively expressed in the stromal. Blood 1996;87:4149–4157.
16. **Mackin A.** Canine immune-mediated thrombocytopenia–Part II. Compend Cont Educ Pract Vet 1995;17:353–364.
17. **Feldman BF, Thomason KJ, Jain NC.** Thrombocytopenia and drugs. Vet Clin North Am Small Anim Pract 1988;18:51–61.
18. **McKeage MJ.** Comparative adverse effect profiles of platinum drugs. Drug Saf 1995;13:228–244.
19. **Ulich TR, del Castillo J, Yin S, et al.** Megakaryocyte growth and development factor ameliorates carboplatin-induced thrombocytopenia in mice. Blood 1995;86:971–976.
20. **Hahn KA, McEntee MF, Daniel GB, et al.** Hematologic and systemic toxicoses associated with carboplatin administration in cats. Am J Vet Res 1997;58:677–679.
21. **Weiss RC, Cox NR, Boudreaux MK.** Toxicological effects of ribavirin in cats. J Vet Pharmacol Ther 1993;16:301–316.
22. **Ahn AH, Cotter SM.** Approach to the anemic patient. In: Robert DVM, Kirk W, Bonagura JD, eds. Current veterinary therapy. XII. Small animal practice. Philadelphia: WB Saunders, 1995;387–493.
23. **Jain NC.** Schalm's veterinary hematology. 4th ed. Philadelphia: Lea & Febiger, 1986.
24. **Aster RH.** Heparin-induced thrombocytopenia and thrombosis. N Engl J Med 1997;332:1374–1376.
25. **Warkentin TE.** Heparin-induced thrombocytopenia. Pathogenesis, frequency, avoidance and management. Drug Saf 1997;17:325–341.
26. **Berndt MC, Castaldi PA.** Drug-mediated thrombocytopenia. Blood Rev 1987;1:111–118.
27. **Christie DJ.** Specificity of drug-induced immune cytopenias. Transfus Med Rev 1993;7:230–241.
28. **Pedersen-Bjergaard U, Andersen M, Hansen PB.** Thrombocytopenia induced by noncytotoxic drugs in Denmark 1968–1991. J Intern Med 1996;239:509–515.
29. **McEwan NA.** Presumptive trimethoprim-sulphamethoxazole associated thrombocytopenia and anaemia in a dog. J Small Anim Pract 1992;33:27–29.
30. **Trimborn A, Vick KP.** Possible side effect of long-term sulfonamide/trimethoprim therapy in dogs. Praktische Tierarzt 1992;73:26–27.
31. **Sullivan PS, Arrington K, West R, et al.** Thrombocytopenia associated with administration of trimethoprim/sulfadiazine in a dog. J Am Vet Med Assoc 1992;201:1741–1744.
32. **Mehta YS, Jijina FF, Badakere SS, et al.** Rifampicin-induced immune thrombocytopenia. Tuber Lung Dis 1996;77:558–562.
33. **Prichard BN.** Adverse reactions to diuretics. Eur Heart J 1992;December:96–103.
34. **Stokol T, Parry BW.** The effect of modified-live virus vaccination on von Willebrand factor antigen concentrations and platelet counts in dogs. Vet Clin Pathol 1997;26:135–137.
35. **Graves TK.** Complications of treatments and concurrent illness associated with hyperthyroidism in cats. In: Robert DVM, Kirk W, Bonagura JD, eds. Current veterinary therapy. XII. Small Anim Pract. Philadelphia: WB Saunders, 1995;387–493.
36. **Edens LM, Robertson JL, Feldman BF.** Cholestatic hepatopathy, thrombocytopenia and lymphopenia associated with iron toxicity in a Thoroughbred gelding. Equine Vet J 1993;25:81–84.
37. **Lewis DC, Bruyette DS, Kellerman DL, et al.** Thrombocytopenia in dogs with anticoagulant rodenticide-induced hemorrhage: eight cases (1990–1995). J Am Anim Hosp Assoc 1997;33:417–422.
38. **Dardik R, Ruggeri ZM, Savion N, et al.** Platelet aggregation on extracellular matrix: effect of a recombinant GPIb-binding fragment of von Willebrand factor. Thromb Haemost 1993;70:522–526.
39. **Coller BS, Gralnick HR.** Studies on the mechanism of ristocetin-induced platelet agglutination. Effects of structural modification of ristocetin and vancomycin. J Clin Invest 1977;60:302–312.
40. **Owens MR, Holme S.** Aurin tricarboxylic acid inhibits adhesion of platelets to. Thromb Res 1996;81:177–185.
41. **Chediak J, Telfer MC, Vander Laan B, et al.** Cycles of agglutination–disagglutination induced by ristocetin. Br J Haematol 1979;43:113–126.
42. **Coller BS.** Polybrene-induced platelet agglutination and reduction in. Blood 1980;55:276–281.
43. **Mills DC, Hunchak K, Karl DW, et al.** Effect of platelet activation on the agglutination of platelets by von Willebrand factor. Mol Pharmacol 1990;37:271–277.
44. **Sullivan PS, Manning KL, McDonald TP.** Association of mean platelet volume and bone marrow megakaryocytopoiesis in thrombocytopenic dogs: 60 cases (1984–1993). J Am Vet Med Assoc 1995;206:332–334.
45. **Northern J Jr, Tvedten HW.** Diagnosis of microthrombocytosis and immune-mediated thrombocytopenia in dogs with thrombocytopenia: 68 cases (1987–1989). J Am Vet Med Assoc 1992;200:368–372.
46. **Jain NC.** Schalm's veterinary hematology. 4th ed. Philadelphia: Lea & Febiger, 1986.
47. **Kristensen AT, Weiss DJ, Klausner JS, et al.** Comparison of microscopic and flow cytometric detection of platelet antibody in dogs suspected of having immune-mediated thrombocytopenia. Am J Vet Res 1994;55:1111–1114.
48. **Weiss DJ.** Aplastic anemia. In: Robert DVM, Kirk W, Bonagura JD, eds. Current veterinary therapy. XII. Small animal practice. Philadelphia: WB Saunders, 1995;479–483.

CHAPTER 68

Immune-Mediated Thrombocytopenia

• MICHAEL A. SCOTT

Immune-mediated thrombocytopenia (IMT) is any thrombocytopenia resulting from immunologic factors, usually antibody-mediated platelet destruction by the mononuclear-phagocyte system. However, cell-mediated immunity may also be involved, and the immune response may be directed against megakaryocytes or even hemopoietic cytokines instead of platelets. Primary IMT (idiopathic or autoimmune) is caused by autoantibodies that are usually reactive with autoantigens on circulating platelets; it is not associated with an underlying condition. Here, secondary IMT refers to any IMT associated with an underlying condition such as systemic lupus erythematosus, neoplasia, infectious disease, or drug exposure. In secondary IMT, platelet-associated antibodies may be bound specifically to platelet autoantigens or to foreign antigens adsorbed to the platelet surface. They may also be nonspecifically bound in the form of immune complexes. Alloimmune thrombocytopenia is caused by alloantibodies that bind to platelet alloantigens. The abbreviation ''ITP'' is not used because it is inconsistently interpreted to mean (a) idiopathic thrombocytopenia, (b) idiopathic thrombocytopenic purpura, (c) IMT (d) immune-mediated thrombocytopenic purpura, and (e) autoimmune thrombocytopenia. Idiopathic thrombocytopenia may not be immune-mediated; IMT may not be associated with purpura; IMT may not be autoimmune.

PRIMARY IMMUNE-MEDIATED THROMBOCYTOPENIA

Primary IMT is most commonly reported in dogs and humans, but idiopathic thrombocytopenias that may be immune mediated occur sporadically in other species.[1-7] Because of imperfect diagnostic criteria and tests, some cases of secondary IMT and even nonimmune thrombocytopenia may be included in this and other reviews of canine primary IMT.

Canine

Pathogenesis

Early case reports describing idiopathic thrombocytopenia in dogs were likely reports of primary IMT.[8-10] The first laboratory evidence for this were positive results of the platelet factor 3 (PF3) release assay with globulin fractions from affected dogs.[11] Direct assays for canine platelet surface-associated immunoglobulin (PSAIg), usually immunoglobulin G (IgG), have since supported clinical diagnoses of canine IMT.[12,13] Acid eluates of platelets from some affected dogs contain Igs that bind to allogeneic platelets and immunoprecipitate the platelet integrin $\alpha_{IIb}\beta_3$ (glycoprotein [GP]IIb/IIIa).[14] Such dogs presumably have accelerated platelet destruction by the mononuclear-phagocyte system because of the presence of antiplatelet antibodies. The antibodies may also bind to megakaryocytes and impair thrombopoiesis. When platelet production does not compensate for accelerated platelet destruction, thrombocytopenia develops. As with the analogous human condition, reasons for anti-platelet antibody production by autoreactive B lymphocytes are poorly understood.[15]

Signalment

Dogs of any breed, age, or gender can suffer from primary IMT. Some investigators have found no breed predisposition,[11,16] whereas others have reported predispositions in toy poodles, miniature poodles, standard poodles, old English sheepdogs, cocker spaniels, and German shepherds.[17-20] Primary IMT appears to be especially prevalent in cocker spaniels.[12,13]

The age of reported dogs that have IMT has ranged from 7 months to 15 years, with 6 to 7 years a consistently reported mean.[11-13,17-21] Although a gender bias has sometimes been inapparent,[13,21,22] the overall number of females reported with IMT is approximately twice the number of males.[11,12,16-22] A similar female bias occurs with chronic, but not acute, IMT in humans.[23]

History and Physical Examination

Clinical signs are usually first noticed within 3 days of presentation,[11] but they may be completely lacking or present for many months.[20] Even dogs that have platelet concentrations as low as $3000/\mu L$ may be bright and alert with no clinical signs of disease. Presenting complaints and findings usually include epistaxis, bruising, gastrointestinal hemorrhage (melena, hematemesis, and hematochezia), oral bleeding, vaginal bleeding, ocular bleeding or blindness (hyphema or subretinal hemorrhage), hematuria, stiffness, lethargy, weakness, collapse, or anorexia.[11,16,19,20,24–26] Prolonged bleeding is sometimes noted with estrus, whelping, surgery, or venipuncture. Careful inspection may be needed to reveal subtle petechiae and ecchymoses, the hallmarks of thrombocytopenic hemorrhage. They are especially common on the ventral abdomen, the inner limbs, and the mucous membranes, and they may be mistaken for a rash.[27] Cerebral bleeding may be reflected by neurologic signs or sudden death. Pallor may accompany substantial hemorrhage or occur in association with concurrent immune-mediated hemolytic anemia (secondary IMT).[16,28]

Because the diagnosis of primary IMT is one of exclusion, the history, physical examination, and laboratory testing must each be thorough enough to exclude secondary IMT and nonimmune thrombocytopenias (Table 68.1). When obtaining historical information about a potential case of IMT, one should inquire about drug exposure, recent vaccinations, recent trips, recent contact with other dogs, previous transfusions, previous and current medical conditions, and confirmed or potential tick exposure. Underlying infections may be suggested by depressed attitude, lymphadenomegaly, ticks, arthritis, or fever. Fever has been reported in as many as two thirds of dogs that have primary or secondary

IMT,[11,19,20] but in fewer than 10% of dogs thought to have primary IMT.[20] Neoplasia may be suggested by the presence of lymphadenomegaly, splenomegaly, other masses, or cachexia. Systemic immune-mediated disease may be suggested by polyarthritis or certain forms of dermatitis. The presence of splenomegaly suggests that thrombocytopenia is a secondary process.[20,23,29]

Diagnostic Testing

CBC Thrombocytopenia may be an unsuspected CBC result, but it is more often an expected finding in patients that have clinical defects in primary hemostasis. True thrombocytopenia should be confirmed before proceeding with further diagnostics, and appropriate reference intervals should be used. Greyhounds may appear to be thrombocytopenic if their lower platelet concentrations are compared with routine reference intervals.[30]

Blood smears should always be evaluated to confirm automated results and to exclude pseudothrombocytopenia, a laboratory artifact occurring when a substantial proportion of the platelets in a sample are not counted. Pseudothrombocytopenia usually occurs when platelets are clumped owing to (1) platelet activation during or after venipuncture, (2) anticoagulant-dependent antibodies reactive to GPIIb/IIIa in the presence of ethylenediaminetetraacetic acid (EDTA) or other anticoagulants, or (3) cold agglutinins.[31–33] Platelet clumps indicate the

---

TABLE 68.1   General Causes of Thrombocytopenia

Decreased platelet production
  chemical toxicants with predictable effects (e.g., chemotherapeutics, estrogens in dogs)
  chemical toxicants with idiosyncratic effects
  myelophthisis
  myelofibrosis
  infections of hemic precursor cells
  hereditary disorders of hemopoiesis
  immune-mediated inhibition of thrombopoiesis or megakaryocytopoiesis
  cytokine-induced suppression of hemopoiesis (with some infections)
  irradiation (whole body)
Decreased platelet survival
  immune-mediated
    primary (idiopathic, autoimmune)
    secondary
      systemic autoimmune disease
      neoplasia
      infection
      drug-induced
    alloimmune
      neonatal alloimmune thrombocytopenia
      posttransfusion purpura
  nonimmune
    vasculitis (e.g., infectious vasculitides, hemolytic uremic syndrome)
    consumptive coagulation/coagulopathy (e.g., DIC, envenomation)
    activation/damage by drugs or infectious agents
    activation by foreign surfaces (e.g., catheters, extracorporeal circulation)
    blood loss from anticoagulant rodenticide toxicosis (probably caused by platelet
      consumption at multiple sites of hemorrhage, not by platelet loss)
Abnormal platelet distribution (e.g., splenic sequestration)

need for a new sample collected with a "clean stick". If anticoagulant-induced clumping is suspected,[34,35] a new sample should be tested promptly after collection into a citrate tube. Pseudothrombocytopenia may also occur if many platelets are larger than the high threshold setting of automated hematology analyzers. Clinically normal cavalier King Charles spaniels may have many large platelets that lead to falsely low values with most automated methods.[36,37] Platelets should be counted manually when many giant platelets are present.

Dogs diagnosed with IMT usually have fewer than 50,000 platelets/μL,[13,16,18,38] and frequently fewer than 10,000/μL.[13,20] On average, their platelet concentrations have been significantly lower than those of dogs that have presumed nonimmune thrombocytopenias.[18,38] However, mild and moderate compensated IMTs may go unrecognized or may be attributed to other causes because they do not fit expected patterns. Most reports associate bleeding with fewer than 30,000 or even 10,000 platelets/μL,[20] but bleeding may occur at higher concentrations.[11] Inconsistent bleeding tendencies among dogs that have similar platelet concentrations may relate to variations in vascular stability, trauma, the rapidity with which thrombocytopenia develops, the age and metabolic activity of the circulating platelets, or the antigenic specificities of antiplatelet antibodies.[39] Binding to functional platelet epitopes[40–42] or shared epitopes on endothelial cells[43,44] may exacerbate hemorrhage in some patients.

Small, normal, or large platelets may be present. The accurate measurement of mean platelet volume (MPV) on clinical samples is problematic, but decreased MPV has been associated with immune-mediated platelet destruction.[20,38,45] In one study, low MPV appeared to be a specific indicator of primary IMT in dogs.[38] However, nonimmune thrombocytopenias of similar severity were not discussed; the analyzer may have had a bias toward low MPVs when few platelets and relatively more background particles were assessed.

Anemia, usually regenerative, has been present in roughly half of all reported cases of primary and secondary IMT.[16,18,20,24] It may occur because of concurrent immune-mediated hemolytic anemia, but it is commonly secondary to blood loss.[11,16,19,20,22,24,46] Leukogram patterns may suggest underlying or concurrent disease, but they are not useful in diagnosing primary IMT.[16,18,24] CBC abnormalities suggesting secondary IMT or nonimmune thrombocytopenia include bicytopenia, pancytopenia, leukemia, an inflammatory leukogram, granular lymphocytosis, significant hyperproteinemia, intracellular organisms (e.g. fungi, ehrlichiae), distemper inclusions, extracellular parasites such as microfilaria, and erythrocyte abnormalities such as spherocytosis, schistocytosis, or dacryocytosis.

Bone Marrow Bone marrow evaluation may be indicated when multiple cytopenias are present or when there is a suspicion of leukemia, multiple myeloma, or any myeloproliferative disorder. Other causes of production failure may be identified, including myelofibrosis, metastatic cancer, and granulomatous infections.

If hypoplasia or aplasia are suspected, a core biopsy should be collected in addition to an aspirate. Thrombocytopenia should not be considered a contraindication to bone marrow aspirations in dogs that have IMT, although prolonged pressure may be needed to achieve hemostasis.

The evaluation of marrow in dogs that have isolated thrombocytopenias is of questionable value and may be more useful prognostically than diagnostically. Megakaryocytes are usually in normal or increased numbers, and an increase in immature megakaryocytes is common.[20,25,47] However, some dogs that have presumed IMT have had absent or significantly reduced numbers of megakaryocytes.[9,20,25,47,48] Megakaryocytic hypoplasia or aplasia suggests a somewhat poorer prognosis and a more delayed response to appropriate therapy.[20,47] Megakaryocytic hyperplasia has generally been interpreted as evidence of accelerated thrombopoiesis, but impaired thrombopoiesis may occur despite stimulated megakaryocytopoiesis. Impaired thrombopoiesis occurs in many human patients who have primary IMT and normal to increased megakaryocyte numbers,[15,49,50] presumably because of cross-reacting antiplatelet antibodies. Canine platelets and megakaryocytes share some reactive sites, including epitopes on GPIIIa.[51,52] Dogs that have IMT or those made thrombocytopenic by injections of rabbit anti-[canine platelet] antiserum have developed significant thrombocytopenia associated with megakaryocyte cytoplasmic vacuolation, foaminess, basophilia, and decreased granularity.[25,47,51] These morphologic changes may be indicative of immune-mediated cell damage and impaired thrombopoiesis.

Other Tests A routine chemistry profile and urinalysis should be done to exclude or identify other diseases. Hemostasis profiles may produce evidence of consumptive coagulation or coagulopathy. Survey radiographs and ultrasonography may reveal splenomegaly or occult neoplasia. Blood cultures may be indicated when findings are suggestive of possible septicemia. Serology and PCR tests may be used to detect exposure to, or infection with, rickettsial agents. If systemic immune-mediated disease is suspected, tests for antinuclear antibodies, rheumatoid factor, LE cells, and erythrocyte- or neutrophil-associated Ig may be indicated.

Platelet Antibody Assays Assays to diagnose "ITP" are frequently requested, and several have been developed; however, the diagnosis of primary IMT remains a diagnosis of exclusion in people and dogs.[53,54] Human and veterinary assays are primarily of investigational value. Early assays such as the PF3 test were insensitive and nonspecific indirect functional assays; they cannot be recommended.[55] Most dogs diagnosed with IMT have had negative PF3 results.[19,20,22,25,56] Most later assays have used labeled antiglobulin reagents to detect platelet- or megakaryocyte-reactive immunoglobulins. These assays include the direct megakaryocyte immunofluorescence assay (D-MIFA),[19,25,51,57] enzyme-linked immunosorbent assays,[12,35,56,58,59] platelet immunoradiometric assays,[13,60–62] and microscopic and flow-cytometric platelet immunofluorescence assays.[57,63–65] Many of these have been indirect assays of serum or plasma and cannot differentiate autoantibodies from confounding circulating immune complexes, aggregates of IgG formed in heated or stored sera, or acquired and naturally occurring alloantibodies to common or platelet-specific antigens.[23,66,67]

Preferable assays are direct assays of patient platelets if they are designed to assess only surface Igs. Total platelet IgG is mostly within platelet α-granules.[68] Unlike PSAIg, total IgG is not a reliable indicator of immune-mediated platelet destruction.[68,69] Direct assays for PSAIg[12,13,35,65] can probably differentiate most cases of IMT from nonimmune thrombocytopenias, but no assay can differentiate primary IMT from secondary IMT. The presence of increased PSAIg is evidence of an immune component to the thrombocytopenia, and it may support a clinician's decision to institute immunosuppressive therapy. However, PSAIg has been increased in human patients who have presumed nonimmune thrombocytopenias.[15] Transport and storage of samples may profoundly and unpredictably affect the results of some assays,[13,35] so valid results may be available only locally where assays are offered.

The D-MIFA is generally done with air-dried smears of patient bone marrow, so transport problems are minimal. However, platelets and megakaryocytes are not antigenically identical, so D-MIFA positivity may not mirror PSAIg positivity.[70] Also, (1) some marrow samples have too few megakaryocytes for confident evaluation,[19,25,57] (2) high background fluorescence may interfere with differentiation of positive from negative,[57,71] and (3) damaged cells may allow detection of intracellular Igs when in fact no relevant surface-bound Ig is present.[69,70] The cumulative sensitivity of D-MIFAs for substantiating reported clinical diagnoses of IMT is approximately 50%.[19,25,57] Other approaches to supporting clinical diagnoses of IMT are insensitive, nonspecific, or impractical for routine use.

Therapy

When treating dogs that have IMT, aspirin and other antiplatelet drugs should be avoided. Medications that may cause or contribute to the thrombocytopenia should be discontinued whenever possible. Trauma (including intramuscular injections) should be minimized, and underlying problems should be treated appropriately. Other therapy should be aimed at raising platelet concentrations enough to protect against clinical hemorrhage, though occasional dogs may do well despite low platelet concentrations and no medical management. Platelet concentrations within the reference interval are the preferred target, but concentrations of 50,000 to 100,000 platelets/μL are probably adequate in the absence of platelet dysfunction.[17,22,29,72,73] Efforts to reach reference values can be frustrating for the client and the veterinarian, and side effects of therapy can be a detriment to the patient.

Specific therapy generally begins with immuno-suppressive corticosteroid therapy (approximately 0.2 mg/kg dexamethasone or 2 mg/kg prednisone or prednisolone every 12 hr), which stabilizes vascular endothelium, decreases macrophage phagocytosis of opsonized platelets, possibly increases platelet production to a small degree, and eventually diminishes antibody production. It is used to stabilize the patient while providing time for spontaneous remission. Therapy is gradually tapered over weeks to months until being withdrawn or maintained at the minimal effective dose as directed by platelet concentrations. Side effects or inadequate response justify other therapeutic approaches. Additional treatments reflect clinical bias, have potential side effects, and are not based on randomized, controlled, clinical trials. The common immunosuppressive options have been reviewed.[74,75] Various combinations of azathioprine, cyclophosphamide, and vincristine have been used with inconsistent success.[16,20,29,46,76–78] Danazol,[62,79] cyclosporine,[80] and human gamma globulin may be useful in refractory cases.[81,82] Combination therapy with reduced doses of individual drugs may reduce unwanted side effects.

Splenectomy removes a major source of antibody production and a major site of platelet destruction, but its clinical usefulness in dogs that have primary IMT is unclear. In dogs, splenectomy has sometimes been associated with clinical improvement[21,22,83,84] and has sometimes appeared to be unhelpful.[16,17,20,46] Similarly, splenectomy of dogs sensitized to allogeneic platelets has inconsistently decreased the survival of transfused allogeneic platelets.[85] It remains to be seen if response to splenectomy can be predicted. Postsplenectomy hemobartonellosis is a recognized complication, though the incidence appears to be low.[86]

Platelet transfusions will likely result in little increment in platelet concentrations, because transfused platelets are rapidly destroyed by circulating antiplatelet antibodies.[67] However, significant transient increments may occur, and they justify transfusions when dogs that have IMT require surgery or when there is severe, life-threatening hemorrhage such as that within the central nervous system (CNS).[11,29,87] Multiple units of platelet concentrates are usually required for an appreciable effect.

Outcome

Dogs appear to suffer from acute and chronic forms of primary IMT, perhaps analogous to the human conditions. As many as half of the dogs that have IMT experience a single, acute bout of thrombocytopenia followed by recovery.[11,16,21,39] Recovery may occur within a week,[39] though others have found that 2 to 35 days (mean of 8) were necessary for platelet concentrations to exceed 100,000/μL.[16] Other dogs respond initially but relapse and require chronic therapy.[11,16,21,39,88] Relapses have reportedly been precipitated by various stressors.[17] Relatively crude estimates from cases at referral institutions suggest that as many as 20% of the dogs die without responding to therapy, often because of hemorrhage.[11,16,39] Deaths may also result from cessation of therapy because of the expense and prognosis of treating relapsing dogs that have an apparently incurable condition. Which outcome a particular dog will have is currently unpredictable.

SECONDARY IMMUNE-MEDIATED THROMBOCYTOPENIA

IMT associated with underlying conditions, including systemic autoimmune disease is generally referred to as secondary IMT. Secondary IMT includes conditions for which PSAIg is not caused by antiplatelet antibodies. PSAIg may instead be the result of antibody binding to adsorbed, non-self-antigens associated with infectious agents, drugs, or neoplasia.[89] It may also include immune complexes bound to platelets by (1) complement-mediated immune adherence,[90–92] (2) Fc receptors for IgG in some species,[90,93] or (3) nonspecific interactions.[66] Circulating immune complexes may arise from infectious diseases, vaccinations, drugs, neoplasia, or systemic autoimmune diseases.

Systemic Autoimmune Diseases

Primary IMT is but one clinical presentation on a spectrum of somewhat indistinct autoimmune disorders with different antibody specificities.[94,95] Systemic lupus erythematosus (SLE) associated with presumed IMT has been reported in dogs, cats, and horses.[96–98] An immune-mediated pathogenesis to the thrombocytopenia in dogs that have SLE has been supported by PSAIg positivity and positive results with D-MIFAs or indirect assays.[11,12,19,56–59,64] Thrombocytopenia frequently accompanies immune-mediated hemolytic anemia in dogs,[16,28,99] and it occasionally does so in cats and horses.[2,5,7] This situation mimics Evans' syndrome,[100] which now defines the co-occurrence of IMT and immune-mediated hemolytic anemia. An immune-mediated pathogenesis to the thrombocytopenia has been supported by assay positivity in some affected dogs.[11,19,22,25,56,57,64] A female gender bias was not found in dogs that had Evans' syndrome.[16,22] Positive indirect results for platelet-bindable Ig have also been reported in a dog that had steroid-responsive idiopathic neutropenia and thrombocytopenia and in a dog that had thrombocytopenia and red cell aplasia.[57] IMT has occasionally been clinically diagnosed or suspected in dogs that have rheumatoid arthritis or pemphigus,[18,58] and thrombocytopenia has accompanied juvenile-onset polyarthritis syndrome in Akitas.[101]

Neoplasia

Thrombocytopenia frequently occurs in association with neoplasia.[3,18,102–104] The pathogenesis of thrombocytopenia associated with neoplasia is multifactorial, but immune-mediated platelet destruction may be an under-recognized contributor.[105] This may help explain shortened platelet survivals without concurrent decreases in fibrinogen survivals in dogs that have various multicentric or metastatic neoplasms.[106–108] A significant positive association has been reported between the diagnosis of lymphosarcoma and the diagnosis of IMT in dogs,[109] and this is supported by results of D-MIFAs and indirect assays for platelet-bindable Ig.[19,57,110] Similar assays, although imperfect, have also been positive in dogs that have various hemic and nonhemic neoplasia.[19,57,106,111] IMT has also been diagnosed in horses that had lymphosarcoma.[112]

Infectious Diseases

Thrombocytopenia is commonly associated with infections caused by viruses, bacteria (especially the rickettsials), protozoa, fungi, and nematodes.[3,18,113,114] The pathogeneses of these infectious thrombocytopenias may be complicated, involving various combinations of suppressed platelet production, altered platelet distribution, increased consumption, or immune-mediated and nonimmune destruction. Many bacterial, viral, fungal, and protozoal diseases have been associated with IMT in humans.[115] In general, infection-associated IMT may be related to cross-reactive antibodies, organism-induced production of autoantibodies, exposure of platelet cryptantigens by the presence of the organisms, binding of antibodies to infectious agents (or their parts) attached to the platelets, or the induction of platelet-associated immune complexes.[115]

Bacteria   PSAIg is elevated in some thrombocytopenic human patients that have bacterial sepsis, and it may represent autoantibodies to cryptantigens induced by bacteria.[116,117] Alternatively, because some bacteria bind directly to platelets,[118,119] antibodies bound to the bacteria may lead to elevated PSAIg. Rickettsial diseases are a common infectious cause of thrombocytopenia in endemic areas, but the pathogeneses of the thrombocytopenias are poorly understood. Immune-mediated platelet destruction is thought to contribute to the thrombocytopenia of acute canine monocytic ehrlichiosis,[120–125] and positive Coombs' tests have suggested that immune-mediated disease may not be restricted to platelets.[126,127] PSAIg or serum platelet-bindable Igs have been increased in some naturally and experimentally infected dogs.[12,19,120,121] However, further studies are needed to document the consistent presence of PSAIg and to characterize the nature and binding specificities of involved Igs. Immune mechanisms may contribute to thrombocytopenias in other ehrlichial infections.

Viruses   Specific platelet autoantibodies, usually directed against GPIIb/IIIa, have been reported in people who have measles, HIV infections, and other viral diseases,[15,128] but the contribution of PSAIg to viral thrombocytopenias in veterinary species is mostly unknown. Cats that have feline immunodeficiency virus (FIV) and feline leukemia virus (FeLV) infections may develop thrombocytopenias with immune components.[97] Immune-mediated platelet destruction appears to contribute to the thrombocytopenia associated with equine infectious anemia, but impaired platelet production is also involved.[129-131] Puppies experimentally infected with canine distemper virus developed significant thrombocytopenia and increased PSAIgG.[132] A complement-independent, immune complex-induced destruction of platelets appeared to contribute to the thrombocytopenia. However, the nature of the proposed complexes and their orientation with respect to the platelet surface are unknown, and thrombocytopenia has not been consistently recognized in older or spontaneously infected dogs. Dogs[133-135] and other species[17] vaccinated with modified-live virus (MLV) distemper vaccines may develop mild to occasionally significant[133] transient decreases in platelet concentrations. Although clinical purpura has reportedly followed 1 to 21 days after routine clinical MLV vaccinations,[17,136] further studies of these clinical observations have not been published. Acute thrombocytopenic purpura has occurred in people vaccinated with a MLV measles, mumps, and rubella vaccine, usually 2 to 3 weeks after vaccination.[137] PSAIg was increased in many of these patients, and circulating antibodies with specificity to GPIIb/IIIa were present in some.[138]

Protozoa, Fungi, and Nematodes

Canine leishmaniasis is commonly associated with thrombocytopenia, sometimes marked.[139] Circulating immune complexes have been related to thrombocytopenia in human leishmaniasis,[140] and they may play an important role in dogs, either directly or secondary to immune-complex vasculitis.[139] Thrombocytopenia occurring in dogs that have babesiosis may also have an immunodestructive component.[12,141] Specific IgG binding to platelet-bound malarial antigen mediates the IMT complicating some human malarial infections.[89] Thrombocytopenia commonly accompanies canine and human histoplasmosis,[113,142,143] and it has been associated with disseminated candidiasis in dogs.[113] The mechanisms are not clear, but there is evidence that increased PSAIgG and immune complexes may accelerate platelet destruction.[144,145] PSAIg may also mediate platelet destruction in dogs that have dirofilariasis.[12]

Drugs

Drugs may produce thrombocytopenia by many mechanisms, including immune-mediated platelet destruction by drug-induced antibodies. Drug-induced antibodies may be drug-dependent and require the presence of the drug or its metabolite[146] for platelet binding, or they may occasionally be drug-independent and behave like autoantibodies that bind in the absence of drug.[147] Some drug-dependent antibodies bind to cells in the form of drug-antibody complexes. Others bind directly to either membrane cryptantigens exposed by the presence of the drug or to drug-protein neoantigens on the cell surface. Whatever the mechanism, drug-induced thrombocytopenias are usually severe. Evidence that thrombocytopenia is immune-mediated and drug-induced includes (1) development of thrombocytopenia and PSAIg at least a few days after drug exposure, (2) in vitro drug dependency of the binding of serum or plasma antibodies to

platelets or platelet GPs, (3) resolution of thrombocytopenia and PSAIg levels after drug withdrawal, and (4) relapse after reexposure to the drug (rarely shown).

In dogs, drug-induced IMT has been suspected in association with several drugs, but strong evidence has often been lacking because of unavailable or inadequate assays for PSAIg. Drugs that have been best incriminated are gold compounds[61] and sulfonamides,[12,45] both of which are also well-documented causes of drug-induced IMT in people.[23] Immune-mediated mechanisms may also have contributed to the multifactorial thrombocytopenia associated with high-dose cefonicid and cefazedone in dogs.[148] However, drug-dependent binding of antibodies has not been reported with any drug in a veterinary species.

With any acute thrombocytopenia of unknown origin, all medications should be withdrawn and replaced with suitable substitutes when necessary. Drug-induced thrombocytopenias usually respond rapidly to drug withdrawal when drug-dependent antibodies are involved. Glucocorticoids may be helpful by improving vascular integrity, but they have not been shown to speed recovery of platelet concentrations in humans. Transfusions are indicated for life-threatening hemorrhage, though transfused platelets are probably destroyed rapidly while drug levels persist. In humans, plasma exchange and high-dose intravenous IgG have been useful. In the long term, the causative drug should be avoided.

Alloimmune Thrombocytopenias

Neonatal Alloimmune Thrombocytopenia

Neonatal alloimmune thrombocytopenia occurs when maternal antibodies to paternal epitopes on neonatal platelets are passively transferred through the placenta or colostrum. These antibodies bind to neonatal platelets and lead to their premature destruction. Neonatal alloimmune thrombocytopenia has been described in pigs, horses, and possibly mules.[149-151] In pigs,[152-156] the condition has been seen after two or more pregnancies, with the antibodies remaining for subsequent litters. One quarter to all the pigs in a litter are affected.[155] They are usually born healthy and develop decreased platelet concentrations at approximately a week of age. Megakaryocytic hyperplasia and hypoplasia have been reported, possibly varying with disease progression. The almost complete lack of megakaryocytes in some pigs indicates suppressed megakaryocytopoiesis.[156] Cross fostering can be used to prevent the disease.

The diagnosis of neonatal alloimmune thrombocytopenia is mostly one of exclusion, sepsis being the most common differential. Where available, antibody assays could document the presence of PSAIg in the neonate, the absence of maternal PSAIg, and the presence of maternal antibody reactivity with paternal and neonatal, but not maternal, platelets. Specific therapy may not be required, but glucocorticoids may be useful in severely affected newborns. Platelet transfusions are indicated if hemorrhage is severe or if CNS hemorrhage is suspected. Compatible platelets are preferred and can be obtained from the dam, but they should be washed to remove plasma antibodies. Future offspring from the same mating pair are at risk of developing the same disease.

Posttransfusion Purpura

Mostly recognized in human patients, posttransfusion purpura usually occurs approximately 1 week after a platelet-incompatible transfusion. It is associated with severe thrombocytopenia and high titers of platelet-reactive alloantibodies. These antibodies mediate destruction of transfused as well as autologous platelets despite the lack of reactivity, after recovery, between the alloantibodies and the autologous platelets.[23] This destruction of autologous platelets is incompletely understood but may relate to the adsorption of soluble antigens on autologous platelets, or to stimulation of autoantibody formation.[15] Posttransfusion purpura may also occur passively within a few hours after alloantibodies are inadvertently transfused. Similar posttransfusion purpuras have been reported in dogs and pigs.[12,85,157–159] Marked posttransfusion thrombocytopenia has also been reported in canine recipients of DEA1-incompatible erythrocytes or plasma containing anti-DEA1 alloantibodies.[160] The thrombocytopenia resolved within a few hours of transfusion, possibly owing to sequestration and immune adherence of platelets to antibody-coated erythrocytes.

REFERENCES

1. **Humber KA, Beech J, Cudd TA, Palmer JE, Gardner SY, Sommer MM.** Azathioprine for treatment of immune-mediated thrombocytopenia in two horses. J Am Vet Med Assoc 1991;199:591–594.
2. **Gaschen FP, Smith Meyer B, Harvey JW.** Amegakaryocytic thrombocytopenia and immune-mediated haemolytic anaemia in a cat. Comp Haematol Int 1992;2:175–178.
3. **Jordan HL, Grindem CB, Breitschwerdt EB.** Thrombocytopenia in cats: a retrospective study of 41 cases. J Vet Intern Med 1993;7:261–265.
4. **Peterson JL, Couto CG, Wellman ML.** Hemostatic disorders in cats: a retrospective study and review of the literature. J Vet Intern Med 1995; 9:298–303.
5. **Lubas G, Ciattini F, Gavazza A.** Immune-mediated thrombocytopenia and hemolytic anemia (Evans syndrome) in a horse. Equine Pract 1997;19:27–32.
6. **Morris DD, Whitlock RH.** Relapsing idiopathic thrombocytopenia in a horse. Equine Vet J 1983;15:73–75.
7. **Sockett DC, Traub-Dargatz J, Weiser MG.** Immune-mediated hemolytic anemia and thrombocytopenia in a foal. J Am Vet Med Assoc 1987; 190:308–310.
8. **Gowing GM.** Idiopathic thrombocytopenic purpura in the dog. J Am Vet Med Assoc 1964;145:987–990.
9. **Brodey RS.** Clinico-pathologic conference. J Am Vet Med Assoc 1964; 144: 628–637.
10. **Magrane HJ Jr, Magrane WG, Ross JR.** Idiopathic thrombocytopenic purpura in a dog—a case report. J Am Vet Med Assoc 1959;520–522.
11. **Wilkins RJ, Hurvitz Al, Dodds-Laffin J.** Immunologically mediated thrombocytopenia in the dog. J Am Vet Med Assoc 1973;163:277–282.
12. **Lewis DC, Meyers KM, Callan MB, Bücheler J, Giger U.** Detection of platelet-bound and serum platelet-bindable antibodies for diagnosis of idiopathic thrombocytopenic purpura in dogs. J Am Vet Med Assoc 1995; 206:47–52.
13. **Scott MA.** Canine immune-mediated thrombocytopenia: assay development, a role for complement, and assessment in a toxicologic study. Michigan State University, PhD, 1995;451.
14. **Lewis DC, Meyers KM.** Studies of platelet-bound and serum platelet-bindable immunoglobulins in dogs with idiopathic thrombocytopenic purpura. Exp Hematol 1996;24:696–701.
15. **George JN, El-Harake MA, Aster RH.** Thrombocytopenia due to enhanced platelet destruction by immunologic mechanisms. In: Beutler E, Lichtman MA, Coller BS, Kipps TJ, eds. Williams hematology. 5th ed. New York: McGraw-Hill, 1995;1315–1355.
16. **Jackson ML, Kruth SA.** Immune-mediated hemolytic anemia and thrombocytopenia in the dog: a retrospective study of 55 cases diagnosed from 1969 through 1983 at the Western College of Veterinary Medicine. Can Vet J 1985;26:245–250.
17. **Dodds WJ.** Immune-mediated diseases of the blood. Adv Vet Sci Comp Med 1983;27:163–196.
18. **Grindem CB, Breitschwerdt EB, Corbett WT, Jans HE.** Epidemiologic survey of thrombocytopenia in dogs: a report on 987 cases. Vet Clin Pathol 1991;20:38–43.
19. **Jain NC, Switzer JW.** Autoimmune thrombocytopenia in dogs and cats. Vet Clin North Am Small Anim Pract 1981;421–433.
20. **Williams DA, Maggio-Price L.** Canine idiopathic thrombocytopenia: clinical observations and long-term follow-up in 54 cases. J Am Vet Med Assoc 1984;185:660–663.
21. **Jans HE, Armstrong PJ, Price GS.** Therapy on immune mediated thrombocytopenia: a retrospective study of 15 dogs. J Vet Intern Med 1990;4:4–7.
22. **Feldman BF, Handagama P. Lubberink AAME.** Splenectomy as adjunctive therapy for immune-mediated thrombocytopenia and hemolytic anemia in the dog. J Am Vet Med Assoc 1985;187:617–619.
23. **Aster RH.** The immunologic thrombocytopenias. In: Kunicki TJ, George JN, eds. Platelet immunobiology: molecular and clinical aspects. Philadelphia: JB Lippincott Company, 1989;387–435.
24. **Jain NC.** Immunohematology. In: Jain NC, ed. Schalm's veterinary hematology. 4th ed. Philadelphia: Lea & Febiger, 1986;990–1039.
25. **Joshi BC, Jain NC.** Detection of antiplatelet antibody in serum and on megakaryocytes of dogs with autoimmune thrombocytopenia. Am J Vet Res 1976;37:681–685.
26. **Halliwell REW.** Autoimmune disease in domestic animals. J Am Vet Med Assoc 1982;181:1088–1096.
27. **Clark HC, Childress RD, Coleman NC.** Idiopathic thrombocytopenic purpura: a review and case report. Vet Med 1980; March:427–430.
28. **Klag AR, Giger U, Shofer FS.** Idiopathic immune-mediated hemolytic anemia in dogs: 42 cases (1986–1990). J Am Vet Med Assoc 1993;202: 783–788.
29. **Feldman BF, Thomason KJ, Jain NC.** Quantitative platelet disorders. Vet Clin North Am Small Anim Pract 1988;18:35–49.
30. **Sullivan PS, Evans HL, McDonald TP.** Platelet concentration and hemoglobin function in greyhounds. J Am Vet Med Assoc 1994;205:838–841.
31. **George JN.** Thrombocytopenia: pseudothrombocytopenia, hypersplenism, and thrombocytopenia associated with massive transfusion. In: Beutler E, Lichtman MA, Coller BS, Kipps TJ, eds. Williams hematology. 5th ed. New York: McGraw-Hill, 1995;1355–1360.
32. **Casonato A, Bertomoro A, Pontara E, Dannhauser D, Lazzaro AR, Girolami A.** EDTA dependent pseudothrombocytopenia caused by antibodies against the cytoadhesive receptor of platelet gpIIB-IIIA. J Clin Pathol 1994;47:625–630.
33. **Schrezenmeier H, Müller H, Gunsilius E, Heimpel H, Seifried E.** Anticoagulant-induced pseudothrombocytopenia and pseudoleucocytosis. Thromb Haemost 1995;73:506–513.
34. **Kubo Y, Amejima S, Miyagi A.** Artifacts: Case A-5. In: Tvedten HW, ed. Multi-species hematology atlas Technicon H·1E system. Tarrytown, NY: Miles Inc., 1993;134–135.
35. **Lewis DC, Meyers KM.** Effect of anticoagulant and blood storage time on platelet-bound antibody concentrations in clinically normal dogs. Am J Vet Res 1994;55:602–605.
36. **Smedile LE, Houston DM, Taylor SM, Post K, Searcy GP.** Idiopathic, asymptomatic thrombocytopenia in Cavalier King Charles Spaniels: 11 cases (1983–1993). J Am Anim Hosp Assoc 1997;33:411–415.
37. **Brown SJ, Simpson KW, Baker S, Spagnoletti MA, Elwood CM.** Macrothrombocytosis in cavalier King Charles spaniels. Vet Rec 1994;135: 281–283.
38. **Northern J Jr, Tvedten HW.** Diagnosis of microthrombocytosis and immune mediated thrombocytopenia in dogs with thrombocytopenia: 68 cases (1987–1989). J Am Vet Med Assoc 1992;200:368–372.
39. **Thompson JP.** Immunologic diseases. In: Ettinger SJ, ed. Textbook of veterinary internal medicine: diseases of the dog and cat. 4th ed. Philadelphia: WB Saunders, 1994;2:2002–2029.
40. **Kristensen AT, Weiss DJ, Klausner JS.** Platelet dysfunction associated with immune-mediated thrombocytopenia in dogs. J Vet Intern Med 1994;8:323–327.
41. **Balduini CL, Bertolino G, Noris P, Piovella F, Sinigaglia F, Bellotti V, Samaden A, Torti M, Mazzini G.** Defect of platelet aggregation and adhesion induced by autoantibodies against platelet glycoprotein IIIa. Thromb Haemost 1992;68:208–213.
42. **Deckmyn H, De Reys S.** Functional effects of human antiplatelet antibodies. Semin Thromb Hemost 1995;21:46–59.
43. **Morrison FS, Baldini MG.** Antigenic relationship between blood platelets and vascular endothelium. Blood 1969;33:46–56.
44. **Hager EB, Burns RO, Carter RD, Merrill JP.** Lesions produced in homografted canine kidneys by prior immunization with donor platelets. Fed Proc 1962;21:37.

45. **Sullivan PS, Arrington K, West R, McDonald TP.** Thrombocytopenia associated with administration of trimethoprim/sulfadiazine in a dog. J Am Vet Med Assoc 1992;201:1741–1744.

46. **Helfand SC, Jain NC, Paul M.** Vincristine-loaded platelet therapy for idiopathic thrombocytopenia in a dog. J Am Vet Med Assoc 1984; 185:224–226.

47. **Hoff B, Lumsden JH, Valli VEO.** An appraisal of bone marrow biopsy in assessment of sick dogs. Can J Comp Med 1985;49:34–42.

48. **Murtaugh RJ, Jacobs RM.** Suspected immune-mediated megakaryocytic hypoplasia or aplasia in a dog. J Am Vet Med Assoc 1985; 186:1313–1315.

49. **Ballem PJ, Segal GM, Stratton JR, Gernsheimer T, Adamson JW, Slichter SJ.** Mechanisms of thrombocytopenia in chronic autoimmune thrombocytopenic purpura: evidence of both impaired platelet production and increased platelet clearance. J Clin Invest 1987;80:33–40.

50. **Tomer A, Hanson SR, Harker LA.** Autologous platelet kinetics in patients with severe thrombocytopenia: discrimination between disorders of production and destruction. J Lab Clin Med 1991;118:546–554.

51. **Joshi BC, Jain NC.** Experimental immunologic thrombocytopenia in dogs: a study of thrombocytopenia and megakaryocytopoiesis. Res Vet Sci 1977;22:11–17.

52. **Darbes J, Colbatsky F, Minkus G.** Demonstration of feline and canine platelet glycoproteins by immuno- and lectin histochemistry. Histochemistry 1993;100:83–91.

53. **George JN, Woolf SH, Raskob GE, Wasser JS, Aledort LM, Ballem PJ, Blanchette VS, Bussel JB, Cines DB, Kelton JG, Lichtin AE, McMillan R, Okerbloom JA, Regan DH, Warrier I.** Diagnosis and treatment of idiopathic thrombocytopenic purpura: recommendations of the American Society of Hematology. Ann Intern Med 1997;126:319–326.

54. **George JN, Raskob GE.** Idiopathic thrombocytopenic purpura: a concise summary of the pathophysiology and diagnosis in children and adults. Semin Hematol 1998;35:5–8.

55. **Mueller-Eckhardt C, Kiefel V.** Laboratory methods for the detection of platelet antibodies and identification of antigens. In: Kunicki TJ, George JN, eds. Platelet immunobiology: molecular and clinical aspects. Philadelphia: JB Lippincott Company, 1989;436–453.

56. **Campbell KL, George JW, Greene CE.** Application of the enzyme-linked immunosorbent assay for the detection of platelet antibodies in dogs. Am J Vet Res 1984; 45:2561–2564.

57. **Kristensen AT, Weiss DJ, Klausner JS, Laber J, Christie DJ.** Detection of antiplatelet antibody with a platelet immunofluorescence assay. J Vet Intern Med 1994;8:36–39.

58. **McVey DS, Shuman WS.** Detection of antiplatelet immunoglobulin in thrombocytopenic dogs. Vet Immuno Immunopathol 1989;22:101–111.

59. **McVey DS, Rudd R, Toshach K, Moore WE, Keeton KS.** Systemic autoimmune disease and concurrent nematode infection in a dog. J Am Vet Med Assoc 1989;195:957–960.

60. **Shulman NR, Leissinger CA, Hotchkiss AJ, Kautz CA.** The nonspecific nature of platelet-associated IgG. Trans Assoc Am Physicians 1982; 95:213–220.

61. **Bloom JC, Blackmer SA, Bugelski PJ, Sowinski JM, Saunders LZ.** Gold-induced immune thrombocytopenia in the dog. Vet Pathol 1985;22:492–499.

62. **Bloom JC, Meunier LD, Thiem PA, Sellers TS.** Use of danazol for treatment of corticosteroid-resistant immune-mediated thrombocytopenia in a dog. J Am Vet Med Assoc 1989;194:76–78.

63. **Thiem PA, Abbott DL, Moroff S, McGrath JP, Bloom JC.** Preliminary findings on the comparison of flow cytometric and solid-phase radioimmunoassay techniques for the detection of serum antiplatelet antibodies in dogs. Vet Clin Pathol 1991;20:18.

64. **Kristensen AT, Weiss DJ, Klausner JS, Laber J, Christie DJ.** Comparison of microscopic and flow cytometric detection of platelet antibody in dogs suspected of having immune-mediated thrombocytopenia. Am J Vet Res 1994;55:1111–1114.

65. **Lewis DC, McVey DS, Shuman WS, Muller WB.** Development and characterization of a flow cytometric assay for detection of platelet-bound immunoglobulin G in dogs. Am J Vet Res 1995;56:1555–1558.

66. **Karpatkin S, Xia J, Patel J, Thorbecke GJ.** Serum platelet-reactive IgG of autoimmune thrombocytopenic purpura patients is not F(ab')$_2$ mediated and a function of storage. Blood 1992;80:3164–3172.

67. **Slichter SJ, O'Donnell MR, Weiden PL, Storb R, Schroeder M-L.** Canine platelet alloimmunization: the role of donor selection. Br J Haematol 1986;63:713–727.

68. **George JN.** Platelet immunoglobulin G: its significance for the evaluation of thrombocytopenia and for understanding the origin of α-granule proteins. Blood 1990;76:859–870.

69. **George JN, Saucerman S.** Platelet IgG, IgA, IgM, and albumin: correlation of platelet and plasma concentrations in normal subjects and in patients with ITP of dysproteinemia. Blood 1988; 72:362–365.

70. **Hyde P, Zucker-Franklin D.** Antigenic differences between human platelets and megakaryocytes. Am J Pathol 1987;127:349–357.

71. **Slappendel RJ.** Interpretation of tests for immune-mediated blood diseases. In: Kirk RW, ed. Current veterinary therapy. IX. Small animal practice. Philadelphia: WB Saunders Company, 1986;498–505.

72. **Handagama P, Feldman BF.** Immune-mediated thrombocytopenia in the dog. Canine Pract 1985;12:25–30.

73. **George JN, Woolf SH, Raskob GE, Wasser JS, Aledort LM, Ballem PJ, Blanchette VS, Bussel AB, Cines DB, Kelton JG, Lichtin AE, McMillan R, Okerbloom JA, Regan DH, Warrier I.** Idiopathic thrombocytopenic purpura: a practice guideline developed by explicit methods for The American Society of Hematology. Blood 1996;88:3–40.

74. **Miller E.** Immunosuppressive therapy in the treatment of immune-mediated disease. J Vet Intern Med 1992;6:206–213.

75. **Lewis DC, Meyers KM.** Canine idiopathic thrombocytopenic purpura. J Vet Intern Med 1996;10:207–218.

76. **Greene CE, Scoggin J, Thomas JE, Barsanti JA.** Vincristine in the treatment of thrombocytopenia in five dogs. J Am Vet Med Assoc 1982;180:140–143.

77. **Sullivan PS.** Immune mediated thrombocytopenia: recent advances in diagnosis and treatment. Proceedings of the 12th Annual Veterinary Medical Forum 1994;149–151.

78. **Golden DL, Langston VC.** Uses of vincristine and vinblastine in dogs and cats. J Am Vet Med Assoc 1988;193:1114–1117.

79. **Holloway SA, Meyer DJ, Mannella C.** Prednisolone and danazol for treatment of immune-mediated anemia, thrombocytopenia, and ineffective erythroid regeneration in a dog. J Am Vet Med Assoc 1990; 197: 1045–1048.

80. **Cook AK, Gregory CR, Stewart AF.** Effects of oral cyclosporine (CS) in dogs with refractory immune-mediated anemia (IMA) or thrombocytopenia (ITP). Proceedings of the 12th Annual Veterinary Medical Forum 1994;1001.

81. **Scott-Moncrieff JC, Reagan WJ.** Human intravenous immunoglobulin therapy. Semin Vet Med Surg (Small Anim) 1997;12:178–185.

82. **Reagan WJ, Scott-Moncrieff JC, Snyder PW, Kelly K, Glickman LT, Bloom JC.** Action of human intravenous gamma globulin on the canine hematopoietic system. Blood 1994;84(10):662a.

83. **Dunayer E, Binkowski G.** Support for closing of experimental head injury laboratory. J Am Vet Med Assoc 1986;188:460–461.

84. **Helfand SC.** Splenectomy: an old issue of current controversy. J Am Vet Med Assoc 1986;188:461–462.

85. **Baldini M.** Acute "ITP" in isoimmunized dogs. Ann N Y Acad Sci 1965;124:543–549.

86. **Kuehn NF, Gaunt SD.** Hypocellular marrow and extramedullary hematopoiesis in a dog: hematologic recovery after splenectomy. J Am Vet Med Assoc 1986;188:1313–1315.

87. **Carr JM, Kruskall MS, Kaye JA, Robinson SH.** Efficacy of platelet transfusions in immune thrombocytopenia. Am J Pathol 1986;80:1051–1054.

88. **Feldman BF, Thomason KJ, Jain NC.** Immune-mediated thrombocytopenia in a dog. Vet Clin North Am Small Anim Pract 1988;18:258–260.

89. **Kelton JG, Keystone J, Moore J, Denomme G, Tozman E, Glynn M, Neame PB, Gauldie J, Jensen J.** Immune-mediated thrombocytopenia of malaria. J Clin Invest 1983;71:832–836.

90. **Nelson DS.** Immune adherence. In: Dixon FJ, Humphrey JH, eds. Advances in immunology, vol 3. New York: Academic Press, 1963;131–180.

91. **Hebert LA.** Physiology and cell biology update: the clearance of immune complexes from the circulation of man and other primates. Am J Kidney Dis 1991;XVII:352–361.

92. **Manthei U, Nickells MW, Barnes SH, Ballard LL, Cui W-Y, Atkinson JP.** Identification of a C3b/iC3 binding protein of rabbit platelets and leukocytes: a CR1-like candidate for the immune adherence receptor. J Immunol 1988;140:1228–1235.

93. **Rosenfeld SI, Anderson CL.** Fc receptors of human platelets. In: Kunicki TJ, George JN, eds. Platelet immunobiology: molecular and clinical aspects. Philadelphia: JB Lippincott, 1989;337–353.

94. **Miescher PA, Tucci A, Beris P, Favre H.** Autoimmune hemolytic anemia and/or thrombocytopenia associated with lupus parameters. Semin Hematol 1992;29:13–17.

95. **Gorman NT, Werner LL.** Immune-mediated diseases of the dog and cat. I. Basic concepts and the systemic immune-mediated diseases. Br Vet J 1986;142:395–402.

96. **Lewis RM, Schwartz R, Henry WB Jr.** Canine systemic lupus erythematosus. Blood 1965;25:143–160.

97. **Werner LL, Gorman NT.** Immune-mediated disorders of cats. Vet Clin North Am Small Anim Pract 1984;14:1039–1064.

98. **Geor RJ, Clark EG, Haines DM, Napier PG.** Systemic lupus erythematosis in a filly. J Am Vet Med Assoc 1990;197:1489–1492.

99. **Lewis RM, Schwartz RS, Gilmore CE.** Autoimmune diseases in domestic animals. Ann N Y Acad Sci 1965;124:178–200.

100. **Evans RS, Duane RT.** Acquired hemolytic anemia. I. The relation of erythrocyte antibody production to activity of the disease. II. The significance of thrombocytopenia and leukopenia. Blood 1949;4:1196–1213.

101. **Dougherty SA, Center SA, Shaw EE, Erb HA.** Juvenile-onset polyarthritis syndrome in Akitas. J Am Vet Med Assoc 1991;198:849–856.

102. **Grindem CB, Breitschwerdt EB, Corbett WT, Page RL, Jans HE.** Thrombocytopenia associated with neoplasia in dogs. J Vet Intern Med 1994; 8:400–405.

103. **Madewell BR, Feldman BF, O'Neill S.** Coagulation abnormalities in dogs with neoplastic disease. Thromb Haemost 1980;44:35–38.

104. **Madewell BR.** Hematological and bone marrow cytological abnormalities in 75 dogs with malignant lymphoma. J Am Anim Hosp Assoc 1986; 22:235–240.

105. **Ey FS, Goodnight SH.** Bleeding disorders in cancer. Semin Oncol 1990; 17:187–197.

106. **Helfand SC, Couto CG, Madewell BR.** Immune-mediated thrombocytopenia associated with solid tumors in dogs. J Am Anim Hosp Assoc 1985;21:787–794.

107. **O'Donnell MR, Slichter SJ, Weiden PL, Storb R.** Platelet and fibrinogen kinetics in canine tumors. Cancer Res 1981;41:1379–1383.

108. **Slichter SJ, Weiden PL, O'Donnell MR, Storb R.** Interruption of tumor-associated platelet consumption with platelet enzyme inhibitors. Blood 1982;59:1252–1258.

109. **Keller ET.** Immune-mediated disease as a risk factor for canine lymphoma. Cancer 1992;70:2334–2337.

110. **Helfand SC.** Neoplasia and immune-mediated thrombocytopenia. Vet Clin North Am Small Anim Pract 1988;18:267–270.

111. **Woods JP, Johnstone IB, Bienzle D, Balson G, Gartley CJ.** Concurrent lymphangioma, immune-mediated thrombocytopenia, and von Willebrand's disease in a dog. J Am Anim Hosp Assoc 1995;31:70–76.

112. **Reef VB, Dyson SS, Beech J.** Lymphosarcoma and associated immune-mediated hemolytic anemia and thrombocytopenia in horses. J Am Vet Med Assoc 1984;184:313–317.

113. **Breitschwerdt EB.** Infectious thrombocytopenia in dogs. Compend Cont Educ Small Anim Pract 1988;10:1177–1186.

114. **Sellon DC, Levine J, Millikin E, Palmer K, Grindem C, Covington P.** Thrombocytopenia in horses: 35 cases (1989–1994). J Vet Intern Med 1996;10:127–132.

115. **Wilson JJ, Neame PB, Kelton JG.** Infection-induced thrombocytopenia. Semin Thromb Hemost 1982;8:217–233.

116. **van der Lelie J, van de Plas-van Dalen CM, von dem Borne AEGKr.** Platelet autoantibodies in septicaemia. Br J Haematol 1984;58:755–760.

117. **Kelton JG, Neame PB, Gauldie J, Hirsh J.** Elevated platelet-associated IgG in the thrombocytopenia of septicemia. N Engl J Med 1979;300:760–764.

118. **Yeaman MR, Sullam PM, Dazin PF, Norman DC, Bayer AS.** Characterization of Staphylococcus aureus-platelet binding by quantitative flow cytometric analysis. J Infect Dis 1992;166:65–73.

119. **Sullam PM, Payan DG, Dazin PF, Valone FH.** Binding of viridans group streptococci to human platelets: a quantitative analysis. Infect Immun 1990;3802–3806.

120. **Waner T, Harrus S, Weiss DJ, Bark H, Keysary A.** Demonstration of serum antiplatelet antibodies in experimental acute canine ehrlichiosis. Vet Immunol Immunopthol 1995;48:177–182.

121. **Harrus S, Waner T, Weiss DJ, Keysary A, Bark H.** Kinetics of serum antiplatelet antibodies in experimental acute canine ehrlichiosis. Vet Immunol Immunopthol 1996;51:13–20.

122. **Smith RD, Hooks JE, Huxsoll DL, Ristic M.** Canine ehrlichiosis (tropical canine pancytopenia): survival of phosphorus-32-labeled blood platelets in normal and infected dogs. Am J Vet Res 1974;35:269–273.

123. **Smith RD, Ristic M, Huxsoll DL, Baylor RA.** Platelet kinetics in canine ehrlichiosis: evidence for increased platelet destruction as the cause of thrombocytopenia. Infect Immun 1975;11:1216–1221.

124. **Codner EC, Roberts RE, Ainsworth AG.** Atypical findings in 16 cases of canine ehrlichiosis. J Am Vet Med Assoc 1985;186:166–169.

125. **Pierce KR, Marrs GE, Hightower D.** Acute canine ehrlichiosis: platelet survival and factor 3 assay. Am J Vet Res 1977;38:1821–1825.

126. **Waddle JR, Littman MP.** A retrospective study of 27 cases of naturally occurring canine ehrlichiosis. J Am Anim Hosp Assoc 1988;24:615–620.

127. **Kuehn NF, Gaunt SD.** Clinical and hematologic findings in canine ehrlichiosis. J Am Vet Med Assoc 1985;186:355–358.

128. **Kaplan C, Morinet F, Cartron J.** Virus-induced autoimmune thrombocytopenia and neutropenia. Semin Hematol 1992;29:34–44.

129. **Tornquist SJ, Oaks JL, Crawford TB.** Elevation of cytokines associated with the thrombocytopenia of equine infectious anaemia. J Gen Virol 1997;78:2541–2548.

130. **Crawford TB, Wardrop K, Tornquist SJ, Reilich E, Meyers KM, McGuire TC.** A primary production deficit in the thrombocytopenia of equine infectious anemia. J Virol 1996;70:7842–7850.

131. **Clabough DL, Gebhard D, Flaherty MT, Whetter LE, Perry ST, Coggins L, Fuller FJ.** Immune-mediated thrombocytopenia in horses infected with equine infectious anemia virus. J Virol 1991;65:6242-6251.

132. **Axthelm MK, Krakowka S.** Canine distemper virus-induced thrombocytopenia. Am J Vet Res 1987;48:1269–1275.

133. **Pineau S, Belbeck LW, Moore S.** Levamisole reduces the thrombocytopenia associated with myxovirus vaccination. Can Vet J 1980;21:82–84.

134. **Straw B.** Decrease in platelet count after vaccination with distemper-hepatitis (DH) vaccine. Vet Med 1978;June:725–726.

135. **Jones B-E.** Platelet aggregation in dogs after live-virus vaccination. Acta Vet Scand 1984;25:504–509.

136. **Dodds WJ.** Immune-mediated blood diseases. Gazette 1987; April:74–76.

137. **Peltola H, Heinonen OP, Valle M, Paunio M, Virtanen M, Karanko V, Cantell K.** The elimination of indigenous measles, mumps, and rubella from Finland by a 12-year, two-dose vaccination program. N Engl J Med 1994;331:1397–1402.

138. **Nieminen U, Peltola H, Syrjälä MT, Mäkipernaa A, Kekomäki R.** Acute thrombocytopenic purpura following measles, mumps and rubella vaccination. A report on 23 patients. Acta Pediatr 1993;82:267–270.

139. **Slappendel RJ.** Canine leishmaniasis: a review based on 95 cases in the Netherlands. Vet Quarterly 1988;10:1–16.

140. **Miescher PA, Belehu A.** Leishmaniasis: hematologic aspects. Semin Hematol 1982;19:93–99.

141. **Taboada J. Babesiosis.** In: Greene CE, ed. Infectious diseases of the dog and cat. 2nd ed. Philadelphia: WB Saunders, 1998;473–481.

142. **Clinkenbeard KD, Tyler RD, Cowell RL.** Thrombocytopenia associated with disseminated histoplasmosis in dogs. Compend Cont Educ Small Anim Pract 1989;11:301–306.

143. **Clinkenbeard KD, Cowell RL, Tyler RD.** Disseminated histioplasmosis in dogs: 12 cases (1981–1986). J Am Vet Med Assoc 1988;193:1443–1447.

144. **Des Prez RM, Steckley S, Stroud RM, Hawiger J.** Pathogenesis: interaction of Histoplasma capsulatum with human platelets. J Infect Dis 1980;142:32–39.

145. **Kucera JC, Davis RB.** Thrombocytopenia associated with histoplasmosis and an elevated platelet associated IgG. J Clin Pathol 1983;79:644–664.

146. **Kiefel V, Santoso S, Schmidt S, Salama A, Mueller-Eckhardt C.** Metabolite-specific (IgG) and drug-specific antibodies (IgG, IgM) in two cases of trimethoprim-sulfamethoxazole-induced immune thrombocytopenia. Transfusion 1987;27:262–265.

147. **Lerner W, Caruso R, Faig D, Karpatkin S.** Drug-dependent and non-drug-dependent antiplatelet antibody in drug-induced immunologic thrombocytopenic purpura. Blood 1985;66:306–311.

148. **Bloom JC, Thiem PA, Sellers TS, Deldar A, Lewis HB.** Cephalosporin-induced immune cytopenia in the dog: demonstration of erythrocyte-, neutrophil-, and platelet-associated IgG following treatment with cefazedone. Am J Hematol 1988;28:71–78.

149. **Buechner-Maxwell V, Scott MA, Godber L, Kristensen A.** Neonatal alloimmune thrombocytopenia in a quarter horse foal. J Vet Intern Med 1997;11:304–308.

150. **Traub-Dargatz JL, McClure JJ, Koch C, Schlipf JW Jr.** Neonatal isoerythrolysis in mule foals. J Am Vet Med Assoc 1995;206:67–70.

151. **Stormorken H, Svenkerud R, Slagsvold P, Lie H.** Thrombocytopenic bleedings in young pigs due to maternal isoimmunization. Nature 1963; 198:1116–1117.

152. **Linklater KA.** The experimental reproduction of thrombocytopenic purpura in piglets. Res Vet Sci 1975;18:127–133.

153. **Saunders CN, Kinch DA, Imlah P.** Thrombocytopenic purpura in pigs. Vet Rec 1966;79:549–550.

154. **Dimmock CK, Webster WR, Shiels IA, Edwards CL.** Isoimmune thrombocytopenic purpura in piglets. Aust Vet J 1982;59:157–158.

155. **Saunders CN, Kinch DA.** Thrombocytopenic purpura of pigs. J Comp Pathol 1968;78:513–523.

156. **Nordstoga K.** Thrombocytopenic purpura on baby pigs caused by maternal isoimmunization. Pathol Vet 1965;2:601–610.

157. **Linklater KA.** Post-transfusion purpura in a pig. Res Vet Sci 1977;22: 257–258.

158. **Cöp WAG.** Blood group antagonism in newborn piglets. Neth J Vet Sci 1969;2:66–73.

159. **Wardrop K, Lewis D, Marks S, Buss M.** Posttransfusion purpura in a dog with hemophilia A. J Vet Intern Med 1997;11:261–263.

160. **Swisher SN, Young LE.** The blood grouping system of dogs. Physiol Rev 1961;41:495–519.

CHAPTER 69

Secondary Thrombocytopenia

• KAREN E. RUSSELL and CAROL B. GRINDEM

Thrombocytopenia is defined as a decrease in circulating platelets and is the most common acquired hemostatic disorder in veterinary and human medicine. Thrombocytopenia results from one or a combination of the following basic mechanisms: decreased or defective platelet production, increased peripheral platelet destruction or consumption, or abnormal distribution. In this chapter, thrombocytopenia that arises secondarily to accelerated destruction or consumption of platelets, complex or undetermined mechanisms, and miscellaneous causes are discussed.

PLATELET KINETICS

Platelets are the second most numerous circulating cell in blood and are essential for coagulation, maintenance of vascular integrity, and control of hemostasis. These small, anucleate cells originate by cytoplasmic fragmentation of mature bone marrow megakaryocytes. Platelet production is regulated by several growth factors. Megakaryocyte colony-stimulating factor (MK-CSF), granulocyte-macrophage-CSF (GM-CSF), interleukin (IL)-3, IL-6, IL-11, and thrombopoietin are major factors controlling megakaryocytopoiesis and thrombocytopoiesis. IL-1, IL-4, IL-6, and granulocyte-CSF (G-CSF) may act synergistically. In vitro, erythropoietin simulates megakaryocytopoiesis.[1]

Each megakaryocyte is capable of generating several thousand platelets. Daily platelet production is approximately $35,000 \pm 4,000$ platelets$/\mu$L.[2] Platelet production is thought to be regulated by total platelet mass rather than platelet numbers. In situations of increased demand, platelet production can increase as much as twofold to eightfold.

PATHOGENESIS

Platelet numbers remain fairly constant within a species, but platelet numbers vary widely between different species. Platelets circulate for approximately 5 to 9 days in most species and are normally removed from circulation by age-dependent attrition. Premature removal of

platelets in pathologic states occurs through consumptive, or nonimmune or immune-mediated destructive processes. When consumption or destruction of platelets exceeds bone marrow production, thrombocytopenia results.

Increased Platelet Loss or Consumption

Thrombocytopenia secondary to rapid, increased consumption or loss of platelets may occur with massive trauma, extensive external hemorrhage, or exchange blood transfusion. In situations of trauma or external hemorrhage, thrombocytopenia is generally mild to moderate, transient, and usually reversible without specific treatment.[3]

Accelerated consumption of platelets can be brought on by widespread activation of the coagulation system or endothelial damage. Disseminated intravascular coagulation (DIC), thrombocytopenic thrombotic purpura (TTP), and hemolytic uremic syndrome (HUS) are complex syndromes characterized by widespread consumption of platelets, resulting in moderate to significant thrombocytopenia. DIC is a common complication seen in both veterinary and human medicine. TTP and HUS occur in humans but are rare in veterinary species. A syndrome resembling HUS has been reported in 3 horses and 1 heifer.[4,5,6] Animal models for TTP have been described.[7]

Disseminated Intravascular Coagulation

DIC occurs secondarily to a wide variety of insults and diseases. DIC can be acute, subacute, or chronic and is characterized clinically by hemorrhage and microthrombosis. The pathophysiology of DIC is discussed in Chapter 86.

Common disorders associated with DIC include vascular damage, septicemia with release of bacterial endotoxins, release of tissue thromboplastin from necrotic or malignant tissue, or release of other procoagulant proteins. Approximately 65% of DIC cases in humans occur secondarily to infection; bacterial infection is the most common. In gram-negative infections, bacterial release of endotoxin (lipopolysaccharide) causes simultaneous activation of the coagulation system and inhibition of coagulation control mechanisms. Endotoxin stimulates intrinsic coagulation directly by activating Factor (F) XII or indirectly by activating FXII via endothelial damage. Endotoxin stimulates the extrinsic coagulation pathway by causing generation and increased surface expression of thromboplastins or tissue factor from inflammatory cells, primarily monocytes. Activated monocytes release IL-1 and tumor necrosis factor alpha (TNF-α), which decreases endothelial expression of thrombomodulin and prevents activation of protein C and thus negates control of an important coagulation inhibitory pathway.

Thrombocytopenic Thrombotic Purpura and Hemolytic Uremic Syndrome

In humans, the thrombotic microangiopathies are exemplified by two syndromes, TTP and HUS. The pathogenesis of both is heterogenous and often the origin is unknown; many consider them to be different expressions of the same disease mechanism. TTP and HUS may occur either as a primary condition or as a secondary complication. Most cases of HUS occur in childhood after bloody diarrhea caused by *Shigella dysenteriae* serotype I or various *Escherichia coli* serotypes. The classical triad of TTP is characterized by severe thrombocytopenia, intravascular hemolysis with schistocytes, and neurologic symptoms. Severe renal dysfunction is also a prominent feature of HUS.

The thrombotic microangiopathies are characterized by endothelial damage and platelet aggregation with resultant thrombocytopenia, hemolytic anemia, and thromboses. High plasma concentrations of thrombomodulin, tissue plasminogen activator, and von Willebrand factor (vWF) are observed in many TTP patients. Plasminogen activator inhibitor type I and urine endothelin concentrations are increased in HUS patients. Concentrations return to normal when patients enter remission.

Platelet aggregation may be caused by the presence in plasma of abnormally large vWF molecules that bind platelets and cause aggregation and activation much more actively than smaller vWF molecules. In TTP, endothelial damage may cause leakage of stored large vWF multimers into subendothelial tissue and plasma. Normal cleavage and clearance of these large vWF multimers is limited, causing increased concentrations and extensive platelet aggregation. This extensive, systemic platelet aggregation causes platelet consumption and moderate to significant thrombocytopenia.

Laboratory Confirmation of Consumptive Thrombocytopenias

Thrombocytopenia and microangiopathic anemia with schistocytes are typical laboratory findings in DIC and TTP-HUS. Differentiation can often be made with the help of coagulation screening tests, including fibrinogen and fibrinogen-fibrin degradation product (FDP) concentrations, one-stage prothrombin time (OSPT), and activated partial thromboplastin time (APTT). In DIC, classical laboratory findings are three or more of the following: thrombocytopenia, decreased plasma fibrinogen concentration, increased plasma FDP concentration, and prolonged APTT and OSPT. In contrast to DIC, coagulation tests and FDP concentrations are usually normal with TTP or HUS.[8]

Platelet Destruction: Immune Mediated, Nonimmune Mediated, and Complex Mechanisms

Immune-mediated thrombocytopenia is covered in Chapter 119. Briefly, immune-mediated destruction of platelets may be primary (idiopathic) or may occur in association with infectious agents, neoplasia, drugs, autoimmune, isoimmune, or neonatal-immune diseases. A diagnosis of idiopathic or primary immune-mediated thrombocytopenia is made after all other potential causes have been eliminated.

Immune destruction of platelets occurs when circulating platelets coated with antibody, antigen-antibody complexes, or complement are phagocytized by macrophages in the spleen, liver, and bone marrow. The result is decreased platelet survival and life span. The spleen is the largest lymphoid organ, and the major site of antibody production and platelet removal.

Platelet aggregation, phagocytosis, or lysis resulting in platelet destruction and thrombocytopenia can occur independently of immune-mediated events. Nonimmune-mediated platelet destruction occurs in some acute bacterial and viral infections and in cardiovascular disease. Thrombocytopenia occurring from venomous snakebites may be secondary to DIC or may result from directing aggregating affects on platelets. Platelet activation with thrombocytopenia is associated with severe and extensive burns.

Platelet destruction in bacterial infections can occur as a result of platelet adherence or aggregation to activated monocytes or neutrophils. In gram-negative infections, monocytes are stimulated by endotoxin, express tissue factor on their surface, and generate thrombin. Thrombin, a potent platelet agonist, causes platelet activation and aggregation. Platelets adhere to monocytes and are phagocytized. Neutrophil stimulation is not believed to be a major cause of platelet removal and is probably more important with regard to platelet function and thrombus formation. Exotoxins released from gram-positive bacteria may directly damage platelets and contribute to thrombocytopenia.

The pathogenesis of thrombocytopenia associated with acute viral infections is often multifactorial, even though one mechanism may predominate. Direct platelet damage or lysis is one proposed mechanism of viral-associated thrombocytopenia. Myxovirus infection (Newcastle disease virus and influenza) decreases platelet survival by removal of platelet membrane sialic acid by viral neuraminidase with resultant platelet lysis. Other viruses in which platelet damage is suspected

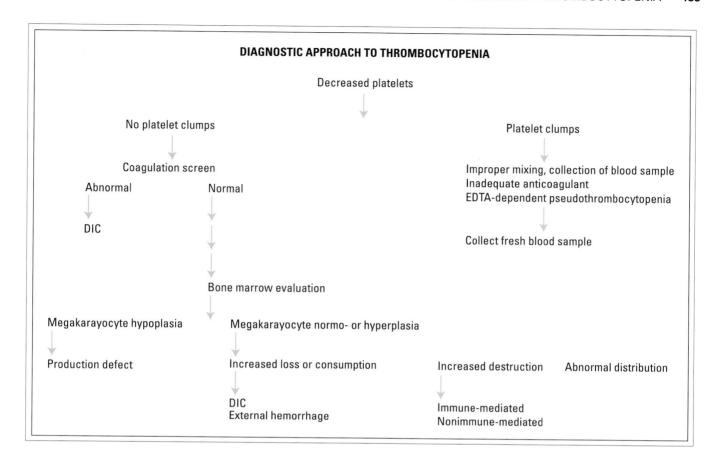

DIAGNOSTIC APPROACH TO THROMBOCYTOPENIA

Decreased platelets

No platelet clumps

Coagulation screen

Abnormal   Normal

DIC

Bone marrow evaluation

Megakarayocyte hypoplasia   Megakarayocyte normo- or hyperplasia

Production defect   Increased loss or consumption   Increased destruction   Abnormal distribution

DIC
External hemorrhage   Immune-mediated
Nonimmune-mediated

Platelet clumps

Improper mixing, collection of blood sample
Inadequate anticoagulant
EDTA-dependent pseudothrombocytopenia

Collect fresh blood sample

---

include bovine viral diarrhea virus and hog cholera virus.

In humans, platelets can be damaged and destroyed by mechanical means in arterial disease with roughened endothelial surfaces and narrowed microcirculation, stenotic or prosthetic heart valves, or cardiac bypass surgery. Turbulent circulation causes membrane damage and microparticle formation.[9] Interactions of platelets with altered or damaged endothelial surfaces cause extensive platelet activation, clumping, and removal of platelets by the mononuclear phagocytic system.[10] This may also occur in viral infections that infect or alter endothelial cells. In vitro, virally transformed endothelial cells show a significant increase in platelet adherence.

Many of the rickettsial diseases are associated with thrombocytopenia. Several mechanisms contribute to thrombocytopenia, including immune-mediated platelet destruction, direct damage, associated vasculitis, and platelet production deficits. DIC may occur as a secondary complication.

Abnormal Platelet Distribution

In health, approximately 30 to 40% of the total circulating platelet pool may be stored in the spleen, which is referred to as physiologic platelet sequestration. The liver and bone marrow are additional tissue sites of platelet sequestration. Hypersplenism is a pathologic condition in which as much as 90% of circulating platelets become sequestered predominately in the spleen. Hypersplenism is characterized by the presence of one or more cytopenias with corresponding bone marrow hyperplasia of the cells type(s) and significant splenomegaly. Splenic size is probably the most important factor that determines the degree of thrombocytopenia; the spleen must be significantly enlarged to cause a severe decrease in circulating platelets. Although hypersplenism is characterized by splenomegaly, the presence of splenomegaly does not always signify hypersplenism.

Thrombocytopenia that results from hypersplenism can be thought of as a displacement of the majority of platelets from peripheral circulation into a reversible, but slowly exchanging, splenic pool.[11] Thrombocytopenia secondary to splenic pooling is different from that seen with idiopathic thrombocytopenic purpura in which there is active removal of platelets by the splenic macrophages.[11] In hypersplenism, thrombocytopenia is evident on a complete blood count (CBC), but the total number of platelets and platelet mass are actually normal. Platelet survival is often or is usually normal, as is platelet production.[12]

Hypersplenism is rare in animals but a few suspected cases have been described.[1,13] All other causes of splenomegaly should be ruled out before a diagnosis of primary hypersplenism is made. Recommended treatment in these cases is splenectomy.

Hypothermia adversely affects platelet morphology and can cause a mild transient thrombocytopenia owing to pooling of platelets in the spleen.[1] Transient thrombocytopenia can also occur with endotoxemia and hypotension.

Artifactual or Spurious Causes

Decreased platelet counts should always be confirmed by microscopic examination of a blood smear and, if necessary, the platelet count repeated on a freshly drawn blood sample. It is imperative that the venipuncture is carefully performed to prevent initiation of platelet activation, aggregation, and clotting that causes artifactual changes on the CBC and makes platelet parameters unreliable. Delayed time of exposure to anticoagulant, improper mixing, or improper collection can all contribute to falsely low platelet counts.

Ethylenediamine tetra-acetic acid (EDTA)-dependent pseudothrombocytopenia, an in vitro phenomenon, has been reported in humans and in one horse and has been suspected in a miniature pig.[11,14,15] Platelet clumping, which is evident on a blood smear, falsely lowers the platelet count and is caused by antibodies that agglutinate platelets in the presence of EDTA.[16,17] To rule out EDTA-dependent pseudothrombocytopenia, a fresh blood sample drawn into a citrate anticoagulant should give platelet counts within a normal reference range and with no microscopic evidence of platelet clumps on a blood film.

CLINICAL SIGNS
OF THROMBOCYTOPENIA
AND RISK OF HEMORRHAGE

Clinical signs leading one to suspect thrombocytopenia include petechiation and ecchymosis in tissues or mucosal membranes, epistaxis, melena, hematochezia, hematuria, prolonged bleeding after venipuncture, or retinal hemorrhage or hyphema. However, the complaint of bleeding is actually uncommon. Frequently, thrombocytopenia is first identified on a routine CBC. Animals having a low platelet count may be asymptomatic or present for lethargy, weakness, fever, or other signs related to the primary underlying disease process. Despite the observation that hemorrhage is not a consistent feature, thrombocytopenic animals are at an increased risk of bleeding.

Hemorrhage solely caused by thrombocytopenia does not usually occur until peripheral platelet numbers are severely depleted (<50,000 platelets/μL). Animals that have platelet counts of 10,000 or less platelets/μL are at great risk of hemorrhage. Abnormal or compromised platelet function or vascular disease in a thrombocytopenic animal enhances the risk of hemorrhage.

DIAGNOSTIC EVALUATION

The first evidence that an animal is thrombocytopenic may be from a routine CBC. Likewise, a CBC should be the first test performed in any animal that is suspected to have a bleeding disorder. Generally, EDTA-anticoagulated blood is acceptable for platelet counts for 5 hours after collection when kept at 20°C and 24 hours when kept at 4°C; however, certain platelet parameters are affected by anticoagulant, time, or refrigeration.[18] Specific platelet parameters available on most automated CBCs include platelet count, mean platelet volume (MPV), and platelet distribution width (PDW). In addition to these automated parameters, microscopic examination of the blood film for platelet morphology and evidence of platelet clumping or adherence to leukocytes should also be included. If the platelet count is normal in an animal that has abnormal bleeding, abnormal platelet function or coagulopathy should be considered.

MPV estimates platelet size and is inversely proportional to platelet number. Increases in MPV suggest responsive thrombopoiesis such as secondary platelet destruction, some myeloproliferative diseases, and hyperthyroidism.[19,20] Decreases in MPV have been reported in some dogs that have early manifestations of immune-mediated thrombocytopenia.[21] Decreases in MPV are more often associated with bone marrow failure. Artifactual increases in MPV arise when platelets are exposed to EDTA, cooled to room temperature (25°C), or refrigerated (4°C), or if there is delayed exposure to an anticoagulant.[18,22] Minimal changes in MPV occur when blood is collected in an anticoagulant containing a citrate anticoagulant and is kept at 37°C.[18,22]

PDW is a value given by some automated particle counters and represents an index of variation in platelet size. PDW may be useful in laboratories that do not routinely perform smear evaluations. A novel platelet parameter recently described is mean platelet component concentration (MPC).[23,24] MPC was determined with a modified two-angle light-scattering technology and found to be sensitive to the activation state of feline platelets.[24]

Microscopic examination of a blood film is necessary to evaluate platelet morphology and to ensure accuracy of automated platelet counts. Although, manual methods are less accurate and precise than automated methods for platelet enumeration, they become necessary, when platelet counts fall below the limit of sensitivity or linearity (5,000 to 20,000 platelets/μL) of the hematology instrument.

Once an animal is found to be thrombocytopenic, additional diagnostic testing is often necessary to elucidate the cause. Additional tests that should be considered include a coagulation panel, bone marrow analysis, serology or DNA analysis for infectious agents, and bacterial cultures. In thrombocytopenic horses, an agar gel immunodiffusion test (Coggins test) or an enzyme-linked immunosorbent assay (ELISA) to rule out equine infectious anemia is indicated.

Bone marrow evaluation of megakaryocytes may be necessary to determine if thrombocytopenia is secondary to a platelet production defect or is caused by peripheral platelet destruction. The typical finding in cases of diminished or defective platelet production is the absence of or the decreased numbers of megakaryocytes. Abnormal morphology and size may also be observed. In most cases of peripheral platelet destruction, megakaryocyte numbers are normal to increased. Often megakaryocytes are increased in size and ploidy as well. Both aspiration and core biopsies of bone marrow should be taken since both approaches offer certain advantages. Cellular morphology is more superior with aspiration biopsies, whereas core biopsies are more useful for evaluation of megakaryocyte numbers, myelofibrosis, or necrosis. For proper and complete bone marrow interpretation, a blood sample should be taken for a CBC at the time of bone marrow sampling.

Antiplatelet or antimegakaryocytic antibody assays, reticulated platelet analyses, and platelet function studies are additional tests that may be considered for the evaluation of platelet disorders. Routine antiplatelet antibody assays measure platelet-associated antibodies and confirm an immune component but do not distinguish between primary and secondary immune-mediated thrombocytopenia. Reticulated platelets are young platelets recently released from bone marrow and that contain increased RNA concentrations.[25,26] In cases of peripheral platelet destruction, the percentage of reticulated platelets is increased in circulation. Thrombocytopenic patients who have compromised platelet production have decreased percentages of reticulated platelets in circulation.[27] The percentage of reticulated platelets was increased in two horses that had DIC and several ponies acutely infected with equine infectious anemia virus.[28] Many platelet function assays are only available at specialized or institutional laboratories and may not be readily available or practical.

Avian and Reptile Thrombocytes

In addition to having a primary role in hemostasis, thrombocytes of birds are also phagocytic. Thrombocyte numbers in most avian species range between 20,000 and 30,000/μL or approximately 10 to 15 thrombocytes per 1000 erythrocytes; one to two thrombocytes per monolayer area under oil immersion (100) is considered normal or adequate in most birds.[29] Thrombocytes in reptiles appear to have the traditional hemostatic role. In normal reptiles, thrombocyte numbers in blood range between 25 and 350 thrombocytes per 100 leukocytes.[30]

THERAPEUTIC PRINCIPLES

Management of platelet disorders includes supportive therapy to control acute shock and control bleeding or ongoing platelet destruction. After patient stabilization, specific therapy such as pathogen-specific drug therapy or immunosuppressive therapy is initiated to treat the underlying disorder. Platelet-rich plasma transfusions or fresh whole blood (if anemia is present) and gastrointestinal protectants can be used to stop or to prevent bleeding. Vincristine, anabolic steroids, erythropoietin, IL-3, or GM-CSF can be used to stimulate platelet production.

SPECIES-SPECIFIC DISORDERS AND DISEASES ASSOCIATED WITH THROMBOCYTOPENIA

Canine

In one large epidemiologic survey, thrombocytopenia was documented in 5.2% of the dogs studied. A total of 987 dogs that had thrombocytopenia were studied, and of these, 5% were primary immune mediated; 23% were due to infectious or inflammatory causes; 13% were associated with neoplasia; and the remaining 59% were of miscellaneous causes that included trauma (12%), clumping (12%), therapy (12%), loss (5%), renal or liver (5%), DIC (1.5%), bone marrow (1%), sequestration (0.5%), or unknown (52%).[31]

Viral-associated thrombocytopenia has been reported with canine distemper virus (CDV), canine herpes virus, canine infectious hepatitis virus (adenovirus type I) and canine parvovirus. Thrombocytopenia occurs in dogs naturally and experimentally infected with CDV and is caused by immune-mediated destruction, defective production, and direct platelet damage by virus.[32] Dogs vaccinated with modified-live adenovirus and myxovirus products become thrombocytopenic within 48 hours after vaccination; thrombocytopenia is mild to moderate, lasting 1 to 3 weeks.[33,34] Thrombocytopenia associated with canine herpes virus and canine infectious hepatitis virus occurs secondary to vascular endothelial damage and DIC.[35,36] Thrombocytopenia caused by bone marrow suppression can occur with canine parvovirus infection.[36]

Thrombocytopenia is common in canine ehrlichiosis (*Ehrlichia canis*, canine granulocytic ehrlichiosis, *Ehrlichia platys*). Megakaryocyte hypoplasia and decreased platelet survival secondary to immunologic and consumptive processes contribute to thrombocytopenia with *E. canis*. Mild thrombocytopenia can occur in dogs that have Rocky Mountain spotted fever (*Rickettsia rickettsii*) and is believed to result secondarily from vasculitis and platelet consumption. The mechanism of thrombocytopenia associated with *E. platys* infections is not known. Decreased platelet production is not likely, since the organism is not found in megakaryocytes, and megakaryocytes are increased in infected dogs.[37]

Spirochetemia has been reported in four dogs presumed to be naturally infected.[38,39,40] Thrombocytopenia was documented in two of the four dogs and suspected in a third.[39,40] Serum from two dogs contained indirect fluorescent antibodies (IFAs) to *Borrelia burgdorferi*, but polymerase chain reaction (PCR) analysis failed to detect *B. burgdorferi* DNA.[40]

Severe bacteremic, septicemic, or endotoxemic vascular damage with fulminant DIC is associated with some bacterial infections and has been observed with canine leptospirosis, salmonellosis, and other aerobic and anaerobic infections.[40] Increased platelet consumption with DIC and possibly increased sequestration infrequently cause thrombocytopenia in dogs that have systemic fungal infections, including severe histoplasmosis and disseminated candidiasis.[40,41] Bone marrow suppression and thrombocytopenia has been associated with chronic heartworm disease.[42] Thrombocytopenia is a consistent finding in canine babesiosis and most likely results from associated endothelial damage and DIC.[36,43] Thrombocytopenia secondary to increased consumption and DIC occurs in some dogs that have leishmaniasis.[43a]

Thrombocytopenia has been reported in approximately 13% of dogs that have neoplasia (lymphoma, multiple myeloma, myelogenous leukemia, and hemangiosarcoma). Immune-mediated platelet destruction, paraprotein-coated platelets, and chemotherapeutic bone narrow suppression are implicated. Chemotherapy-associated thrombocytopenia can be severe but is usually transient, and platelet numbers rebound when the drug regimen is discontinued.

Feline

The overall prevalence of thrombocytopenia is cats is approximately 2%.[44] Thrombocytopenia secondary to decreased or defective platelet production occurs with feline leukemia virus (FeLV), feline immunodeficiency virus (FIV), and feline panleukopenia virus. The prevalence of thrombocytopenia in FIV-positive cats ranges from 6 to 16%.[45,46,47] Cats that have concurrent FIV and FeLV infections are more likely to have thrombocytopenia caused by a greatly increased risk of developing myeloproliferative disease with myelophthisis.[46,48] Vasculitis, increased destruction (through immune-complex deposition and direct viral effects), and DIC contribute to thrombocytopenia observed in cats infected with feline infectious peritonitis virus.[49] Thrombocytopenia is observed in cats that have suspected ehrlichiosis and antibody titers to E. canis and Escherichia risticii.[50] Thrombocytopenia occurs in cytauxzoonosis and is mostly likely to be caused by DIC and possibly platelet phagocytosis.[51]

Equine

In a recent retrospective study, thrombocytopenia was documented in 1.5% of the horses studied; thrombocytopenia was prevalent in horses that had gastrointestinal, inflammatory, or infectious diseases.[52] Thrombocytopenia in horses is most commonly associated with DIC, or endotoxemia and septicemia. The DIC in horses may occur secondarily to gram-positive or gram-negative bacteremia, viremia, neoplasia, hepatic disease, renal disease, burns, vasculitides, fetal death in utero, or circulating immune complexes or immune thrombocytopenia.[53]

In horses, viral diseases associated with thrombocytopenia include equine infectious anemia virus (EIAV),

equine viral arteritis (EVA), African horsesickness virus (AHSV), and Venezuelan encephalitis virus (VEE). Thrombocytopenia is common in horses acutely infected with virulent strains of EIAV and may occur in chronically infected horses[54,55] Multiple mechanisms, including immune-mediated destruction, impaired production, and possibly nonimmune destruction, are likely involved.[54,56,57] Thrombocytopenia is less common in EVA and is most likely secondary to vasculitis.[58] Significant thrombocytopenia occurs in horses experimentally infected with VEE; immune-mediated destruction and decreased production are suspected.[3,59] Endothelial cell infection and intravascular coagulation are thought to contribute to decreased platelet numbers in horses experimentally infected with AHSV.[60,61]

Thrombocytopenia, leukopenia, and mild anemia are consistent hematologic abnormalities in equine granulocytic ehrlichiosis (Ehrlichia equi). The mechanism(s) causing thrombocytopenia has not been elucidated. E. equi also infects sheep, cattle, dogs, cats, goats, and nonhuman primates; infections are mild or asymptomatic. Thrombocytopenia may occur in horses infected with Ehrlichia risticii (Potomac horse fever, equine ehrlicial colitis).[62,63] Mechanisms of thrombocytopenia are not fully elucidated but most likely involve DIC.[63]

Bovine

Thrombocytopenia in cattle acutely infected with bovine viral diarrhea virus is believed to be caused by a direct virus effect on platelets. Megakaryocytic hyperplasia, rapid rebound, and recovery of platelet counts occur and failure to detect immunoglobulin on platelet surfaces argues against a platelet production deficit or an immune-mediated platelet destruction. Evidence for a direct viral effect includes finding viral antigen on platelets and the recovery of virus in tissue culture inoculated with washed platelets.[64] Pulmonary edema and thrombocytopenia with petechial hemorrhages are seen in cattle infected with Theilera parva, the causal agent of East coast fever. Experimental infections with Trypanosoma congolense and Trypanosoma vivax in cattle consistently cause thrombocytopenia. Multiple mechanisms, including reduced platelet life span, decreased platelet production, and DIC are implicated. In experimental infections, cattle and water buffalo in the terminal stages of acute infection with Theilera lawrencei become leukopenic and thrombocytopenic.

Ovine

Thrombocytopenia occurs in sheep infected with blue tongue virus (BTV).[65] The suggested mechanism is platelet consumption caused by widespread vascular lesions and vascular thrombosis. In an earlier study, the virus was isolated from platelets from infected sheep and cattle, but thrombocytopenia was not reported.[66] Sheep and cattle infected with Ehrlichia phagocytophilia, a tickborne disease, become transiently and severely neutropenic and thrombocytopenic.

Caprine

In African trypanosomiasis, thrombocytopenia is a consistent finding in goats and other species.[67] The degree of thrombocytopenia and development of hemorrhage correlates to the degree of parasitemia.

Camelid

Hyperthermia in South American camelids (llama, alpaca, vicuna, and guanaco) causes hemoconcentration, increased erythrocyte fragility, leukocytosis, thrombocytopenia, and coagulation abnormalities leading to DIC.[68]

Cervids

Hemorrhagic diathesis, thrombosis, and DIC occur in white-tailed deer infected with BTV. Viral infection, replication, and damage to endothelium occurs. Platelets or megakaryocytes are not directly damaged, however, ultrastructural evidence for platelet activation is observed. Viral-induced endothelial damage is the inciting cause of DIC in BTV-infected deer.[69]

Porcine

African swine fever (ASF) and hog cholera in swine are hemorrhagic diseases and are associated with severe thrombocytopenia. In ASF, viral antigen-antibody immune complexes cause in vitro platelet aggregation, suggesting that immune-mediated destruction is one mechanism of thrombocytopenia.[70] The virus also infects megakaryocytes.[71] In pigs infected with hog cholera virus, thrombocytopenia is associated with viremia and is probably caused by direct platelet damage, viral damage of endothelial cells, and bone marrow suppression.

Ferrets

Thrombocytosis and neutrophilia occur initially and are followed by thrombocytopenia, neutropenia, lymphopenia, anemia and a hypocellular bone marrow with prolonged estrus in ferrets.[72,73] Thrombocytopenia also occurs in ferrets given exogenous estrogen.[74]

Avian

Thrombocytopenia in birds is most commonly associated with severe septicemia; the mechanism is most likely multifactorial, involving a combination of increased peripheral demand and depressed thrombocyte production.[75] Thrombocytopenia can be seen with artifactual clumping and DIC secondary to septicemia, hemopoietic neoplasia, and bone marrow toxicity.[76] Thrombocytes in birds can be difficult to differentiate from lymphocytes, and thrombocytopenia may be misdiagnosed when cells are not properly identified.

Species Disorders, Diseases Associated with Secondary Thrombocytopenia

Canine

Infectious: CDV and vaccination, canine herpes virus, canine infectious hepatitis virus, canine parvovirus, *E. canis,* canine granulocytic ehrlichiosis, *E. platys* (canine infectious cyclic thrombocytopenia), *R. rickettsii* (Rocky Mountain spotted fever), spirochetosis, leptospirosis, salmonellosis, histoplasmosis, disseminated candidiasis, chronic heartworm disease, leishmaniasis, babesiosis, and hemobartonellosis

Neoplasia: Lymphoma, multiple myeloma, myelogenous leukemia, hemangiosarcoma, and cancer chemotherapy

Miscellaneous: DIC, snakebites, endotoxemia, septicemia, and vasculitis

Feline

Infectious: FeLV, FIV, feline panleukopenia virus, feline infectious peritonitis, cytauxzoonosis, and ehrlichiosis

Equine

Infectious: EIAV, EVA, African horsesickness, Venezuelan encephalitis virus, *E. equi* (equine granulocytic ehrlichiosis), *E. risticii* (Potomac horse fever)

Miscellaneous: DIC, endotoxemia, septicemia, gastrointestinal disease, and neoplasia

Bovine

Infectious: bovine viral diarrhea virus, *T. parva* (East coast fever), *T. congolense, T. vivax,* and *T. lawrencei* in water buffalo

Miscellaneous: DIC, septic mastitis, or metritis

Ovine

BTV and *E. phagocytophilia*

Caprine

African trypanosomiasis

Camelid

Hyperthermia

Cervids

BTV

Porcine

ASF and hog cholera

Ferrets

Estrogen induced

Avian

Septicemia, DIC, hemopoietic neoplasia, artifactual clumping, and misidentification

REFERENCES

1. **Jain NC.** Essentials of veterinary hematology. Philadelphia: Lea & Febiger, 1993;105–132.
2. **Jandl JH.** Blood: textbook of hematology. 2nd ed. Boston: Little, Brown and Company, 1996;1301–1360.
3. **Sellon DC, Grindem CB.** Quantitative platelet abnormalities in horses. Compend Cont Educ Pract Vet 1994;16:1335–1347.
4. **MacLachlan NJ, Divers TJ.** Hemolytic anemia and fibrinoid change of renal vessels in a horse. J Am Vet Med Assoc 1982;181:716–717.

5. **Morris CF, Robertson JL, Mann PC, Clark S, Divers TJ.** Hemolytic uremic-like syndrome in two horses. J Am Vet Med Assoc 1987;191:1453–1454.

6. **Roby KW, Bloon JC, Becht JL.** Postpartum hemolytic-uremic syndrome in a cow. J Am Vet Med Assoc 1987;190:187–190.

7. **Sanders WE, Reddick RL, Nichols TC, Brinkhous KM, Read MS.** Thrombotic thrombocytopenia induced in dogs and pigs: The role of platelet and platelet vWF in animal models of thrombotic thrombocytopenic purpura. Arterioscler Throm Vasc Biol 1995;15:793–800.

8. **Moake JL.** Thrombotic thrombocytopenic purpura and the hemolytic uremic syndrome. In: Hoffman R, Benz EJ, Shattil SJ, Furie B, Cohen HJ, Silberstein LE, eds. Hematology: basic principles and practice. 2nd ed. New York: Churchill Livingstone, 1995;1879–1889.

9. **George JN, El-Harake M.** Thrombocytopenia due to enhanced platelet destruction by nonimmunologic mechanisms. In: Beutler E, Lichman MA, Coller BS, Kipps TJ, eds. Williams hematology. 5th ed. New York: McGraw-Hill, 1995;1290–1315.

10. **Bithell TC.** Thrombotic thrombocytopenic purpura and other forms of nonimmunologic platelet destruction. In Lee GR, Bithell TC, Foerster J, Athens JW, Lukens JN, eds. Wintrobe's clinical hematology. 9th ed. Philadelphia: Lea & Febiger, 1993;1356–1362.

11. **George JN.** Thrombocytopenia: pseudothrombocytopenia, hypersplenism, and thrombocytopenia associated with massive transfusion. In: Beutler E, Lichman MA, Coller BS, Kipps TJ, eds. Williams hematology. 5th ed. New York: McGraw-Hill, 1995;1335–1360.

12. **Hill-Zoebel RL, McCandless B, Kang SA, Chikkappa G, Tsan MF.** Organ distribution and fate of human platelet: Studies of asplenic and splenomegalic patients. Am J Hematol 1986;23:231–238.

13. **Kuehn NF, Gaunt SD.** Hypocellular marrow and extramedullary hematopoiesis in a dog: Hematologic recovery after splenectomy. J Am Vet Med Assoc 1986;188:1313–1315.

14. **Ragan HA.** Platelet agglutination induced by ethylenediaminetetraacetic acid in blood samples from a miniature pig. Am J Vet Res 1972;33:2601–2603.

15. **Hinchchliff KW, Kociba GJ, Mitten LA.** Diagnosis of EDTA-pseudothrombocytopenia in a horse. J Am Vet Med Assoc 1993;203:1715–1716.

16. **Berkman N, Michaeli Y, Or R, Eldor A.** EDTA-dependent pseudothrombocytopenia: A clinical study of 18 patients and a review of the literature. Am J Hematol 1991;36:195–201.

17. **Warkentin TE, Trimble MS, Kelton JG.** Thrombocytopenia due to platelet destruction and hypersplenism. In: Hoffman R, Benz EJ, Shattil SJ, Furie B, Cohen HJ, Silberstein LE, eds. Hematology: basic principles and practice. 2nd ed. New York: Churchill Livingstone, 1995;1889–1909.

18. **Morris MW, Davey FR.** Basic examination of blood. In Henry JB, ed. Clinical diagnosis and management by laboratory methods. 19th ed. Philadelphia: WB Saunders, 1996;549–593.

19. **Small SM, Bettigole RE.** Diagnosis of myeloproliferative disease by analysis of platelet volume distribution. Am J Clin Pathol 1981;76:685–691.

20. **Ford HC, Toomath RJ, Carter JM, Delahunt JW, Fagerstrom JN.** Mean platelet volume is increased in hyperthyroidism. Am J Hematol 1988;27:190–193.

21. **Northern J, Tvedten HW.** Diagnosis of microthrombocytosis and immune-mediated thrombocytopenia in dogs with thrombocytopenia: 68 cases (1987–1989). J Am Vet Med Assoc 1992;200:368–372.

22. **Handagama P, Feldman B, Kono C, Farver T.** Mean platelet volume artifacts: The effect of anticoagulants and temperature on canine platelets. Vet Clin Pathol 1986;15:13–17.

23. **Chapman ES, Hetherington EJ, Zelmanovic D.** A simple automated method for determining ex-vivo platelet activation state. Blood 1996;88(suppl 2):50b.

24. **Zelmanovic D, Hetherington EJ.** Automated analysis of feline platelets in whole blood, including platelet count, mean platelet volume, and activation state. Vet Clin Pathol. 1998;27:2–9.

25. **Ault KA, Knowles C.** In vivo biotinylation demonstrates that reticulated platelets are the youngest platelets in circulation. Exp Hematol 1995;23:996–1001.

26. **Dale GL, Friese P, Hynes LA, Burstein SA.** Demonstration that thiazole orange-positive platelets in the dog are less than twenty four hours old. Blood 1995;85:1822–1825.

27. **Kienast J, Schmitz G.** Flow cytometric analysis of thiazole orange uptake by platelets: A diagnostic aid in the evaluation of thrombocytopenic disorders. Blood 1990;75:116–121.

28. **Russell KE, Perkins PC, Grindem CB, Walker KM, Sellon DC.** A flow cytometric method for detecting thiazole orange positive platelets (reticulated platelets) in thrombocytopenic horses. Am J Vet Res 1997;58:1092–1096.

29. **Campbell TW.** Avian hematology and cytology. 2nd ed. Ames, IA: Iowa State University Press, 1995;3–19.

30. **Sypek J, Borysenko M.** Reptiles. In: Rowley AF, Ratcliffe NA, eds. Vertebrate blood cells. Cambridge, UK: Cambridge University Press, 1988;211–256.

31. **Grindem CD, Breitschwerdt EB, Corbett WT, Jans HE.** Epidemiologic survey of thrombocytopenia in dogs: a report on 987 cases. Vet Clin Pathol 1991;20:38–43.

32. **Axthelm MK, Krakowka S.** Canine distemper virus-induced thrombocytopenia. Am J Vet Res 1987;48:1269–1275.

33. **Pineau S, Belbeck LW, Moore S.** Levamisole reduces the thrombocytopenia associated with myxovirus vaccination. Can Vet J 1980;21:82–84.

34. **Straw B.** Decrease in platelet count after vaccination with distemper-hepatitis (DH) vaccine. Vet Med Small Anim Clin 1978;73:725–726.

35. **Wigton DH, Kociba GJ, Hoover EA.** Infectious canine hepatitis: animal model for viral-induced disseminated intravascular coagulation. Blood 1976;47:287–296.

36. **Breitschwerdt EB.** Infectious thrombocytopenia in dogs. Compend Cont Educ Pract Vet 1988;10:1177–1190.

37. **Gaunt SD, Baker DC, Babin SS.** Platelet aggregation studies in dogs with acute Ehrlichia platys infection. Am J Vet Res 1990;51:290–293.

38. **Schalm OW.** Uncommon hematologic disorders: spirochetosis, trypanosomiasis, leishmaniasis, Pelger-Heut anomaly. Canine Pract 1979;6:46–49.

39. **Moreland KJ, Wilson EA, Simpson RB.** Concurrent Ehrlichia canis and Borrelia burgdorferi infections in a Texas dog. J Am Anim Hosp Assoc 1990;26:635–639.

40. **Breitschwerdt EB, Nicholson WL, Kiehl AR, Steers C, Meuten DJ, Levine JF.** Natural infections with Borrelia spirochetes in two dogs from Florida. J Clin Microbiol 1994;32:352–357.

41. **Clinkenbeard KD, Tyler RD, Cowell RL.** Thrombocytopenia associated with disseminated histoplasmosis in dogs. Compend Cont Educ Pract Vet 1989;11:301–306.

42. **Davenport DJ, Breitschwerdt EB, Carakostas MC.** Platelet disorders in the dog and cat. Part I: Physiology and pathogenesis. Compend Cont Educ Pract Vet 1982;4:762–772.

43. **Jacobson LS, Clark IA.** The pathophysiology of canine babesiosis: new approaches to an old puzzle. J S Afr Vet Assoc 1994;65:134–145.

43a. **Slappendel RJ, Ferrer L.** Leishmaniasis. In: Greene CE, ed. Infectious diseases of the dog and cat. 2nd ed. Philadelphia: WB Saunders, 1998;450–458.

44. **Jordan HL, Grindem CB, Breitschwerdt EB.** Thrombocytopenia in cats: a retrospective study of 41 cases. J Vet Intern Med 1993;7:261–265.

45. **Yamamoto JK, Hansen H, Ho EW, Morishita TY, Okuda T, Sawa TR, Nakamura RM, Pedersen NC.** Epidemiological and clinical aspects of feline immunodeficiency virus infections in cats from the continental United States and Canada and possible mode of transmission. J Am Vet Med Assoc 1989;194:213–220.

46. **Shelton GH, Linenberger ML, Grant CK, Abkowitz JL.** Hematologic manifestations of feline immunodeficiency virus infection. Blood 1990;76:1104–1109.

47. **Hart SW, Nolte I.** Hemostatic disorders in feline immunodeficiency virus-seropositive cats. J Vet Intern Med 1994;8:355–362.

48. **Shelton GH, Cotter SM, Gardener MB, Hardy WD, DiGiacomo RF.** Feline immunodeficiency virus and feline leukemia virus infections and their relationship to lymphoid malignancies in cats: A retrospective study (1968–1988). J Acquir Immune Defic Syndr 1990;3:623–630.

49. **Boudreaux MK, Weiss RC, Toivio-Kinnucan M, Spano JS.** Potentiation of platelet responses in vitro by feline infectious peritonitis virus. Vet Pathol 1990;27:261–268.

50. **Peavy GM, Holland CJ, Dutta SK, Smith F, Moore A, Rich LJ, Lappin MR, Richter K.** Suspected ehrlichial infection in five cats from a household. J Am Vet Med Assoc 1997;210:231–234.

51. **Franks PT, Harvey JW, Sheilds RP, Lawman MJP.** Hematological findings in experimental feline cytauxzoonosis. J Am Anim Hosp Assoc 1988;24:395–401.

52. **Sellon DC, Levine J, Millikin E, Palmer K, Grindem C, Covington P.** Thrombocytopenia in horses: 35 cases (1989–1994). J Vet Intern Med 1996;10:127–132.

53. **Feldman BF.** Disseminated intravascular coagulation. Compend Cont Educ Pract Vet 1981;3:46–57.

54. **Clabough DL, Gebhard D, Flaherty MT, Whetter LE, Perry ST, Coggins L, Fuller FJ.** Immune-mediated thrombocytopenia in horses infected with equine infectious anemia virus. J Virol 1991;65:6242–6251.

55. **Cohen ND, Carter GK.** Persistent thrombocytopenia in a case of equine infectious anemia. J Am Vet Med Assoc 1991;199:750–752.

56. **Crawford TB, Wardrop KJ, Tornquist SJ, Reilich E, Meyers KM, McGuire TC.** A primary production deficit in the thrombocytopenia of equine infectious anemia. J Virol 1996;70:7842–7850.

57. **Russell KE, Perkins PC, Hoffman MR, Miller RT, Walker KM, Fuller FJ, Sellon DC.** Platelets from thrombocytopenic ponies acutely infected with equine infectious anemia virus are activated in vivo and hypofunctional. Virology 1999;259:7–19.

58. **Sellon DC.** Diseases of the hematopoietic system. In Kobluk CN, Ames TR, Gear RJ, eds. The horse: diseases and clinical management. Philadelphia: WB Saunders, 1995;1073–1110.

59. **Walton TE, Alvarez O, Buckwalter RM, Johnson KM.** Experimental infection of horses with enzootic and epizootic strains of Venezuelan equine encephalitis virus. J Infect Dis 1973;128:271–278.

60. **Laegrid WW, Burrage TG, Stone-Marschat M, Skowronek A.** Electron microscopic evidence for endothelial infection by African Horsesickness Virus. Vet Pathol 1992;29:554–556.

61. **Skowronek AJ, LaFranco L, Stone-Marschat MA, Burrage TG, Rebar AH, Laegreid WW.** Clinical pathology and hemostatic abnormalities in experimental African Horsesickness. Vet Pathol 1995;32:112–121.

62. **Ziemer EL, Whitlock RH, Palmer JE, Spencer PA.** Clinical and hematologic variables in ponies with experimentally induced equine ehrlichial colitis (Potomac horse fever). Am J Vet Res 1987;48:63–67.

63. **Morris DD, Messick J, Whitlock RH, Palmer J, Ward MV, Feldman BF.** Effect of equine ehrlichial colitis on the hemostatic system in ponies. Am J Vet Res 1988;49:1030–1036.

64. **Corapi WV, French TW, Dubovi EJ.** Severe thrombocytopenia in young calves experimentally infected with noncytopathic bovine viral diarrhea virus. J Virol 1989;63:3934–3943.

65. **McColl KA, Gould AR.** Bluetongue virus infection in sheep: haematological changes and detection by polymerase chain reaction. Aust Vet J 1994; 71:97–101.

66. **Ellis JA, Luedke AJ, Davis WC, Wechsler SJ, Mecham JO, Pratt DL, Elliott JD.** T lymphocyte subset alterations following bluetongue virus infection in sheep and cattle. Vet Immun Immunopathol 1990; 24:49–67.

67. **Davis CE.** Thrombocytopenia a uniform complication of African trypanosomiasis. Acta Trop 1982;39:123–134

68. **Fowler ME.** Medicine and surgery of South American camelids. 2nd ed. Ames, IA: Iowa State University Press, 1998;231–249.

69. **Howerth EW, Tyler DE.** Experimentally induced bluetongue virus infection in white-tailed deer: Ultrastructural findings. Am J Vet Res 1988;49:1914–1922.

70. **Edwards JF, Dodds J, Slausson DO.** Mechanism of thrombocytopenia in African swine fever. Am J Vet Res 1985;46:2058–2063.

71. **Edwards JF, Dodds JW, Slausson DO.** Megakaryocytic infection and thrombocytopenia in African swine fever. Vet Pathol 1985;22:171–176.

72. **Kociba GJ, Caputo CA.** Aplastic anemia associated with estrus in pet ferrets. J Am Vet Med Assoc 1981;178:1293–1294.

73. **Sherrill A, Gorham JR.** Bone marrow hypoplasia associated with estrus in ferrets. Lab Anim Sci 1985;35:280–286.

74. **Bernard SL, Leathers CW, Brobst DF, Gorham JR.** Estrogen-induced bone marrow depression in ferrets. Am J Vet Res 1983;44:657–661.

75. **Campbell TW.** Hematology. In: Ritchie BW, Harrison GJ, Harrison LR, eds. Avian medicine: principles and application. Lake Worth, TX: Wingers Publishing, 1997;176–198.

76. **Rosskopf WJ, Woerpel RW.** Using clinical pathology results in avian clinical medicine with case reports. In: Rosskopf WJ, Woerpel RW, eds. Disease of cage and aviary birds. 3rd ed. Baltimore: Williams & Wilkins, 1996;838.

CHAPTER 70

Acquired Platelet Dysfunction

• MARY K. BOUDREAUX

Acquired platelet function disorders can occur secondary to a variety of causes, including organ dysfunction, drug treatment, infection, and malignancies. Platelet function disorders may be manifested as a decrease in function (hyporeactive platelets) or an increase in function (hyperresponsive platelets). Reduced platelet reactivity is often not apparent in the form of spontaneous hemorrhage unless other hemostatic problems co-exist. However, although animals may not spontaneously hemorrhage, they may be more susceptible to excessive hemorrhage after trauma or surgery. Animals suspected of having reduced platelet function but do not have spontaneous hemorrhage, should be evaluated with a buccal mucosa bleeding time (BMBT) prior to surgical procedures.[1] Although the BMBT will not always determine which animals are at risk for excessive hemorrhage during surgery, the BMBT is the most reliable clinical test available for determining in vivo platelet function.

Enhanced platelet reactivity may promote a prothrombotic state in a variety of disorders. In vitro platelet function studies in certain disease states may be warranted to determine the need for anti-platelet medication as part of the overall treatment regimen.

Whether platelet hyporesponsiveness or hyperresponsiveness exists, identification and treatment or removal of the underlying cause will be the most beneficial in terms of returning platelet function to normal.

REDUCED PLATELET FUNCTION

Uremia

Platelet adhesion is impaired resulting in a prolonged bleeding time. In a study involving induced renal failure in dogs, platelet numbers, volume, and aggregation did not change, however, platelet adhesion, platelet retention on glass beads, and buccal mucosa bleeding time were impaired or prolonged.[2] Although altered von Willebrand factor (vWF) function and structure have been implicated as causes of bleeding in uremia in human beings, this has not been documented in dogs.[3] Plasma of uremic human beings contain low molecular weight degradation products of adhesive proteins which can bind to platelet glycoprotein IIb/IIIa complexes (integrin $\alpha_{IIb}\beta_3$) and inhibit fibrinogen binding.[4] Studies have not been performed to determine if these degradation products are present in uremic dogs. Other possible mechanisms described in humans who have chronic renal failure include increased secretion of prostacyclin and nitric oxide which induce a rise in platelet cAMP and inhibition of platelet reactivity.[5,6] Thrombomodulin levels are also increased in chronic renal failure which implies systemic endothelial damage.[7] Other types of platelet defects described in uremia in human beings, such as platelet storage pool defects, are likely secondary to platelet activation during dialysis.[8]

Drugs

Antiinflammatory Agents

Cyclooxygenase inhibitors, such as aspirin, irreversibly inactivate the cyclooxygenase enzyme resulting in inhibition of thromboxane A_2 generation. In dogs, aspirin inhibits collagen-induced platelet aggregation but has little to no effect on ADP- or thrombin-induced platelet aggregation.[9] Nonaspirin nonsteroidal antiinflammatory agents (NSAID) reversibly inactivate the cyclooxygenase enzyme. Platelet inhibition is transitory and mild and usually does not last for more than 6 hours depending on the half-life of the agent involved.[10] As cyclooxygenase-2 (COX-2)-selective NSAIDs become more readily available, inhibition of platelet function will not be a concern because platelets contain cyclooxygenase-1 (COX-1).[11] Although aspirin and other NSAIDs are documented to inhibit platelet reactivity, animals treated with recommended dosages usually do not spontaneously bleed unless an underlying disorder is present. In dogs, the most common underlying disorder unmasked by cyclooxygenase-inhibiting drugs is von Willebrand's disease. Elective surgical procedures should be avoided in animals receiving cyclooxygenase-inhibiting medications.

Antibiotics

β-lactam antibiotics such as penicillin bind to platelet membranes resulting in reversible inhibition of agonist

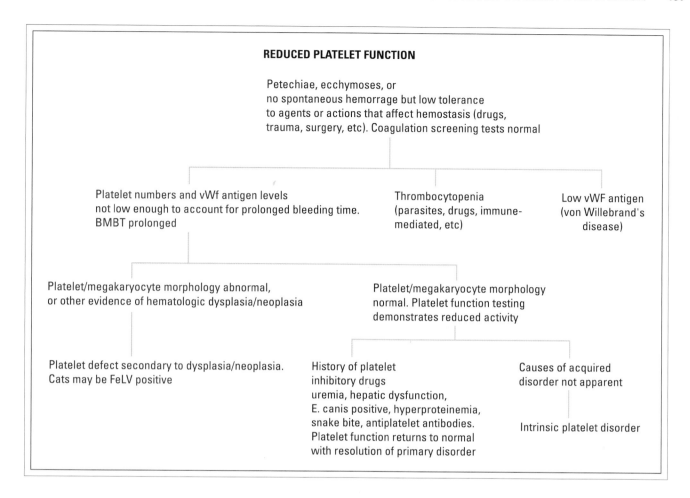

receptors but irreversible impairment of agonist-induced calcium influx across the platelet membrane. In vivo inhibition of platelet function in humans usually requires 48 hours to develop but may persist for 3 to 10 days.[12] A study evaluating cephalothin effects on platelets in dogs indicated a mild, transient prolongation in the buccal mucosa bleeding time (BMBT) and short-term impairment of ADP-induced platelet aggregation.[13] Cephalothin-induced inhibition of human platelet aggregation was more pronounced in patients with hypoalbuminemia.[14] The effect of albumin on β-lactam antibiotic inhibition of platelet function has not been evaluated in dogs.

Calcium Channel Blockers

Agents such as barbiturates and cardiovascular drugs, including diltiazem, nifedipine, and verapamil may inhibit platelet reactivity. These agents primarily prevent calcium fluxes across platelet membranes which are necessary for platelet activation events, however, other effects are also likely.[15] Platelet inhibitory effects vary between species and with type of drug and dosage.

Antiplatelet Antibodies

Antibodies to the platelet glycoprotein complex IIb-IIIa (integrin $\alpha_{IIb}\beta_3$) have resulted in an acquired thrombas-

thenia without thrombocytopenia in human beings.[16] An in vitro study in dogs suggested that dogs that have ITP may have circulating antibodies that inhibit platelet reactivity.[17] Acquired thrombasthenia should be ruled out in an animal suspected of having an intrinsic platelet function disorder. This may require isolation of bound antibody and/or demonstration of adequate levels of glycoprotein IIb/IIIa complexes on the surface of platelets.

Infectious Agents

Ehrlichia Canis Platelet function may be diminished in the absence of thrombocytopenia. A possible cause is hyperproteinemia resulting in inhibition of platelet adhesion and/or aggregation.[18,19] Similar inhibition of platelet function has been observed in myelomas with accompanying hyperproteinemias.

Yersinia Pestis Organisms have an outer membrane protein similar in structure to a portion of the thrombin-binding and von Willebrand-binding domain of glycoprotein Ib. This protein inhibited thrombin- and ristocetin-induced human platelet aggregation and may play a role in early stages of plague infection by preventing platelet activation.[20]

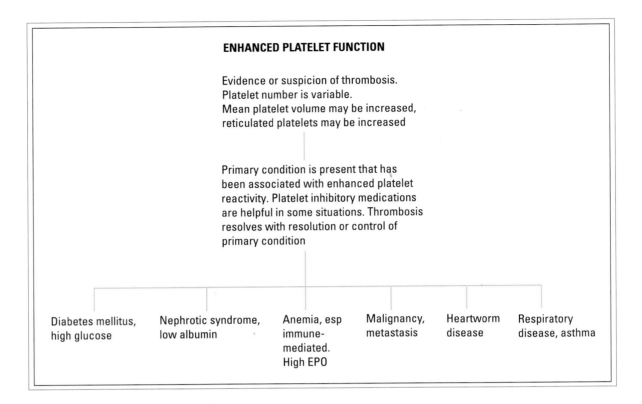

ENHANCED PLATELET FUNCTION

Evidence or suspicion of thrombosis.
Platelet number is variable.
Mean platelet volume may be increased,
reticulated platelets may be increased

Primary condition is present that has
been associated with enhanced platelet
reactivity. Platelet inhibitory medications
are helpful in some situations. Thrombosis
resolves with resolution or control of
primary condition

| Diabetes mellitus, high glucose | Nephrotic syndrome, low albumin | Anemia, esp immune-mediated. High EPO | Malignancy, metastasis | Heartworm disease | Respiratory disease, asthma |

Feline Leukemia Virus   Platelet reactivity can be enhanced or inhibited and can be accompanied by thrombocytosis, thrombocytopenia, or normal platelet numbers. Effects observed are likely related to viral effects at the stem cell level resulting in production of dysplastic/neoplastic megakaryocytes as seen in myelodysplastic and myeloproliferative disease states.[21]

Snake Venoms   The venom of some snakes contain platelet inhibitory peptides which may cause systemic platelet dysfunction. Types of inhibitory compounds identified include disintegrin-like proteins which bind to the platelet glycoprotein complex IIb-IIIa (integrin $\alpha_{IIb}\beta_3$) and competitively inhibit fibrinogen binding.[22] Venom from the South American pit viper *Bothrops jararaca* contains a high molecular weight hemorrhagic metalloproteinase, Jararhagin, which causes the loss of platelet collagen receptors and degrades von Willebrand factor.[23]

Neoplasia   A variety of defects can occur in platelets of patients with leukemia or myeloproliferative disease. These defects may involve platelet membrane glycoproteins, platelet granules, and/or signal transduction pathways. Platelet numbers may be increased, decreased, or normal and platelet function may be enhanced or diminished. In people who have myeloproliferative disorders, the pattern of platelet-related dysfunction may change with time; ie, enhanced platelet reactivity early in disease may change to impaired platelet function later in disease.[24] Megakaryoblastic leukemias are rare and difficult to definitively diagnose.[25]

Liver Disease   In human beings who have advanced cirrhosis, platelet aggregation is impaired secondary to an acquired defect in signal transduction.[26] The liver is also the clearing site for degradation products of fibrinolysis such as fibrin/fibrinogen degradation products (FDP). FDP can competitively inhibit the binding of fibrinogen to platelet receptors resulting in an inhibition of platelet aggregation. Diminished whole-blood platelet aggregation responses were documented in a group of 20 dogs that had liver disease. Six of the dogs had platelet-type bleeding patterns; FDP levels were not increased in any of the dogs evaluated.[27]

ENHANCED PLATELET FUNCTION

Diabetes Mellitus

Large, activated platelets are present in humans that have insulin-dependent and noninsulin-dependent diabetes.[28,29] This finding suggests that platelets may contribute to a prothrombotic state as well as be involved in the development of diabetic vasculopathy.

Nephrotic Syndrome

Human beings who have hypoalbuminemia and nephrotic syndrome have enhanced ADP-induced platelet aggregation and increased circulating levels of β-thromboglobulin suggesting a hyperaggregable state and increased in vivo platelet activation.[30,31] Dogs that have nephrotic syndrome have also been shown to have enhanced ADP platelet responses.[32] In human beings and dogs, platelet hyperresponsiveness in vitro can be corrected by increasing the albumin concentration of plasma. Platelet hyperresponsiveness may play a role in the prothrombotic state observed in patients with nephrotic syndrome.

Hormone Treatment

Erythropoietin administration in dogs has been shown to result in an increase in reticulated platelet number and platelet hyperreactivity.[33] High physiologic EPO levels in dogs that have autoimmune-hemolytic anemia may contribute to the prothrombotic state often observed in this condition.

Malignancies

A study in dogs that have varying types of malignancies, including carcinomas and sarcomas, indicated a general enhancement in platelet reactivity. More studies are needed to determine which types of neoplasias are more likely to be associated with enhanced platelet reactivity and whether enhanced platelet reactivity is associated with tumor metastasis.[34]

Infectious Agents/Parasites

Feline Infectious Peritonitis Virus (FIPV) FIPV has been shown to enhance platelet reactivity both in vitro and in vivo.[35,36] Although FIPV was shown to potentiate and activate platelets in vitro, enhanced platelet reactivity in vivo may be owing to direct viral effects or secondary to virus-induced endothelial or inflammatory cell changes.

Heartworm Disease Heartworm-infected dogs were found to have enhanced ADP-induced platelet aggregation and release.[37] Excreted parasite products, erythrocyte hemolysis, and/or endothelial changes may be responsible for enhanced platelet reactivity. Aspirin, at recommended dosages, was found to be ineffective in inhibiting platelet reactivity in some heartworm-infected dogs.[9]

Asthma Platelets of human beings who have bronchial asthma release increased calcium from internal stores suggesting a potentiation of the phosphatidylinositol (Pl) pathway. In vitro platelet activation is also enhanced. During asthmatic attacks, platelet factor 4 (PF-4) and β-thromboglobulin are released into the circulation and into bronchoalveolar lavage (BAL) fluid suggesting platelet activation and contribution to the overall inflammatory process. Theophylline inhibits the platelet hyperresponsiveness suggesting that increased cAMP levels successfully prevent enhanced calcium release from patient platelets.[38] The role of platelets in chronic obstructive pulmonary disease or allergic respiratory disease in horses, cats, or dogs has not been investigated.

REFERENCES

1. **Jergens AE, Turrentine MA, Kraus KH, et al.** Buccal mucosa bleeding times of healthy dogs and of dogs in various pathologic states, including thrombocytopenia, uremia, and von Willebrand's disease. Am J Vet Res 1987;48(9):1337–1342.
2. **Brassard JA, Meyers KM, Person M, et al.** Experimentally induced renal failure in the dog as an animal model of uremic bleeding. J Lab Clin Med 1994;124:48–54.
3. **Brassard JA, Meyers KM.** Von Willebrand factor is not altered in azotemic dogs with prolonged bleeding time. J Lab Clin Med 1994;124:55–62.
4. **Walkowiak B, Michalak E, Borkowska E, et al.** Concentration of RGDS-containing degradation products in uremic plasma is correlated with progression in renal failure. Thromb Res 1994;76:133.
5. **Kyrle PA, Stockenhuber F, Brenner B, et al.** Evidence for an increased generation of prostacyclin in the microvasculature and an impairment of the platelet alfa-granule release in chronic renal failure. Thromb Haemost 1988;60:205–208.
6. **Noris M, Benigni A, Boccardo P, et al.** Enhanced nitric oxide synthesis in uremia: implications for platelet dysfunction and dialysis hypotension. Kidney Int 1993;44:445–450.
7. **Mezzano D, Tagle R, Pais E, et al.** Endothelial cell markers in chronic uremia: relationship with hemostatic defects and severity of renal failure. Thromb Res 1997;88:465–472.
8. **Zachee P, Vermylen J, Boogaerts MA.** Hematologic aspects of end-stage renal failure. Ann Hematol 1994;69:33–40.
9. **Boudreaux MK, Dillon AR, Ravis WR, et al.** Effects of treatment with aspirin or aspirin/dipyridamole combination in heartworm-negative, heartworm-infected and embolized heartworm-infected dogs. Am J Vet Res 1991;52(12):1992–1999.
10. **Schafer AI.** Effects of nonsteroidal antiinflammatory drugs on platelet function and systemic hemostasis. J Clin Pharmacol 1995;35:209–219.
11. **Kawai S, Nishida S, Kato M, et al.** Comparison of cyclooxygenase-1 and -2 inhibitory activites of various nonsteroidal anti-inflammatory drugs using human platelets and synovial cells. Eur J Pharmacol 1998;347:87–94.
12. **Burroughs SF, Johnson GJ.** Beta-lactam antibiotics inhibit agonist-stimulated platelet calcium influx. Thromb Haemost 1993;69(5):503–508.
13. **Schermerhorn T, Barr SC, Stoffregen DA, et al.** Whole-blood platelet aggregation, buccal mucosa bleeding time, and serum cephalothin concentration in dogs receiving a presurgical antibiotic protocol. Am J Vet Res 1994;55(11):1602–1607.
14. **Sloand EM, Klein HG, Pastakia P, et al.** Effect of albumin on the inhibition of platelet aggregation by β-lactam antibiotics. Blood 1992;79(8):2022–2027.
15. **Rostagno C, Abbate R, Gensini GF, et al.** In vitro effects of two novel calcium antagonists (nitrendipine and nisoldipine) on intraplatelet calcium redistribution, platelet aggregation and thromboxane A2 formation. Comparison with diltiazem, nifedipine and verapamil. Thromb Res 1991;63:457–462.
16. **Niessner H, Clemetson KJ, Panzer S, et al.** Acquired thrombasthenia due to GPIIb/IIIa-specific platelet autoantibodies. Blood 1986;68(2):571–576.
17. **Kristensen AT, Weiss DJ, Klausner JS.** Platelet dysfunction associated with immune-mediated thrombocytopenia in dogs. J Vet Intern Med 1994;8(5):323–327.
18. **Varela F, Font X, Valladares JE, et al.** Thrombocytopathia and light-chain proteinuria in a dog naturally infected with Ehrlichia canis. J Vet Intern Med 1997;11(5):309–311.
19. **Kuehn NF, Gaunt SD.** Clinical and hematologic findings in canine ehrlichiosis. J Am Vet Med Assoc 1985;186(4):355–358.
20. **Leung KY, Reisner BS, Straley SC.** YopM inhibits platelet aggregation and is necessary for virulence of *Yersinia pestis* in mice. Infect Immun 1990;58(10):3262–3271.
21. **Blue JT, French TW, Kranz JS.** Non-lymphoid hematopoietic neoplasia in cats: a retrospective study of 60 cases. Cornell Vet 1988;78:21–42.
22. **Rahman S, Lu X, Kakkar V, et al.** The integrin $\alpha_{IIb}\beta_3$ contains distinct and interacting binding sites for snake-venom RGD (Arg-Gly-Asp) proteins. Biochem J 1995;312:223–232.
23. **Kamiguti AS, Hay CRM, Theakston RDG, et al.** Insights into the mechanism of haemorrhage caused by snake venom metalloproteinases. Toxicon 1996;34(6):627–642.
24. **Baker RI, Manoharan A.** Platelet function in myeloproliferative disorders: characterization and sequential studies show multiple platelet abnormalities, and change with time. Eur J Haematol 1988;40:267–272.
25. **Pucheu-Haston CM, Camus A, Taboada J, et al.** Megakaryoblastic leukemia in a dog. J Am Vet Med Assoc 1995;207(2):194–196.
26. **Laffi G, Cominelli F, Ruggiero M, et al.** Altered platelet function in cirrhosis of the liver: Impairment of inositol lipid and arachidonic acid metabolism in response to agonists. Hepatology 1988;8(6):1620–1626.

27. **Willis SE, Jackson ML, Meric SM, et al.** Whole blood platelet aggregation in dogs with liver disease. Am J Vet Res 1989;50(11):1893–1897.

28. **Tschoepe D, Roesen P, Esser J, et al.** Large platelets circulate in an activated state in diabetes mellitus. Semin Thromb Hemost 1991;17(4):433–438.

29. **Tschoepe, Rauch U, Schwippert B.** Platelet-leukocyte-cross-talk in diabetes mellitus. Horm Metab Res 1997;29:631–635.

30. **Goubran F, Maklady F.** In vivo platelet activity and serum albumin concentration in nephrotic syndrome. Blut 1988;57:15–17.

31. **Machleidt C, Mettang T, Starz E, et al.** Multifactorial genesis of enhanced platelet aggregability in patients with nephrotic syndrome. Kidney Int 1989;36:1119–1124.

32. **Green RA, Russo EA, Greene RT, et al.** Hypoalbuminemia-related platelet hypersensitivity in two dogs with nephrotic syndrome. J Am Vet Med Assoc 1985; 186(5):485–488.

33. **Wolf RF, Peng J, Friese P, et al.** Erythropoietin administration increases production and reactivity of platelets in dogs. Thromb Haemost 1997; 78:1505–1509.

34. **McNiel EA, Ogilvie GK, Fettman MJ, et al.** Platelet hyperfunction in dogs with malignancies. J Vet Intern Med 1997;11(3):178–182.

35. **Boudreaux MK, Weiss RC, Toivio-Kinnucan M, et al.** Enhanced platelet reactivity in cats experimentally infected with feline infectious peritonitis virus. Vet Pathol 1990;27:269–273.

36. **Boudreaux MK, Weiss RC, Toivio-Kinnucan M, et al.** Potentiation of platelet responses in vitro by feline infectious peritonitis virus. Vet Pathol 1990; 27:261–268.

37. **Boudreaux MK, Dillon AR, Spano JS.** Enhanced platelet reactivity in heartworm-infected dogs. Am J Vet Res 1989;50(9):1544–1547.

38. **Moritani C, Ishioka S, Haruta Y, et al.** Activation of platelets in bronchial asthma. Chest 1998;113(2):452–458.

CHAPTER 71

Essential Thrombocythemia and Reactive Thrombocytosis

• CAROL P. MANDELL

Thrombocytosis is defined as an increase in platelet numbers in peripheral blood in excess of the reference range.[1-3] Thrombocytosis may be caused by a primary bone marrow disorder or may be secondary to a wide variety of diseases and physiologic states.

Essential thrombocythemia, a persistent primary thrombocytosis, is a rare chronic myeloproliferative disorder; one of several other myeloproliferative disorders that includes polycythemia vera, chronic myelogenous leukemia, and myelofibrosis. In addition to essential thrombocythemia, the other myeloproliferative disorders and the myelodysplastic syndromes may manifest thrombocytosis. The myeloproliferative disorders are closely related to each other and are distinguished from one another based on specific diagnostic criteria developed for humans who have these disorders.[4,5] Some synonyms for essential thrombocythemia are idiopathic thrombocythemia, primary hemorrhagic thrombocythemia, and thromboasthenia.

Secondary thrombocytosis or reactive thrombocytosis is characterized by transiently increased platelet counts in patients who have conditions other than the myeloproliferative disorders. With the advent of routine electronic platelet counting in veterinary clinical laboratories, thrombocytosis is being identified with increasing frequency.[1,2] In this chapter, essential thrombocythemia and secondary or reactive thrombocytosis are characterized and differentiated. Differential diagnoses and diagnostic criteria for these two entities are presented, and the pathogenesis, clinical presentation, clinical laboratory findings, and therapy of essential thrombocythemia in domestic animals in comparison with the disease in humans are reviewed.

THROMBOCYTOSIS

Platelet reference ranges vary among the domestic animals. In fact, healthy small laboratory rodents have platelet counts in excess of 1,000,000 platelets/μL. Thrombocytosis, from nonmalignant causes, is usually modest, transient, asymptomatic and less than 1,000,000 platelets/μL. However, exceedingly high platelet counts (greater than 1,000,000/μL) may be life threatening and associated with clinical signs of bleeding or thrombosis.

In humans, thrombocytosis, regardless of the origin, is associated with spurious elevations of serum potassium, lactate dehydrogenase, phosphorus, uric acid, zinc, acid phosphatase and mucopolysaccharide concentrations.[6,7] The spurious elevation in these serum analytes is believed to be caused by release of cellular substances from platelets during in vitro platelet aggregation, secretion, and coagulation before harvesting of the serum. Spurious hyperkalemia or pseudohyperkalemia has been reported in dogs that have both reactive thrombocytosis and myeloproliferative disorders.[8,9,10] Serum potassium concentrations are significantly higher than plasma potassium values in dogs that have normal and increased platelet counts. It is suggested that in patients that have thrombocytosis, increased serum potassium concentrations should be confirmed with simultaneous plasma potassium determinations.

Physiologic thrombocytosis results from increased mobilization of platelets from splenic and nonsplenic (mainly pulmonary) platelet pools. The nonsplenic platelet pool is mobilized during mild exercise. Epinephrine injection or endogenous release mobilize the splenic pool. During vigorous exercise, both splenic and pulmonary pools are mobilized and contribute to thrombocytosis. Species differences exist; 10-minutes of exercise caused no significant changes in platelet counts in ponies.[11]

Reactive thrombocytosis is associated with various conditions. Increased megakaryocytopoiesis and thrombocytosis can occur after peripheral loss of platelets caused by immunologic, infectious, neoplastic, or traumatic causes. In addition, hypoxemia caused by blood loss, respiratory, or cardiac compromise can lead to increased thrombocytopoiesis. In human patients who have reactive thrombocytosis, megakaryocyte (MK) numbers and MK ploidy are increased.[12] Secondary or reactive thrombocytosis may be related to increased pro-

TABLE 71.1   Causes of Reactive Thrombocytosis in Humans and Domestic Animals

Humans	Domestic Animals	
	Horses [a]	Dogs and Cats [b]
Physiologic—excitement, exercise	Gastrointestinal inflammation	Neoplasia
Blood loss	Colitis	
Iron-deficiency anemia	Infectious/inflammatory disease	Lymphoma, melanoma, nasal adenocar-
Acute and chronic hemorrhage	Respiratory infections—pleuritis, pneu-	cinoma, CNS neoplasia, mast cell tu-
Postpartum disease	monia	mor, mesothelioma
Immunologic	Septic arthritis or polyarthritis	Gastrointestinal disorders
Hemolytic anemia	Abdominal abscess	Pancreatitis, hepatitis, gingivitis, coli-
Rebound after thrombocytopenia	*Rhodococcus equi* lymphadenitis	tis, inflammatory bowel disease
Rheumatoid arthritis	Trauma/fractures	Endocrine disease
Acute and chronic infection/inflammation		Immunologic
Tuberculosis, septic arthritis, chronic		Immune-mediated hemolytic anemia
pneumonia, gastrointestinal disorders		Immune-mediated thrombocytopenia
Postsplenectomy		Systemic lupus erythematosus
Cardiopulmonary bypass surgery		Blood loss/hemorrhage
		Iron-deficiency anemia
Neoplasia		Trauma/surgery
Mesothelioma, acute lymphoblastic leu-		Fractures
kemia, hepatocellular carcinoma, sarco-		
mas, CNS tumors		Drug therapy
Drug therapy		Corticosteroids, antineoplastic drugs
Epinephrine, corticosteroids,		Postsplenectomy
cyclosporine, vinca alkaloids, mico-		
nazole		
Young children		

[a]Data from Sellon DC, Levine JF, Palmer K, Millikin E, et al. Thrombocytosis in 24 horses (1989–1994). J Vet Intern Med 1997;11:24–29, with permission.
[b]Data from Hammer AS. Thrombocytosis in dogs and cats: a retrospective study. Comp Haematol Int 1991;1:181–186.

duction of thrombopoietic factors that increase platelet production by MKs. The clinical conditions associated with reactive thrombocytosis in humans and domestic animals are chronic hemorrhage, trauma, fractures, surgery, splenectomy, hyposplenic states, acute or chronic infections, inflammatory conditions, malignancies, iron deficiency, hyperadrenocorticism, and therapy with glucocorticoids and Vinca alkaloids (Tables 71.1 and 71.2).

Human patients who have reactive thrombocytosis may have altered levels of cytokines and inflammatory mediators that may be positive modulators for megakaryocytopoiesis.[13,14] In contrast to human patients who have essential thrombocythemia, patients that have reactive thrombocytosis and rheumatoid arthritis had increased levels of interleukin (IL)-6, IL-1β, and IL-4.[15,16] In a second study on a group of consecutively tested human patients that had thrombocytosis, IL-6 and C-reactive protein were increased in 81% of patients that had reactive thrombocytosis. No increases in IL-6 were detected in patients that had clonal thrombocythemia associated with the myeloproliferative disorders. In nonhuman primates (Macaca mulatta), administered human recombinant IL-6, platelet counts increased twofold to threefold above baseline.[17] Acute phase proteins also increased in these IL-6-treated macaques. Similar increases in platelet counts have also been noted in mice administered IL-6.[14] It is not known whether serum cy-

tokine levels are increased in cases of thrombocytosis in domestic animals. Knowledge of serum IL-6 concentrations may be a useful adjunct in the differential diagnosis of essential thrombocythemia versus reactive thrombocytosis (see Table 71.3).

Two retrospective studies in domestic animals address the issue of reactive thrombocytosis. Sellon and colleagues[2] studied the disorders associated with thrombocytosis in horses presented to a veterinary medical teaching hospital. For the study, thrombocytosis was defined as a platelet count greater than 400,000 platelets/μL. Thrombocytosis was an uncommon occurrence. Only 24 (1%) of 2346 horses presented with a platelet count greater than 400,000 platelets/μL. Mean and standard deviation (SD) platelet count of this population was 505,000 +/− 159,000 platelets/μL. Of the 24 horses, 20 (83%) had platelet counts between 400,000 and 500,000 platelets/μL. The one horse that had a platelet count of 1,100,000 platelets/μL was diagnosed with a pulmonary thrombosis and possible marrow dysplasia. The most common conditions associated with mild thrombocytosis in these horses were inflammatory and infectious conditions such as abdominal abscess, pleuritis, peritonitis, pneumonia, septic arthritis, and *Rhodococcus equi* lymphadenitis (Table 71.1). In addition, thrombocytosis was more common in young, male horses. The clinical pathologic findings most strongly

TABLE 71.2 **Selected Examples of Thrombocytosis in the Dog, Cat, and Horse from the UCDavis Veterinary Medical Teaching Hospital***

Species	Platelet Count/μL of Blood	Clinical Diagnosis or Symptoms
Dog	200,000–500,000	Reference Range
	2,073,000	Vincristine and immunosuppressive therapy for immune-mediated thrombocytopenia
	1,988,000	Suppurative bronchitis, enteritis
	1,148,000	Iron deficiency anemia
	828,000	Iron deficiency anemia
	755,000	Hyperadrenocorticism
	738,000	Squamous cell carcinoma
	737,000	Adenocarcinoma
	713,000	Prednisolone and immunosuppressive therapy for immune-mediated hemolytic anemia
	673,000	Mast cell tumor
	618,000	Nasal trauma
	613,000	Chronic inflammation/infection
Cat	300,000–800,000	Reference Range
	2,046,000	Lymphocytic leukemia
	1,470,000	Anemia and bleeding
	1,432,000	Mast cell tumor
	1,378,000	Myelogenous leukemia
	1,256,000	Myeloproliferative disorder
	1,163,000	6 days after therapy for thrombocytopenia
	876,000	Erythemic myelosis
	872,000	Lymphocytic leukemia
Horse	100,000–350,000	Reference Range
	632,000	Pleuritis
	611,000	Foal pneumonia
	510,000	Fluctuating temperature
	474,000	Combine immune deficiency
	472,000	CNS ataxia, abscess
	450,000	Strangles
	405,000	Pleuritis, heparin therapy for DIC

*After Jain, 1986, p. 470.

TABLE 71.3 **Comparison of the Features of Reactive Thrombocytosis (RT) and Essential Thrombocythemia (ET) in Humans***

	Reactive Thrombocytosis	Essential Thrombocythemia
Patient age	children <2 years	adults
Platelet count	$<1000 \times 10^3/\mu L$	$>1000 \times 10^3/\mu L$
Complications	usually none	thrombosis/bleeding
Splenomegaly	rare	frequent
Durations thrombocytosis	transient	persistent
Platelet morphology	normal but large	large but dysplastic
PDW	within reference range	increased
Platelet function	normal	abnormal
Spontaneous megakaryocyte colony growth	yes	no
Pathogenesis	secondary to other disorders (see Table 71.1)	clonal stem cell disorder
Other abnormal cell lines	no	possible
Serum IL-6	increased	not increased
Serum thrombopoietin	increased	normal or increased

*(Kutti, 1996 #3; Sutor, 1995 #274.)

associated with thrombocytosis were hyperfibrinogenemia, leukocytosis, and anemia. The study found that thrombocytosis is a rare condition in horses, is often mild, and is not associated with a poor prognosis.

A similar retrospective study was performed for dogs and cats.[1] Of 2180 complete blood counts performed on dogs at a university veterinary medical teaching hospital, 118 (5.4%) had elevated platelet counts greater than 500,000 platelets/μL. In cats, 17 (2.8%) of 605 complete blood counts showed increased platelet counts. Similar to the equine study, the majority of feline and canine platelet counts were only mildly to moderately increased (less than 700,000 platelets/μL). The most common disorders associated with thrombocytosis in dogs and cats are neoplasia, gastrointestinal disorders, and endocrine diseases (Table 71.1). In addition, platelet count increases were noted in dogs treated with corticosteroids and antineoplastic agents.

Corticosteroids may increase platelet counts by decreasing phagocytosis of platelets by macrophages.[18] Reactive thrombocytosis also occurs in Cushing's patients that have high endogenous levels of glucocorticoids. Although the effect of vincristine on augmenting platelet production is well documented in humans and animals,[19,20] the mechanism of action is not entirely known. It is believed that vincristine binds to platelet microtubules and helps localize the drug to phagocytes that destroy the platelets. In mice, vincristine increases colony-forming unit-MKs (CFU-MKs) in the spleen, and increases the number of splenic MKs and platelets.[21]

After splenectomy, platelet counts increase in humans within 2 to 10 days, peak after 2 weeks and gradually decrease to baseline within 2 to 3 months.[22] The rise in platelet counts is because platelet destruction is decreased. Splenectomized dogs also show a similar pattern as illustrated in Table 71.4.

ESSENTIAL THROMBOCYTHEMIA

Essential thrombocythemia is a myeloproliferative disorder characterized by the proliferation of a pluripotent hemopoietic stem cell, leading to expansion of the MK compartment in bone marrow, growth and maturation to large, mature MKs, and the excessive and presumably autonomous production of structurally and functionally abnormal platelets.[23] In humans, it is well established as a clonal disorder of the multipotent hematopoietic stem cell. In women who have essential thrombocythemia that were heterozygous for X-linked glucose-6-phosphate dehydrogenase isoenzymes B and A, only a single isoenzyme type was detected in their platelets, neutrophils, and red blood cells. However, both isoenzymes, types A and B, were detected in nonhemopoietic tissues from these patients. These data indicated the clonal nature of essential thrombocythemia, and it was subsequently classified as a myeloproliferative disorder along with polycythemia vera, chronic myelogenous leukemia, and myelofibrosis.[24,25] Similar genetic studies to determine clonality have not been performed on the few

cases of essential thrombocythemia reported in domestic animals.

In humans, typical bone marrow histologic features include hypercellularity, increased number and size of MKs with mature cytoplasm, and multilobated nuclei with irregular chromatin. MKs tend to cluster in small aggregates adjacent to sinuses. Masses or sheets of platelets are also seen in bone marrow smears. Stainable bone marrow iron stores are adequate.[26,27] Culture of bone marrow or blood shows spontaneous and autonomous erythroid (burst-forming unit-erythroid [BFU-E]) and CFU-MK colony growth with increased numbers of MK colonies in the absence of exogenously added hemopoietic growth factors.[4,27]

In humans, platelet structure and function are abnormal. Table 71.5 lists the platelet abnormalities identified in humans who have essential thrombocythemia.[27,28] However, no particular platelet abnormality is pathognomic or diagnostic for essential thrombocythemia. Because so few cases of essential thrombocythemia have been identified in domestic animals, a similar list has not been developed.

The main clinical signs in humans who have essential thrombocythemia are related to microvascular thrombosis or bleeding. Thrombosis is manifested as digital ischemia, acrocyanosis, and microvascular occlusion in the central nervous system (CNS), coronary circulation, or skin leading to CNS ischemia, myocardial infarction, and ulceration and necrosis of the skin, respectively.[26,29] The pathogenesis of thrombosis remains unclear. Several studies have determined that thrombosis is associated with increased platelet turnover as determined by counting reticulated platelets by flow cytometry[30,31] and increased platelet activation assessed by platelet aggregation and flow-cytometric studies.[32] Bleeding in essential thrombocythemia is characterized by platelet or vascular-type bleeding rather than bleeding caused by a coagulation factor deficiency. Thus, bleeding time and platelet aggregation tests may be abnormal.

Recently, thrombopoietin, the ligand for the gene product of the proto-oncogene c-mpl has been cloned and identified as a major regulator of megakaryocytopoiesis.[33] Paradoxically, patients that have essential thrombocythemia have normal to increased concentrations of thrombopoietin in the presence of extreme thrombocytosis. This suggests dysregulation of feedback mechanisms regulating thrombopoietin concentrations in patients that have essential thrombocythemia.[23]

The myeloproliferative disorders include essential thrombocythemia, polycythemia vera, chronic myelogenous leukemia, and myelofibrosis. Thrombocytosis is also a feature of the other myeloproliferative disorders and some myelodysplastic syndromes in humans. The Polycythemia Study Group[5] has stated that essential thrombocythemia is a diagnosis of exclusion, where all other causes of thrombocytosis are excluded to make a diagnosis. Recently, other groups[4,34] suggest that positive markers for essential thrombocythemia such as increased DNA ploidy of MKs by flow-cytometric analysis, cytokine levels (i.e., IL-6 and thrombopoietin), bone marrow histology, and megakaryocytic and erythrocytic

TABLE 71.4   Example of Postsplenectomy Reactive Thrombocytosis in a Dog With Idiopathic Anemia*

Status	Platelet Count/μL of Blood
Pre-splenectomy	377,000
Days postsplenectomy	
2 days	1,197,000
5 days	1,395,000
12 days	1,305,000
26 days	1,061,000
40 days	617,000

*After Jain, 1986, p. 470.

TABLE 71.5   Platelet Abnormalities in Humans With Essential Thrombocythemia*

Bleeding time

Abnormal platelet aggregation with epinephrine, collagen, and ADP

Acquired storage pool disease

Abnormalities of platelet membranes
  Surface glycoprotein abnormalities
    Decreased gp Ib, IIb, IIIa
    Increased gp IV
  Cell receptor abnormalities
    Reduced α2 adrenergic receptors
    Reduced prostaglandin D2 receptors
    Decreased procoagulant activity
    Increased Fc receptors

Acquired von Willibrand's disease
  Decreased in large multimers of VWF leading to Type II VWD
    Possibly due to adsorption of VWF to platelet surfaces

Abnormal arachidonic acid metabolism
  12-lipoxygenase deficiency
  Abnormal 12-lipoxygenase lacking functional enzyme activity (Tomo, 1997 #140)

*Adapted from Rosenthal in *Blood Principles and Practice of Hematology*, 1995.

TABLE 71.6   Two Schemes of Diagnostic Criteria for Essential Thrombocythemia in Human Beings*

Polycythemia Study Group (Murphy, 1997 #142)
  I. Platelet count greater than 600,000/μL
  II. Hematocrit less than 40% or normal RBC mass
  III. Stainable iron in bone marrow or normal serum ferritin or normal MCV
  IV. No Philadelphia chromosome or bcr/abl gene rearrangement (not applicable to domestic animals)
  V. Collagen fibrosis of marrow
    A. Absent or
    B. Less than 1/3 biopsy area without both marked splenomegaly and leukoerythroblastic reaction
  VI. No cytogenetic or morphologic evidence for a myelodysplastic syndrome
  VII. No cause for reactive thrombocytosis

Criteria Proposed by Kutti and Wadenvtk (Kutti, 1996 #3)**
  A1   Platelet count greater than 600,000/μL
  A2   No increase in RBC mass in the presence of stainable iron in bone marrow or failure of iron trial
  A3   No Philadelphia chromosome
  A4   Megakaryocytic hyperplasia (i.e., increased megakaryocyte number and size) in histologic bone marrow sections and/or increased megakaryocytic ploidy (by 2 color flow cytometric analysis), no collagen fibrosis
  B1   Splenomegaly on isotope scan or ultrasound examination
  B2   Unstimulated growth of BFU-E and/or CFU-Meg present
  B3   Normal ESR/Fibrinogen

*Diagnosis is considered established if A1, A2, A3, and A4 are fulfilled, OR A1, A2, A3, plus 2 B criteria are met.
**This scheme incorporated bone marrow histology, bone marrow culture, and flow cytometric studies of megakaryocyte ploidy (1996).

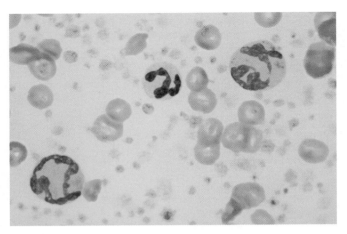

FIGURE 71.1 Peripheral blood smears from a canine patient with ET show many macroplatelets and a population of hypogranular platelets. Two basophils that stain poorly with Wright's stain are also present. (Wright's stain, 1000).

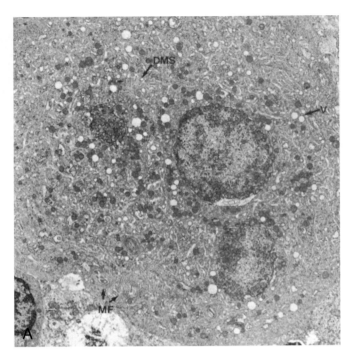

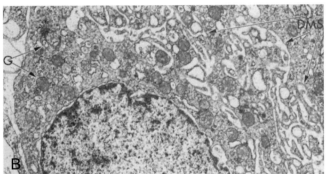

FIGURE 71.2 Electron micrographs of megakarocytes from a canine patient with ET. **A.** Abnormal MK contains abundant heterochromatin. Cytoplasm has large amounts of the demarcation membrane system that is vacuolated (V) in some areas and reduplicated in others. Note whorled arrangements of demarcation membrane systems (DMS) forming myelin figures (MF). **B.** Higher magnification of abnormal MK shows the extensive DMS and a population of alpha and dense granules (G). Magnification ×18,400.

colony growth may be of importance in the diagnosis of essential thrombocythemia. Table 71.6 presents the diagnostic criteria from the Polycythemia Study Group and the diagnostic criteria proposed by Kutti et al.[4] These criteria for essential thrombocythemia in humans have been helpful in making a diagnosis of essential thrombocythemia in domestic animals. Essential thrombocythemia is differentiated from megakaryoblastic leukemia by the presence of malignant MKs in other lymphoid organs in addition to bone marrow (i.e., lymph nodes, spleen, liver, etc.). Patients that have megakaryoblastic leukemia may present with either thrombocytopenia or thrombocytosis.

Few cases of essential thrombocythemia have been reported in domestic animals. Only six canine and two feline cases have been identified in the recent literature.[35,36,37,38,39] Thrombocytosis has also been reported in a dog that had a myeloproliferative disorder that was diagnosed as a chronic myelogenous leukemia potentially in transition to essential thrombocythemia.[40] The dogs that were diagnosed with essential thrombocythemia were between 4 and 11 years old and presented to the referral hospitals with lethargy, pale mucus membranes, weight loss, pica, anorexia, and exercise intolerance. One cat that had essential thrombocythemia was an 8-year-old domestic long hair with weight loss, lethargy, polyphagia, and pica. No cases showed signs of hemorrhage or thromboembolism. Splenomegaly caused by significant extramedullary hematopoiesis was noted in only one of the six dogs. Presenting hematologic findings were nonregenerative anemia or regenerative anemia attributed to either hemorrhage or hemolysis. Platelet counts at presentation ranged from 925,000/μL to 4,950,000/μL or were merely estimated as significantly increased on blood smears. Platelets were often increased in size or occasionally showed hypogranularity or disparate shapes. Bone marrow cytologic findings among the cases had some similar features. Most notable were megakaryocytic hyperplasia with less than 30%

megakaryoblasts, increased platelet budding; multiple, large platelet masses or sheets; erythroid hypoplasia; and myeloid hyperplasia. In general, bone marrow iron stains showed adequate bone marrow iron. In the 2 cases in which thrombopoietin was measured, it was within reference range in a dog[35] and a cat.[37]

A unique hematologic feature in one dog that had essential thrombocythemia was hyperplasia of the basophilic myelocytes in bone marrow and a significant basophilia in peripheral blood. Basophilia and eosinophilia has also been noted rarely in children who have essential thrombocythemia.[26] Interestingly, the mature basophils in this canine case were unusual in that their granules

TABLE 71.7	Summary of CBC and Bone Marrow Findings in Selected Cases With Essential Thrombocythemia at Presentation				
Reference	**Species**	**Age/Sex Breed**	**Pertinent Hemogram & Chemistry Findings**	**Bone Marrow Cytology**	**Therapy**
Hopper et al (Hopper, 1989 #233)	Canine	11 yr/FS Airedale	Nonregenerative anemia (PCV 15%) Thrombocytosis (4.9 × $10^6/\mu L$) Basophilia (4836/μL) Spurious hyperkalemia Hypogranular and macro-platelets	Megakaryocytic hyper-plasia Increased megakaryo-blasts (<20%) Dysmegakaryocyto-poiesis Multiple platelet masses Basophilic hyperplasia Erythroid hypoplasia	^{32}P Normal platelet count 4 weeks post-therapy
Simpson et al (Simpson, 1990 #317)	Canine	8 yr/F Irish Setter	Nonregenerative anemia (PCV 14%) Thrombocytosis (957 × $10^3/\mu L$) Unclassified blasts (7.1 × $10^3/\mu L$)	Megakaryocytic hyper-plasia Multiple platelet masses Megakaryocytes sur-rounded by platelet masses	Cyclophosphamide Vincristine Cytosine arabinoside Prednisone Platelet count nor-mal post-therapy
Bass et al (Bass, 1998 #126)	Canine	10.5 yr/MC Shih Tzu	Regenerative anemia (AIHA) Thrombocytosis (925 × $10^3/\mu L$) Macroplatelets Plasma thrombopoietin—normal	Normal distribution of megakaryocytic cells Myeloid hyperplasia Erythroid hypoplasia Iron stores adequate	Hydroxyurea No response
Hammer et al (Hammer, 1990 #221)	Feline	8 yr/MC DSH	Marked neutrophilia with left shift Thrombocytosis (1.965 × $10^6/\mu L$) Occasional macro-platelets Plasma thrombopoietin—not increased	Megakaryocytic hyper-plasia Myeloid hyperplasia Multiple platelet masses Iron stores adequate	Therapeutic iron trial No response Melphalan Died of sepsis

stained poorly with Wright's stain but well with Giemsa and toluidine blue (Fig. 71.1). Cytochemical stains and electron microscopy were performed on bone marrow from this patient. The blasts in bone marrow stained strongly positive for eserine-sensitive acetylcholinesterase, a MK-specific enzyme marker; mildly diffusely positive for alpha-naphthyl acetate esterase; and negative for the myeloid markers, alkaline phosphatase, myeloperoxidase, and chloroacetate esterase. A similar pattern of cytochemical stains is seen in human patients who have essential thrombocythemia.[41] The ultrastructure of the canine platelets and MKs in this case with essential thrombocythemia were similar to those reported in human beings.[42,43,44] Platelets were dysplastic, significantly pleomorphic with increased and distended open canalicular systems; these morphologic changes, however, are nonspecific and can be noted in other myeloproliferative disorders. MKs were dysmorphic and showed abnormal maturation with a lack of cytoplasmic organization, reduplication, and poorly organized demarcation membranes. Maturing MKs lacked well-demarcated platelet fields because of the abnormal demarcation membrane system (Fig. 71.2). Platelet aggregation with arachidonic acid and adenosine diphosphate (ADP) showed hypoaggregability of platelets with less than 20% aggregation.

Mean platelet volume was within reference range. Table 71.7 compares the presenting hemograms and bone marrow findings in four recent cases of essential thrombocythemia.

THERAPY OF ESSENTIAL THROMBOCYTHEMIA

Humans who have essential thrombocythemia may not have a shortened life expectancy, and many may not require specific therapy. Patients who have a high risk of thrombosis are treated. Hydroxyurea is considered standard therapy in humans. Two new platelet-lowering drugs used in humans are interferon-α and anagrelide, a drug that lowers platelet counts by altering MK maturation.[45]

Four cases of essential thrombocythemia have been treated in veterinary medicine. Two dogs[38,39] were successfully treated (i.e., reduction of the platelet count to the reference range) with either ^{32}P or a combination chemotherapeutic regimen of cyclophosphamide, vincristine, cytosine arabinoside, and prednisone. The other two cases did not respond to hydroxyurea or melphalan.[35,37]

REFERENCES

1. **Hammer AS.** Thrombocytosis in dogs and cats: a retrospective study. Comp Haematol Int 1991;1:181–186.
2. **Sellon DC, Levine JF, Palmer K, Millikin E, et al.** Thrombocytosis in 24 horses (1989–1994). J Vet Intern Med 1997;11:24–29.
3. **Yohannan MD, Higgy KE, al-Mashhadani SA, Santhosh-Kumar CR.** Thrombocytosis. Etiologic analysis of 663 patients. Clin Pediatr 1994;33:340–343.
4. **Kutti J, Wadenvik H.** Diagnostic and differential criteria of essential thrombocythemia and reactive thrombocytosis. Leuk Lymphoma 1996;1:41–45.
5. **Murphy S, Peterson P, Iland H, Laszio J.** Experience of the Polycythemia Vera Study Group with essential thrombocythemia: a final report on diagnostic criteria, survival, and leukemic transition by treatment. Semin Hematol 1997;34:29–39.
6. **Ladenson JH, Tsai L-MB, Michael JM, Kessler G, et al.** Serum versus heparinized plasma for eighteen common chemistry tests: is serum the appropriate specimen? Am J Clin Pathol 1974;62:545–552.
7. **Lutomski DM, Bower RH.** The effect of thrombocytosis on serum potassium and phosphorus concentrations. Am J Med Sci 1994;307:255–258.
8. **Degen MA.** Correlation of spurious potassium elevation and platelet count in dogs. Vet Clin Pathol 1987;15:20–22.
9. **Mandell CP, Goding B, Degen MA, Hopper PE, et al.** Spurious elevation of serum potassium in two cases of thrombocythemia. Vet Clin Pathol 1988;17:32–33.
10. **Reimann KA, Knowlen GG, Tvedten HW.** Factitious hyperkalemia in dogs with thrombocytosis. The effect of platelets on serum potassium concentration. J Vet Intern Med 1989;3:47–52.
11. **Lephard EE.** Effect of exercise on platelet size and number in ponies. Vet Record 1977;101:488.
12. **Kutti J.** The management of thrombocytosis. Eur J Haematol 1990;44:81–88.
13. **Crosier PS, Clark SC.** Basic biology of the hematopoietic growth factors. Semin Oncol 1992;19:349–361.
14. **Hill RJ, Warren MK, Stenberg P, Levin J, et al.** Stimulation of megakaryocytopoiesis in mice by human recombinant interleukin-6. Blood 1991;77:42–48.
15. **Ertenli I, Haznedaroglu IC, Kiraz S, Celik I, et al.** Cytokines affecting megakaryocytopoiesis in rheumatoid arthritis with thrombocytosis. Rheumatol Int 1996;16:5–8.
16. **Haznedaroglu IC, Ertenli I, Ozcebe OI, Kiraz S, et al.** Megakaryocyte-related interleukins in reactive thrombocytosis versus autonomous thrombocythemia. Acta Haematol 1996;95:107–111.
17. **Mayer P, Geissler K, Valent P, Ceska M, et al.** Recombinant human interleukin 6 is a potent inducer of the acute phase response and elevates the blood platelets in nonhuman primates. Exp Hematol 1991;19:688–696.
18. **Frye JL, Thompson DF.** Drug-induced thrombocytosis. J Clin Pharm Ther 1993;18:45–48.
19. **Greene CE, Scoggin J, Thomas JE, Barsanti JA.** Vincristine in the treatment of thrombocytopenia in five dogs. J Am Vet Med Assoc 1982;180:140–143.
20. **Helfand SC, Jain NC, Paul M.** Vincristine-loaded platelet therapy for idiopathic thrombocytopenia in a dog. J Am Vet Med Assoc 1984;185:224–226.
21. **Robertson JH, Crozier EH, Woodend BE.** The effect of vincristine on the platelet count in rats. Br J Haematol 1970;19:331–337.
22. **Triplett DA, ed.** Qualitative or functional disorders of platelets (Chapter 5). Platelet function: laboratory and clinical application. Chicago: American Society of Clinical Pathologists, 1978;123–159.
23. **Griesshammer M, Bangerter M, Schrezenmeier H.** A possible role for thrombopoietin and its receptor c-mpl in the pathobiology of essential thrombocythemia. Semin Thromb Hemost 1997;23:419–423.
24. **Fialkow PJ, Faguet GB, Jacobson RJ, Vaidya K, et al.** Evidence that essential thrombocythemia is a clonal disorder with origin in a multipotent stem cell. Blood 1981;58:916–919.
25. **Singal U, Prasad AS, Halton DM, Bishop C.** Essential thrombocythemia: a clonal disorder of hematopoietic stem cell. Am J Hematol 1983;14:193–196.
26. **Michiels JJ, Van GP.** Essential thrombocythemia in childhood. Semin Thromb Hemost 1997;23:295–301.
27. **Rosenthal DS, Murphy S.** Thrombocytosis. In: Handin RI, Lux SE, Stossel TP, eds. Blood: principles and practice of hematology. Philadelphia: JB Lippincott Company, 1995;439–455.
28. **Tomo K, Takayama H, Kaneko Y, Fujita J, et al.** Qualitative platelet 12-lipoxygenase abnormality in a patient with essential thrombocythemia. Thromb Haemost 1997;77:294–297.
29. **Wirth K, Schoepf E, Mertelsmann R, Lindemann A.** Leg ulceration with associated thrombocytosis: healing of ulceration associated with treatment of the raised platelet count. Br. J Dermatol 1998;138:533–535.
30. **Rinder HM, Schuster JE, Rinder CS, Wang C, et al.** Correlation of thrombosis with increased platelet turnover in thrombocytosis Blood 1998;91:1288–1294.
31. **Robinson MS, Harrison C, Mackie IJ, Machin SJ, et al.** Reticulated platelets in primary and reactive thrombocytosis [letter]. Br J Haematol 1998;101:388–389.
32. **Nurden P, Bihour C, Smith M, Raymond JM, et al.** Platelet activation and thrombosis: studies in a patient with essential thrombocythemia. Am J Hematol 1996;51:79–84.
33. **Kaushansky K.** Thrombopoietin: the primary regulator of platelet production. Blood 1995;86:31–40.
34. **Michiels JJ, Juvonen E.** Proposal for revised diagnostic criteria of essential thrombocythemia and polycythemia vera by the Thrombocythemia Vera Study Group. Semin Thromb Hemost 1997;23:339–347.
35. **Bass MC, Schultze AE.** Essential thrombocythemia in a dog: case report and literature review. J Am Anim Hosp Assoc 1998;34:197–203.
36. **Evans RJ, Jones DRE, Gruffydd-Jones TJ.** Essential thrombocythaemia in the dog and cat: a report of four cases. J Small Anim Pract 1982;23:457–467.
37. **Hammer AS, Couto CG, Getzy D, Bailey MQ.** Essential thrombocythemia in a cat. J Vet Intern Med 1990;4:87–91.
38. **Hopper PE, Mandell CP, Turrel JM, Jain NC, et al.** Probable essential thrombocythemia in a dog. J Vet Intern Med 1989;3:79–85.
39. **Simpson JW, Else RW, Honeyman P.** Successful treatment of suspected essential thrombocythaemia in the dog. J Small Anim Pract 1990;31:345–348.
40. **Degen MA, Feldman BF, Turrel JM, Goding B, et al.** Thrombocytosis associated with a myeloproliferative disorder in dog. J Am Vet Med Assoc 1989;194:1457–1459.
41. **Koike T.** Megakaryoblastic leukemia: the characterization and identification of megakaryoblasts. Blood 1984;64:683–692.
42. **Murphy S.** Thrombocytosis and thrombocythemia. Clin Hematol 1983;12:89–106.
43. **Tablin F, Jain NC, Mandell CP, Hopper PE, et al.** Ultrastructural analysis of platelets and megakaryocytes from a dog with probable essential thrombocythemia. Vet Pathol 1989;26:289–293.
44. **Thiele J, Jansen B, Orth KH, Orth H, et al.** Ultrastructure of megakaryocytes in the human bone marrow of patients with primary (essential) thrombocythemia [see comments]. J Submicrosc Cytol Pathol 1988;20:671–681.
45. **Tefferi A, Elliott MA, Solberg LJ, Silverstein MN.** New drugs in essential thrombocythemia and polycythemia vera. Blood Rev 1997;11:1–7.

CHAPTER 72

von Willebrand Disease

• MARJORY BROOKS

Von Willebrand disease (vWD) is the most common canine hereditary bleeding disorder. The disease is heterogeneous, with subtype classifications based on severity of clinical signs, mode of inheritance, and biochemical abnormalities of von Willebrand factor protein (vWF). Appropriate diagnostic and management strategies must take into account this clinical variability.

DISEASE MECHANISM

The pathognomonic feature of vWD is a lack of functional vWF that causes abnormal primary hemostasis and prolongation of in vivo bleeding time. vWF is a multimeric plasma glycoprotein that plays a central role in hemostasis by supporting platelet adhesion at sites of vessel injury. Endothelial cells are the major site of vWF synthesis and storage. Platelets provide a secondary pool of vWF in some species, however, canine platelets contain barely any vWF.[1] vWF undergoes extensive intracellular processing and assembly. Two subunit vWF molecules join to form dimers, followed by the association of dimers to form multimers. Multimers consist of from 2 to more than 100 vWF subunits and range in molecular weight size from 500,000 to 20 million d. vWF is secreted from endothelial cells via a steady-state (constitutive) pathway or stored in endothelial cell organelles and released in response to stimuli such as thrombin and epinephrine. In plasma, vWF forms a non-covalent complex with coagulation Factor (FVIII) and appears to stabilize the functional half-life of FVIII. On exposure to subendothelium, vWF binds to collagen and then undergoes a conformation change that facilitates its interaction with platelets by means of platelet surface glycoprotein lb (Fig. 72.1). Intraplatelet bridging is also mediated by vWF. High-molecular weight vWF multimers are most effective in promoting platelet adhesion. Deficiency of vWF, or preferential loss of high-molecular weight forms, results in failure of platelet adhesion and aggregation, especially under high shear in the microcirculation.[2]

DISEASE CLASSIFICATION

On the basis of clinical severity, plasma vWF concentration, and vWF multimer structure, vWD is classified into one of three general types (Table 72.1).[3] Type 1 vWD is defined as a partial quantitative deficiency of vWF. Plasma vWF concentration is low (<50% of normal), but the vWF that is present has normal multimer structure and supports platelet interactions in vitro. In general, clinical severity correlates with reduction in plasma vWF concentration. Most type 1 vWD-affected dogs that express a bleeding tendency have plasma vWF concentration of less than 20%.[4,5]

Type 2 vWD includes qualitative abnormalities of vWF structure and function. Although comprising as much as 15% of vWD cases in humans, type 2 vWD is unusual in animals. The biochemical characterization of type 2 vWD in animals consists of low plasma vWF concentration, a disproportionate loss of high-molecular weight multimers, and significant reduction of in vitro vWF-dependent platelet agglutination. This form of vWD is analogous to the subtype classification of 2A vWD in humans. Type 2B vWD, not yet identified in animals, refers to variants with increased vWF affinity for platelet surface GPlb.[3]

Type 3 vWD is a severe quantitative deficiency of vWF. Affected animals have virtually no plasma or platelet vWF (<0.1%). In humans, type 3 vWD is associated with a concomitant significant reduction in plasma FVIII activity (FVIII:C) to less than 5% of normal. The reduction in FVIII:C is less pronounced in dogs, with values typically greater than 30%.[6] Spontaneous hemarthrosis, a sign associated with FVIII:C deficiency, is therefore rarely seen in canine type 3 vWD.

CLINICAL SIGNS

The most common clinical signs of vWD include mucosal hemorrhage, cutaneous bruising, and prolonged bleeding from surgical or traumatic wounds. These signs are typical of primary hemostatic defects and are clinically indistinguishable from inherited or acquired platelet dysfunction. Reports of vWD describe epistaxis, hematuria, gastrointestinal hemorrhage, prolonged estral bleeding and gingival bleeding at tooth eruption sites.[4] Petechiae do not appear to be signs of vWD in dogs. Types 2 and 3 vWD cause a severe bleeding tendency, and one or more episodes of hemorrhage typically occur by the time the animal is 1 year old. Neonatal

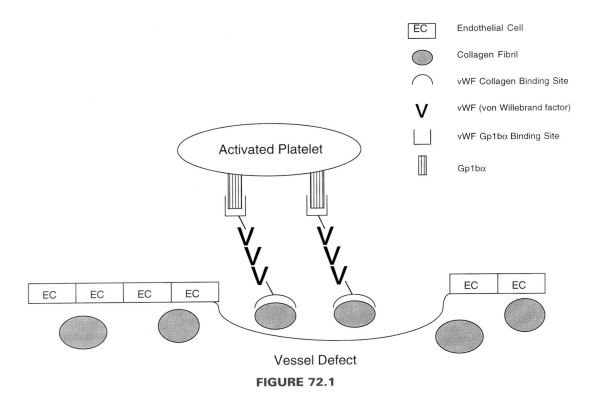

FIGURE 72.1

Legend:
- EC — Endothelial Cell
- Collagen Fibril
- vWF Collagen Binding Site
- V — vWF (von Willebrand factor)
- vWF Gp1bα Binding Site
- Gp1bα

Activated Platelet

Vessel Defect

deaths caused by hemorrhage occur, but many animals affected with severe vWD survive to adulthood. The bleeding tendency associated with type 1 vWD ranges from mild to severe. Mildly affected dogs experience clinically relevant hemorrhage only if they undergo extensive surgery or trauma. The anatomic site of tissue injury influences the consequences of hemorrhage. Oronasal and urinary tract tissues are rich in fibrinolysins, and injuries to these tissues often lead to more severe bleeding complications than skin incisions or superficial wounds. Minor bleeds into critical sites such as the central nervous system (CNS) or respiratory tract may cause severe morbidity and mortality in vWD-affected dogs.

The bleeding tendency of vWD is exacerbated by concurrent thrombocytopenia or by disease conditions or drug administration that impairs platelet function.[7] Nonsteroidal anti-inflammatory drugs (NSAIDs) and plasma expanders are commonly used drugs that have antiplatelet effects. All NSAIDs interfere with intraplatelet prostaglandin metabolism, causing reduced production of thromboxane, a potent platelet agonist. Synthetic colloids like dextran and hydroxyethyl starch (hetastarch) cause in vitro abnormalities of platelet aggregation, believed to be mediated by means of interference with platelet membrane receptors. Platelet dysfunction accompanies common disease conditions, including uremia, hyperproteinemia, anemia, and liver disease, by means of multifactorial and complex mechanisms. Animals having concurrent vWF deficiency may experience clinical signs of hemorrhage that complicate management of these disorders.

INHERITANCE AND EXPRESSION PATTERNS

As males and females transmit and express the defect with equal frequency, vWD is an autosomal trait. The human gene for vWF is on chromosome 12. The canine vWF gene has been localized to an autosome, however, consensus nomenclature for individual linkage groups comprising the canine karyotype has not yet been established.

Recessive Forms

Recessive inheritance and expression patterns are characteristic of loss-of-function mutations, where absence of a gene product in homozygotes causes clinical signs, and heterozygotes are clinically normal. All affected individuals have two abnormal vWF alleles, one transmitted from the dam and one from the sire. Types 2 and 3 vWD in dogs are recessive traits. Obligate heterozygotes are clinically normal, but have low (<50%) plasma concentration of vWF.[4,8]

Dominant Forms

Dominant inheritance and expression patterns are associated with gain-of-function mutations, where the presence of an abnormal gene product interferes with critical functional sites or pathways. Clinical signs may be identical for dogs homozygous and heterozygous for disease-causing mutations. Incomplete dominance implies variability of disease expression between individuals carrying the same mutation. The inheritance of type 1 vWD in most human families is reported to be dominant or incompletely dominant.[3] On the basis of breeding studies between Doberman pinschers and mixed breed dogs, type 1 vWD was reported to be a recessive trait.[9] Certain clinical features of canine type 1 vWD are compatible with incomplete dominance, including a range of severity for dogs having comparable values of plasma vWF concentration and the fact that all affected dogs have readily detectable levels of structurally normal plasma vWF. More detailed studies, combining molecular genetic analyses with biochemical and clinical characterization of vWD pedigrees are needed to clarify mode of inheritance in most affected breeds.

Breed Prevalence in Dogs

Estimates of breed prevalence of vWD are difficult to determine accurately. In general, diagnosis bias favors identification of clinically severe forms. The characteristics of animals chosen for screening are often influenced by monetary concerns and dynamics of breed clubs, rather than random selection methods. On the basis of clinical reports, however, it is apparent that prevalence of vWD varies between breeds, and within each affected breed a single type of vWD predominates (Table 72.1).

Acquired von Willebrand Disease

An acquired hemostatic defect with features typical of vWD (mucosal bleeding, long bleeding time, low plasma vWF concentration, and abnormal cofactor activity) has been described in humans as a rare complication of autoimmune and lymphoproliferative disorders, hypothyroidism, and the use of ciprofloxacin and hetastarch.[7] Various pathogenetic mechanisms are believed to cause vWF deficiency in these disorders, including inhibition, decreased synthesis, and increased proteolysis of vWF. Acquired vWD is not well characterized in dogs. Hypothyroidism has been associated with expression of vWD, however differentiation between acquired vWF deficiency or concurrent hypothyroidism and congenital vWF deficiency is difficult to determine.[10] Experimentally induced hypothyroidism did not cause low plasma vWF in normal dogs.[11] Regardless of inherited or acquired origin, dogs having low plasma vWF and apparent spontaneous episodes of mucosal hemorrhage (epistaxis, hematuria, and gingival hemorrhage) should be carefully evaluated to detect any endocrinopathy or infection that may have precipitated the bleeding event.

DIAGNOSTIC TESTS

vWD should be considered in the differential diagnosis of bleeding diatheses (Algorithm). Although vWD is uncommon in species other than dogs, isolated cases have been identified in cats, horses, and cattle.

If platelet count and coagulation panel are within normal limits, bleeding time determination is useful as a screening test for vWD. Prolongation of buccal mucosal bleeding time (BMBT) is specific for primary hemostatic defects, and animals clinically affected with vWD have long bleeding times. In general, finite bleeding times of 5 to 10 minutes are seen in mild to moderate type 1 vWD (reference range of 2 to 4 minutes), whereas ani-

TABLE 72.1	Type Classification of Canine von Willebrand Disease		
Classification	Plasma vWF Concentration/Multimer Structure	Clinical Severity	Reported Breeds
Type 1	Low concentration/proportional decrease all multimer forms	variable	Airedale, Akita, Dachshund, Doberman pinscher, German shepherd, Golden retriever, Greyhound, Irish Wolfhound, Manchester terrier, Schnauzer, PW Corgi, Poodle, Shetland sheepdog
Type 2	Low concentration/absence of high molecular weight multimers	severe	German shorthaired pointer, German wirehaired pointer
Type 3	Plasma vWF absent	severe	Familial: Chesapeake retriever, Dutch Kooiker, Scottish terrier, Shetland sheepdog Sporadic: Border collie, Bull terrier, Cocker spaniel, Labrador retriever, Mixed breed, Pomeranian

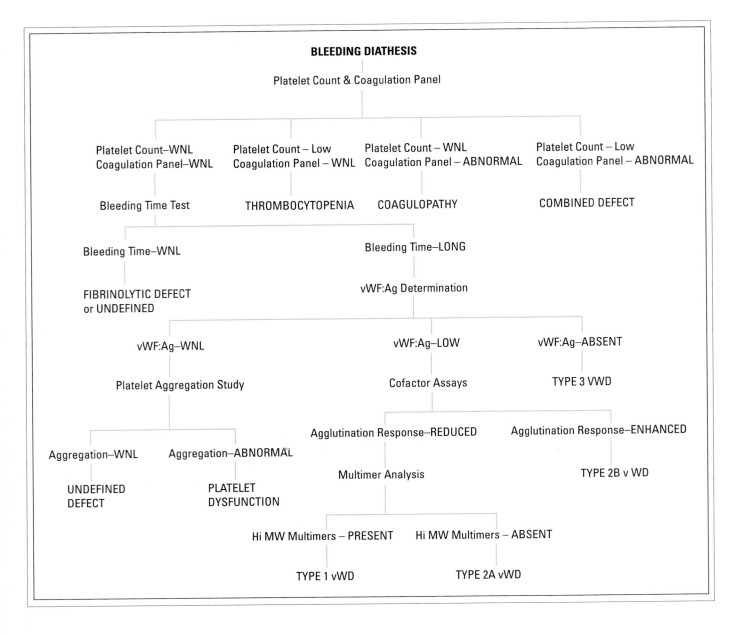

mals having the most severe forms typically have BMBT of >12 minutes.[12]

Definitive diagnosis of vWD requires specific assay of plasma vWF. Canine and feline vWF are antigenically and functionally distinct from human vWF, and samples must be analyzed with methods validated for use in these species.[13] Plasma separated from whole blood drawn into sodium citrate or ethylenediamine tetra-acetic acid (EDTA) anticoagulant is suitable for vWF analyses. Samples that are hemolyzed or clotted during the collection process are often depleted of vWF, and do not represent accurate measures of in vivo vWF levels.

Quantitative Assays

vWF antigen (vWF:Ag) assay is a quantitative measure of plasma vWF. The enzyme-linked immunosorbent assay (ELISA) technique is the most rapid, sensitive, and reproducible test method for determining plasma vWF concentration and is the most widely used screening test for detecting vWF deficiency.[2] Test results are usually reported as units per deciliter or percent, compared with the laboratory's standard plasma having an assigned value of 100 U/dL or 100%. Reference ranges for each species assayed should be established by each testing laboratory. In most laboratories, plasma vWF:Ag values of less than 50% (<50 U/dL) fall below reference range and are considered vWF deficient.[5,8,14]

Functional Assays

Cofactor assays are semiquantitative, functional tests of vWF-dependent platelet agglutination. Comparisons

SECTION VIII
Hemostasis
Rafael Ruiz de Gopegui

CHAPTER 73

Hemostasis: Introduction, Overview, Laboratory Techniques

• REINHARD MISCHKE and INGO J.A. NOLTE

The hemostatic system carries out important functions when the vascular wall is damaged. First, the integrity must be restored as quickly as possible, thus primarily minimizing blood loss. It is also involved in creating the conditions for growth of fibroblasts in the course of wound healing. The combination of numerous control mechanisms prevents, under physiologic conditions, blood coagulation far beyond the affected area and thus a narrowing of intact blood vessels.

Hemostatic disorders can be caused by a shifting of this balance in the direction of hypercoagulability accompanied by a tendency toward thrombosis.[1] More important in veterinary medicine, however, is an imbalance toward the opposite side with an increased tendency toward bleeding (hemorrhagic diathesis). This is often caused by reduced coagulation factor activity or a reduced number (thrombocytopenia) or malfunction of the blood platelets (thrombopathia), sometimes in connection with a hyperfibrinolysis, which, in most of the cases, appears secondary after a disseminated intravascular coagulation ([DIC], consumption coagulopathy). The clinically important syndrome of DIC includes both possible defective variations of the hemostatic system. After systemic activation by numerous different pathomechanisms (e.g., tissue thromboplastin release through injury or tumor), there is excessive coagulation in the area of the capillaries, which can lead to hypocoagulability by immense consumption of the hemostatic potential.[2]

Hemostatic disorders are rarely hereditary (e.g., hemophilia A, hemophilia B, and Willebrand's disease) but are more often acquired (e.g., coumarin poisoning, hepatogen-mediated coagulopathy, DIC, and immune-mediated thrombocytopenia).

Study of the hemostatic system in animals is important when one considers scientific questions in various disciplines (e.g., internal medicine, oncology, surgery); numerous animal models also make it immensely important for humans.[3,4] With the progress of diagnostic and therapeutic possibilities in veterinary medicine, blood coagulation diagnosis has in the meantime also received great attention in clinical veterinary medicine.

An indication of hemostatic diagnosis is, for example, heavy external bleeding, an extensive hematoma or a body cavity effusion of unclear origin. Study of the hemostatic system is also advisable for checking the degree of severity of changes in the blood coagulation status in diseases that often cause acquired, partly subclinical, progressing hemostatic disorders. In addition, it is required for preoperative screenings and for control of an anticoagulant and fibrinolytic therapy.

A hemostatic disorder is suspected when there is lengthy or even nonstanched hemorrhage after venipuncture, when there is hemorrhage in several locations at the same time, or when the level of hemorrhage bears no relation to the injury. In hereditary blood coagulation disorders, the case history already supplies indications. For example, hemophilic dogs regularly experience severe bleeding complications during teething.[5]

If there is systemic functional impairment of the blood coagulation, usually only a differentiated study of the hemostatic system can provide an explanation of its origin. It provides the basis for targeted treatment.

OVERVIEW, PHYSIOLOGY OF HEMOSTASIS

The process of hemostasis is a diverse interplay among the vascular wall, the blood platelets, and the coagulation system. When blood comes into contact with subendothelial structures (collagen fibers or the basal membrane) or tissue (release of tissue thromboplastin or phospholipids), the mechanisms are set in motion within a short period.[6,7,8]

Stanching of capillary hemorrhage is also supported by a few seconds contraction of the smooth muscle cells of the arteries and arterioles in the afferent region after vessel injury. This ensures a decrease in blood flow and loss. At the same time, the first blood platelets adhere on the exposed collagen fibers.[6] The adhesion of the thrombocytes on subendothelial structures results from the Willebrand factor, synthesized and secreted by the endothelial cells. On one hand, the secretor thrombus, rich in platelets, grows rapidly because an electric signal steers the platelets to the vascular lesion. On the other hand, there is a positive feedback mechanism whereby the thrombocytes release, among other things, secondary platelet activators during aggregation (e.g., thromboxane A_2, adenosine diphosphate, platelet-activating factor). The thrombocyte aggregate results in an initial, if only labile closure of the wound and thus stops the bleeding.

The platelet thrombus is stabilized by a fibrin network that is the end product of the coagulation system, which weaves itself around the platelet aggregate and connects it to the vascular wall. The retraction of the fibrin, supported by a centripetal contraction of the actomyosin of the thrombocytes, also leads to a reduction in the size of the thrombus and thus also in the size of the blood flow blockage. The further breakdown of the clot, which is finally replaced by repair tissue, is carried out with the aid of lysosomal enzymes of the thrombocytes and the fibrinolytic system.

Fibrin results from the effect of thrombin, the most important coagulation protease. Thrombin splits the fibrinopeptides A and B from fibrinogen molecules, producing fibrin monomers that polymerize spontaneously into strands and finally into a net. Transglutaminase factor XIII then ensures that the fibrin net is connected together by means of a covalent cross-linking between lysine and glutamic acid of different fibrin strands.

Formation of thrombin from prothrombin occurs by means of activated factor X in connection with factor V as cofactor and phospholipid. The reactions that lead to the activation of factor X and thus to thrombin formation are usually divided into two reaction paths, the intrinsic and the extrinsic (see Algorithm). This differentiation should be retained in the following for didactic reasons, although it does not exist in vivo because of numerous connecting points.

The extrinsic activation path, which is considered the most important today, starts when factor VII is activated by adsorption on the ubiquitously occurring tissue thromboplastin (a protein-phospholipid complex), released in tissue injury or from damaged blood cells. Shortly after adsorption, activated factor VII (factor VIIa) activates factor X.[7]

The contact of blood with negative-laden foreign surfaces, on which factor XII is adsorbed and activated, leads to the initial reaction of the intrinsic system.[8] As such, collagen exposed by endothelial defects or pathologically altered vessel endothelium (e.g., in the hemangioendothelioma) have an effect as does in vitro or extracorporeal circulation (e.g. dialysis and cell separator),

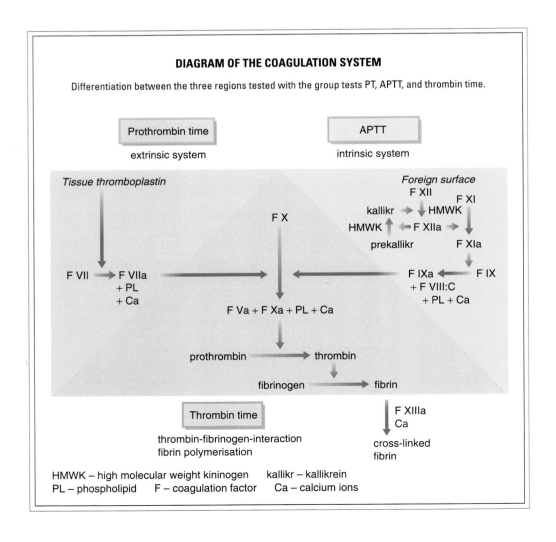

DIAGRAM OF THE COAGULATION SYSTEM

Differentiation between the three regions tested with the group tests PT, APTT, and thrombin time.

Prothrombin time — extrinsic system

APTT — intrinsic system

Tissue thromboplastin

Foreign surface
F XII
F XI
kallikr → ↓ HMWK
HMWK ↑ ← F XIIa → ↓
prekallikr
F XIa

F X

F VII → F VIIa + PL + Ca

F IXa ← F IX
+ F VIII:C
+ PL + Ca

F Va + F Xa + PL + Ca

prothrombin → thrombin

fibrinogen → fibrin

Thrombin time
thrombin-fibrinogen-interaction
fibrin polymerisation

F XIIIa
Ca

cross-linked fibrin

HMWK – high molecular weight kininogen   kallikr – kallikrein
PL – phospholipid   F – coagulation factor   Ca – calcium ions

glass, kaolin, sulfatides, and to a much lesser extent, plastic and steel. Factor XIIa activates prekallikrein into kallikrein, which then contributes to the further activation of factor XII molecules. High-molecular-weight kininogen (HMWK) is involved as cofactor in the subsequent activation of factor XI into factor XIa by factor XIIa. Ca^{2+} ions are involved in the factor XIa-induced activation of factor IX into factor IXa. The following transformation of factor X into factor Xa through factor IXa is greatly accelerated by the presence of factor VIII in connection with phospholipid and calcium. Factor VIII acts thus as a cofactor without its own enzymatic activity like factor V, whereby both of them have to be activated then by thrombin in a positive feedback. Factor VIII characterizes a small subunit of the factor VIII molecule, which is lacking in patients that have hemophilia A, whereas a larger subunit corresponds to Willebrand factor (see above). The cascade-shaped activation of serine proteases from proenzymes, together with the positive feedback mechanisms, results in a vast potentiation of the initial signal. However, the importance of the factors XII and XI as well as prekallikrein and HMWK, involved initially in the contact activation, for the physiologic hemostasis is considered to be small today. Thus, a severely increased tendency to hemorrhage is described neither in animals nor in humans who suffer from an inherited lack of one of these factors. The reason for this is that factor VIIa, through the so-called Josso's loop, is able to activate factor IX, too.

The presence of phospholipids is important for the coagulation process. The coagulation factors (II, V, VIII, IX, X) bind to their surface so that there is local accumulation and the factors are thus more easily accessible for an enzymatic reaction. Mainly membranes of the blood platelets are available as a phospholipid surface, which emphasizes how important the functioning of all components and their interaction is for normal hemostasis.

The binding of the coagulation factors to phospholipids occurs mainly by means of Ca^{2+} ions whose presence is necessary for most enzymatic reactions. This connection provides the basis on which to keep the blood samples incoagulable until the coagulation analysis, which is achieved by adding the chelating agent ethylenediamine tetra-acetic acid (EDTA) or Na citrate and thus neutralizing the calcium effect.

As with an increased tendency to hemorrhage after hemostatic disorder, a threatening situation also occurs with blood coagulation far beyond the affected area, with formation of thromboses or DIC. On the one hand, numerous thrombophobic characteristics of the intact endothelial cells ensure the hemostatic process that is clearly confined to the affected area. The system also provides a guard against this with numerous antiregulatory factors, such as inhibitors of coagulation factors and the fibrinolytic system (see Chapter 78, Fibrinolytic System).

Amongst the inhibitors of the coagulation system, protein C, which after its activation mainly proteolyses factors Va and VIIIa and also increases the fibrinolytic activity, and particularly antithrombin are of importance. Antithrombin inhibits the serine proteases thrombin and factor Xa, and to a lesser extent also factors

IXa, XIa, XIIa and plasmin, by forming irreversible 1:1 complexes. This complex formation is a slow process taking minutes, but when heparin is present it takes only seconds.[9]

LABORATORY TECHNIQUES

Blood Sampling and Collection of Sample Material

Significant analysis results of hemostasis tests make higher demands on blood sampling techniques than most other parameters in the clinical laboratory. An inexpertly carried out technique and the choice of unsuitable sample container are the most common causes of activation of the coagulation system already in the sample container, leading to false analysis results. For measuring the number of thrombocytes, EDTA blood is required. On the other hand, the screening tests of the coagulation system, like the activity of the individual coagulation factors, single components of the fibrinolytic system, and the relevant inhibitors, are measured from citrated plasma or citrated blood.

Sample Containers

To produce citrated plasma, first obtain citrated blood; prefabricated sample containers are available for this procedure from various manufacturers. In the sample containers, which are graduated accordingly, sufficient volume of 0.11 mol/L Na citrate solution is used so that the ratio between citrate solution and blood is 1:9 (e.g., 0.2 mL citrate + 1.8 mL blood). As an alternative to the commercially available collection systems, a disposable 2- or 5-mL syringe can be filled with 0.2 or 0.5 mL of commercially prepared 0.11 mol/L Na citrate solution. Then, if there is not too great a vacuum in the syringe, blood can be aspirated.

Should there be clear deviations in the mixture ratio between blood and anticoagulant, false test results are achieved owing to a deviating dilution of the coagulation factor content and a fluctuating citrate concentration. In patients that have highly fluctuating hematocrit, this situation requires that the above-mentioned regulation for the mixture ratio, which is valid for animals that have physiologic hematocrit, be varied by use of controlled underfilling (decreased hematocrit) or overfilling (increased hematocrit) of the tube with blood.

Use of the Vacutainer system cannot be recommended. Because the mixture ratio cannot be exactly controlled, incomplete siliconization of the glass tube can lead to contact activation and, depending on the sampling technique, contamination with tissue thromboplastin cannot be excluded.

Blood Collection and Citrated Plasma Acquisition

Blood collection should be carried out if possible without or after careful and brief (<30 seconds) congestion, since a congestion in the vascular system activates the hemostasis and fibrinolysis system. For quick and least stressful puncture, an extremely sharp disposable syringe with a wide lumen should be used. The first drops of blood (approximately 0.5 to 1 mL) should be disposed of or kept, for example, for clinicochemical tests. In this way, a contamination of the samples for hemostaseologic tests by tissue thromboplastin can be avoided. Repetition of the accumulation process or puncture of the same vein is only recommended after at least 30 minutes.

When sterile tubes are used, the blood should flow carefully along the wall of the tube into the sample container. If citrated blood is obtained with a syringe, aspiration should be carefully performed, since frothing can lead to activation of the coagulation factors. In obtaining citrated blood, particular importance must also be attached to a rapid and intensive mixing of the collected blood with the Na citrate so that sample coagulation is avoided. To do this, the sample container must be tipped and revolved carefully several times. If tubes are used, it is recommended that they already are shaken carefully while the blood is being collected.

Centrifugation of the sample and subsequent immediate removal by pipette of the platelet-poor plasma supernatant should be performed as quickly as possible, at the latest within 2 hours after blood collection. Immediately before centrifugation for 10 minutes at 1500 to 2000 g, the sample should be checked for possible clots. Clinicians should dispose of coagulated samples.

Test Procedure

Global Tests

Global tests give global information on the hemostatic potential of a blood sample and thus on the functioning of the interaction between thrombocytic (preparation of platelet factor 3 or phospholipids) and plasmatic components. Although the coagulation time of an additive-free whole blood sample (spontaneous coagulation time according to Lee and White)[10] and the recalcification time, i.e., the fibrin formation time after recalcification of a citrated blood sample, are classic diagnostic tests, they are only seldom used today, even in animals.

Activated Coagulation Time   In the modification activated coagulation time (ACT), native blood is put into a sample tube with contact activator.[11] The test thus gives a quick result, and since it is simple to perform, it is also widely used in veterinary practices. For better standardization, the tube containing the sample either can be placed in a heating block at a temperature of 37°C or can be held in the hand until clots have formed.

The causes for an extended ACT can be a significant deficiency of one of the coagulation factors involved in the course of the intrinsic system (HMWK; prekallikrein; factors XII, XI, IX, VIII, X, V, II; and fibrinogen) and can also be clear thrombocytopenia or the presence of inhibitors, heparin, or anticoagulants.

Thrombelastography, Resonance Thrombography   Thrombelastography and resonance thrombography are procedures, which record the whole course of coagulation, including a possible hyperfibrinolysis, in a curve. The curve, particularly of the resonance thrombography, as opposed to the coagulation times mentioned above, allows a certain differentiation in the origin of the hemostatic disorder.

In thrombelastography, native blood or immediately previously recalcified citrated blood is placed in a stainless steel cuvette heated to 37°C, which moves with a motorized slow-turning motion. A frictionless hanging steel cylinder is dipped into the blood. It is then connected by the resulting clot to the wall of the cuvette and incorporated into the turning movement. The turning movement of the cylinder supplies the measurement signal, leading physiologically to a spindle-shaped curve.

As a further development of thrombelastography, resonance thrombography is more user-friendly and offers, in particular, a differentiated issue of results, which allows a difference to be made between the effect of fibrin formation and blood platelet activity (Fig. 73.1).[12]

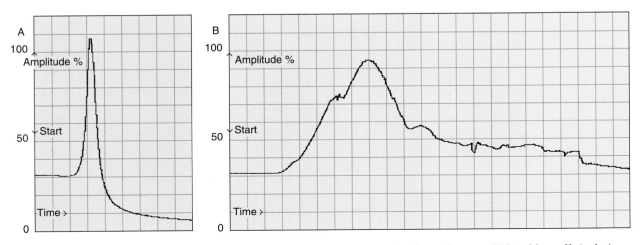

FIGURE 73.1 Severely altered resonance thrombogram (RTG) of a 2-year-old male collie with severe DIC and hyperfibrinolysis caused by polytrauma, **B** (Fibrinogen concentration, 0.55 g/L; and soluble fibrin, 34 μg/mL) in comparison with a normal RTG, **A.**

However, as all other global-screening tests,[12] resonance thrombography has the disadvantage of having low sensitivity, e.g., with regard to the recognition of the lack of a single factor or thrombocytopenia. The procedure is particularly suitable, however, as a screening test for fibrin formation defects, which are demonstrated much more sensitively than in the group tests. It is therefore much more advantageous for use in the diagnosis and the control of the course of the DIC-hyperfibrinolysis complex, where it also gives fast and summarized information on the changes in the plasmatic and thrombocytic hemostasis potential and its influence by fibrin (fibrinogen) degradation products and anticoagulants used therapeutically.

In resonance thrombography, a metal pendulum sunken in a cuvette with recalcified citrated blood performs an orbital oscillation. The elasticity of the clot that is forming creates an increase in the frequency of the oscillation of the pendulum itself to the resonance level of the exciting oscillation and thus to the increase in the oscillation radius of the pendulum (rise in the curve, fibrin leg), which serves as a parameter. The subsequent decrease in the radius of the pendulum oscillation (drop in the curve, thrombocyte leg) reflects the contraction tension caused by the thrombocytes within the clot.

Number of Thrombocytes (see Clinical Platelet Disorders Section)

Plasmatic Hemostasis Components
Test Procedure

The measurement of the activity of the individual coagulation factors and of the group tests is performed mainly by classical coagulation methods and the measurement of the coagulation inhibitors partly by these methods. The occurrence of the first fibrin clot, which can be detected manually, mechanically, or optically with coagulometers, forms the measurement signal.

Manually, the time point of coagulation can be recorded either with a previously annealed platinum hook (hook method), which is pulled through the test substance at regular interval or by the tilting method, whereby the tube with the plasma-reagent mixture is moved rhythmically until the test substance sets. Of the various coagulometer methods, the coagulometer according to Schnitger and Gross, based on the hook method, has proved successful. A sphere coagulometer is also suitable for the veterinary practice. It records the clot formation by a magnetic sensor that registers changes in location of a ball in the test substance due to the clot. Other coagulometers record the increase in turbidity intensity during the coagulation process.

An instrument working on the basis of dry chemistry has also proved to be basically suitable, with certain modifications, for hemostasis diagnosis in the dog and with limitations in the cat.[13] The disadvantages compared with conventional methods are a low sensitivity and a limited test spectrum.

For some years, alternative chromogenic substrates have been available for the measurement of group tests and various individual factors, but also for plasminogen,

inhibitors and activation markers, and these are also partly used in veterinary medicine.[14] These are synthetic peptides that demonstrate a specific amino acid frequency for certain proteases of the hemostasis system, coupled with a color indicator (p-nitroaniline). The cleavage of the indicator can be recorded photometrically.

Group Tests   To check the plasmatic coagulation system rationally, the screening tests prothrombin time (PT) and activated partial thromboplastin time (APTT) are widely used, and as so-called group tests, they each record several coagulation factors of the extrinsic or intrinsic system (see Algorithm).[15] When there is a pathologic result in these two tests, the complementary measurement of thrombin time is shown, with the help of which defects in the thrombin-fibrinogen interaction and fibrin polymerization by fibrinogen degradation products or heparin can be detected.

Together, these three tests record the whole plasmatic coagulation system with the exception of the fibrin cross-linking that depends on factor XIII (see Algorithm). By combining the findings from several group tests, one can often make a tentative diagnosis by also considering the number of thrombocytes and if necessary the capillary bleeding time, which can then be confirmed by individual factor analyses.

The in vitro imitation of the exogenous activation path during measurement of the PT succeeds by addition of the reagent components of tissue thromboplastin and Ca^{2+} ions to citrated plasma. In APTT, a reagent to activate the intrinsic system and which contains a surface activator and a phospholipid component, is first added to the citrated plasma, and then Ca^{2+} ions are added as starting reagent after an incubation period. For measuring the thrombin time, a reagent containing thrombin is added to citrated plasma.

For the group tests, commercial test kits are available from various manufacturers. These are optimized for the measurement of human plasma and can also be used basically for animals. For the APTT, significant differences exist between the individual factor sensitivity of the various reagents. With a sensitive APTT reagent, even mild individual factor deficits can be detected in the plasma of various animal species, despite an APTT that is much shorter than in humans, by an APTT prolongation so that it becomes an almost ideal screening test. In contrast, the PT insensitively exhibits a decreased activity in a coagulation factor in animal species that have high activity of the accelerator factor V, such as dog and cat.[16,17] Thus, in those laboratories in which coagulation analyses are often carried out on certain species, it is recommended to use an adaptation of the test according to the animal species-specific requirements. In this connection, for example, a 1:20 predilution of the test plasma with buffer solution is considered suitable with simultaneous fibrinogen substitution.[16,17]

The use of animal species-, method-, and reagent-specific reference ranges is important for the interpretation of the results of groups tests and also of other hemostaseologic test procedures. These reference ranges

TABLE 73.1	Reference Ranges of the Activated Partial Thromboplastin Time (Sec) Measuring Plasma of Different Species with Different Reagents			
Reagent		Dog	Cat	Human
Pathromtin (Dade Behring, Liederbach, Germany)		14.5–19	14.5–22	26–40
PTT reagent (Roche Diagnostics GmbH, Mannheim, Germany)		10–13	10.5–14	30–40

are best achieved in the laboratory when based on a sufficiently large number of volunteers ($n \geq 40$). Alternatively, as a rough guide, one or, better, several controls from healthy individuals from the relevant animal species can also be used. The measurement of sample material from animals in a laboratory specializing in the measurement of human plasma regularly leads to false interpretations when a comparison is carried out with the reference ranges for humans given by the laboratory, when the coagulation time (in the case of prothrombin time) is calculated with a reference curve of human reference plasma in percent activity, or when a comparison is made as a ratio with a human control. The clear differences exist between the reference ranges of different species and between different reagents are shown in Table 73.1, with APTT used as an example.

Fibrinogen Concentration Because the liver synthesis rate of fibrinogen in connection with its role as acute phase protein can be greatly increased, a lack of fibrinogen remains limited to rare cases of extreme hyperfibrinolysis. Measurement of the fibrinogen concentration is therefore much less often required for diagnosis than is commonly thought.

The numerous different methods record either the coagulable part of the protein, which is also effective in vivo (e.g., Clauss method, kinetic, photometric fibrinogen detection, and gravimetry after complete coagulation), or the molecule independent of its function (e.g., immunologic evidence and heat precipitation). In veterinary medicine, the Clauss method[18] is most commonly used with commercial test kits, and this represents a modification of the thrombin time. By prediluting the sample, the fibrinogen concentration is placed in an area where, with standardized thrombin level, the fibrin formation rate is proportional to the fibrinogen concentration. Although the test kit calculation tables or the commercial human standards can be closely used for samples from dog and cat, with horse plasma the values measured are far too low.

If necessary, a species-specific fibrinogen standard can be produced with a gravimetric determination of the fibrinogen content of a relevant reference plasma. The addition of thrombin to the diluted sample transforms the fibrinogen into fibrin, which one can collect by rolling it on a small rod and then weigh by drying it at 100°C on an analytical balance.

Individual Factor Activity The activity of individual coagulation factors is mainly measured coagulo-

metrically by modification of the test instructions for PT (factors II, V, VII, and X) or APTT (factors VIII, IX, XI, XII, prekallikrein, and HMWK). Instead of the sample, in this test a combination of a prediluted sample and a deficiency plasma is used. Commercial, usually immunoadsorbed deficiency plasmas of human origin are available, in which the relevant factor to be determined is reduced to an activity <1%, whereas the rest of the factors lies in the human reference range. Therefore, according to the basic principle of the method, an excess of all other factors exists, so that the coagulation time of the test substance only depends on the activity of the factor to be measured in the sample.

In various animal species, different levels of coagulation factor activity are measured, compared with humans (Table 73.2).[19–21] In particular, the activity level of the accelerators, factors V and VIII, lies often many times higher than that of humans. Thus, in comparison with humans, the factor V activity is eight times higher in the dog and five times higher in the cat and in cattle. Factor VIII activity in cats is 13 times higher (in dogs, 8 times; in cattle, 5 times) than in humans. Therefore, the measurement results of other factors were influenced by the fluctuations of these factors when the measurement of the coagulation activity in the respective animal species is carried out with human deficiency plasma and the usual low sample dilution used for humans (1:5 to 1:20, depending on the coagulation factor). To maintain the basic principle of activity measurement of individual factors also in the samples from these animal species, a higher sample dilution is therefore necessary ($1:5 \geq 40$).

The species differences in the activity of individual coagulation factors emphasize the necessity for standardization with a species- and also reagent-batch-specific calibration curve. For this, different dilutions of a pool of citrated plasma from at least 40 healthy individuals of the relevant species are measured instead of the sample.

Willebrand Factor The function of the Willebrand factor as an adhesion protein in the adhesion and aggregation of thrombocytes leads to defective primary hemostasis, when there is an extreme, inherited, or ac-

TABLE 73.2	Activity of Various Individual Coagulation Factors (% of Normal Human Plasma) in Plasma of Different Animal Species		
Coagulation Factor	Cattle	Dog	Cat
II	40	100	100
V	550	900	500
VII	5	300	125
X	25	100	60
VIII	450	800	1300
IX	200	200	100
XI	70	300	170
XII	200	200	140

quired Willebrand factor deficiency. This can be seen by an extended capillary bleeding time, a simple-to-perform screening test of choice that can be carried out under clinical conditions.[22] Measurement of the plasma level of the Willebrand factor can be done in special laboratories with different commercial immunologic test systems (enzyme-linked immunosorbent assay [ELISA], latex test, and Laurell electroimmunoassay) for human blood, since a partial cross-reactivity exists with the Willebrand factor of different animal species.[23] Detection with functional tests, e.g., a reagent on the basis of lyophilized human thrombocytes and ristocetin is also indicated. For an exact classification, a multimeric analysis is necessary in some cases.

Inhibitors, Antithrombin   As the most important inhibitor of the blood coagulation system, the measurement of antithrombin activity is of clinical importance as an additional test in consumptive coagulopathy, particularly in cases with heparin therapy. The use of commercial test kits on the basis of factor II or factor-X-dependent chromogenic substrates is preferred. In animal species that have an antithrombin activity that is higher than that in humans (horse, 170%; cattle, 130%; and dog, 120%), modifications of the test instructions (predilution of the plasma, variation of the sample–reagent ratio or concentrated dissolution of the reagents) are often necessary. The measurement of other inhibitors such as protein C, α_2-macroglobulin and α-antitrypsin, for which there are also commercial test kits available on the basis of chromogenic substrates is particularly reserved for scientific questions.

Soluble Fibrin   Demonstration of increased activation of the blood coagulation system is often unnecessary in routine diagnostics. However, it is of enormous importance for scientific questions.

The method of choice for animal plasma is the measurement of the concentration of the soluble fibrin with a commercially available chromogenic substrate test.[24] The function principle of the test is based on the presence of fibrin having an accelerating effect on the activation of plasminogen through the plasminogen activator that is also present in the reagent. The extent of plasminogen activation into plasmin is then determined with a plasmin-dependent chromogenic substrate. For the dog, the reference values are <10 $\mu g/mL$ plasma.

To prove an increased concentration of soluble fibrin in individual samples of different species (e.g., dog, cat, and horse), a semiquantitative agglutination test is also suitable (e.g., FM [fibrin monomer]-test, Roche Diagnostics GmbH, Mannheim, Germany).[25] This test is based on human erythrocytes, which are laden with human fibrin monomers, agglutinating if an increased concentration of soluble fibrin is present in the sample.

REFERENCES

1. **Greene RA, Kabel, AL.** Hypercoagulable state in three dogs with nephrotic syndrome: role of acquired antithrombin III deficiency. J Am Vet Med Assoc 1982;181:914–917.
2. **Slappendel RJ.** Disseminated intravascular coagulation. Vet Clin North Am Small Anim Pract 1988;18:169–184.
3. **Tanaka H, Kobayashi N, Maekawa T.** Studies on production of antithrombin III with special reference to endotoxin—induced DIC in dogs. Thromb Haemost 1986;56:137–143.
4. **Kay MA, Landen CN, Rothenberg SR, Taylor LA, Leland F, Wiehle S, Fang B, Bellinger D, Finegold M, Thompson AR, Read M, Brinkhous KM, Woo SLC.** In vivo hepatic gene therapy. Complete albeit transient correction of factor IX deficiency in hemophilia B dogs. Proc Natl Acad Sci USA 1994;91:2353–2357.
5. **Littlewood JD.** Haemophilia A (factor VIII deficiency) in German Shepherd dogs. J Small Anim Pract 1988;29:117–128.
6. **White JG.** Morphological and functional aspects of cellular hemostatic mechanisms. Hämostaseologie 1996;16:78–87.
7. **Bauer KA.** Activation of the factor VII-tissue factor pathway. Thromb Haemost 1997;78:108–111.
8. **Schmaier AH.** Contact activation: a revision. Thromb Haemost 1997;78:101–107.
9. **Holmer E.** Anticoagulant properties of heparin and heparin fractions. Scand J Haematol 1980;25(suppl 36):25–39.
10. **Osbaldiston GW, Stowe EC, Griffith PR.** Blood coagulation: comparative studies in dogs, cats, horses and cattle. Br Vet J 1970;126:512–521.
11. **Middleton DJ, Watson ADJ.** Activated coagulation times of whole blood in normal dogs and dogs with coagulopathies. J Small Anim Pract 1978;19:417–422.
12. **Hartert H.** Biorheology in the practice of medicine: resonance thrombography. Biorheology 1984;21:19–32.
13. **Monce KA, Atkins CE, Loughman CM.** Evaluation of a commercially available prothrombin assay kit for use in dogs and cats. J Am Vet Med Assoc 1995;207:581–584.
14. **Lanevschi A, Kramer JW, Greene SA, Meyers KM.** Evaluation of chromogenic substrate assays for fibrinolytic analytes in dogs. Am J Vet Res 1996;57:1124–1130.
15. **Feldman BF.** Diagnostic approaches to coagulation and fibrinolytic disorders. Semin Vet Med Surg (Small Anim) 1992;7:315–322.
16. **Mischke R, Nolte I.** Optimization of prothrombin time measurements in canine plasma. Am J Vet Res 1997;58:236–241.
17. **Mischke R, Deniz A, Nolte I.** Influence of sample predilution on the sensitivity of prothrombin time in feline plasma. J Vet Med A 1996;43:155–162.
18. **Clauss A.** Gerinnungsphysiologische Schnellmethode zur Bestimmung des Fibrinogens. Acta Haematol 1957;17:237–246.
19. **Lewis JH.** Comparative hematology. Studies on cats including one with factor XII (Hageman) deficiency. Comp Biochem Physiol 1981;68A:355–360.
20. **Zondag ACP, Kolb AM, Bax NMA.** Normal values of coagulation in canine blood. Haemostasis 1985;15:318–323.
21. **Karges HE, Funk KA, Ronneberger H.** Activity of coagulation and fibrinolysis parameters in animals. Arzneim-Forsch Drug Res 1994;44:793–797.
22. **Nolte I, Niemann C, Bowry SK, Failing K, Müller-Berghaus G.** A method for measuring capillary bleeding time in non-anaesthetized dogs: prolongation of the bleeding time by acetylsalicylic acid. J Vet Med A 1997;44:625–628.
23. **Johnson GS, Turrentine MA, Kraus KH.** Canine von Willebrand's disease. A heterogeneous group of bleeding disorders. Vet Clin North Am Small Anim Pract 1988;18:195–229.
24. **Wiman B, Ranby M.** Determination of soluble fibrin in plasma by a rapid and quantitative spectrophotometric assay. Thromb Haemost 1986;55:189–193.
25. **Largo R, Heller V, Straub PW.** Detection of soluble intermediates of the fibrinogen-fibrin conversion using erythrocytes coated with fibrin monomers. Blood 1976;46:991–1002.

CHAPTER 74

Vascular Wall: Endothelial Cell

• RAFAEL RUIZ DE GOPEGUI and TOMÁS NAVARRO

The hemostatic response may be considered a defensive function that avoids blood loss from damaged vasculature (hemorrhage) and that ensures adequate blood flow, maintaining the vascular tree free of obstruction (thrombosis). The adequate equilibrium between activation and inhibition of hemostasis depends on interactions between endothelial cells, platelets, blood cells, coagulation activators, and coagulation inhibitors.

Vascular endothelial cells (EC) are the lining cells of blood vessels. In the past, vascular endothelium was considered the nonthrombogenic internal cover of blood vessels. However, these cells interact actively with plasma proteins and cells, playing a key role on hemostasis equilibrium. ECs are now recognized to have an important role in hemostasis, inflammatory reactions, and immunity. Hemostatic function of the EC is discussed in this chapter.

The EC possesses antithrombotic properties that maintain blood fluidity and prevent thrombus formation on the normal vascular wall. These properties change when endothelial cell activation occurs (Table 74.1). EC activation may be induced by loss of vascular integrity; expression of leukocyte adhesion molecules; cytokine production; or upregulation of major histocompatibility antigens (human leukocyte antigen [HLA]) molecules, originally termed human lymphocyte system A.[1]

Tissue factor (TF) synthesis may be enhanced by interleukin 1, tumor necrosis factor, mitogens, insulin, interferon, endotoxins, viruses, thrombin, immune complexes, phorbol esters, and occupancy of cell adhesion molecules.[2] Platelet, EC, and monocyte interaction induces or amplifies TF synthesis through P-selectin, E-selectin, and integrins. Phosphatidylserine is crucial for TF activity, acting as a cofactor of TF-factor VIIa complex.[3,4]

Von Willebrand's factor (vWf) is mainly synthesized in EC and stored in secretory vesicles termed Weibel–Palade bodies. ECs may release the factor into the vascular tree or into the subendothelial matrix where it is bound to collagen. Functionally active vWf release may be induced by thrombin, histamine, and fibrin.[5]

Plasminogen activator inhibitor type 1 (PAI 1) is the major physiologic inhibitor of tissue plasminogen activator (tPA). Endothelial synthesis and release may be increased by endotoxins,[6] stress, hormonal changes, and hypertriglyceridemia.[7]

The antithrombotic properties of EC depend on prostacyclin (PGI$_2$), thrombomodulin (TM), heparinlike molecules, tPA, ectoenzymes, protease nexins, TF pathway inhibitors, and nitric oxide synthesis.

Prostacyclin (PGI$_2$) is a metabolite of the arachidonic acid in the cyclooxygenase pathway that inhibits platelet activation, adhesion, secretion, aggregation, and maintains vascular relaxation. Prostacyclin synthesis and release may be stimulated by shear stress, interleukin-1, and thrombin.[8]

Thrombomodulin (TM) is an acidic integral membrane protein expressed on the luminal surface of EC. Thrombin bound to TM activates protein C and loses its procoagulant activity. Activated protein C (APC) with its cofactor protein S digests factors Va and VIIIa, thus inhibiting tenase and prothrombinase complexes. Protein S is a vitamin-K-dependent glycoprotein synthesized by the liver, the megakaryocytes, and the endothelium. Protein S duplicates APC-dependent inactivation of factors VIIIa and Va. Thrombin-cleaved protein S has also an APC-independent anticoagulant effect: It inhibits the prothrombinase reaction and the intrinsic factor X activation by means of a specific interaction with factor VIII. Plasma protein S circulates free or bound to the complement system inhibitor C4b-binding protein, which enhances the inhibitory effect on factor X.[9]

Heparinlike molecules include heparan sulfate proteoglycans (HSPG) and dermatan sulfate proteoglycans (DSPG). HSPGs catalyze thrombin inhibition by antithrombin III. They are bound to the luminal surface of the endothelium and present in the extracellular matrix. Microvascular endothelium synthesizes larger amounts of HPSG than endothelium of large vessels.[10] DSPGs are deposited in the extracellular matrix and expressed on the cell surface;[11] DSPGs are also synthesized by fibroblasts and smooth muscle cells. Dermatan sulfate may be considered the most potent heparin cofactor II activator,[12] which efficiently inhibits clot-bound thrombin.

Plasminogen activators catalyze the conversion of plasminogen to plasmin. EC synthesizes tissue tPA. It binds to fibrin and catalyzes plasminogen activation. It is considered the most important fibrinolytic system activator.[13]

Ectoenzymes (adenosine diphosphatase [ADPase],

TABLE 74.1	**Prothrombotic Modifications of Vascular Endothelium**	
Function	**Effect**	**Mechanism**
Coagulation	Activation	Expression of tissue factor
Coagulation inhibition	Impaired	Thrombomodulin and heparan sulfate proteoglycans loss
Fibrinolysis	Inhibition	Plasminogen activator inhibitor type I release
Platelets	Activation	Platelet activating factor release
Platelet aggregation inhibition	Impaired	Prostacyclin downregulation and ecto-ADPase loss

adenosine triphosphatase [ATPase], and angiotensin-converting enzyme) are located on the luminal surface of EC membrane. ADPase degrades adenosine diphosphate (ADP), which is a major mediator of platelet aggregation and vasoconstriction.

Platelet activation and adhesion to damaged vasculature are suppressed by PGI_2 and endothelium-dependent relaxing factor-nitric oxide (EDRF-NO or NO). Both molecules act synergistically on vasorelaxation and platelet aggregation inhibition.[14]

Annexin V is a nonglycosylated protein present in plasma, arterial EC, and venous EC. Anticoagulant activity of annexin V is based on its capability to bind to negatively charged phospholipids, displacing phospholipid-dependent coagulation factors.[15]

Protease nexin 1 (PN1) is a serpin synthesized by fibroblasts, muscle cells, nervous tissue, and platelets. PN1 acts as a suicide substrate for thrombin and urokinase (uPA). PN1 forms 1:1 stoichiometric complexes with these proteases, which are then rapidly bound, internalized, and degraded. Its inhibitory activity is accelerated by glycosaminoglycans.[16,17]

PN2 is a potent, reversible, and competitive inhibitor of factors IXa and XIa. High-molecular-weight heparin potentiates the ability of PN2 to inhibit factor XIa.[18,19]

Direct inhibitors of TF-factor VIIa complex include tissue factor pathway inhibitor 1 (TFPI 1), TFPI 2, annexin V, antithrombin III, sphingosine, and platelet factor 4. TFPI 1 is synthesized in the endothelium (mainly), the megakaryocytes, and the macrophages.[20] Plasma TFPI 1 circulates bound to low-density lipoproteins, but there is also an endothelial pool. Unfractionated heparin and, specifically, low-molecular-weight heparin enhances TFPI 1 release.[21] Inflammation enhances TF synthesis, whereas only a slight increase in TFPI 1 synthesis occurs.[22]

REFERENCES

1. **Hunt BJ, Jurd KM.** Endothelial cell activation. A central pathophysiological process. BMJ 1998;316:1328–1329.
2. **Mantovani A, Sozzani S, Vecchi A, Introna M, Allavena P.** Cytokine activation of endothelial cells: new molecules for an old paradigm. Thromb Haemost 1997;78:406–414.
3. **Adams DH, Shaw S.** Leucocyte-endothelial interactions and regulation of leucocyte migration. Lancet 1994;343:831–836.
4. **Bach R, Gentry R, Nemerson Y.** Factor VII binding to tissue factor in reconstituted phospholipid vesicles: induction of cooperativity by phosphatidylserine. Biochem 1986;25:4007–4020.
5. **Ruiz de Gopegui R, Feldman BF.** Von Willebrand factor. Comp Haematol Int 1997;7:187–196.
6. **Collatos C, Barton MH, Schleef R, Prasse KW, Moore JN.** Regulation of equine fibrinolysis in blood and peritoneal fluid on a study of colic cases and induced endotoxaemia. Equine Vet J 1994;26:474–481.
7. **Takada A, Takada Y, Urano T.** The physiological aspects of fibrinolysis. Thromb Res 1994;76:1–31.
8. **Wu KK.** Endothelial cells in hemostasis, thrombosis, and inflammation. Hosp Pract (Off Ed) 1992;27:145–166.
9. **Koppelman SJ, Hackeng TM, Sixma JJ, Bouma BN.** Inhibition of the intrinsic factor X activating complex by protein S: evidence for a specific binding of protein S to factor VIII. Blood 1995;86:1062–1071.
10. **Marcum JA, Rosenberg RD.** Heparin-like molecules with anticoagulant activity are synthesized by cultured endothelial cells. Biochem Biophys Res Commun 1985;126:365–372.
11. **Cavari S, Vannucchi S.** Glycosaminoglycans exposed on the endothelial cell surface. Binding of heparin-like molecules derived from serum. FEBS Lett 1993;323:155–161.
12. **Sié P, Dupoy D, Caranobe C, Petitou M, Boneu B.** Antithrombotic properties of a dermatan sulfate hexasaccharide fractionated by affinity for heparin cofactor II. Blood 1993;81:1771–1777.
13. **Blombäck B.** Fibrinogen and fibrin–proteins with complex roles in hemostasis and thrombosis. Thromb Res 1996;83:1–75.
14. **Wu KK.** Endothelial nitric oxide synthase (eNOS) and cyclooxygenase (COX) in vasoprotection: a paradigm for vascular gene therapy. Thrombose 1998;2:3–7.
15. **Bombeli T, Mueller M, Haeberli A.** Anticoagulant properties of the vascular endothelium. Thromb Haemost 1997;77:408–423.
16. **Donovan FM, Vaughan PJ, Cunningham DD.** Regulation of protease nexin-1 target protease specificity by collagen type IV. J Biol Chem 1994;269:17199–17206.
17. **Knauer MF, Kridel SJ, Hawley SB, Knauer DJ.** The efficient catabolism of thrombin-protease nexin 1 complexes is a synergistic mechanism that requires both the LDL receptor-related protein and cell surface heparins. J Biol Chem 1997;272:29039–29045.
18. **Schmaier AH, Dahl LD, Rozemuller AJM, Roos RAC, Wagner SL, Chung R, van Nostrand WE.** Protease nexin-2/amyloid beta-protein precursor. A tight binding inhibitor of coagulation factor IXa. J Clin Invest 1993;92:2540–2548.
19. **Zhang Y, Scandura JM, Van Nostrand WE, Walsh PN.** The mechanism by which heparin promotes the inhibition of coagulation factor XIa by protease nexin-2. J Biol Chem 1997;272:16268–16273.
20. **Drew AF, Davenport P, Apostolopoulos J, Tipping PG.** Tissue factor pathway inhibitor expression in atherosclerosis. Lab Invest 1997;77:291–298.
21. **Hoppensteadt DA, Walenga JM, Fasanella A, Jeske W, Fareed J.** TFPI antigen levels in normal human volunteers after intravenous and subcutaneous administration of unfractionated heparin and low molecular weight heparin. Thromb Res 1995;77:175–183.
22. **Camerer E, Kolstø AB, Prydz H.** Cell biology of tissue factor, the principal initiator of blood coagulation. Thromb Res 1996;81:1–41.

CHAPTER 75

Congenital and Acquired Vascular Wall Diseases

• RAFAEL RUIZ DE GOPEGUI

Vascular endothelium plays a key role in the development of thrombosis, disseminated intravascular coagulation (DIC), defective hemostasis, atherosclerosis, and inflammation. Endothelial injury may be induced by infectious agents, prolonged hypotension, hypoxia, acidosis, inflammation, and immune mechanisms.

INHERITED VASCULAR WALL DISEASE

Ehlers–Danlos Syndrome

Ehlers–Danlos syndrome is also termed cutaneous asthenia and dermatosparaxis. It is an inherited connective tissue disease induced by an abnormal collagen synthesis. Increased vascular fragility has been described in human collagen diseases such as *pseudoxanthoma elasticum,* Marfan's syndrome, Rhendu–Ossler, and Ehlers–Danlos. However, the vascular fragility and subsequent bleeding tendency are not confirmed in veterinary medicine. The disease is characterized by joint laxity and skin hyperextensibility or fragility. As a result, affected animals may present with large skin tears, with little or no bleeding, secondary to slight trauma. The lacerations heal readily leaving visible cigarette paper scars. Some animals present subcutaneous hematomas as well. The disease has been reported in dogs, cats, sheep, cattle, minks, and humans.[1] Diagnosis is based on a clinical history of easily torn skin in absence of severe trauma, increased skin extensibility, and skin biopsy.[2] Prognosis is poor, and euthanasia is elected in most cases. Therapy consisting in vitamin C administration has been attempted, since it is necessary in collagen synthesis.[3]

von Willebrand's Disease

von Willebrand's disease can be considered an endothelial cell defect resulting in thrombopathia. (See Section XIII, Genetic Hematologic Disease.)

Familial Vasculopathy

Inherited disorders of blood vessels are rare in veterinary medicine. However, four canine breeds (German shepherd, beagle, Scottish terrier, and greyhound) may present an idiopathic and inherited vasculopathy. Vasculitis and collagenolysis have been observed in affected German shepherd dogs. Despite high concentrations of platelet factor (PF) 3 having been reported, hemorrhage or thrombocytopenia has not been observed.[4]

Cutaneous and renal glomerular vasculopathy of the greyhound is characterized by multifocal skin ulcerations often accompanied of limb edema and acute renal failure. Renal afferent arteriolar thrombosis, dermal arterial thrombosis, microangiopathy-induced hemolytic anemia, and thrombocytopenia, without abnormal coagulation screening tests, have been reported in affected greyhounds.[5]

ACQUIRED VASCULAR WALL DISEASE

Rocky Mountain Spotted Fever

Rickettsia ricketsii, a gram-negative bacterium in the family Rickettsiaceae and transmitted by tick vectors *Dermacentor andersoni, Dermacentor variabilis, and Amblyomma americanum* causes Rocky Mountain spotted fever. Clinical infection is recognized almost exclusively in the spring and summer months, when tick vectors are most active.[6] Acute disease develops during 2 weeks after infection.

R ricketsii replicates in endothelial cells, inducing necrotizing vasculitis. The altered endothelium induces platelet and fibrinolytic activation, causing thrombocytopenia and DIC. Clinical signs may include fever, depression, petechiae, ecchymosis, edema, lameness, dyspnea, nasal and ocular discharge, cough, vomiting, diarrhea, lymphadenopathy, splenomegaly, cardiac arrhythmia, and renal failure. Central nervous system involvement, often as vestibular disease, is caused by diffuse meningoencephalitis.[7]

Clinical diagnosis of RMSF is based on clinical history, physical examination, laboratory data, serum indirect immunofluorescence (IFA) assay or enzyme linked immunosorbent assay (ELISA), and response to therapy. Serologic testing can be negative in acute cases.

Effective treatment may be achieved with doxycycline 5 mg/kg q12h, orally, 14 to 21 days. Chloramphenicol, oxytetracycline, and enrofloxacin may also be considered. Severe cases may require intravenous fluid or transfusion therapy as well.

Heartworm Disease

Heartworm disease is caused by the nematode *Dirofilaria immitis* and is transmitted by *Culex* and *Anopheles* genus mosquitoes. Heartworm infection is common in endemic areas, affecting dogs more frequently than cats.

Clinical presentations vary among minimal respiratory signs to severe right congestive cardiac failure and multisystemic disease.

Adult worms reside in the right ventricle and pulmonary artery but, with high numbers of adult worms, they may reach the right atrium and the caudal *vena cava*. Adult *D immitis* have been identified in aberrant locations such as systemic arterial system, aorta, liver, eyes, central nervous system, skin, muscles, peritoneum, and bronchioles.[8] Severe parasite burden may induce caval syndrome, due to partial obstruction of blood flow into the right ventricle and interference with tricuspid valve closure. Caval syndrome is characterized by acute disease course, severe anemia, liver disease, renal disease, cardiac congestion, intravascular hemolysis, and hemoglobinuria.[9]

Endothelial damage by adult worms leads to villous myointimal proliferation and subendothelial exposition. *Dirofilariae* depress endothelium-dependent relaxation and induce pulmonary arterial endothelium proliferation and thickening of *tunica media*.[10] Microfilariae induce antigen-antibody formation, immune-mediated sensitization and pulmonary eosinophilic infiltrates. As a result, cardiopulmonary lesions such as pulmonary hypertension, pulmonary infiltrates with eosinophilia, allergic pneumonitis, pulmonary thromboembolism, or right ventricle hypertrophy may develop.

Hemostasis is activated because of the endothelial damage leading to platelet activation and hypercoagulability. Depending on the severity of the case, thrombocytopenia, DIC or pulmonary thromboembolism may occur.

Diagnosis requires direct identification of microfilariae (Knott test) or ELISA for adult filarial antigen (occult antigen). Microfilaremia is seldom found in feline heartworm disease.[11] Therapy requires cage rest and hospitalization and comprises symptomatic therapy and elimination of the parasites. Adulticide therapy may be achieved with thiacetarsamide 2.2 mg/kg (4 doses in 48 hours) intravenously (IV) or melarsomine 2.5 mg/kg (two doses in 2 days) intramuscularly (IM). Individual evaluation is mandatory. Surgical extraction of adult worms should be considered if adult worms are present in right atrium and vena cava. Prophylaxis consisting of ivermectin, milbemycin oxime, or diethylcarbamazine is strongly recommended. Microfilaricide therapy must be administered 4 weeks after adulticide therapy.[12]

Leishmaniasis

Leishmaniasis are a group of infections caused by an intracellular protozoa of the genus *Leishmania* belonging to the family of Trypanosomatidae. With some exceptions, leishmaniasis are zoonotic diseases with transmission between sand fly vectors of the genus *Phlebotomus* or *Sergentomyia* (Africa, Asia, and Europe), *Lutzomyia* (America), and mammalian reservoirs in sylvatic or peridomestic cycles.[13]

In endemic areas, leishmaniasis is frequent in dogs and infrequent in cats and horses. Most dogs develop viscerocutaneous leishmaniasis and the cutaneous form is considered a manifestation of dissemination of the parasites. The classic form causes chronic wasting, decreased activity, anemia, anorexia, fever that waxes and wanes, diarrhea, conjunctivitis, rhinitis, lameness, epistaxis, splenomegaly, and renal failure. Most common dermatologic clinical signs include alopecia, nonpruritic diffuse dry seborrhea, scaling on the nose, face and extremities, erosions, and onychogryphosis. Cutaneous nodules also can be present, but they are less common. Ocular manifestations include conjunctivitis, keratitis, anterior uveitis, blepharitis, and retinitis.[14] Analytic results reveal hypochromic normocytic anemia, hyperproteinemia, dysproteinemia (decrease of albumin and increase of γ globulin). The increase of γ globulins is caused by polyclonal activation of B lymphocytes and dysregulation of T lymphocytes.[15] Monoclonal gammopathy has seldom been reported.[16] Thrombocytopenia, thrombopathia, prolonged thrombin time, and increased fibrin or fibrinogen degradation products indicate that *Leishmania* infection may affect primary hemostasis, coagulation, and fibrinolysis. The compromise of hemostasis is multiple, and *Leishmania* infection may potentially induce DIC.[17] The mechanism of the altered hemostasis remains unclear, but multiple factors may be involved. Disseminated intravascular coagulation may be triggered by the endothelial damage induced directly by *Leishmania* protozoa or by the deposition of circulating immunocomplex.[18] Renal disease caused by canine leishmaniasis may induce thrombosis owing to protein-losing glomerulopathy or aggravated DIC.[19]

The presence of *Leishmania* sp. amastigotes has been described within macrophages cytoplasm of mononuclear phagocyte system and other locations including spleen, lymph nodes, tonsils, bone marrow, liver, urinary bladder, intestinal lamina propria, lung alveolar macrophages, choroid plexus,[20] cerebrospinal fluid,[21] urine, semen,[22] and peritoneal fluid[23]; *Leishmania* sp. amastigotes have also been observed in other phagocyte cell types than macrophages, including monocytes, neutrophils, eosinophils, endothelial cells, and fibroblasts.[24]

Diagnosis of leishmaniasis has been traditionally

based on cytologic or histopathologic observation of *Leishmania* sp. amastigotes. In cytologic preparations, several staining methods, such as Giemsa, Romanowsky and Wright, or Diff-Quik, can be used to recognize amastigotes. Immunoperoxidase staining is more sensitive for the identification of *Leishmania* spp. in tissues.[25] The application of polymerase chain reaction (PCR) allows to identify *Leishmania* more accurately and even with sparse diagnostic samples.[26] Identification of anti-*Leishmania* antibodies, in serum, may be attempted by several methods, including indirect IFA, ELISA, immunoblot analysis (Western blot), direct agglutination test (DAT), or indirect immunoperoxidase assay (IPA). Serologic testing should be attempted if visceral leishmaniasis is suspected and parasitologic diagnosis is negative. However, a positive serologic titer does not imply that the dog will develop clinical leishmaniasis. In localized cutaneous leishmaniasis, serologic diagnosis can be unreliable in both dogs and people and direct diagnosis is required.[27]

There is no a unique or universally effective therapy for leishmaniasis. Canine leishmaniasis has a worse prognosis than human forms of the disease, and relapses are frequently observed. Allopurinol (10 to 15 mg/kg q12h orally) can be used for long-term administration (6 months) in canine leishmaniasis, as a single drug or combined with pentavalent antimonial compounds as sodium stibogluconate or meglumine antimonate (50 to 100 mg/kg q12h subcutaneously 15 to 20 days).

Treatment of leishmaniasis in both people and dogs can be unrewarding, making prevention the key for long-term success. Prevention of leishmaniasis depends on the knowledge of the parasite life cycle and the control of the vector. The use of permethrin treated screens,[28] or dog collars impregnated with deltamethrin have been used to control sand flies.[29]

Equine Viral Arteritis

Equine viral arteritis is a contagious infection caused by the equine arteritis virus of the family Arteriviridae. The virus replicates in macrophages and endothelial cells, but may have a predilection for the media of small muscular arteries. Clinical signs may include fever, depression, abdomen and limb edema, stomatitis, and petechiae. In severe cases, hematology alterations include neutrophilia, lymphopenia, eosinopenia, and thrombocytopenia. Diagnosis may be achieved by ELISA.[30]

Feline Infectious Peritonitis

Feline infectious peritonitis virus (Coronaviridae) replicates in the cytoplasm of macrophages. Infected macrophages migrate in the blood to venules in serosal and pleural surfaces, meninges, ependyma, and uveal tissue. Infected macrophages tend to congregate around small vessels, inducing disseminated vasculitis that may involve multiple organs.[31] Vascular endothelium damage increases vascular permeability and compromises hemostasis. Direct effects of the virus on platelets, mono-

nuclear inflammatory cells, and vascular endothelium induce a procoagulant state.[32] Severe thrombosis and vasculitis may occur owing to feline infectious peritonitis virus infection; associated with immune-complex deposition in vascular lesions, thrombocytopenia, and DIC.

Clinical presentation depends on the virulence of the causal agent, host immune response, and organ systems affected. Clinical signs may include hyperthermia; anorexia; depression; abdominal or pleural effusions (exudative form); pyogranulomas in omentum, intestine, and kidneys (dry form); mesenteric lymphadenopathy; uveitis; and neurologic involvement. Laboratory abnormalities vary depending on clinical presentation and severity. However, nonregenerative anemia, neutrophilia, lymphopenia, thrombocytopenia, and increased $\alpha2$ globulin and γ globulin (albumin : globulin ratio less than 0.81) are common.[33] Hyperglobulinemia may occur in plasma, abdominal and pleural effusions. Diagnostic procedures include serum indirect IFA and ELISA,[34] direct IFA of cytocentrifuged pleural and peritoneal effusions, PCR,[35] and immunoperoxidase of histopathologic sections of tissues.[36] Although, differentiation among enteric coronaviruses and feline infectious peritonitis virus is still challenging. Therapy is based on supportive care, immunosuppression, antiviral agents, and immunomodulation; but results are inconsistent and prognosis should be guarded.[37] An intranasal vaccine is available, but avoiding exposure to the virus is the best prophylactic measure.

Neoplasia

Neoplasia may induce vascular lesions and subsequent hemorrhage. Vascular neoplasia, such as hemangiosarcoma may induce severe hemostatic compromise. (See Chapter 83, Acquired Coagulopathy III: Neoplasia.)

Endocrinopathy

In severe cases of hypoadrenocorticism, gastrointestinal hemorrhage has also been described.[38] Ecchymosis may also occur with hypoadrenocorticism, most probably caused by diminished muscular support of the vascular tree. Direct vascular involvement by tumor growth may occur owing to Cushing's disease.[39]

Equine Purpura Hemorrhagica

Equine purpura hemorrhagica is a vasculitis syndrome that may follow *Streptococcus equi* or influenza virus infection. Clinical signs include subcutaneous edema and mucosal petechiae, but dyspnea, colic, dysphagia, laminitis, or renal disease may occur. Diagnosis is based on clinical history and observation of leukocytoclastic venulitis in skin biopsy.[40]

Other

Other causes of acquired vascular lesion are immune-mediated disease, drug reaction,[41] trauma, gastrointestinal ulcer, and vitamin C deficiency. Vascular involvement has also been suggested in equine exercise-induced pulmonary hemorrhage.[42]

REFERENCES

1. **Hegreberg GA, Padgett GA.** Ehlers-Danlos syndrome in animals. Bull Pathol 1967;8:247.
2. **Barnett KC, Cottrell BD.** Ehlers-Danlos syndrome in a dog. J Small Anim Pract 1987;28:941.
3. **Scott DW, Muller WH, Griffin CE.** Congenital and hereditary defects. Muller & Kirk's small animal dermatology. 5th ed. Philadelphia: WB Saunders, 1995;736–805.
4. **Weir JAM, Yager JA.** Familial cutaneous vasculopathy of German Shepherd dogs. Vet Dermatol 1993;4:41.
5. **Cowan LA, Hertzke DM, Fenwick BW, Andreasen CB.** Clinical and clinicopathologic abnormalities in Greyhounds with cutaneous and renal glomerular vasculopathy: 18 cases (1992–1994). J Am Vet Med Assoc 1997;210:789–793.
6. **Greene CE.** Rocky Mountain spotted fever. J Am Vet Med Assoc 1987;191:666–671.
7. **Lappin MR.** Rickettsial diseases. In: Leib MS, Monroe WE, eds. Practical small animal internal medicine. Philadelphia: WB Saunders, 1997;861–872.
8. **Goggin JM, Biller DS, Rost CM, DeBey BM, Ludlow CL.** Ultrasonographic identification of *Dirofilaria immitis* in the aorta and liver of a dog. J Am Vet Med Assoc 1997;210:1635–1637.
9. **Kitagawa H, Kitoh K, Iwasaki T, Sasaki Y.** Comparison of laboratory data in dogs with heartworm caval syndrome surviving and nonsurviving after surgical treatment. J Vet Med Sci 1997;59:609–611.
10. **Matsukura Y, Washizu M, Kondo M, Motoyoshi S, Itoh A, Nakajyo S, Shimizu K, Urakawa N.** Decreased pulmonary arterial endothelium-dependent relaxation in heartworm-infected dogs with pulmonary hypertension. Am J Vet Res 1997;58:171–174.
11. **Atkins CE, Atwell RB, Dillon R, Genchi C, Hayasaki M, Holmes RA, Knight DH, Lukof DK, McCall JW, Slocombe JOD.** American Heartworm Society Guidelines. Compend Cont Educ Pract Vet. 1997;19:422–429.
12. **Bond BR.** Heartworm disease. In: Leib MS, Monroe WE, eds. Practical small animal internal medicine. Philadelphia: WB Saunders, 1997;235–252.
13. **Hommel M, Jaffe CL, Travi B, Milon G.** Experimental models for leishmaniasis and for testing anti-leishmanial vaccines. Ann Trop Med Parasitol 1995;89:S55–S73.
14. **Roze M.** Histopathology and serology studies in ocular leishmaniasis of the dog. Proc Am Coll Vet Ophtalmol, 1986.
15. **Bunn-Moreno MM, Madeira ED, Miler K, et al.** Hypergammaglobulinemia in Leishmania donovani infected hamsters: possible association with a polyclonal activator of B cells and with suppression of T cell function. Immunology 1985;59:427–34.
16. **Font A, Closa JM, Mascort J.** Monoclonal gammopathy in a dog with visceral leishmaniasis. J Vet Intern Med 1994;8:233–235.
17. **Valladares JE, Ruiz de Gopegui R, Riera C, Alberola J, Gállego M, Espada Y, Portús M, Arboix M.** Study of haemostatic disorders in experimentally induced leishmaniasis in Beagle dogs. Res Vet Sci 1998;64:195–198.
18. **Pumarola M, Brevik L, Badiola J, et al.** Canine leishmaniasis associated with systemic vasculitis in two dogs. J Comp Pathol 1991;105:279–286.
19. **Font A, Gines C, Closa JM, Mascort J.** Visceral leishmaniasis and disseminated intravascular coagulation in a dog. J Am Anim Hosp Assoc 1994;204:1043–1044.
20. **Nieto CG, Viñuelas J, Blanco A, et al.** Detection of Leishmania infantum amastigotes in canine choroid plexus. Vet Rec 1996;139:346–347.
21. **Prasad LS, Sen S.** Migration of *Leishmania donovani* amastigotes in the cerebrospinal fluid. Am J Trop Med Hyg 1996;55:652–654.
22. **Riera C, Valladares E.** Viable Leishmania infantum in urine and semen of experimentally infected dogs. Parasitol Today 1996;12:412.
23. **Ruiz de Gopegui R, Espada Y.** What is your diagnosis? Peripheral blood and abdominal fluid from a dog with abdominal distention. Vet Clin Pathol 1998;27:64–67.
24. **Hervas-Rodriguez J, Mozos E, Mendez A, et al.** Leishmania infection of canine skin fibroblasts in vivo. Vet Pathol 1996;33:469–473.
25. **Sells PG, Burton M.** Identification of *Leishmania* amastigotes and their antigens in formalin fixed tissue by immunoperoxidase staining. Trans R Soc Trop Med Hyg 1981;75:461–468.
26. **Mathis A, Deplazes P.** PCR and in vitro cultivation for detection of *Leishmania* spp. in diagnostic samples from humans and dogs. J Clin Microbiol 1995;33:1145–1149.
27. **Mengistu G, Akuffo H, Fehniger TE, et al.** Comparison of parasitological and immunological methods in the diagnosis of leishmaniasis in Ethiopia. Trans R Soc Trop Med Hyg 1992;86:154–157.
28. **Basimike M, Mutinga MJ.** Effects of permethrin-treated screens on phlebotomine sand flies, with reference to *Phlebotomus martini*. J Med Entomol 1995;32:428–432.
29. **Killickkendrick R, Killickkendrick M, Focheux C, Dereure J, Puech MP, Cadiergues MC.** Protection of dogs from bites of phlebotomine sandflies by deltamethrin collars for control of canine leishmaniasis. Med Vet Entomol 1997;11:105–111.
30. **Monreal L, Villatoro AJ, Hooghuis H, Ros I, Timoney PJ.** Clinical features of the 1992 outbreak of equine viral arteritis in Spain. Equine Vet J 1995;27:301–304.
31. **Hoskins JD.** Update on feline coronavirus disease. In: August JR, ed. Consultations in feline internal medicine. 3rd ed. Philadelphia: WB Saunders, 1997;44–50.
32. **Boudreaux MK, Weiss RC, Toivio-Kinnnucan M, Cox N, Spano JS.** Enhanced platelet reactivity in cats experimentally infected with feline peritonitis virus. Vet Med 1990;27:269–273.
33. **Lappin MR.** Viral diseases. In: Leib MS, Monroe WE, eds. Practical small animal internal medicine. Philadelphia: WB Saunders, 1997.
34. **Troy GC, Becker MJ, Greene RT.** Proficiency testing of selected antigen and antibody tests for use in dogs and cats. J Am Vet Med Assoc 1996;209:914–917.
35. **Gamble DA, Lobbiani A, Gramegna M, Moore LE, Colucci G.** Development of a nested PCR assay for detection of feline infectious peritonitis virus in clinical specimens. J Clin Microbiol 1997;35:673–675.
36. **Kennedy MA, Brenneman K, Millsaps RK, Black J, Potgieter LN.** Correlation of genomic detection of feline coronavirus with various diagnostic assays for feline infectious peritonitis. J Vet Diagn Invest 1998;10:93–97.
37. **Watari T, Kaneshima T, Tsujimoto H, Ono K, Hasegawa A.** Effect of thromboxane synthetase inhibitor on feline infectious peritonitis in cats. J Vet Med Sci 1998;60:657–659.
38. **Medinger TL, Williams DA, Bruyette DS.** Severe gastrointestinal hemorrhage in three dogs with hypoadrenocorticism. J Am Vet Med Assoc 1993;202:1869–1872.
39. **Vandenbergh AGGD, Voorhout G, van Sluijs FJ, Rijnberk A, van den Ingh TSGAM.** Haemorrhage from a canine adrenocortical tumour: a clinical emergency. Vet Rec 1992;131:539–540.
40. **Morris DD.** Diseases of the hemolymphatic system. In: Reed SM, Bayly WM, eds. Equine internal medicine. Philadelphia: WB Saunders, 1998;558–607.
41. **Morris DO.** Cutaneous vasculitides. Proceedings of the 16th ACVIM Forum San Diego, CA, 1998.
42. **Weiss DJ, McClay CB, Smith CM, Rao CHR, White JG.** Platelet function in the racing thoroughbred: implication for exercise-induced pulmonary hemorrhage. Vet Clin Pathol 1990;19:35–39.

CHAPTER 76

Coagulation Activators

• FRANCISCO J. RONCALÉS and JUAN MANUEL SANCHO

The mechanism of blood coagulation constitutes a complex and dynamic process of platelets, plasma, and blood vessel endothelium interaction. Blood coagulation is part of the hemostatic process. It is usually initiated through vessel wall damage and subsequent protease enzymes activation, ending with soluble fibrinogen into insoluble fibrin transformation. On the other hand, the natural anticoagulant mechanisms limit and localize hemostatic plug (thrombus) formation at the injured blood vessel site. The procoagulant system is composed of serine protease enzymes and cofactors. It requires the interaction with phospholipids provided by platelets or damaged endothelial cells. The blood coagulation system has classically been divided into intrinsic and extrinsic pathways for factor X activation (Fig. 76.1). The extrinsic pathway may be the form of initial fibrin formation. Actually, some authors propose the concept of two stages rather than two pathways: the first phase, initiation, depends on tissue factor, and the second phase, augmentation, includes the components of the previously termed intrinsic pathway.[1] However, the concept of two pathways is useful in clinical practice since the most used coagulation tests are prothrombin time and activated partial thromboplastin time, which explore extrinsic and intrinsic pathways, respectively.[2]

PLASMATIC COAGULATION BIOCHEMISTRY

The plasmatic phase of blood coagulation involves a group of serine protease enzymes (coagulation factors) that are in inactive form and undergo activation after coagulation initiation. These coagulation factors are outlined in the text that follows.[3-4]

Contact Pathway Factors

Factor XII (Hageman factor) is a single chain glycoprotein of 80,000 d codified in human chromosome 5, with a plasmatic concentration of 30 μg/mL. Activated factor XII is a two-chain enzyme with light and heavy chains.

The light chain has the enzymatic activity. Factor XII belongs to the contact pathway and initiates the intrinsic blood coagulation pathway. However, factor XII also has an effect on the extrinsic pathway (factor VII can be activated by factor XIIa), on the complement (activates the classical pathway of complement by interacting with macromolecular C1), and on fibrinolysis (suggested by the homology of factor XII with tissue plasminogen activator and urokinase).[5] Factor XII has not been detected in avians and cetaceans.[6]

Prekallikrein (Fletcher factor) is a glycoprotein of 85,000 d, synthesized in the liver as a single-chain protein. It is activated to kallikrein (two-chain enzyme) by factor XIIa. The light chain has catalytic activity: activates soluble factor XII and cleaves high-molecular-weight kininogen (HMWK). Concentration in human plasma is 50 μg/mL.[4-5]

HMWK is an α globulin with a plasmatic concentration of 80 μg/mL. Kallikrein cleaves HMWK and releases a nonapeptide and a kinin-free protein with two peptidic chains (62,000 and 56,000 d). Factor XIIa cleaves HMWK similarly to kallikrein.[4-5] The light chain has procoagulant activity.

Factor XI (Rosenthal factor, plasma thromboplastin antecedent [PTA]) is a serine protease with two identical sulfide-linked chains of 160,000 d codified in human chromosome 4 and synthesized by the liver. Plasma factor XI forms a complex with HMWK and has a concentration of 5 to 6 μg/mL in humans. Factor XI activity in birds and horses is lower than in humans.[6]

Vitamin-K-Dependent Factors

Besides protein C (PC) and protein S, there are four blood factors that require vitamin K to be functional. They are serine proteases with catalytic domains at their carboxyl-terminal end. These factors are synthesized in the liver as proteins with a signal peptide in their amino-terminal end, which is removed after glycosylation. Probably, this peptide affects the glutamic acid (Gla) residues (Gla domain) carboxylation. This reaction, catalyzed by γ glutamylcarboxylase (vitamin-K-dependent enzyme), occurs within the hepatocyte. Most vitamin-

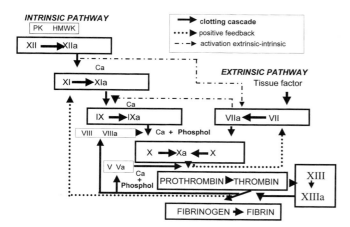

FIGURE 76.1 Regulation of blood coagulation. PK: prekallikrein; HMWK: high-molecular-weight kininogen; Phosphol: phospholipids.

K-dependent factors have an activation peptide in their molecule that is released after the activation. Thus, an active two-chain enzyme exposes its catalytic domains.[3]

Factor IX (Christmas factor, plasma thromboplastin component [PTC]) is a 57,000-d, single-chain glycoprotein with plasmatic concentration of 5 μg/mL and is codified in chromosome X.

Factor VII (proconvertin) is a 48,000-d, single-chain glycoprotein with a low plasmatic concentration (0.5 μg/mL) caused by its short life span and codified in human chromosome 13.

Factor II (prothrombin) is a 70,000-d, single-chain serine protease with plasmatic concentration of 100 μg/mL, codified in human chromosome 11. The active form, thrombin, is constituted by two sulfide-linked chains.

Factor X (Stuart-Prower factor) is a 55,000-d, two-chain, vitamin K-dependent glycoprotein, codified in human chromosome 13 with a plasmatic concentration of 10 μg/mL.

Cofactors and Other Factors

Factor V (proaccelerin) is a 350,000-d, single-chain, nonenzymatic cofactor with a plasmatic concentration of 10 μg/mL and is codified in human chromosome 1. Its structure is similar to factor VIII. Factor V has three regions termed A, B, and C (domain organization A1-A2-B-A3-C1-C2). The region A has homology with ceruloplasmin and may bind calcium; the region C binds to platelet phospholipids; and the function of domain B is unknown. Factor V is activated to factor Va by thrombin, which cleaves away the B domain, leaving a heterodimeric structure composed of a heavy chain (A1-A2) and a light chain (A3-C1-C2).[3,7]

Factor VIII or antihemophilic factor A (AHF) is a 250,000-d, glycoprotein nonenzymatic cofactor codified in chromosome X. Plasma factor VIII circulates complexed with von Willebrand factor (vWf) with a concentration of 0.1 μg/mL and a life span of 10 hours. However, in absence of vWf, its plasma half-life is sig-

nificantly reduced. Activation of factor VIII by thrombin results in a heterotrimer with an A1, A2, and A3-C1-C2 subunit.[3–4]

vWF factor is a multimeric adhesive glycoprotein composed of 270-kd polypeptide subunits linked by disulfide bonds and synthesized by endothelial cells and megakaryocytes. It is codified in human chromosome 12. Plasma vWf also forms high-molecular-weight (between 800,000 and 12.5 × 10⁹ d) multimers and has a concentration of 10 μg/mL. vWF is required for platelet adhesion and aggregation through the platelet's glycoprotein Ib/IX receptor complex and integrin $\alpha_{IIb}\beta_3$.[3,4,8]

Tissue factor (TF) is a single-chain glycoprotein complexed with phospholipids and synthesized as a 295 amino acid polypeptide. Its mature form has three regions: a 21 amino acid intracellular domain, a 23 amino acid transmembrane segment, and a 219 amino acid extracellular region. TF has been found in vascular adventitia, skin epithelium, mucosa, and connective tissue surrounding most organs; but it has not been found in unperturbed endothelium. This support the hypothesis that TF would constitute a hemostatic envelope, ready to initiate the blood coagulation after a disruption of the vascular wall.[1,9] TF synthesis by endothelial and monocyte cells can be induced by cytokines (interleukin [IL]-1, INF, tumor necrosis factor α [TNF α], virus, endotoxins, thrombin, immune complexes, phorbol esters, mitogens (platelet-derived growth factor, epidermal growth factor, insulin) and occupancy of cell adhesion molecules.[1]

Factor I (fibrinogen) is a 340,000-d glycoprotein with three pairs of chains disposed in two subunits. Its mean plasma concentration in people is 300 mg/dL and its life span ranges from 48 to 72 hours. Recently, a 420,000-d new form of fibrinogen has been described. This fibrinogen constitutes 1 to 2% of the total fibrinogen pool and appears more resistant to proteolytic degradation.[10,11]

Factor XIII (fibrin-stabilizing factor) is a 340,000-d protein composed of two subunits: A and B. One fragment from subunit A is released by thrombin in presence of calcium during activation to factor XIIIa.

EXTRINSIC PATHWAY

The extrinsic pathway is activated when TF, in the vascular adventitia or expressed on damaged cells, contacts and complexes with circulating factor VII. Complex formation of factor VII and TF is enhanced in the presence of calcium and phospholipids.[1,12,13] Factor VII is activated by factors Xa and IXa or by factor XIIa. Factor VIIa-TF complex then activates factor X, which then activates factor IX. Then extrinsic activation is considered the initiating way of blood coagulation. This fact may explain the relevance of factors VII, VIII, IX, and XI deficiencies.[1,14,15] The hemostatic effect of the extrinsic pathway is short lived because of the presence of several inhibitors of the TF-factor VII complexlike TF pathway inhibitor (TFPI)-1, TFPI-2, annexin V, antithrombin III (ATIII), sphingosine, and platelet factor 4.[1,16,17] TFPI-1 is mainly synthesized in vascular endothelium and appears to be the most active inhibitor of factor VIIa-TF complex. The effectiveness of TFPI decreases if factors IX and VIII are present. Disseminated intravascular coagulation (DIC) has been studied in rabbits that have reduced TFPI-1 levels.[18,19] The anticoagulant effect of low-molecular-weight heparin (LMWH) depends on both TFPI-1 and ATIII.[17,20–22] The importance of the extrinsic pathway has been demonstrated in different thrombosis models in rabbits, baboons, and dogs.[20,23]

INTRINSIC PATHWAY

The intrinsic activation of factor X is induced by factor IXa. It is initiated through a negatively charged surface or an endotoxin contact. Factor XII complexes with factor XI and HMWK, undergoing factor XII activation. Factor XIIa activates factor XI and prekallikrein. Kallikrein accelerates the process by factor XII activation increase: positive feedback. Kallikrein catalyzes also an autolytic cleavage, producing β kallikrein, with decreased coagulant activity and HMWK cleavage.[5] HMWK binds to prekallikrein and factor XI as cofactor for the contact system surface-mediated reactions. The significance of contact pathway in the physiologic blood coagulation process remains controversial because isolated deficiencies of factor XII, prekallikrein, or HMWK do not induce hemorrhagic tendency.

Factor IX is activated by factor XIa. The newly generated factor IXa activates factor X. This activation is significantly enhanced by factor IXa and factor VIII (activated by traces of thrombin) complex formation in presence of calcium and phospholipid. The endothelium provides a specific 140-kd membrane protein for factor IXa. This protein enhances the union of IXa-VIIIa-X complex on the endothelial surface, where the coagulation process occurs.

PHASE OF THROMBUS FORMATION

The result of both pathways, intrinsic and extrinsic, is the conversion of the factor X to Xa. Factor Xa binds to factor Va, calcium, and phospholipid, constituting the prothrombinase complex that rapidly activates prothrombin to thrombin.

Thrombin, a trypsinlike enzyme, cleaves fibrinogen releasing fibrinopeptides A and B from α and β chains, respectively, and one fibrin monomer. The released fibrinopeptides activate fibrinogen. Thrombin has primarily affinity for Aα chain. The sequence 8–23 and 34–51 of the Aα chain are of prime importance for the fibrinogen-thrombin interaction. Thus, fibrinopeptide A is released at the fastest rate and, after clot formation, fibrinopeptide B is released.[10] Polymerization of activated fibrinogen molecules involves interactions of domains A and B of the fibrinogen and complementary sites a and b (located in the fragment D domain and in the fragment D or αC domain, respectively). Polymerization initiates by interaction between the A do-

main of one molecule and the a site of another. Initial polymerization continues by fibrinopeptide B release, cleaved by thrombin, and interaction between the B domain and the b site.[10] The last step is the formation of covalent cross-linked fibrin, that involves factor XIIIa. Factor XIII is also activated by thrombin. It is a calcium-dependent transglutaminase that catalyzes the formation of peptidic links between glutamine and lysine residues of α and γ chains, releasing ammonia. Fibrin dimers are formed by cross-linked fragment D domains; α chains link at several levels. Stabilized fibrin is insoluble in urea or monochloroacetic acid that can dissolve nonstabilized fibrin or γ–γ crosslinked fibrin.[10] Factor XIII also induces fibrinogen polymerization[24] and catalyzes link formation between fibrinogen and fibronectin.[25] Other plasma proteins such as albumin may modulate the clot network formation.[10]

COAGULATION FACTORS IN DIFFERENT SPECIES

In early evolution periods hemostatic problems were solved in primitive animals by conversion of clotting protein called coagulogen into insoluble coagulin. Fibrinogen probably arises from a structurally related coagulogen of these primitive arthropods.[26] The development of higher organized animals lead finally to the complete clotting cascade with some variations.

Studies of reptilian hemostasis performed in *Python molurus bivittatus* demonstrate the presence of both extrinsic and intrinsic pathways. Fibrinogen plasma levels are similar to that of people, but there were only detected small levels of factors XII and VIII, whereas factors IX and VII, prekallikrein, and HMWK were undetectable. The activated short partial thromboplastin time, suggests the existence of prothrombin. However, the prothrombin time is shorter than in people.[27]

Activities of factors X and IX and vWf are lower in rat plasma than in human plasma, whereas factors V, VIII, XII, and ATIII activities were higher[28]; fibrinogen, prothrombin, and factors VII and XIII activities were equivalent.[29]

Rabbit plasma has equivalent factors VII and XII activities of human plasma. However, the rest of the factors have increased activities.[29]

Pigs have higher concentrations of factors V, VIII, IX, XI, and XII than humans. Yet, factor X, prothrombin, and fibrinogen levels are identical.[29,30]

Similar concentrations of fibrinogen and factor VIII have been demonstrated in human and baboon plasmas.[29,31]

Feline plasma has higher activities of factors V, VIII, IX, and XI; equivalent activities of factors VII and XIII; and lower activity of factor X than human plasma.[29]

Canine plasma has similar activity of prothrombin and higher activities of fibrinogen, factor VIII, and contact factors than human plasma.[29,31] Factor activities in disease behave similarly in the dog than in people. Dogs that have liver cirrhosis have decreased levels of factors VII and X, but normal factor VIII.[32] Increased concentrations of fibrinogen and higher activity of the coagulation factors V, VII, X, VIII, and IX have been observed in canine chronic renal failure.[33] Decreased activity of factors II, X, and XI has been described in dogs suffering from acute lymphoblastic leukemia, which is probably related to DIC.[34]

Factors I, V, VIII, IX, and IX levels are higher in sheep than in human plasma. Conversely, factors II, VII, X, XI, and XIII are lower in sheep than in human plasma.

In horses, activity of factors I, II, V, and X is higher than in people. Recently, the use of chromogenic assays to determine coagulation proteins such as factors VII, VIII, IX, and X and C1-esterase inhibitor in horses has been described.[35] Equine fibrinogen and C1-esterase inhibitor behave also as acute-phase proteins.[36]

MARKERS OF COAGULATION ACTIVATION

The recent advances in the knowledge of blood coagulation have yielded new methods for prethrombotic states diagnosis. These methods are based on the detection of coagulation activation markers. Increased levels of these markers suggests activation of the hemostatic mechanism but may not predict thrombosis. Their clinical application is yet limited since these techniques are not available in laboratory routine. These markers can be classified in several groups (Table 76.1).[37–39]

1. Activated blood factors
   Factor VIIa. Factor VIIa is the activation marker of the extrinsic pathway. The activity of factor VIIa can be measured in plasma by a functional assay that detects free factors.
   Factor XIIa. Factor XIIa may be determined by immunologic technique to evaluate the contact system activation.

TABLE 76.1 Activation Markers of Coagulation and Fibrinolysis

Activated Blood Factors
—Factor VIIa
—Factor XIIa
Peptides of Activation
—Factor IX activation peptide
—Factor X activation peptide
—Prothrombin fragment 1 + 2 (F 1 + 2)
—Fibrinopeptides A and B
—Peptide of activation of the protein C
Complexes Enzyme-Inhibitor
—Factor X-inhibitor
—Factor XI-inhibitor
—Thrombin-antithrombin complex (TAT)
—Protein C-inhibitor
Markers of Fibrinolytic Activation
—Plasmin-antiplasmin complexes
—D-dimer
—E fragment
—Bβ peptide 15-42

2. Activation peptides
   Factor IX activation peptide. Factor IX releases a 35 amino acid residue peptide in activation. Its life span is 15 minutes and can be determined by enzyme-linked immunosorbent assay (ELISA) or radioimmunoassay (RIA).
   Factor X activation peptide. Factor X releases a 52 amino acid residue peptide during activation. Its life span is 30 minutes and can be measured by ELISA or radioimmunoassay.
   Prothrombin fragment 1 + 2 (F1 + 2). F1 + 2 is the prothrombin activation peptide. It is a molecule of 273 amino acid residues with a life span of 90 minutes. It can be measured by immunoassays. Normal plasmatic concentration ranges from 0.67 to 1.97 nmol/L in humans. Determination of plasmatic concentration in New Zealand rabbits by ELISA was unrewarding.[40]
   Fibrinopeptide A. Fibrinopeptide A is the 16 amino acid residue peptide released from chain α of fibrinogen. Its life span is 3 to 5 minutes. Fibrinopeptide A concentration in human plasma determined by ELISA are approximately 1 pmol/L and by radioimmunoassay is 0.64 pmol/L. Accurate determination requires prior fibrinogen elimination of the sample. Fibrinopeptide A has been detected in baboons, mice, dogs, pigs, and sheep.[41]
   PC activation peptide. PC is a vitamin-K-dependent serin-protease glycoprotein. It inactivates factors Va and VIIIa by limited proteolysis. PC is activated by the thrombin-thrombomodulin complex and releases a polypeptide with a 5-minute life span.
3. Enzyme-inhibitor complexes
   Factor X-inhibitor. The concentration of factor Xa-ATIII complex may be measured by immunologic assay. This marker correlates with factor X activation.
   Factor XI-inhibitor. Complexes formed by factor XI and several inhibitors such as α1-antitrypsin (α1-AT), PC inhibitor, ATIII, and C1 inhibitor may be measured by ELISA.
   Thrombin-antithrombin III complex (TAT). Physiologically, thrombin is mostly inhibited by ATIII, forming a TAT complex, whose life span is 15 minutes. TAT complex concentration is determined by ELISA or RIA. This determination constitutes a thrombin formation indicator. TAT complexes have been determined in mice, rats, rabbits, dogs, pigs, horses, sheep, and baboons but not in avians.[41] In horses affected by carbohydrate-induced acute laminitis, measurement of TAT complexes did not indicate systemic activation of coagulation.[42] However, plasma TAT levels in horses that have colic reflected the systemic activation of hemostasis.[43]
   PC inhibitors (PCIs). The plasma concentration of PC-PCI is undetectable, but concentration of PC-α1-AT determined by ELISA is 7.5 ng/mL. The life span of these complexes is 40 and 140 minutes.
4. Markers of fibrinolytic activation
   Plasmin-antiplasmin complexes. The detection of plasmin-inhibitor complexes is a good fibrinolysis activation marker. The life span of these com-

plexes is 12 hours and can be measured by ELISA or RIA. The levels in human plasma range from 80 to 470 ng/mL.

D-dimers and other fibrinogen-fibrin degradation products. Plasmin has fibrinogen and fibrin as its major substrates, leading to the production of specific fragments called fibrinogen-fibrin degradation products. The most important is D-dimer, which is characteristic of fibrin breakdown and may be measured by ELISA or latex techniques.

The development of these markers provides a more precise knowledge of the hemostasis mechanisms and improves the prethrombotic states diagnosis. Thus, an increase of activation peptides and TAT complexes has been described in DIC, sepsis, neoplasia, surgical procedures, and liver diseases.[44,45] Fibrinogen and fibrin degradation products (FDPs) are routinely used for DIC diagnosis. Commercial test kits that contain latex particles coated with rabbit antihuman FDP antiserum constitute a rapid semiquantitative method for serum FDPs determination. In dog serum, a concentration of 10 μg/mL or more is considered evidence of increased fibrinolytic activity.[46,47] Coagulation and fibrinolysis activation markers are being widely studied in human and veterinary medicine. Increased levels have been described in myeloproliferative disease, lymphoproliferative disease, obstetric complications, thromboembolism,[48] venous thrombosis,[49] coumarin therapy,[50] inherited thrombophilic syndromes,[51] ulcerative colitis and Crohn's disease,[52] aortic aneurysm,[53] and exercise.[54] In conclusion, these markers provide information, in certain clinical situations, as regards thrombotic process initiation.

REFERENCES

1. **Camerer E, Kolstff AB, Prydz H.** Cell biology of tissue factor, the principal initiator of blood coagulation. Thromb Res 1996;81:1–41.
2. **Jesty J, Nemerson Y.** The pathways of blood coagulation. In: Beutler E, Lichtman MA, Coller BS, Kipps T, eds. Williams hematology. 5th ed. New York: Mc Graw Hill, 1995.
3. **Roberts HR, Lozier JN.** New perspectives on the coagulation cascade. Hosp Pract (Off Ed) 1992;27:97–112.
4. **Hathaway WE, Goodnight SH Jr.** Physiology of hemostasis and thrombosis. In: Pennington J, Finn S, eds. Disorders of hemostasis and thrombosis. A clinical guide. New York: McGraw-Hill, 1993.
5. **Wachtfogel YT, DeLa Cadena RA, Colman RW.** Structural biology, cellular interactions and pathophysiology of the contact system. Thromb Res 1993;72:1–21.
6. **Vergnes C, Pontois M.** La coagulation sanguine. Pratique médicale et chirurgicale de l'animal de compagnie 1985;20:265–277.
7. **Villoutreix BO, Dahlback B.** Structural investigation of the A domains of human blood coagulation factor V by molecular modeling. Protein Sci 1998;7:1317–1325.
8. **Ruiz de Gopegui R, Feldman BF.** Von willebrand's disease. Comp Haematol Int 1997;7:187–196.
9. **Solovey A, Gui LH, Key NS, Hebbel RP.** Tissue factor expression by endothelial cells in sickle cell anemia. J Clin Invest 1998;101:1899–1904.
10. **Blömback B.** Fibrinogen and fibrin-proteins with complex roles in hemostasis and thrombosis. Thromb Res 1996;83:1–75.
11. **Fu Y, Grieninger G.** Fib$_{420}$: a normal human variant with two extended α chains. Proc Natl Acad Sci U S A 1994;91:2625–2628.
12. **Sabharwal AK, Birktoft JJ, Gorka J, Wildgoose P, Petersen LC, Bajaj SP.** High affinity Ca(2+)-binding site in the serine protease domain of human factor VIIa and its role in tissue factor binding and development of catalytic activity. J Biol Chem 1995;270:15523–15530.
13. **Ruf W, Rhemtulla A, Morrisey JH, Edgington TS.** Phospholipid-independent and -dependent interactions required for tissue factor receptor and cofactor function. J Biol Chem 1991;266:16256.
14. **Bauer KA, Kass BL, Cate H, Hawiger JJ, Rosenberg RD.** Factor IX is activated in vivo by the tissue factor mechanism. Blood 1990;76:731–736.
15. **Nemerson Y.** The tissue factor pathway of blood coagulation. Semin Hematol 1992;29:170.
16. **Sprecher CA, Kisiel W, Mathewes S, Foster DC.** Molecular cloning, expression, and partial characterization of a second human tissue-factor-pathway inhibitor. Proc Natl Acad Sci U S A 1994;91:3353–3357.
17. **Rao LV, Rapaport SI, Hoang AD.** Binding of factor VIIa to tissue factor permits rapid ATIII/heparin inhibition of factor VIIa. Blood 1993;81:2600–2607.
18. **Sandset PM, Warn-Cramer BJ, Maki SL, Rapaport SI.** Immunodepletion of extrinsic pathway inhibitor sensitizes rabbits to endotoxin-induced intravascular coagulation and the generalized Shwartzman reaction. Blood 1991;78:1496–1502.
19. **Sandset PM, Warn-Cramer BJ, Rao LV, Maki SL, Rapaport SI.** Depletion of extrinsic pathway inhibition (EPI) sensitizes rabbits to DIC induced with tissue factor: Evidence supporting a physiological role for EPI as a natural anticoagulant. Proc Natl Acad Sci U S A 1991;88:708–712.
20. **Holst J, Lindblad B, Bergqvist D, Nordfang O, Ostergaard PB, Petersen JG, Nielsen G, Hedner U.** Antithrombotic effect of recombinant truncated tissue factor pathway inhibitor (TFPI1-161) in experimental venous thrombosis. A comparison with low molecular weight heparin. Thromb Haemost 1994;71:214–219.
21. **Kijowski R, Hoppenstead D, Walenga J, Borris L, Lassen MR, Fareed J.** Role of tissue factor pathway inhibitor in post surgical deep venous thrombosis (DVT) prophylaxis in patients treated with low molecular weight heparin. Thromb Res 1994;74:53–64.
22. **Rao LV, Nordfang O, Hoang AD, Pendurthi UR.** Mechanism of antithrombin III inhibition of factor VIIa/tissue factor activity on cell surfaces. Comparison with tissue factor pathway inhibitor/factor Xa-induced inhibition of factor VIIa/tissue factor activity. Blood 1995;85:121–129.
23. **Van'T Veer C, Hackeng TM, Delahaye C, Sixma JJ, Bouma BN.** Activated factor X and thrombin formation triggered by tissue factor on endothelial cell matrix in a flow model: effect of the tissue factor pathway inhibitor. Blood 1994;84:1132–1142.
24. **Blömback B, Procyk R, Adamson L, Hessel B.** Factor XIII induced gelation of human fibrinogen-An alternative thiol enhanced, thrombin independent pathway. Thromb Res 1985;37:613–628.
25. **Procyk R, Adamson L, Block M, Blömback B.** Factor XIII catalyzed formation of fibrinogen-fibronectin oligomers-a thiol enhanced process. Thromb Res 1985;40:833–852.
26. **Bergner A, Oganessyan V, Muta T, et al.** Crystal structure of a coagulogen, the clotting protein from horseshoe crab: a structural homologue of nerve growth factor. EMBO J 1996;15:6789–6797.
27. **Ratnoff OD, Rosenberg MJ, Everson B, et al.** Notes on clotting in a Burmese python (Python molurus bivittatus). J Lab Clin Med 1990;115:629–635.
28. **Lewis JH, Van Thiel DH, Hasiba U, et al.** Comparative hematology and coagulation: studies on rodentia (rats). Comp Biochem Physiol A 1985;82:211–215.
29. **Dodds WJ.** Hemostasis. In: Kaneko JJ, Harvey JW, Bruss ML, eds. Clinical biochemistry of domestic animals. 5th ed. San Diego: Academic Press, 1997;241–283.
30. **Roussi J, André P, Samama M, et al.** Platelet functions and haemostasis parameters in pigs: absence of side effects of a procedure of general anaesthesia. Thromb Res 1996;81:297–305.
31. **Feingold HM, Pivacek LE, Melaragno AJ, et al.** Coagulation assays and platelet aggregation patterns in human, baboon, and canine blood. Am J Vet Res 1986;47:2197–2199.
32. **Mischke R, Pohle D, Schoon HA, Fehr M, Nolte I.** Alterations of hemostasis in liver-cirrhosis of the dog. DTW 1998;105:43–47.
33. **Mischke R.** Alterations of hemostasis in dogs suffering from chronic renal-insufficiency. Berl Munch Tierarztl Wochenschr 1997;110:445–450.
34. **Mischke R, Freund M, Leinemannfink T, Eisenberger B, Casper J, Nolte I.** Hemostatic abnormalities in dogs suffering from acute lymphoblastic leukemia. Berl Munch Tierarztl Wochenschr 1998;111:53–59.
35. **Topper MJ, Prasse KW.** Chromogenic assays for equine coagulation factors VII, VIII:C, IX, and X, and C1-esterase inhibitor. Am J Vet Res 1998;59:538–541.
36. **Topper MJ, Prasse KW.** Analysis of coagulation proteins as acute-phase reactants in horses with colic. Am J Vet Res 1998;59:542–545.
37. **Kenneth A, Bauer MD.** New markers for in vivo coagulation. Curr Opin Hematol 1994;1:341–346.
38. **Manucci PM.** Diagnosis of the hypercoagulable state. Sangre (Barc) 1993;38:26–27.
39. **Páramo JA, López Y, Muñoz MC, et al.** Diagnosis of hypercoagulability states. Sangre (Barc) 1997;42:493–502.
40. **Monreal L, Angles AM, Ruiz de Gopegui R, et al.** Normal values for hematological and hemostatic parameters in the rabbit. Determination of new parameters for experimental models of thrombosis and hemostasis. Sangre (Barc) 1993;38:365–369.
41. **Ravanat C, Freund M, Dol F, Cadroy Y, Roussy J, Incardona F, et al.** Cross-reactivity of human molecular markers for detection of prethrombotic states in various animal species. Blood Coagul Fibrinolysis 1995;6:446–455.

42. **Weiss DJ, Monreal L, Angles AM, Monasterio J.** Evaluation of thrombin-antithrombin complexes and fibrin fragment D in carbohydrate-induced acute laminitis. Res Vet Sci 1996;61:157–159.

43. **Topper MJ, Prasse KW.** Use of enzyme-linked immunosorbent assay to measure thrombin-antithrombin III complexes in horses with colic. Am J Vet Res 1996;57:456–462.

44. **Payen JF, Baruch M, Horvilleur E, Richard M, Gariod T, Polack B.** Changes in specific markers of haemostasis during reduction mammoplasty. Br J Anaesth 1998;80:464–466.

45. **Novacek G, Kapiotis S, Jilma B, Quehenberger P, Michitsch A, Traindl O, Speiser W.** Enhanced blood coagulation and enhanced fibrinolysis during hemodialysis with prostacyclin. Thromb Res 1997;88:283–290.

46. **Feldman BF, Madewell BR, O'Neill S.** Disseminated intravascular coagulation: antithrombin, plasminogen and coagulation abnormalities in 41 dogs. J Am Vet Med Assoc 1981;179:151.

47. **Slappendel RJ.** Disseminated intravascular coagulation. Vet Clin North Am Small Anim Pract 1988;18:169–184.

48. **Bounameaux H, de Moerlose P, Perrier A, Reber G.** Plasma measurement of D-dimer as diagnostic aid in suspected venous thromboembolism: an overview. Thromb Haemost 1994;71:1–6.

49. **Monreal M, Angles AM, Monreal L, Roncalés J, Monasterio J.** Effects of recombinant hirudin on D dimer levels before and after experimental venous thrombosis. Haemostasis 1994;24:338–343.

50. **Elias A, Bonfils S, Doud Elias M, Gauthier B, Sie P, Boccalon H, et al.** Influence of long term oral anticoagulants upon prothrombin fragment 1+2, thrombin-antithrombin III complex and D-dimer levels in patient affected by proximal deep vein thrombosis. Thromb Haemost 1993;69:302–305.

51. **Manucci PM, Tripodi A, Botasso B, Baudo F, Finazzi G, De Stefano V, et al.** Markers of procoagulant imbalance in patients with inherited thrombophilic syndromes. Thromb Haemost 1992;67:200–202.

52. **Kjeldsen J, Lassen JF, Brandslund I, DeMuckadell OBS.** Markers of coagulation and fibrinolysis as measures of disease activity in inflammatory bowel disease. Scand J Gastroenterol 1998;33:637–643.

53. **Yamazumi K, Ojiro M, Okumura H, Aikou T.** An activate state of blood coagulation and fibrinolysis in patients with abdominal aortic aneurysm. Am J Surg 1998;175:297–301.

54. **Prisco D, Paniccia R, Bandinelli B, Fedi S, Cellai AP, Liotta AA, Gatteschi L, Giusti B, Colella A, Abbate R, Gensini GF.** Evaluation of clotting and fibrinolytic activation after protracted physical exercise. Thromb Res 1998; 89:73–78.

CHAPTER 77

Coagulation Inhibitors

• IAN B. JOHNSTONE

The blood coagulation mechanism consists of a series of proteolytic reactions in which inactive proenzymes (zymogens) are converted to active enzymes. Each serine protease is responsible for a subsequent proenzyme-to-enzyme conversion. The activation events take place on the surface of cells such as platelets, white cells, and endothelial cells. These reactions are catalyzed by nonenzymatic cofactors that either alter the conformation of the zymogen or bind converting enzymes and zymogens in proximity on the cell surface. It is the activity of these macromolecular complexes of converting enzyme, zymogen, and cofactor on a phospholipid membrane that form the basis of the major events in coagulation. Traditionally, the coagulation mechanism is divided into intrinsic (contact activated) and extrinsic (tissue factor [TF] activated) pathways.[1-3]

Factors V and VIII are cofactors in the coagulation mechanism and function in a similar manner. Activated factors Va and VIIIa bind to negatively charged phospholipid and serve as high-affinity receptors or cofactors for factors Xa and IXa, respectively, increasing their rates of activation.[4] Thrombin is central to the coagulation system, and its unopposed action results in blood clotting through the conversion of fibrinogen to fibrin. In addition, thrombin can act upon factors V, VIII, XI, and XIII; protein C; and blood platelets.

The activity of the coagulation mechanism is regulated in part by several events designed to attenuate the major events in the coagulation process by inhibiting converting enzymes, destroying protein cofactors, or preventing the availability of surface receptors necessary for the formation of the macromolecular complexes. These inhibitory agents are known as coagulation inhibitors.

The natural coagulation inhibitors consist of two major groups; the components of the antithrombin III (ATIII)–heparin pathway and the components of the thrombomodulin (TM)–protein C (PC)–protein S (PS) pathway. The ATIII–heparin pathway is a major system for the neutralization of activated factors of the intrinsic pathway. In the TM–PC–PS pathway, PS functions as a phospholipid-bound cofactor to activated PC (APC) in the degradation of factors VIIIa and Va, an effect that results in inhibition of tenase (factor VIIIa–factor IXa/Ca^{++}–phospholipid) and prothrombinase (factor Xa–factor Va–Ca^{++}–phospholipid) activities.[4] The effects of these two major inhibitory pathways is complimented by other natural plasma coagulation inhibitors.

The objective of the inhibitory pathways is to regulate the proteinases formed at the various steps in the amplification events of coagulation, and to downregulate a procoagulant stimulus as it passes down the coagulation cascade so that only a large procoagulant stimulus is capable of triggering fibrin production in sufficient amounts to generate an obstructive thrombus.[3] The ATIII–heparin and the TM–PC–PS inhibitory pathways play a particularly central role in modulating the thrombogenic status of the endothelium.[5] Disturbances in the normally delicate balance between procoagulation and the anticoagulation mechanisms through a reduction in the activity of coagulation inhibitors may result in hemostatic disorders known as thrombophilias.[6,7]

Much of the current information relating to coagulation inhibitors has been developed through investigations of acquired or inherited deficiency states in humans. However, coagulation inhibitors and their function and relative importance in nonhuman mammals is an expanding area of interest in veterinary medicine.[8,9]

ANTITHROMBIN III-HEPARIN SYSTEM

Antithrombin III

ATIII is a member of the serine-proteinase inhibitor family of proteins and was initially named the heparin cofactor when it was shown to be necessary for the anticoagulant activity of heparin. ATIII is now recognized to account for approximately 80% of the thrombin-inhibitory capacity of plasma.

Human ATIII is a single-chained alpha-2 globulin with a molecular weight of approximately 58 kD. Its structural and functional domains have been well defined.[3,10-13] It is synthesized in the liver[14] and in endothelial cells[15] and is normally present in human plasma at a concentration of approximately 150 μg/mL.[2,16] Many similarities of ATIII exist in mammalian antithrombins.[10]

The primary action of this glycoprotein is to bind to thrombin, preventing its action in converting fibrinogen to fibrin. ATIII neutralizes thrombin by forming a 1:1 stoichiometric complex by means of a reactive site (arginine) and an active site (serine) interaction.[2] This inhibitory effect of ATIII is catalyzed by heparin and by proteoglycans such as heparan sulfate (HS), which may be present in high concentrations locally at the endothelial surface. Exposure of HS and the receptor, TM on the surface off the vascular endothelium, likely helps to maintain fluidity at the vessel wall.[3,16]

Heparin-induced acceleration is caused by heparin binding to the lysine site on the ATIII molecule in such a way that the arginine site is allosterically modified and is more readily available for interaction with thrombin.[2] The arginine reactive site of ATIII irreversibly binds to the serine site on the activated clotting factor, rendering it inactive. Trace amounts of heparin can catalyze the interaction of large amounts of hemostatic enzyme and ATIII. Neutralization of hemostatic enzymes by the ATIII–heparin complex results in the release of the mucopolysaccharide from the protease inhibitor on a one-to-one molar basis (Fig. 77.1). Heparin is therefore capable of initiating multiple episodes of protease–protease inhibitor complex formation.

The activated hemostatic enzymes of the intrinsic coagulation pathway (factors XIIa, XIa, Xa, and IXa) are neutralized by ATIII in a manner similar to that of thrombin. Factor VIIa is only slowly inactivated by the ATIII–heparin complex.[17]

Thrombin–ATIII complexes (TAT) are formed on inactivation of thrombin by ATIII, and these complexes are cleared by the mononuclear phagocytic system. On release into the circulation, TAT complexes may bind to the protein, vitronectin (VT), and these TAT–VT complexes may then bind to endothelial HS proteoglycans and be subsequently internalized.[18] Increases in plasma concentrations of TAT complexes are useful indicators of latent activation of the clotting mechanism.[19–21] Increases in TAT complexes have been observed in conditions such as sepsis,[22] deep venous thrombosis,[19] disseminated intravascular coagulation (DIC),[23] and pregnancy.[24] Methods of quantifying plasma TAT complexes in animal plasmas are currently being investigated.[25]

Species differences in plasma concentrations of ATIII activity have been described, with the amounts being somewhat higher in the equine and bovine compared with the canine and man. Age- and breed-related differences in plasma ATIII activity have been reported in horses.[26–28]

Inherited deficiencies of ATIII are a common cause of spontaneous or recurrent venous thromboembolic disease in humans. Many variant forms that fall into two major categories have been described: Type I (classical) where there is a corresponding reduction in both ATIII antigen and ATIII activity caused by impaired synthesis of the protein and Type II (dysantithrombinemia) characterized by normal amounts of functionally deficient ATIII protein.[16,29] In inherited ATIII deficiency, it has been suggested that failure to regulate the coagulation mechanism is most evident after a major trigger to the system (i.e., pregnancy, surgery, or injury) that causes the impaired inhibitory mechanisms to be overwhelmed.[3]

Acquired deficiencies of plasma ATIII activity are common in DIC in humans[29,30] and in many species of domestic animals,[8,31,32] and with liver disease in horses and cattle.[32,33] Increases in plasma ATIII concentrations have been reported as part of the acute-phase inflammatory reaction in humans[34,35] and in cats.[9]

Heparin

Heparin is a highly sulfated glycosaminoglycan with a molecular weight ranging from 3 to 100 kD. It is synthesized by mast cells and is widely distributed in mammalian tissues, including the lung, liver, kidneys, heart, and intestine.[36] The structure of heparin is significantly heterogeneous and varies with respect to sequence and ratio of its hexose units, the extent of sulfation, and the degree of N-acetylation. Specific domains on the heparin molecule are responsible for its ability to form complexes with ATIII and to modulate the biological activity of this protease inhibitor.[37] Heparin is the only complex carbohydrate capable of binding to an antithrombin, activating the protease inhibitor and accelerating the neutralization of hemostatic enzymes. The pharmacokinetics of heparin in man and many species of animals has been well documented.[38–41]

The primary mechanism of action of heparin was described above. Heparin is an anticoagulant mainly by virtue of its ability to bind to and enhance the activity of ATIII, with the net effect being suppression of the

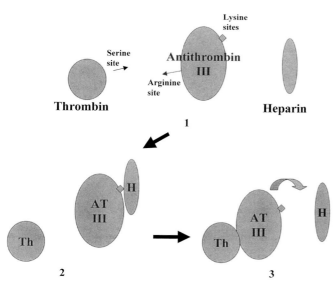

FIGURE 77.1 Proposed mechanism of action of ATIII and heparin. (Adapted from **Rosenberg RD.** The molecular basis of blood diseases. In: Stamatoyannopoulos G, Nienhuis AW, Leder P, Majerus PW, eds. Regulation of the hemostatic mechanism. Philadelphia: WB Saunders, 1987;534–574, with permission.) The presence of heparin facilitates the binding of ATIII to thrombin. Heparin is then released from the TAT complex and is available to interact with other thrombin molecules.

thrombin-dependent amplification of the coagulation mechanism and the inhibition of thrombin-mediated conversion of fibrinogen to fibrin.

Other mechanisms contributing to the anticoagulant effect of heparin have been described. Heparin can enhance release of TF pathway inhibitor (TFPI) from endothelial cells.[41] The latter inhibits the factor VIIa–TF complex and prevents activation of the extrinsic pathway of coagulation. It has been suggested that ATIII and factor X may bind to heparin at distinct sites on the heparin molecule, resulting in a transient complex of ATIII–heparin–factor X, and that factor X may guide the complex to a phosphatylserine-rich site on the cell surface in proximity to the factor VIIa–TF complex where it facilitates rapid neutralization of factor VIIa.[42]

Heparin and activated PC (APC) may act synergistically in decreasing thrombin generation by prothrombinase. These synergistic mechanisms include heparin enhancement of ATIII-dependent inhibition of factor V activation by thrombin, inactivation of membrane-bound factor Va by APC, and proteolytic inactivation of membrane-bound factor V by APC, an event enhanced by heparin.[43]

Heparin may also be useful as an antithrombotic agent in high shear-stress (arterial) environments because of its ability to interfere with platelet–von Willebrand factor (vWf) hemostatic mechanisms. Some forms of heparin (usually higher-molecular-weight forms) bind to the platelet glycoprotein Ib receptor, a receptor to which vWf normally binds when platelets adhere at sites of vascular injury. Chemical modification of heparin has been used to separate its vWf-binding and ATIII-binding properties.[44] Such intervention may be of future therapeutic benefit in treating thrombotic disease if different heparins can be selectively produced for their anticoagulant and antiplatelet effects.

Heparin, especially low-molecular-weight forms, is an important therapeutic agent in the prevention and treatment of hypercoagulable conditions and in the treatment of thromboembolic disease in both humans and animals.[2,41,45,46]

THROMBOMODULIN–PROTEIN C–PROTEIN S ANTICOAGULANT PATHWAY

Protein C

PC, a vitamin-K-dependent serine-protease zymogen, is a central protein in one of the major regulatory pathways of coagulation. Like all K-dependent factors, vitamin K is required for the posttranslational carboxylation of the N terminal; without carboxylation, the functional potential of the protein is lost.[28] Upon activation, PC becomes a potent inhibitor of the coagulation mechanism and a stimulator of the fibrinolytic system. The net effect of PC activation is therefore to limit the size of a thrombus by inhibition of fibrin generation and enhancement of fibrin dissolution.[47]

Protein C is a 62-kD glycoprotein that occurs in minute amounts in human plasma (approximately 4 to 5 μg/mL) and is composed of disulfide-linked heavy

(40 kD) and light (20 kD) chains.[47] Both human and bovine PC appear to have similar functional and physiochemical properties.[48,49] PC is activated by the removal of a small peptide from the amino-terminal end of the heavy chain. The major physiologic activator of PC is thrombin (Fig. 77.2). Thrombin itself acts slowly; however, when thrombin forms a complex with the endothelial cell cofactor, TM, the rate of activation increases more than 20,000-fold.[50,51] A unique aspect of TM's action is that on binding thrombin there is a loss of thrombin's procoagulant function (fibrinogen cleavage, factor V activation, and platelet activation).[50] Antiphospholipid antibodies can inhibit PC activation through an effect on TM.[52]

The major action of APC is to inactivate factors Va and VIIIa, cofactors of the rate-limiting steps of coagulation, the formation of tenase and prothrombinase. This inactivation involves the enzymatic degradation of factors Va and VIIIa, and requires phospholipid, calcium ions, and PS.[53–55] Native (nonactivated) PC inactivates these procoagulant factors approximately 40 to 80 times more slowly.[53] APC specifically degrades membrane-bound factors Va and VIIIa, whereas nonactivated forms of factors V and VIII are poor substrates for APC.[55]

The plasma serine-protease inhibitor, PC inhibitor, inhibits APC (as well as thrombin and factor Xa), and this inhibitory effect is greatly enhanced by heparin.[56] Beta 2-glucosephosphate isomerase (GPI) competitively inhibits the action of APC possibly by inhibiting the binding of APC to the phospholipid surface.[57]

The mechanism of the profibrinolytic effect of APC is uncertain. APC may interact with endothelial cells

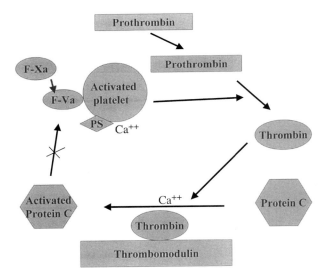

FIGURE 77.2 Proposed mechanism of inhibition of prothrombinase formation by TM-PC-PS. (Adapted from **Rosenberg RD.** The molecular basis of blood diseases. In: Stamatoyannopoulos G, Nienhuis AW, Leder P, Majerus PW, eds. Regulation of the hemostatic mechanism. Philadelphia: WB Saunders, 1987;534–574, with permission.) Activated PC inactivates platelet-bound factor Va, and this inhibition is enhanced by the cofactor, PS.

to increase the release of tissue plasminogen activator (tPA),[58] or may inactivate the major inhibitor of tPA.[59]

Techniques are now available for quantitation of both PC antigen and PC activity in human and animal plasmas.[28,60-64] Barton et al[28] found that neonatal foals had more PC but with less functional activity than did older foals (25 to 30 days of age) or adult light breed horses. In human infants, decreases in both functional and antigenic activity have been reported.[63,64] Normal plasma concentrations of PC range from approximately 65 to 130% in horses, dogs, and humans.[60,65]

Downregulation of the TM–PC–PS system has been reported in association with the acute-phase inflammatory response.[35] DIC-induced consumption of PC has been described in humans,[47,61] dogs,[60] and other species.[66,67] The lupus-like anticoagulants may facilitate thrombosis by inhibiting PC and its cofactor, PS, through an effect of phospholipid.[52] PC activity and gamma-carboxylated PC concentrations decrease in vitamin K deficiency, whereas PC antigen concentrations are reduced to a lesser extent. In such circumstances, functionally defective decarboxylated PC protein induced by vitamin K absence-PC (PIVKA-PC) is present.[68] A deficiency of PC activity (in the presence of normal concentrations of plasma PC antigen) has been described in a thoroughbred foal exhibiting clinical signs of hypercoagulability.[65]

Recently, increased resistance to APC has been identified as a major risk factor for venous thromboembolism in humans, with a reported 2 to 10% incidence in the population.[69] This APC resistance appears most often to be related to a single-point mutation in the factor V gene that results in a lifelong hypercoagulable state caused by impaired inactivation of the mutated factor Va by APC.[70,71]

Protein S

PS is a single-chained polypeptide[4,49] with a molecular weight of 69 to 84 kD that is synthesized in liver cells, endothelial cells, and megakaryocytes.[68,72,73] The structure of PS is similar to that of other vitamin-K-dependent proteins; however, this protein has a much higher avidity for phospholipid and calcium ions.[2] Binding with calcium protects PS from degradation by thrombin and induces a conformational change required for its activity.[18]

Unlike most of the other vitamin-K-dependent plasma proteins, PS is not the zymogen of a serine protease (Fig. 77.2). Rather, it functions as a cofactor to enhance the inactivation of factors Va and VIIIa by APC.[2,74] APC and PS form a 1:1 stoichiometric complex on the surface of phospholipids and in the presence of calcium ions. This enzyme–cofactor interaction drastically accelerates the rate of inactivation of factors Va and VIIIa.[2] This action is localized to the surface of platelets, peripheral blood cells, or endothelial cells that bear specific receptors for these factors.[2,55] The importance of PS is demonstrated by the anticoagulant activity of APC being significantly reduced after removal of PS from plasma.[75] A deficiency of PS, either acquired or heredi-

tary, predisposes to thrombotic tendencies. Recently, it has been proposed that PS may also exert an APC-independent anticoagulant effect by inhibiting both the intrinsic tenase and the prothrombinase complexes directly.[18]

PS exists in the plasma in two forms: free PS and PS bound to a high-molecular-weight protein known as C4b-binding protein.[76] Present information suggests that the free PS is a more effective cofactor of APC than is the C4b-bound form.[68,75] Consequently, a high concentration of C4b-binding protein in a patient's blood could cause an acquired defect in free PS and thus form a risk factor for developing thrombotic complications. Although the total PS concentration may not change significantly in vitamin K deficiency, a considerable amount of free PS is converted to the complex form, probably because of a change in C4b-binding properties caused by the conversion of gammacarboxylated PS to PIVKA-PS (decarboxylated PS).[68]

HEPARIN COFACTOR II

Heparin cofactor II (HC-II) is a plasma thrombin inhibitor antigenically different from ATIII and with different pharmacokinetics.[29,77] HC-II is secreted by the liver into the blood where it is present at a concentration of approximately 1.2 μM. The physiologic importance of HC-II is still unclear. Like ATIII, HC-II's inhibitory action on thrombin is greatly enhanced by heparin and other sulfated glycosaminoglycans in the circulation or localized on the vascular endothelium. However, unlike ATIII, its thrombin-inhibitory action is also greatly enhanced (approximately 1000×) by dermatan sulfate proteoglycans (DSPGs).[29] Its action on thrombin is likely mediated by interaction with DSPG in the vessel wall, and since most DSPG are located in the extracellular matrix, it has been proposed that HC-II may act essentially in the extravascular environment.[18] Tran and Duckert[29] suggested that HC-II might function as a thrombin-inhibitor reserve when ATIII levels become subnormal (as in DIC).

TISSUE FACTOR PATHWAY INHIBITOR

TFPI is a heterogeneous group of plasma proteins (molecular weight, 36 to 43 kD) found at low concentrations (approximately 2.7 μM) bound to lipoproteins. Approximately 10% of blood TFPI is carried within platelets and can be released locally when these cells are stimulated.[1] Heparin increases plasma TFPI concentrations severalfold indicating the presence of an additional TFPI pool, probably in endothelial cells.[18,78] Functional domains on the protein serve as binding sites for heparin, lipoproteins, and phospholipids and are essential for its anticoagulant activity. TFPI is a potent inhibitor of factor VIIa–TF-catalyzed factor X activation. Factor Xa generated by factor VIIa–TF binds irreversibly to TFPI with the formed complex binding in a calcium-dependent

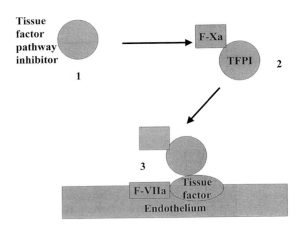

FIGURE 77.3 Proposed mechanism of inhibition of factor Xa and TF-factor VIIa by TFPI on the surface of endothelial cells. TFPI binds to and inhibits factor Xa, and the binary complex then binds to membrane-associated TF-factor VIIa.

manner to membrane-bound factor VIIa–TF (Fig. 77.3). The TFPI–factor Xa complex has a high affinity for negatively charged phospholipids.[79] Other clotting factors can affect TFPI concentrations; for example, factors VIII and IX significantly reduces the ability of TFPI to inhibit factor VIIa–TF (18). Recently a second human TFPI (TFPI-2) has been isolated from human plasma.[80] Its importance has yet to be established.

OTHER COAGULATION INHIBITORS

Annexin V

Annexin V is one of a family of nonglycosylated proteins (annexins) sharing the common feature of binding to calcium and phospholipids. It occurs in human plasma at a concentration of approximately 20 to 80 nM, and has been detected in the cytoplasm of venous and arterial endothelial cells, in erythrocytes, in lymphocytes, in monocytes, and in platelets. Annexin V has anticoagulant properties. It is likely that annexin V acts by displacing phospholipid-dependent coagulation factors, thus inhibiting the formation of thrombin by factors Va and Xa, and factor Xa by factor VIIa–TP and by factor IXa–factor VIIIa. Its physiologic importance as a natural anticoagulant is not yet established.[18]

REFERENCES

1. **Broze GJ.** The role of tissue factor pathway inhibitor in a revised coagulation cascade. Semin Hematol 1992;29:159–169.
2. **Rosenberg RD.** The molecular basis of blood diseases. In: Stamatoyannopoulos G, Nienhuis AW, Leder P, Majerus PW, eds. Regulation of the hemostatic mechanism. Philadelphia: WB Saunders, 1987;534–574.
3. **Boisclair MD, Philippou H, Lane DA.** Thrombogenic mechanisms in the human: fresh insights obtained by immunodiagnostic studies of coagulation markers. Blood Coagul Fibrinolysis 1993;4:1007–1021.
4. **Dahlback B.** Purification of human vitamin K-dependent protein S and its limited proteolysis by thrombin. Biochem J 1983;209:837–846.
5. **Cadroy Y, Diquelou A, Dupouy D, et al.** The thrombomodulin/protein C/protein S anticoagulant pathway modulates the thrombogenic properties of the normal resting and stimulated endothelium. Arterioscler Thromb Vasc Biol 1997;17:520–527.
6. **Haslar RNH.** Thrombophilia: some recent advances in understanding. J R Nav Med Serv 1995;81:203–206.
7. **Humphries JE.** Thrombophilia and complex acquired deficiencies of antithrombin, protein C, and protein S. Semin Hematol 1995;32:8–18.
8. **Green RA.** Pathophysiology of antithrombin III deficiency. Vet Clin North Am Small Anim Pract 1988;18:95–104.
9. **Welles E.** Antithrombotic and fibrinolytic factors. A review. Vet Clin North Am Small Anim Pract 1996;26;1111–1127.
10. **Tyler-Cross R, Sobel M, McAdory LE, et al.** Structure-function relations of antithrombin III-heparin interactions as assessed by biophysical and biological assays and molecular modeling of peptide-pentasaccharide-docked complexes. Arch Biochem Biophys 1996;334:206–213.
11. **Lane DA, Kunz G, Olds RJ, et al.** Molecular genetics of antithrombin deficiency. Blood Rev 1996;10:59–74.
12. **Tsiang M, Jain AK, Gibbs CS.** Functional requirements for inhibition of thrombin by antithrombin III in the presence and absence of heparin. J Biol Chem 1997;272;12024–12029.
13. **Niessen RW, Lamping RJ, Peters M, et al.** Fetal and neonatal development of antithrombin III plasma activity and liver messenger RNA levels in sheep. Pediatr Res 1996;39:685–691.
14. **Fair DS, Bahnak BR.** Human hepatoma cells secrete single chain factor X, prothrombin and antithrombin III. Blood 1984;64:194–204.
15. **Chan V, Chan TK.** Antithrombin III in fresh and cultured human endothelial cells-a natural anticoagulant from the vascular endothelium. Thromb Res 1979;15:209–213.
16. **Beresford CH.** Antithrombin III deficiency. Blood Rev 1988;2:239–250.
17. **Godal HC, Rygh M, Laake K.** Progressive inactivation of purified FVII by heparin and antithrombin III. Thromb Res 1974;5:773–775.
18. **Bombeli T, Mueller M, Haeberli A.** Anticoagulant properties of the vascular endothelium. Thromb Haemost 1997;77:402–423.
19. **Pelzer H, Schwarz A, Heimburger N.** Determination of human thrombin-antithrombin III complex in plasma with an enzyme-linked immunosorbent assay. Thromb Haemost 1988;59:101–106.
20. **Tengborn L, Palmblad S, Wojeiechowski J, et al.** D-dimer and thrombin/antithrombin III complex-Diagnostic tools in deep venous thrombosis? Haemostasis 1994;24;344–350.
21. **Wada H, Wakita Y, Nakase T, et al.** Diagnosis of pre-disseminated intravascular coagulation stage with hemostatic molecular markers. The Mie DIC study group. Pol J Pharmacol 1996;48:225–228.
22. **Lorente JA, García-Frade LJ, Landin L, et al.** Time course of hemostatic abnormalities in sepsis and its relation to outcome. Chest 1993;103:1536–1542.
23. **Takahashi H, Tatewaki W, Wada K, et al.** Thrombin vs plasmin generation in disseminated intravascular coagulation associated with various disorders. Am J Hematol 1990;3:90–95.
24. **van Wersch JWJ, Ubachs JMH.** Blood coagulation and fibrinolysis during normal pregnancy. Eur J Clin Chem Clin Biochem 1991;29:45–50.
25. **Ravanat C, Freund M, Dol F, et al.** Cross-reactivity of human molecular markers for detection of prothrombotic states in various animal species. Blood Coagul Fibrinolysis 1995;6:446–455.
26. **Bernard W, Morris D, Divers T, et al.** Plasma antithrombin III values in healthy horses: effect of sex and/or breed. Am J Vet Res 1987;48:866–868.
27. **Johnstone IB, Physick-Sheard P, Crane S.** Breed, age and gender differences in plasma antithrombin-III activity in clinically normal young horses. Am J Vet Res 1989;50;1751–1753.
28. **Barton MH, Morris DD, Crowe N, et al.** Hemostatic indices in healthy foals from birth to one month of age. J Vet Diagn Invest 1995;7:380–385.
29. **Tran Tri H, Duckert F.** Heparin cofactor II determination-Levels in normals and patients with hereditary antithrombin III deficiency and disseminated intravascular coagulation. Thromb Haemost 1984;52:112–116.
30. **Bick RL.** Disseminated intravascular coagulation and related syndromes. Boca Raton: CRC Press, 1983.
31. **Welch RD, Watkins JP, Taylor TS, et al.** Disseminated intravascular coagulation associated with colic in 23 horses (1984–1989). J Vet Intern Med 1992;6:29–35.
32. **Pusterla N, Braun U, Forrer R, et al.** Antithrombin III activity in plasma of healthy and sick cattle. Vet Rec 1997;140:17–18.
33. **Johnstone IB, Petersen D, Crane S.** Antithrombin III (ATIII) activity in plasmas from normal and disease horses, and in normal canine, bovine and human plasmas. Vet Clin Pathol 1987;16:14–18.
34. **Plesca LA, Bodizs G, Cucuianu M, et al.** Hemostatic balance during the acute inflammatory reaction; with special reference to antithrombin III. Rom J Physiol 1995;32:71–76.
35. **Cucuianu M, Plesca L, Bodiza G, et al.** Acute phase and the hemostatic balance. Rom J Intern Med 1996;34:13–18.
36. **Engelberg H.** Heparin: Metabolism, physiology and clinical application. Springfield: Charles C Thomas, 1963.
37. **Rosenberg R, Lam L.** Correlation between structure and function of heparin. Proc Natl Acad Sci U S A 1979;76:1218–1222.

38. **McAvoy T.** Pharmacokinetic modeling of heparin and its clinical implications. J Pharmacokinet Biopharm 1979;7:331–354.

39. **Beguin S, Lindhout T, Hemker C.** The mode of action of heparin in plasma. Thromb Haemost 1988;60:457–462.

40. **Gerhands H.** Low dose calcium heparin in horses: plasma heparin concentration, effects on red cell mass and on coagulation variables. Equine Vet J 1991;23:37–43.

41. **Moore BR, Hinchcliff KW.** Heparin: a review of its pharmacology and therapeutic use in horses. J Vet Intern Med 1994;8:26–35.

42. **Hamamoto T, Foster DC, Kisiel W.** The inhibition of human factor VIIa-tissue factor by antithrombin III-heparin is enhanced by factor X on a human bladder carcinoma cell line. Int J Hematol 1996;63:51–63.

43. **Petaja J, Fernández JA, Gruber A, et al.** Anticoagulant synergism of heparin and activated protein C in vitro. Role of a novel anticoagulant mechanism of heparin, enhancement of inactivation of factor V by activated protein C. J Clin Invest 1997;99:2655–2663.

44. **Sobel M, Bird KE, Tyler-Cross R, et al.** Heparins designed to specifically inhibit platelet interaction with von Willebrand factor. Circulation 1996; 93:992–999.

45. **Parker J, Fubini S, Car B, et al.** Prevention of intraabdominal adhesions in ponies by low-dose heparin therapy. Vet Surg 1987;16:459–462.

46. **Frydman A.** Low-molecular-weight heparins: an overview of their pharmacodynamics, pharmacokinetics and metabolism in humans. Haemostasis 1996;26:24–38.

47. **Marlar RA.** Protein C in thromboembolic disease. Semin Thromb Haemost 1985;11:387–393.

48. **Kisiel W, Davie W.** Protein C. Methods Enzymol 1981;80:320–332.

49. **Stenflo J, Jonsson M.** Protein S, a new vitamin K-dependent protein from bovine plasma. FEBS Lett 1979; 101:377–381.

50. **Esmon CT, Esmon NL.** Protein C activation. Semin Thromb Haemost 1984;10:122–130.

51. **Esmon CT, Fukudome K.** Cellular regulation of the protein C pathway. Semin Cell Biol 1995;6:259–268.

52. **Malia RG, Kitchen S, Greaves M, et al.** Inhibition of activated protein C and its cofactor protein S by antiphospholipid antibodies. Br J Haematol 1990;76:101–107.

53. **Marlar RA, Kleiss AJ, Griffin JH.** Mechanism of action of human activated protein C, a thrombin-dependent anticoagulant enzyme. Blood 1982;59: 1064–1072.

54. **Stenflo J.** Structure and function of protein C. Semin Thromb Haemost 1984; 10:109–121.

55. **Dahlback B.** Factor V and protein S as cofactors to activated protein C. Haematologica 1997;82:91–95.

56. **Rezaie AR, Cooper ST, Church FC, et al.** Protein C inhibitor is a potent inhibitor of the thrombin-thrombomodulin complex. J Biol Chem 1995; 270:25336–25339.

57. **Mori T, Takeya H, Nishioka J, et al.** Beta 2-glycoprotein modulates the anticoagulant activity of activated protein C on the phospholipid surface. Thromb Haemost 1996;75:49–55.

58. **Comp PC, Esmon CT.** Generation of fibrinolytic activity by infusion of activated protein C into dogs. J Clin Invest 1981;8:1221–1228.

59. **van Hinsbergh VWM, Bertina RM, van Wijngaarden A, et al.** Activated protein C decreases plasminogen activator inhibitor activity in endothelial cell conditioned medium. Blood 1985;65:444–451.

60. **Madden RM, Ward M, Marlar RA.** Protein C activity in endotoxin-induced disseminated intravascular coagulation in a dog model. Thromb Res 1989;55:297–307.

61. **Pabinger I.** Clinical relevance of protein C. Blut 1986;53:63–75.

62. **Welles E, Prasse K, Duncan A, et al.** Antigenic assay for protein C determination in horses. Am J Vet Res 1990;51:1075–1078.

63. **Karpatkin M, Mannucci P, Bhogal M, et al.** Low protein C in the neonatal period. Br J Haematol 1986;62:137–142.

64. **Ankola P, Nardi M, Karpatkin M.** Functional activity of protein C in newborn infants. Am J Pediatr Hematol Oncol 1992;14:140–143.

65. **Edens LM, Morris DD, Prasse KW, et al.** Hypercoagulable state associated with a deficiency of protein C in a thoroughbred colt. J Vet Intern Med 1993;7:190–193.

66. **Taylor FB, Chang A, Esmon CT, et al.** Protein C prevents the coagulopathic and lethal effects of *Escherichia coli* infusion in the baboon. J Clin Invest 1987;79:918–925.

67. **Emekli NB, Ulutin ON.** The protective effect of autoprothrombin II-anticoagulant on experimental DIC formed animals. Haematologica 1980;65: 644–651.

68. **Matsuzaka T, Tanaka H, Fukuda M, et al.** Relationship between vitamin K dependent coagulation factors and anticoagulants (protein C and protein S) in neonatal vitamin K deficiency. Arch Dis Child 1993;68:297–302.

69. **Chrobak L, Dulicek P.** Resistance to activated protein C as pathogenic factor of venous thromboembolism. Acta Medica Hradec Kralove 1996; 39:55–62.

70. **Hillarp A, Dahlback B, Zoller B.** Activated protein C resistance: from phenotype to genotype and clinical practice. Blood Rev 1995;9:201–212.

71. **Samama MM, Simon D, Horellou MH, et al.** Diagnosis and clinical characteristic of inherited activated protein C resistance. Haemostasis 1996; 26:315–330.

72. **F1air DS, Marlar RA, Levin EG.** Human endothelial cells synthesize protein S. Blood 1986;67:1168–1171.

73. **Ogura M, Tanabe N, Nishioka J.** Biosynthesis and secretion of functional protein S by a human megakaryocytic cell line (MEG-01). Blood 1987; 70:301–306.

74. **Walker FJ.** Protein S and the regulation of activated protein C. Semin Thromb Haemost 1984;10:131–134.

75. **Bertina RM, van Wijngaarden A, Reinalda-Poot J, et al.** Determination of plasma protein S—The protein cofactor of activated protein C. Thromb Haemost 1985;53:268–272.

76. **Dahlback B.** Interaction between vitamin K-dependent protein S and the complement protein, C4b-binding protein. A link between coagulation and the complement system. Semin Thromb Haemost 1984;10:139–148.

77. **Hatton MW, Hoogendoorn H, Southward SM, et al.** Comparative metabolism and distribution of rabbit heparin cofactor II and rabbit antithrombin in rabbits. Am J Physiol 1997;272:824–831.

78. **Sandset P, Abildgaard U, Larsen M.** Heparin induces release of extrinsic coagulation pathway inhibitor (EPI). Thromb Res 1988;50:803–813.

79. **Lindout T, Salemink I, Valentin S, et al.** Tissue factor pathway inhibitor: regulation of its inhibitory activity by phospholipid surfaces. Haemostasis 1996;26:89–97.

80. **Sprecher CA, Kisiel W, Mathewes S, et al.** Molecular cloning, expression, and partial characterization of a second human tissue-factor-pathway inhibitor. Proc Natl Acad Sci U S A 1994;91:3353–3360.

CHAPTER 78

Fibrinolytic System

• BENJAMIN J. DARIEN

The fibrinolytic system in mammalian blood plays an important role in the dissolution of blood clots and the maintenance of a patent vascular system.[1-3] Fibrin is also formed during inflammation and plays an important temporary role in tissue injury, but must be removed when normal tissue structure and function is restored.[4,5] Thus, a fibrin clot that forms in a vessel to stop hemorrhage or in a joint or tissue in response to inflammation, is remodeled and then removed to restore normal blood flow or tissue function, respectively. In addition, the fibrinolytic system also plays a vital role in normal physiologic reproduction, wound repair, angiogenesis, tissue remodeling, and in the pathogenesis of neoplastic diseases.[6] The fibrinolytic system is the principle effector of clot (or fibrin) removal and controls the enzymatic degradation of fibrin. Its action is coordinated (in a manner similar to that of coagulation) through the interaction of activators, zymogens, enzymes, and inhibitors to provide local activation (and regulation) at sites of fibrin deposition. Disorders of the fibrinolytic system may result either from impaired activation (thrombotic complications) or from excessive activation (bleeding tendency) of the fibrinolytic system.[7-10]

The fibrinolytic system (see Algorithm) comprises an inactive proenzyme, plasminogen, which can be converted to the active enzyme, and plasmin, which degrades fibrin (and fibrinogen) into soluble fibrin (fibrinogen) degradation products (FDPs) in the process of fibrinolysis (fibrinogenolysis).[1,2,6] Two immunologically distinct physiologic plasminogen activators have been identified in blood: tissue plasminogen activator (tPA) and urokinase (UK) plasminogen activator (uPA). Inhibition of the fibrinolytic system may occur either at the level of the plasminogen activators (see Algorithm), by specific plasminogen activator inhibitors ([PAI] 1 and PAI 2) or at the level of plasmin, by α_2-antiplasmin (also referred to as α_2-plasmin inhibitor, α_2-PI). Some of the main components of the fibrinolytic system are summarized in Table 78.1. An intrinsic pathway involving several proteins, including factor XII and high-molecular-weight kininogen (HMWK), and prekallikrein (PK) may also induce plasminogen activation. Kallikrein generated from PK by the action of activated factor XII (XIIa) and HMWK may activate uPA.

PLASMINOGEN AND PLASMIN

Activation of the circulating zymogen plasminogen yields the fibrinolytic enzyme plasmin. Plasminogen is synthesized in hepatic cells and the major pathway for elimination is by means of catabolic degradation rather than by conversion to plasmin.[4,8,11] Activators convert plasminogen to the two-chain plasmin molecule by cleaving it into a heavy (A) and a light (B) chain. The effector sites on the A chain, known as lysine binding sites, mediate the interaction of plasmin with fibrin and the plasma inhibitor α_2-antiplasmin. The B chain contains the active site of the plasmin molecule that is homologous in structure and function to other serine proteases (e.g., thrombin and factor Xa), cleaving esters of lysine, and arginine. Although the principal physiologic substrate of plasmin is fibrin, it is a nonspecific endopeptidase that can attack any peptide containing an arginine-lysine residue sequence. Consequently, plasmin inactivates other elements of the coagulation cascade, including fibrinogen into FDPs, factors VIII and V, and degrades PK, HMWK, and elements of the complement cascade.[1,2,6] Additionally, plasmin can cleave plasminogen to produce a small activation peptide, lysine plasminogen, which has a higher affinity for binding fibrin and a greater reactivity with plasminogen activators. This later action serves to accelerate plasminogen conversion to plasmin, since the lysine-plasminogen form is more susceptible to activator cleavage than the parent plasminogen. The capacity of lysine analogs such as ε-aminocaproic acid (EACA) to bind to these sites on plasminogen and compete with lysine-like sites on fibrin forms the basis of their fibrinolytic-inhibitory potential.[6]

ENDOGENOUS ACTIVATORS OF FIBRINOLYSIS

Several substances are known to possess the ability to convert plasminogen to plasmin and are known generically as plasminogen activators. Endogenous plasminogen activators are physiologic constituents of the homeostatic system and are classified as either intrinsic

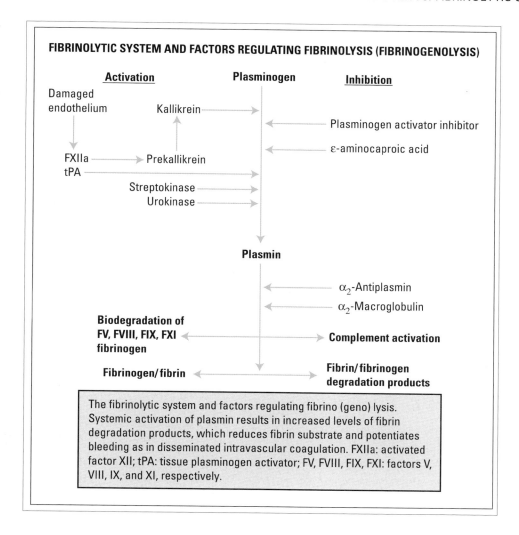

FIBRINOLYTIC SYSTEM AND FACTORS REGULATING FIBRINOLYSIS (FIBRINOGENOLYSIS)

The fibrinolytic system and factors regulating fibrino (geno) lysis. Systemic activation of plasmin results in increased levels of fibrin degradation products, which reduces fibrin substrate and potentiates bleeding as in disseminated intravascular coagulation. FXIIa: activated factor XII; tPA: tissue plasminogen activator; FV, FVIII, FIX, FXI: factors V, VIII, IX, and XI, respectively.

or extrinsic activators. Exogenous plasminogen activators, such as streptokinase, are nonphysiologic activators that can convert plasminogen to plasmin.

Intrinsic Activators

The intrinsic activators consist of the plasma proteins that exist as inactive (zymogen) precursors in the circulation. Many of these substances are central to the mediation of coagulation and inflammation. The pathways of intrinsic plasminogen activation center on the activation of factor XII (Hageman factor), which not only participates in the contact phase of the intrinsic coagulation pathway but also has been shown to induce fibrinolysis.[3,4,6,8] Although the physiologic activation of factor XII involves contact with collagen or negatively charged surfaces, several of the coagulation factors are known to induce factor XII activation, including HMWK (Fitzgerald factor), kallikrein (Fletcher factor), and plasmin itself. Since plasmin can, in turn, activate factor XII, amplification of fibrinolysis is possible. Upon activation,

TABLE 78.1	Pathophysiologic Factors That Regulate Fibrinolysis/Thrombolysis
Promote	**Limit**
Plasminogen incorporation into a thrombus via fibrin binding	Fibrin crosslinking by factor XIIIa
Platelet clot retraction	Low ratio of tPA to plasminogen activator inhibitor (PAI 1 or PAI 2)
Endothelial cell and macrophage biosynthesis of tPA	Low ratio of endothelial surface to thrombus volume in large vessels
Binding of tPA to fibrin	Efficient inhibition of free plasmin to α_2-antiplasmin
Enhanced tPA or uPA activity in the presence of fibrin	α_2-antiplasmin impairs plasmin binding to fibrin
Protection of plasmin (bound to fibrin) from α_2-antiplasmin binding	Binding of α_2-antiplasmin to fibrin

factor XIIa can activate plasminogen directly or indirectly by means of PK and HMWK activation, which may convert plasminogen to plasmin via the generation of Kallikrein or urokinase plasminogen activator (uPA).

Extrinsic Activators

Central to the plasmin-based fibrinolytic system is the essential conversion of the circulating proenzyme plasminogen into the active serine protease plasmin. Plasminogen activators, of which there are two types, include tPA and uPA.[4,6,8,12] Both types of activators are serine proteases that have a high specific activity in converting plasminogen to plasmin. Tissue type activators have been isolated from normal tissues, endothelial cells, and malignant cell lines.[6,11] Released tPA has a high affinity for fibrin or fibrin-bound plasminogen and increased activity in the presence of fibrin, properties that both localize tPA activity and enhance fibrinolytic potential at sites of fibrin deposition. In addition, tPA increases the binding of plasminogen to fibrin clots, a process that ensures a continuous supply of plasminogen during tPA-mediated lysis.

Another group of the extrinsic plasminogen activators is the uPA (or UK).[6,8] UK is a glycoprotein produced mainly by the renal parenchymal cells and excreted in small quantities into the urine. Although uPA synthesis occurs mainly in the kidney, other cells, including fibroblasts, epithelial cells pneumocytes, and placental cells produce this substance. Bovine endothelial cells in culture have been shown to secrete uPA.[13] It is believed that uPA plays an important role in tissue remodeling, inflammation, tumor invasion, fertilization, and embryogenesis.

ENDOGENOUS INHIBITORS OF FIBRINOLYSIS

Several substances, both endogenous and synthetic have been identified as inhibitors of fibrinolysis. Inhibition of fibrinolysis results either through inhibition of plasmin directly or by inhibition of plasminogen activation. The endogenous substances that inhibit plasmin are members of a group of serine proteases and serine-protease inhibitors (serpins) that inactivate a wide variety of plasma enzymes, including components of the coagulation pathway.

Plasmin and Plasminogen Activator Inhibitors

The principal physiologic inhibitor of plasmin is α_2-antiplasmin, which is present in plasma as well as in platelets.[6,8,12,14] The plasmin-antiplasmin interaction is central to the physiologic control of fibrinolysis, which must provide for intermittent activation at local sites of fibrin deposition without initiating a systemic proteolytic state. In plasma, α_2-antiplasmin reacts exceedingly fast with plasmin, irreversibly inhibiting the enzyme by forming a stable 1:1 bimolecular complex. In the process, α_2-antiplasmin is partly degraded by plasmin. Other plasmin inhibitors such as α_2-macroglobulin may exert a limited role, particularly if the capacity of α_2-antiplasmin is exceeded by a high concentration of free plasmin. Other plasma protease inhibitors such as antithrombin III, α_1-antitrypsin, and C_1-inactivator have some antiplasmin activity in vitro but exert minimal physiologic effect in the blood.

Inhibitors of tPAs also play an important role in the control of fibrinolysis.[2,4,12] Multiple mechanisms are involved in the rapid inhibition of tPA in plasma. PAI 1 and PAI 2 are specific rapid-reacting inhibitors of tPA, which is present at low concentration in normal plasma, but at higher concentrations in many clinical conditions (see below). PAI 1 inhibits its target proteases by formation of a 1:1 stoichiometric reversible complex. PAI 1 is synthesized by endothelial cells and hepatocytes and is also present in platelets where it is found in the α granules. PAI 1 is secreted or released by endothelial cells and platelets in response to thrombin, endotoxin, tumor necrosis factor α, and interleukin 1. It rapidly inactivates tPA, thereby inhibiting fibrinolysis (by means of decreased plasmin activity). Activated protein C also modulates the fibrinolytic system by decreasing PAI 1 activity.

MEASUREMENTS

Pathologic activation of free plasminogen in primary fibrinolysis or disseminated intravascular coagulation (DIC) results in circulating levels of plasmin that supersede the inactivating capacity of the various antiplasmins.[4-8] Pathologic fibrinolysis (fibrinogenolysis) constitutes a medical emergency because circulating fibrin monomers and FDPs can cause uncontrollable bleeding.[4,7] Fibrinolytic activation can be assessed by direct measurement of plasminogen or plasmin and plasminogen activator and inhibitor levels by commonly available synthetic substrate (chromogenic) techniques. The euglobulin lysis test is a clot-based assay that tests the fibrinolytic mechanism (plasminogen activation) in plasma and offers some clinically useful information for assessing fibrinolytic system in clinical disorders, including DIC.[15] Direct measurement of plasmin in plasma can be difficult because it is rapidly inactivated by complexing with fast-acting α_2-antiplasmin and slow-acting α_2-macroglobulin. If these two fibrinolytic system inhibitors are significantly elevated, there may be an ineffective fibrinolytic response with resultant enhanced fibrin monomer precipitation, fibrin deposition, and vascular thrombosis (see Chapter 85, Acquired Coagulopathy V: Thrombosis). Tests of fibrinogen and fibrin catabolism include the immune-based FDPs procedure.[16-23] FDPs are potent inhibitors of coagulation and, like other anticoagulants, they cause abnormalities in the global coagulation assays prothrombin time (PT), activated partial thromboplastin time (APTT), and thrombin time (TT).[24-26]

Most recent studies that report on alterations of the fibrinolytic system have measured plasminogen and plasmin, tPA or uPA, and their inhibitors (PAI 1 and PAI 2, and α_2-antiplasmin, respectively) by use of chromogenic assays with computer-assisted analyzers.[7,16–20,22,23,27–31] Other less commonly used assays include spontaneous clot lysis, euglobulin lysis time, fibrin slide incubation technique or ^{131}I-labeled fibrinogen.[7,15,18,32] The euglobulin lysis test or whole-blood clot lysis time can be used to estimate the degree of fibrinolytic activity. For the euglobulin lysis time, plasma is acidified and on refrigeration, a precipitate forms that contains fibrinogen, plasminogen, active plasmin, and plasminogen activators. This precipitate is termed the euglobulin fraction. Excluded from the precipitate are most plasma antiplasmins, so that fibrinolysis may proceed unchecked. The precipitate can be isolated and redissolved in buffer containing calcium-binding anticoagulant. A timer is started when excess calcium is added to the euglobulin fraction to precipitate a clot (which forms almost immediately). The clot undergoes dissolution as a result of newly formed plasmin generated by its activators during the incubation period. The quantity of circulating plasminogen activators present in the original plasma sample and the rate at which the clot dissolves are related. The euglobulin lysis time or measurement of plasma fibrinolytic activity is the time required for the euglobulin fraction to dissolve. A shortening of the euglobulin lysis time implies greater fibrinolytic activity. Normal fibrinolysis proceeds slowly in the euglobulin system, so that a firm clot in sera is present after 24 hours in rabbits, cows, horses, pigs, sheep, chickens, turkeys, ducks, and frogs; after 5 to 24 hours in monkeys, cats, mice, and fish; after 1 to 5 hours in dogs; and almost immediately in hamsters.[33–35]

CLINICAL OBSERVATIONS

Fibrin formation (coagulation) and dissolution (fibrinolysis) are thought to occur simultaneously during hemostasis, with the balance of these forces influencing the occurrence and clinical course of thrombohemorrhagic disease.[4–8,26,36–38] Disruption of control of fibrinolysis can shift the balance of clot formation and dissolution and lead to bleeding if there is excessive fibrinolysis or to thrombosis if there is inappropriate fibrinolytic inhibition.

Primary disorders of fibrinolysis are poorly defined in the veterinary literature. Because the overall plasma fibrinolytic activity is the result of the balance between activators and inhibitors, thrombosis can occur as a result of excessive inhibitory activity and subsequent deficient fibrinolysis. In this condition, referred to as hypercoagulation, coagulation has been activated and the threshold resistance to thrombosis decreased.[37] Hypercoagulation is a pathophysiologic state that precedes clinical DIC. Because hypocoagulation is not present (as in cases of DIC), a clinicopathologic diagnosis of hypercoagulation is poorly defined. Consequently, a diagnosis of hypercoagulation is made by correlating the clinical progression (or deterioration) of a patient with an understanding of the pathomorphologic pro-

cesses of diseases that can result in hemostatic alterations or DIC. Determining that a patient is at risk of developing DIC provides the clinician an opportunity to treat the coagulopathy and possibly avert a bleeding diathesis or DIC. Hypercoagulation in the horse and cow is most commonly associated with inflammatory, infectious, and ischemic intestinal disorders.[22,24,25,29,39,40] In horses with strangulating obstructions and inflammatory disorders, plasminogen and plasminogen activators, protein C, and antithrombin III decreased and FDPs increased.[16,17,19,29] Protein C has anticoagulant effects by inactivating factors V or Va and VIII or VIIIa, and potentiates fibrinolysis by neutralizing the effects of PAI. Antithrombin III has anticoagulant activity by inactivating several serine proteases, including factor Xa and thrombin (IIa).[4,5,25,29,36] Consumption of protein C and antithrombin III diminishes the host anticoagulant response to coagulation. The thrombotic condition that often follows these disorders is the result of impaired systemic fibrinolysis and anticoagulation, which are characterized by a relative lack of plasminogen activators secondary to increased PAIs and by the consumption of circulating anticoagulants, respectively.

Bleeding in veterinary patients is primarily the result of excessive fibrinolysis caused by increased levels of tPA or to $\alpha2$-antiplasmin or PAI 1 deficiency concomitant with the antihemostatic effects of FDPs, as in DIC.[16–18,23,29,30] Secondary fibrinolysis is an appropriate physiologic response to systemic large-vessel and microvascular thrombosis that occurs during hypercoagulation and in DIC. Primary fibrinolysis, which results from excess fibrin forming independent of activation of the coagulation cascade, has not been documented yet in veterinary species. In hypercoagulation and DIC, treatment is directed at restoring the hemostatic balance. Therefore, the patients are usually given whole blood or fresh platelet-rich plasma, to replace consumed platelets and coagulation proteins, and heparin to decelerate the coagulopathy.[4,5,26,37,41] In patients that have a single isolated bleed, such as a uterine artery tear, EACA is an effective inhibitor of fibrinolysis. EACA is contraindicated in the treatment of hypercoagulation because it potentiates microvascular thrombosis.

REFERENCES

1. **Corriveau DM.** Major elements of hemostasis. In: Corriveau DM, Fritsma GA, eds. Hemostasis and thrombosis in the clinical laboratory. Philadelphia: JB Lippincott, 1988;1.
2. **Corriveau DM.** Plasma proteins: factors of the hemostatic mechanism. In: Corriveau DM, Fritsma GA, eds. Hemostasis and thrombosis in the clinical laboratory. Philadelphia: JB Lippincott, 1988;34.
3. **Rappaport SI.** Introduction to hematology. 2nd ed. Philadelphia: JB Lippincott, 1987;432.
4. **Green RA, Thomas JS.** Hemostatic disorders: coagulation and thrombosis. In: Ettinger SJ, Feldman EC, eds. Textbook of veterinary internal medicine diseases of the dog and cat. 4th ed. Philadelphia: WB Saunders, 1995;1946.
5. **Ruiz de Gopegui R, Feldman F.** Hemostatic diseases. In: Leib MS, Monroe WE, eds. Practical Small Animal Internal Medicine. Philadelphia: WB Saunders, 1997;973.
6. **Collen D, Lijnen JD.** Basic ands clinical aspects of fibrinolysis and thrombolysis. Blood 1991;78:3114–3124.
7. **Tvedten H.** Hemostatic abnormalities. In: Willard MD, Tvedten H, Turnwald GH, eds. Small animal clinical diagnosis by laboratory methods. 2nd ed. Philadelphia: WB Saunders, 1994;81.
8. **Bennet B, Ogston D.** Fibrinolytic bleeding syndromes. In: Ratnoff OD,

Forbes CD, eds. Disorders of hemostasis. 2nd ed. Philadelphia: WB Saunders, 1991;327.

9. **Vervloet MG, Thijs LG, Hack E.** Derangements of coagulation and fibrinolysis in critically ill patients with sepsis and septic shock. Semin Thromb Hemost 1998;24:33–44.

10. **Bick RL.** Disseminated intravascular coagulation: Pathophysiological mechanisms and manifestations. Semin Thromb Hemost 1998;24:3–18.

11. **Stack MS, Madison EL, Pizzo SV.** Tissue-type plasminogen activator. In: High KA, Roberts HR, eds. Molecular basis of thrombosis and hemostasis. New York: Marcel Dekker, 1995;479.

12. **Lawrence DA, Ginsburg D.** Plasminogen activator inhibitors. In: High KA, Roberts HR, eds. Molecular basis of thrombosis and hemostasis. New York: Marcel Dekker, 1995;517.

13. **Levin EG, Loskutoff DJ.** Cultured bovine endothelial cells produce both urokinase and tissue-type plasminogen activators. J Cell Biol 1982;94:631–637.

14. **Aoki N.** α_2-Plasmin inhibitor. In: High KA, Roberts HR, eds. Molecular basis of thrombosis and hemostasis. New York: Marcel Dekker, 1995;545.

15. **Fritsma GA.** Clot-based assays of coagulation. In: Corriveau DM, Fritsma GA, eds. Hemostasis and thrombosis in the clinical laboratory. Philadelphia: JB Lippincott, 1988;92.

16. **Baxter GM, Parks AH, Prasse KW.** Effects of exploratory laparotomy on plasma and peritoneal coagulation/fibrinolysis in horses. Am J Vet Res 1991;52:1121–1127.

17. **Collatos C, Barton MH, Prasse KW, Moore JN.** Intravascular and peritoneal coagulation and fibrinolysis in horses with acute gastrointestinal tract diseases. J Am Vet Med Assoc 1995;207:465–470.

18. **Grubbs ST, Olchowy TWJ.** Bleeding disorders in cattle: A review and diagnostic approach. Vet Med 1997;8:737–743.

19. **Welles EG, Williams MA, Tyler JW, Lin HC.** Hemostasis in cows with endotoxin-induced mastitis. Am J Vet Res 1993;54:1230–1234.

20. **Green RA, Kabel AL.** Hypercoagulable state in three dogs with nephrotic syndrome: role of acquired antithrombin III deficiency. J Am Vet Med Assoc 1982;181:914–918.

21. **Kitoh K, Watoh K, Kitagawa H, Saski Y.** Blood coagulopathy in dogs with shock induced by injection of heartworm extract. Am J Vet Res 1994;55:1542–1563.

22. **Peterson JL, Couto CG, Wellman ML.** Hemostatic disorders in cats: a retrospective study and review of the literature. J Vet Intern Med 1995;9:298–303.

23. **Wells EG, Boudreaux MK, Tyler JW.** Platelet, antithrombin, and fibrinolytic activities in taurine-deficient and taurine-replete cats. Am J Vet Res 1993;54:1235–1243.

24. **Feldman BF.** Coagulopathies in small animals. J Am Vet Med Assoc 1981;179:559–563.

25. **Drazner FH.** Clinical implications of disseminated intravascular coagulation. Compend Cont Educ Pract Vet 1982;4:974–981.

26. **Boudreaux MK.** Platelet and coagulation disorders. In: Morgan RV, ed. Handbook of small animal practice. 3rd ed. Philadelphia: WB Saunders, 1997;698.

27. **Boudreaux MK, Weiss RC, Cox N, Spano JS.** Evaluation of antithrombin III activity as an indicator of disseminated intravascular coagulation in cats with induced feline infectious peritonitis virus infection. Am J Vet Res 1989;50:1910–1913.

28. **Barton MH, Collatos C, Moore JN.** Endotoxin induced expression of tumour necrosis factor, tissue factor and plasminogen activator inhibitor activity by peritoneal macrophages. Equine Vet J 1996;28:382–389.

29. **Prasse KW, Topper MJ, Moore JN, Welles EG.** Analysis of hemostasis in horses with colic. J Am Vet Med Assoc 1993;203:685–693.

30. **Kawcak CE, Baxter GM, Getzy DM, Stashak TS, Chapman PL.** Abnormalities in oxygenation, coagulation, and fibrinolysis in colonic blood of horses with experimentally induced strangulation obstruction. Am J Vet Res 1995;56:1642–1650.

31. **Darien BJ, Potempa J, Moore JN, Travis J.** Antithrombin III activity in horses with colic: An analysis of 46 cases. Equine Vet J 1991;23:211–214.

32. **Trent AM, Bailey JV.** Bovine peritoneum: fibrinolytic activity and adhesion formation. Am J Vet Res 1986;47:653–660.

33. **Irfan M.** Fibrinolytic activity in animals of different species. Q J Exp Physiol 1968;53:374.

34. **Niewiarowski S, Latollo Z.** Comparative studies of the fibrinolytic system on sera of various vertebrates. Thromb Haemost 1959;3:404.

35. **Ogston D, Bennett B.** Surface-mediated reactions in the formation of thrombin, plasmin, and kallikrein. Br Med Bull 1978;34:107–112.

36. **Darien BJ.** Haemostasis—a clinical review. Equine Vet Educ 1993;5:33–36.

37. **Darien BJ.** Hypercoagulation: pathophysiology, diagnosis and treatment. Equine Vet Educ 1993;5:37–40.

38. **Morris DD.** Thrombophlebitis in horses: the contribution of hemostatic dysfunction to pathogenesis. Compend Cont Educ Pract Vet 1989;11:1386–1395.

39. **Darien BJ, Williams MA.** Possible hypercoagulation in 3 foals with septicaemia. Equine Vet Educ 1993;5:19–22.

40. **Carr EA, Carlson GP, Wilson MD, Read DH.** Acute hemorrhagic pulmonary infarction and necrotizing pneumonia in horses: 21 cases (1967–1993). J Am Vet Med Assoc 1997;210:1774–1778.

41. **Darien BJ.** Heparin therapy: rationale and clinical indications. Compend Cont Educ Pract Vet 1993;15:1273–1276.

CHAPTER 79

Inflammation, Kinins, and Complement System Interaction With Hemostasis

• CARMEN JIMÉNEZ and FRANCISCO FERNÁNDEZ

The inflammatory response is a complex series of events directed to protect the organism against injuries or infectious agents. The vascular reaction at the site of damage is a characteristic feature of inflammation. The coordinated actions of local resident cells, vascular endothelium, plasma mediator systems, platelets, and leukocytes combine to protect the body against injury. Despite this beneficial and indispensable role, the inflammatory response could cause harm. The inappropriate or unregulated response constitutes the basis of a wide variety of disease processes.[1]

Inflammation occurs in two phases: acute and chronic. The acute phase is characterized by local hemodynamic and microvascular changes; leukocyte accumulation, with adhesion and transmigration, is followed by activation and toxic products release. The entire process is regulated by various plasma- and cell-derived mediators. Conversely, chronic inflammation persists more and is less stereotypic. Cellular infiltration is composed primarily of lymphocytes and monocytes and is often accompanied by resident fibroblasts proliferation and capillaries growth.[1,2]

Activation of the coagulation cascade during the inflammatory response is an essential component of the host response to injury.[3] Coagulation represents a double-edged sword. It is necessary for hemostasis and acute containment of an injured or infective focus. Coagulation also amplifies the inflammatory response, decreases bacterial and toxic products clearance and, in the critically ill host, contributes to end-organ damage and death.[4-6] Four main systems in the blood that interact with the coagulation system are almost always involved in development of tissue inflammation:

1. The complement system. Plasma proteins that can give rise to chemotaxis mediators, increased vascular permeability, opsonin activity, phagocytic activation, and cytolysis comprise the complement system. Fibrin is responsible for the activation of Hageman factor (factor XIIa), and factor XIIa fragments (factor XIIf or β-XIIa) activate C1 to C1 esterase. Kallikrein lysates C1 components and activates the alternative pathway. Plasmin and thrombin can convert C3 to C3a, and C4b-binding protein indirectly regulates protein S.[1,7]

2. The contact system. Factor XIIa converts plasma prekallikrein into kallikrein. Kallikrein cleaves high-molecular-weight kininogen (HMWK) to produce bradykinin. Bradykinin induces vasodilatation, increased vascular permeability, smooth muscle contraction, and cellular glucose uptake.[1,8]

3. The acute-phase reaction. The induction of procoagulant activity in endothelial cells exposed to interleukins (IL)-1 and IL-6 and secondary cytokines such as tumor necrosis factor α (TNFα) links the coagulation system to the inflammatory response as well. Several factors such as fibrinogen, factors V and VIII, von Willebrand factor, tissue plasminogen activator, plasminogen activator inhibitor, and α_1-antitrypsin increase in acute inflammation.[9]

4. The inflammatory cellular response. Neutrophils, monocytes macrophages, eosinophils, basophils, lymphocytes, mast cells, and platelets interact with plasma components and release cytokines or their inhibitors (fibronectin and thrombospondin).[2,4]

In this chapter, we focus on the kinins and the complement system. The plasma kinin-forming system consists of three essential plasma proteins that interact on binding to certain negatively charged surfaces or macromolecular complexes. The pathway consists of a complex loop of interaction in which two zymogen factors, factor XII and prekallikrein, become activated to trypsinlike proteases in the presence of the nonenzymatic cofactor HMWK. Once factor XII is activated to factor XIIa, it converts plasma prekallikrein to kallikrein and kallikrein digests HMWK to liberate the vasoactive peptide bradykinin, which is an important component of the inflammatory response (Fig. 79.1).

Factor XIIa converts coagulation factor XI to factor XIa to continue the intrinsic blood clotting; it is known as contact activation. Thus, bradykinin is a cleavage product of the initiating step of this cascade. However, for optimal activation of factor XII, both prekallikrein

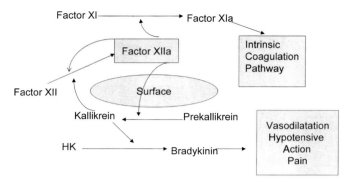

FIGURE 79.1 Kinin and contact system interaction.

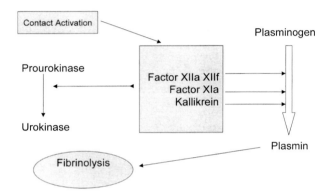

FIGURE 79.2 Fibrinolysis activation by contact system.

and HMWK must be present. This intrinsic coagulation- or kinin-forming cascade appears to be in equilibrium in plasma, even in the absence of any exogenous surface.[6] It has recently become evident that certain blood cells and vascular wall endothelial cells are capable of binding the proteins of the kinin-forming cascade.[5,10] Kinins are proinflammatory peptides released from plasma proteins. Their involvement in the inflammatory response has been demonstrated by dry sponge implantation in rats.[11]

The contact system (factor XII-dependent pathway) induces plasminogen activation to plasmin. This intrinsic fibrinolytic system activation is impaired in factor XII, prekallikrein or HMWK deficient plasmas. In a baboon sepsis model, it has been observed that factor XII and the contact system play an important role in both fibrinolysis and complement activation (Fig. 79.2). Administration of monoclonal antifactor XII to baboons suffering lethal sepsis partially prevented hypotension and prolonged survival. Activation of factor XII by lipopolysaccharide (LPS) or bacterial proteinases contributes to the kallikrein-kinin axis and to activation of the classic C1-esterase-dependent cascade. Therefore, it may promote the septic hypotensive response in people and animals.[4]

Factor XI is one protein of the coagulation contact activation system that assembles on the surface of circulating neutrophils. In one study, the in vitro responses of neutrophils from normal and factor XI deficient cattle (homozygous with less than 2% of normal plasma factor XI activity) were compared. The results indicated that differences in the in vitro neutrophil function were related with the quantity of factor XI.[12]

The complement system comprises approximately 24 plasma and cell membrane proteins. The contact phase of blood coagulation interacts with the complement system. It has been reported that factor XIIf, initiates the classical pathway of complement through direct activation of C1. The complement pathway may also be activated by kallikrein with the release of C5a-like chemotactic peptide from C5. The activation of the alternative pathway factor B by kallikrein has also been reported. Furthermore, the inhibitor of the first component of complement (C1-INH) is the major inhibitor of the factor XIIa and is not active against other coagulation enzymes except kallikrein and factor XIa. In C1 inhibitor deficiencies, the activation of the contact and complement system may contribute to angioedema attack secondary to kinin release.[13,14]

Complement activation results from local generation of active coagulation factor XIIa, cellular damage, direct induction by the alternative route, or LPS or bacterial proteinases exposure. The nine major components, C1 to C9, are sequentially activated, forming a cascade. C3 is the most abundant and pivotal complement protein present in plasma. The early (opsonizing) stages leading to cell coating with C3b can occur by two different pathways: (1) the classical pathway, usually activated by gamma immunoglobulin (Ig) G or IgM cell coating; and (2) the alternative pathway, which is quicker, activated by IgA, endotoxin (from gram-negative bacteria) and the other complement system factors. This alternative pathway in vertebrates is important in inflammatory reactions, and may be activated by bacterial substances such as LPS or zymosan. Macrophages and neutrophils have C3b receptors degraded to C3d, which is detected by the antiglobulin test by use of an anticomplement agent. Only five proteins of the complement pathway participate directly in cell lysis. These proteins form a functional complex of the complement component C5b-9, membrane attack complex (MAC), the common effector arm for both pathways. However, the terminal complement complexes C5b-7, C5b-8 and C5b-9 also can generate nonlethal signals. In vivo, the result of the C5a and C5b-9 attack complex is the increase of tissue factor expression; C5b also leads to prothrombinase-containing vesicles generating from platelets and endothelial cell membrane. This sequence not only increases the generation of thrombin but disseminates circulating, coagulation-inducing particles. Finally, products of activated cells such as neutrophils, platelets, and mast cells exert proinflammatory effects on both endothelial cells and macrophages, further amplifying the local alterations.[15]

Humans and animals that have complement deficiencies are susceptible to bacterial infections and diseases mediated by immune complexes. The pathogenesis of lesions has been studied in experimental animal models that induced activation and depletion of complement. There are evidences as regards complement involvement in the immune response of the hyperacute xenograft rejection, microvascular disease, and the thrombotic microangiopathy or the demyelination.[16–19]

REFERENCES

1. **Vaporciyan AA, Ward PA.** Inflammatory response. In: Beutler E, Lichtman MA, Coller BS, Kipps TJ, eds. Williams hematology. 5th ed. New York: McGraw-Hill, 1995.
2. **Altieri DC.** Inflammatory cell participation in coagulation. Semin Cell Biol 1995;6:269–274.
3. **Davie EW.** The coagulation cascade: Initiation, maintenance, and regulation. Biochemistry 1991;30:1036–1040.
4. **McGilvray ID, Rotstein OD.** Role of the coagulation system in the local and systemic inflammatory response. World J Surg 1998;22:179–186.
5. **Rock G, Wells P.** New concepts in coagulation. Crit Rev Clin Lab Sci 1997;34:475–501.
6. **Kaplan AP, Joseph K, Shibayama Y, Reddigari S, Ghebrehiwet B, Silverberg M.** The intrinsic coagulation/kinin-forming cascade: assembly in plasma and cell surfaces. Adv Immunol 1997;66:225–272.
7. **Johnston RB Jr.** The complement system in host defense and inflammation: the cutting edges of a double edged sword. Pediatr Infect Dis J 1993;12:933–941.
8. **Hewarld H, Morgelin M, Olsen A, Rhen M, Dalhback B, Muller-Esterl W, et al.** Activation of the contact system on bacterial surfaces a clue to serious complications in infectious diseases. Nat Med 1998;4:298–302.
9. **Johnson K, Aarden L, Choi Y, De Groot E, Creasey A.** The proinflammatory cytokine response to coagulation and endotoxin in whole blood. Blood 1996;87:5051–5060.
10. **Hasan AAK, Cines DB, Ngaiza JR, Jaffe EA, Shmaier AH.** High-molecular-weight kininogen is exclusively membrane bound on endothelial cells to influence activation of vascular endothelium. Blood 1995;85:3134–3143.
11. **Damas J, Bourdon V, Remacle-Volon G, Adam A.** Proteinase inhibitors, kinins and inflammatory reaction induced by sponge implantation in rats. Eur J Pharmacol 1990;175:341–346.
12. **Coomber BL, Galligan CL, Gentry PA.** Comparison of in vitro function of neutrophils from cattle deficient in plasma factor XI activity and from normal animals. Vet Immunol Immunopathol 1997;58:121–131.
13. **Morgan BP.** Physiology and pathophysiology of complement: progress and trends. Crit Rev Clin Lab Sci 1995;32:265–298.
14. **Cugno M, Cicardi M, Bottasso B, Coppola R, Paonessa R, Mannucci PM, et al.** Activation of the coagulation cascade in C1-inhibitor deficiencies. Blood 1997;89:3213–3218.
15. **Nicholson-Weller A, Halperin JA.** Membrane signaling by complement C5b-9, the membrane attack complex. Immunol Res 1993;12:244–257.
16. **Candina D, Lenikoski BA, Robson SC, Miyatake T, Scesney SM, et al.** Effect of repetitive high-dose treatment with soluble complement receptor type 1 and cobra venom on discordant xenograft survival. Transplantation 1996;62:336–342.
17. **Nangaku M, Alpers CE, Pippin J, Shankland SJ, Adler S, Jonhson RJ, et al.** Renal microvascular injury induced by antibody to glomerular endothelial cells is mediated by C5b-9. Kidney Int 1997;52:1570–1578.
18. **Piddesden JI, Stordh MK, Hobbs M, Freeman AM, Lassman H, et al.** Soluble recombinant complement receptor type 1 inhibits inflammation and demyelination in antibody mediated demyelinating experimental allergic encephalomyelitis. J Immunol 1994;152:5477–5484.
19. **Jakobs FM, Davis EA, Qian Z, Liu DY, Baldwin WM, Sanfilippo F.** The role of CD11b/CD18 mediated neutrophil adhesion in complement deficient xenograft recipients. Clin Transplant 1997;11:516–521.

CHAPTER 80

Avian Hemostasis

• YVONNE ESPADA

Physiology of blood coagulation is less known in avian than in mammalian species. Numerous studies on avian hemostasis have been carried out mixing avian plasma with human deficient plasma, to determine specific factor activities.[1]

Blood coagulation has traditionally been understood as a cascade of proteolytic reactions initiated in two pathways that meet in a common pathway to form an insoluble fibrin net. Although it has been controversial, now the extrinsic pathway combined with the common pathway is considered more important than intrinsic pathway in avian coagulation. Electron microscopy has shown that in vivo hemostasis is fast; fibrin formation occurs 10 seconds after vascular injury.[2] Contamination of a blood sample with tissue fluid significantly reduces blood clotting time, supporting the effectiveness of the extrinsic pathway.[3]

Avian thrombocytes may have less involvement than mammal platelets in the coagulation initiation. Thrombocyte-specific granules contain serotonin and constitute a source of thromboplastin of lower concentration than in mammalian platelets. Thrombocytes have also phagocytic function.[4] They are involved in hemostasis through a fibrinogen-mediated process. Fibrinogen-dependent aggregation has been inhibited in vitro by an antiglycoprotein IIb antibody. Fibrinogen acts as a molecular bridge for thrombocyte aggregation.[5] Thrombocyte aggregation may be induced with thrombin, collagen, arachidonic acid, and serotonin. Avian thrombocytes may be unresponsive to other aggregating agents such as ristocetin and adenosine diphosphate (ADP).[2]

COAGULATION

Intrinsic Pathway

Chicken whole-blood coagulation (Algorithm) accelerates in contact with surface activators such as kaolin or glass.[6] Therefore, certain contact activation occurs in avian hemostasis.[7] Clotting times of abnormal avian plasma can be corrected with reagents containing human factors VIII and IX, suggesting analogous activities between human and chicken factors. However, factor XII has not been detected in avian plasma, and factor XI activity may be significantly reduced[8] or absent.[6] Plasma prekallikrein and high-molecular-weight kininogen are, apparently, absent as well. Conversely, avian plasma may be activated in vitro by reptilian or mammalian factor XIIa. Thereafter, avian kinin system differs from the mammalian system and acts independently of factor XII.[9]

Vitamin-K-Dependent Factors

Coagulation factors II, VII, IX, and X are present in avian plasma and their activities are significantly reduced by vitamin K depletion. In addition, the prolonged clotting time observed in affected birds could be corrected by the addition of normal serum that is free of factors I, V, and VIII.[10] Similar factors VII and X levels were detected in humans and in avians.[2] However, factors II and IX activities were lower than in human plasma.[8]

Factor V

With similar activity in human plasma, factor V has been detected in avian plasma.[2]

Tissue Factor

Avian tissue factor interacts with mammalian factor VII.[11] When homologous tissue thromboplastin is used, the prothrombin time (PT) of avian plasma is no longer than that of many mammalian species. In general, the shortest plasma PT of a given specie is obtained when the thromboplastin source is brain tissue of the same or closely related species.[9]

Fibrinogen

Fibrinogen concentration is similar in birds and mammals, and behaves as an acute-phase protein as well.[8,12–14] Avian plasma fibrinogen may be activated with bovine

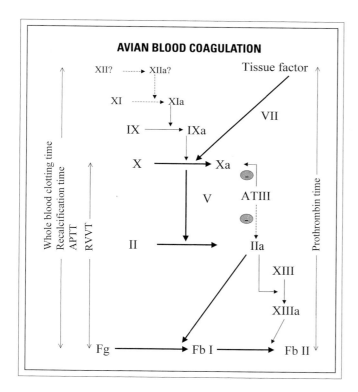

AVIAN BLOOD COAGULATION

thrombin for fibrinogen determination by von Clauss method.[13]

Coagulation Inhibitors

Antithrombin III (ATIII) activity has been determined in broiler plasma by use of the chromogenic technique. Since heparin avoids avian blood coagulation in vitro, the presence of a heparin-dependent coagulation inhibitor can be suspected. Avian ATIII can inhibit purified bovine factor Xa in the presence of heparin. The residual quantity of factor Xa is determined by the rate of hydrolysis of the chromogenic substrate S-2765. Results may be calculated by comparison (linear regression analysis) with a human plasma standard curve and expressed as percent ATIII activity. Avian ATIII also behaves as an acute-phase reactant.[13]

Fibrinolysis

Fibrinolysis in birds might be compared with that of Hageman-factor-deficient people whose intrinsic fibrinolytic pathway, factor XII dependent, is absent. The euglobulin lysis time is unaffected by the addition of a kaolin suspension.[2] Avian urokinase-type plasminogen activator (uPA) has been detected in cultures of normal and transformed chicken cells. Conversion of single-chain prourokinase (pro-uPA) to two-chain active uPA may occur in plasmin absence, suggesting an autoactivation mechanism, whereas mammalian uPA is synthesized in zymogen form, single-chain pro-uPA, and is activated to two-chain uPA by plasmin.[15] Antiplasmin activity has also been detected in avian plasma.[2]

SAMPLES AND TECHNIQUES

Avian blood samples can be obtained by several methods: (1) jugular venipuncture (the right jugular vein is substantially larger than the left),[16] wing vein, medial metatarsal vein, toenail clipping, and cardiac puncture.[4] Toenail clipping is not recommended because contamination with tissue thromboplastin and cardiac puncture is only indicated before necropsy. Hemorrhage and hematoma formation often occur after sampling. This may be prevented by use of the smallest needle available and by compression of the venipuncture site.[7] Blood samples should not exceed 10% of total blood volume[4] or 1% of the body weight.[16] Samples taken for coagulation studies must be collected in 3.8% sodium citrate (one part of sodium citrate solution and nine parts of blood) with plastic or siliconized glass to avoid contact activation.

Thrombocytes

When samples are difficult to obtain, thrombocytes may occasionally aggregate, in spite of the anticoagulant.[4,7] Thrombocytes can be counted by the Natt and Herrick's method or may be estimated in the blood smear. Normal thrombocytes counts are 20,000 to 30,000/μL.[7] See Chapter 178, Normal Avian Hematology (Chicken and Turkey).

Whole-Blood Clotting Time

It is a general screening test of coagulation. Blood is collected into nonsiliconized tubes, and they are tilted every 15 seconds until a firm clot is observed.[17] Contamination of blood samples with tissue thromboplastin may shorten clotting time.[18]

Prothrombin Time

Avian origin thromboplastin source is required for PT assay. Homologous, species-specific thromboplastin sources give more accurate results. Tissue thromboplastin can be prepared by repeated extraction of brain tissue with acetone.[19] The second saline extracts of the acetone-dehydrated brain powder have more thromboplastic activity.[20] Alternate techniques are extraction of brain powder[21] with 0.025 M $CaCl_2$ at 42° C and phenol-saline extraction.[22] Different sources of brain thromboplastin or determination techniques (semiautomated, manual, etc.), and frozen or fresh plasma samples may give different results of PT. Fibrinogen may precipitate in frozen plasma samples with subsequent prolongation of PT.[22] Normal values of PT in chickens are 9 to 11 sec.[21]

Recalcification Time

Intrinsic pathway is evaluated with recalcification time. Reagents used are $CaCl_2$ and crushed glass or Celite, as contact activators.[6]

Activated Partial Thromboplastin Time

Platelet factor substitute prepared from chicken brain can be used as cephalin source. Plasma must be preincubated with kaolin for 3 minutes before $CaCl_2$ is added.[6]

Modified Russell's Viper Venom Time

The common pathway is evaluated with Russell's viper venom time (mRVVT). It has been described with purified factor-X-activating enzyme (RVV-X) and diluted in $CaCl_2$. A mixture of turkey plasma and rabbit-brain cephalin was incubated 1 minute at 37°C before the RVV-X addition.[23]

Fibrinogen

Fibrinogen can be determined by the micro heat-precipitation test in 3 minutes at 56°C or by the von Clauss method with bovine thrombin.[13] Normal levels are from 100 to 400 mg/dL.[7]

Antithrombin III

ATIII activity has been determined by chromogenic assay. Plasma ATIII activities were significantly lower in chickens than in mammals.[13]

HEMOSTASIS MODIFICATION IN DISEASE

Vitamin K Absence or Antagonism

Poisoned rodents, with anticoagulant rodenticides, may lead to secondary poisoning of predatory birds.[24,25] Coumarin intoxication caused by contaminated wood straw in transport boxes has also been described.[26] Chickens were more resistant to coumarin intoxication than mammals.

Vitamin K depletion in breeder hens may induce hemorrhages in chicks. Sulfaquinoxaline administration may aggravate avitaminosis K.[27] Administration of vitamin K_1 is recommended for avitaminosis K, whereas vitamin K_3 (menadione) has not been effective against high doses of dicoumarol-type anticoagulants.[24]

Disseminated Intravascular Coagulation

DIC has been described in several infections, as *Borrelia anserina*[28]; hemorrhagic enteritis by adenoviruslike particles in turkeys[29]; turkeys exposed to *Pasteurella multocida*[23]; infectious bursal disease virus (IBVD)[30,31] *Salmonella pullorum*, *Escherichia coli*, laryngotracheitis virus[32]; and *Erysipelotrix rhusiopathiae*.[14] The presence of disseminated microthrombi has been observed. Chemical mediators release, tissue thromboplastin release from tissue necrosis, antigen-antibody complexes, products of inflammation, and endotoxin are involved in pathogenesis of DIC in birds.

Mycotoxins

Aflatoxin is a potent hepatotoxin. It induces a dose-dependent PT prolongation, which may denote the severity of aflatoxicosis.[33,34] The PT prolongation observed in turkeys correlates with hypoprothrombinemia and hypofibrinogenemia.[35] Aflatoxicosis in broilers induces factors II,[36] VIII, and IX depletion.[37] Experimental administration of T-2 toxin and ochratoxin may induce hepatotoxicity and prolonged prothrombin time as well.[17,38]

Parasites

Coccidiosis may induce hemorrhagic gastroenteritis. Prolonged PT and reduced factor V activity have been reported with *Eimeria adenoeides*,[35] *Eimeria acervulina*, *Eimeria necatrix*,[39] and *Eimeria tenella* infection in poultry.[36]

REFERENCES

1. **Archer RK.** Blood coagulation. In:Bell DJ, Freeman BM, ed. Physiology and biochemistry of the domestic fowl. London: Academic Press, 1971;897–911.
2. **Belleville J, Cornillon B, Baguet PJ, Clendinnen G, Eloy R.** Haemostasis, blood coagulation and fibrinolysis in the Japanese quail. Comp Biochem Physiol A Physiol 1982;71A:219–230.
3. **Tahira N, Dube B, Agrawal GP.** Blood coagulation studies in some wild indian birds: effect of different tissue thromboplastins. J Comp Pathol 1977;87:451–457.
4. **Campbell TW, Dein FJ.** Avian hematology: the basics. Vet Clin North Am Small Anim Pract 1984;14:223–248.
5. **O'Toole ET, Hantgan RR, Lewis JC.** Localization of fibrinogen during aggregation of avian thrombocytes. Exp Mol Pathol 1994;61:175–190.
6. **Doerr JA, Hamilton PB.** New evidence for intrinsic blood coagulation in chickens. Poultry Sci 1981;60:237–242.
7. **Zinkl JG.** Avian hematology. In: Jain NC, ed. Schalm's veterinary hematology. 4th ed. Philadelphia: Lea & Febiger, 1986;256–273.
8. **Dodds WJ.** Hemostasis. In: Kaneko JJ, Harvey JW, Bruss ML, eds. Clinical biochemistry of domestic animals. 5th ed. San Diego: Academic Press, 1997;281–283.
9. **Spurling NW.** Comparative physiology of blood clotting. Comp Biochem Physiol A Physiol 1981;68A:541–548.
10. **Horrox NE.** Congenital vitamin K dependant blood clotting factors deficiency in day-old turkey poults. Vet Rec 1979;104:604–605.
11. **Kase F, Butchers J, Spurling NW.** Comparison of the rate-limiting influence of factor VII on mammalian plasma coagulation following extrinsic activation by avian and mammalian tissue thromboplastins. Comp Biochem Physiol A Physiol1980;65A:421–426.
12. **Hawkey C, Hart MG.** An analysis of the incidence of hyperfibrinogenaemia in birds with bacterial infections. Avian Pathol 1988;17:427–432.
13. **Espada Y, Ruiz de Gopegui R, Cuadradas C, Cabañes FJ.** Fumonisin mycotoxicosis in broilers: plasma proteins and coagulation modifications. Avian Dis 1997;41:73–79.
14. **Shibatani M, Suzuki T, Chujo M, Nakamura K.** Disseminated intravascular coagulation in chickens inoculated with *Erysipelothrix rhusiopathiae*. J Comp Pathol 1997;117:147–156.
15. **Alexander DS, Sipley JD, Quigley JP.** Autoactivation of avian urokinase-type plasminogen activator (uPA)- A novel mode of initiation of the uPA/plasmin cascade. J Biol Chem 1998;273:7457–7461.
16. **Murray MJ.** Diagnostic techniques in avian medicine. Semin Avian Exotic Pet Med 1997;6:48–54.
17. **Doerr JA, Huff WE, Tung HT, Wyatt RD, Hamilton PB.** A survey of T-2 toxin, ochratoxin, and aflatoxin for their effects on the coagulation of blood in young broiler chickens. Poult Sci 1974;53:1728–1734.
18. **Bigland CH.** Blood clotting times of five avian species. Poult Sci 1964; 43:1035–1039.
19. **Griminger P, Shum YS, Budowski P.** Effect of dietary vitamin K on avian brain thromboplastin activity. Poult Sci 1970;49:1681–1686.
20. **Shum YS, Griminger P.** Thromboplastic activity of acetone-dehydrated chicken brain powder extracts after repeated extraction and dilution. Poult Sci 1972;51:402–407.
21. **Doerr JA, Wyatt RD, Hamilton PB.** Investigation and standardization of prothrombin times in chickens. Poult Sci 1975;54:969–980.
22. **Timms L.** The estimation of prothrombin time of chicken and turkey plasma using a phenol-saline thromboplastin or Russell viper venom. Br Vet J 1977;133:623–628.

23. **Friedlander RC, Olson LD.** Consumptive coagulopathy in turkeys exposed to *Pasteurella multocida.* Avian Dis 1995;39:141–144.

24. **Griminger P.** Blood coagulation. In: Sturkie PD, ed. Avian Physiology. 4th ed. New York: Springer-Verlag, 1986;121–129.

25. **Massey JG, Valutis L, Marzluff J, Powers LV.** The anticoagulant diphacinone's effect on crow prothrombin time. Proceedings Assoc Avian Vet 1997;97–98.

26. **Munger LL, Su JJ, Barnes HJ.** Coumafuryl (Fumarin®) toxicity in chicks. Avian Dis 1993;37:622–624.

27. **Sauter EA, Petersen CF, Steele EE.** Dietary and management procedures for development of consistent hemorrhagic symptoms in chicks. Poult Sci 1975;54:1433–1437.

28. **Nikolov ND, Lozeva T.** Effect of inoculating *Borrelia anserina,* disintegrated ultrasonically, on blood coagulation and haemodynamics in chicks. Veterinarnomeditsinski-Nauki 1987;24:50–54.

29. **Gómez-Villamandos JC, Carranza J, Sierra MA, Carrasco L, Hervás J, Blanco A, Fernández A.** Hemorrhagic enteritis by adenovirus-like particles in turkeys: a possible pathogenic mechanism. Avian Dis 1994;38:647–652.

30. **Skeeles JK, Lukert PD, De Buyssacher EV, Fletcher OJ, Brown J.** Infectious bursal disease viral infections. II. The relationship of age, complement levels, virus-neutralizing antibody, clotting and lesions. Avian Dis 1979;23:107–117.

31. **Skeeles JK, Slavik M, Beasley JN, Brown AH, Meinecke CF, Maruca S, Welch S.** An age-related coagulation disorder associated with experimental infection with infectious bursal disease virus. Am J Vet Res 1980;41:1458–1461.

32. **Yassein S, Shaker MH, Aly AA.** Laboratory evaluation of haemostasis in some diseases of fowls. Egyptian J Comp Pathol Clin Pathol 1992;5:97–107.

33. **Fernández A, Verde MT, Gómez J, Gascón M, Ramos JJ.** Changes in the prothrombin time, haematology and serum proteins during experimental aflatoxicosis in hens and broiler chickens. Res Vet Sci 1995;58:119–122.

34. **Espada Y, Gómez J, Lavin S.** Alteraciones hematológicas y del tiempo de protrombina en pollitos broiler intoxicados con aflatoxina B1. VIII. Eur Poult Conf Proc 1990;537–540.

35. **Witlock DR, Wyatt RD, Anderson WI.** Relationship between *Eimeria adenoeides* infection and aflatoxicosis in turkey poults. Poult Sci 1982;61:1293–1297.

36. **Witlock DR, Wyatt RD.** Effects of Eimeria tenella infection and dietary aflatoxin on blood coagulation of young broiler chicks. Avian Dis 1978;22:481–486.

37. **Doerr JA, Hamilton PB.** Aflatoxicosis and intrinsic coagulation function in broiler chickens. Poult Sci 1981;60:1406–1411.

38. **Huff WE, Doerr JA, Wabeck CJ, Chaloupka GW, May JD, Merkley JW.** Individual and combined effects of aflatoxin and ochratoxin A on bruising in broiler chickens. Poult Sci 1983;62:1764–1771.

39. **Ruff MD, Wyatt RD, Witlock DR.** Effect of coccidiosis on blood coagulation in broilers. J Parasitol 1978;64:23–26.

CHAPTER 81

Acquired Coagulopathy I: Avitaminosis K

• M. RENEE PRATER

VITAMIN K

Vitamin K is an important cofactor in the intrinsic, extrinsic, and common pathways of the clotting system, where it is required for activation of vitamin-K-dependent coagulation factors. Factor activation is conferred by means of postribosomal carboxylation of the glutamyl residues on coagulation factors II, VII, IX, and X. Vitamin K is also required for synthesis of the anticoagulant proteins C and S, which specifically inhibit factors V and VIII in the clotting process.[1] Therefore, deficiency or antagonism of vitamin K can result in severe or fatal acquired coagulopathies.

Vitamin K is a fat-soluble vitamin, which is found in three forms: K_1 (phylloquinone), K_2 (menaquinone) and synthetic K_3 (menadione). Vitamin K_1 is found primarily in green leafy vegetables and vegetable oils, and is absorbed via the lymphatics in the anterior small intestine.[2] Vitamin K is synthesized by bacterial microflora in the ileum and colon, and its absorption via the lymphatics is facilitated by bile salts and fats. Vitamin K_3 is a synthetic product, which is thought to be absorbed via capillaries of the colon.

The daily requirements of vitamin K are small, and the liver stores several days' supply, so deficiency in health is rare; however, several inflammatory and toxic disorders may lead to an absolute or relative vitamin K deficiency, which may result in an acquired coagulopathy. To maintain adequate levels of vitamin K, human beings must daily absorb approximately 2 μg of vitamin K per kilogram of body weight; in the United States, a normal human diet provides approximately 300 to 500 μg of vitamin K per day.[3] The daily requirement of vitamin K in the dog has been reported to be 1.25 μg/kg of body weight.[4] Vitamin K deficiencies can be caused by

1. Dietary insufficiency, which is rarely observed in domestic animals that are fed modern commercial diets, but may occur in association with parenteral nutrition. Neonatal animals are thought to occasionally express a mild and transient vitamin K deficiency, caused by either insufficient protein synthesis in the immature liver or a malnourished mother.
2. Decreased intestinal production by intestinal microflora owing to administration of broad-spectrum (especially oral) antibiotics.
3. Decreased absorption secondary to underlying gastrointestinal, hepatic, renal, or pancreatic disorders.
4. Antagonism by warfarin or other anticoagulant rodenticides.[5]

CLOTTING FACTORS

The liver is the site of production of all clotting factors except factor VIII and calcium. Factor VIII is synthesized in hepatic sinusoidal endothelial cells (but not in other endothelial cells) and also in scattered mononuclear cells in the spleen, kidney, lung, and lymph nodes. Factors II, VII, IX, and X (procoagulant serine proteases) and proteins C and S (anticoagulant serine proteases) depend on vitamin K for activation.[6] Factors II, VII, IX, and X are produced in the hepatocyte as inactive precursors. These precursors contain 10 to 16 gamma glutamyl amino acid groups that must be carboxylated in the presence of vitamin K for calcium binding and for activation in clot formation.[7] During the carboxylation of factor precursor proteins, the active, reduced form of vitamin K is oxidized by vitamin K epoxidase to its epoxide form, which then must be regenerated by vitamin K epoxide reductase back to its reduced form to once again be active. The inhibition of vitamin K epoxide reductase by anticoagulant rodenticides results in depletion of active vitamin K_1 and an accumulation of vitamin K epoxide in the blood.[8] This causes decreased transformation of the precursors of factors II, VII, IX, and X to their active forms, which quickly leads to a coagulopathy. Because factors II, VII, IX, and X have short plasma half-lives in the dog (41, 6.2, 13.9, and 16.5 hours, respectively), they are rapidly depleted in vitamin K antagonism.[9]

Vitamin K is also required for synthesis of a group of anticoagulant proteins known as protein C.[10,11] Protein C is a single-chain glycoprotein that is complimentary in its anticoagulant actions to antithrombin III (ATIII), and functions where active clotting is taking place. Protein C is activated by the thrombin–thrombomodulin complex and neutralizes activated forms of factors V and VIII in plasma. Specifically, activated protein C–phospholipid complex competes with factor IXa–phospholipid complex for factor VIIIa, and with a factor Xa–phospholipid complex for factor Va, which prevents activation of factors V and VIII, inhibiting further thrombin production. Protein C may also enhance the induction of fibrinolytic activity by proteolytic inactivation of tissue plasminogen activator inhibitor.[12,13] A factor C deficiency puts the patient at increased risk of venous thrombosis.[11] Protein S is another soluble protein, which depends on vitamin K for its activation. Protein S, in the presence of calcium, is required for the binding of protein C to phospholipid on the surface of platelets and other cells and so acts as an anticoagulant cofactor in the inhibition of factors V and VIII.[14–16]

GENERAL INFORMATION ON ANTICOAGULANT RODENTICIDES

Domestic animals may develop various acquired coagulopathies. One of the most common causes of acquired coagulopathy in veterinary species is ingestion of toxic quantities of anticoagulant rodenticides. Approximately 8.4% of 41,854 calls to human poison control centers involve dog or cat anticoagulant rodenticide poisoning, and 9.2% of 454 anticoagulant rodenticide deaths were reported by 37 poison control centers in 1990.[17] Comparable incidences of exposure, toxicity, and death are also observed in veterinary teaching hospitals and state veterinary diagnostic laboratories,[18] and are the most commonly used rodenticide in rodent control.[19]

Coumarin anticoagulants were originally discovered in relation to reports of moldy sweet clover poisoning in cattle. Sweet clover contains a coumarin derivative that is converted to dicoumarol by the fungus and causes acquired coagulopathy in cattle who ingest moldy sweet clover.[20] From this research, first-generation rodenticides such as warfarin and pindone were developed for control of unwanted vermin and for therapeutic use in human medicine for prevention of thrombosis and pulmonary embolism in patients that have atrial fibrillation and prosthetic heart valves or after orthopedic surgery. Warfarin acts indirectly on coagulation by competitively inhibiting the enzyme vitamin K epoxide reductase, which causes an accumulation of the inactive form of vitamin K (vitamin K epoxide) in the blood and prevents posttranslational carboxylation of the vitamin-K-dependent coagulation precursor proteins.[21] The first-generation rodenticides demonstrate low toxicity in nontarget species, require repeated ingestion to become toxic, and demonstrate a relatively short biologic half-life of approximately 14.5 hours in domestic species.[22]

Variable ingestion of first-generation rodenticides has led to drug resistance in rodents, which spurred the development of second-generation 4-hydroxy coumarins (bromadiolone and brodifacoum) and indan-1,3-dione rodenticides (pindone and diphacinone). These newer anticoagulant rodenticides are more potent, have a longer duration of action, and rely on a single dose

for toxicity. The longer biologic half-life is caused in part by plasma protein binding of the compound and slow release into the blood, which makes relay toxicosis a concern for domestic and wild animals that ingest previously poisoned rodents.[5,21,23–27]

Species and individual variations in susceptibility to the effects of anticoagulant rodenticides are seen, and predisposing factors to the development of a coagulopathy include a high-fat diet, concurrent medications, and underlying disease.[2,21,28] A high-lipid diet not only facilitates increased rodenticide absorption from the gastrointestinal tract, but it also increases plasma concentration of the rodenticide by decreasing the amount of protein-bound warfarin in lipemic plasma. High dietary vitamin E levels are thought to interfere with vitamin-K-dependent coagulation.[29] Drugs can specifically or nonspecifically affect the potency of anticoagulant rodenticides. The coccidiostat sulfaquinoxaline has similar mechanism of action to the anticoagulant rodenticides, and cephalosporins such as cefmetazole, which have an N-methylthiotetrazole (NMTT), chain have been theorized to also inhibit vitamin K epoxide reductase.[30,31] Drugs such as oxyphenbutazone, diphenylhydantoin, sulfonamides, corticosteroids, and phenylbutazone displace albumin-bound warfarin, and increase free (active) rodenticide concentration in the blood. High plasma concentrations increase the severity of the coagulopathy but also cause a slightly faster rate clearance of the toxin from the body. Broad-spectrum antibiotics indirectly affect the potency of the anticoagulant rodenticides by decreasing vitamin K production by the intestinal microflora. This results in an exaggerated decrease in the availability of active vitamin K necessary for hemostasis. Aspirin, promazine-type tranquilizers, sulfonamides, nitrofurans, local anesthetics, antihistamines, testosterone, anderolone, anabolic steroids, corticosteroids, and epinephrine inhibit hemostasis by other mechanisms, and their concurrent administration may contribute to the severity of the acquired coagulopathy. Since warfarin is metabolized by hepatic microsomal enzymes, drugs such as carbamazepine, rifampin, and barbiturates, which induce hepatic microsomal enzyme synthesis, can help in decreasing the hypothrombinemic effect of warfarin and thus diminish the severity of the toxicosis.

Certain disease states may also exacerbate the severity of an acquired coagulopathy in anticoagulant rodenticide poisoning. Uremia causes decreased serum protein binding of warfarin, and renal failure may slow the excretion of the unbound fraction, thus affecting the potency or duration of action of the compound. Viremia and live virus vaccines cause a relative thrombocytopenia, which can also magnify the severity of the coagulopathy. Preexisting liver disease, chronic biliary obstruction, exocrine pancreatic insufficiency, intestinal malabsorption, and DIC may also play an important role in the clinical manifestation of an acquired coagulopathy through decreased production of clotting factors, decreased clearance or metabolism of the drug, decreased absorption of vitamin K, or interference in platelet numbers or function.[32–37]

VITAMIN K DEFICIENCY OR ANTAGONISM

In veterinary species, bleeding disorders have many causes that can be grouped into two broad categories: disorders of platelet numbers or function and hereditary or acquired deficiencies of clotting factors. A relative or absolute deficiency in vitamin-K-dependent coagulation factors is a fairly common cause of acquired coagulopathy in domestic animals. Its development may be multifactorial, and may include diet; diseases of the alimentary tract, kidney, liver, or pancreas; and concurrent administration of other drugs. Treatment in these cases includes administration of parenteral vitamin K_1, and when this treatment is ineffective in normalizing the clotting times, an underlying hepatocellular necrosis or dysfunction resulting in decreased protein synthesis or activation of coagulation factors must be considered. Vitamin K antagonism is much more common than vitamin K deficiency and often is caused by ingestion of an anticoagulant rodenticide.[21,31]

DIAGNOSIS

Clinical signs associated with vitamin K antagonism are broad and nonspecific and are related to organ dysfunction secondary to hemorrhage and hypovolemia. The onset of clinical signs is often several days after ingestion of the anticoagulant when all or many of the vitamin-K-dependent coagulation factors have been inactivated. Clinical signs may include acute death due to massive hemorrhage, dyspnea associated with hypovolemia or bleeding into the thoracic cavity, excessive bleeding at venipuncture sites, external hematomas, bleeding into joint spaces, and other nonspecific signs such as anemia, weakness, pallor, hematemesis, epistaxis, hematuria, melena, and hematochezia.[17,23,26,38,39] Diagnosis of vitamin K deficiency or antagonism is based on history, physical examination, laboratory evaluation of clotting abnormalities, and response to vitamin K_1 therapy. Because of the relatively short biologic half-life of factor VII in circulation (approximately 4 to 6 hours in veterinary species), initial clinical signs and prolongation of prothrombin time (PT) stem almost exclusively from a factor VII deficiency, and this prolongation in PT typically peaks at 36 to 72 hours. And, in the first few days, the concurrent inhibition of the anticoagulant protein C (half-life of approximately 8 to 10 hours) may mask the factor VII deficiency or even cause a short period of potential hypercoagulability until the activity of factor X falls and tips the balance in favor of bleeding. The clinical signs often worsen over time, and prolonged activated partial thromboplastin time (APTT) is seen as active forms of factors II, IX, and X sequentially disappear from circulation in accordance with their half-lives (41, 13.9, and 16.5 hours, respectively).[40] The World Health Organization has developed an international reference preparation of tissue factor from human brain in an attempt to standardize PT testing. The International Normalized Ratio is obtained from determining the PT with this international standard. Additional measures of hemostasis such as platelet count, plasma ATIII and fibrinogen concentrations, and thrombin time usually remain normal. Increased fibrinolysis of extravasated blood leads to mild increases in fibrin degradation products (FDPs), which may cause platelet dysfunction and an exacerbation of hemostatic impairment.[41] The synthesis of the active forms of the vitamin-K-dependent clotting factors remains inhibited until the antagonist is metabolized and excreted, and this time can vary from several days to months, according to the specific type and amount of rodenticide exposure.

In vitamin K deficiency or antagonism, the liver produces inactive proteins antigenically similar to factors II, VII, IX, and X. These are known as proteins induced by vitamin K absence or antagonism (PIVKA), and quantification of these proteins have been used in the diagnosis of suspected rodenticide poisoning. Elevation in circulating PIVKA concentrations may even be detected in the blood before prolongation of the PT and APTT.[42] Circulating PIVKAs are quickly converted to their functional forms after vitamin K administration, and carboxylation of the factors often occurs within 8 to 12 hours of administration of vitamin K.

Additional testing may include quantification of vitamin K epoxide levels. The inactive, oxidized form of the vitamin accumulates in the blood when the enzyme vitamin K epoxide reductase is inhibited in anticoagulant rodenticide poisoning.[43,44] Use of the ratio of serum vitamin $K_1 : K_1$ epoxide has been shown to be variably effective in determining exposure and duration of action of vitamin K_1 epoxide reductase inhibitors.[18] These tests can be used not only to diagnose anticoagulant rodenticide toxicity but also to determine the length of vitamin K therapy.

THERAPY

Therapy for anticoagulant rodenticide toxicosis includes correction of hypovolemia and the coagulopathy. Fluid and oxygen therapy may minimize organ dysfunction caused by hypovolemia and hemorrhage, and fresh plasma may be required (as much as 10% of the total blood volume) for replacement of active coagulation factors in severe cases. Emetics, adsorbents, and cathartics may minimize absorption of the ingested product if treatment begins shortly after exposure to the toxin. Vitamin K_1 is given first subcutaneously and then orally until the toxin is sufficiently metabolized and excreted. Initial loading dose is 5 mg/kg, given subcutaneously in multiple sites, followed in 6 to 12 hours with 1.25 to 2.5 mg/kg subcutaneously or orally at 12-hour intervals. Accurate identification of the type of rodenticide from blood, tissue, or urine samples may be helpful in determining the duration of vitamin K_1 therapy, and repeated coagulation panels are used to assess the efficacy and duration of therapy. The PT and APTT should be checked every 2 to 3 days after cessation of therapy, and therapy may need to be reinstituted with reemergent prolongation in PT and APTT.[21,23,24,45–48] Administration of intravenous vitamin K is not recommended because of its association with anaphylaxis, and use of the synthetic vitamin K_3 is not advised because of a slow patient response time and questionable safety and efficacy.[49] Heinz-body anemia is a potential adverse reaction to high doses of vitamin K_1 (>5 mg/kg).[50] Treatment with vitamin K_1 may be ineffective if there is underlying hepatic disease causing decreased production of coagulation proteins.

Acquired coagulopathies associated with vitamin K deficiency or antagonism can provide a challenging, yet rewarding, diagnostic and therapeutic opportunity for veterinary practitioners. Determination of the cause of the coagulopathy through coagulation panels, other diagnostics, and response to treatment can result in a favorable prognosis for the animal.

REFERENCES

1. **Mount M.** Vitamin K and its therapeutic importance. J Am Vet Med Assoc 1982;180:1354.
2. **Ettinger S, Feldman E.** Diseases of the small intestine. Textbook of veterinary internal medicine. 4th ed. Philadelphia: WB Saunders, 1995;1169–1232.
3. **Rapaport S.** Acquired coagulation disorders. In: Introduction to hematology. 2nd ed. Philadelphia: JB Lippincott, 1987;541–557.
4. **Griminger P.** Nutritional requirements for vitamin K-animal studies. In: The biochemistry assay, and nutritional value of vitamin K and related compounds. Chicago, IL: Association of Vitamin Chemists, 1971;39–59.
5. **Feldman B.** Coagulopathies in small animals. J Am Vet Med Assoc 1981;179:559–563.
6. **Furie BC, Furie B.** Vitamin K-dependent blood coagulation proteins. In: Arias I, Boyer JL, Fausto N, et al, eds. The liver: biology and pathobiology. 3rd ed. New York: Raven Press, 1994;1217–1225.
7. **Green D.** Disorders of the vitamin K-dependent coagulation factors. In: Beutler E, Lichtman M, Coller B, Kipps T, eds. Williams hematology. 5th ed. New York: McGraw-Hill, 1995;1481–1485.
8. **Craciun A, Groenen-van Dooren M, Thijssen M, Vermeer C.** Induction of prothrombin synthesis by K-vitamins compared in vitamin K-deficient and in brodifacoum-treated rats. Biochem Biophys Acta 1998;1380:75–81.
9. **Hellemans J, Vorlat M, Verstraete M.** Survival time of prothrombin and factors VII, IX, and X after complete synthesis of blocking doses of coumarin derivatives. Br J Haematol 1963;9:506–512.
10. **Gallop P, et al.** Carboxylated calcium-binding proteins and vitamin K. N Engl J Med 1980;302:1460.
11. **Marder V.** Molecular bad actors and thrombosis. N Engl J Med 1984;310:588.
12. **Baboir B, Stossel T.** The clotting cascade and its regulations: congenital and acquired clotting factor disorders. In: Hematology: a pathophysiological approach. 2nd ed. New York: Churchill Livingstone, 1990;181–201.
13. **Barton M, Morris D, Norton N, Prasse K.** Hemostatic and fibrinolytic indices in neonatal foals with presumed septicemia. J Vet Intern Med 1998;12:26–35.
14. **Esmon C.** Protein C: biochemistry, physiology, and clinical implication. Blood 1983;62:1155.
15. **Rosenberg R, Rosenberg J.** Natural anticoagulant mechanisms. J Clin Invest 1984;74:1.
16. **Shattil S, Bennett J.** Platelets and their membranes in hemostasis: physiology and pathophysiology. Ann Intern Med 1981;94:108.
17. **Murphy M.** Toxin exposures in dogs and cats: pesticides and biotoxins. J Am Vet Med Assoc 1994;205:414–421.
18. **Felice J, Murphy M.** CVT update: anticoagulant rodenticides. In: Bonagura J, Kirk R, eds. Current veterinary therapy. 12th ed. Philadelphia: WB Saunders, 1995;228–232.
19. **Guitart R, Manosa S, Guerrero X, Mateo R.** Animal poisonings: the 10-year experience of a veterinary analytical toxicology laboratory. Vet Hum Toxicol 1999;41:331–335.
20. **Smith W.** Relation of bitterness to the toxic principle in sweet clover. J Agr Res 1938;56:145.
21. **Mount M, Feldman B.** Mechanism of diphacinone rodenticide toxicosis in the dog and its therapeutic importance. Am J Vet Res 1983;44:2009.
22. **Neff-Davis C, Davis L, Gillette E.** Warfarin in the dog: pharmacokinetics as related to clinical response. J Vet Pharmacol Ther 1981;135–140.
23. **DuVall M, Murphy M, Ray A, Reagot J.** Case studies on second-generation anticoagulant rodenticide toxicities in nontarget species. J Vet Diagn Invest 1989;1:66.
24. **Feldman B, Mount M, Roemer O, Wills G.** Diphacinone (2-diphenylacetyl-1, indandione; diphenadione) coagulopathy in California dogs. California Vet 1981;9:15–22.
25. **Murphy J, Gerken D.** The anticoagulant rodenticides. In: Kirk R, Bonagura J, eds. Current veterinary therapy. 10th ed. Philadelphia: WB Saunders, 1989;143–146.
26. **Schulman A, Lusk R, Lippincott C, Ettinger S.** Diphacinone-induced coagulopathy in the dog. J Am Vet Med Assoc 1986;188:402.
27. **Travlos G, Carson T, Ross P.** Diagnostic evaluation of acute diphenadione toxicosis in the dog. American Association of Veterinary Laboratory Diagnosticians, 27th annual proceedings, 1984:403–412.
28. **Wintrobe M, et al.** Acquired coagulation disorders. Clinical hematology. 8th ed. Philadelphia: Lea & Febiger, 1981;1206–1246.
29. **Frank J, Weiser H, Biesalski H.** Interaction of vitamins E and K: effect of high dietary vitamin E on phylloquinone activity in chicks. Int J Vitam Nutr Res 1997;67:242–247.
30. **Breen G, St Peter W.** Hypoprothrombinemia associated with cefmetazole. Ann Pharmacother 1997;31:180–184.
31. **Neer T, Savant R.** Hypoprothrombinemia secondary to administration of sulfaquinoxaline to dogs in a kennel setting. J Am Vet Med Assoc 1992;200:1344.
32. **Furie B, Furie B.** Molecular and cellular biology of blood coagulation. N Engl J Med 1992;326:800.
33. **Hardy R.** Diseases of the liver and their treatment. In: Ettinger S, ed. Textbook of veterinary internal medicine. 3rd ed. Philadelphia: WB Saunders, 1989;1479–1527.
34. **Neer T, Hedlund C.** Vitamin K-dependent coagulopathy in a dog with bile and cystic duct obstructions. J Am Anim Hosp Assoc 1989;25:461.
35. **Payne J.** Fulminant liver failure. Med Clin North Am 1986;70:1067.
36. **Perry L, et al.** Exocrine pancreatic insufficiency with associated coagulopathy in a cat. J Am Anim Hosp Assoc 1991;27:109.
37. **Strombeck D, Guilford W.** Maldigestion, malabsorption, bacterial overgrowth, and protein-losing enteropathy. In: Small animal gastroenterology. 2nd ed. Davis, CA: Stonegate Publishing, 1990;296–319.
38. **Franz S, et al.** A study of accidents, illnesses, and deaths resulting from the use of commensal rodenticides. EPA public hearing on rodenticide bait stations, Sacramento, CA, 1984.
39. **Green R, et al.** Laboratory evaluation of coagulopathies due to vitamin K antagonism in the dog: three case reports. J Am Anim Hosp Assoc 1979;15:691.
40. **Mount M.** Diagnosis and therapy of anticoagulant rodenticide intoxications. Vet Clin North Am Small Anim Pract 1988;18:115.
41. **McCaw D, et al.** Effect of internal hemorrhage on fibrinogen degradation products in canine blood. Am J Vet Res 1986;47:1620.
42. **Mount M.** Proteins induced by vitamin K absence or antagonists ("PIVKA"). In: Kirk R, ed. Current veterinary therapy. 9th ed. Philadelphia: WB Saunders, 1986;513–515.
43. **Jensen R.** *Optimizing the INR.* Clin Hemost Rev 1997;11:1–9.
44. **Mount M, Kass P.** Diagnostic importance of vitamin K1 and its epoxide measured in serum of dogs exposed to an anticoagulant rodenticide. Am J Vet Res 1989;10:1704.
45. **Mount M.** Toxicology. In: Ettinger S, ed. Textbook of veterinary internal medicine. 3rd ed. Philadelphia: WB Saunders, 1989;456–483.
46. **Scott E, et al.** Warfarin: effects of intravenous loading doses and vitamin K on warfarin anticoagulation in the pony. Am J Vet Res 1978;39:1888.
47. **Scott E, et al.** Warfarin: effects of anticoagulant, hematologic, and blood enzyme values in normal ponies. Am J Vet Res 1979;40:142.
48. **Woody B, Murphy M, Ray A, Green R.** Coagulopathic effects and treatment of brodifacoum toxicosis in dogs. J Vet Intern Med 1992;6:23.
49. **Nangerone L.** Injectable vitamin K3 (Letter). J Am Vet Med Assoc 1986;189:85.
50. **Fernandez F, et al.** Vitamin K-induced Heinz body formation in dogs. J Am Vet Med Assoc 1984;20:711.

CHAPTER 82

Acquired Coagulopathy II: Liver Disease

• M. RENEE PRATER

The liver is pivotal in the maintenance of coagulation homeostasis. The liver biosynthesizes many procoagulant, anticoagulant, and fibrinolytic proteins in the initiation and control of coagulation.[1] The liver is also involved in the clearance of soluble and particulate activated clotting factors and products of fibrinolysis. Bleeding tendencies and abnormalities in the coagulation test results are not common in animals that have mild to moderate hepatic disease for several reasons:

1. The liver produces large quantities of coagulation factors and is efficient in clearing circulating anticoagulants.[2]
2. There must be a rapid loss of greater than 70% functional hepatic mass for a significant decrease in production of clotting factors to occur, and even with this severe loss of hepatic parenchyma, often clinical bleeding is not observed.[3,4] The liver is quick to regenerate hepatocytes after hepatocellular injury or necrosis.
3. Hepatic disease can also cause increased production of certain clotting factors, including fibrinogen in bovine inflammatory diseases,[5] factors I and V in human obstructive jaundice,[6] and von Willebrand factor (vWf) in canine hepatitis and human hepatocellular necrosis.[7,8] This may serve either to mask a bleeding tendency or to predispose the patient to a thrombotic episode.

Clinically observed disorders of hemostasis, however, can be observed in association with other conditions. These conditions are as follows: massive hepatocellular necrosis; cirrhosis; terminal phases of chronic liver disease; other concurrent disease or drug treatment; in association with surgery or trauma; and with disturbances in levels of erythropoietin, cytokines such as tumor necrosis factor and interleukin-6, and thrombopoietin.[9,10]

COAGULATION FACTORS AND LIVER DISEASE

Clotting factors produced by the hepatocytes include fibrinogen (factor I); prothrombin (factor II); factors V, VII, IX, X, XI, and XIII; prekallikrein; and high-molecular-weight kininogen. vWF is synthesized by endothelial cells and megakaryocytes, whereas factor VIII is thought to be produced in the liver vascular endothelium. Consequently, decreased functional hepatic mass may result in a diminishing of clotting factor activity in proportion to the degree of hepatocellular damage, leading to prolonged coagulation times and possible bleeding tendencies. Loss of greater than 70 to 80% of the functional hepatic mass is considered sufficient to cause a clinical coagulopathy, but the nature of the disease, the rate of its onset, and the degree of severity may cause variability in the observed clinical signs of bleeding.

Factor deficiency in liver disease may be attributable to decreased factor synthesis, abnormal factor synthesis, excessive consumption, or proteolysis,[11,12] and their decreased activity correlates well with the degree of hepatocellular necrosis and the concomitant decrease in production of albumin. However, the factor deficiency is often noted clinically before a peripheral hypoalbuminemia caused by the relative short half-lives of the coagulation factors.[13] In human liver disease, factor VII shows the greatest reduction in activity, factor IX shows the least severe depletion, and changes in factors II and X are intermediate.[14] An acute-phase response causes elevation of factor VIII and increased risk of venous thromboembolism in acute hepatitis caused by an interleukin-6-mediated increased expression of factor VIII messenger RNA (mRNA), but the factor VIII that is produced is often qualitatively abnormal.[14-17]

The liver is responsible for removing many of the activated products of coagulation. Soluble coagulation proteins are removed by hepatocytes, and particulate products, such as prothrombinase, tissue thromboplastin, fibrin, fibrin monomers, and fibrin degradation products (FDPs), are cleared by the mononuclear phagocyte system. These particulate products may also be cleared by phagocytes in the lungs, tissue, and by blood leukocytes.[5] The hepatocytes and macrophages remove activated coagulation factors by way of endocytosis through clathrin-coated pits, and this action is facilitated by the removal of sialic acid residues from carbohydrate chains of the glycoprotein clotting factors.[18] This removal of coagulation products may serve to protect the body from thrombosis or the development of disseminated intravascular coagulation (DIC).

ANTICOAGULATION FACTORS AND LIVER DISEASE

The liver is also responsible for synthesis of clotting inhibitors, including antithrombin III (ATIII), α_2-macroglobulin, α_1-antitrypsin, and α_1-acid glycoprotein. Acute or severe liver disease can cause variations in the biosynthesis, consumption, and destruction of these anticoagulants, which may predispose the patient to an acquired coagulopathy. ATIII is a single-chain α_2 glycoprotein, whose actions as the primary physiologic inhibitor of coagulation are modified at least 1000-fold by heparin. It is produced in the liver, is found in circulation and in extravascular sites, and has a half-life of approximately 42 hours. ATIII inhibits coagulation by forming an irreversible, equimolar complex with clotting factors XII, XI, IX, X, and II.[19] It also inhibits plasmin, an important fibrinolytic agent, and kallikrein, which activates factors XII, XI, and VII. The levels of ATIII decline in hepatic disease,[20,21] owing to reduced hepatic synthesis and increased use. Mild to moderate ATIII deficiency may just shorten coagulation times that have been prolonged by liver disease-induced coagulation deficiencies, thus confounding an accurate diagnosis of a hemostatic disorder.[5] More significant ATIII deficiency results in increased risk of renal or pulmonary thrombosis in liver disease. Decreased circulating ATIII is used as an indicator of severity of liver disease, and significant ATIII deficiencies of greater than 50% tend to be associated with poor survival rates in human liver disease patients.[22]

By forming irreversible complexes with thrombin, kallikrein, plasmin, and other proteolytic enzymes, the glycoprotein α_2-macroglobulin inhibits their activities. This glycoprotein has been identified in cell membranes and is thought to be produced in liver fibroblasts. The plasma concentrations of α_2-macroglobulin tend to decrease in severe liver disease, contributing to clotting and fibrinolytic deficits.[18] The glycoprotein α_1-antitrypsin is an alpha globulin that is produced in the liver, is present both in plasma and on platelets, and functions as an acute-phase reactant and as the major trypsin inhibitor in plasma. It also inhibits chymotrypsin, urokinase, and plasmin, as well as factor XIa.[23] The glycoprotein α_1-acid glycoprotein is another acute-phase reactant protein that is also active in the modulation of coagulation. Its circulating half-life is 5 days, and its plasma concentration increases in proportion to the severity of human and animal hepatic inflammatory and neoplastic conditions.[24-27]

FIBRINOLYSIS AND LIVER DISEASE

The liver is also involved in the regulation of fibrinolysis, and functions both in the synthesis of fibrinolytic agents (plasminogen, plasminogen activators, and plasmino-

gen proactivators) and in the synthesis of fibrinolytic inhibitors (antiplasmins and inhibitors of plasminogen activators and proactivators).[28-30] The liver is also active in clearing activators and products of fibrinolysis. Increased production of proteins involved in fibrinolysis or decreased availability of their inhibitors may lead to excessive fibrinolysis and bleeding tendencies.

Plasminogen is an alpha-globulin that is produced by hepatocytes and the endothelium and is present in plasma and extravascular spaces. It complexes with fibrinogen and fibrin during clot formation, where it is converted to the active serine-protease plasmin. Here it proteolyses fibrinogen and fibrin, causing local fibrinolysis of FDPs or fibrin split products. Plasmin also hydrolyzes factors V and VII, complement components, and certain hormones. The rate of fibrinolysis may be increased in liver disease in three ways: (1) diminished synthesis of fibrinolytic inhibitors such as α_2-antiplasmin and others, (2) enhanced production of plasmin, and (3) reduced clearance of plasminogen activators from the blood as it flows through the liver. This increased fibrinolysis may cause oozing from sites of surgery, venipuncture, and trauma.[31,32] Additionally, enhanced plasmin production in liver disease promotes the activation of kinins that cause hypotension, shock, and end-organ damage.[33]

CONTRIBUTING FACTORS TO COAGULOPATHIES

Bleeding problems associated with hepatic disease in dogs and cats are rare. Although 66 to 85% of patients that have hepatopathies display abnormalities in their coagulograms, fewer than 2% of patients develop coagulopathies.[11] Typically, clinically observed hemostatic disorders are associated with a combination of derangements in coagulation, fibrinolysis, and other contributing factors. Contributing factors may include concurrent infectious or inflammatory diseases such as fulminant hepatitis,[2] primary amyloidosis,[34] biliary obstruction and cholestasis,[35] thrombocytopenia or thrombocypathias, or DIC.[36] Surgery, trauma, transplantation, congenital hemostatic disorders,[13] exposure to drugs such as anticoagulant rodenticides or antibiotics, and acute exacerbations of chronic disorders may also contribute to severe or fatal hemostatic problems. Because of the interactions among the coagulation, complement, kinin, and fibrinolytic systems identification of the primary cause of the coagulopathy is often challenging.

The liver has limited ways that it responds to injury, and the specific hepatic response dictates the type of coagulopathy that is observed clinically. It is thought that hepatocyte specialization is based on its location within the hepatic lobule, and proteins produced in the richly oxygenated zone 1 (periportal) include many metabolic enzymes, structural proteins, and coagulation proteins, whereas the proteins produced in the poorly oxygenated zone 3 (centrilobular) are different qualitatively and quantitatively. Therefore, a zonal inflammatory or infiltrative hepatic lesion may result in a specific type of coagulation disorder.[37]

Hepatocellular degeneration, cholestasis, fibrosis, biliary hyperplasia, and hepatocellular regeneration are typical hepatic responses to injury; several of these may occur simultaneously, and their combined effects determine the nature and the extent of the hemostatic disorder.[38] For example, bacterial hepatitis and resulting hepatocellular necrosis typically causes a decrease in factor V production.[6] However, bacterial hepatitis also elicits inflammation and cholestasis, which result in hyperfibrinogenemia and increased plasma factor V concentration.[39]

Changes in quantitative or qualitative platelet activity may also contribute to an acquired coagulopathy in liver disease. Pseudothrombocytopenia secondary to congestive splenomegaly and platelet sequestration is often observed in cases of advanced cirrhosis, and a true thrombocytopenia caused by increased consumption can be observed in secondary complications such as DIC. The expansive endothelial surface of the hepatic sinusoids provides ideal interaction for gastrointestinal infectious agents and their endotoxins to cause vascular injury, and a decrease in clearance of these toxins or agents caused by hepatocellular disease can lead to development of DIC. It is thought that increased plasma levels of E-selectin reflect the activation of endothelial cells induced by cytokines, which may lead to DIC and subsequent organ failure.[28,40] Other pathogenic mechanisms for the development of DIC include release of coagulation proteins from damaged hepatocytes, impaired hepatic clearance of activated coagulation factors, reduced concentration or activity of ATIII, and stagnation of blood flow in mesenteric collaterals.[41] DIC causes increased production of FDPs and increased use of coagulation factors and ATIII in liver sinusoids. The specific hemostatic clinical signs that are observed depend on the disease process, its severity and chronicity, the presence of concurrent disorders, and also on the individual's response to these underlying disorders.

DIAGNOSIS

Clinical signs of coagulopathies related to liver disease may range from asymptomatic to life-threatening thrombotic or hemorrhagic disorders and may include spontaneous bleeding, excessive or prolonged bleeding after surgical procedures or trauma, petechiae, purpuras, ecchymoses, hematomas, hemarthroses, hematuria, epistaxis, hematochezia, and melena.[32] Capillary refill time, buccal mucosal bleeding time, and coagulation tests (prothrombin time [PT], activated partial thromboplastin time [APTT], and individual coagulation factor concentrations) are typically performed to help identify the cause of the coagulopathy.[7] A blood smear may help to identify abnormalities in platelet numbers and platelet morphology and may help in the identification of anemia caused by disease-induced alterations in red cell lipid metabolism and red cell morphologic abnormalities, such as presence of schistocytes.[10] Generally,

severe acute canine hepatopathies tend to prolong both PT and APTT, whereas chronic or low-grade canine hepatic diseases may cause slightly prolonged APTT and normal PT.[42] Disorders associated with coagulopathies in cats include liver disease, neoplasia, and feline infectious peritonitis.[43] A recent study of cats that had liver disease showed the presence of at least one coagulation abnormality in 82% of cats studied, and prolonged PT caused by a vitamin-K-responsive factor VII deficiency was the most commonly observed deficiency. Those cats with significant increases in alkaline phosphatase (ALP) activity were more likely to demonstrate hemostatic derangements than those that had only mildly increased ALP.[44]

Decreases in plasma clotting factors are typically due either to diminished synthesis, increased destruction or consumption, or production of abnormal forms of the proteins.[45] Factor VII deficiency is usually demonstrated first in acute or chronic liver disease, because of its short half-life in domestic species (4 to 6 hours), and factor VII deficiency and prolonged PT have been associated with the highest prognostic value in the diagnosis of acute liver disease.[42] Typically, abnormalities in the PT and APTT are detected before or in the absence of clinical bleeding, and these tests are considered unreliable indicators in the risk of bleeding; hence they have limited value in determining contraindications for the performance of surgical procedures such as obtaining a liver biopsy.[46-48] In acute viral hepatitis, there is a slight to moderate increase in PT without serious bleeding. However, a rapid rise in PT with clinical signs of bleeding such as ecchymoses and bleeding from injection sites may indicate massive hepatocellular necrosis.[32] Decreases in certain factors tend to be associated with specific hepatopathies: canine plasma levels of factor VIII decrease with hepatic neoplasia, factors VII and X tend to decrease with human hepatic neoplasms and primary amyloidosis, and factors IX and X tend to diminish in dogs that have hepatic disease.[34,49] A low fibrinogen concentration in the absence of DIC offers an unfavorable prognosis in patients that have underlying hepatic disease.[42]

In addition to decreased production and increased use of clotting factors in liver disease, production of abnormal factors suggest the presence of hepatic disease. High quantities (>300 mg/mL) of abnormal prothrombin antigen differentiate primary human hepatocellular carcinoma from hepatitis, cirrhosis, and metastatic carcinoma with 91% specificity.[50] Qualitative alterations in the hepatic synthesis of the vitamin-K-dependent coagulation factors are seen in patients that have hepatic disease, and abnormal prothrombin and α_1-fetoprotein antigens are diagnostic in 84% of human patients who have hepatoma. The abnormal prothrombin is called proteins induced by vitamin K absence or antagonism (PIVKA) -II, and is produced in the liver in a relative absence of active vitamin K, where inhibition of the vitamin K epoxide cycle leads to defective gamma carboxylation of prothrombin.[51,52]

Quantitative or qualitative platelet abnormalities are also seen in patients that have liver diseases. Human and canine patients that have liver disease have a decreased ability to aggregate platelets in response to certain agonists.[6,35,39,49,53–55] Reduced platelet numbers may be caused by splenic sequestration, reduced production or increased destruction, as in DIC, or increased circulation of older and less active platelets. Qualitative platelet defects are seen in cholestatic liver disease caused by increased production or decreased clearance of FDPs in DIC, and may help to explain a coagulopathy in a patient that has normal coagulation tests and normal platelet numbers.[35]

TREATMENT

Treatment for coagulopathies related to liver disease depends on the patient's individual clinical signs. Vitamin K therapy is often helpful in converting inactive vitamin-K-dependent coagulation factors (PIVKAs) back to their functional forms and are given in hemostatic disorders secondary to obstructive jaundice. Hepatopathies involving massive hepatocellular necrosis are not vitamin K responsive owing to decreased production of coagulation proteins. Additional treatment for severe bleeding disorders may involve the use of fresh whole blood, which contains functional platelets and minimal amounts of ammonia compared with stored blood, thus minimizing an exacerbation of a hepatic encephalopathy. Platelet concentrates may also be used as a source of functional platelets. Fresh frozen plasma or cryoprecipitate can be administered as a source of fibrinogen replacement. Prothrombin complex concentrates are not often given for replacement of vitamin-K-dependent clotting factors, as they are thought to contain activated clotting intermediates that may trigger DIC and secondary fibrinolysis in patients that have advanced liver disease, but specific recombinant factor concentrates have been used successfully in the treatment of coagulopathies in human cirrhosis patients.[32,56] Replacement of ATIII with fresh plasma or ATIII concentrates to minimize the severity of developing DIC is commonly done in human patients, but use of heparin to potentiate the effects of ATIII is often avoided because of the possibility of excessive bleeding.[57] Therapeutic intervention for hepatopathy-induced coagulopathies should generally be reserved for the more severe cases and for those patients that have a reasonable chance for correction of the underlying defect.[42,58]

Because of wide variabilities in the liver's hemostatic response to injury or inflammation, it is wise to use history, clinical signs, physical examination, quantitative and qualitative estimates of coagulation factor activity and platelet numbers and function, and response to therapy together in the diagnostic and prognostic evaluation of the patient that has liver disease.

REFERENCES

1. Whitney M, Boon G, Rebar M, et al. Ultracentrifugal and electrophoretic characteristics of the plasma lipoproteins of miniature schnauzer dogs with idiopathic hyperlipoproteinemia. J Vet Intern Med 1993;7:253.
2. Wigton D, Kociba G, Hoover E. Infectious canine hepatitis: animal model for viral-induced disseminated intravascular coagulation. Blood 1976;47:287–293.
3. Furnival C, Mackenzie R, MacDonald G, Blumgart L. The mechanism of impaired coagulation after partial hepatectomy in the dog. Surg Gynecol Obstet 1976;143:81–86.
4. Williams W, Beutler E, Ersley A. Hematology. 2nd ed. New York: McGraw-Hill, 1977;1644.
5. Schalm O, Jain N, Carroll E. Veterinary hematology. 3rd ed. Philadelphia: Lea & Febiger, 1975;682.
6. Deutsch E. Blood coagulation changes in liver disease. Prog Liver Dis 1965;2:69–83.
7. Badylak S, Dodds W, Van Vleet J. Plasma coagulation factor abnormalities in dogs with naturally occurring hepatic disease. Am J Vet Res 1983;44:2336–2340.
8. Biland L, Duckert F, Prisender S. Quantitative estimation of coagulation factors in liver disease. The diagnostic and prognostic value of factor XIII, factor V, and plasminogen. Thromb Haemost 1978;3:646–656.
9. Lindblad G, Backgren A. Megakaryocytes, thrombocytes and blood clotting times in dogs with experimental hepatitis contagiosa canis. Acta Vet Scand 1964;5:370.
10. Mehta A, McIntyre N. Haematological disorders in liver disease. Forum (Genova) 1998;8:8–25.
11. Badylak S. Coagulation disorders and liver disease. Vet Clin North Am Small Anim Pract 1988;18:87–93.
12. Furie BC, Furie B. Vitamin K-dependent blood coagulation proteins. In: Arias I, Boyer JC, Fausto N, et al, eds. The liver biology and pathobiology. 3rd ed. New York: Raven Press, 1994;1217–1225.
13. Bloom A, Peake I. Molecular genetics of factor VIII and its disorders. Semin Hematol 1977;14:319–339.
14. Wintrobe M, et al. Acquired coagulation disorders. In: Clinical hematology. 8th ed. Philadelphia: Lea & Febiger, 1981;1206–1246.
15. O'Donnell J, Tuddenham E, Manning R, et al. High prevalence of elevated factor VIII levels in patients referred for thrombophilia screening: role of increased synthesis and relationship to the acute phase response. Thromb Haemost 1997;77:825–828.
16. Stirling D, Hannant W, Ludlam C. Transcriptional activation of the factor VIII gene in liver cell lines by interleukin-6. Thromb Haemost 1998;79:74–78.
17. Strombeck D, Guilford W. Hepatic necrosis and acute hepatic failure. In: Small animal gastroenterology. 2nd ed. Davis, CA: Stonegate Publishing, 1990;574–592.
18. Jain N. Essentials of veterinary hematology. Philadelphia: Lea & Febiger, 1993;417.
19. Mammen E. Antithrombin: its physiological importance and role in DIC. Semin Thromb Hemost 1998;2:19–25.
20. Booth D, et al. Dimethylnitrosamine-induced hepatotoxicosis in dogs as a model of progressive canine hepatic disease. Am J Vet Res 1992;53:411.
21. Johnstone I, Petersen D, Crane S. Antithrombin III (ATIII) activity in plasmas from normal and diseased horses, and in normal canine, bovine and human plasma. Vet Clin Pathol 1987;16:14.
22. Rodzynek J, Preut C, Leautard P, et al. Diagnostic value of antithrombin III and aminopyrine breath test in liver disease. Arch Intern Med 1986;146:677.
23. Baboir B, Stossel T. Antithrombic therapy-anticoagulants, antiplatelet drugs, and fibrindritic agents. In: Hematology: a pathophysiological approach. 2nd ed. New York: Churchill Livingstone, 1990;231–250.
24. Routledge P. Clinical relevance of alpha-1-acid glycoprotein in health and disease. Prog Clin Biol Res 1989;300:185.
25. Motoi Y, Itoh H, Tamura K, et al. Correlation of serum concentration of alpha-1 acid glycoprotein with lymphocyte blastogenesis and development of experimentally-induced or naturally acquired hepatic abscesses in cattle. Am J Vet Res 1992;53:574.
26. Taira T, Fujinaga T, Tamura K, et al. Isolation and characterization of alpha-1 acid glycoprotein from horses, and its evaluation as an acute-phase reactive protein in horses. Am J Vet Res 1992;53:961.
27. Tamura K, Yatsu T, Itoh H, et al. Isolation, characterization, and quantitative measurement of serum alpha-1 acid glycoprotein in cattle. Jpn J Vet Sci 1989;51:987.
28. Carr J. Disseminated intravascular coagulation in cirrhosis. Hepatology 1989;10:103.
29. Furie B, Furie B. Molecular and cellular biology of blood coagulation. N Engl J Med 1992;326:800.
30. Green R. Clinical implications of antithrombin III deficiency in animal diseases. Comp Cont Educ Vet Pract 1984;6:537.
31. Hersch S, Kunelis T, Francis R Jr. The pathogenesis of accelerated fibrinolysis in liver cirrhosis: a critical role for tissue plasminogen activator inhibitor. Blood 1987;69:1319.
32. Rapaport S. Acquired coagulation disorders. In: Introduction to hematology. 2nd ed. Philadelphia: JB Lippincott, 1987;541–557.
33. Kaplan A, Silverberg M. The coagulation-kinin pathway of human plasma. Blood 1987;70:1.
34. Greipp P, Kyle R, Bowie E. Factor X deficiency in primary amyloidosis. N Engl J Med 1972;287:388–397.
35. Meyer D, Chiapella A. Cholestasis. Vet Clin North Am Small Anim Pract 1985;15:215.

36. **Hamilton P, Stalker A, Douglas A.** Disseminated intravascular coagulation. A review. J Clin Pathol 1978;31:609–619.
37. **Gumucio J, Miller D.** Functional implications of liver cell heterogeneity. Gastroenterology 1981;80:393–403.
38. **Cheville N.** Cell pathology. Ames, IA: Iowa State University Press, 1976;22.
39. **Lowsowksy M, Simmons A, Miloszewski K.** Coagulation abnormalities in liver disease. Postgrad Med 1973;53:147–152.
40. **Okajima K, Uchiba M, Murakami K, Okabe H, Takatsuki K.** Plasma levels of soluble E-selectin in patients with disseminated intravascular coagulation. Am J Hematol 1997;54:219–224.
41. **Fiore L, et al.** Alterations of hemostasis in patients with liver disease. In: Zakim D, Boyer T, eds. Hepatology: a textbook of liver disease. 2nd ed. Philadelphia: WB Saunders, 1990;546–571.
42. **Center SA, Johnson SE, Bunch SE.** Pathophysiology, laboratory diagnosis, and diseases of the liver. In: Ettinger S, Feldman E, eds. Textbook of veterinary internal medicine. 4th ed. Philadelphia: WB Saunders, 1995.
43. **Peterson J, Couto C, Wellman M.** Hemostatic disorders in cats: a retrospective study and review of the literature. J Vet Intern Med 1995;9:298–303.
44. **Lisciandro S, Hohenhaus A, Brooks M.** Coagulation abnormalities in 22 cats with naturally occurring liver disease. J Vet Intern Med 1998;12:71–75.
45. **Lechner K, et al.** Coagulation abnormalities in liver disease. Semin Thromb Hemost 1977;4:40.
46. **Ahmed M, Mutimer D, Elias E, et al.** A combined management protocol for patients with coagulation disorders infected with hepatitis C virus. Br J Haematol 1996;95:383–388.
47. **Ewe K.** Bleeding after liver biopsy does not correlate with indices of peripheral coagulation. Dig Dis Sci 1981;26:388.
48. **Inabnet W, Deziel D.** Laparoscopic liver biopsy in patients with coagulopathy, portal hypertension, and ascites. Am Surg 1995;61:603–606.
49. **Walls W, Losowsky M.** The hemostatic defect of liver disease. Gastroenterology 1971;60:108–119.
50. **Liebman H, Furie B, Tong M, et al.** Des-gamma-carboxy (abnormal) prothrombin as a serum marker of primary hepatocellular carcinoma. N Engl J Med 1984;310:1427–1431.
51. **Blanchard R, Furie B, Jorgensen M.** Acquired vitamin K-dependent carboxylation deficiency in liver disease. N Engl J Med 1981;305:242–248.
52. **Nakao A, Virji A, Iwaki Y, Carr B, Iwatsuki S, Starzl E.** Abnormal prothrombin (DES-gamma-carboxy prothrombin) in hepatocellular carcinoma. Hepatogastroenterology 1991;38:450–453.
53. **Bick R.** Platelet function defects: a clinical review. Semin Thromb Hemost 1992;18:167.
54. **Bowen D, et al.** Platelet functional changes secondary to hepatocholestasis and elevation of serum bile acids. Thromb Res 1988;52:649.
55. **Willis S, et al.** Whole blood platelet aggregation in dogs with liver disease. Am J Vet Res 1989;50:1893.
56. **Bernstein D, Jeffers L, Erhardtsen E, et al.** Recombinant factor VIIa corrects prothrombin time in cirrhotic patients: a preliminary study. Gastroenterology 1997;113:1930–1937.
57. **Inthorn D, Hoffmann J, Hartl W, Muhlbayer D, Jochum M.** Antithrombin III supplementation in severe sepsis: beneficial effects on organ dysfunction. Shock 1997;8:328–334.
58. **Staudinger T, Locker G, Frass M.** Management of acquired coagulation disorders in emergency and intensive-care medicine. Semin Thromb Hemost 1996;22:93–104.

CHAPTER 83

Acquired Coagulopathy III: Neoplasia

• DOUGLAS H. THAMM and STUART C. HELFAND

Patients that have cancer may present with inappropriate bleeding or thrombosis from various causes. These include direct tumor invasion through vessel walls, alterations in tumor-associated vascular endothelium, the release of factors from tumor cells or tumor-associated cells, tumor-induced organ dysfunction, and the effects of cytotoxic chemotherapy. Although large studies of hemostatic abnormalities in veterinary cancer patients are sparse, numerous case reports have documented the presence of alterations in hemostasis associated with various tumor types.[1-9] The incidence of altered laboratory hemostatic parameters in humans with neoplasia has been as high as 98% in some studies[10] and in one series of canine cancer patients, 83% of untreated dogs had laboratory evidence of abnormal hemostasis. The most common manifestations were thrombocytopenia (36%), prolonged activated partial thromboplastin time (APTT) (32%), and high or low levels of fibrinogen (25% each).[11] A study of cats with coagulation disorders identified neoplasia in 20% of all affected animals.[12] Various cancers in veterinary patients have been associated with a spectrum of hemostatic abnormalities (Table 83.3).

Abnormal coagulation may be caused by perturbations in primary or secondary hemostasis or in the pathways responsible for clot dissolution (fibrinolysis). Primary hemostasis involves the interactions of platelets with the vascular endothelium and fibrinogen, whereas secondary hemostasis refers to the activation of soluble coagulation factors leading to the generation of thrombin and the polymerization of fibrin monomers. Subtle changes in the balance of procoagulant and anticoagulant factors as a result of neoplasia can lead to the development of thrombosis or hemorrhage. In addition, disseminated intravascular coagulation (DIC), a systemic uncontrolled activation of the coagulation cascade, may also be a consequence of neoplasia.

Uncontrolled hemorrhage is a serious and potentially life-threatening consequence of cancer and its treatment, which may be refractory to standard forms of therapy.[13] Abnormal bleeding can be the presenting complaint in animals that have certain malignancies such as hemangiosarcoma[14] and multiple myeloma.[15]

Thrombosis is another serious and potentially fatal paraneoplastic condition that may be clinically silent in some patients. Thrombosis usually occurs at sites distant from the tumor mass,[16] although intratumoral thrombosis occurs and may be partially responsible for the heterogeneity in oxygenation observed in some solid tumors. Pulmonary thromboembolism (PTE) is becoming more frequently recognized in animals. A recent case series of dogs that had PTE documented the presence of neoplasia in approximately 30% of cases.[17]

The pathogenesis of DIC in cancer is multifactorial, but the result is systemic generation of thrombin and plasmin, leading to concurrent fibrin polymerization and fibrinolysis, with depletion of coagulation factors, platelets, and fibrinogen.[13] In patients that have severe DIC, uncontrolled bleeding is often the most prominent clinical feature, although postmortem examination can reveal striking thrombosis at multiple sites.[18] DIC may be acute or uncompensated or chronic and compensated. In uncompensated DIC, prolongation of the prothrombin time (PT) and APTT, hypofibrinogenemia, thrombocytopenia, increased levels of fibrin degradation products (FDPs), decreased antithrombin III (ATIII), and clinical evidence of abnormal bleeding are present.[19] Compensated DIC is more common in patients that have neoplasia, and may manifest itself with thrombosis rather than hemorrhage. Compensated DIC is often more difficult to detect clinically, as APTT and PT may be normal or even shortened, and fibrinogen concentration and platelet counts may be normal.[18] Many patients that have compensated DIC may have elevations in FDPs and elevated levels of fibrinopeptide A (fpA), which is a protein fragment liberated by thrombin from the Aα chain of fibrinogen and a marker for intravascular thrombin activation.[16] Although measurement of fpA is possible in dogs,[20] serum fpA levels have not been measured in veterinary cancer patients to our knowledge.

PRIMARY HEMOSTASIS

Platelets

Thrombocytopenia is the most common platelet abnormality observed in small-animal patients[21] (Table 83.1). A retrospective study of almost 1000 thrombocytopenic

TABLE 83.1   Neoplastic Conditions Associated With Thrombocytopenia

Decreased platelet production
  Myelophthisis
  Myelodysplasia
  Estrogen secreting tumors
  Feline leukemia virus
  Antitumor drugs
Increased platelet destruction
  Immune-mediated thrombocytopenia
  Shortened platelet survival
  Microangiopathy
Increased platelet utilization
  Disseminated intravascular coagulation
  Tumor-associated hemorrhage
Increased platelet sequestration

TABLE 83.2   Antineoplastic Drugs Which May Alter Hemostasis

Proposed Mechanism	Drug(s)
Thrombocytopenia	Bleomycin, CCNU, Cytosine Arabinoside, Melphalan, Methotrexate, Platinum, Doxorubicin, Actinomycin D
Thrombocytosis	Vincristine, Vinblastine
Thrombocytopathia	Melphalan, Vincristine
Inhibition of factor synthesis	L-Asparaginase
Vitamin K antagonism	Actinomycin-D
Dysfibrinogenemia	Melphalan
Hyperfibrin(ogen)olysis	Doxorubicin, Daunorubicin

dogs identified neoplasia in 13%, excluding those patients that had chemotherapy-related thrombocytopenia[21] (Table 83.2), and a study of thrombocytopenic cats revealed neoplasia in 40%.[22] Retrospective studies of canine cancer patients have identified thrombocytopenia in 10 to 36%.[11,23]

Multiple causes for thrombocytopenia associated with neoplasia have been identified (Table 83.1). These include (1) consumption, seen in DIC or chronic bleeding[13]; (2) sequestration within an enlarged spleen, such as that seen with diffuse infiltrative disease,[24] or sequestration within blood-filled sinuses, such as that associated with canine hemangiosarcoma[8,14]; (3) decreased production as a result of myelophthisis, a mechanism responsible for thrombocytopenia in many patients that have hemolymphatic neoplasia.[25] Contemporary thoughts are that this is caused by the direct crowding of marrow elements by infiltrating cancer cells, but tumor cell secretion of soluble factors that suppress hemopoiesis may also play a role[26,27]; (4) direct suppression of platelet production caused by the effects of cytotoxic chemotherapy agents, such as Lomustine (CCNU) and other alkylating agents, cytosine arabinoside, methotrexate, mitomycin C, bleomycin, doxorubicin, actino-

mycin D, and the platinum drugs[18,28] (Table 83.2); (5) shortened platelet life span, which has been documented in both human and canine cancer patients[29,30]; and (6) immune-mediated platelet destruction. Cancer patients may have circulating antibodies that are reactive with epitopes present on the surface of platelets or their precursors. Antiplatelet and antimegakaryocyte antibodies have been demonstrated in the serum of canine and human patients that have cancer.[31–33]

Treatment of thrombocytopenias, depending on cause, may include transfusion of platelets or whole blood, immunosuppressive drugs, or the Vinca alkaloids, which are capable of increasing platelet counts in certain species.[34] Recently, recombinant human thrombopoietin (rh-Tpo) has become available. Although limited data regarding its use in animals have been generated, rh-Tpo appears to increase platelet counts significantly in normal dogs, although the development of anti-rh-Tpo antibodies in the dog could potentially affect endogenous platelet production adversely[35] (J. Modiano, personal communication, 1998). The use of rh-Tpo in veterinary medicine is the subject of ongoing studies.

Thrombocytosis may occur in animals that have cancer as well, although it is less common than thrombocytopenia, being seen in only 3% of canine cancer patients in one study.[11] However, a prospective study of humans who have cancer documented thrombocytosis in 57%.[10] In one survey, 30% of human thrombocytosis cases were associated with neoplastic disease.[36] Cancer-associated thrombocytosis may be a consequence of increased platelet production from the bone marrow in the face of shortened platelet life span[29,30] or may be caused by a neoplastic proliferation of platelet precursors.[36,37] Abnormal bleeding is a possible consequence, especially if the platelet count exceeds 600,000 to 1,000,000 cells per microliter, although thrombosis is also possible.[38] A primary neoplastic overproduction of platelets or megakaryocytes (megakaryoblastic leukemia) associated with a thrombocytosis has been experimentally induced in a dog. Platelet morphology and function were significantly altered in this animal.[9]

The platelets of some cancer patients, although normal in number, may be hyperfunctional. McNeil et al[39] demonstrated that platelets from dogs that have malignancies had significantly shorter delays in aggregation response, increased maximal aggregation, and increased adenosine triphosphate (ATP) secretion in response to collagen, and responded by aggregation to lower concentrations of adenosine diphosphate (ADP) than platelets from clinically normal dogs. The ability to increase platelet aggregability may confer a selective advantage upon tumor cells. Coating of tumor cells with platelets may enhance their survival in circulation and aid their arrest in blood vessels of distant organs, enhancing their metastatic potential.[40,41]

Platelet function may instead be impaired, resulting in an abnormal buccal mucosal bleeding time (template bleeding time) in the face of otherwise normal coagulation studies. This may occur owing to coating of platelets with malignant paraprotein or to coating by FDPs.[13] Acquired von Willebrand's disease (vWD) has been documented in humans who have leukemias, lymphomas, myeloproliferative syndromes, and dysproteinemias. Possible mechanisms that have been suggested include inhibition of cofactor activity, binding of von Willebrand factor (vWF) to tumor cells, or abnormal proteolysis of the vWF molecule.[18] A case of concurrent thrombocytopenia, vWD and lymphangiosarcoma was recently reported in a dog; however, it was suspected that this dog's vWD was congenital rather than acquired.[7] In the dog, platelet aggregation can be impaired secondary to vincristine treatment,[34] but this is probably not of clinical significance (Table 83.2).

Vascular Endothelium

The interaction between platelets and vascular endothelium is of major importance to primary hemostasis. It has been well documented that tumor vasculature differs significantly from normal tissue vasculature in ways that promote abnormal hemostasis. Tumor vasculature commonly contains blind-ended or irregular tortuous vessels, incomplete endothelial linings and basement membranes, and arteriovenous shunts.[42] Platelet-tumor aggregates around tumor vessel endothelium and separation of endothelial cell junctions have been demonstrated in vivo in various tumors. Additionally, circulating tumor emboli may damage normal endothelium, leading to decreased production of vasodilator and anticoagulant agents by the damaged cells.[43]

Canine hemangiosarcoma (HSA) is probably the most striking example of abnormal blood vessel endothelium and its consequences in veterinary oncology. HSA is a neoplasm of immature vascular endothelial cells characterized by multiple abnormal blood-filled channels and spaces, and often containing intratumoral thrombi.[44] Many animals that have HSA suffer from moderate to severe consumptive coagulopathy, which may be characterized by thrombocytopenia, prolongation of APTT, increased concentrations of FDPs, and clinical evidence of bleeding. In one retrospective study, 50% of HSA patients had clinicopathologic evidence of DIC, and 25% died as a result of hemostatic abnormalities.[14] However, another study documented coagulation abnormalities in only 5% of dogs that had cutaneous HSA.[45]

Treatment for the consumptive coagulopathy associated with vascular neoplasms in humans has consisted of surgery or radiation when possible, transfusions of multiple units of platelets, plasma, or both; heparin; or steroids.[46] In dogs that have consumptive coagulopathy associated with neoplasia, the first line of treatment is to control the tumor through surgery, radiotherapy, or chemotherapy. Adjunctive treatments that may be of benefit include whole-blood or plasma transfusions and low-dose subcutaneous heparin therapy (5 to 10 IU/kg subcutaneously q8h), although 75 IU/kg subcutaneously q8h is also commonly used in veterinary practice.[47]

SECONDARY HEMOSTASIS

Secondary hemostasis is initiated with the activation of clotting factors, usually in response to exposed subendo-

thelial collagen or to a soluble factor (tissue factor or thromboplastin). Progressive activation of the coagulation cascade ensues, culminating in the conversion of prothrombin to thrombin and the subsequent polymerization of fibrin. Balanced against this are the actions of antithrombotic molecules such as ATIII, which binds to and inactivates certain clotting factors (serine proteases), and the action of plasmin that is primarily responsible for fibrinolysis. Tumors are capable of perturbing many components of the coagulation cascade, which can result in excessive bleeding, clot formation, or DIC.

Clotting Factor Abnormalities

Hemorrhagic Tendencies

Decreases in concentrations of specific clotting factors have been reported in numerous cancers in humans, but individual factor analysis has rarely been performed in veterinary patients. The most common single factor deficiencies encountered in humans who have cancer include deficiencies in factors V, VIII, X, and XIII.[13,16] An isolated deficiency of prekallikrein has been described in a dog that had transitional cell carcinoma,[6] and an isolated factor V deficiency was reported in a dog that had nasal carcinoma.[2] Antineoplastic drugs such as L-asparaginase (L-ASP) that inhibit protein synthesis may produce transient decreases in multiple clotting factors[48] (Table 83.2), although the clinical significance of these findings in veterinary cancer patients is unknown. A decrease in the vitamin-K-dependent factors (II, VII, IX, X), caused by a relative deficiency in vitamin K, can be seen in cancer patients, although this is probably of little clinical significance in veterinary patients.[16] In addition, the antineoplastic drug Actinomycin D is also capable of direct vitamin K antagonism.[49] Functional inhibition of clotting factor activity by antibodies may be responsible in part for the bleeding diathesis encountered with the malignant paraproteinemias. Reports have documented decreased activity of factors II, V, VII, VIII, and X associated with human multiple myeloma.[13,50] Plasmapheresis has been effective in resolving bleeding tendencies in human and veterinary myeloma patients,[51,52] although the majority improve clinically after initiation of chemotherapy.[15]

Production of nonspecific heparinlike anticoagulants has been documented in humans who have multiple myeloma, and rarely, solid tumors.[18,53,54] It is well known that canine mast cell tumors (MCTs) are capable of secreting clinically relevant quantities of heparin as well,[55] and this finding has relevance especially when approaching MCT surgically (Table 83.3). Obtaining adequate hemostasis during surgery can be a challenge in certain MCTs, and this may be caused in part by the local secretion of large quantities of heparin. The release of other inflammatory mediators from malignant mast cells may also activate the clotting cascade, leading to changes consistent with DIC.[56] Increases in serum thrombomodulin have been documented in human patients who have end-stage cancer and may serve as a marker for endothelial cell damage, as well as being an

TABLE 83.3 **Veterinary Tumor Types Commonly Associated With Hemostatic Abnormalities**

Tumor Type	Alteration(s)	Laboratory Findings
Hemangiosarcoma	Consumptive Coagulopathy (DIC)	↑ PT, APTT, FDPs, ACT
	Thrombocytopenia	↓ ATIII, Fg, Plt
Multiple Myeloma	Thrombopathia	↑ BMBT
	Decreased Factor Activity	↑ PT, APTT, ACT
	Enhanced Fibrinolysis	↑ FDPs
Lymphoma	Thrombocytopenia	↓ Plt
Mast Cell Tumor	Local Heparin Release	↑ PT, APTT, FSP, ACT
	DIC	↓ ATIII, Fg, Plt
Inflammatory mammary CA	DIC	↑ PT, APTT, FDPs, ACT
		↓ ATIII, Fg, Plt

Abbreviations: APTT—Partial thromboplastin time; PT—Prothrombin time; ACT—Activated clotting time; FDPs—Fibrin(ogen) degradation products; ATIII—Antithrombin III; Fg—Fibrinogen; Plt—Platelets; BMBT—Buccal mucosal bleeding time

extremely potent inactivator of thrombin and potentiator of protein C (PC) activity, which is important in regulating antithrombotic pathways.[57]

Thrombotic Tendencies

Increases in certain coagulation factors may be seen with tumors in humans, and presumably, veterinary patients. The most common coagulation factor increases in human oncology are in factors V, VIII, IX, XI and tissue factor (TF).[13,58] These increases may be caused by direct secretion of coagulation factors by the tumor cells or by tumor-associated inflammatory cells and endothelial cells.[58-60] The activation of the clotting cascade as a result of enhanced factor production may lead to thrombotic disease or DIC and may also serve to enhance tumor cell survival in circulation and increase metastatic potential, as discussed above. In fact, enhanced expression of TF by tumor cells has been shown to be an independent prognostic indicator for survival in human breast cancer patients.[61] Increased TF production by tumor-associated inflammatory cells may be in part responsible for the abnormal coagulation parameters observed in some dogs that have so-called inflammatory mammary carcinomas, rapidly growing carcinomas commonly associated with a moderate to significant inflammatory cell component[62] (Table 83.3).

Decreases in the concentration of anticoagulant molecules such as thrombomodulin, ATIII, and PC may have the same prothrombotic effect as increases in procoagulant molecules. In one study, roughly 10% of newly diagnosed cancer cases in humans had measurable decreases in ATIII concentrations, and 70% had decreased PC concentrations.[63] L-ASP has the potential to temporarily inhibit synthesis of not only clotting factors but also ATIII.[64] In veterinary medicine, dogs that have lymphoma that received L-ASP had a significantly greater decrease in ATIII levels than normal dogs receiving L-ASP,[65] and one report documents cerebral thrombosis after L-ASP administration to a dog with lymphoma, presumably caused at least in part by a decrease in ATIII.[1] Protein loss, from diffuse neoplastic

gastrointestinal infiltration or glomerulopathy, may also result in a net decrease in ATIII concentration. Assays to measure serum ATIII levels in canine serum are available, and these may help to identify animals at risk for developing thrombosis. In addition, animals that have low ATIII levels are less likely to respond to heparinization, as heparin's role in antithrombotic therapy is through potentiation of ATIII's activity.[66] Measurement of coagulation inhibitors has not been performed in large numbers of veterinary cancer patients.

Fibrin or Fibrinogen Abnormalities

The pathway of secondary hemostasis culminates in the polymerization of fibrin, and its subsequent depolymerization during clot lysis. Neoplasms have the potential to alter both arms of this process. Hyperfibrinogenemia, which could be a consequence of chronic antigenic stimulation, can be detected in approximately 40% of human cancers and 25% of canine cancers.[10,11] Hypofibrinogenemia was also documented in 25% of the patients in one study of canine cancer.[11] Increased consumption, as seen with DIC, may play a role in this hypofibrinogenemia. In vivo studies have demonstrated a shortened fibrinogen life span in dogs that have neoplasia compared with normal canine control subjects.[30]

Alterations in fibrin monomer polymerization (dysfibrinogenemia) or enhanced fibrinolysis may also occur. Acquired dysfibrinogenemia has been documented in human patients who have multiple myeloma[67] and renal cell carcinoma.[68] Hyperfibrinolysis, presumably as a result of enhanced plasmin activity, has been demonstrated in human patients who have multiple myeloma, multiple carcinomas, and soft tissue sarcomas.[13] This may be because of elaboration of molecules such as tissue plasminogen activator or urokinase-like plasminogen activator or by direct cleavage of fibrinogen by tumor-derived proteases.[18] Doxorubicin also directly causes increases in fibrinolysis; this has led to clinical bleeding in some human patients[69] (Table 83.2). Finally, a decrease in fibrinolytic activity (hypofibrinolysis) has been observed after combination chemotherapy in human patients who have lung cancer; this decreased activity may have led to an increase in thrombotic events after initiation of therapy.[70]

In summary, although clinically significant perturbations in the coagulation system may be uncommon in veterinary cancer patients, the recognition and identification of such problems when they occur can have great importance in terms of patient survival. It is important to remember that appropriate antineoplastic therapy (surgery, chemotherapy, and radiotherapy) remains the mainstay of treatment for coagulation disorders in cancer patients.

REFERENCES

1. **Swanson JF, Morgan S, Green RA, et al.** Cerebral thrombosis and hemorrhage in association with L-asparaginase administration. J Am Anim Hosp Assoc 1986;22:749–755.
2. **Prasse KW, Hoskins JD, Glock RD, et al.** Factor V deficiency and thrombocytopenia in a dog with adenocarcinoma. J Am Vet Med Assoc 1972;160:204–207.
3. **Shepard VJ, Dodds-Laffin WJ, Laffin RJ.** Gamma A myeloma in a dog with defective hemostasis. J Am Vet Med Assoc 1972;160:1121–1127.
4. **Jones DRE, Gruffydd-Jones TK, McCullagh KG.** Disseminated intravascular coagulation in a dog with thoracic neoplasia. J Small Anim Pract 1980;21:303–309.
5. **Ihle SL, Baldwin CJ, Pifer SM.** Probable recurrent femoral artery thrombosis in a dog with intestinal lymphosarcoma. J Am Vet Med Assoc 1996;208:240–242.
6. **Chinn DR, Dodds WJ, Selcer BA.** Prekallikrein deficiency in a dog. J Am Vet Med Assoc 1986;188:69–71.
7. **Woods JP, Johnstone IB, Bienzle D, et al.** Concurrent lymphangioma, immune-mediated thrombocytopenia, and von Willebrand's disease in a dog. J Am Anim Hosp Assoc 1995;31:70–76.
8. **Rishniw M, Lewis DC.** Localized consumptive coagulopathy associated with cutaneous hemangiosarcoma in a dog. J Am Anim Hosp Assoc 1994;30:261–264.
9. **Cain R, Feldman BF, Kawakami TG, et al.** Platelet dysplasia associated with megakaryoblastic leukemia in a dog. J Am Vet Med Assoc 1986;188:529–530.
10. **Sun NJ, McAfee WM, Hum GJ, et al.** Hemostatic abnormalities in malignancy, a prospective study of one hundred eight patients. Part I: coagulation studies. Am J Clin Pathol 1979;71:10–16.
11. **Madewell BR, Feldman BF, O'Neill S.** Coagulation abnormalities in dogs with neoplastic disease. Thromb Haemost 1980;44:35–38.
12. **Peterson JL, Couto GC, Wellman ML.** Hemostatic disorders in cats: a retrospective study and review of the literature. J Vet Intern Med 1995;9:298–303.
13. **Bick RL.** Alterations of hemostasis associated with malignancy: etiology, pathophysiology, diagnosis and management. Semin Thromb Hemost 1978;5:1–26.
14. **Hammer AS, Couto CG, Swardson C, et al.** Hemostatic abnormalities in dogs with hemangiosarcoma. J Vet Intern Med 1991;5:11–14.
15. **Vail DM.** Plasma cell neoplasms. In: Withrow S, MacEwen E, eds. Small animal clinical oncology. 2nd ed. Philadelphia: WB Saunders, 1996;509–520.
16. **Ratnoff OD.** Hemostatic emergencies in malignancy. Semin Oncol 1989;16:561–571.
17. **LaRue MJ, Murtaugh RJ.** Pulmonary thromboembolism in dogs: 47 cases (1986–1987). J Am Vet Med Assoc 1990;197:1368–1372.
18. **Rosen PJ.** Bleeding problems in the cancer patient. Hematol Oncol Clin North Am 1992;6:1315–1328.
19. **Pasquini E, Gianni L, Aitini E, et al.** Acute disseminated intravascular coagulation syndrome in cancer patients. Oncology 1995;52:505–508.
20. **Wilner GD.** Measurement of fibrinopeptide A in canine blood—an interim report. Thromb Res 1979;15:601–610.
21. **Grindem CB, Breitschwerdt EB, Corbett WT, et al.** Epidemiologic survey of thrombocytopenia in dogs: a report on 987 cases. Vet Clin Pathol 1991;20:38–43.
22. **Jordan HL, Grindem CB, Breitschwerdt EB.** Thrombocytopenia in cats: a retrospective study of 41 cases. J Vet Intern Med 1993;7:261–265.
23. **Grindem CB, Breitschwerdt EB, Corbett WT, et al.** Thrombocytopenia associated with neoplasia in dogs. J Vet Intern Med 1994;8:400–405.
24. **Harker LA, Finch CA.** Thrombokinetics in man. J Clin Invest 1969;48:963–974.
25. **Madewell BR.** Hematological and bone marrow cytological abnormalities in 75 dogs with malignant lymphoma. J Am Anim Hosp Assoc 1986;22:235–240.
26. **Selleri C, Maciejewski JP, Sato T, et al.** Interferon-gamma constitutively expressed in the stromal microenvironment of human marrow cultures mediates potent hematopoietic inhibition. Blood 1996;87:4149–4157.
27. **Sawada K, Sato N, Koike T.** Inhibition of GM-CSF production by recombinant human interleukin-4: negative regulator of hematopoiesis. Leuk Lymphoma 1995;19:33–42.
28. **Handagama P, Feldman BF.** Thrombocytopenia and drugs. Vet Clin North Am Small Anim Pract 1988;18:51–65.
29. **Tranum BL, Haut A.** Thrombocytosis: platelet kinetics in neoplasia. J Lab Clin Med 1974;84:615–619.
30. **O'Donnell MR, Slichter SJ, Weiden PL, et al.** Platelet and fibrinogen kinetics in canine tumors. Cancer Res 1981;41:1379–1383.
31. **Schwartz KA, Slichter SJ, Harker LA.** Immune-mediated platelet destruction and thrombocytopenia in patients with solid tumors. Br J Hematol 1982;51:17–24.
32. **Kristensen AT, Weiss DJ, Klausner JS, et al.** Detection of antiplatelet antibody with a platelet immunofluorescence assay. J Vet Intern Med 1994;8:36–39.
33. **Helfand SC, Couto CG, Madewell BR.** Immune-mediated thrombocytopenia associated with solid tumors in dogs. J Am Anim Hosp Assoc 1984;21:787–794.
34. **Mackin AJ, Allen DG, Johnstone IB.** Effects of vincristine and prednisone on platelet numbers and function in clinically normal dogs. Am J Vet Res 1995;56:100–108.
35. **Peng J, Friese P, Wolf RF, et al.** Relative reactivity of platelets from thrombopoietin- and interleukin-6-treated dogs. Blood 1996;87:4158–4163.
36. **Levin J, Conley CL.** Thrombocytosis associated with malignant diseases. Arch Intern Med 1964;114:497–500.
37. **Degen MA, Feldman BF, Turrel JM, et al.** Thrombocytosis associated with a myeloproliferative disorder in a dog. J Am Vet Med Assoc 1989;194:1457–1459.
38. **Silverstein MN.** Primary or hemorrhagic thrombocythemia. Arch Int Med 1968;122:18–22.
39. **McNeil EA, Ogilvie GK, Fettman MJ, et al.** Platelet hyperfunction in dogs with malignancies. J Vet Intern Med 1997;11:178–182.
40. **Nierodzik ML, Klepfish A, Karpatkin S.** Role of platelets, thrombin, integrin IIb-IIIa, fibronectin and von Willebrand factor on tumor adhesion in vitro and metastasis in vivo. Thromb Haemost 1995;74:282–290.
41. **Mogi Y, Kogawa K, Takayama T, et al.** Platelet aggregation induced by adenosine diphosphate released from cloned murine fibrosarcoma cells is positively correlated with the experimental metastatic potential of the cells. Jpn J Cancer Res 1991;82:192–198.
42. **Brown JM, Giaccia AJ.** The unique physiology of solid tumors: opportunities (and problems) for cancer therapy. Cancer Res 1998;58:1408–1416.
43. **Naschitz JE, Yeshurun D, Lev LM.** Thromboembolism in cancer: changing trends. Cancer 1993;71:1384–1390.
44. **Pulley LT, Stannard AA.** Skin and soft tissues. In: Moulton J, ed. Tumors in domestic animals. 3rd ed. Los Angeles: University of California Press, 1990;47–48.
45. **Hargis AM, Feldman BF.** Evaluation of hemostatic defects secondary to vascular tumors in dogs: 11 cases. J Am Vet Med Assoc 1991;198:891–894.
46. **White CW, Wolf SJ, Korones DN, et al.** Treatment of childhood angiomatous diseases with recombinant interferon α-2a. J Pediatr 1991;118:59–66.
47. **Ruehl WD, Mills C, Feldman BF.** Rational therapy in disseminated intravascular coagulation. J Am Vet Med Assoc 1982;181:76–78.
48. **Gralnick HR, Henderson E.** Hypofibrinogenemia and coagulation factor deficiencies with L-asparaginase treatment. Cancer 1971;27:1313–1320.
49. **Olson RE.** Vitamin K-induced prothrombin formation antagonism by actinomycin-D. Science 1964;145:926–928.
50. **Colwell NS, Tollefsen DM, Blinder MA.** Identification of a monoclonal thrombin inhibitor associated with multiple myeloma and a severe bleeding disorder. Br J Hematol 1997;97:219–226.
51. **Godal HC, Borchgrevink CF.** The effect of plasmapheresis on the hemostatic function in patients with macroglobulinemia Waldenstrom and multiple myeloma. Scand J Clin Lab Invest 1965;17 (suppl 84):133–138.
52. **Shull RM, Osborne CA, Barrett RE, et al.** Serum hyperviscosity syndrome associated with IgA multiple myeloma in two dogs. J Am Anim Hosp Assoc 1978;14:58–70.
53. **Kaufman PA, Gockerman JP, Greenberg CS.** Production of a novel anticoagulant by neoplastic plasma cells: report of a case and review of the literature. Am J Med 1989;86:612–616.
54. **Chapman GS, George CB, Danley DL.** Heparin-like anticoagulant associated with plasma cell myeloma. Am J Clin Pathol 1985;83:764–766.
55. **Hottendorf GH, Nielsen SW, Kenyon AJ.** Canine mastocytoma. I. Blood coagulation time in dogs with mastocytoma. Pathol Vet 1965;2:129–141.
56. **O'Keefe DA, Couto CG, Burke-Schwartz C, et al.** Systemic mastocytosis in 16 dogs. J Vet Intern Med 1987;1:75–80.
57. **Lindahl AK, Boffa MC, Abildgaard U.** Increased plasma thrombomodulin in cancer patients. Thromb Haemost 1993;69:112–114.
58. **Naschitz JE, Yeshurun D, Eldar S, et al.** Diagnosis of cancer-associated vascular disorders. Cancer 1996;77:1759–1767.
59. **Moore KL, Esmon CT, Esmon NL.** Tumor necrosis factor leads to the

internalization and degradation of thrombomodulin from the surface of bovine aortic endothelial cells in culture. Blood 1989;73:159–165.

60. **Helin H.** Macrophage procoagulant factors–mediators of inflammatory and neoplastic tissue lesions. Med Biol 1986;64:167–176.

61. **Kakkar AK, Ellis IO, Blamey RW, et al.** Tissue factor: a new independent prognostic marker in breast cancer. Proc Am Assoc Cancer Res 1996;201.

62. **Susaneck SJ, Allen TA, Hoopes J, et al.** Inflammatory mammary carcinoma in the dog. J Am Anim Hosp Assoc 1983;19:971–976.

63. **Nand S, Fisher SG, Salgia R, et al.** Hemostatic abnormalities in untreated cancer: incidence and correlation with thrombotic and hemorrhagic complications. J Clin Oncol 1987;5:1998–2003.

64. **Mitchell L, Hoogendorn H, Giles AR, et al.** Increased endogenous thrombin generation in children with acute lymphoblastic leukemia: risk of thrombotic complications in L'Asparaginase-induced antithrombin III deficiency. Blood 1994;83:386–391.

65. **Rogers KS, Barton CL, Benson PA, et al.** Effects of single-dose L-asparaginase on coagulation values in healthy dogs and dogs with lymphoma. Am J Vet Res 1992;53:580–584.

66. **Green RA.** Pathophysiology of antithrombin III deficiency. Vet Clin North Am Small Anim Pract 1988;18:95–104.

67. **O'Kane MJ, Wisdom GB, Desai ZR, et al.** Inhibition of fibrin monomer polymerisation by myeloma immunoglobulin. J Clin Pathol 1994;47:266–268.

68. **Dawson NA, Barr CF, Alving BM.** Acquired dysfibrinogenemia–paraneoplastic syndrome in renal cell carcinoma. Am J Med 1985;78:682–686.

69. **Bick RL, Fekete LF, Wilson WL.** Adriamycin and fibrinolysis. Thromb Res 1976;8:467–469.

70. **Gabazza EC, Taguchi O, Yamakami T, et al.** Alteration of coagulation and fibrinolysis systems after multidrug anticancer therapy for lung cancer. Eur J Cancer 1994;30A:1276–1281.

CHAPTER 84

Acquired Coagulopathy IV: Acquired Inhibitors

• RAFAEL RUIZ DE GOPEGUI

Acquired anticoagulants have been described in humans, laboratory animals, and small animals. These pathologic inhibitors of coagulation are also termed circulating anticoagulants and consist primarily of immunoglobulins directed against functional epitopes of hemostasis components. Clinical expression of acquired inhibitors is variable. In severe cases, either hemorrhage or thrombosis or merely altered coagulation screening tests without hemorrhage may occur.

The presence of acquired inhibitors is suspected when an altered coagulation screening test cannot be explained by single or multiple coagulation factor deficiency. The mixture of normal species-specific plasma with the deficient plasma corrects the prolonged coagulation test result. However, when an acquired inhibitor is present, the addition of normal plasma to the problem plasma results in a lack of correction of the prolonged coagulation tests. Once the abnormality of the screening procedure has been identified, it must be proved that this abnormality has been induced by an acquired inhibitor. The use of antithrombotic drugs or inadequate technique must be ruled out. The screening coagulation test is performed in the patient, in normal (species-specific) pooled plasma, and in a 1:1 mixture of the two samples immediately and after 1 hour of incubation at 37°C. If the patient's coagulation test is prolonged and does not normalize by the addition of normal pooled plasma, either immediately or after incubation, the presence of an inhibitor is suggested. If the abnormality consists in a single or multiple coagulation factor deficiency, the 1:1 mixture coagulation test result is normal. Weak inhibitors may require serial dilutions up to one part of pooled plasma and four parts of problem plasma to perform more accurate mixing studies. In people who have antiphospholipid-protein antibodies (APA), the abnormal coagulation test result is accentuated in the mixing study.

COAGULATION FACTORS INHIBITORS

Factor VIII Acquired Inhibitor

The development of factor VIII inhibitors is a serious complication of hemophilia A replacement therapy. Re-peated transfusions of homologous factor VIII may induce an immune response against factor VIII in both humans and dogs. Affected patients produce antibodies against factor VIII, which inactivate the transfused factor.[1] Inhibitor development propensity appears to be genetically based. Genetic predisposition has been proposed in individuals who have gross gene deletion where the absence of any gene product could result in the recognition of transfused factor VIII as a nonself protein. However, point mutation is observed in the majority of hemophilia A people developing factor VIII inhibitor.[2] Factor VIII inhibitors present variable severity among individuals, as well. Factor VIII inhibitory activity may be quantified in Bethesda units per mL.[3] If the plasma that has an inhibitor potency of 1 Bethesda unit per milliliter is mixed 1:1 with a normal species-specific pooled plasma (100% factor VIII activity), the resultant functional factor VIII activity of the mixture is 50% factor VIII activity.

Factor IX Acquired Inhibitor

Because of repeated transfusions, factor IX inhibitor has been described in human hemophilia B. It has also been reported for people who have immune-mediated disease and in gene therapy research in which adenoviral vectors in rodents and dogs have been studied.[4]

Factor XI Acquired Inhibitor

Because of repeated transfusions, factor XI inhibitor has been described in human hemophilia C, in people who have immune-mediated disease, and in a 5-year-old male cat. The cat presented severe epistaxis that ceased after transfusion of fresh whole blood. Prolonged activated partial thromboplastin time (APTT) and low factor XI activity were observed. The inhibitory effect was enhanced by incubation at 37°C.[5]

INTERFERENCE INHIBITORS

Interference inhibitors block more than one single coagulation factor. This type of acquired inhibitor affects activating complexes (APAs) or fibrin formation and polymerization (fibrin or fibrinogen degradation products). These inhibitors may be observed in immune-mediated diseases, lymphoproliferative disease, and disseminated intravascular coagulation (see Chapter 86, Acquired Coagulopathy VI: Disseminated Intravascular Coagulation).

Lupus Anticoagulant

Antiphospholipid antibodies or APAs are a family of autoimmune or alloimmune immunoglobulins that recognize protein phospholipid complexes in in vitro laboratory test systems. These molecules were firstly detected in human syphilis in 1906 by Dr A. Wassermann.[6] Forty five years later, the presence of a peculiar circulating anticoagulant in human systemic lupus erythematosus (SLE) was described as lupus anticoagulant (LA).[7] Most of these patients did not have hemorrhages. However, several clinical complications, including arterial or venous thrombosis, unexplained thrombocytopenia, or recurrent spontaneous abortion were described in LA patients. Venous or arterial thrombosis may affect 30 percent of LA patients. The increased thrombotic risk may be explained by several mechanisms, including reduced plasma concentration of functional coagulation inhibitors (antithrombin III, protein C, or protein S), inhibition of prostacyclin production, inhibition of protein C system, antiendothelial cell antibodies, or anti-β_2 glycoprotein 1 antibodies.[8]

APAs (LAs) have been described in canine SLE. Prolonged activated partial thromboplastin time among other coagulation screening tests was observed. However, the dog developed fatal pulmonary thromboembolism.[9]

Animal models have also been developed for the study of APA. Thrombosis, thrombocytopenia, or obstetric complications induced by APA were observed in experimentation mice.[10,11]

Diagnosis of APA in human medicine includes anticardiolipin antibody and LA testing. LAs diagnosis requires a prolonged coagulation screening test (such as activated partial thromboplastin time, kaolin clotting time, plasma clotting time, or Textarin time), demonstration that the prolongation is caused by an inhibitor rather than a factor deficiency (mixing study), and demonstration that the inhibitor is phospholipid dependent (dilute Russell's viper venom time or dilute prothrombin time, or platelet neutralization procedure). Therapy should be directed to the primary disease inducing LA, but antithrombotic therapy with heparin or aspirin may be considered as well.

Monoclonal Immunoglobulins

Multiple myeloma and Waldenström's macroglobulinemia are systemic proliferations of malignant plasma cells or their precursors arising as a clone of a single cell that usually involves multiple bone marrow sites. These neoplasms are characterized by the production of monoclonal or biclonal gammaglobulins.[12] Complications associated with multiple myeloma include hypercalcemia, hyperviscosity syndrome, renal failure, immunosuppression, spinal cord compression, and hemostasis abnormalities.[13] Spontaneous hemorrhages, epistaxis and gingival bleeding, are frequently observed.[14] They can be induced by thrombocytopenia and thrombopathia, reduction or inhibition of plasma coagulation proteins, and disseminated intravascular coagulation. The presence of a monoclonal protein appears to interfere von Willebrand's factor–glycoprotein Ib binding, resulting in diminished platelet adhesiveness. Thereafter, the myeloma paraprotein may also act as an interference inhibitor on coagulation factors and fibrin polymerization.[15,16] Interference inhibitors induced by myeloma and Waldenström's macroglobulinemia have been widely described in humans; paraproteins exert the inhibitory activity on primary hemostasis and most coagulation factors, particularly on factor VIII.

HEPARIN

Canine mast cell neoplasia may induce several paraneoplastic syndromes such as coagulopathy, eosinophilia, basophilia, nonregenerative anemia, delayed wound healing or wound heal dehiscence, ulceration, pruritus, vascular lesion, hypotensive shock, and gastrointestinal ulcer. These syndromes, may be induced by mast cell degranulation and release of granule contents, including heparin, histamine, serotonin, eosinophil chemotactic factor, tryptase, and chimase.[17,18] Mast-cell paraneoplastic coagulopathy is characterized by prolonged thrombin time, prolonged activated partial thromboplastin time, and hemorrhagic tendency.[19]

REFERENCES

1. **Giles AR, Tinlin S, Hoogendoorn H, et al.** Development of factor VIII: C antibodies in dogs with hemophilia A (factor VIII: C deficiency). Blood 1984;63:451–456.
2. **Tinlin S, Webster S, Giles AR.** The development of homologous (canine/anti-canine) antibodies in dogs with haemophilia A (factor VIII deficiency): a ten-year longitudinal study. Thromb Haemost 1993;69:21–24.
3. **Kaper CK, Aledort LM, Counts RB, et al.** A more uniform measurement of factor VIII inhibitors. Thromb Diath Haemorrh 1975;34:869–872.
4. **Fang B, Wang H, Gordon G, Bellinger DA, Read MS, Brinklaus KM, Woo SLC, Eisensmith RC.** Lack of persistence of E1-recombinant adenoviral vectors containing a temperature sensitive E2a mutation in immunocompetent mice and hemophilia B dogs. Gene Ther 1996;3:217–222.
5. **Feldman BF, Soares CJ, Kitchell BE, et al.** Hemorrhage in a cat caused by inhibition of factor XI (plasma thromboplastin antecedent). J Am Vet Med Assoc 1983;182:589–591.
6. **Wassermann A, Neisser A, Bruck C.** Eine serodiagnostische Reaktion bei Syphilis. Dtsch Med Wochenschr 1906;32:745–746.
7. **Mueller JF, Ratnoff O, Heinle RW.** Observations on the characteristics of an unusual circulating anticoagulant. J Lab Clin Med 1951;38:254–261.
8. **Triplett DA.** Antiphospholipid-protein antibodies: laboratory detection and clinical relevance. Thromb Res 1995;78:1–31.
9. **Stone MS, Johnstone IB, Brooks M, et al.** Lupus-type "anticoagulant" in a dog with hemolysis and thrombosis. J Vet Intern Med 1994;8:57–61.
10. **Hashimoto Y, Kawamura M, Ichikawa K, Suzuki T, et al.** Anticardiolipin antibodies in (NZW × BXSB) F1 mice: a model of antiphospholipid syndrome. J Immunol 1992;149:1063–1068.
11. **Branch DW, Dudley DJ, Mitchell MD,** Creighton KA, et al. Immunoglobulin G fractions from patients with antiphospholipid antibodies cause fetal death in Balb/c mice: a model for autoimmune fetal loss. Am J Obstet Gynecol 1990;163:210–216.

12. **Peterson EN, Meininger AC.** Immunoglobulin A and immunoglobulin G biclonal gammopathy in a dog with multiple myeloma. J Am Anim Hosp Assoc 1997;33:45–47.
13. **Hammer AS, Couto CG.** Complications of multiple myeloma. J Am Anim Hosp Assoc 1994;30:9–14.
14. **Campbell KL, Latimer KS.** Polysystemic manifestations of plasma cell myeloma in the dog: a case report and review. J Am Anim Hosp Assoc 1985;21:59–66.
15. **Ruiz de Gopegui R, Espada Y, Vilafranca M, et al.** Paraprotein-induced defective haemostasis in a dog with IgA (kappa-light chain) forming myeloma. Vet Clin Pathol 1994;23:70–71.
16. **Vail DM.** Plasma cell neoplasms. In: Withrow SJ, MacEwen EG, eds. Small animal oncology. 2nd ed. Philadelphia: WB Saunders, 1996;509–520.
17. **Caughey GH, Viro NF, Calonico LD, et al.** Chymase and tryptase in dog mastocytoma cells: asynchronous expression as revealed by enzyme cytochemical staining. Histochem Cytochem 1988;36:1053–1060.
18. **Fox LE, Rosenthal RC, Twedt DC, et al.** Plasma histamine and gastrin concentrations in 17 dogs with mast cell tumors. J Vet Intern Med 1990;4:242–246.
19. **Hottendorf GH, Nielson SW, Kenyon AJ.** Canine mastocytoma. I. Blood coagulation in dogs with mastocytoma. Pathologica Veterinaria 1965;2:219–241.

CHAPTER 85

Acquired Coagulopathy V: Thrombosis

• BENJAMIN J. DARIEN

The last 10 years have presented us with a better understanding of the pathogenesis of arterial and venous thrombosis.[1] Alteration in Virchow's triad (changes in blood coagulation factors and abnormalities in blood flow and endothelial damage), provide the basis for thromboembolic disease.[2] It is now well understood that a derangement to the physiologic hemostasis system of procoagulant and fibrinolytic factors and their respective regulatory mechanisms, can not only lead to bleeding but also to thrombosis (Table 85.1). The term thrombophilia (hypercoagulability or prethrombotic states) denotes a predisposition to an increased risk of thrombosis. Thrombophilia comprises several congenital, familial, and acquired disorders of the hemostatic system that predispose a patient to thromboembolic events. Deficiencies in the regulatory mechanisms of clotting, such as antithrombin III (ATIII) and protein C, are known to potentiate thrombosis.[3–7] Impaired fibrinolysis may also be associated with thrombosis by means of a release disturbance of tissue plasminogen activator (tPA) or elevated levels of plasminogen activator inhibitor (PAI 1).[4,8,9] Other factors that have been associated with thrombophilia include abnormalities of factor XII, prekallikrein and fibrinogen, acquired platelet dysfunction, and circulating inhibitors.[10–12]

A coordinated interaction and regulation between coagulation, fibrinolysis, platelets, and endothelium normally maintain hemostasis. Any disorder within one of these systems can influence the physiologic balance toward a prethrombotic state. [Many authors use the term hypercoagulable state and prethrombotic state interchangeably].[2,13] Because abnormalities at the cellular level are undetectable ex vivo (or detectable only with extraordinary laboratory efforts) our knowledge of thrombophilic conditions is at present based mainly on abnormal coagulation and fibrinolysis. Hypercoagulation should designate a condition in which a patient's blood is actually clotting in vivo, whether clinically evident or not. The most extreme case is acute disseminated intravascular coagulation (DIC) (also known as consumptive coagulopathy), a serious disorder of hemostasis with deposition of microthrombi with concurrent hemorrhage in the capillary bed.[2,14]

The onset of thrombin generation initiates platelet aggregation, clotting of fibrinogen and activation of factors V and VIII, which accelerates or amplifies thrombin generation. During the clotting process, thrombin is incorporated into the forming thrombus, where it is not fibrin bound but rather is entrapped in fibrin matrices.[15,16] The most common coagulopathies resulting in thrombosis include ATIII and protein C consumption, with the former leading to unregulated activation of factor Xa and thrombin and the latter to unimpeded availability of complex assembly-activated cofactors.[2,11,17,18] Within a thrombus, thrombin can then activate factor XIII for cross-linking fibrin and for consuming any trapped protease inhibitors. Also included in fibrin rich thrombi are red blood cells, referred to as coagulation or red thrombi, which form in areas of complete blood stasis such as the intestinal microvasculature after ischemia and reperfusion injury. Mixed platelet thrombi occur in areas of slow-to-moderate flow and are composed of red blood cells and neutrophils, which play a pivotal role in thrombus maturation, as in lung injury. High blood flow systems (arteries) develop thrombi that are composed primarily of aggregated platelets surrounding a fine fibrin mesh and are referred to as platelet or white thrombi.

The most common causes of thrombotic episodes recognized in animals are underlying disease states that result in aberrant coagulation mechanisms, such as infectious diseases (bacteria, viruses, and fungi), tissue injury (smoke inhalation, burns, and trauma) or obstetric complications.[3,19] Other causes of thrombosis in animals include infection with certain parasites, immune-mediated diseases, neoplasia, and the use of indwelling catheters in patients that have altered hemostasis.[8,13,17,20–23] The pathogenic mechanism shared by these individual causes is their ability to affect the coagulation cascade. However, it seems likely that hypercoagulability alone is not sufficient to induce thrombosis and that additional risk factors are required, such as platelet activation and enhanced endothelial cell tissue factor activity and reduced thrombomodulin function.

DIAGNOSIS

Thrombosis may occur in the arteries, veins, capillaries, or chambers of the heart. The clinical manifestations of thrombosis are caused by localized vascular obstruction

574

TABLE 85.1	Pathophysiologic Predisposing Factors Associated with Thromboembolization		
Vascular Disorders	**Alteration in Hemostasis**	**Alterations in Blood Flow**	
Immune-mediated (vasculitis, phlebitis, arteritis and amyloidosis) Infection (septicemia, endotoxemia, granulomatous diseases and abscesses) Parasitism [Heartworm (*Dirofilaria immitis*) pulmonary arterial disease and visceral leishmaniasis] Neoplasia (e.g., hemangiosarcoma and angiomatosis) Immune-mediates diseases (AIHA, IMTP and nephrotic syndrome) Ischemia reperfusion injury (visceral strangulation and obstruction) Necrotizing pneumonia (bacterial and toxic) Trauma (intravenous catheters, irritating or hyperosmolar substances and burns)	Hypercoagulation (nephrotic syndrome, septicemia, neoplasia and DIC) Platelet disorders (IMHA, IMTP, uremia and thrombocytosis) Metabolic/immune disorders (Cushing's syndrome and glomerulopathies)	Hypovolemia and/or dehydration (shock, trauma and burns) Cardiac (vegetative endocarditis, valvular insufficiency and vascular anomalies) Hemodynamic (congestive heart failure, cardiac tamponade and pulmonary hypertension)	

and embolization of the thrombi. They are variable in nature and severity, depending on the location and size of the thrombus. Acute onset of dyspnea is often associated with pulmonary thrombosis and occasionally patients may develop hemoptysis. Infarction or embolization within the genitourinary system can present with hematuria, abdominal pain, and splinting. Similarly, embolization to the viscera may have similar clinical signs, although small animals may vomit or become incontinent. Distal aortic emboli, as in cats, often display great pain in the affected limb, which on palpation is cool, lacks a pulse and is pale.[22-26] Acute changes in mentation or gait may reflect embolization of the central nervous system.

Thromboembolization can be a difficult diagnosis clinically and usually requires sophisticated diagnostic techniques such as digital subtraction angiography, ascending contrast venography, angiography, impedance plethysmography, ^{125}I-fibrinogen scanning, and Doppler ultrasonography.[3,21-23,27] A high suspicion of thromboembolic disease can be inferred from an abnormal scintigraphic ventilation or perfusion scan. Consequently, the diagnosis of hypercoagulation is essential for the identification of individuals at high risk for thrombosis and for early treatment of thrombotic disorders. Routine global screening tests, such as the prothrombin time (PT) and activated partial thromboplastin time (APTT), are useful for the detection of hypocoagulable (DIC) states or a bleeding tendency but not for detection of hypercoagulability. Because the clotting factors are present in great excess in the circulation and only a small portion of these factors are activated during thrombus formation in vivo, the measurement of their plasma levels (via routine clotting tests), is not a good monitor for thrombophilic disorders. In fact, the ability of the laboratory to perform hemostasis testing beyond routine PT and APTT is the secret for effective prethrombotic state screening, such as ATIII. Listed below are brief descriptions of a few of the commercially available hemostasis assays that are useful for detecting potential abnormalities that can indicate protrombotic states.

Chromogenic Factor VII Assay

The extrinsic pathway of blood coagulation is initiated by the formation of a complex between tissue factor on cell surfaces and activated factor VII (fVIIa). This enzyme complex activates factor X to factor Xa. The chromogenic assay of fVII is based on the end-point determination of generated factor Xa in plasma following activation by tissue thromboplastin and calcium.

Platelet Aggregation Assays

Aggregation of platelets is measured photometrically by recording changes in light transmission of a suspension of platelets in plasma following the addition of selected agonists. Commonly used reagents (agonists) include adenosine diphosphate (ADP), epinephrine, and collagen. The most important use of these assays is the monitoring of antiplatelet therapy. The principle of the assays is to evaluate agonist-induced platelet adherence to surfaces or aggregation to each other. Because each agonist induces a characteristic aggregation scan, pharmacologic or pathologic altered platelet function can be determined.

Protein C Assays

Protein C is an important regulator of activated factors V and VIII, and it enhances fibrinolysis by neutralizing the effects of PAI. Both functional (chromogenic and clot-based) and antigenic (Laurell rocket) assays are available. Protein C deficiency is most commonly associated with septicemia-induced coagulopathies.

Antithrombin III Assays

Similar chromogenic (functional) and immunologic (antigen) assays are available for the coagulation inhibitor antithrombin III (ATIII).[18,28,29] A decrease in plasma ATIII activity is associated with thromboembolic tendencies. Currently, ATIII quantitation for clinical patients is only available at a few veterinary teaching hospitals (e.g., Comparative Hemostasis Laboratory, School of Veterinary Medicine, University of Wisconsin-Madison). This circulating anticoagulant is probably most important for its suppression of thrombin and factor Xa. ATIII inhibition is only effective in conjunction with heparin or heparinlike substances; as ATIII activity drops to less than 70% (caused by acquired deficiencies), heparin therapy becomes essentially ineffective. In the horse and dog, plasma ATIII activity between 60 and 75% of normal species control are associated with increased risk of thrombosis, whereas ATIII activity less than 60% of normal in these species are associated with irreversible organ (e.g., after intestinal lischemia and reperfusion injury, protein losing gastroenteropathies and nephropathies) or multi-organ mortality.

Fibrin (Fibrinogen) Degradation Products Assays

Fibrin degradation products (FDPs), also known as fibrinogen split products, are the result of plasminogen digestion of both cross-linked and non-cross-linked fibrin and fibrinogen.[9,30] Increased concentrations (or titer ratios) helps establish the diagnosis of hypercoagulation, and DIC and can be used in monitoring fibrinolytic therapy. Products of fibrinolysis (plasminogen, α_2-antiplasmin, tPA, and PAI-1), have been discussed previously and the reader should see Chapter 78, Fibrinolytic System.

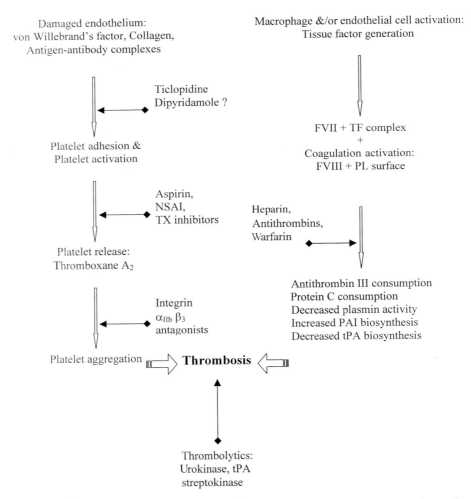

FIGURE 85.1 The hemostatic system and factors central to thrombogenesis. Systemic activation of platelets and coagulation proteins concomitant with vascular activation/injury results in thrombin generation. Vascular intimal injury (arterial) or disturbances in blood flow (venule) increase the risk of thrombus formation. NSAI: nonsteroidal antiinflammatory; $\alpha_{IIb}\beta_3$: glycoprotein $\alpha IIb/\beta III$; FVII: factor VII; TF: tissue factor; PL: phospholipid surface; PAI: plasminogen activator inhibitor; t-PA: tissue plasminogen activator; TX: thromboxane.

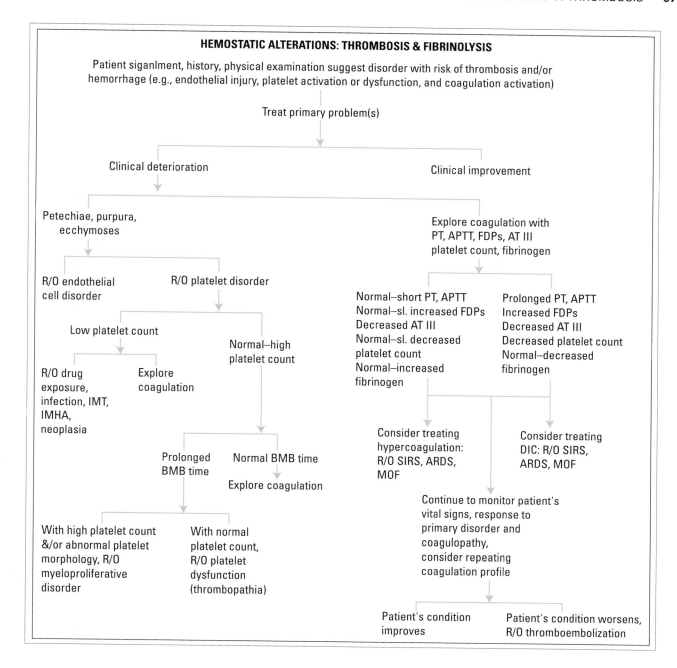

HEMOSTATIC ALTERATIONS: THROMBOSIS & FIBRINOLYSIS

Patient siganlment, history, physical examination suggest disorder with risk of thrombosis and/or hemorrhage (e.g., endothelial injury, platelet activation or dysfunction, and coagulation activation)

Treat primary problem(s)

Clinical deterioration / Clinical improvement

Petechiae, purpura, ecchymoses

Explore coagulation with PT, APTT, FDPs, AT III platelet count, fibrinogen

R/O endothelial cell disorder

R/O platelet disorder

Low platelet count

Normal–high platelet count

R/O drug exposure, infection, IMT, IMHA, neoplasia

Explore coagulation

Prolonged BMB time

Normal BMB time

Explore coagulation

With high platelet count &/or abnormal platelet morphology, R/O myeloproliferative disorder

With normal platelet count, R/O platelet dysfunction (thrombopathia)

Normal–short PT, APTT
Normal–sl. increased FDPs
Decreased AT III
Normal–sl. decreased platelet count
Normal–increased fibrinogen

Prolonged PT, APTT
Increased FDPs
Decreased AT III
Decreased platelet count
Normal–decreased fibrinogen

Consider treating hypercoagulation: R/O SIRS, ARDS, MOF

Consider treating DIC: R/O SIRS, ARDS, MOF

Continue to monitor patient's vital signs, response to primary disorder and coagulopathy, consider repeating coagulation profile

Patient's condition improves

Patient's condition worsens, R/O thromboembolization

THERAPY

Because Virchow's triad is central to the etiopathogenesis of thrombosis or thromboembolism, therapy is directed at correcting abnormalities of blood flow, regulation of coagulation (hemostasis) and endothelial cell activation or injury (in conjunction with therapy for the underlying disorder).[2,19,31] Thus, the major thrombolytic goals are divided between diminishing continual thrombogenesis and correcting the hemostatic imbalance and administering thrombolytic (preferably site specific) therapy. The former is achieved with a combination of anticoagulant (heparin, warfarin, or both) or antiplatelet therapies (aspirin, dipyridamole, and ticlopidine), whereas the latter is achieved with thrombolytic agents such as tPA, streptokinase (SK), and urokinase (UK) (Fig. 85.1).[25,32–40] Irrespective of the therapeutic regimen, the patients' hemostatic mechanisms must be closely monitored to avoid serious bleeding or thrombotic complications.

Anticoagulants

These drugs act by primarily inhibiting thrombogenesis and rely on the patient's circulating fibrinolytic activity to reduce the size of the existing thrombi and reestablish blood flow. From a pathophysiologic perspective, these drugs are most useful in treating low blood flow venous thrombosis because of the underlying coagulopathy.[33,39,40] Therapeutic management of most thromboembolic disorders involves the short-term use of heparin and thrombolytic therapy to achieve systemic anticoagulation and initiate fibrinolysis, respectively, during the acute stages. Long-term antiplatelet therapy is used most widely for prophylactic measures and prevention of recurrence.[23,24,32] Heparin and low-molecular-weight heparin, potent inhibitors of thrombin and of thrombin generation, act by catalyzing the inactivation of thrombin and factor Xa by ATIII. Depending on the base line APTT, an intravenous loading dosage of 100 to 200 U/kg is recommended to achieve the desired antithrombotic effect (to prolong the APTT to 1.5 to 2-fold normal). Because these compounds accelerate the consumption of ATIII, patients are at risk of developing thromboembolism when plasma ATIII activity is less than 60%.[2,5] The risk of thromboembolism is increased in patients that have hypercoagulable conditions. Therefore, administering fresh (or fresh-frozen) plasma while the patient is receiving heparin should restore ATIII activity. To prevent the systemic activation of the clotting proteins upon entry into the circulation, it is recommended that the plasma be pretreated with the initial heparin dose (100 to 200 U/kg) and incubated at room temperature for 30 minutes to ensure the ATIII is adequately activated. Because heparin administration reduces plasma ATIII activity, heparin therapy should be gradually tapered off through 48 hours to prevent rebound hypercoagulation.[29]

As a vitamin K antagonist, warfarin inhibits the synthesis of the vitamin-K-dependent blood-clotting proteins, prothrombin, and factors VII and IX, required for normal blood coagulation.[2,24,25] In addition, the vitamin-K-dependent regulatory proteins, protein C and S, are also affected caused by a decrease in vitamin-K-dependent posttranslational modification. The anticoagulant effect of warfarin depends on the reduction in the synthesis of biologically active vitamin-K-dependent blood-clotting proteins and the normal clearance from the circulation of fully active vitamin-K-dependent blood-clotting proteins synthesized before the introduction of the vitamin K antagonist. As such, the administration of warfarin does not induce immediate anticoagulation but rather requires 4 to 5 days to achieve its therapeutic goal.

Because factor VII is at the beginning of the extrinsic pathway and has the shortest half-life and is suppressed more quickly than the other vitamin-K-dependent blood-coagulation proteins, the PT is sensitive to factor VII activity. Tissue factor initiates the extrinsic pathway of blood coagulation by activating the vitamin-K-dependent proteins, factors II (prothrombin), VII, IX, and X. Warfarin administration prolongs the PT from the normal range (approximately 10 to 12 seconds, depending on the species) into the therapeutic range (1.5 to 2.0 times the control PT) by inhibiting the formation of functional vitamin-K-dependent proteins. Because warfarin does not prolong the PT for 1 to 2 days after the initiation of therapy and because its anticoagulant action is achieved only after 4 or 5 days, heparin is usually administered concomitantly to achieve immediate anticoagulation.[23-25] Coumadin (warfarin sodium) is usually started at a dosage of 0.5 mg/kg q24h by mouth and tapered to achieve the desired state of anticoagulation. Because of high individual patient variability, close monitoring of the PT is important. However, since rebound hypercoagulability has not been reported coumarin therapy may be stopped abruptly. For treating acute thromboembolization heparin is administered at an initial dosage of 200 U/kg intravenously (IV), followed 2 hours later by 100 to 130 U/kg q6h subcutaneously, adjusting the dosage to maintain APTT values 1.5 to 2 times the base line. The discontinuation of warfarin therapy and the administration of vitamin K1 (initial loading dosage of 3 mg/kg, followed by a daily dosage of 1 mg/kg) may treat moderate complications, such as hematomas or mild gastrointestinal bleeding.

Antiplatelet Therapy

By inhibiting platelet aggregation and adhesion, antiplatelet drugs prevent the formation and subsequent fibrin mesh central to establishing the primary platelet plug.[14,23,32] Arterial thrombi, which form under conditions of abnormal circulatory patterns and damaged vascular endothelium, are the most susceptible to antiplatelet therapy. A wide variety of agonists can induce platelet activation and subsequent integrin $\alpha_{IIb}\beta_3$ expression. Integrin $\alpha_{IIb}\beta_3$ is responsible for ligating platelets to fibrinogen, thus initiating the second phase of platelet aggregation.[34-37] Agents that block the binding between integrin $\alpha_{IIb}\beta_3$ and fibrinogen have a profound effect on thrombus formation; thus the target of many of the newer platelet inhibitors is the platelet integrin $\alpha_{IIb}\beta_3$ receptor. These compounds contain the 3-amino acid sequence, arginine-glycine-aspartic acid (RGD), which are identical to specific binding residues on fibrinogen. In contrast, selective cyclooxygenase inhibitors like aspirin only prevent the biosynthesis of thromboxane A2. Because platelet activation can occur through other pathways, aspirin has a more limited effect on inhibiting platelet function than integrin $\alpha_{IIb}\beta_3$ inhibitors.

Aspirin predictably induces impaired platelet aggregation with epinephrine, ADP, arachidonic acid, and low concentrations of collagen and thrombin.[32,38] These alterations are a direct result of inhibition of cyclooxygenase, with the resulting deficient biosynthesis of platelet arachidonic acid metabolism, thromboxane A2. Thromboxane A2 induces platelet aggregation after binding to specific platelet membrane receptors and promoting α-granule and dense granule secretion. With cyclooxygenase inhibition, only the primary, reversible wave of platelet aggregation occurs, but not the secondary wave and platelet secretion, after stimulation by epinephrine and low concentrations of ADP, thrombin, and collagen. Because cats lack glucuronyl transferase, the enzyme needed to metabolize aspirin, they are particularly sensitive to aspirin-induced platelet dysfunction.[32] A dosage of 0.5 mg/kg q 12 hour in the dog and 25 mg/kg twice weekly in the cat is effective in decreasing platelet aggregation. In the horse, a dose of 60 grain, by mouth, once daily is effective in altering platelet function. In the cow, 100 mg/kg, by mouth, q12 hour is an effective antiinflammatory dose.

Dipyridamole is a nonnitrate coronary vasodilator that increases coronary blood flow.[35,36] The mechanism by which dipyridamole inhibits platelet aggregation is not fully known but may be related to inhibition of platelet phosphodiesterase, which leads to increased cAMP within platelets. High cyclic adenosine monophosphate (cAMP) concentrations are inhibitory to platelet function.

Ticlopidine is used to reduce the risk of thromboembolism in patients who have cardiovascular disease or who are intolerant to aspirin.[35–37] It is being studied for its effect in preventing myocardial infarction and restrictive cardiomyopathy. Ticlopidine impairs fibrinogen binding to integrin $\alpha_{IIb}\beta_3$ and inhibits platelet aggregation induced by many agonists, including ADP and collagen. The effect of ticlopidine on platelet function occurs by 48 hours after ingestion, and the degree of bleeding time prolongation is equivalent to aspirin, but has the advantage of not affecting prostacyclin production. Minor side affects include bruising and epistaxis, whereas major complications include neutropenia, aplastic anemia, and thrombocytopenia.

Thrombolytic Therapy

In contrast to anticoagulants and antiplatelet therapy, which prevent thrombus formation and the extension and propagation of a preformed thrombus, fibrinolytic agents digest and dissolve arterial and venous thromboemboli.[1] The dissolution of thrombi and emboli results in the reperfusion distal to the site of obstruction and return of nutrients and oxygen to tissues previously deprived of blood flow. Thrombolytic agents (SK, UK, and tPA) are administered by intravenous systemic infusion and by local intravenous or intra-arterial perfusion.[23,27,31] Although modest differences characterize these agents, all generate the proteolytic enzyme plasmin by means of plasminogen activation and none activate or interact with plasminogen at only the site of thrombus formation. Thrombolytic therapy should be initiated as close to diagnosis as possible as fibrinolysis is less successful when initiated on older well-organized thrombi.[2,3] Systemic intravenous infusion of SK can be administered for 30 to 60 minutes at a rate of 90,000 IU, followed by 45,000 IU/hr, for a total of 6 to 12 hours.[23] When local perfusion of a thrombus is achievable, a catheter is placed adjacent to or into it. The local perfusion technique is most successful when performed on arterial thrombi. One benefit of employing the local perfusion technique is significantly lower doses of thrombolytic agent are used. When employing low-dosage schedules (5000 to 7500 U/hr SK; 15,000 to 20,000 U/

hr UK), significant systemic effects may not be observed until after 6 to 8 hours of infusion. Excessive activation of the fibrinolytic system increases the risk of hemorrhage. A convenient assay for monitoring activation of fibrinolysis is the thrombin time (TT), which should be measured before the initiation of thrombolytic therapy. The TT is fairly simple to perform, the results are rapidly available and accurately reflect fibrinolytic activity. Initiating heparin therapy early has been advocated on the premise that it will regulate thrombosis growth and augment fibrinolysis. However, heparin therapy should be discontinued at the time of thrombolytic therapy, as it can significantly prolong the TT.

REFERENCES

1. **Runge MS.** The future of thrombolytic therapy. Frontier 1992;39–42.
2. **Green RA, Thomas JS.** Hemostatic disorders: coagulopathies and thrombosis. In: Ettinger SJ, Feldman EC, eds. Textbook of veterinary internal medicine. Diseases of the dog and cat. 4th ed. Philadelphia: WB Saunders, 1995;1946.
3. **Triplett EA, O'Brien RT, Wilson DG, Steinberg H, Darien BJ.** Thrombosis of the brachial artery in a foal. J Vet Intern Med 1996;10:330–332.
4. **Williamson LH.** Antithrombin III: a natural anticoagulant. Compend Cont Educ Pract Vet 1991;13:100–107.
5. **Green RA, Kabel AL.** Hypercoagulable state in three dogs with nephrotic syndrome: role of acquired antithrombin III deficiency. J Am Vet Med Assoc 1982;191:914–917.
6. **Kawcak CE, Baxter GM, Getzy DM, Stashak TS, Chapman PL.** Abnormalities in oxygenation, coagulation, fibrinolysis in colonic blood of horses with experimentally induced strangulation obstruction. Am J Vet Res 1995; 56:1642–1650.
7. **Collatos C, Barton MH, Prasse KW, Moore JN.** Intravascular and peritoneal coagulation and fibrinolysis in horses with acute gastrointestinal tract diseases. J Am Vet Med Assoc 1995;207:465–470.
8. **Bunch SE, Metcalf MR, Crane SW, Cullen JM.** Idiopathic pleural effusion and pulmonary thromboembolism in a dog with autoimmune hemolytic anemia. J Am Vet Med Assoc 1989;195:1748–1753.
9. **Lanevshi A, Kramer JW, Greene SA, Meyers KM.** Evaluation of chromogenic substrate assays for fibrinolytic analytes in dogs. Am J Vet Res 1996;57:1124–1130.
10. **Hammer AS, Couto CG, Swardson C, Getzy D.** Hemostatic abnormalities in dogs with hemangiosarcoma. J Am Vet Med Assoc 1991;5:11–14.
11. **Greco DS, Green RA.** Coagulation abnormalities associated with thrombosis in a dog with nephrotic syndrome. Compend Cont Educ Pract Vet 1987;9:653–658.
12. **Welles EG, Boudreaux MK, Tyler JW.** Platelet, antithrombin, and fibrinolytic activities in taurine-deficient and taurine-replete cats. Am J Vet Res 1993;54:1235–1243.
13. **Stone MS, Johnstone IB, Brooks M, Bollinger TK, Cotter SM.** Lupus-Type "Anticoagulant" in a dog with hemolysis and thrombosis. J Am Vet Med Assoc 1994;8:57–61.
14. **Boudreaux MK.** Platelet and coagulation disorders. In: Morgan RV, ed. Handbook of small animal practice. 3rd ed. Philadelphia: WB Saunders, 1997;698.
15. **Dennis JS.** The pathophysiologic sequelae of pulmonary thromboembolism. Compend Cont Educ Pract Vet 1991;13:1811–1818.
16. **Stump DC, Mann KG, Vermont B.** Mechanisms of thrombus formation and lysis. Ann Emerg Med 1988;17:1138–1147.
17. **Rasedee A, Feldman BF.** Nephrotic Syndrome: a platelet hyperaggregability state. Vet Res Commun 1985;9:199–211.
18. **Darien BJ, Potempa J, Moore JN, Travis J.** Antithrombin III activity in horses with colic: an analysis of 46 cases. Equine Vet J 1991;23:211–214.
19. **Collatos C.** Hemostatic dysfunction. In: Robinson NE, ed. Current therapy in equine medicine 4. Philadelphia: WB Saunders, 1997;286.
20. **Morris DD.** Thrombophlebitis in horses: the contribution of hemostatic dysfunction to pathogenesis. Compend Cont Educ Pract Vet 1989;11:1386–1395.
21. **Klein MK, Dow SW, Rosychuk R.** Pulmonary thromboembolism associated with immune-mediated hemolytic anemia in dogs: ten cases (1982–1987). J Am Vet Med Assoc 1989;195:246–250.
22. **LaRue MJ, Murtaugh RJ.** Pulmonary thromboembolism in dogs: 47 cases (1986–1987). J Am Vet Med Assoc 1990;197:1368–1372.
23. **Bonagura JD, Fox PR.** Restrictive cardiomyopathy. In: Bonagura JD, Kirk RW, eds. Kirk's current veterinary therapy. XII. Small animal practice. Philadelphia: WB Saunders, 1995;863.
24. **Kittleson MD.** CVT update: feline hypertrophic cardiomyopathy. In: Bona-

gura JD, Kirk RW, eds. Kirk's current veterinary therapy. XII. Small animal practice. Philadelphia: WB Saunders, 1995;854.

25. **Harpster NK, Baty CJ.** Warfarin therapy of the cat at risk of thromboembolism. In: Bonagura JD, Kirk RW, eds. Kirk's current veterinary therapy. XII. Small animal practice. Philadelphia: WB Saunders, 1995;868.

26. **Flanders JA.** Feline aortic thromboembolism. Compend Cont Educ Pract Vet 1986;8:473–482.

27. **Ramsey CC, Burnery DP, Macintire DK, Finn-Bodner S.** Use of streptokinase in four dogs with thrombosis. J Am Vet Med Assoc 1996;209: 780–785.

28. **Topper MJ, Prasse KW, Morris MJ, Duncan A, Crowe NA.** Enzyme-linked immunosorbent assay for thrombin-antithrombin III complexes in horses. Am J Vet Res 1996;57:427–431.

29. **Hellebrekers LJ, Slappendel RJ, Van den Brom WE.** Effect of sodium heparin and antithrombin III concentration on activated partial thromboplastin time in the dog. Am J Vet Res 1985;46:1460–1462.

30. **Hauptman JG, Feldman BF, O'Neill SL, Lippert AC, Davis AT.** A turbidimetric method for fibronectin assay in the dog. Am J Vet Res 1998;49:1935–1936.

31. **Suter PF, Fox PR.** Peripheral vascular disease. In: Bonagura JD, Kirk RW, eds. Kirk's current veterinary therapy. XII. Small animal practice. Philadelphia: WB Saunders, 1995.

32. **Holland M, Chastain CB.** Uses and misuses of aspirin. In: Bonagura JD, Kirk RW, eds. Kirk's current veterinary therapy. XII. Small animal practice. Philadelphia: WB Saunders, 1995;70.

33. **Vrins A, Carlson G, Feldman B.** Warfarin: a review with emphasis on its use in the horse. Can Vet J 1983;24:211–213.

34. **Weiss DJ, Evanson OA, Wells RE.** Evaluation of arginine-glycine-aspartate-containing peptides as inhibitors of equine platelet function. Am J Vet Res 1997;58:457–460.

35. **Fernandez-Ortiz A, Jang I-K, Fuster V.** Antiplatelet and antithrombin therapy. Coron Artery Dis 1994;5:297–305.

36. **Schafer AI.** Antiplatelet therapy. Am J Med 1996;101:199–209.

37. **Nichols AJ, Ruffolo RR Jr, Huffman WF, Poste G, Samanen J.** Development of GPIIb/IIIa antagonists as antithrombotic drugs. TIPS 1992;13:413–417.

38. **Grauer GF, Rose BJ, Toolan L, Hull Thrall MA, Colgan SP.** Effects of low-dose aspirin and specific thromboxane synthetase inhibition on whole blood platelet aggregation and adenosine triphosphate secretion in healthy dogs. Am J Vet Res 1992;53:1631–1636.

39. **Monreal L, Villatoro AJ, Monreal M, Espada Y, Anglés AM, Ruiz de Gopegui R.** Comparison of the effects of low-molecular-weight and unfractioned heparin in horses. Am J Vet Res 1995;56:1281–1285.

40. **Darien BJ.** Heparin therapy: rationale and clinical indications. Compend Contin Educ Pract Vet 1993;15:1273–1276.

Acquired Coagulopathy VI: Disseminated Intravascular Coagulation

• REBECCA KIRBY and ELKE RUDLOFF

Platelets and clotting factors are stimulated within the blood vessel at the site of injury by structural changes within that vessel and by substances released into that vessel as a consequence of tissue damage in adjacent areas. A tough fibrin clot is formed over the site of injury, which maintains vascular integrity and minimizes blood loss (Fig. 86.1). The fibrin clot is modified by the fibrinolytic system and the size of the clot controlled by endogenous anticoagulants (Fig. 86.2). This restricts the coagulation process to a focal area of the vessel and aids in the production of a tight fibrin seal over the damaged site. This local phenomenon is called hemostasis and is life saving.

When these same structural changes occur in multiple blood vessels simultaneously or when procoagulant substances resulting from tissue damage are released in significant quantities into the systemic circulation, coagulation occurs randomly within vessels throughout the body. Microthrombi are produced throughout the capillary network, obstructing blood flow and resulting in tissue hypoxia and cell death. This continuous activation of the coagulation cascade eventually results in depletion of the platelets, natural anticoagulants, and coagulation proteins. Fibrinolysis is now ongoing and systemic. Uncontrolled hemorrhage can result. Animals can die from thrombosis or hemorrhage before the initiating cause has been eliminated. This generalized phenomenon is called disseminated intravascular coagulation (DIC) and is life threatening.

Intravascular coagulation was reported to occur after transfusion with incompatible blood as early as 1876. A bleeding diathesis, most likely DIC, was reported by Hardaway and McKay in a wounded soldier in Korea in 1951.[1] However, it was not until the mid-1960s that DIC become a recognized clinical syndrome.[2] The syndrome of DIC can be a complication of many disease processes with the clinical signs varying with the duration and intensity of the coagulation changes. DIC is a recognized clinical syndrome in dogs.[3] It is rarely diagnosed or described in the cat.

Anticipation of the initiating causes and diagnosis of DIC early in any disease process allows early and aggressive treatment of this secondary but life-threatening complication. The goal is to change the meaning of DIC from "Death Is Coming" into a "Darn Inconvenient Complication".

PATHOPHYSIOLOGY

Normal Hemostasis

By understanding the normal mechanisms of coagulation and anticoagulation (Figs. 86.1, 86.2, and 86.3), it is possible to recognize initiators of the syndrome and to anticipate DIC as a complication of disease or trauma. Platelets play a key role in hemostasis and provide the initial, but temporary plug. Platelets are activated and adhere to exposed subendothelial collagen at the site of vascular injury. Once a platelet adheres, it releases adenosine diphosphate (ADP) and thromboxane A2, which recruit more platelets to aggregate at the site of injury. The adjacent endothelial cells release prostacyclin once the platelet plug has bridged the gap between the endothelial cells. Vasodilation occurs and platelets are no longer stimulated to aggregate at that site, controlling the size of the plug. In addition to forming the platelet plug, platelets, together with calcium, provide phospholipids that interact with activated factors V and X of the common and activated factors VIII and IX of the intrinsic coagulation pathways (Fig. 86.3).

When there is injury to the vessel and its surrounding tissues, chemical mediators are released locally that stimulate coagulation for effective hemostasis and recruit white blood cells (WBC) for removal of debris. Tissue thromboplastin (TTP) is released into the blood at the site of injury and activates factor VII (extrinsic pathway). Activated factor VII can then activate factor XII (intrinsic pathway) and factor X (common pathway). Contact tissue factor (CTF) is in the tissues at the site of injury. Direct contact with this tissue factor stimulates the fibrinolytic system and activates factor XII. Recruited WBCs release cytokines such as tumor necrosis factor (activates factor VII) and interleukin-1 (activates factors

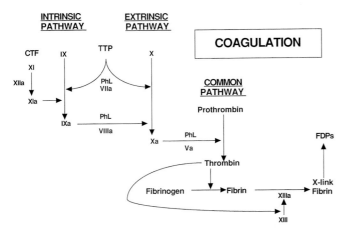

FIGURE 86.1 Coagulation cascade. There are multiple initiators of the coagulation cascade. When exposed to the blood, TTP converts factors IX to IXa and X to Xa in the presence of factor VIIa and phospholipid (PhL). Within the intrinsic pathway, CTF converts factor XI to XIa under the influence of factor XIIa–activated high-molecular-weight kininogen (HMWK) complex. Factor XIa also converts factor IX to IXa. Factor IXa converts factor X to Xa in the presence of factor VIIIa and phospholipid. Once factor Xa has formed, it converts prothrombin to thrombin under the influence of factor Va and PhL. Thrombin influences the conversion of fibrinogen to fibrin, and it converts factor XIII to XIIIa. Factor XIIIa allows cross-linking of the fibrin clot. The fibrin clot is eventually dissected into FDPs.

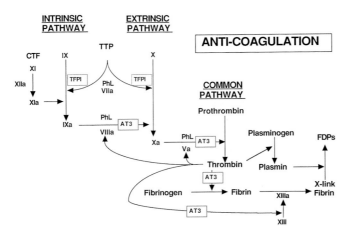

FIGURE 86.2 Natural anticoagulants. ATIII blocks factors IXa, Xa, and thrombin activity. Tissue factor pathway inhibitor (TFPI) blocks factor VIIa–TTP complex. Thrombin activates protein C, which degrades Factors Va and VIIIa. Thrombin also converts plasminogen to plasmin, which regulates fibrin cross-linking, forming FDPs.

VII and XII). Platelet-activating factor, a strong promoter of platelet aggregation, is also released from inflammatory cells.

The fibrinolytic system is activated (plasminogen to plasmin) to regulate clot formation and to tighten the fibrin meshwork of the final clot. Fibrin degradation products (FDPs) are produced during this process,

which further inhibit coagulation. The action of plasmin is regulated by plasminogen activator inhibitor (PAI). Anticoagulants such as antithrombin III (ATIII) and thrombomodulin-protein C-protein S complex are important in regulating the amplification of the coagulation cascade and inhibiting the actions of thrombin. ATIII irreversibly binds with and inactivates thrombin, plasmin, and activated factors XII, XI, X, and IX. Antithrombin III action is accelerated by the binding of endogenous heparins to antithrombin (Fig. 86.4).

Disseminated Intravascular Coagulation

The process of DIC is a complex syndrome involving a transition between accelerated activation of platelets, coagulation proteins and plasmin evolving into consumption of coagulation proteins, endogenous anticoagulants, and inhibitors of fibrinolysis. Coagulation is accelerated systemically when (1) the blood comes into contact with large areas of tissue or vascular endothelial damage with exposed subendothelial collagen, TTP and CTF, (2) when there are significant quantities of WBC, circulating inflammatory mediators, and cytokines (Table 86.1), (3) when there is significant contact of coagulation proteins with circulating platelet or red blood cell phospholipids, (4) when there is circulating cellular debris such as heartworm segments or red blood cell carcasses that act as contact factors, and (5) any combination of the above. The clinical syndrome of DIC is a secondary event and can be initiated by various underlying or primary disorders.[4-6] A list of disease entities known to have DIC as a complication and the potential initiators of accelerated coagulation are listed in Table 86.2.

As coagulation becomes accelerated, the natural anticoagulants are consumed. Plasmin is activated and fibrinolysis is ongoing. PAI is consumed. The now unregulated plasmin enzymatically degrades factors XI, IX, VIII, and V, contributing to the decrease in these clotting factors.[2,4] It becomes apparent that the transition from accelerated coagulation to consumption of coagulants and anticoagulants corresponds with the clinical consequences of microthrombosis and vascular occlusion followed by uncontrolled hemorrhage.

In summary, DIC results from a systemic exposure of the platelets and coagulation proteins to initiators of coagulation. Thrombosis of the microcirculation leads to capillary stasis and tissue hypoxia. This perpetuates the syndrome by providing additional opportunities for platelet adhesion and aggregation, and ample stimulation by CTF, TTP, and circulating mediators of both the intrinsic and extrinsic coagulation cascade. Uncontrolled coagulation leads to a rapid consumption of platelets, PAI, and natural anticoagulants and to consumption or degradation of coagulation factors.

Diagnosis of Disseminated Intravascular Coagulation

The diagnosis of DIC is based on (1) clinical suspicion, (2) knowledge of the pathophysiologic mechanisms re-

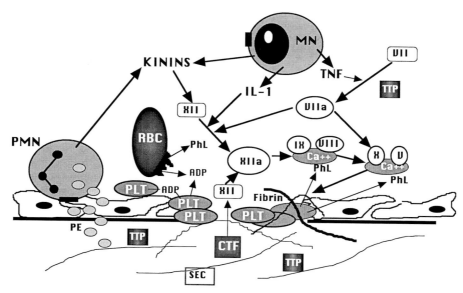

FIGURE 86.3 Initiators of coagulation in DIC. Platelets adhere to exposed subendothelial collagen and release ADP, which attracts more platelets. Inflammatory cells migrate to the area of tissue damage and release their cytokines and proteolytic enzymes. The cytokines activate circulating coagulation factors, and the proteolytic enzymes can induce more damage to the capillary structure. Contact tissue factors are released from the damaged subendothelial tissues and activate circulating factor XII. Damaged tissues release TTP, which activates circulating factor VII. Factors IX, VIII, X, and V are activated by platelet phospholipids and calcium, leading to the formation of fibrin. Damaged red blood cells release ADP that attracts platelets, phospholipids that can activate factors IX and VIII and X and V, and the red blood cell carcass acts as a contact factor to stimulate the coagulation cascade. PLT , platelet; TTP, tissue thromboplastin; SEC, subendothelial collagen; CTF, contact tissue factors; PE, proteolytic enzymes; PMN, polymorphonuclear cell; RBC, red blood cell; PhL, phospholipid; ADP, adenosine triphosphate; MN, monocyte; IL-1, interleukin 1; TNF, tumor necrosis factor; XII, factor XII; XIIa, activated factor XII; VII, factor VII; VIIa, activated factor VII; X, IX, VIII, V, factors X, IX, VIII, V; Ca++, calcium.

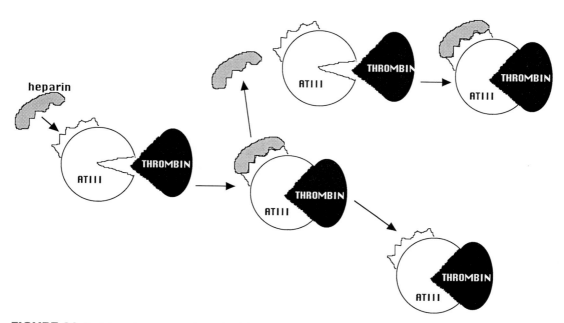

FIGURE 86.4 Interactions among heparin, ATIII, and thrombin. ATIII is a natural anticoagulant that binds and inactivates thrombin. The configuration of the ATIII–thrombin binding site is obscure, making the joining of the two molecules a slow process. Heparin temporarily binds with ATIII, changes its configuration, and makes the ATIII–thrombin binding site readily available. The ATIII–thrombin joining is accelerated 1000 times with heparin present. Once the ATIII–thrombin complex is formed, the heparin detaches from that ATIII molecule and is available to accelerate another ATIII–thrombin binding.

TABLE 86.1   Chemical Mediators Initiating DIC

Mediator	Activity
Platelet activating factor	Platelet activation, platelet aggregation
Kinins	Activation of factor XII
Complement	Red cell and platelet lysis
	Activates factor XII
	Kinin production
Tissue thromboplastin	Activates factor VII
Contact tissue factor	Activates factor XII
Phospholipids	Activate factor X, V, IX, VIII
Proteolytic enzymes	Activate factor VII
Thromboxane A$_2$	Platelet aggregation, vasoconstriction
Leukotrienes	White cell aggregation and activation
Cytokines	
Tumor necrosis factor	Contact tissue factor activation of factor XII
	Downregulation of thrombomodulin
	Inhibition of tissue plasminogen activation
	Upregulation of tissue plasminogen activator inhibitor
	Stimulation of platelet activating factor
Interleukin-1	Stimulation of factors VII and XII
Interleukin-6	Stimulates inflammatory cascade

sponsible in associated diseases, and (3) abnormal serial coagulation tests indicative of the syndrome. The clinical signs of DIC and results of coagulation testing vary in animals, depending on what phase of the syndrome the animal is experiencing (Table 86.3). The phase of DIC depends on the intensity of the underlying disease, the concentration and variety of initiators present, and the length of time the coagulation mechanisms are exposed to the initiators.

Minimal laboratory evaluation involves platelet number estimation and an activated clotting time (ACT). In the average clinical practice, serial evaluation of platelet numbers and ACT can provide immediate indicators of the diagnosis and phase of DIC. Ideally, activated partial thromboplastin time (APTT), prothrombin time (PT), and platelet count, with fibrinogen, FDPs, and ATIII quantification should be done. These coagulation profiles should be serially evaluated to determine coagulation trends in any animal thought to have a disease likely to initiate DIC but with nondiagnostic test results.

In the peracute (hypercoagulable) phase of DIC, there may be no overt clinical signs attributable to DIC, but accelerated coagulation, fibrinolysis, and consumption of anticoagulants are occurring. PT, APTT, and ACT may be normal or shortened. Platelet counts are beginning to decline but may still be within the normal range, requiring serial platelet counts over several hours to detect the declining trend.

As coagulation continues, the animal moves into the acute (consumptive) phase of DIC. Clinical signs include

oozing of blood from venipuncture sites or actual hemorrhage. The coagulation factors become consumed, prolonging the APTT, PT, and ACT. Fibrinogen is converted to fibrin, decreasing the fibrinogen. However, systemic inflammation can bring the fibrinogen level to normal or slightly elevated. The anticoagulation system breaks down the fibrin clots, resulting in increased amounts of circulating FDPs. However, the liver may remove them and bring the FDP concentration back to normal.

Chronic DIC can cause continuous, but tolerable, activation of the coagulation system. The liver and bone marrow may be able to increase production of coagulation factors, fibrinogen, and platelets and maintain an accelerated coagulation-anticoagulation steady state. The PT, APTT, and ACT is normal or prolonged. The platelet count is decreased. Fibrinogen is normal or low, and FDPs may be absent or elevated, depending on the liver function.

Plasmin activity is directed toward the degradation of fibrinogen and fibrin, producing peptide products called fibrin-related antigens. Fragments of these peptides are known as FDPs. When plasmin directs its enzyme activity on cross-linked fibrin monomers, in the presence of fibronectin, D-dimers are produced. The quantitation of D-dimers plays an important role in the diagnosis of DIC in human medicine.[2,4]

Plasma antithrombin activity is a key test for the diagnosis and monitoring of DIC.[2,7–9] The activity of ATIII declines early in the DIC process as this endogenous anticoagulant is consumed. Activity levels less than 80% are presumed diagnostic for DIC in humans. When antithrombin level falls to less than 60% in critically ill humans, a 96% mortality rate is expected.[10,11] Clinical experience in the dog and cat has shown that ATIII levels less than 80% are indicative of DIC. Levels less than 60% require replacement of ATIII as part of the treatment plan (Table 86.4).

Treatment of Disseminated Intravascular Coagulation

Successful therapy of DIC depends on early suspicion and detection in a critically ill animal. There is a five-step approach to treatment: (1) promotion of capillary flow; (2) elimination of the initiating cause; (3) support of target organs of microthrombi, ischemia and hemorrhage; (4) replacement therapy; and (5) heparin administration, as needed.

Once DIC is suspected, the first treatment priority is to fill the microvasculature and promote capillary blood flow and tissue oxygenation. Aggressive intravascular volume resuscitation is required. During the peracute (hypercoagulable) phase of DIC, the use of dextran is considered in conjunction with crystalloids because of its ability to decrease platelet adherence and increase flow through small vessels. However, if the animals has a systemic inflammatory response syndrome disease,

TABLE 86.2	Clinical Diseases and Their Initiators of the DIC Syndrome
Clinical Disease	**Initiators**
Systemic Inflammatory Response Syndrome[a]	Exposure subendothelial collagen
	Accelerated immune response
	Cytokine and inflammatory mediators
	Release of trypsin (pancreatitis)
Uncontrolled immune-mediated cellular destruction[b]	Red cell membrane phospholipids
	Circulating cellular debris
	Cytokine release
Trauma/Burns	Exposure subendothelial collagen
	Accelerated immune response
	Cytokine and inflammatory mediators
	Circulating cellular debris
	Circulating tissue thromboplastin
	Contact tissue factor activation of factor XII
Metabolic acidosis	Exposure subendothelial collagen
Severe shock	Exposure subendothelial collagen
	Accelerated immune response
	Cytokine and inflammatory mediators
	Poor clearance of activating clotting factors
	Poor delivery of fresh inhibitors
Disseminated neoplasia	Exposure subendothelial collagen
	Increased tissue thromboplastin/factor
	Accelerated immune response
	Expression of procoagulant and fibrinolytic activating factors
Hepatosplenic disease	Increased tissue thromboplastin
	Contact tissue factor activation of factor XII
	Increased plasmin
	Decreased production of clotting factors
	Poor endotoxin clearance
	Decreased production of coagulation inhibitors (liver)
	Insufficient clearance of activated factors and inhibitor complexes (liver)
Heartworm disease	Increased tissue thromboplasin
	Contact tissue factor activation of factor XII
Envenomation	Enzymatic activation of factor X

[a] Pancreatitis, peritonitis, gastroenteritis, pyometra, pneumonia, burns, trauma, neoplasia, vasculitis, rickettsial infection, hyperthermia, hypothermia, rickettsial, fungal and viral diseases
[b] Immune-mediated hemolytic anemia, incompatible blood transfusion, autotransfusion.

TABLE 86.3	Clinical Signs and Diagnostic Indicators of DIC	
Phase of DIC	**Clinical Signs**	**Coagulation Test**
Peracute phase (hypercoagulable)	No overt signs	PT, APTT, ACT or fast, normal platelet numbers, declining fibrinogen, normal or elevated FDPs <10, ATIII decreased FDPs <10, ACTII
Acute phase (consumptive)	Oozing blood or hemorrhage	Prolonged PT, normal or prolonged APTT, ACT, decreased platelet numbers, fibrinogen normal or low, FDPs >10, decreased ATIII
Chronic phase	No signs or oozing blood	Prolonged PT, APTT, ACT, decreased platelet numbers, normal or decreased fibrinogen, normal or elevated FDPs, decreased or normal ATIII

hydroxyethyl starch would be the synthetic colloid of choice in any phase of DIC (10 to 20 mL/kg intravenously to dogs; 5 to 15 mL/kg intravenously and slowly in cats) to improve blood pressure and cardiac output. Stroma-free hemoglobin (10 to 30 mL/kg to dogs; 5 to 15 mL/kg intravenously and slowly in cats) has the potential to provide oncotic pressure similar to heta-

starch while carrying oxygen to the tissues distal to the microthrombus.

The use of positive inotropic agents or vasodilators are indicated if fluids and colloids do not adequately improve capillary flow. Dobutamine (5 to 10 mg/kg/min, dogs; 2.5 to 5 mg/kg/min, cats) or dopamine (2 to 5 mg/kg/min) can be used for their

TABLE 86.4 Using Antithrombin III Values to Guide Therapy for DIC		
Antithrombin III Activity	**Interpretation**	**Therapy**
>90%	Normal	Continue to monitor
<80%	Low—concern for hypercoagulation	Monitor closely consider heparin
<60%	Very low—at risk for thrombosis and DIC	Requires heparin and ATIII replacement
<30%	Critical—immediate risk for thrombosis, DIC, and death	Requires heparin and aggressive, immediate ATIII replacement

Reprinted with permission from Feldman BF, Kirby R, Caldin M: Recognition and treatment of disseminated intravascular coagulation, Kirk's Current Veterinary Therapy XIII, Philadelphia: WB Saunders, 1996;190–194.

positive inotropic effect and little chronotropic effect. Should there be adequate intravascular volume with hypertension and inadequate tissue blood flow, nitroprusside (0.5 to 10 mg/kg/min) is titrated to effect. Careful blood pressure and central venous pressure monitoring is required.

Rapid elimination of the underlying disease state is the second priority. Body fluids should be cultured and appropriate antibiotics employed to treat sepsis. Septic foci should be drained or removed. Debridement of dead tissue or removal of the inciting cancer mass is done as early as possible. Unfortunately, many causes such as acute pancreatitis, heat stroke, heartworm disease, and hematologic diseases take time for correction, requiring patient support in the interim. When DIC is associated with a cause that cannot be successfully treated, the owner should be appraised of the grim prognosis.

The lungs, kidneys, liver, spleen, gut, and pancreas are targets for microthrombosis and ischemia or hemorrhage owing to their large capillary networks or ability to produce vasoactive substances. These organs must be supported while definitive therapy is employed. Oxygen supplementation and ventilatory support can be required for pulmonary insufficiency. Afferent glomerular arteriolar dilation by dopamine (1 to 3 mg/kg/min) is frequently necessary for renal support. Enteral nutrition and sucralfate give some additional protection to the gut, and appropriate antibiotic therapy should be employed when breakdown of the gut mucosal barrier is suspected.

Blood component replacement is the fourth priority. Theoretically, the addition of coagulation factors to the blood vascular system could "add fuel to the fire" by providing more coagulation factors. However, clinical experience in human and veterinary medicine does not support this premise. When the animal is compromised from loss of red blood cells, transfusion with washed packed red blood cells is ideal. Uncontrolled bleeding caused by consumption of coagulation factors (acute phase) may be stabilized with whole blood or plasma transfusions. It is not uncommon that multiple units are required. Cryoprecipitate can provide fibronectin, fibrinogen, factor VIII, and ATIII. The administration of fresh whole blood is needed when red blood cells, platelets, coagulation proteins, and oncotic components are required.

Animal studies have shown that when ATIII is ad-

ministered to subjects infused with a potent thromboplastin, the natural anticoagulant abilities of the blood were maintained and were protective against DIC and death.[12] Fresh frozen plasma, frozen plasma, fresh whole blood, cryoprecipitate, and stored whole blood are currently the only clinically available source of ATIII in veterinary medicine, in contrast to human medicine in which ATIII concentrates are available. Antithrombin III levels can be used to guide plasma replacement and heparin therapy (Table 86.4). It may require as many as 2 to 5 plasma infusions to bring the ATIII level back into therapeutic range.

Heparin administration is the fifth step of therapeutics and must be closely associated with ATIII replacement therapy. Heparin is best used early in the DIC process, when ATIII levels are adequate. The ATIII–thrombin complex inactivates thrombin and prevents fibrin formation. Heparin binds with ATIII, changes its configuration, and accelerates the ATIII–thrombin binding 1000 times faster than what occurs without heparin (Fig. 86.4).

When given alone, heparin can diminish ATIII levels.[13] It is therefore vital for the therapeutic actions of heparin that there is adequate ATIII present. Because acidosis inactivates heparin, tissue perfusion must be established and pH corrected prior to heparinization.

Several methods have been described to activate ATIII with heparin, and at time of publication the most appropriate method had not been identified. Heparin therapy has been reported as ineffective in the treatment of DIC,[14] and often the cause of severe hemorrhagic complications. It is anticipated that most of the poor responses to heparin are the result of heparin being administered when there is inadequate ATIII. In the absence of ATIII, heparin has only weak antithrombotic effects related to heparin cofactor II activity against thrombin.[15]

Initial heparin dose and route of administration remains a controversy. One technique is to add the first heparin dose (50 to 200 IU/kg) to the plasma or whole blood bag prior to transfusion administration. This is meant to activate ATIII prior to administering coagulation proteins while providing the first heparinizing dose. However, therapeutic heparin levels are not immediately achieved, and there are no clinical studies supporting the pharmacokinetic accuracy of this technique. A second method of heparinization is more commonly described: 100 IU/kg injection administered subcutaneously at the time of transfusion administration. Absorption time may be affected by inadequate tissue perfusion. A third method of heparinization is by administering the first dose intravenously as a 50 IU/kg bolus. Clinical trials are required to define the pharmacokinetics of heparin injections in animals.

Once the ATIII levels are more than 60%, heparin is continued alone at 50 to 100 U/kg subcutaneously every 8 hours. Should more plasma or blood be required, additional heparin in the bag should not be necessary since the animal is already heparinized. Heparin administration is continued until the source of DIC is removed and the animal is hemodynamically stabilized. Heparin therapy must be tapered over 48 hours before stopping to prevent rebound thrombosis.

REFERENCES

1. **Hardaway RM, McKay DG, Williams JH.** Lower nephron nephrosis. Amer J Surg 1954;87:41–46.
2. **Bick RL.** Disseminated intravascular coagulation and related syndromes: a clinical review. Semin Thromb Hemost 1988;14:299–338.
3. **Bateman SW, Mathews KA, Abrams-Ogg ACG.** Disseminated intravascular coagulation in dogs: review of the literature. J Vet Emerg Crit Care 1998;8:29–44.
4. **Bell WR.** The pathophysiology of disseminated intravascular coagulation. Semin Hematol 1994;31:19–25.
5. **Bell WR, Braine HG, Ness PM, Kickler TS.** Improved survival in thrombotic thrombocytopenic-hemolytic uremic syndrome: clinical experience in 108 patients. N Engl J Med 1991;325:398–403.
6. **Bick RL.** Coagulation abnormalities in malignancy: a review. Semin Thromb Hemost 1991;18:353–371.
7. **Bick R, Baker WF.** Disseminated intravascular coagulation. Hematol Pathol 1992;6:1.
8. **Bick R, Dukes M, Wilson W, Fekete L.** Antithrombin III as a diagnostic aid in disseminated intravascular coagulation. Thromb Res 1977;10:721.
9. **Kirby R:** Septic shock. In: Bonagura JD, Kirk RW, eds. Kirk's current veterinary therapy. XII. Philadelphia: WB Saunders, 1996;139–146.
10. **Helgren M, Egberg N, Eklund J.** Blood coagulation and fibrinolytic factors and their inhibitors in critically ill patients. Intensive Care Med 1984;10:23–28.
11. **Wilson R, Mammen E, Robson M, Heggers J, Soullier G, Depoli P.** Antithrombin, prekallikrein and fibronectin levels in surgical patients. Arch Surg 1986;121:635–640.
12. **Taylor FB Jr, Emerson TE Jr, Jordan R, et al.** Antithrombin-III prevents the lethal effects of *Escherichia coli* infusion in baboons. Circ Shock 1988;26:227.
13. **Hardaway RM, Adams WH.** Thrombosis. In: Hardaway RM, Adams WH, eds. Blood problems in critical care. I. Philadelphia: JB Lippincott Co, 1989;139–174.
14. **Bang NU.** Diagnosis and management of thrombosis. In: Shoemaker WC, Ayres S, Grenvik A, et al, eds. Textbook of critical care. Philadelphia: WB Saunders, 1989;886–895.
15. **Demers C, Henderson P, Blajchman MA, et al.** An antithrombin III assay based on factor Xa inhibition provides a more reliable test to identify congenital antithrombin III deficiency than an assay based on thrombin inhibition. Thromb Haemost 1993;69:231.

CHAPTER 87

Anticoagulant and Fibrinolytic Drugs

• RAFAEL RUIZ DE GOPEGUI and LUIS MONREAL

Thrombotic disorders are frequent complications of severe diseases in small animal and equine medicine. The efficacy of several antithrombotic drugs, currently used in people, has been evaluated for their application in veterinary medicine. But there are differences in the effectiveness of antithrombotics among animal species owing to their different hemostatic physiology as regards activator and inhibitor activities, platelet activation, and protein metabolism. In addition, the importance of human antithrombotic therapy has focused research on new molecules with antithrombotic activity, so that their efficacy is improved with the lowest detrimental effects. Therefore, new products are being tested in clinical human trials and experimental models. Antithrombotic therapy includes three groups of drugs based on their main action: antiplatelets, anticoagulants, and fibrinolytics.

ANTIPLATELETS

Antiplatelet drugs inhibit platelet activation and aggregation, and are administered to prevent human arterial thrombosis. In veterinary medicine, they have been used to prevent thrombosis in endotoxemia, verminous colic, cardiomyopathy, and heartworm disease. Although clinical efficacy has yet to be confirmed in these diseases,[1] antiplatelets have been effective, during prodromal stages, in prevention of carbohydrate-induced equine laminitis.[2]

Aspirin

Aspirin is the best-known antiplatelet drug. Aspirin irreversibly acetylates the active site of platelet and endothelial cyclooxygenase, disrupting prostaglandin and thromboxane synthesis. However, other platelet activators such as thrombin, ADP, platelet-activating factor (PAF), collagen, or epinephrine can still induce platelet aggregation. PAF and thrombin are more important mediators of platelet aggregation in horses than thromboxane A_2 (TxA_2).[3,4] Then, thromboxane inhibitors would be less effective than in people, and thrombin inhibitors would be more effective. Moderate doses of aspirin may inhibit platelet aggregation and secretion. Low-dose aspirin is administered for prophylaxis and treatment of thrombosis in human and veterinary medicine. Effectiveness of aspirin administration and dosage regimens for thromboprophylaxis in *Dirofilaria immitis* infection and other causes of pulmonary thromboembolism remain controversial.[5-9] Recommended aspirin doses for antiplatelet activity are 25 mg/kg orally twice a week in the cat[10,11] 0.5 to 10 mg/kg once or twice a day in the dog,[6,12,13] and 4 to 12 mg/kg in the horse.[1] Low doses may be equally effective than high doses and may reduce adverse effects such as gastrointestinal bleeding.[14]

Antiplatelets in Development

The limitations and adverse events associated with aspirin have prompted the search for other antiplatelet agents. Many new, more potent, antiplatelet agents are now available for clinical evaluation.[15,16] At present, most of them are under investigation to evaluate clinical efficacy in people.

Antagonist of Adenosine Diphosphate

Ticlopidine is considered an effective antithrombotic drug. It has a different spectrum of side effects than aspirin, being recommended in cases in which aspirin is contraindicated (gastrointestinal bleeding). It exerts maximal inhibitory effect after three days of administration.

Clopidogrel binds to adenylate cyclase-coupled ADP receptors on the platelet surface, preventing ADP-dependent platelet activation. In animal models, it has reduced arterial and venous thrombus formation, with higher efficacy and lower gastrointestinal upset than aspirin.[16,17]

Dipyridamole acts as a phosphodiesterase inhibitor, increasing prostacyclin activity and delaying ADP clearance from plasma. It has been used in association with other antithrombotic drug.[18]

Platelet Integrin $\alpha_{IIb}\beta_3$ Blockers

These molecules block the platelet receptor of fibrinogen, and are now considered promising antiplatelet agents.[19,20]

Abciximab is a monoclonal antibody fragment that blocks the integrin $\alpha_{IIb}\beta_3$. It induces almost complete and reversible inhibition of platelet function.[21] It may potentially have greater clinical efficacy and be safer than other antiplatelet drugs.[19,20]

Integrilin is a potent inhibitor of the fibrinogen binding function of integrin $\alpha_{IIb}\beta_3$, with a rapid onset of action, and a short half-life.[19,20]

RGDS and RPR 110885 are integrin $\alpha_{IIb}\beta_3$ receptor antagonists that contain an amino acid sequence, arginine-glycine-aspartate (RGD). This sequence is identical to residues 572–574 of the fibrinogen molecule. Addition of a fourth amino acid such as serine (RGDS), valine, or tryptophane substantially increases activity. RGDS inhibition of platelet aggregation has been studied in humans, dogs, rhesus monkeys, guinea pigs, and rats. RGDS and RPR 110885 inhibit platelet aggregation and platelet adhesion to subendothelial collagen and may be useful for thrombotic diseases therapy in horses.[8]

Others to Be Evaluated

Thromboxane synthase inhibitors
Thromboxane receptor blockers
Prostacyclin
Antagonists of serotonin
Ajoene[22]
Angelitriol and angelol[23]
Eugenol and acetyl eugenol[24,25]
Dauricoside, dauricine and daurisoline[26,27]

ANTICOAGULANTS

Anticoagulants are indicated to control the hypercoagulable states. Some anticoagulants may also act as antiplatelets, since platelet recruitment is primarily mediated by thrombin.[28] In veterinary medicine, hypercoagulability may occur in exercise, severe gastrointestinal disease, endotoxemia, sepsis, neoplasia, dirofilariasis, pancreatitis, cardiomyopathy, and different disseminated intravascular coagulation (DIC) causes.[29,30]

Vitamin K Antagonists

These products are represented by coumarin compounds. They inhibit hepatic synthesis of vitamin-K-dependent clotting factors (factors II, VII, IX, and X). Thus, they induce prothrombinopenia, instead of reducing hypercoagulability.[31] Proteins C and S are vitamin-K-dependent proteins as well; they are reduced during coumarin administration. Since thrombotic risk can be increased during initiation (first 3 to 4 days) and termination of coumarin therapy, simultaneous heparin administration should be considered in these moments.

Warfarin is still widely used as anticoagulant in humans because it is effective and allows oral administration. In small-animal medicine, it can be recommended to prevent thromboembolism in feline cardiomyopath-

ies.[32] However, there are many factors that can influence the individual response to warfarin, making the dosing protocol variable (0.1 to 0.2 mg/kg q24h initially) and difficult to maintain constant. The risk of spontaneous bleeding is also high and requires a closed monitor of clotting times; maintain prothrombin time 1.5 to 2 times over baseline or international normalization ratio (INR) 2 to 3.[31-33]

Heparin

Heparin has been the most important antithrombotic drug up to now. It has anticoagulant effect and inhibits thrombin-mediated platelet recruitment and aggregation as well. Although heparin is a polysaccharide with a molecular weight varying from 4 to 40 kd, only a small fraction of this molecule is responsible for its anticoagulant effect. The active site of heparin contains a specific pentasaccharide sequence that binds to antithrombin III (ATIII), the main inhibitor of coagulation, and accelerates its activity by 2000-fold. Therefore, heparin induces inhibition of factors Xa and factor IIa.[29,34]

Different studies have evaluated heparin efficacy for hypercoagulable states in humans, horses, dogs, and cats.[29,34] However, some undesirable effects, such as bleeding complications, thrombocytopenia, individual variability in dosage response,[34] and dose-dependent erythrocyte agglutination in horses, have been observed.[35] Long-term heparin administration have also induced osteoporosis[36] and a steady decrease of plasma ATIII activity.

Dosage protocols proposed for heparin therapy in veterinary medicine are variable. Based on experimental models, the therapeutic range is achieved when the anti-factor Xa activity in plasma ranges 0.2 to 0.4 U/mL.[34] But this level of heparinemia has frequently induced hemorrhage. Lower doses (0.05 to 0.2 U/mL) have been recommended for thromboprophylaxis, maintaining effectiveness and reducing bleeding risk.[29] Since plasma heparin concentration and prolongation of clotting times during heparin therapy has high correlation (as much as $r = 0.92$),[37,38] activated partial thromboplastin time (APTT) has normally been used to monitor heparin therapy. Appropriate heparin concentrations have been achieved with APTT increases of 1.5 to 2.5 times over the reference value. Thus, an effective heparin dosage to prevent thrombosis would correspond to this prolongation of the patient's APTT[34]; lower doses could diminish its efficacy, and higher doses would increase bleeding tendency. Currently, this may be achieved with 80 to 100 U/kg bodyweight q8h or q12h. Note that modifications on APTT determination (different thromboplastins and contact activators) may potentially affect the sensitivity of the determination to heparin. Different dosages are proposed in veterinary literature, but they should achieve sufficient heparinemia for an effective thromboprophylaxis with low bleeding risks.[39] Further clinical trials should be conducted to obtain more accurate dosages in veterinary medicine. In addition, the specific undesirable effects associated with heparin conducted to develop new safer and more convenient anti-thrombotic drugs.

Low-Molecular-Weight HEPARIN

Standard heparin can be fragmented in different portions containing the unit responsible of ATIII affinity and binding. Low-molecular-weight heparin (LMWH) fractions (4 to 5 kd) have been developed and their suitability as antithrombotic drugs investigated. It has been shown that reducing the molecular weight of heparin, bioavailability, affinity for ATIII, anti-factor Xa effect, and thrombin inhibition duration increases, whereas affinity for heparin cofactor II, interaction with platelets and endothelial cells, bleeding tendency, and prolongation of clotting times diminishes.[34,40,41] Furthermore, LMWH does not produce thrombocytopenia and erythrocyte agglutination in horses.[38] LMWHs have advantages over unfractioned heparin, including anti-thrombotic efficacy, longer half-life, more predictable anticoagulant response, and fewer bleeding complications.[40,42,43]

Different studies confirmed that LMWH are effective as antithrombotic drugs in experimental models and clinical trials in people; even more effective than unfractioned heparin.[40,44,45] In the veterinary literature, there are no reports as regards the use of LMWH and its efficacy as yet, but its use in clinical cases has started.

The recommended dosage for thromboprophylaxis depends on which LMWH is used (dalteparin, enoxaparin, fraxiparine, etc), but it corresponds to those to achieve the anti-Xa activity desired for thromboprophylaxis with lesser bleeding risk (0.05 to 0.2 U/mL).[42] Dalteparin can be administered 50 U/kg q24h subcutaneously.[38]

In contrast to unfractionated heparin, low doses of LMWH do not prolong, significantly, clotting times. Thus, clotting times are not suitable to monitor LMWH therapy. Only an anti-Xa activity test can be recommended to check heparinemia.[38,40,46]

Other Heparinoids and Heparin Fragments

Pentasaccharides are the newest synthetic fragments from the molecule of heparin that contain the active unit to bind to ATIII. They have shown higher affinity to ATIII than other heparins, and more selective inhibition of factor Xa. It has been reported that they strongly inhibited thrombus formation in experimental models of venous thrombosis, without inducing thrombocytopenia and hemorrhage.[47] Clinical trials in humans have demonstrated antithrombotic effectiveness and long bioavailability, even with once a week administration.[47,48]

Pentosan polysulfate is a low-molecular-weight sulfated heparinoid polysaccharide derived from *Fagus sylvatica* (beechwood) shavings. It has been used as antithrombotic drug for nearly 30 years in Europe. However, its antithrombotic efficacy was lower than other compounds and has been substituted. However, it has been reported effective in canine and equine cystitis and osteoarthritis therapy, owing to its high affinity to the bladder and chondroprotective activity.[49–51]

Other glycosaminoglycans are being considered. Glycosaminoglycans are heparinoids with certain anticoagulant properties. Several polysulfated glycosaminoglycans are being marketed for the treatment of osteoarthritis and degenerative joint disease. As anticoagulants, they prolong clotting times,[52–54] but this activity seems to be related with an activation of heparin cofactor II, with potent thrombin-inhibitory activity in the vessel wall.[55] Dermatan sulfate has been effective in a DIC model, with lower hemorrhage risk than other anticoagulants.[55,56]

Direct Thrombin Inhibitors

These new antithrombotic drugs have become the focus of interest of clinicians and researchers because their antithrombin activity is independent of ATIII. This advantage may permit use of them in ATIII-depleted patients, especially in DIC.[57] As direct antithrombin drugs, they have also shown important antiplatelet action.[58,59] Some of them are now available.

Hirudin is a direct thrombin inhibitor derived from the leech *Hirudo medicinalis*. A recombinant form of hirudin (r-hirudin) and a synthetically designed hirudin (hirulog) have been produced for therapeutic use. At present, both forms are available in Europe and America respectively.[57]

Hirudin is the most potent thrombin-specific inhibitor, which forms equimolar complexes with thrombin, among thrombin inhibitors.[60] In contrast to heparin, hirudin is not inactivated by antiheparin proteins and have no direct effects on platelets avoiding the heparin-induced thrombocytopenia. Furthermore, hirudin seems to be a more effective anticoagulant than heparin in both arterial and venous thrombosis, given its ability to inactivate clot or subendothelium-bound thrombin.[61]

Different studies have been performed to compare its efficacy with aspirin, heparin, and LMWH in experimental thrombosis models and clinical trials. Hirudin has been considered a promising antithrombotic, at least as effective as LMWH, for thromboprophylaxis.[57,61–63] However, patients should be monitored to avoid hemorrhage induced by hirudin therapy. Hirudin induces a dose-dependent prolongation of APTT,[64] therefore, it can be considered an appropriate test to monitor hirudin therapy.[46,65]

Other Anticoagulants in Study

Other Antagonists to Thrombin

Argatroban is a synthetic highly specific and reversible thrombin inhibitor. It has shown a safe and potent antithrombotic effect when administered as intravenous infusion. Thus, it could be indicated in cases in which heparin is contraindicated (such as heparin-induced thrombocytopenia).[66,67]

Inogatran is a new selective active site inhibitor of thrombin, which has shown to be also effective as antithrombotic agent both in the venous and arterial thrombosis experimental models, with weak prolongation of bleeding time.[68]

Efegatran has also shown that is effective as antithrombotic with a high therapeutic index.[69]

Melagatran is another new potent, competitive, and rapid inhibitor of thrombin, with a high oral bioavailability in the dog.[70]

Factor Xa Inhibitors

The factor Xa inhibitors may be effective in inhibiting the generation of thrombi, compared with other antithrombotics.[71,72]

Antistasin is a factor Xa inhibitor isolated from the salivary glands of the Mexican leech *Haementeria officinalis* and synthesized by recombinant methods. In a DIC model, it was shown to be fully effective as an anticoagulant drug, at least as effective as heparin.[71,73]

Others

New therapeutic strategies include inactivation of bound thrombin, inhibition of thrombin receptors activation by thrombin, and interruption of thrombin generation.[28,55] Some examples are:

- PPACK, a synthetic thrombin inhibitor, which irreversibly blocks the active site of thrombin
- Tissue factor pathway inhibitors
- Recombinant protein C
- Recombinant thrombomodulin

Different compounds with anticoagulant activity (mainly anti-Xa or antithrombin) have been found from the salivary glands of different species of mosquitoes, flies, *Hemiptera*, ticks, and leeches.[74]

FIBRINOLYTICS

Fibrinolysis is an important mechanism of hemostasis inhibition. It is initiated by activation of the inactive zymogen plasminogen into an active serin protease, plasmin. Plasmin has similar substrates to thrombin (factors V and VIII, fibrinogen, and fibrin), but an opposite effect; plasmin proteolytic action inactivates factors V and VIII and generates fibrinogen degradation products (FgDP) and fibrin degradation products (FDP) with further inhibitory effects on fibrin polymerization and platelet aggregation.

Aortic thromboembolism is a common sequela of feline cardiomyopathy. Medical therapy comprises vasodilators, anticoagulants, aspirin, serotonin antagonists, and thrombolytic drugs.[75] Treatment of feline aortic thromboembolism remains difficult and acute reperfusion syndrome may induce further complications.

Plasminogen activators are enzymes that catalyze the conversion of plasminogen to plasmin. Streptokinase (SK) and urokinase plasminogen activator (uPA) may convert plasminogen to plasmin in the circulating blood as well as on the fibrin surface of thrombus. The activation of circulating plasminogen induces a proteolytic state that predisposes to hemorrhage. As a result, systemic use of streptokinase and uPA involves an important risk.

SK is isolated from the broth of group C β-hemolytic streptococci cultures. SK activates plasminogen indirectly by forming complex with free plasminogen. SK administration (90,000 IU intravenously as loading dose and 45,000 IU/h diluted in saline for 3 hours) induced systemic fibrinolysis but was unsuccessful in terms of thrombus reduction and reperfusion in feline aortic thromboembolism.[76] However, the same dosage regimen was effective and had minor adverse effects in four dogs that had thrombosis.[77]

Recombinant tissue plasminogen activator (rtPA) is a single- or double-chain polypeptide serine protease. It has low affinity for circulating plasminogen, but in the presence of fibrin, enzymatic activity is enhanced 1000-fold.[78] As a result, tissue plasminogen activator (tPA) and plasminogen would bind fibrin-activating fibrinolysis in the site of interest and may potentially avoid a systemic proteolytic state.[79] However, hemorrhage risk increases with high FDP concentration and hypofibrinogenemia that may result from thrombolysis and prolonged tPA infusion. Multiple bolus intravenous injection (0.25 to 1 mg/kg every 60 minutes; total dose 1 to 10 mg/kg) appears to be safer and more effective in terms of earlier recanalization of thrombosed vessels and lower bleeding tendency.[80] In cats that had aortic thromboembolism, rtPA effectively decreased the reperfusion time and recovery. However, a 50% acute mortality rate during therapy was observed owing to hyperkalemia, congestive heart failure, and coronary thrombosis.[81] Thrombolytic therapy has been also attempted in experimentally induced canine pulmonary thromboembolism.[82] Thrombolytic therapy with rtPA may be improved with LMWH administration as adjunctive therapy.[83]

Recombinant pro-urokinase (r-pro-UK) is a single-chain precursor of high-molecular-weight urokinase (UK). It is a second-generation plasminogen activator that directly activates fibrin-bound plasminogen to plasmin. Plasmin converts pro-UK to high-molecular-weight UK in a positive feedback reaction. Then, high-molecular-weight UK increases the activation of plasminogen to plasmin. Administration of 80,000 IU/kg of r-pro-UK to beagle dogs restored arterial flow and did not induce a systemic proteolytic state in an experimental thrombosis model.[84]

REFERENCES

1. **Cambridge H, Lees P, Hooke RE, Russell CS.** Antithrombotic actions of aspirin in the horse. Equine Vet J 1991;23:123–127.
2. **Weiss DJ, Evanson OA, McClenahan D, Fagliari JJ, Jenkins K.** Evaluation of platelet activation and platelet-neutrophil aggregates in ponies with alimentary laminitis. Am J Vet Res 1997;58:1376–1380.
3. **Heath MF, Evans RJ, Poole AW, Hayes LJ, McEvoy RJ, Littler RM.** The effects of aspirin and paracetamol on the aggregation of equine blood platelets. J Vet Pharmacol Ther 1994;17:374–378.
4. **Jarvis GE, Evans RJ.** Platelet-activating factor and not thromboxane A$_2$ is an important mediator of endotoxin-induced platelet aggregation in equine heparinised whole blood *in vitro*. Blood Coagul Fibrinolysis 1996;7:194–198.

5. **Rawlings CA, Farrell RL, Mahood RM.** Morphological changes in the lungs of cats experimentally infected with *Dirofilaria immitis:* response to aspirin. J Vet Intern Med 1990;4:292–300.
6. **Watari T, Takeda K, Goitsuka R, Hasegawa A.** Platelet aggregation in dogs infected with Dirofilaria immitis. J Jpn Vet Med Assoc 1993;46:42–45.
7. **Hart S, Deniz A, Sommer B, Kietzmann M, Nolte I.** Wirkung von Acetyl-salicylsäure auf Thrombozyten-aggregation und kapillare Blutungszeit bei gesunden Katzen. DTW 1995;102:476–480.
8. **Weiss DJ, Evanson OA, Wells RE.** Evaluation of arginine-glycine-aspartate-containing peptides as inhibitors of equine platelet function. Am J Vet Res 1997;58:457–460.
9. **Gentry PA, Tremblay RRM, Rose ML.** Failure of aspirin to impair bovine platelet function. Am J Vet Res 1989;50:919–922.
10. **Greene CE.** Effects of aspirin and propanolol on feline platelet aggregation. Am J Vet Res 1985;46:1820–1823.
11. **Behrend EN, Grauer GF, Greco DS, Rose BJ, Thrall MAH.** Comparison of the effects of diltiazem and aspirin on platelet aggregation in cats. J Am Anim Hosp Assoc 1996;32:11–18.
12. **Grauer GF, Rose BJ, Toolan L, Thrall MAH, Colgan SP, Hull Thrall MA.** Effects of low-dose aspirin and specific thromboxane synthetase inhibition on whole blood platelet aggregation and adenosine triphosphate secretion in healthy dogs. Am J Vet Res 1992;53:1631–1635.
13. **Rackear D, Feldman BF, Farver T, Lelong L.** The effect of three different dosages of acetylsalicylic acid on canine platelet aggregation. J Am Anim Hosp Assoc 1988;24:23–26.
14. **Hawkey CJ, Somerville KW, Marshall S.** Prophylaxis of aspirin induced gastric mucosal bleeding with ranitidine. Aliment Pharmacol Ther 1988; 2:245–252.
15. **Kawamura M, Imura Y, Moriya N, Kita S, Fukushi H, Sugihara H, Nishikawa K, Terashita Z.** Antithrombotic effects of TAK-029, a novel GPIIb/IIIa antagonist, in guinea pigs: comparative studies with ticlopidine, clopidogrel, aspirin, prostaglandin E1 and argatroban. J Pharmacol Exp Ther 1996; 277:502–510.
16. **Joseph JE, Machin SJ.** New antiplatelet drugs. Blood Rev 1997;11:178–190.
17. **Coukell AJ, Markham A.** Clopidogrel. Drugs 1997;54:745–750.
18. **Gibbs CR, Lip GY.** Do we still need dipyridamole? Br J Clin Pharmacol 1998;45:323–328.
19. **Tcheng JE.** Platelet glycoprotein IIb/IIIa integrin blockade: recent clinical trials in interventional cardiology. Thromb Haemost 1997;78:205–209.
20. **Van de Werf F.** Clinical trials with glycoprotein IIb/IIIa receptor antagonists in acute coronary syndromes. Thromb Haemost 1997;78:210–213.
21. **Coller BE, Scudder LE.** Inhibition of dog platelet function in *in vivo* infusion of F(ab′)2 fragments of a monoclonal antibody to the platelet glycoprotein IIb/IIIa receptor. Blood 1985;66:1456–1459.
22. **Rendu F.** L'ajoene, un antiagregant efficace et subtil. Acta Botanica Gallica 1996;143:149–154.
23. **Liu JH, Xu SX, Yao XS, Kobayashi H.** Two new 6-alkylcoumarins from Angelica pubescens f. biserrata. Planta Med 1995;61:482–484.
24. **Srivastava KC.** Antiplatelet principles from a food spice clove (Syzygium aromaticum L.). Prostaglandins Leukot Essent Fatty Acids 1993;48:363–372.
25. **Saeed SA, Simjee RU, Shamim G, Gilani AH.** Eugenol: a dual inhibitor of platelet-activating factor and arachidonic acid metabolism. Phytomedicine 1995;2:23–28.
26. **Hu SM, Xu SX, Yao XS, Cui CB, Tezuka Y, Kikuchi T.** Dauricoside, a new glycosidal alkaloid having an inhibitory activity against blood-platelet aggregation. Chem Pharm Bull 1993;41:1866–1868.
27. **Zhou JA, Ding YX, Gu SF, Ye XM, Zeng FD, Tu YS, Yang YH.** Investigation on platelet aggregation of dauricine in patients with cardiovascular diseases. Chin Pharmacol Bull 1994;10:33–36.
28. **Harker LA, Hanson SR, Kelly AB.** Antithrombotic strategies targeting thrombin activities, thrombin receptors and thrombin generation. Thromb Haemost 1997;78:736–741.
29. **Moore BR, Hinchcliff KW.** Heparin: a review of its pharmacology and therapeutic use in horses. J Vet Intern Med 1994;8:26–35.
30. **Monreal L, Anglés AM, Monreal M, Espada Y, Monasterio J.** Changes in haemostasis in endurance horses: detection by highly sensitive ELISA-tests. Equine Vet J Suppl 1995;18:120–123.
31. **Ansell JE.** Oral anticoagulant therapy. In: Hull R, Raskob G, Pineo G, eds. Venous thromboembolism: an evidence-based atlas. Armonk: Futura Publishing Co, 1996.
32. **Harpster NK, Baty CJ.** Warfarin therapy of the cat at risk of thromboembolism. In: Bonagura JD, Kirk RW, eds. Kirk's current veterinary therapy. XII. Philadelphia: WB Saunders, 1995;868–873.
33. **Scott EA, Byars TD, Lamar AM.** Warfarin anticoagulation in the horse. J Am Vet Med Assoc 1980;177:1146–1151.
34. **Hirsh J, Fuster V.** Guide to anticoagulant therapy. Part 1: Heparin. Circulation 1994;89:1449–1468.
35. **Moore JN, Mahaffey EA, Zboran M.** Heparin-induced agglutination of erythrocytes in horses. Am J Vet Res 1987;48:68–71.
36. **Monreal M, Viñas L, Monreal L, Lavín S, Lafoz E, Anglés AM.** Heparin-related osteoporosis in rats. A comparative study between unfractionated and a low-molecular-weight heparin. Haemostasis 1990;20:204–207.
37. **Bounameaux H, Marbet GA, Lammle B, Eichlisberger R, Duckert F.** Monitoring of heparin treatment. Comparison of thrombin time, activated partial thromboplastin time, and plasma heparin concentration and analysis of the behaviour of antithrombin III. Am J Clin Pathol 1980;74:68–73.
38. **Monreal L, Villatoro AJ, Monreal M, Espada Y, Anglés AM, Ruiz de Gopegui R.** Comparison of the effects of low-molecular-weight and unfractioned heparin in horses. Am J Vet Res 1995;56:1281–1285.
39. **Gerhards H, Eberhardt C.** Plasma heparin values and hemostasis in equids after subcutaneous administration of low-dose calcium heparin. Am J Vet Res 1988;49:13–18.
40. **Dunn CJ, Sorkin EM.** Dalteparin sodium. A review of its pharmacology and clinical use in the prevention and treatment of thromboembolic disorders. Drugs 1996;52:276–305.
41. **Verhaeghe R.** The use of low-molecular-weight heparins in cardiovascular disease. Acta Cardiol 1998;53:15–21.
42. **Caen JP.** A randomized double-blind study between a low molecular weight heparin Kabi 2165 and standard heparin in the prevention of deep vein thrombosis in general surgery. A french multicenter trial. Thromb Haemost 1988;59:216–220.
43. **Kakkar VV, Cohen AT, Edmonson RA, Phillips MJ, Cooper DJ, Das SK, Maher KT, Sanderson RM, Ward VP, Kakkar S.** Low molecular weight versus standard heparin for prevention of venous thromboembolism after major abdominal surgery. Lancet 1993;341:259–265.
44. **Monreal M, Silveira P, Monreal L, Monasterio J, Angles AM, Lafoz E, Lorente L.** Comparative study on the antithrombotic efficacy of four low-molecular-weight heparins in three different models of experimental venous thrombosis. Haemostasis 1991;21:91–97.
45. **Schumacher WA, Heran CL, Steinbacher TE.** Low-molecular-weight heparin (fragmin) and thrombin active-site inhibitor (argatroban) compared in experimental arterial and venous thrombosis and bleeding time. J Cardiovasc Pharmacol 1996;28:19–25.
46. **Ruiz de Gopegui R, Espada Y, Monreal M, Anglés AM, Monreal L, Feldman BF, Viñas L.** Biological monitoring of three antithrombotic drugs: single dose therapy. Comp Haematol Int 1997;7:42–46.
47. **Herbert JM, Herault JP, Bernat A, van Amsterdam RG, Lormeau JC, Petitou M, van Boeckel C, Hoffman P, Meuleman DG.** Biochemical and pharmacological properties of SANORG 34006, a potent and long-acting synthetic pentasaccharide. Blood 1998;91:4197–4205.
48. **Hoppensteadt DA, Jeske WP, Walenga JM, Fu K, Yang LH, Ing T, Herbert JM, Fareed J.** Efficacy of pentasaccharide in a dog model of hemodialysis. Thromb Res 1997;88:159–170.
49. **Smith MM, Ghosh P, Numata Y, Bansal MK.** The effects of orally administered calcium pentosan polysulfate on inflammation and cartilage degradation produced in rabbit joints by intraarticular injection of a hyaluronate-polylysine complex. Arthritis Rheum 1994;37:125–136.
50. **Little C, Ghosh P.** Potential use of pentosan polysulfate for the treatment of equine joint disease. In: McIlwraith CW, Trotter GW, eds. Joint disease in the horse. Philadelphia: WB Saunders, 1996;281–292.
51. **Read RA, Cullis-Hill D, Jones MP.** Systemic use of pentosan polysulphate in the treatment of osteoarthritis. J Small Anim Pract 1996;37:108–114.
52. **Beale BS, Goring RL, Clemmons RM, et al.** The effect of semi-synthetic polysulfated glycosaminoglycans on the hemostatic mechanism in the dog. Vet Surg 1990;19:57.
53. **De Haan JJ, Beale BS, Clemmons RM, et al.** The effects of polysulfated glycosaminoglycan (Adequan R) on activated partial thromboplastin time, prothrombin time, complete blood count, biochemical profile and urinalysis in cats. Vet Comp Orthop Traum 1994;7:77–81.
54. **Trotter GW.** Polysulfated glycosaminoglycan (Adequan). In: McIlwraith CW, Trotter GW, eds. Joint disease in the horse. Philadelphia: WB Saunders, 1996;270–280.
55. **Bombeli T, Mueller M, Haeberli A.** Anticoagulant properties of the vascular endothelium. Thromb Haemost 1997;77:408–423.
56. **Onaya J, Kyogashima M, Sunose A, Miyauchi S, Mizuno S, Horie K.** Effects of dermatan sulfate, a heparin cofactor II mediated thrombin inhibitor, on the endotoxin-induced disseminated intravascular coagulation model in the rat: comparison with low-molecular weight heparin, nafamostat mesilate and argatroban. Jpn J Pharmacol 1998;76:397–404.
57. **Verstraete M.** Direct thrombin inhibitors: appraisal of the antithrombotic/hemorrhagic balance. Thromb Haemost 1997;78:357–363.
58. **Yamashita T, Yamamoto J, Sasaki Y, Matsuoka A.** The antithrombotic effect of low molecular weight synthetic thrombin inhibitors, argatroban and PPACK, on He-En laser-induced thrombosis in rat mesenteric microvessels. Thromb Res 1993;69:93–100.
59. **Verstraete M.** Modulating platelet function with selective thrombin inhibitors. Haemostasis 1996;26 Suppl 4:70–77.
60. **Callas DD, Hoppensteadt D, Fareed J.** Comparative studies on the anticoagulant and protease generation inhibitory actions of newly developed site-directed thrombin inhibitory drugs. Efegatran, argatroban, hirulog, and hirudin. Semin Thromb Hemost 1995;21:177–183.
61. **Monreal M, Costa J, Salva P.** Pharmacological properties of hirudin and its derivatives. Potential clinical advantages over heparin. Drugs Aging 1996;8:171–182.
62. **Monreal M, Galego G, Monreal L, Anglés AM, Monasterio J, Oller B.** Comparative study on the antithrombotic efficacy of hirudin, heparin and a

low-molecular weight heparin in preventing experimentally induced venous thrombosis. Haemostasis 1993;23:179–183.

63. **Meyer BJ, Badimon JJ, Chesebro JH, Fallon JT, Fuster V, Badimon L.** Dissolution of mural thrombus by specific thrombin inhibition with r-hirudin: comparison with heparin and aspirin. Circulation 1998;97:681–685.

64. **Lidon RM, Theroux P, Juneau M, Adelman B, Maraganore J.** Initial experience with a direct antithrombin, hirulog, in unstable angina: anticoagulant, antithrombotic, and clinical effects. Circulation 1993;88:1495–1501.

65. **Monreal M, Monreal L, Ruiz de Gopegui R, Espada Y, Angles AM, Monasterio J.** Effects of two different doses of hirudin on APTT, determined with eight different reagents. Thromb Haemost 1995;73:219–222.

66. **Duval N, Lunven C, O'Brien DP, Grosset A, O'Connor SE, Berry CN.** Antithrombotic actions of the thrombin inhibitor, argatroban, in a canine model of coronary cyclic flow: comparison with heparin. Br J Pharmacol 1996;118:727–733.

67. **Matsuo T, Koide M, Kario K.** Development of argatroban, a direct thrombin inhibitor, and its clinical application. Semin Thromb Hemost 1997;23:517–522.

68. **Gustafsson D, Elg M, Lenfors S, Borjesson I, Tejer-Nilsson AC.** Effects of inogatran, a new low-molecular-weight thrombin inhibitor, in rat models of venous and arterial thrombosis, thrombolysis and bleeding time. Blood Coagul Fibrinolysis 1996;7:69–79.

69. **Smith GF, Shuman RT, Craft TJ, Gifford DS, Kurz KD, Jones ND, Chirgadze N, Hermann RB, Coffman WJ, Sandusky GE, Roberts E, Jackson CV.** A family of arginal thrombin inhibitors related to efegatran. Semin Thromb Hemost 1996;22:173–183.

70. **Gustafsson D, Antonsson T, Bylund R, Eriksson U, Gyzander E, Nilsson I, Elg M, Mattsson C, Deinum J, Pehrsson S, Karlsson O, Nilsson A, Sorensen H.** Effects of melagatran, a new low-molecular-weight thrombin inhibitor, on thrombin and fibrinolytic enzymes. Thromb Haemost 1998; 79:110–118.

71. **Dunwiddie CT, Nutt EM, Vlasuk GP, Siegl PK, Schaffer LW.** Anticoagulant efficacy and immunogenicity of the selective factor Xa inhibitor antistasin following subcutaneous administration in the rhesus monkey. Thromb Haemost 1992;67:371–376.

72. **Prasa D, Svendsen L, Sturzebecher J.** Inhibition of thrombin generation in plasma by inhibitors of factor Xa. Thromb Haemost 1997;78:1215–1220.

73. **Theunissen HJ, Dijkema R, Swinkels JC, de Poorter TL, Vink PM, van Dinther TG.** Mutational analysis of antistasin, an inhibitor of blood coagulation factor Xa derived from the Mexican leech *Haementeria officinalis*. Thromb Res 1994;75:41–50.

74. **Stark KR, James AA.** Anticoagulants in vector arthropods. Parasitol Today 1996;12:430–437.

75. **Behrend EN, Grauer GF, Greco DS.** Feline hypertrophic cardiomyopathy, part 3. Feline Pract 1997;25:22–25.

76. **Killingsworth CR, Eyster GE, Adams T.** Streptokinase treatment of cats with experimentally induced aortic thrombosis. Am J Vet Res 1986;47:1351–1359.

77. **Ramsey C, Burney DP, Macintire DK, Finn-Bodner S.** Use of streptokinase in four dogs with thrombosis. J Am Vet Med Assoc 1996;209:780–785.

78. **Coller BS.** Platelets and thrombolytic therapy. N Engl J Med 1990;322:33–42.

79. **Yokoyama M, Ichikawa Y, Yatani A, Matsui K, Nakahara H, Kaneko M, Sakurama T, Ueshima S, Matsuo O.** Comparative studies of thrombolysis with single-chain and two-chain recombinant tissue-type plasminogen activators in canine coronary thrombosis. J Cardiovasc Pharmacol 1996;7:571–572.

80. **Clare AC, Kraje BJ.** Use of recombinant tissue-plasminogen activator for aortic thrombolysis in a hypoproteinemic dog. J Am Vet Med Assoc 1998;212:539–543.

81. **Pion PD.** Aortic thromboembolism and thrombolytic therapy. Vet Clin North Am Small Anim Pract 1988;18:79–86.

82. **Ikeda T, Nakatani S, Takata H, Nosaka M, Yoshikawa A, Tanaka H, Yukawa S.** Effect of tPA on regional lung perfusion in unilobar canine pulmonary thromboembolism. Am J Respir Crit Care Med 1997;156:1483–1486.

83. **Leadley RJ, Kasiewski CJ, Bostwick JS, Bentley R, McVey MJ, White FJ, Perrone MH, Dunwiddie CT.** Comparison of enoxaparin, hirulog, and heparin as adjunctive antithrombotic therapy during thrombolysis with rtPA in the stenosed canine coronary artery. Thromb Haemost 1997;78:1278–1285.

84. **Burke SE, Lubbers NL, Nelson RA, Henkin J.** Comparison of dose regimens for the administration of recombinant pro-urokinase in a canine thrombosis model. Thromb Haemost 1997;77:1025–1030.

SECTION IX

Hematologic or Hemopoietic Neoplasia–Lymphoid Neoplasia

Karen M. Young

CHAPTER 88

Oncogenesis

• E. GREGORY MacEWEN

Cancer development is a complex process involving multiple changes in genotype and phenotype. Although the individual steps in tumorigenesis are not completely understood, in simplistic terms, cells in a neoplastic clone undergo a series of successive genetic changes, each of which alters the cell genome in a way that confers selective growth advantage to cells in the clone. Characterization of the biochemical changes underlying each of these genetic alterations contributes a better understanding of tumorigenesis, provides better information about prognosis, and leads to improved strategies for the diagnosis and treatment of cancer.

CELL PROLIFERATION AND CELL DEATH

In normal tissues that undergo cell renewal there is a balance among cell proliferation, growth arrest, differentiation, and programmed cell death or apoptosis. Characterization of the molecular events that regulate cell proliferation and permit transformed cells to escape control mechanisms is essential to an understanding of cancer.

Cell Cycle

The cell cycle comprises four phases (Fig. 88.1). The gaps between mitosis (M) and DNA synthesis (S) are called the G_1 (intermediate) and G_2 (premitotic) phases; the duration of individual phases of the cell cycle varies depending on the cell population. Nonproliferating cells are usually arrested between the M and S phases and are referred to as G_0 cells. Most cells in normal tissues are in a quiescent or G_0 state.[1] Many oncogenes (Table 88.1) promote progression through G_1, because their expression results in inappropriate production of growth factors (e.g., v-sis/PDGF), constitutive activation of growth factor receptors (e.g., v-fms/CSF-1-R, v-erbB/EGF-R, trk/NGF-R, and met/HGF-R), or activation of signal transduction pathways (ras and raf).[2]

A family of cyclin-dependent kinases (cdks) controls the cell cycle. Cyclins (A to H) are the regulatory subunits, and their levels fluctuate during the cell cycle and are tightly regulated. Kinases are the catalytic component. The complex has enzymatic activity that controls progression of a cell through the cycle. For example, passage through G_1 is regulated by cyclin D-dependent kinase (cdk4). D-type cyclins associate with cdks 2, 4, 5, and 6, and these kinases control reentry of cells into the proliferation cycle.[3] A primary role for cyclin D-associated kinases in vivo appears to be phosphorylation of the retinoblastoma susceptibility protein, pRb, which is required during G_1 to permit progression to S phase in normal cells.[4]

There are two families of cdk inhibitory proteins. Kinase inhibitory proteins (KIP) include p21, p27, and p57. KIPs bind to and inhibit a wide range of cdks, including cdks 1 to 6. The protein p27 can act throughout the cell cycle and is under control of the tumor suppressor gene protein, p53. Inhibitors of kinases (INK) comprise the second family of inhibitory proteins, and INK4 proteins (p15, p16, p18, and p19) specifically inhibit the cyclin D-dependent kinases. Both the development and progression of cancer involve processes that target the cyclins, cdks, and cdk inhibitors.[3]

Cell Death

There are two major mechanisms of cell death: necrosis and apoptosis. Necrosis is a passive process of injury, resulting in cell swelling and lysis. In contrast, apoptosis is an adenosine triphosphate (ATP)-dependent process and involves activation of numerous intracellular genetically programmed cellular pathways leading to DNA fragmentation, cell shrinkage, and loss of cell contact. Mammalian cells contain numerous effectors of apoptosis, including interleukin-1β converting enzyme (ICE), a cysteine protease that cleaves and inactivates poly (ADP-ribose) polymerase, a DNA repair enzyme. Cysteine proteases, including ICE proteases and caspases, are activated by cleavage of precursor molecules, leading to apoptosis.[5]

A family of related gene products that interact with each other to influence apoptotic tendencies does exist.[5] The first of the negative regulators of apoptosis to be identified was the bcl-2 gene. The anti-apoptotic bcl-2 protein was originally recognized in follicular lympho-

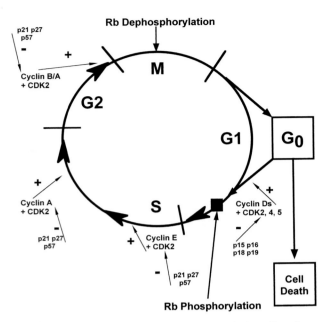

FIGURE 88.1 Cell cycle. Progression through the cell cycle is controlled by a series of cdks and cdk inhibitors. The cdks (cdk 2,4,5) positively regulate progression, and the cdk inhibitors (p15, p21, p27, etc.) negatively regulate the cycle. Phosphorylation and dephosphorylation of the retinoblastoma susceptibility protein (pRb) is also necessary for progression through the cycle.

TABLE 88.1	Some Oncogene Groups
Oncogene	**Function**
Growth Factors	
int-1	Matrix protein
int-2	Fibroblast growth factor-related protein
sis	Platelet-derived growth factor
Growth Factor Receptors	
erbB-1	Epidermal growth factor receptor
fms	CSF-1 receptor
Kit	Stem cell growth factor
met	Hepatocyte growth factor
neu/erbB-2	Heregulin receptor
trk	Nerve growth factor receptor
G proteins	
H-ras	GTPase
K-ras	GTPase
N-ras	GTPase
Cytoplasmic Kinases	
bcr-abl	Tyrosine kinase
src	Tyrosine kinase
raf/mil	Serine-threonine kinase
mos	Serine-threonine kinase
Other cytoplasmic proteins	
bcl-2	Anti-apoptosis
Nuclear Proteins	
erbA	Thyroid hormone receptor
ets	Transcription factor
fos	Transcription factor
jun	Transcription factor
myb	Transcription factor
myc	Transcription factor
rel	Transcription factor

mas associated with a 14:17 chromosomal translocation. These lymphomas are indolent and difficult to cure with chemotherapy. Korsmeyer and others have developed a model in which the bcl-2 family member, bax, can drive the cell toward apoptosis when the protein forms complexes with itself.[6–9] When bcl-2 is expressed in high levels it forms complexes with bax, preventing bax from complexing with itself and thereby impeding apoptosis. When *bcl-2* and *bcl-xL* (another anti-apoptotic gene) are overexpressed, these cells are resistant to chemotherapy.

Apoptosis mediated by anticancer drugs may involve activation of death-inducing ligand or receptor systems such as the CD95 ligand (FasL) and the CD95 receptor (Fas).[10] The CD95 system is related to the tumor necrosis factor receptor (TNFR), another important component of the apoptotic response. Death-promoting signaling depends on FasL engaging the Fas receptor, leading to activation of a cytoplasmic death domain.[11] This pathway plays a major role in modulating the responsiveness of the immune system: FasL expressed by activated T cells binds the Fas receptor on other lymphocytes, resulting in apoptosis of these latter cells, thereby regulating suppression of the immune system. Some tumor cells that express Fas receptors are somehow resistant to Fas-mediated apoptosis. Furthermore, these cells can mount a Fas counterattack by expressing FasL, leading to local immune suppression through receptor-mediated apoptosis of T cells (Fig. 88.2).[12] This represents one method by which tumor cells effectively evade the immune system.

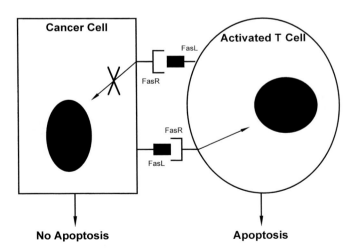

FIGURE 88.2 Fas counterattack. The tumor cell expresses Fas (CD95) receptor but is somehow resistant to Fas-mediated T cell cytotoxicity. The cancer cell expresses functional Fas-L, which induces apoptosis in Fas-sensitive-activated T cells that infiltrate the tumor. (Modified from O'Connell J, O'Sullivan GC, Collins K, Shanahan F. The Fas counterattack: Fas-mediated T cell killing by colon cancer cells expressing Fas ligand. J Exp Med 1996;184: 1075–1082; with permission.)

ONCOGENES

Studies of viral oncogenesis have identified various genetic events important in the development of mammalian tumors. These include activation of specific genes carried by viruses or of cellular genes, referred to as viral or cellular oncogenes, respectively (Table 88.1).[13] Cells contain proto-oncogenes that are essential to normal biological processes, encoding products that regulate cell growth and differentiation. Oncogenes result from genetic alterations in proto-oncogenes and are typically positive regulators of the cell cycle. When activated, oncogenes promote cellular function and enhance malignant transformation. Many of the originally isolated oncogenes encode elements of mitogenic signal transduction pathways (e.g., *ras*, *src*, and *raf*), transcription factors (e.g., *myc*, *myb*, *fos*, *erbA*), or growth factors and their receptors (e.g., *sis*, *erbB*, *kit*, *met*, and *fms*). These factors function by altering the expression of key proteins or families of proteins that regulate the transformed phenotype. Ultimately, one aspect of the transformed phenotype must, at least at some level, involve dysregulation of the cell cycle.

TUMOR SUPPRESSOR GENES

In contrast to the oncogenes described above, various genes referred to as tumor suppressor genes or antioncogenes have been identified. Tumor suppressor genes are negative regulators and promote cell transformation through their loss of function. Although activated oncogenes act in a dominant manner, tumor suppressor genes act in a recessive manner. Thus, mutations in tumor suppressor genes figure prominently in the development of familial cancers, but mutations also occur commonly in sporadic (noninherited) forms of cancers. Knudsen's hypothesis states that in familial cancers one mutation is transmitted through the germline, and the second mutation occurs somatically. In sporadic cancers, both mutations have to occur within the same somatic cell.[14] Numerous mutations identified in tumor suppressor genes are associated with certain disease processes. For example, mutations in *Rb*, *WT-1*, *APC*, *BRCA2*, and *p53* are linked with retinoblastoma, Wilms' tumor, familial colonic polyposis, familial breast cancer, and Li-Fraumeni syndrome, respectively.[15] Tumor suppressor genes encode proteins involved in suppressing cell proliferation, promoting cell death, and maintaining genome integrity. The most common tumor suppressor mutation has been identified in the *p53* gene.

p53 gene

The *p53* tumor suppressor gene has been referred to as the guardian of the genome and plays a critical role in the cellular response to DNA damage leading to cell cycle arrest in G_1 or apoptosis (Fig. 88.3A). Transient arrest in G_1 allows time for repair of damaged DNA. In cells exposed to agents, including γ-irradiation and various chemotherapeutic drugs that cause DNA strand breaks, the p53 protein has been shown to initiate apoptosis. Two important genes activated by p53 are *GADD45* (growth arrest and DNA damage inducible) and *p21/WAF1*. Expression of *GADD45* results in growth inhibition as measured by the reduced capacity of recipient cells to generate colonies in culture.[16] The *p21/WAF1* gene encodes the protein p21 that inhibits the cdks required for cells to enter into the G_1-S transition.[17] Apoptosis induced by oncogenes, such as c-*myc* and *E1A*, is also p53 dependent. Recently, a novel gene has been identified whose products are structurally and functionally similar to *p53*. This gene is termed *p73* and appears to share the growth inhibiting and apoptosis-promoting effects of *p53*.[18]

In many human and animal tumors, there are recessive mutations in the *p53* gene.[19,20] Cells that lack wild-type expression of *p53* because of mutation have a selective advantage as they may enter S phase inappropriately after treatment with metabolic inhibitors that normally arrest cells in G_1. These cells have a higher incidence of genetic instability and gene amplification.

In mice overexpression of *MDM2* (murine double minute 2), which encodes a p53-binding protein, negatively affects the functions of p53 that relate to transcription, G_1 arrest, and apoptosis. A human homologue of this gene has been identified. *MDM2* amplification has been described in cells from low-grade B cell lymphomas, osteosarcomas, and a number of soft tissue sarcomas, and its anti-p53 effect may explain the tumorigenesis in neoplasms that lack abnormalities in the *p53* gene.[21]

DOMINANT ONCOGENES

Most oncogenes act through direct intervention in normal cell cycle regulation. Gain-of-function mutations result in activation of proto-oncogenes (e.g., *ras*) that constitutively express components of signaling cascades, including growth factors or their receptors.

Growth Factor Receptors

Receptors for growth factors share the capacity to phosphorylate tyrosine residues on proteins, thereby activating a signaling cascade. Receptor protein tyrosine kinases (RPTKs) contain several discrete domains, including an extracellular ligand-binding domain, a transmembrane domain, a protein tyrosine kinase domain, and a carboxyl-terminal domain.[2,22] Interaction of a growth factor with its receptor at the cell surface leads to a tight association, so that growth factors are capable of mediating their activities at nanomolar concentrations (Table 88.2). After binding of the growth factor ligand, a conformational change results in dimerization of the receptor, permitting the two intracellular catalytic domains to phosphorylate each other and activate signal

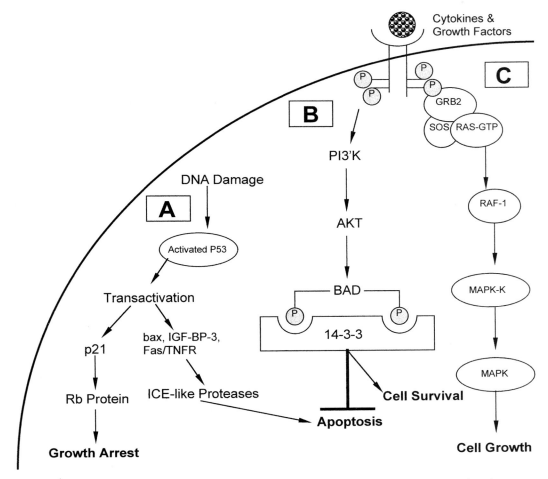

FIGURE 88.3 Interactions among p53 activation, apoptosis, growth factor-induced survival, and proliferation. **A.** DNA damage leads to activation of p53. If the DNA damage is irreversible, then apoptotic pathways are activated; bax homodimerization leads to activation of ICE proteases (and caspases), leading to apoptosis. Additional pro-apoptotic events under control of p53 include increases in insulin growth factor-binding protein-3 (IGF-BP-3), CD95 (Fas–FasL) interactions, and activation of the tumor necrosis factor receptor (TNFR). With reversible DNA damage, p53 induces G_1 arrest via activation of p21 and inhibition of Rb phosphorylation. **B.** Growth factors can promote cell survival by activating the PI3'K and AKT signaling pathway, leading to phosphorylation of BAD, a bcl-2 protein, and binding to 14-3-3 protein, which blocks apoptosis and leads to cell survival. **C.** *Auto-* or *trans*-phosphorylation of the receptor tyrosine kinases allows binding of GRB2 and son-of-sevenless (SOS), resulting in exchange of guanosine diphosphate (GDP), activation of the ras protein, and subsequent activation of raf-1. The ERK kinases (MAPK-K and MAPK) are activated by raf-1 leading to activation of transcription factors that coordinate cell growth.

TABLE 88.2   Properties of Some Selected Growth Factors in Malignancy

Growth Factor	Receptor	Action
Platelet-Derived Growth Factor (PDGF)	PDGF-R	Mesenchymal/smooth muscle proliferation
Epidermal Growth Factor (EGF) and Transforming Growth Factor-α (TGFα)	EGF-R	Epithelial cell growth
Fibroblast Growth Factor (FGF) 1 & 2 acidic and basic	FGF-R	Pro-angiogenesis
Transforming growth factor-β (TGFβ) family	TGFβ-R$_{(1-3)}$	Immunosuppression Inhibition of cell proliferation
Insulin-Like Growth Factors (IGF-1, IGF-2)	IGF-1R	Proliferation Anti-apoptosis
Stem Cell Factor (SCF)	c-Kit	Mast cell growth
Hepatocyte Growth Factor (HGF), formerly Scatter-Factor (SF)	c-Met	Mesenchymal cell growth/proangiogenesis Plasma cell growth
Interleukin-7	IL-7R	Proliferation of ALL cells
Interleukin-6	IL-6R	Proliferation of myeloma cells

transduction pathways. The mitogenic pathway is mediated through the growth factor receptor binding protein (GRB2) and subsequent activation of the ras and mitogen-activated protein kinase (MAPK) signaling pathways (Fig. 88.3C).[23] Some growth factors, particularly insulin-like growth factor-1 (IGF-1), can promote cell survival by activating phosphatidylinositide-3-OH kinase (PI3'K) and its downstream target, serine-threonine kinase AKT, also known as protein kinase B.[24] Activation of the PI3'K–AKT signaling pathway results in complexing of the bcl-2 proteins, ultimately promoting cell survival (Fig. 88.3B).[25]

TELOMERE-TELOMERASE HYPOTHESIS

Telomeres, defined as the ends of eukaryotic chromosomes that contain multiple repeats of specific DNA sequences and associated proteins, are necessary to prevent DNA degradation, end-to-end fusion, and chromosome instability.[26] In humans telomeres contain the repeated sequences $(TTAGGG)_n$ comprising several kilobases in length. Telomerase, an enzyme that mediates replication of telomeres, is a multisubunit ribonucleoprotein enzyme that synthesizes TTAGGG repeats onto chromosome ends by use of RNA components as a template. Telomerase, therefore, compensates for progressive telomere erosion. The telomere-telomerase hypothesis states that most somatic cells lack significant telomerase expression, whereas, in contrast, tumor cells have short telomeres and increased telomerase activity, which prolongs cell survival.[27]

Numerous investigators have studied the influence of telomere length, telomerase expression, or both on clinical outcome. In a recent study of 58 human patients with B-cell chronic lymphocytic leukemia (CLL), telomere length was inversely correlated with telomerase activity, and short telomere length and high telomerase activity were associated with a significantly shorter median survival time. Furthermore, compared with other clinical features (e.g., clinical stage, organomegaly, lymph node involvement, etc.), telomerase activity was the most significant prognostic factor.[28] In addition, telomere length and telomerase activity may serve as diagnostic markers, as well as potential therapeutic targets.

MOLECULAR BIOLOGY OF LYMPHOID NEOPLASMS

Lymphoid malignancies represent an extremely heterogeneous group of neoplastic diseases and are characterized by proliferation of lymphocytes and their precursors. A model of multistep tumorigenesis for human lymphoid tumors is shown in Figure 88.4.[29] The most common lesions detected in human lymphoid neoplasms are chromosomal translocations. Many translocations represent rearrangements in the antigen receptor gene, namely the immunoglobulin (Ig) and T cell receptor (TCR) genes in B and T cells, respectively. These

chromosomal translocations may result from errors in Ig or TCR recombination, so that sequences from different chromosomes are linked instead of sequences within the same antigen receptor locus. These translocations result in proto-oncogene activation and involve c-*myc* and, less commonly, *ras* translocations. Finally, disruption of tumor suppressor genes by chromosomal deletion of one allele and inactivation of the other allele represents another mechanism of tumorigenesis in lymphoid tumors. Mutation of the *p53* tumor suppressor gene is the most common lesion identified. Table 88.3 summarizes the frequency of genetic lesions detected in human lymphoid tumors.

In canine lymphoma, most chromosomal aberrations are numerical and less structural compared with human lymphoid tumors. In one series of 61 dogs that had lymphoma, 18 had reciprocal chromosomal translocation resulting from the centric fusion of two acrocentric chromosomes, and the remainder were numerical aberrations with a trisomy of chromosome 13 being the most common.[30] Interestingly, analysis of first remission and survival times demonstrated that those dogs that had trisomy 13 had the best prognosis after chemotherapy.[13] In another study of canine lymphoma, 1 of 28 dogs evaluated showed activation of the proto-oncogene, N-*ras*.[31] Mutation of *p53* is more common, and in one small study of 8 cases, 3 dogs exhibited p53 gene mutations.[32]

ONCOGENIC VIRUSES

The infection of tumor cells by oncogenic viruses is considered a mechanism of inducing genetic lesions since viruses introduce foreign genes into target cells. In people, three distinct viruses are associated with the development of specific subtypes of lymphoma: Epstein-Barr virus (EBV), human T cell lymphotropic virus-I (HTLV-I), and human herpesvirus-8 (HHV-8).[33–35] No oncogenic tumor viruses have been identified in dogs; however, in cats the feline leukemia virus (FeLV) has been well characterized. FeLV is a chronic leukemia virus that is replication-competent. This virus alters cells through a mechanism known as insertional mutagenesis, in which proviral integration leads to the aberrant activation of adjacent cellular genes.[36] FeLV has been shown to activate mutant *myc* function in T cells.[37] After infection there is a long latency before tumors develop, and the tumors are clonal.

In contrast, HTLV-I, HTLV-II, and the bovine leukemia virus (BLV) belong to a distinct group of retroviruses that have been referred to as *trans*-regulating retroviruses. HTLV-I initiates a multistep process leading to acute T cell leukemia. Infection results in translation of two proteins, Tax and Rex. Tax is critical for viral replication and functions as a transcriptional coactivator of viral and cellular genes. Cellular genes that are responsive to transcriptional activation by Tax include the genes encoding IL-2, the α subunit of the IL-2 receptor, granulocyte-macrophage-colony-stimulating-factor

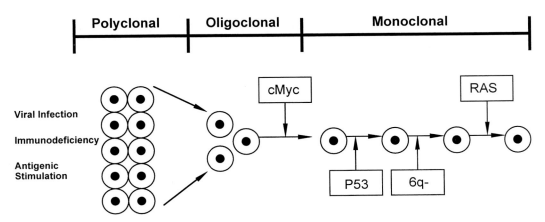

FIGURE 88.4   Multistep tumorigenesis in human B cell non-Hodgkin's lymphoma. Viral infection (e.g., with EBV) in association with immunosuppression (e.g., induced by HIV) or chronic antigenic stimulation leads to a polyclonal expansion of lymphocytes. Multiple genetic lesions (c-*myc* activation and *p53* mutation) within a single clone leads to neoplastic transformation. Chromosomal deletions and *ras* activation contribute to unregulated cell growth and survival, leading to expansion of lymphoid tissue. (Modified from **Gaidano G, Dalla-Favera R.** Molecular biology of lymphoid neoplasms. In: Mendelsohn J, Howley PM, Israel MA, Liotta LA, eds. The molecular basis of cancer. Philadelphia: WB Saunders, 1995;251–279; with permission).

TABLE 88.3   Frequency of Genetic Lesions in Human Lymphoid Neoplasms

Lymphoid Tumors	bcl-2	c-myc	bcl-1	bcl-6	p53	6q-	ras
Low Grade							
Small lymphocytic	—	—	—	—	—	20%	—
Mantle zone lymphoma	—	—	50%	—	—	NA	—
Follicular, small cell	70–90%	—	—	—	—	20%	—
Follicular, mixed	70–90%	—	—	—	—	20%	—
Intermediate Grade							
Follicular, large cell	70–90%	—	—	—	—	20%	—
Diffuse, small cell	—	5–20%	—	30%	—	20%	—
Diffuse, mixed	—	5–20%	—	30%	—	20%	—
Diffuse, large cell	—	5–20%	—	30%	—	20%	—
High Grade							
Immunoblastic	—	20%	—	—	—	20%	—
Lymphoblastic	—	NA	—	—	NA	NA	—
Small noncleaved	—	100%	—	—	30%	20%	—
Transformed[a]	90%	10%	—	—	70%	NA	—
B-CCL	—	—	—	—	15%	—	—
B-ALL	—	100%	—	—	60%	—	—
T-ALL	—	<5%	—	—	<5%	—	10%
Myeloma	—	25%	—	—	15%	—	30%

[a] B cell non-Hodgkin's lymphomas that have undergone histologic progression from a follicular to a diffuse pattern.
B-CLL, B cell chronic lymphocytic leukemia.
B-ALL, B cell acute lymphoblastic leukemia.
T-ALL, T cell acute lymphoblastic leukemia.
NA, not assessed.
—, no lesion detected.
Modified after Gaidano G, Dalla-Favera R. Molecular biology of lymphoid neoplasms. In: Mendelsohn J, Howley P, Israel MA, Liotta LA, eds. The molecular basis of cancer. Philadelphia: WB Saunders, 1995;251–279; with permission.

(GM-CSF), and the proto-oncogenes, c-*sis* and c-*fos*. For example, after infection of CD4-positive lymphocytes by HTLV-I, these T cells develop IL-2 receptors. The Rex protein is essential for viral replication.

Infection with BLV leads to persistent lymphocytosis characterized by a significant increase in circulating B lymphocytes. These lymphocytes have increased expression of major histocompatibility complex (MHC) class II molecules and the α subunit of the IL-2 receptor.[38] The progression to overt leukemia is associated with the upregulation of *myc* expression and point mutations in *p53*.[39,40]

SUMMARY

The evidence that cancer results from alterations in cells at the level of the genome is overwhelming. The development of tumors requires two or more mutations in stem cells, leading to activation of cellular oncogenes and loss of function of tumor suppressor genes. Tumor growth depends on growth kinetics, expression of appropriate growth factor receptors, and availability of autocrine or paracrine growth factors. Continued growth and metastasis require development of a blood supply (angiogenesis) and activation of invasive mechanisms. Most lymphoid tumors are associated with chromosomal abnormalities, leading to the activation of oncogene products that cause unchecked cell proliferation and to the loss of tumor suppressor genes. The next generation of cancer therapy will depend on a better understanding of the molecular events associated with tumor development.

REFERENCES

1. **Pardee A.** G1 events and regulation of cell proliferation. Science 1989; 246:603–608.
2. **Van der Geer P, Hunter T.** Receptor protein-tyrosine kinases and their signal transduction pathways. Ann Rev Cell Biol 1994;10:251–337.
3. **Sherr CJ, Roberts JM.** Inhibitors of mammalian G1 cyclin-dependent kinases. Genes Dev 1995;9:1149–1163.
4. **Kouzarides T.** Transcriptional control by the retinoblastoma protein. Semin Cancer Biol 1995;6:91–98.
5. **Kroemer G, Petit P, Zamzami N, Vayssiere JL, Mignotte B.** The biochemistry of programmed cell death. FASEB J 1995;9:1277–1287.
6. **Korsmeyer S.** Regulators of cell death. Trends Genet 1995;11:101–105.
7. **Korsmeyer SJ.** Programmed cell death: bcl-2. In: DeVita VT, Hellman S, Rosenberg SA, eds. Important advances in oncology. Philadelphia: JB Lippincott Co, 1993;19–28.
8. **Hu Z, Minden MD, McCulloch EA.** Direct evidence for the participation of bcl-2 in the regulation by retinoic acid of the Ara-C sensitivity of leukemic stem cells. Leukemia 1995;9:1667–1673.
9. **Vaux D, Strasser A.** The molecular biology of apoptosis. Proc Natl Acad Sci U S A 1996;93:2239–2244.
10. **Friesen C, Herr I, Krammer PH, Debatin KM.** Involvement of the CD95 (APO-1/Fas) receptor/ligand system in drug-induced apoptosis in leukemia cells. Nature Med 1996;2:574–577.
11. **Owen-Schaub LB, Angelo LS, Radinsky R, Ware CF, Gesner TG, Bartos DP.** Soluble Fas/APO-1 in tumor cells: a potential regulator of apoptosis. Cancer Lett 1995;94:1–8.
12. **O'Connell J, O'Sullivan GC, Collins JK, Shanahan F.** The Fas counterattack: Fas-mediated T cell killing by colon cancer cells expressing Fas ligand. J Exp Med 1996;184:1075–1082.
13. **Benchimol S, Minden MD.** Viruses, oncogenes, and tumor suppressor genes. In: Tannock I, Hill RP, eds. The basic science of oncology. 3rd ed. New York: McGraw-Hill, 1998;79–105.
14. **Moolgavkar S, Knudson AG Jr.** Mutation and cancer: a model for human carcinogenesis. J Natl Cancer Inst 1981;66:1037–1053.
15. **Levine A.** Tumor suppressor genes. In: Mendelsohn J, Howley PM, Israel MA, Liotta LA, eds. The molecular basis of cancer. Philadelphia: WB Saunders Co, 1995;86–104.
16. **Kasten M, Zhan Q, El-Deiry WS, Carrier F, Jacks T, Walsh WV, Plunkett BS, Vogelstein B, Fornace AJ Jr.** A mammalian cell cycle checkpoint utilizing p53 and GADD45 is defective in ataxia-telangiectasia. Cell 1992;71: 587–597.
17. **El-Deiry WS, Harper JW, O'Connor PM, Velculescu VE, Carman CE, Jackman J, Pietenpol JA, Burrell M, Hill DE, Wang Y, et al.** WAF1/CIP1 is induced in p53-mediated G1 arrest and apoptosis. Cancer Res 1994;54:1169–1174.
18. **Oren M.** Lonely no more: p53 finds its kin in a tumor suppressor haven. Cell 1997;90:829–832.
19. **Hollstein M, Sidransky D, Vogelstein B, Harris C.** p53 mutations in human cancers. Science 1991;253:49–53.
20. **Smith ML, Fornace AJ Jr.** The two faces of tumor suppressor p53. Am J Pathol 1996;148:1019–1022.
21. **Chen J, Wu X, Lin J, Levine AJ.** MDM-2 inhibits the G1 arrest and apoptosis functions of the p53 tumor suppression protein. Mol Cell Biol 1996;16:2445–2452.
22. **Radinsky R.** Growth factors and their receptors in metastasis. Cancer Biol 1991;2:169–177.
23. **Davis RJ.** The mitogen-activated protein kinase signal transduction pathway. J Biol Chem 1993;268:14553–14556.
24. **Datta R, Dudek H, Tao X, Masters S, Fu H, Gotoh Y, Greenberg ME.** AKT phosphorylation of BAD couples survival signals to the cell-intrinsic death machinery. Cell 1997;91:231–241.
25. **Yaffe M, Rittinger K, Volinia S, Caron PR, Aitken A, Leffers H, Gamblin SJ, Smerdon SJ, Cantley LC.** The structural basis of 14-3-3: phosphopeptide binding specificity. Cell 1997;91:961–971.
26. **Harley C, Futcher A, Greider C.** Telomeres shorten during aging of human fibroblasts. Nature 1990;345:458–460.
27. **Ezzell C.** The telomere-cancer connection: will exceptions make a new rule? J NIH Res 1995;7:41.
28. **Bechler O, Eisterer W, Pall G. et al.** Telomere length and telomerase activity predicts survival in patients with B-cell CLL. Cancer Res 1998;58:4918–4922.
29. **Gaidano G, Dalla-Favera R.** Molecular biology of lymphoid neoplasms. In: Mendelsohn J, Howley PM, Israel MA, Liotta LA, eds. The molecular basis of cancer. Philadelphia: WB Saunders, 1995;251–279.
30. **Hahn K, Richardson RC, Hahn EA, Chrisman CL.** Diagnostic and prognostic importance of chromosomal aberrations identified in 61 dogs with lymphosarcoma. Vet Pathol 1994;31:528–540.
31. **Edwards M, Pazzi KA, Gumerlock PH, Madewell BR.** c-N-ras is activated infrequently in canine malignant lymphoma. Toxicol Pathol 1993;21: 288–291.
32. **Vedhoen N, Stewart J, Brown R, Milner J.** Mutations of the p53 gene in canine lymphoma and evidence for germ line p53 mutations in the dog. Oncogene 1998;16:249–255.
33. **Hamilton-Dutoit S, Pallersen G.** A survey of Epstein-Barr virus gene expression in spontaneous non-Hodgkin's lymphoma. Am J Pathol 1992;140: 1315–1325.
34. **Ballerini P, Gaidano G, Gong JZ, Tassi U, Saglio G, Knowles DM, Dalla-Favera R.** Multiple genetic lesions in acquired immunodeficiency syndrome-related non-Hodgkin's lymphoma. Blood 1993;81:166–176.
35. **Cesarman E, Chang Y, Moore PS, Said WM, Knowles DM.** Kaposi's sarcoma-associated herpesvirus-like DNA sequences in AIDS-related body-cavity-based-lymphomas. N Engl J Med 1995;332:1186–1191.
36. **Pantginis J, Beaty RM, Levy LS, Lenz J.** The feline leukemia virus long terminal repeat contains a potent determinant of T-cell lymphomagenicity. J Virol 1997;71:9786–9791.
37. **Fulton R, Gallagher R, Crouch D, Neil JC.** Apparent uncoupling of oncogenicity from fibroblast transformation and apoptosis in a mutant myc gene transduced by feline leukemia virus. J Virol 1996;70:1154–1162.
38. **Stone D, Hof AJ, Davis WC.** Up-regulation of IL-2 receptor alpha and MHC class II expression on lymphocyte subpopulations from bovine leukemia virus infected lymphocytotic cows. Vet Immunol Immunopathol 1995; 48:65–76.
39. **Stone D, Norton LK, Magnuson NS, Davis WC.** Elevated pim-1 and c-myc proto-oncogene induction in B lymphocytes from BLV-infected cows with persistent B lymphocytosis. Leukemia 1996;10:1629–1638.
40. **Ishiguro N, Furuoka H, Matsui T, Horiuchi M, Shinagawa M, Asahina M, Okada K.** p53 mutations as a potential cellular factor for tumor development in enzootic bovine leukosis. Vet Immunol Immunopathol 1997; 55:351–358.

CHAPTER 89

Classification of Lymphomas

• JOANNE B. MESSICK and MARON B. CALDERWOOD MAYS

Lymphomas are a diverse group of lymphoid neoplasms that originate in lymph nodes, other primary lymphoid organs, or extranodal sites. Lymphoid neoplasms that predominantly involve the bone marrow and peripheral blood are considered leukemias. Lymphomas represent a clonal expansion of an anatomic or developmental compartment of lymphoid cells that have distinct morphologic and immunophenotypic characteristics (Fig. 89.1). Classification of lymphomas in both human and veterinary medicine has generated considerable controversy and confusion over the past 3 decades. The ultimate goal of a classification system is to correlate the variety of cell subtypes (Table 89.1) and architectural features of lymphoma with clinical behavior in terms of responsiveness to therapy and outlook for the patient. The morphologic criteria, therefore, must be sufficiently distinct to permit different observers to reach the same conclusions. Several serially proposed classification schemes have attempted to correlate with cytologic, histologic, or immunophenotypic features of non-Hodgkin's lymphoma (NHL) in people who have prognosis and response to therapy. Veterinary pathologists have adapted three of these classification schemes to characterize canine and bovine nodal lymphomas.

The first widely accepted classification scheme for human NHL was proposed in 1956 by Rappaport and colleagues.[1,2] The pattern of growth, whether follicular or diffuse, and cytologic features of the malignant lymphocytes, whether well differentiated or poorly differentiated or histiocytic, were evaluated with this scheme. However, unlike in people,[3] a follicular growth pattern is seen in only a few canine NHLs.[4-7] By use of the Rappaport scheme, most canine lymphomas have been classified as either diffuse poorly differentiated lymphocytic or diffuse histiocytic lymphomas.[4-7] Not only is the term histiocytic confusing, as it was applied when the estimated number of large transformed lymphocytes exceeded 50%, but the diffuse histiocytic subgroup in dogs and humans has been found to be heterogenous, consisting of different morphologic and immunologic cell types.[8] Therefore, it is not surprising that the Rappaport classification appears to be of little value for predicting tumor behavior or influencing treatment selection in canine lymphoma.[4]

Since morphology alone was insufficient to define and reliably distinguish the majority of lymphoma types, many attempts were made during the 1970s to develop new classification schemes with other criteria. The Kiel classification was the first scheme to include the immunophenotype (B or T cell) of the malignant lymphocytes in addition to morphology.[9] However, no attempt was made to correlate the grade of lymphoma with the natural history, response to therapy, or patient survival. This system of classification was favored in Europe, yet by the late 1970s at least six different schemes were in use throughout the world.

In an effort to "translate among the various classification systems and to facilitate clinical comparisons of case reports and therapeutic trials," an international multi-institutional study was sponsored by the National Cancer Institute (NCI).[10] The subsequent Working Formulation (WF) attempted to correlate survival data obtained in clinical trials with morphologic criteria alone. The subtypes defined by the WF and applied to lymphomas in humans relate to biology of the tumor and survival of the patient; however, the system does not account for the cell of origin of the lymphoma.

The most current classification in human pathology, the Revised European-American Classification of Lymphoid Neoplasms (REAL),[11] has not yet been evaluated for animal species. The major problem with the REAL is that it is a list of lymphoproliferative entities rather than a classification system and fails to provide the clinician with information about biology or progression of the tumor. Since cytogenetic analysis and detailed phenotyping are required for defining these entities, the REAL scheme is unlikely to be of value in the near future for classification of lymphomas in veterinary medicine.

The main basis for classification of lymphomas by the veterinary pathologist is still the architecture, mitotic rate, and cellular morphology of the tumor. Recent studies have demonstrated the usefulness of immunohistochemistry.[12] In the WF and other classification systems, lymphomas of small cells (nuclei ≤1.5 red blood cells in diameter) with a low mitotic rate (<5/HPF) have a slow rate of progression. The cells are generally small with clumped chromatin and inconspicuous nucleoli. The growth pattern may be follicular, pseudofollicular, or diffuse; however, the growth is relatively nondestructive. Although these low-grade lymphomas are associ-

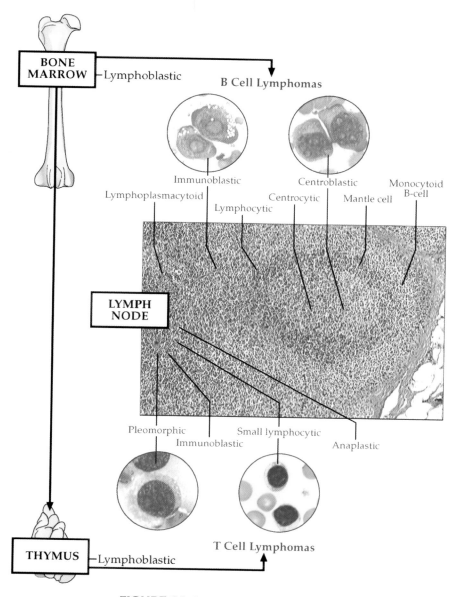

FIGURE 89.1 Histogenesis of lymphoma.

ated with long survival times, they are virtually incurable and may not be treated initially. On the other hand, high-grade lymphomas with a high mitotic rate (>10/ HPF) are potentially curable, yet if left untreated they are rapidly progressive and deadly. The cells often have large nuclei (>2.0 red blood cells in diameter) containing an open or vesicular chromatin pattern and prominent nucleoli. Some of the lymphocytes in high-grade lymphomas have moderate amounts of cytoplasm. The growth pattern is almost always diffuse and destructive. Between these two extremes are the intermediate-grade lymphomas. A low to medium mitotic rate is characteristic of these neoplasms, although the tumor cell size may be variable. These lymphomas typically show some differentiated characteristic, such as a follicular or mantle zone architecture.

Using the Working Formulation or the updated Kiel classification (Table 89.2), the most striking features of NHLs in dogs and cattle are: (1) follicular lymphomas are rare, (2) low-grade lymphomas occur infrequently, (3) the majority of low-grade, small cell lymphomas are T cell derived (canine lymphomas only), (4) high-grade lymphomas occur frequently, if the diffuse large cell subtype is included, and (5) the majority of high-grade canine lymphomas and all enzootic (bovine leukemia virus-positive) bovine lymphomas are a B cell phenotype. Almost all subtypes of low-, intermediate-, and high-grade lymphomas have been described in these animal species. A previously developed algorithm for classification of canine lymphomas,[13] which is based on the WF and accounts for histologic (architecture and mitotic rate) and cytologic features (size and shape of the

TABLE 89.1   Lymphocyte Subtypes

Lymphocyte Subtype	Cytologic Features
Low or Intermediate Grade	
Small Lymphocytic	Small size, round nucleus, coarse chromatin, scant pale cytoplasm. Variants include centrocytic-like (irregular or notched nuclei), clear cell (extended and pale cytoplasm that may contain fine azurophilic granules), and prolymphocytic-like (fine chromatin and distinctly nucleolated). Mitoses are absent or very low.
Small Cleaved Cell (Centrocytic)	Small to medium size (cells from 6 to 12 μ or slightly larger than normal lymphocytes), cleaved or irregular nucleus, clumped chromatin, nucleoli absent or small, and inconspicuous, scant cytoplasm.
Mantle Cell (Intermediate Lymphocyte)	Small to medium size, round to slightly irregular nucleus (shape of the nucleus is intermediate between the small lymphocytic and centrocytic), abundant and weak-staining cytoplasm.
Monocytoid B cell	Small to medium size, nuclear chromatin varies from moderately clumped to vesicular, nucleoli are small and inconspicuous, consistently abundant pale cytoplasm.
High Grade	
Lymphoblast	Small to medium size, average 15 μ in diameter (range = 10 to 20 μ), nucleus convoluted but may be nonconvoluted, fine chromatin, absent or small inconspicuous nucleoli.
Small Noncleaved Cell (Burkitt's)	Medium size, uniform, round nucleus, multiple central nucleoli, intensely staining cytoplasm.
Centroblastic (Large Cell, Cleaved or Noncleaved)	Large size (13 to 30 μ in diameter), round nucleus with vesicular chromatin, 1 to 3 nucleoli that are often apposed to the nuclear membrane, scant basophilic cytoplasm. Mitoses are frequent.
Immunoblast	Large size (greater than 20 μ), round nucleus, single large central nucleolus, basophilic cytoplasm.
Pleomorphic Large Cell (Large Cell Immunoblastic)	Large pleomorphic cells, some of which are multinucleated. The cytoplasm is abundant and often deeply basophilic. Nucleoli are large and prominent.

nucleus and presence, number, and location of nucleoli), has been modified to emphasize these tumor grades and is included to facilitate the discussion that follows.

LOW-GRADE NODAL LYMPHOMAS

The reported prevalence of low-grade lymphomas varies from a low of 5.3 and 7.0% for dogs and cows, respectively,[13–15] to a high of 26.1% for dogs.[12] Low-grade tumors account for 8 to 11% of feline lymphomas. (VE Valli, personal communication, July 1999). The majority of low-grade lymphomas in both dogs and cattle have a diffuse pattern with effacement of the normal nodal architecture. Either the mitotic index is characteristically low (≤ 5/HPF) or no mitotic figures are observed at all, and a starry sky pattern (arising from by the presence of numerous macrophages) is not present. A true follicular tumor, which is considered composed of germinal center-derived B lymphocytes, is rare in animal species. However, paracortical expansion of small cells compressing residual benign follicles may mimic a nodular pattern (pseudofollicular). The presence of a pseudofollicular pattern has been reported in association with chronic lymphocytic leukemia (CLL). Based on recent immunologic studies, a T lymphocyte phenotype (CD3+, mb 1−) was found in approximately half of all low-grade lymphomas in dogs. The cells in the majority of the small cell, low-grade malignancies had a T lymphocyte phenotype, whereas in all cases of centrocytic and mac-

ronucleolated medium-sized cell (MMC) low-grade malignancies, the cells had a B lymphocyte phenotype.[12] The cellular morphology of diffuse, small cell lymphomas is variable. The nuclei are approximately the same size as an erythrocyte or slightly larger (usually <1.5 red blood cells in diameter). In the typical small lymphocyte, the nucleus is uniformly round with a coarsely aggregated chromatin pattern, and nucleoli are absent or small and inconspicious (Fig. 89.2).[13] These cells resemble well-differentiated lymphocytes, however, variant small cell types recently have been reported in dogs. Variant small lymphocytes include a small cell type with irregular or notched nuclei (centrocytic-like), eccentric nuclei with pale cytoplasm often containing azurophilic granules (clear cells), or nuclei with fine chromatin and distinct nucleoli (prolymphocytic-like).[12] The category of low-grade, B cell lymphoma designated as a MMC[12] is characterized by lymphocytes with nuclei approximately 1.5 to 2 times the diameter of a red blood cell and with a low mitotic index. Many of the nuclei have a prominent large central nucleolus. These cells appear to have been identified by others as small-sized immunoblasts.[13,16] It remains to be determined whether this tumor fits best into the low- or high-grade category.

Mantle cell lymphoma was first established as a clinicopathologic entity in human medicine in the early 1990s,[17] but it is not a well recognized entity in animal species. This tumor is thought to arise from a subset of small B cells that reside in the mantle zone of secondary follicles. The immunoreactivity of malignant lympho-

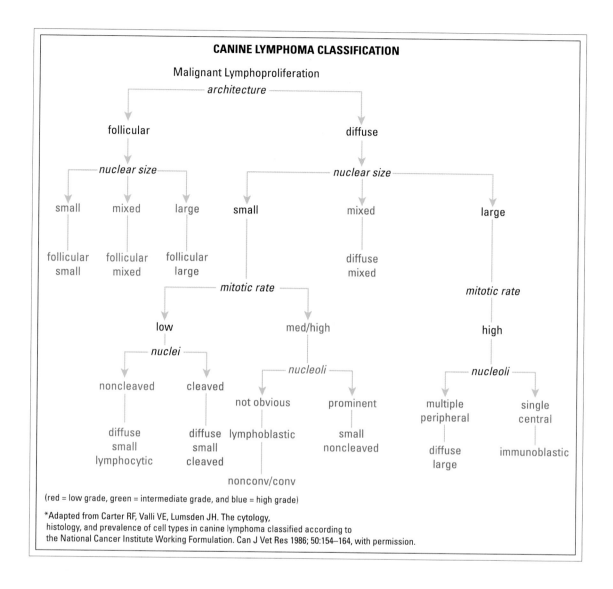

CANINE LYMPHOMA CLASSIFICATION

Malignant Lymphoproliferation

(red = low grade, green = intermediate grade, and blue = high grade)

*Adapted from Carter RF, Valli VE, Lumsden JH. The cytology, histology, and prevalence of cell types in canine lymphoma classified according to the National Cancer Institute Working Formulation. Can J Vet Res 1986; 50:154–164, with permission.

cytes for CD5 and cyclin D_1, but failure to react with either CD10 or CD23, are characteristic of mantle cell lymphomas in humans.[18] These cells are small with nuclei that vary in shape from round to slightly irregular. The malignant lymphocytes expand the mantle of the follicle and grow around or replace germinal centers. Thus, in early stages the lymphoma has a mantle zone or nodular pattern, whereas in later stages it may have a more diffuse pattern with only a few areas of nodularity. Although mantle cell lymphoma is believed to be a low-grade indolent type of lymphoma, recent studies suggest it may behave in a more aggressive manner. Thus, the clinical course and survival cannot be inferred based on its tumor grade alone.

Another well-recognized low-grade malignant B cell lymphoma in people is the marginal zone lymphoma.[19] When marginal zone lymphomas involve lymph nodes they are called monocytoid B cell lymphomas (MBcL) (Fig. 89.3A and 89.3B), and when they involve extranodal sites they are called mucosal-associated lymphatic tissue (MALT) lymphomas. The pattern and architectural features of this neoplasm are variable since the neoplastic population may arise from more than one anatomic compartment of the lymph node. The neoplastic monocytoid B cells may vary in size and shape; however, their cytoplasm is consistently abundant and pale staining, and these cells usually fail to express CD5 and CD10.[20] It has been speculated that lymphomas of MMCs are the equivalent of lymphomas that develop in the marginal zones in people. The acceptance of mantle cell and marginal zone lymphomas as distinct histologic or clinical entities in human medicine is based on the characteristic immunoreactivity or cytogenetic markers of the neoplastic populations.

INTERMEDIATE-GRADE NODAL LYMPHOMAS

Diffuse lymphomas of small cleaved (centrocytic) or mixed small cleaved and large cells (centrocytic cen-

TABLE 89.2 Classification of Nodal Lymphomas

KIEL (Updated) Classification	NCI-Working Formulation 1992
Low grade (slow rate of progression/indolent)	

Diffuse, small cell
  Lymphocytic, CLL & PLL[a]; B or T diffuse
Variants,[b] small cell
  T—Clear
  Prolymphocytic-like
  T—Centrocytic-like (Pleomorphic)
Lymphoplasmacytic/Immunocytoma
Plasmacytic
Follicular
  Centrocytic
Follicular
  Centrocytic-centroblastic
Centrocytic
 	
Macronucleolated medium-sized[b,c]
	Diffuse, small cell
	  Small lymphocytic, CLL
	  Small lymphocytic, plasmacytoid
	
	Plasmacytoid lymphocytic
	Plasmacytoma
	Follicular
	  Small cleaved cell
	Follicular
	  Mixed small cleaved & large cell
	Mantle cell
	Monocytoid B-cell
	
	Diffuse
	  Macronucleolated medium-sized[c]

Intermediate grade (intermediate rate of progression)	

Diffuse
  Centrocytic
Diffuse
  Centroblastic-centrocytic
Follicular
  Centroblastic/centrocytic
 	
Diffuse
  Centroblastic
	Diffuse
	  Small cleaved cell
	Diffuse
	  Mixed small & large cell
	Follicular
	  Predominately large cell
	
	Diffuse
	  Large cell, cleaved/noncleaved[c]

High grade (rapid rate of progression/aggressive)	

B-Immunoblastic
T-Large cell anaplastic
Small cell unclassifiable
  Burkitt's-type
  B or T-Plasmacytoid[b]
B or T-Lymphoblastic
 	
Miscellaneous
  T-Pleomorphic, mixed or large cell
  Mycosis fungoides
	Immunoblastic
	Large cell anaplastic
	Diffuse (Burkitt's/non-Burkitt's)
	  Small noncleaved cell
	
	Lymphoblastic
	  Convoluted & non-convoluted
	
	Miscellaneous
	  Pleomorphic, mixed or large cell
	  Mycosis fungoides

[a] PLL = prolymphocytic leukemia.
[b] Canine malignant lymphomas with no known human counterparts.
[c] Lymphocyte subtype is the same but grade designation is different.
(red = low grade, green = intermediate grade, and blue = high grade)

troblastic) are encountered infrequently in dogs and cattle. These neoplasms possess a B lineage phenotype and are derived from follicular center cells but do not form follicles and have a low mitotic rate. The nucleus of the small cleaved cell is approximately the same size as a red blood cell and has a deep cleft or linear indentation. The nucleus usually has a clumped chromatin pattern that obscures one or two small nucleoli. Only a scant amount of cytoplasm is found in the centrocyte. Except for one report,[8] a follicular pattern in intermediate-grade lymphomas is an uncommon finding in animal species. When present, the nuclei of the proliferating cells are at least two red blood cells in diameter with multiple nucleoli, and the mitotic rate is high in the follicles (Fig.

89.4A–C). In addition to the proportion of large cells, the proportions of follicular versus diffuse areas may vary in this subtype. Human patients who have follicular predominantly large cell lymphoma, having only focally follicular areas, are often treated as having a diffuse large cell lymphoma.

HIGH-GRADE NODAL LYMPHOMAS

Diffuse large cell cleaved or noncleaved lymphomas are classified as intermediate-grade lymphomas according to the WF. However, these neoplasms (diffuse centroblastic) represent a high-grade lymphoma in the Kiel

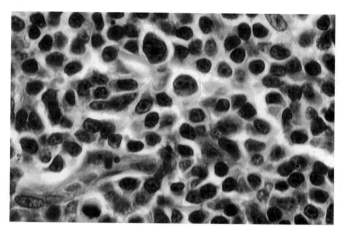

FIGURE 89.2 Canine low-grade T cell small lymphocytic lymphoma/chronic lymphocytic leukemia (SLL/CLL). The tumor cells have scant to moderate cytoplasm with small round nuclei (<1.5 red blood cell diameters) and darkly stained clumped chromatin. Nucleoli are either absent or inconspicuous. There are rare immunoblasts and many hyperplastic venules. H&E, 1000×. Contributors: Drs. Ted Valli and Lisa Miller.

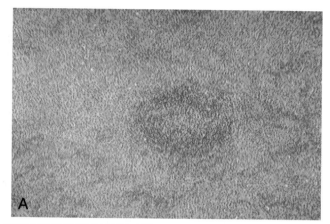

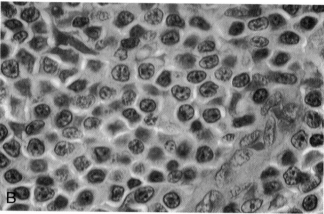

FIGURE 89.3 Canine low-grade monocytoid B cell lymphoma. **A.** Note diffuse to vaguely nodular pattern of growth of small to medium-sized cells. The tumor cells surround residual foci of benign small lymphocytes in a fading germinal center. H&E, 100×. **B.** Tumor nuclei are small to medium (slightly larger than a red blood cell) and round to slightly irregular with an abundant amount of light-staining cytoplasm. The chromatin has mild vesiculation with rimming of chromatin against the nuclear membrane and retention of chromacenters with parachromatin clearing. Small nucleoli are present in approximately one third of the cells. H&E, 1000×. Contributors: Drs. Ted Valli and H. L. Goettsche.

Classification. In dogs, the reported frequency of this subtype varies from 20%[13] to as much as 48.5%.[12] This is the most common subtype of lymphoma reported in cattle. The cleaved variant of the diffuse large cell type with a high mitotic index and B cell origin is characteristic of enzootic bovine lymphoma.[15,21]

Of the high-grade lymphomas (Kiel classification), the majority are classified as either diffuse centroblastic (large cell cleaved or noncleaved) (Fig. 89.5) or immunoblastic.[8,12,16,22] The population of lymphocytes in the centroblastic subtype is often heterogeneous, and at times centroblasts may be in the minority. The nucleus of the centroblast is large, often two or more red blood cells in diameter, the chromatin pattern is open and vesicular, and nucleoli are usually peripheral and may impinge on the nuclear membrane (Fig. 89.6A and B). A medium to high mitotic rate, prominence of nucleoli, and frequent occurrence of a starry sky pattern are also reported in this subtype.[19] These findings are reminiscent of the high-grade, small, noncleaved cell lymphomas in the study of Carter et al[13] and may account for the higher percentage (24.2%) they reported in this category. Variations in the size of nuclei are common in the small noncleaved lymphomas, and thus diffuse large (centroblastic) and small noncleaved cells overlap in size. For the designation large noncleaved to be applied, the percentage of large noncleaved cells (centroblasts) must be greater than 25%.

Recent immunologic studies have established that a B cell phenotype is involved in all the canine[12] and bovine lymphomas[21] with a diffuse large cell (centroblastic) component. This B cell neoplasm is believed to be of germinal center origin. The other category of diffuse, high-grade, B cell neoplasms, immunoblastic lymphoma,[12] is believed to arise from B cells that mature outside the germinal center (see Fig. 89.1). However, in human medicine there is no convincing evidence based on survival and immunohistological studies for the validity of the distinction between centroblastic and immunoblastic lymphomas. It has been suggested that these two categories be replaced by a single group known as large cell B cell lymphomas.[23] Further studies will be necessary to determine the validity of using a single group to define the diffuse large cell B cell lymphomas in dogs and other animal species.

The occurrence of immunoblastic lymphoma in dogs varies from 14.9% to 25.6%, except that Teske et al[8] classified only 6% as this subtype. Immunoblastic lymphomas consist of large cells with high nuclear volumes. The immunoblast has a single prominent nucleolus or several nucleoli in a paracentral location, an eccentrically placed nucleus, and deeply basophilic cytoplasm (Fig. 89.7A and B).[13] A lower frequency of 2.4 to 8.5% has been reported for the occurrence of immunoblastic lymphomas in cattle.[15,21]

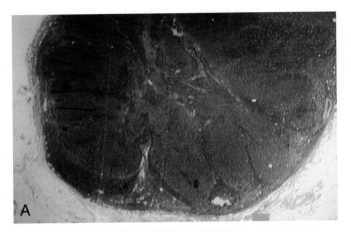

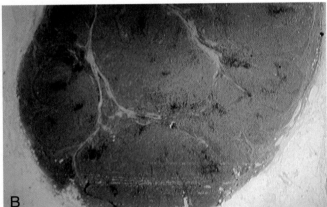

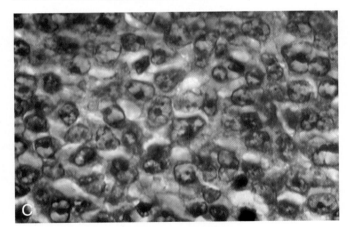

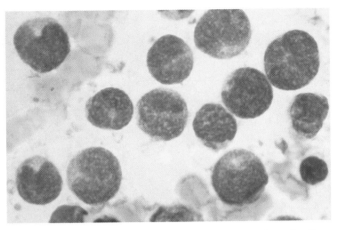

FIGURE 89.5 Touch preparation of canine large cleaved cell lymphoma. The cells have nuclear diameters of as much as 2 red blood cells with a deep cleft. Wright–Giemsa stain, 500×. Contributor: Dr. Rose Raskin.

FIGURE 89.4 Canine intermediate-grade follicular large B cell lymphoma. **A** and **B.** Tumor cells did not express the pan T cell antigen CD3, however, small arteries, high endothelial venules, and benign positively stained T lymphocytes are compressed between the expanding nodular structures. **A.** H&E, 12.5×. **B.** Immunoperoxidase for CD3, 12.5×. **C.** Tumor cells, which expressed the pan B cell antigen, CD79, have large noncleaved nuclei varying from 2 to 3 red blood cell diameters. Prominent nucleoli are often central and joined to thickened nuclear membranes by a coarsely branched chromatin structure. H&E, 1000×. Contributors: Drs. Ted Valli and Dale Webb.

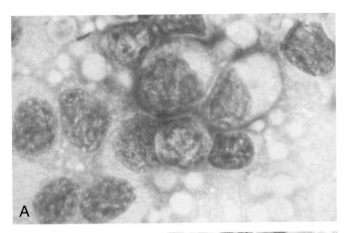

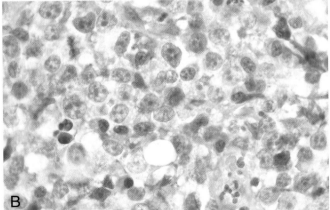

FIGURE 89.6 Canine high-grade diffuse large cell lymphoma. The cells have nuclei >2 red blood cell diameters with multiple medium to large, sometimes peripheral, nucleoli and moderate amounts of pale cytoplasm. **A.** Touch preparation. Wright–Giemsa stain, 500×. Contributor: Dr. Rose Raskin. **B.** Formalin-fixed tissue section. H&E, 250×.

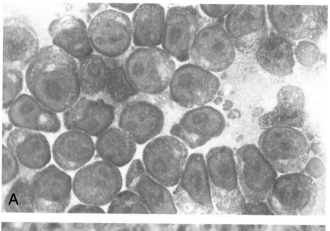

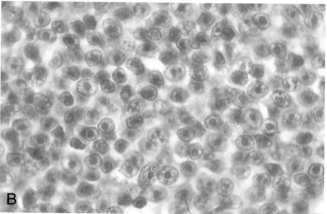

FIGURE 89.7 Canine high-grade, diffuse immunoblastic lymphoma. The cells have nuclear diameters of >2 red blood cells with a large central nucleolus or multiple paracentral nucleoli and moderate amounts of cytoplasm. **A.** Touch preparation. Wright-Giemsa stain, 400×. Contributor: Dr. John Harvey. **B.** Formalin-fixed tissue section. H&E, 250×.

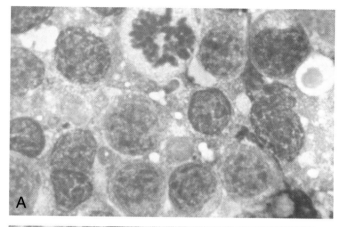

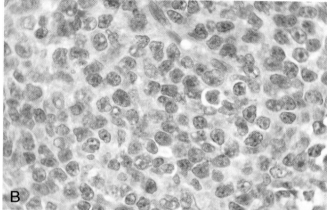

FIGURE 89.8 Canine high-grade, diffuse lymphoblastic lymphoma. The cells have nuclear diameters of approximately 1.5 red blood cells with small or indistinct nucleoli and moderate to scant cytoplasm. **A.** Touch preparation. Wright-Giemsa stain, 500×. Contributor: Dr. Rose Raskin. **B.** Formalin-fixed tissue section. H&E, 250×.

Except for one report,[13] lymphoblastic lymphomas are uncommon in studies of canine, feline, and bovine lymphoma. As in other high-grade subtypes, the architecture is diffuse and the mitotic rate is usually high. However, the round to oval or irregularly shaped nuclei are only approximately 1.5 red blood cells in diameter. The chromatin pattern is hyperchromatic with a fine to cribriform pattern. Nucleoli are generally absent or obscured by the chromatin pattern. The cytoplasm is scant to moderately abundant, pale staining, and almost undetectable (Fig. 89.8A and B).

EXTRANODAL LYMPHOMAS

One major criticism of all the lymphoma classification schemes currently used in veterinary medicine is that no distinction is made between nodal and extranodal lymphomas. It has been known for years that there are differences in the pathogenesis and prognosis of extranodal and nodal lymphomas, yet it was assumed that these tumors were similar in their histogenesis. Recent studies, however, suggest that many of the extranodal lymphomas may arise from cells of the MALT, rather than lymphoid cells of the lymph nodes.[19] In humans, the immunophenotype of MALT lymphomas is used to distinguish them from other neoplastic proliferations of small lymphoid cells. In contrast to most small lymphocytic or intermediate cell lymphomas (mantle cell) and small cleaved cell lymphomas (centrocytic) that are positive for CD5 and CD10, respectively, the lymphocytes comprising MALT lymphomas are negative for these markers.[11,24]

Extranodal lymphomas in animal species have been identified in various sites, including large and small intestine, stomach, skin, eye, central nervous system, kidney, and others. Extranodal lymphomas often have particular clinical characteristics, and the prognosis depends primarily on the stage or extent of disease. Thus, the extent of disease as determined by penetration of the stomach or intestinal wall and spread to lymph nodes may be of more prognostic importance than the grade of tumor.

Cutaneous lymphoid neoplasms are a heterogenous

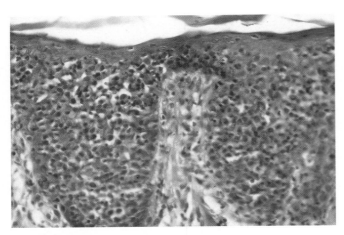

FIGURE 89.9 Canine epitheliotropic cutaneous or mucocutaneous lymphoma. Pleomorphic yet homogenous lymphoid cells invade the epithelium. H&E, 100×. Contributor: Dr. Thelma Lee Gross.

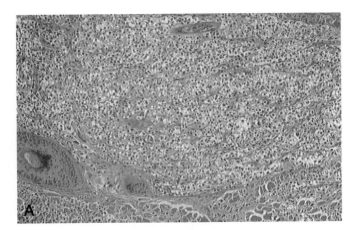

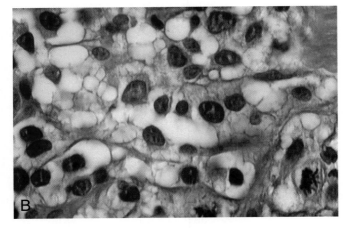

FIGURE 89.10 Canine pleomorphic large T cell cutaneous lymphoma. **A.** The mononuclear tumor cell population is separated into nests, islands, and individual cells by collagen fibers and connective tissue strands. H&E, 100×. **B.** The tumor cells, which stained positively for the pan T cell antigen CD3, have round to indented nuclei and moderate to abundant pale staining or clear cytoplasm. Nucleoli are large, prominent, and often multiple. The mitotic rate is high, and some of the tumor cells are multinucleated. H&E, 1000×. Contributors: Drs. John Andrews and John Hintermeister.

group of disorders. An epitheliotropic form of cutaneous lymphoma is more commonly recognized in dogs than in cats and closely resembles human mycosis fungoides (MF) (Fig. 89.9).[25] Recent studies have demonstrated that canine MF is a T cell lymphoma characterized by a clonal infiltrate of lymphocytes usually having a CD3+ and CD8+ phenotype.[26] The nonepitheliotropic variant of cutaneous lymphomas in dogs and cats is also predominantly of a T cell phenotype.[25] Cutaneous lymphomas with pleomorphic cells, whose morphology and T cell phenotype are similar to peripheral T cell lymphomas in humans, have been reported in dogs (Fig 89.10A and B).[12]

Alimentary lymphoma is another extranodal form of the disease and in both dogs and cats may be preceded by lymphocytic-plasmacytic enteritis. Although both B and T cell phenotypes have been described in cats,[27–29] gastrointestinal lymphoma is recognized less commonly in dogs, and the phenotype of the tumors is not well documented. Alimentary lymphoma is usually a disease of older feline leukemia virus-negative cats.[29] Lymphomas composed of large granular lymphocytes (LGLs) have also been reported to occur in the small intestine, particularly the jejunum of cats.[30,31] In humans, immunophenotypic results indicate that LGLs have either a natural killer or a cytotoxic T lymphocyte phenotype. The perforin-like,[32] CD3, and CD57-like[31] immunoreactivity of the tumor cells in some cats suggests that this neoplasm is composed of cytotoxic T lymphocytes. Severe necrosis and perforation of the intestine in cats may be responsible for the poor prognosis associated with this disease.

REFERENCES

1. **Rappaport H, Winter WJ, Hicks EB.** Follicular lymphoma. A re-evaluation of its position in the scheme of malignant lymphoma, based on a survey of 253 cases. Cancer 1956;9:792–821.
2. **Rappaport H.** Tumors of the hematopoietic system. In: Atlas of tumor pathology, section 3, fascile 8. Washington, DC: US Armed Forces Institute Pathology, 1966;270.
3. **Lieberman PH, Filippa DA, Straus DJ, Thaler HT, Cirrincione C, Clarkson BD.** Evaluation of malignant lymphomas using three classifications and the working formulation. 482 cases with median follow-up of 11.9 years. Am J Med 1986;81:365–380.
4. **Weller RE, Holmberg CA, Theilen GH, Madewell BR.** Histologic classification as a prognostic criterion for canine lymphosarcoma. Am J Vet Res 1980;41:1310–1314.
5. **Squire RA, Bush M, Melby EC, Neeley LM, Yarbrough B.** Clinical and pathologic study of canine lymphoma: clinical staging, cell classification and therapy. J Natl Cancer Inst 1973;41:566–574.
6. **Holmberg CA, Manning JS, Osburn BI.** Canine malignant lymphomas: comparison of morphologic and immunologic parameters. J Natl Cancer Inst 1976;56:125–135.
7. **Moulton JE, Harvey JW.** Tumors of lymphoid and hematopoietic tissue. In: Moulton JE, ed. Tumors of domestic animals. 3rd ed. Berkeley, CA: University of California Press, 1990;231–307.
8. **Teske E, van Heerde P, Rutteman GR, Kurzman ID, Moore PF, MacEwen EG.** Prognostic factors for treatment of malignant lymphoma in dogs. J Am Vet Med Assoc 1994;205:1722–1728.
9. **Lennert K, Stein H, Kaiserling E.** Cytological and functional criteria for the classification of malignant lymphomata. Br J Cancer 1975;31(suppl 2):29–43.
10. **National Cancer Institute.** Study of classifications of non-Hodgkin's lymphomas: summary and description of a working formulation for clinical usage. The Non-Hodgkin's Lymphoma Pathologic Classification Project. Cancer 1982;49:2112–2135.
11. **Harris NL, Jaffe ES, Stein H, Banks PM, Chan JK, Cleary ML, Delsol G, De Wolf-Peeters C, Falini B, Gatter KC, Grogan TM, Isaacson PG, Knowles DM, Mason DY, Muller-Hermelink HK, Pileri SA, Piris MA, Ralfkiaer E, Warnke RA.** A revised European-American classification of lymphoid

neoplasms: a proposal from the International Lymphoma Study Group. Blood 1994;84:1361–1392.

12. **Fournel-Fleury C, Magnol JP, Bricaire P, Marchal T, Chabanne L, Delverdier A, Bryon PA, Felman P.** Cytohistological and immunological classification of canine malignant lymphomas: comparison with human non-Hodgkin's lymphomas. J Comp Pathol 1997;117:35–59.

13. **Carter RF, Valli VE, Lumsden JH.** The cytology, histology and prevalence of cell types in canine lymphoma classified according to the National Cancer Institute Working Formulation. Can J Vet Res 1986;50:154–164.

14. **Appelbaum FR, Sale GE, Storb R, Charrier K, Deeg HJ, Graham T, Wulff JC.** Phenotyping of canine lymphoma with monoclonal antibodies directed at cell surface antigens: classification, morphology, clinical presentation and response to chemotherapy. Hematol Oncol 1984;2:151–168.

15. **Vernau W, Valli VE, Dukes TW, Jacobs RM, Shoukri M, Heeney JL.** Classification of 1,198 cases of bovine lymphoma using the National Cancer Institute Working Formulation for human non-Hodgkin's lymphomas. Vet Pathol 1992;29:183–195.

16. **Greenlee PG, Filippa DA, Quimby FW, Patnaik AK, Calvano SE, Matus RE, Kimmel M, Hurvitz AI, Lieberman PH.** Lymphomas in dogs. A morphologic, immunologic, and clinical study. Cancer 1990;66:480–490.

17. **Duggan MJ, Weisenburger DD, Ye YL, Bast MA, Pierson JL, Linder J, Armitage JO.** Mantle zone lymphoma. A clinicopathologic study of 22 cases. Cancer 1990;66:522–529.

18. **Dorfman DM, Pinkus GS.** Distinction between small lymphocytic and mantle cell lymphoma by immunoreactivity for CD23. Mod Pathol 1994;7: 326–331.

19. **Nathwani BN, Brynes RK, Lincoln T, Hasmann ML.** Classifications of non-Hodgkin's lymphomas. In: Knowles DM, ed. Neoplastic hematopathology. Baltimore: Williams & Wilkins, 1992;555–600.

20. **Zukerberg LR, Medeiros LJ, Ferry JA, Harris NL.** Diffuse low-grade B-cell lymphomas. Four clinically distinct subtypes defined by a combination of morphologic and immunophenotypic features. Am J Clin Pathol 1993; 100:373–385.

21. **Vernau W, Jacobs RM, Valli VEO, Heeney JL.** The immunophenotypic characterization of bovine lymphomas. Vet Pathol 1997;34:222–225.

22. **Parodi AL, Dargent F, Crespeau F.** Histological classification of canine malignant lymphomas. Zentralbl Veterinarmed A 1988;35:178–192.

23. **Stein H, Lennert K, Feller AC, Mason DY.** Immunohistological analysis of human lymphoma: correlation of histological and immunological categories. Adv Cancer Res 1984;42:67–147.

24. **Hiddemann W, Longo DL, Coiffier B, Fisher RI, Cabanillas F, Cavalli F, Nadler LM, De Vita VT, Lister TA, Armitage JO.** Lymphoma classification-the gap between biology and clinical management is closing. Blood 1996;88: 4085–4089.

25. **Day MJ.** Immunophenotypic characterization of cutaneous lymphoid neoplasia in the dog and cat. J Comp Pathol 1995;112:79–96.

26. **Moore PF, Olivry T, Naydan D.** Canine cutaneous epitheliotropic lymphoma (mycosis fungoides) is a proliferative disorder of CD8+ T cells. Am J Pathol 1994;144:421–429.

27. **Holmberg CA, Manning JS, Osburn BI.** Feline malignant lymphomas: comparison of morphologic and immunologic characteristics. Am J Vet Res 1976;37:1455–1460.

28. **Mahony OM, Moore AS, Cotter SM, Engler SJ, Brown D, Penninck DG.** Alimentary lymphoma in cats: 28 cases (1988–1993). J Am Vet Med Assoc 1995;207:1593–1598.

29. **Zwahlen CH, Lucroy, MD, Kraegel SA, Madewell BR.** Results of chemotherapy for cats with alimentary malignant lymphoma: 21 cases (1993–1997). J Am Vet Med Assoc 1998;213:1144–1149.

30. **Wellman ML, Hammer AS, DiBartola SP, Carothers MA, Kociba GJ, Rojko JL.** Lymphoma involving large granular lymphocytes in cats: 11 cases (1982–1991). J Am Vet Med Assoc 1992;201:1265–1269.

31. **Darbes J, Majzoub M, Breuer W, Hermanns W.** Large granular lymphocyte leukemia/lymphoma in six cats. Vet Pathol 1998;35:370–379.

32. **Kariya K, Konno A, Ishida T.** Perforin-like immunoreactivity in four cases of lymphoma of large granular lymphocytes in the cat. Vet Pathol 1997;34:156–159.

CHAPTER 90

Bovine Leukemia Virus-Associated Lymphoproliferative Disorders

• GARY L. COCKERELL and RICHARD A. REYES

Bovine leukemia virus (BLV) is a common, worldwide infection of cattle that causes two lymphoproliferative disorders, persistent lymphocytosis (PL) and malignant lymphoma (ML) or lymphocytic leukemia (LL). BLV is not only an important cause of naturally occurring disease in cattle, but also provides a valuable animal model to study analogous diseases caused by similar viruses in human beings. In this chapter we highlight prominent features of BLV as well as the infection and spectrum of lymphoproliferative disorders with which it is associated in cattle. In addition, reference is given to several recently published comprehensive reviews and symposia on the biology of BLV.[1-4]

THE AGENT: BOVINE LEUKEMIA VIRUS

BLV is a member of the family Retroviridae, subfamily Oncovirinae. It is morphologically similar to C-type leukemia viruses, but because of its complex genomic structure, BLV has been classified in a separate group with human T cell lymphotropic virus (HTLV).[4] The BLV genome consists of a dimer of identical, single-stranded RNA molecules and a virion-associated magnesiumdependent reverse transcriptase. The integrated pro-virus is 8.7 kbases in length and has been sequenced in its entirety.[5] In addition to *gag, pol,* and *env* genes typical of other retroviruses, BLV and other members of this complex group contain a 3' region, designated *pX*, that encodes viral regulatory proteins. The most thoroughly studied of these is the *trans*-regulatory protein, Tax, which increases the rate of viral transcription by activating the promoter in the viral long terminal repeat (LTR). Tax is also postulated to play a critical role in BLV-associated lymphoproliferative disorders by influencing the expression of normal host genes. Compared with other members of Retroviridae, BLV is genetically stable, making it unlikely that different manifestations of BLV infection are the result of differences in strains of virus.

EPIDEMIOLOGIC CONSIDERATIONS

Host Range

Cattle are the most common and the only unequivocal natural host for BLV. Sheep are highly susceptible to experimental infection with BLV and progress through the same stages of infection and disease as naturally infected cattle.[6]

Prevalence

The reported seroprevalence of BLV infection varies widely, but rates of as much as 50% of cattle and greater than 75% of herds are common in the United States.[7] All breeds are equally susceptible to infection, although, owing to differences in management and animal husbandry practices, disease is more frequent in dairy breeds compared with beef breeds. There is an association between bovine major histocompatibility complex (MHC) class II haplotype and resistance to the development of PL, indicating a host genetic component in determining disease progression.[8]

Transmission

Transmission of BLV takes place by the horizontal route. True vertical transmission (through gametes) does not occur. Transmission by contamination of semen, ova, or embryos derived from BLV-infected sires or dams does not occur; however, in utero transmission occurs in as much as 10% of newborn calves from infected dams. In addition, approximately 15% of calfhood infections are from ingestion of colostrum contaminated with BLV-

BOVINE LEUKEMIA VIRUS-ASSOCIATED LYMPHOPROFILERATIVE DISORDERS

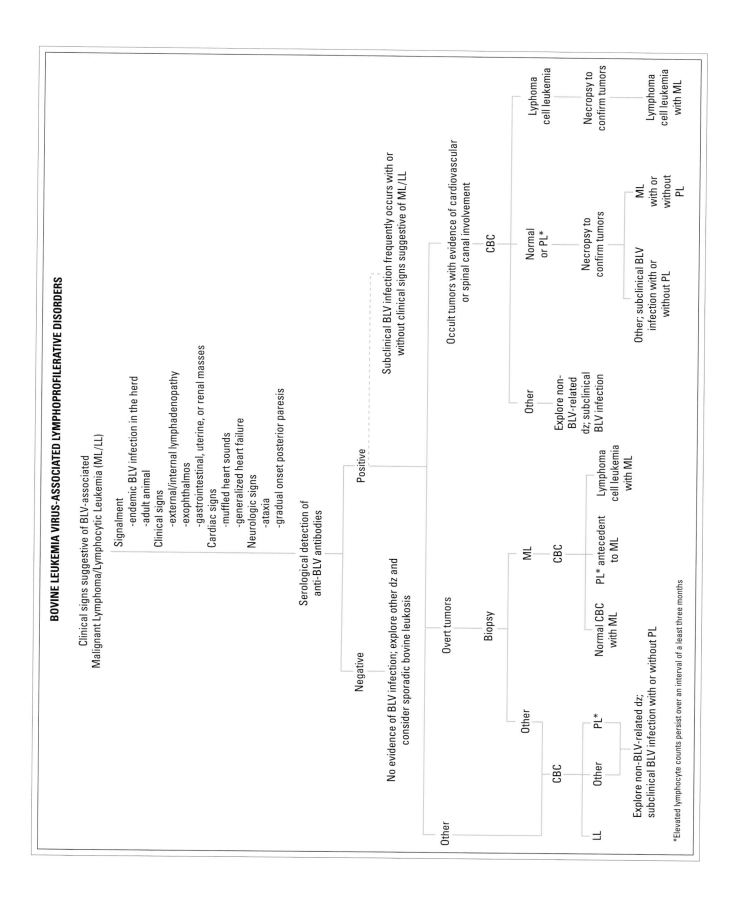

Clinical signs suggestive of BLV-associated
Malignant Lymphoma/Lymphocytic Leukemia (ML/LL)

Signalment
-endemic BLV infection in the herd
-adult animal
Clinical signs
-external/internal lymphadenopathy
-exophthalmos
-gastrointestinal, uterine, or renal masses
Cardiac signs
-muffled heart sounds
-generalized heart failure
Neurologic signs
-ataxia
-gradual onset posterior paresis

Serological detection of
anti-BLV antibodies

Negative → No evidence of BLV infection; explore other dz and
consider sporadic bovine leukosis

Positive → Subclinical BLV infection frequently occurs with or
without clinical signs suggestive of ML/LL

Overt tumors

Other

Biopsy → ML → CBC → PL* antecedent to ML → Lymphoma cell leukemia with ML

Normal CBC with ML

Other → CBC → PL*

Other

LL

Explore non-BLV-related dz;
subclinical BLV infection with or without PL

Other → Explore non-BLV-related
dz; subclinical
BLV infection

Occult tumors with evidence of cardiovascular
or spinal canal involvement

CBC → Normal or PL* → Necropsy to confirm tumors → ML with or without PL

Other; subclinical BLV infection with or without PL

Lymphoma cell leukemia

Necropsy to confirm tumors → Lymphoma cell leukemia with ML

*Elevated lymphocyte counts persist over an interval of a least three months

615

infected lymphocytes. The simultaneous presence of anti-BLV antibodies in this colostrum provides some degree of protection.[9,10]

Because BLV remains highly cell-associated, transmission requires transfer of whole cells, especially lymphocytes. The most common source of infectious material is blood, and as little as 0.1 μL is sufficient to transfer infection. Increased rates of natural transmission occur when there is close contact between cattle, although the exact mode of transmission under these conditions remains unclear. Iatrogenic transmission potentially can occur in situations in which there is the probability for transfer of infected blood, e.g., the use of common injection needles, dehorning, and rectal palpation. BLV can be recovered from hematophagous insects after feeding on infected cattle; however, mechanical transmission of BLV by insects has not been proved under natural conditions.[10,11]

PATHOGENESIS

Stages of Infection

After horizontal transmission, BLV establishes a subclinical, low-level infection of B lymphocytes. Less than 5% of peripheral blood mononuclear cells (PBMC) contain randomly integrated provirus. The infection persists for the lifetime of the animal, but does not progress beyond this stage in the majority (~65%) of BLV-infected cattle.

During the next 3 to 5 years, approximately 30% of BLV-infected cattle develop PL, a subclinical, polyclonal, persistent increase in total circulating lymphocytes.[12] The percentage of infected PBMC in cattle with PL increases to as much as 50%. PL is a preneoplastic condition since BLV-infected cattle with PL have at least a twofold greater risk to develop ML or LL compared with BLV-infected cattle with normal hemograms.[13]

Within 3 to 10 years after infection, ≤5% of BLV-infected cattle develop ML or LL, a fatal, monoclonal or oligoclonal, B cell lymphoproliferative disease. Tumor cells contain one to four copies of clonally integrated provirus that are usually transcriptionally active[14-16]; however, as much as 25% of tumors contain 5'-deleted provirus and are replication-defective.[17]

Cellular Tropism

The principal target cell of BLV is the B lymphocyte. Virus has been detected in various other cell types, but the pathogenic significance of these cellular tropisms remains unknown. The expanded lymphocyte population in BLV-infected cattle with PL has a peculiar phenotype with elevated levels of expression of MHC class II, immunoglobulin M (IgM), CD5, and the interleukin 2 receptor, indicating they are activated, cycling B cells.[18-20]

Neoplastic lymphocytes from BLV-infected cattle with ML display a mature B cell phenotype.[21] They most often express surface IgM, frequently in association with another immunoglobulin (Ig) isotype, suggesting transformation during isotype switching late in B cell ontogeny.[22]

Antiviral Immune Response

BLV-infected cattle develop antibodies against all major viral proteins, but the antiviral immune response cannot control the infection. Antiviral antibody titers progressively increase in cattle with PL and reach maximal levels with the development of ML or LL, suggesting increased virus expression with advancing stages of disease. BLV-infected cattle develop a CD4+ helper T cell response to the external glycoprotein (GP) GP51 and the major core antigen p24. Impaired proliferation of CD4+ T cells in response to viral antigens correlates with progressive disease.[23]

Host-Virus Interaction

The BLV envelope GP complex, GP51-GP30, is critical for infectivity.[4] The external subunit, GP51, serves as the binding domain to the host target cell. The transmembrane subunit, GP30, anchors the complex in the viral envelope and the plasma membrane of infected cells. Amino acid motifs in the cytoplasmic tail of GP30 that are important for viral infectivity have also been implicated in signal transduction pathways in other cell systems. Both GP51 and GP30 mediate cell fusion. The BLV receptor has only begun to be studied and remains to be fully characterized.[24]

BLV replicates minimally in vivo and remains highly cell-associated, thus there is a low level of viremia. However, the vigorous antiviral antibody response in BLV-infected cattle indicates there is at least limited or intermittent viral expression in vivo. This has now been confirmed with polymerase chain reaction (PCR) methodology.[15] For reasons that are not clear, viral transcription and translation are significantly upregulated after short-term in vitro incubation of infected PBMC. There is evidence for the presence of a non-Ig factor(s) in the plasma of cattle that regulates BLV expression in vivo, but the biological significance of this finding remains unresolved.[25]

Viral load in persistently infected cattle gradually increases with advancing stages of infection. Early evidence suggested that BLV replication was transcriptionally linked to host cell activation and proliferation.[26] It is now known that BLV transcription can be induced through normal B cell signaling pathways, such as protein kinase C.[27] Further, transcriptional regulatory elements in the BLV LTR-binding proteins, such as cyclic adenosine monophosphate (cAMP) response element binding protein[28] and NF-κB,[29] that also regulate the transcription of genes critical to host cell activation and proliferation. This suggests that BLV replication and disease progression may be enhanced by non-BLV-related events that are mediated by multigene activating transcription factors.

When cultured in vitro, there is an incremental delay in the onset of apoptosis of lymphocytes from BLV-infected cattle that correlates with advancing stages of disease.[30] Apoptosis is preferentially delayed in the expanded B cell populations that progressively accumulate in BLV-infected cattle with PL and ML or LL. This delay in B cell apoptosis further correlates with an increase in the reciprocal expression of *bcl-2:bax*,[31] two members of a recently recognized family of oncogenes that regulate apoptosis.[32] Taken together, these results suggest BLV imparts a survival advantage on infected cells and that prolonged cell survival contributes to the progressive expansion of B cell populations in BLV-infected cattle.

Mechanisms of Transformation

The ultimate mechanism of BLV-induced cellular transformation remains unknown. The virus does not contain a recognized *onc* gene characteristic of acute transforming sarcoma retroviruses, nor does it have preferred sites of integration characteristic of *cis*-acting chronic leukemia viruses.[4] By analogy to HTLV-I, the BLV *trans*-acting viral regulatory gene, *tax*, is suspected to play a role in leukemogenesis.[33] Once cells are transformed, viral transcription is not necessary to maintain the transformed phenotype; however, the 3′ portion of the genome, including *tax*, is probably important in the transformation process since it is retained even in tumors harboring deleted proviruses.[17]

Karyotypic analysis of neoplastic cells from cattle with ML or LL has revealed numerous chromosomal abnormalities,[34] but these have not been associated with the location of known proto-oncogenes. Given the altered structure or expression of several proto-oncogenes, including *p53*,[35,36] *bcl-2*, and *bax*,[30,31] in BLV-infected cattle, this is obviously an important area for future study.

PATHOLOGY AND HEMATOLOGY

Subclinical Infection

BLV-seropositive cattle have normal hematologic profiles. However, increased numbers of B cells are present in a proportion of these animals without an absolute increase in the number of circulating lymphocytes.[37]

Persistent Lymphocytosis

Although PL is defined on the basis of hematologic abnormalities, PL is also a subclinical stage of BLV infection. The usual hematologic definition of PL is a lymphocyte count that exceeds the mean plus 3.00 standard deviations for the respective breed and age and persists over an interval of at least 3 months. This definition differentiates PL from transient lymphocytosis associated with conditions unrelated to BLV infection in cattle. An example of age- and breed-adjusted criteria for the

diagnosis of PL is given in Table 90.1.[38] The absolute increase in circulating lymphocytes in BLV-infected cattle with PL is caused by an increase in CD5+/IgM+ B cells, resulting in an inverted B:T cell ratio.[18–20] Morphologically atypical circulating lymphocytes may be present in PL, but these may occasionally be observed in normal cattle or cattle with various non-BLV-related conditions.

Malignant Lymphoma or Lymphocytic Leukemia

Historically, BLV-associated ML or LL has been referred to as enzootic bovine leukosis or the adult form of bovine lymphoma to differentiate it from the less common sporadic bovine leukosis. The latter usually occurs in younger animals, is not associated with BLV, and includes calf, thymic, and cutaneous forms.

BLV-associated ML occurs as solid tissue tumors, most frequently involving lymph nodes. Numerous nonlymphoid tissues are commonly involved, including (in decreasing order of frequency) heart, abomasum, kidney, uterus, spinal canal, and intestine. Bone marrow is infrequently involved. Several histologic classification systems used in human hemopoietic neoplasia have been successfully applied to bovine ML.[39,40]

Hemograms and cytology of blood are extremely variable in bovine ML or LL. A normal hemogram is present in 10 to 30% of cases. Anemia (normocytic, normochromic) is frequently present and usually results in part from blood loss in the gastrointestinal tract from neoplastic involvement. An absolute lymphocytosis is also frequently present and often reflects preexisting PL superimposed on the development of ML. Circulating atypical or immature lymphocytes may be present in as many as 50% of the cases of ML (sometimes referred to as lymphoma cell leukemia), but this may not be reflected in increased total lymphocyte counts. The presence of abnormal lymphocytes in the blood, especially in adult cattle, is highly suspicious of ML (Fig. 90.1). BLV-associated LL occurs in 5 to 10% of cases and is manifest as massive increases in circulating neoplastic lymphoblasts (Fig. 90.2).

TABLE 90.1	Criteria for Determination of PL in California Holstein-Fresian Cattle	
	Absolute Lymphocyte Count/μL	
Age	**Normal**	**PL**[a]
0–6 months	<9,000	>9,000
6–12 months	<11,000	>11,000
1–2 years	<11,000	>11,000
2–3 years	<8,000	>8,000
3–4 years	<7,000	>7,000
4 ≥ 5 years	<6,500	>6,500

[a] Elevated lymphocyte counts persist over an interval of at least 3 months.

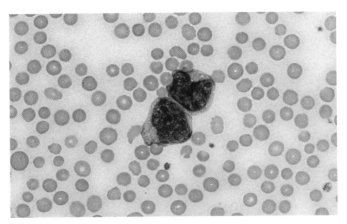

FIGURE 90.1 Blood from a BLV-infected cow with ML, showing atypical lymphocytes. Note large lymphocytes, with or without asymmetrically indented nuclei and prominent nucleoli. Magnification 1500×. (Photomicrograph courtesy of Dr. Karen M. Young.)

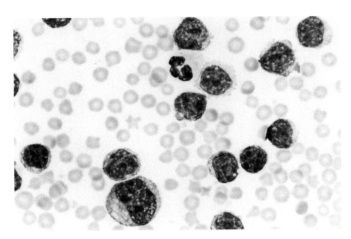

FIGURE 90.2 Blood from a BLV-infected cow with LL and a total white blood cell count (WBC) of 300,000/μL, 97% of which were lymphocytes. Note anisocytosis, anisokaryosis, and prominent nucleoli. A normal neutrophil (top, center) is included for size comparison. Magnification 1450×. (Case courtesy of Dr. Duane Lassen.)

CLINICAL SIGNS

The only stage of BLV infection associated with clinical signs is ML or LL. Adult cattle (5 to 8 years of age) are most frequently affected, and once ML or LL is diagnosed, the disease progresses rapidly with anorexia, wasting, decreased milk production, and death within 1 to 4 months. At least half of cattle with ML or LL present with lymphadenopathy affecting single or multiple external or internal lymph nodes. Depending on the involvement of other organs in the neoplastic process, other common clinical signs include chronic indigestion, melena or diarrhea (gastrointestinal tract), heart failure (myocardium), posterior paralysis (spinal canal), and exophthalmos (retrobulbar tissue).

DIAGNOSIS

Detection of a humoral anti-BLV antibody response, especially against GP51, is the most commonly used indicator of infection. The most common procedures used are the agar gel immunodiffusion (AGID) test, radioimmunoassay, and enzyme-linked immunosorbent assay.[41] Of these, the AGID test is most frequently used. It is available as a commercial kit, is inexpensive and relatively easy to perform, and yields quick, easily interpretable results that correlate well with infection.

The presence of antiviral antibodies is only an indirect indication of BLV infection and assumes that once the cow is infected it remains so for life. It does not indicate that the cow has PL, ML, or LL nor that these conditions will develop in the future. Anti-BLV antibodies may not be detectable for several months post-infection, may decline at parturition owing to concentration in colostrum, and in calves as old as 6 months of age may give a false-positive result as a result passive absorption from colostrum from seropositive dams.

Direct detection of BLV is a less common means of diagnosis. Since minimal viral replication occurs in vivo, more laboratory-intensive procedures, such as tissue culture, PCR, immunohistochemistry, and electron microscopy, are required to detect the virus directly.[42]

TREATMENT OR PREVENTION OR ERADICATION

No effective antiviral treatment exists for cattle in any stage of BLV infection. Treatment of cattle with ML or LL is only palliative. Similarly, there is currently no effective vaccine for prevention of BLV infection, although attempts are ongoing. A BLV vaccine must not only be efficacious, but must also allow for differentiation between an immune response induced as a result of vaccination versus naturally acquired infection. Because BLV is transmitted in a cell-associated form, it is not highly contagious and, therefore, can be fairly easily eradicated. Eradication procedures require that infected animals be identified and either segregated or slaughtered, and that corrective management practices be implemented.[7]

REFERENCES

1. **Burny A, Cleuter Y, Kettmann R, et al.** Bovine leukemia virus: facts and hypotheses derived from the study of an infectious cancer. Vet Microbiol 1988;17:197–218.
2. **Trainin Z.** Special issue: bovine leukemia virus. Vet Immunol Immunopathol 1989;22:199–305.
3. **Evermann J.** Special symposium on bovine leukemia virus. Vet Med 1992;87:185–278.
4. **Kettmann R, Burny A, Callebut I, et al.** Bovine leukemia virus. In: Levy JA, ed. The retroviridae. New York: Plenum Press, 1994;39–81.
5. **Sagata N, Yasunaga T, Tsuzuku-Kawamura J, Ohishi K, Ogawa Y, Ikawa Y.** Complete nucleotide sequence of the genome of bovine leukemia virus: its evolutionary relationship to other retroviruses. Proc Natl Acad Sci U S A 1985;82:677–681.
6. **Djilali S, Parodi A-L, Levy D, Cockerell GL.** Development of leukemia and lymphosarcoma induced by bovine leukemia virus in sheep: a hematopathological study. Leukemia 1987;1:777–781.
7. **DiGiacomo RF.** The epidemiology and control of bovine leukemia virus infection. Vet Med 1992;87:248–257.

8. **Anlong X, van Eijk MJT, Park C, Lewin HA.** Polymorphism in *BoLa-drb3* exon 2 correlated with resistance to persistent lymphocytosis caused by bovine leukemia virus. J Immunol 1993;151:6977–6985.
9. **DiGiacomo RF.** Vertical transmission of the bovine leukemia virus. Vet Med 1992;87:258–261.
10. **Hopkins SG, DiGiacomo RF.** Natural transmission of bovine leukemia virus in dairy and beef cattle. Vet Clin North Am Food Anim Pract 1997;13:107–128.
11. **DiGiacomo RF.** Horizontal transmission of the bovine leukemia virus. Vet Med 1992;87:263–271.
12. **Depelchin A, Letesson JJ, Lostrie-Trussart N, Mammerickx M, Portetelle D, Burny A.** Bovine leukemia virus (BLV)-infected B cells express a marker similar to the CD5 T cell marker. Immunol Lett 1989;20:69–76.
13. **Ferrer JF, Marshak RR, Abt DA, Kenyon SJ.** Relationship between lymphosarcoma and persistent lymphocytosis in cattle: a review. J Am Vet Med Assoc 1979;175:705–708.
14. **Cockerell GL, Rovnak J.** The correlation between the direct and indirect detection of bovine leukemia virus infection in cattle. Leuk Res 1988;12:465–469.
15. **Jensen WA, Rovnak, J, Cockerell GL.** *In vivo* transcription of the bovine leukemia virus *tax/rex* region in normal and neoplastic lymphocytes of cattle and sheep. J Virol 1991;65:2484–2490.
16. **Reyes RA, Cockerell GL.** Unintegrated bovine leukemia virus DNA: association with viral expression and disease progression. J Virol 1996;70:4961–4965.
17. **Tajima S, Ikawa Y, Aida Y.** Complete bovine leukemia virus (BLV) provirus in conserved in BLV-infected cattle throughout the course of B-cell lymphosarcoma development. J Virol 1998;72:7569–7576.
18. **Matheise JP, Delcommenne M, Mager A, Didembourg CH, Letesson JJ.** CD5+ B cells from bovine leukemia virus infected cows are activated cycling cells responsive to interleukin 2. Leukemia 1992;6:304–309.
19. **Schwartz I, Bensaid A, Polack B, Perrin B, Berthelemy M, Levy D.** *In vivo* leukocyte tropism of bovine leukemia virus in sheep and cattle. J Virol 1994;68:4589–4596.
20. **Mirsky ML, Olmstead CA, Da Y, Lewin HA.** The prevalence of proviral bovine leukemia virus in peripheral blood mononuclear cells at two subclinical stages of infection. J Virol 1996;70:2178–2183.
21. **Vernau W, Jacobs RM, Valli VE, Heeney JL.** The immunophenotypic characterization of bovine lymphomas. Vet Pathol 1997;34:222–225.
22. **Heeney JL, Valli VEO.** Transformed phenotype of enzootic bovine leukosis lymphoma reflects differentiation-linked leukemogenesis. Lab Invest 1990;62:339–346.
23. **Orlik O, Splitter GA.** Progression to persistent lymphocytosis and tumor development in bovine leukemia virus (BLV)-infected cattle correlates with impaired proliferation of CD4+ T cells in response to *gag*- and *env*-encoded BLV proteins. J Virol 1996;70:7584–7593.
24. **Suzuki T, Ikeda H.** The mouse homolog of the bovine leukemia virus receptor is closely related to the δ subunit of the adapter-related protein complex AP-3, not associated with the cell surface. J Virol 1998;72:593–599.
25. **Zandomeni RO, Estaban E, Carrera-Zandomeni M, Ferrer JF.** Host soluble factors with blocking and stimulating activity on the expression of the bovine leukemia virus. J Infect Dis 1994;170:787–794.
26. **Villouta G, Botto G, Rudolph W.** Spontaneous and mitogen-induced RNA synthesis by blood lymphocytes from bovine leukemia virus virus-infected and normal cows. Vet Immunol Immunopathol 1988;18:287–291.
27. **Jensen WA, Wicks-Beard BJ, Cockerell GL.** Inhibition of protein kinase C results in decreased expression of bovine leukemia virus. J Virol 1992;66:4427–4433.
28. **Willems L, Kettmann R, Chen G, Portetelle D, Burny A, Derse D.** A cyclic AMP-responsive DNA-binding protein (CREB2) is a cellular transactivator of the bovine leukemia virus long terminal repeat. J Virol 1992;66:766–772.
29. **Brooks PA, Nyborg JK, Cockerell GL.** Identification of an NF-κB binding site in the bovine leukemia virus promoter. J Virol 1995;69:6005–6009.
30. **Reyes RA, Cockerell GL.** Bovine leukemia virus-associated leukemogenesis is correlated with suppression of programmed cell death and increased expression of *bcl-2*. 2000; submitted.
31. **Reyes RA, Cockerell GL.** Increased ratio of *bcl-2/bax* expression is associated with bovine leukemia virus-induced leukemogenesis in cattle. Virology 1998;242:184–192.
32. **Yang E, Korsmeyer SJ.** Molecular thanatopsis: a discourse on the BCL2 family and cell death. Blood 1996;88:386–401.
33. **Green P, Chen ISY.** Regulation of human T cell leukemia virus expression. FASEB J 1990;4:169–175.
34. **Schnurr MW, Carter RF, Dubé ID, Valli VE, Jacobs RM.** Nonrandom chromosomal abnormalities in bovine lymphoma. Leuk Res 1994;18:91–99.
35. **Dequiedt F, Ketmann R, Burny A, Willems L.** Mutations in the p53 tumor-suppressor gene are frequently associated with bovine leukemia virus-induced leukemogenesis in cattle but not in sheep. Virology 1995;209:676–683.
36. **Tajima S, Zhuang WZ, Kato MV, Okada K, Ikawa Y, Aida Y.** Function and conformation of wild-type p53 protein are influenced by mutations in bovine leukemia virus-induced B-cell lymphosarcoma. Virology 1998;243:235–246.
37. **Fossum C, Burny A, Portetelle D, Mammerickx M, Morein B.** Detection of B and T cells, with lectins or antibodies, in healthy and bovine leukemia virus-infected cattle. Vet Immunol Immunopathol 1988;18:269–278.
38. **Theilen GH, Dungworth DL, Lengyel J, Rosenblatt LS.** Bovine lymphosarcoma in California: epizootiologic and hematologic aspects. Health Lab Sci 1;96–106.
39. **Parodi A-L, Mialot M, Crespeau F, et al.** Attempt for a new cytological and cytoimmunological classification of bovine malignant lymphoma (BML) (lymphosarcoma). In: Straub OC, ed. 4th International Symposium on Bovine Leukosis. The Hague, Netherlands: Martinus Nijhoff, 1982;561–572.
40. **Vernau W, Valli VEO, Dukes TW, Jacobs RM, Shoukri M, Heeney JL.** Classification of 1,198 cases of bovine lymphoma using the National Cancer Institute Working Formulation for human non-Hodgkin's lymphomas. Vet Pathol 1992;29:183–195.
41. **Evermann JF.** A look at how bovine leukemia virus infection is diagnosed. Vet Med 1992;87:272–278.
42. **Evermann JF, Jackson MK.** Laboratory diagnostic tests for retroviral infections in dairy and beef cattle. Vet Clin North Am Food Anim Pract 1997;13:87–106.

CHAPTER 91

Lymphoma

• DAVID M. VAIL

Lymphoma (lymphosarcoma) is the most common hematopoietic tumor of all domestic species and is defined as a proliferation of malignant lymphoid cells that primarily affects lymph nodes or solid visceral organs such as the liver or spleen. Although lymphoma has been reported in all domestic and nearly all mammalian species, the discussions herein are confined to dogs, cats, and to a lesser extent horses.

ORIGIN

The origin of lymphoma in companion animals is for the most part unknown. In cats, certain forms have been directly and indirectly associated with feline leukemia virus (FeLV) and feline immunodeficiency virus (FIV), respectively; however, no strong evidence exists for a retroviral origin in dogs. A weak association between lymphoma in dogs and the use of pesticides or exposure to strong magnetic fields has been observed in preliminary epidemiologic studies, however, more thorough studies are necessary to evaluate these associations further.[1-3] In rare cases a familial component has been suggested by occasional clustering of lymphoma in related dogs.[4]

CLASSIFICATION OF LYMPHOMA

Lymphoma can be classified by anatomical site, histologic or cytologic phenotype, and immunophenotype. Clinical stage is assigned according to criteria established by the World Health Organization (WHO) as outlined in Table 91.1.

Canine Classification

The multicentric form, typically WHO stage III or IV, accounts for the majority of cases (80 to 85%) in the dog.[5-7] Alimentary (~7%), cutaneous (~6%), mediastinal (~3%), and miscellaneous extranodal forms (central nervous system, bone, heart, nasal cavity, primary ocular) are less frequently encountered. Regardless of the histologic classification scheme used (e.g., Kiel, NCI-Working Formulation), the majority (80%) of canine lymphomas are similar to medium- and high-grade non-Hodgkin's lymphomas in humans.[5,8-10] Approximately 70 to 80% of canine lymphomas are of B cell immunophenotypic derivation, with the remainder being primarily of T cell derivation.[5,8-10]

Feline Classification

In the past 10 to 15 years, the availability of widespread FeLV testing and vaccination programs has resulted in a shift in the frequency of anatomical type, immunophenotypic derivation, and retroviral association in cats that have lymphoma.[11,12] Before this era, the mediastinal and multicentric forms predominated, and lymphoma was associated with younger, FeLV-positive cats. Today, lymphoma primarily effects older FeLV-negative cats, and the alimentary form predominates (Table 91.2). The majority of affected cats (80 to 90%) are negative for FeLV antigenemia, in direct contrast to reports published before widespread availability of the FeLV test and vaccine when nearly 70% were FeLV-positive. As one would predict, along with a shift away from FeLV antigen-associated tumors has come a shift away from traditional signalment and relative frequency of anatomical sites. The median age of 9 to 10 years now reported is considerably higher than the 4 to 6 year medians reported before this era. The median age of cats within various anatomical tumor groupings has not changed, and sites traditionally associated with FeLV (i.e., mediastinal and multicentric) still usually occur in younger, FeLV antigenemic cats, whereas the alimentary form occurs most often in older, FeLV-negative cats. This change in the epidemiology of lymphoma in cats could be caused by FeLV vaccination itself, or the procedure of FeLV antigen testing prior to vaccination followed by separation of potentially infective cats from the susceptible population. Either situation would result in the observed reduction in the number of FeLV-positive cats that have lymphoma. A distinct class of lymphoma in cats, large granular lymphoma, has more recently been reported and is discussed in Chapter 95, Lymphoproliferative Disorders of Large Granular Lymphocytes.

CLINICAL PRESENTATION AND SIGNS

Canine Multicentric Lymphoma

Lymphoma affects primarily middle-aged to older dogs of either sex, and many different breeds are represented. The majority of dogs present with incidental generalized lymphadenopathy and are otherwise healthy. Only 10 to 20% of dogs are clinically ill (WHO substage b), with nonspecific signs, such as inappetence, anorexia, weight loss, and lethargy.[5–7] Paraneoplastic hypercalcemia may result in polyuria and polydipsia. In Stage V disease, if bone marrow involvement is significant, peripheral cytopenias and consequent neutropenic sepsis, thrombocytopenic hemorrhage, or anemia may be present.

Canine Lymphoma of Other Sites

Clinical signs at presentation reflect the anatomical form present in each individual case. The alimentary forms result in signs specific to the gastrointestinal tract, including vomiting, diarrhea, weight loss, and inappetence. Respiratory signs, including dyspnea and muffled heart sounds, may be seen in dogs that have mediastinal lymphoma. Precaval syndrome, i.e., pitting edema of the head, neck, and forelimbs secondary to tumor compression or invasion of the vena cava, may also be observed with this form. Paraneoplastic hypercalcemia is present in nearly half of the dogs that have mediastinal lymphomas[13]; therefore, polydipsia and polyuria are common presenting complaints in those cases. Cutaneous lymphoma is discussed at length in Chapter 96, Cutaneous Lymphoma. Tumors involving other sites result in signs attributable to the location (i.e., lameness with bone lesions, neurologic compromise with central nervous system [CNS] lymphoma).

Feline Lymphoma

No breed or sex predilections have been identified. Age and its association with FeLV status have been discussed previously. Cats that have FeLV-associated lymphoma are more likely to have pale mucous membranes caused by anemia. Unlike dogs that have lymphoma, cats are more likely to be ill at presentation, and 75% or more present in substage b.[11,12] The clinical presentation of lymphoma in cats depends on the anatomic site involved. Cats that have alimentary lymphoma have variable degrees of weight loss, unkempt hair coats, inappetence, chronic diarrhea, and vomiting. Mediastinal disease often results in severe respiratory distress from the presence of a large intrathoracic mass or pleural effusion. Cats that have renal lymphoma may have polyuria or polydipsia secondary to renal failure. Chronic serosanguinous nasal discharge, exophthalmos, and facial deformity are common signs in cats that have nasal lymphoma.

DIAGNOSIS

Physical Examination

Palpation of all assessable lymph nodes, including a rectal examination in the dog should be undertaken. The mucous membranes should be inspected for pallor or petechia indicative of anemia or thrombocytopenia secondary to significant bone marrow involvement and to detect icterus or uremic ulcers that develop from major organ infiltration. Abdominal palpation may reveal organomegaly, intestinal wall thickening, or mesenteric lymphadenopathy. Thoracic compression in cats

---

TABLE 91.1	World Health Organization Clinical Staging for Domestic Animals With Lymphoma
Stage	**Criteria**
I	Single lymph node
II	Multiple lymph nodes in a regional area
III	Generalized lymphadenopathy
IV	Liver and/or spleen (with or without stage III)
V	Bone marrow or blood involvement and/or any nonlymphoid organ (with or without stage I to IV)
Substage	
a	Without clinical signs of disease
b	With clinical signs of disease

From: World Health Organization. *TNM Classification of Tumors in Domestic Animals.* Geneva, World Health Organization; 1980.

TABLE 91.2	Characteristics of Feline Lymphoma by Anatomical Site			
Anatomical Site	**Relative Frequency**	**Age**	**T Cell Association**	**FeLV Positivity**
Alimentary	50–70%	Aged (~10–14 yrs)	Low	Low (≤5%)
Multicentric	10–25%	Depends on FeLV status[a]	Depends on FeLV status[a]	Approximately one-third
Mediastinal/Thymic	10–20%	Young	High	High (>80%)
Nasal	~10%	Aged	Low	Low
Renal	5–10%	Middle-aged	Low to moderate	Low to moderate
Other	5–25%	Mixed	Mixed	Mixed

[a] FeLV-positive cats tends to be younger, and their tumors are more frequently of T cell derivation.

and auscultation in both dogs and cats may suggest the presence of a mediastinal mass or pleural effusion. Funduscopic and ocular assessment may reveal abnormalities (e.g., uveitis, hemorrhage, ocular infiltration) in as many as half the dogs that have lymphoma.[14]

Hematologic Evaluation

A complete blood count (CBC), including a platelet count, is a necessary part of any evaluation of dogs or cats suspected of having lymphoma as hematologic abnormalities occur in the majority of cases.[15] Anemia, when present, is usually normocytic, normochromic (nonregenerative), reflecting anemia of chronic disease. If concurrent blood loss or paraneoplastic hemolysis are present, regenerative anemias may be observed. Cats that have FeLV-associated disease often have a macrocytic anemia. The anemia may be accompanied by thrombocytopenia and leukopenia and circulating atypical lymphocytes if significant myelophthisis is present. It is important to differentiate multicentric lymphoma with bone marrow involvement (i.e., Stage V disease) from acute lymphoblastic leukemia (see Chapter 93, Acute Lymphocytic Leukemia) as the prognosis for each is entirely different. Hypoproteinemia is most commonly observed in animals that have alimentary lymphoma secondary to chronic diarrhea.

Bone marrow aspiration is a diagnostic test in some cases and is required for clinical staging. In addition to neoplastic infiltration (Fig. 91.1), increased myeloid:erythroid ratios may be observed.

Serum Biochemical Testing

Test results may reflect the anatomical site involved (e.g., liver-specific enzyme activity or bilirubin eleva-

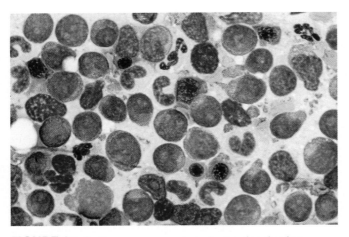

FIGURE 91.1 Bone marrow aspirate from a dog that has multicentric lymphoma and infiltration of bone marrow. Majority of cells are large lymphoid cells with high nuclear:cytoplasmic ratios, fine chromatin, prominent nucleoli, and basophilic cytoplasm. Occasional granulocytic and erythroid precursors are present. Wright–Giemsa stain. Original magnification 600×. Photomicrograph courtesy of Karen M. Young, University of Wisconsin-Madison.

tions may result from hepatic parenchymal infiltration). Approximately 15% of dogs that have lymphoma (40% of those that have mediastinal involvement) have hypercalcemia secondary to a paraneoplastic syndrome.[13,15] In cases of hypercalcemia of unknown origin, lymphoma should always be considered high on the differential disease list and thorough diagnostics directed at this possibility should ensue. In addition, the presence of hypercalcemia can serve as a marker for response to therapy or recrudescence of disease. Azotemia can occur secondary to renal infiltration with tumor, hypercalcemic nephrosis, or prerenal dehydration. Monoclonal globulin elevations may occur infrequently with B cell-derived lymphoma.

Retroviral Status

Retroviral screening (i.e., FeLV and FIV) is important in cats from a diagnostic and prognostic standpoint. The relative frequency of FeLV associations are presented in Table 91.2.

Imaging

Imaging by radiography, ultrasonography, or computed tomography (CT) may be of diagnostic importance in those cases lacking peripheral lymphadenopathy or limited to intracavitary or extranodal sites. Imaging is equally important for clinical staging (i.e., determining extent of disease), which may have a significant affect on the overall prognosis and alter the caregiver's willingness to pursue therapy. Abnormal findings, including pulmonary infiltrates (typically a diffuse interstitial pattern) or thoracic lymphadenopathy, are noted on thoracic radiographs in approximately two-thirds to three-quarters of dogs that have lymphoma.[16,17] Importantly, cranial mediastinal lymphadenopathy correlates negatively with both remission and survival duration.[16] For the more typical cases of multicentric lymphoma in dogs, imaging in the author's practice is limited to thoracic radiographs, as there is no prognostic difference between dogs with stage III versus IV disease (absence or presence of hepatic and splenic involvement), however, cranial mediastinal lymphadenopathy is of prognostic significance.[16] Special studies, including contrast imaging of the gastrointestinal tract, CT or myelographic studies of the CNS, and skeletal surveys are reserved for those cases in which the appropriate anatomical site is suspected.

However, involvement of sublumbar lymph nodes, spleen, or liver may be found by abdominal radiography or ultrasonography in approximately half of the cases in dogs. Abdominal ultrasonographic examination is most important in cats when intestinal lymphoma is suspected.

Cytologic and Histopathologic Diagnosis

Microscopic confirmation of lymphoma is the cornerstone of diagnosis in both the cat and dog. Cytologic

TABLE 91.3 Common Differential Diagnoses for Lymphoma

Anatomical Form	Differential List
Generalized Lymphadenopathy	Disseminated infections (e.g., bacterial, viral, rickettsial, parasitic, and fungal)
	Immune-mediated disorders (e.g., systemic lupus erythematosus, polyarthritis, vasculitis, and dermatopathy)
	Other hemopoietic tumors (e.g., leukemia, multiple myeloma, malignant and systemic histiocytosis)
	Tumors metastatic to lymph nodes
	In cats, many benign reactive hyperplastic conditions of lymph nodes (see text)
Alimentary	Infiltrative enteritis (e.g., lymphocytic and plasmacytic enteritis)
	Nonlymphoid intestinal neoplasms
	Granulomatous enteritis
	Gastrointestinal mast cell tumor in cats
Cutaneous	Infectious dermatitis (e.g., advanced pyoderma)
	Immune-mediated dermatitis (e.g., pemphigus)
	Other cutaneous neoplasms
Mediastinal	Thymoma
	Heart base tumor (chemodectoma)
	Ectopic thyroid tumor
	Pulmonary lymphomatoid granulomatosis
	Granulomatous disease (e.g., hilar lymphadenopathy with blastomycosis)

evaluation of fine-needle aspirates (FNA) by a skilled clinical pathologist may be adequate to make a diagnosis of lymphoma in dogs, however, conclusive histologic confirmation is recommended. Predominance of a homogenous population of immature lymphoid cells is suggestive of lymphoma. Avoidance of nodes draining reactive areas (e.g., submandibular nodes in the presence of periodontal disease) is recommended as reactive hyperplasia may mask (or mimic) the true neoplastic condition.

In the cat, cytologic evaluation of FNA of lymph nodes is insufficient for a diagnosis of lymphoma owing to difficulties encountered in distinguishing lymphoma from benign hyperplastic lymph node syndromes unique to the species. These include idiopathic peripheral lymphadenopathy, plexiform vascularization of lymph nodes, and peripheral lymph node hyperplasia of young cats.[18-21] Rather, whole lymph node excision is necessary, as the orientation and architectural abnormalities are necessary for diagnosis.

Histologic and cytologic samples can be analyzed by various histochemical and immunohistochemical techniques to determine immunophenotype (B versus T cell), tumor proliferation rates (e.g., Ki-67, proliferating cell nuclear antigen [PCNA], argyrophilic nucleolar organizer regions [AgNOR]), and histologic subtype (high-, intermediate-, or low-grade tumors).[5,8,10,22-24] At present only immunophenotype in dogs is consistently predictive of prognosis. Histologic markers of multidrug resistance and apoptotic pathways (e.g., P-glycoprotein, p53) are currently undergoing evaluation in dogs that have lymphoma; however, their significance requires further evaluation.[25-28]

Additional cytologic or histologic assessments may be warranted when extranodal sites are suspected. Thoracocentesis and cytologic evaluation of pleural fluid is often diagnostic in cats that have mediastinal lymphoma, however, it is less likely to be diagnostic in dogs that have effusions secondary to mediastinal involvement because tumor cells are often not found in the fluid. Conversely, cerebrospinal fluid (CSF) analysis is more helpful in dogs than cats that have CNS lymphoma owing to its extradural location in the latter species.[29,30] In cats suspected of having CNS lymphoma, bone marrow and renal involvement are often present concomitantly, and cytologic sampling of these organs is easier than sampling spinal sites.

DIFFERENTIAL DIAGNOSIS

The differential diagnosis for lymphoma varies with the anatomical form of the disease. Common differential diagnoses are presented in Table 91.3.

PROGNOSIS

Prognostic Factors in Dogs

Factors known to affect or suspected of affecting remission rates or remission and survival durations in dogs that have lymphoma are presented in Table 91.4. Most studies fail to correlate age, body weight, or breed with prognosis. Clinical stage, with the exception of significant stage V disease, does not appear to significantly affect prognosis in dogs. The exception would include those cases in which bone marrow is heavily infiltrated, in which obvious leukemia is present, or in which peripheral cytopenias exist secondary to myelophthisis. Two factors that consistently correlate with prognosis in dogs are immunophenotype and WHO substage status.[5-9,16] Many reports have confirmed that dogs that have CD3 immunoreactive tumors (i.e., T cell derivation) are associated with significantly shorter remission and survival durations. Similarly, dogs that have sub-

TABLE 91.4 Factors Known or Suspected to Affect Prognosis in Dogs with Lymphoma

Factor	Strength of Association	Comments
WHO[a] clinical stage	Weak	Likely only predictive of outcome in Stage V disease with marked marrow involvement.
WHO[a] substage	Strong	Dogs with substage b experience shorter remission and survival durations.
Immunophenotype	Strong	Dogs with T cell lymphoma experience shorter remission and survival durations than dogs with B cell tumors.
Hypercalcemia	Moderate	Poorer prognosis is not independent, more likely due to T cell association.
Prolonged steroid pretreatment	Moderate	Most studies show previous steroid use shortens response durations.
Sex	Moderate	Several large studies report that males experience shorter remission and survival durations. Other reports contradictory.
Proliferation rate	Moderate	High proliferation may confer better response. Other reports contradictory.
Cranial mediastinal lymphadenopathy	Moderate to strong	Large compilation of cases reports association with shorter remission and survival durations. Other reports contradictory.
Histologic grade	Weak	Low-grade tumors less likely to respond to chemotherapy but may have a longer natural course.
P-glycoprotein expression	Moderate	Associated with poor response rates and shorter remission and survival durations.

[a] WHO = World Health Organization

stage b disease (i.e., clinically ill) also do poorly compared with dogs with substage a disease.

Various other factors have been reported to correlate with prognosis but should be considered in light of the following. Some are not found to correlate in all studies, others are preliminary reports, or contradictory reports exist in the literature. Several indices correlate only following univariate analysis, however, when scrutinized by multivariate analysis (where all factors are considered together), they are no longer significant. Hypercalcemia is such an example. In several reports, it is associated with a poor prognosis, however, if multivariate analysis is performed, it is no longer predictive, primarily because dogs that have hypercalcemia are more likely to have T cell-derived lymphoma, which is a much stronger correlate.

Prognostic Factors in Cats

Unlike the dog, CD3 immunoreactivity has not been established as a negative prognostic index in the cat and may reflect the wider variations in frequency of different anatomical forms of lymphoma and the difficulty in separating out differences.[11] Factors most strongly associated with a more positive outcome in cats are complete response to therapy (unfortunately this cannot be determined before therapy), negative FeLV status, early clinical stage, substage a, and the addition of doxorubicin to the treatment protocol.[11,31,32] In general, cats that are not FeLV antigenemic and that achieve a complete response on combination-based chemotherapy protocols have a higher likelihood of long-term survival, with approximately one third surviving 1.5 years after diagnosis. Overall, cats that have nasal lymphoma have the best prognosis, as local radiotherapy (or chemotherapy if radiotherapy is not available) results in excellent control with median survivals approaching 1.5 years.

LYMPHOMA OF HORSES

Lymphoma is much less common in horses than in dogs and cats, with a reported frequency of between 0.4 and 5% of all neoplasms in the horse.[33,34] As in other species, several anatomical forms can occur, with multicentric or generalized lymphoma involving peripheral and internal lymph nodes occurring most frequently.[35,36] The alimentary form appears to be the next most common form followed by extranodal cutaneous, respiratory, and ocular forms. Most are intermediate- or low-grade histologic forms, and high-grade forms are encountered less commonly than in other domestic species.

Presenting signs are variable, depending on the anatomical site involved. However, nonspecific signs of chronic disease, including weight loss, inappetence, lethargy, and anemia, are most commonly reported. Diagnosis results from cytologic or histologic assessment of affected lymphoid or extranodal tissues or malignant effusions from the pleural or peritoneal space.

Little objective data exist on the prognosis and outcome of horses with lymphoma. Short-term survival appears to be the norm for the multicentric and alimentary forms, although long-term survivals have been reported for solitary alimentary forms treated by surgical resection alone.[37] The cutaneous form of lymphoma in horses can wax and wain in its clinical course, and horses can survive for many months or years with the disease.

REFERENCES

1. **Hayes HM, Tarone RE, Cantor KP, et al.** Case-control study of canine malignant lymphoma: positive association with dog owner's use of 2,4-dichlorophenoxyacetic acid herbicides. J Natl Cancer Inst 1991;83:1226–1231.
2. **Zahm SH, Blair A.** Pesticides and non-Hodgkin's lymphoma. Cancer Res 1992;52:5485S–5488S.
3. **Reif JS, Lower KS, Ogilvie GK.** Residential exposure to magnetic fields and risk of canine lymphoma. Am J Epidemiol 1995;141:352–359.
4. **Teske E, de Vos JP, Egberink HF, Vos JH.** Clustering in canine malignant lymphoma. Vet Quarterly 1994;16:134–136.
5. **Vail DM, Kisseberth WC, Obradovich JE, et al.** Assessment of potential doubling time (Tpot), argyrophilic nucleolar organizer regions (AgNOR), and proliferating cell nuclear antigen (PCNA) as predictors of therapy response in canine non-Hodgkin's lymphoma. Exp Hematol 1996;24:807–815.
6. **Keller ET, MacEwen EG, Rosenthal RC, et al.** Evaluation of prognostic factors and sequential combination chemotherapy for canine lymphoma. J Vet Intern Med 1993;7:289–295.
7. **Valerius KD, Susaneck SJ, Withrow SJ et al.** Doxorubicin alone or in combination with asparaginase, followed by cyclophosphamide, vincristine, and prednisone for treatment of multicentric lymphoma in dogs: 121 cases (1987–1995). J Am Vet Med Assoc 1997;210:512–516.
8. **Teske E, van Heerde P, Rutteman GR, et al.** Prognostic factors for treatment of malignant lymphoma in dogs. J Am Vet Med Assoc 1994;205:1722–1728.
9. **Greenlee PG, Filippa DA, Quimby FW, et al.** Lymphomas in dogs. Cancer 1990;66:480–490.
10. **Fournel-Fleury C, Magnol JP, Bricaire P, et al.** Cytohistological and immunological classification of canine malignant lymphomas: comparison with human non-Hodgkin's lymphomas. J Comp Pathol 1997;117:35–59.
11. **Vail DM, Moore A Ogilvie GK, et al.** Feline lymphoma (145 cases): proliferation indices, CD3 immunoreactivity and their association with prognosis in 90 cats receiving therapy. J Vet Intern Med 1998;12:349–354.
12. **Mauldin GE, Mooney SC, Meleo KA, et al.** Chemotherapy in 132 cats with lymphoma: 1988–1994. Proceedings of the 15th Annual Conference of the Veterinary Cancer Society, Tucson, AZ, 1995;35–36 (abstract).
13. **Rosenberg MP, Matus RE, Patnaik AK.** Prognostic factors in dogs with lymphoma and associated hypercalcemia. J Vet Intern Med 1991;5:268–271.
14. **Krohne SDG, Henderson NM, Richardson RC, Vestre WA.** Ocular involvement in canine lymphoma, a retrospective study. Proceedings of the 7th Annual Conference of the Veterinary Cancer Society, Madison, WI, 1987;27 (abstract).
15. **Madewell BR.** Hematological and bone marrow cytological abnormalities in 75 dogs with malignant lymphoma. J Am Anim Hosp Assoc 1986;22:235–240.
16. **Starrak GS, Berry CR, Page RL, et al.** Correlation between thoracic radiographic changes and remission/survival duration in 270 dogs with lymphosarcoma. Vet Radiol Ultrasound 1997;38:411–418.
17. **Blackwood L, Sullivan M, Lawson H.** Radiographic abnormalities in canine multicentric lymphoma: a review of 84 cases. J Small Anim Pract 1997;38:62–69.
18. **Moore FM, Emerson WE, Cotter SM, DeLellis RA.** Distinctive peripheral lymph node hyperplasia of young cats. Vet Pathol 1986;23:386–391.
19. **Mooney SC, Patnaik AK, Hayes AA, MacEwen EG.** Generalized lymphadenopathy resembling lymphoma in cats: six cases (1972–1976). J Am Vet Med Assoc 1987;190:897–900.
20. **Lucke VM, Davies JD, Wood CM, Whitbread TJ.** Plexiform vascularization of lymph nodes: An unusual but distinctive lymphadenopathy in cats. J Comp Pathol 1987;97:109–119.
21. **Kirkpatrick CE, Moore FM, Patnaik AK, Whiteley HE:** Argyrophilic, intracellular bacteria in some cats with idiopathic peripheral lymphadenopathy. J Comp Pathol 1989;101:341–349.
22. **Fournel-Fleury C, Magnol JP, Chabanne L, et al.** Growth fractions in canine non-Hodgkin's lymphoma as determined in situ by the expression of the Ki-67 antigen. J Comp Pathol 1997;117:61–72.
23. **Vail DM, Kravis LD, Kissiberth WC, et al.** Application of rapid CD3 immunophenotype analysis and argyrophilic nucleolar organizer region (AgNOR) frequency to fine needle aspirate specimens from dogs with lymphoma. Vet Clin Pathol 1997;26:66–69.
24. **Teske E, Rutteman GR, Kuipers-Dijkshoorn NJ, et al.** DNA ploidy and cell kinetic characteristics in canine non-Hodgkin's lymphoma. Exp Hematol 1993;21:579–584.
25. **Moore AS, Leveille CR, Reimann KA, et al.** The expression of P-glycoprotein in canine lymphoma and its association with multidrug resistance. Cancer Invest 1995;13:475–479.
26. **Bergman PJ, Ogilvie GK, Powers BE.** Monoclonal antibody C219 immunohistochemistry against P-glycoprotein: Sequential analysis and predictive ability in dogs with lymphoma. J Vet Intern Med 1996;10:354–359.
27. **Lee JJ, Hughes CS, Fine RL, et al.** P-glycoprotein expression in canine lymphoma. Cancer 1996;77:1892–1898.
28. **Gamblin RM, Sagartz JE, Couto CG.** Overexpression of p53 tumor suppressor protein in spontaneously arising neoplasms of dogs. Am J Vet Res 1997;58:857–863.
29. **Lane SB, Kornegay JN, Duncan JR, Oliver JE Jr.** Feline spinal lymphosarcoma: a retrospective evaluation of 23 cats. J Vet Intern Med 1994;8:99–104.
30. **Spodnick GJ, Berg J, Moore FM, Cotter SM.** Spinal lymphoma in cats: 21 cases (1976–1989). J Am Vet Med Assoc 1992;200:373–376.
31. **Moore AS, Cotter SM, Frimberger AE, et al.** A comparison of doxorubicin and COP maintenance of remission in cats with lymphoma. J Vet Intern Med 1996;10:372–375.
32. **Mooney SC, Hayes AA, MacEwen EG, et al.** Treatment and prognostic factors in lymphoma in cats: 103 cases (1977–1981). J Am Vet Med Assoc 1989;194:696–702.
33. **Priester WA, Mantel N.** Occurrence of tumors in domestic animals. Data from 12 United States and Canadian colleges of veterinary medicine. J Natl Cancer Inst 1971;47:1333–1339.
34. **Baker JF, Leyland A.** Histologic survey of tumors of the horse with particular reference to those of the skin. Vet Rec 1975;96:419–422.
35. **Rebhun WC, Bertone A.** Equine lymphosarcoma. J Am Vet Med Assoc 1984;184:720–721.
36. **Schneider DA.** Lymphoproliferative and myeloproliferative disorders. In: Robinson NE, ed. Current therapy in equine medicine. 4th ed. Philadelphia: WB Saunders, 1997;295–299.
37. **Dabareiner RM, Sullens KE, Goodrich LR.** Large colon resection for treatment of lymphosarcoma in two horses. J Am Vet Med Assoc 1996;208:895–897.

CHAPTER 92

Lymphoma: Principles of Management

• DAVID M. VAIL

The management of lymphoma in companion animal species can be gratifying initially as response rates approaching 90% in dogs and 70% in cats result after various chemotherapeutic approaches. Unfortunately, most animals eventually succumb to disseminated recurrence of their disease in a more chemotherapy-resistant form.

THERAPY

Once a diagnosis is established, untreated dogs and cats generally live an average of 4 to 6 weeks after diagnosis. Lymphoma, typically a systemic disease, requires a systemic approach to therapy (i.e., chemotherapy). Exceptions to this include lymphoma in solitary sites or extranodal lymphomas in which localized therapy, involving either surgery or radiotherapy, may be indicated.

Systemic Chemotherapy in Dogs that have Lymphoma

Various chemotherapeutic approaches have been reported in the veterinary literature for the treatment of lymphoma. This likely reflects our inability to achieve cure in the majority of cases. Although remission rates approach 80 to 90% with available combination chemotherapeutic protocols and the quality of life of our patients is generally excellent during the period of remission, the majority of dogs eventually die from recurrence of multidrug-resistant disease.[1]

Prior to initiating therapy, caregivers should be educated about the advantages and disadvantages of various chemotherapeutic protocols. Several factors should be considered and discussed, including the cost, time commitment, efficacy, toxicity, and experience of the clinician with the protocols in question. The availability of generic drugs provides more affordable protocols to a larger segment of our veterinary clientele. In general, more complex drug combinations represent a greater expense, are more time consuming (i.e., repeated office visits, closer monitoring), and are more likely to result in toxicity than simpler, single-agent protocols. However, as a general rule, more complex combination protocols result in longer remission and survival durations than single-agent protocols.

A complete listing of all available protocols for dogs that have lymphoma is beyond the scope of this chapter, and the reader is referred to a recent review and other reports.[1-3] Rather, an example of the combination protocol used by the author and the most widely used single-agent protocol are presented.

Combination protocols used in veterinary practice are usually modifications of combinations of cyclophosphamide (C), doxorubicin (H, hydroxydaunarubicin), vincristine (O, Oncovin®), and prednisone (P) or CHOP protocols initially designed for treating people who have lymphoma. Regardless of which CHOP-based protocol is used, overall median remission and survival times are approximately 8 and 12 months, respectively.[1] Approximately 20 to 25% of treated dogs are alive 2 years or longer after initiation of therapy. Response rates and length of response vary according to the presence or absence of prognostic factors previously discussed in Chapter 91, Lymphoma. Historically, after an induction period during which drugs are given weekly, treatment intervals are slowly spread out, and drugs are given less frequently in what is termed the maintenance phase of the protocol. Important questions yet to be answered in veterinary medicine are how long the maintenance phase should last and whether maintenance therapy should be used at all. In most human protocols, no benefit to continued maintenance therapy has been shown after the typical 6 month induction phase of therapy. Therefore, therapy is discontinued until recurrence is observed. In veterinary medicine, no definitive studies exist to support or refute maintenance therapy. Presently, the author prefers a modified version of the University of Wisconsin-Madison lymphoma protocol outlined in Table 92.1.[4] Chemotherapy is discontinued at 6 months if the dog is in complete remission at that time. This protocol results in remission in approximately 90% of dogs treated, and remission and survival lengths are similar to those historically observed when long-term maintenance is used. After therapy is discontinued, dogs are reevaluated monthly by physical examination with special attention to lymph node size. If recurrence is suspected, the diagnostic steps outlined in Chapter 91, Lymphoma are reinstituted.

TABLE 92.1	Combination Chemotherapy Protocol for Dogs With Lymphoma		
Treatment Week	**Drug, Dosage, and Route**	**Treatment Week**	**Drug, Dosage, and Route**
1	Vincristine, 0.5–0.7 mg/m^2, IV L-Asparaginase, 400 Units/kg, SC Prednisone, 2.0 mg/kg, PO, daily	11	Vincristine, 0.5–0.7 mg/m^2, IV
2	Cyclophosphamide 200 mg/m^2, IV Prednisone, 1.5 mg/kg, PO, daily	13	Cyclophosphamide, 200 mg/m^2, IV
3	Vincristine, 0.5–0.7 mg/m^2, IV Prednisone, 1.0 mg/kg, PO, daily	15	Vincristine, 0.5–0.7 mg/m^2, IV
4	Doxorubicin, 30 mg/m^2, IV Prednisone, 0.5 mg/kg, PO, daily	17	Doxorubicin, 30 mg/m^2, IV
6	Vincristine, 0.5–0.7 mg/m^2, IV	19	Vincristine, 0.5–0.7 mg/m^2, IV
7	Cyclophosphamide, 200 mg/m^2, IV	21	Cyclophosphamide, 200 mg/m^2, IV
8	Vincristine, 0.5–0.7 mg/m^2, IV	23	Vincristine, 0.5–0.7 mg/m^2, IV
9[a]	Doxorubicin, 30 mg/m^2, IV	25[b]	Doxorubicin, 30 mg/m^2, IV

[a] If in complete remission at week 9, continue to week 11.
[b] If in complete remission at week 25, therapy is discontinued, and monthly reevaluations are instituted.

Doxorubicin is the most effective and commonly used single agent available for dogs that have lymphoma[2,5,6] and is given at a dosage of 30 mg/m^2 intravenously every 3 weeks for a total of 5 treatments. Response rates of 75 to 80% result, and median remission and survival durations of 5 and 7 months, respectively, are reported. Advantages of this single-agent protocol include a shorter time commitment, fewer hospital visits, and side effects that are attributable to one drug.

Alternatives should be offered to caregivers who, for financial or other concerns, decline more aggressive systemic chemotherapy. In these cases prednisone (2 mg/kg by mouth daily) often results in short remissions of approximately 1 to 2 months. It is important for clients to understand that, should more aggressive therapy subsequently be pursued, dogs receiving prior prednisone therapy are more likely to develop multiple-drug resistance and to experience shorter remission and survival durations with combination protocols. This is particularly true if prednisone has been used long term or if dogs have experienced recurrence of disease while on prednisone.[7] Therefore, the earlier clients opt for more aggressive therapy, the more likely a durable response will result.

Systemic Chemotherapy in Cats that have Lymphoma

Several combination chemotherapeutic protocols for cats have been reported and reviewed.[1,8–10] It is now clear that in cats the addition of doxorubicin to cyclophosphamide (C), Oncovin (O) or vincristine, prednisone (P) (COP)-based protocols results in longer remission and survival durations than does COP alone.[8,10] In general, cats do not experience the same response rates or remission and survival durations as dogs that have lymphoma; complete response rates in cats are between 50 and 70%, and overall median remission and survival durations are approximately 4 and 6 months, respectively. This is tempered somewhat with the knowledge that of those cats achieving a complete response with combination chemotherapy, a larger proportion (30 to 40%) experience more durable remission and survival times (i.e., ≥2 years) than do dogs. The response rate and length of response vary according to the presence or absence of prognostic factors discussed previously in Chapter 91, Lymphoma. The modified CHOP-based protocol preferred by the author for cats is presented in Table 92.2.

Reinduction or Rescue Therapy

Unfortunately, most dogs and cats that have lymphoma experience recurrence of their disease after initially successful chemotherapy, and at this time the disease usually is more resistant to chemotherapy. There is recent evidence that tumor cells from dogs that have recurrent lymphoma are more likely to express the gene encoding the P-glycoprotein transmembrane drug pump that is often associated with multiple-drug resistance.[11–13] At the first recurrence, it is recommended that reinduction be attempted with the protocol that was initially successful. Although second remissions usually can be achieved, the length of responses are, in general, half that encountered in the initial therapy. A subset of animals, however, enjoy long-term responses.

If reinduction fails, the use of so-called rescue agents or protocols may be attempted. Rescue agents are drugs or drug combinations that are not found in the standard CHOP protocol and are specifically reserved for use in the drug-resistant setting. Various rescue protocols have been reported and reviewed in the veterinary literature.[1,14] The most common protocols include single agent or combination usage of actinomycin D, mitoxantrone, doxorubicin (if doxorubicin was not part of the original induction protocol), a combination of doxorubicin and dacarbazine, and mechlorethamine (M), Oncovin (O) or vincristine, procarbazine (P), and prednisone (P) (MOPP). Mitoxantrone, doxorubicin, and MOPP have also been advocated in cats that have resistant relapse.

TABLE 92.2 **Combination Chemotherapy Protocol for Cats With Lymphoma**

Treatment Week	Drug, Dosage, and Route	Treatment Week	Drug, Dosage, and Route
1	Vincristine, 0.5–0.7 mg/m^2, IV L-Asparaginase, 400 Units/kg, SC Prednisone, 2.0 mg/kg, PO, daily	11	Vincristine, 0.5–0.7 mg/m^2, IV
2	Cyclophosphamide 200 mg/m^2, IV Prednisone, 2.0 mg/kg, PO, daily	13	Chlorambucil, 1.4 mg/kg, PO
3	Vincristine, 0.5–0.7 mg/m^2, IV Prednisone, 1.0 mg/kg, PO, daily	15	Vincristine, 0.5–0.7 mg/m^2, IV
4	Doxorubicin, 25 mg/m^2, IV Prednisone, 1.0 mg/kg, PO[a]	17	Methotrexate, 0.5–0.8 mg/kg IV
6	Vincristine, 0.5–0.7 mg/m^2, IV	19	Vincristine, 0.5–0.7 mg/m^2, IV
7	Cyclophosphamide 200 mg/m^2, IV	21	Chlorambucil, 1.4 mg/kg, PO
8	Vincristine, 0.5–0.7 mg/m^2, IV	23	Vincristine, 0.5–0.7 mg/m^2, IV
9[b]	Doxorubicin, 25 mg/m^2, IV	25[c]	Doxorubicin, 25 mg/m^2, IV

[a] Prednisone is continued (1 mg/kg, PO) every other day from this point on.
[b] If in complete remission at week 9, continue to week 11.
[c] If in complete remission at week 25, therapy is continued at 3 week intervals following the same sequence of drugs used in weeks 11 through 25 until week 51. If in complete remission at week 51, continue treatments at 4 week intervals using the same sequence of drugs with the exception that methotrexate is substituted for doxorubicin from this point forward.

Overall rescue response rates of 40 to 50% are reported; however, most responses are not durable, typically lasting for 1.5 to 2 months. A small subset of animals will enjoy longer remissions after rescue.

Therapy for Extranodal Lymphoma

If extranodal involvement is part of multicentric disease, then a systemic protocol previously discussed should be instituted. However, if the extranodal site is solitary and not part of a multicentric presentation, localized therapy may be used without systemic chemotherapy. In these cases strict adherence to staging procedures, including bone marrow evaluation and radiographic or ultrasonographic imaging of the thorax and abdomen, is warranted to ensure the disease is confined to a single site. Localized therapy, i.e., surgical resection, radiotherapy, or both, is often effective. Clients should be forewarned, however, that systemic disease is likely to occur months to years later, and the animal should be monitored regularly. In the author's opinion, systemic therapy should be withheld until systemic disease is documented.

If central nervous system (CNS) involvement is part of a more generalized process, the penetration of chemotherapeutic drugs through the blood–brain barrier (BBB) may be of concern, and additional drugs are recommended. In standard CHOP protocols, only prednisone consistently penetrates the BBB. The addition of cytosine arabinoside, which does achieve therapeutic levels in cerebrospinal fluid, to a CHOP-based protocol is recommended in such cases. Radiotherapy, either directed to the entire neural axis in the case of multifocal CNS lymphoma or to specific CNS locations in cases of solitary central or spinal lymphoma, can also be effective. Cytoreductive surgery has been attempted in a small number of cases of extradural lymphoma in both cats

and dogs with mixed results.[15–17] Therapy for cutaneous lymphoma is discussed in Chapter 96, Cutaneous Lymphoma.

Ancillary Therapy for Paraneoplastic Hypercalcemia

As with any paraneoplastic condition, removing the inciting disease is the treatment of choice. This is relatively straight-forward when dealing with naive (previously untreated) lymphoma or multiple myeloma as response rates of 90% are typical. In cases in which the primary tumor is less likely to be dealt with satisfactorily in the short term (e.g., metastatic anal sac adenocarcinoma) or the degree of hypercalcemia is significantly affecting the quality of life of the patient, ancillary therapy directed specifically at lowering serum calcium levels should be instituted. An algorithm for selecting appropriate treatment for hypercalcemia of malignancy is presented in Figure 92.1.

For the acute treatment of hypercalcemia, saline diuresis (typically at twice maintenance levels) with a high sodium crystalloid (e.g., 0.9% NaCl) is the cornerstone of therapy. If clinical signs are significant or the magnitude of hypercalcemia is great (>15 mg/dL), the addition of calcitonin (4 to 8 U/kg intramuscularly or subcutaneously twice daily to effect) is effective in the short term. Animals treated in this way should be monitored closely for overhydration and hypocalcemia. It is important to stress that prednisone, or other corticosteroids, should not be used as a means of lowering serum calcium until a diagnosis has been established. Instituting corticosteroid therapy without a diagnosis in cases of lymphoma or myeloma can result in difficulty in making a diagnosis and in subsequent short-lived remissions. Additionally, when the tumor recurs, the likelihood of multidrug resistance is much higher when the patient

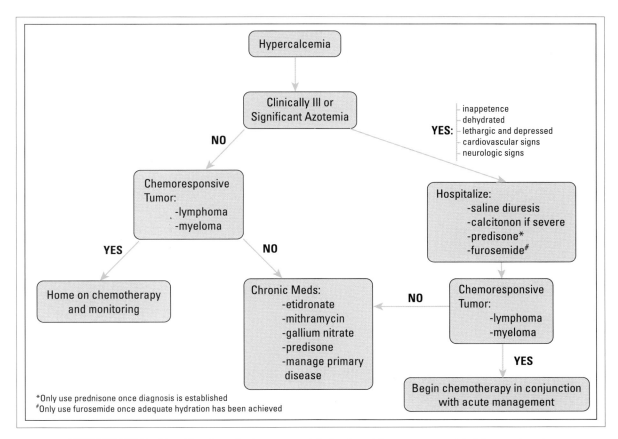

FIGURE 92.1 Algorithm for selecting appropriate treatment for cancer-associated hypercalcemia.

is on single-agent prednisone therapy.[7] Also, the use of furosemide is overstated in most references as its addition to saline diureses adds little benefit to diuresis alone. If furosemide is initiated prior to establishing adequate hydration, decrease in renal blood flow may occur and exacerbate hypercalcemia.

If the primary tumor is not chemoresponsive, chronic therapy for hypercalcemia may be instituted. The bisphosphonate etidronate (Didronel; for dogs, 5 mg/kg/d by mouth; for cats, 10 mg/kg/d by mouth) is the most effective therapy in the author's experience. Other drugs that have been used infrequently in veterinary practice for treating hypercalcemia include mithramycin (25 μg/kg intravenously every 5 to 21 days, depending on response) and gallium nitrate (2.5 μg/kg intravenously once a day for 5 days). Long-term prednisone therapy may also be of benefit in these cases.

Therapy of Lymphoma in Horses

Information regarding therapy in horses that have lymphoma is limited. Systemic approaches have been derived mainly from modifications of combination chemotherapeutic protocols used in dogs and cats.[18] Remission rates and survival times are not reported, although anecdotally approximately 50% of cases respond for periods of months or more. Single-agent corticosteroids

have been used for palliation. If the disease is found to be solitary, localized approaches (e.g., surgical resection or radiotherapy) may be of benefit. Long-term survival has been reported for solitary alimentary forms treated by surgical resection alone.[19]

The Future of Lymphoma Therapy

Based on the similarity of results reported with the many varied combination chemotherapy protocols, it appears that the veterinary profession has gone as far as possible with available protocols. All combination protocols reported to date are arriving at the same 10- to 12-month median survival brick wall. Advances in remission and survival durations await the development of new chemotherapeutic drugs or novel treatment modalities. Active areas of investigation in both human and veterinary medicine include the exploration of novel immunomodulatory approaches and mechanisms of avoiding or abrogating multidrug resistance, enhancing tumor apoptosis (programmed cell death), and targeting therapy with immunoconjugates (i.e., antibody-directed therapies). As a practitioner who experiences both the gratification that comes with high initial response rates and the frustration of equally high relapse rates in my patients, I eagerly await new advances.

REFERENCES

1. **Vail DM.** Recent advances in chemotherapy for lymphoma of dogs and cats. Compend Cont Educ Pract Vet 1993;15:1031–1037.
2. **Valerius KD, Susaneck SJ,** Withrow SJ, et al. Doxorubicin alone or in combination with asparaginase, followed by cyclophosphamide, vincristine, and prednisone for treatment of multicentric lymphoma in dogs: 121 cases (1987–1995). J Am Vet Med Assoc 1997;210:512–516.
3. **Teske E, van Heerde P, Rutteman GR, et al.** Prognostic factors for treatment of malignant lymphoma in dogs. J Am Vet Med Assoc 1994;205:1722–1728.
4. **Keller ET, MacEwen EG, Rosenthal RC, et al.** Evaluation of prognostic factors and sequential combination chemotherapy for canine lymphoma. J Vet Intern Med 1993;7:289–295.
5. **Carter RF, Harris CK, Withrow SJ, et al.** Chemotherapy of canine lymphoma with histopathological correlation: Doxorubicin alone compared to COP as first treatment regimen. J Am Anim Hosp Assoc 1987;23:587–596.
6. **Postorino NC, Susaneck SJ, Withrow SJ, et al.** Single agent therapy with adriamycin for canine lymphosarcoma. J Am Anim Hosp Assoc 1989;25:221–225.
7. **Price GS, Page RL, Fischer BM, et al.** Efficacy and toxicity of doxorubicin/cyclophosphamide maintenance therapy in dogs with multicentric lymphosarcoma. J Vet Intern Med 1991;5:259–262.
8. **Vail DM, Moore AS, Ogilvie GK, et al.** Feline lymphoma (145 cases): proliferation indices, CD3 immunoreactivity and their association with prognosis in 90 cats receiving therapy. J Vet Intern Med 1998;12:349–354.
9. **Mauldin GE, Mooney SC, Meleo KA, et al.** Chemotherapy in 132 cats with lymphoma: 1988–1994. Proc 15th Annual Conference of the Veterinary Cancer Society, Tucson, AZ, 1995;35–36 (abstract).
10. **Moore AS, Cotter SM, Frimberger AE, et al.** A comparison of doxorubicin and COP maintenance of remission in cats with lymphoma. J Vet Intern Med 1996;10:372–375.
11. **Moore AS, Leveille CR, Reimann KA, et al.** The expression of P-glycoprotein in canine lymphoma and its association with multidrug resistance. Cancer Invest 1995;13:475–479.
12. **Bergman PJ, Ogilvie GK, Powers BE.** Monoclonal antibody C219 immunohistochemistry against P-glycoprotein: sequential analysis and predictive ability in dogs with lymphoma. J Vet Intern Med 1996;10:354–359.
13. **Lee JJ, Hughes CS, Fine RL, et al.** P-glycoprotein expression in canine lymphoma. Cancer 1996;77:1892–1898.
14. **Mauldin GE, Mooney SC, Mauldin GN.** MOPP chemotherapy as rescue for cats with refractory lymphoma. Proc Annual Conference of the American College of Veterinary Radiology and Veterinary Cancer Society, Chicago, IL, 1997;98 (abstract).
15. **Lane SB, Kornegay JN, Duncan JR, Oliver JE Jr.** Feline spinal lymphosarcoma: A retrospective evaluation of 23 cats. J Vet Intern Med 1994;8:99–104.
16. **Spodnick GJ, Berg J, Moore FM, Cotter SM.** Spinal lymphoma in cats: 21 cases (1976–1989). J Am Vet Med Assoc 1992;200:373–376.
17. **Couto CG, Cullen J, Pedroia V, Turrel JM.** Central nervous system lymphosarcoma in the dog. J Am Vet Med Assoc 1984;184:809–813.
18. **Schneider DA.** Lymphoproliferative and myeloproliferative disorders. In: Robinson NE, ed. Current therapy in equine medicine. 4th ed. Philadelphia: WB Saunders, 1997;295–299.
19. **Dabareiner RM, Sullens KE, Goodrich LR.** Large colon resection for treatment of lymphosarcoma in two horses. J Am Vet Med Assoc 1996;208:895–897.

CHAPTER 93

Acute Lymphocytic Leukemia

• JAIME F. MODIANO and STUART C. HELFAND

Acute lymphocytic or lymphoblastic leukemia (ALL) is a neoplastic disease characterized by the clonal proliferation of malignant lymphoid progenitors in the bone marrow. Unlike chronic lymphocytic leukemia (CLL), the malignant cells in ALL exhibit little differentiation potential. Blast cells and pro-lymphocytes are the predominant cells in ALL (Fig. 93.1). Lymphocytic leukemias of large granular lymphocytes that may be distinct from ALL and CLL, or a variant of either, also have been identified in dogs,[1,2] cats,[3,4] rats,[5] and ferrets.[6] Like other leukemias, ALL arises from the bone marrow, in contrast to lymphomas that arise from lymphoid cells outside the bone marrow.

ALL can present in a leukemic phase (leukocytosis with large numbers of circulating blast cells in the peripheral blood), subleukemic phase (normal to reduced leukocyte concentrations with few circulating blast cells in the peripheral blood), or aleukemic phase (leukopenia with no detectable circulating blast cells in the peripheral blood). The presence of circulating blast cells may reflect their stage of transformation and the presence on these cells of adhesion molecules or receptors for cytokines or chemokines that promote entry into the vasculature. ALL cells can infiltrate solid organs, including the spleen, liver, and lymph nodes. In these cases, it is virtually impossible to distinguish between ALL and stage V lymphoma.

BIOLOGY OF ALL

The terminology used to distinguish acute and chronic leukemias was initially established based on the survival time of affected patients.[7] This classification was then adapted to reflect the finding that in acute leukemias there is usually a preponderance of immature proliferating cells, whereas most cells in chronic leukemias appear well differentiated. In human patients, ALL is the most common leukemia of children, but it is seen less frequently in adults.[7,8] In animals, ALL can occur in most domestic and exotic species. At present, ALL is probably most significant as a veterinary clinical entity in dogs and cats. The bovine leukemia complex is an important model of retroviral-induced tumors, but it is not generally deemed to be an economically significant disease.

Recent improvements in diagnostic methodologies will allow us to recognize ALL more frequently in exotic animals kept as pets or within zoologic collections.

The incidence of ALL in dogs and cats is uncertain. Studies performed 2 decades ago by Dorn, cited in previous editions of this textbook, identified leukemia as a rare condition (224/100,000 cats, and 30/100,000 dogs). Moreover, it has been suggested that the ratio of lymphoma to leukemia seen at referral institutions may be skewed, as veterinarians in general practice may be more likely to refer cases of leukemia and treat cases of lymphoma in their own practices.[9] We recently evaluated 23 consecutive cases of canine and feline leukemia referred for diagnosis to the Texas Veterinary Medical Center between 1996 and 1998.[10] This study showed that dogs had a bimodal age distribution, with 6/16 being 1 to 4 years old and 8/16 being >8 years old. Most of the dogs were female (11/16), and 10 were spayed. No breed predilection was observed. Six of 7 cats were domestic breeds, but there was no age or sex predilection.

Our experience suggests that the dynamics of leukemia in small animals may be changing. As more veterinarians routinely use complete blood counts in health maintenance programs, cases of leukemia may be identified more often. This alone suggests that the incidence of cases seen at referral centers should be increasing. However, the historically poor prognosis associated with leukemia in small animals also may influence an owner's decision to not pursue treatment and opt for euthanasia. This may artificially decrease the incidence of leukemia seen at veterinary referral centers. Furthermore, improved control of retroviral diseases in cats through preventive measures also may have reduced the incidence of feline leukemia. The recent advent of large, centralized diagnostic pathology centers that are used by representative populations of practicing veterinarians may permit the design of studies to address the dynamics of the incidence and prevalence of leukemia in domestic animals.

CLASSIFICATION OF ALL

The French-American-British (FAB) cooperative group has established three distinct morphologic classifica-

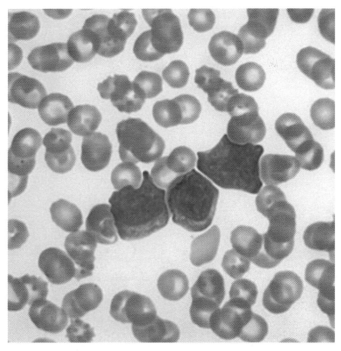

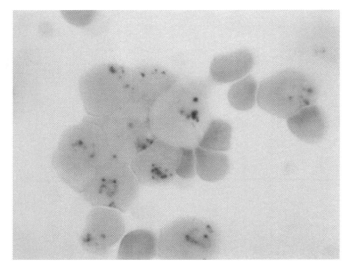

FIGURE 93.2 Enzyme cytochemistry of blast cells from a case of B cell ALL. Photomicrograph of blast cells from the same dog as in Figure 93.1 after cytochemical staining for NBE. Note the focal distribution of the cytoplasmic staining in the blast cells and the nonstaining erythrocytes. Original magnification 500×.

FIGURE 93.1 Morphologic appearance of blast cells from a case of B cell ALL. Photomicrograph showing three lymphoid blast cells in the peripheral blood of a dog that has ALL. Original magnification 500×.

tions for ALL in human patients. These three forms, ALL-L1, ALL-L2, and ALL-L3, are classified based on the age of the patient, the nuclear and cytoplasmic features of the cells, and the presence of prominent versus inconspicuous nucleoli . However, the FAB classification does not appear to have any prognostic significance in cases of ALL.

Cytochemical analysis has been the gold standard used to identify the origin of hematopoietic tumor cells.[7,11–13] Among the commonly used cytochemical reactions, lymphocytes can exhibit N-butyrate esterase (NBE) activity, with a focal distribution of the cytoplasmic staining (Fig. 93.2), acid phosphatase activity, and alkaline phosphatase activity.[11,13] However, there are several shortcomings to the use of cytochemistry to classify leukemic cells, including the loss of activity of the enzymes over time and the small numbers of cells that can be examined visually.

It has been estimated that cytochemical analysis could result in revisions of the final diagnosis in many cases of canine and feline leukemias based on morphology alone.[9] More recently, it was shown that more than 20% of the cytochemical diagnoses of human leukemias are discordant with the immunologic diagnoses.[14] It has been our experience that immunologic detection of leukocyte markers can eliminate problems associated with decreased enzyme activity in stored samples. Some of the markers that have been used to identify the ontogeny of lymphocytic leukemic cells in humans and in animals include cytoplasmic CD3ε (a component of the T cell

receptor complex), surface or cytoplasmic immunoglobulin (Ig), cytoplasmic CD79a (Igα, a component of the B cell receptor complex), CD21 (a B cell-restricted component of the complement receptor), CD45RA (a lymphocyte-restricted isoform of the CD45 common leukocyte antigen present in naive cells), CD5 (a scavenger receptor found in most T cells and in certain B cells that localize to the peritoneal and pleural cavities), and DR (an antigen of the class II major histocompatibility complex found in B cells and some activated T cells). Conversely, myeloid cells can be identified by the expression of L1- calprotectin, CD14 (the receptor for the bacterial lipopolysaccharide-binding protein, LPS-BP), and lysosomal enzymes such as lysozyme, α_1-antitrypsin, and α_1-antichymotrypsin.[10,15] Since some of these molecules are shared by cells committed to differentiate along dissimilar lineages, it is often necessary to examine the concomitant expression of two or more of these selective markers (Figs. 93.3 and 93.4).

A classification that relies on the immunophenotype of blast cells and on the presence of specific genetic abnormalities has been developed and used extensively for human lymphoblastic leukemias.[7] Using this as a fundamental starting point, Pui and Evans[8] proposed a risk-classification system in which children aged 1 to 9 with B cell precursor ALL, a leukocyte count <50,000/μL, hyperdiploidy or a characteristic chromosomal rearrangement (resulting in the fusion of portions of the *ETV6* and *CBFA2* genes), and a good early response comprise a low-risk (or good predicted response) group, showing as much as 90% survival at 5 years. Patients who have T cell leukemia, who have failure of induction or poor early response, or who have rearrangements involving the *MLL* gene or resulting in fusion of the *BCR* and *ABL* genes, comprise a high-risk group with <40% survival at 5 years. The remaining patients comprise a standard-risk group with intermediate survival times.

Although cytogenetic abnormalities are powerful predictors for response to therapy in human ALL,[16] only a few studies have documented cytogenetic abnormalities in dogs and cats that have lymphoma and leukemia.[17-19] Trisomy of chromosome 13 is a favorable prognostic indicator in dogs that have lymphoma[20]; however, the nature of cytogenetic abnormalities and their prognostic significance in dogs and cats that have leukemia are unclear. In our experience, aneuploidy has not been a common finding in canine leukemias, but additional work is necessary to clarify the nature of the genetic lesions leading to ALL in domestic animals.

In the foreseeable future, immunophenotyping of ALL in dogs and cats may prove to be a fruitful diagnostic tool. In one study of 9 cases of dogs that had ALL, the immunophenotype indicated B cell origin (surface immunoglobulin or sIg+) in 2 dogs, T cell origin (defined by monoclonal antibody 8.358 that reacts with a pan-T cell marker) in 3 dogs, and null cell origin (non-B–non-T) in 4 dogs.[21] Two studies examined clonal rearrangements of the Ig heavy (IgH) chain gene, the T cell receptor β (TCRβ) gene, or the TCR gene in dogs that had lymphoma or leukemia.[22,23] One of these studies[23] evaluated 13 dogs that had lymphoma and 1 dog that

had ALL by Southern blot analysis of DNA. Four dogs that had stage V lymphoma had IgH rearrangements, and the dog that had ALL had a TCRβ rearrangement. The other study evaluated lymphocyte antigen receptor gene rearrangements by polymerase chain reaction amplification in dogs that were diagnosed with leukemia at one of 3 referral centers.[22] This study included 19 dogs that had lymphoid leukemia other than CLL and multiple myeloma. Of these dogs, 10 had clonal IgH rearrangements, 6 had clonal TCR rearrangements, 1 had clonal rearrangements of both IgH and TCR, and 2 had no detectable rearrangement of either gene (although one of these had evidence of cytoplasmic CD79a, suggesting a B cell lineage). Rearrangements of the IgH gene or the TCR gene were undetectable in non-lymphoid leukemias. Finally, our group documented the immunophenotype of 23 consecutive cases of canine and feline leukemia referred for diagnosis to the Texas Veterinary Medical Center. ALL was diagnosed in 5/16 dogs and 2/7 cats[10]; all 5 dogs also were included in the study by Avery.[22] Immunophenotyping showed 3 of the 5 canine ALL cases were of B cell origin (defined by expression of sIg, CD79a, CD21, or IgH rearrangement), and 2 were of T cell origin (defined by expression of cytoplasmic CD3 or TCR rearrangement). One T cell leukemia was positive for CD8, the other was negative for both CD4 and CD8. Both of the feline ALL cases were of T cell origin (CD3+), and neither was associated with FeLV infection.

The prognostic significance of the ALL immunophe-

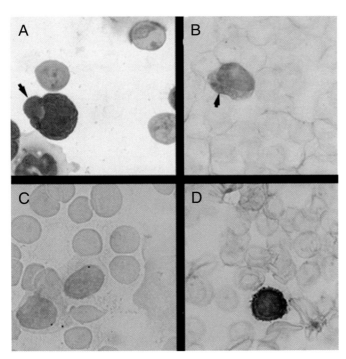

FIGURE 93.3 Immunocytochemistry of blast cells from a case of B cell ALL. Photomicrographs of blast cells from the same dog as in Figure 93.1 after immunocytochemical staining for (**A**) sIg and cytoplasmic Ig; (**B**) CD79a; and (**C**) CD3. Staining for CD3 in a normal peripheral blood lymphocyte is shown in (**D**). Note the focal accumulation of staining for Ig and CD79a (arrows) characteristic of many B cell ALLs (**A** and **B**). Original magnification 500×.

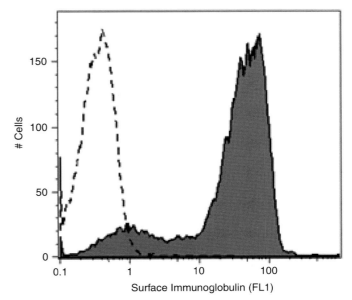

FIGURE 93.4 Flow cytometric analysis of sIg expression in blast cells from a case of B cell ALL. Peripheral blood cells from the same dog as in Figure 93.1 were stained with a biotinylated rabbit anticanine Ig antibody followed by avidin conjugated to fluorescein isothiocyanate (FITC) and analyzed flow cytometrically. The solid histogram represents staining for sIg on the blast cells. The dashed line represents background staining with an irrelevant control antibody. The blast cells in this case uniformly expressed high levels of sIg.

notype remains to be determined. In our study, one dog that had T cell ALL had extensive central nervous system involvement at presentation, as is common for human patients who have T cell ALL,[24] whereas none of the dogs that had B cell ALL had this manifestation. The dogs in this study were either not treated or did not achieve lasting remission times. One of the cats that had ALL was treated with prednisone and achieved partial remission, with the blast cells in the peripheral circulation decreasing from 21,600/μL to 12,400/μL. This cat was still alive 3 months after diagnosis. None of the other studies that examined ALL immunophenotypes reported quantifiable remission times in these patients.

PATHOGENESIS OF ALL

As with other cancers, ALL can be considered a genetic disease, regardless of the inciting cause. Mutations in genes that disable the normal growth control mechanisms of lymphoid cells provide cells with a selective growth advantage. Thus, tumors arise frequently from cells with a high turnover rate, such as lymphocytes that undergo mitosis frequently both in the course of differentiation and in their unending fight against invading pathogens.

The inciting cause for the genetic lesion leading to leukemia can be heritable or acquired, with viral infections being especially important in the development of some animal leukemias. A feature of retroviruses is their capacity to incorporate host DNA during their life cycle. This host DNA may include growth-associated genes (oncogenes) that are inappropriately expressed on infection of new cells, leading to transformation.[25] Alternatively, the integration of proviral DNA adjacent to normal cellular proto-oncogenes may similarly lead to inappropriate expression of these genes resulting in transformation.[26,27] Additionally, proteins encoded by retroviruses (e.g., human T cell lymphotropic virus-I [HTLV-I] Tax) and transforming DNA viruses (e.g., SV40 T antigen and adenovirus E1A) also can inactivate important tumor suppressor proteins, such as p16/Ink-4a, a potent inhibitor of cell proliferation, or Rb, the retinoblastoma susceptibility gene product, respectively.[28–32]

At present, FeLV- and bovine leukemia virus (BLV)-induced leukemias are still occasionally seen in the United States. Despite the implications of its name, FeLV infection is not commonly associated with leukemia in cats, and in the cases in which it occurs, nonlymphoid leukemias (and especially erythremic myelosis) may be more common than lymphoid leukemias. Yet, there is one report of FeLV integration upstream from the endogenous c-myc, resulting in the activation of this gene in a case of T cell leukemia.[26] Bovine leukemia is almost invariably associated with BLV infection, but the role of BLV in leukemogenesis is unclear. The possibility that BLV-infected cells elude apoptosis is supported by evidence of mutations in p53 (a gene that promotes apoptosis) and increased expression of bcl-2 (a gene that prevents apoptosis) in cases of BLV-induced neoplasia.[33,34] The possibility that the BLV Tax protein may increase expression of growth-associated genes, such as those encoding cytokine receptors, or inactivate other tumor suppressor proteins, such as p16/Ink-4a, remains to be determined.

Not all genetic alterations associated with lymphoproliferative diseases are associated with viral infections. Amplification of growth-promoting proto-oncogenes[35] or spontaneous mutations that inactivate tumor suppressor genes[30] also can result in the development of lymphoid leukemia. Moreover, numerous nonrandom chromosomal translocations have been defined in human leukemias that result in the untimely activation of various oncogenes that promote cell growth or impair apoptosis.[16,36,37] It is generally believed that a second hit beyond the initial mutation is required for progression to overt leukemia. However, recent studies performed in transgenic mice bearing a mutation seen frequently in human ALL strongly support the overwhelming proneoplastic effect some of these genetic lesions can have in immature lymphocytes.[38]

DIAGNOSIS OF ALL

Animals affected with ALL have a spectrum of nonspecific signs, including lethargy, fever, anorexia, weight loss, bruising, and altered mentation. In addition, physical examination may reveal pale mucous membranes and organomegaly. In most cases of ALL, a leukocytosis with circulating blasts occurs, but subleukemic and aleukemic forms also can be seen. In the latter cases hematologic abnormalities, including nonregenerative anemia, neutropenia, and thrombocytopenia, are often present.

Examination of the bone marrow is essential for establishing a diagnosis of ALL. If >40 to 50% of the total nucleated cells in the bone marrow resemble lymphoblasts or if a homogeneous population of lymphoblasts has effaced the normal hematopoietic architecture, ALL should be considered in the differential diagnosis. A presumptive diagnosis of ALL should be confirmed by phenotyping, as the final diagnosis is frequently altered when the ontogeny of the malignant cells is confirmed by methods other than morphologic examination of blood smears and bone marrow specimens.

Various factors must be considered in the selection of additional tests after a presumptive diagnosis of ALL. The usefulness of a definitive diagnosis in patient management must be considered. We believe that the phenotype of the leukemic cells may have prognostic significance and may influence therapeutic decisions. We have developed a simple panel that, with enzyme cytochemistry, immunohistology, and flow cytometry, can be used to establish the phenotype of most leukemias within 48 to 72 hours. Each of these tests provides distinct information that has an effect on the diagnostic decision; thus, these tests are not mutually exclusive. The availability of a suitable sample(s) may be a limiting factor in test selection. In the ideal situation, the patient would be available to allow sufficient diagnostic material to be obtained with minimal risk to perform all the necessary tests irrespective of cost. Unfortunately, extended transport time, financial constraints, limited availability of sample material, and experience in sample collection and preparation may dictate test selection.

Table 93.1 lists the panel we have used to phenotype leukemias of dogs and cats after a morphologic diagnosis is established by microscopic examination of blood and bone marrow specimens. The selection of diagnostic tests is a fluid process, with each answer determining the next step until a definitive diagnosis is achieved, or until the diagnostic possibilities are exhausted. Each test

serves to narrow the list of differentials and lead to a specific branch along the decision tree.

TREATMENT OF ALL

Treatment of ALL in dogs and cats by use of standard chemotherapeutic approaches is unrewarding.[39,40] Conversely, some subtypes of pediatric ALL have a response rate of >80% with a high proportion of complete responders surviving longer than 5 to 10 years.[8] The greater success in the treatment of human ALL is at least in part due to the use of intensive myeloablative chemotherapy and bone marrow transplantation. This has not been a feasible alternative in most cases of canine

TABLE 93.1 Panel of Tests to Phenotype Canine and Feline Leukemias

Method	Enzyme or Antigen	Expression	Priority
Cytochemistry	Myeloperoxidase	Myeloid cells	All leukemias
Cytochemistry	Chloroacetate esterase	Granulocytes	All leukemias
Cytochemistry	N-butyrate esterase	Monocytes (diffuse distribution) Lymphocytes (focal distribution)	All leukemias
Immunocytochemistry	Vimentin (intermediate filament)	Mesenchymal cells (presence and subcellular distribution are helpful to establish degree of leukocyte maturation)	All leukemias
Immunocytochemistry	CD18 (β integrin)	Panleukocyte marker (in lymphocytes it may be restricted to specific subsets or activated cells)	All leukemias
Immunocytochemistry	L1-calprotectin (calcium binding cytoplasmic protein involved in cellular defense)	Myeloid cells	All leukemias
Immunocytochemistry	CD45RA (isoform of the CD45 protein tyrosine phosphatases)	Subset of naïve lymphocytes (B cells > T cells)	All leukemias
Immunocytochemistry	CD3ε (component of the CD3 signaling complex of the T cell receptor)	T cells	All leukemias
Immunocytochemistry	CD79a (component of the immunoglobulin-signaling complex of the B cell receptor)	B cells	All leukemias
Immunocytochemistry	CD21 (complement receptor [CR2, C3dR])	B cells	All leukemias
Immunocytochemistry	FEr2 (antigen with restricted expression to erythroid cells)[a]	Erythroid cells	All leukemias
Flow cytometry	CD45RB (isoform of the CD45 protein tyrosine phosphatases)	All leukocytes	All leukemias
Flow cytometry	sIg (surface immunoglobulin)	B cells	All leukemias
Flow cytometry	CD14 (LPS-binding protein)	Monocytes	All leukemias
Immunocytochemistry or flow cytometry	CD4 (adhesion molecule that interacts with MHC class II)	Helper T cells (also neutrophils in the dog)	T cell leukemias
Immunocytochemistry or flow cytometry	CD8 (adhesion molecule that interacts with MHC class I)	Cytotoxic T cells	T cell leukemias

[a] Reactivity of anti-FEr2 antibody has only been demonstrated in cells of feline origin.

and feline leukemia. However, the recent availability of cytokines, such as erythropoietin and granulocyte-colony-stimulating factor (G-CSF), that support hematopoiesis may permit the use of more aggressive protocols, drugs with narrow therapeutic indices, and possibly allogeneic bone marrow transplantation to treat dogs and cats that have ALL.[41-45] In addition to these aggressive modalities, the possibility of using approaches that take advantage of the expression of molecules restricted to ALL cells (for example, the α chain of the interleukin-2 receptor) may allow veterinarians to improve the outcome of therapy for dogs and cats that have ALL.[2,46]

Efforts to treat ALL in animal species have relied on those chemotherapeutic agents that are effective in treating lymphoma. Most experience has been in the dog. Despite intensive regimens combining L-asparaginase, vincristine, cyclophosphamide, doxorubicin, cytosine arabinoside (given by continuous infusion at 100 mg/m² once daily for 4 days), and prednisone, responses generally have been disappointing. Chemotherapy is highly effective in reducing the leukemic cell count quickly and correlates with improvement in clinical signs. However, based on examination of the bone marrow and peripheral blood smear, leukemic cells persist and invariably predict early relapse. Thus, without total myeloablation it has not been possible to achieve remissions appreciably longer than 6 months in most canine patients. The severe toxicity associated with total myeloablative regimens has been unacceptable in veterinary practice and is the major obstacle to improving the duration of remission achieved through the use of chemotherapy. With this in mind, it may be safest to treat ALL with standard (and less toxic) lymphoma protocols until appropriate ancillary supportive protocols have been established for animal patients subjected to intensive bone marrow ablative chemotherapeutic regimens.

REFERENCES

1. **Wellman ML, Couto CG, Starkey RJ, et al.** Lymphocytosis of large granular lymphocytes in three dogs. Vet Pathol 1989;26:158–163.
2. **Helfand SC, Modiano JF, Moore PF, Soergel SA, MacWilliams PS, Dubielzig RR, Hank JA, Sondel PM.** Functional interleukin-2 receptors are expressed on natural killer-like leukemic cells from a dog with cutaneous lymphoma. Blood 1995;86:636–645.
3. **Franks PT, Harvey JW, Mays MC, Senior DF, Bowen DJ, Hall BJ.** Feline large granular lymphoma. Vet Pathol 1986;23:200–202.
4. **Wellman ML, Hammer AS, DiBartola SP, et al.** Lymphoma involving large granular lymphocytes in cats: 11 cases (1982–1991). J Am Vet Med Assoc 1992;201:1265–1269.
5. **Losco PE, Ward JM.** The early stage of large granular lymphocyte leukemia in the F344 Rat. Vet Pathol 1984;21:286–291.
6. **Boone LI, Barthel R, Helman RG, et al.** Large granular lymphocyte leukemia in a ferret. Vet Clin Pathol 1995;24:6–10.
7. **Goasguen JE, Bennet JM, Henderson ES.** Biologic diagnosis of leukemias. In: Henderson ES, Lister TA, Greaves MF, eds. Leukemia. 6th ed. Philadelphia: WB Saunders, 1996;8–33.
8. **Pui Ch, Evans WE.** Acute lymphoblastic leukemia. Eng J Med 1998; 339:605–615.
9. **Couto CG.** Leukemias. In: Nelson RW, Couto CG, eds. Essentials of small animal internal medicine. St. Louis: Mosby Year Book, 1992;871–878.
10. **Modiano JF, Wojcieszyn J, Avery AC.** Timely and accurate diagnosis of leukemias in small animals: the first step towards successful therapy. Proc Ann Mtg Vet Cancer Soc 1998;18:28.
11. **Facklam NR, Kociba GJ.** Cytochemical characterization of leukemic cells from 20 dogs. Vet Pathol 1985;22:363–369.
12. **Facklam NR, Kociba GJ.** Cytochemical characterization of feline leukemic cells. Vet Pathol 1986;23:155–161.
13. **Grindem CB, Stevens JB, Perman V.** Cytochemical reactions in cells from leukemic dogs. Vet Pathol 1986;23:103–109.
14. **Kheiri SA, MacKerrell T. Bonagura V, et al.** Flow cytometry with or without cytochemistry for the diagnosis of acute leukemias? Cytometry 1998; 34:82–86.
15. **Modiano JF, Smith R III, Wojcieszyn J, et al.** The use of cytochemistry, immunophenotyping, flow cytometry, and in vitro differentiation to determine the ontogeny of a canine monoblastic leukemia. Vet Clin Pathol 1998;27:40–49.
16. **Look AT.** Oncogenic transcription factors in the human acute leukemias. Science 1997;278:1059–1064.
17. **Grindem CB, Buoen LC.** Cytogenetic analysis of leukaemic cells in the dog. A report of 10 cases and a review of the literature. J. Comp Pathol 1986;96:626–635.
18. **Nolte M, Werner M, Nolte I, et al.** Different cytogenetic findings in two clinically similar leukaemic dogs. J Comp Pathol 1993;108:337–342.
19. **Goh K, Smith RA, Proper JS.** Chromosomal aberrations in leukemic cats. Cornell Vet 1981;71:43–46.
20. **Hahn KA, Richardson RC, Hahn EA, et al.** Diagnostic and prognostic importance of chromosomal aberrations identified in 61 dogs with lymphosarcoma. Vet Pathol 1994;31:528–540.
21. **Reuslander DA, Gebhard DH, Tompkins MB, et al.** Immunophenotypic characterization of canine lymphoproliferative disorders. In Vivo 1997; 11:169–172.
22. **Avery AC.** Diagnosis of canine lymphocytic neoplasia using clonal rearrangements of antigen receptor genes. Proc 1st Conference on Canine Immunogenetics and Immunologic Diseases; Davis, CA, July 31–Aug 2, 1998.
23. **Momoi Y, Nagase M, Okamoto Y, et al.** Rearrangements of immunoglobulin and T-cell receptor genes in canine lymphoma/leukemia cells. J Vet Med Sci 1993;55:775–780.
24. **Hoelzer D.** Acute lymphoblastic leukemia in adults. In: Henderson ES, Lister TA, Greaves MF, eds. Leukemia. 6th ed. Philadelphia: WB Saunders, 1996;446–478.
25. **Schulz TF, Neil JC.** Viruses and leukemia In: Henderson ES, Lister TA, Greaves MF, eds. Leukemia. 6th ed. Philadelphia: WB Saunders, 1996; 160–178.
26. **Miura T, Shibuya M, Tsujimoto H, et al.** Molecular cloning of a feline leukemia provirus integrated adjacent to the c-myc gene in a feline T-cell leukemia cell line and the unique structure of its long terminal repeat. Virology 1989;169:458–461.
27. **Holbrook NJ, Gulino A, Durand D, et al.** Transcriptional activity of the gibbon ape leukemia virus in the interleukin 2 gene of MLA 144 cells. Virology 1987;159:178–182.
28. **Yamada Y, Hatta Y, Murata K, et al.** Deletions of p15 and/or p16 genes as a poor-prognosis factor in adult T-cell leukemia. J Clin Oncol 1997; 15:1778–1785.
29. **Hatta Y, Yamada Y, Tomonaga M, et al.** Extensive analysis of the retinoblastoma gene in adult T cell leukemia/lymphoma (ATL). Leukemia 1997; 11:984–989.
30. **Cayuela JM, Madani A, Sanhes L, et al.** Multiple tumor-suppressor gene 1 inactivation is the most frequent genetic alteration in T-cell acute lymphoblastic leukemia. Blood 1996;87:2180–2186.
31. **Cayuela JM, Gardie B, Sigaux F.** Disruption of the multiple tumor suppressor gene MTS1/p16(INK4a)/CDKN2 by illegitimate V(D)J recombinase activity in T-cell acute lymphoblastic leukemias. Blood 1997;90:3720–3726.
32. **Schroder M, Mathieu U, Dreyling MH, et al.** CDKN2 gene deletion is not found in chronic lymphoid leukaemias of B- and T-cell origin but is frequent in acute lymphoblastic leukaemia. Br J Haematol 1995;91:865–870.
33. **Reyes RA, Cockerell GL.** Increased ratio of bcl-2/Bax expression is associated with bovine leukemia virus-induced leukemogenesis in cattle. Virology 1998;242:184–192.
34. **Dequiedt F. Kettmann R, Burny A, et al.** Mutations in the p53 tumor-suppressor gene are frequently associated with bovine leukemia virus-induced leukemogenesis in cattle but not in sheep. Virology 1995;209: 676–683.
35. **Mina RB, Tateyama S, Miyoshi N, et al.** Amplification of a c-yes-1-related oncogene in canine lymphoid leukemia. J Vet Med Sci 1994;56:773–774.
36. **Hagemeijer A, Grosveld G.** Molecular cytogenetics of leukemia. In: Henderson ES, Lister TA, Greaves MF, eds. Leukemia 6th ed. Philadelphia: WB Saunders, 1996;131–144.
37. **Nowell PC.** Cancer, chromosomes, and genes. Lab Invest 1992;66:407–417.
38. **Honda H, Oda H, Suzuki T, et al.** Development of acute lymphoblastic leukemia and myeloproliferative disorder in transgenic mice expressing p210bcr/abl: a novel transgenic model for human Ph1-positive leukemias. Blood 1998;91:2067–2075.
39. **Couto CG.** Clinicopathologic aspects of acute leukemias in the dog. J Am Vet Med Assoc 1985;186:681–685.
40. **Helfand SC.** Low-dose cytosine arabinoside-induced remission of lymphoblastic leukemia in a cat. J Am Vet Med Assoc 1987;191:707–710.
41. **Storb R, Raff RF, Appelbaum FR, et al.** DLA-identical bone marrow grafts after low-dose total body irradiation: the effect of canine recombinant hematopoietic growth factors. Blood 1994;84:3558–3566.

42. **Nash RA, Schuening FG, Seidel K, et al.** Effect of recombinant canine granulocyte-macrophage colony-stimulating factor on hematopoietic recovery after otherwise lethal total body irradiation. Blood 1994;83:1963–1970.

43. **Schuening FG, Storb R, Goehle S, et al.** Recombinant human granulocyte colony-stimulating factor accelerates hematopoietic recovery after DLA-identical littermate marrow transplants in dogs. Blood 1990;76:636–640.

44. **Schuening FG, Appelbaum FR, Deeg HJ, et al.** Effects of recombinant canine stem cell factor, a c-kit ligand, and recombinant granulocyte colony-

stimulating factor on hematopoietic recovery after otherwise lethal total body irradiation. Blood 1993;81:20–26.

45. **Schuening FG, Nemunaitis J, Appelbaum FR, et al.** Hematopoietic growth factors after allogeneic marrow transplantation in animal studies and clinical trials. Bone Marrow Transplant 1994;14:S74–S77.

46. **Waldmann TA, White JD, Carrasquillo JA, et al.** Radioimmunotherapy of interleukin-2R alpha-expressing adult T-cell leukemia with Yttrium-90-labeled anti-Tac. Blood 1995;86:4063–4075.

CHAPTER 94

Chronic Lymphocytic Leukemia

• STUART C. HELFAND and JAIME F. MODIANO

BIOLOGY, IMMUNOPHENOTYPE, AND CLONALITY

Chronic lymphocytic leukemia (CLL) is a disease of uncontrolled proliferation of a malignantly transformed lymphoid stem cell in which the progeny have a strong tendency to differentiate within the bone marrow and migrate widely throughout tissues and blood. Circulation of these cells is prolonged and gives rise to peripheral blood lymphocytosis, ranging from 10,000 to >100,000 cells/μL of blood. The ontogeny of CLL is complicated, and it has now become apparent, through the use of antibodies that distinguish B cells from T cells, that CLL is a heterogeneous group of diseases in the dog and, probably, the horse. In contrast to acute lymphoblastic leukemia (ALL) in which there is failure of differentiation within an early stem cell compartment leading to progressive increase of cell numbers within this compartment, CLL is characterized by increased cell numbers not only within the stem cell compartment, but also within the more differentiated, naturally larger compartments that follow. Thus, in CLL, there is a wider range of cell types expressed within the malignant clone than in ALL.[1] Variation in proliferation rates between malignant cells within the multiple differentiation compartments may account for differences in response to therapy. It is not known why malignant cells differentiate in CLL, although the nature of the specific genetic lesion in CLL likely accounts for this behavior.

The development of monoclonal antibodies to type canine lymphocytes represents one of the most important advances in veterinary oncology. These reagents are helping to clarify the lineage of lymphocytes in canine and equine CLL. Compared with malignant lymphoma, CLL is an infrequently encountered variation of lymphoid cancer in animal species. Thus, accruing a large series of CLL patients for study is difficult, and one must always be cautious of overinterpreting results based on small populations.

T lymphocytes typically express a membrane antigen receptor, the T cell receptor (TCR), that is unique to cells of this lineage. This receptor exists in two forms as a heterodimer, each composed of two distinct subunits. The $\alpha\beta$ TCR predominates on most circulating T cells,

with lesser numbers of $\gamma\delta$ TCR lymphocytes. Other distinct T cell markers include accessory molecules that aid T cells in antigen recognition. For example, helper T lymphocytes express CD4, whereas cytotoxic T cells express CD8. A complex of membrane proteins associated with the TCR, known as CD3, is common to all T lymphocytes. Identification of B cells has been facilitated by use of antibodies that recognize surface immunoglobulin (Ig), characteristically expressed on the cell membranes of B lymphocytes, or other unique B cell membrane proteins, such as B5,[2] CD21, and CD79a; the latter is also known as Igα and functions as a membrane anchor for surface Ig.[3,4] In contrast to unactivated T lymphocytes, B cells express surface major histocompatibility complex class II molecules for which unique antibodies are also available in several animal species.

In recent studies, monoclonal antibodies against these lymphocyte surface molecules have been used to type the lymphocytes in canine CLL. Ruslander and colleagues reported that in 8 of 12 dogs that had CLL, the lymphocytes were of the CD8$^+$ T cell phenotype, whereas B cell markers were expressed in 3 dogs. The lymphocytes in one dog did not express recognizable markers (null cell).[2] In a study of 14 cases of canine leukemia by one of the authors, immunophenotyping of the cells in 3 cases of CLL revealed the malignant lymphocytes to be T cells in two cases and B cells in one case.[5] A larger case series of canine leukemias studied by Vernau and Moore[6] further supported the predominance of T cell-derived lineage in canine CLL, with the leukemic cells in 73% of 54 dogs exhibiting CD3 positivity. So-called large granular lymphocytes (LGLs), technically an enlarged small lymphocyte containing cytoplasmic granules, comprised the malignant population of 54% of the dogs that had CLL in this study.[6] These cells were almost exclusively CD8$^+$ and expressed the $\alpha\beta$ TCR (69%) more often than the $\gamma\delta$ TCR (31%). B cell CLL (CD21$^+$ or CD79a$^+$) comprised 26% of the cases of canine CLL in the study. Seemingly, in contrast to human CLL in which malignant B cells constitute the dominant immunophenotype, CLL in the dog appears to be primarily a T cell cancer. There has been one report of a dog with a CD3$^-$ Igα^- chronic leukemic blood profile associated with cutaneous infiltrates in which the cells were shown to be natural killer lymphocytes.[7] Immunophenotyping of CLL in two horses indicated one animal had T cell CLL and the other B cell CLL.[8] Typing lymphocytes in (canine) CLL is not an inconsequential exercise, because, as in malignant lymphoma, the immunophenotype of CLL may be prognostic of responsiveness to therapy.

CLL is often an indolent disease, and the diagnosis may be incidental to routine blood studies done for other purposes. Because the cells in CLL are morphologically indistinguishable from normally differentiated lymphocytes, CLL is diagnosed in part by eliminating other causes of lymphocytosis. Indeed, the differential diagnosis for CLL is limited, as there are few conditions that cause lymphocytosis of mature lymphocytes. Immune responses can occasionally cause mature lymphocytosis (e.g., postvaccinal responses in young dogs). One of the authors has observed mature lymphocytosis ($\geq 10,000/\mu L$) in dogs treated with human recombinant interleukin-2.[9] Clonality is the hallmark of a malignant cell population, and the use of the polymerase chain reaction to analyze gene rearrangements within cell populations for clonality has provided a powerful means to demonstrate clonal expansion of malignant cells. During the development of thymus-derived T lymphocytes, various rearrangements of genes encoding TCR subunits take place, ensuring a wide repertoire of TCR specificity in each individual. Similarly, Ig genes are rearranged during B cell ontogeny, ensuring development of diverse B cell clones that have a wide range of surface Ig specificity. Demonstrating identical gene rearrangements within the presumed neoplastic cell population proves all the cells were derived from the same precursor, confirming clonality, and supports the diagnosis of malignancy. This strategy has been used in veterinary medicine by Avery and colleagues to examine peripheral blood cells from dogs that had mature lymphocytosis, as well as other lymphoproliferative diseases.[10] Of 10 dogs presumed to have CLL, 7 that had B cell CLL and 3 that had T cell CLL had rearranged Ig (heavy chain) and TCR genes, respectively. Thus, there was 100% correlation between immunophenotype and distinct gene rearrangements appropriate for each immunophenotype. This type of analysis now provides an important tool for proving malignancy as a cause for mature lymphocytosis versus polyclonal immune reactivity to an immunologic stimulus.

CLINICAL PRESENTATION AND DIAGNOSIS

The presenting signs of CLL are vague, nonspecific, or nonexistent. In the dog, CLL is most commonly seen in older animals (e.g., median age 10.5 years)[11] and constitutional disturbances such as lethargy, inappetence, and vomiting predominate. Less often diarrhea, polyuria or polydipsia, and intermittent lameness have been seen.[11] Physical findings, including splenomegaly, mild to moderate lymphadenopathy, and hepatomegaly, also vary and are typical of lymphoproliferative disorders. Abdominal organomegaly with distention of

the splenic capsule may incite nausea and vomiting. In the horse, cutaneous edema and peripheral lymphadenopathy have been observed in a small number of patients that had CLL.[8] The striking hematological abnormality in most cases of CLL is leukocytosis caused by mature lymphocytosis (Fig. 94.1). Peripheral blood lymphocyte counts are usually elevated ($>6000/\mu L$ to $>100,000/\mu L$). Mild nonregenerative normocytic normochromic anemia is common, and platelet counts are normal to moderately reduced. Bone marrow aspiration cytology demonstrates significantly increased numbers of small lymphocytes comprising $>30\%$ of the nucleated cells within bone marrow. Generally, because the marrow is not completely effaced by malignant lymphocytes, erythroid and myeloid precursors are adequately represented or mildly decreased.

Hyperglobulinemia resulting from monoclonal gammopathy has been observed in dogs that had CLL.[2,11] One case series of 22 dogs that had CLL indicated hyperglobulinemia was present in approximately 30% of the dogs, and serum protein electrophoresis performed on serum from 21 of these dogs revealed monoclonal gammopathy in 15 (68%).[11] Immunoglobulin M (IgM) gammopathy was identified most often, followed by immunoglobulin A (IgA) and G (IgG). Given the programming of B cells to produce Ig, such a finding in CLL is not surprising. However, the presence of monoclonal gammopathies suggests that the majority of cases in this study were caused by B cell CLL, which is unexpected given the more recent studies indicating T cell prevalence in canine CLL. Lymphocyte immunophenotyping was not a component of that report. Despite the high frequency of gammopathies, it is interesting that clinical signs secondary to gammopathy (e.g., hemorrhage, central nervous system [CNS] signs, renal dysfunction) were not observed. Two cases of equine CLL reportedly had IgG gammopathies, despite a T cell phenotype in

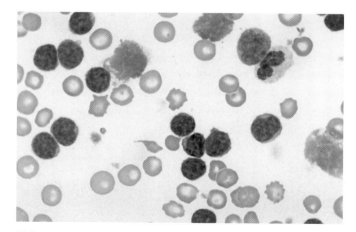

FIGURE 94.1 Photomicrograph of peripheral blood from a dog that has CLL. The predominant nucleated cell is a well-differentiated small lymphocyte. There are increased numbers of disintegrated cells, which are seen frequently on blood films from animals that have high numbers of lymphocytes. Wright's stain; original magnification 400×. (Photomicrograph courtesy of Dr. Karen M. Young).

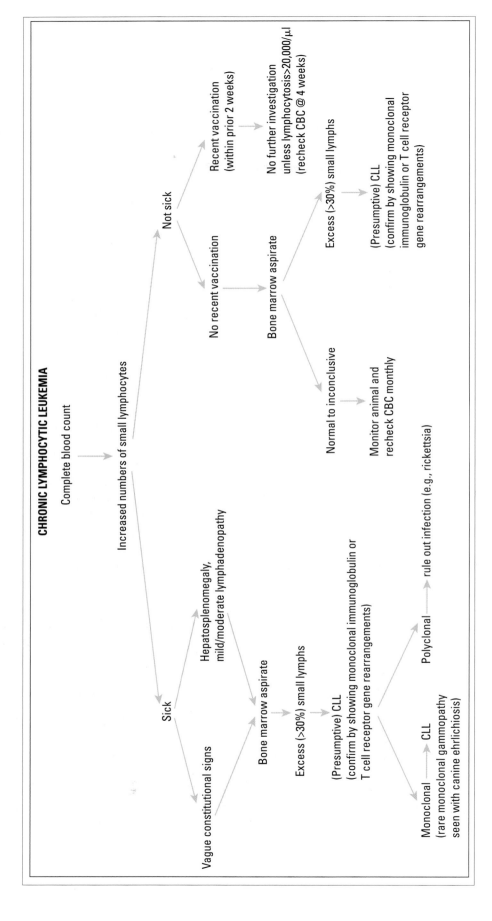

CHRONIC LYMPHOCYTIC LEUKEMIA

Complete blood count

Increased numbers of small lymphocytes

Sick

Not sick

Sick:

Hepatosplenomegaly, mild/moderate lymphadenopathy

Vague constitutional signs

Bone marrow aspirate

Excess (>30%) small lymphs

(Presumptive) CLL
(confirm by showing monoclonal immunoglobulin or T cell receptor gene rearrangements)

Monoclonal → CLL
(rare monoclonal gammopathy seen with canine ehrlichiosis)

Polyclonal → rule out infection (e.g., rickettsia)

Not sick:

Recent vaccination (within prior 2 weeks)

No further investigation unless lymphocytosis>20,000/μl (recheck CBC @ 4 weeks)

No recent vaccination

Bone marrow aspirate

Excess (>30%) small lymphs

(Presumptive) CLL
(confirm by showing monoclonal immunoglobulin or T cell receptor gene rearrangements)

Normal to inconclusive

Monitor animal and recheck CBC monthly

640

one horse and B cell in the other.[8] It is reasonable to perform serum protein electrophoresis as part of the workup for CLL, as this may provide another marker of disease activity that can be used to monitor therapeutic response. Immunoelectrophoresis, as well as Ig quantitation, can help to determine if the paraprotein is truly monoclonal and of a single isotype. Lymphocyte immunophenotyping is becoming more widely available to clinicians and should also be requested when feasible.

THERAPY

In contrast to ALL in which the goal of therapy is to eliminate all neoplastic stem cells, the objective of therapy in CLL is to slow proliferation of the neoplastic clone(s) without total ablation of the bone marrow. Seemingly, this is a reasonable goal as dogs that have CLL can enjoy a somewhat good quality of life while coexisting with their cancer, despite impaired lymphocyte immune responses.[8,12] Indeed, one report described a 2-year course of CLL in a dog that did not receive therapy and experienced a good quality of life.[12] Thus, when indicated, chemotherapy is used to control, not cure, CLL.

Animals presenting with signs of clinical illness should receive chemotherapy in an effort to reduce the neoplastic cell count and lessen the organomegaly. Therapy can be given intermittently (e.g., 1 to 2 months followed by observation) as dictated by clinical signs and cell counts. Compared with high-grade lymphoma and ALL, CLL is most likely a disease with a low growth fraction, thus responses to chemotherapy often take longer to be observed. Typically the alkylating agent, chlorambucil, is used in combination with prednisone, which induces apoptosis of lymphocytes. Chlorambucil has been used at 0.2 mg/kg/d by mouth for 7 to 14 days followed by reduction to 0.1 mg/kg/d or at 2 mg/m^2 every other day. As there may be an advantage to administering alkylating agents in pulse doses, the authors favor 20 mg/m^2 by mouth once every 14 days. Standard doses of prednisone used to treat lymphoid cancers suffice; an effective protocol is 30 mg/m^2 by mouth once daily for 7 days followed by 20 mg/m^2 by mouth for 7 days, then tapering to 10 mg/m^2 by mouth once daily for 7 days (or continued every other day).[11] Standard doses of vincristine (0.5 to 0.7 mg/m^2 intravenously once every 7 days in the dog) can be added to potentially accelerate therapeutic response. For refractory cases, cyclophosphamide (200 to 250 mg/m^2 intravenously once every 7 days or 50 mg/m^2/d by mouth for 4 days per week) or, rarely, more intensive lymphoma chemotherapy (e.g., adding doxorubicin, L-asparaginase) can be used if necessary, but typically is not employed for initial treatment. Failure to respond, as measured by lack of improvement in cell counts, bone marrow cytology, protein dyscrasias, and clinical signs, may portend a poor prognosis. Recently, efforts to correlate clinical response with lymphocyte immunophenotype have suggested a worse prognosis for T cell CLL in the dog, which is in agreement with responses observed in canine lymphoma.[2,13,14] Generally, CLL in the dog is considered a slowly progressive disease with inexorable progression of lymphocyte proliferation. Median survival times have been favorable, reported to range from 1 to longer than 2 years.[11,15,16] Most dogs that have CLL survive for 1 year.

In summary, CLL is an uncommon oddity within the complex of lymphoproliferative diseases. It invariably has a better prognosis than other forms of leukemia, and its recognition is important to providing clients with accurate information required for making informed decisions about the care of their animals.

REFERENCES

1. **Magrath IT.** Lymphocyte differentiation: an essential basis for the comprehension of lymphoid neoplasia. J Natl Cancer Inst 1981;67:501–513.
2. **Ruslander DA, Gebhard DH, Thompkins MB, Grindem CB, Page RL.** Immunophenotypic characterization of canine lymphoproliferative disorders. In Vivo 1997;11:169–172.
3. **Jones M, Cordell JL, Beyers AD, Tse AGD, Mason DY.** Detection of T and B cells in many animal species using cross-reactive anti-peptide antibodies. J Immunol 1993;150:5429–5435.
4. **Pleiman CM, D'Ambrosio D, Cambier JC.** The B-cell antigen receptor complex: structure and signal transduction. Immunol Today 1994;15:393–399.
5. **Modiano JF, Wojcieszyn J, Avery AC.** Timely and accurate diagnosis of leukemias in small animals: the first step towards successful therapy. In: 18th Annual Conference of the Veterinary Cancer Society. 1998;18:28.
6. **Vernau W, Moore PF.** An immunophenotypic study of canine leukemias and preliminary assessment of clonality by polymerase chain reaction. Vet Immunol Immunopathol 1999;69:145–164.
7. **Helfand SC, Modiano JF, Moore PF, Soergel SA, MacWilliams PS, Dubielzig RR, Hank JA, Sondel PM.** Functional interleukin-2 receptors are expressed on natural killer-like leukemic cells from a dog with cutaneous lymphoma. Blood 1995;86:636–645.
8. **Dascanio JJ, Zhang CH, Antczak DF, Blue JT, Simmons TR.** Differentiation of chronic lymphocytic leukemia in the horse. J Vet Intern Med 1992;6:225–229.
9. **Helfand SC, Soergel SA, MacWilliams PS, Hank JA, Sondel PM.** Clinical and immunological effects of human recombinant interleukin-2 given by repetitive weekly infusion in normal dogs. Cancer Immunol Immunother 1994;39:84–92.
10. **Burnett R, Vernau W, Moore P, Avery A.** Diagnosis of canine lymphocytic neoplasia using clonal rearrangements of antigen receptor genes. In: International Canine Immunogenetics and Immunologic Diseases Conference. 1998;1:21.
11. **Leifer CE, Matus RE.** Chronic lymphocytic leukemia in the dog: 22 cases (1974–1984). J Am Vet Med Assoc 1986;189:214–217.
12. **Harvey JW, Terrell TG, Hyde DM, Jackson RI.** Well-differentiated lymphocytic leukemia in a dog: long-term survival without therapy. Vet Pathol 1981;18:37–47.
13. **Teske E, van Heerde P, Rutteman GR, Kurzman ID, Moore PF, MacEwen EG.** Prognostic factors for treatment of malignant lymphoma in dogs. J Am Vet Med Assoc 1994;205:1722–1728.
14. **Vail DM, Kisseberth WC, Obradovich JE, Moore FM, London CA, MacEwen EG, Ritter MA.** Assessment of potential doubling time (T_{pot}), argyrophilic nucleolar organizer regions (AgNOR), and proliferating cell nuclear antigen (PCNA) as predictors of therapy response in canine non-Hodgkin's lymphoma. Exp Hematol 1996;24:807–815.
15. **Hodgkins EM, Zinkl JG, Madewell BR.** Chronic lymphocytic leukemia in the dog. J Am Vet Med Assoc 1980;117:704–707.
16. **Couto CG, Sousa C.** Chronic lymphocytic leukemia with cutaneous involvement in a dog. J Am Anim Hosp Assoc 1986;22:374–379.

CHAPTER 95

Lymphoproliferative Disorders of Large Granular Lymphocytes

• MAXEY L. WELLMAN

DEFINITION

Large granular lymphocytes (LGL) are a morphologically unique population of lymphocytes characterized by the presence of azurophilic granules in the cytoplasm.[1] Some LGL resemble large lymphocytes with abundant cytoplasm, which initially led to the designation large granular lymphocytes. Although it is now recognized that not all granular lymphocytes are large or have abundant cytoplasm, most literature still refers to this population of lymphocytes as large granular lymphocytes. In humans, LGL are described as lymphoid cells with at least three clearly defined azurophilic granules, each of which is 0.5 μm or greater in diameter.[2] This morphologic description has been applied to LGL in other species.

CLASSIFICATION

LGL develop from CD34+ bone marrow stem cells and constitute only a minority (1 to 15%) of peripheral blood lymphocytes in healthy individuals.[1,3–5] There are two subsets of LGL in humans, based on expression of leukocyte differentiation (cluster of differentiation [CD]) antigens and the T cell receptor (TCR) complex and on in vitro cytotoxicity. With these criteria, some LGL appear to be activated cytotoxic T lymphocytes (T cell LGL), and others appear to be natural killer (NK) cells (NK cell LGL).[1] Although there are some exceptions, this classification seems to be clinically relevant in humans because several syndromes are associated with clonal proliferations of specific subsets of LGL.[1,6] Similar syndromes likely exist in animals, as has been proposed recently for cats that have LGL leukemia and lymphoma.[7]

IMMUNOPHENOTYPE

In humans, T cell LGL express the CD3/TCR complex on their cell membranes, rearrange TCR genes, and have weak or negligible cytotoxic activity in vitro.[1] Most T cell LGL are negative for the helper T cell phenotype (CD4) and are either positive or negative for the cytotoxic T cell phenotype (CD8).[8] Rarely, T cell LGL are positive for both CD4 and CD8.[9] NK cell LGL do not express the CD3/TCR

complex and have a germline configuration of TCR genes. NK cell LGL have strong cytotoxicity in vitro that is not restricted by the major histocompatibility complex.[1] Several other leukocyte differentiation antigens such as CD16, CD56, and CD57, also have been used in classifying LGL, but there appears to be some lineage infidelity in expression of these markers in clonal proliferations of LGL (Fig. 95.1).

LGL from a few dogs and cats that had LGL leukemia or lymphoma have been immunophenotyped. LGL from some of these cases have been positive for CD3, which suggests that they are T cell LGL (PF Moore, personal communication, 1993–1994).[7,10,11] In some cats that have LGL leukemia or lymphoma, tumor cells also have been positive for CD57, which occurs on some NK cell and T cell LGL in humans.[7] In rats that have LGL leukemia, the neoplastic lymphocytes appear to be NK cell LGL.[12,13] The immunophenotype of LGL in other animals that have LGL lymphoproliferative disorders has not been clearly documented.

TISSUE DISTRIBUTION

In healthy individuals, LGL have been identified in many tissues, including blood, bone marrow, spleen, stomach, small and large intestine, lung, liver, gall bladder, uterus, and placenta. Some species variation in tissue distribution seems to exist, although this assumption may result from lack of extensive studies involving multiple tissues in many species. Synonyms for LGL include intraepithelial lymphocytes and globule leukocytes for LGL in the intestine and Pit cells for LGL in the liver. These cells have been shown to be lymphoid cells, based on expression of T cell or NK cell markers and the content of the granules (e.g., perforin). Tissue LGL likely develop from circulating LGL that originate in bone marrow.[14,15]

FUNCTION

The function of LGL is incompletely characterized and likely depends on tissue distribution. In general, cytotoxic T lymphocytes and NK cells mediate cytotoxicity in tumors, viral infection, autoimmune reactions, and trans-

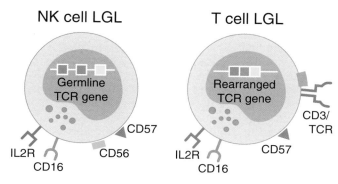

FIGURE 95.1 Immunophenotype and characteristics of the TCR gene in NK cell LGL and T cell LGL from humans. (Adapted from Loughran TP. Clonal diseases of large granular lymphocytes. Blood 1993;82:1–14, with permission.)

plant rejection.[16] In the intestine, LGL may be involved in antigen recognition and regulation of mucosal immunity. In the uterus, LGL may be involved in early events in placentation.[17] LGL express interleukin (IL) 2 and stem cell factor receptors.[16,18] Human LGL secrete several ILs, hemopoietic growth factors, and cytokines, including IL-1, IL-2, α and γ interferon, granulocyte-macrophage colony stimulating factor (GM-CSF), and tumor necrosis factor.[16,19–22] Therefore, LGL may have multiple effects on the immune system and hemopoiesis.

The granules in LGL resemble lysosomes and contain substances that mediate cell lysis, including perforin, a pore-forming protein unique to cytotoxic T lymphocytes and NK cells.[23,24] Perforin has been identified in LGL from humans, rats, mice, cats, and guinea pigs.[14] Several serine proteases and high molecular weight proteoglycans also have been identified in LGL granules.[25] The extensive necrosis that occurs in some LGL tumors may be caused by perforin and serine proteases released from neoplastic LGL.[14]

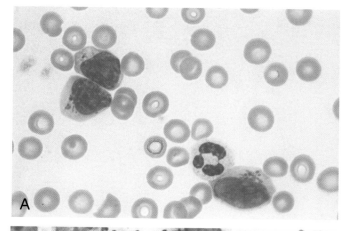

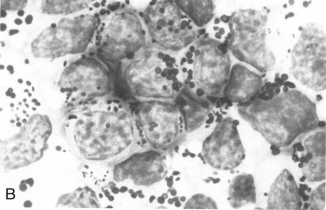

FIGURE 95.2 Morphology of LGL from a dog and a cat that had lymphoproliferative disorders of LGL. Notice the difference in tinctorial quality, size, number, and distribution of the granules. **A.** Peripheral blood from a dog that had LGL leukemia. LGLs were positive for CD3. **B.** Mesenteric lymph node from a cat that had LGL lymphoma. (Wright–Giemsa stain, ×1000)

LIGHT MICROSCOPY

LGL have a characteristic microscopic appearance because of the presence of distinct cytoplasmic granules when stained with Romanowsky-type stains like Wright–Giemsa stain. In most species, there appears to be wide variation in cell size; nuclear morphology; tinctorial quality of the granules; and granule number, size, shape, and distribution (Fig. 95.2). LGL may resemble small, medium, or large lymphocytes and range in size from 8 to 18 μm in diameter. Nuclei may be round, indented, or irregularly shaped and have fine, moderately clumped, or densely clumped chromatin. Nucleoli may be present or inconspicuous.[4,5,11]

LGL granules may appear azurophilic (magenta), eosinophilic, or basophilic with Wright–Giemsa stain. The granules usually stain well with Romanowsky-type stains, but may not stain with some commercial quick stains.[11] The granules often are not apparent with H&E staining, except in some intestinal LGL tumors in cats, in which the granules are quite prominent. There may be

three to more than ten granules per cell as well as significant variation in the number of granules in normal or neoplastic LGL from the same animal. Granule size varies from 0.5 to 2 μm.[2,4,5,11] Granules may be round, oval, or irregular in shape and may appear to be surrounded by a halo. The granules usually are located in a perinuclear region, near the nuclear indentation if the nucleus is reniform, but they also may be dispersed throughout the cytoplasm. LGL from guinea pigs and several South American rodents contain only a single, large, eosinophilic cytoplasmic inclusion called a Kurloff body. Guinea pig LGL have been shown to exhibit NK cell activity.[27]

ULTRASTRUCTURE

Ultrastructurally, LGL are characterized by the presence of membrane-bound cytoplasmic granules (Fig. 95.3).[4,25] In most cases, the granules appear electron-dense. Granules with parallel tubular arrays or a double-density appearance have been described in LGL from humans, but

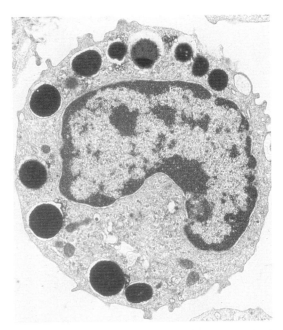

FIGURE 95.3 Ultrastructure of LGL from a dog that had LGL leukemia. Notice the distinct membrane-bound granules with an electron-dense core. (Reprinted with permission from Wellman ML, Couto CG, Starkey RJ, Rojko JL. Lymphocytosis of large granular lymphocytes in three dogs. Vet Pathol 1989;26:158–163).

these have not been clearly documented in LGL from other species. The cytoplasm also may contain mitochondria, free ribosomes, short strands of rough endoplasmic reticulum, and a prominent Golgi apparatus. The cell surface is covered with short microvilli.[25]

CYTOCHEMICAL AND HISTOCHEMICAL STAINING

The cytochemical and histochemical staining pattern of LGL varies with species, and reported results are not consistent within a species. Most LGL from humans stain positively with β-glucuronidase and acid phosphatase (ACP),[6] but these stains are not used routinely in veterinary medicine. Most LGL are negative for toluidine blue (except in guinea pigs) and histamine, which may be useful in distinguishing these cells from mast cells.[14,28] Some LGL are focally positive when stained with α-naphthyl butyrate esterase (αNBE), which is different from the diffuse staining in monocytes.[4] There are reports of both positive and negative staining with chloracetate esterase (CAE). Peroxidase activity usually is absent, which may be useful in distinguishing these cells from myeloid precursors. Results of staining with Periodic acid-Schiff (PAS) and phosphotungstic acid hematoxylin (PTAH) are variable.

LGL LYMPHOPROLIFERATIVE DISORDERS

Lymphoproliferative disorders involving LGL have been described in many species, including humans, cats, dogs,

horses, rats, ferrets, and birds.[1,4,5,29–32] LGL lymphoproliferative disorders may be transient or chronic. Transient proliferations likely are polyclonal or reactive, whereas chronic proliferations may be polyclonal or clonal. There is controversy over the use of the term clonal to imply neoplasia or malignancy because spontaneous remission and absence of disease progression have been reported in people who have clonal proliferations of LGL.[33] The diagnosis of LGL lymphoproliferative disorders in humans used to be based on peripheral blood LGL counts of greater than $2 \times 10^9/L$ that persisted for 6 months. However, not all LGL lymphoproliferative disorders involve increased numbers of circulating LGL, and some aggressive forms of LGL lymphoproliferative diseases have a short clinical course.[33,34] In animals, LGL lymphoproliferative disorders have been recognized by increased numbers of circulating LGL or the presence of masses or enlarged organs infiltrated with LGL.

Clonal proliferations of LGL have been documented in humans and in cats by demonstrating rearranged TCR genes.[1,28] Currently, it is difficult to document clonality of NK cell LGL. Although clonality has not been established for LGL lymphoproliferative disorders in most animals, it often is implied based on clinical findings and disease progression. Clonal proliferations of LGL in humans have been associated with Epstein-Barr virus, human immunodeficiency virus, and human T cell lymphotropic virus.[3,35,38] Although feline leukemia provirus genomes have been cloned from LGL tumor cells in cats,[37] there is no clear documentation of virus-associated LGL proliferations in other species.

It is important to recognize that not all LGL proliferations indicate leukemia or lymphoma. Polyclonal (reactive) proliferations of LGL have been reported in people who have cytomegalovirus infection and in patients that have been splenectomized or have nephrotic syndrome. LGL proliferations that presumably are polyclonal have been reported in dogs that have *Ehrlichia canis* infection and in birds that have coccidiosis.[32,38]

LGL LYMPHOPROLIFERATIVE DISORDERS IN HUMANS

Several clinical syndromes are associated with clonal proliferations of T cell LGL in humans. The most common syndrome is chronic T cell LGL leukemia, which typically is associated with significant neutropenia, recurrent infections, a high incidence of rheumatoid arthritis, and a prolonged clinical course.[1] Neoplastic LGL infiltrate bone marrow, liver, and spleen and usually are small lymphocytes with round nuclei, condensed chromatin, and a CD4−, CD8+, CD56−, and CD57+ immunophenotype.[1] In an aggressive form of T cell leukemia or lymphoma, neoplastic LGL are found in bone marrow, liver, and spleen, and numerous other organs. Neoplastic cells often exhibit significant nuclear pleomorphism or have a blastic appearance and usually are CD4−, CD8+, CD56+, and CD57−. Other syndromes include intestinal T cell lymphomas, in which the jejunum and mesenteric lymph nodes are infiltrated with CD4−, CD8+/− tumor

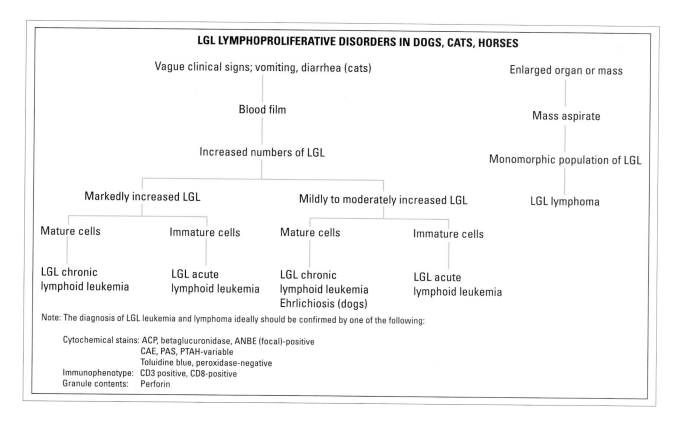

LGL LYMPHOPROLIFERATIVE DISORDERS IN DOGS, CATS, HORSES

cells, and hepatosplenic T cell LGL lymphomas, in which the hepatic sinusoids and spleen are infiltrated with CD4−, CD8+, CD56+ / − tumor cells.[1,33] Some T cell LGL proliferations have been associated with pure red cell aplasia.

Lymphoproliferative disorders of NK cell LGL include chronic proliferations that do not require specific treatment, aggressive disorders associated with Epstein-Barr virus, NK cell lymphoma, and acute leukemia of NK-LGL. NK cell lymphomas occur in the nasal cavity, are characterized by angiocentric tumor infiltrates and necrosis, and may be associated with Epstein-Barr virus.[3] The neoplastic cells are CD4−, CD8+, CD56+, and CD57−. NK cell LGL leukemia appears to be an aggressive clonal proliferation with massive hepatosplenomegaly and coagulopathies. The neoplastic cells are CD4−, CD8+, CD56+, and CD57−.[1,3,39]

LGL LYMPHOPROLIFERATIVE DISEASE IN CATS

There is confusion in the terminology of LGL proliferative disorders in cats. Similar tumors involving large mononuclear cells with prominent cytoplasmic granules have been called globule leukocyte tumors, LGL lymphomas, or granulated round cell tumors.[5,7,14,40–47] In many of these reports, convincing evidence of the origin of the tumor cells was not presented. However, results from recent studies suggest that these cells are either T cell LGL or NK cell LGL, based on expression of CD3, positive staining for perforin, and rearrangement of TCR genes.[7,14,28,45]

Most cats that have LGL lymphoproliferative disorders have lymphoma. LGL lymphoma appears to occur in older cats, but there is no apparent sex predilection.[5,28] Affected cats typically present with vague clinical signs such as lethargy, anorexia, weight loss, vomiting, diarrhea, and a palpable abdominal mass. Occasionally, cats have pleural or abdominal effusion.[5,7] Hematologic abnormalities include significant neutrophilia with a left shift, circulating neoplastic LGL, and mild nonregenerative anemia, but these changes are variable. Serum biochemical abnormalities include hypoproteinemia, hypoalbuminemia, hypocalcemia, and hyperbilirubinemia, but in some cats, only minimal laboratory abnormalities are present.[5]

The diagnosis of LGL lymphoma in cats frequently can be made cytologically from a fine-needle aspirate of involved tissue. Most abdominal masses involve the jejunum, ileum, or mesenteric lymph nodes but infiltration by neoplastic LGL has been described for bone marrow, peripheral lymph nodes, mediastinal lymph nodes, heart, lung, liver, spleen, kidney, adrenal medulla, omentum, mesentery, salivary gland, thyroid gland, pancreas, skin, urinary bladder, spinal cord, and brain.[5,7,14,28,40–47] Neoplastic cells also have been identified in pleural and abdominal fluid. Significant necrosis has been reported in the spleen, intestinal mucosa, and lymph nodes.

The granules in feline LGL are prominent with Wright-Giemsa stain. The granules from some tumors may stain brightly eosinophilic with H&E, but in other tumors the granules are difficult to identify with H&E. Cytochemical staining of LGL from cats is variable.

LGL may be positive or negative for αNBE and CAE activity but usually are negative for peroxidase activity and positive for ACP and β-glucuronidase activity. Feline LGL appear to be negative when stained with toluidine blue and positive when stained with PAS and PTAH.[5,10,28,41–44,46] LGL in neoplastic proliferations in cats are positive for CD3 with anti-human CD3 antibodies, and some LGL tumors in cats also express CD57.[7] Some LGL lymphomas appear to have clonal rearrangements of TCR genes.[28]

Although most cats that have LGL lymphoma that have been evaluated for feline leukemia virus infection by conventional methods have been negative, feline leukemia provirus genomes have been cloned from tumor cells isolated from cats that have LGL lymphoma.[37] These findings suggest that there may be integration of feline leukemia provirus in the nuclei of neoplastic LGL from some cats. Most cats that have been evaluated for feline immunodeficiency virus have been negative. The clinical course in cats that have LGL lymphoma is variable. Most cats have been euthanized without treatment, but some cats appear to have responded to combination chemotherapy or to surgical resection of the abdominal mass.[7,47]

LGL LYMPHOPROLIFERATIVE DISEASES IN DOGS

Lymphoproliferative diseases of LGL in dogs include neoplastic and nonneoplastic disorders. In dogs that have neoplastic proliferations of LGL, clinical signs are vague and include lethargy, anorexia, polydipsia, and polyuria.[4,11] Peripheral lymph nodes may be mildly enlarged, and there may be splenomegaly or hepatosplenomegaly. Pleural effusion and a cranial mediastinal mass have been reported. In some dogs the disease behaves like an aggressive form of lymphoid leukemia, and these dogs may have significant lymphocytosis. Lymphocyte counts of 67 to $138 \times 10^9/L$ have been reported. The majority (80 to 97%) of the circulating lymphocytes in these dogs are LGL, and there is infiltration of bone marrow, spleen, and liver.[4] Other cases have been recognized that clinically behave like chronic lymphoid leukemia. These dogs may have significant lymphocytosis and bone marrow involvement, but with a clinical course that progresses slowly over several years.[11] Other hematologic abnormalities in dogs that have LGL leukemia may include mild nonregenerative anemia, thrombocytopenia, and neutropenia or neutrophilia. Complete remission with normalization of the leukocyte count and CD4:CD8 ratio has been reported with chemotherapy in a dog that had chronic lymphoid leukemia involving LGL.[11]

LGL in dogs that have LGL leukemia may be small, medium, or large with a minimal to moderate amount of cytoplasm. Nuclei are round, oval, indented, or clover-leaf shaped with finely stippled to coarsely clumped chromatin, and nucleoli may be present or absent.[4,11] Granule number and size are variable. The granules may not be visible with some commercial quick stains but are apparent with Wright–Giemsa stain.[11] Neoplastic LGL appear to be negative for CAE, Sudan black B, peroxidase, ACP, PAS, and toluidine blue and focally positive for αNBE activity with and without sodium fluoride.[4,11] LGL from some dogs that have LGL leukemia are positive for CD3 and CD8 (PF Moore, personal communication, 1993–1994).[11]

Nonneoplastic proliferations of LGL have been described in dogs that have chronic ehrlichiosis. Laboratory abnormalities in these dogs include hyperproteinemia and moderate lymphocytosis. Lymphocyte counts were less than $20 \times 10^9/L$. The majority of circulating lymphocytes had a morphologic appearance compatible with LGL. Hematologic abnormalities resolved after appropriate antibiotic therapy.[38]

LGL LYMPHOPROLIFERATIVE DISEASES IN HORSES

There are few reports of horses that have LGL lymphoproliferative disorders.[29,48,49] These horses were old (14 to 18 years) and presented for depression, anorexia, weight loss, diarrhea, and abdominal discomfort. Hematologic findings were unremarkable except for increased numbers of LGL in two horses. There was infiltration of multiple tissues, including bone marrow, liver, kidney, abdominal lymph nodes, intestine, pancreas, and lung. LGL also were present in abdominal fluid. Neutropenia was reported in one horse. LGL in horses appear to have a morphology typical of LGL in other species except that multinucleate LGL have been described only in the horse. The granules are apparent with Wright–Giemsa stain but stain poorly with H&E. Positive staining with PTAH appears to be typical for equine LGL.

RATS

LGL leukemia occurs in aged Fisher rats. Affected rats are emaciated, have massive splenomegaly and have severe hemolytic anemia in the late stage of the disease.[30] Leukocytosis is characterized by variable numbers of abnormal LGL. Thrombocytopenia occurs in some rats. Neoplastic lymphocytes infiltrate the spleen, lymph nodes, and hepatic sinusoids. Lung, heart, kidneys, and bone marrow may be involved in advanced cases. Erythrophagocytosis by neoplastic LGL has been described. The granules in the neoplastic cells are visible with Wright–Giemsa stain but are inapparent with H&E staining. The leukemic cells originate from NK cells and stain positively with β-glucuronidase and ACP.[12,30]

MICE

Experimentally-induced LGL proliferations have been described in mice transgenic for the *tax* gene of the human T cell lymphotropic virus.[50] LGL proliferations have also been described in mice transgenic for the human GM-CSF receptor that are treated with GM-CSF.[21]

FERRETS

LGL lymphoma has been reported in a ferret that presented with a nonspecific clinical history, peripheral lymphadenopathy, and splenomegaly.[31] There was mild leukopenia with lymphopenia, normocytic normochromic anemia, and thrombocytopenia. Small numbers of LGL with atypical morphology were present in the peripheral blood. Atypical LGL were present in an aspirate from the prescapular lymph node. On histologic examination, there was infiltration of LGL in the spleen, liver, lung, and kidney. LGL stained lightly eosinophilic with Giemsa stain, and rare cells were positive with PTAH.

BIRDS

Lymphoproliferative disease involving LGL in the small intestine has been described in goldfinches and warblers that have intestinal coccidial infections. This may represent an exaggerated immunologic or inflammatory cellular response rather than a neoplastic proliferation.[32]

REFERENCES

1. **Loughran TP.** Clonal diseases of large granular lymphocytes. Blood 1993;82:1–14.
2. **Cerezo L, Shuster JJ, Pullen DJ, et al.** Laboratory correlates and prognostic significance of granular acute lymphoblastic leukemia in children. Am J Clin Pathol 1991;95:526–531.
3. **Oshimi K.** Lymphoproliferative disorders of natural killer cells. Int J Hematol 1996;63:279–309.
4. **Wellman ML, Couto CG, Starkey RJ, et al.** Lymphocytosis of large granular lymphocytes in three dogs. Vet Pathol 1989;26:158–163.
5. **Wellman ML, Hammer AS, DiBartola SP, et al.** Lymphoma involving large granular lymphocytes in cats: 11 cases (1982–1991). J Am Vet Med Assoc 1992;201:1265–1269.
6. **Chan WC, Link S, Mawle A, et al.** Heterogeneity of large granular lymphocyte proliferations: delineation of two major subtypes. Blood 1986;68:1142–1153.
7. **Darbès J, Majzoub M, Breuer W, et al.** Large granular lymphocyte leukemia/lymphoma in six cats. Vet Pathol 1998;35:370–379.
8. **Sun T, Cohen NS, Marino J, et al.** CD3+, CD4−, CD8− large granular T-cell lymphoproliferative disorder. Am J Hematol 1991;37:173–178.
9. **Sala P, Tonutti E, Feruglio C, et al.** Persistent expansions of CD4+ CD8+ peripheral blood T cells. Blood 1993;82:1546–1552.
10. **Cheney CM, Rojko JL, Kociba GJ, et al.** A feline large granular lymphoma and its derived cell line. In Vitro 1990;26:455–463.
11. **Goldman EE, Grindem CB.** What is your diagnosis? Seven-year-old dog with progressive lethargy and inappetence. Vet Clin Pathol 1997;26:187, 195–197.
12. **Van den Brink MR, Palomba ML, Basse PH, et al.** In situ localization of 3.23+ natural killer cells in tissues from normal and tumor-bearing rats. Cancer Res 1991;51:4931–4936.
13. **Ward JM, Reynold CW.** Large granular lymphocyte leukemia: a heterogeneous lymphocytic leukemia in F344 rats. Am J Pathol 1983;111:1–10.
14. **Kariya K, Konno A, Ishida T.** Perforin-like immunoreactivity in four cases of lymphoma of large granular lymphocytes in the cat. Vet Pathol 1997;34:156–159.
15. **Wisse E, Graet F, Luo D, et al.** Structure and function of sinusoidal lining cells in the liver. Toxicol Pathol 1996;24:100–111.
16. **Berke G.** Functions and mechanisms of lysis induced by cytolytic T lymphocytes and natural killer cells. In: Paul WE, ed. Fundamental immunology. New York: Raven Press, 1989;735–764.
17. **Orvieto R, Bar-Hava I, Schwartz A, et al.** Interleukin-2 production by human pre-implantation embryos. Gynecol Endocrinol 1997;11:331–334.
18. **Carson WE, Fehniger TA, Caligiuri MA.** CD56 bright natural killer subsets: Characterization of distinct functional responses to interleukin-2 and the c-kit ligand. Eur J Immunol 1997;27:354–360.
19. **Blanchard DK, Michelini-Norris MB, Djeu JY.** Production of granulocyte-macrophage colony stimulating factor by large granular lymphocytes stimulated with Candida albicans: role in activation of human neutrophil function. Blood 1991;77:2259–2265.
20. **Michelini-Norris MB, Blanchard DK, Friedman H, et al.** Involvement of large granular lymphocytes in the induction of tumor necrosis factor by Mycobacterium avian-intracellulare complex. J Leukoc Biol 1991;550:529–538.
21. **Nishajima I, Nakahata T, Watanabe S, et al.** Hematopoietic and lymphopoietic responses in human granulocyte-macrophage colony-stimulating factor (GM-CSF) receptor transgenic mice injected with human GM-CSF. Blood 1997;90:1031–1038.
22. **Young HA.** Regulation of interferon-gamma gene expression. J Interferon Cytokine Res 1996;16:563–568.
23. **Yagita H, Nakahata M, Kawasaki A, et al.** Role of perforin in lymphocyte-mediated cytolysis. Adv Immunol 1992;511:215–242.
24. **Podack ER, Hengartner H, Lichtenheld MG.** A central role of perforin in cytolysis? Annu Rev Immunol 1991;9:124–157.
25. **Vollenweider I, Groscurth P.** Ultrastructure of cell mediated cytotoxicity. Electron Microsc Rev 1991;4:249–267.
26. **Jain NC.** Essentials of veterinary hematology. Philadelphia: Lea & Febiger, 1993;68–69.
27. **Taouji S, Debout C, Izard J.** Arylsulfatase B in Kurloff cells: increased activity of anionic isoforms in guinea pig acute lymphoblastic leukemia. Leuk Res 1996;20:259–264.
28. **Endo Y, Cho K, Nishigaki K, et al.** Clinicopathological and immunological characteristics of six cats with granular lymphocytes tumors. Comp Immunol Microbiol Infect Dis 1998;21:27–42.
29. **Grindem DB, Roberts MC, McEntee MF, et al.** Large granular lymphocyte tumor in a horse. Vet Pathol 1989;26:86–88.
30. **Stromberg PC.** Large granular lymphocyte leukemia in F344 rats. Model for human Tγ lymphoma, malignant histiocytosis, and T-cell chronic lymphocytic leukemia. Am J Pathol 1985;119:517–519.
31. **Boone LI, Barthel R, Helman RG, et al.** Large granular lymphocyte leukemia in a ferret. Vet Clin Pathol 1995;24:6–10.
32. **Swayne DE, Getzy D, Slemons RD, et al.** Coccidiosis as a cause of transmural lymphocytic enteritis and mortality in captive Nashville warblers (Vermivora ruficapilla). J Wildl Dis 1991;27:614–620.
33. **Dhodapkar MV, Li C-Y, Lust JA, et al.** Clinical spectrum of clonal proliferations of T-large granular lymphocytes: a T-cell clonopathy of undetermined significance. Blood 1994;84:1620–1627.
34. **Macon WR, Williams ME, Greer JP, et al.** Natural killer-like T-cell lymphomas: Aggressive lymphomas of T-large granular lymphocytes. Blood 1996;87:1474–1483.
35. **Martin MP, Biggar RJ, Hamlin-Green G, et al.** Large granular lymphocytosis in a patient infected with HTLV-II. AIDS Res Hum Retroviruses 1993;9:715–719.
36. **Pulik M, Lionnet F, Genet P, et al.** CD3+ CD8+ CD56- clonal large granular lymphocytes leukemia and HIV infection. Br J Haematol 1997;98:447–445.
37. **Matsumoto Y, Tsujimoto H, Fukasawa M, et al.** Molecular cloning of feline leukemia provirus genomes integrated in the feline large granular lymphoma cells. Arch Virol 1990;111:177–185.
38. **Weiser MG, Thrall MA, Fulton R, et al.** Granular lymphocytosis and hyperproteinemia in dogs with chronic ehrlichiosis. J Am Anim Hosp Assoc 1991;27:84–88.
39. **Jaffe E.** Classification of natural killer (NK) and NK-like T-cell malignancies. Blood 1998;87:1207–1210.
40. **Drobatz KJ, Rogers F, Waddle J.** Globule leukocyte tumor in six cats. J Am Anim Hosp Assoc 1993;29:391–396.
41. **Finn J, Schwartz LW.** A neoplasm of globule leukocytes in the intestine of a cat. J Comp Pathol 1972;82:323–328.
42. **Franks PT, Harvey JW, Mays MC, et al.** Feline large granular lymphoma. Vet Pathol 1986;23:200–202.
43. **Goitsuka R, Tsuji M, Matsumoto Y, et al.** A case of feline large granular lymphoma. Jpn J Vet Sci 1988;50:593–595.
44. **Honor DJ, DeNicola DB, Turek JJ, et al.** A neoplasm of globule leukocytes in a cat. Vet Pathol 1986;23:287–292.
45. **Konno A, Hashimoto Y, Kon Y, et al.** Perforin-like immunoreactivity in feline globule leukocytes and their distribution. J Vet Med Sci 1994;56:1101–1105.
46. **McEntee MF, Horton S, Blue J, et al.** Granulated round cell tumor of cats. Vet Pathol 1993;30:195–203.
47. **Mcpherron MA, Chavkin MJ, Powers BE, et al.** Globule leukocyte tumor involving the small intestine in a cat. J Am Vet Med Assoc 1994;204:241–245.
48. **Kramer J, Tornquist S, Erfle J, et al.** Large granular lymphocyte leukemia in a horse. Vet Clin Pathol 1993;22:126–128.
49. **Quist CF, Harmon BG, Mahaffey EA, et al.** Large granular lymphocyte neoplasia in an aged mare. J Vet Diagn Invest 1994;6:111–113.
50. **Grossman WJ, Ratner L.** Cytokine expression and tumorigenicity of large granular lymphocyte leukemia cells from mice transgenic for the tax gene of human T-cell leukemia virus type I. Blood 1997;90:783–794.

CHAPTER 96

Cutaneous Lymphoma and Variants

• KAREN A. MORIELLO

Cutaneous lymphoma is broadly divided into the histopathologic subgroups of epitheliotropic cutaneous lymphoma (ECL) and nonepitheliotropic cutaneous lymphoma (NECL). Cutaneous lymphoma has several different clinical presentations and can be confused with many non-neoplastic skin diseases.

EPITHELIOTROPIC CUTANEOUS LYMPHOMA

ECL is an uncommon T cell neoplasm and has been reported in dogs, cats, horses, ferrets, rats, cattle, and hamsters. In dogs, the reported incidence varies from 1 to 8% of all skin malignancies. The origin is unknown. In humans, there is controversy as to whether the cellular proliferation begins as a reactive or neoplastic process. There is preliminary evidence in one cat that feline leukemia virus (FeLV) may be involved in the cause of feline ECL even though cats test negative for FeLV antigens.[1] Canine ECL is predominantly a $\gamma\delta$ T cell lymphoma in which T cells express CD8.[2]

Clinical Features

ECL is divided into several syndromes based on clinical signs, laboratory testing, and historical findings. The clinical features tend to blend with time, suggesting these syndromes represent a spectrum of the disease. ECL is a disease of older animals with a mean age of onset of 9 to 12 years. There is no sex or breed predilection.

Mycosis Fungoides

ECL is usually limited to the skin and is commonly called mycosis fungoides (MF). The term MF is an archaic and confusing misnomer (being confused with mycotic skin disease) and refers to the initial presentation of skin tumors that resemble mushrooms. As early signs are nonspecific, occurring in many other skin diseases, MF is often referred to as the great impersonator. In dogs and cats, four clinical presentations have been described:

1. Pruritic erythroderma and scaling. Many patients are examined for the complaint of idiopathic seborrhea or pruritus that is nonresponsive to treatment. Hair loss is common (Figs. 96.1 and 96.2).
2. Mucocutaneous ulceration or depigmentation of the nose, mucous membranes, or footpads. This is a rare presentation, and lesions may be localized to one or more of these regions. This form can be confused with pemphigus vulgaris, canine uveodermatologic syndrome, bullous pemphigoid, or lupus erythematosus.
3. Solitary or multiple plaques and tumors. The pruritic erythroderma form progresses to coalescing areas of thickened plaques and, eventually, to discrete tumors.
4. Infiltrative and ulcerative oral mucosal disease. An initial misdiagnosis of chronic stomatitis is common.

Pruritic erythroderma and scaling represent the early form of ECL. In people this stage may last for months or years before progressing to the stage of plaque and subsequently tumor. In dogs, this progression occurs over a period of months. In cats, early signs may also include areas of hair loss and mild scaling suggestive of dermatophytosis or demodicosis (see Alopecia mucinosa, below).

In ferrets, ECL begins as a pruritic scaling dermatosis. Alopecia, variable pruritus, depigmentation of nose and footpads, ulcerated plaques, onychogryposis, and diffuse erythema have been seen. Peripheral lymphadenopathy is variable.

Other findings include clinical signs of systemic illness (depression, weight loss, anorexia, fever, and lethargy) and peripheral lymphadenopathy, particularly in advanced cases. Internal organs usually are not affected, but may be involved late in the disease.

Sézary Syndrome

A rare variant of ECL seen in dogs, cats, and humans, Sézary syndrome is characterized by exfoliative erythroderma, multiple skin plaques and nodules, pruritus, peripheral lymphadenopathy, and the presence of Sézary cells (see Sézary Cells, below) in the cutaneous infiltrate and the peripheral blood (i.e., lymphocytic leukemia). In one case, a discrete neoplastic lung lesion was found.[3]

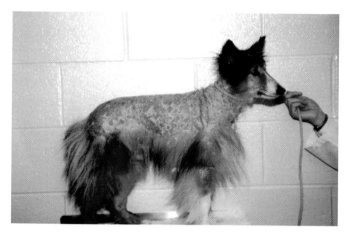

FIGURE 96.1 ECL in a Shetland sheep dog.

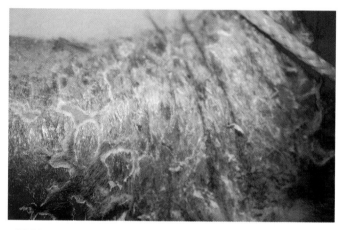

FIGURE 96.2 Close-up of the skin of the dog in Figure 96.1.

but there is no evidence of neoplasia. Histologic findings consistent with ECL develop over a period of months.

Laboratory Features

Skin Biopsy

Definitive diagnosis of ECL is made by histologic examination of multiple skin biopsies.[5] In patients that have early disease or that have unusual presentations, multiple biopsies over time may be needed before compatible histologic findings are found. Histologic findings typical of ECL include epitheliotropism of atypical lymphocytes, Pautrier microabscesses (focal accumulations of pleomorphic and atypical lymphocytes within the epithelium), the presence of mycosis cells (large 20- to 30-μm-diameter lymphocytes with hyperchromatic, indented, or folded nuclei), and a lichenoid band of pleomorphic lymphoid cells with or without plasma cells, neutrophils, and eosinophils in the superficial dermis and surrounding appendages (Figs. 96.3 and 96.4). In the early stages of the disease, histologic findings may be confused with lupoid skin disease or sebaceous adenitis.[5]

Immunohistochemical Staining

Cells are positive for CD3, indicating that they are of T cell lineage.[2] See Chapter 41, Lymphoid Markers: Use for Diagnosis, Treatment, and Prognosis, for a more detailed discussion of cell markers.

Sézary Cells

Sézary cells or Lutzner cells are found in the peripheral blood and characterize Sézary syndrome. These cells are small, 8- to 20-μm-diameter lymphocytes with hyperconvoluted nuclei that exhibit numerous fingerlike projections producing a cerebriform appearance.

Histologically, Sézary syndrome is indistinguishable from ECL limited to the skin.

Rare Presentations of Epitheliotropic Cutaneous Lymphoma

In the *tumor d'emblee variant* of ECL, solitary or multiple tumors develop without preexisting patch or plaque lesions.[4,5] *Pagetoid reticulosis* (Woringer-Kolopp disease) is a variant of localized ECL in which minimal dermal involvement occurs and lesions do not progress beyond the plaque stage.[4,5] Three cases of presumed pagetoid reticulosis have been described in dogs,[2] but no cases have been reported in cats. *Alopecia mucinosa* is a prodromal form of ECL in cats that have symptomatic, well-demarcated areas of alopecia and scaling on the head and neck.[4,5] On initial skin biopsy mucinosis of the epidermis and outer root sheath of the hair follicle is found,

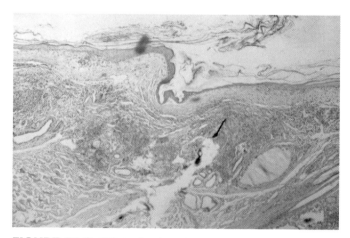

FIGURE 96.3 ECL in the skin of a dog. Note the intense cellular infiltrate at the dermal-epidermal junction. Courtesy of Dr. D. J. DeBoer, University of Wisconsin (original magnification 40×).

Direct Immunofluorescence

Skin biopsy specimens may show an intercellular pattern of deposition of immunoglobulin suggestive of pemphigus. False positive direct immunofluorescence (DIF) findings are common.

Cutaneous Cytology

Fine-needle aspirates of plaques or nodules often show pleomorphic atypical lymphocytes.

Lymph Node Aspirate

Reactive lymphoid hyperplasia with or without atypical lymphocytes is characteristic.

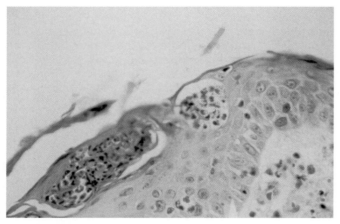

FIGURE 96.4 Pautrier microabscesses (focal accumulations of pleomorphic, atypical lymphocytes within the epithelium). Courtesy of V. Fadok, University of Florida (original magnification 100×).

Complete Blood Count

Hematologic findings may be normal or abnormal, depending on how early the disease is diagnosed.

Bone Marrow

Cytologic examination of bone marrow aspirates usually reveals no abnormalities.

Treatment

To date, therapy for ECL has resulted in sporadic responses. Chemotherapeutic protocols for systemic lymphoma have occasionally produced some degree of clinical improvement for 1 to 5 months. Topical mechlorethamine (nitrogen mustard) has been recommended for treatment of early lesions; however, there are no studies to document that mechlorethamine increases survival time.[4] Oral retinoids (isotretinoin or etretinate 1 to 8 mg/kg by mouth once daily) in conjunction with oral prednisone (2 to 4 mg/kg once daily) may produce clinical improvement.[6] Peg-l-asparaginase 30 U/kg intramuscularly or intraperitoneally weekly or biweekly produces a decrease in erythema and scaling in 50% of dogs treated; this therapy has no effect on the plaque or tumor stage.[7] Liposomal doxorubicin (Doxil) has resulted in remission in approximately 40% of cases, with some remissions being durable (Dr. David Vail, University of Wisconsin, personal communication, 1998).

Prognosis

The prognosis for ECL is grave. Many animals are euthanized as the intense pruritus is poorly responsive to

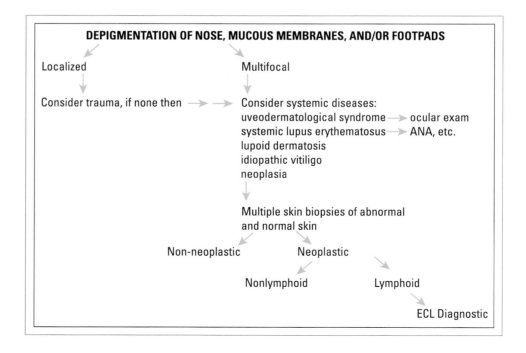

MUCOCUTANEOUS ULCERATION OR STOMATITIS

Azotemia or irritant reaction   No azotemia or irritant reaction

Localized to oral cavity   Involving multiple mucous
membranes

Consider dental disease,   Consider drug eruption, infections
if none then → →   (candidiasis, herpes, bacteria),
autoimmune disease (e.g., bullous
pemphigoid, pemphigus vulgaris,
systemic lupus erythematosus,
erythema multiforme)

Cytological examination of mucous membranes to
rule out yeast infection
Discontinue medications, if any
CBC, chemistry panel, UA, ANA,
multiple biopsies of lesions (particulary vesicles
and bullae)

Non-neoplastic   Neoplasia/proliferative

Nonlymphoid   Lymphoid

NECL   ECL

medical therapy. The survival time from diagnosis to death or euthanasia is 5 to 10 months. Some animals, however, have lived as long as 3 years, and the disease can wax and wane. Death is usually from septicemia, metastatic lymphoma, or euthanasia.

NONEPITHELIOTROPIC CUTANEOUS LYMPHOMA

The origin of NECL in animals is unknown; however epidemiologic studies suggest that environmental, infectious, and genetic influences may be involved.[8] This is the least common form of cutaneous lymphoma in the dog and the most common form in the cat.[2,4] Although rare, this tumor can occur in horses, guinea pigs, mice, and rabbits. The disease occurs in older animals (9 to 10 years of age) with no sex predilection. In dogs, boxers, St. Bernards, basset hounds, Irish setters, cocker spaniels, German shepherd dogs, golden retrievers, Weimeraners, and Scottish terriers may be predisposed.[4] There is no recognized breed predilection in other species.

Clinical Features

Skin

Tumors can be solitary, but are usually multifocal or generalized. The masses usually appear as firm dermal

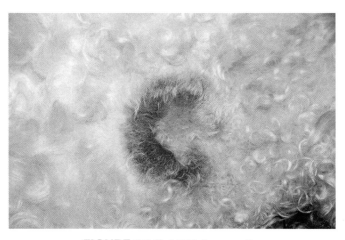

FIGURE 96.5 NECL in a poodle.

or subcutaneous nodules and are often red to purple (Fig. 96.5). Sometimes the lesions appear as serpiginous or irregular masses. Alopecia is variable. Exfoliative erythema is present in less than 20% of cases. Pruritus is rare, in contrast to ECL where it is very common and may be the presenting complaint. Involvement of the oral cavity (tongue and oropharynx) is uncommon but has been observed in dogs.

PRURITIC ERYTHRODERMA AND SCALING

↓

Visual examination for ectoparasites, skin scrapings, flea combings, impression smears of skin for bacteria and/or yeast dermatitis, dermatophyte culture, if negative

↘

Therapeutic trials: flea control, ivermectin, systemic antibiotics, systemic antifungals, if negative or no response

↘

Multiple skin biopsies of representative lesions

↙ ↘

Non-neoplastic, inflammatory skin disease   Proliferative/neoplastic skin disease

↙ ↘

Nonlymphoid   Lymphoid

↙ ↘

NECL   ECL

Other Organs

Affected animals often have signs of systemic involvement. Progression of the disease is rapid with lymph node and systemic metastasis. Lymphadenopathy is present in approximately two-thirds of patients. Splenomegaly may be present. Two cases of canine NECL associated with pulmonary vasoinvasive lymphoma have been described; respiratory distress was the presenting complaint in both cases.[2]

Laboratory Features

Immunophenotyping

Recent studies have shown that NECL are almost exclusively T cell lymphomas involving proliferation of $\alpha\beta$ or $\gamma\delta$ T cells with a CD8+ or CD4-/CD8-phenotype.[2] Previously, these tumors were believed to be of B lymphocyte origin.[4]

Cutaneous Cytology

Fine-needle aspirates of NECL typically show a uniform population of large histiocytic lymphocytes. These lymphocytes have ovoid to folded vesicular nuclei and abundant cytoplasm that may be vacuolated.

Skin Biopsies

Multiple skin biopsies of representative lesions are recommended; diagnostic excisional biopsy of small lesions is optimum.[5] Histologic findings typical of NECL include diffuse sheets or nodular aggregates of homogeneous lymphocytes in the deep dermis and subcutaneous tissue, a Grenz zone (area without cells) between the epithelium and the lymphoid infiltrate, and rare neoplastic lymphocytes in the epidermis. Cells are inter-mediate in size between small lymphocytes and macrophages and have scant, amphophilic cytoplasm. Large vesicular nuclei are round to ovoid, folded, or irregular with one or more nucleoli found along the nuclear membrane. The mitotic index is moderate to high. An eosinophilic infiltrate is common in 50% of cases, making it difficult to distinguish these cells from poorly differentiated cutaneous mast cell tumors or histiocytic proliferative skin diseases. Immunohistochemical staining techniques may be needed to differentiate NECL from these disorders.

Other Findings

In cats, FeLV and feline immunodeficiency virus tests are commonly negative. In dogs, hypercalcemia and increased serum viscosity may be present in rare cases; some cases are associated with monoclonal or biclonal gammopathies. Serum chemistry findings often are normal. Complete blood counts may be normal or abnormal, depending on how early the disease is diagnosed. Abnormal findings include normocytic normochromic anemia, leukocytosis, and circulating atypical lymphocytes.

Treatment

Many animals are euthanized because of poor prognosis, poor response to therapy, or aggressive progression of disease.[2,4,9,10] Solitary nodules may be excised, but recurrence is common. Some solitary nodules respond to radiation therapy. Concurrent chemotherapy enhances the chances of a rapid clinical remission; however, remission times for primary cutaneous lymphoma are shorter than for multicentric lymphoma.[10] The mean survival time from onset of skin lesions to death (usually euthanasia) is approximately 4 months.[10]

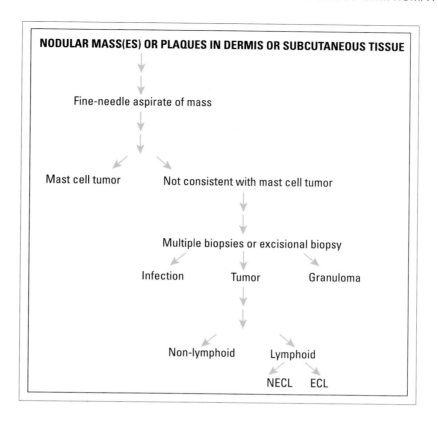

NODULAR MASS(ES) OR PLAQUES IN DERMIS OR SUBCUTANEOUS TISSUE

Fine-needle aspirate of mass

Mast cell tumor   Not consistent with mast cell tumor

Multiple biopsies or excisional biopsy

Infection   Tumor   Granuloma

Non-lymphoid   Lymphoid

NECL   ECL

REFERENCES

1. **Tobey JC, Houston DM, Breur GJ, et al.** Cutaneous T-cell lymphoma in a cat. J Am Vet Med Assoc 1994;204:606–609.
2. **Moore PF, Affolter VK, Olivry T, Schrenzel MK.** The use of immunological reagents in defining the pathogenesis of canine skin diseases involving proliferation of leukocytes. In: Kwochka KW, Willemse T, von Tscharner C, eds. Advances in veterinary dermatology, vol 3. Oxford: Butterworth Heinemann, 1998;77–94.
3. **Foster AP, Evans E, Kerlin R, et al.** Cutaneous T-cell lymphoma with Sézary syndrome in a dog. Vet Clin Pathol 1997;26:188–192.
4. **Scott DW, Miller WH, Griffin CE.** Lymphohistiocytic neoplasms. In: Small animal dermatology. 5th ed. Philadelphia: WB Saunders, 1995;1064–1072.
5. **Gross TL, Ihrke PJ, Walder EJ.** Lymphocytic tumors. In: Veterinary dermatopathology. A macroscopic and microscopic evaluation of canine and feline skin disease. St. Louis: Mosby Year Book, 1992;476–481.
6. **White SD, Rosychuk RAW, Scott KV, et al.** Use of isotretinoin and etretinate for the treatment of benign cutaneous neoplasia and cutaneous lymphoma in dogs. J Am Vet Med Assoc 1993;202:387–391.
7. **Moriello KA, MacEwen G, Schultz KT.** Peg L-asparaginase in the treatment of canine epitheliotropic lymphoma and histiocytic proliferative dermatitis. In: Ihrke PJ, Mason IS, White SD, eds. Advances in veterinary dermatology, vol 2. Oxford: Pergamon Press, 1993;293–299.
8. **Misdorp W.** Veterinary cancer epidemiology. Vet Q 1996;18:32–36.
9. **Moore PF, Olivry T.** Cutaneous lymphomas in companion animals. Clin Dermatol 1994;12:499–505.
10. **Beale KM, Bolon B.** Cutaneous lymphosarcoma: epitheliotropic and nonepitheliotropic, a retrospective study. In: Ihrke PJ, Mason IS, White SD, eds. Advances in veterinary dermatology, vol 2. Oxford: Pergamon Press, 1993;273–284.

CHAPTER 97

Plasma Cell Tumors and Macroglobulinemia

• DAVID M. VAIL

Plasma cell tumors result from neoplastic proliferation of cells of the B-lymphocyte or plasma cell lineage. Proliferation is believed in most instances to be monoclonal (i.e., derived from a single cell) in nature as homogeneous immunoglobulin (Ig) typically is produced. Plasma cell tumors include multiple myeloma (MM), immunoglobulin M (IgM) (Waldenström) macroglobulinemia, and solitary plasmacytoma (including solitary osseous plasmacytoma and extramedullary plasmacytoma). Based on incidence and severity, MM is the most clinically important plasma cell neoplasm.

MULTIPLE MYELOMA

Multiple myeloma (MM) represents 8% of all hematopoietic tumors in the dog.[1,2] The incidence in the cat is unknown; however, it is diagnosed much less frequently in this species.[3,4] MM is rare in other domestic species. In most cases the malignant plasma cells produce excessive amounts of a single type of Ig or Ig fragment, referred to as the M-component. Rarely, production of biclonal Ig has been reported.[5] The M-component can represent any class of Ig or fragments of the molecule, including the light chains (Bence Jones protein) or heavy chains (heavy chain disease).

Origin

The origin of MM is unknown. In humans, genetic predisposition, viral infection, chronic immune stimulation, and exposure to carcinogens have all been suggested as contributing factors.[6–8] MM has not been associated with either feline leukemia virus (FeLV) or feline immunodeficiency virus (FIV) infection in cats.

Pathophysiology

Neoplastic infiltration of organ systems or the presence of high circulating levels of M-component result in a wide array of abnormalities and related clinical syndromes. Animals that have MM are immunocompromised, and infectious diseases are often the ultimate cause of death. Normal Ig, as well as albumin, levels are usually depressed, and neutropenia may be present secondary to marrow infiltration (myelophthisis).

Myelophthisis, blood loss from coagulation disorders, anemia of chronic disease, and increased erythrocyte destruction secondary to high serum viscosity can result in variable cytopenias in animals that have MM. Normocytic normochromic (nonregenerative) anemia is encountered in two-thirds of affected dogs, and thrombocytopenia and leukopenia are observed in 25 to 30%.[1,9]

Several abnormalities can lead to a bleeding diathesis in animals that have MM. Hemorrhage may result from thrombocytopenia or interference with coagulation by M-component. Decreased platelet aggregation and release of platelet factor-3, adsorption of minor clotting proteins, generation of abnormal fibrin polymerization, and a functional decrease in calcium may all play roles in hemostatic defects.

Hypercalcemia, although rare in the cat, occurs in 15 to 20% of dogs that have MM and results primarily from the production of factors by the neoplastic cells that induce resorption of bone.[1,9,10,11] Osteolysis may also result in skeletal lesions. Elevated circulating N-terminal parathyroid hormone-related protein was noted in two dogs that had MM and hypercalcemia, although its relative contribution to hypercalcemia is unknown.[10] Hypercalcemia may also be exacerbated by associated renal disease.

Hyperviscosity syndrome (HVS) represents one of several clinicopathologic abnormalities resulting from greatly increased serum viscosity. HVS occurs in approximately 20% of dogs that have MM, but is less commonly observed in the cat. The extent of HVS is related to the type, size, shape, and concentration of the M-component in the blood. It is more likely when IgM macroglobulinemia is present owing to the higher molecular weight of IgM; however, IgA- and IgG-related HVS can occur.[1,9,12–19] The high serum viscosity can result in a bleeding diathesis, neurologic signs (e.g., dementia, depression, seizure activity, and coma), ophthalmic abnormalities (e.g., dilated and tortuous retinal vessels, retinal hemorrhage, retinal detachment), and increased cardiac workload with the potential for subsequent development of cardiomyopathy.[1,9,12–15] These consequences are thought to result from sludging of blood in small vessels, ineffective delivery of oxygen and nutrients, and coagulation abnormalities. The high protein concentration may also cause rouleaux formation by erythrocytes.

Evidence of renal disease is documented in 30 to 50% of dogs that have MM.[1] Nephropathy can result from Bence Jones (light-chain) proteinuria (BJP), tumor infiltration of renal tissue, hypercalcemia, amyloidosis, diminished perfusion secondary to hyperviscosity syndrome, dehydration, or ascending urinary tract infections, alone or in combination. The incidence of BJP is not established in the cat; however, it occurs in approximately 25 to 40% of dogs that have MM.

Cardiac disease, if present, usually results from excessive cardiac workload and myocardial hypoxia secondary to hyperviscosity. Anemia and amyloid deposition in the myocardium may be complicating factors.

Clinical Presentation and Signs

MM occurs in aged dogs and cats, and no breed or sex predilection has been consistently reported. Clinical signs are variable owing to the wide range of previously discussed pathologic effects occurring with MM[1] and are listed in decreasing order of frequency in Table 97.1. Lameness associated with osteolytic lesions is seen in approximately half the dogs that have MM. A bleeding diathesis is usually manifested as epistaxis and gingival bleeding. Central nervous system signs may include dementia, seizure activity, and deficiencies in midbrain or brainstem localizing reflexes secondary to HVS or extreme hypercalcemia. Signs reflective of transverse myelopathies secondary to vertebral column infiltration, pathologic fracture, or compression from an extradural mass compression can also occur.

In cats, anorexia and weight loss are the most common clinical signs, and a history of chronic respiratory infections may be present.[4,20] Hind-limb paresis secondary to osteolysis of lumbar vertebral bodies has been reported,[21] but skeletal lesions are uncommon in cats. Rather, organomegaly from organ infiltration with tumor is seen more commonly. Epistaxis, pleural and peri-

toneal hemorrhagic effusions, retinal hemorrhage, and central neurologic signs have been reported.[4,9,16–19] Polydipsia and polyuria can occur secondary to renal disease, and dehydration may develop.

Diagnosis

A diagnosis of multiple myeloma follows demonstration of bone marrow plasmacytosis, osteolytic bone lesions (primarily in the dog), and serum or urine myeloma proteins (M-component). In the absence of osteolytic bone lesions, a diagnosis also can be made if marrow plasmacytosis is associated with a progressive increase in M-component.

When MM is suspected, a complete blood count (CBC), platelet count, serum biochemistry profile, and urinalysis should be performed. Particular attention should be paid to renal function tests and serum calcium levels. If clinical hemorrhage is evident, evaluation of hemostasis (e.g., platelet count and prothrombin and partial thromboplastin times) and serum viscosity measurements should be undertaken.

Serum electrophoresis and immunoelectrophoresis determine the presence of a monoclonal gammopathy (Fig. 97.1) and categorize the class of Ig involved. In the dog, the incidence of immunoglobulin G (IgG) or immunoglobulin A (IgA) gammopathy is nearly equal, whereas the majority of cases of MM in the cat involve IgG.[1,4,9,16–19] If IgM constitutes the M-component, the term macroglobulinemia (Waldenström) is applied. Biclonal gammopathy has also been reported.[5,22] Occasionally,

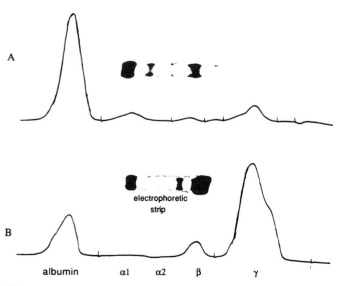

FIGURE 97.1 **A.** Serum protein electrophoresis from a normal dog and a stained cellulose acetate electrophoretic strip with accompanying densitogram. **B.** Serum protein electrophoresis from a dog that has MM. Note large M-component spike (representing an IgA monoclonal gammopathy) present in the γ region. Reprinted with permission from Vail DM. Plasma cell neoplasms. In: Withrow SJ, MacEwen EG, eds. Small animal clinical oncology. 2nd ed. Philadelphia: WB Saunders, 1996;512.

TABLE 97.1	Frequency of Clinical Signs in Dogs With Multiple Myeloma
Clinical Sign	**Frequency Reported (%)**
Lethargy and weakness	62
Lameness	47
Bleeding	37
Fundoscopic abnormalities	35
Polyuria/polydipsia	25
CNS deficit	12

cryoglobulinemia has been demonstrated in dogs that have MM.[9,23,24] Cryoglobulins are paraproteins that are insoluble at temperatures below 37°C and require blood collection and clotting to be performed at 37°C prior to serum separation. Electrophoresis, or heat precipitation, of urine is necessary to detect Bence Jones proteins as commercial urine dipstick methods do not detect these proteins.

Definitive diagnosis usually requires a bone marrow aspirate or core biopsy. Sometimes multiple aspirates are required for obtaining a diagnostic specimen. Normal marrow contains less than 5% plasma cells, whereas in myelomatous marrow the percentage is typically much higher (Fig. 97.2). The degree of differentiation and, therefore, the microscopic appearance of malignant plasma cells can vary from that of normal plasma cells to those in early stages of differentiation. Bizarre forms may also be observed.

The presence and extent of osteolytic lesions have diagnostic, prognostic, and therapeutic implications and should be determined by skeletal survey radiography. Rarely, biopsy of osteolytic lesions (i.e., Jamshidi core biopsy) is necessary for diagnosis. Bony lesions can be isolated discrete lesions (including pathologic fractures) or diffuse osteopenias. Approximately 25 to 30% of dogs that have MM have evidence of bony lysis or diffuse osteoporosis. Bones engaged in active hematopoiesis (e.g., vertebrae, ribs, pelvis, skull, and proximal long bones) are more commonly affected. Skeletal lesions are rare in cats that have MM and in dogs that have IgM (Waldenström) macroglobulinemia.[1,4,9,20] In macroglobulinemia, malignant cells are more likely to infiltrate the spleen, liver, and lymphoid tissue than bone.[8,24]

All animals should undergo a careful funduscopic exam. Abnormalities may include retinal hemorrhage, venous dilatation with sacculation and tortuosity, retinal detachment, and blindness.

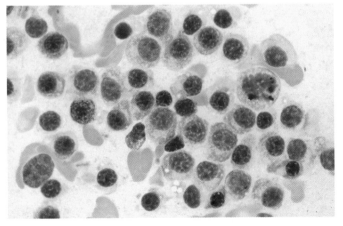

FIGURE 97.2 Bone marrow aspirate from a dog that has MM. Plasma cells comprise >50% of the nucleated-cell population. A mitotic figure is present. Occasional late erythroid precursors are scattered among the plasma cells. Wright-Giemsa Stain. Original magnification 600×. Photomicrograph courtesy of Karen M. Young, University of Wisconsin-Madison.

Differential Diagnosis

Syndromes other than MM can be associated with monoclonal gammopathies and should be considered in the list of differential diagnoses. These include other lymphoproliferative disorders (e.g., lymphoma and chronic and acute lymphocytic leukemia), chronic infections (e.g., ehrlichiosis, leishmaniasis, and feline infectious peritonitis), and monoclonal gammopathy of unknown significance (MGUS). MGUS (also referred to as benign, essential, or idiopathic monoclonal gammopathy) is a benign monoclonal gammopathy that is not associated with osteolysis, bone marrow infiltration, or BJP.[25,26] Ehrlichiosis may also cause bone marrow plasmacytosis and should be eliminated from the diagnosis based on serology and a history of exposure.

Treatment

Initial Therapy of Multiple Myeloma

Therapy should be directed at both the tumor cell mass and the secondary systemic effects. Chemotherapy is highly effective at reducing myeloma cell burden, relieving bone pain, initiating skeletal healing, and reducing levels of serum Igs.[1,9] Its use significantly enhances the quality of most patients' lives and prolongs their survival. Complete elimination of neoplastic myeloma cells is rarely achieved, however, and although MM remains a gratifying disease to treat, eventual relapse is to be expected.

The treatment of choice for MM in dogs is a combination of melphalan, an alkylating agent, and prednisone. The initial starting dosage of melphalan is 0.1 mg/kg by mouth once daily for 10 days; it is then reduced to 0.05 mg/kg by mouth once daily continuously. Prednisone is initiated at a dosage of 1.0 mg/kg by mouth once daily for 10 days, then reduced to 0.5 mg/kg every other day. Therapy is continued until clinical relapse occurs or myelosuppression, in particular thrombocytopenia, necessitates a dose reduction. CBCs, including platelet counts, should be performed biweekly for 2 months after initiation of therapy and monthly thereafter. If significant thrombocytopenia or neutropenia occurs, reduction of the dose or treatment frequency may be necessary. An alternative pulse dosing regimen for melphalan (7 mg/m² by mouth daily for 5 consecutive days every 3 weeks) has been used successfully in a small number of cases in which thrombocytopenia resulted from the use of more conventional continuous low-dose therapy. Melphalan and prednisone therapy has also been used in cats that have MM; however, response rates are low and durations of response are short-lived.

Cyclophosphamide has been advocated as an alternative alkylating agent for the treatment of MM; however, there is no evidence to suggest it is superior. In the author's practice, cyclophosphamide is limited to those animals that present with severe hypercalcemia or with widespread systemic involvement in which a faster-acting alkylating agent theoretically would alleviate systemic effects of the disease more quickly. In those situations, cyclophosphamide is initiated at a dosage of 200 mg/m^2 intravenously once at the same time oral melphalan therapy is started. Chlorambucil, another alkylating agent, has been used successfully for the treatment of IgM macroglobulinemia in dogs at a dosage of 0.2 mg/kg by mouth once daily.[9]

Evaluation of Response to Therapy

Evaluations of response should be based on improvement in clinical signs, clinicopathologic parameters, and radiographic appearance of skeletal lesions. Subjective improvement in bone pain, lameness, lethargy, and anorexia should be evident within 3 to 4 weeks. Resolution of laboratory abnormalities, including reduction in serum Ig levels or BJP, is usually noted within 3 to 6 weeks. Alleviation of osteolytic bone lesions may take months of therapy, and radiographic resolution may only be partial.

Complete resolution of MM rarely occurs with therapy, and a reduction in measured M-component (i.e., Ig or Bence Jones proteins) to at least 50% of pretreatment values would be classified as a good response.[9] Quantification of serum Ig or urine Bence Jones protein is performed monthly until a good response is noted and then every 2 to 3 months thereafter. Bone marrow evaluation is performed if M-component levels again rise or if clinical signs recur. Additionally, if clinicopathologic evidence of cytopenias (thrombocytopenia in particular) occurs during therapy, a bone marrow aspirate is indicated to differentiate between myelophthisis and chemotherapy-induced myelosuppression.

Therapy Directed at Complications of Multiple Myeloma

Reduction of neoplastic plasma cells results in long-term control of complications, including hypercalcemia, HVS, bleeding diatheses, renal disease, immunosuppression, and pathologic skeletal fractures. Therapy directed more specifically at these complications may, however, be indicated in the short term.

If hypercalcemia is severe and causes significant clinical signs, standard therapies specifically directed at lowering serum calcium are indicated (see Chapter 92, Lymphoma: Principles of Management). Moderate hypercalcemia typically resolves within 2 to 3 days after initiation of melphalan or prednisone chemotherapy.

Plasmapheresis is used for managing clinically significant hyperviscosity syndrome. Whole blood is collected from the patient, centrifuged to separate plasma from packed cells, and the latter is then resuspended in normal saline and reinfused back into the patient. Bleeding diathesis usually resolves along with HVS, however, platelet-rich plasma transfusions may be necessary in the face of thrombocytopenia.

Renal impairment may necessitate aggressive fluid therapy, careful attention to secondary urinary tract infections, and appropriate antimicrobial therapy. Patients that have multiple myeloma are often immunosuppressed; however, although prophylactic antibiotic therapy in dogs that have MM has been recommended,[9] no benefit to this approach over diligent monitoring for infection and subsequent aggressive antimicrobial therapy has been observed in people who have MM.[27] When indicated, cidal antimicrobial agents with low nephrotoxic potential are preferred.

Pathologic fractures of weight-bearing long bones or of vertebrae with resulting spinal cord compression may require immediate surgical intervention in conjunction with systemic chemotherapy. Stabilization of fractures and spinal cord decompression should be undertaken when necessary and may be followed with external beam radiotherapy. Etidronate, a biphosphonate used to inhibit bone resorption, is presently being investigated for use in cases of widespread bony lysis to palliate bone pain. Further investigations are warranted to determine its efficacy.

Rescue Therapy

Rescue therapy is initiated at the time of relapse when melphalan or prednisone combinations are ineffective or in cases that are initially resistant to standard therapy. The author has had, in a few cases, success with a combination of doxorubicin (30 mg/m^2 intravenously q 21 days), vincristine (0.7 mg/m^2 intravenously days 8 and 15), and prednisone (1.0 mg/kg by mouth daily), given in 21-day cycles. Most dogs initially respond to this rescue protocol, however, the response tends to be short-lived, lasting only a few months. High-dose cyclophosphamide (300 mg/m^2 intravenously q 7 days) has also been used with limited success as a rescue agent. A durable rescue with liposome-encapsulated doxorubicin has been reported in a dog that had MM.[28]

Prognosis

In the short term, the prognosis for dogs that have MM is good with respect to initial control of the tumor and a return to good quality of life, and a median survival of 540 days is reported. In a group of 60 dogs that had MM, 43% achieved a complete remission (i.e., serum Ig levels normalized) and 49% achieved a partial remission (i.e., Ig levels were <50% pretreatment values), whereas only 8% did not respond to combination chemotherapy with melphalan or prednisone.[1] The long-term prognosis for dogs that have MM is poor, however, as recurrence is expected. Eventually, the tumor is no longer responsive to available chemotherapeutic agents. Death results from either renal failure or sepsis, or owners choose euthanasia owing to the animal's intractable bone or spinal pain. The presence of hypercalcemia, BJP, and extensive bony lysis are known negative prognostic indices in the dog. Less is understood about the prognosis for dogs that have IgM macroglobulinemia. In a report of 9 cases, response to chlorambucil occurred in the majority of dogs, and a median survival of 11 months was reported.[9]

The prognosis for multiple myeloma in cats is poor

compared with that for dogs.[4,18,20] Most cats transiently respond to melphalan or prednisone or cyclophosphamide-based protocols; however, responses are not durable, and most animals succumb within 2 to 3 months after diagnosis. One case of long-term survival has been reported in a cat.[11]

SOLITARY PLASMACYTOMA

Focal monoclonal plasmacytic tumors can originate in bone or soft tissues and are referred to as solitary osseous plasmacytoma (SOP) and extramedullary plasmacytoma (EMP), respectively. The majority of SOP eventually progresses to systemic MM.[29,30] The biological behavior of EMP varies with the anatomical location. Cutaneous and oral cavity EMPs are typically benign disorders in the dog. In contrast, noncutaneous EMP, in particular alimentary tract tumors, are associated with a much more aggressive natural behavior and have been reported to involve the esophagus, stomach, and small and large intestine.[31–36] Although bone marrow involvement and gammopathies are less common in these alimentary cases, metastasis to regional lymph nodes is common. There is one report of subcutaneous EMP in a cat that had IgG gammopathy that progressed to lymph node and distant metastasis.[37]

Clinical Signs

Anatomical location of involvement is reflected by clinical signs associated with solitary plasmacytomas. In rare cases there are significant elevations in M-component proteins, and hyperviscosity syndromes may occur. SOP is usually associated with pain and lameness if the appendicular skeleton is affected or neurologic signs if vertebrae are involved. The more benign cutaneous form of EMP usually is not associated with clinical signs. In contrast, animals that have alimentary EMP often present with signs suggestive of gastrointestinal disease. Ataxia and seizure activity secondary to tumor-associated hypoglycemia have been reported in one dog that had extramedullary plasmacytoma.[38]

Diagnosis

Biopsy and histopathologic evaluation of tissue are necessary for the diagnosis of SOP and EMP. Immunohistochemical analysis to detect Ig, light and heavy chains, and thioflavin T may be helpful in confirming a diagnosis in more poorly differentiated tumors. In these cases thorough staging of the disease, including evaluation of bone marrow, serum protein electrophoresis, and skeletal survey radiographs, is required for ensuring confinement of the disease to a single site prior to initiation of therapy.

Therapy

If thorough clinical staging fails to identify systemic involvement, animals that have solitary forms of plasma cell tumors may be treated with local therapy in the absence of systemic chemotherapy. Local therapy can include surgical excision or external beam radiotherapy, alone or in combination. Most dogs that have SOP and noncutaneous EMP eventually develop systemic MM, and whether systemic chemotherapy should be initiated at the time of local therapy is controversial. In humans who have solitary plasmacytomas, systemic spread may not occur for many months to years after diagnosis, and there is no advantage to initiating systemic chemotherapy before documentation of systemic spread.[27] In the author's opinion, the same reasoning should be applied to animal patients: after local control of the tumor, the animal should be monitored regularly. If recurrence of disease and systemic spread are detected, systemic therapy described above for MM is warranted.

Prognosis

Cutaneous plasmacytomas in dogs are usually cured after surgical excision. Dogs that have SOP or EMP of the alimentary tract treated by surgical excision in combination with systemic chemotherapy once systemic disease is documented enjoy long-term survival in the majority of cases.

REFERENCES

1. **Matus RE, Leifer CE, MacEwen EG, Hurvitz AI.** Prognostic factors for multiple myeloma in the dog. J Am Vet Med Assoc 1986;188:1288–1291.
2. **Liu S-K, Dorfman HD, Hurvitz AI, et al.** Primary and secondary bone tumors in the dog. J Small Anim Pract 1977;18:313–326.
3. **Engle GC, Brodey RS.** A retrospective study of 395 feline neoplasms. J Am Anim Hosp Assoc 1969;5:21–31.
4. **Carpenter JL, Andrews LK, Holzworth J.** Tumors and tumor like lesions. In: Holzworth J, ed. Diseases of the cat. Medicine and surgery. Philadelphia: WB Saunders, 1987:406–596.
5. **Larsen AE, Carpenter JL.** Hepatic plasmacytoma and biclonal gammopathy in a cat. J Am Vet Med Assoc 1994;205:708–710.
6. **Potter M, Morrison S, Weiner F.** Induction of plasmacytomas with silicone gel in genetically susceptible strains of mice. J Natl Cancer Inst 1994;86:1058–1065.
7. **Imahori S, Moore GE.** Multiple myeloma and prolonged stimulation of RES. N Y State J Med 1972;72:1625–1628.
8. **Porter DD.** The development of myeloma-like condition in mink with Aleutian disease. Blood 1967;25:736–741.
9. **MacEwen EG, Hurvitz AI.** Diagnosis and management of monoclonal gammopathies. Vet Clin North Am Small Anim Pract 1977;7:119–132.
10. **Shull RM, Osborne CA, Barrett RE, et al.** Serum hyperviscosity syndrome associated with IgA multiple myeloma in two dogs. J Am Anim Hosp Assoc 1978;14:58–70.
11. **Hurvitz AI, Haskins SC, Fischer CA.** Macroglobulinemia with hyperviscosity syndrome in a dog. J Am Vet Med Assoc 1970;157:455–460.
12. **Center SA, Smith JF.** Ocular lesions in a dog with hyperviscosity secondary to an IgA myeloma. J Am Vet Med Assoc 1982;181:811–813.
13. **Kirschner SE, Niyo Y, Hill BL, Betts DM.** Blindness in a dog with IgA-forming myeloma. J Am Vet Med Assoc 1988;193:349–350.
14. **Hawkins EC, Feldman BF, Blanchard PC.** Immunoglobulin A myeloma in a cat with pleural effusion and serum hyperviscosity. J Am Vet Med Assoc 1986;188:876–878.
15. **Williams DA, Goldschmidt MH.** Hyperviscosity syndrome with IgM monoclonal gammopathy and hepatic plasmacytoid lymphosarcoma in a cat. J Small Anim Pract 1982;23:311–323.
16. **Forrester SD, Greco DS, Relford RL.** Serum hyperviscosity syndrome associated with multiple myeloma in two cats. J Am Vet Med Assoc 1992;200:79–82.
17. **Hribernik TN, Barta O, Gaunt SD, Boudreaux MK.** Serum hyperviscosity syndrome associated with IgG myeloma in a cat. J Am Vet Med Assoc 1982;181:169–170.
18. **Rosol TJ, Nagode LA, Couto CG, et al.** Parathyroid hormone (PTH)-related protein, PTH, and 1,25-dihydroxyvitamin D in dogs with cancer associated hypercalcemia. Endocrinology 1992;131:1157–1164.

19. **Sheafor SE, Gamblin RM, Couto CG.** Hypercalcemia in two cats with multiple myeloma. J Am Anim Hosp Assoc 1996;32:503–508.
20. **Drazner FH.** Multiple myeloma in the cat. Compend Cont Educ Pract Vet 1982;4:206–216.
21. **Mitcham SA, McGillivray SR, Haines DM.** Plasma cell sarcoma in a cat. Can Vet J 1985;26:98–100.
22. **Jacobs RM, Couto CG, Wellman ML.** Biclonal gammopathy in a dog with myeloma and cutaneous lymphoma. Vet Pathol 1986;23:211–213.
23. **Braund KG, Everett RM, Bartels JE, DeBuysscher E.** Neurologic complications of IgA multiple myeloma associated with cryoglobulinemia in a dog. J Am Vet Med Assoc 1979;174:1321–1325.
24. **Hurvitz AI, MacEwen EG, Middaugh CR, Litman GW.** Monoclonal cryoglobulinemia with macroglobulinemia in a dog. J Am Vet Med Assoc 1977;170:511–516.
25. **Hoenig M, O'Brien JA.** A benign hypergammaglobulinemia mimicking plasma cell myeloma. J Am Anim Hosp Assoc 1988;24:688–690.
26. **Dewhirst MW, Stamp GL, Hurvitz AI.** Idiopathic monoclonal (IgA) gammopathy in a dog. J Am Vet Med Assoc 1977;170:1313–1316.
27. **Anderson K.** Plasma cell tumors. In: Holland JF, Frei E, Bast RC, Kufe DW, Morton DL, Weichselbaum RR, eds. Cancer medicine. 3rd Ed. Philadelphia: Lea & Febiger, 1993:2075–2092.
28. **Kisseberth WC, MacEwen EG, Helfand SC, et al.** Response to liposome-encapsulated doxorubicin (TLC D-99) in a dog with myeloma. J Vet Intern Med 1995;9:425–428.
29. **MacEwen EG, Patnaik AK, Hurvitz, Bradley R.** Nonsecretory multiple myeloma in two dogs. J Am Vet Med Assoc 1984;184:1283–1286.
30. **Meis JM, Butler JJ, Osborne BM, Ordonez NG.** Solitary plasmacytomas of bone and extramedullary plasmacytomas. Cancer 1987;59:1475–1485.
31. **Hamilton TA, Carpenter JL.** Esophageal plasmacytoma in a dog. J Am Vet Med Assoc 1994;204:1210–1211.
32. **MacEwen EG, Patnaik AK, Johnson GF, Hurvitz AI.** Extramedullary plasmacytoma of the gastrointestinal tract in two dogs. J Am Vet Med Assoc 1984;184:1396–1398.
33. **Brunnert SR, Dee LA, Herron AJJ, Altman NH.** Gastric extramedullary plasmacytoma in a dog. J Am Vet Med Assoc 1992;200:1501–1502.
34. **Jackson MW, Helfand SC, Smedes SL, et al.** Primary IgG secreting plasma cell tumor in the gastrointestinal tract of a dog. J Am Vet Med Assoc 19194;204:404–406.
35. **Lester SJ, Mesfin GM.** A solitary plasmacytoma in a dog with progression to a disseminated myeloma. Can Vet J 1980;21:284–286.
36. **Trevor PB, Saunders GK, Waldron DR, Leib MS.** Metastatic extramedullary plasmacytoma of the colon and rectum in a dog. J Am Vet Med Assoc 1993;203:406–409.
37. **Carothers MA, Johnson GC, DiBartola SP, et al.** Extramedullary plasmacytoma and immunoglobulin-associated amyloidosis in a cat. J Am Vet Med Assoc 1989;195:1593–1597.
38. **DiBartola SP.** Hypoglycemia and polyclonal gammopathy in a dog with plasma cell dyscrasia. J Am Vet Med Assoc 1982;180:1345–1348.

CHAPTER 98

Cancer-Associated Hypercalcemia

• THOMAS J. ROSOL and CHARLES C. CAPEN

CANCER-ASSOCIATED HYPERCALCEMIA

The most common cause of clinically relevant hypercalcemia in animals and humans is cancer-associated hypercalcemia (CAH). There are three principal pathogenic mechanisms (Fig. 98.1): (1) humoral hypercalcemia of malignancy (HHM), (2) local bone resorption induced by hematologic malignancies that grow primarily in the bone marrow, and (3) local osteolysis of bone by metastatic tumors.[1]

Humoral Hypercalcemia of Malignancy: Pathogenesis and Associated Neoplasms

HHM is the most common form of CAH and is associated with diverse malignant neoplasms.[1] It occurs most often in dogs and sporadically in cats, horses, and other animals.[2] Clinical findings include hypercalcemia (total and ionized), hypophosphatemia, hypercalciuria (often with decreased fractional calcium excretion), increased excretion of phosphorus, and increased osteoclastic bone resorption. It results from the release of humoral factors by cancer cells that induce osteoclastic bone resorption, renal reabsorption of calcium, or increased calcium absorption from the intestine.[3]

The most important humoral factor is parathyroid hormone-related protein (PTHrP), but other factors may act alone or in concert with PTHrP (Fig. 98.2). Such factors include interleukin-1, tumor necrosis factors, transforming growth factors, and 1,25-dihydroxyvitamin D (calcitriol). PTHrP binds to the N-terminal PTH/PTHrP receptor in bone and kidney, but does not cross-react immunologically with native parathyroid hormone (PTH) (Fig. 98.3). PTHrP results in stimulation of osteoclastic bone resorption, increased renal tubular calcium reabsorption, and decreased renal tubular phosphate reabsorption. Cytokines act synergistically or additively with PTHrP by stimulating osteoclastic bone resorption. Interleukin-1 stimulates bone resorption in vivo and in vitro and is synergistic with PTHrP.[4] Transforming growth factors-α and -β can stimulate bone resorption in vitro and have been identified in tumors associated with HHM, including adenocarcinomas derived from apocrine glands of the anal sac in dogs.[5] In some forms of HHM, there are increased serum levels of 1,25-dihydroxyvitamin D that may increase calcium absorption from the intestine.[6]

The humoral factors represent proteins or hormones that are produced by cells of the body from which the malignancy is derived and typically act locally (paracrine action). For example, PTHrP is produced by normal tissues, including epidermis, endocrine glands, lymphocytes, bone, brain, cardiac and smooth muscle, and epithelial cells in many organs where it functions as a paracrine factor.[2,7] Despite the widespread production of PTHrP in the body, serum PTHrP concentrations are low (<2 pmol/L). In HHM, tumor cells secrete excessive amounts of the humoral factors that function distant to the tumor in bone and kidney (endocrine action). Before PTHrP was identified it was understood that tumors associated with HHM induced a syndrome that mimicked primary hyperparathyroidism owing to secretion of a PTH-like factor. Purification of the PTH-like activity from human and animal tumors associated with HHM resulted in the characterization of PTHrP.[1]

The kidney plays a critical role in the pathogenesis of hypercalcemia, because calcium reabsorption is stimulated by PTHrP. The level of renal function in the patient may contribute to development of hypercalcemia. Animals that suffer from dehydration or impaired renal function are more susceptible to developing hypercalcemia or have worse hypercalcemia owing to decreased renal excretion of calcium.

Malignancies that are commonly associated with HHM include T cell lymphoma and adenocarcinomas derived from apocrine glands of the anal sac.[1,8] In addition, sporadic cases of HHM occur with thymoma or carcinomas originating in diverse tissues, such as lung, pancreas, thyroid gland, skin, mammary gland, nasal cavity, and adrenal medulla.[1,3]

Lymphoma

Lymphoma is the most common cause of HHM in dogs.[9,10] Approximately 30% of dogs that have lymphoma develop clinically relevant hypercalcemia. Most dogs that have lymphoma and hypercalcemia have the clinical syndrome of HHM, since increased osteoclastic

Cancer-Associated Hypercalcemia

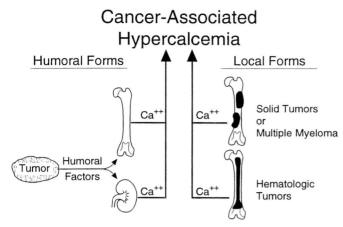

FIGURE 98.1 Pathogenesis of CAH. Humoral and local forms of CAH increase circulating concentrations of calcium by stimulation of osteoclastic bone resorption and increased renal tubular reabsorption of calcium.

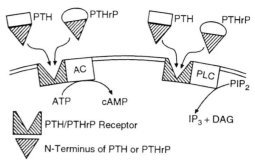

FIGURE 98.3 PTHrP induces many of the effects of PTH by interacting with the PTH receptor in bone and kidney and activating adenylate cyclase (AC) to form cAMP and phospholipase C (PLC) to form inositol triphosphate (IP_3) and diacylglycerol (DAG) from phosphatidylinositol (PIP_2). Stimulation of the PTH receptor results in increased osteoclastic bone resorption and renal tubular reabsorption of calcium, inhibition of renal tubular reabsorption of phosphorus, and stimulation of renal production of 1,25-dihydroxyvitamin D (calcitriol).

Humoral Factors and HHM

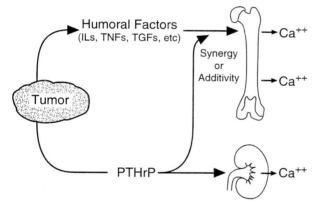

FIGURE 98.2 Humoral factors, such as PTHrP, interleukin-1 (IL-1), tumor necrosis factors (TNF), or transforming growth factors (TGF), produced by tumors induce HHM by acting as systemic hormones and stimulating osteoclastic bone resorption or increasing tubular reabsorption of calcium.

resorption is present in bones without evidence of tumor metastasis. Lymphomas associated with HHM are usually of the T cell subset.[8] Most dogs that have lymphoma and HHM have significantly increased circulating PTHrP concentrations, but levels are lower (2 to 15 pmol/L, normal is <2) than in dogs that have carcinomas and HHM (Fig. 98.4), and there is no correlation with serum calcium concentration.[6] This indicates that PTHrP is an important hormone in dogs that have HHM and lymphoma but that it is not the sole humoral factor responsible for the stimulation of osteoclasts and development of hypercalcemia. It is likely that cytokines, such as interleukin-1 and tumor necrosis factor, and 1,25-dihydroxyvitamin D may function synergisti-

cally with PTHrP to induce HHM in dogs that have lymphoma (Fig. 98.2).[1]

Lymphoma is an uncommon cause of HHM in cats,[11] ferrets,[12] horses,[13] and humans. There is a subset of lymphoma in humans (adult T cell lymphoma or leukemia [ATL]) that is caused by human T cell lymphotropic virus (HTLV-I) infection and has a high incidence of HHM. The ATL cells secrete PTHrP and other cytokines. Neoplastic ATL cells from humans have increased PTHrP and cytokine production resulting from stimulation of gene transcription by tax, the virally encoded transcription factor.[14] Dogs that have HHM and lymphoma may have a pathogenesis of hypercalcemia similar to that occurring in humans who have HTLV-I-induced lymphoma or leukemia.

Some dogs and humans that have lymphoma and hypercalcemia have increased serum 1,25-dihydroxyvitamin D (calcitriol) levels that may be responsible for or contribute to the development of hypercalcemia.[6,15] Certain lymphocytes contain the 1α-hydroxylase (similar to renal tubules) that converts 25-hydroxyvitamin D to the active metabolite, 1,25-dihydroxyvitamin D. Therefore, neoplastic lymphocytes that retain this capability can synthesize excessive 1,25-dihydroxyvitamin D, inducing increased calcium absorption from the intestinal tract and facilitate the development of hypercalcemia. In some cases of lymphoma this may be the principal humoral factor causing hypercalcemia.

Carcinoma

Carcinomas are the second most common cause of HHM in dogs. HHM occurs most frequently in dogs that have adenocarcinoma derived from apocrine glands of the anal sac (approximately 60% of cases) and sporadically with other carcinomas. Secretion of PTHrP plays the major role in the pathogenesis of HHM in patients that have carcinoma, and plasma PTHrP may be as great as

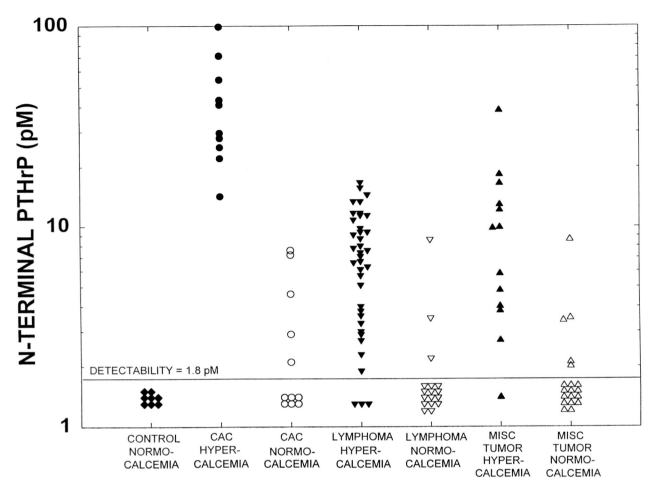

FIGURE 98.4 Circulating N-terminal PTHrP concentrations in normal dogs (CONTROL); dogs that have hypercalcemia (>12 mg/dl) and carcinomas of anal sac (CAC), lymphoma, or miscellaneous tumors (MISC TUMOR); and dogs that have normocalcemia (<12 mg/dl) and CAC, lymphoma, or miscellaneous tumors. (From Rosol TJ, Nagode LA, Couto CG, Hammer AS, Chew DJ, Peterson JL, Ayl RD, Steinmeyer CL, Capen CC. Parathyroid hormone (PTH)-related protein, PTH, and 1,25-dihydroxyvitamin D in dogs with cancer-associated hypercalcemia. Endocrinology 1992;131:1157-1164, with permission.)

100 pmol/L.[6] Carcinoma with HHM also occurs sporadically in cats and horses (e.g., squamous cell carcinoma).[3,13]

The adenocarcinoma derived from apocrine glands of the anal sac of dogs consistently fulfills the criteria for HHM.[16] This unique tumor appears primarily in middle-aged (mean of 10 years) female dogs and rarely metastasizes to bone. Dogs that have this tumor and HHM have hypercalcemia (12 to 24 mg/dL), hypophosphatemia, decreased immunoreactive PTH, increased osteoclastic bone resorption, and increased urinary excretion of calcium, phosphorus, and cyclic adenosine monophosphate (cAMP).[16]

Hypercalcemia was present at the time of diagnosis in 80 to 100% of affected dogs in early studies.[16,17] With earlier detection, the incidence of hypercalcemia can be lower (33%) in dogs.[18] Surgical removal or radiation therapy of the adenocarcinoma results in a rapid return of serum calcium and phosphorus to normal.[6] Metastasis to sublumbar lymph nodes occurs in a high percentage

(94%) of the dogs and is associated with a recrudescence of the biochemical alterations in serum and urine.[16]

Most dogs that have HHM have increased circulating concentrations of PTHrP (Fig. 98.4). Plasma concentrations of PTHrP are greatest in dogs that have apocrine adenocarcinomas of the anal sac and sporadic carcinomas associated with HHM (10 to 100 pM).[6] The serum calcium concentrations in these dogs correlate well with circulating PTHrP concentrations and are consistent with the concept that PTHrP plays a primary role in the pathogenesis of HHM in these dogs. Some dogs that have apocrine adenocarcinomas and normocalcemia can have increased plasma PTHrP concentrations (2 to 10 pM), but the concentrations are lower than in dogs that have hypercalcemia.

Some dogs that have apocrine adenocarcinomas have inappropriate levels of 1,25-dihydroxyvitamin D (in the normal range or increased) for the degree of hypercalcemia.[6] This suggests that the humoral factors produced by the neoplastic cells are capable of stimulating renal 1α-hydroxylase and increasing the formation of 1,25-dihydroxyvitamin D even in the presence of increased blood calcium. Plasma immunoreactive PTH is not increased in hypercalcemic dogs and is significantly less than that in dogs that have primary hyperparathyroidism.

Hematologic Malignancies

Some forms of hematologic malignancies grow preferentially in the bone marrow environment and induce hypercalcemia by inducing bone resorption locally.[1] This occurs most commonly with multiple myeloma and lymphoma or leukemia. Hypercalcemia has been reported in 17% of dogs and occasionally in cats that have multiple myeloma.[19,20] Numerous paracrine factors or cytokines act as stimulators of tumor-cell proliferation and are responsible for the stimulation of local bone resorption. The cytokines most often implicated in the pathogenesis of bone resorption include interleukin-1, tumor necrosis factor-α, and tumor necrosis factor-β (lymphotoxin).[21] Other cytokines or factors that may play a role include interleukin-6, transforming growth factor-α and -β, and PTHrP.[22] Production of low levels

of PTHrP by a tumor in bone may stimulate local bone resorption without inducing a systemic response since circulating concentrations of PTHrP are not increased. Prostaglandins (especially prostaglandin E2) also may be responsible for the local stimulation of bone resorption.

Some dogs that have lymphoma and hypercalcemia have localized bone resorption associated with growth of tumor in the medullary cavities of bones without evidence of increased bone resorption at sites distant from the tumor metastases.[23] The mediator of local bone resorption has not been identified; however, prostaglandin E2 may be an important primary or secondary local mediator of bone resorption in these dogs. Other potential mediators include cytokines, such as interleukin-1 or tumor necrosis factors. In some cases of lymphoma both HHM and bone metastases may contribute to the pathogenesis of hypercalcemia.[24,25]

Tumors Metastatic to Bone

Solid tumors that metastasize widely to bone can produce hypercalcemia by the induction of local bone resorption associated with tumor growth. This is not common in animals, but it is an important cause of CAH in humans.[1] Tumors that often metastasize to bone and

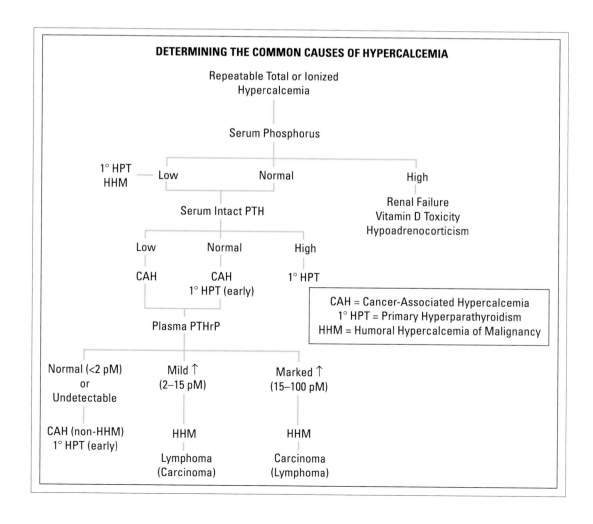

induce hypercalcemia in human patients include breast and lung carcinoma. Metastasis to bone in dogs has been reported most frequently with carcinoma of mammary gland, prostate, liver, and lung, and the humerus, femur, and vertebrae are the most likely sites of metastasis.[26] Primary bone tumors are not often associated with hypercalcemia in dogs or cats.

The pathogenesis of enhanced bone resorption is not well understood, but the two primary mechanisms are: (1) secretion of cytokines or factors that stimulate local bone resorption and (2) indirect stimulation of bone resorption by tumor-induced cytokine secretion from local immune or bone cells.[27] Cytokines or factors that may be secreted by tumor cells and stimulate local bone resorption include PTHrP,[28] transforming growth factors-α and -β, and prostaglandins (especially prostaglandin E2). PTHrP often is not secreted in high enough concentrations to induce HHM, but local production of PTHrP by tumor cells increases bone resorption and may enhance the capacity of tumors to metastasize to bone.[28] Bone resorbing activity can be inhibited by indomethacin in some cases, which suggests that prostaglandins are either directly or indirectly associated with the stimulation of bone resorption. The cytokines most often implicated in indirect stimulation of bone resorption by local immune cells include interleukin-1 and tumor necrosis factor.

Effects of Hypercalcemia

Ionized calcium is the serum calcium fraction that is important for the pathophysiologic effects of calcium.[29] Excess circulating levels of calcium ion are toxic to cells[30] and can result in cell death owing to deranged cell function and reduced energy production. Effects on the central nervous system, gastrointestinal system, heart, and kidney are of most importance clinically.

Polydipsia, polyuria, anorexia, depression, and weakness are the most common clinical signs in animals that have hypercalcemia.[31,32] Individual animals often have remarkable differences in clinical signs despite a similar magnitude of hypercalcemia. The severity of clinical signs and development of lesions from hypercalcemia depend not only on the magnitude of hypercalcemia, but also on its rate of development and duration. Anorexia, vomiting, and constipation result from hypercalcemia by reducing the excitability of gastrointestinal smooth muscle, as well as from direct effects on the central nervous system. Dehydration is common owing to increased fluid loss from vomiting and polyuria. Acidosis increases the proportion of serum calcium that is ionized, worsening clinical signs, whereas alkalosis lessens toxicity and clinical signs by decreasing the proportion of calcium that is ionized.

Abnormal renal function frequently accompanies hypercalcemia. The frequency of azotemia is higher in dogs that have a malignant neoplasm (71%) than in those that have hypercalcemia from primary hyperparathyroidism (11%).[33] Azotemia caused by hypercalcemia can result from prerenal reduction in extracellular fluid volume, renal vasoconstriction, decreased permeability of the glomerulus, acute tubular necrosis from ischemic and toxic effects of hypercalcemia, and chronic renal failure.[32]

Calcium ion has the unique capacity to regulate its own renal excretion. This action is mediated by the recently identified Ca^{2+}-sensing receptors on the renal epithelial cells.[34] Direct effects of hypercalcemia on the kidney include reduced tubular calcium and sodium reabsorption, antagonism to the actions of PTH, and inhibition of antidiuretic hormone action on cells of the collecting duct. This results in decreased urine concentration, polyuria, and hypercalciuria.[33] These responses by the kidney facilitate calcium excretion and help to alleviate the toxic effects of hypercalcemia on the kidney. Dehydration or renal failure significantly impairs the capacity of the kidney to excrete calcium and results in drastic worsening of the hypercalcemia.

Removal of the underlying cause is the definitive treatment for hypercalcemia, but this is not always immediately possible. In animals that have multicentric neoplasia or a nonresectable malignancy, the tumor burden and hypercalcemia may be decreased by appropriate chemotherapy, radiation therapy, and immunotherapy. Chemotherapy may disrupt neoplastic cellular metabolism so that the tumor can no longer synthesize enough humoral factors to sustain the hypercalcemia. Amelioration of the serum calcium concentration can occur despite lack of obvious reduction in tumor size in these patients. The principal agents used for symptomatic therapy of hypercalcemia include 0.9% NaCl infusion, sodium bicarbonate, furosemide, and bisphosphates (inhibitors of bone resorption).[9] See Chapter 92, Lymphoma: Principles of Management, for additional information.

Diagnosis

Serum Total and Ionized Calcium and Phosphorus

Discovery of increased serum total calcium concentration should be verified by repeated measurements. Total calcium concentration is more commonly measured than is serum ionized calcium (Ca^{2+}) concentration. In many clinical conditions, the total calcium concentration can be used as an indirect measure of Ca^{2+} concentration, but this can lead to a misinterpretation of calcium status in some patients. In dogs that have lymphoma and hypercalcemia, serum Ca^{2+} and total calcium concentrations correlate well, and serum Ca^{2+} measurement does not have an advantage compared to total calcium.[35] However, measurement of only total calcium concentration in dogs that have lymphoma and normocalcemia can result in overlooking mild ionized hypercalcemia. In cats, serum Ca^{2+} concentrations are only moderately well correlated to total calcium concentrations.[36] However, it is ideal to measure Ca^{2+} directly, and Ca^{2+} measurements may be superior to total calcium measurements in clinical conditions such as hyperparathyroidism, renal disease, hypoproteinemia and hyper-proteinemia, acid-base disturbances, and critical illnesses.[9,37] Serum phosphorus concentrations are usually low or in the low normal range in animals that have HHM owing to inhibition of renal reabsorption of phosphate by PTHrP. If the animals have azotemia, serum phosphorus can be increased secondary to renal failure.

Parathyroid Hormone-Related Protein

PTHrP is a 141 amino acid, single chain protein hormone. Two-site immunoradiometric assay (IRMA) and N-terminal radioimmunoassay (RIA) are available for the measurement of human PTHrP. These assays are useful in measuring biologically active PTHrP levels in the dog.[6,38,39] Because of the high degree of sequence homology in PTHrP between species, especially in the first 111 amino acids,[40] these assays likely will be useful for cats as well. An N-terminal RIA for human PTHrP has not proved useful to measure circulating PTHrP in a small number of horses.[13] PTHrP is susceptible to degradation by serum proteases; therefore, PTHrP concentrations must be measured in fresh or frozen plasma by use of ethylenediamine tetra-acetic acid (EDTA) as an anticoagulant. EDTA complexes with plasma calcium, which is required for the function of some proteases. The addition of protease inhibitors, such as aprotinin and leupeptin may provide further inhibition of proteolysis in plasma.[41] PTHrP concentrations measured in serum are inaccurate because of proteolysis during clotting and sample handling.

The circulating forms of PTHrP are not completely understood, because the molecule rapidly undergoes proteolysis intracellularly and extracellularly after secretion into blood.[41] The forms of PTHrP that are present in vivo include intact PTHrP, an N-terminal peptide, a combined N-terminal and midregion peptide, a midregion peptide, and a C-terminal peptide.[42,43] The fragments that would be expected to have PTH-like biologic activity in vivo include N-terminal PTHrP (1–36), N-terminal and midregion PTHrP (1–86), and intact PTHrP (1–141). The two-site immunologic assays measure intact PTHrP (1–141) and PTHrP (1–86) because antibodies binds to the N-terminus and midregion. N-terminal RIAs measure intact PTHrP (1–141), PTHrP (1–86), and N-terminal PTHrP (1–36). C-terminal PTHrP accumulates in the serum of human patients who have renal failure, suggesting that C-terminal PTHrP peptides, like PTH, are excreted by the kidney.[44]

Parathyroid Hormone

PTH circulates predominantly as intact PTH (1–84) and carboxyl-terminal fragments. Only intact PTH is biologically active, so it is best to measure this form in serum or plasma. Owing to homology between PTH from humans and animals, commercial assays developed for human PTH have been used successfully in certain animal species.[39] A two-site IRMA for intact human PTH has been validated in the dog and cat.[45,46] Cancer-associated hypercalcemia is associated with a low or below normal

PTH concentration.[6] Serum PTH is increased in most patients that have primary hyperparathyroidism, resulting from an adenoma of chief cells in the parathyroid gland.[6] Early in the course of disease of some animals that have primary hyperparathyroidism, serum PTH may be in the high normal range and serum Ca^{2+} concentration will be mildly increased. This is an inappropriate response of PTH to high serum calcium and is indicative of hyperparathyroidism. Animals that have late-stage renal failure and secondary hyperparathyroidism will have increased serum PTH concentrations.[47]

1,25-dihydroxyvitamin D (Calcitriol)

Measurement of vitamin D metabolites, although not commonly performed in clinical veterinary medicine, occasionally is helpful in the diagnosis of disorders of calcium homeostasis. The metabolites are stable during refrigeration and freezing, but samples should not be exposed to light for long periods. The metabolites of vitamin D are chemically identical in all mammals; therefore, receptor-binding assays and RIAs developed for use in humans are satisfactory for the measurement of the circulating vitamin D metabolites in animals.[48,49] Most reference laboratories do not perform assays for 1,25-dihydroxyvitamin D, so it will be necessary to identify a large medical center with an endocrinology division or a research laboratory that performs the assay.

REFERENCES

1. **Rosol TJ, Capen CC.** Biology of disease: mechanisms of cancer-induced hypercalcemia. Lab Invest 1992;67:680–702.
2. **Rosol TJ, Capen CC.** Calcium-regulating hormones and diseases of abnormal mineral (calcium, phosphorus, magnesium) metabolism. In: Kaneko JJ, Harvey JW, Bruss ML, eds. Clinical biochemistry of domestic animals. 5th ed. San Diego: Academic Press, 1997:619–702.
3. **Rosol TJ, Capen CC.** Pathogenesis of humoral hypercalcemia of malignancy. Domest Anim Endocrinology 1988;5:1–21.
4. **McCauley LK, Rosol TJ, Stromberg PC, Capen CC.** In vivo and in vitro effects of interleukin-1α and cyclosporin A on bone and lymphoid tissues in mice. Toxicol Pathol 1991;19:1–10.
5. **Merryman JI, Rosol TJ, Brooks CL, Capen CC.** Separation of parathyroid hormone-like activity from transforming growth factor-α and -β in the canine adenocarcinoma (CAC-8) model of humoral hypercalcemia of malignancy. Endocrinology 1989;124:2456–2563.
6. **Rosol TJ, Nagode LA, Couto CG, Hammer AS, Chew DJ, Peterson JL, Ayl RD, Steinmeyer CL, Capen CC.** Parathyroid hormone (PTH)-related protein, PTH, and 1,25-dihydroxyvitamin D in dogs with cancer-associated hypercalcemia. Endocrinology 1992;131:1157–1164.
7. **Philbrick WM, Wysolmerski JJ, Galbrath S, Holt E, Orloff JJ, Yang KH, Vasavada RC, Weir EC, Broadus AE, Stewart AF.** Defining the roles of parathyroid hormone-related protein in normal physiology. Physiol Rev 1996;76:127–173.
8. **Weir EC, Norrdin RW, Matus RE, Brooks MB, Broadus AE, Mitnick M, Johnston SD, Insogna KL.** Humoral hypercalcemia of malignancy in canine lymphosarcoma. Endocrinology 1988;122:602–608.
9. **Rosol TJ, Chew DJ, Nagode LA, Schenck PA.** Disorders of calcium: hypercalcemia and hypocalcemia. In: DiBartola SP, ed. Fluid therapy in small animal practice. 2nd ed. Philadelphia: WB Saunders, 2000:108–162.
10. **Rosenberg MP, Matus RE, Patnaik AK.** Prognostic factors in dogs with lymphoma and associated hypercalcemia. J Vet Intern Med 1991;5:268–271.
11. **Engelman RW, Tyler RD, Good RA, Day NK.** Hypercalcemia in cats with feline-leukemia-virus-associated leukemia-lymphoma. Cancer 1985;56:777–781.
12. **Kawasaki T.** Creatinine: unreliable indicator of renal failure in ferrets. J Small Anim Med Exotics 1991;1:28–29.
13. **Rosol TJ, Nagode LA, Robertson JT, Leeth BD, Steinmeyer CL, Allen CM.** Humoral hypercalcemia of malignancy associated with ameloblastoma in a horse. J Am Vet Med Assoc 1994;204:1930–1933.
14. **Ikeda K, Inoue D, Okazaki R, Kikuchi T, Ogata E, Matsumoto T.** Parathyroid hormone-related peptide in hypercalcemia associated with adult T cell leukemia/lymphoma: molecular and cellular mechanism of parathyroid

hormone-related peptide overexpression in HTLV-I-infected T cells. Miner Electrolyte Metab 1995;21:166–170.

15. **Seymour JF, Gagel RF.** Calcitriol: the major humoral mediator of hypercalcemia in Hodgkin's and non-Hodgkin's lymphomas. Blood 1993;82:1383–1394.

16. **Meuten DJ, Segre GV, Capen CC, Kociba GJ, Voelkel EF, Levine L, Tashjian AH, Chew DJ, Nagode LA.** Hypercalcemia in dogs with adenocarcinoma derived from apocrine glands of the anal sac: biochemical and histomorphometric investigations. Lab Invest 1983;48:428–435.

17. **Rijnberk A, Elsinghorst AM, Koeman JP, Hackeng WHL, Lequin RM.** Pseudohyperparathyroidism associated with perirectal adenocarcinomas in elderly female dogs. Tijdschr Diergeneeskd 1978;103:1069–1075.

18. **Ross JT, Scavelli TD, Matthiesen DT, Patnaik AK.** Adenocarcinoma of the apocrine glands of the anal sac in dogs: a review of 32 cases. J Am Anim Hosp Assoc 1991;27:349–355.

19. **Matus RE, Leifer CE, MacEwen EG, Hurvitz AI.** Prognostic factors for multiple myeloma in the dog. J Am Vet Med Assoc 1986;188:1288–1292.

20. **Sheafor SE, Gamblin RM, Couto CG.** Hypercalcemia in two cats with multiple myeloma. J Am Anim Hosp Assoc 1996;32:503–508.

21. **Martin TJ, Grill V.** Hypercalcemia and cancer. J Steroid Biochem Mol Biol 1992;43:123–129.

22. **Black KS, Mundy GR.** Other causes of hypercalcemia: Local and ectopic secretion syndromes. In: Bilezikian JP, Marcus R, Levine MA, eds. The parathyroids. New York Raven Press, 1994;341–358.

23. **Meuten DJ, Kociba GJ, Capen CC, Chew DJ, Segre GV, Levine L, Tashjian AH Jr, Voelkel EF, Nagode LA.** Hypercalcemia in dogs with lymphosarcoma: biochemical, ultrastructural, and histomorphometric investigations. Lab Invest 1983;49:553–562.

24. **Barthez PY, Davis CR, Pool RR, Hornof WJ, Morgan JP.** Multiple metaphyseal involvement of a thymic lymphoma associated with hypercalcemia in a puppy. J Am Anim Hosp Assoc 1995;31:82–85.

25. **Henry CJ, Lanevschi A, Marks SL, Beyer JC, Nitschelm SH, Barnes S.** Acute lymphoblastic leukemia, hypercalcemia, and pseudohyperkalemia in a dog. J Am Vet Med Assoc 1996;208:237–239.

26. **Meuten DJ.** Hypercalcemia. Vet Clin North Am Small Anim Pract 1984; 14:891–910.

27. **Garrett IR.** Bone destruction in cancer. Semin Oncol 1993;20:4–9.

28. **Powell GJ, Southby J, Danks JA, Stillwell RG, Hayman JA, Henderson MA, Bennett RC, Martin TJ.** Localization of parathyroid hormone-related protein in breast cancer metastases: increased incidence in bone compared to other sites. Cancer Res 1991;51:3059–3061.

29. **Rosol TJ, Capen CC.** Pathophysiology of calcium, phosphorus, and magnesium metabolism in animals. Vet Clin North Am Small Anim Pract 1996;26:1155–1184.

30. **Rasmussen H, Barrett P, Smallwood J, Bollag W, Isales C.** Calcium ion as an intracellular messenger and cellular toxin. Environ Health Perspect 1990;84:17–25.

31. **Feldman EC, Nelson RW.** Hypercalcemia and primary hyperparathyroidism. In: Feldman EC, ed. Canine and feline endocrinology and reproduction. 2nd ed. Philadelphia: WB Saunders, 1996;455–496.

32. **Chew DJ, Carothers MA.** Hypercalcemia. Vet Clin North Am Small Anim Pract 1989;19:265–288.

33. **Kruger JM, Osborne CA, Nachreiner RF, Refsal KR.** Hypercalcemia and renal failure: etiology, pathophysiology, diagnosis, and treatment. Vet Clin North Am Small Anim Pract 1996;26:1417–1445.

34. **Brown EM, Hebert SC.** Calcium-receptor-regulated parathyroid and renal function. Bone 1997;20:303–309.

35. **Teachout DJ, Taylor SM, Archer PJ.** A comparison of serum ionized calcium concentrations and serum total calcium concentrations in dogs with lymphoma. Zentralbl Veterinarmed A 1997;44:195–200.

36. **Deniz A, Mischke R.** Ionized calcium and total calcium in the cat. Berl Munch Teirarztl Wochenschr 1995;108:105–108.

37. **Schenck PA, Chew DJ, Brooks CL.** Effects of storage on normal canine serum ionized calcium and pH. Am J Vet Res 1995;56:304–307.

38. **Weir EC.** Hypercalcemia and malignancy. Proc 10th ACVIM Forum 1992; 10:604–612 (abstract).

39. **Chew DJ, Nagode LA, Rosol TJ, Carothers MA, Schenck P.** Utility of diagnostic assays in the evaluation of hypercalcemia and hypocalcemia: parathyroid hormone, vitamin D metabolites, parathyroid hormone-related protein, and ionized calcium. In: Bonagura JD, ed. Kirk's current veterinary therapy. XII. Small animal practice. Philadelphia: WB Saunders, 1995: 378–383.

40. **Burtis WJ.** Parathyroid hormone-related protein: structure, function, and measurement. Clin Chem 1992;38:2171–2183.

41. **Pandian MR, Morgan CH, Carlton E, Segre GV.** Modified immunoradiometric assay of parathyroid hormone-related protein: Clinical application in the differential diagnosis of hypercalcemia. Clin Chem 1992;38:282–288.

42. **Yang KH, dePapp AE, Soifer NE, Dreyer BE, Wu TL, Porter SE, Bellantoni M, Burtis WJ, Insogna KL, Broadus AE, Philbrick WM, Stewart AF.** Parathyroid hormone-related protein: evidence for isoform- and tissue-specific posttranslational processing. Biochemistry 1994;33:7460–7469.

43. **Burtis WJ, Dann P, Gaich GA, Soifer NE.** A high abundance midregion species of parathyroid hormone-related protein: Immunological and chromatographic characterization in plasma. J Clin Endocrinol Metab 1994; 78:317–322.

44. **Burtis WJ, Brady TG, Orloff JJ, Ersbak JB, Warrell RP Jr, Olson BR, Wu TL, Mitnick ME, Broadus AE, Stewart AF.** Immunochemical characterization of circulating parathyroid hormone-related protein in patients with humoral hypercalcemia of malignancy. N Engl J Med 1990;322:1106–1112.

45. **Torrance AG, Nachreiner R.** Intact parathyroid hormone assay and total calcium concentration in the diagnosis of disorders of calcium metabolism in dogs. J Vet Intern Med 1989;3:86–89.

46. **Barber PJ, Elliott J, Torrance AG.** Measurement of feline intact parathyroid hormone: Assay validation and sample handling studies. J Small Anim Pract 1993;34:614–620.

47. **Nagode LA, Chew DJ.** The use of calcitriol in treatment of renal disease of the dog and cat. Proc 1st Purina International Nutrition Symposium 1991;1:39–49.

48. **Horst RL, Reinhardt TA, Hollis BW.** Improved methodology for the analysis of plasma vitamin D metabolites. Kidney Int 1990;38:S28–S35.

49. **Hollis BW, Kamerud JQ, Kurkowski A, Beaulieu J, Napoli JL.** Quantification of circulating 1,25-dihydroxyvitamin D by radioimmunoassay with an ^{125}I-labeled tracer. Clin Chem 1996;42:586–592.

CHAPTER 99

Thymoma

• KAREN M. YOUNG

THYMIC DEVELOPMENT AND FUNCTION

The thymus is an immune organ, located in the cranial mediastinum, that is derived from the endoderm of the third and fourth branchial pouches. Lymphocytes from bone marrow home to the thymus where they encounter a microenvironment essential for T cell differentiation. During their development T cells acquire a wide functional repertoire owing to rearrangements of genes encoding the subunits of the T cell receptor. The thymus is surrounded by a thin connective tissue capsule and is divided into ill-defined lobules by septa. A cytoreticulum of stellate epithelial cells (reticular cells) along with a few reticular fibers provide a scaffolding for the small lymphocytes that densely pack the cortex and thin out somewhat in the medulla where some larger lymphocytes are found. There are no discrete lymphatic nodules. In the medulla concentric whorls of flattened epithelium, sometimes keratinized, swollen, or calcified in the center, are termed Hassall's corpuscles. Other cells that comprise the thymic cellular population are macrophages, interdigitating or dendritic cells, eosinophils, and mast cells, which can be numerous in the aged thymus. In some species myoid cells are found, and erythroblasts and plasma cells may also be present. The thymus achieves its maximal weight early in life, at approximately 4 to 5 months of age in dogs, and then undergoes a slow atrophy or involution, ultimately replaced by fatty fibrous tissue and existing as only a remnant in adults.[1,2]

THYMIC TUMORS

Neoplasms of thymic tissue, termed thymomas, arise from the epithelial component of the gland even though mature lymphocytes may be the predominant cell type. These tumors are rare, but have been reported in various species, including dogs, cats, horses, pigs, cattle, sheep, and goats. In the latter there is a higher incidence, reaching 25% in a closed herd of Saanen dairy goats in Montana.[3–7] The average age of dogs that have thymomas is 8.7 years (range 3 to 15 years). No breed or gender predilection has been defined, although there is a sug-

gestion that female dogs, as well as medium- and large-sized dogs, may be more affected.

Pathogenesis and Biologic Behavior

The etiology or cause of thymomas is not characterized. Well-encapsulated noninvasive thymomas are typically slow growing and have a benign behavior. Malignancy is characterized by local invasion of great vessels, the visceral and parietal pleura, the pericardium, or the rib cage. Distant metastases to the lung, regional lymph nodes, liver, spleen, bone, or brain are rare.[8–12]

Associated Syndromes

Of the paraneoplastic syndromes reported to occur in animals that have thymomas, the most common one is myasthenia gravis (MG), occurring in up to 30 to 40% of dogs that have thymomas.[13] However, MG is rarely reported in cats.[14] Acquired MG associated with thymomas or thymic cysts results from production of anti-acetylcholine receptor (anti-AChR) antibodies, possibly because thymic myoid cells and muscle cells at the neuromuscular junction have antigenic similarities. Antibodies may possibly block the acetylcholine receptor, increase the rate of receptor degradation, promote receptor lysis through complement activation, or act by a combination of these mechanisms. The principal clinical manifestations are muscle weakness and megesophagus. Definitive diagnosis of MG is made by measuring serum levels of anti-AChR antibodies with a radioimmunoassay. After thymectomy, antibody titers may fall slowly.

Nonthymic neoplasms, possibly arising because of decreased immune surveillance, occur in approximately 30% of dogs that have thymomas and include lymphoma, osteosarcoma, adenocarcinomas, and lung tumors.[11] Autoimmune disorders, such as immune-mediated hemolytic anemia and polymyositis, also may be present in animals that have thymomas.[11] Uncommonly, hypercalcemia of malignacy is associated with this neoplasm[9,15] (see Chapter 98, Humoral Hypercalcemia of Malignancy). In people who have thymomas, hyperglobulinemic purpura and pure red cell aplasia have been reported.[16,17] The true incidence of these para-neoplastic syndromes is difficult to quantify as some thymomas undoubtedly go undetected, and reported cases tend to be those with interesting findings of an associated disorder.

Clinical Signs

Animals develop signs related to the physical presence of the tumor or associated with a paraneoplastic syndrome.[4,7,9,11] In small dogs and cats, the tumor may result in decreased compressibility of the cranial thorax. Pleural effusion, which can be chylous, is present in some animals that have consequent dyspnea, tachypnea, and muffled lung sounds. Lethargy, cough, caudodorsal displacement of heart sounds, and pericardial effusion can also occur. The tumor may cause swelling of the face, neck, and forelimbs, so-called precaval syndrome, from obstruction of vessels and lymphatics.[18] In animals that have MG, muscle weakness and megesophagus may be evident, resulting in dysphagia or regurgitation with consequent aspiration pneumonia. Clinical signs of other paraneoplastic syndromes may be present and may constitute the presenting signs.

Diagnostic Tests and Differential Diagnoses

Imaging

On survey radiographs of the thorax, a mass in the cranial mediastinum is seen.[7,11] On the lateral view the trachea may be displaced dorsally, whereas the heart may be located in a caudodorsal position depending on the size of the mass. In the dorsoventral projection, the mediastinum appears widened, and the heart may be displaced laterally. Possible causes of a cranial mediastinal mass in addition to thymoma include other neoplasms, inflammatory lesions, ectopic tissue, or cysts. Tumors may arise from structures within the mediastinum (e.g., lymph nodes, esophagus, and ectopic thyroid), extend into the mediastinum from adjacent tissues (e.g., heart, lung, chemoreceptors), or be part of metastatic or multicentric disease (e.g., lymphoma). Inflammatory diseases include fungal or bacterial diseases causing granuloma formation, abscesses, or lymphadenopathy. Nonseptic eosinophilic inflammation may be present. Ectopic tissues of the third and the fourth branchial pouches include thyroid and parathyroid glands. Finally, branchial cysts can occur.[19]

Ultrasonographic imaging is useful if pleural effusion is present or if fine-needle aspiration or needle biopsy of the mass is to be attempted.[20] Typically, thymomas display mixed echogenicity with cavitations and indistinct borders, whereas lymphoma appears as a solid, round, discrete lesion that is diffusely hypoechoic. Computed tomography (CT) is useful not only in detecting the lesion but in characterizing its invasiveness.[21] Magnetic resonance imaging (MRI) is an excellent imaging modality for soft tissue lesions and is also potentially

useful, but with older scanners respiratory motion interferes with the image owing to the time required to acquire an image (Dr. Lisa Forrest, University of Wisconsin, personal communication).

Laboratory Features and Cytology

Typically, there are no significant findings on the complete blood count, serum biochemical profile, or urinalysis. If the animal has aspiration pneumonia associated with MG and megesophagus, an inflammatory leukogram may be evident. Cytologic evaluation of fine-needle aspirates, or imprints, of thymomas can be useful.[22-24] Small lymphocytes comprise the major cellular component of samples obtained by transthoracic fine-needle aspiration. Occasionally, the epithelial component is present, and round, oval, or stellate epithelial cells may be seen. In most cases of canine thymomas, mast cells are visualized. Cytologic evaluation may not give a definitive diagnosis in all cases but is useful in ruling out lymphoma, an important differential diagnosis that is treated systemically with combination chemotherapy rather than surgical excision.

Pathology

Needle biopsies of thymomas may be attempted, taking care to avoid great vessels in proximity to the mass. Typically, the diagnosis is made from tissue obtained at the time of surgical resection (see Treatment, below). If the tumor is invasive or nonresectable, wedge biopsies should be obtained if therapy is to be attempted. Multiple areas of the mass should be sampled owing to the cystic nature of the lesion. Thymomas vary widely in size. The gross appearance is characteristically a nodular, encapsulated mass that is grayish white and can be either firm or soft. Cystic areas are common, and there may be hemorrhagic or necrotic foci. On histopathologic examination, epithelial cells that are round, oval, or spindle-shaped arranged in solid, trabecular, cribriform, whorled, or rosette patterns are present. Aggregates of cells resembling Hassall's corpuscles may be evident. Mitotic figures and anaplastic changes are uncommon. Small lymphocytes are the other major cellular element, and the proportion of epithelial and lymphoid cells is variable.[3,8,12] Morphologic patterns vary among and within tumors and do not seem to correlate with biological behavior. In goats, myoid cells, which comprise part of the normal thymus, may be present in the thymoma. Rarely in canine thymoma, the epithelial cells contain melanin, and this pigmented variant can be confused with melanoma (Dr. Gary Hogge, University of Wisconsin, personal communication, 1998). The most important consideration is to distinguish thymoma from lymphoma, as systemic therapy is warranted in the latter.

Cytochemistry

Histochemical analyses of thymomas provide definitive evidence of the epithelial origin of this neoplasm, as tumor cells are strongly positive for various cytokeratins.[25] In human thymomas, there is an association between the expression of adhesion molecules and histologic subtype, but no correlation exists with biological behavior regarding invasiveness of the tumor or the presence of paraneoplastic syndromes.[26]

Treatment

The essence of treatment is local control. Surgical resection is potentially curative if the tumor is small, encapsulated, and noninvasive.[7,11,27] At the time of surgery care should be taken to avoid tearing the capsule and damaging associated vessels and nerves. If surgical resection is not possible, other modalities may be employed. Combination chemotherapy, typically using a protocol used in the treatment of lymphoma (see Chapter 91, Lymphoma), is cytoreductive and decreases the lymphoid component (Dr. David Vail, University of Wisconsin, personal communication). The same is true for radiation therapy.[11,28] Either one of these modalities can be used prior to surgical resection to decrease the size of large tumors in animals.[29] The response of the neoplastic epithelial component is less well characterized. Using radiation therapy as a single modality is of concern owing to the inclusion of normal tissues (heart and lung) in the field.

Prognosis

With complete resection of the thymoma and the absence of megesophagus, the prognosis is good.[8,11] The prognosis is worse for animals that have paraneoplastic syndromes or invasive thymomas. In one study, dogs that had megesophagus had a mean survival time of 16 days postoperatively.[9]

REFERENCES

1. **Weiss L.** The thymus. In: Weiss L, ed. Cell and tissue biology. A textbook of histology. 6th ed. Baltimore: Urban & Schwarzenberg, 1988;479–495.
2. **Evans HE, Christensen GC.** Miller's anatomy of the dog. 2nd ed. Philadelphia: WB Saunders, 1979;839.
3. **Moulton JE, Harvey JW.** Tumors of the lymphoid and hematopoietic tissues. Thymoma. In: Moulton JE, ed. Tumors in domestic animals. 3rd ed. Berkeley: University of California Press, 1990;267–268.
4. **Carpenter JL, Holzworth J.** Thymoma in 11 cats. J Am Vet Med Assoc 1982;181:248–251.
5. **Parker GA, Casey HW.** Thymomas in domestic animals. Vet Pathol 1976; 13:353–364.
6. **Sandison AT, Anderson LJ.** Tumors of the thymus in cattle, sheep and pigs. Cancer Res 1969;29:1146–1150.
7. **Aronsohn M.** Canine thymoma. Vet Clin North Am Small Anim Pract 1985;15:755–767.
8. **Aronsohn MG, Schunk KL, Carpenter JL, King NW.** Clinical and pathologic features of thymoma in 15 dogs. J Am Vet Med Assoc 1984;184:1355–1362.
9. **Atwater SW, Powers BE, Park RD, et al.** Thymoma in dogs: 23 cases (1980–1991). J Am Vet Med Assoc 1994;205:1007–1013.
10. **Bellah JR, Stiff ME, Russell RG.** Thymoma in the dog: two case reports and review of 20 additional cases. J Am Vet Med Assoc 1983;183:306–311.
11. **Withrow SJ.** Thymoma. In: Withrow SJ, MacEwen EG, eds. Small animal clinical oncology. 2nd ed. Philadelphia: WB Saunders, 1996;530–533.
12. **Day MJ.** Review of thymic pathology in 30 cats and 36 dogs. J Small Anim Pract 1997;38:393–403.
13. **Braund KG.** Peripheral nerve disorders: myasthenia gravis. In: Ettinger SJ, Feldman EC, eds. Textbook of veterinary internal medicine. Diseases of the dog and cat. Philadelphia: WB Saunders, 1995;712–713.
14. **Scott-Moncrieff JC, Cook JR, Lantz GC.** Acquired myasthenia gravis in a cat with thymoma. J Am Vet Med Assoc 1990;196:1291–1293.
15. **Harris CL, Klausner JS, Caywood DD, Leininger JR.** Hypercalcemia in a dog with thymoma. J Am Anim Hosp Assoc 1991;27:281–284.
16. **Schneiderman P.** The vascular purpuras. In: Beutler E, Lichtman MA, Coller BS, Kipps T, eds. Williams hematology. 5th ed. New York: McGraw-Hill, 1995;1401–1412.
17. **Erslev AJ.** Pure red cell aplasia. In: Beutler E, Lichtman MA, Coller BS, Kipps T, eds. Williams hematology. 5th ed. New York: McGraw-Hill, 1995;448–456.
18. **Peaston AE, Church DB, Allen GS, Haigh S.** Combined chylothorax, chylopericardium, and cranial vena cava syndrome in a dog with thymoma. J Am Vet Med Assoc 1990;197:1354–1356.
19. **Liu SK, Patnaik AK, Burk RL.** Thymic branchial cysts in the dog and cat. J Am Ved Med Assoc 1983;182:1095–1098.
20. **Konde LJ, Spaulding K.** Sonographic evaluation of the cranial mediastinum in small animals. Vet Radiol 1991;32:178–184.
21. **Burk RL.** Computed tomography of thoracic disease in dogs. J Am Vet Med Assoc 1991;199:617–621.
22. **Cowell RL, Tyler RD, Baldwin CJ.** The lung parenchyma. In: Cowell RL, Tyler RD, Meinkoth JH, eds. Diagnostic cytology and hematology of the dog and cat. St. Louis: Mosby, 1999;174–182.
23. **Mills JN, Shaw SE, Kabay MJ.** The cytopathological features of thymoma in a dog. J Small Anim Pract 1985;26:167–175.
24. **Rae CA, Jacobs RM, Couto CG.** A comparison between the cytological and histological characteristics in thirteen canine and feline thymomas. Can Vet J 1989;30:497–500.
25. **Gonzalez M, Rodriguez A, Pizarro M, Llorens P.** Immunohistochemical study of a non-invasive canine thymoma: a case report. Zentralblatt fur Veterinarmedizin 1997;44:309–406.
26. **Pan CC, Ho DM, Chen WY, Chiang H, Fahn HJ, Wang LS.** Expression of E-cadherin and alpha- and beta-catenins in thymoma. J Pathol 1998;184:207–211.
27. **Gores BR, Berg J, Carpenter JL, Aronsohn MG.** Surgical treatment of thymoma in cats: 12 cases (1987–1992). J Am Vet Med Assoc 1994;204:1782–1785.
28. **Hitt ME, Shaw DP, Hogan PM.** Radiation treatment for thymoma in a dog. J Am Vet Med Assoc 1987;190:1187–1190.
29. **Meleo KA.** The role of radiotherapy in the treatment of lymphoma and thymoma. Vet Clin North Am Small Anim Pract 1997;27:115–129.

SECTION X

Hematologic or Hemopoietic Neoplasia–Nonlymphoid Hemopoietic Neoplasia

Carol B. Grindem

CHAPTER 100

Classification and Biology of Myeloproliferative Disorders

• JANICE M. ANDREWS

CLASSIFICATION

Leukemias are malignant diseases of hemopoietic tissue characterized by replacement of the normal bone marrow with an abnormal clonal proliferation of blood cells. Often but not always there is a concomitant increase of the neoplastic blood cells in peripheral blood. Additionally, the neoplastic blood cells commonly infiltrate other hemic and lymphoid tissue such as spleen, lymph nodes, and liver.

Leukemias are broadly classified into two principal groups according to cell lineage: myeloproliferative or lymphoproliferative. Myeloproliferative disorders include myeloid, monocytic, megakaryocytic, and erythrocytic leukemias along with the myelodysplastic syndromes (Table 100.1). Each group is subclassified as chronic or acute and denotes the clinical course of the disease and also suggests the degree of cell immaturity observed. Acute and chronic were originally used to define and classify leukemias when no treatment was available. Without therapy patients that have acute leukemias typically die within days to weeks of diagnosis, whereas those that have chronic forms may survive for months to years. Acute leukemias are defined as malignancies of immature hemopoietic cells or blasts. The blasts may represent different stages of maturation and are recognized by use of morphologic characteristics and cytochemical stains. Chronic leukemias are characterized by more mature hemopoietic cells infiltrating the bone marrow and blood. Another subclassification of myeloproliferative disorders includes myelodysplastic syndromes. Myelodysplastic syndromes are a group of disorders (Table 100.1) clinically characterized by anemia, leukopenia, or thrombocytopenia, with maturation defects present in one or more cell lines in the bone marrow.

In human medicine myeloid and lymphoid leukemias are further subclassified according to the French-American-British (FAB) system.[1] The criteria rely on morphology to identify cell lineage and degree of differentiation present, and cytochemistry to differentiate and subclassify into lymphoid and myeloid. Because leukemias differ in their clinical features, response to therapy, and prognoses, it is mandatory that an accurate diagnosis be established before treatment is initiated.

A scheme for classification of acute myeloid leukemias (AML) and myelodysplastic syndromes has been established in dogs and cats patterned after the FAB criteria for classification of AML in humans.[2] The criteria and individual categories are further discussed in greater detail in Chapter 106, Acute Myeloid Leukemia.

Recent advances in the application of newer techniques are now employed to improve the accuracy of classification. These include immunophenotyping (see Chapter 103, CD Antigens and Immunophenotyping) and cytogenetics. Immunophenotyping uses specific monoclonal antibodies to differentiation antigens. The advent of flow cytometry has provided a powerful tool for analysis of immunophenotyped cells and is becoming an essential component in the study of leukemias and complements morphology and cytochemical stains.

CLONALITY

A fundamental feature of leukemic cells are their monoclonality, implying they are derived from a single stem cell that has become neoplastic. Clonal marker systems are used to determine not only the presence of clonality but to investigate at what stage of hemopoietic cell development the neoplastic cells originate. In humans who have AML, the neoplastic cell may arise from any step of the proliferating bone marrow pool, from the pluripotent stem cell to promyelocyte.[3,4] This likely explains the morphologic and clinical variations observed in patients who have AML. Molecular markers used to investigate clonality in myeloproliferative disorders include X-linked gene polymorphisms, acquired chromosomal markers, acquired DNA changes, and immunophenotyping.

MOLECULAR MECHANISMS OF LEUKEMOGENESIS

One important understanding is that the progression from normal cells to malignancy represents a multistep process. Now that more is understood about the molecular mechanisms that regulate normal cell growth, it is clear that failure of one or more of these is a fundamental step leading to malignant transformation. Cell proliferation and differentiation is regulated by proteins encoded by proto-oncogenes (growth promoting) and tumor suppressor genes (growth suppressing). It is recognized that oncogenesis involves specific molecular events resulting in genetic alterations of these two classes of genes with subsequent dysregulation of cell growth. Genetic abnormalities include chromosomal translocations, point mutations, amplifications, and deletions (Table 100.2). These genetic changes usually result in activation of proto-oncogenes (oncogenes) or inactivation of tumor suppressor genes. Although the exact origin of these genetic abnormalities is unknown, several environmental inciting factors are known that include radiation, chemical agents, and retroviral infections.

RADIATION-INDUCED LEUKEMIAS

Radiation exposure is considered an important environmental mutagen in humans. An increase incidence of leukemias has been reported in atomic bomb survivors,[5] patients given low-dose radiation for ankylosing spondylitis,[6] and radium dial painters.[7]

Dogs exposed to protracted whole-body irradiation have been found to have an increased incidence of myeloproliferative disorders.[8–10] Specifically, these included both myelogenous leukemias and erythroleukemias.

Ionizing radiation induces DNA strand breaks, resulting in chromosomal aberrations that may ultimately result in malignant transformation of the cell.

RETROVIRAL LEUKEMOGENESIS AND ONCOGENES

Retroviruses are RNA viruses that infect both animals and humans. Each virion or infectious particle contains two identical copies of positive sense, single-stranded RNA molecules that is reversed transcribed into double-stranded DNA and subsequently randomly integrates into the infected cells host genome as a provirus. The proviral genome contains genes essential for viral replication (*gag, pol,* and *env*) flanked on each side by long

TABLE 100.1 Classification of Myeloproliferative Disorders

Acute Myeloproliferative Disorders
AUL: Acute undifferentiated leukemia
MO: Minimally differentiated leukemia with restricted myeloid differentiation by electron microscopy and/or by immunophenotyping
M1: Myeloblastic leukemia without maturation
M2: Myeloblastic leukemia with maturation
M3: Promyelocytic leukemia
M4: Myelomonocytic leukemia
M5: Monocytoid leukemia
  M5a: Monoblastic leukemia
  M5b: Monocytic leukemia
M6: Erythroleukemia
M7: Megakaryocytic leukemia

Chronic Myeloproliferative Disorders
Chronic myeloid leukemia
  Chronic myelogenous leukemia
  Chronic basophilic leukemia
  Chronic eosinophilic leukemia
  Chronic monocytic leukemia
  Chronic myelomonocytic leukemia
Polycythemia vera
Essential thrombocythemia
Idiopathic myelofibrosis with myeloid metaplasia
Mast-cell leukemia

Myelodysplastic Syndromes
Myelodysplastic syndrome, refractory cytopenia (MDS-RC)
Myelodysplastic syndrome with excess blasts (MDS-EB)
Myelodysplastic syndrome with erythroid predominance (MDS-Er)
Chronic myelomonocytic leukemia

TABLE 100.2 Mechanism of Activation of Proto-Oncogenes

Alteration Type	Definition and Result	Oncogene Example
Chromosomal Translocations	Translocation of portions of one chromosome to another, resulting in overexpression of oncoprotein	c-*myc*
Point Mutations	Substitution of one nucleotide by another, resulting in altered protein function	c-*ras*
Amplification	Increase in the number of copies of a gene per cell, resulting in overexpression of oncoprotein	c-*myc*, N-*myc*
Transduction	Incorporation of proto-oncogenes into a retroviral genome, resulting in expression of an abnormal protein	v-*src*
Insertion	Retroviral integration is located nearby or within a proto-oncogene, resulting in overexpression	c-*myc*, *erb*B, *wnt*-1
Protein–protein interaction	Results in stabilization and altered function of oncoprotein	pp60[c-src] and middle T antigen

terminal repeats (LTRs). The LTRs carry *cis*-acting signals that direct transcription and RNA processing.

Many oncogenes were initially discovered on studying the pathogenesis of retroviruses that induce tumors in animals. In particular, first described was the Rous sarcoma virus (RSV), an avian type C retrovirus that induces tumors quickly in susceptible birds.[11] Tumorigenesis required a viral gene termed *src*, which was later found to be homologous to a normal cellular gene.[12] Retroviruses, like RSV that induce tumors rapidly are known as acutely transforming viruses. Acutely transforming viruses possess not only *gag, pol,* and *env* genes but incorporate cellular oncogenes from the host genome through a recombination process called transduction. These genes are referred to as viral oncogenes (v-*onc*) derived from their cellular homologs termed proto-oncogenes (c-*onc*). Examples of other acutely transforming retroviruses include avian erythroblastosis and avian myeloblastosis viruses that both induce leukemia and lymphoma within days of inoculation.

Additionally, the retroviral provirus may alter the expression of a host cell proto-oncogene by insertional mutagenesis. This involves integration of a provirus in the vicinity of a proto-oncogene, leading to aberrant expression of that gene. The first example of insertional mutagenesis was the avian leukosis virus that often integrates within the proto-oncogene, *c-myc*.[13] The pathogenesis of animal models of leukemias and lymphomas are described in greater detail in Chapter 107, Feline Leukemia Virus and Feline Immununodeficiency Virus.

TUMOR SUPPRESSOR GENES

Cell proliferation is regulated by a balance between proto-oncogenes (growth promoting) and tumor suppressor genes (growth constraining). Therefore, inactivation or loss of function of tumor suppressor genes contributes to oncogenesis. The most extensively studied tumor suppressor genes are p53 and retinoblastoma. Retroviral insertional inactivation and rearrangements of p53 have been observed in mouse erythroleukemias, supporting that loss of function may contribute to leukemogenesis.[14]

REFERENCES

1. **Handin RI, Lux SE, Stossel TP.** Blood: principles and practice of hematology. Philadelphia: JB Lippincott,1995.
2. **Jain NC, Blue JT, Grindem CB, et al.** Proposed criteria for classification of acute myeloid leukemia in dogs and cats. Vet Clin Pathol 1991;20(3):63–82.
3. **Fialkow PJ, Singer JW, Raskind WH, et al.** Clonal development stem cell differentiation, and clinical remissions in a acute nonlymphocytic leukemia. N Engl J Med 1987;317:468–473.
4. **Fialkow PJ, Rasland WR, Singer JW, Dow LW, Najfeld V, Veith R.** Clonal development of the acute leukemias. Bone Marrow Transplant 1989;4(1):76–78.
5. **Ichimaru M, Ishimaru T, Belsky JL.** Incidence of leukemia in atomic bomb survivors belonging to a fixed cohort in Hiroshima and Nagasaki, 1950–1971: radiation dose, years after exposure, age at exposure, and type of leukemia. J Radiat Res 1978;19:262–282.
6. **Court–Brown WM, Doll R.** Mortality from cancer and other causes after radiotherapy for ankylosing spondylitis. Br Med J 1965;2:1327–1332.
7. **Berlin NI, Wassermann RL.** The association between systemically administered radioisotopes and subsequent malignant disease. Cancer 1976;37:1097–1101.
8. **Tolle DV, Fritz TE, Norris WP.** Radiation-induced erythroleukemia in the beagle dog. Amer J Patholo 1977;87:499–506.
9. **Dungworth DL, Goldman M, Switzer JW, McKelvie DH.** Development of a myeloproliferative disorder in beagles continuously exposed to ^{90}Sr. Blood 1969;34:610–632.
10. **Seed TM, Tolle DV, Fritz TE, Devine RL, Poole CM, Norris WP.** Irradiation-induced erythroleukemia and myelogenous leukemia in the beagle dog: hematology and ultrastructure. Blood 1977;50:1061–1079.
11. **Rous P.** A sarcoma of the fowl transmissible by an agent separable from the tumor cells. J Exp Med 1911;13:397–411.
12. **Stehelin D, Varmus HE, Bishop JM, Vogt PK.** DNA related to the transforming gene(s) of avian sarcoma viruses is present in normal avian DNA. Nature 1976;260:170–173.
13. **Hayward WS, Neel BG, Astrin SM.** Activation of a cellular onc gene by promoter insertion in ALV-induced lymphoid leukosis. Nature 1981;290:475–480.
14. **Hicks GG, Mowat M.** Integration of friend murine leukemia virus into both alleles of the p53 oncogene in an erythroleukemic cell line. J Virol 1988;62:4752–4755.

CHAPTER 101

Hematologic Abnormalities Associated With Cancer Therapy

• ANNE M. BARGER and CAROL B. GRINDEM

Cancer therapy is most effective against cells that are initiating DNA synthesis or are actively dividing. Unfortunately this is a nondiscriminatory process that also affects actively renewing tissues of the body, specifically hemopoietic cells, epidermis and intestinal epithelium. These cells generally have a short lifespan and are therefore fairly sensitive to cancer therapy.

The complete blood cell count (CBC) is an excellent reflection of the bone marrow and is used to monitor the affects of cancer therapy. Deleterious side effects of cancer therapy are often reflected in the bone marrow cells with the shortest half-life (i.e., neutrophils with $T_{1/2}$ = 6 to 10 hours, platelets $T_{1/2}$ = 5 to 10 days.) Not surprisingly, neutropenia followed by thrombocytopenia are the most common and dose-limiting hematologic abnormalities. Anemia is an uncommon sequelae.

Cancer therapy involves multiple modalities. A wide range of chemotherapeutic agents, site specific or whole-body radiation therapy, and hyperthermia have been used to treat cancer. Combination therapeutic protocols have led to less toxic, more efficacious treatment of cancers. Neoplastic cell populations are targeted during specific stages of the cell cycle with agents that work by different mechanisms. To avoid overlapping toxicity, it is therefore important to understand the pharmacokinetics as well as the deleterious side effects associated with individual therapies.

Discussions in this chapter are limited to the direct effects of cancer therapy on hemopoietic cells, but the reader needs to be aware that gastrointestinal (GI), renal, liver and cardiac toxicities are equally important and may be therapy limiting or life threatening. Also, secondary drug effects such as immune-mediated neutropenia, thrombocytopenia, and hemolytic anemia occur but are not discussed in this chapter.

CHEMOTHERAPY

Systemic chemotherapy is used in the treatment of metastatic or disseminated neoplasia.[1] Chemotherapeutic agents can have multiple toxic effects, especially in rapidly dividing cells (Table 101.1). Neutropenia can occur 5 to 10 days after administration, and the most important complication observed is sepsis.[2] The degree of toxicity associated with drug administration may vary based on the degree of tumor destruction, the level of systemic disease associated with the neoplasia, the tumor-induced changes in metabolism and the competency of the immune system.[2]

Multiple categories of chemotherapuetic drugs are being used in veterinary medicine. Each has a slightly different mode of action and different hematologic derangement.

Alkylating Agents

Mechanistically, these drugs form covalent bonds with organic compounds by replacing a hydrogen atom with an alkyl radical. The alkylation produces breaks in the DNA and cross-links the twin strands to interfere with DNA replication and transcription of RNA. Effects vary from interference with mitosis to mutagenesis and immunosuppression.[1]

Disruption of mitosis results in myelosuppression. Manifestations of this myelosuppression are neutropenia, thrombocytopenia and, less often, anemia.[2]

Cyclophosphamides are one of the most common alkylating agents used in veterinary medicine. Hematologic abnormalities observed include possibly severe neutropenia[3] (nadir of 7 to 14 days) and thrombocytopenia[4] though cyclophosphamides, considered a platelet sparing drug. With chronic therapy, a reticulocytopenia can occur, resulting in a nonregenerative anemia.[1] Generally, however, the neutropenia is considered the dose-limiting effect. After toxicity to the marrow has occurred, it requires 18 to 25 days to recover.[4] In cats, a combined therapy with cyclophosphamides and mitoxantrone induces a neutropenia that has a nadir of 2 to 10 days.[5]

Busalfan is myelosuppressive. However, it primarily

TABLE 101.1   Chemotherapeutic Agents and Bone Marrow Toxicity in Dogs and Cats

Chemotherapeutic Agent	Myelosuppression	Neutropenia	Thrombocytopenia	Anemia
Alkylating Agents				
Cyclophophamide	yes	yes	—	—
Chloroambucil	yes	—	—	—
Melphalan	yes	—	—	—
Busulfan	yes	—	yes	—
Antimetabolites				
5-Fluorouracil	yes	yes	yes	yes[a]
Methotrexate	yes	yes	—	—
Cytosine	yes	yes	—	—
Arabinoside	—	—	—	—
6-mercaptopurine	yes	—	—	—
6-thioguanine	yes	yes[b]	yes[b]	
Antineoplastic Antibiotics				
Doxorubicin	yes	yes	yes	yes
Daunomycin	yes	yes	yes	—
Idarubicin	yes	yes	—	—
Bleomycin	no	—	—	—
Actinomycin-D	no	—	—	—
Naturally Occuring Compounds				
Vincristine	yes	yes	—	yes[c,d]
Vinblastine	yes	yes	—	—
L-asparaginase	no	—	—	—
Miscellaneous				
Cisplatin	yes	yes	yes	yes
Carboplatin	yes	yes	yes	—
Dacarbazine	yes	—	—	—
Procarbazine	yes	yes	—	—
Hydroxyurea	yes	—	—	—
Hormones				
Glucocorticoids	no	—	—	—
Estrogen compounds	yes	yes	yes	yes[e]

[a] If administered IV
[b] Cats
[c] Dogs
[d] Mild
[e] Severe

affects megakaryocytes, resulting in a thrombocytopenia.[2]

Chlorambucil is the least toxic of the alkylating agents. At doses used in veterinary medicine toxicity rarely occurs. However, if an animal is overdosed, myelosuppression occurs.[1]

Melphalan's myelosuppressive action is manifested as a neutropenia. The toxic effects of melphalan are exacerbated in renal failure because this drug is excreted via the kidneys.[2]

Various hemopoietic effects exist for other alkylating agents. These agents and their hemopoietic effects are summarized in Table 101.1.

Antimetabolites

The antimetabolite drugs each have a slightly different mechanism of action but they all function by interfering or inhibiting a specific enzyme that is necessary for purine or pyrimidine synthesis.[1] Because these drugs inhibit DNA synthesis, they are specific for the S phase of the cell cycle. Leukopenia, characterized specifically by neutropenia, is frequently observed.

5-fluorouracil (5-FU) is a pyrimidine analog that inhibits thymidylate synthetase, an enzyme necessary for the formation of thymidylic acid.[1] A mild depression in myeloid and platelet numbers is associated with 5-FU administration 2 to 4 days after exposure.[2] When administered via the intravenous route a decrease in red blood cells, hematocrit, and hemoglobin may be observed.[6] In humans, 7 to 20 days after administration, there is a leukopenia and thrombocytopenia. In chickens a heteropenia has been observed with 5-FU administration.[7] Use of this drug in cats is contraindicated because of severe neurologic signs.[2]

Cytosine arabinoside is another pyrimidine analog that blocks the conversion of cytidine to deoxycytidine, thus blocking DNA synthesis. Rapidly dividing bone marrow cells are affected, resulting in neutropenia with a nadir of 5 to 7 days.[1] Neutropenia is usually associated with long-term use. The bone marrow requires 7 to 14 days to recover.

6-mercaptopurine (6-MP) is a purine analog. Other closely related drugs in this category include 6-thioguanine and azathioprine. Azathioprine is actually a derivative of 6-MP that is broken down to 6-MP by the liver.[1] Nonfunctional nucleic acid strands are formed because these purine antagonists compete with purines in the synthesis of nucleic acids.[8] These three drugs are myelosuppressive. In normal cats, 6-thioguanine can cause a significant neutropenia and thrombocytopenia. The thrombocytopenia can become so severe as to result in hemorrhage with a secondary decrease in hematocrit and hemoglobin. Bone marrow myeloid and megakaryocytic hypoplasia were documented in these cats.[9] In contrast animals treated with methotrexate (MTX), another antimetabolite drug, have bone marrow hyperplasia.[10]

MTX is an antagonist of folic acid. It inhibits dihydrofolate reductase, the enzyme responsible for reducing folic acid to its active form.[1] Administration of MTX maintains folic acid in its inactive form. Because MTX is excreted primarily by the kidney, the effects of toxicity are more severe in animals that have renal failure.[1] Common toxic side effects of MTX include myelosuppression and severe GI disease. Myelosuppression is characterized by a severe neutropenia that can be dose limiting.[11] However, it is the duration of exposure rather than the actual dose that results in toxicity. MTX-induced macrocytic anemia has been reported in humans but not in dogs and cats. Lack of development of macrocytic anemia in animals may be caused by the short duration of MTX's use in a cyclic protocol or by species variation.

Antineoplastic Antibiotics

The antitumor antibiotics form stable complexes with DNA inhibiting either DNA or RNA synthesis. The primary antibiotics in this category include the anthracycline antibiotics (doxorubicin, daunorubicin, mitoxantrone, and idarubicin), bleomycin, and actinomycin-D. Because the latter two antibiotics have not been shown to have a significant toxic effect on the marrow, the focus in this section is on the anthracycline antibiotics. These antibiotics appear to intercalate between nucleotide pairs within the DNA helix that hinders DNA, RNA, and protein synthesis.[12] Although antineoplastic antibiotics do not appear to be cell-cycle specific, they are consistently myelosuppressive.

Doxorubicin is most well known for its cardiotoxicity; however, with chronic administration, it also causes significant myelosuppression manifested as a leukopenia, thrombocytopenia, and a regenerative anemia.[13] Acute, short-term effects of doxorubicin are bone marrow hypoplasia and lymphoid atrophy.[14] The myelosuppression in short-term treatment is dose dependent. At higher doses, the leukopenia and thrombocytopenia occur in approximately 7 to 14 days and resolve approximately 17 to 20 days posttreatment. Leukopenia is not observed at lower doses.[15] Poikilocytosis has also been reported in dogs, cats, and humans undergoing doxorubicin treatment. In humans, burr cells, stomatocytes, and schizocytes have been observed.[16] A study in cats revealed that neutropenia was the most significant finding. Poikilocytosis consisting of ovalocytes, echinocytes, and, less commonly, keratocytes was also reported.[17]

Mitoxantrone is a derivative of anthracene and thereby related to doxorubicin. Mitoxantrone, however, is not cardiotoxic.[18] In humans the myelosuppressive effects of mitoxantrone (neutropenia and thrombocytopenia) are mild and readily reversible. In dogs the more critical dose-limiting effect appears to be neutropenia that can be severe.[18] Sepsis secondary to neutropenia is a concern with this drug. The simultaneous administration of granulocyte-macrophage-colony-stimulating factor (GM-CSF) decreases the duration of neutropenia associated with mitoxantrone in animals.[19] Although the frequency of leukopenia is uncommon in cats, the white blood cell count drops because of a decrease in neutrophil count.[5,20] Therefore, a differential count in the CBC is important for detection of this declining neutrophil count.

Daunomycin reportedly causes myelosuppression in dogs and humans.[10] However the hemograms remained within reference range in one study in cats pretreated with glucocorticoids and antihistamines. Nonetheless, there was still a decline in the total white blood cell count.[9]

Idarubicin is a synthetic anthracycline analog that is more lipophilic than doxorubicin. In humans the most common toxicity is myelosuppression. In cats leukopenia is frequently observed. Occasionally, the neutropenia is so severe that the affected animal dies of sepsis.[21]

Naturally Occurring Compounds

Three naturally occurring compounds used as chemotherapeutic agents are vincristine, vinblastine, and asparaginase. Decreased hemopoiesis with L-asparaginase is unlikely because most normal cells can produce their own L-asparagine, and hence there is no suppression.[2,10]

Vincristine and vinblastine are vinca alkaloids. By inhibiting mitotic spindle function these drugs arrest cells at metaphase of mitosis, resulting in increased numbers of mitosis within the bone marrow.[22] Other atypical cellular configurations include irregular nuclear shape and nuclear fragmentation.[23] Nuclear blebbing and binucleation can be seen within both myeloid and erythroid cell lines, but it is much more common within the erythroid cell line.[23] In the dog, binucleated metarubricytes are a frequent finding and increased bone marrow mitosis have been reported to occur as early as 6 hours after one therapeutic dose of 0.01 mg/kg, intravenously.[23] (Fig. 101.1) These changes occur in the bone marrow early and are generally transient.

Vincristine has varying and dose-dependent effects

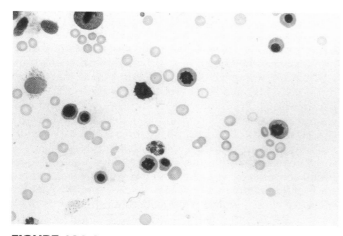

FIGURE 101.1 Increased mitosis and nuclear blebbing observed in bone marrow from a dog 8 hours after vincristine therapy.

on platelets. Low doses (therapeutic) cause an initial decrease in platelet numbers followed by a transient thrombocytosis.[24] Platelet function has been examined and even at a low dose, the ability of platelets to aggregate is decreased. However, the clot retraction and buccal mucosal bleeding times are most affected.[24]

Cats treated with vincristine can have a significant neutropenia within 1 week of administration.[25] However, dogs experience mild myelosuppression with a moderate neutropenia and slight anemia.[25,26]

Vinblastine is similar in action to vincristine.[22] Therefore, the toxicities observed are similar, although the myelosuppressive effects occur at the therapeutic doses with vinblastine.[2]

Miscellaneous Drugs

Cisplatin and carboplatin are platinum-containing compounds that act by cross-linking strands of DNA; hence DNA synthesis is inhibited.[2] Both drugs are myelosuppressive. Cisplatin causes neutropenia and thrombocytopenia.[27] Neutropenia is far more prevalent than thrombocytopenia.[28] A bimodal nadir for dogs is observed on day 6 and 15 for the neutrophil count.[29] A mild to moderate normocytic, normochromic, nonregenerative anemia has been reported 3 to 4 weeks after therapy.[30]

Cisplatin's use in cats is limited owing to severe pulmonary toxicity.[31] Carboplatin is much more tolerable in cats and dogs. Neutropenia is observed in dogs with a nadir of 14 days.[32] Thrombocytopenia has also been reported in these species and can be severe.[32]

Hydroxyurea interferes with DNA synthesis by inhibiting ribonucleotide reductase and has been reported to cause bone marrow suppression.[2] It has been used to treat polycythemia and chronic granulocytic leukemia in dogs.[1]

Hormones

Glucocorticoids (prednisone and dexamethasone) are frequently used drugs in cancer therapy, predominantly

in the treatment of lymphoma. They have no myelosuppressive affects.[1] In fact, they may stimulate hemopoiesis. Classic hematologic changes of glucocorticoid therapy include neutrophilia, lymphopenia, eosinopenia and in dogs, monocytosis.[33]

Estrogen-related compounds such as estradiol and diethylstilbestrol (DES) have been used in the treatment of mammary tumors as well as prostatic hyperplasia. Estradiol is more likely to result in bone marrow toxicity than DES.[1] Hematologic abnormalities include thrombocytopenia and aplastic anemia.[33] Estrogen consistently causes a transient decrease in the platelet count with an increase in the neutrophil count approximately 10 to 20 days after administration.[34] Aplastic anemia takes weeks to develop and is idiosyncratic. Bone marrow core biopsy is necessary to confirm a diagnosis of aplastic anemia.

HYPERTHERMIA AND TOTAL-BODY IRRADIATION

Hyperthermia

Hyperthermia has been used alone and in combination with other treatment modalities such as chemotherapy or radiation. Hyperthermia is directly cytotoxic at temperatures exceeding 41°C. Indirectly, hyperthermia causes microcirculatory damage.[1] Whole-body hyperthermia is more likely to cause hematologic changes than site-specific treatment. Whole-body hyperthermia actually causes a transient increase in platelet number in mice.[35] This helps alleviate the dose-limiting effects of thrombocytopenia observed with total-body irradiation. Examination of blood smears in patients treated with hyperthermia at North Carolina State University, College of Veterinary Medicine revealed atypically hypersegmented neutrophils with a pinwheel appearance (Fig. 101.2) and unclassified poikilocytosis. The overall neutrophil number, however, remained within reference range.

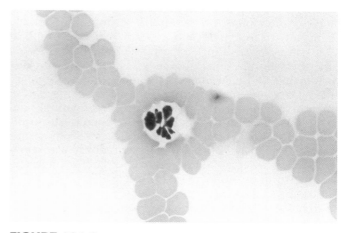

FIGURE 101.2 Atypically hypersegmented neutrophil from a dog treated with whole-body hyperthermia.

Total-Body Irradiation

Proliferating bone marrow cells are sensitive to radiation treatment. Ionizing radiation kills proliferating cells or at least disrupts their reproductive ability. In contrast to most cell-cycle-specific chemotherapeutic agents, radiation can kill the marrow stem cells.[1] Thrombocytopenia, which is often dose limiting,[35] and severe neutropenia are the most common hematologic complications of total-body irradiation.

ADJUNCT THERAPY

In response to the cytopenias associated with cancer treatment as well as to the neoplasia that directly affects the marrow, erythropoietin, thrombopoietin, and GM-CSF are used in human medicine to stimulate marrow hemopoietic response. In veterinary medicine GM-CSF is one of the most prevalent drugs to alleviate marrow suppression.

In human studies, GM-CSF therapy resulted in a transient rise in blood leukocytes within 3 days after initial administration[36] and reduced the severity of thrombocytopenia in chemotherapy recipients. In dogs, recombinant canine GM-CSF has been used in conjunction with chemotherapeutics to reduce the severity and duration of neutropenia.[20] An increase in the neutrophil count occurs within 24 hours after administration of the drug.[37] Dogs receiving this drug also had a significant elevation in monocyte numbers within 48 hours.

DIAGNOSTIC APPROACH TO MYELOSUPPRESSIVE DRUG TOXICITIES

Before initiating cancer therapy, a complete physical examination should be performed and a minimum database that includes a CBC, serum biochemical profile, and urinalysis should be analyzed. Preexisting factors such as cytopenias or renal disease need to be identified and incorporated into the selection of an anticancer therapeutic protocol.

Serious complications of cancer therapy can occur rapidly after onset of therapy. It is important for the clinician to anticipate and recognize these complications. Acute side effects of cancer therapy can include anaphylactic reactions, tumor lysis syndrome and disseminated intravascular coagulation (DIC). Development of severe neutropenia, thrombocytopenia, or hemolytic anemia at any point during treatment should alert the clinician to reevaluate therapeutic protocols and to institute supportive therapy. The most dangerous myelosuppressive effects of cancer therapy are sepsis caused by severe neutropenia and hemorrhage, resulting from thrombocytopenia (platelet counts usually $<20,000/\mu L$). Close monitoring of CBCs alerts the clinician to these potential problems and allows early therapeutic intervention (i.e., decreasing the dose or delaying the administration of the chemotherapeutic drug).

Assessing the toxic effects of cancer therapy may be especially challenging in the leukemic patient because of leukemia-associated cytopenias (neutropenia, thrombocytopenia and anemia) and decreased hematopoietic precursors in the bone marrow. It is imperative to establish a pretreatment baseline CBC and bone marrow in these patients and to evaluate sequential CBCs on a routine basis. Frequency of monitoring CBCs and biochemical profiles depends on the patient's physical condition, the type of cancer, preexisting laboratory abnormalities, and the anticancer therapy selected.

Development of therapy-related leukemia is an additional complication of cancer therapy in humans treated for hematopoietic malignancies. These secondary leukemias are clinically and prognostically different from de novo acute myeloid leukemia (AML) and are often preceded by a myelodysplastic syndrome.[38] Alkalizing agents, nitrosoureas, and procarbazine are most frequently incriminated.

REFERENCES

1. **Theilin GH, Madewell BR.** Veterinary cancer therapy. 2nd ed. Philadelphia: Lea and Febiger, 1987.
2. **O'keefe DA, Harris CL.** Toxicology of oncologic drugs. Vet Clin North Am 1990;20:483–503.
3. **Medleau L, Dawe DL, Calvert CA.** Immunosuppressive effects of cyclophosphamide, vincristine and L-asparaginase in dogs. Am J Vet Res 1983;44:176–180.
4. **Stanton ME, Legendre AM.** Effects of cyclophosphamide in dogs and cats. J Am Vet Med Assoc 1986;188:1319–1322.
5. **Henry CJ, Brewer WG, Royer NS.** Hematological and clinical responses to combined mitoxantrone and cyclophosphamide administration to normal cats. Can Vet J 1994;35:706–708.
6. **Dorman DC, Coddington KA, Richardson RC.** 5-Fluorouracil toxicosis in the dog. J Vet Intern Med 1990;4:254–257.
7. **Dhinakar R, Savage CE, Jones RC.** Effect of heterophil depletion by 5-FU on infectious bronchitis infection in chickens. Avian Pathol 1997;26:427–432.
8. **Dowling PM.** Immunosuppressive drug therapy. Can Vet J 1995;36:781–783.
9. **Henness AM, Theilen GH, Lewis JP.** Clinical investigation of doxorubicin, daunomycin and 6-thioguanine in normal cats. Am J Vet Res 1977; 38:521–524.
10. **Bortnowskin HB, Rosenthal RC.** Preclinical evaluation of L-asparaginase and methotrexate administered at intermediate doses in dogs. Am J Vet Res 1991;52:1636–1638.
11. **Cotter SM, Leroy PM.** High-dose methotrexate and leucovorin rescue in dogs with osteogenic sarcoma. Am J Vet Res 1978;39:1943–1945.
12. **Susaneck SJ.** Doxorubicin therapy in the dog. J Am Vet Med Assoc 1983;182:70–72.
13. **Van Vleet JF, Ferrans VJ.** Clinical observations, cutaneous lesions and hematologic alterations in chronic adriamycin intoxication in dogs with and without vitamin E and selenium supplementation. Am J Vet Res 1980;41:691–699.
14. **Ogilvie GK, Richardson RC, Curtis CR, et al.** Acute and short-term toxicoses associated with the administration of doxorubicin to dogs with malignant tumors. J Am Vet Med Assoc 1989;195:1584–1587.
15. **Burrow JP, Favora BE, Brenman J, et al.** Effect of adriamycin on circulating erythrocytes. Proc Am Assoc Cancer Res Am Soc Clin Oncol. 1977;18:6–11.
16. **Badylak SF, Van Vleet JF, Herman EH, Ferrans VJ, Myers CE.** Poikilocytosis in dogs with chronic doxorubicin toxicosis. Am J Vet Res 1985;46:505–508.
17. **O'keefe DA, Schaeffer DJ.** Hematologic toxicosis associated with doxorubicin administration in cats. J Vet Intern Med 1992;6:276–282.
18. **Ogilvie GK, Obradovich JE, Elmslie RE, et al.** Toxicosis associated with administration of mitoxantrone to dogs with malignant tumors. J Am Vet Med Assoc 1991;198:1613–1617.
19. **Kochevor DT, Middendorf DL, Mealey KL, et al.** Pharmacokinetics and haematological effects of a single intravenous dose of mitoxantrone in cats. J Vet Pharmacol Ther 1995;18:471–475.
20. **Ogilvie GK, Obradovich JE, Cooper MF, et al.** Use of recombinant canine granulocytic colony-stimulating factor to decrease myelosuppression associated with the administration of mitoxantrone in the dog. J Vet Intern Med 1992;6:44–47.
21. **Moore AS, Ruslander D, Cotter SM, et al.** Efficacy of, and toxicoses associated with, oral idarubicin administration in cats with neoplasia. J Am Vet Med Assoc 1995;296:1550–1554.
22. **Jordan MA, Thrower D, Wilson L.** Mechanism of inhibition of cell proliferation by vinca alkaloids. Cancer Res 1991;51:2212–2222.

23. **Alleman AR, Harvey JW.** The morphologic effects of vincristine sulfate on canine bone marrow cells. Vet Clin Pathol 1993;22:36–41.
24. **Mackin AJ, Allen DG, Johnstone IB.** Effects of vincristine and prednisone on platelet numbers and function in clinically normal dogs. Am J Vet Res 1995;56:100–108.
25. **Hahn KA, Fletcher CM, Legendre AM.** Marked neutropenia in five tumor-bearing cats one week following single-agent vincristine sulfate chemotherapy. Vet Clin Pathol 1996;25:121–123.
26. **Hahn KA.** Vincristine sulfate as single-agent chemotherapy in a dog and a cat with malignant neoplasms. J Am Vet Med Assoc 1990;197:504–506.
27. **Moore AS, Cardona A, Shapiro W, Madewell BR.** Cisplatin (cisdiamine-dichloroplatinum) for treatment of transitional cell carcinoma of the urinary bladder or urethra. J Vet Intern Med 1990;4:148–152.
28. **Knapp DK, Richardson RC, Bonney PL, Hahn K.** Cisplatin therapy in 41 dogs with malignant tumors. J Vet Intern Med 1988;2:41–46.
29. **Ogilvie GK, Krawiec DK, Gelberg HB, et al.** Evaluation of a short-term saline diuresis protocol for the administration of cisplatin. Am J Vet Res 1988;49:1076–1078.
30. **Page RL, Leifer CE.** Cisplatin, a new antineoplastic drug in veterinary medicine. J Am Vet Med Assoc 1985;186:288–290.
31. **Knapp DW, Richardson RC, Denicola DB, et al.** Cisplatin toxicity in cats. J Vet Intern Med 1987;1:29–35.
32. **Page RL, McEntee MC, George SL, et al.** Pharmacokinetic and phase 1 evaluation of carboplatin in dogs. J Vet Intern Med 1993;7:235–240.
33. **Jain NC.** Essentials of veterinary hematology. Philadelphia: Lea and Febiger, 1993;128–129.
34. **Ettinger SJ, Feldman EC.** Textbook of veterinary internal medicine. 4th ed. Philadelphia: WB Saunders, 1995;1889.
35. **Robins HI, Longo WL, Steeves RA, et al.** Adjunctive therapy (whole body hyperthermia versus lonidamine) to total body irradiation for the treatment of favorable B-cell neoplasms: a report of two pilot clinical trials and laboratory investigations. Int J Radiat Oncol Biol Phys 1990;18:909–920.
36. **Edmonson JH, Hartmann MD, Long HJ, et al.** Granulocyte-macrophage colony-stimulating factor. Cancers 1992;70:2529–2539.
37. **Obradovich JE, Oglivie GK, Powers BE, Boone T.** Evaluation of recombinant canine granulocyte colony-stimulating factor as an inducer of granulopoiesis. J Vet Intern Med 1991;5:75–79.
38. **Miller KM.** Clinical manifestations of acute myeloid leukemia. In: Hoffman R, Benz ES, et al, eds. Hematology principles and practice. 2nd ed. New York: Churchill, Livingston, 1995;993–1014.

CHAPTER 102

Myelodysplastic Syndromes and Myelofibrosis

• JULIA T. BLUE

MYELODYSPLASTIC SYNDROMES

Myelodysplastic syndromes (MDSs) are a group of clonal hematologic disorders that originate, as do the acute myeloid leukemias (AML) and chronic myeloproliferative disorders (MPD), from hemopoietic stem cells. MDSs are heterogeneous with regard to presenting signs and laboratory abnormalities but share the common features of ineffective hemopoiesis and morphologic evidence of disturbed maturation in blood and bone marrow cells.[1] Myelodysplasia can evolve into AML and for this reason is viewed as a preleukemic disorder. MDSs are neoplastic, clonal hemopathies, and lethal in many cases without progression to AML owing to severe cytopenias consequent to reduced ability of affected marrow to produce mature blood cells. Failure to maintain normal numbers of mature blood cells results from multiple defects in growth and differentiation and increased apoptosis of hemopoietic cells.[2]

Causes and Incidence

Evidence for the clonal nature of myelodysplasia was first inferred from observation of maturation abnormalities in multiple cell lines (erythroid, myeloid, and megakaryocytic). Clonality was subsequently confirmed by studies of human patients in which cytogenetic and molecular diagnostic methods were used.[2] Various cytogenetic aberrations and point mutations in cellular oncogenes and tumor suppressor genes have been identified in human patients who have MDS.[3,4] None of the cytogenetic abnormalities are specific for MDS but some are highly associated with certain subtypes of MDS and have prognostic significance.

A specific mutagenic event is unknown for the majority of human patients who have MDS, but in approximately 20%, MDSs are secondary to previous chemotherapy, especially alkylating agents, or exposure to radiation or chemicals such as benzene and its derivatives.[2] Feline leukemia virus (FeLV), an oncogenic retrovirus, is the probable cause of MDS in most cats. MDS and AML have been induced by experimental infection with FeLV[5] and approximately 80% of cats that have MDS are positive for FeLV in tests for viral antigen in blood. Initiating causes have not been identified in dogs and horses that have spontaneous MDS, but hematologic disorders with characteristics of myelodysplasia and AML have been reported in dogs exposed experimentally to continuous gamma radiation.[6]

Quantitative data on the incidence and epidemiologic characteristics of MDS in domestic animals are not available because pertinent studies have not been undertaken. In the past, MDSs were fairly common in cats, but the incidence seems to have decreased in recent years, presumably owing to vaccination against FeLV infection. MDSs are even less frequently recognized in dogs and rarely in horses.

Classification of Myelodysplastic Syndromes

Guidelines for the cytomorphologic recognition and classification of MDS in humans were developed by the French-American-British (FAB) cooperative group to improve diagnostic consistency and prognostic accuracy.[7] Five MDSs, called refractory anemia (RA) or refractory cytopenias (RC), refractory anemia with ringed sideroblasts (RARS), refractory anemia with excess blasts (RAEB), refractory anemia with excess blasts in transformation (RAEB-t) and chronic myelomonocytic leukemia (CMMoL) were defined on the basis of characteristics identified by quantitative and morphologic evaluation of blood and bone marrow.[1] Further refinement of diagnosis and prognosis for individual syndromes and their variants has been accomplished through application of immunophenotyping and identification of cytogenetic and molecular lesions. Many factors are used to determine prognosis, but, generally, high bone marrow blast cell counts and multiple, severe cytopenias are predictors of short survival and high probability of progression to AML.

The FAB guidelines for the diagnosis of myelodysplasia are applicable to animals, but modifications of the classification scheme have been recommended by veterinary hematologists.[8–10] In the proposed veterinary scheme the categories MDS erythroid predominant (MDS-Er), MDS refractory cytopenia (MDS-RC), and MDS excess blasts (MDS-EB) replace RA, RARS, RAEB, and RAEB-t as more representative of disease in animals.[10] CMMoL is included in the MDS because it is characterized by the presence of multilineage dyspoiesis and cytopenias and a high rate of progression to AML,[11] even though it resembles chronic granulocytic leukemia in its propensity to cause leukocytosis and infiltration of extramedullary tissue.

An unknown number of cats included in earlier reports of myeloproliferative disorders undoubtedly had MDS if contemporary criteria for diagnosis were applied. A few reports specifically address cases of MDS in cats,[9,12–14] dogs,[15,16] and horses.[17]

Clinical Features

Presenting signs in cats, dogs, and horses that have MDS are varied and not specific. Usually, clinical signs are related to cytopenias, especially anemia, and include lethargy, weakness, decreasing appetite, rapid or labored breathing, decreased grooming activity, and pica.[12] Recurrent or chronic bacterial and fungal infections, related to decreased neutrophil number or function, are the chief problems in some patients. Manifestations of abnormal primary hemostasis, secondary to thrombocytopenia or platelet dysfunction, include epistaxis and petechiae. Duration of clinical signs before diagnosis is variable, ranging from days to months, but usually the onset appears to be sudden. In some cases, myelodysplasia is diagnosed incidental to evaluation for unrelated problems. Pallor, increased heart and respiratory rates, fever, and poor body condition are common physical findings related to MDS. Enlargement of spleen, liver, and lymph nodes is present in most animals that have CMMoL but is not associated with other forms of myelodysplasia.

Hematologic Features

Myelodysplasia is suggested by abnormalities in blood but, in most cases, the diagnosis requires examination of well-prepared smears of bone marrow aspirates. The hallmark features are decreased numbers of mature blood cells in one or more cell lines, morphologic evidence of dysplastic maturation (Table 102.1), and a marrow blast cell count of less than 30% of hemopoietic cells.

Blood

The patterns of peripheral abnormalities in individual patients are highly variable.[12] Multiple cytopenias are

TABLE 102.1	Morphologic Features of Dysplastic Hemopoiesis
Cell Line	**Bone Marrow and/or Peripheral Blood Findings**
Erythroid	Increased percentage of rubriblasts and prorubricytes in marrow
	Megaloblastic rubricytes (large, with nuclei less mature than cytoplasm)
	Nuclear changes: multiple, fragmented, lobulated nuclei; disorganized mitoses; abnormal chromatin patterns; visible nucleoli in rubricytes
	Sideroblasts and siderocytes
	Normochromic macrocytes
Megakaryocytic	Dwarf megakaryocytes with one or more round nuclei
	Large, hypolobulated forms
	Hypergranulated and hypogranulated giant platelets
	Circulating dwarf megakaryocytes and nuclei
Granulocytic	Increased percentage of myeloblasts and progranulocytes in marrow
	Hypersegmented and hyposegmented nuclei
	Giant size
	Decreased number, size, and/or staining of eosinophil granules

common, but decreased numbers of mature cells of one or two cell lines can be accompanied by normal or increased numbers of other cells. Almost all animals are anemic, many are macrocytic, and most are reticulocytopenic. Normochromic macrocytes can be found by examination of blood smears in most cases, even those with a mean cell volume (MCV) within reference limits. Anemia is often severe in cats and is usually mild to moderate in dogs. Slight to moderate reticulocytosis is present in a few cases. Nucleated red cells, including basophilic and megaloblastic rubricytes, are often found in blood; in some patients the number of nucleated red blood cells (nRBCs) exceeds the leukocyte count. Some cats are Coombs' positive. The majority of patients are slightly to severely thrombocytopenic, but a few have normal to increased platelet counts. Giant, abnormally granulated platelets are frequently found, regardless of the count. Dwarf megakaryocytes and their nuclei, which resemble lymphocyte nuclei with a fringe of cytoplasm, circulate in many animals that have CMMoL (Fig. 102.1). Patients that have MDS-Er, MDS-RC, and MDS-EB are likely to have low to normal neutrophil and monocyte counts with or without mild left shift. Those that have CMMoL typically have leukocytosis, which can exceed 100,000 cells/μL, with neutrophilia and monocytosis and pronounced left shift in both series. Immature and dysplastic eosinophils are present in many dogs and cats that have CMMoL. Circulating myeloid blast cells are less than 5% of blood leukocytes in all forms of MDSs except CMMoL in which blasts may be 5 to 10% of the blood leukocytes. Hypersegmented

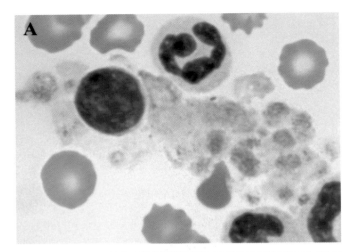

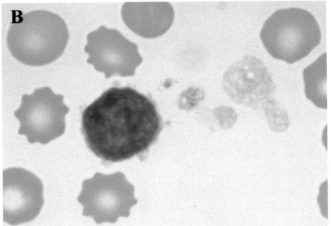

FIGURE 102.1 Photomicrographs of dwarf megakaryocytes in blood from a dog that has CMMoL. Megakaryocyte-shedding platelets is shown in **A** and a nucleus with a fringe of cytoplasmic projections, which distinguishes it from a lymphocyte, is shown in **B**.

granulocytes and monocytes are more frequently found in CMMoL than in the other forms.

Bone Marrow

Bone marrow is typically normocellular to hypercellular in patients that have MDS-Er, MDS-RC, and MDS-EB, but cellularity in some patients is decreased or patchy. Significant hypercellularity and a high myeloid cells relative to erythroid cells (M:E) ratio are consistent findings in CMMoL. A simplified differential count of at least 200 hemopoietic cells should be performed to distinguish MDS from AML and non-neoplastic hyperplasias. Stromal and accessory cells, such as macrophages, lymphocytes, and plasma cells, are not included in the differential count. Cells should be sorted into the following categories: erythroid cells, myeloid blast cells, and differentiating neutrophils (progranulocytes through segmented neutrophils). Cells of other series (monocytes, eosinophils, basophils, or megakaryocytes) should be

counted separately. Rubriblasts should be counted separately if erythroid cells are greater than 50% of the hemopoietic cells; otherwise they are included in the total erythroid-cell category. Type I myeloblasts and monoblasts have similar appearance in smears stained with Romanowsky stains but usually can be distinguished from rubriblasts (Fig. 102.2). Myeloblasts with fewer than 15 red-pink granules are type II myeloblasts; more heavily granulated cells should be considered progranulocytes and included in the differentiating neutrophil category. Myeloblasts and monoblasts can be differentiated by cytochemical procedures. Promonocytes have irregularly shaped nuclei and deep blue, usually agranular cytoplasm (Fig. 102.2).

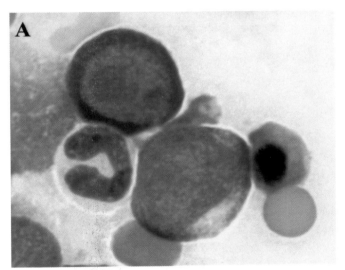

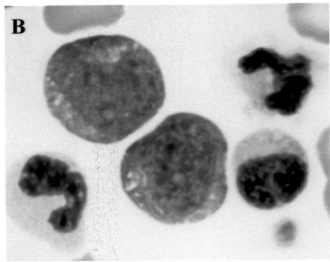

FIGURE 102.2 Features of rubriblasts and myeloblasts are compared in **A**, a field in marrow from a cat that has MDS-EB. The rubriblast has deeper blue cytoplasm and rounder nucleus than the cell beside it, which could be either a myeloblast or monoblast. **B.** Promonocytes in blood from a dog that has CMMoL have nuclei with more irregular contours, coarser chromatin, and lower N:C than myeloid blast cells. The field shown in **B** includes two promonocytes and three neutrophils.

The differential count is used to classify MDS. MDS-Er is the diagnosis if the M:E ratio is less than 1, and blast cells, including rubriblasts, are less than 30% of all nucleated hemopoietic cells (ANC). MDS-RC is diagnosed if the M:E ratio is greater than 1 and blast cells, excluding rubriblasts, are less than 6% of ANC. MDS-EB is indicated by an M:E ratio greater than 1 and a blast cell count, excluding rubriblasts, between 6 and 29% of ANC. CMMoL is recognized by a pattern comprising significant increases in both granulocytes and cells of monocytic lineage in marrow and blood, with blast cell count greater than 5% and less than 30% of ANC in marrow. Typically, cells in the monocyte series compose 20 to 60% of the marrow cells with a significant increase in promonocytes. MDS-EB is the most common form of myelodysplasia in cats, whereas CMMoL is the most common form in dogs.

Evidence of dysplastic hemopoiesis (dyspoiesis) is required for a diagnosis of myelodysplasia. Dysplastic erythroid cells and megakaryocytes are numerous in most animals that have MDS unless cells of these series are scarce. Megaloblastic rubricytes (Fig. 102.3) are typically found in all forms of MDS. Sideroblasts and siderocytes (Fig. 102.3) are numerous in some cases. Dwarf megakaryocytes, large hypolobulated megakaryocytes, and giant platelets with abnormal granulation (Figs. 102.1 and 102.4) are common findings. Increased percentage of myeloid blast cells and a left shift in neutrophils and monocytes are the main indicators of dysmyelopoiesis in many cases. Abnormal nuclear shapes in granulocytes and monocytes and hypogranular eosinophils are sometimes seen in MDS-RC and MDS-EB but are most common in CMMoL (Fig. 102.5).

Abnormalities of stromal and accessory marrow cells are associated with MDS.[18] Myelofibrosis develops secondary to MDS in some cats. Increased numbers of small lymphocytes in aspirate smears and lymphoid nodules in sections of marrow are found in some cats that have myelodysplasia. Hemosiderin is present in most cats, a species that normally lacks hemosiderin in marrow. Hemophagocytic macrophages are present in many animals.

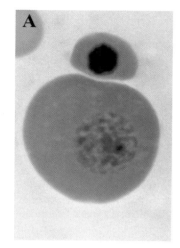
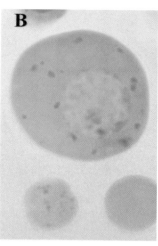
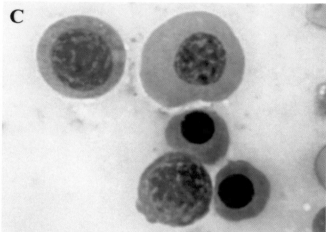

FIGURE 102.3 Common manifestations of dyserythropoiesis are shown in these photomicrographs of marrow from cats that have MDS-EB. A strikingly megaloblastic rubricyte in **A** abuts a rubricyte of normal size. A megaloblastic sideroblast and normocytic siderocyte, containing granules of iron stained blue by Perl's stain, are shown in **B**. The three megaloblastic rubricytes in **C** show more subtle changes reflecting asynchrony of nuclear and cytoplasmic maturation. The two small rubricytes with pyknotic nuclei and polychromatophilic cytoplasm have matured normally.

Outcome and Treatment

Survival time after diagnosis ranges from a few days to a few months for most animals because of the advanced stage of disease and severity of cytopenias at the onset of clinical signs. Many patients are euthanatized soon after diagnosis. Progression to AML does occur, but data are insufficient to estimate the probability of progression in an individual animal or for the different classes of MDS. Personal observations indicate that animals that have low blast counts and mild to moderate cytopenias can live for months to years with supportive treatment, such as blood component and antimicrobial therapy, administered as needed. Recognition of myelodysplasia in these patients is usually incidental to examination for other problems. Intensive cytoreductive chemotherapy is of little benefit to most MDS patients, particularly

those that have low blast cell counts, and can exacerbate life-threatening cytopenias.[2] Administration of hemopoietic growth factors alleviates the effects of cytopenias.[2,19] Combinations of recombinant human erythropoietin (rhEpo), recombinant granulocyte-colony-stimulating factor (rhG-CSF), and recombinant granulocyte-macrophage-CSF (rhGM-CSF) appear to have synergistic effects in human patients, reducing transfusion requirements and risk of infections. Allogeneic bone marrow transplantation is the most effective treatment for hemopoietic neoplasia in human and animal patients but is feasible for only a few patients.[19,20]

Differential Diagnosis

An experienced hematopathologist can diagnose most cases of MDS by careful examination of marrow and blood, but the diagnosis can be questionable in patients that lack pronounced evidence of multilineage dyspoiesis or excess blast cells. Benefit of doubt should be extended to such patients, and other benign or potentially reversible disorders should be excluded by diagnostic testing and response to treatment. Nutritional or drug-induced deficiencies of folate, pyridoxine, and cobalamin are potential explanations for dyserythropoiesis that can be excluded by measurement of serum concentrations of these vitamins or by consideration of treatment and dietary history. Chloramphenicol, vincristine, and lead poisoning can produce siderocytes and nuclear abnormalities in erythroid cells. Immune-mediated (both idiopathic and drug induced), ineffective hemopoiesis should be considered in patients that have selective or multiple cytopenias and cellular marrow without multilineage dyspoiesis. Congenital (mac-

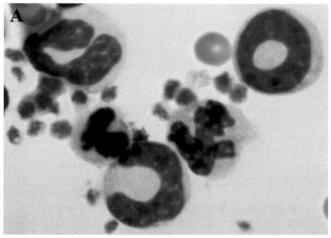

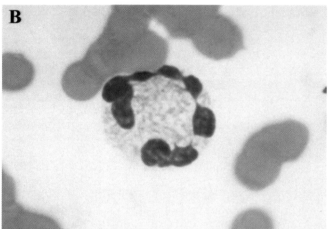

FIGURE 102.5 Dysmyelopoiesis can be manifested as abnormalities of size, granulation, and nuclear shapes. In a field of marrow from a cat that has MDS-EB, **A,** two segmented neutrophils of normal size are flanked by three giant bands, one with a ring nucleus. A hypersegmented and sparsely granulated eosinophil in the blood of a cat that has CMMoL is shown in **B.**

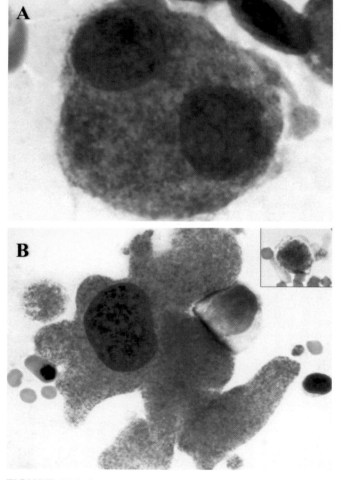

FIGURE 102.4 Dysmegakaryopoiesis can result in dwarf megakaryocytes with one or more round nuclei, **A,** and larger cells with hypolobulated nuclei, **B.** The cytoplasm of the megakaryocyte in **B** appears to be breaking into large fragments, which can circulate as giant, hypergranular platelets as shown in the inset of **B.** The cells shown here are in marrow of cats; megakaryocytes in blood are shown in Figure 102.1. (The magnification of **A** is 2.5 times greater than **B.**)

rocytosis of toy and miniature poodle dogs) and idiopathic syndromes of dyserythropoiesis[21] are recognized in dogs. Neutrophilia, monocytosis, and myeloid hyperplasia induced by infection, inflammation, or paraneoplastic effects can usually be distinguished from CMMoL by complete diagnostic evaluation. In contrast to CMMoL, the monocytic component of marrow in reactive hyperplasias is virtually always less than 10%, and the blast count is less than 5%.

MYELOFIBROSIS

Myelofibrosis is an increase in collagen and other proteins of the extracellular matrix in marrow, a process that involves increased proliferation and synthetic activity of marrow fibroblasts. Transforming growth factor β (TGF-β), platelet derived growth factor (PDGF), and epidermal growth factor (EGF) are fibrogenic cytokines

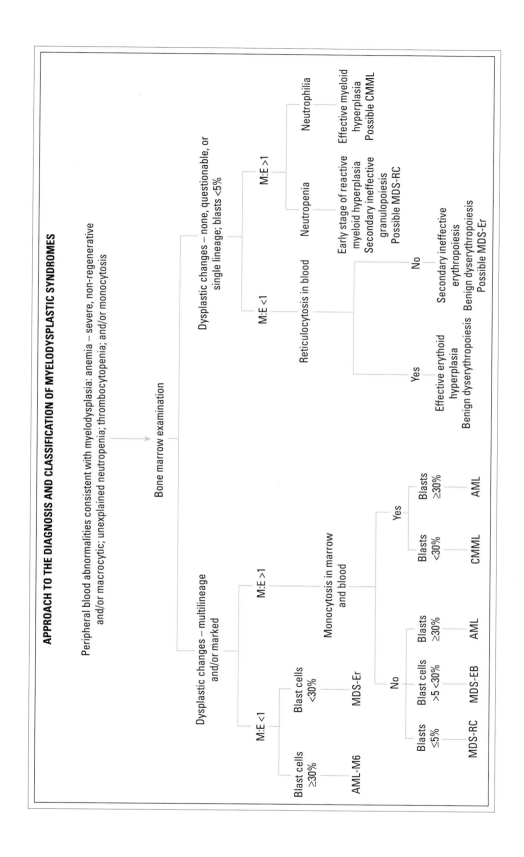

APPROACH TO THE DIAGNOSIS AND CLASSIFICATION OF MYELODYSPLASTIC SYNDROMES

Peripheral blood abnormalities consistent with myelodysplasia: anemia – severe, non-regenerative and/or macrocytic; unexplained neutropenia; thrombocytopenia; and/or monocytosis

Bone marrow examination

Dysplastic changes – multilineage and/or marked

Dysplastic changes – none, questionable, or single lineage; blasts <5%

M:E <1

Blast cells ≥30% → AML-M6

Blast cells <30% → MDS-Er

M:E >1

Monocytosis in marrow and blood

No:
Blasts ≤5% → MDS-RC
Blast cells >5 <30% → MDS-EB
Blasts ≥30% → AML

Yes:
Blasts <30% → CMML
Blasts ≥30% → AML

M:E <1

Reticulocytosis in blood

Yes → Effective erythoid hyperplasia
Benign dyserythropoiesis

No → Secondary ineffective erythropoiesis
Benign dyserythropoiesis
Possible MDS-Er

M:E >1

Neutropenia → Early stage of reactive myeloid hyperplasia
Secondary ineffective granulopoiesis
Possible MDS-RC

Neutrophilia → Effective myeloid hyperplasia
Possible CMML

687

that have been implicated as important modulators of proliferation and synthesis in marrow fibroblasts and endothelial cells.[22] Myelofibrosis is a reactive process associated with various diseases and can resolve with correction of the primary disease. Hematologic abnormalities in animals that have myelofibrosis are those of the primary disease.

A pivotal role for megakaryocytes in the pathogenesis of myelofibrosis has been established by studies of human patients who have a chronic myeloproliferative disorder called, misleadingly, idiopathic myelofibrosis (IMF), which is a clonal hemopathy characterized by abnormal megakaryocytes, severe myelofibrosis, and splenic enlargement by extramedullary hemopoiesis. This syndrome is also known as primary myelofibrosis and agnogenic myeloid metaplasia with myelofibrosis. Excessive production or intramedullary release of fibrogenic cytokines by megakaryocytes is thought to underlie myelofibrosis in IMF, acute megakaryoblastic leukemia (AML-M7), and MDS with prominent dysmegakaryopoiesis.[22] An animal model of myelofibrosis and osteosclerosis has been created by inducing mice to overexpress thrombopoietin (TPO) by retroviral-mediated gene transfer.[23] Constant high levels of TPO induce megakaryocytic hyperplasia and myelofibrosis, which is reversed by transplantation with normal marrow. The role of marrow macrophages and the mechanisms leading to myelofibrosis secondary to diseases that do not feature abnormalities of megakaryocytes have been less intensively investigated, but activated monocytes and macrophages are known to produce high levels of TGF-β and PDGF.[24]

Myelofibrosis develops in dogs and cats that have AML-M7, as in human patients. IMF, closely resembling the human disease in presentation and lesions, has been reported in an aged marmoset.[25] In cats, MDS and AML are the most common diseases underlying myelofibrosis. Myelofibrosis accompanied an inherited hemopoietic disorder in young, related pygmy goats.[26] The syndrome was manifested from birth as anemia with diminishing hematocrits, reticulocyte counts, neutrophils, and platelets until death at 6 to 12 weeks of age. Extramedullary hemopoiesis, hyperplasia of atypical megakaryocytes, and severe myelofibrosis were identified at necropsy. Personal observations indicate that myelofibrosis in dogs is most commonly associated with immune-mediated, nonregenerative anemia. Affected dogs are anemic and reticulocytopenic despite significant, but ineffective, erythroid hyperplasia. Fibrosis resolves if effective erythropoiesis is restored by immunosuppressive therapy. Myelofibrosis also occurs in dogs that have hemolytic anemia because of pyruvate kinase

deficiency. Other disorders associated with focal or diffuse fibrosis include infectious diseases, radiation, drugs, and cancer with and without marrow metastases.[27]

REFERENCES

1. **Kouides PA, Bennett JM.** Morphology and classification of the myelodysplastic syndromes and their pathologic variants. Semin Hematol 1996;33:95–110.
2. **Fenaux P.** Myelodysplastic syndromes. Hematol Cell Ther 1996;38:363–380.
3. **Bartram CR.** Molecular genetic aspects of myelodysplastic syndromes. Semin Hematol 1996;33:139–147.
4. **Fenaux P, Morel P, Lai JL.** Cytogenetics of myelodysplastic syndromes. Semin Hematol 1996;33:127–138.
5. **Toth SR, Onions DE, Jarret O.** Histopathological and hematological findings in myeloid leukemia induced by a new feline leukemia virus isolate. Vet Pathol 1986;23:462–470.
6. **Tolle DV, Cullen SM, Seed TM, Fritz TE.** Circulating micromegakaryocytes preceding leukemia in three dogs exposed to 2.5 R/day gamma radiation. Vet Pathol 1983;20:111–114.
7. **Bennett JM, Catovsky D, Daniel MT, et al.** Proposals for the classification of the myelodysplastic syndromes. Br J Haematol 1982;51:189–199.
8. **Jain NC, Blue JT, Grindem CB, et al.** Proposed criteria for classification of acute myeloid leukemia in dogs and cats. Vet Clin Pathol 1991;20:63–82.
9. **Jain NC.** Classification of myeloproliferative disorders in cats using criteria proposed by the animal leukemia study group: a retrospective study of 181 cases. Comp Haematol Int 1993;3:125–134.
10. **Raskin RE.** Myelopoiesis and myeloproliferative disorders. Vet Clin North Am Small Anim Pract 1996;26:1023–1042.
11. **Rosati S, Anastasi J, Vardiman J.** Recurring diagnostic problems in the pathology of the myelodysplastic syndromes. Semin Hematol 1996;33:111–126.
12. **Blue JT, French TW, Scarlett JS.** Non-lymphoid hematopoietic neoplasia in cats: a retrospective study of 60 cases. Cornell Vet 1988;78:21–42.
13. **Baker RJ, Valli VEO.** Dysmyelopoiesis in the cat: a hematological disorder resembling refractory anemia with excess blasts in man. Can J Vet Res 1986;50:3–6.
14. **Raskin RE.** Myelodysplastic changes in a cat with myelomonocytic leukemia. J Am Vet Med Assoc 1985;187:171–174.
15. **Couto CG, Kallet AJ.** Preleukemia syndrome in a dog. J Am Vet Med Assoc 1984;184:1389–1392.
16. **Weiss DJ, Raskin RE, Zerbe C.** Myelodysplastic syndrome in two dogs. J Am Vet Med Assoc 1985;187:1038–1040.
17. **Durando MM, Alleman AR, Harvey JW.** Myelodysplastic syndrome in a quarter horse gelding. Equine Vet J 1994;26:83–85.
18. **Blue JT.** Myelofibrosis in cats with myelodysplastic syndrome and acute myelogenous leukemia. Vet Pathol 1988;24:154–160.
19. **Anderson JE, Appelbaum FR.** Myelodysplasia and myeloproliferative disorders. Curr Opin Hematol 1997;4:261–267.
20. **Gasper PW, Rosen DK, Fulton R.** Allogeneic marrow transplantation in a cat with acute myeloid leukemia. J Am Vet Med Assoc 1996;208:1280–1284.
21. **Weiss D, Reidarson TH.** Idiopathic dyserythropoiesis in a dog. Vet Clin Pathol 1989;18:43–46.
22. **Reilly JT.** Pathogenesis of idiopathic myelofibrosis: role of growth factors. J Clin Pathol 1992;45:461–464.
23. **Yan X-Q, Lacey D, Hill D, Chen Y.** A model of myelofibrosis and osteosclerosis in mice induced by overexpressing thrombopoietin (mpl ligand): reversal of disease by bone marrow transplantation. Blood 1996;88:402–409.
24. **Rameshawar P, Denny TN, Stein D, Gascon P.** Monocyte adhesion in patients with bone marrow fibrosis is required for the production of fibrogenic cytokines. J Immunol 1994;153:2819–2830.
25. **Khan KNM, Logan AC, Blomquist EM.** Idiopathic myelofibrosis (agnogenic myeloid metaplasia) in a marmoset (*Callithrix jacchus*): hematologic and histopathologic changes. Vet Pathol 1997;34:341–345.
26. **Cain GR, East N, Moore PF.** Myelofibrosis in young pygmy goats. Comp Haematol Int 1994;4:167–172.
27. **Reagan WJ.** A review of myelofibrosis in dogs. Toxicol Pathol 1993;21:164–169.

CHAPTER 103

CD Antigens and Immunophenotyping

• GREGG A. DEAN

Before the mid-1970s few tools existed for exploring cell surface molecules. During this time, the relative simplicity of the erythrocyte was exploited to study the anatomy and composition of the cell membrane. Electron microscopy and radiolabeling were used to develop the cell membrane model of a lipid bilayer spanned by proteins. Two of the first proteins observed to span the lipid bilayer were erythrocyte glycophorin and band 3. Development of techniques to solubilize cell membranes with detergents and separate proteins by affinity chromatography provided powerful tools for the identification of many membrane-associated proteins. Monoclonal antibody techniques drastically accelerated the characterization of cell surface molecules. By immunizing mice with cells of another species, a shotgun approach was used to generate monoclonal antibodies to various molecules. With many investigators generating antibodies, often against the same antigens, and using various names for antibodies and their antigen specificity, it was difficult to correlate results from different laboratories. Eventually, it was clear that a common nomenclature was needed to make sense of the growing number of cell surface molecules and antibodies against them.

CLUSTER OF DIFFERENTIATION NOMENCLATURE

International workshops were organized to cluster monoclonal antibodies labeling specific cellular antigens. Flow cytometry was used to characterize the pattern of labeling on various cell types for each antibody. Antibodies with the same pattern of labeling were considered to label the same antigen. The antigens identified by clusters of antibodies were often indicators of the differentiation state of the cells and, thus were given a cluster of differentiation (CD) antigen designation. The workshops assign new antibodies to existing CD numbers or, if an antibody recognizes a previously unidentified antigen, a new CD number is assigned to the novel antigen.

Many monoclonal antibodies against human leukocyte antigens have been characterized and assigned to a CD through a series of six international workshops. There are over 200 human cell surface antigens identified by antibodies that have been clustered through the workshops. These antigens have been assigned as CD1 through CD166 with families of similar antigens being assigned a CD number followed by a letter (i.e., CD1a and CD1b). Workshops have been organized for several domestic veterinary species, including mice, ruminants, horses, swine, and dogs, but not for cats.[1-4] These workshops have assigned antibodies to a CD number consistent with the human nomenclature when the antigen identified is proved to be an orthologue to the human antigen. Antigens found to be unique to a veterinary species are assigned a species-specific designation such as swine workshop cluster 1 (SWC1). A summary of antigens characterized by veterinary workshops and feline antigens identified in the literature are presented in Table 103.1.[1-14]

IMMUNOPHENOTYPING HEMOPOIETIC NEOPLASMS

Cell surface molecules provide a means by which the origin of hemopoietic cells may be determined. Immunophenotyping employs antibodies to label antigens that may characterize or identify a cell or a tissue type. Immunophenotyping can be performed on tissue sections, cells on glass slides, or cells in suspension. The technique applied to tissues or cells on slides is immunohistochemistry or immunocytochemistry, respectively. Cells in suspension are most easily evaluated by flow cytometry. Hemolymphatic cells express numerous cell surface molecules, and distribution of these antigens can be broad or may be present only on specific cell types (Table 103.2). The antigens of greatest use are those surface proteins found only on a single lineage and that are characteristic of the stage of maturation.

The purpose of immunophenotyping is to provide an objective and reproducible method for the diagnosis of hematologic malignancies. The diagnosis is based on the immunologic identification and characterization of clonally expanded abnormal hemopoietic precursor cells. Although to date, the clinical applications of im-

TABLE 103.1   Summary of CD Antigens Identified in Veterinary Species

Antigen	Equine	Ruminant	Swine	Canine	Feline	Distribution[a]
CD1	—	X	X	—	X	cortical thymocytes, B-cell subset, dendritic cells, Langerhans cells
CD2	X	X	X	—	—	T cells, NK cells
CD3	X	X	X	—	—	T cells
CD4	X	X	X	X	X	T-helper cells, monocytes, macrophages
CD5	X	X	X	X	X	T cells, B-cell subset
CD6	—	X	X	—	—	T cells, B-cell subset
CD8	X	X	X	X	X	T-cytotoxic cells
CD9	—	—	—	—	X	platelets, monocytes, pre-B cells
CD10	—	—	—	—	—	pre-B cells, granulocytes
CD11a	X	X	—	X	—	leukocytes
CD11b	—	X	—	X	—	granulocytes, monocytes, NK cells
CD11c	—	X	—	X	—	granulocytes, monocytes, NK cells, T-cell subset, B-cell subset
CD13	X	—	—	—	—	monocytes, granulocytes
CD14	—	X	X	—	—	monocytes
CD16	—	—	X	—	—	NK cells, macrophages, granulocytes
CD18	—	X	X	—	—	leukocytes
CD19	—	—	—	—	—	B cells
CD20	—	—	—	—	—	B cells
CD21	—	X	X	X	X	B cells
CD25	—	X	X	—	X	activated T cells
CD28	X	—	—	—	—	leukocytes
CD29	—	—	X	—	—	leukocytes
CD34	—	—	—	—	—	hemopoietic pregenitor cells
CD41/61	—	X	—	X	—	platelets, megakaryocytes
CD44	X	X	X	X	—	leukocytes, erythrocytes
CD45	—	X	—	X	X	leukocytes
CD45R	—	X	—	X	—	B cells, T-cell subset
CD45RA	—	—	X	—	—	B cells, T-cell subset, monocytes
CD45RC	—	—	X	—	—	B cells, T-cell subset
CD45RO	—	X	—	—	—	B cells, T-cell subset, monocytes
CD49	—	—	—	X	—	B cells, activated T cells, monocytes, platelets
CD58	—	X	—	—	—	broad
CD62L	—	X	—	—	—	lymphocytes, monocytes, NK cells
CD69	—	—	X	X	—	activated T and B cells, NK cells
CD71	—	X	—	—	—	proliferating cells
	Eq MHC 1	WC1	SWC1	THY-1	Ly1	
	Eq MHC II	WC4	SWC2	MHCII	My1	
	B Lymphocytes	WC5	SWC3	Cluster A	Er1	
	Thymocytes	WC6	SWC4	Cluster H	Er2	
	Granulocytes	WC7	SWC5	Cluster K	—	
	Macrophages	WC8	SWC6	—	—	
	EqWC1	WC9	SWC7	—	—	
	EqWC2	WC10	SWC8	—	—	
	—	WC11	SWC9	—	—	
	—	WC13	—	—	—	
	—	WC14	—	—	—	
	—	WC15	—	—	—	

[a]Additional information on antigen distribution for each species and for distribution of antigens not assigned to a CD can be found in indicated references. Equine[4]; Ruminant[1]; Swine[3]; Canine[2]; Feline.[5–14]

munophenotyping have been limited in veterinary medicine, experimental applications have been instrumental in studies of the immune system and neoplasia. Conversely, in human medicine, flow cytometry has become the preferred clinical method for lineage assignment and for maturational analysis of malignant cells in acute leukemias and lymphomas.[15] It is also used to monitor therapy and detect minimal residual disease. In many cases of hemolymphatic neoplasia, flow cytometry may identify clonality and aberrant features of a malignant cell population. Note that immunophenotyping is only useful if it extends the cytologic or histopathologic evaluation. The final diagnostic classification of hemopoietic neoplasia is based on clinical findings, morphologic features, and cytochemical and immunologic characterization.

TABLE 103.2 Surface Molecules on Hematopoietic Progenitor Cells

	Pluripotent SC	CFU-GEMM	CFU-GM	CFU-G	Myelocyte	CFU-M	Promonocyte	CFU-Eo	Myelocyte-Eo	CFU-Baso	Myelocyte-Baso	CFU-Meg	Megakaryocyte	BFU-E	CFU-E	Lymphoid	Molecule
CD11B	–	–	–	–	–	–	–	X	X	–	–	–	–	–	–	X	αM Intergin, CR3
CD13	–	–	X	X	X	X	X	X	X	–	–	–	–	–	–	–	aminopeptidase N
CD14	–	–	–	–	–	–	X	–	–	–	X	–	–	–	–	–	Binds LPS
CD15	–	–	–	X	X	X	X	–	X	–	–	–	–	–	–	–	Lewis X antigen
CD32	–	–	–	–	–	–	–	–	X	–	–	–	–	–	–	X	FcRIII
CD33	–	X	X	X	X	X	X	X	X	–	X	–	–	X	–	–	Sialic acid binding protein
CD34	–	X	X	–	–	–	–	X	–	X	–	X	–	–	–	X	E- and L-selectin ligand
CD35	–	–	–	–	–	–	–	–	X	–	–	–	–	–	–	X	CR1
CD36	–	–	–	–	–	–	–	–	–	–	–	–	–	X	–	–	GPIV (IIIb)
CD42a	–	–	–	–	–	–	–	–	–	–	–	–	X	–	–	–	GPIX
CD42b	–	–	–	–	–	–	–	–	–	–	–	–	X	–	–	–	GPIB-α
CD42c	–	–	–	–	–	–	–	–	–	–	–	–	X	–	–	–	GPIB-β
CD42d	–	–	–	–	–	–	–	–	–	–	–	–	X	–	–	–	GPV
CD49f	–	–	–	–	–	–	–	–	–	–	–	–	X	–	–	X	α6-integrin
CD51	–	–	–	–	–	–	–	–	–	–	–	–	X	–	–	–	α4-integrin
CD61	–	–	–	–	–	–	–	–	–	–	–	–	X	–	–	–	β3-integrin
CD90	X	–	–	–	–	–	–	–	–	–	–	–	–	–	–	–	Thy-1
CD114	–	–	–	–	X	–	–	–	X	–	X	–	–	–	–	–	G-CSF receptor
CD115	–	–	X	–	–	X	X	–	–	–	–	–	–	X	–	–	M-CSF receptor
CD116	–	X	X	X	X	X	X	X	X	–	–	–	–	X	X	–	GM-CSF receptor α chain
CD117	X	X	–	–	–	–	–	–	–	–	–	–	–	–	–	X	SCF-receptor
CD123	X	X	X	X	X	–	X	X	–	X	X	X	X	X	X	–	IL-3 receptor α chain
CD131	–	–	X	X	X	–	X	X	X	–	–	–	X	X	X	–	Common β chain for IL3, IL5, GM-CSF receptor
CD135	X	X	–	–	–	–	–	–	–	–	–	–	–	–	–	–	Flt3

Abbreviations: SC, stem cell; CFU, colony forming units; GEMM, granulocyte, erythrocyte, monocyte, megakaryocyte; GM, granulocyte, monocyte; G, granulocyte; M, monocyte; Eo, eosinophil; Baso, basophil; e, erythrocyte, BFU, burst-forming unit; IL, interleukin; SCF, stem cell factor; CR, complement receptor; FcR, antibody receptor; LPS, lipopolysaccharide; GP, glycoprotein.

PREPARATION OF SAMPLES FOR IMMUNOPHENOTYPING

Samples from many sources, including blood, bone marrow, mass or organ aspirate, mass or organ biopsy, or cavity fluid can be used in immunophenotyping assays. Cytologic or histopathologic evaluation is recommended prior to flow cytometric analysis. The presence of the suspected neoplastic population must be confirmed to avoid analyzing and misinterpreting a sample that does not contain the population in question. This error may occur in three ways:

1. If therapy is initiated between collection of the sample for microscopy and flow cytometry
2. If a different site or organ (i.e. lymph node) is aspirated for microscopy versus flow cytometry
3. If neoplastic cells are shed intermittently into an effusion

Caution must also be exercised during performance of flow cytometry on old samples (>30 hours) as neoplastic cells may preferentially die or lyse over time.

Appropriate handling of the sample is critical to gain accurate and useful information from immunophenotyping. Polypropylene syringes and tubes should be used for collection and storage of the specimen because some cells can adhere to uncoated glass or polystyrene. Preservative-free heparin (50 U/ml) is generally the preferred anticoagulant, particularly if nucleated cells are to be harvested by density-gradient separation. Use of ethylenediamine tetra-acetic acid (EDTA) may reduce platelet aggregation and loss of myeloid cells caused by adhesion, and therefore, may be advantageous in some situations. Samples should be stored at room temperature (18 to 22°C) until analysis, as storage at less than 10°C often leads to adsorption of immunoglobulins to cells and a selective loss of cells or antigens. Diluting the sample 1:2 in a buffered tissue culture medium containing 2% fetal calf serum (FCS) or bovine serum albumin (BSA) helps preserve nucleated cells. Ultimately, each laboratory must verify the optimal anticoagulant and storage temperature for detecting antigens of interest.

Preparation of a sample for flow cytometry consists of erythrocyte elimination and antibody labeling of nucleated cells. Erythrocytes may be lysed either before or after incubation with the antibodies. Commercially available lysing kits and automated sample processing stations have been used successfully. Alternatively, mononuclear cells can be purified by density-gradient separation with ficoll hypaque solution (density of 1.077), and then stained with antibody. Erythrocyte lysis techniques are less time consuming and result in minimal loss of nucleated cells. Density-gradient separation results in an enrichment of blasts, which may be advantageous when one performs single-color fluorescent antibody analysis. If density-gradient separation is used, the sample must again be evaluated microscopically to document the presence of cells of interest. The appropriate technique for sample preparation varies depending on the nature of the sample (degree of erythrocyte contamination, nucleated cell count, volume of specimen, and absolute and relative number of cells of interest) and type of antibody labeling (single versus multiple antibody).

Directly fluorochrome-conjugated monoclonal antibodies are preferred for the labeling of cellular antigens. Furthermore, simultaneous use of two or more different monoclonal antibodies conjugated to different fluorochromes yields the most information. Directly conjugated monoclonal antibodies reduce time and expense for sample labeling while also reducing the level of background staining that is frequently introduced by indirect labeling techniques. Antibodies should be diluted in phosphate-buffered saline with 1 to 5% protein (BSA or FCS) and sodium azide (0.1 to 0.2%). This same solution should be used for washing cells during the labeling procedure. The azide reduces capping and internalization of antibody-bound cell surface antigens. After labeling, samples can be fixed in buffered paraformaldehyde (2%) and remain stable for days to weeks.

Positive and negative controls should be included for each staining procedure. Labeling of one antigen that is expected to be highly expressed on many nucleated cells (such as CD45 or major histocompatibility complex I [MHC I]) serves as a positive control. Negative controls vary, depending on whether direct or indirect and single-antibody or multiple-antibody labeling is performed. Minimally, isotype-matched fluorochrome-conjugated antibodies of irrelevant specificity should be used as negative controls. Quality assurance can be accomplished by phenotyping normal samples.

During analysis of a specimen by use of flow cytometry, the population of interest must be identified by light scatter or immunophenotypic characteristics. Forward light scatter is roughly correlated to cell size, and side light scatter is roughly correlated to intracellular complexity (i.e., granularity). An abnormal population may be obvious as a distinct population not normally observed for a particular tissue. If the total cell population is mixed and the abnormal population has light scatter characteristics that overlap with normal cell populations, it can be difficult to identify the abnormal population solely by light-scatter features. In such cases the abnormal population may be revealed by an atypical immunophenotype such as dual expression of markers that are normally lineage specific. After the population is identified, it can be further characterized regarding lineage and state of maturation.

APPLICATION OF HEMOPOIETIC NEOPLASM IMMUNOPHENOTYPING

In veterinary species as well as in humans, one of the most important applications of immunophenotyping is to differentiate lymphoid versus nonlymphoid leukemia or neoplasia. The majority of available monoclonal antibodies for veterinary species identify lymphocyte markers. It is essential to employ a panel of monoclonal antibodies for immunophenotyping because some antigens associated with differentiation may be lost during neoplastic transformation. Unfortunately, once lymphocytic neoplasia is eliminated, few reagents are available to characterize neoplasia of hemopoietic precursors. To assist in the classification of human acute myeloid leukemias according to the French-American-British (FAB) system, a study group has recommended a large panel of monoclonal antibodies.[15] No such consensus exists for veterinary species. However, the recommended system for immunophenotyping in human medicine provides a diagnostic starting point with available reagents and identifies many important reagents for future development. The majority of clinical cases evaluated in veterinary species have been canine and feline.[16–18]

GUIDELINES FOR CASE SELECTION AND APPROACH TO FLOW CYTOMETRY DATA INTERPRETATION

1. Criteria for case selection
   a. Neoplasia of lymphoid or hemopoietic origin is highly suspected.
   b. Suspect population comprises a significant percentage of total nucleated cells (>5%) or suspect cell type is larger than other nucleated elements, thus allowing identification on light-scatter histograms.
   c. Sample is a single-cell suspension or can be processed to a single-cell suspension.
   d. Adequate sample can be obtained (>10^7 cells).
2. Identify suspect population on flow-cytometry histograms
   a. Identify based on abnormal light-scatter characteristics (Figs. 103.1 and 103.2)
   b. Identify by a combination of light-scatter and fluorescent-antibody labeling (Fig. 103.3A, B, C)

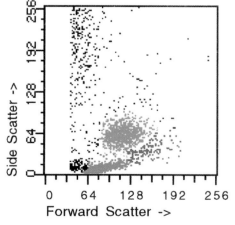

FIGURE 103.1 Light-scatter histogram of normal canine peripheral blood cells. Red identifies lymphocytes, green identifies granulocytes, and blue identifies monocytes.

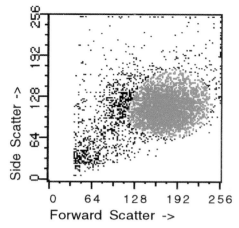

FIGURE 103.2 Light-scatter histogram of leukemic canine peripheral blood. The abnormal (neoplastic) population predominates with a loss of normal leukocyte populations. Setting an analysis gate (shown in red) is straightforward when the abnormal population is this apparent.

3. Characterize surface antigen expression
   a. Identify the presence of abnormal antigen expression, abnormal combinations of antigens, or lack of normal antigen expression compared with normal hemopoietic cells.
   b. When evaluating a population of cells by flow cytometry, it is impossible to tell whether all cells within an analysis gate are part of the population of interest. In fact, it is most likely they are not. Analysis gates may also include normal cells, platelet clumps, and cell debris. Therefore, simple percentages of positive staining (i.e., 75% of cells express CD4) are not useful and can be misleading. In the dog, a CD4+ population could be compatible with a lymphocytic, granulocytic, or monocytic phenotype. It is most useful to use double- or triple-antibody labeling to determine what other antigens are on the CD4+ cells. Thus a CD4+/CD3+/CD14− phenotype would indicate lymphoid origin, a CD4+/CD3−/CD14+ phenotype would indicate monocytic origin, and CD4+/CD3−/CD14− phenotype would indicate a granulocytic origin.
   c. In veterinary medicine, the lack of antibodies conjugated to various fluorochromes may prohibit double- or triple-antibody labeling. In such cases, combining light-scatter characteristics with antibody labeling is the next best approach. Although there will be no direct demonstration that two or three specific antigens occur on the same cells, additional confidence is gained by knowing that the individually labeled antigens appear on populations with identical light-scatter characteristics.
   d. Knowing the limitations of the techniques and reagents is essential. For example, cell surface immunoglobulin has been used as an indicator of a B-lymphocyte phenotype. Although it is true that B

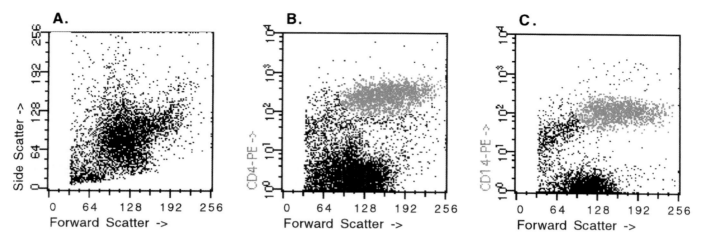

FIGURE 103.3 Light-scatter and fluorescence histograms of leukemic canine peripheral blood. The light-scatter histogram is clearly abnormal, however the abnormal cell population appears to overlap with other, possibly normal cell populations, **A.** By evaluating fluorescence versus light scatter, the abnormal population is revealed to be large, based on forward light scatter and CD4+, and CD14+, based on fluorescence (populations shown in red on **B** and **C**). In this case antibodies were conjugated to phycoerythrin (PE). These histograms identify the neoplastic cell population as CD4+ CD14+, which is consistent with a monocytic origin.

lymphocytes express surface immunoglobulin, in vivo or in vitro coating of normal or neoplastic cells often occurs. Therefore, the presence of surface immunoglobulin is supportive of a B-lymphocyte phenotype in the presence of other lineage-specific markers (i.e., CD19, CD20, CD21, or CD22) but is in no way diagnostic of B-lymphocyte neoplasia per se.

4. Correlate data, make diagnosis
   a. Determine significance of each piece of data.
   b. Make diagnosis based on clinical findings, morphology, cytochemistry, and immunophenotype.

BEYOND IMMUNOPHENOTYPING

A cluster designation is no longer simply a designation for antibody reactivity. To classify the reactivity of an antibody through a workshop, one must also determine the nature of the antigen labeled. This includes determining the molecular weight of the antigen and if a new CD is created, the antigen must be sequenced. The sequence can then be compared with existing databases to biologically characterize the specific role of the antigen. This process has revealed the biological significance of many CD antigens found on various populations of cells. Ultimately, this enhances our understanding of the biology of hemopoiesis and hemopoietic neoplasms and may suggest potential therapeutic approaches. For example a hemopoietic neoplasm may be immunophenotyped and found positive for CD13, CD14, CD33, CD64, CDw65, and CD115. This immunophenotype and supportive morphologic criteria would characterize the neoplasm as M5 (monoblastic origin) by the FAB system. With the additional knowledge that CD115 is the receptor for M-CSF, the M5 FAB classification makes sense biologically, as well as morphologically. Furthermore,

therapeutic options such as the use of macrophage-colony-stimulating factor (M-CSF) to force neoplastic cells to differentiate or the use of cytotoxic compounds that specifically target CD115 expressing cells have a rational basis. Although these types of strategies are in their infancy, immunophenotyping is essential for the evolution of a more sophisticated and efficacious therapeutic approach to hemopoietic neoplasia.

REFERENCES

1. **Naessens J, Howard CJ, Hopkins J.** Nomenclature and characterization of leukocyte differentiation antigens in ruminants. Immunol Today. 1997;18:365–368.
2. **Cobbold S, Metcalfe S.** Monoclonal antibodies that define canine homologues of human CD antigens: summary of the First International Canine Leukocyte Antigen Workshop (CLAW). Tissue Antigens. 1994;43:137–154.
3. **Saalmuller A.** Characterization of swine leukocyte differentiation antigens. Immunol Today. 1996;17:352–354.
4. **Lunn DP, Holmes MA, Antczak DF.** Summary report of the Second Equine Leucocyte Antigen Workshop. Vet Immunol Immunopathol 1996;54:159–161.
5. **Woo JC, Moore PF.** A feline homologue of CD1 is defined using a feline-specific monoclonal antibody. Tissue Antigens. 1997;244–251.
6. **Willett BJ, Hosie MJ, Jarrett O, Neil JC.** Identification of a putative cellular receptor for feline immunodeficiency virus as the feline homologue of CD9. Immunology 1994;81:228–233.
7. **Ackley CD, Cooper MD.** Characterization of a feline T-cell-specific monoclonal antibody reactive with a CD5-like molecule. Am J Vet Res 1992;53:466–471.
8. **Ackley CD, Hoover EA, Cooper MD.** Identification of a CD4 homologue in the cat. Tissue Antigens 1990;35:92–98.
9. **Tompkins MB, Gebhard DH, Bingham HR, Hamilton MJ, Davis WC, Tompkins WA.** Characterization of monoclonal antibodies to feline T lymphocytes and their use in the analysis of lymphocyte tissue distribution in the cat. Vet Immunol Immunopathol 1990;26:305–317.
10. **Ohno K, Goitsuka R, Kitamura K, Hasegawa A, Tokunaga T, Honda M.** Production of a monoclonal antibody that defines the alpha-subunit of the feline IL-2 receptor. Hybridoma 1992;11:595–605.
11. **Klotz FW, Cooper MD.** A feline thymocyte antigen defined by a monoclonal antibody (FT2) identifies a subpopulation of non-helper cells capable of specific cytotoxicity. J Immunol 1986;136:2510–2514.
12. **Willett BJ, de Parseval A, Peri E, Rocchi M, Hosie MJ, Randall R, Klatzmann D, Neil JC, Jarrett O.** The generation of monoclonal antibodies recognising novel epitopes by immunisation with solid matrix antigen-antibody complexes reveals a polymorphic determinant on feline CD4. J Immunol Methods 1994;176:213–220.

TABLE 104.2	**Generalized Histiocytoses Infiltrating Bone Marrow (*continued*)**			
Disease Name	**Characteristic/Diagnostic Features**	**Differentials**	**Special Stains**	**Cell Type of Origin**
Monocytic leukemia (Mol, M5)	Features include transient/fluctuating monocytosis, nonregenerative anemia, normoblastemia. Bone marrow: phthisis of erythrocytic and megakaryocytic lines, hypercellularity. AMol: low to normal leukocyte counts. Monomorphic population of immature monocytoid cells resembling cleaved lymphoblasts. CMoL: High leukocyte counts with well-differentiated monocytes predominating. Middle-aged, large breed dogs, and FeLV positive cats at risk.	Acute lymphocytic leukemia: AMoL or AMMoL lack positivity for lymphoid markers. MMol: in MoL, fewer than 20% of cells should show positivity for SBB or myeloperoxidase. SH: AMoL cells are poorly differentiated. CMoL not associated with cutaneous lesions. MH: MoL lacks erythrophagia.	Positive NSE (with and without fluoride inhibition). Variable PAS, peroxidase, SBB.	Mol: Monocytic precursor. MMoL: Myeloid/monocytic precursor.
Hemophagic histiocytosis (HH)	Associated with concurrent infectious, neoplastic, or metabolic disease. Features include cytopenia of two or more cell lines, schizocytes, circulating activated macrophages. Infiltration of bone marrow—less often liver, spleen, lymph nodes—within mature, erythrophagic and hemosiderin-laden histiocytes.	MH: histiocytes of HH are well differentiated. SH: SH lacks prominent erythrophagia, and HH lacks cutaneous involvement. IMHA: HH not associated with agglutination or spherocytes as with IMHA. Granulomatous inflammation/marrow necrosis: Cytophagia is not characteristic of these disorders, as with HH.	Positive Prussian Blue (iron within macrophages).	Nonneoplastic macrophage.
Storage disorders includes: Gaucher Disease, Niemann–Pick Disease, Sea Blue Histiocytosis	Inherited disorders of defective cellular catabolism caused by lysosomal enzyme deficiencies. Typically manifest in juvenile to young adult animals. May see hepatosplenomegaly, anemia, leukopenia, thrombocytopenia, and, less consistently, cutaneous, skeletal, and neural accumulations of distended, well-differentiated histiocytes.	Granulomatous disease, SH, or secondary to various conditions, including chronic myelogenous leukemia, chronic lymphocytic leukemia, AIDS. Distinguish storage disorders by demonstrating enzyme deficiency.	Varies with disorder. Gaucher: PAS, SBB, AP. Niemann–Pick: Lipid stains. Sea Blue Histiocytosis: PAS, SBB, acid-fast stains.	Nonneoplastic monocyte, or macrophage.

a MNGC = multinucleated giant cell, BMD = Bernese Mountain dog, IMHA = immune mediated hemolytic anemia, NSE = nonspecific esterase, AP = acid phosphatase, PAS = periodic acid Schiff, αAT = α-1-antitrypsin, Mac-2 = a galactose-specific lectin that binds IgE[15], αCT = α-1-antichymotrypsin, SBB = Sudan black B.
Data from Ward JM, Sheldon W. Expression of mononuclear phagocyte antigens in histiocytic sarcoma of mice. Vet Pathol 1993;30:560–565 with permission.

MALIGNANT FIBROUS HISTIOCYTOMA

MFH is a soft tissue mesenchymal neoplasm of older dogs, cats, and horses characterized by an infiltrate of mixed fibroblastic and histiocytic cellular morphology. Diagnosis is controversial, as some pathologists believe MFH merely represents a diagnostic catch-all for poorly differentiated sarcomas.[17] A more appropriate name for these morphologically mixed neoplasms may be malignant spindle cell tumors until definitive phenotypic identification is determined.[4]

MFH typically manifests as single or multiple, firm, smooth to nodular, subcutaneous masses, most often occurring on the hindlimbs, dorsal thorax, and pelvic region. These masses are locally aggressive and frequently recur after surgical excision. Although metasta-

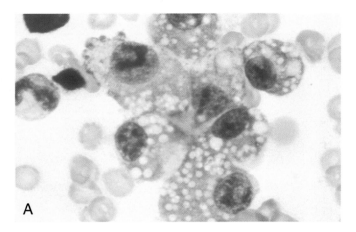

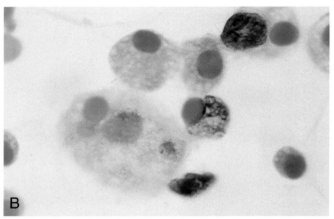

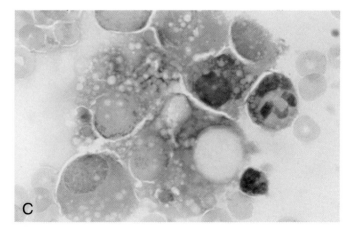

FIGURE 104.1 **A.** Canine bone marrow aspirate. Neoplastic cells from malignant histiocytosis. Large cells with moderate to abundant, basophilic staining, vacuolated cytoplasm. Nuclei vary from round to ovoid and exhibit immature features such as open chromatin, and multiple nucleoli. Wright–Giemsa, 400×. (Courtesy of F. Fernandez) **B.** Canine bone marrow aspirate. Malignant histiocytes stained with lysozyme, a cytochemical marker of histiocytic cells. A positive reaction is indicated by the patchy orange cytoplasmic staining. Lysozyme, 400×. (Courtesy of F. Fernandez) **C.** Canine bone marrow aspirate. Malignant histiocytes stained with NSE, a cytochemical marker of histiocytic cells. Diffuse red cytoplasmic staining indicates a positive reaction. NSE, 400×. (Courtesy of F. Fernandez)

sis is uncommon in cats[18] and horses,[19] several published reports cite high rates of metastasis, particularly of the giant cell variant of MFH, in dogs.[20, 21] Sites common for distant metastasis of MFH in dogs include spleen, liver, lung, lymph nodes, and, less commonly, the adrenals, nasal cavity and skeleton. Among purebred dogs, increased incidence of MFH has been reported in the golden retriever and Rottweiler.[22] No sex predilection has been identified for MFH in dogs or cats.

Clinical presentation is vague and nonspecific and may include lethargy, anorexia, and weight loss. Clinicopathologic features are also variable and of little diagnostic value. Anemia[20, 21] hypoalbuminemia,[21] and increased liver enzymes[21] have been reported. Cytologically, MFH is composed of a variable ratio of two main cell types with overlapping morphologic features: one mononuclear and one mesenchymal. Multinucleated giant cells are frequently present. Mononuclear cells resemble those described for MH, except that cytophagia is uncommon. A mixed inflammatory component[22] or collagenous matrix[17] may also be evident.

Histiogenesis of MFH is controversial. The most common hypothesis is that the cell of origin is a fibroblast or other mesenchymal precursor, with the capacity to exhibit histiocytic differentiation.[22] Differentials are summarized in Table 104.2. MFH is generally distinguished from MH by a lack of erythrophagia and the usually prominent fibrous component seen in MFH. Variable positivity for cytokeratin,[23] S-100 protein,[23] lysozyme,[24] αAT,[25] α-chymotrypsin (ACT),[24] desmin,[20, 23, 24] actin,[22] and vimentin[20] have been reported in MFH.

MONOCYTIC AND MYELOMONOCYTIC LEUKEMIA

Both monocytes and granulocytes are derived from a common stem cell, colony-forming unit-granulocyte macrophage (CFU-GM). Therefore, neoplastic transformation of this cell or of an earlier multipotential stem cell, results in myelomonocytic leukemia (MMoL), which may exhibit features of monocytic cells, granulocytic cells, or both. Neoplastic transformation of committed monocytic precursor cells (CFU-macrophage [CFU-M] or later) in the bone marrow of domestic animals is uncommon, but has been reported in the canine,[26–29] feline,[30] equine,[27] and bovine.[26] MoL most often affects middle-aged animals, and no specific breed or sex predilection has been identified, although large breed dogs may be at increased risk.[26] In the cat, MoL has been reported in association with concurrent feline leukemia virus (FeLV) infection.[27] Disease is characterized by an acute onset of clinical signs and rapid progression. Prognosis, despite chemotherapy and supportive measures, is poor.

Clinical signs are nonspecific and include dullness, anorexia, weight loss, and fever. Lymphadenopathy, tonsillar enlargement, and hepatosplenomegaly are common findings in the canine[26–28] but are infrequently reported in the feline.[27] Less commonly, respiratory, gastrointestinal, ocular, and genitourinary signs may be

DISTINGUISHING BONE MARROW HISTOCYTOSIS/MONOCYTOSIS*

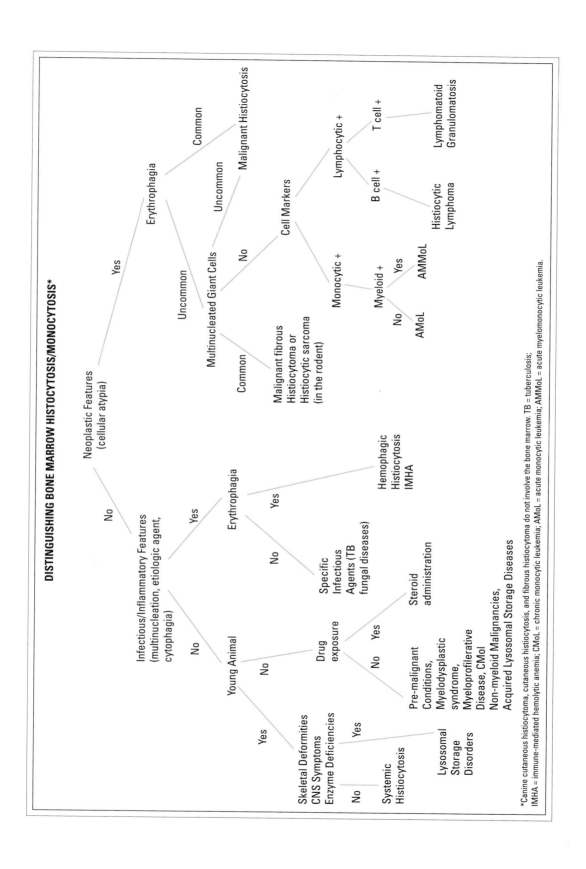

*Canine cutaneous histiocytoma, cutaneous histiocytosis, and fibrous histiocytoma do not involve the bone marrow. TB = tuberculosis; IMHA = immune-mediated hemolytic anemia; CMoL = chronic monocytic leukemia; AMoL = acute monocytic leukemia; AMMoL = acute myelomonocytic leukemia.

701

observed. Hematologic features typical of MoL include a mild nonregenerative anemia, normoblastemia, and a variable degree of leukocytosis. Anemia of MoL is typically milder than in other forms of leukemia. Platelet counts are generally normal to decreased, and disseminated vascular coagulation (DIC) may occur late in the course of disease. Clinical chemistry changes are less consistent but may include elevated liver serum enzyme levels, likely attributable to neoplastic infiltration of the liver or to hypoxic hepatocellular injury.

Histopathologic findings characteristic of MoL include diffuse infiltration of bone marrow, lymph nodes, spleen, liver, and, less consistently, other organs and tissues by a uniform population of neoplastic mononuclear cells. In chronic MoL (CMoL), the neoplastic monocytes are well differentiated and may be indistinguishable from normal monocytes. In contrast, the immature to blastic neoplastic cells typical of acute MoL (AMoL) are large, with large, round to cleaved to lobulated nuclei, irregularly clumped chromatin and a scant to moderate amount of palely basophilic cytoplasm that occasionally contains uniform small vacuoles (Fig. 104.2). N:C ratio is generally high, and fine azurophilic cytoplasmic granulation has been reported.[26] Monoblasts are characterized by a lack of nuclear indentation and the presence of nucleoli.[26] Mitotic index is high. Perivascular accumulations of neoplastic monocytes and hemorrhagic infarcts are common within infiltrated tissues.[26, 27]

Cytochemical staining (nonspecific esterase [NSE]), and cell surface markers (CD14 and major histocompatibility complex [MHC] class II) may be necessary to identify or confirm the monocytic lineage of neoplastic cells in AMoL or acute MMoL (AMMoL).[31] Ultrastructural features are unreliable in distinguishing leukemic monocytes from other neoplastic leukocytes, or from nonneoplastic circulating monocytes.[29] For this reason it is essential to consider morphologic appearance, cytochemical staining properties, cell surface markers, in addition to EM features to identify the lineage of neoplastic leukocytes.

HEMOPHAGIC HISTIOCYTOSIS

HH is a nonneoplastic proliferation of histiocytes with increased cytophagic activity occurring principally within the bone marrow and less reliably within the lymph nodes, spleen, and liver. It has been reported in both humans and small animals in association with concurrent infectious, neoplastic, or metabolic disease.[32, 33] The pathophysiology of HH may relate to an immunoregulatory T-cell disorder, resulting in the increased release of lymphokines and the subsequent histiocyte proliferation and cytophagia.[34] Clinical signs include fever, anemia, lymphadenopathy, and hepatosplenomegaly. In humans, coagulopathies, liver disease, and skin rash may accompany HH.[32] Other clinical signs vary and are often related to underlying disease.

Characteristic hematological features of HH include cytopenia of at least two cell lines and the observation of schizocytes as well as activated or erythrophagic macrophages in circulation.[32, 33] Bone marrow aspiration typically reveals a hypocellular marrow,[32] although this finding was inconsistent among the documented veterinary cases of HH.[33] A more reliable finding was the infiltration of variable numbers of well-differentiated cytophagic macrophages. Phagocytosis of hematopoietic elements from all cell lines and all stages of maturation is possible in HH. Normal to increased hemosiderin deposits may also be observed.

Bone marrow histologic examination is characterized by a variably cellular marrow with proliferation of benign-appearing, erythrocytophagic macrophages. In humans, histopathology is reported to be less sensitive at detecting the characteristic histiocytic hemophagia of HH than is bone marrow cytopathology.[32]

MH and SH are the veterinary diseases most resembling HH.[33] Criteria that are useful in identifying HH include the well-differentiated appearance of the histiocytes, the lack of cutaneous involvement, prominent erythrophagia, and multiple cytopenias consistently observed. Other differentials include granulomatous inflammation of the bone marrow and bone marrow necrosis. With either of these disorders, increased numbers of macrophages may be seen consuming cellular debris, but cytophagia is not reported.[35]

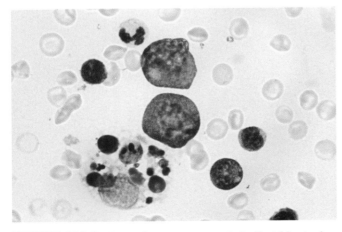

FIGURE 104.2 Canine bone marrow aspirate. Variably sized, neoplastic monoblasts in AMoL. Cytoplasm is scant to moderate in amount and stains basophilic. Nuclei are large, round to cleaved, and contain irregularly clumped chromatin. A segmented neutrophil (top left) and a leukophagic macrophage (bottom left) are also visible. Wright–Giemsa, 400×.

STORAGE DISORDERS OF MONOCYTIC OR HISTIOCYTIC CELLS: GAUCHER DISEASE, NIEMANN–PICK DISEASE, SEA BLUE HISTIOCYTOSIS, FABRY'S DISEASE, TAY–SACHS DISEASE

Storage disorders of monocytic or histiocytic cells are uncommon diseases of defective cellular catabolism.

First described in humans, many of these same disorders have subsequently been reported in various animal species.[36] The disease is usually attributable to inherited lysosomal enzyme deficiencies, resulting in the accumulation of enzyme substrates within histiocytic cell cytoplasm. Consequently, macrophages distended with nondigested material accumulate in various tissues; most often in bone marrow, spleen, liver, lung, skin, nervous, and skeletal tissues. Clinical symptoms of disease are generally referable to diminished organ function and pain associated with the proliferation of nonneoplastic macrophages displacing normal organ parenchyma and not directly to the enzyme deficiency or substrate accumulation. Symptoms classically associated with storage disorders include hepatosplenomegaly; anemia; leukopenia; thrombocytopenia; petechia; and less consistently, cutaneous, skeletal, and neural accumulations of distended histiocytes. Therefore, these storage disorders may resemble more commonly diagnosed inflammatory or neoplastic histiocytoses. (See Table 104.2.)

Cellular features of macrophages in storage disorders are characteristic for each of the specific diseases and aid in diagnosis. For example, in Gaucher disease, large proliferating macrophages are characterized by abundant, palely basophilic staining cytoplasm with a wrinkled paper appearance. These cells stain positively with periodic acid Schiff (PAS) and Sudan black B (SBB). By electron microscopy, secondary phagosomes fill the cytoplasm and appear as elongated bodies that react with acid phosphatase (AP).[37] In Niemann–Pick disease, histiocytes appear foamy cytologically and are distended with variably sized clear vacuoles that appear to be lipid-containing cytosomes by electron microscopy.[37] Sea Blue histiocytosis is aptly named for the proliferation of bone marrow, liver, and splenic histiocytes containing cytoplasmic granules that stain a characteristic blue-green with Wright's or Giemsa stain. These granules also stain positively with PAS, SBB, and acid-fast stains, as well as exhibit autofluorescence.[37]

Diseases that overwhelm catabolic enzyme capacity may be cytologically indistinguishable from these inherited storage diseases. For example, Gaucher's cells have been identified in patients that have chronic myelocytic leukemia, chronic lymphocytic leukemia, acquired immunodeficiency syndrome (AIDS) and in other diseases associated with increased leukocyte turnover in which the mononuclear phagocytic system is overwhelmed, causing catabolic substrates to accumulate within macrophages.[37] Confirmation of a storage disorder requires documentation of decreased enzymatic activity or demonstration of a genetic mutation responsible for a particular enzyme defect.

CANINE CUTANEOUS HISTIOCYTOMA

CCH is a common, cutaneous mass lesion of young dogs. It represents a focal proliferation of epidermotropic Langerhans cells.[38] CCH is characterized by the sudden appearance and rapid growth of generally solitary, 0.5- to 2.0-cm, round, raised, hairless, erythematous, dermal nodules. Lesions often occur on the face, ears, head, neck, forelimbs, and feet. Spontaneous regression of these masses has perpetuated debate as to whether they are truly neoplastic or are inflammatory.

Cytologically, these masses are composed of round to ovoid, uniform mononuclear cells. Nuclei are eccentrically located and vary in shape from round to cleaved to reniform. Binucleate cells are seen occasionally. Cytoplasm is smooth, stains palely basophilic, and varies from scant to moderate in amount (Fig. 104.3). Lymphocytic inflammation may be admixed with increasing intensity as the tumor regresses. Cellular features are sufficiently unique to suggest a diagnosis, particularly when considered together with gross appearance and clinical history.

The histologic appearance of CCH has been well documented elsewhere.[17] Differentials include other cutaneous inflammatory and neoplastic lesions such as mast cell tumor (MCT), cutaneous histiocytosis, plasmacytoma, and epidermotropic lymphoma. Unfortunately, no reliable special stains that definitively identify CCH exist. Lysozyme and αAT are both reported to be inconsistent in positively staining the histiocytic cells of CCH.[39]

CUTANEOUS HISTIOCYTOSIS

CH is a benign disorder characterized by cutaneous histiocytic masses and plaques grossly resembling those seen in CCH. However, in CH, these proliferations are multiple, may involve the mucus membranes, often have a waxing-waning course unresponsive to treatment, and only rarely spontaneously regress.[40] Like CCH, CH typically occurs in younger dogs. Its origin is speculative, but it is thought to be inflammatory, given that the occasional spontaneous regression of CH lesions is not anticipated with true neoplasms. In some in-

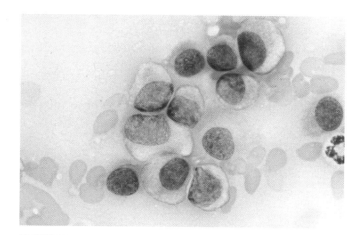

FIGURE 104.3 CCH. Uniform, round to ovoid, mononuclear cells with eccentric, round nuclei and scant to moderate, palely basophilic, smooth cytoplasm. A segmented neutrophil is also visible at the right margin of the photograph. Wright–Giemsa, 400×.

stances, steroid administration may induce remission of lesions.[41]

Cytologically, CH is distinguished from CCH by an infiltrate of larger, more vesicular histiocytic cells.[41] Convincing criteria of malignancy are not observed. A variable degree of admixed lymphocytic and neutrophilic inflammation is possible, as is rare erythrophagia.

Two histologic patterns are described for CH: a superficial dermal pattern resembling a more pleomorphic variant of CCH, and a second more invasive pattern characterized by periadnexal and perivascular histiocytic infiltrates within the deep dermis and panniculus.[41] These patterns are not distinct, and a continuous spectrum of histologic appearance is possible, even within the same animal.

Differentials are the same as those for CCH. Most difficult to distinguish from CH is epitheliotropic lymphoma, particularly in those cases exhibiting a diffuse infiltration focused on adnexal structures. The histiocytes of CH have been reported to stain positively with NSE and negatively for AP.[41] Recent findings of CD4 and Thy-1 expression by these cells suggest a Langerhans or dendritic origin.[4]

FIBROUS HISTIOCYTOMA

FH most often refers to a disorder of dogs and cats characterized by unilateral or bilateral ocular masses that are slowly progressive and benign in behavior. The masses are grossly pale, fleshy, and typically arise from the corneal-scleral junction. Less commonly, FH nodules may be associated with nictitans, eyelids, or periorbital tissues. Among affected dogs, young to middle-aged collies are overrepresented.[42] Cytologically, FH is not distinctive, resembling granulomatous inflammation, often with multinucleated giant cells seen.

The pathophysiology of FH is unknown, and cell type of origin is as yet uncertain because proliferation of cells with both histiocytic and fibrocytic features are observed.[42] Histologic features and results of implant and explant studies are more suggestive of reactive hyperplasia than of neoplasia or infection.[42] Despite this, lesions are often refractory to anti-inflammatory doses of topically or systemically administered steroids and tend to recur after excision.[43] Azathioprine has been used in the management of FH with success in four dogs.[43]

REFERENCES

1. **Cline MJ.** Histiocytes and histiocytosis. Blood 1994;84:2840–2853.
2. **Moore PF.** Systemic histiocytosis of Bernese Mountain dogs. Vet Pathol 1984;21:554–563.
3. **Padgett GA, Madewell BR, Kellert ET, Jodar L, Packard M.** Inheritance of histiocytosis in Bernese Mountain dogs. J Small Anim Pract 1995;36:93–98.
4. **Affolter VK, Moore PF.** Histiocytosis. In Proceedings of the 14th Annual Congress European Society of Veterinary Dermatologists-European Congress of Veterinary Dermatologists, Pisa, Italy, 1997.
5. **Paterson S, Boydell P, Pike R.** Systemic histiocytosis in the Bernese Mountain dog. J Small Anim Pract 1995;36:233–236.
6. **Scherlie PH, Smedes SL, Feltz T, Dougherty SA, Rus RC.** Ocular manifestations of systemic histiocytosis in a dog. J Am Vet Med Assoc 1992;201:1229–1232.
7. **Lester GD, Alleman AR, Raskin RE, Calderwood-Mays MB.** Malignant histiocytosis in an Arabian filly. Equine Vet J 1993;25:471–473.
8. **Moore PF, Rosin A.** Malignant histiocytosis of Bernese Mountain dogs. Vet Pathol 1986;23:1–10.
9. **Hayden DW, Waters DJ, Burke BA, Manivel JC.** Disseminated malignant histiocytosis in a Golden Retriever: clinicopathologic, ultrastructural, and immunohistochemical findings. Vet Pathol 1993;30:256–264.
10. **Ramsey IK, McKay JS, Rudorf H, Dobson JM.** Malignant histiocytosis in three Bernese Mountain dogs. Vet Rec 1996;138:440–444.
11. **Visonneau S, Cesano A, Tran T, Jeglum KA, Santoli D.** Successful treatment of canine malignant histiocytosis with the human major histocompatibility complex nonrestricted cytotoxic T-cell Line TALL-104[1]. Clin Can Res 1997;3:1789–1797.
12. **Freeman L, Stevens J, Loughman C, Tompkins M.** Malignant histiocytosis in a cat. J Vet Intern Med 1995;9:171–173.
13. **Walton RM, Brown DE, Burkhard MJ, Donnelly KB, Frank AA, Obert LA, Withrow SJ, Thrall MA.** Malignant histiocytosis in a domestic cat: cytomorphologic and immunohistochemical features. Vet Clin Pathol 1997;26:56–60.
14. **Newlands CE, Houston DM, Vasconelos DY.** Hyperferritinemia associated with malignant histiocytosis in a dog. J Am Vet Med Assoc 1994;205:849–851.
15. **Ward JM, Sheldon W.** Expression of mononuclear phagocyte antigens in histiocytic sarcoma of mice. Vet Pathol 1993;30:560–565.
16. **Hsu SM, Ho YS, Hsu PL.** Lymphomas of true histiocytic origin. Am J Pathol 1991;138:1389–1404.
17. **Pulley LT, Stannard AA.** Tumors of the skin and soft tissues. In: Moulton JE, ed. Tumors in domestic animals. 3rd ed. Berkley, CA: University of California Press, 1990;23–38.
18. **Gibson KL, Blass CE, Simpson M, Gaunt SD.** Malignant fibrous histiocytoma in a cat. J Am Vet Med Assoc 1989;194:1443–1445.
19. **Render JA, Harrington DD, Wells RE, Dunstan RW, Turek JJ, Boosinger TR.** Giant cell tumor of soft parts in six horses. J Am Vet Med Assoc 1983;183:790–793.
20. **Rogers KS, Hellman RG, Hurley KJ, Earley JW.** Splenic malignant fibrous histiocytoma in two dogs. J Am Vet Med Assoc 1994;30:253–256.
21. **Waters CB, Morrison WB, DeNicola DB, Widmer WR, White MR.** Giant cell variant of malignant fibrous histiocytoma in dogs: 10 cases (1986–1993). J Am Vet Med Assoc 1994;205:1420–1424.
22. **Kerlin RL, Hendrick MJ.** Malignant fibrous histiocytoma and malignant histiocytosis in the dog—convergent or divergent phenotypic differentiation? Vet Pathol 1996;33:713–716.
23. **Pace LW, Kreeger JM, Miller MA, Turk JR, Fischer JR.** Immunohistochemical staining of feline malignant fibrous histiocytomas. Vet Pathol 1994;31:168–172.
24. **Thoolen RJMM, Vos JH, VanDerLinde-Sipman JS, DeWeger RA, VanUnmk JAM, Misdorp W, VanDijk JE.** Malignant fibrous histiocytoma in dogs and cats: an immunohistochemical study. Res Vet Sci 1992;53:198–204.
25. **Pires MA.** Malignant fibrous histiocytoma in a puppy. Vet Rec 1997;140:234–235.
26. **Mackey LJ, Jarrett WFH, Lauder IM.** Monocytic leukemia in the dog. Vet Rec 1975;96:27–30.
27. **Jain NC.** The leukemia complex. Essentials of veterinary hematology. Philadelphia, PA: Lea & Febiger, 1993;838–908.
28. **Couto CG.** Clinicopathologic aspects of acute leukemias in the dog. J Am Vet Med Assoc 1985;186:681–685.
29. **Grindem CB, Stevens JB, Perman V.** Cytochemical reactions in cells from leukemic dogs. Vet Pathol 1986;23:103–109.
30. **Facklam NR, Kociba GJ.** Cytochemical characterization of feline leukemic cells. Vet Pathol 1986;23:155–161.
31. **Modiano JF, Smith R, Wojcieszyn J, Thomas JS, Rosenbaum BA, Ball C, Nicholds EA, Anthony MA, Barton CL.** The use of cytochemistry, immunophenotyping, flow cytometry, and in vitro differentiation to determine the ontogeny of a canine monoblastic leukemia. Vet Clin Pathol 1998;27:40–49.
32. **Reiner AP, Spivak JL.** Hematophagic histiocytosis: a report of 23 new patients and a review of the literature. Medicine 1988;67:369–388.
33. **Walton RM, Modiano JF, Thrall MA, Wheeler SL.** Bone marrow cytologic findings in four dogs and a cat with hematophagocytic syndrome. J Vet Intern Med 1996;10:7–14.
34. **Woda BA, Sullivan JL.** Reactive histiocytic disorders. Am J Clin Pathol 1993;99:459–463.
35. **Weiss DJ.** Histopathology of canine nonneoplastic bone marrow. Vet Clin Pathol 1992;21:71–84.
36. **Haskins M, Giger U.** Lysosomal storage diseases. In: Kaneko JJ, Harvey JW, Bruss ML, eds. Clinical biochemistry of domestic animals. 5th ed. San Diego, CA: Academic Press, 1997;741–760.
37. **Athens JW.** Disorders involving the monocyte-macrophage system—the "storage diseases." In: Lee GR, Bithell TC, Foerster J, Athens JW, Lukens JN, eds. Wintrobe's clinical hematology. 9th ed. Philadelphia, PA: Lea & Febiger, 1993.
38. **Moore PF, Schrenzel MD, Affolter VK, Olivry T, Naydan D.** Canine cutaneous histiocytoma is an epidermotropic langerhans cell histiocytosis that

expresses CD1 and specific B$_2$-integrin molecules. Am J Pathol 1996;148:1699–1708.

39. **Moore PF.** Utilization of cytoplasmic lysozyme immunoreactivity as a histiocytic marker in canine histiocytic disorders. Vet Pathol 1986;23:757–762.

40. **Carpenter JL, Thornton GW, Moore FM, King NW Jr.** Idiopathic periadnexal multinodular granulomatous dermatitis in twenty-two dogs. Vet Pathol 1987;24:5–10.

41. **Calderwood-Mays MB, Bergeron JA.** Cutaneous histiocytosis in dogs. J Am Vet Med Assoc 1986;188:377–381.

42. **Smith JS, Bistner S, Riis R.** Infiltrative corneal lesions resembling fibrous histiocytoma: clinical and pathologic findings in six dogs and one cat. J Am Vet Med Assoc 1976;169:722–726.

43. **Latimer CA, Wyman M, Szymanski C, Winston SM.** Azathioprine in the management of fibrous histiocytoma in two dogs. J Am Anim Hosp Assoc 1983;19:155–158.

CHAPTER 105

Clinical Diagnosis and Management of Acute Nonlymphoid Leukemias and Chronic Myeloproliferative Disorders

• ELIZABETH E. GOLDMAN and JOANNE C. GRAHAM

I n domestic animals and humans, acute and chronic myeloproliferative disorders (MPDs) are less frequently reported than lymphoproliferative disorders (LPDs).[1,2] Few reports of successful therapies for acute nonlymphoid leukemias can be found in the veterinary literature because many animals die shortly after or are euthanized at the time of diagnosis. However, several different chemotherapeutic protocols have been used successfully to treat patients that have chronic nonlymphoid leukemias. New adjunctive therapies are currently being explored. Goals of therapy include eradication of the leukemic cell population with a return to normal, regulated hemopoiesis and palliative supportive care for those patients that have poor response to chemotherapeutic protocols.

Nonlymphoid leukemias can be classified according to cell origin and include clonal proliferation of neutrophils, eosinophils, basophils, monocytes, megakaryocytes, erythrocytes, and mast cells (Table 105.1). Occasionally, nonlymphoid leukemias may be of mixed-cell lineage, including myelomonocytic leukemia, consisting of immature myelocytes and monocytes, and erythroleukemia, consisting of neoplastic erythrocytes and granulocytes. Cytochemical stains are often needed to determine cell lineage. Specific cytomorphologic criteria adapted from the French-American-British group and the National Cancer Institute definitions of acute myelogenous leukemias in people have already been described to classify acute nonlymphoid leukemias in dogs and cats.[3-9]

No age, breed, or sex predilection has been identified for animals that have nonlymphoid leukemia. Myeloproliferative disorders in dogs are of unknown origin, although environmental, viral,[10] and genetic causes have been postulated.[1,11] In contrast, MPDs have been associated with feline leukemia virus (FeLV) and feline immunodeficiency virus (FIV) infection in cats.[12-17]

Unfortunately, as previously alluded, the prognosis for animals that have acute nonlymphoid leukemia is poor. Therefore, at the time of diagnosis, frank discus-

sion with the owner regarding prognosis, cost, and time commitment is critical, because there are few cases of successful therapies reported.[18-20] This may be owing to the rapidly progressive nature of acute leukemia or the insidious onset of nonspecific signs associated with leukemia, making earlier diagnosis difficult. The prognosis for animals that have primary erythrocytosis and chronic granulocytic leukemia is guarded, but these diseases may be controlled for long periods with appropriate therapy. Accurate diagnosis is essential, because the type of leukemia determines the next course of action for the clinician and owners.

TREATMENT PRINCIPLES FOR THE PATIENT THAT HAS LEUKEMIA

Before discussing chemotherapeutic options with clients, it is prudent to explain additional key aspects of managing a patient that has leukemia. First, it is important to communicate that chemotherapy in veterinary medicine is generally palliative and rarely curative but that long-term remission and a good quality of life may be achieved with this treatment modality. Also, although therapy is directed to improve the health and well-being of the patient, there can be minor to potentially life-threatening complications associated with chemotherapy. Care must be taken when administering myelosuppressive chemotherapeutic agents to patients that have acute myeloid leukemias because cytopenias are usually already present at the time of diagnosis. Sepsis caused by profound neutropenia and bleeding caused by thrombocytopenia are common sequelae.

However, chemotherapy is still efficacious against leukemic cells. Cancer cell populations are heterogeneous in regard to the percentage of cells in any stage of the cell cycle.[21] This has therapeutic implications. Many chemotherapeutic agents have anticancer activities during a limited phase of the cell cycle. Combination drug protocols use chemotherapeutic agents proved to have efficacy against cancer when used alone. Therefore, combination protocols may be more advantageous for treating leukemia because each drug used can attack a different neoplastic cell population by different mechanisms over different stages of the cell cycle (Table 105.2). It is important, however, that the chemotherapeutic agents are given at consistent intervals; therefore, owner and patient compliance is critical for success.

Additionally, managing veterinary patients that have leukemia requires a commitment to provide supportive care and nutritional support (Table 105.3). Supportive care includes keeping the patient well hydrated, keeping electrolytes in balance, and providing nursing care for

the animal's comfort.[22–26] Intravenous or subcutaneous fluids may be necessary periodically to maintain adequate hydration. Hypoproteinemic patients may require plasma transfusions or synthetic colloid administration. Anemic patients may require blood transfusions when the anemia is causing clinical signs of illness. Patients that have leukemia may also be immunosuppressed from chemotherapy or secondary to the disease process itself. Prophylactic broad-spectrum antibiotics may be necessary and are recommended in severely neutropenic patients to help reduce the risk of infection.

Nutritional support is often overlooked but is essential in patients that have leukemia who are refusing to eat and drink or are losing weight, skeletal muscle mass, and fat stores. Nutritional needs can be determined by calculating the resting energy requirement (RER) and then multiplying that value by an illness factor from 1.25 to 2.0 (Table 105.3). Nutrition can be temporarily provided enterally by means of forced or tube feeding or parenterally through intravenous administration. Enteral nutrition is the preferred route because it is more physiologic and provides needed nutrients to the enterocytes of the gastrointestinal tract. Appetite stimulants such as cyproheptadine, diazepam, or oxazepam may be used short term in anorexic patients. Thus, informing your clients of potential complications and additional care is an essential part of the decision-making process before long-term time and financial commitments are made for treatment.

TABLE 105.1	Classification of Myeloproliferative Disorders by Cell Origin

Preleukemic syndrome
  Myelodysplastic syndrome
Granulocytes
  Acute myeloblastic/myelocytic leukemia
  Myelomonocytic leukemia
  Erythroleukemia
  Eosinophilic leukemia
  Basophilic leukemia
  Chronic myelogenous/granulocytic leukemia
Megakaryocytes
  Acute megakaryoblastic leukemia
  Essential thrombocythemia
Monocytes
  Monocytic leukemia
  Myelomonocytic leukemia
Erythrocytes
  Erythroleukemia
  Primary erythrocytosis
Miscellaneous
  Mast-cell leukemia/systemic mastocytosis

DIAGNOSTIC APPROACH

Diagnostic evaluation and staging of animals suspected of having leukemia should follow a systematic approach and should be performed before initiation of chemother-

---

TABLE 105.2	Chemotherapeutic Agents Used to Treat Nonlymphoid Leukemias	
Class	**Drug Name**	**Mode of Action**
Antitumor antibiotic	Doxorubicin	Inhibits DNA duplication and dependent RNA synthesis by forming stable complexes (intercalation) with DNA Free radical formation Topoisomerase II inhibitor allowing lethal DNA strand breaks
Alkylating agent	Cyclophosphamide Melphalan Busulfan Hydroxyurea	Cell-cycle nonspecific Cross-links DNA to prevent DNA template function Breaks DNA strands Forms linkages on same strand of DNA inhibiting DNA synthesis
Plant alkaloid	Vincristine	Arrests cell division by binding to the microtubules of the mitotic spindle Cytolytic effects on nonproliferating cells in early mitosis
Synthetic antimetabolite	Cytosine arabinoside	Cell-cycle specific: S phase or DNA synthesis Incorporates into DNA and disrupts DNA template function Inhibits DNA polymerase and interferes with enzyme biosynthesis of nucleic acids
Purine analog	6-thioguanine	Inhibits synthesis of DNA and RNA
Glucocorticoid	Prednisone	Interferes with cell growth receptors Causes DNA fragmentation

TABLE 105.3	Supportive Care for the Patient with Leukemia
Treatment	**Dosages**
Crystalloid fluids (maintenance rate)	24–30 ml/pound body weight/day IV divided as an hourly rate
Lactated Ringer's solution	24–30 mL/pound body weight/day SQ divided BID-QID
0.9% NaCl	
KCl supplementation	20 mEq KCl/liter of fluid
Whole blood transfusion	Milliliters of donor blood = 2.2 × (recipient weight in kg) × 40 (dog) or 30 (cat) × $\dfrac{\text{HCT desired} - \text{HCT of recipient}}{\text{HCT of donor blood}}$
Calories (Resting energy requirement)	RER (kcal) = 30 × (Body weight in kg) + 70 [for dogs and cats >2 kg]
Force feeding	RER = 70 (Body weight in kg)$^{0.75}$
Nasogastric tube	[for dogs and cats <2 kg]
Pharyngostomy tube	Mild illness: RER × 1.25
Gastrostomy tube	Moderate illness: RER × 1.5
	Severe illness: RER × 2.0
Total parenteral nutrition	
Antibiotics	
Amoxicillin/ Clavulanic acid	10–22 mg/kg PO BID
Cephalexin	10–22 mg/kg PO BID
Enrofloxacin	2.5–5.0 mg/kg PO once to twice/day

apy. The evaluation should start with a thorough history that may help differentiate between acute and chronic forms of leukemia. It is an important distinction because acute leukemias may carry a much poorer prognosis for long-term survival compared with the potentially less rapidly aggressive forms of chronic leukemia. Acute leukemias are usually characterized by clinical signs lasting from a few days to weeks versus the weeks to months of clinical signs often noted by owners of animals that have chronic nonlymphoid leukemias. However, both disorders can have an acute clinical presentation because of existing pancytopenias. Disease associated with both acute and chronic leukemias is manifested by nonspecific signs of illness, including lethargy, weakness, anorexia, weight loss, shifting leg lameness, vomiting, and diarrhea.[8,9,27,28]

A complete physical examination should be performed on all suspect patients. Physical abnormalities reported include peripheral lymphadenomegaly, abdominal organomegaly, particularly hepatosplenomegaly, fever, tachycardia, tachypnea or respiratory distress, poor body condition, mucous membrane pallor or petechiae, and neurologic abnormalities associated with central and peripheral polyneuropathies.[8,9,27–32]

A minimum database should include a complete blood count with blood smear evaluation, serum biochemistry profile, and urinalysis. A complete blood count with differential confirms the presence of cytopenias detected by an automated machine and may be used to look for abnormal cell morphology and peripheral

blastemia. A blood smear from an animal that has acute leukemia may be characterized by blast-cell proliferation without significant differentiation, whereas a smear from a patient that has chronic leukemia may reveal proliferation of more differentiated cells with partial, but incomplete maturation. In both cases, normal hematopoiesis is adversely affected. Blood smears should be carefully scrutinized for blood cell parasites, such as *Hemobartonella* and *Ehrlichia* sp. Serum chemistries and urinalyses may be used to evaluate the overall health status of the animal and alert the clinician to other organ involvement. Clinicopathologic abnormalities commonly reported in dogs and cats that have acute and chronic nonlymphoid leukemias include leukocytosis, leukopenia (in association with myelodysplastic syndrome), nonregenerative anemia, thrombocytopenia, thrombocytosis, macrocytosis, metarubricytosis, azotemia, hyperphosphatemia, and elevated serum alkaline phosphatase and serum alanine transaminase levels.[1,8,9,33]

Serologic testing of animals for infectious organisms, particularly cats, is recommended and should include serum enzyme-linked immunosorbent assay (ELISA) or indirect fluorescent antibody (IFA) testing for FeLV and FIV. Bone marrow samples may also be submitted for IFA testing for FeLV. The clinician should consider running rickettsial titers on pancytopenic dogs and cats in endemic regions.

Additional diagnostic tests may be indicated on an individual case basis. Staging, or determining the extent of disease, generally includes thoracic and abdominal radiographs and abdominal ultrasound. In those animals that have peripheral lymphadenomegaly or abdominal organomegaly, evaluation of enlarged organs and lymph nodes by fine-needle aspiration or biopsy with cytologic evaluation might prove helpful in confirming a diagnosis and differentiating myeloproliferative from lymphoproliferative disorders. Direct Coombs' testing to rule out immune-mediated destruction of red blood cells may be indicated. Heartworm and gastrointestinal parasite testing is recommended for animals suspected of having eosinophilic leukemia. Buffy coat smear evaluation concentrates atypical cells for further cytologic interpretation and is especially recommended when systemic mastocytosis is suspected.

The eventual diagnosis, however, does rely on the examination of peripheral blood cells in concert with a bone marrow aspirate or core biopsy. Special cytochemical stains and criteria to describe cell morphology are often needed to identify cell origin. Rarely is electron microscopy a necessary tool for determining the origin of leukemic cells, except in cases of highly undifferentiated leukemias. This diagnostic tool is not readily available, but it may be performed at certain institutions.

MYELODYSPLASTIC SYNDROME

Leukemia is defined as the unregulated, clonal proliferation of neoplastic hemopoietic cells that originate in the bone marrow. Most commonly leukemia is diagnosed by the presence of dysplastic or atypical immature hemopoietic cells circulating in the peripheral blood and also in the bone marrow. However, a preleukemic, aleukemic, or bone marrow myelodysplastic phase may precede recognizable leukemia. This condition, termed myelodysplastic syndrome (MDS), is characterized by peripheral cytopenias of two to three cell lines and abnormal red blood-cell morphology, such as macrocytosis and metarubricytosis. The bone marrow remains normocellular to hypercellular, with features of dyserythropoiesis, dysgranulopoiesis, and dysthrombopoiesis, and less than 30% of all nucleated cells as blasts.[1,3,33] Plasma cells and macrophages may be increased in the bone marrow of animals that have this condition.[34]

This syndrome is rarely reported in dogs and other species[34-37] and may be a retrospective diagnosis once a recognizable leukemic phase occurs. Acute leukemic transformation of a myelodysplastic state has been reported to occur 5 to 12 weeks after diagnosis of MDS in dogs.[34] However, MDS may not progress to overt leukemia in all cases. Therefore, the prognosis for animals that have MDS may be better than for those that have overt leukemia. Unfortunately, it is not possible to predict which patients will develop recognizable leukemia.

MDS and acute leukemia have been reported in cats in association with natural and experimental FeLV infection.[14,33] The progression from MDS to leukemia may occur rapidly, within 1 week to several months in cats.[36,38] In addition, many cats are ill at the time of diagnosis. Therefore, the prognosis in cats may not be as favorable as in dogs.

Currently, because of a lack of strong evidence to suggest that chemotherapy delays the development of leukemia, no standard treatment protocol exists for animals that have MDS. Treatment includes supportive care with intravenous or subcutaneous fluids, whole-blood transfusions, vitamin supplementation, caloric support, and antibiotics when indicated to treat secondary infections (Table 105.3).[21-26] In people, treatment is not usually initiated until acute leukemia is seen, although occasional positive response to androgens or corticosteroids has been reported.[39,40] The goal in investigational therapy in human medicine is to induce differentiation of hematopoietic cells during the myelodysplastic period by use of pharmaceuticals such as etretinate, cis-retinoic acid, granulocyte-colony-stimulating factors, interleukin-3, erythropoietin, and low-dose cytosine arabinoside.[33,41,42]

ACUTE MYELOPROLIFERATIVE DISORDERS

Acute Myeloid Leukemias

Acute myeloblastic leukemia (M1 and M2) and myelomonocytic leukemia (M4) are the most commonly reported acute myeloid leukemias in dogs.[1,28,33,43] Various myelodysplastic conditions and acute leukemias, including erythroleukemia, and myelomonocytic leuke-

mia have been reported in cats, particularly in association with FeLV and FIV infections.[29,33] However, the distinction between these different types of acute nonlymphoid leukemias may not be as important as differentiating them from acute lymphoid leukemia, because most of the acute nonlymphoid leukemias are treated with similar therapeutic regimens and often with limited success.

Reports of myelomonocytic leukemia in dogs,[43-49] cats,[50,51] horses,[52] and cattle,[53] seem the most abundant of the acute myeloid leukemias. This MPD is characterized by increased numbers of monoblasts and myeloblasts with neutrophilic differentiation together in the bone marrow and peripheral blood. Clinicopathologic changes include an increased peripheral white blood cell count, consisting of a neutrophilia and monocytosis with atypical blast forms, accompanied by anemia and normal to low platelet numbers.

Acute monocytic leukemia may be more common in dogs than cats.[54-56] This MPD is characterized by a significant peripheral blood monocytosis and mild to moderate anemia. Monocytic leukemia is further subdivided into two categories, including M5a characterized by a greater percentage of immature monoblasts and promonocytes compared with M5b in which leukemic cells are more differentiated.[3]

Acute erythroblastic leukemia or erythroleukemia is thought to arise from neoplastic proliferation of a common pluripotential progenitor cell with differentiation to both red and white blood cells. This acute myeloid leukemia is reported in cats and is characterized by disorderly stages of red and white cell maturation in the peripheral blood. Erythroid cells in the bone marrow constitute greater than 50% of all bone marrow cells, and myeloblasts are greater than or equal to 30% of the nonerythroid cells.[3] A subcategory of this acute myeloid leukemia is erythroleukemia with erythroid predominance, which historically has been recognized as erythremic myelosis. Erythremic myelosis is characterized by excessive production of erythroid elements and is characterized by a moderate to severe anemia with normoblastemia (rubriblasts to metarubricytes), macrocytosis, significant anisocytosis with few to no reticulocytes, and a bone marrow with increased numbers of normal-appearing erythroid precursors.[3,57,58] This condition may undergo blast transformation to granulocytic, poorly differentiated, or erythroleukemia.[59] Transformation of erythremic myelosis to erythroleukemia and then acute granulocytic leukemia has been reported in humans.[33]

Different chemotherapeutic drugs alone or in combination have been used to treat acute myeloid leukemia and include doxorubicin, cyclophosphamide, vincristine, cytosine arabinoside, 6-thioguanine, busulfan, melphalan, and prednisone (Table 105.2).[15,21] In addition, supportive care, including whole blood or platelet-rich plasma transfusions and broad-spectrum antibiotics when indicated must be given. Various induction and maintenance protocols have been suggested for use in dogs and cats (Table 105.4) with survival times of treated animals ranging from 4 to 78 days.[1,7,15,33,44-46,56] The most common side effects associated with these chemothera-

TABLE 105.4   Protocols Reported for the Treatment of Acute Nonlymphoid Leukemias

Chemotherapeutic Agent	Dose	Route of Administration
Protocol #1[*1,7,33,45]		
Induction		
Cytosine arabinoside	100 mg/m²	IV for 30–60 minutes q 12 hr × 3–6 d
6-thioguanine	40–50 mg/m²	PO × 4d
Doxorubicin‡	10–15 mg/m²	IV daily for 3 days, pretreat with diphenhydramine 2 mg/kg IM or SQ
		or
	30 mg/m²	IV q 21d, pretreat with diphenhydramine 2 mg/kg IM or SQ
Prednisone	40 mg/m²	PO divided BID × 7d
Maintenance		
Cytosine arabinoside	100 mg/m²	SQ or IV once to twice weekly
6-thioguanine	40 mg/m²	PO twice weekly
Doxorubicin‡	30 mg/m²	IV q 21 days, pretreat as above
Prednisone	20 mg/m²	PO QOD
Protocol #2[*1,45,46]		
Induction		
Cytosine arabinoside	100–200 mg/m²	Slowly IV for 12–24 hours/day × 3d and repeated weekly
Doxorubicin‡	30 mg/m²	IV q 2–3 weeks alternating with cytosine arabinoside
Maintenance (COAP)		
Cyclophosphamide	50 mg/m²	PO daily QOD × 4 days/week or for 4 consecutive days/week
Vincristine	0.5 mg/m²	IV once weekly for 8 weeks
Prednisone	20 mg/m²	PO divided BID × 7d, then 10 mg/m² PO daily
Cytosine arabinoside	100 mg/m²	IV daily × 4d of the first week only
Protocol #3[*44]		
Doxorubicin‡	30 mg/m²	IV q 21d, pretreat as above
Cyclophosphamide	50 mg/m²	PO QOD
Prednisone	40 mg/m²	PO divided BID × 7d, then 20 mg/m² PO QOD
Protocol #4[†56,70]		
Cytosine arabinoside	100 mg/m²	SQ q 8 hr for 3–4 injections repeated q 5–9 d

Data from references 1, 7, 33, 44–46, 56 and 70 with permission.
* Protocols #1–3 reported in dogs.
† Protocol #4 reported in cats.
‡ For animals ≤20 pounds, doxorubicin dose recommended is 1 mg/kg.

peutic agents include myelosuppression, particularly leukopenia and thrombocytopenia, and gastrointestinal toxicity, including anorexia, vomiting, and diarrhea.

Acute Megakaryoblastic Leukemia

The differentiation between megakaryoblastic or megakaryocytic leukemia and primary or essential thrombocythemia may be confusing because earlier literature presents overlapping criteria for the diagnosis of both conditions. Megakaryoblastic leukemia is a variant of acute myelogenous leukemia (M7) characterized by the clonal proliferation of megakaryocytes in the bone marrow with evidence of morphologic abnormalities, including dwarf or micromegakaryocytes and megakaryoblasts with few to no nuclear lobations and decreased ploidy. More than 30% of all nucleated cells within the bone marrow are megakaryoblasts in the leukemic condition. Bone marrow fibrosis may be seen.[3,60–69] The peripheral blood picture is variable, showing evidence of pancytopenia or leukocytosis with a normal, decreased or, more commonly, increased platelet population. Platelets may be morphologically abnor-

mal, with giant forms and variable granulation. In the classic definition of megakaryocytic leukemia, megakaryoblasts are seen in the peripheral blood. Neoplastic cells may also infiltrate other tissues, including liver, spleen, lymph nodes, lungs, kidneys, and meningeal vessels.[3,60,61]

The chemotherapeutic agent cytosine arabinoside has been used to treat cats with megakaryoblastic leukemia. Peripheral blastemia was eliminated within 4 days in one cat treated with cytosine arabinoside at a dosage of 100 mg/m² divided 4 times subcutaneously daily for 6 days. Unfortunately, bone marrow hypoplasia developed within 6 days, such that the drug was temporarily discontinued. A maintenance protocol was attempted with cytosine arabinoside (100 mg/m² divided 3 times daily subcutaneously on day 1 and day 4 of each week) and cyclophosphamide (100 mg/m² orally on day 6 weekly for 3 weeks) until the cat became severely neutropenic, and the drugs were withdrawn. Six weeks later the cat developed thrombocytosis, and maintenance therapy was restarted. The cat's condition continued to deteriorate, and it was euthanized on day 122.[70] Therapies employed in the treatment of human megakaryoblastic leukemia include granulocyte-colony-stimulating factor, cytosine arabinoside, etoposide, and bone marrow allografts.[67]

CHRONIC MYELOPROLIFERATIVE DISORDERS

Chronic Myeloid Leukemias

Definitive diagnostic criteria for chronic myeloid leukemias in animals is currently lacking. In humans, this condition is associated with a chromosomal abnormality, the Philadelphia chromosome (Ph), which has not yet been identified in domestic animal species.[1,33,71–74] This group of hematologic disorders encompasses chronic myelogenous or granulocytic (CML or CGL), chronic monocytic (CMoL), and chronic myelomonocytic (CMMoL) leukemias. These leukemias are differentiated from the MDS by a lack of moderate bone marrow dysplasia and the presence of a profound predominantly mature leukocytosis rather than the peripheral cytopenias seen with MDS.[3]

Chronic myelogenous or granulocytic leukemia is characterized by a profound leukocytosis consisting of a significant well-differentiated neutrophilia with a disorderly left shift. White blood cell counts ranging from 41,000 to 169,000 cells/μL have been reported in dogs.[73,74] Remaining clinicopathologic data is variable, with mild to moderate anemia, thrombocytopenia, and thrombocytosis noted. Other organs may be infiltrated by the neoplastic cells. Bone marrow samples demonstrate a significant myeloid cells relative to erythroid cells (M:E) ratio,[73,74] ranging from 3.5 to 23.7:1, with myeloid hyperplasia and relative maturity of cells. A relative or absolute erythroid hypoplasia may be evident. Cats are often positive for FeLV.[1,33]

Because leukocytosis is the only consistent finding in cases of CML, the clinician must rule out other causes for a profound neutrophilia. These disorders include bacterial, fungal, and parasitic infections, a chronic inflammatory process, such as immune-mediated disease, and acute myeloid leukemia. A complete diagnostic workup should be performed as previously discussed, but additional diagnostic tests, including urine and blood cultures, protein electrophoresis, and an antinuclear antibody titer may be useful in excluding infectious, inflammatory, and immune-mediated causes.

Treatment of this condition is controversial in both veterinary and human medicine, because animals and people can live for months to years without treatment before a terminal blast crisis occurs.[1,71,72] Variable survival times have been reported in untreated dogs and have ranged from 80 days to 4.5 years.[73,74] It is uncertain whether chemotherapy is efficacious in reducing the risk of a blast crisis, so supportive care may be the only treatment necessary.

Treatment in people has been directed at reducing and eradicating Ph-positive clones in the chronic phase of disease. Therapies employed include splenic irradiation and splenectomy, radioactive phosphorus, bone marrow transplantation, and chemotherapeutic agents such as busulfan, hydroxyurea, mercaptopurine, thioguanine, cytosine arabinoside, and prednisone. Unfortunately, once a myeloid blast crisis occurs, chemotherapeutic protocols may be ineffective, and death usually occurs in 2 to 3 months.[72]

Hydroxyurea and busulfan have been used to treat dogs that have CML. One dog was splenectomized.[74] Dosages of busulfan include 2 to 8 mg per dog per day orally.[27] Various protocols include hydroxyurea at doses of 20 to 25 mg/kg orally twice daily until the white blood cell count decreases to 15,000 to 20,000 cells/μL. The dose is then decreased by 50% on a daily basis or to 50 mg/kg orally biweekly or triweekly.[73] Another protocol includes hydroxyurea at 50 mg/kg orally once daily for 14 days until the white blood cell count is within normal reference range, and then reduces the frequency of administration to every other day and then to every 3 days.[73] Survival times in treated dogs range from 41 days to longer than 690 days. Despite therapy with hydroxyurea, some dogs still succumb to a terminal blast crisis.[73]

Eosinophilic Leukemia and Idiopathic Hypereosinophilic Syndrome

Eosinophilic leukemia is considered a chronic MPD and a variant of granulocytic leukemia. This condition develops when disorderly proliferation of eosinophils occurs with an increase in immature forms in the peripheral blood and bone marrow. Eosinophilic leukemia is difficult to differentiate from the idiopathic hypereosinophilic syndrome recognized in cats, and it is questionable whether this type of leukemia occurs in dogs.[75,76] Eosinophilic leukemia occurs naturally and can be induced experimentally by FeLV infection in cats,[13,77] and has been recognized as an eosinophilic MPD in a young standardbred horse[78] and in a Syrian hamster.[79] A diagnosis is often made by the exclusion of other causes for hypereosinophilia.

This MPD is recognized predominantly in feline patients and is characterized by a mature eosinophilia (range of 3200 to 130,000 cells/μL) with a disproportionate number of immature forms of eosinophils.[1,33] The bone marrow contains an increased M:E ratio with increased numbers of eosinophil precursors. Lymph nodes, spleen, and liver are often infiltrated by increased numbers of eosinophils.

Cats affected with eosinophilic leukemia are usually adults (range of 10 months to 10 years), with the median age at diagnosis being 8 years. Females seem overrepresented. Clinical signs and physical examination findings include vomiting, diarrhea, hepatosplenomegaly, and peripheral lymphadenomegaly. Clinicopathologic abnormalities include eosinophilia, often with absolute counts of >1.5 × 10^3 cells/μL, hypogranular immature eosinophils, anemia, and thrombocytopenia.[80,81] Authors of one report of a leukemic cat that had a moderate increase in alkaline phosphatase (ALP) without evidence of hepatic disease suggested that the increased

ALP was released from eosinophils rich in this enzyme; however, this is an inconsistent finding.[13]

Conditions that commonly cause eosinophilia need to be excluded before a diagnosis of eosinophilic leukemia can be made. These conditions include allergic bronchitis; internal and external parasitism, including heartworm disease; hypersensitivity reactions, including inhalant, flea, and food allergies; eosinophilic enteritis; eosinophilic granuloma complex; and the paraneoplastic syndrome associated with tumors, especially mast cell tumors.[82–84] A complete blood count, serum biochemical analysis, urinalysis, FeLV, FIV, and heartworm test, fecal flotation, and skin scraping should be performed. Consideration of thoracic and abdominal radiography and abdominal ultrasound should be given in cases for which mast cell neoplasia, allergic bronchitis, eosinophilic granulomas, and atypical parasitism are suspected. Endoscopic evaluation with biopsy of the gastrointestinal tract may also be required for ruling out underlying gastrointestinal causes of hypereosinophilia.

True distinction between eosinophilic leukemia and idiopathic hypereosinophilic syndrome is unclear. In general, eosinophilic leukemia is believed to be associated with a more rapid progression of disease characterized by a greater number of immature eosinophil precursors, a higher M:E ratio and dysgranulopoiesis of the eosinophil line in the bone marrow, and a more notable anemia compared with the more chronic course and lack of identifiable cause for the more mature eosinophilic hyperplasia appreciated with hypereosinophilic syndrome.[1,33,81] Further differentiation between these two syndromes in people has been made using chromosome markers, such as the Ph-chromosome present in pluripotential stem cells of patients that have chronic myelogenous leukemia. Other diagnostic aids include gamma E immunoglobulin (IgE) levels, used to predict response to treatment in people, cultures of bone marrow nucleated cells, and leukocyte ALP levels.[81]

Generally, cats that have eosinophilic leukemia respond poorly to treatment and experience rapid progression of their disease state. Corticosteroids as a single agent have been used to treat this condition with variable success with most cats dying within 6 months of diagnosis.[81–85] Prednisone at a dose of 2 mg/kg orally twice daily resulted in an 8-month remission for one cat. When the cat relapsed, hydroxyurea (15 mg/kg/day orally) was added to the treatment regimen with no effect.[84] Hydroxyurea at a dose of 40 mg/kg/day orally, then every other day, then every third day as needed to prevent the development of neutropenia, in combination with prednisone, was successful in two cats reported to be alive at 40 and 30 months past diagnosis.[85] Dexamethasone and a whole-blood transfusion used to treat a 10-month-old standardbred foal resulted in a positive clinical response, but the foal was euthanized before complete evaluation of treatment response.[78]

Basophilic Leukemia

Basophilic leukemia is a rare variant of chronic granulocytic leukemia. This MPD must be differentiated from mast cell leukemia cytologically. Mature basophils can be recognized by the presence of segmented nuclei with variable numbers of dark purple cytoplasmic granules, whereas mast cells contain round to oval nuclei with abundant small, round metachromatic-staining cytoplasmic granules. Basophilic leukemia is characterized by a leukocytosis of mature basophils with a synchronous left shift consisting predominantly of basophilic metamyelocytes, a variable degree of anemia, and possible thrombocytosis.[1,33,61] Basophilic leukemia must also be differentiated from a basophilia secondary to a hypersensitivity reaction, inflammation, or the paraneoplastic syndrome associated with systemic mastocytosis. A left shift is atypical for most hypersensitivity reactions.[85] Hepatic and splenic enlargement and lymphadenomegaly have been noted in the few reports of dogs that have basophilic leukemia.[18,19,86] A single case of acute myeloid leukemia with basophilic differentiation was reported in a 4-year-old FeLV- and FIV-positive domestic short-hair cat.[87]

Protocols used to treat basophilic leukemia in dogs have been reported. Chemotherapeutic agents used to treat this form of granulocytic leukemia include busulfan and hydroxyurea. Busulfan (0.1 mg/kg/day orally) was initially used as a single agent to treat a dog that had basophilic leukemia. However, no significant change of the complete blood count and bone marrow samples was seen after 2 weeks. Next, hydroxyurea (50 mg/kg twice daily orally) was added with significant reduction in white blood cell and basophil counts and in lymph node and splenic sizes within 4 weeks.[19] An additional report of hydroxyurea use indicated that remission may be achieved within 1 week of administration.[18] These reports of dogs that have basophilic leukemia treated with hydroxyurea have indicated remission times of 8 and 21 months, even after hydroxyurea was withdrawn owing to severe drug-induced leukopenia. The most commonly reported side effect of hydroxyurea is myelosuppression, resulting in leukopenia that may require withdrawal of the drug. Other side effects have included pruritus, erythema, alopecia, and hyperglycemia.[18]

Essential Thrombocythemia

In contrast to megakaryoblastic leukemia, essential thrombocythemia is a chronic MPD characterized by an abnormal proliferation of megakaryocytes that are morphologically normal in the bone marrow. This condition is characterized by a profound thrombocytosis (usually greater than 600,000 platelets/μL) and increased numbers of giant platelets with abnormal granulation. No circulating blast forms are seen in the peripheral blood.[3,20,61,88–91] Often, a spurious serum hyperkalemia, caused by release of potassium from platelets during clot formation, may be present in the chemistry panel. This pseudohyperkalemia can be avoided by measuring plasma potassium concentrations instead. Diseases or conditions that cause a reactive thrombocytosis should be ruled out. Such conditions include iron-deficiency anemia, chronic inflammation, hemolytic anemia, rebound thrombocytosis secondary to correction of immune-mediated thrombocytopenia, excitement-induced splenic contraction, drug-induced thrombocytosis, and rebound thrombocytosis postsplenectomy.[33,85]

The Polycythemia Vera Study Group has proposed the following criteria for diagnosing essential thrombocythemia in people: (1) platelet count >600,000 cells/μL, (2) a normal initial hematocrit or packed cell volume (PCV) that does not increase with iron supplementation, (3) a normal serum iron concentration, (4) no evidence of collagen fibrosis in the bone marrow, and (5) no identifiable cause for reactive thrombocytosis.[88]

In an earlier report, one 15-mg dose of nandrolone decanoate given by intramuscular injection to a cat diagnosed with essential thrombocythemia resulted in remission, and the cat was still alive 4 years after diagnosis.[20] More recently, a cat that had essential thrombocythemia was treated with 0.5 mg of melphalan orally for 4 days and then 0.5 mg of melphalan orally every other day, but it lived only 39 days.[88] Hydroxyurea and radiophosphorus were found to be unsuccessful in treating two dogs that had presumptive essential thrombocythemia.[85,89] A dog that had suspected essential thrombocythemia was treated successfully with the cyclophosphamide, vincristine, cytosine arabinoside, and prednisone (COAP) protocol until the dog was euthanized 8 months after diagnosis when hemorrhagic cystitis developed.[90]

Treatment of essential thrombocythemia in people is controversial, because some patients are asymptomatic. Chemotherapeutic agents used to treat people who have essential thrombocythemia include hydroxyurea, radioactive phosphorus, and melphalan.[88]

Primary Erythrocytosis

Primary erythrocytosis or polycythemia vera is a chronic MPD characterized by a neoplastic clonal proliferation of well-differentiated red blood cells irrespective of erythropoietin levels, with a resultant rise in the PCV, hematocrit, hemoglobin concentration, and red blood cell count. The clinician must differentiate between relative polycythemia, caused by dehydration or splenic contraction, and absolute polycythemia, caused by increased levels of erythropoietin or by primary erythrocytosis. Systemic hypoxemia secondary to cardiopulmonary diseases, high altitudes, and hemoglobinopathies is a condition that may lead to elevated erythropoietin levels and resultant secondary absolute polycythemia. Likewise, renal neoplasia sometimes results in an overproduction of erythropoietin, leading to polycythemia.[1,33,61]

Primary erythrocytosis is a rare neoplastic disorder. Most cases have been reported in middle-aged dogs,[92,93] with fewer cases identified in middle-aged cats (median age of 6 years).[94-96] Male cats seem overrepresented.[94-96] Clinical signs in both species are related to the hyperviscosity syndrome, resulting in impaired blood flow and tissue hypoxia (owing to the increased numbers of red blood cells in the vascular beds). Abnormal signs and

physical examination findings include brick red or dark red mucous membranes; neurologic manifestations, such as blindness, mental depression, ataxia, or seizures; increased bleeding tendencies; polyuria; polydipsia; vomiting; anorexia; dilated retinal vessels; and mild splenomegaly.[92-96] Nonspecific signs may be present for weeks to months prior to diagnosis. Packed cell volumes in dogs and cats that have primary erythrocytosis range from 65 to 85% and bone marrow samples may show evidence of erythroid hyperplasia. White blood cell and platelet counts may also be increased.[92-96]

Diagnostic evaluation should include a complete blood count, serum biochemistry profile, and urinalysis. Further diagnostic tests to rule out causes of secondary polycythemia include thoracic and abdominal radiographs, electrocardiogram, echocardiogram, abdominal ultrasound, and arterial blood gas analysis. Bone marrow should be sampled and a serum erythropoietin level obtained. Patients that have primary erythrocytosis usually have a normal to low serum erythropoietin level in conjunction with an elevated red blood cell count. Primary erythrocytosis is diagnosed when causes for relative and secondary absolute polycythemia have been disproved and the PCV remains elevated in the face of a low-normal erythropoietin level.[92-96]

Treatment initially includes supportive care, often including 2 to 3 times maintenance rates (60 to 90 ml/pound body weight/day) of a crystalloid fluid given intravenously to correct dehydration within the first 12 to 24 hours (Table 105.3). Of course, the clinician must use judgment to determine an appropriate fluid load for each individual patient, because some patients may be cardiovascularly compromised.

Further treatment may require therapeutic phlebotomy. The goal of this procedure is to reduce the PCV by 15% or by one sixth of the starting value, such that the PCV remains between 50 and 60% or close to a normal reference range, with elimination of abnormal clinical signs. This may be accomplished by removal of 20 ml of whole blood per kilogram of body weight from the patient and replacing the blood volume removed with an equivalent volume of crystalloid solution. A PCV should be checked every 2 to 4 weeks as needed, and plebotomy may be performed at such time intervals as necessary. If phlebotomy is required more often than every 2 months, chemotherapy should be considered.

Hydroxyurea is the preferred treatment for animals that have this hematologic disorder. In the dog, a loading dose of 30 mg/kg/day orally for 7 to 10 days, followed by a maintenance dose of 15 mg/kg/day orally is recommended. Dogs may reach remission in 2 to 6 weeks on this protocol and may be maintained in remission for months to years.[33,93] If the dog comes out of remission, it is recommended that the animal be reloaded with hydroxyurea at the higher dose. Once the dog has reached remission, the owners should be informed to watch for return of clinical signs and monitor PCVs every 1 to 3 months. Complete blood counts should also be monitored periodically for myelosuppression.

Because cats appear to have a greater sensitivity to hydroxyurea at higher doses, it is recommended to increase the dose of the drug slowly. The recommended starting dose for an average 10-lb cat is 125 mg per cat orally every other day for 2 weeks increased to 250 mg per cat orally twice weekly for 2 weeks and then to 500 mg per cat orally weekly or as often as needed to keep the PCV within target range.[94] When a toxic level is reached, methemoglobinemia and Heinz-body hemolytic anemia have been reported to occur in cats.[33,94] Because of this potential risk, it may be prudent to hospitalize the cat for 24 hours at the time of incremental dose increases to observe for adverse side effects.[33] In a recent report, three cats that had primary erythrocytosis were successfully treated with hydroxyurea and are alive 7, 5, and 4 years after initial diagnosis.[85]

Radiophosphorus (^{32}P) has been shown to have some long-term effect in the treatment of primary erythrocytosis. ^{32}P accumulates in bone and causes bone marrow irradiation. Doses of 1.5 (total dose) to 3.25 mCi/m^2 have been tried in dogs in combination with phlebotomy or busulfan at 2 mg orally daily.[33,92,97]

ADJUNCTIVE TREATMENTS FOR NONLYMPHOID LEUKEMIAS

Additional treatment methodologies are continually being explored in veterinary and human medicine for the treatment of nonlymphoid leukemias. These include the use of terminal growth differentiators, immunomodulators and growth factors, and allogeneic bone marrow transplantation.

Retinoic acids (RAs) have been used to induce differentiation of cancer cells in patients that have acute promyelocytic leukemia (APL). Cancer can block normal growth of a cell, arresting it at an immature, poorly regulated phase. Theoretically, if this growth blockade can be overcome, then cell maturation and cell death could proceed. Vitamin A derivatives (retinoic acids) are believed to induce terminal maturation of cancer cells and have been shown to induce granulocytic differentiation in vitro.[98] An isomer of all-*trans* RA, 13-*cis* RA or isotretinoin, has been used to treat a few patients that have APL with limited success. Dosages used in people range from 45 to 100 mg/m^2 orally divided twice daily. Side effects include headache, skin dryness, hepatotoxicity, and acute respiratory distress.[98]

Immunomodulators have been used in veterinary medicine for many years as adjunctive therapies for immunocompromised cats infected by FeLV and FIV. Although they have little to no efficacy against most tumors, they may offer some immunostimulatory and antiviral effects, improving quality of life. Acemannan is a complex mannose polymer, an active principle of aloe vera extracts, which is taken up by macrophages and enhances the release of interferon, interleukin-1, tumor necrosis factor (TNF), and prostaglandin E$_2$.[99] *Propionibacterium acnes* preparation is a killed bacterial culture that stimulates interleukin-1 and promotes natural-

killer-cell activity through release of TNF and interferon. Interleukin-1 has antitumor activity and may stimulate hemopoietic activity.[99] Granulocyte-colony-stimulating factor and erythropoietin might be used to stimulate hemopoiesis. Use of these products may improve clinical and hematologic abnormalities in clinically ill patients.

Allogenic bone marrow transplantation has had reported success in cats.[100] Bone marrow transplantation in a cat that had erythroleukemia resulted in a 72-day survival time posttransplantation.[101] Successful bone marrow engraftment in a 2-year-old domestic short-hair cat that had acute myeloid leukemia resulted in a remission time of 4 years after bone marrow transplantation.[100] This procedure has the potential to offer a cure for certain neoplastic conditions.

Until more cases of acute nonlymphoid leukemia and chronic MPDs are correctly identified and treated and successful therapies are reported in the veterinary literature, the prognosis for most of these conditions will continue to remain guarded to poor. Therapy for nonlymphoid leukemia in people continues to be extensively explored, and perhaps in the future our veterinary patients may benefit from these medical advances.

REFERENCES

1. **Young KM, MacEwen EG.** Canine myeloproliferative disorders. In: Withrow SJ, MacEwen EG, eds. Small animal clinical oncology. 2nd ed. Philadelphia: WB Saunders, 1996;495–509.
2. **Jain NC.** The leukemias: general aspects. In: Jain NC, ed. Essentials of veterinary hematology. Philadelphia: Lea and Febiger, 1993;307–318.
3. **Jain NC, Blue JT, Grindem CB, et al.** A report of the animal leukemic study group. Proposed criteria for classification of acute myeloid leukemias in dogs and cats. Vet Clin Pathol 1991;20(3):63–82.
4. **Facklam NR, Kociba GJ.** Cytochemical characterization of feline leukemic cells. Vet Pathol 1986;23:155–161.
5. **Facklam NR, Kociba GJ.** Cytochemical characterization of leukemic cells in 20 dogs. Vet Pathol 1985;22:363–369.
6. **Grindem CB, Stevens JB, Perman J.** Cytochemical reactions in cells from leukemic dogs. Vet Pathol 1986;23:103–109.
7. **Jain NC, Madewell BR, Weller RE, et al.** Clinical-pathological findings and cytochemical characterization of myelomonocytic leukaemia in 5 dogs. J Comp Pathol 1981;91:17–31.
8. **Grindem CB, Stevens JB, Perman V.** Morphological classification and clinical and pathological characteristics of spontaneous leukemia in 17 dogs. J Am Anim Hosp Assoc 1985;21:219–226.
9. **Grindem CB, Perman V, Stevens JB.** Morphological classification and clinical and pathological characteristics of spontaneous leukemia in 10 cats. J Am Anim Hosp Assoc 1985;21:227–236.
10. **Sykes GP, King JM, Cooper BC.** Retrovirus-like particles associated with myeloproliferative disease in the dog. J Comp Pathol 1985;95:559–564.
11. **Felsburg PJ, Somberg RL, Krakowka GS.** Acute monocytic leukemia in a dog with x-linked severe combined immunodeficiency. Clin Diagn Lab Immunol 1994;1(4):379–384.
12. **Toth SR, Onions DE, Jarrett O.** Histopathological and hematological findings in myeloid leukemia induced by a new feline leukemia virus isolate. Vet Pathol 1986;23:462–470.
13. **Swenson CL, Carothers MA, Wellman ML, et al.** Eosinophilic leukemia in a cat with naturally acquired feline leukemia virus infection. J Am Anim Hosp Assoc 1993;29:497–501.
14. **Evans RJ, Gorman NT.** Myeloproliferative disease in the dog and cat: definition, aetiology, and classification. Vet Rec 1987;121:437–443.
15. **Yates RW, Weller RE, Feldman BF.** Myeloproliferative disease in a cat. Mod Vet Pract 1984;65:753–757.
16. **Reinacher M.** Diseases associated with spontaneous feline leukemia virus (FeLV) infection in cats. Vet Immunol Immunopathol 1989;21:85–95.
17. **Hutson CA, Rideout BA, Pederson NC.** Neoplasia associated with feline immunodeficiency virus infection in cats of Southern California. J Am Vet Med Assoc 1991;199(10):1357–1362.
18. **Mears EA, Raskin RE, Legendre AM.** Basophilic leukemia in a dog. J Vet Intern Med 1997;11(2):92–94.

19. **MacEwen EG, Drazner FH, McClelland AJ, et al.** Treatment of basophilic leukemia in a dog. J Am Vet Med Assoc 1975;166(4):376–380.
20. **Evans RJ, Jones DRE, Gruffydd-Jones TJ.** Essential thrombocythaemia in the dog and cat. J Small Anim Pract 1982;23:457–467.
21. **Morrison WB.** Chemotherapy. In: Morrison WB, ed. Cancer in dogs and cats: medical and surgical management. Baltimore: Williams & Wilkins, 1998;351–358.
22. **Salisbury SK, LaFond E, Morrison WB.** Blood transfusion and management of pain, infection, and nutritional needs in the postoperative cancer patient. In: Morrison WB, ed. Cancer in dogs and cats: medical and surgical management. Baltimore: Williams & Wilkins, 1998;323–350.
23. **DiBartola SP.** Introduction to fluid therapy. In: DiBartola SP, ed. Fluid therapy in small animal practice Philadelphia: WB Saunders, 1992;321–340.
24. **Authement JM.** Blood transfusion therapy. In: DiBartola SP, ed. Fluid therapy in small animal practice Philadelphia: WB Saunders, 1992;371–383.
25. **Lippert AC, Tony Buffington CA.** Parenteral nutrition. In DiBartola SP, ed. Fluid therapy in small animal practice. Philadelphia: WB Saunders, 1992;384–418.
26. **Abood SK, Dimski DS, Tony Buffington CA, et al.** Enteral nutrition. In: DiBartola SP, ed. Fluid therapy in small animal practice. Philadelphia: WB Saunders, 1992;419–435.
27. **Gorman NT, Evans RJ.** Myeloproliferative disease in the dog and cat: clinical presentations, diagnosis and treatment. Vet Rec 1987;121:490–496.
28. **Couto CG.** Clinicopathologic aspects of acute leukemias in the dog. J Am Vet Med Assoc 1985;186(7):681–685.
29. **Fraser CJ, Joiner GN, Jardine JH, et al.** Acute granulocytic leukemia in cats. J Am Vet Med Assoc 1974;165(4):355–359.
30. **Carpenter JL, King NW Jr, Abrams KL.** Bilateral trigeminal nerve paralysis and horner's syndrome associated with myelomonocytic neoplasia in a dog. J Am Vet Med Assoc 1987;191(12):1594–1596.
31. **Christopher MM, Metz AL, Klauser J, et al.** Acute myelomonocytic leukemia with neurologic manifestations in a dog. Vet Pathol 1986;23:140–147.
32. **Weller RE, Gessler M, Jain NC.** Myeloblastic leukemia and leukemic meningitis in a dog. Mod Vet Pract 1981;61:42–46.
33. **Ogilvie GK, Moore AS.** Bone marrow neoplasia. In: Ogilvie GK, Moore AS, eds. Managing the veterinary cancer patient: a practice manual. Trenton, NJ: Veterinary Learning Systems, 1995;260–279.
34. **Weiss DJ, Raskin RH, Zerbe C.** Myelodysplastic syndrome in two dogs. J Am Vet Med Assoc 1985;187(10):1038–1040.
35. **Couto CG, Kallet AJ.** Preleukemic syndrome in a dog. J Am Vet Med Assoc 1984;184(11):1389–1392.
36. **Madewell BR, Jain NC, Weller RE.** Hematologic abnormalities preceding myeloid leukemia in three cats. Vet Pathol 1979;16:510–519.
37. **Saarni MI, Linman JW.** Preleukemia: the hematologic syndrome preceding acute leukemia. Am J Med 1973;55:38–47.
38. **Blue JT, French TW, Kranz JS.** Non-lymphoid hematopoietic neoplasia in cats: a retrospective study of 60 cases. Cornell Vet 1988;78:21–42.
39. **Koeffler HP, Golde DW.** Human preleukemia. Ann Intern Med 1980; 93:347–353.
40. **Greenberg PL.** The smoldering myeloid leukemic states: clinical and biologic features. Blood 1983;61(6):1035–1044.
41. **Tricot G, Dekker AW, Boogaerts MA, et al.** Low dose cytosine arabinoside (Ara C) in myelodysplastic syndromes. Br J Haematol 1984;58:231–240.
42. **Vincent PC, Buck M, Young GAR, et al.** Low dose cytosine in acute nonlymphoblastic leukemia or myelodysplastic syndrome: report of six cases and review of the literature. Aust N Z J Med 1985;15:10–15.
43. **Barthel CH.** Acute myelomonocytic leukemia in a dog. Vet Pathol 1974;11:79–86.
44. **Hamlin RH, Duncan RC.** Acute nonlymphoid leukemia in a dog. J Am Vet Med Assoc 1990;196(1):110–112.
45. **Rohrig KE.** Acute myelomonocytic leukemia in a dog. J Am Vet Med Assoc 1983;182(2):137–141.
46. **Graves TK, Swenson CL, Scott MA.** A potentially misleading presentation and course of acute myelomonocytic leukemia in a dog. J Am Anim Hosp Assoc 1997;33:37–41.
47. **Ragan HA, Hackett PL, Dagle GE.** Acute myelomonocytic leukemia manifested as myelophthistic anemia in a dog. J Am Vet Med Assoc 1976; 169(4):421–425.
48. **Linnabary RD, Holscher MA, Glick AD, et al.** Acute myelomonocytic leukemia in a dog. J Am Anim Hosp Assoc 1978;14:71–75.
49. **Green RA, Barton CL.** Acute myelomonocytic leukemia in a dog. J Am Anim Hosp Assoc 1977;13:708–712.
50. **Raskin RE, Krehbiel JD.** Myelodysplastic changes in a cat with myelomonocytic leukemia. J Am Vet Med Assoc 1985;187(2):171–174.
51. **Stann SE.** Myelomonocytic leukemia in a cat. J Am Vet Med Assoc 1979;174(7):722–725.
52. **Brumbaugh GW, Stitzel KA, Zinkl JG, et al.** Myelomonocytic myeloproliferative disease in a horse. J Am Vet Med Assoc 1982;180:313–316.
53. **Woods PR, Gossett RE, Jain NC, et al.** Acute myelomonocytic leukemia in a calf. J Am Vet Med Assoc 1993;203(11):1579–1582.
54. **Latimer KS, Dykstra MJ.** Acute monocytic leukemia in a dog. J Am Vet Med Assoc 1984;184(7):852–855.
55. **Schalm OW.** 1. Acute monocytic leukemia 2. Reticulum cell sarcoma. Canine Pract 1976; Aug:19–21.
56. **Henness AM, Crow SE, Anderson BC.** Monocytic leukemia in three cats. J Am Vet Med Assoc 1977;170(11):1325–1328.
57. **Harvey JW, Shields RP, Gaskin JM.** Feline myeloproliferative disease: changing manifestations in the peripheral blood. Vet Pathol 1978;15: 437–448.
58. **Schalm OW.** Myeloproliferative disorders in the cat: 2. Erythremic myelosis. Feline Pract 1975;5:20–23.
59. **Schalm OW.** Myeloproliferative disorders in the cat: 3. Progression from erythroleukemia into granulocytic leukemia. Feline Pract 1975;5:31–33.
60. **Messick J, Carothers M, Wellman M.** Identification and characterization of megakaryoblasts in acute megakaryoblastic leukemia in a dog. Vet Pathol 1990;27:212–214.
61. **Harvey JW.** Myeloproliferative disorders in dogs and cats. Vet Clin North Am Small Anim Pract 1981;11:349–381.
62. **Holscher MA, Collins RD, Cousar JB, et al.** Diagnosis using anti-factor viii immunoperoxidase technique: megakaryocytic leukemia in a cat. Feline Pract 1983;13(4):8–12.
63. **Colbatzky F, Hermanns W.** Acute megakaryoblastic leukemia in one cat and two dogs. Vet Pathol 1993;30:186–194.
64. **Shull RM, DeNovo RC, McCracken MD.** Megakaryoblastic leukemia in a dog. Vet Pathol 1986;23:533–536.
65. **Harvey JW, Henderson CW, French TW, et al.** Feature case: myeloproliferative disease with megakaryocytic predominance in a dog with occult dirofilariasis. Vet Clin Pathol 1990;11(1):5–11.
66. **Bolon B, Buergelt CD, Harvey JW, et al.** Megakaryoblastic leukemia in a dog. Vet Clin Pathol 1990;18(3):69–72.
67. **Pucheu-Haston CM, Camus A, Taboada J, et al.** Megakaryoblastic leukemia in a dog. J Am Vet Med Assoc 1995;207(2):194–196.
68. **Holscher MA, Collins RD, Glick AD, et al.** Megakaryocytic leukemia in a dog. Vet Pathol 1978;15:562–565.
69. **Schmidt RE, Letscher RM, Toft JD II.** Megakaryocytic myelosis in cats: review and case report. J Small Anim Pract 1983;24:759–762.
70. **Hamilton TA, Morrison WB, DiNicola DB.** Cytosine arabinoside chemotherapy for acute megakaryocytic leukemia in a cat. J Am Vet Med Assoc 1991;199(3):359–361.
71. **Koeffler HP, Golde DW.** Chronic myelogenous leukemia—new concepts (first of two parts). N Engl J Med 1981;304(20):1201–1209.
72. **Koeffler HP, Golde DW.** Chronic myelogenous leukemia—new concepts (second of two parts). N Engl J Med 1981;304(21):1269–1274.
73. **Leifer CE, Matus RE, Patnaik AK, et al.** Chronic myelogenous leukemia in the dog. J Am Vet Med Assoc 1983;183(6):686–689.
74. **Joiner GN, Fraser CJ, Jardine JH, et al.** A case of chronic granulocytic leukemia in a dog. Can J Comp Med 1976;40:153–160.
75. **Jensen AL, Nielson OL.** Eosinophilic leukemoid reaction in a dog. J Small Anim Pract 1992;33(7):337–340.
76. **Ndikuwera J, Smith DA, Obwolo MJ, et al.** Chronic granulocytic leukaemia/eosinophilic leukaemia in a dog. J Small Anim Pract 1992; 33(11):553–557.
77. **Lewis MG, Kociba GJ, Rojko JL, et al.** Retroviral-associated eosinophilic leukemia in the cat. Am J Vet Res 1985;46(5):1066–1070.
78. **Morris DD, Bloom JC, Roby KA, et al.** Eosinophilic myeloproliferative disorder in a horse. J Am Vet Med Assoc 1984;185(9):993–996.
79. **Port CD, Richter WR.** Brief communications: eosinophilic leukemia in a Syrian hamster. Vet Pathol 1977;14:283–286.
80. **Neer TM.** Hypereosinophilic syndrome in cats. Compend Cont Educ Pract Vet 1991;13:549–555.
81. **Huibregtse BA, Turner JL.** Hypereosinophilic syndrome and eosinophilic leukemia: a comparison of 22 hypereosinophilic cats. J Am Anim Hosp Assoc. 1994;30:591–599.
82. **Center SA, Randolph JF, Erb HN, et al.** Eosinophilia in the cat: a retrospective study of 312 cases (1975–1986). J Am Anim Hosp Assoc. 1990; 26:349–358.
83. **Hendrick M.** A spectrum of hypereosinophilic syndromes exemplified by six cats with eosinophilic enteritis. Vet Pathol 1981;18:188–200.
84. **Harvery RG.** Feline hypereosinophilia with cutaneous lesions. J Small Anim Pract 1990;31:453–456.
85. **Hamilton TA.** The leukemias. In: Morrison WB, ed. Cancer in dogs and cats: medical and surgical management. Baltimore: Williams & Wilkins, 1998;721–729.
86. **Alroy J.** Basophilic leukemia in a dog. Vet Pathol 1972;9:90–95.
87. **Bounous DI, Latimer KS, Campagnoli RP, et al.** A brief communication: acute myeloid leukemia with basophilic differentiation (AML, M-2B) in a cat. Vet Clin Pathol 1994;23(1):15–18.
88. **Hammer AS, Couto CG, Getzy D, et al.** Essential thrombocythemia in a cat. J Vet Intern Med 1990;4(2):87–91.
89. **Hopper PE, Mandell CP, Turrel JM, et al.** Probable essential thrombocythemia in a dog. J Vet Intern Med 1989;3(2):79–85.
90. **Simpson JW, Else RW, Honeyman P.** Successful treatment of suspected essential thrombocythemia in the dog. J Small Anim Pract 1990; 31(7):345–348.

91. **Bass MC, Schultze AE.** Essential thrombocythemia in a dog: case report and literature review. J Am Anim Hosp Assoc. 1998;34:197–203.

92. **McGrath CJ.** Polycythemia vera in dogs. J Am Vet Med Assoc 1974; 164:1117–1122.

93. **Peterson ME, Randolph JF.** Diagnosis of canine primary polycythemia and management with hydroxyurea. J Am Vet Med Assoc 1982;180:415–418.

94. **Watson ADJ, Moore AS, Helfand SC.** Primary erythrocytosis in the cat. Treatment with hydroxyurea. J Small Anim Pract 1994;35:320–325.

95. **Reed C, Ling GV, Gould D, et al.** Polycythemia vera in a cat. J Am Vet Med Assoc 1970;157:85–91.

96. **Hasler AH, Giger U.** Serum erythropoietin values in polycythemic cats. J Am Anim Hosp Assoc 1996;32:294–301.

97. **Smith M, Turrel JM.** Radiophosphorus (32P) treatment of bone marrow disorders in dogs: 11 cases (1970–1987). J Am Vet Med Assoc 1982; 194:98–102.

98. **Warrell RP Jr.** Retinoic acid and acute promyelocytic leukemia. Biol Ther Cancer 1991;1(3):1–12.

99. **Tizard I.** Use of immunomodulators as an aid to clinical management of feline leukemia virus-infected cats. J Am Vet Med Assoc 1991;199(10):1482–1485.

100. **Gasper PW, Rosen DK, Fulton R.** Allogeneic marrow transplantation in a cat with acute myeloid leukemia. J Am Vet Med Assoc 1996;208(8):1280–1284.

101. **Raskin RE, Medley JM, Reimann KA.** Allogeneic bone marrow transplantation for the treatment of acute feline leukemia. Vet Clin Pathol 1986;15:5.

CHAPTER 106

Acute Myeloid Leukemia

• CAROL B. GRINDEM

Acute myeloid leukemias (AML) are neoplastic myeloproliferative disorders (MPD) originating from hematopoietic stem cells that control granulocytic, monocytic, erythrocytic, and megakaryocytic production. In contrast to chronic leukemias and myelodysplastic MPDs, AMLs are characterized by numerous (≥30%) blast cells in the bone marrow. Typically, the white blood cell (WBC) count is elevated and atypical blast cells are circulating in high numbers.[1-9]

ORIGIN AND PREVALENCE

Viruses, chemicals, ionizing radiation and antineoplastic drugs have been associated with AML.[3-9] Other than feline leukemia virus (FeLV) and feline immunodeficiency virus (FIV) in cats, natural causal agents for AML have not been identified in domestic animals. Additionally, except for the cat, MPDs are uncommon in domestic animals.[1,2] Acute lymphocytic leukemia (ALL) is more prevalent than AML, and lymphomas occur more frequently than any type of leukemia in most animal species.[1,2,6,7]

The hospital prevalence rates for myeloid versus lymphoid leukemia from the Veterinary Medical Data Base at Purdue University for 1987–1997 were as follows: cat −0.05% (75/165,835) versus 0.06% (99/165,836); dog—0.02% (85/531,388) versus 0.08% (424/531,388); avian—0.01% (2/32,268) versus 0.01% (3/32,268); and horse—0.001% (2/155,636) versus 0.004%(7/155,636). However, this data must be interpreted cautiously because the majority of leukemias in the cat were subclassified as just feline leukemia (3,344/165,836). Also, 0.02% (29/165,388) cat and 0.02% (91/531,388) dog leukemias were subclassified as unspecified leukemia. No myeloid leukemias were reported for cows, sheep, goats, pigs, or other large animals. Age-related differences between myeloid and lymphoid leukemia are not apparent in domestic animals. However, in humans, ALL is more common than AML in childhood, but this pattern reverses in adulthood.[8,9]

CLINICAL SIGNS AND LABORATORY FINDINGS

Clinical signs associated with AML are nonspecific and similar to clinical signs associated with ALL or other systemic hematopoietic disorders.[1,2] Lethargy, weakness, inappetence, fever, splenomegaly, hepatomegaly, and mild lymphadenopathy are frequently observed. Additional clinical signs and physical findings of leukemia in the horse are dependent edema of the ventrum, limbs, or genitalia; epistaxis; dyspnea, or increased lung sounds; and ulceration of the skin and mucous membranes.[10,11]

Leukocytosis, severe anemia, and thrombocytopenia are common laboratory findings (see Chapter 109, Hematologic Abnormalities Accompanying Leukemia). Blast cells are usually, but not always, present in high numbers in the peripheral blood. AML blast cells generally have more abundant cytoplasm that may contain fine granules compared with the scant, agranular cytoplasm from ALL blast cells (Tables 106.1 and 106.2). However, morphology alone is an unreliable way to identify cell lineage in AML. Aleukemic leukemia and subleukemic leukemia are terms that have been used to describe leukemias in which no or few, respectively, recognizable neoplastic cells are present in circulation. Bone marrow findings in AML include ≥30% blast cells with or without megaloblastic red cells, abnormal myeloid maturation, and increased numbers of eosinophilic or basophilic precursors.

Histologic morphology and infiltration patterns may be helpful in distinguishing lymphoma from AML, but they are generally not helpful in differentiating AML from ALL or subclassifying AML. In AML, neoplastic cells infiltrate the bone marrow and usually infiltrate the red pulp of the spleen, the sinusoidal and portal areas of the liver, the subcapsular sinuses and medullary rays of the lymph nodes, and the vascular structures in other organs.[6,7] Immunophenotypic markers, cytochemical staining, and ultrastructural morphology are indispensible in classifying AML.

Differential features that are more typical of lymphoma than AML or ALL include severe lymphade-

TABLE 106.1   Bone Marrow Classification of Acute Myeloid Leukemia

Type of Leukemia	FAB Classification	Characteristic Features
Acute undifferentiated leukemia	AUL	All BM cells are blast cells that lack any identifiable morphologic, cytochemical, or immunologic markers. Blasts in the cat may have the appearance of the outdated term, reticuloendotheliosis cells, having an eccentric nuclei, distinct nucleoli, pseudopodia, some azurophilic cytoplasmic granules, and moderately basophilic cytoplasm.
Myeloid leukemia without maturation	MO	All BM cells are myeloblasts. Myeloid lineage is established by ultrastructural demonstration of myeloperoxidase positive granules or immunologic detection of myeloid antigen(s).
Myeloid leukemia with minimal maturation	M1	≥90% of BM cells are myeloblasts and <10% are maturing granulocytes or monocytes. >3% of blast cells stain positively with myeloid markers such as myeloperoxidase, Sudan black B, chloroacetate esterase, and/or alkaline phosphatase.
Myeloid leukemia with maturation	M2	≥30% but <90% of BM cells are myeloblasts and >10% of cells are maturing granulocytes. <20% of cells are monoblasts or monocytes. Blast cells and maturing granulocytes stain positively with myeloid markers (myeloperoxidase, Sudan black B, chloroacetate esterase, and/or alkaline phosphatase). Basophilic or eosinophilic (M2-B or M2-Eo) maturation rarely occurs.
Promyelocytic leukemia	M3	≥30% but <90% of BM cells are myeloblasts. >10% of cells are maturing granulocytes, predominately atypical promyelocytes. Not yet reported in dogs or cats.
Myelomonocytic leukemia	M4	≥30% of BM cells are myeloblasts and monoblasts. Also, >20% of cells are maturing granulocytes and >20% of cells are monoblasts and maturing monocytes. Myeloid cells stain with myeloid markers and monocytic cells stain with CD14 and nonspecific esterase that is inhibited by fluoride. M4 with eosinophilia (M4-Eo) reported in humans.
Monoblastic leukemia	M5a	≥80% of BM cells are monoblasts and <20% of cells are myeloblasts and maturing granulocytes. Monoblasts are large, delicate cells with round to irregular nuclear outline, stippled chromatin, 1 or more prominent nucleoli, and a moderate amount of basophilic agranular cytoplasm. Monoblasts stain with CD14 and nonspecific esterase that is inhibited by fluoride.
Monocytic leukemia	M5b	≥30% but ≤80% of BM cells are monoblasts, and <20% of cells are myeloblasts and maturing granulocytes. >80% of cells are monoblasts and maturing monocytes. Monoblasts and monocytes stain with nonspecific esterase and are inhibited by fluoride. CD14 also stains monocytes.
Erythroleukemia	M6	≥50% of BM cells are nucleated erythroid cells, and ≥30% of the nonerythroid cells are myeloblasts. Myeloblasts stain with myeloid markers. No reliable cytochemical markers are available for red cell precursors. Ultrastructure and cell surface markers may be helpful.
Erythroleukemia with erythroid predominance	M6-Er	≥50% of BM cells are nucleated erythroid cells, and ≥30% of all nucleated cells are myeloblasts and rubriblasts. Myeloblasts stain with myeloid markers. No reliable cytochemical markers are available for red cell precursors. Ultrastructure and cell surface markers may be helpful.
Megakaryocytic leukemia	M7	≥30% of BM cells are megakaryoblasts. Dwarf megakaryocytes and myelofibrosis may occur. Megakaryoblasts stain positively for platelet glycoprotein IIb-IIIa, acetylcholinesterase, alpha-naphthyl acetate esterase, and periodic acid-Schiff and stain negatively for myeloperoxidase, Sudan black B, and alpha-naphthyl butyrate esterase.

nopathy, mild anemia rather than severe anemia, and leukopenia or lack of circulating neoplastic cells. Late-stage lymphoma with bone marrow infiltration may have similar clinical and laboratory findings to AML or ALL.

MORPHOLOGIC FEATURES OF HEMATOPOIETIC PRECURSOR CELLS

Classification of acute leukemias is based on the presumed cell of origin. Tentative identification of cell lineage is done by examination of morphologic features of blast cells on Romanowsky-stained smears (Table 106.2). Accurate assessment of cell lineage and maturation, however, requires additional confirmation such as cytochemical staining, immunophenotyping, and ultrastructural studies.

Because the diagnosis and classification of AML is based on the number and the type of blast cells, it is important to have guidelines for cell identification. Two types of myeloblasts have been described in animals,[2,4,5] and four types of myeloblasts have been proposed in man.[8,12,13] The primary reason for subtyping myeloblasts is to distinguish them from promyelocytes. Remember, promyelocytes and promonocytes are not included in the blast count in the French-American-British (FAB) classification. Also, rubriblasts are only included if the myeloid-to-erythroid (M:E) ratio in bone marrow is less

than one.[2,4,5] General features of the various blasts are as follows. Megakaryoblasts usually are the largest followed by monoblasts, myeloblasts, lymphoblasts, and rubriblasts. Monoblasts may have the most abundant cytoplasm and the most delicate chromatin pattern, but some of the cells in acute monocytic leukemias in animals have lacked these features and have appeared similar to ALL or AML blastic cells. The rubriblast is distinctive because of its intensely basophilic cytoplasm, coarser nuclear chromatin, and large prominent nucleolus.

Auer rods are pink-staining, needlelike dysplastic cytoplasmic lysosomes derived from the incorporation of primary azurophilic granules into autophagic vacuoles.[9] Phi bodies are small fusiform or spindle-shaped rods similar to Auer rods that stain with hydroperoxidases.[14] Auer rods or Phi bodies are pathognomic for AML in humans but are not features of AML in animals.[1,2,9]

Myeloblast Type I

Large (diameter of 1.5 to 3 times the size of a red cell) and round, the myeloblast type I cell has a round to oval nucleus that is centrally located. The cell's chromatin pattern is delicate, finely stippled or lacy, and nucleoli may be prominent. The nuclear-to-cytoplasmic (N:C) ratio is high (>1.5), and the cytoplasm is pale to moderately blue. Infrequently, a few small cytoplasmic vacuoles may be observed (Fig. 106.1).[1,3,15]

TABLE 106.2   Cytologic and Cytochemical Features of Blood and Bone Marrow Cells in Leukemia[a]

Characteristic	Lymphocytic[b]	Granulocytic[b]	Monocytic[b]
Cell size	Usually small	Usually large	Usually large
Nuclear shape	Round to oval, smooth contour, rare clefting or slight indentation	Round to oval, smooth contour	Irregular, smooth, or clefted contour; nuclear folds may be present
Nuclear chromatin	Fine to coarsely granular (gravel-like) or clumped	Finely stippled (sand-like)	Finely stippled or reticular (linearly fibrillar)
Nucleoli	One or more; distinct or inconspicuous	One or more; distinct or inconspicuous	One or more; distinct or inconspicuous
Amount of cytoplasm	Scant to moderately abundant	Moderately abundant	Moderately abundant
Nuclear:cytoplasmic ratio	High	Low to high	Low to high
Cytoplasmic basophilia	Slight to significant	Moderate	Moderate
Cytoplasm	Smooth, featureless, rarely vacuolated	Ground glasslike; no vacuoles unless toxic	Grayish blue, foamy, or vacuolated
Azurophilic granules	Generally absent; rarely, few and large	Many, small but distinct	Usually absent; sometimes fine and indistinct
Specific granules	−	+	−
Cytochemical markers			
Peroxidase	−	+, usually strong	+, usually weak
Alkaline phosphatase	−	+, some cells	−
Lipase	−	−	+
Nonspecific esterase	−	−	+
Cell rafts	−	+	+
Proliferative cell line	Recognizable lymphocytic	Maturation toward neutrophilic series	Maturation toward monocytic cells

[a] Cell morphology varies with the patient and with time in the same patient. All cytologic criteria do not manifest in every case; mixed leukemias are sometimes encountered.
[b] −, absent; +, present.
Reprinted with permission from Essentials of Veterinary Hematology. Jain NC, ed. Philadelphia: Lea & Febiger, 1993; 308.

Myeloblast Type II

With similar features to type I myeloblast, the myeloblast type II has some (less than 15) tiny azurophilic granules that are scattered in the cytoplasm, and its N:C ratio is lower. Although usually centrally located, the nucleus may be eccentrically placed (Fig. 106.2)[1,3,15]

Myeloblast Type III

With more than 20 cytoplasmic azurophilic granules, the myeloblast type III is a hypergranular myeloblast.[12,13] A delicate chromatin pattern and a higher N:C ratio are features that help distinguish a myeloblast type III from a promyelocyte.

Myeloblast Type IV

Hypogranular Auer rod containing cells have a Golgi zone and round to slightly indented nuclei, delicate nu-

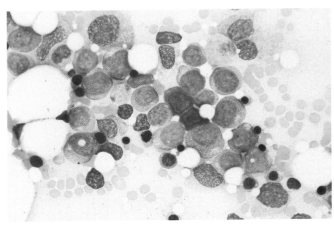

FIGURE 106.3 Myeloblasts with scant cytoplasm; promyelocytes with more abundant cytoplasm, containing azurophilic granules; two rubriblasts; donut-shaped myelocyte; and a pale-staining eosinophilic precursor.

clear chromatin, and deeply basophilic cytoplasm.[13] These cells are not reported in animals.

Promyelocyte

Increased chromatin clumping and numerous dispersed azurophilic cytoplasmic granules and lower N:C ratio differentiate the promyelocyte from the myeloblast. Eccentric nucleus, prominent nucleoli, and a clear Golgi zone may occur. The acute promyelocytic leukemia blasts in humans may have abnormally large and prominent granules (Fig. 106.3).[8,9]

Monoblast

With a large round cell, the monoblast has a similar or lower N:C ratio than the myeloblast. The nucleus is round to moderately irregular in shape with a stippled to finely reticular nuclear chromatin pattern, one or more prominent nucleoli, and a moderate amount of basophilic agranular cytoplasm. Some of the monoblasts from animals that have M5 have been readily confused with myeloblasts or lymphoblasts, reinforcing the need for cytochemistry or immunophenotyping (Fig. 106.4).

Promonocyte

Compared with the monoblast, this large cell has more abundant, less basophilic cytoplasm (a cerebriform nucleus with prominent nuclear folds), lacy chromatin and no distinct nucleoli. Cytoplasmic vacuoles and fine azurophilic granulation may be present.

Lymphoblast

Although variable, certain key features are helpful in distinguishing lymphoblasts from myeloblasts. These

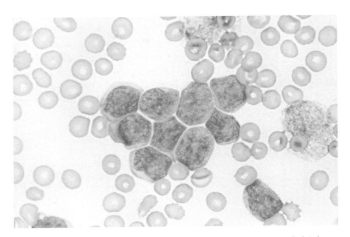

FIGURE 106.1 Delicate, pale-staining myeloblasts with high N:C ratio from a dog that has AML (M1) (Wright–Giemsa).

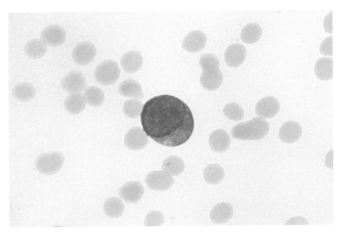

FIGURE 106.2 Large myeloblast with eccentric nucleus and indistinct nucleolar membrane from the peripheral blood of a cat that has AUL (Wright–Giemsa).

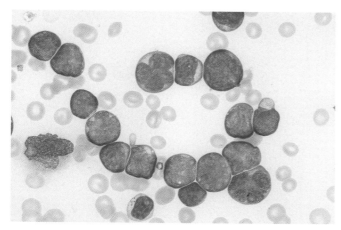

FIGURE 106.4 Large monoblasts with finely stippled chromatin, round to irregular shaped nuclei, and scant basophilic cytoplasm from the bone marrow of a dog that has acute monoblastic leukemia (M5a).

similar to myeloblasts or lymphoblasts to atypical multi-nucleated blasts. Cytoplasm is deeply basophilic, may have vacuoles and a few granules, and may form cyto-plasmic projections (Fig. 106.6).[1–3,15]

CLASSIFICATION OF ACUTE MYELOID LEUKEMIAS

In 1991, the FAB criteria used in human oncology were adapted for the classification of AML and myelodysplas-tic syndromes in the dog and cat. See Figure 106.7 and Table 106.2).[3–5,16–21]

Optimally, the diagnosis of leukemia is based on ex-amination of Romanowsky-stained blood and bone marrow films and a core bone marrow biopsy. A mini-mum 200-cell differential bone marrow count is needed to determine the percentage of blast cells (myeloblasts, monoblasts, and megakaryoblasts), to evaluate myeloid,

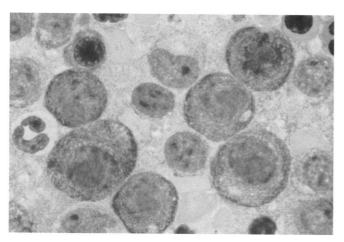

FIGURE 106.5 Large rubriblasts with prominent nucleoli, coarse nuclear chromatin, and dark blue cytoplasm from the bone marrow of a cat that has erythroleukemia (M6-Er) (Wright–Giemsa).

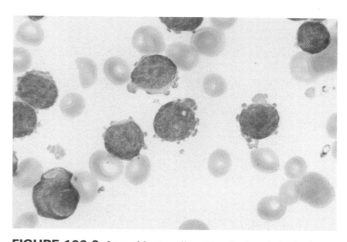

FIGURE 106.6 Large blastic cells with cytoplasmic blebs from the bone marrow of a dog that has acute megakaryoblastic leukemia (M7) (Wright–Giemsa).

features are higher N:C ratio, usual lack of cytoplasmic granules, and coarser chromatin pattern of lym-phoblasts.

Rubriblasts

Smaller cell size, deeply blue cytoplasm, slightly more condensed chromatin, and prominent nucleoli are fea-tures of rubriblasts rather than myeloblasts. Pro-rubricytes (not included in the FAB blast cell count) have increased nuclear condensation and nucleoli or nucleolar rings are absent (Figs. 106.3 and 106.5).

Megakaryoblasts

Morphologically, megakaryoblasts from leukemic pa-tients are heterogeneous, varying from small round cells

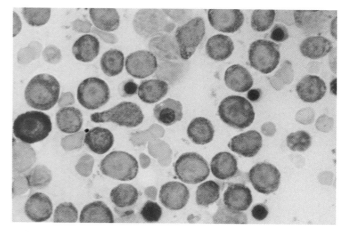

FIGURE 106.7 Undifferentiated blast cells with scant cytoplasm and one cell forming a pseudopod. Bone marrow from a cat that has AUL (Wright–Giemsa).

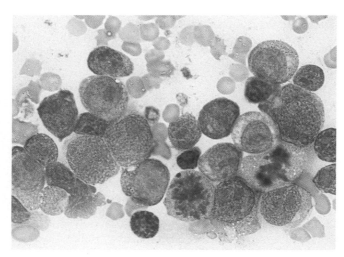

FIGURE 106.8 Myeloblasts, two mitotic figures, and two erythroblasts from the bone marrow of a cat that has AML (M1) (Wright–Giemsa).

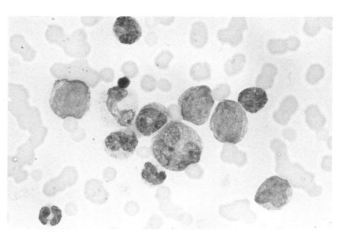

FIGURE 106.9 Myeloblasts, immature granulocytes and monocytoid cell from blood of a dog that has acute myelomonocytic leukemia (Wright–Giemsa).

erythroid, and megakaryocyte morphology and maturation patterns, and to calculate a M:E ratio. Lymphocytes, plasma cells, mast cells, and macrophages are excluded from the calculation of blast-cell percentages and M:E ratios. A core biopsy is needed to confirm myelofibrosis or a possible hypocellular bone marrow with AML. Confusion about myeloid disorders and specific terminology has been decreased by use of a uniform classification system. For example, the terms reticuloendotheliosis and erythremic myelosis are no longer recommended for classification of animal leukemias. By use of the FAB criteria, most cases of reticuloendotheliosis would be classified as acute undifferentiated leukemia (AUL), and erythremic myelosis would be either acute erythroleukemia with erythroid predominance (M6-Er) or MDS with erythroid predominance (MDS-Er), depending on the percent of blast cells in the bone marrow. AUL, AML (M0,M1,M2), acute promyelocytic leukemia (M3), acute myelomonocytic leukemia (M4), acute monoblastic leukemia (M5a, M5b), acute erythroleukemia (M6, M6-Er) and acute megakaryocytic leukemia (M7) are defined below.

Acute Undifferentiated Leukemia

AUL refers to acute leukemias lacking morphologic and immunologic characteristics of either lymphoid or myeloid lineage. See Figure 106.7.

Acute Myeloid Leukemia Without Maturation

The blast cells of AML without maturation (M0) are undifferentiated by light microscopy and cytochemical reactions. Myeloid lineage is established by ultrastructural demonstration of myeloperoxidase-positive granules or the detection of one or more lineage-specific myeloid antigens. Lymphoid differentiation should be excluded by immunophenotyping.

Acute Myeloid Leukemia With Minimal Maturation

Characterized morphologically by undifferentiated blast cells ≥90%, AML with minimal maturation (M1), is accompanied by scant azurophilic granules (Fig. 106.8). No more than 10% of cells show evidence of myeloid or monocytic maturation. Cytochemical stains are required for differentiating these cells from lymphoblasts. At least 3% of M1 blast cells should be myeloperoxidase (MPO) or Sudan black B (SBB) positive. See Figure 106.1.

Acute Myeloid Leukemia With Maturation

Distinguished from M1 by clear evidence of maturation (See Fig. 106.3), AML with maturation (M2) myeloblasts account for more than 30% but less than 90% of nucleated cells, whereas monocyte precursors comprise less than 20% of cells. In humans, increased numbers of eosinophilic (M2-Eo) or basophilic (M2-B) precursors, pseudo-Pelger-Huet cells and hypogranular neutrophils may be seen. The MPO-staining reaction is strongly positive and nonspecific esterase staining (NSE) is negative in most cells. AML with basophilic differentiation (M2-B) has been reported in a cat.[22]

Acute Promyelocytic Leukemia

Although acute promelyocytic leukemia (M3) is rare in animals, it has been reported in pigs, but not yet in dogs or cats.[23] Criteria for M3 are ≥30% but <90% myeloblasts in the bone marrow. Greater than 10% of cells are maturing granulocytes, predominantly (often >50%) abnormal hypergranular, hypogranular, or microgranular promyelocytes. Abundant Auer rods may be arranged in bundles (faggots). Disseminated intravascular coagulation often occurs in M3 patients.[9]

Acute Myelomonocytic Leukemia

The presence of both granulocytic and monocytic precursors characterizes acute myelomonocytic leukemia (M4) (Fig. 106.9). Each cell line accounts for at least 20% but not more than 80% of the nucleated bone marrow cells. Reliable identification of M4 requires use of special stains such as MPO and NSE. M4 with eosinophilia (M4-Eo) has been recognized in humans.[8]

Acute Monoblastic Leukemia

There are two forms of acute monoblastic leukemia: M5a and M5b. In acute monoblastic leukemia without differentiation (M5a), ≥80% of the bone marrow cells are monoblasts (See Fig. 106.4). These are large cells with delicate lacy nuclear chromatin and agranular basophilic cytoplasm. Acute monoblastic leukemia with maturation (M5b) has more bone marrow promonocytes and monocytes. Nuclear folding, gray-blue cytoplasm and azurophilic cytoplasmic granulation are indications of monocytic maturation. Between 30 and 80% of the bone marrow nucleated cells are monoblasts, and >80% of the cells are monoblasts and monocytes. Monocytosis may be significant in the peripheral blood (Fig. 106.10). Monocytes stain with NSE. This reaction is inhibited by sodium fluoride. MPO staining is usually negative or only slightly positive.

Acute Erythroleukemia

Except for in cats and birds, acute erythroleukemia (M6 and M6-Er) is rare in animals and humans.[3,5,21,24,25] The

key feature that distinguishes M6 or M6-Er from other types of acute leukemia is that the erythroid precursors comprise greater than 50% of nucleated bone marrow cells with an M:E ratio of less than one. Prominent megaloblastic or atypical erythroid precursors are common (Fig. 106.5 and 106.11). For either M6 or M6-Er, myeloblasts and monoblasts are <30% of all nucleated cells (ANC) in the bone marrow. If blasts are ≥30% of ANC, the leukemia is an AML (Fig. 106.7) such as M2, M4, or M5. M6 is characterized by an M:E ratio of <1, and ≥30% of all nonerythroid cells (NEC) are myeloblasts. In M6-Er, the myeloblast (present in decreased proportion to M6) and rubriblast numbers are combined and account for ≥30% ANC in the bone marrow. Unfortunately, no reliable cytochemical markers are available for red cell precursors. Immunologic markers are being developed but are not readily available.

Acute Megakaryocytic Leukemia

Rare in animals and in humans, acute megakaryocytic leukemia (M7) may be associated with myelofibrosis.[26–28] Megakaryoblasts (≥30% of ANC) are pleomorphic and may resemble lymphoblasts or myeloblasts. Micromegakaryocytes are often found in the blood and bone marrow. Cytoplasmic blebs or platelet shedding help identify megakaryoblasts (see Fig. 106.6). Cytochemical, ultrastructural, and immunophenotypic features are necessary for definitive diagnosis of M7. Megakaryoblasts are acetylcholine esterase and factor-VIII-related

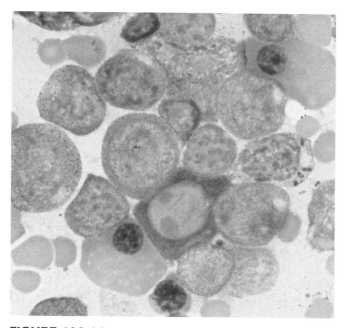

FIGURE 106.11 Megaloblasts and rubriblasts with prominent nucleoli from the bone marrow of a cat that has erythroleukemia (M6-Er) (Wright–Giemsa). Reprinted with permission from Grindem CB. Classification of myeloproliferative diseases. In: August JR, ed. Consultations in feline internal medicine 3. Philadelphia: WB Saunders, 1997;504.

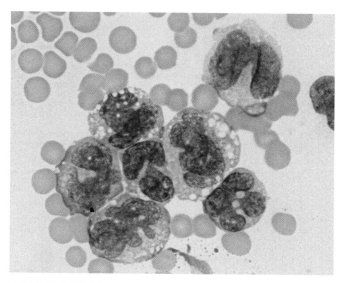

FIGURE 106.10 Atypical monocytes from the peripheral blood of a cat that has acute monocytic leukemia (M5b) (Wright–Giemsa).

antigen positive, platelet peroxidase positive on ultrastructure and glycoproteins IIb-IIIa positive on immunophenotyping.[15,26–28]

MISCELLANEOUS ACUTE LEUKEMIAS

A limitation of the FAB classification is the lack of criteria for some types of acute nonlymphocytic leukemias (ANLL), but all of them are uncommon in animals. AUL, mixed lineage ANLL, hypocellular ANLL, and acute basophilic, acute eosinophilic and acute mast cell leukemias have not be identified by the FAB classification. Acute basophilic, eosinophilic, and mast cell leukemias are rare in animals and in humans.[1,2,6,22,29] Also, they may be difficult to differentiate from the more chronic forms of these leukemias as well as from AMLs with basophilic or eosinophilic maturatiion (M2-B or M2-Eo).[22]

Immunophenotypic and molecular markers have demonstrated human leukemias that are heterogeneous and appear to be of mixed lineage with individual cells expressing both myeloid and lymphoid features.[8,9,30] These have been referred to as mixed lineage, biphenotypic or hybrid leukemias. Proposed mechanisms for these clonal or biclonal mixed-lineage leukemias with cell marker overlap include: (1) abnormal cell development with inappropriate expression of a combination of lymphoid and myeloid antigens, (2) clonal expansion of cells that have retained features that cross over cell lineages, (3) malignancies involving neoplastic proliferation of more than one clone of cells.[8,9] Imperatively, before diagnosing a mixed-lineage leukemia, remember that the majority of monoclonal antibodies are neither tumor specific nor lineage restricted. Therefore, significant overlap in their reactivity with various lymphoid and myeloid cells may occur. The extent of overlap of antigenic expression must be considered during a diagnosis of acute biphenotypic or mixed leukemia.

SPECIES-SPECIFIC FINDINGS

All types of AML (M1 to M7) have been reported in dogs and cats except acute promyelocytic leukemia (M3). Acute myeloid, myelomonocytic, and monocytic leukemias are most frequently reported.[1–7,31–35] Acute megakaryocytic leukemia (M7) is rare in both dogs and cats.[26–28] Erythroleukemia (M6 and M6-Er), which is fairly common in cats, is uncommon in dogs.[1,2,4,5,24]

Myelomonocytic leukemia is the most frequently reported nonlymphoid leukemia in the horse.[10,11] Monocytic leukemia, chronic granulocytic leukemia, and eosinophilic leukemia have also been reported.[1,2,10,11,36]

Published reports of myeloid leukemias in cattle,[7,37,40] sheep[41] and goats[42] are rare. Promyelocytic leukemia, which has not been reported in dogs or cats, has been reported in pigs.[23,37] Other types of myeloid leukemia (granulocytic leukemia, erythremic myelosis, erythroleukemia, and eosinophilic leukemia) have been reported, but they are uncommon in the pig.[7,23,37–39]

Avian retroviruses cause a wide variety of hematopoietic neoplasms in poultry, including erythroblastosis, myeloblastosis, and myelocytomatosis.[25] Variables that affect the type of neoplasm that develops are viral strain, route of inoculation, and age and sex of the bird.[25] Although leukemia is uncommon in pet birds, granulocyte leukemia may be more common in the macaw whereas lymphocyte leukemia is more common in budgerigars, canaries and Amazon parrots.[42a]

Myeloid leukemias have been reported in various laboratory animals, including mice,[43–47] rats,[44,47] rabbits,[37] hamsters,[48,49] and monkeys.[50] Most types of nonlymphoid hematopoietic neoplasms (histiocytic sarcoma, granulocytic leukemia, erythroid leukemia, and mast cell tumors) are more common in mice than rats.[44] Histiocytic sarcoma is the most common nonlymphoid hematopoietic neoplasm in the mouse.[43,44] In both the mouse and the rat, granulocytic leukemia seems rare, and it must be distinguished from myeloid metaplasia.[44] Incidence and type of hematopoietic tumor are characteristic for each mouse or rat strain, and sex and age differences have been reported.[43,45]

Myeloid leukemias appear to be uncommon in reptiles. Granulocytic leukemia has been reported in a tortoise.[51]

DIAGNOSIS OF ACUTE MYELOID LEUKEMIA

Diagnosis of AML begins with a routine complete blood cell (CBC) count that includes examination of a blood smear. Acute leukemia may be immediately obvious if high numbers of delicate blasts with little or no maturation are present. Without excess blast cells, hematologic abnormalities, especially those involving more than one cell line coupled with vague clinical signs of lethargy, weakness, and organomegaly, should trigger the clinician to evaluate the bone marrow for leukemic infiltration. If ≥30% of the nucleated bone marrow cells are blastic cells, acute leukemia is likely. The major precaution is that a bone marrow in the early phase of recovery (such as that in a cat recovering from acute panleukopenia virus infection) could have a bone marrow that looks like leukemia.[52]

To confirm AML, the excess blast population must be identified as nonlymphoid blast cells, either myeloblasts, monoblasts, erythroblasts, or megakaryoblasts. (See the Algorithm). Identification may be possible on morphology alone if the blastic cells are showing some differentiating. However, cytochemical staining, immunophenotyping, or ultrastructural morphology are needed to confirm cell of origin and to subclassify the AML.[5,33] Use of a battery of specific markers that includes myeloid (MPO, SBB, chloroacetate esterase), and monocytic (NSE, CD14) markers is recommended. Acetylcholine esterase, factor-VIII-related antigen, platelet peroxidase, and platelet glycoprotein IIb-IIIa are helpful markers of megakaryocytic differentiating. To eliminate ALL, at least one T-cell marker (such as CD3) and one B-cell marker (such as CD21) should be used. Antigenic B-cell markers are preferred to surface immunoglobulin testing. Unfortunately, CD markers for myeloid and erythroid cells are not readily available in veterinary medicine.

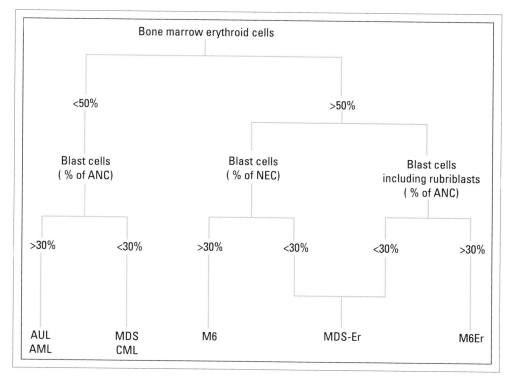

Schematic to classification of acute myeloid leukemias and myelodysplastic syndromes in dogs and cats. Blast cells include myeloblasts, monoblasts, and megakaryoblasts. ANC, all nucleated cells in bone marrow excluding lymphocytes, plasma cells, macrophages, and mast cells; NEC, nonerythroid cells in bone marrow; AUL, acute undifferentiated leukemia; AML, acute myeloid leukemias M1 to M5 and M7; CML, chronic myeloid leukemias including chronic myelogenous, chronic myelomonocytic, and chronic monocytic leukemias; MDS, myelodysplastic syndrome; MDS-Er, myelodysplastic syndrome with erythroid predominance; M6, erythroleukemia; M6Er, erythroleukemia with erythroid predominance. (From Jain NC et al. A report of the animal leukemia study group: Proposed criteria for classification of acute myeloid leukemias in dogs and cats. Vet Clin Pathol 1991;20:63.)

Cytogenetic studies of human AML have revealed that greater than 50% of patients have acquired chromosomal abnormalities. These chromosomal aberrations constitute tumor markers of diagnostic and prognostic value.[8,9] Documentation of chromosomal abnormalities in animal leukemias is difficult, and the significance of cytogenetic aberrations is unknown. However, a recurrent cytogenetic abnormality in acute canine leukemia of trisomy 1 was recently documented.[53]

DIFFERENTIAL DIAGNOSES FOR INCREASED BONE MARROW BLAST CELLS

Arrested maturation patterns characterized by excessive blast cells occurs in leukemia, with immune destruction of more mature cells or with early bone marrow repopulation (for example, recovery from panleukopenia and canine parvovirus infection). Scrutinizing the history (vaccinations, drugs, previous illness, and clinical signs), having the blood and bone marrow examined by an experienced veterinary hematologist, and sequential monitoring of the blood and bone marrow should distinguish benign maturation arrest patterns from leukemia. To distinguish leukemia from bone marrow in the acute stage of recovery, sequential CBCs and bone marrows should be performed. A recovering bone marrow shows an orderly maturation pattern with time (3 to 5 days), whereas acute leukemia has a persistence of excess blasts, and maturation is not orderly.

Chronic leukemias and MDSs are differentiated from AML by bone marrow blast cell counts of less than 30%. However, both of these conditions may terminate in AML. Additionally, whereas the AML are typically associated with numerous blast cells in the peripheral blood, chronic myeloid leukemias are associated with marked increases in well differentiated leukocytes (neutrophils, monocytes, eosinophils, or basophils). Myelodysplastic syndromes are characterized by peripheral cytopenias, hyperplastic bone marrows, and prominent dysplastic cellular changes. See Chapter 102, Myelodysplastic Syndromes and Myelofibrosis; Chapter 108, Chronic Myeloid Leukemias; and the algorithm at the end of this chapter for greater details.

With bone marrow hyperplasia (myeloid hyperplasia with inflammation or erythroid hyperplasia with regenerative anemia), the percent of blast cells is less than 30%, maturation is orderly, and no or few dysplastic cells are observed. Differentiation from chronic leukemias and MDSs may be more challenging. Sequential monitoring and identification of a cause for the hyperplasia are important.

PROGNOSIS AND THERAPY

Prognosis for AML in animals is poor. Most animals die or are euthanized shortly after diagnosis. Therapeutic options include supportive therapy, chemotherapy, immunotherapy, radiation, and bone marrow transplantation (see Chapters 105, Clinical Diagnosis and Management of Acute and Chronic Myeloproliferative Disorders, and 17, Hemopoietic Stem Cell Transplantation). Encouragingly, significant progress has been made in the treatment and cure of AML in humans in the past 20 years. This information should provide insights into the treatment of leukemias in animals.

REFERENCES

1. **Jain NC.** The leukemia complex. In: Jain NC, ed. Schalm's veterinary hematology. 4th ed. Philadelphia: Lea and Febiger, 1986;838–908.
2. **Jain NC.** The leukemias. In: Jain NC, ed. Essentials of veterinary hematology. Philadelphia: Lea and Febiger, 1993, 319–348.
3. **Jain NC.** The leukemias: general aspects. In: Jain NC, ed. Essentials of veterinary hematology. Philadelphia: Lea and Febiger, 1993, 307–318.
4. **Jain NC, Blue JT, Grindem CB, et al.** Proposed criteria for classification of acute myeloid leukemia in dogs and cats: a report of the Animal Leukemia Study Group. Vet Clin Pathol 1991;20:63–82.
5. **Jain NC.** Classification of myeloproliferative disorders in cats using criteria proposed by the Animal Leukemia Study Group: a retrospective study of 181 cases (1969–1992). Comp Haematol Int 1993; 3:25–134.
6. **Moulton JE, Harvey JW.** Tumors of the lymphoid and hematopoietic tissues. In: Moulton JE, ed. Tumors in domestic animals. 3rd ed. Berkeley, CA: University of California Press, 1990, 231–307.
7. **Valli VEO.** The hematopoietic system. In: Jubb KVF, Kennedy PC, Palmer N, eds. Pathology of domestic animals. 4th ed. San Diego, CA: Academic Press, 1993;3:114–133.
8. **Lukens JN.** Classification and differentiation of the acute leukemias. In: Lee GR, Bithell TC, Foerster J, et al. Wintrobe's clinical hematology. 9th ed. Philadelphia: Lea and Febiger. 1993;2:1873–1891.
9. **Miller KB.** Clinical manifestations of acute myeloid leukemia. In: Hoffman R, Benz EJ Jr, Shattil SJ, et al. Hematology, basic principles and practice. 2nd ed. New York: Churchill Livingston 1995;993–1014.
10. **Latimer KS, White SL.** Acute monocytic leukaemia (M5a) in a horse. Comp Haematol Int 1996;6:111–114.
11. **Ringger NC, Edens L, Bain P, et al.** Acute myelogenous leukaemia in a mare. Aust Vet J 1997;75:329–331.
12. **Goasguen JE, Bennett JM.** Classification of acute myeloid leukemia. Clin Lab Med 1990;10:661–81.
13. **Wong KF, Chan JK.** Proposal for a type IV blast in the FAB classification [letter]. Am J Hematol 1995;49:168.
14. **Hanker JS, Laszlo J, Moore JO.** The light microscopic demonstration of hydroperoxidase-positive Phi bodies and rods in leukocytes in acute myeloid leukemia. Histochemistry 1978;58:241–252.
15. **Raskin RE.** Myelopoiesis and myeloproliferative disorders. Vet Clin North Am Small Anim Pract 1996;26:1023–1042.
16. **Bennett JM, Catovsky D, Daniel MT, et al.** Proposals for the classification of the acute leukemias. French-American-British (FAB) Cooperative Group. Br J Haematol 1976;33:451–458.
17. **Bennett JM, Catovsky D, Daniel MT, et al.** Proposed revised criteria for the classification of acute myeloid leukemia. Ann Intern Med 1985;103:620–625.
18. **Bennett JM, Catovsky D, Daniel MT, et al.** Criteria for the diagnosis of acute leukemia of megakaryocyte lineage (M7). Ann Intern Med 1985;103:460–462.
19. **Bennett JM, Catovsky D, Daniel MT, et al.** Proposal for the recognition of minimally differentiated acute myeloid leukaemia. Br J Haematol 1991; 78:325–329.
20. **Buddle R.** Enzyme and immunohistochemical studies on acute monocytic leukemia (FAB M5): proposal for a new immunohistochemical subclassification. Acta Haematol 1996; 95:102–106.
21. **Goldberg SL, Noel P, Klumpp TR, Dewald GW.** The erythroid leukemias: a comparative study of erythroleukemia (FAB M6) and Di Guglielmo disease. Am J Clin Oncol 1998; 21:42–47.
22. **Bounous DI, Latimer KS, Campagnoli RP, Hynes PF.** Acute myeloid leukemia with basophilic differentiation (AML, M-2B) in a cat. Vet Clin Pathol 1994;23:15–18.
23. **Breuer W, Heinritzi K, Hermanns W.** Acute myeloid-leukemia (promyelocytic leukemia) with demonstration of virus-particles in a boar—light-microscopic, histochemical and ultrastructural findings. Berl Munch Tierarztl Wochenschr 1995;108:380–384.
24. **Shimada T, Matsumoto Y, Okuda M, et al.** Erythroleukemia in two cats naturally infected with feline leukemia virus in the same household. J Vet Med Sci 1995;57:199–204.
25. **Payne LN, Purchase HG.** Neoplastic diseases: leukosis/sarcoma group. In: Calnek BW, Barnes JH, Beard CW, Reid WM, Yoder HW Jr, eds. Diseases of poultry. 9th ed. Ames, IA: Iowa State University Press, 1991:386–439.
26. **Messick J, Carothers M, Wellman M.** Identification and characterization of megakaryoblasts in acute megakaryoblastic leukemia in a dog. Vet Pathol 1990;27:212–214.
27. **Colbatzky F, Hermanns W.** Acute megakaryoblastic leukemia in one cat and two dogs. Vet Pathol 1993;30:186–194.
28. **Burton S, Miller L, Horney B, et al.** Acute megakaryoblastic leukemia in a cat. Vet Clin Pathol 1996;25:6–9.
29. **Peterson LC, Parkin JL, Arthur DC, Brunning RD.** Acute basophilic leukemia. A clinical, morphologic and cytogenetic study of eight cases. Am J Clin Pathol 1991;96:160–170.
30. **Khalidi HS, Medeiros LJ, Chang KL, et al.** The immunophenotype of adult acute myeloid leukemia: high frequency of lymphoid antigen expression and comparison of immunophenotype, French-American-British classification, and karyotypic abnormalities. Am J Clin Pathol 1998;109:211–220.
31. **Jain NC, Madewell BR, Weller RE, Geissler MC.** Clinical-pathological findings and cytochemical characterization of myelomonocytic leukaemia in 5 dogs. J Comp Pathol 1981;91:17–31.
32. **Grindem CB, Stevens JB, Perman V.** Morphological classification and clinical and pathological characteristics of spontaneous leukemia in 17 dogs. J Am Anim Hosp Assoc 1985;21:219–226.
33. **Graves TK, Swenson CL, Scott MA.** A potentially misleading presentation and course of acute myelomonocytic leukemia in a dog. J Am Anim Hosp Assoc 1997;33:37–41.
34. **Blue JT, French TW, Kranz JS.** Non-lymphoid hematopoietic neoplasia in cats: a retrospective study of 60 cases. Cornell Vet 1988;78:21–42.
35. **Grindem CB.** Classification of myeloproliferative diseases. In: August JR, ed. Consultations in feline internal medicine 3. Philadelphia: WB Saunders, 1997;499–508.
36. **Morris DD, Bloom JC, Roby KA, et al.** Eosinophilic myeloproliferative disorder in a horse. J Am Vet Med Assoc 1984;185(9):993–996.
37. **Marcato PS.** Swine lymphoid and myeloid neoplasms in Italy. Vet Res Commun 1987;11:325–337.
38. **Magaki G.** Hematopoietic neoplasms of slaughter animals. Natl Cancer Inst Monogr 1969;32:121–151.
39. **Squire RA.** Hematopoietic tumors of domestic animals. Cornell Vet 1964;54:97–149.
40. **Woods PR, Gossett RE, Jain NC, et al.** Acute myelomonocytic leukemia in a calf. J Am Vet Med Assoc 1993;203(11):1579–1582.
41. **Monlux AW, Anderson WA, Davis CL.** A survey of tumors occurring in cattle, sheep, and swine. Am J Vet Res 1956;27:647–677.
42. **Puette M, Latimer KS.** Acute granulocytic leukemia in a slaughter goat. J Vet Diagn Invest 1997;9:318–319.
42a. **Fudge AM, Joseph V.** Disorders of avian leukocytes. In: Fudge AM, ed. Laboratory medicine. Avian and exotic pets. Philadelphia: WB Saunders, 2000;19–25.
43. **Frith CH, Ward JM, Frederickson T, Harleman JH.** Neoplastic lesions of the hematopoietic system. In: Mohr U, Dungworth DL, Capen CC, Carlton WW, Sundberg JP, Ward JM, eds. Pathobiology of the aging mouse. Washington, DC: ILSI Press, 1996;1:219–235.
44. **Frith CH, Ward JM, Chandra M.** The morphology, immunohistochemistry, and incidence of hematopoietic neoplasms in mice and rats. Toxicol Pathol 1993;21:206–218.
45. **Jones TC, Ward JM, Mohr U, Hunt RD,** eds. Hemopoietic system. Berlin: Springer-Verlag, 1990.
46. **Davis LA, Morton DG.** Granulocytic leukemia and uterine adenocarcinoma in a white-footed mouse (peromyscus leucopus). Lab Anim Sci 1993; 43:367–369.
47. **Heath JE.** Granulocytic leukemia in rats: a report of two cases. Lab Anim Sci 1981;31:504–506.
48. **Benjamin SA, Brooks AL.** Spontaneous lesions in Chinese hamsters. Vet Pathol 1977;14:449–462.
49. **Port DC, Richter WR.** Eosinophilic leukemia in a syrian hamster. Vet Pathol 1977;14:283–286.
50. **Loeb WF, Gard EA, Valerio MG.** Acute monocytic leukemia in an African green monkey. Lab Anim Sci 1982;32:428 [Abstract].
51. **Roskof WJ, Howard EB, Gendron AP.** Granulocytic leukemia in a tortoise. Mod Vet Pract 1981;701–702.
52. **Messick JB, McCullough SM, Treadwell NG, et al.** What is your diagnosis? Dysmyelopoiesis secondary to severe leukopenic episode. Vet Clin Pathol 1997;26:23–25,36–37.
53. **Reimann N, Bartnitzke S, Bullerdick J, et al.** Trisomy 1 in a canine acute leukemia indicating the pathogenetic importance of polysomy 1 in leukemias of the dog. Cancer Genet Cytogenet 1998;101:49–52.

CHAPTER 107

Feline Leukemia Virus and Feline Immunodeficiency Virus

• HOLLY JORDAN

Two of the most common infectious causes of feline illness and death, feline leukemia virus (FeLV) and feline immunodeficiency virus (FIV), are frequently associated with hemolymphatic disease. Characterization of these retroviral infections has had a significant effect on feline health and has also provided valuable contributions to our understanding of the pathogenesis of related human disorders, such as acquired immunodeficiency syndromes and leukemogenesis. First described by Jarrett et al in 1964,[1] FeLV is a C-type oncornavirus (e.g., oncogenic or tumor-causing RNA virus) in the family Retroviridae similar to avian and murine leukemia viruses. It causes not only neoplastic disorders such as, leukemia and lymphoid neoplasia, but is also associated with nonneoplastic diseases that include cytopenias and immune dysfunction. The first report of FIV, also a retrovirus, appeared in 1987.[2] Owing in part to its prolonged clincial course, the nononcogenic FIV is classified in the lentivirus (from Latin *lentus,* slow) subfamily and causes progressive debilitation of the immune system.

PREVALENCE

Both viruses have a worldwide distribution. In healthy domestic cat populations within the United States, the seroprevalence of FeLV and FIV infections are similar (approximately 2 to 5%).[3-5] Infection rates may be twofold to threefold higher in other countries, particularly some parts of Europe, Australia, and Japan.[6-8] Not surprisingly, sick cat populations maintain a two to four times greater infection rate, compared with healthy cats.[4,6-10] This is particularly true of cats that have hematologic abnormalities. In one Canadian survey, nearly half of the patient group that had severe cytopenias were FeLV seropositive, whereas 87% of patients that had hematopoietic neoplasms were FeLV infected.[11] Outdoor males are typically at greatest risk of infection, most likely owing to territorial fighting and biting behavior.[10] Many nondomestic cat species appear to be susceptible to FIV infection, although it is uncertain whether clinical illness results.[12,13] Interestingly, genetic analyses have so far demonstrated that nondomestic cat FIV isolates are usually distinct from the domestic cat FIV, suggesting that FIV-related viruses have been endemic in some of these species for a considerable time and that cross-species transmission is a rare event.[13] FeLV infection is apparently uncommon in exotic felids.[14]

PATHOGENESIS: FELINE LEUKEMIA VIRUS

FeLV is currently classified into three subgroups (A, B, and C) on the basis of envelope protein characteristics.[15] Preliminary data shows that these subgroups use different receptors. Subgroup A, which is present in all isolates and is transmitted in natural infections, putatively binds a 70-kD molecule that remains to be fully characterized.[16] Subgroup B is present in approximately half of virus isolates. It evolves from recombination of ectropic FeLV A and endogenous FeLV envelope gene elements.[17] Similar to gibbon ape leukemia virus, Subgroup B binds a Na^+-dependent phosphate symporter called Pit1.[18] Found in approximately 1% of isolates, subgroup C also arises de novo from FeLV A through mutation or recombination with endogenous FeLV sequences.[15] Current evidence suggests its receptor is homologous to a D-glucarate transporter molecule in the major facilitator superfamily.[19] The surface envelope glycoprotein, SU, is an important determinant of cell tropism and receptor recognition. SU mutations influence pathogenicity, for example, virus variant 61C causes fatal immunodeficiency, whereas the variant, FeLV-Sarma-C, causes aplastic anemia.[20]

Transmission most frequently occurs through direct contact with saliva and nasal secretions by means of licking, grooming, biting, or through shared food or water dishes.[21] Vertical transmission can also occur and sexual transmission is likely.[21] Subsequent to oropharyngeal exposure, the virus initially replicates in macrophages and CD4+ T, CD8+ T, and B lymphocytes in regional lymph nodes.[22] The virus then distributes throughout the lymphoid system, including thymus, spleen, lymph nodes, gut-associated lymphoid tissue, and bone marrow, where replication proceeds in follicular center cells, intestinal crypt cells, marrow stromal fibroblasts and myeloid, erythroid, and megakaryocytic precursors.[21,22] Most cats (approximately 60%) develop adequate immunity and either a transient or self-limiting infection.[21] Thirty percent of cats fail to contain viral replication and become persistently viremic.[21,22] In such cats the virus disseminates widely throughout epithelial tissues, including the salivary glands, oropharynx, nasal passages, trachea, esophagus, stomach, intestines, pancreas, uterus, and urinary bladder. This typically occurs within 4 to 6 weeks after exposure, though in a small proportion of cats persistent viremia may not be detectable until 3 months after exposure.[5] Virus shedding via these tissues can begin as early as 3 weeks after infection.[15] Chronically viremic cats usually succumb to progressive immune suppression, lymphoid and myeloid cell depletion, or neoplasia within 2 to 4 years. In a small proportion of cats (5 to 10%), FeLV is sequestered in select tissues for weeks to years.[21,22] Such latent infections may potentially be reactivated by immunosuppressive drugs or other stressors, although this appears to be uncommon.[22]

Researchers initially studied FeLV as a model of virally induced leukemia endemic in an outbred mammalian species.[1,15] However, lymphoma, particularly T-cell origin, is the most common malignancy associated with infection.[23,24] Myeloproliferative diseases and fibrosarcoma have also been reported in infected cats.[21] In recent years the presence of at least three genetic determinants of FeLV-induced transformation have been elucidated: (1) transcriptional regulatory sequences in the viral long terminal repeat, (2) insertional mutagenesis or transduction of host cellular proto-oncogenes such as c-*myc*, *pim-1*, *flvi-1*, or *fit-1*, and (3) functional virally encoded structural proteins.[25] Transformed cells may express a unique neoantigen called feline oncornavirus-associated cell membrane antigen (FOCMA). This molecule likely represents FeLV-related envelope antigens.[22] Antibody responses to this antigen confer protection to tumor development.[26]

Despite its recognition as a leukemogenic virus, a minority of naturally FeLV-infected cats actually go on to develop neoplasia.[27,28] Most cats succumb to cachexia, secondary infections, or degenerative blastopenic processes in association with progressive immune suppression.[21,29] The majority of FeLV isolates eventually cause immune deficiency,[21] although FeLV feline AIDS (FAIDS), a naturally occurring isolate derived from the thymic lymphoma of a domestic cat, causes an accelerated acquired immunodeficiency syndrome (AIDS).[30] Animals infected with FeLV FAIDS develop leukopenia, lymphopenia, and persistent loss of CD4+ and CD8+ T-cells.[21] These cats also have delayed skin allograft rejection, impaired gamma M immunoglobulin (IgM) and gamma G immunoglobulin (IgG) responses to T-dependent antigens, and defective T-helper activity.[30] Lymphocyte loss is thought to be caused by direct cytopathicity through cell killing and fusion.[20] Apoptotic

mechanisms may also be involved.[31] Immune dysfunction and tumor development may be interrelated in FeLV infection through impaired immune recognition of transformed cells and possibly through activation of other latent oncogenic viruses.[32]

PATHOGENESIS: FELINE IMMUNODEFICIENCY VIRUS

In community-acquired infections, FIV is most likely transmitted most frequently via saliva or blood through biting.[33] Sexual transmission may also occur[34] and offspring can be infected in utero, peripartum, and through nursing.[35] Lymphoid tissues, bone marrow, and salivary glands are the primary targets for initial viral replication.[36,37] The virus can subsequently be detected in various nonlymphoid tissues, including the brain, kidney, lung.[37] The molecular receptor(s) for FIV are uncertain. CD4 is not a receptor.[38] CD9, initially thought to be a receptor, now appears to function in postentry events.[38,39] Like the human lentivirus, human immunodeficiency virus type 1 (HIV-1), the chemokine receptor, CXCR4, may also play a role in FIV entry.[40] Cellular targets of FIV include T lymphocytes (CD4+ and CD8+), B lymphocytes, macrophages, megakaryocytes, and astrocytes. CD4+ T lymphocytes appear to be predominant targets during primary infection, CD8+ T lymphocytes and B lymphocytes harbor higher provirus levels during chronic infection.[41]

Feline lentivirus infection is similar to that seen in HIV-1-infected people.[42] Acute infection is characterized by transient high plasma virus loads, mild to moderate panlymphopenia, and nonspecific illnesses, such as fever and lymphadenopathy. Concomitant with the appearance of an antibody response 2 to 6 weeks after infection, circulating virus levels decline and cats usually become asymptomatic for months to years. Despite the presence of humoral and cellular immune activity, however, most cats do not clear virus and remain persistently infected. Indeed, progressive immune dysfunction may continue during the asymptomatic phase, and patients may ultimately develop diseases associated with acquired immune deficiency (e.g., progressive generalized lymphadenopathy, cachexia, opportunistic infections, chronic infections, etc.).[41,42] Interestingly, provirus-positive cats without detectable antibodies have been described,[43] suggesting that a small proportion of exposed cats either contain viral replication or encounter a defective virus variant. FIV-related immunologic changes also parallel those seen in HIV-1 infection.[37] CD4+ T-cell numbers decline, CD8+ T-cell populations expand, particularly CD8α+β and CD8α+β[10] subpopulations, and CD4+:CD8+ T-cell ratios decrease.[41,44] Like FeLV, the mechanisms of CD4+ T-cell loss appear to involve direct cell killing, cell fusion, and apoptotic pathways.[37,45] Seropositive cats also demonstrate reduced proliferative responses to mitogens and interleukin (IL) -2, decreased responses to T-dependent, but not T-independent antigens, polyclonal B-cell activation, and hypergammaglobulinemia.[41,46] Cytokine production is frequently altered. Plasma tumor necrosis factor α (TNF-α) concentrations may be elevated, and production of IL-1 and IL-6 by stimulated peripheral blood leukocytes is enhanced.[46] Experimental evidence suggests that overexpression of IL-10 in conjunction with decreased IL-2 and IL-12 expression influences loss of resistance to opportunistic intracellular pathogens.[47]

CLINICAL DISEASE

Because of the broad range of clinical illnesses seen in retrovirus infections, the presence of FeLV or FIV infection is generally considered in the diagnostic workup for all sick cats. FeLV and FIV cause many similar presenting clinical signs, such as fever, weight loss, lymphadenopathy, lethargy, gingivitis, and diarrhea.[5] FeLV is also associated with leukemia, lymphoid and myeloid malignancies, cytopenias, myelodysplastic syndromes, glomerulonephritis, neurologic disease, immune complex disease, reproductive failure, and failure to thrive in kittens.[5] Additional clinical illnesses observed in FIV patients include stomatitis, respiratory disease, anterior uveitis, neurologic disorders, as well as lymphoid and nonlymphoid malignancies.[37] Because both retroviruses can cause immune dysfunction, infected cats may present initially with illnesses referable to secondary pathogens (e.g., other viruses, bacteria, fungi, parasites, or protozoa).[48]

HEMATOLOGIC DISORDERS ASSOCIATED WITH FELINE RETROVIRAL INFECTIONS

Feline Leukemia Virus

Nonregenerative anemia is common in FeLV-seropositive cats.[49] Mild to moderate, normocytic to macrocytic, normochromic anemia with little polychromasia and reticulocytopenia is frequently seen. With the exception of macrocytosis, this general pattern is characteristic of the anemia of chronic inflammatory conditions and may be attributed to the presence of the virus, other secondary infections, or neoplasia.[28] Such cats often exhibit erythroid hypoplasia[50] and decreased blast-forming unit-erythroid (BFU-E) and colony-forming unit-erythroid[51] (CFU-E) with elevated erythropoietin levels.[51,52] The mechanism of normocytic macrocytosis (MCV >55 fl) in the absence of reticulocytosis is uncertain, but is likely related to defective erythrocytic maturation.[53] Hemolytic changes, e.g., regenerative anemia, erythroid hyperplasia, or normoblastemia, are apparent in approximately 10% of FeLV anemias and have been associated with the opportunistic hemoparasite, *Hemobartonella felis*, or an immune-mediated cause.[5] Interestingly, a positive Coomb's test result may be seen in FeLV-positive cats in the absence of hemolytic disease.[54] A profound, fatal anemia known as pure red cell aplasia develops in a small proportion (<1%) of FeLV-infected cats.[19,28] This condition is characterized by a severe, progressive depletion of red blood cells at all maturation

stages. Hematocrits are typically less than 10%, and cats lack circulating reticulocytes. Diagnosis is confirmed by the absence of erythroid precursors in bone marrow specimens with persistence of myeloid and megakaryocytic populations. These cats have normal erythrocyte survival times and elevated erythropoietin levels.[28] FeLV subgroup C isolates are usually associated with this condition, and Abkowitz[55] has hypothesized that viral proteins, such as gp70, directly inhibit BFU-E differentiation.

Total leukocyte concentrations may be high, normal, or decreased during FeLV infection. Elevated neutrophil counts can be observed in patients that have concomitant inflammatory illness. Absolute lymphopenia or neutropenia are common, although they usually occur in conjunction with other hematologic deficiencies.[28] Both CD4+ and CD8+ T-lymphocyte populations decline during FeLV infection; CD4+:CD8+ T-cell ratios may be normal or decreased.[56,57] Low neutrophil concentrations may be transient, persistent, or cyclical.[28] The mechanism of neutropenia is unknown, although some cats respond to steroid administration implicating an immune-mediated component. Bone marrow studies have shown that the frequencies of CFU-granulocyte-macrophage (CFU-GM) are typically normal, but maturation arrest at the metamyelocyte stage in some animals points to a developmental blockade.[28] Loss of neutrophil function has been documented in FeLV-infected cats.[5] Deficient granulocytic defense is likely one mechanism that predisposes cats to secondary infections. Indeed, 9% of FeLV deaths may be attributed to sepsis secondary to a generalized panleukopenia. This panleukopenic syndrome appears clinically and histologically similar to feline parvovirus infection.[5] Cats typically present with vomiting, diarrhea, and anemia and bone marrow aspirates demonstrate myeloblastopenia. This syndrome is particularly devastating in kittens infected with FeLV-FAIDS variants.[30]

FeLV infects megakaryocytes and platelets, thus it is not surprising that infected cats may become thrombocytopenic.[58] Thrombocytopenia is likely caused by several mechanisms, including direct cytopathicity, defective platelet production, and immune-mediated destruction. Platelet function may also be subnormal in infected patients.[5] Morphologic platelet abnormalities are not uncommon; giant platelets have been attributed to a virally induced demarcation defect.[58] However, a predisposition to hemorrhage has not been clearly documented. Transient thrombocytosis occurs in some viremic cats.[28]

Pancytopenia has been described in FeLV-infected cats.[28] Patients present with severe nonregenerative anemia, neutropenia, lymphopenia, and thrombocytopenia. All cell lines are deficient in bone marrow specimens. In some cases, this likely represents progressive infection with FeLV subtype C.[28] Pancytopenia may also appear in cats with myeloproliferative disease, leukemia, or FeLV-associated myelofibrosis or osteosclerosis. Not surprisingly, FeLV subtype C has been associated with medullary osteosclerosis wherein viral infection of osteocytes and osteoblasts is associated with defective bone resorption and remodeling, resulting in excessive boney trabecule within the marrow cavity.[5,59]

Cats presenting with myeloproliferative disease are highly suspect for FeLV infection—nearly 80% of patients that have this condition are FeLV positive.[60] These cats often develop moderate to severe nonregenerative, macrocytic anemia, and other cytopenias. Marrow cellularity is normal to increased with increased immaturity.[5] Megaloblastic erythroid cells and giant platelets have been described,[28] and medullary sclerosis may be observed.[59]

FeLV has been associated with nearly all types of acute lymphoid and myeloid leukemia in the cat with the exception of eosinophilic leukemia.[28] Indeed, the frequency of FeLV infections among cats that have acute myeloid leukemia reportedly approaches 90%.[60] These patients have normal or increased total leukocyte numbers and circulating blasts are usually evident. In addition to leukemia, patients may develop nonregenerative anemia or thrombocytopenia. Bone marrow specimens are hypercellular with greater than 30% blasts. FeLV is also highly associated with lymphoid malignancies.[27,61] Most cats (70%) with lymphoblastic leukemia and a similar proportion of cats with lymphosarcoma are FeLV positive.[62] Jackson and colleagues[62] found that a large majority of feline lymphosarcomas contain FeLV DNA (74%) and most (54%) express viral proteins. T-lymphocyte tumors are most common, though B-lymphocyte tumors are also reported in FeLV-infected cats.[61,62] Interestingly, cats that have chronic lymphocytic leukemia are usually FeLV negative.[28]

Feline Immunodeficiency Virus

With the exception of lymphopenia or neutropenia, hematologic abnormalities are frequently not detected in cats that have naturally acquired FIV infection until they become ill at which point peripheral blood-cell changes are common and varied.[28,63–65] The mechanisms underlying these changes remain to be clarified. Hematologic responses to the sequela of generalized immune dysfunction (e.g., concurrent infections, malnutrition, cachexia, neoplasia) are likely to be major factors, but it is uncertain to what extent the virus mediates these effects directly. Indeed, FIV does not replicate in erythroid or granulocytic precursors, unlike FeLV.[66] Furthermore, Linenberger, et al[66] have shown that hematologically normal FIV-positive cats exhibit normal frequencies of CFU-E, BFU-E, and CFU-GM, cell-cycle kinetics, and in vitro growth characteristics. Nonetheless, the virus can be found in bone marrow within lymphocytes, macrophages, and megakaryocytes. Morphologic marrow changes have been reported, including increased concentrations of lymphocytes and plasma cells, and occasionally the presence of lymphoid aggregates or follicles. Increased eosinophils, megaloblastic dysmorphic features, and hyperplasia of individual cell lines have also been described.[28,63,67,68] Thus, it is possible that the feline lentivirus may be similar to HIV-1 for which there is strong evidence that infection of auxillary cells (T cells,

macrophages, and endothelial cells) and viral gene products indirectly influence hematopoietic activity.[69]

In some surveys, anemia has been detected in nearly 40% of FIV seropositive cats.[64,68,70,71] Most patients manifest mild, nonregenerative anemia.[8,28,64,72] Low hematocrits (<24%) may be identified in seropositive cats that lack a concurrent disease, but are more common in sick patients, suggesting that anemia in FIV AIDS patients may be caused, in part, by the mechanisms underlying anemia of chronic inflammation.[28] Decreased frequency of BFU-E have been reported in chronically infected cats.[63] H. felis, has been detected in as many as 10% of blood samples from FIV-positive cats, though hemolytic anemia is uncommon in these patients.[64] Interestingly, Walker and Canfield[68] found that healthy infected cats have fewer type 1 reticulocytes and fewer mature erythroid cells, compared with uninfected healthy cats, indicating that the potential for virally induced erythroid effects cannot be excluded.

Lymphopenia is one of the most consistently identified leukocytic changes in seropositive cats.[28,64,68] As mentioned, this is primarily attributed to both a relative and absolute CD4+ T-cell loss. Neutropenia is evident in as much as 34% of FIV-infected patients.[64,72] It tends to be mild and transient, although it may be pronounced in some experimental infections.[73–76] Severe neutropenia has been reported also in naturally FIV-infected cats treated with the antifungal drug, griseofulvin.[71] Although this drug-associated neutropenia is likely to have an immune-mediated component, other suggested factors related to low neutrophil counts in FIV infection include a serum inhibitor of myeloid progenitor growth, accessory cell dysfunction, alterations in cell-cycle and growth characteristics, and reduced frequencies of CFU-GM.[73,75] Other leukocytic abnormalities, e.g., leukocytosis, neutrophilia, monocytosis, and transient lymphocytosis,[63–65,72] have been reported in seropositive cat populations with variable frequencies and probably depend on health status and stage of infection.

Platelet concentrations are typically within normal reference ranges in FIV-infected cats.[72] As many as 16% of patients have mild thrombocytopenia caused by an undetermined mechanism.[28] Immune-mediated thrombocytopenia has not been reported and platelet function does not appear to be altered in infected animals.[77] Prolonged activated partial thromboplastin time and thrombin time have been described in seropositive cats, however, hemorrhagic tendencies are rare.[28,77]

Although FIV has not been shown to be directly oncogenic, infection is associated with an increased likelihood of malignancy, including lymphoid and myeloid neoplasias, and various carcinomas and sarcomas.[41] Shelton et al[61] calculated that seropositive cats have a 5.6 times greater relative risk of developing leukemia or lymphoma than seronegative cats. Lymphosarcoma is the most common neoplasm in seropositive animals.[61] These tumors are usually extranodal and most commonly express a B-lymphocyte phenotype, although T and non-B or non-T lymphoid tumors have been described.[78,79] In contrast to FeLV, it is uncommon to find viral constituents in these neoplasms.[78–80]

DIAGNOSIS

The American Association of Feline Practitioners and the Academy of Feline Medicine have jointly issued comprehensive guidelines pertaining to diagnostic testing for feline retroviruses that emphasize the importance of patient risk, confirmatory testing, and follow-up.[81] In clinical practice cats are screened for FeLV infection most commonly with enzyme-linked immunosorbent assay (ELISA) technology that detects circulating FeLV protein in serum, plasma, whole blood, tears, or saliva. Currently, the recommended confirmatory test for FeLV infection is an immunofluorescence assay (IFA) that detects FeLV antigens in leukocytes or platelets on blood smears, buffy coat smears, or bone marrow aspirates. In contrast to FeLV, cats that have FIV infection often have low levels of circulating virus, thus most commercial FIV diagnostic tests detect antibodies against the virus rather than viral proteins. However, because it is unlikely that FIV-infected cats clear infection, despite the presence of an antibody response, seropositive cats are usually considered to have lifelong infections.[82] An FIV ELISA is typically used as a screening test. It is recommended that positive ELISA results be confirmed with a Western blot or IFA. Alternative tests for feline retroviruses are currently under development and future detection methodologies will likely exploit molecular techniques currently used by research laboratories, for instance, polymerase chain reaction to detect viral nucleic acids.[11]

PATIENT MANAGEMENT

Most persistently viremic FeLV-infected cats die within 3 to 4 years after initial diagnosis.[83] Asymptomatic FIV-infected cats can survive for many years; however, once cats develop AIDS-like diseases, the prognosis shortens to approximately six months.[84] Therapeutic options for feline retroviral infections have been reviewed elsewhere.[5] Currently, most retroviral therapies in cats are experimental with no consistently effective regimens. Immunomodulators (e.g., acemannan, *Propionibacterium acnes*), cytokines, and antiviral drugs have been investigated with variable success.[5,85] Promising results have been reported in FeLV-infected cats receiving adoptive transfer of activated T lymphocytes in conjunction with zidovudine and interferon (IFN)-α.[86] Prevention of retroviral infections is key and is accomplished through testing and quarantine, as well as vaccination. There are no commercially available FIV vaccines at the present, despite intensive research in this area. FeLV vaccines have been available for numerous years and considerations for their use have been reviewed.[5,87]

REFERENCES

1. Jarrett WFH, Crawford EM, Martin WB, Davie F. Leukemia in the cat. A virus-like particle associated with leukaemia (lymphosarcoma). Nature 1964;202:567–569.
2. Pederson NC, Ho EW, Brown ML, Yamamoto JK. Isolation of a T-lymphotropic virus from domestic cats with an immunodeficieny-like syndrome. Science 1987;235:790–793.
3. Glennon PJ, Cockurn T, Stark DM. Prevalence of feline immunodeficiency virus and feline leukemia virus infections in random-source cats. Lab Anim Sci 1991;41:545–547.
4. Grindem CB, Corbett WT, Ammerman BE, Tompkins MT. Seroepidemiological survey of feline immunodeficiency virus infection in cats of Wake County, North Carolina. J Am Vet Med Assoc 1989;194:226–228.
5. Rojko JL, Hardy WD Jr. Feline leukemia virus and other retroviruses. In: Scherding RG, ed. The cat: diseases and clinical management. New York: Churchill Livingstone, 1994;263–432.
6. Braley J. FeLV and FIV: survey shows prevalence in the United States and Europe. Feline Pract 1994;22:25–28.
7. Ishida T, Washizu T, Toriyabe K, Motoyoshi S, Tomoda I. Feline immunodeficiency virus infection in cats of Japan. J Am Vet Med Assoc 1989; 194:221–225.
8. Walker C, Canfield PJ, Love DN, McNeil DR. A longitudinal study of lymphocyte subsets in a cohort of cats naturally-infected with feline immunodeficiency virus. Aust Vet J 1996;73:218–224.
9. Hosie MJ, Robertson C, Jarrett O. Prevalence of feline leukemia virus and antibodies to feline immunodeficiency virus in cats in the United Kingdom. Vet Rec 1989;128:293–297.
10. O'Connor TP, Tonelli QJ Scarlett JM. Report of the National FeLV/FIV awareness project. J Am Vet Med Assoc 1991;199:1348–1353.
11. Jackson ML, Haines DM, Taylor SM, Misra V. Feline leukemia virus detection by ELISA and PCR in peripheral blood from 68 cats with high, moderate, or low suspicion of having FeLV-related disease. J Vet Diagn Invest 1996; 8:25–30.
12. Plotnick AN, Larsen RS. Feline lentivirus infection in nondomestic felids. Semin Vet Med Surg (Small Anim) 1995;10:251–255.
13. VandeWoude S, O'Brien SJ, Langelier K, Hardy WD, Slattery JP, Zuckerman EE, Hoover EA. Growth of lion and puma lentiviruses in domestic cat cells and comparisons with FIV. Virology 1997;233:185–192.
14. Lutz H, Isenbugel E, Lehmann R, Sabapara RH, Wolfensberger C. Retrovirus infection in non-domestic felids: serological studies and attempts to isolate a lentivirus. Vet Immunol Immunopathol 1992;35:215–224.
15. Jarrett O. Overview of feline leukemia virus research. J Am Vet Med Assoc 1991;199:1279–1281.
16. Ghosh AK, Bachmann MH, Hoover EA, Mullins JI. Identification of a putative receptor for subgroup A feline leukemia virus on feline T cells. J Virol 1992;66:3707–3714.
17. Chen H, Bechtel MK, Shi Y, Phipps A, Mathes LE, Hayes KA, Roy-Burman P. Pathogenicity induced by feline leukemia virus, Rickard strain, subgroup A plasmic DNA (pFRA). J Virol 1998;72:7048–7056.
18. Tailor C, Kabat D. Variable regions A and B in the envelope glycoproteins of feline leukemia virus subgroup B and amphotropic murine leukemia virus interact with discrete receptor domains. J Virol 1997;71:9383–9391.
19. Quigley JG, Burns CC, Anderson MM, Lynch ED, Sabo KM, Overbaugh J, Abkowitz JL. Cloning of the cellular receptor for feline leukemia virus subgroup C (FeLV-C), a retrovirus that induces red cell aplasia. Blood 2000;95:1093–1099.
20. Rohn JL, Overbaugh J. Feline leukemia virus and feline immunodeficiency virus. In: Chen ISY, Ahmed R, eds. Persistent viral infections. New York: John Wiley and Sons, 1999;379–408.
21. Hoover EA, Mullins JI. Feline leukemia virus infection and diseases. J Am Vet Med Assoc 1991;199:1287–1297.
22. Rojko JL, Kociba GJ. Pathogenesis of infection by the feline leukemia virus. J Am Vet Med Assoc 1991;199:1305–1310.
23. Hardy WD Jr. Oncogenic viruses of cats: the feline leukemia and sarcoma viruses. In: Holzworth J, ed. Diseases of the cat: medicine and surgery. Philadelphia: WB Saunders, 1987;246–268.
24. Cotter SM. Feline leukemia virus: pathophysiology, prevention, and treatment. Cancer Invest 1992;10:173–181.
25. Levy LS, Starkey CR, Prabhu S, Lobelle-Rich PA. Cooperating events in lymphomagenesis mediated by feline leukemia virus. Leukemia 1997; 11(suppl 3);239–241.
26. Essex M, Sliski AH, Cotter SM, Jakowski RR, Hardy WD Jr. Immunosurveillance of naturally occurring feline leukemia. Science 1975;190:790–792.
27. Reinacher M. Disease associated with spontaneous feline leukemia virus (FeLV) infection in cats. Vet Immunol Immunopathol 1989;21:85–94.
28. Shelton GH, Linenberger ML. Hematologic abnormalities associated with retroviral infections in the cat. Semin Vet Med Surg 1995;10:220–233.
29. Hardy WD Jr, McClelland JA. Feline leukemia virus: its related diseases and control. Vet Clin North Am 1977;7:93–103.
30. Hoover EA, Mullins JI. FeLV/FAIDS immunodeficiency syndrome. In: Willett BJ, Jarrett O, eds. Feline immunology and immunodeficiency. New York: Oxford University Press, 1995;318–350.
31. Rojko JL, Fulton RM, Resanka LF, Williams LL, Copelan E, Cheney CM, Reichel GS, Neil JC, Mathes LE, Fisher TG, Cloyd MW. Lymphocytotoxic strains of feline leukemia virus induce apoptosis in feline T4–thymic lymphoma cells. Lab Invest 1992; 66:418–426.
32. Rohn JL, Gwynn SR, Lauring AS, Lineberger ML, Overbaugh J. Viral genetic variation, AIDS, and the multistep nature of carcinogenesis: the feline leukemia virus model. Leukemia 1996;10:1867–1869.
33. Yamamoto JK, Sparger E, Ho EW, Andersen PR, O'Connor TP, Mandell

CP, Lowenstine L, Munn R, Pedersen NC. Pathogenesis of experimentally induced feline immunodeficiency virus infection in cats. Am J Vet Res 1988; 49:1246–1258.

34. Jordan H, Howard J, Sellon R, Wildt D, Tompkins W, Kennedy-Stoskopf S. Transmission of feline immunodeficiency virus in domestic cats via artificial insemination. J Virol 1996;70:8224–8228.

35. O'Neil LL, Burkhard MJ, Diehl JL, Hoover EA. Vertical transmission of feline immunodeficiency virus. Semin Vet Med Surg (Small Anim) 1995; 10:267–278.

36. Beebe AM, Dua N, Faith TG, Moore PF, Pedersen NC, Dandekar S. Primary stage of feline immunodeficiency virus infection: viral dissemination and cellular targets. J Virol 1994;68:3080–3091.

37. Bendinelli M, Pistello M, Lombardi S, Poli A, Garzelli C, Matteucci D, Ceccherini-Nelli L, Malvaldi G, Tozzini F. Feline immunodeficiency virus: an interesting model for AIDS studies and an important cat pathogen. Clin Microbiol Rev 1995;8:87–112.

38. Willett BJ, Hosie MJ, Jarrett O, Neil JC. Identification of a putative cellular receptor for feline immunodeficiency virus as the feline homologue of CD9. Immunology 1994;81:228–233.

39. de Parseval A, Lerner DL, Borrow P, Willett BJ, Elder JH. Blocking of feline immunodeficiency virus infection by a monclonal antibody to CD9 is via inhibition of virus release rather than interference with receptor binding. J Virol 1997;71:5742–5749.

40. Willett BJ, Picard L, Hosie MJ, Turner JD, Adema K, Clapham PR. Shared usage of the chemokine receptor CXCR4 by the feline and human immunodeficiency viruses. J Virol 1997;71:6407–6415.

41. English RV, Tompkins MB. Effect of FIV infection on the peripheral immune system. In: Willett BJ, Jarrett O, eds. Feline immunology and immunodeficiency. New York: Oxford University Press, 1995;131–150.

42. Pedersen NC. Clinical overview of feline immunodeficiency virus. J Am Vet Med Assoc 1991;199:1298–1305.

43. Dandekar S, Beebe AM, Barlough J, Phillips T, Elder J, Torten M, Pedersen NC. Detection of feline immunodeficiency virus (FIV) nucleic acids in FIV-seronegative cats. J Virol 1992;66:4040–4049.

44. Shimojima M, Miyazawa T, Kohmoto M, Ikeda Y, Nishimura Y, Maeda K, Tohya Y, Mikami T. Expansion of CD8α+β− cells in cats infected with feline immunodeficiency virus. J Gen Virol 1998;79:91–94.

45. Johnson CM, Benson NA, Papadi GP. Apoptosis and CD4+ lymphocyte depletion following feline immunodeficiency virus infection of a T-lymphocyte cell line. Vet Pathol 1996;33:195–203.

46. Willett BJ, Flynn JN, Hosie MJ. FIV infection of the domestic cat: an animal model for AIDS. Immunol Today 1997;18:182–189.

47. Levy JK, Ritchey JW, Rottman JB, Davidson MG, Liang Y-H, Jordan HL, Tompkins WA, Tompkins MB. Elevated interleukin-10-to-interleukin-12 ratio in feline immunodeficiency virus-infected cats predicts loss of type1 immunity to Toxoplasma gondii. J Infect Dis 1998;178:503–511.

48. Lappin M. Opportunistic infections associated with retroviral infections in cats. Semin Vet Med Surg (Small Anim) 1995;10:244–250.

49. Cotter SM. Anemia associated with FeLV infection. J Am Vet Med Assoc 1979;175:1191–1194.

50. Hoover EA, Kociba GJ, Hardy WD, Yohn DS. Erythroid hypoplasia in cats inoculated with feline leukemia virus. J Natl Cancer Inst 1974;53:1271–1276.

51. Wardrop KJ, Kramer JW, Abkowitz JL, Clemons G, Adamson JW. Quantitative studies of erythropoiesis in the clinically normal, phlebotomized, and feline leukemia virus-infected cat. Am J Vet Res 1986;47:2274–2277.

52. Kociba GJ, Lange RD, Dunn CD. Serum erythropoietin changes in cats with FeLV-induced erythroid aplasia. Vet Pathol 1983;20:48–52.

53. Weiser MG, Kociba GJ. Erythrocyte macrocytosis in feline leukemia virus-associated anemia. Vet Pathol 1983;20:687–697.

54. Dunn JK, Searcy GP, Hirsch VM. The diagnostic significance of a positive direct antiglobulin test in anemic cats. Can J Comp Med 1984;48:349–353.

55. Abkowitz JL. Retrovirus-induced feline pure red cell aplasia: pathogenesis and response to suramin. Blood 1991;77:1442–1451.

56. Hoffmann-Fezer G, Bauer M, Hartmann K, Mysliwieta J, Thefeld S, Beer B, Thum I, Kraft W. Comparison of T-cell subpopulations in cats naturally infected with feline leukaemia virus or feline immunodeficiency virus. Res Vet Sci 1996;61:222–226.

57. Tompkins MB, Nelson PD, English RV, Novotney C. Early events in the immunopathogenesis of feline retrovirus infections. J Am Vet Med Assoc 1991;199:1311–1315.

58. Boyce JT, Kociba Gj, Jacobs RM, Weiser RM. Feline leukemia virus-induced thrombocytopenia and macrothrombocytosis in cats. Vet Pathol 1986;23:16–20.

59. Hoover EA, Kociba GJ. Bone lesions in cats with anemia induced by feline leukemia virus. J Natl Cancer Inst 1974;53:1277–1284.

60. Blue JT, French TW, Kranz JS. Non-lymphoid hematopoietic neoplasia in cats: a retrospective study of 60 cases. Cornell Vet 1988;78:21–42.

61. Shelton GH, Grant CK, Cotter SM, Abkowitz JL. Feline immunodeficiency virus and feline leukemia virus infections and their relationships to lymphoid malignancies in cats: a retrospective study (1968–1988). J Acquir Immun Defic Synd Hum Retrovirol 1990;3:623–630.

62. Jackson ML, Wood SL, Misra V, Haines DM. Immunohistochemical identification of B and T lymphocytes in formalin-fixed, paraffin-embedded feline lymphosarcomas: relation to feline leukemia virus status, tumor site and patient age. Can J Vet Res 1996;60:199–204.

63. Shelton GH, Linenberger ML, Persik MT, Abkowitz JL. Prospective hematologic and clinicopathlogic study of asymptomatic cats with naturally acquired feline immunodeficicency virus infection. J Vet Intern Med 1995; 9:133–140.

64. Sparkes AH, Hopper CD, Millard WG, Gruffydd-Jones TJ, Harbour DA. Feline immunodeficiency virus infection. Clinicopathologic findings in 90 naturally occurring cases. J Vet Intern Med 1993;7:85–90.

65. Thomas JB, Robinson WF, Chadwick BJ, Robertson ID, Jones PS. Leukogram and biochemical abnormalities in naturally occurring feline immunodeficiency virus infection. J Am Anim Hosp Assoc 1993;29:272–278.

66. Linenberger ML, Shelton GH, Persik MT, Abkowitz JL. Hematopoiesis in asymptomatic cats infected with feline immunodeficiency virus. Blood 1991;78:1963–1968.

67. Beebe AM, Gluckstern TG, George J, Pedersen NC, Dandekar S. Detection of feline immunodeficiency virus infection in bone marrow of cats. Vet Immunol Immunopathol 1992;35:37–49.

68. Walker C, Canfield P. Haematological findings in cats naturally infected with feline immunodeficiency virus. Comp Haematol Intl 1996;6:77–85.

69. Moses A, Nelson J, Bagby GC Jr. The influence of human immunodeficiency virus-1 on hematopoiesis. Blood 1998;91:1479–1495.

70. Hopper CD, Sparks AH, Gruffyd-Jones TJ, et al. Clinical and laboratory findings in cats infected with feline immunodeficiency virus. Vet Rec 1989; 125:341–346.

71. Shelton GH, Grant CK, Linenberger ML, Abkowitz JL. Severe neutropenia associated with griseofulvin therapy in cats with feline immunodeficiency virus infection. J Vet Intern Med 1990;4:317–319.

72. Shelton GH, Linenberger ML, Abkowitz JL. Hematologic abnormalities in cats seropositive for feline immunodeficiency virus. J Am Vet Med Assoc 1991;199:1353–1357.

73. Linenberger ML, Beebe AM, Pedersen NC, Abkowitz JL, Dandekar S. Marrow accessory cell infection and alterations in hematopoiesis accompany severe neutropenia during experimental acute infection with feline immunodeficiency virus. Blood 1995;85:941–951.

74. Mandell CP, Parger EE, Pedersen NC, Jain NC. Long-term haematological changes in cats experimentally infected with feline immunodeficiency virus (FIV). Comp Haematol Intl 1992;2:8–17.

75. Shelton GH, Abkowitz JL, Linenberger, ML, Russell RG, Grant CK. Chronic leukopenia associated with feline immunodeficiency virus infection in a cat. J Am Vet Med Assoc 1989;194:253.

76. Shelton GH, Linenberger ML, Grant CK, Gardner MB, Hardy WD Jr, DiGiacomo GF. Hematologic manifestations of feline immunodeficiency virus infection. Blood 1990;76:1104–1109.

77. Hart SW, Nolte I. Hemostatic disorders in feline immunodeficiency virus-seropositive cats. J Vet Intern Med 1994;8:355–362.

78. Callanan JJ, Jones BA, Irvine J, Willett BJ, McCandlish IAP, Jarrett O. Histologic classification and immunophenotype of lymphosarcomas in cats with naturally and experimentally acquired feline immunodeficiency virus infections. Vet Pathol 1996;33:264–272.

79. Endo Y, Cho K, Nishigaki K, Momoi Y, Nishimura Y, Mizuno T, Goto Y, Watari T, Tsujimoto H, Hasegawa A. Molecular characteristics of malignant lymphomas in cats naturally infected with feline immunodeficiency virus. Vet Immunol Immunopathol 1997;57:153–167.

80. Beatty JA, Callanan JJ, Terry A, Jarrett O, Neil JC. Molecular and immunophenotypical characterization of a feline immunodeficiency virus (FIV)-associated lymphoma: a direct role for FIV in B-lymphocyte transformation. J Virol 1998;72:767–771.

81. American Association of Feline Practitioners and the Academy of Feline Medicine. Recommendations for FeLV and FIV testing. Compend Contin Educ Pract Vet. 1997;19:1105–1107.

82. Barr MC. FIV, FeLV, and FIPV: interpretation and misinterpretation of serological test results. Semin Vet Med Surg (Small Anim) 1996;11:144–153.

83. Macy DW. Management of the FeLV-positive patient. In: Kirk RW, Bonagura JD, eds. Current veterinary therapy. Philadelphia: WB Saunders, 1989;10: 1069–1076.

84. Macy DW. Feline immunodeficiency virus. In: Scherding RG, ed. The cat: diseases and clinical management. New York: Churchill Livingstone, 1994; 433–448.

85. McCaw D. Caring for the retrovirus infected cat. Semin Vet Med Surg (Small Anim) 1995;10:216–219.

86. Zeidner NS, Mathiason-DuBard CK, Hoover EA. Reversal of feline leukemia virus infection by adoptive transfer of activated T lymphocytes, interferon alpha, and zidovudine. Semin Vet Med Surg (Small Anim) 1995; 10:256–266.

87. Elston T, Rodan H, Flemming D, Ford RB, Hustead DR, Richards JR, Rosen DK, Scherk-Nixon MA, Scott PW. 1998 Report of the American Association of Feline Practitioners and Academy of Feline Medicine Advisory Panel on Feline Vaccines. J Am Vet Med Assoc 1998;212:227–241.

CHAPTER 108

Chronic Myeloid Leukemias

• JOANNE B. MESSICK

Chronic myeloid leukemias (CMLs) are a group of clonal proliferative disorders that include chronic granulocytic leukemias (CGLs) that may be of the neutrophil, eosinophil, or basophil type, as well as chronic monocytic leukemia (CMoL), chronic myelomonocytic leukemia (CMMoL), polycythemia vera (PV), essential thrombocythemia (ET) and myelofibrosis with myeloid metaplasia (MMM) (Fig. 108.1). These disorders arise from the neoplastic transformation of a multipotent bone marrow stem cell (Fig. 108.2). Support for the clonal origin of CMLs is based on the discovery that human patients who have CGL possess the Philadelphia (Ph1) chromosome abnormality in not only the granulocytic cells but also in megakaryocytic, monocytic, and erythroid cells.[1] Moreover, analysis of restriction fragment length polymorphisms of several X chromosome-linked genes in human patients who have CMLs have recently been used to confirm the clonal nature of these disorders.[2] In veterinary species the clonal nature of the proliferative population is often unknown, and malignancy is based on a progressive clinical course that is unresponsive to therapy, aberrant cellular morphology, and absence of an underlying cause. CMLs are characterized by gradually increasing numbers of differentiated hemopoietic cells that results in a significant leukocytosis, erythrocytosis, or thrombocytosis. The exact reason why a particular cell population has a proliferative advantage is not known. It has been suggested that the primary defect in chronic leukemias may not be unregulated proliferation of leukemic stem cells but rather discordant maturation such that a slight delay in cell maturation results in the increased myeloid mass.[3]

CMLs are predominantly diseases of the older dog and cat, but they may occur at any age and has been reported in other species.[4] Typically, the onset of a CML is insidious, with a gradual increase in peripheral cell numbers, splenomegaly, hepatomegaly, and increasing systemic signs such as anorexia, weight loss, and anemia. At any time during the course of a CML, there may be a fairly abrupt change from a disease characterized by excessive production of functional, well-differentiated cells to a disorder associated with bone marrow failure or a terminal blast phase. Transformation into acute leukemia is common in human CGL patients and has also been reported in dogs and cats. Death may be related to organ infiltration and dysfunction or may occur because of hemorrhage and severe infection during chronic or terminal phases. In dogs and cats, the survival is months to years for CGL compared with a survival of only weeks to months for acute myelogenous leukemias patients.[5]

CMLs may be difficult to distinguish from hyperplastic responses and myelodysplastic syndromes (MDSs). Low or normal numbers of blast cells in the bone marrow accompanied by a peripheral blood neutrophilia more than twice normal are more consistent with myeloid hyperplasia. Features such as neutrophil toxicity, increased inflammatory proteins, and identification of an underlying cause for the response (i.e., inflammatory nidus and tumor) are also helpful in identifying a severe hyperplastic response. The rebound hemopoietic changes characteristic of dogs and cats after chemical or viral insults to the bone marrow may also be confused with an AML or CML and are ruled out by sequential examinations of blood and marrow. CMLs may be distinguished from MDSs by the absence of prominent dysplastic changes in the bone marrow and by the presence of a significant increase in cell counts in the peripheral blood.

CHRONIC GRANULOCYTIC LEUKEMIA

CGL results from a neoplastic transformation occurring in a single multipotent bone marrow stem cell. In humans CGL is associated with a characteristic chromosome abnormality known as Ph1.[3] The chromosomal abnormality found in all dividing hemopoietic cells involves the loss of chromosomal material from the long arm of one member of chromosome 22. In this translocation, cytogenetic materials from the breakpoint cluster region of chromosome 22 are fused with the cellular oncogene, c-alb, from chromosome 9 to form a hybrid gene (bcr-alb). This reciprocal translocation plays an important role in initiating neoplastic transformation and is associated with enhanced tyrosine kinase activity.[3] The abnormal kinase activity is believed to function in the regulation of cell growth, perhaps as the result of

FIGURE 108.1 CMPDs.

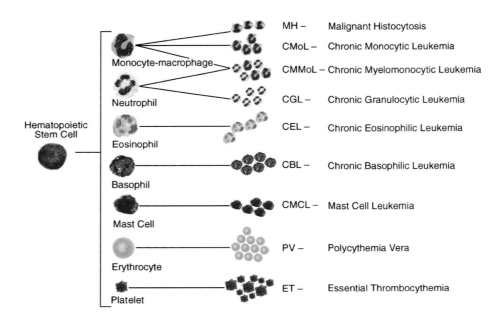

FIGURE 108.2 Origin of MPDs from a multipotent stem cell and transformations that may occur.

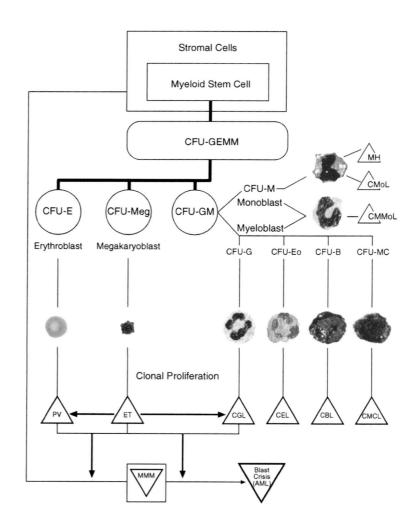

transcription activation of genes that rescue the cell from programmed cell death (apoptosis).

CGL is a rare myeloproliferative disorder in veterinary species. In the majority of dogs and cats that have CGL, a causative factor cannot be identified. However, a significantly increased risk of developing granulocytic leukemias, in both the acute and chronic forms, has been reported to occur in dogs and miniature swine subjected to high doses of radiation.[6] Often, a history of weight loss that may occur over several months exists, with depression and weakness associated with anemia. Myelophthisic or hemopoietic inhibition by cytokines may play a role in the pathogenesis of this anemia. In the peripheral blood, there is a variable degree of a granulocytosis, with a predominance of mature granulocytes; however, some or all other granulocytic precursors stages may also be found.[7] (Fig. 108.3) Leukocyte counts in dogs that have CGL may range from 16,000 to 169,000 cell/μL and in the cat, counts as high as 389,000/μL have been reported.[7] The neoplastic granulocytes may have enhanced cellular functions, including significantly increased phagocytic capacity, superoxide generation, and secretion of enzymes.[8] Enhanced granulocyte-macrophage-colony-stimulating factor (GM-CSF) synthesis has been hypothesized to be the cause for the observed cellular hyperresponsiveness. Further, it has been shown that CML in mice may be induced by retroviral transduction of the gene for GM-CSF, suggesting that excessive synthesis of this factor may induce leukemia.[9]

Hepatosplenomegaly is also a common finding in both dogs and cats that have CGL and is caused by organ infiltration by the neoplastic cells or extramedullary hematopoiesis. Examination of the bone marrow serves mainly to confirm the diagnosis already suspected from the peripheral blood findings. On bone marrow aspiration cytology, particles are densely hypercellular with almost complete obliteration of normal fat spaces. The myeloid-to-erythroid (M:E) ratio may range from 3:1 to as high as 24:1 and an abnormal myeloid maturation with increased numbers of myeloblasts, promyelocytes, and neutrophilic myelocytes is usually observed.[7] The granulocyte precursors may be abnormally large in size and display a bizarre nuclear shape, and in mature neutrophils, hypersegmentation may be a prominent feature. A bone marrow core biopsy is valuable for documenting the degree of fibrosis that may develop in the later stages of CGL.

CHRONIC BASOPHILIC LEUKEMIA

Basophilic leukemia is a rare chronic myeloproliferative disorder characterized by excessive production of basophils. Seven cases of basophilic leukemia have been reported in the dog.[10] These dogs had a significant splenomegaly, anemia, and leukocytosis in which most of the circulating leukocytes were basophils. In humans, basophilic leukemia has been associated with a specific chromosomal abnormality, uncommon clinical presentation, and occurrence in infancy. The clinical signs in these patients are consistent with a hyperhistaminemia syndrome and include urticarial rashes, gastrointestinal disorders, and peptic ulceration.[11]

In the majority of the canine cases, morphologic evidence of basophilic lineage was provided by light microscopy. However, cytochemical stains such as omega-exonuclease, a specific marker for basophils, in combination with the granulocyte marker, chloracetate esterase (CAE), have also been shown to be helpful in establishing a diagnosis.[12] The neoplastic basophilic population may be sensitive to hydroxyurea; however, hydroxyurea may also produce severe bone marrow suppression.[13]

MAST-CELL LEUKEMIA

Since the mast cell is derived from a myeloid stem cell, mast cell leukemia, can be regarded as a myeloproliferative disorder.[14] Mast-cell leukemia is a rare and aggressive proliferative disorder characterized by the presence of large numbers of atypical mast cells in the peripheral blood. The events responsible for mast cell proliferation in the leukemic process are largely unknown, however, in humans and dogs a derangement the *c-kit* receptor or its ligand is likely to play a primary role in this disease.[15–17] In contrast to the basophil, the development and secretory function of mast cells depends on stem cell factor, which is the ligand for the receptor encoded by *c-kit*.

Systemic mastocytosis may occur as a de novo leukemia or may be associated with one or more solid tumors in dogs, cats, and horses.[4] Whether the mastocytosis is associated with a leukemia or solid tumor, the result is often the same; there is an uncontrolled and progressive proliferation and infiltration of mast cells into various organs. In humans the criteria required for establishing a diagnosis of mast cell leukemia included:

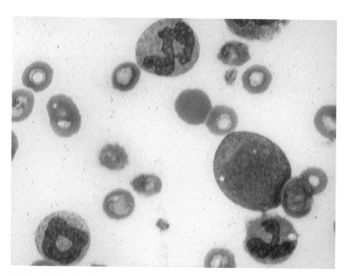

FIGURE 108.3 Peripheral blood from a dog that has CGL; myeloid cells are found at all stages of differentiation.

1. the percentage of mast cells in the peripheral blood differential being greater than 10%
2. the mast cells displaying cellular atypia
3. cytochemical staining of the leukemic cells being consistent with a mast cell lineage.[18]

The use of basic dyes such as Giemsa and toluidine blue may be helpful to demonstrate the specific metachromatic granules of the mast cells in tissue sections, whereas peroxidase and CAE staining may be used to help distinguish mast cell leukemia from other leukemias in which blast cells may contain cytoplasmic granules. Mild, transient peripheral blood mastocytosis has been reported in acute inflammatory conditions and increased numbers of mast cells have been described in hypoplastic or aplastic marrows of animals. These conditions must not be mistaken for a neoplastic process.

When dissemination occurs in the dog and cat, it is often associated with signs of systemic illness, including anorexia, vomiting, and diarrhea. Ulceration of the stomach and duodenum with subsequent perforation and peritonitis may also occur owing to the release of large amounts of mediators, such as histamine, from the mast cells. The most common gross lesion in mast cell leukemia is a significant splenomegaly. Mast-cell tumors can be found throughout the alimentary tract.

CHRONIC EOSINOPHILIC LEUKEMIA

Chronic eosinophilic leukemia (EL) is a rare myeloproliferative disorder in the cat. Typically, the patient has a significant proliferation of mature eosinophils in the peripheral blood. The differential diagnoses must include reactive eosinophilia and hypereosinophilic syndrome (HES). A reactive eosinophilia is defined as an absolute eosinophil count of $1.5 \times 10^3/\mu L$ or greater and that in which an underlying cause for the eosinophilia is recognized. The most common underlying causes of eosinophilia are parasitism, feline asthma, eosinophilic granuloma complex, eosinophilic enteritis, and neoplasia, in particular mast cell tumors.[19] However, the distinction between HES and EL is less clear and it has been suggested that these two conditions are variants of the same disorder. Both HES and EL are associated with a prolonged idiopathic peripheral and tissue eosinophilia and organ dysfunction[19–21] in which the overproduction of interleukin (IL)-5 may play a primary role in the disease process.[22] The presence of rare blasts in the peripheral blood, morphological abnormalities in eosinophils (intermediate forms containing both eosinophilic and basophilic granules), and immature eosinophilic infiltrates in the tissues have been used to confirm the diagnosis of EL.[19,23] Cats diagnosed with EL have a higher average M:E ratio with abnormal and immature eosinophils occurring more frequently and in higher proportions in the peripheral blood.[19] The hematocrit of leukemic cats was also significantly lower than in HES cats. A slight female predisposition was noted in the HES population.

CHRONIC MYELOMONOCYTIC LEUKEMIA, CHRONIC MONOCYTIC LEUKEMIA, AND MALIGNANT HISTIOCYTOSIS

Monocyte or macrophage malignancies are, for the most part, rare clonal disorders in veterinary species. These disorders are associated with proliferation of cells displaying enzymatic, functional or immunophenotypic characteristics of a histiocytic lineage. The suspicion of malignancy is also based on an aggressive clinical course or aberrant cellular morphology. The proliferative disorders involving the monocyte or macrophage series include (1) CMMoL, (2) CMoL, and (3) malignant histocytosis. Guidelines have been proposed for distinguishing, based on the peripheral blood findings, chronic granulocytic leukemia from myelomonocytic leukemia in humans (Table 108.1).[24]

CMMoL is a clonal stem cell disorder characterized by an excessive proliferation of mature and immature cells of both the granulocytic and monocytic series (Fig. 108.4). The clinical course of this disease is characterized by refractory anemia often with an unexplained leukopenia that gradually evolves to CMMoL. Based on multivariant analysis of clinical, hematologic, and biochemical features of CMMoL in humans, high monocyte counts, and spleen enlargement were identified as poor prognostic indicators for survival.[25] As with other chronic MPDs (CMPD), this disease may transform into an acute leukemia. Repeated examinations of blood and marrow with special stains or immunophenotyping are needed to confirm the diagnosis of CMMoL.

CMoL is a rare CMPD that is characterized by an excessive proliferation of cells of the monocytic series. This disease is frequently indolent with a clinical coarse that is characterized by a persistent monocytosis that is unresponsive to therapeutic agents. Splenomegaly of uncertain origin is a common finding, and initial hematologic evaluation may only reveal an anemia with a normal or low white cell count.[26] In humans, dermal lesions in which the malignant cells invade the skin before they appear in the peripheral blood or bone marrow, have been described.[27] Over time, the patient develops monocytosis, usually with an accompanying leukocytosis. There is a corresponding myeloid hyperplasia and an increase in the number of mature monocytes in the bone marrow. CMoL may terminate in blast crisis

---

TABLE 108.1 Peripheral Blood Findings that Distinguish Chronic Granulocytic Leukemia and Chronic Myelomonocytic Leukemia.[26]

Finding	CGL	CMMoL
Basophils	≥2%	<2%
Monocytes	<3%	≥3–10%; usually >10%
Granulocytic dysplasia	none	present
Immature granulocytes	>20%	≤10%
Blasts	≤2%	<2%

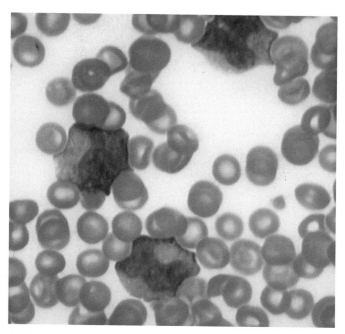

FIGURE 108.4 Peripheral blood smear from a cat demonstrating the spectrum of granulocytic and monocytic maturation found in CMMoL.

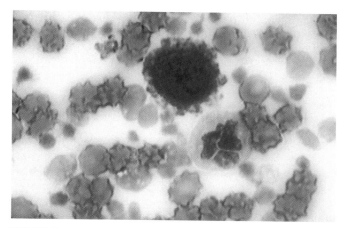

FIGURE 108.5 Peripheral blood of a dog that has ET. A persistently elevated platelet count that cannot be explained by a known cause was found. A rare micromegakaryoblast and bizarre, giant platelets were also noted.

with rapidly increasing numbers of immature cells of the monocyte lineage. As with CMMoL, repeated examinations of blood and marrow are necessary, in addition to special stains or immunophenotyping to confirm the diagnosis.

Malignant histiocytosis (MH) is a common proliferative disorder in the Bernese Mountain dog.[28] MH has a familial association in Bernese Mountain dogs, and in flat-coated retrievers and golden retrievers the incidence of this disorder may also be increased.[29] In other breeds the disorder is rare. MH is characterized by systemic proliferation and infiltration of tissues by morphologically atypical cells of the macrophage lineage. Splenic, liver, lymph node, lung, and bone marrow infiltration by malignant histiocytes typifies a majority of the canine cases.[29,30] Since the clonality of the neoplastic population is unknown, malignancy as applied to MH in the canine is based on the rapidly progressive clinical course and bizarre morphology of histocytes that have a propensity for phagocytosis, especially of erythrocytes. Staining for lysozyme, a marker for mononuclear phagocytic differentiation, is frequently positive in MH cases in the canine. Light and electron microscopic findings that include cytoplasmic vacuoles, lipid droplets, numerous lysosomes, phagocytic activity, and absence of junctional complexes, also support the histiocytic origin of this disorder.[30]

ESSENTIAL THROMBOCYTHEMIA (MEGAKARYOCYTIC MYELOSIS)

Essential thrombocythemia (ET) is an uncommon MPD in dogs and cats. The leukemic process is characterized by a persistently elevated platelet count that cannot be explained by a known cause (Fig. 108.5). Secondary or reactive thrombocytosis that may occur in malignancy, infection, iron-deficiency anemia, chronic inflammatory disease, or other MPD must be excluded before a diagnosis of ET can be established.[31] The PV study group have proposed the following criteria for supporting a diagnosis of ET in humans: more than 600×10^9 platelets/L, normal hemoglobin, stainable iron in marrow with normal values for ferritin and mean corpuscular volume, and absence of Ph-chromosome, marrow fibrosis and underlying cause for reactive thrombocytosis.[32] Recent reports suggests that ET may arise as a consequence of a mutation(s) in the gene that encodes for thrombopoietin or its receptor.[33,34]

ET is generally a disease of older animals and has been reported in three cats and six dogs.[35–37] Platelet counts often exceed $1.0 \times 10^6/\mu L$ in the peripheral blood. The platelets vary greatly in size, some of which are extremely large and show variable granulation and basophilia. Both hemorrhagic and thrombotic tendencies in this disorder have been reported. The most striking abnormality in the bone marrow is a significant increase in numbers of normal or atypical megakaryocytic cells. The megakaryocytes in ET are mature but distinguished by their larger than normal size and highly lobulated, high-ploidy, dense nuclei.

POLYCYTHEMIA VERA

Polycythemia vera (PV) is a clonal proliferative disorder characterized by erythropoietin-independent growth of primitive precursors, leading to a greatly expanded red cell mass. In humans the disease is often accompanied by a slight leukocytosis and thrombocytosis. This is an unusual finding in animals. The clinical course is indolent, however in the later stages of this disorder there may be increasing marrow fibrosis and eventual failure or transformation to an acute leukemia may occur in a low percentage of patients. The disease in animals is rare, although it has been described in cats, dogs, mice, and cattle.[38-40]

The diagnosis of PV requires an assessment of both plasma volume and red cell blood mass. Patients that have an increased red cell mass and decreased plasma volume have a relative polycythemia. Conditions such as shock and dehydration, which are commonly encountered in veterinary species, may induce relative polycythemia; in addition, this disease may develop in patients that are receiving diuretic or cardiac medications. On the other hand, patients that have an increased red cell mass that do not have a significant decrease in plasma volume have an absolute polycythemia that may be either a primary or a secondary disorder. Absolute polycythemia is classified as secondary if the patient is hypoxic or has a tumor and their serum concentrations of erythropoietin are increased.[41] Whereas, in the absence of hypoxia, polycythemia in a patient that has no other tumors and that has normal or decreased serum erythropoietin concentrations is classified as a primary MPD or PV.[42,43] Bone marrow examination is rarely helpful in making the diagnosis of PV.

MYELOFIBROSIS WITH MYELOID METAPLASIA (AGNOGENIC WITH MYELOID METAPLASIA)

MMM is a CMPD characterized by splenomegaly, extramedullary hematopoiesis, immature granulocytes, and erythroblasts in the blood (leukoerythroblastosis), teardrop-shaped red blood cells, and significant fibroblastic proliferation in the bone marrow. The primary disease process involves the neoplastic transformation and clonal proliferation of a single pluripotent hematopoietic stem cell. However, the myelofibrosis is a result of a nonclonal fibroblastic proliferation. Thus, the bone marrow fibrosis is a secondary or reactive process induced by growth factors released from abnormally proliferating hematopoietic cells, principally megakaryocytes.[44,45] The origin of MMM is unknown; however, animal models of the disease have been produced by the use of saponin, lead acetate, radiation, and benzene.[45] A single case report of this disorder occurring in a marmoset is found in the veterinary literature.[46]

In humans, MMM is interrelated to other CMPDs. Approximately 12 to 15% of patients that have PV and essential thrombocythemia may transform into a disorder simulating MMM, whereas 5% of patients that have CGL evolve into a state indistinguishable from MMM. Terminally, approximately 7% of human patients who have MMM will transform into an acute myelogenous leukemia. Rare examples of familial myelofibrosis have also been reported.[47]

REFERENCES

1. **Whang J, Frei E III, Tijo JH, Carbone PP, Brecher G.** The distribution of the Philadelphia chromosome in patients with chronic myelogenous leukemia. Blood 1963;22:664–673.
2. **Anger B, Janssen JWG, Schrezenmeier H, Hehlmann R, Heimpel H, Bar-** tram CR. Clonal analysis of chronic myeloproliferative disorders using X-linked DNA polymorphisms. Leukemia 1990;4:258–261.
3. **Clarkson BD, Strife A, Wisniewski D, Lambek C, and Carpino N.** New understanding of the pathogenesis of CML: a prototype of early neoplasia. Leukemia 1997;11:1404–1428.
4. **Valli VEO.** Pathology of domestic animals. In: Jubb KVF, Kennedy PC, Palmer N, eds. The hematopoietic system. 4th ed. San Diego: Academic Press, 1993;114–133.
5. **Raskin RE.** Myelopoiesis and myeloproliferative disorders. Vet Clin North Am Small Anim Pract 1996;26:1032–1042.
6. **Dungworth DL, Goldman M, Switzer JW, McKelvie DH.** Development of a myeloproliferative disorder in beagles continuously exposed to ⁹⁰SR. Blood 1969;34:610–632.
7. **Jain NC.** The neutrophils. In: Jain NC, ed. Schalm's veterinary hematology. 4th ed. Philadelphia, PA: Lea and Febiger, 1986;676–730.
8. **Thomsen MK, Jensen AL, Skar-Nielsen T, Flemming K.** Enhanced granulocyte function in a case of chronic granulocyte leukemia in a dog. Vet Immunol Immunopathol 1991;28:143–156.
9. **Daley GQ, Van Etten RA, Baltimore D.** Induction of chronic myelogenous leukemia in mice by P210bcr/alb gene of the Philadelphia chromosome. Science 1990;247:824–830.
10. **Mears EA, Raskin RE, Legendre AM.** Basophilic leukemia in a dog. J Vet Intern Med 1997;11:92–94.
11. **Dastugue N, Duchayne E, Kuhlein E, Ribie H, Demur C, Aurich J, Robert A, Sie P.** Acute basophilic leukaemia and translocation t(X;6)(p11;q23) Br J Haematol 1997;98:170–176.
12. **Mahaffey EA, Brown TP, Duncan JR,** et al. Basophilic leukemia in a dog. J Comp Pathol 1987;97:393–399.
13. **MacEwen EG, Drazner FH, McClelland AJ, Wilkins RJ.** Treatment of basophilic leukemia in a dog. J Am Vet Med Assoc 1975;166:376–380.
14. **Travis WD, Li CY, Hoagland HC, Travis LB, Banks PM.** Mast-cell leukemia: report of a case and review of the literature. Mayo Clin Proc 1986;61:957.
15. **Galli SJ, Hammel I.** Mast cell and basophil development. Curr Opin Hematol 1994;1:33–39.
16. **London CA, Kisseberth WC, Galli SJ, Geissler EN, Helfand SC.** Expression of stem cell factor receptor (*c-kit*) by the malignant mast cells from spontaneous canine mast cell tumours. J Comp Pathol 1996;115:399–414.
17. **Morimoto M, Tsujimura T, Kanakura Y, Kitamura Y, Matsuday H.** Expression of *c-kit* and stem cell factor mRNA in liver specimens from healthy dogs. Am J Vet Res 1998;59:363–366.
18. **Torrey E, Simpson K, Wilbur S, Munoz P, Skikne B.** Malignant mastocytosis with circulating mast cells. Am J Hematol 1990;34:283–286.
19. **Huibregtse BA, Turner JL.** Hypereosinophilic syndrome and eosinophilic leukemia: a comparison of 22 hypereosinophilic cats. J Am Anim Hosp Assoc 1994;30:591–599.
20. **McEwen SA, Valli VEO, Hulland TJ.** Hypereosinophilic syndrome in cats: a report of three cases. Can J Comp Med 1984;49:248–253.
21. **Saxon B, Hendrick M, Waddle J.** Restrictive cardiomyopathy in a cat with hypereosinophilic syndrome. Can Vet J 1991;32:367–369.
22. **Schrezenmeier H, Thome SD, Tewald F, Fleischer B, Raghavachar A.** Interleukin-5 is the predominant eosinophilopoietin produced by cloned T lymphocytes in hypereosinophilic syndrome. Exp Hematol 1993;21,358–365.
23. **Finlay D.** Eosinophilic leukemia in the cat: a case report. Br Vet J 1985;141:74.
24. **Bennett JM, Catovsky D, Daniel MT, Flandrin G, Galton DAG, Gralnick H, Sultan C, Cox C.** The chronic myeloid leukaemias: guidelines for distinguishing chronic granulocytic, atypical chronic myeloid, and chronic myelomonocytic leukaemia. Proposals by the French-American-British Cooperative Leukaemia Group. Br J Haematol 1994;87:746–754.
25. **Ribera JM, Cervantes F, Rozman C.** A multivariate analysis of prognostic factors in chronic myelomonocytic leukaemia according to the FAB criteria. Br J Haematol 1987;65:307–311.
26. **Bearman RM, Kjeldsberg CR, Pangalis GA, Rappaport H.** Chronic monocytic leukemia in adults. Cancer 1981;48:2239–2255.
27. **Daoud MS, Snow JL, Gibson LE, Daoud S.** Aleukemic monocytic leukemia cutis. Mayo Clin Proc 1996;71:161–168.
28. **Padget GA, Madewell BR, Keller ET, Jordar L, Packard M.** Inheritance of histiocytosis in Bernese mountain dogs. J Small Anim Pract 1995;36:93–98.
29. **Brown DE, Thrall MA, Getzy DM, Weiser GM, Ogilvie GK.** Cytology of canine malignant histiocytosis. Vet Clin Pathol 1994;23:118–122.
30. **Moore PF, Rosin A.** Malignant histiocytosis of Bernese Mountain dogs. Vet Pathol 1986;23:1–10.
31. **Jain NC.** The platelets. In: Essentials of veterinary hematology. Malvern, PA: Lea & Febiger, 1993;124.
32. **Murphy S, Peterson P, Iland H.** Experience of the Polycythemia Vera Study Group with essential thrombocythemia: a final report on diagnostic criteria, survival, and leukemic transition by treatment. Semin Haematol 1997;34:29–39.
33. **Kondo T, Okabe M, Sanada M, Kurosawa M, Suzuki S, Kobayashi M, Hosokawa M, Asaka M.** Familial essential thrombocythemia associated with one-base deletion in the 5'-untranslated region of the thrombopoietin gene. Blood 1998;92:1091–1096.
34. **Wang JC, Chen C, Novetsky AD, Lichter SM, Ahmed F, Friedberg NM.**

Blood thrombopoietin levels in clonal thrombocytosis and reactive thrombocytosis. Am J Med 1998;104:451–455.

35. **Evans RJ, Jones DRE, Gruffydd-Jones TJ.** Essential thrombocytothaemia in the dog and cat: a report of four cases. J Small Anim Pract 1982;23:457–467.
36. **Hammer AS, Couto CG, Getzy D, Bailey MQ.** Essential thrombocythemia in a cat. J Vet Intern Med 1990;4:87–91.
37. **Harvey JW, Henderson CW, French TW, Meyer DJ.** Myeloproliferative disease with megakaryocytic predominance in a dog with occult dirofilariasis. Vet Clin Pathol 1980;11:5–11.
38. **Kaneko JJ.** Iron metabolism in familial polycythemia of Jersey calves. Am J Vet Res 1968;29:949–952.
39. **McGrath CJ.** Polycythemia vera in dogs. J Am Vet Med Assoc 1974;164:1117–1121.
40. **Khanna C, Bienzle D.** Polycythemia vera in a cat: bone marrow culture in erythropoietin-deficient medium. J Am Anim Hosp Assoc 1994;30:45–49.
41. **Giger U.** Serum erythropoietin concentrations in polycythemic and anemic dogs. Proc 9th Ann Col Vet Intern Med Forum, New Orleans, LA, 1991;143–145.
42. **Cook SM, Lothrop CD Jr.** Serum erythropoietin concentrations measured by radioimmunoassay in normal, polycythemic, and anemic dogs and cats. J Vet Intern Med 1994;8:18–25.
43. **Hasler AH, Gieger U.** Serum erythropoietin values in polycythemia cats. J Am Anim Hosp Assoc 1996;32:294–301.
44. **Tefferi A, Silverstein MN.** Current perspective in agnogenic myeloid metaplasia. Leuk Lymphoma 1996;1(suppl 22):169–171.
45. **Silverstein MN.** Agnogenic myeloid metaplasia. In: Cancer medicine. 3rd ed. Malvern: Lea & Febiger. 1993;1943–1946.
46. **Khan KNM, Logan, AC, Blomquist EM.** Idiopathic myelofibrosis (agnogenic myeloid metaplasia) in a marmoset (*Callithrix jacchus*): hematologic and histopathologic changes. Vet Pathol 1997;34:341–345.
47. **Mallouh AA, Sa'di AR.** Agnogenic myeloid metaplasia in children. Am J Dis Child 1992;146:965–967.

Hematologic Abnormalities Accompanying Leukemia

• PAULA PERKINS

Quantitative and qualitative abnormalities in the cells of the peripheral blood are commonly seen in conjunction with the leukemic process, and these changes often have diagnostic and therapeutic implications. Though these changes are nonspecific and may be caused by diseases other than neoplasia, documentation of the persistence and gradual worsening of these abnormalities, along with the elimination of other potential causes, leads the astute clinician to consider neoplasia in the list of differential diagnoses. Then, once the disease is diagnosed, the hematologic changes that accompany leukemia pose a therapeutic challenge, as the patient may succumb to infectious agents or hemorrhage. Identifying and monitoring these changes provide valuable clues to the disease process itself and the therapy necessary for correct treatment and maintenance of the leukemic patient.

GENERAL CONCEPTS

Gorman and Evans[1] lists the following as the hallmarks of potential myeloproliferative disease:

- The presence of a refractory anemia in which, although there is no evidence of a marrow response in the form of reticulocytosis, there is either increased mean cell volume (MCV) or large numbers of nucleated red blood cells (NRBCs) in the peripheral circulation.
- The presence of an unexplained cytopenia, particularly a neutropenia.
- The presence of morphologically abnormal white blood cells (WBCs). Commonly there may be giant neutrophils, abnormal nuclear morphology, abnormal neutrophil granulation or evidence of neutrophil dysfunction despite adequate or increased neutrophil numbers.
- The presence of unexplained thrombocytopenia or large and abnormally granulated platelets (shift platelets). Granulation may be reduced or excessive or show abnormal granule size, staining, or variability.

The formation of platelet pseudopods is often excessive.
- The presence of a persistent significant thrombocytosis.
- The presence of a grossly increased buffy coat or significant leukocytosis.
- The presence of a grossly increased packed cell volume (PCV) and red cell count.

In summary, therefore, myeloproliferative disease should be included in the list of differential diagnoses in any patient that shows an unexplained and unresolving increase or decrease in any of the hemic cell lines, especially if morphologic abnormalities accompany the change in number. Note that the number and function of the normal components of one or more cell lines are generally decreased in any leukemic process.[2] For example, a progressively worsening, nonregenerative anemia is commonly noted, which may be normocytic normochromic or, occasionally, macrocytic normochromic.[2-5] Potential mechanisms for this decrease in RBC mass include myelophthisis, ineffective erythropoiesis, immune-mediated destruction, and hemorrhage.[2] Neutropenia is common and predisposes the patient to sepsis.[2,3] Thrombocytopenia is frequently noted.[5,6] In a study of 15 dogs with nonlymphoid hemic tumors, the average platelet count was $128,733 \pm 46,825/\mu L$, with 24% being thrombocytopenic.[6] These patients are predisposed to hemorrhage owing to decreased platelet numbers and abnormal cell function.[2,7]

The astute clinician, therefore, should be keenly aware of these abnormalities and their potential ties to leukemia. Patients demonstrating these disorders should be closely monitored with routine complete blood cell counts (CBCs), and appropriate diagnostic and therapeutic measures should be quickly and vigorously instituted.

MYELODYSPLASTIC SYNDROME

Myelodysplastic syndrome (MDS) or preleukemia refers to the condition preceding the development of overt leukemia in which the patient exhibits one or more cytopenias and abnormalities in cell morphology and function.[8-11] These changes are reflective of dyshematopoiesis. In the bone marrow, erythroid precursors may be large and megaloblastic (having mature, fully hemoglobinized cytoplasm with an immature nucleus). Binucleated rubricytes and fragmented nuclei may be prominent. Myeloid cells may be giant forms or have unusually prominent granulation. Megakaryocytes may be immature with small fragmented nuclei.[12] Overall cellularity of the bone marrow may be increased or decreased. In the peripheral blood, there is typically a nonregenerative anemia, and there may be an inappropriate normoblastemia with occasional immature cells having multiple or fragmented nuclei.[5,10,11] Macrocytosis not associated with reticulocytosis is well documented in cats that have MDS[5] and has also been reported in dogs.[12] Dysgranulopoiesis may be evidenced by hypersegmentation or hyposegmentation of the nucleus, giant neutrophils or bands, monocytoid nuclei, or granules present in abnormal quantities or shapes.[5] Platelets may also be abnormally large or have abnormal granulation.[5,10]

A recent retrospective study of nonlymphoid hematopoietic neoplasia in cats[5] supports the diagnostic usefulness of cytopenias in myelodysplastic conditions. In this study, 60 cats having either MDS ($n = 21$) or acute myelogenous leukemia ($n = 38$) were evaluated. Of the 60, 96% of the MDS cats were anemic, with the majority (62%) being moderately affected (PCV 10 to 20%). The anemia was nonregenerative (aggregate reticulocyte counts of <1.5%) in 81% of the MDS cats, and 48% had MCVs >55 fL. Total leukocyte counts tended to be low or low normal in MDS, with 43% of the cats having counts <5500 WBCs/μL and 52% having WBC counts between 5500 and 19,500/μL. Only 5% had leukocyte counts greater than 19,500/μL. Neutropenia (neutrophils <3000/μL) was noted in 43% of the MDS cats. Thrombocytopenia was not as prevalent as anemia or neutropenia in these cats; platelet counts varied considerably, with the 21 MDS cats being divided evenly among <50,000 platelets/μL (7 cats), 50,000 to 200,000/μL (7 cats), and >200,000/μL (7 cats).

Pancytopenia with significant macrocytosis was reported in one horse that had MDS diagnosed by bone marrow examination.[13] The horse was presented for evaluation of a 4-week history of exercise intolerance, tachycardia, tachypnea, and petechial hemorrhages on the oral and nasal mucosae. A severe pancytopenia was noted (PCV 0.05 L/L; normal range 0.32 to 0.47 L/L; WBC 1.1×10^3/μL, normal range 5.2 to 13.9×10^3/μL; platelets $<2 \times 10^3$/μL, normal range 100 to 270×10^3/μL). There was also a significant macrocytosis (80 fl, normal range 43 to 54 fl) and a moderate anisocytosis. Bone marrow examination revealed a maturation arrest in the myeloid series and severe dyserythropoiesis without concurrent erythroid hyperplasia. A diagnosis of MDS was made. The horse's condition deteriorated over the following 2 days, and euthanasia was elected before the disease could progress further. The macrocytosis in this case was remarkable. In the horse, macrocytosis

may be associated with a regenerative response, but the magnitude of the increase is usually less than 10 to 15%.[13] In this case, the macrocytic RBCs probably formed from megaloblastic precursors in the bone marrow rather than from a response to the anemia.

ACUTE MYELOPROLIFERATIVE DISEASES

As the disease progresses from myelodysplasia to overt neoplasia, the peripheral quantitative and qualitative abnormalities become progressively worse. The total WBC count may be decreased, within normal limits, or elevated to greater than 500,000 cells/μL, depending on the contribution of the neoplastic component.[2,14] Nonregenerative anemia and thrombocytopenia are once again common features. In one study of MDS and MPD in dogs and cats,[15] 51.7% of all cases examined had a leukocytosis. Only 18.4% were leukopenic. Anemia was present in 87.5% of these animals, and 18.4% had circulating NRBCs. Thrombocytopenia was noted in 85.7% of the cases[15] and was typically moderate to severe[16] with macrothrombocytes being common.[17]

As with MDS, these abnormalities lead to difficulties in patient management. Leukopenia or loss of normal leukocyte function leads to recurrent infections, febrile episodes, and delays in wound healing.[11,18] Neoplastic cells in large numbers may form leukemic thrombi, leading to vascular damage and hemorrhage in such diverse sites as the central nervous system, the eyes, or the lungs.[11] Thrombocytopenia or lack of normal platelet function predisposes the leukemic patient to formation of petechia or ecchymoses, epistaxis, hematuria, or gastrointestinal bleeding. Myelogenous leukemia in humans is associated with microvascular thrombosis and disseminated intravascular coagulation (DIC), caused by the release of a procoagulant substance from lysosomal granules.[11] Recognition of these potentially life-threatening sequelae to leukemia is crucial to successful patient management.

Acute Myeloblastic Leukemia (AML-M1/M2)

In both dogs and cats, the majority of cases of acute myeloblastic leukemia (AML) show a leukocytosis with a disorderly left shift extending to the blast cell (Fig. 109.1).[8,11] Some cases, however, may have a white cell count that is decreased or within normal limits,[2,19] and pancytopenia has also been reported.[17] The total WBC count may also fluctuate over time from a significant leukocytosis to a count that approaches reference range. This phenomenon has been reported in human AML and is hypothesized to be caused by cyclic production and release from the bone marrow.[8] In cats, the mean WBC count in 22 cases of AML-M1 was $50,545 \pm 20,861$ cells/μL, with a significant left shift to blast forms. The neutrophil count in 21 of these cats, however, was either within reference range or decreased.[16] AML-M2 in 34 cats showed a pattern similar to M1. The mean WBC

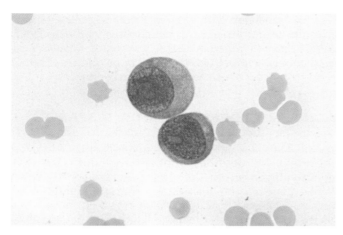

FIGURE 109.1 Large atypical myeloblasts from the peripherial blood of a cat that has AML-M1. (Wright–Giemsa stain, ×400)

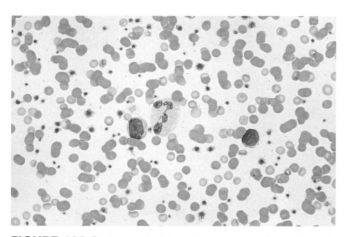

FIGURE 109.2 Peripherial blood from a cat that has AML-M2. Two myeloblasts, a giant neutrophil, and numerous hyperchromic platelets from the peripheral blood of a cat that has AML-M2. (Wright–Giemsa stain, ×70)

count was 19,924 ± 30,701 cells/μL, with a left shift similar to M1 but occurring in proportionally smaller numbers. Leukopenia was present in approximately one third of these cats.[16]

Morphologic abnormalities in the granulocytes in AML-M1 and M2 may include variations in the size and shape of the cell or the nucleus. Nuclear hypersegmentation is an occasionally prominent finding,[8] and giant forms with abnormal nuclear chromatin are common (Fig. 109.2).[20,21] One case of AML-M2 in a 2-year-old German Shepherd reported giant metamyelocytes and bands (greater than twice normal size), neutrophils with Pelger-Huet-like nuclear morphology, binucleated cells, and loss of normal cytoplasmic granulation.[20] Cells with evidence of asynchronous nuclear-to-cytoplasmic maturation have also been noted.[19,22]

The erythroid cell line in AML-M1 and M2 is usually depressed in both dogs and cats. In 23 cases of granulo-

cytic leukemia in dogs, the average PCV was 21%.[23] Twenty of 21 cats (95.2%) with AML-M1 and 28 of 34 cats (82.4%) with M2 had PCVs less than 24%.[16] In both species, the anemia is nonregenerative, although circulating erythroid precursors may be noted.[4,16] Four of 21 cats (19%) with AML-M1 and five of 34 cats (14.7%) with M2 had >10 NRBCs/100 WBCs. Erythrocyte indices are typically within normal limits or macrocytic normochromic,[14] and anisocytosis may be significant.[24,25]

Platelet counts in AML-M1 and M2 are often decreased. In the cat, 12 of 21 cases of M1 (57.1%) and 15 of 34 cases of M2 (44.1%) had thrombocytopenia of <100,000 cells/μL. Giant forms are common,[14,20,26] and platelets larger than erythrocytes have been reported in the dog. Platelets may also be vacuolated or have abnormally large granules[20] or may appear overly basophilic.[26]

Acute Myelomonocytic Leukemia (AML-M4)

Acute myelomonocytic leukemia is characterized by a leukocytosis with a left shift, a monocytosis that often includes immature forms, anemia, and thrombocytopenia.[8,17,27] In the dog, a persistent monocytosis may be noted before the onset of overt leukemia.[17]

In five dogs that had AML-M4,[27] leukocytosis was present in four of five animals, and immature granulocytes extending to the blast stage were noted in all cases. Total WBC counts in these dogs ranged from 10,400 to 422,400, with a mean WBC of 103,900 cells/μL. Neutrophils may be hypersegmented,[28] and giant toxic-appearing bands may be noted.[29] Both mature and immature monocytes may be present and may show atypical morphology or erythrophagocytosis.[28,30] Anemia is a common finding, with PCVs averaging 18–33% in 14 reported cases.[23,27] The anemia is typically nonregenerative, and MCV may be normal or increased. Anisocytosis, poikilocytosis, and leptocytosis are reported, and the anisocytosis may be significant.[27,30] Immature erythroid cells are often seen, and in some cases normoblastemia is the primary abnormality.[27,31] Thrombocytopenia is common and is often severe, and large forms may be present.[10,27,28,30]

In the cat, there is a moderate to significant leukocytosis[8] characterized by neutrophilia, a left shift extending to blasts, and a significant monocytosis.[8,11,32] The total WBC count frequently exceeds 100,000 cells/μL.[16] Neutrophils may be basophilic with Döhle bodies, and giant hypersegmented forms (macropolycytes) may comprise a large proportion of the total neutrophil population.[32] These abnormal cells are also reported to be erythrophagocytic.[32] A mild to severe nonregenerative anemia is common, with a normal to increased MCV[8,32] and a slight to significant anisocytosis.[33] Thrombocytopenia is common, and platelets may be large with abnormal morphology or irregular granulation.[8,32,33]

Five cases of AML-M4 in the horse[34–38] describe hematologic abnormalities similar to those seen in the dog and cat. Anemia, neutropenia, and thrombocytopenia are typical, whereas the total WBC count is variable.[34] Neutrophils may show abnormal morphology, including toxic change,[34,38] hypersegmentation, cytoplasmic blebbing, asynchronous nuclear-to-cytoplasmic maturation, vacuolization, and fragmented or ringed nuclei.[37]

Acute Monocytic Leukemia (AML-M5)

This form of leukemia is characterized by a less severe anemia than other types and a variable total WBC count with a significant monocytosis.[7,15,39] Seven cases of both canine and feline acute monocytic leukemia showed 22 to 88% monocytes, and six of the seven had monocyte counts exceeding 5000 cells/μL.[15] In three reports of AML-M5 in the dog, the total WBC count ranged from 16,800 to 800,000 cells/μL, with the leukocytosis being caused primarily by the increase in the number of monocytes. Granulocyte and lymphocyte counts were within normal limits.[40] The total WBC count in a second report of three dogs that had AML-M5 ranged from 90,700 to 146,000 cells/μL, with an average WBC of 96,300. Again, the significant leukocytosis was due to the presence of neoplastic cells (Fig. 109.3).[17] The PCV is generally in the low 30s, as contrasted to the more severe anemia seen in AML-M4 (PCV ~25%) or granulocytic leukemia (PCV ~20%).[23] It may also be within normal limits.[17,23] The anemia is typically nonregenerative, but significant extramedullary hematopoiesis in the spleen contributes to a more efficient maintenance of the red cell mass. Large numbers of immature erythroid cells may also be present,[40,41] and the mature erythrocytes may show anisocytosis and poikilocytosis.[41] Platelet counts are generally decreased, but the thrombocytopenia is less severe than M1, M4, or acute lymphocytic leukemia. The mean platelet count in three reported cases of AML-M5 was 102,000, with a range of 39,000 to 133,000 cells/μL.[17] The majority of these cases had giant forms present.

In the cat, AML-M5 tends to produce high WBC counts. In a study of 179 cats that had various types of leukemia and myelodysplasia, the cats with AML-M5

had the highest mean WBC count (197,317 cells/μL) and the most significant monocytosis (180,140 cells/μL).[16] Overall, the WBC count may be moderately to significantly elevated, with a left shift extending to blasts, and the monocytosis typically includes many immature forms.[8,11] Neutrophils may show toxic change as evidenced by cytoplasmic basophilia and Döhle bodies.[11,42] As in the dog, cats that have AML-M5 are typically anemic but to a lesser degree than in other leukemias. Hematocrits in five published cases of feline AML-M5 averaged 23.4%,[29,42,43] and a retrospective study that included six cases of AML-M5 reported all six cats as having PCVs of less than 24%.[16] The anemia may be normocytic or macrocytic and is nonregenerative. Platelet counts tend to be significantly decreased. In a retrospective study of 179 cats with AML and MDS, the mean platelet count for the six M5 cats was approximately 6000 cells/μL.[16] This degree of thrombocytopenia was the most pronounced of all the leukemias evaluated.

Erythroleukemia (AML-M6) and Erythremic Myelosis (M6-Er)

Erythremic myelosis and erythroleukemia are considered by most authorities to be different manifestations of the same illness, beginning with a predominance of immature erythroid cells in the peripheral blood in erythremic myelosis (M6-Er) and progressing to a mixture of neoplastic myeloid and erythroid cells in AML-M6.[8,39] A study by the Animal Leukemia Group has recommended that erythremic myelosis now be considered either a subcategory of erythroleukemia or a myelodysplastic syndrome (MDS-Er), depending on the percentage of blast cells in the bone marrow.[15] Naturally occurring AML-M6 and erythremic myelosis have only been reported in the cat.[2] In the dog, erythroleukemia has been induced by exposure to radiation.[44]

In both disorders, a moderate to severe nonregenera-

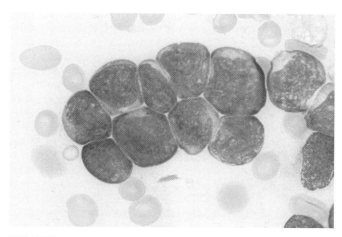

FIGURE 109.3 Large monoblasts from a dog that has AML-M5. (Wright–Giemsa stain, ×400)

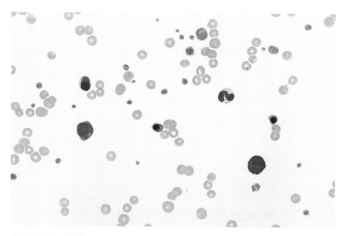

FIGURE 109.4 Peripheral blood from a cat that has erythroleukemia. Two blast cells, three nucleated red cells, giant platelets, and a macrocytic nonregenerative anemia are present. (Wright–Giemsa stain, ×70)

tive anemia with large numbers of circulating erythroid precursors is typical (Fig. 109.4).[7,16,45] In a retrospective study of feline myeloproliferative diseases, 20 of 21 cats with AML-M6 (95%) and 10 of 10 cats with M6-Er had PCVs less than 24%.[16] Sixty-seven percent of the AML-M6 cats and 100% of the M6-Er cats had more than 10 nucleated RBCs (NRBCs) per 100 WBCs in peripheral blood.[16] The normoblastemia is variable in degree of immaturity and in the number of cells observed. Erythroid precursors may number only a few, or there may be hundreds per 100 WBCs.[46,47] Cells may be as immature as the rubriblast or may be primarily the more mature forms.[19,48] Morphologic abnormalities may include large forms, double nuclei, or there may be asynchrony in nuclear-to-cytoplasmic maturation.[19,39,48] Some cases of erythremic myelosis, however, may show only anemia with a significant anisocytosis.[48] It is theorized that the macrocytic red cells in this disorder are the result of megaloblastic precursors in the bone marrow. A defect in nucleic acid synthesis or mitosis leads to asynchronous maturation of the nucleus and cytoplasm, forming megaloblasts and giant metarubricytes and eventually macrocytic red cells in circulation.[49] Siderocytes or sideroblasts have also been reported.[45,50] Total WBC counts and platelet counts are variable in both disorders.[16]

Megakaryocytic Leukemia (AML-M7)

Severe nonregenerative anemia, a variable white cell count, and quantitative and qualitative platelet abnormalities characterize megakaryocytic leukemia in both dogs and cats.[7,8,47] In the dog, the platelet count is variable but is usually significantly decreased. Giant or bizarre forms and hypogranulation or hypergranulation may be noted.[47] Dwarf megakaryocytes or megakaryoblasts are often found in circulation[2,15] and may contain vacuoles or cytoplasmic blebs.[2] The platelets are dysfunctional, leading to bleeding episodes in the patient.[47] In the cat, there is typically a significant increase in the number of circulating platelets with giant and bizarre forms predominating.[51]

CHRONIC MYELOPROLIFERATIVE DISEASES

The chronic leukemias are distinguished from the acute MPDs by the degree of differentiation of the neoplastic component. In the chronic diseases, the predominent cell type is the more mature form, as opposed to the large numbers of circulating blasts seen in the acute leukemias.

Chronic Myelogenous Leukemia (CML)

A significant leukocytosis consisting primarily of neutrophils and bands is the hallmark of chronic myelogenous leukemia. The WBC count may be in excess of 100,000 cells/μL, and although mature and immature

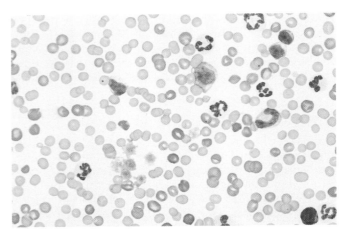

FIGURE 109.5 Blast cells, segmented neutrophils, band neutrophil, giant platelets and a regenerative anemia from a dog that has chronic myelogenous leukemia. (Wright–Giemsa stain, ×70)

neutrophils are generally present, the mature forms predominate (Fig. 109.5).[2,15] In some cases, however, the left shift may be more disorderly, and cells at the same level of maturation may show variation in size and shape.[2] Hypersegmentation of the nucleus, pyknosis, and nuclear fragmentation are also reported.[52] A moderate anemia is common, and the platelet count may be increased or decreased.[2,33] The diagnostic dilemma with this disease is distinguishing the neoplastic proliferation from a leukemoid reaction secondary to infectious, immune-mediated, or neoplastic diseases. In man, the presence of the Philadelphia chromosome is used to differentiate CML from a leukemoid response. In the dog, however, specific chromosomal abnormalities have not been reported.[52,53] The diagnosis of CML is usually one of exclusion, after all other causes of the significant leukocytosis are eliminated.

Eosinophilic Leukemia (EL)

Eosinophilic leukemia has been reported only in cats, and the majority of cases have been feline leukemia virus (FeLV) negative.[2,11] EL is characterized by a significant peripheral eosinophilia, eosinophilic hyperplasia of the bone marrow, and eosinophilic infiltration into multiple organs.[54] Eosinophil counts in five reported cases ranged from 29,900 to 109,500 cells/μL, with an average count of 54,500.[55] In some cases, the cells were poorly granulated and difficult to identify. The diagnostic dilemma associated with this condition is distinguishing EL from hypereosinophilic syndrome (HES), a disease of unknown origin that also causes a significant eosinophilia and organ infiltration in cats. Two criteria may be of use in differentiating these two diseases: the immaturity of the eosinophils, and the degree of concurrent anemia. Eosinophil precursors are more commonly noted in the blood of EL cats than in those with hypereosinophilic syndrome. In one retrospective study of EL and HES,[54] five of six cats with EL had circulating immature eosinophils, whereas only three of 13 HES cats showed this pattern. The immature cells also comprised a higher percentage of the total WBC count in EL cats than in cats with hypereosinophilic syndrome. Anemia was more severe in EL than in HES. The mean hematocrit for the cats with EL was 25.4%, compared with a mean of 34% for the HES cats. Evaluation of the bone marrow may also aid in differentiating these two diseases. Eosinophilic hyperplasia is present in the bone marrow in both EL and HES, but the myeloid-to-erythroid (M:E) ratio tends to be lower in HES. In three of three cases of EL in which an M:E ratio was reported, the ratio exceeded 10:1. The average ratio was 16.4:1. In eight of nine cases of HES, however, the M:E ratio was less than 10.1 and averaged 7.27:1. Maturation may be orderly or disorderly in either disease.[54]

Basophilic Leukemia

This condition is characterized by a significant peripheral basophilia. The more mature forms usually predominate, but there may also be a significant left shift extending to the blast.[7,56–59] In six cases reported in the literature, the absolute basophil count ranged from 2200 to 45,212 cells/μL.[56–58] In the majority of cases, there was also a mild to moderate nonregenerative anemia and eosinophilia, and platelet counts varied from normal to a significant thrombocytosis. The diagnostic dilemma related to this disease is differentiating it from mast cell neoplasia, but morphologic characteristics generally distinguish the two cell types.

Polycythemia Vera (PV)

A neoplastic proliferation of the erythroid cell line, polycythemia vera causes a significant increase in hematocrit (PCV 65 to 80%), total RBC mass, and hemoglobin concentration.[7] Leukocytosis and thrombocytosis, seen commonly in the human variant of PV, are rare in veterinary species.[7,47] In a retrospective study of 11 dogs that had PV, the RBC mass was increased in six of six dogs measured, and the total blood volume was increased in five of six dogs. Leukocytosis was present in only three of 11 dogs, however, and thrombocytopenia was noted in only four of eight.[60] The bone marrow in dogs with PV is hypercellular, but the M:E ratio is within normal limits, and the erythroid cell line shows orderly maturation. The erythrocytes in circulation are typically normal in morphology and function, though microcytic hypochromic cells may develop as increased erythropoiesis and therapeutic phlebotomies deplete iron stores. Clinical signs are attributable to hyperviscosity caused by the increased red cell mass. Hyperemia of the mucous membranes and tortuous retinal blood vessels are the most frequently recognized signs, and neurologic abnormalities may occur owing to central nervous system hypoxia.[61]

Essential Thrombocythemia (ET)

Well-documented cases of essential thrombocythemia are rare and must be distinguished from thrombocytosis secondary to various inflammatory, traumatic, or neoplastic disorders. ET is characterized by a significant, persistent thrombocytosis and defects in platelet function. In one case of ET in a dog, platelet counts over the course of 72 weeks ranged from 577,000 to 1,200,000 cells/μL, and morphologic abnormalities such as giant forms and serpentine shapes were noted.[61] Thrombosis, hemorrhage, and microcytic hypochromic anemia caused by chronic bleeding are reported sequelae to this disease.[39,47,62]

Primary Myelofibrosis

Collagen deposition and abnormal proliferation of all cell lines in the bone marrow are the hallmarks of this myeloproliferative disease.[7,47] A normocytic normochromic anemia with anisocytosis and poikilocytosis, typically dacryocytes and ovalocytes, is common, as are circulating erythroid and myeloid precursors.[2,39,47] Platelets counts are variable,[2,47] and there may be abnormalities of platelet function.[39]

REFERENCES

1. **Gorman NT, Evans RJ.** Myeloproliferative disease in the dog and cat: clinical presentations, diagnosis and treatment. Vet Rec 1987;121:490–496.
2. **Young KM, MacEwen EG.** Canine myeloproliferative disorders. In: Withrow SJ, MacEwen EG, ed. Clincal Veterinary Oncology. Philadelphia: JB Lippincott, 1989.
3. **Hardy WD, MacEwen EG.** Feline retroviruses. In: Withrow SJ, MacEwen EG, ed. Clincal veterinary oncology. Philadelphia: JB Lippincott, 1989.
4. **Theilen GH, Madewell BR.** Hematopoietic neoplasms, sarcomas and related conditions. Part II—Feline. In: Theilen GH, Madewell BR, ed. Veterinary cancer medicine. Philadelphia: Lea and Febiger, 1987.
5. **Blue JT, French TW, Kranz JS.** Non-lymphoid hematopoietic neoplasia in cats: a retrospective study of 60 cases. Cornell Vet 1988;78:21–42.
6. **Grindem CB, Breitschwerdt EB, Corbett WT, Page RL, Jans HE.** Thrombocytopenia associated with neoplasia in dogs. J Vet Intern Med 1994;8(6):400–405.
7. **Young KM.** Myeloproliferative disorders. Vet Clin North Am 1985;15(4):769–781.
8. **Jain NC.** The leukemia complex. In: Jain NC, ed. Schalm's veterinary hematology. 4th ed. Philadelphia: Lea and Febiger, 1986.
9. **Toth SR, Onions DE, Jarrett O.** Histopathological and hematological findings in myeloid leukemia induced by a new feline leukemia virus isolate. Vet Pathol 1986;23:462–470.
10. **Couto CG, Kallet AJ.** Preleukemic syndrome in a dog. J Am Vet Med Assoc 1984;184(11):1389–1392.
11. **Jain NC.** The leukemias. In: Jain NC, ed. Essentials of veterinary hematology. Philadelphia: Lea and Febiger, 1993.
12. **Weiss DJ.** Myelodysplastic syndrome in two dogs. J Am Vet Med Assoc 1985;187(10):1038–1040.
13. **Durando MM, Alleman AR, Harvey JW.** Myelodysplastic syndrome in a Quarter Horse gelding. Equine Vet J 1994;26(1):83–85.
14. **Madewell BR, Theilen GH.** Hematopoietic neoplasms, sarcomas and related conditions. Part IV—Canine. In: Theilen GH, Madewell BR, ed. Veterinary cancer medicine. Philadelphia: Lea and Febiger, 1987.
15. **Jain NC, Blue JT, Grindem CB, et al.** Proposed criteria for classification of acute myeloid leukemia in dogs and cats: a report of the Animal Leukemia Study Group. Vet Clin Pathol 1991;20(3):63–82.
16. **Jain NC.** Classification of myeloproliferative disorders in cats using criteria proposed by the Animal Leukemia Study Group: a retrospective study of 181 cases (1969–1992). Comp Haematol Int 1993;3:125–134.
17. **Couto CG.** Clinicopathologic aspects of acute leukemias in dogs. J Am Vet Med Assoc 1985;186(7):681–685.
18. **Weller RE, Geissler M, Jain NC.** Myeloblastic leukemia and leukemic meningitis in a dog. Mod Vet Pract 1980;61(1):42–46.
19. **Gilmore CE, Holzworth J.** Naturally occurring feline leukemia: clinical,

pathologic and differential diagnostic features. J Am Vet Med Assoc 1971;158(6):1013–1030.

20. **Keller P, Sager P, Freudiger U, Speck B.** Acute myeloblastic leukemia in a dog. J Comp Pathol 1985;95:619–632.

21. **Schalm OW, Switzer JW.** Bone marrow disease in the cat. I. Atypical granulocytic leukemia. California Vet 1968;22 (4):24–28.

22. **Cooper BJ, Watson AJ.** Myeloid neoplasia in a dog. Aust Vet J 1975;51:150–154.

23. **Latimer SK, Dykstra MJ.** Acute monocytic leukemia in a dog. J Am Vet Med Assoc 1984;184(7):852–855.

24. **Evans RJ, Gorman NT.** Myeloproliferative disease in the dog and cat: definition, aetiology and classification. Vet Rec 1987;121:437–443.

25. **Rouse BT, Osborne AD, Grunsell CS.** Acute granulocytic leukemia in a bitch. Vet Rec 1967;80(13):408–410.

26. **Sutton RH, McKellow AM, Bottrill MB.** Myeloproliferative disease in the cat: a granulocytic and megakaryocytic disorder. N Z Vet J 1978;26:273–274.

27. **Jain NC, Madewell BR, Weller RE, Geissler MC.** Clinical-pathological findings and cytochemical characterization of myelomonocytic leukaemia in 5 dogs. J Comp Pathol 1981;91:17–31.

28. **Green RA, Barton CL.** Acute myelomonocytic leukemia in a dog. J Am Anim Hosp Assoc 1977;13:708–712.

29. **Grindem CB, Stevens JB, Perman V.** Morphological classification and clinical and pathological characteristics of spontaneous leukemia in 17 dogs. J Am Anim Hosp Assoc 1985;21:219–226.

30. **Ragan HA, Hackett PL, Dagle GE.** Acute myelomonocytic leukemia manifested as myelophthisic anemia in a dog. J Am Vet Med Assoc 1976;169(4):421–425.

31. **Christopher MM, Metz AL, Klausner J, Polzin D, Hayden DW.** Acute myelomonocytic leukemia with neurologic manifestations in the dog. Vet Pathol 1986;23:140–147.

32. **Raskin RE, Krehbiel JD.** Myelodysplastic changes in a cat with myelomonocytic leukemia. J Am Vet Med Assoc 1985;187(2):171–174.

33. **Madewell BR, Jain NC, Weller RE.** Hematologic abnormalities preceding myeloid leukemia in three cats. Vet Pathol 1979;16:510–519.

34. **Spier SJ, Madewell BR, Zinkl JG, Ryan AM.** Acute myelomonocytic leukemia in a horse. J Am Vet Med Assoc 1986;188(8):861–863.

35. **Buechner-Maxwell V, Zhang C, Robertson J, Jain NC, et al.** Intravascular leukostasis and systemic aspergillosis in a horse with subleukemic acute myelomonocytic leukemia. J Vet Intern Med 1994;8(4):258–263.

36. **Bienzle D, Hughson SL, Vernau W.** Acute myelomonocytic leukemia in a horse. Can Vet J 1993;34:36–37.

37. **Mori T, Ishida T, Washizu T, Yamagami T, et al.** Acute myelomonocytic leukemia in a horse. Vet Pathol 1991;28:334–336.

38. **Brumbaugh GW, Stitzel KA, Zinkl JG, Feldman BF.** Myelomonocytic myeloproliferative disease in a horse. J Am Vet Med Assoc 1982;180(3):313–316.

39. **Harvey JW.** Myeloproliferative disorders in dogs and cats. Vet Clin North Am Small Anim Pract 1981;11(2):349–381.

40. **Mackey LJ, Jarrett WH, Lauder IM.** Monocytic leukemia in a dog. Vet Rec 1975;96(1):27–30.

41. **Tolle DV, Seed TM, Fritz TE, Lombard LS, Poole CM, Norris WP.** Acute monocytic leukemia in an irradiated beagle. Vet Pathol 1979;16:243–254.

42. **Henness AM, Crow SE, Anderson BC.** Monocytic leukemia in three cats. J Am Vet Med Assoc 1977;170(11):1325–1328.

43. **Tsujimoto H, Shirota K, Hayashi T, Hasegawa A, et al.** Monocytic leukemia in a cat. Jpn J Vet Sci 1981;43:957–961.

44. **Tolle DV, Fritz TE, Norris WP.** Radiation-induced erythroleukemia in the beagle dog. Am J Pathol 1977;87(3):499–506.

45. **Yoshimitsu M, Murata H.** Erythroleukemia in a cat with special reference to the fine structure of primitive cells in its peripheral blood. Jpn J Vet Sci 1980;42:531–541.

46. **Schalm OW.** Myeloproliferative disorders in the cat. California Vet 1976;30(6):32–37.

47. **Fournel-Fleury C, Magnol JP, Guelfi JF.** Leukemias and myeloid dysplasias. In: Fournel-Fleury C, Magnol JP, Guelfi JF, ed. Atlas of cancer cytology in the dog and cat. Conference Nationale des Veterinaries Specialises en Petits Animaux, Paris, 1994.

48. **Sodikoff DH, Schalm OW.** Primary bone marrow disease in the cat. III. Erythremic myelosis and myelofibrosis, a myeloproliferative disorder. California Vet 1968;22:16–20.

49. **Hirsch V, Dunn J.** Megaloblastic anemia in the cat. J Am Anim Hosp Assoc 1983;19:873–880.

50. **Zawidzka ZZ, Janzen E, Grice HC.** Erythremic myelosis in a cat. Vet Pathol 1964;1:530–541.

51. **Michel RL, O'Handley P.** Megakaryocytic myelosis in a cat. J Am Vet Med Assoc 1976;168(11):1021–1025.

52. **Leifer CE, Matus RE, Patnaik AK, MacEwen EG.** Chronic myelogenous leukemia in the dog. J Am Vet Med Assoc 1983;184(7):686–689.

53. **Pollett L, vanHove W, Mattheeuws D.** Blastic crisis in chronic myelogenous leukaemia in a dog. J Small Anim Pract 1978;19:469–475.

54. **Huibregtse BA, Turner JL.** Hypereosinophilic syndrome and eosinophilic leukemia: a comparison of 22 hypereosinophilic cats. J Am Anim Hosp Assoc 1994;30:591–599.

55. **Swensen CL, Carothers MA, Wellman ML, Kociba GJ.** Eosinophilic leukemia in a cat with naturally acquired feline leukemia virus infection. J Am Anim Hosp Assoc 1993;29:497–501.

56. **Mahaffey EA, Brown TP, Dunca JR, Latimer KS, et al.** Basophilic leukemia in a dog. J Comp Pathol 1987;97:393–399.

57. **Mears EA, Raskin RE, Legendre AM.** Basophilic leukemia in a dog. J Vet Intern Med 1997;11(2):92–94.

58. **MacEwen EG, Drazner FH, McClelland AJ, Wilkins RJ.** Treatment of basophilic leukemia in a dog. J Am Vet Med Assoc 1975;166(4):376–380.

59. **Bounous DL, Latimer KS, Campagnoli RR, Hynes PF.** Acute myeloid leukemia with basophilic differentiation (AML, M-2B) in a cat. Vet Clin Pathol 1994;23:15–18.

60. **McGrath CJ, Krawiec DR, Johnston SD.** Canine polycythemia vera: a review of diagnostic features. Vet Med 1982;77(4):611–613.

61. **Wysoke JM, van Heerden J.** Polycythaemia vera in a dog. J S Afr Vet Assoc 1990;61(4):182–183.

62. **Bass MC, Schultze AE.** Essential thrombocythemia in a dog: case report and literature review. J Am Anim Hosp Assoc 1998;34:197–203.

CHAPTER 110

Systemic Mastocytosis and Mast Cell Leukemia

• MICHELLE L. PLIER and PETER S. MACWILLIAMS

Various mast cell diseases have been documented and studied in animals and in humans. For the latter, several classification schemes have been proposed to describe benign and malignant systemic mast cell disorders.[1-3] In domestic animals, mast cell proliferation can be associated with inflammatory and allergic disorders as well as mast cell neoplasia. Mast cell neoplasia manifests as either a cutaneous proliferation of mast cells in the skin and subcutis, or less frequently as a systemic disorder in which mast cells invade internal organs. Terminology used to describe systemic mast cell neoplasia in the veterinary medical literature includes systemic mastocytosis, splenic mastocytosis, visceral mastocytosis, disseminated mastocytosis, malignant mastocytosis, disseminated mastocytoma, malignant mastocytoma, anaplastic mastocytoma, multicentric mast cell tumor, and systemic mast cell disease.[4] As used in this chapter, systemic mastocytosis refers to infiltration of internal organs or hemolymphatic tissue by neoplastic mast cells.

Systemic mastocytosis with or without concurrent mast cell leukemia is more often diagnosed in domestic cats. Disseminated mast cell disease and mast cell leukemia have also been documented in dogs and other domestic and exotic animals.[5-13] Systemic mastocytosis may be accompanied by cutaneous mast cell tumors or may develop some time after diagnosis of cutaneous mast cell neoplasia (Fig. 110.1a). Solitary or disseminated visceral organ involvement alone has also been observed in several species, particularly cats. Whereas the extent of invasion varies among individuals, neoplastic mast cell infiltrates are found most frequently in the lymph nodes (Fig. 110.1b), the spleen (Fig. 110.2), the liver (Fig. 110.3), the gastrointestinal tract, and the bone marrow. Infiltrates have been observed in virtually all organs and also within body cavities.

Known in earlier reports as mast myelocyte leukemia or as basophilic leukemia,[5,14] mast cell leukemia is a rare myeloproliferative sequela to systemic mastocytosis. In human patients, mast cell leukemia is considered an acute myeloid leukemia.[3]

ORIGIN AND PATHOGENESIS

Neither the origin nor the pathogenesis of proliferative mast cell disorders in humans or animals is completely understood. A consistent association with feline leukemia, feline immunodeficiency, or feline infectious peritonitis has not been demonstrated,[15,16] although mast cell neoplasia has been reported in two feline immunodeficiency virus positive cats.[17,18] Systemic mastocytosis has also been identified in a bovine leukemia virus positive Holstein cow; however, viral particles were not detected in the mast cell infiltrates.[7]

Studies in mast cell-deficient mice as well as human patients who had systemic mastocytosis and mast cell leukemia have confirmed a hematopoietic origin for mast cells and their precursors.[19-21] As mentioned in Chapter 48: Basophils and Mast Cells, c-kit ligand (stem cell factor, mast cell growth factor) promotes mast cell proliferation and, in concert with other hematopoietic growth factors, stimulates growth of other progenitor cells and melanocytes.[1,22,23] The proto-oncogene, c-kit, encodes for a transmembrane tyrosine kinase receptor expressed by mast cells, hematopoietic precursors, and leukemic myeloid cells.[22,23] Several mechanisms could lead to unregulated mast cell growth and survival. These include (1) mutations or deregulation of either the c-kit gene, its receptor, or its ligand or (2) c-kit-ligand-independent processes that affect other mast cell growth factors or their receptors.[24] Point mutations of the c-kit gene in a human mast cell leukemia cell line and a human patient who had an aggressive form of systemic mastocytosis have been discovered.[22,25] Induction of a lethal systemic mast cell disease in mice transplanted with bone marrow cells expressing the v-erbB oncogene[9] as well as mast cell proliferation in people who have

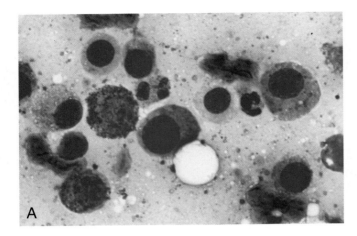

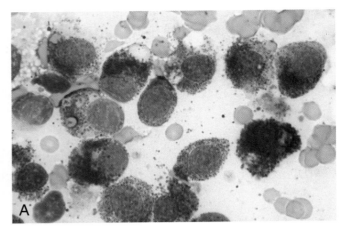

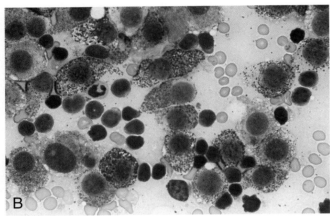

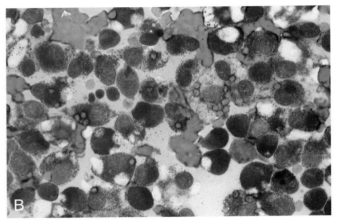

FIGURE 110.1 Fine-needle aspirate of cutaneous mast cell tumor and regional lymph node from a dog (Wright's-Giemsa stain). **A.** Cutaneous mast cell tumor. Anisocytosis, anisokaryosis, and variable amounts of cytoplasmic granulation are evident in the mast cell population. (400×). **B.** Regional lymph node. The presence of numerous mast cells with only a few remaining small lymphocytes indicates metastatic disease. Although not visible in this sample, an increase in eosinophils may be observed in lymph nodes with mast cell tumor metastasis. (165×)

FIGURE 110.2 Fine-needle aspirate of spleen from a case of mast cell leukemia in a cat (Wright–Giemsa stain). **A.** Numerous mast cells are present at the expense of lymphoid cells that normally populate the spleen. Mast cells are characterized by distinct cell margins, variable numbers of small basophilic granules, and pale blue round nuclei (400×). **B.** Pleomorphic mast cells are numerous and contain intracytoplasmic erythrocytes (165×).

myelodysplastic and blast crisis of chronic myeloid leukemia[23] offer insights into *c-kit* ligand independent mechanisms.

CLINICAL SIGNS AND PHYSICAL EXAMINATION

Many of the clinical signs and paraneoplastic syndromes associated with disseminated mast cell disease are attributed to release of vasoactive substances elaborated by mast cells.[1,16,26] Animals may present with vague systemic signs consisting of lethargy, depression, anorexia, and weight loss. Vomiting, hematemesis, diarrhea, and melena as a result of gastrointestinal ulceration are common in cats and dogs.[15,26,27] Splenomegaly, hepatomegaly, lymphadenopathy, and intestinal or other intraabdominal masses are often detected on physical examination of small animal patients. Significant splenomegaly is common in cats. Palpation should be done carefully to avoid mast cell degranulation and histamine release. Other findings noted include cutaneous tumors, hemorrhage, dyspnea, pleural or peritoneal effusions, hypotensive shock, pale mucous membranes, and sudden death as a consequence of splenic rupture or perforation of gastrointestinal ulcers.[5,15,26,28] Systemic mastocytosis has been diagnosed in humans after anaphylactic reactions to *Hymenoptera* stings.[29]

LABORATORY FINDINGS

Although hemograms and results of other laboratory tests are often unremarkable, various hematologic abnormalities may be encountered in animals that have systemic mastocytosis or mast cell leukemia. Notable findings include mastocytemia (circulating mast cells),

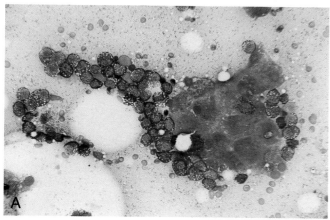

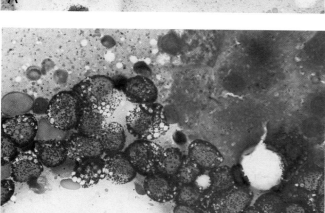

FIGURE 110.3 Fine-needle aspirate of liver from a dog that has systemic mastocytosis (Wright–Giemsa stain). **A.** Numerous mast cells surround a sheet of normal hepatocytes (80×). **B.** Well-granulated mast cells have infiltrated the hepatic parenchyma. Normal hepatocytes are located in the upper right quadrant (165×).

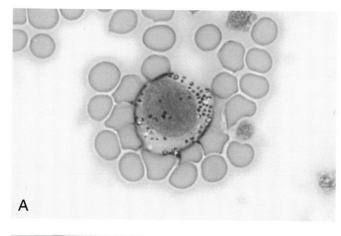

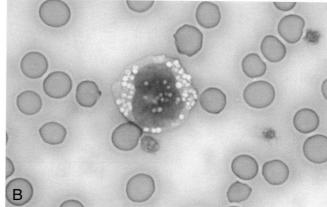

FIGURE 110.4 Blood film from a cat that has mast cell leukemia (Wright–Giemsa stain, 500×). Mast cells were most frequent on the feathered edge of the blood smear. **A.** In this case, mast cell granules are sparse and do not obscure nuclear morphology. **B.** Degranulation has left clear, distinct, cytoplasmic vacuoles in this mast cell.

eosinophilia, basophilia, and bone marrow infiltration (marrow mastocytosis).

Circulating mast cells may be observed at the time systemic mastocytosis is diagnosed. The number of mast cells detected on peripheral blood smears can vary, ranging from 0–32% in reported cases.[15] Mast cells may appear intermittently or as many as several months after splenectomy or removal of cutaneous mast cell tumors.[15,26] Mast cells are frequently observed at the feathered edge of peripheral blood smears (Fig. 110.4). Buffy coat smears facilitate detection when mast cell numbers are low. Animals that have concurrent mast cell leukemia can have moderate to significant leukocytoses with substantial numbers of mast cells in the leukocyte differential, although percentages have ranged from 3 to 74% in reported cases.[4,8] Recognizable mast cells may be accompanied by poorly differentiated mast cells or blasts that require cytochemical staining or electron microscopy for further identification.[11,30]

Elevated peripheral eosinophil and basophil counts have been noted in cats and dogs regardless of mastocytemia.[4,26,30–32] Although usually associated with hypereo-

sinophilic syndrome and eosinophilic leukemia, significant to extreme eosinophilia (24,210/μL and 93,624/μL), in the absence of mastocytemia, has been documented in two cats that had disseminated gastrointestinal mast cell tumors.[31]

Mast cell infiltrates may or may not be observed on marrow aspirates from animals that have systemic mastocytosis, despite concurrent peripheral blood or buffy coat smear findings.[26] Eosinophilic hyperplasia without mast cell hyperplasia has accompanied moderate to extreme peripheral eosinophilia.[31,32] Bone marrow specimens from animals that progress to mast cell leukemia contain mast cell infiltrates; however, mast cells may or may not predominate. Mast cells infiltrating marrow may appear as well differentiated, heavily granulated cells or as large primitive cells that contain few purple granules.

Erythrophagocytosis by neoplastic mast cells may be observed in peripheral blood smears, bone marrow aspirates, and cytologic preparations (Fig. 110.2).[11,33] This is not a feature unique to mast cells but has also been associated with feline myeloproliferative disorders and canine malignant histiocytosis.[5]

Simultaneous myeloid (granulocytic) and mast cell proliferation has been reported in a dog that had systemic mastocytosis.[34] Hematopoietic or lymphoproliferative disorders have developed concurrently in human patients who had systemic mastocytosis or mast cell leukemia.[35,36]

Other significant findings include lymphopenia associated with stress or exogenous corticosteroids; a left shift accompanying inflammatory processes such as gastrointestinal ulceration or tumor abscessation; anemia; neutrophilia; neutropenia; and leukopenia.[5,26,27] Abnormal hemostatic profiles or evidence of disseminated intravascular coagulation have been noted in cats and dogs[4,26,27,30] No consistent abnormalities have been reported on routine biochemical profiles. Elevated histamine and decreased gastrin concentrations have been documented in dogs that had mast cell tumors regardless of the clinical stage of disease.[37]

DIAGNOSIS

Animals may be evaluated because of a history of cutaneous mast cell neoplasia or as part of the clinical staging of mast cell disease at the time of diagnosis (Algorithms 1 and 2). Identification of mast cell infiltration of internal organs or hemolymphatic tissue establishes a diagnosis of systemic mastocytosis. Although the diagnosis is frequently made from cytologic specimens, mast cell proliferation can incite a pronounced eosinophil response in tissue and peripheral blood that can mask the underlying neoplasia. In such cases, exploratory surgery and biopsy are necessary for a definitive diagnosis. Further evaluation, including a complete blood count, biochemical profile, coagulation profile, urinalysis, buffy coat smear, bone marrow aspirate, survey radiographs or ultrasound followed by fine-needle aspiration or biopsy of suspicious lesions, and analysis of pleural or peritoneal effusion provide valuable information for clinical staging, treatment, and prognosis. When gastrointestinal hemorrhage is suspected, a fecal occult blood test may also be warranted. Complete blood counts, evaluation of multiple buffy coat smears, and aspirates or biopsies of new masses or bone marrow can also be used to monitor disease progression and development of mast cell leukemia.

On peripheral blood or cytologic preparations, normal and neoplastic mast cells exhibit affinity for various stains. Granule size, number, and contents such as heparin, glycosaminoglycans, and esterases determine many of the staining characteristics.[38-40] When stained with Romanovsky-type stains, individual mast cells are medium to large, 10 to 20 μm, round cells that possess numerous purple granules that surround and often obscure a single centrally located round to oval nucleus. Mast cell granules may not stain sufficiently with quick-staining methods, on hematoxyin and eosin stained tissue sections, or after decalcification of bone marrow tissue sections.[41,42] Poorly differentiated mast cells may

also stain less intensely.[11,30,39,40] In either case, mast cells can be mistaken for macrophages, vacuolated epithelial cells, plasma cells, or undifferentiated round cells (Fig 110.4b).

Additional cytochemical staining can differentiate leukemic mast cells from other poorly differentiated cells bearing cytoplasmic granules.[19,43,44] Positive cytochemical and histochemical reactions with Giemsa, toluidine blue, alcian blue, periodic acid-Schiff, naphthyl AS-D chloroacetate esterase, acid phosphatase, and α-naphthyl butyrate esterase as well as negative staining with peroxidase, α-naphthyl acetate esterase, and Sudan black IV have been documented in animals that had systemic mastocytosis and mast cell leukemia.[8,30,45,46] Electron microscopy and immunohistochemical staining for CD 68 can provide further positive identification for poorly differentiated mast cells.[40,41]

In the absence of inflammatory or allergic disease, mastocytemia likely reflects disseminated disease in animals diagnosed with mast cell neoplasia (McManus personal communication, 1998).[47] However, mastocytemia and bone marrow mastocytosis must be interpreted cautiously in animals not diagnosed or suspected of having systemic mastocytosis. Mature mast cells are rarely seen on peripheral blood smears and bone marrow aspirates from healthy animals.[20,38,48] Circulating mast cells have been observed in association with regenerative anemias, inflammatory or allergic disorders, and non-mast cell neoplasias as well as systemic mastocytosis and mast cell leukemia in dogs (Table 110.1), (McManus personal communication, 1998).[47,49-51] In some instances, the number of mast cells observed on buffy coat smears approached or surpassed those typically observed with neoplastic mast cell disease (McManus personal communication, 1998). Many of the dogs that had inflammatory disease had concurrent inflammatory leukograms with or without left shifts and toxicity. Mastocytemia has also been noted in severely stressed animals: in two cats, one that had hypereosinophilic syndrome and another that had severe flea allergic dermatitis, and in healthy and diseased golden hamsters (McManus personal communication, 1998).[38,52]

Bone marrow mastocytosis is not pathognomonic for mast cell neoplasia and has also been associated with various disorders in dogs (Table 110.2), (McManus personal communication, 1998).[49,51] Increased mast cell numbers, ranging from 2 to 20% of all cells seen, including stromal cells and adipocytes, were noted in dogs that had aplastic anemia.[51] Bone marrow mast cell hyperplasia has also been documented in mice as a consequence of busulfan-induced marrow hypoplasia and osteoporosis[53]; in rats fed vitamin and mineral deficient diets[54,55]; and in a foal that had generalized cutaneous mastocytosis resembling urticaria pigmentosa, a benign mast cell disorder of infants and young children.[3,56] In people, marrow mastocytosis may precede myelofibrosis or may accompany chronic liver and kidney disease, hematopoietic and lymphoproliferative disorders, and osteoporosis.[2,51]

Systemic mastocytosis has been diagnosed in dogs according to the following criteria[26]: (1) mast cells pres-

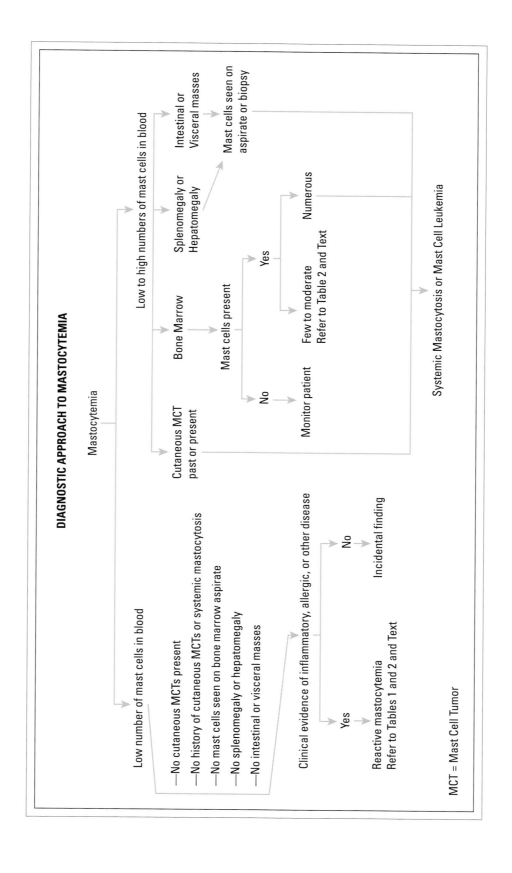

DIAGNOSTIC APPROACH TO MASTOCYTEMIA

Mastocytemia

Low number of mast cells in blood

—No cutaneous MCTs present
—No history of cutaneous MCTs or systemic mastocytosis
—No mast cells seen on bone marrow aspirate
—No splenomegaly or hepatomegaly
—No intestinal or visceral masses

Clinical evidence of inflammatory, allergic, or other disease

Yes → Reactive mastocytemia
Refer to Tables 1 and 2 and Text

No → Incidental finding

Low to high numbers of mast cells in blood

Cutaneous MCT past or present

Bone Marrow

Splenomegaly or Hepatomegaly

Intestinal or Visceral masses

Mast cells seen on aspirate or biopsy

Mast cells present

No → Monitor patient

Yes → Few to moderate
Refer to Table 2 and Text

Numerous

Systemic Mastocytosis or Mast Cell Leukemia

MCT = Mast Cell Tumor

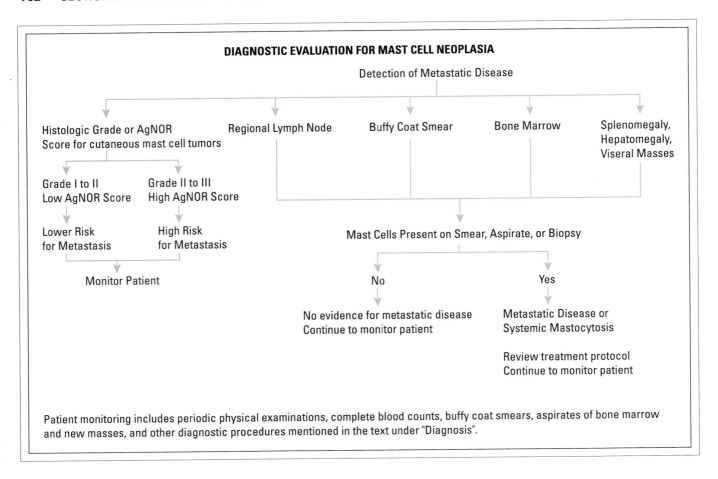

DIAGNOSTIC EVALUATION FOR MAST CELL NEOPLASIA

Patient monitoring includes periodic physical examinations, complete blood counts, buffy coat smears, aspirates of bone marrow and new masses, and other diagnostic procedures mentioned in the text under "Diagnosis".

TABLE 110.1	Disease Conditions Associated with Masto-cytemia in Dogs

Allergy
   atopy, flea allergic dermatitis, sarcoptic mange, and food allergy

Regenerative Anemias
   immune-mediated hemolytic anemia and hemorrhage

Inflammation/Infection/Tissue Injury
   parvoviral enteritis, aspiration pneumonia, bacterial infection,
   acute pancreatic necrosis, acute renal insufficiency, trauma-
   induced tissue injury and gastric torsion

Neoplasia
   systemic mastocytosis
   mast cell leukemia
   non-mast cell neoplasia

TABLE 110.2	Disease Conditions Associated with Bone Marrow Mastocytosis in Dogs

Anemia
   regenerative and nonregenerative anemias, aplastic anemia
   and iron deficiency anemia

Marrow Hypoplasia

Myelofibrosis

Lymphoma

Systemic Mastocytosis

Mast cell Leukemia

ent on peripheral blood or buffy coat smears; (2) evidence of bone marrow involvement (>10 mast cells/1000 nucleated cells); (3) hepatic or splenic involvement (Figs. 110.2 and 110.3); and (4) involvement of lymph nodes distant from the primary tumor (Fig. 110.1). In light of new information that dogs, especially, can have mastocytemia or marrow mastocytosis for reasons not associated with mast cell neoplasia, the first two diag-

nostic criteria are general guidelines at best. Diagnosing systemic mastocytosis or mast cell leukemia based solely on these two features may be misleading, particularly in animals that have inflammatory or allergic diseases or when mast cell numbers are low. In these and all cases, it becomes imperative to document organ infiltration and to rule out other causes of mastocytemia and bone marrow mastocytosis. Finding mast cell infiltration of a visceral mass or organ such as spleen, liver, or intestine, suffices for a diagnosis of systemic mastocytosis without peripheral blood or marrow involvement. If the bone marrow contains neoplastic mast cell aggregates, other organs are infiltrated as well.

Considerable overlap exists between systemic mastocytosis and mast cell leukemia in animals and humans. Specific criteria for diagnosing concurrent mast cell leukemia in animals that have systemic mastocytosis have not been established. However, most veterinary cases reported have documented ≥10% mast cells in peripheral blood and significant marrow infiltration. In human patients who have systemic mastocytosis, the following criteria must be fulfilled before mast cell leukemia is diagnosed: (1) mast cell circulation of ≥10% mast cells on a peripheral blood leukocyte differential; (2) evident morphologic atypia in the leukemic mast cells; (3) cytochemical features characteristic of mast cells; and (4) diffuse bone marrow infiltration by atypical mast cells.[3,43,44] Whereas every requirement may not apply to all cases of mast cell leukemia in animals, definite criteria for the diagnosis of mast cell leukemia in veterinary patients may evolve as additional case material accumulates.

TREATMENT AND PROGNOSIS

Treatment and prognosis depend on the histologic grade and argyrophillic nucleolar organizer region (AgNOR) score of cutaneous mast cell tumors, clinical stage of disease, and presence of systemic signs.[16,57] The AgNOR score is determined by staining cytologic preparations or tissue sections with a silver colloid stain and counting the number of argyrophilic sites of ribosomal transcription in nucleoli. High scores indicate greater proliferative activity of the cells and correlate with the histologic grade and biologic behavior of cutaneous mast cell tumors.[57] Various treatment options are available for mast cell neoplasia, including surgical excision, radiotherapy, chemotherapy, or a combination of these. Antihistamines (diphenhydramine, cimetidine, ranitidine) and gastrointestinal protectants (sucralfate, misoprostol) may be used to alleviate systemic signs.[16]

Animals that have systemic mastocytosis or mast cell leukemia have a guarded to poor prognosis. Most animals survive only a few months after diagnosis.[16,26] Cats that have mast cell neoplasia limited to the spleen, on the other hand, enjoy longer median survival times after splenectomy. In a study of splenic mast cell tumors, the prognosis for cats that had positive buffy coat smears or bone marrow aspirates did not differ significantly from those cats that did not have mastocytemia or evidence of bone marrow involvement.[27]

REFERENCES

1. **Golkar L, Bernhard JD.** Mastocytosis. Lancet 1997;349:1379–1385.
2. **Lichtman MA.** Basophilopenia, basophilia, and mastocytosis. In: Beutler E, Lichtman MA, Coller BS, Kipps TJ, eds. Williams hematology. 5th ed. New York: McGraw-Hill, 1995;852–858.
3. **Stone RM, Bernstein SH.** Mast cell leukemia and other mast cell neoplasms. In: Holland JF, Bast RC, Morton DL, Frei E, Kufe DW, Weichselbaum RR, eds. Cancer medicine. 4th ed. Baltimore: Williams & Wilkins, 1997;2829–2834.
4. **Davies AP, Hayden DW, Klausner JS, et al.** Noncutaneous systemic mastocytosis and mast cell leukemia in a dog: case report and literature review. J Am Anim Hosp Assoc 1981;17:361–368.
5. **Jain NC.** The leukemia complex. In: Jain NC, ed. Schalm's veterinary hematology. 4th ed. Philadelphia: Lea & Febiger, 1986;838–908.
6. **Hill JE, Langheinrich KA, Kelley LC.** Prevalence and location of mast cell tumors in slaughter cattle. Vet Pathol 1991;28:449–450.
7. **Shaw DP, Buoen LC, Weiss DJ.** Multicentric mast cell tumor in a cow. Vet Pathol 1991;128:450–452.
8. **Bean-Knudsen DE, Caldwell CW, Wagner JE, et al.** Porcine mast cell leukemia with systemic mastocytosis. Vet Pathol 1989;26:90–92.
9. **von Ruden R, Kandels S, Radaszkiewicz T, et al.** Development of a lethal mast cell disease in mice reconstituted with bone marrow cells expressing the *v-erb* B oncogene. Blood 1992;79:3145–3158.
10. **Brown SA.** Neoplasia. In: Hillyer EV, Quesenberry KE, eds. Ferrets, rabbits, and rodents: clinical medicine and surgery. Philadelphia: WB Saunders, 1997;99–114.
11. **Khan KNM, Sagartz JE, Koenig G, et al.** Systemic mastocytosis in a goat. Vet Pathol 1995;32:719–721.
12. **Guzman-Silva MA.** Systemic mast cell disease in the Mongolian gerbil, *Meriones unguiculatus*: case report. Lab Anim 1997;31:373–378.
13. **Winter VH, Saar C, Goltenboth R.** Mastzellenleukose und duodenumkarzinom bei einem gepard (*Azinonyx jubatus schraber*). Kleintierpraxis 1980;25:499–504.
14. **Lillie RD.** Mast myelocyte leukemia in a cat. Am J Pathol 1931;7:713–721.
15. **Liska WD, MacEwen EG, Zaki FA, et al.** Feline systemic mastocytosis: a review and results of splenectomy in seven cases. J Am Anim Hosp Assoc 1979;15:589–597.
16. **Vail DM.** Mast cell tumors. In: Withrow SJ, MacEwen EG, eds. Small animal clinical oncology. 2nd ed. Philadelphia: WB Saunders, 1996;192–210.
17. **Shelton GH, Waltier RM, Connor SC, et al.** Prevalence of feline immunodeficiency virus and feline leukemia virus infections in pet cats. J Am Anim Hosp Assoc 1989;25:7–12.
18. **Barr MC, Butt MT, Anderson KL, et al.** Spinal lymphosarcoma and disseminated mastocytoma associated with feline immunodeficiency virus infection in a cat. J Am Vet Med Assoc 1993;202:1978–1980.
19. **Dalton R, Chan L, Batten E, et al.** Mast cell leukaemia: evidence for bone marrow origin of the pathological clone. Br J Haematol 1986;64:397–406.
20. **Galli SJ.** New insights into "the riddle of the mast cells": Microenvironmental regulation of mast cell development and phenotypic heterogeneity. Lab Invest 1990;62:5–33.
21. **Kirshenbaum AS, Kessler SW, Goff JP, et al.** Demonstration of the origin of human mast cells from CD34+ bone marrow progenitor cells. J Immunol 1991;146:1410–1415.
22. **Furitsu T, Tsujimura T, Tono T, et al.** Identification of mutations in the coding sequence of the proto-oncogene *c-kit* in a human mast cell leukemia cell line causing ligand-independent activation of *c-kit* product. J Clin Invest 1993;92:1736–1744.
23. **Valent P, Spanblochl E, Bankl HC, et al.** *Kit* ligand / mast cell growth factor-independent differentiation of mast cells in myelodysplasia and chronic myeloid leukemic blast crisis. Blood 1994;84:4322–4332.
24. **Galli SJ.** New concepts about the mast cell. N Engl J Med 1993;328:257–265.
25. **Pignon JM, Giraudier S, Duquesnoy P, et al.** A new *c-kit* mutation in a case of aggressive mast cell disease. Br J Haematol 1997;96:374–376.
26. **O'Keefe DA, Couto CG, Burke-Schwartz C, et al.** Systemic mastocytosis in 16 dogs. J Vet Intern Med 1987;1:75–80.
27. **Feinmehl R, Matus R, Mauldin GN, et al.** Splenic mast cell tumors in 43 cats (1975–1992). [Abstract] Proc Annu Conf Vet Cancer Soc 1992;12:50.
28. **Gilmore CE, Holzworth J.** Naturally occurring feline leukemia: clinical, pathologic, and differential diagnostic features. J Am Vet Med Assoc 1971;158:1013–1031.
29. **Kors JW, Van Doormaal JJ, De Monchy JGR.** Anaphylactoid shock following Hymenoptera sting as a presenting symptom of systemic mastocytosis. J Intern Med 1993;233:255–258.
30. **Lester SJ, McGonigle LF, McDonald GK.** Disseminated anaplastic mastocytoma with terminal mastocythemia in dog. J Am Anim Hosp Assoc 1981;17:355–360.
31. **Bortnowski HB, Rosenthal RC.** Gastrointestinal mast cell tumors and eosinophilia in two cats. J Am Anim Hosp Assoc 1992;28:271–275.
32. **Pollack MJ, Flanders JA, Johnson RC.** Disseminated malignant mastocytoma in a dog. J Am Anim Hosp Assoc 1991;27:435–440.
33. **Madewell BR, Munn RJ, Phillips LP.** Endocytosis of erythrocytes *in vivo* and particulate substances *in vitro* by feline neoplastic mast cells. Can J Vet Res 1987;51:517–520.
34. **Bronstad A, Jenssen M, Espenes A, et al.** Systemic mastocytosis and myeloid proliferation in a dog. A case report. Norsk Veterinaertidsskrift 1994;106:289–296.
35. **Travis WD, Li CY, Yam LT, et al.** Significance of systemic mast cell disease with associated hematologic disorders. Cancer 1988;62:965–972.
36. **Horny HP, Ruck M, Wehrmann M, et al.** Blood findings in generalized mastocytosis: evidence of frequent simultaneous occurrence of myeloproliferative disorders. Br J Haematol 1990; 76:186–193.
37. **Fox LE, Rosenthal RC, Twedt DC, et al.** Plasma histamine and gastrin concentrations in 17 dogs with mast cell tumors. J Vet Intern Med 1990;4:242–246.
38. **Jain NC.** The basophil and the mast cell. In: Jain NC, ed. Schalm's veterinary hematology. 4th ed. Philadelphia: Lea & Febiger, 1986;756–767.
39. **Klatt EC, Lukes RJ, Meyer PR.** Benign and malignant mast cell prolifera-

tions. Diagnosis and separation using a pH-dependent toluidine blue stain in tissue section. Cancer 1983;51:1119–1124.

40. **Simoes JPC, Schoning P.** Canine mast cell tumors: A comparison of staining techniques. J Vet Diag Invest 1994;6:458–465.

41. **Bain BJ, Clark DM, Lampert IA.** Myeloproliferative disorders. In: Bone marrow pathology. 2nd ed. Oxford: Blackwell Scientific Publications, 1996;126–152.

42. **Clinkenbeard KD.** Diagnostic cytology: Mast cell tumors. Compend Contin Educ Pract Vet 1991;13:1697–1701.

43. **Li CY, Yam LT.** Cytochemical characterization of leukemic cells with numerous cytoplasmic granules. Mayo Clin Proc 1987;62:978–985.

44. **Travis WD, Li CY, Hoagland HC, et al.** Mast cell leukemia: report of a case and review of the literature. Mayo Clin Proc 1986;61:957–966.

45. **Guerre R, Millet P Groulade P.** Systemic mastocytosis in a cat: remission after splenectomy. J Small Anim Pract 1979;20:769–772.

46. **Holscher M, McCurley T, Eisinberg K, et al.** Mast cell leukemia in a cat. Feline Pract 1986;16:11–14.

47. **Cayatte SM, McManus PM, Miller WH, et al.** Identification of mast cells in buffy coat preparations from dogs with inflammatory skin diseases. J Am Vet Med Assoc 1995;206:325–326.

48. **Bookbinder PF, Butt MT, Harvey HJ.** Determination of the number of mast cells in lymph node, bone marrow, and buffy coat cytologic specimens from dogs. J Am Vet Med Assoc 1992;200:1648–1650.

49. **McManus P.** Canine mastocytemia and marrow mastocytosis: disease associations, incidence and severity. [Abstract] Vet Pathol 1997;34:474.

50. **Stockham SL, Basel DL, Schmidt DA.** Mastocytemia in dogs with acute inflammatory diseases. Vet Clin Pathol 1986;15:16–21.

51. **Walker D, Cowell RL, Clinkenbeard KD, et al.** Bone marrow mast cell hyperplasia in dogs with aplastic anemia. Vet Clin Pathol 1997;26:106–111.

52. **Fulton GP, Joftes DL, Kagan R, et al.** Hematologic findings in the total body x–irradiated hamster. Blood 1954;9:622–631.

53. **McManus PM, Weiss L.** Busulfan-induced chronic bone marrow failure: changes in cortical bone, marrow stromal cells, and adherent cell colonies. Blood 1984;64:1036–1041.

54. **Belanger LF.** Variations in the mast cell population of skin and bone marrow in magnesium-deprived rats. The influence of sex hormones. J Nutr 1977;107:2164–2170.

55. **Belanger LF.** The influence of zinc-deprivation on the mast cell population of the bone marrow and other tissues. J Nutr 1978;108:1315–1321.

56. **Prasse KW, Lundvall RL, Cheville NF.** Generalized mastocytosis in a foal, resembling urticaria pigmentosa of man. J Am Vet Med Assoc 1975;166:68–70.

57. **Kravis LD, Vail DM, Kisseberth WC, et al.** Frequency of argyrophilic nucleolar organizer regions in fine-needle aspirates and biopsy specimens from mast cell tumors in dogs. J Am Vet Med Assoc 1996;209:1418–1420.

CHAPTER 111

Cytochemical Tests for Diagnosis of Leukemia

• ROSE E. RASKIN and AMY VALENCIANO

GENERAL CONSIDERATIONS FOR STAINING NEOPLASTIC CELLS

The first step in the identification and classification of hematopoietic neoplasia is a morphologic characterization of the poorly differentiated blast cell population and accompanying cells. This may be followed by special tests to better define the cell of origin. Poorly differentiated cells are indistinguishable by morphology alone but may be better identified by their cytochemical characteristics. This is critical for acute leukemias and especially useful in domestic animals like the dog, cat, and horse. The use of cytochemical staining can improve the diagnosis and sometimes change the initial morphologic interpretation.[1-6]

The general premise of cytochemistry for hematopoietic malignancies is that the neoplastic cells contain the same enzymes or cellular products as are found in cells from healthy individuals. However, occasional irregularities may occur related to the altered development of neoplastic or dysplastic cells.[7] Cytochemical staining is best interpreted when a panel rather than one or two stains are performed since discrepancies may occur with neoplastic cells. The reader should refer to Chapter 51, Cytochemistry of Normal Leukocytes, for a more complete description of the stains and their mechanism of activity.

In general, lymphoid cells do not stain with many cytochemical stains. However, negative staining does not automatically indicate a lymphoid neoplasm. Rather it may represent an undifferentiated myeloid malignancy. Stain intensity is often very weak or absent in the most undifferentiated cells because they contain few of the necessary enzymes or cellular constituents found within lysosomal granules, cytoplasm, or the plasma membrane. On the other hand, some enzymes such as myeloperoxidase found in the primary granules of granulocytes are present to a greater extent in the earlier stages. In cytochemistry, it is best to interpret the results of positive staining rather than the lack of staining. Positive staining is meaningful, whereas negative staining leads to uncertainty.

In addition to stain intensity, the pattern of staining may be diagnostic. T lymphocytes bearing focal lysosomal granules often produce a focal or discrete localization of nonspecific esterase enzyme activity compared with the diffuse or granular nature found in some nonlymphoid cells. Lymphoid cells are better classified with immunologic markers but lineage- and species-specific monoclonal antibodies are limited in availability. Until this situation is fully remedied, it remains worthwhile to use cytochemical staining to identify T lymphocytes from non-T lymphocytes.

In the interpretation of staining data, additional factors are considered. One factor is the species involved. Reactions seen within one species cannot be extended readily to other species. For example, feline eosinophils normally do not stain with either peroxidase (PER) or Sudan black B (SBB) whereas it is present in other species.[8] Another factor involves the extent of staining within the sample. The percentage of stained blast cells in the bone marrow should be sufficient to establish a positive reaction with a given stain. Generally, this is greater than 3%. In the case of myeloperoxidase or SBB, greater than 3% of the blast cells present should be positive to identify the human M1 or myeloblastic leukemia without maturation.[9] It is best to count a minimum of 200 bone marrow cells when calculating this figure to avoid an overestimation or an underestimation.[1]

Cytochemistry is applicable to nonlymphoid cells and ideal as a diagnostic tool as it involves minimal cost and is readily performed at many veterinary colleges. This stain methodology may be applied to hemolymphatic tissues such as blood, bone marrow, lymph nodes, spleen, thymus, or liver in the form of fresh, frozen,[10] or plastic embedded tissues.[11] In addition to light microscopy, cytochemical staining has been applied to electron microscopic specimens.[12]

COMMON CYTOCHEMICAL STAINS FOR THE IDENTIFICATION OF HEMATOPOIETIC NEOPLASIA

The use of these stains in classifying acute leukemias in veterinary medicine is provided as an algorithm. A

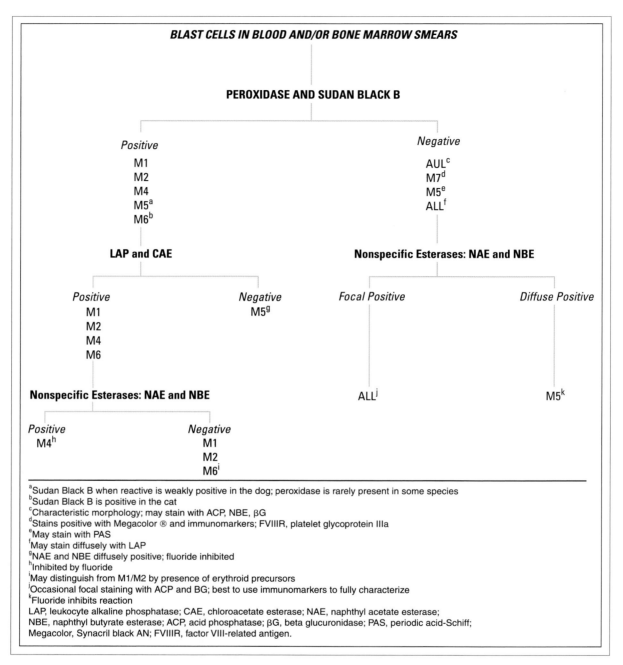

Algorithm for distinguishing blast cells in blood or bone marrow using cytochemical stains.

summary of 171 selected cases in the literature demonstrates the range of stain reactions in nonlymphoid neoplasia for several animal species in Table 111.1.

Peroxidase

PER is an enzyme found in several nonlymphoid cells and is present within different sites of the cell. For example, it is found within the primary or lysosomal granules of neutrophils, the crystalloid matrix of the secondary eosinophil granules, and, to a lesser extent, within the lysosomal granules of the monocyte. The blast cells within the bone marrow should stain positive with PER for the following subtypes of acute myeloid leukemia: M1 (myeloblastic leukemia without maturation), M2 (myeloblastic leukemia with maturation), M4 (myelomonocytic leukemia), and M6 (erythroleukemia). Rare positive staining in M5a (monoblastic leukemia without maturation) is possible but has only been documented in veterinary medicine.[13] The intensity of staining within mature neutrophils reflects the level of activity within

TABLE 111.1 Summary of Cytochemical Staining in 171 Selected Cases of Nonlymphoid Malignancies

Disease/Subtype/Species	# Cases	PER	SBB	CAE	LAP	NAE	NBE	Fluoride	ACP	ACP/T	βG	PAS
Acute Undifferentiated Leukemia												
Cat	1	neg	neg	ND	ND	ND	pos/neg	ND	pos/neg	ND	pos	ND
Myeloblastic/M1 or M2												
Dog	5	pos	pos/neg	pos	pos	neg	neg	ND	pos	neg	ND	neg
Cat	7	pos/neg	pos	pos	pos/neg	neg	neg	ND	pos	pos	ND	pos
Horse	1	pos	pos	pos	neg	ND	neg	neg	pos	ND	ND	pos
Swine	6	pos	ND	ND	ND	ND	ND	ND	ND	ND	ND	ND
Eosinophilic/Chronic or M2												
Cat	2	neg	neg	pos/neg	pos	ND	pos/neg	ND	pos	pos	ND	pos
Horse	1	ND	pos	ND	ND	ND	ND	ND	ND	ND	ND	ND
Basophilic/Chronic or M2												
Dog	2	neg	neg	pos/neg	neg	pos	neg	ND	pos	ND	ND	pos/neg
Cat	1	neg	neg	pos	pos/neg	pos	ND	ND	pos	ND	ND	ND
Myelomonocytic/M4												
Dog	20	pos/neg	pos	pos	pos	pos	pos	neg	pos	neg	ND	pos/neg
Cat	2	pos	pos	pos	pos/neg	pos	pos	neg	neg	ND	ND	pos/neg
Horse	4	pos	pos	pos	neg	pos	pos	neg	ND	ND	ND	ND
Cattle	1	neg	pos	pos	ND	pos	ND	ND	ND	ND	ND	ND
Monocytic/M5												
Cattle	10	pos/neg	pos/neg	neg	neg	pos	ND	neg	ND	ND	ND	pos/neg
Cat	3	neg	neg	neg	neg	pos	pos	neg	neg	neg	ND	pos
Horse	1	ND	ND	pos/neg	pos/neg	pos	ND	ND	ND	ND	ND	ND
Erythroleukemia/M6 or M6Er												
Cat M6	4	neg	pos	pos	pos	neg	pos/neg	neg	pos	pos	ND	pos/neg
Cat M6Er	4	neg	neg	pos/neg	pos/neg	ND	neg	ND	pos/neg	pos/neg	ND	pos/neg
Dog M6Er	1	neg	pos/neg	neg	pos/neg	ND	ND	ND	pos	pos	ND	neg
Megakaryoblastic/M7 or ET												
Dog M7/ET	10	neg	pos/neg	pos/neg	neg	pos	pos/neg	pos/neg	pos/neg	neg	ND	pos
Cat M7	2	neg	ND	neg	neg	neg	neg	ND	neg	ND	ND	pos
Malignant Histiocytosis												
Dog	3	neg	pos/neg	pos	neg	pos	neg	ND	pos	pos/neg	ND	pos/neg
Horse	1	ND	ND	ND	ND	ND	pos	ND	ND	ND	ND	ND
Cat	2	ND	ND	ND	ND	ND	pos	neg	pos	ND	ND	ND
Mast Cell Neoplasia												
Dog	39	neg	neg	pos	neg	ND	pos/neg	ND	pos/neg	ND	ND	pos/neg
Cat MCT/Leukemia	2	neg	neg	pos	neg	ND	pos/neg	ND	pos/neg	pos/neg	ND	pos/neg
Goat	1	ND	ND	ND	ND	ND	ND	ND	ND	ND	ND	pos
Cattle	1	ND	ND	ND	ND	ND	ND	ND	ND	ND	ND	ND
Pig	4	ND	ND	pos	ND	ND	pos	ND	pos	ND	ND	pos/neg
Horse	30	ND	ND	ND	ND	ND	ND	neg	ND	ND	ND	ND

PER = peroxidase, SBB = Sudan black B, CAE = chloroacetate esterase, LAP = leukocyte alkaline phosphatase, NAE = naphthyl acetate esterase, NBE = naphthyl butyrate esterase, ACP = acid phosphatase, ACP/T = acid phosphatase with tartrate, βG = beta glucuronidase, PAS = periodic acid-Schiff, ET = essential thrombocythemia, neg = no reaction; pos = easily detectable; pos/neg = weak or occasional reactivity, ND = not determined.

myeloblasts. There is a deficiency of PER activity for myelogenous leukemia in human medicine but during remission after chemotherapy, the activity increases and can be better detected in the mature neutrophil. Therefore monitoring PER activity may provide prognostic information regarding the efficacy of treatment in people.

Lymphoid malignancies traditionally lack PER staining; however, occasional reports in human medicine have identified molecular expression of the enzyme.[14] There are no known reports of PER staining in veterinary cases of acute undifferentiated leukemia, basophilic leukemia, megakaryoblastic leukemia, acute lymphoid leukemia, lymphoma, malignant histiocytosis, or mast cell neoplasia. PER staining was helpful in the diagnosis of several canine, feline, equine, and porcine cases of myeloblastic leukemia (Fig. 111.1) and myelomonocytic leukemia.[3,5,12,15–24]

Sudan Black B

SBB dye binds with intracellular lipids by an unknown mechanism. Lipids are generally found within the secondary granules of neutrophils and eosinophils and to a lesser extent within primary granules. Although these granulocytes present with a moderate to strong reaction, monocytes produce a weak positive reaction. The blast cells within the bone marrow should stain positive with SBB (Fig. 111.2) in the following subtypes of acute myeloid leukemia: M1 (myeloblastic leukemia without maturation), M2 (myeloblastic leukemia with maturation), M4 (myelomonocytic leukemia), M5 (monocytic leukemia), and M6 (erythroleukemia). Lymphoid malignancies traditionally lack positive reactions with SBB. However, one case of canine acute lymphoblastic leukemia displayed slight sudanophilia.[4] One case of canine malignant histiocytosis had positive SBB staining.[4] There are no known reports of SBB staining in veterinary cases of acute undifferentiated leukemia, basophilic leukemia, megakaryoblastic leukemia, or mast cell neoplasia. SBB

staining was helpful in the diagnosis of several canine, feline, equine, and bovine cases of myeloblastic leukemia, eosinophilic leukemia, monocytic leukemia, myelomonocytic leukemia, and erythroleukemia.[4,6,16,19,25–30]

Chloroacetate Esterase

Found within the primary and the secondary granules of neutrophils and within the specific granules of basophils is the enzyme chloroacetate esterase (CAE). The stain is sometimes referred to as a specific esterase, which relates to its resistance to fluoride inhibition to alter its stain reaction. CAE may be performed together with a nonspecific esterase stain for monocytes to detect both neutrophil and monocyte populations simultaneously.[31] The mechanism of stain reaction is similar to that of nonspecific esterases in that liberated naphthol compounds when coupled with a diazonium salt form a highly colored product near the site of enzyme activity. Although CAE is generally specific for neutrophils, other cell types have weak reactions. For example, mild positive reactions may occur within the monocytes of horses and ruminants. In addition, slight reactions within normal megakaryocytes of dogs and cats have been noted.[4,6]

Positive reactions with CAE (Fig. 111.3) occur in the following subtypes of acute myeloid leukemia: M1 (myeloblastic leukemia without maturation), M2 (myeloblastic leukemia with maturation), M4 (myelomonocytic leukemia), and M6 (erythroleukemia). CAE is less sensitive but more specific than PER in distinguishing granulocytic and monocytic precursors. In addition to its specificity for neutrophils, it is regarded as a marker for basophilic leukemia and mast cell tumors. Lymphoid malignancies generally lack positive reactions with CAE. However, one case each of canine and feline acute lymphoblastic leukemia (ALL) displayed a slight reaction.[6] This is similar to human medicine in which rare cases of positive staining have occurred in ALL. In addition CAE staining was noted in several feline lymphoma

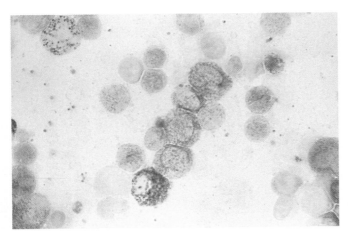

FIGURE 111.1 Diffuse PER staining of blast cells in canine AML-M2. Bone marrow cytology. 250× original magnification.

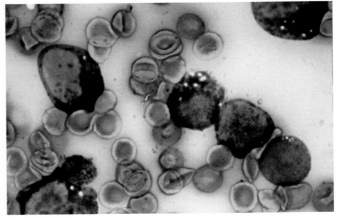

FIGURE 111.2 Diffuse SBB staining of blast cells in canine AML-M4. Bone marrow cytology. 500× original magnification.

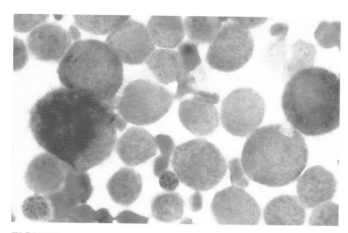

FIGURE 111.3 Granulocytic blast cells stain CAE positive in feline AML-M4. Bone marrow cytology. 500× original magnification.

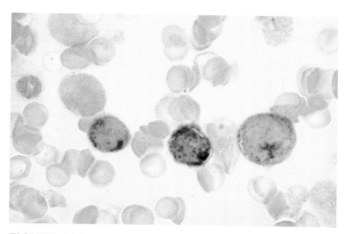

FIGURE 111.4 Diffuse LAP staining of blast cells in canine AML-M4. Bone marrow cytology. 500× original magnification.

cases, many of which involved large granular lymphocytes.[32–34] One case of feline eosinophilic leukemia was positive for CAE.[6] Occasional weak to moderate staining was noted in three cases of canine megakaryoblastic leukemia.[35,36] One case of weak CAE staining occurred in a horse that had monocytic leukemia.[37] There are no known reports of CAE staining in canine or feline cases of monocytic leukemia. CAE staining was helpful in the diagnosis of several canine, feline, bovine, equine, and porcine cases of myeloblastic leukemia, basophilic leukemia, myelomonocytic leukemia, malignant histiocytosis, mast cell tumor, and erythroleukemia.[4,6,16,18–24,26–29,38–43]

Leukocyte Alkaline Phosphatase

The mechanism of the leukocyte alkaline phosphatase (LAP) stain reaction is similar to that of the esterases with the enzyme hydrolyzing the reaction to produce liberated naphthol compounds that bind with a colored dye while in an alkaline medium. This enzyme is present within several cells in veterinary medicine, and its stain reaction differs from that observed in people. In humans, the concentration of the enzyme is intense in the secondary granules of the neutrophil, but LAP is lacking in normal late-stage neutrophil forms in the dog and cat. In contrast, the horse has positive staining in mature neutrophils. In addition to neutrophils, LAP is present between the specific granules of eosinophils and feline basophils.[8] Generally lymphocytes and monocytes lack positive staining.

Because LAP may be found in neutrophil precursors, it has been suggested that the presence of enzyme activity is a specific marker for myelogenous origin of canine and feline leukemia.[8] Specific subtypes of acute myeloid leukemia that display LAP (Fig. 111.4) activity include M1 (myeloblastic leukemia without maturation), M2 (myeloblastic leukemia with maturation), M4 (myelomonocytic leukemia), and M6 (erythroleukemia). Posi-

tive staining has been documented in cases of feline eosinophilic leukemia.[6,44] One feline case involving basophilic differentiation of an acute myeloid leukemia exhibited cytoplasmic LAP staining.[39] Lymphoid malignancies generally lack positive reactions with LAP. However, positive reactions in lymphoid malignancies have been noted.[4,10,45,46] One case of weak LAP staining was documented in a horse that had monocytic leukemia.[47] LAP staining has been observed in monoblasts from normal dogs and dogs that have monoblastic leukemia (Julia Blue, personal communication, 1998). There are no known reports of LAP staining in feline cases of monocytic leukemia or in canine and feline cases of malignant histiocytosis, megakaryoblastic leukemia, and mast cell tumor. LAP staining was helpful in the diagnosis of several canine and feline cases of myeloblastic leukemia, myelomonocytic leukemia, and erythroleukemia.[3–6,15,18,24,27,48]

Nonspecific Esterases

This group of enzymes is frequently termed nonspecific since sodium fluoride treatment changes the cell specificity for the stain. The activity of α-naphthyl acetate esterase (NAE) and α-naphthyl butyrate esterase (NBE) are the nonspecific esterases most commonly tested. Both react similarly with the mechanism of the stain reaction comparable with that of the specific esterase CAE in which the enzyme hydrolyzes the reaction to produce liberated naphthol compounds that then bind to a colored dye. These enzymes are present within several cells, which occasionally must be differentiated by fluoride inhibition incorporated into the stain procedure. Cells of monocytic origin particularly, as well as lymphocytes, megakaryocytes, and occasionally plasma cells and granulocytes stain positive.[8,49] NBE staining is considered more specific to detect the monocytic line but less sensitive to other cell types and therefore may not require differential inhibition with fluoride.

The nonspecific esterase reaction is used to differentiate monocytic from granulocytic malignancies. Specific subtypes of acute myeloid leukemia that display non-specific esterase positive activity include M4 (myelomonocytic leukemia), M5 (monocytic leukemia), and M7 (megakaryoblastic leukemia). Positive staining has been documented in cases of canine, feline, and equine malignant histiocytosis.[40,50–52] Weak stain reactions with NAE occurred in feline and canine cases involving basophil proliferation.[38,39] In addition, occasional positive NBE reactions have been documented in canine, feline, and porcine mast cell tumors.[6,41,43] One case of feline eosinophilic leukemia reported occasional positive staining with NBE.[6] A cat with an acute undifferentiated leukemia, formerly termed reticuloendotheliosis, had diffuse NBE staining in some of the leukemic cells.[37] One case of feline erythroleukemia was positive for NBE.[6] Lymphoid malignancies may stain with nonspecific esterases, giving a focal rather than diffuse appearance. Some examples of positive staining of lymphoid neoplasia may be found in dogs, cats, cattle, and sheep.[4–6,10,32–34,45,46,49,53,54] There are no known reports of nonspecific esterase staining in canine, feline, or equine cases of myeloblastic leukemia. In summary, NAE has been helpful in diagnosing M4, M5 (Fig. 111.5), M7, blast cells of essential thrombocythemia, and malignant histiocytosis, whereas NBE has been helpful in diagnosing M4, M5, and malignant histiocytosis.[3–6,17–22,24,26–29,35,36,40,47,50–52,55–62]

Acid Phosphatase

The lysosomal enzyme, acid phosphatase (ACP) has a mechanism of stain reaction similar to that of the esterases. The enzyme hydrolyzes the substrate in an acidic medium to produce liberated naphthol compounds, which then bind to a colored dye. ACP is present within several cells, which may be differentiated by tartrate incubation, particularly in human medicine, to detect tartrate-resistant hairy cells. Hairy-cell leukemia is not recognized in veterinary medicine, therefore tartrate inhibition is not routinely performed. However, canine and feline eosinophils and basophils are tartrate-resistant.[4,6] Cells of monocytic origin, megakaryocytes, platelets, granulocytes, and erythroid precursors stain positive in a diffuse manner compared with the focal manner within some lymphocytes.[4,6,8] Since it is found within the primary granules of neutrophils, immature cells contain more activity than later stages.

ACP may be used to detect many different types of blast cells. Specific subtypes of acute myeloid leukemia that display positive activity include M1 or M2 (myeloblastic leukemia), M4 (myelomonocytic leukemia), M6 (erythroleukemia), and M7 (megakaryoblastic leukemia).[4,6,16,35] Positive staining has been documented in cases of canine and feline malignant histiocytosis.[4,40,51] Eosinophilic and basophilic differentiation of acute and chronic myeloid leukemia in the cat and dog display positive staining.[6,38,39] In addition, occasional positive ACP reactions have been documented in canine, feline, and porcine mast cell tumors.[6,41,43] The amoeboid blast cells in a cat that had an acute undifferentiated leukemia had occasional ACP staining.[37] There are no known reports of ACP staining in feline cases of monocytic leukemia. ACP is used in veterinary medicine primarily to detect focal staining in T lymphocytes. Some examples of positive ACP staining in lymphoid malignancies may be found in dogs, cats, cattle, sheep, and pigs.[4,6,10,32–34,46,49,53,63–65]

β Glucuronidase

The hydrolytic enzyme β glucoronidase (βG) has a mechanism of stain reaction similar to that of the esterases. The enzyme hydrolyzes the substrate to produce liberated naphthol compounds, which then bind to a colored dye. βG is present within lymphocytes and monocytes but may be differentiated by focal staining pattern in T lymphocytes and diffuse pattern of staining in some B lymphocytes and monocytes. Diffuse positive staining has been documented in a case of feline acute undifferentiated leukemia.[37] βG is used in veterinary medicine primarily to detect focal staining in T lymphocytes. Three cats that had large granular lymphocyte lymphoma were noted to have positive staining with βG.[34,53]

Periodic Acid-Schiff

Periodic acid oxidizes carbohydrate substances forming an aldehyde that reacts with Schiff's reagent to produce a colored dye. Carbohydrates detected commonly with periodic acid-Schiff (PAS) stain include monosaccharides, glycogen, starch, cellulose, and protein conjugates with carbohydrates such as glycoproteins or mucoproteins. Mature forms of neutrophilic granulocytes and platelets or megakaryocytes stain the most intense with monocytes, eosinophils, and basophils producing a weak positive reaction. Myeloblasts and promyelocytes stain negative and weakly positive with PAS, respec-

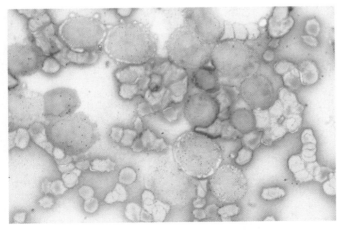

FIGURE 111.5 Diffuse naphthyl acetate esterase staining of monocytoid blast cells that were fluoride sensitive in equine AML-M5a. Bone marrow cytology. 250× original magnification.

tively.[4,6] Lymphocytes usually do not stain positive, or if they do it is a very weak reaction, especially in plasmacytic forms.

In general, PAS staining in veterinary medicine is used to differentiate granulocytic or megakaryocytic precursors from lymphoid precursors. Specific subtypes of acute myeloid leukemia that may display PAS positive activity include M1 or M2 (myeloblastic leukemia), M4 (myelomonocytic leukemia), M5 (monocytic leukemia), M6 or M6Er (erythroleukemia or erythroleukemia with erythroid predominance), and M7 (megakaryoblastic leukemia).[3,4,6,16,28,36,57,58,60,61,66–68] Positive staining has been documented in canine malignant histiocytosis.[4,66] One case of feline eosinophilic leukemia displayed positive PAS reaction.[6] A weak stain reaction with PAS occurred in a case of basophilic leukemia.[38] Mast-cell tumors in the dog, cat, goat, and pig have demonstrated positive PAS reaction.[41–43,69] Infrequent or weak PAS staining has occurred with some feline and equine lymphoid malignancies.[6,33,34,70]

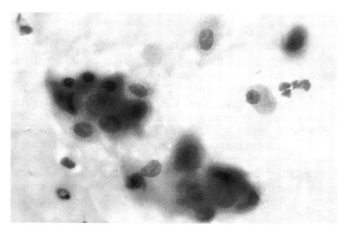

FIGURE 111.6 Strong cytoplasmic staining of cells from a canine mast cell tumor with OEN. Skin mass cytology. 250× original magnification.

MISCELLANEOUS CELL MARKERS FOR ACUTE MYELOID LEUKEMIA

Toluidine blue (TB) is specific for visualizing the granules in mast cells, basophils, and their precursors. It is a basic dye that reacts with acid mucopolysaccharides, forming metachromatic complexes that are products colored other than blue (usually pink to purple) with this stain. When basophilia is present, TB should be used to determine the extent of basophilic precursor involvement for blast cells in an acute myeloid leukemia. TB staining was helpful in the diagnosis of two cases of basophilic leukemia in the dog and for mast cell identification in tumors from the dog, cat, goat, cow, pig, and horse.[38,41–43,69,71–74] Several cases of large granular lymphoma or large granular lymphocyte leukemia in the dog, cat, horse, and ferret were evaluated with TB.[33,34,45,53,70,75] Of the 13 cases stained in the cat, only one demonstrated a positive reaction.[53]

Omega-exonuclease (OEN) is an enzyme stain for basophils or mast cells and their precursors in several species, particularly dogs, cats, primates, and humans. It is an alkaline phosphodiesterase found within the cytoplasm and not in the specific granules; therefore it is said to be more helpful than TB in poorly differentiated or degranulated cells. In addition, it can be helpful to determine the extent of involvement with basophil precursors in cases of acute myeloid leukemia with peripheral basophilia. OEN was used for this purpose in one case of basophilia leukemia in the dog.[38] Also, OEN was used to identify mast cells in tumors (Fig. 111.6) from a dog and cat.[41]

Luna is a specific stain for eosinophil granules that can be used to identify atypical granulocytes or blast cells with eosinophilic differentiation. It was helpful in confirming the presence of eosinophilic precursor cells in a case of leukemia in a horse in which there was a predominance of positive stained cells.[25]

Acetylcholinesterase staining was helpful in the iden-

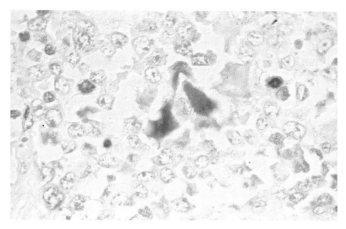

FIGURE 111.7 Immature and mature megakaryocytic precursor cells stain positive with Synacril black AN (Megacolor) in canine AML-M7. Bone marrow histopathology. 250× original magnification.

tification of megakaryocytic precursors in canine cases of megakaryoblastic leukemia and essential or primary thrombocythemia.[59,62] Synacril black AN[76] is a stain useful in the horse and dog (Fig. 111.7) to detect both immature and mature forms of the megakaryocytic series. This textile dye available commercially as Megacolor (Cytocolor, Inc.) selectively stains the acid mucopolysaccharides found in the cytoplasm of megakaryocytes in a metachromatic fashion. It was used to distinguish megakaryocytic precursors from histiocytes in a case of equine malignant histiocytosis.[52] Immunohistochemical staining with antibodies against human von Willebrand factor (factor-VIII-related antigen) and human platelet glycoprotein (GP IIIa) helped characterize the neoplastic cells in several cases of canine and feline megakaryoblastic leukemia.[35,36,77]

SECTION XI
Immunohematology
K. Jane Wardrop

CHAPTER 112

Red Blood Cell Antigens and Blood Groups in the Dog and Cat

• GORDON A. ANDREWS

Inherited characteristic cell surface antigens located on the red-cell membrane are referred to as blood-group antigens. Their detection and description is based on polyclonal or monoclonal antibody serology. The antigens can vary in immunogenicity, and therefore, clinical significance. These antigens participate in recognition of self, and in some cases can serve as markers of disease. In humans for example, neoplastic cells sometimes express altered blood-group antigens. In veterinary medicine, the clinical significance of blood-group antigens is usually in the areas of transfusion reactions and neonatal isoerythrolysis. Blood-group antigens are genetic markers and can be used to resolve some cases of disputed parentage. Though not yet proved in veterinary medicine, blood-group antigens may play a role in immune-mediated hemolytic anemia and may serve as markers of disease. In this chapter our current understanding of the nomenclature, serology, biochemistry, inheritance, incidence, and transfusion significance of the dog and cat blood groups is reviewed.

RED BLOOD CELL ANTIGENS AND BLOOD GROUPS IN THE DOG

Historical Background

The discovery of the human ABO blood-group system in 1900 by Landsteiner stimulated the search for blood-group systems in domestic animals. Canine blood groups were first recognized by Von Dungern and Hirszfeld in 1910, who defined four different blood groups based on immune isoagglutinins.[1]

Swisher and Young[1,2] at the University of Rochester, New York, used dogs as animal models to study in vivo mechanisms of red-cell destruction. In a series of reports they described antigens A, B, C, D, E, F, and G, named in order of their discovery; determined the frequencies of the antigens in a random population of dogs; and characterized the in vivo and in vitro behavior of the isoantibody systems. Their systematic approach to studying the canine blood-group systems was reviewed in 1961 and 1962.[1,2]

Nomenclature

The blood-group antigens were first given letter designations A, B, C, D, E, F, and G, in the order of their discovery. Two categories of A cells were recognized, a strongly reactive group (A) and a series of less strongly reacting cells that could only be detected by the Coomb's antiglobulin test designated as A′ to distinguish them from A. This designation was later changed to A1 and A2.[1] Anti-E- and anti-G-typing sera were lost, so no future comparisons could be made.[3-5] International workshops met in 1972 and 1974 to standardize canine blood groups as defined by isoimmune sera, and to standardize canine blood-group system nomenclature.[6,7] The first workshop designated the terminology canine erythrocyte antigen (CEA) followed by a number to indicate the blood-group antigen. The second workshop adopted the designation dog erythrocyte antigen (DEA) followed first by a number from 1 onward for a locus; second, by a (.); and third, by another number for each allele recognized at a locus. The new terminology was adopted to avoid confusion with the carcinoembryonic antigen system.

A nomenclature system has been proposed that conforms with that used in other species.[3,8] This system would return to an alphabetical designation to name blood-group systems (loci) and would also identify factors, alleles, genotypes, and phenotypes. Based on the last international cooperative effort at defining canine blood-group antigens,[7] general usage among veterinary immunohematologists, and the availability of typing sera, the nomenclature system currently used in the United States is the DEA that includes DEA 1.1, DEA 1.2, DEA 3, DEA 4, DEA 5, and DEA 7. However, the DEA nomenclature system has not been accepted worldwide, and some authors use the newer genetic nomenclature system in reporting new blood-group specificities.[9,10] Until there is worldwide acceptance of a single

TABLE 112.1   Canine Blood Group System Nomenclature

1951[1]	1961[2]	1973[3]	1973[4]	1976[5]	1979[6] (proposed) Blood Group System	1980[7] Blood Factors	1991[8] (proposed) Blood Factors	Alleles	Phenotypes	Genotypes
A	A1	A1	CEA 1	DEA 1.1	A	Aa_1	Aa_1	A^{a1}	$A(a_1)$	$A^{a1}A^{a1}$ $A^{a1}A^{a2}$ $A^{a1}A^{a3}$ $A^{a1}A^-$
A'	A2	A2	CEA 2	DEA 1.2	—	Aa	Aa_2	A^{a2}	$A(a_2)$	$A^{a2}A^{a2}$ $A^{a2}A^{a3}$ $A^{a2}A^-$
—	—	—	—	—	—	—	Aa_3	A^{a3}	$A(a_3)$	$A^{a3}A^{a3}$ $A^{a3}A^-$
—	—	—	—	—	—	—	—	A^-	$A(-)$	A^-A^-
B	B	B	CEA 3	DEA 3	B	Ba	Ba	B^a	$B(a)$	B^aB^a B^aB^-
—	—	—	—	—	—	—	—	B^-	$B(-)$	B^-B^-
C	C	C	CEA 4	DEA 4	C	Ca	Ca	C^a	$C(a)$	C^aC^a C^aC^-
—	—	—	—	—	—	—	—	C^-	$C(-)$	C^-C^-
D	D	D	CEA 5	DEA 5	D	Da	Da	D^a	$D(a)$	D^aD^a D^aD^-
—	—	—	—	—	—	—	—	D^-	$D(-)$	D^-D^-
—	E	—	—	—	—	—	—	—	—	—
—	F	F	CEA 6	DEA 6	F	Fa	Fa	F^a	$F(a)$	F^aF^a F^aF^-
—	—	—	—	—	—	—	—	F^-	$F(-)$	F^-F^-
—	G	—	—	—	—	—	—	—	—	—
—	—	Tr	CEA 7	DEA 7	Tr	Tr^{tr}	Tr^{tr}	Tr^{tr}	$Tr(tr)$	$Tr^{tr}Tr^{tr}$ $Tr^{tr}Tr^0$ $Tr^{tr}Tr^-$
—	—	—	—	—	—	Tr^0	Tr^0	Tr^0	$Tr(0)$	Tr^0Tr^0 Tr^0Tr^-
—	—	—	—	—	—	—	—	Tr^-	$Tr(-)$	Tr^-Tr^-
—	—	He	CEA 8	DEA 8	?[9]	—	—	—	—	—

Data from references 1, 3, 5–9 and 57 with permission.
References: [1] (57), [2] (1), [3] (5), [4] (6), [5] (7), [6] (8), [7] (3), [8] (9)
Notes: [9] Was not designated.

nomenclature system, it is necessary to be familiar with both nomenclature systems. The changes in nomenclature of the dog blood-group systems are summarized in Table 112.1. Typing sera is commercially available in the United States only for DEA 1.1, 1.2, 3, 4, 5, and 7.[11] From a practical standpoint, therefore, these are the antigens that the veterinary practitioner should be most familiar. However, many other blood-group systems have been described, and the lack of commercially available typing sera does not diminish the potential significance of these other systems in transfusion medicine.

Dog Erythrocyte Antigen System

Dog Erythrocyte Antigen System 1.1, 1.2, 1.3 (A System)

This system is a three-factor, four-phenotype system that contains the antigens DEA 1.1, 1.2, 1.3, (equivalent to Aa_1, Aa_2, and Aa_3) and a null type.[9] Breeding studies suggest an autosomal dominant pattern of inheritance with the order of dominance being DEA 1.1, 1.2, 1.3, and null.[2,9,12] Individual dogs exhibit only one phenotype. The antigens are described as subtypes of a linear series.[13] A subtypic series has the characteristic that isoimmune antisera produced to one of the antigens can exhibit grades of cross-reactivity with other antigens in the series. Anti-A (anti-DEA 1.1, 1.2, 1.3) antisera is produced by immunizing an A (DEA 1.1, 1.2, 1.3)-negative dog with red cells from a DEA-1.1-positive dog. Anti-A antisera strongly agglutinates and hemolyzes (in the presence of fresh complement) red cells having DEA 1.1 and causes variable agglutination, does not cause hemolysis, and sensitizes red cells having DEA 1.2 and 1.3 in the antiglobulin test. Anti-A antisera is therefore a mixture of anti-DEA 1.1, 1.2, and 1.3. Anti-DEA 1.1 antisera is produced by immunizing a DEA-1.2-positive dog with red cells from a DEA-1.1-positive dog.[2,11] Anti-

DEA 1.1 antisera reacts only with red cells having DEA 1.1. When an A (DEA 1.1, 1.2, 1.3)-negative dog is immunized with Aa_3 (DEA 1.3) positive cells, the initial antiserum contains antibodies that strongly agglutinate and hemolyze Aa_1 and Aa_2 (DEA 1.1 and DEA 1.2) cells and weakly agglutinate Aa_3 cells. Repeated exposure to Aa_3 cells results in antisera that are strongly reactive with all three cell types.[9] Attempts to produce specific anti-DEA 1.2 and anti-DEA 1.3 have been unsuccessful without performance of red-cell absorption procedures.[1,9]

Incidence

The incidence of DEA 1.1 in the United States is approximately 45%[1,11] and that of DEA 1.2 is approximately 20%.[1,11] DEA 1.3 has been evaluated only in Australia.

Molecular Identity

Immunoprecipitation experiments with polyclonal antisera to DEA 1.2 isolate a protein with a molecular weight of 85 kD.[14] Western blotting experiments with monoclonal antibody specific for DEA 1.1 identify two membrane proteins with molecular weights of 50 and 200 kD.[15]

Transfusion Reactions

The A system is the most important blood-group system from a practical standpoint for transfusion in the dog. Anti-DEA 1.1 is a strong agglutinin and hemolysin in vitro and in vivo. Naturally occurring antibody to DEA 1.1 and 1.2 has not been documented, so first-time transfusion reactions do not occur. However, once sensitized by previous transfusion, subsequent incompatible transfusions can result in severe hemolytic transfusion reactions with hemoglobinuria, hyperbilirubinemia, and removal of the transfused red cells in less than 12 hours.[16]

Transfusion of plasma containing anti-DEA 1.1 antibody results in a hemolytic transfusion reaction in the recipient.[16] Therefore, donor dogs should be determined to be free of this antibody for whole-blood or plasma transfusions. DEA-1.2-negative dogs, once sensitized with DEA-1.2-positive red cells will on subsequent exposure remove the transfused red cells in 12 to 24 hours. DEA-1.2-positive dogs produce a strong anti-DEA 1.1 antibody when exposed to DEA 1.1 red cells and experience an immediate hemolytic transfusion reaction when subsequently exposed to DEA 1.1 red cells.[11] The third factor in this system, Aa_3 (or DEA 1.3) has been described, but transfusion experiments have not been performed.[9] However, the serologic characteristics described above make the transfusion significance of this antigen obvious.

Neonatal Isoerythrolysis

Hemolytic disease in neonatal pups proposed to be naturally occurring neonatal isoerythrolysis has been reported.[17] Experimental neonatal isoerythrolysis caused by blood group A incompatibility has been produced in pups by immunization of an A-negative bitch by transfusion with A-positive red cells, followed by mating to an A-positive sire.[18-20] Sensitization of a DEA-1.1-negative pregnant bitch by previous transfusion or pregnancy can result in neonatal isoerythrolysis in DEA-1.1-positive pups.[18]

Dog Erythrocyte Antigen 3 (B System)

This is currently understood to be a one-factor, two-phenotype system with the antigen DEA 3 and a null phenotype, with DEA 3 being dominant. Naturally occurring anti-DEA 3 antibody has been reported in as much as 20% of DEA-3-negative dogs.[11,17] In the United States, approximately 6% of the general dog population is DEA 3 positive.[1] However, 23% of greyhounds typed at Michigan State University between 1990 and 1995 were DEA 3 positive.[11] Administration of DEA 3 positive red cells to a sensitized dog results in loss of the transfused red cells within 5 days and can result in severe acute transfusion reactions.[2,21]

In Japan, two reagents, a heteroimmune antisera produced in rabbits designated anti-D1 and an isoimmune antisera designated anti-E, were found in comparison tests with DEA reagents to be identical to anti-DEA 3.[22] Western blotting experiments with monoclonal antibody to DEA 3 identify five bands with molecular weights of 34, 53, 59, 64, and 71 kD.[23]

Dog Erythrocyte Antigen 4 (C System)

This is a one-factor, two phenotype system with the antigen DEA 4 and a null phenotype, with DEA 4 being dominant. Naturally occurring antibody to DEA 4 has not been documented. As much as 98% of the general dog population in the United States expresses this antigen.[2] However, the incidence of DEA 4 may be significantly lower in some breeds and geographic locations.[11] DEA-4-negative dogs produce antibody to this antigen when exposed by transfusion, but sensitized dogs did not show red-cell loss or hemolysis when transfused with DEA-4-positive cells.[2] Attempts to induce neonatal isoerythrolysis with blood group C (DEA 4) incompatibility were unsuccessful.[24] The transfusion significance of this antigen is considered incomplete.[11] Immunoprecipitation experiments with polyclonal antisera to DEA 4 isolate a protein with a molecular weight of 32 to 40 kD.[14]

Dog Erythrocyte Antigen 5 (D System)

This is a one-factor, two-phenotype system with the antigen DEA 5 and a null type, with DEA 5 being dominant. Naturally occurring antibody to this antigen has been reported in 10% of random nontransfused dogs in the United States.[2,17] The incidence of this antigen is generally low, but there is breed and geographic variation. As much as 30% of greyhounds in the United States are DEA 5 positive.[11] Transfusion of DEA-5-positive red cells to sensitized dogs results in red-cell sequestration and loss within 3 days.[2] Experimental attempts to induce neonatal isoerythrolysis with blood group D (DEA 5) incompatibility were unsuccessful.[24]

Dog Erythrocyte Antigen 6 (F System)

This is a one-factor, two-phenotype system with the antigen DEA 6 and a null phenotype, with DEA 6 being dominant. Although reported in almost 100% of dogs in the United States,[1] this antigen also exhibits significant breed and geographic variation in expression.[6,25,26] Naturally occurring anti-DEA 6 has not been documented. Transfusion studies in one DEA-6-negative dog showed moderately rapid removal of transfused red cells after sensitization.[1] Typing sera for DEA 6 no longer exists.

Dog Erythrocyte Antigen 7 (Tr System)

A naturally occurring isoantibody and an identically reacting antiserum produced by isoimmunization defines the Tr antigen antibody system.[27] Factor O is an allele in the Tr system, resulting in the Tr system being a two-factor, three-phenotype (Tr, O, and null) system with the order of dominance being Tr, O, and null.[28] The Tr antigen is not an integral red-cell membrane antigen, but rather is believed to be produced elsewhere in the body, secreted into the plasma, and adsorbed onto the red-cell surface.[29] The Tr antigen is expressed in approximately 40 to 54% of dogs.[3,6,27] Naturally occurring, weak, low-titered, nonhemolytic anti-DEA 7 is present in 20 to 50% of DEA-7-negative dogs, and sensitized DEA-7-negative dogs, when transfused with DEA-7-positive red cells, show sequestration and loss of red cells within 72 hours.[11] Immunoprecipitation experiments with polyclonal antisera to DEA 7 isolate three proteins with molecular weights of 53, 58, and 66 kD.[14]

Dog Erythrocyte Antigen 8

This canine red-cell antigen, originally designated as He, was discovered by antiserum raised by isoimmunization, and the antigen reported to exist in 40 to 45% of a random population of dogs.[30] Typing sera for DEA 8 no longer exists.

Other Specificities

N-acetyl-neuraminic acid (NAN) and N-glycolyl-neuraminic acid (NGN) present on gangliosides (hematoside) of the red-cell membrane define an unnamed blood-group system described in Japan.[31,32] Sera from dogs that have NAN hematoside contain an isoantibody that agglutinates red cells of dogs that have NGN hematoside, and the agglutination is inhibited by NGN hematoside. Comparison studies with standardized canine blood-typing reagents have not been performed. Several Oriental breeds express NGN hematoside, especially native breeds of northern China, Korea, and southern Japan, including Japanese mongrel dogs, Kai dogs, Kishu dogs, Japanese spaniels, and Shiba dogs.

A blood-group system referred to as the D system is described in Japan. The D system is composed of two antigens, D1 and D2, with 3 phenotypes, D1, D2, and D1D2. The phenotypes are based on agglutination testing with two rabbit heteroimmune antisera, anti-D1 and anti-D2. Anti-D1 is identical to anti-DEA 3.[22] The D1

and D2 antigens in the D system are codominant factors.[22] The counterpart of D2 has not been described outside of Japan. The incidence of D1 and DEA 3 is high in purebred dogs indigenous to Japan such as the Akita, Shiba, Kishu, Shikoku, and native Japanese mongrel and mixed breeds.[21,22,25] Most Western and European breeds are negative for DEA 3 and D1.[21,22,25] Repeated transfusion of D2-type blood into a D1-type patient or of D1-type blood into a D2-type patient results in severe acute transfusion reactions, indicating the importance of this system in transfusion medicine.[21]

The lectin extracted from seeds of *Clerodendron tricotomum* preferentially agglutinates red cells of some dogs at titers as much as 128, (designated type C), whereas it is completely negative for other dogs (type C).[33] Genetic studies in beagle dogs (62 offspring from 18 matings) indicate the characteristic is inherited as an autosomal dominant trait.[34] This system, designated the C system was compared with the DEA system and found to be different.[22,34-36]

Numerous other specificities have been reported and proposed to represent new blood-group systems.[3,7,10,22,37-40] In most cases, however, comparisons with established blood group systems were not performed, and reagents are not available for comparative studies.

RED BLOOD CELL ANTIGENS AND BLOOD GROUPS IN THE CAT

Historical Background

Ingelbringsten (cited by Ottenburg and Thalhimer)[41] first described naturally occurring isoagglutinins in cats, but did not find evidence of groups similar to the human ABO types. Holmes[42] reported two groups of cats, one designated as group O that contained an isoagglutinin in the serum, and a group that had the corresponding antigen on the red cells, named group EF.[42] Eyquem[43] described two antigens, A and B, and stated that these antigens were identical to the EF and the O reported by Holmes.

Auer and Bell[44] used two naturally occurring antibodies, anti-A and anti-B to characterize the cat blood-group system, which they designated the AB system, and first reported the rare AB phenotype for which both antigens were present on the red cell. They were also the first to describe immediate experimental and naturally occurring transfusion reactions in previously unsensitized cats of known incompatible blood type.[45]

Feline AB Blood-Group System

The AB blood-group system characterized by Auer and Bell is the only blood-group system currently recognized in cats.[44] Three phenotypes occur, type A, which is most common, Type B, which is less common, and type AB, which is rare. A null phenotype does not occur.

The types are defined by naturally occurring isoantibody against the antigen they lack. Type A cats have

TABLE 112.2 Blood Type Frequencies in Domestic Shorthair and Domestic Longhair Cats

Country	n	% A	% B	% AB	Reference
USA (by region)					
northeast	1450	99.7	0.3	0.0	(58)
north central/rocky mountain	506	99.4	0.4	0.2	(58)
southeast	534	98.5	1.5	0.0	(58)
southwest	483	97.5	2.5	0.0	(58)
west coast	812	94.8	4.7	0.5	(58)
Australia	1895	73.3	26.3	0.4	(44)
Virgin Gorda	32	100	0.0	0.0	(59)
Japan	207	90.3	9.7	0.0	(60)
	220	90.0	10.0	0.0	(61)
	299	89.3	1.0	9.7	(62)
England	477	97.0	3.0	0.0	(42)
France	350	85.0	15.0	0.0	(43)
Switzerland	1014	99.6	0.4	0.0	(63)
Germany	600	94.0	6.0	0.0	(64)
Germany	404 dsh/dlh cats	94.1	5.9	0.0	(65)
Germany	868 total cats	92.6	6.7	0.7	(65)
Finland	61	100	0.0	0.0	(64)
Italy	401	88.8	11.2	0.0	(64)
Netherlands	95	95.8	4.2	0.0	(64)
Netherlands	96	94.8	4.2	1.0	(63)
Scotland	70	97.1	2.9	0.0	(63)
Austria	101	97.0	3.0	0.0	(64)
Denmark	105	98.1	1.9	0.0	(66)

n: number of cats blood typed; dsh/dlh: domestic shorthair/domestic longhair.
Data from references 42–44 and 58–66 with permission.

low-titered anti-B hemagglutinins of the gamma M immunoglobulin (IgM) class and hemolysins consisting of equal amounts of gamma G immunoglobulin (IgG) and IgM.[46] Approximately one third of type-A cats have macroscopic agglutinins and hemolysins. Microscopic examination or the antiglobulin test is needed to detect the weak agglutination reactions in the remaining two thirds of the cats. Type-B cats have high-titered anti-A hemagglutinins and hemolysins mainly of the IgM class with lesser amounts of IgG.[46,47] It is the presence of these naturally occurring isoantibodies that is responsible for transfusion reactions and neonatal isoerythrolysis in blood-type-incompatible cats. Type-AB cats do not possess isoantibodies against either A or B.

Genetics

The blood-group antigens A and B are inherited as simple autosomal Mendelian traits, with A being dominant over B.[4,48] All type-B cats are homozygous for the B allele (genotype B/B) and type-A cats can be either homozygous (genotype A/A) or heterozygous (genotype A/B). Blood type AB is not the result of codominant inheritance of type A and B, nor is it the result of chimerism.[44] In spite of extensive breeding studies and pedigree analysis, the mode of inheritance of the AB phenotype remains unknown.[44,49]

Incidence of the Antigens

Type A is the most common blood type. Type B is less common, and type AB is rare. The percentage distribution of types A and B can vary significantly with geographic location within the United States and the world (Table 112.2). The breed incidence of type B ranges from 0 to as much as 60% among different purebred cats (Table 112.3). Type AB is exceedingly rare. In a survey of cats in the United States and Canada, 13 of 9239 cats

TABLE 112.3 Blood Type B Frequencies in Purebred Cats in the United States[48,58,67]

Type-B Frequency	Breeds
0%	Siamese, Burmese, Tonkinese, Russian Blue, Ocicat and Oriental Shorthair
<5%	Maine Coon, Norwegian Forest and DSH/DLH
5–25%	Abyssinian, Himalayan, Birman, Persian, Somali, Sphinx, Scottish Fold and Japanese Bobtail
25–50%	Exotic and British Shorthair, Cornish Rex and Devon Rex

DSH/DLH: Domestic shorthair/domestic longhair.
Data from References 48, 58 and 67 with permission.

(0.14%) were type AB.[49] In Australia, 7 of 1895 cats (0.4%) were type AB.[44] Type AB occurs only in breeds in which type B is detected. Type AB has been found in domestic shorthair (DSH)/domestic longhair (DLH) cats and in Abyssinian, Birman, British short hair, Norwegian forest, Persian, Scottish fold, and Somali purebred cats.[49]

Molecular Characterization of the Antigens

The form of neuraminic acid (sialic acid) on the red-cell membrane glycolipids and glycoproteins determines the blood-group antigens in the cat.[50,51] N-glycolylneuraminic acid (NeuGc) is the determinant of the A antigen. Type-A red cells have NeuGc-NeuGc-Galactose-Glucose-Ceramide ($[NeuGc]_2G_{D3}$) as the major disialoganglioside, and it is the predominant blood type determining ganglioside detected by feline anti-A antisera.[50] Type A red cells also have NeuAc-NeuGc-G_{D3}, for which NeuAc represents N-acetylneuraminic acid, NeuGc-NeuAc-G_{D3}, and a minor amount of $[NeuAc]_2G_{D3}$. Homozygous and heterozygous type-A cats have some differences in their ganglioside profiles, and these differences can be used to determine the genotype of type-A cats.[51]

N-acetylneuraminic acid is the determinant of the B antigen. Type-B red cells have $[NeuAc]_2G_{D3}$ as the only form of the disialoganglioside. Type-B red cells do not contain any detectable NeuGc. Agglutination testing with the lectin of *Triticum vulgaris*, a lectin that binds sialoglycoproteins containing NeuAc, demonstrates selective agglutination of type-B red cells.[52] Type-AB red cells have features of both type A and type B. They are agglutinated by both anti-A and anti-B feline antisera and by the lectin of *T. vulgaris*. Data from two studies suggest the possibility that there is more than one biochemical phenotype in the AB type, a phenotypic difference undetected by feline typing sera, which may explain the reason that investigators have been unable to provide a single genetic mechanism for the inheritance of the AB type.[49-51]

Transfusion Reactions

The presence of naturally occurring isoantibodies is responsible for transfusion reactions in previously unsensitized cats. Virtually all type-B cats have highly titered anti-A agglutinins and hemolysins that can result in severe transfusion reaction and death when as little as 1 mL of type-A blood is administered to a type-B cat.[45,53-55] Rapid intravascular destruction of the type-A red cells occurs within minutes to hours and is complement and IgM mediated. Type-B red cells administered to type-A cats have a half-life of approximately 2 days, and minor transfusion reactions can occur.[55] Removal of type-B cells occurs mostly extravascularly, involving IgG and IgM without significant complement activity.[56]

Neonatal Isoerythrolysis

Neonatal isoerythrolysis occurs in type-A or type-AB kittens born to a type-B queen.[49] The colostrum of type-

B queens contains high concentrations of anti-A antibodies, and colostral antibody is detectable in the serum of newborns as early as 4 hours after birth.[46] Clinical signs in affected kittens can be variable, ranging from inapparent to severe hemolytic anemia with hemoglobinuria, jaundice, and death. Neonatal isoerythrolysis is believed to be a major cause of the fading kitten syndrome.[48]

REFERENCES

1. **Swisher SN, Young LE.** The blood grouping systems of dogs. Physiol Rev 1961;41:495–520.
2. **Swisher SN, Young LE, Trabold N.** In vitro and in vivo studies of the behavior of canine erythrocyte-isoantibody systems. Ann N Y Acad Sci 1962;97:15–25.
3. **Colling DT, Saison R.** Canine blood groups. 1. Description of new erythrocyte specificities. Anim Genet 1980;11:1–12.
4. **Bell K.** The blood groups of domestic mammals. In: Agar NS, Board PG, eds. Red blood cells of domestic mammals. Amsterdam: Elsevier Science Publishers BV, 1983;133–164.
5. **Swisher SN, Bull R, Bowdler J.** Canine erythrocyte antigens. Tissue Antigens 1973;3:164–165.
6. **Vriesendorp HM, Westbroek DL, D'Amaro J, van der Does JA, van der Steen GJ, van Rood JJ, Albert E, Bernini L, Bull RW, Cabasson J, Epstein RB, Erikson V, Feltkamp TEW, Flad HD, Hammer C, Lang R, Largiader F, von Loringhoven K, Los W, Meera Khan P, Saison R, Serrou B, Schnappauf H, Swisher SN, Templeton JW, Uhlschmidt G, Zweibaum A.** Joint report of 1st international workshop on canine immunogenetics. Tissue Antigens 1973;3:145–172.
7. **Vriesendorp HM, Albert E, Templeton JW, Belotsky S, Taylor B, Blumenstock DA, Bull RW, Cannon FD, Epstein RB, Ferrebee JW, Grosse-Wilde H, Hammer C, Krumbacher K, Leon S, Meera Khan P, Mickey MR, Motola M, Rapaport FT, Saison R, Schnappauf H, Scholz S, Schroeder ML, Storb R, Wank R, Westbroek DL, Zweibaum A.** Joint report of the second international workshop on canine immunogenetics. Transplant Proc 1976; VIII:289–314.
8. **Saison R, Colling D.** A proposed nomenclature for canine red blood cell groups. Proceedings of the XVIth International Conference on Animal Blood Groups and Biochemical Polymorphisms, Leningrad, 1979;III:225–228.
9. **Symons M, Bell K.** Expansion of the canine A blood group system. Anim Genet 1991;22:227–235.
10. **Symons M, Bell K.** Canine blood groups: description of 20 specificities. Anim Genet 1992;23:509–515.
11. **Hale AS.** Canine blood groups and their importance in veterinary transfusion medicine. Vet Clin North Am Small Anim Pract 1995;25:1323–1332.
12. **Cohen C, Fuller JL.** The inheritance of blood types in the dog. J Hered 1953;44(6):225–228.
13. **Stormont C.** A note on linear subtyping relationships. In: Papers dedicated to Johannes Moustgaard on the occasion of his 70th birthday, 26 September 1981. Copenhagen: The Royal Danish Agricultural Society, 1981;190–193.
14. **Corato A, Mazza G, Hale AS, Barker RN, Day MJ.** Biochemical characterization of canine blood group antigens: immunoprecipitation of DEA 1.2, 4 and 7 and identification of a dog erythrocyte membrane antigen homologous to human Rhesus. Vet Immunol Immunopathol 1997;59:213–223.
15. **Andrews GA, Chavey PS, Smith JE.** Production, chacterization, and applications of a murine monoclonal antibody to dog erythrocyte antigen 1.1. J Am Vet Med Assoc 1992;201:1549–1552.
16. **Young LE, Ervin DM, Yuile CL.** Hemolytic reactions produced in dogs by transfusion of incompatible dog blood and plasma I. Serologic and hematologic aspects. Blood 1949;4(11):1218–1231.
17. **Young LE, O'Brien WA, Swisher SN, Miller G, Yuile CL.** Blood groups in dogs—their significance to the veterinarian. Am J Vet Res 1952;13:207–213.
18. **Young LE, Christian RM, Ervin DM, Davis RW, O'Brien WA, Swisher SN, Yuile CL.** Hemolytic disease in newborn dogs. Blood 1951;6(4):291–313.
19. **Young LE, Ervin DM, Christian RM, Davis RW.** Hemolytic disease in newborn dogs following isoimmunization of the dam by transfusions. Science 1949;109:630–631.
20. **Christian RM, Ervin DM, Swisher SN, O'Brien WA, Young LE.** Hemolytic anemia in newborn dogs due to absorption of isoantibody from breast milk during the first day of life. Science 1949;110:443.
21. **Ejima H, Nomura K, Bull RW.** Breed differences in the phenotype and gene frequencies in canine D blood group system. J Vet Med Sci 1994;56:623–626.
22. **Ejima H, Kurokawa K.** Comparison test of antibodies for dog blood grouping. Jpn J Vet Sci 1980;42:435–441.
23. **Hara Y, Ejima H, Aoki S, Tagawa M, Motoyoshi S, Sugiyama M, Ikemoto S.** Preparation of monoclonal antibodies against dog erythrocyte antigen D1 (DEA-3). J Vet Med Sci 1991;53:1105–1107.
24. **Young LE, O'Brien WA, Miller G, Swisher SN, Ervin DM, Christian RM, Yuile CL.** Erythrocyte-isoantibody reactions in dogs. Trans N Y Acad Sci 1951;13(series II):209–213.

25. **Ejima H, Kurokawa K, Ikemoto S.** Phenotype and gene frequencies of red blood cell groups in dogs of various breeds reared in Japan. Jpn J Vet Sci 1986;48(2):363–368.

26. **Han BK, Lee CG, Ikemoto S.** Studies on the blood groups of Jindo dogs by dog erytrocyte antigen system. Korean J Anim Sci 1988;30(11):643–651.

27. **Bowdler AJ, Bull RW, Slating R, Swisher SN.** Tr: A canine red cell antigen related to the A-antigen of human red cells. Vox Sang 1971;20:542–554.

28. **Colling DT, Saison R.** Canine blood groups. 2. Description of a new allele in the Tr blood group system. Anim Genet 1980;11:13–20.

29. **Bull RW, Vriesendorp HM, Zweibaum A, Swisher SN.** The inapplicability of CEA-7 as a canine bone marrow transplantation marker. Transplant Proc 1975;7(4):575–577.

30. **Bull RW, Bowdler AJ, Swisher SN.** Two additional antigens in the canine blood group system. Bull Am Soc Vet Clin Pathol 1973;II(3):10–11.

31. **Yasue S, Handa S, Miyagawa S, Inoue J, Hasegawa A, Yamakawa T.** Difference in form of sialic acid in red cell glycolipids of different breeds of dogs. J Biochem 1978;83:1101–1107.

32. **Hashimoto Y, Yamakawa T, Tanabe Y.** Futher studies on the red cell glycolipids of various breeds of dogs. A possible assumption about the origin of Japanese dogs. J Biochem 1984;96:1777–1782.

33. **Yoshida H.** Individual difference of dog blood groups detected by *Clerodendron trichotomum* extract. J Vet Med Sci 1979;691:85–87.

34. **Ikemoto S, Yoshida H.** Genetic studies of new blood group C system on red cells of beagles. Jpn J Vet Sci 1981;43:429–431.

35. **Ikemoto S, Haruhiro Y, Watanabe Y, Suzuki S.** Individual differences within animal blood groups detected by lectins. Proceedings of the XVIth International Conference on Animal Blood Groups and Biochemical Polymorphisms, Leningrad, 1979;2:8–11.

36. **Andrews GA, Chavey PS, Smith JE.** Reactivity of seed lectins with blood typed canine erythrocytes. Comp Haematol Int 1992;2:68–74.

37. **Hall DE.** A naturally occurring red-cell antigen-antibody system in beagle dogs. J Small Anim Pract 1970;11:543–551.

38. **Ikemoto S, Sakurai Y, Ejima H.** Genetic marker in beagle blood: Individual difference within blood groups detected by isohemagglutinin. Jpn J Vet Sci 1976;38:647–649.

39. **Rubinstein P, Morgado F, Blumenstock DA, Ferrebee JW.** Isohemagglutinins and histocompatibility in the dog. Transplantation 1968;6(9):961–969.

40. **Suzuki Y, Stormont C, Morris BG, Shifrine M, Dobrucki R.** New antibodies in dog blood groups. Transplant Proc 1975;7(3):365–367.

41. **Ottenberg R, Thalhimer W.** Studies in experimental transfusion. J Med Res 1915;28:213–229.

42. **Holmes R.** Blood groups in cats. Abstract. J Physiol 1950;111:61P.

43. **Eyquem A, Podliachouk L, Milot P.** Blood groups in chimpanzees, horses, sheep, pigs, and other mammals. Abstract. Ann N Y Acad Sci 1962;97:320–328.

44. **Auer L, Bell K.** The AB blood group system of cats. Anim Genet 1981;12:287–297.

45. **Auer L, Bell K, Coates S.** Blood transfusion reactions in the cat. J Am Vet Med Assoc 1982;180:729–730.

46. **Bücheler J, Giger U.** Alloantibodies against A and B blood types in cats. Vet Immunol Immunopathol 1993;38:283–295.

47. **Wilkerson MJ, Meyers KM, Wardrop KJ.** Anti-A isoagglutinins in two blood type B cats are IgG and IgM. Vet Clin Pathol 1991;20:10–14.

48. **Giger U, Bücheler J, Patterson DF.** Frequency and inheritance of A and B blood types in feline breeds of the United States. J Hered 1991;82:15–20.

49. **Griot-Wenk ME, Callan MB, Casal ML, Chisholm-Chait A, Spitalnik SL, Patterson DF, Giger U.** Blood type AB in the feline AB blood group system. Am J Vet Res 1996;57:1438–1442.

50. **Andrews GA, Chavey PS, Smith JE, Rich L.** N-glycolylneuraminic acid and N-acetylneuraminic acid define feline blood group A and B antigens. Blood 1992;79:2485–2491.

51. **Griot-Wenk M, Pahlsson P, Chisholm-Chait A, Spitalnik PF, Spitalnik SL, Giger U.** Biochemical characterization of the feline AB blood group system. Anim Genet 1993;24:401–407.

52. **Butler M, Andrews GA, Smith JE.** Reactivity of lectins with feline erythrocytes. Comp Haematol Int 1991;1:217–219.

53. **Giger U, Akol KG.** Acute hemolytic transfusion reaction in an Ayssinian cat with blood type B. J Vet Intern Med 1990;4:315–316.

54. **Wilkerson MJ, Wardrop KJ, Giger U, Myers KM.** Two cat colonies with A and B blood types and a clinical transfusion reaction. Feline Pract 1991;19:22–26.

55. **Auer L, Bell K.** Transfusion reactions in cats due to AB blood group incompatibility. Abstract. Res Vet Sci 1983;35:145–152.

56. **Giger U, Bücheler J.** Transfusion of type-A and type-B blood to cats. Abstract. J Am Vet Med Assoc 1991;198:411–418.

57. **Christian RM, Ervin DM, Young LE.** Observations on the in-vitro behavior of dog isoantibodies. J Immunol 1951;66:37–50.

58. **Giger U, Griot-Wenk M, Bücheler J, Smith S, Diserens D.** Geographical variation of the feline blood type frequencies in the United States. Feline Pract 1991;19:21–27.

59. **Bird MS, Cotter SM, Gibbons G, Harris S.** Blood groups in cats. Comp An Pract 1988;2(8):31–33.

60. **Ikemoto S, Sakurai Y.** Individual difference within the cat blood group detected by isohemagglutinin. Jpn J Vet Sci 1981;43:433–435.

61. **Hirota J, Usui R, Oyamada T, Ikemoto S.** The phenotypes and gene frequencies of genetic markers in the blood of Japanese crossbred cats. J Vet Med Sci 1995;57:381–383.

62. **Ejima H, Kurokawa K, Ikemoto S.** Feline red blood cell groups detected by naturally occurring isoantibody. Jpn J Vet Sci 1986;48(5):971–976.

63. **Hubler M, Arnold S, Casal M, Fairburn A, Nussbaumer M, Rusch P.** The distribution of blood groups in cats in Switzerland. Schweiz Arch Tierheilkd 1993;135:231–235.

64. **Giger U, Gorman NT, Hubler M, Leidinger JI, Leidinger EF, Lubas G, Niini T, Slappendel RJ.** Frequencies of feline A and B blood types in Europe. Abstract. Anim Genet 1992;23(suppl 1):17–18.

65. **Haarer M, Grunbaum EG.** Blood group serology in cats in Germany. Kleintierpraxis 1993;38:195–204.

66. **Jensen AL, Olesen AB, Arnbjerg J.** Distribution of feline blood types detected in the Copenhagen area of Denmark. Acta Vet Scand 1994;35:121–124.

67. **Griot-Wenk ME, Giger U.** Feline transfusion medicine: blood types and their clinical importance. Vet Clin North Am Small Anim Pract 1995;25:1305–1322.

CHAPTER 113

Red Blood Cell Antigens and Blood Groups in the Horse

• ANN T. BOWLING

After the discovery of the human ABO blood group system with naturally occurring hemagglutinating antibodies, similar studies were undertaken in animals, including horses. Although such studies identified a few factors, the comprehensive understanding of horse blood groups was obtained with planned immunizations to produce blood grouping antisera (reagents), based on the successful application of such techniques to cattle and sheep. Through isoimmunization and heteroimmunization followed by both hemagglutination and hemolysis testing, Stormont and Suzuki[1] produced reagents that identified 16 factors and formed the basis of horse blood group information as currently defined. Research by laboratories worldwide has led to the definition of 34 factors distributed in seven systems (EAA, EAC, EAD, EAK, EAP, EAQ, EAU) that are briefly described in this chapter. Extensive family studies have shown that the factors or combinations of factors in each system are transmitted as a unit (phenogroup) and inherited as codominant traits. Allelic frequencies for blood groups vary between breeds.[2] Along with tests of protein polymorphisms, blood group testing has been one of the components of highly effective horse parentage verification programs worldwide, but such tests are gradually being phased out in favor of methodologies based on assays of DNA sequence with hair (root cells), not gene products from blood. However, blood grouping has continuing clinical applications for selecting appropriate transfusion donors and for the diagnosis and prevention of the maternal-fetal blood incompatibility problem of newborn foals (neonatal isoerythrolysis [NI]).

REAGENTS AND SEROLOGIC PROCEDURES FOR HORSE BLOOD GROUP TESTING

Although no detailed chemical studies have been undertaken, on the basis of human blood group research it is assumed that the horse blood group antigens are glycolipids or -proteins and that the antigenic sites are carbohydrate moieties. Antisera are generated by isoimmunization. The donor-recipient pairs are chosen to differ by as few known factors as possible, preferably by a single factor, so that the natural immune process of the recipient potentially raise a monospecific blood grouping antiserum. Complex antisera are rendered functionally monospecific by absorptions with red blood cells (RBCs) of an appropriate phenotype. The antiserum may provide a reagent that can be used to test thousands of horses and properly stored reagents (frozen or freeze dried) can last for years.

For serologic testing, an aliquot of a 2% saline suspension of RBCs from each horse is mixed with an aliquot of each antiserum in the reagent battery. The presence of a factor is recognized either by agglutination or by lysis with the complement enzyme cascade. The choice of procedure is not arbitrary, but is determined by the intrinsic properties of the reagent antibodies. Rabbit serum is used as a complement source, but it must first be absorbed at 4°C with horse RBCs to remove the natural heterolysins and agglutinins present in the heterologous serum. Nonreactive samples are scored as negative for the particular factor. Details of serologic testing procedures are provided in Chapter 114, Red Blood Cell Antigens and Blood Groups in the Cow, Pig, Sheep, Goat, and Llama.

Although horse blood grouping reagents are not commercially available, laboratories worldwide that are members of the International Society for Animal Genetics (ISAG) offer standardized testing and use a uniform nomenclature. Participation in the biennial Comparison Tests organized by the Horse Standing Committee provide laboratories the opportunity to identify suitable locally produced reagents and procedures that match results of other laboratories.

HORSE BLOOD GROUPS

The systems, factors, and alleles recognized by the ISAG Horse Standing Committee at its most recent review of blood groups (August 1994) are presented in Table 113.1.

TABLE 113.1	**Seven Loci of Horse Blood Groups, the Factors Detected by Antisera and the Alleles (Phenogroups) That are Recognized by ISAG**	
Locus[b]	**Factors**	**Recognized Alleles**
EAA	abcdefg	A^a A^{adf} A^{adg} A^{abdf} A^{abdg} A^b A^{bc} A^{bce} A^c A^{ce} A^e A^-
EAC	a	C^a C^-
EAD	abcdefghik lmnopqr	D^{adl} D^{adlnr} D^{adlr} D^{bcmq} D^{cefgmq} $D^{cegimnq}$ D^{cfgkm} D^{cfmqr} D^{cgm} D^{cgmp} D^{cgmq} D^{cgmqr} D^{cgmr} D^{deklr} D^{deloq} D^{delq} D^{dfklr} D^{dghmp} D^{dghmq} D^{dghmqr} D^{dkl} D^{dlnq} D^{dlnqr} D^{dlqr} D^q (D^-)
EAK	a	K^a K^-
EAP	abcd	P^a P^{ac} P^{acd} P^{ad} P^b P^{bd} P^d P^-
EAQ	abc	Q^{abc} Q^{ac} Q^a Q^b Q^c Q^-
EAU	a	U^a U^-

[a] The standard nomenclature, based on that of pigs, describes each allele by a capitol letter designation for the system, followed by lower case letters for the factor or factors detected. The absence of detectable factors is designated by the system letter followed by a dash (−).

[b] Although horse blood group systems have historically been designated by a single letter, the loci of horse blood groups are referred to here by the more recent convention for nomenclature of blood groups in which the two letters "EA" for *erythrocyte antigen* precede the traditional system designation.

EAA. Reagents detect seven factors for this open system (includes a recessively inherited null with no detectable product) of 12 alleles. The factors are detected by either agglutination or lysis. Naturally occurring antibodies of specificities anti-Aa and anti-Ac are occasionally found in the sera of horses lacking factor Aa (in any of its allelic combinations), usually as agglutinins. In mares anti-Aa may also be present as a lysin, apparently engendered by a blood-group-incompatible pregnancy. Hemolytic screening for this antibody (and others) before foaling can provide an effective test to identify mares whose foals are at risk for NI.

EAC. This is a simple one-factor, two-allele open system detected by reagents acting as lysins or agglutinins. Horses lacking Ca typically have a low- to moderately high-titered anti-Ca antibody of low avidity that can be the source of mild transfusion reactions in unmatched transfusions. The frequency of C^-/C^- horses is breed dependent but is generally in the range of 1 horse in 20. Risk of NI involving this blood-group system seems low.

EAD. This is a highly polymorphic blood group system detected by reagents, nearly always behaving as agglutinins, for 17 factors that define 25 recognized alleles. Although a null allele occurs, it seems rare and for most breeds the system can be considered genetically closed, providing a very effective system for parentage verification. Naturally occurring antibodies are rare, possibly limited to a specificity similar to Da. Only rarely has this system been implicated in NI cases.

EAK. This is a simple one-factor, two-allele open system detected by reagents acting as lysins or agglutinins. Naturally occurring antibodies are infrequent,

possibly only as a rare occurrence in blood-group-incompatible pregnancies.

EAP. This a four-factor, eight-allele open system detected by reagents acting as lysins or agglutinins. Naturally occurring antibodies are infrequent, possibly only as a rare occurrence in blood-group-incompatible pregnancies.

EAQ. This is a three-factor, six-allele open system detected by reagents acting as lysins. Most of the analyzed cases of NI can be accounted for by incompatibilities of factors between stallion and mare at either *EAA* or *EAQ*. Typically for *EAQ* sensitization, the mare is negative for factor Qa (for most breeds this means negative for Q^{abc}) although the stallion possesses it. The detectable antibody response for Qa has only been reported as a lysin and would be missed by antibody screening based solely on agglutination testing. Occasionally, the antibody presence can be detected only very late in pregnancy.

EAU. This is a simple one-factor, two-allele open system detected by reagents acting as lysins. Naturally occurring antibodies are infrequent, possibly only as a rare occurrence in blood-group-incompatible pregnancies.

The blood-group loci are genetically independent (unlinked); four of the seven have been assigned to linkage groups.[3] *EAK* is in linkage group I (the first linkage group defined for the horse) along with the gene for the red-cell enzyme 6-phosphogluconate dehydrogenase; *EAA* is assigned to linkage group III along with the major histocompatibility complex; *EAU* is assigned to linkage group V with the gene for the enzyme protease inhibitor; and *EAQ* is assigned to an unnamed linkage group along with an anonymous microsatellite marker.[4] Chromosome assignment is available only for *EAA*, on chromosome 20.

BLOOD GROUPS AND BLOOD TRANSFUSIONS

Horses seldom need blood transfusions, but even when needed, few veterinary diagnostic laboratories can perform blood-group testing to identify a matched or closely matched donor since the blood-grouping reagents are not commercially available. Diagnostic laboratories performing hemagglutination cross-match procedures should identify a large percentage of potential transfusion problems, even if the tests cannot identify the specificity. The standard blood typing test report provided by parentage verification tests might be available for some horses requiring transfusion, but it does not identify anti-blood group activity in a horse's blood. However, if a blood group report is available, it is reasonable to assume that any horse negative for factors Aa in the *EAA* system or Ca in the *EAC* system will have anti-Aa or anti-Ca activity in its serum. To avoid a transfusion reaction, such a horse should not receive whole blood from a donor that is positive for those factors.

Probably more than 90% of horses lack naturally occurring anti-blood group antibodies (breeds may be different from each other in this frequency), so a first unmatched whole-blood transfusion is usually well tolerated, without adverse reaction. The recipient will generate antibodies against the blood-group antigens of the foreign RBCs, so a second transfusion either may be ineffective because of the rapid removal of the administered RBCs or may cause an immune system crisis (anaphylaxis) that could lead to sudden death. A transfusion that did not introduce the most highly antigenic factors (particularly Aa) to a recipient that lacked such factors could probably be repeated if needed, because antibody production might only occur at low levels in response to the primary immunization.[5] It is important to remember that whenever a mare is given a RBC transfusion, she is potentially being sensitized to blood-group factors that may subsequently lead to NI problems for her foals.

PLASMA TRANSFUSION

Often a blood transfusion is needed to restore fluid loss, but the RBC component is not essential. In this case, a plasma transfusion may fulfill the clinical requirements. Serum from potential donors can be screened against an RBC panel from selected blood-group-defined horses to identify those without naturally occurring anti-blood group activity. Plasma can be collected and stored frozen to administer as needed.

NEONATAL ISOERYTHROLYSIS

NI is an acute hemolytic disease of newborn foals, a maternal-fetal blood group incompatibility, caused by immunologically mediated RBC destruction. Affected foals are healthy at birth but within 2 to 5 days develop signs of lethargy, elevated pulse and respiration rates and clinical evidence of anemia. NI foals are usually from the second or later pregnancies of a mare, but (rarely) first foals can be affected. The antibody molecules that sensitize the RBCs of the foal have been passively acquired from the dam's colostrum. Recovery may be spontaneous or the disease may progress to severe anemia and death.

The most common blood-group factors involved in NI are anti-Aa and anti-Qa, although other specificities are found. Not all Aa-negative or Qa-negative mares become sensitized, although they may have produced Aa-positive or Qa-positive foals. One source of sensitization is whole-blood transfusion, but this probably accounts for only a small number of cases. Mares negative for both Aa and Ca may be protected from sensitization to Aa by naturally produced anti-Ca antibodies.[6] At present, no simple hypothesis explains why blood-group sensitization occurs in only a few percent of mares at risk.

A serum sample from the pregnant mare taken approximately 3 weeks before she is due to foal can be screened to see if evidence of a blood-group incompati-

bility is found. If the test results are positive for hemolytic anti-blood group activity, it would be strongly advised to withhold the foal from its dam's colostrum before putting it back to its dam's milk after 36 to 48 hours. An alternative colostrum and milk source must be provided to the foal during that period.

Identification of the antibody specificity can be an important component of the diagnosis of NI in a foal. This identification is achieved by screening the pregnant mare's serum against an RBC panel from selected blood-group defined horses. As well, such identification may allow an owner to prevent its recurrence in the mare's subsequent foals by breeding her to stallions negative for the problem blood factor. For example, if the mare has anti-Aa antibodies a stallion lacking the Aa factor would be an appropriate mate. However, the Aa factor is very common; it may be difficult to find a stallion that lacks it and would suit as well for other traits. In such cases, an appropriate management scheme allows the mare to be bred to any stallion deemed suitable, coupled with close monitoring of parturition and the availability of an alternative colostrum for the foal. If the problem is Qa (or any other specificity), it is probably not as difficult to find a blood-group compatible stallion. Identifying the specificity of an alleged sensitization may not be possible by looking at the blood-group reports of a parental pair purported to have produced an NI foal. Because of the high likelihood that any breeding pair will be discordant for several factors, correctly identifying the sensitizing factor is most productively achieved though identification of the antibody specificity from tests of the mare's serum or colostrum.

Neonatal Isoerythrolysis Disease in Mule Foals

Mule breeders are keenly aware that mares bred to jacks (male donkeys) can become sensitized to blood-group factors of donkeys.[7] Monitoring of a pregnant mare's serum for antibodies against the RBCs of the jack to which she is bred is a prudent precaution to identify mule neonates at risk for NI.

Red Blood Cell Donor for the Foal with Neonatal Isoerythrolysis

Appropriate management for a severely anemic NI foal might be to provide a RBC transfusion to alleviate the anemia and prevent death. The best blood donor for the foal is one whose cells lack the factor to which its dam is making antibodies. The sire of the foal is the worst possible donor since he has the factor to which the mare's immune system has responded. The best cell donor is the mare. The mare's RBCs should be administered to the foal in a suitable transfusion solution, but first they must be separated from the plasma that contains the antibodies reacting with the foal's cells. This transfusion donor is unlikely to match the blood-group type of the foal, but it provides the foal with vital RBCs that will not be destroyed as a result of antibodies it received with colostrum from the dam. It is hoped that within a short time the dam's anti-blood group antibodies will be eliminated from the foal's system and that the foal can make sufficient RBCs of its own to prevent a recurrence of the anemia crisis.

REFERENCES

1. **Stormont C, Suzuki Y.** Genetic systems of blood groups in horses. Genetics 1964;50:915–929.
2. **Bowling AT, Clark RS.** Blood group and protein polymorphism gene frequencies for seven breeds of horses in the United States. Animal Blood Groups and Biochemical Genetics 1985;16:93–108.
3. **Bowling AT.** Horse Genetics. Wallingford, UK: CAB International, 1996.
4. **Bowling AT, Millon LV, Eggleston-Stott ML.** Linkage mapping using equine half-sib families. Anim Genet 1996;27(suppl 2):73.
5. **Wong PL, Nickel LS, Bowling AT, Steffey EP.** Clinical survey of anti-red blood cell antibodies in horses after homologous blood transfusion. Am J Vet Res 1986;47:2566–2571.
6. **Bailey E, Albright DG, Henney PJ.** Equine neonatal isoerythrolysis: evidence for prevention by maternal antibodies to the Ca blood group antigen. Am J Vet Res 1988;49:1218–1222.
7. **Traub-Dargatz JL, McClure JJ, Koch C, Schlipf JW Jr.** Neonatal isoerythrolysis in mule foals. J Vet M Assoc 1995;206:67–70.

CHAPTER 114

Red Blood Cell Antigens and Blood Groups in the Cow, Pig, Sheep, Goat, and Llama

• MARIA CECILIA T. PENEDO

Red blood cell antigens and blood groups have been extensively studied in most domestic animals. The identification of blood-group factors expressed on the surface of red-cell membranes and analysis of the patterns of genetic inheritance of these factors have been the subject of intense investigation for the past 50 years. Production of isoimmune and heteroimmune antisera by immunization and the use of absorption procedures for isolation of monospecific antibodies (blood-typing reagents) have been critical for the expansion of the knowledge regarding genetic variation of blood groups in domestic animals. The function of these antigens is not known, but it is likely to be similar to those of humans. In humans, blood-group antigens have been shown to belong to five functional categories:

1. channels and transporters
2. receptors and ligands
3. adhesive molecules
4. enzymes
5. structural proteins

Developments in the human field will certainly stimulate research in animals for elucidation of the role of red-cell antigens.

In this chapter the blood-group systems (or loci) are described for five domestic species: cows, pigs, sheep, goats, and llamas (and the related alpaca). The literature in blood group research is extensive and cannot be fully represented in this chapter. Several excellent reviews of the subject are available.[1-4]

SEROLOGIC ASSAYS FOR BLOOD GROUPS

Hemolytic and agglutination techniques are used to assay blood-group factors. The choice of procedure is determined by characteristics of the red cells of the species of interest, nature of the antigen, and class of antibody. Blood-grouping assays for cattle, sheep, goat and llama are hemolytic tests. In contrast, blood-group factors in pigs are assayed by saline agglutination, the antiglobulin test (Coombs' test), or by hemolytic tests. Some pig factors require addition of dextran (Sigma, St. Louis, MO) to facilitate agglutination and improve scoring of reactions.

Hemolytic tests are typically set up in round-bottom, 96-well microtiter plates. A standard procedure consists of combining, in order, 50 μL of blood-typing reagent with 25 μL of a 2 to 2.5% saline suspension of washed, packed red blood cells and 25 μL of undiluted rabbit complement. After addition of complement, the plate is shaken in a vibrating plate mixer. Reactions are read twice to record the degree of hemolysis; the first reading occurs 30 to 45 minutes after setup; and the second reading occurs 3 hours later. A concave mirror is used for visual determination of hemolysis. Degrees of reactions are classified as 0 (negative, no visible hemolysis), 1 (partial hemolysis), 2 (intermediate), 3 (strong, almost complete) and 4 (complete hemolysis). In negative reactions, red cells remain intact and settle in a pellet at the bottom of the well. When hemolysis is complete, red cells are not visible and the reaction fluid is clear and reddish in color. A complement control consisting of 50 μL of saline, 25 μL of red-cell suspension, and 25 μL of complement is run in parallel with the test reactions.

Rabbit serum is widely used as the source of complement for hemolytic tests. Because rabbits are negative for the heterophile Forssman antigen, they can have Forssman antibodies in high titers. Cattle and camelids are Forssman-negative and therefore hemolytic tests in these species are not affected by Forssman antibodies. For the Forssman-positive red cells of sheep, goats, and pigs, rabbit serum must be absorbed with red cells from these species prior to use as source of complement. Absorptions are carried out at a cold temperature (4°C). Two serial absorptions of 15 to 20 minutes each and a ratio of 1 volume of washed, packed red cells to 2 volumes of rabbit serum are usually sufficient to remove heterophile antibodies without affecting complement function.

Saline agglutination tests are set up in the same way as hemolytic tests, except that complement is omitted.

Reactions proceed at room temperature for 2 to 3 hours. Plates are then shaken briefly to loosen red cells from the bottom of the wells. Reactions are recorded 5 to 10 minutes after resuspension. Degrees of agglutination are recorded as 0 (no agglutination), 1 (partial clumping), 2 (intermediate clumping) and 3 (total clumping of red cells). A microscope can be used to help distinguish between negative and weak positive reactions.

Antiglobulin tests are used with incomplete antibodies that require the addition of rabbit antiglobulin sera to produce agglutination. This procedure is used to detect some blood-group factors in pigs. Addition of dextran to a saline agglutination reaction at a final concentration of 1.5% has been used with some incomplete antibodies in pigs as an alternative to the antiglobulin test.

SOURCE OF BLOOD-TYPING REAGENTS

Blood-typing reagents for domestic animals are not commercially available. They are prepared by laboratories providing blood-typing services. The standardization of reagents for purposes of exchange of blood-type records between laboratories is made by participation in international comparison tests held biannually under the auspices of the International Society of Animal Genetics. The purpose of these tests is to help define specificities of reagents produced by laboratories worldwide and to provide a standard nomenclature for factors and reagents.

CATTLE BLOOD GROUPS

The blood groups of cattle were the first to be studied in detail and provided a model for investigation in other species. The early studies in the 1940s demonstrated the value of isoimmunizations and heteroimmunizations for development of antibodies for blood-group factors. They also defined procedures for preparation of mono-specific antibodies and for assaying blood groups with hemolytic tests that are still in use with few modifications.

Cattle blood groups remain as the primary example of extreme genetic variation of red-cell antigens as evidenced by the extensive list of alleles known in the complex B and C systems. There are currently more than 70 blood-group factors internationally recognized in cattle. Factors are identified by an alphabetical designation (e.g., A, L, S, Z). A numerical subscript is added to letters to describe factors serogically related as subtypes (e.g., A_1, A_2, Y_1, Y_2). The inclusion of the symbols ' and " to a letter (e.g., A', B', A", G") indicates second and third rounds of use of alphabet letters, respectively. One of the most important contributions regarding the genetic inheritance of cattle blood groups was the demonstration that multiple factors co-segregated in specific combinations.[5] Each such combination defined an allele. The term phenogroup was proposed to describe the combinations of factors.[6]

There are 11 genetic systems of blood groups de-scribed in cattle: A, B, C, F, J, L, M, S, Z, R' and T'. It is of interest to note that the J system is not an intrinsic component of the red-cell membrane. J is a tissue and serum antigen that attaches to red cells as serum concentrations become sufficiently high. The J factor is serologically related to human A, sheep R, and pig A factors. Blood-group loci have been mapped to cattle chromosomes by linkage analysis.[7] A summary of cattle blood-group systems, factors, and allelic variants is given in Table 114.1.

PIG BLOOD GROUPS

Development and expansion of pig blood groups is largely because of work carried out in Denmark, Germany, Poland, and Russia. The source of blood-typing reagents is primarily from isoimmune sera. In contrast with cattle, blood-typing reagents for pigs are mostly agglutinins and a few are lysins. Sixteen genetic systems of blood groups are internationally recognized: A, B, C, D, E, F, G, H, I, J, K, L, M, N, O, and P. Some of these, for example, E and M, approach the B and C systems of cattle in complexity. The nomenclature of blood groups designates each system by a capital letter (e.g., B, C) and factors within the system are assigned lowercase letters in order of discovery (e.g., Ba, Bb, Ca). An exception is the A system, still reported with capital letters for the locus and alleles. The A system is related to cattle J, human A, and sheep R systems. Pig A and O factors are not intrinsic components of the cell membrane; they occur as soluble substances in the serum and saliva of A^+ and O^+ animals and attach to red-cell membranes a few weeks after birth. The genetic inheritance of A and O is similar to sheep R system. A is dominant to O and their expression on red cells is under the control of the suppressor gene, S. Antigens of the N system also occur as soluble substances in the serum and milk but are not secreted into the saliva. Blood-group loci have been mapped to pig chromosomes by linkage analysis.[8] A summary of pig blood-group systems, factors, and alleles is given in Table 114.2.

SHEEP BLOOD GROUPS

Developments in the identification of sheep blood-group factors followed closely those in cattle. It was observed early on that certain cattle blood-typing reagents cross-reacted with sheep red cells and detected differences between individuals. Expansion of sheep blood groups occurred during the 1950s and 1960s and resulted in the identification of seven genetic systems: A, B, C, D, M, R, and X. The B and C systems are the more complex and variable. Although no new systems have been discovered, additional factors have been identified. Many of these, however, await official designations. The nomenclature of systems and factors in sheep follows the same rules as those used for pigs. Factors are assigned lowercase letters in order of discovery. There are currently 22 blood-group factors internation-

TABLE 114.1 Cattle Blood Groups

System[a]	Map Location[b]	Blood Factors	Number of Alleles	Alleles[c]
EAA	15	A_1, A_2, H, D, Z'	>10	−, A_1, A_2, A_1D, H, A_1H, A_1Z', etc
EAB	12	B_1, B_2, G_1, G_2, G_3, K, I_1, I_2, O_1, O_2, O_3, Ox, P_1, P_2, Q, T_1, T_2, Y_1, Y_2, A', B', D'E_1', E_2', E_3', F', G', I_1', I_2', J_1', J_2', K', O', P', Q', Y', A", B", G", I"	>600	−, $B_1GKOxY_2A'O'A"$, B_1O_1, $B_1O_1Y_2D'$, B_1I_1Q, $B_2GOxA'A"$, O_1Q', $I_1Y_2E_1'Y'$, I_1Q', $Y_1D'I'$, $GY_2E_1'Q'$, $O_1T_1E_3'F'K'$, $O_1T_1E_3'F'G'K'G"$, $OxQA'E_1'O'$, etc
EAC	18	C_1, C_2, E, R_1, R_2, W, X_1, X_2, C', L', X', C"	>60	−, C_1, C_1EW, C_1R_1W, C_1WL', C_2, C_2WX_2, R_1WL', R_2WX_2L', WX_2, etc
EAF	17	F_1, F_2, V_1, V_2, N'	7	−, F_1, F_2, FN', V_1, V_2, V_1N'
EAJ	11	J	2	−, J
EAL	3	L	2	−, L
EAM	23	M_1, M_2, M'	3	−, M_1, M'
EAS	21	S, H', U_1, U_2, U_1', U_2', S", H", U"	>15	−, SH', H', U_1, $U_1H'H"$, U', U", $U"U_1H'H"$, $U_2'U"$, etc
EAZ	10	Z	2	−, Z
EAR'	16	R', S'	2	R', S'
EAT'	19	T'	2	−, T'

[a] Prefix EA (erythrocyte antigen) is used to indicate type of genetic marker in catalogs of genetic databases.
[b] Map location is from Kappes SM, Bishop MD, Keele JW, et al. Linkage of bovine erythrocyte antigen loci B, C, L, S, Z, R' and T' and the serum protein loci post-transferrin 2 (PTF2), vitamin-D binding protein (Gc) and albumin (ALB) to DNA microsatellite markers. Anim. Genet 1994;25:133–140, with permission and from ArkDB genome database developed by The Roslin Institute Bioinformatics Group (*http://www.ri.bbsrc.ac.uk*).
[c] − (negative) indicates presence of recessive null allele.

ally recognized in sheep. Blood groups in sheep are detected by hemolytic tests with exception of the D system, whose antigens are detected by agglutination test. The B, C, and R systems of sheep are homologous to cattle B, C, and J systems. Features of several sheep blood-group systems are noteworthy. The R system is not an intrinsic component of the red-cell membrane. The antigens are soluble substances found in the serum and saliva. The *R* allele is dominant to *O*. Expression of R and O antigens is under the control of the suppressor gene *I*. Sheep that have genotype i/i do not express R or O antigens in red cells, serum, or saliva. The *C* gene is closely linked to the amino acid transport gene. This association is of interest in light of the fact that erythrocytes with defective transport are never Cb negative. The *M* gene is associated with red-cell potassium transport such that low-potassium (LK) cells are always Mb positive and high-potassium (HK) cells are always Mb negative. It has been postulated that Mb inhibits active potassium transport into cells. Several sheep blood-group systems have been mapped by linkage analysis. A summary of sheep blood-group systems, factors, and allelic variants is given in Table 114.3.

GOAT BLOOD GROUPS

Blood groups in goats are less developed than those of other farm animals. On the basis of cross-reactivity of

sheep blood-typing reagents with goat red cells, it has been shown that goats have blood-group systems homologous to sheep A, B, C, M, and R. Nguyen[9] presented evidence for the existence of six genetic systems of blood groups in goats. The A system, with a single specificity A1, is homologous to sheep Aa. In the B system, 14 specificities were identified. Four are homologous to sheep factors Bb, Be, Bd, and Bi. The C system has a single specificity related to sheep Ca. The E system contains 2 specificities E6 and E18. The F system is defined by a single specificity F19. The R system of goats is defined by a single specificity R related to the R factor of sheep. All systems have a recessive allele "−".

LLAMA BLOOD GROUPS

Blood-group variation in the two domestic South American camelids, llama and alpaca, was investigated by Penedo et al.[10] Isoimmune and heteroimmune sera were developed for these animals. Six blood-group factors were identified and given alphabetical designations in order of discovery: A, B, C, D, E, and F. Factors A and B are inherited as codominant alleles and assigned to blood-group system A. Factors C, D, E, and F were assigned to four separate systems as they seemed transmitted independently from each other and from the A

TABLE 114.2   Pig Blood Groups

System	Map Location[a]	Test Method[b]	Blood Factors	Number of Alleles	Alleles[c]
EAA	1	a, h	A, O	2	A, O
EAB	Unknown	a	a, b	2	a, b
EAC	7[d]	h	A	2	−, a
EAD	12	a	a, b	2	a, b
EAE	9	a	a, b, e, e, f, g, h, I, j, k, l, m, n, o, p, r, s, t	17	aeglns, bdgkmps, defhkmnps, deghkmnps, aeflns, etc
EAF	8	a	a, b, c, d	4	ac, ad, bc, bd
EAG	15	a	a, b	2	a, b
EAH	6	h	a, b, c, d, e	7	−, a, b, ab, bd, cd, be
EAI	18	c	a, b	2	a, b
EAJ	7	c	a, b	3	−, a, b
EAK	9	h	a, b, c, d, e, f, g	6	−, acf, acef, ade, adeg, bf
EAL	4	c, d	a, b, c, d, f, g, h, i, j, k, l, m	6	adhi, bcgi, bdfi, agim, adhjk, adhjl
EAM	11	c, h	a, b, c, d, e, f, g, h, I, j, k, m	20	−, ab, ade, aem, b, bd, bcdi, cd, etc
EAN	9	c	a, b, c	3	a, b, bc
EAO	6	d	a, b	2	a, b
EAP	Unknown	c	a	2	−, a

[a] Chromosome assignments are from Rohrer GA, Vögeli P, Stranzinger G, et al. Mapping 28 erythrocyte antigen, plasma protein and enzyme polymorphisms using an efficient genomic scan of the porcine genome. Anim Genet 1997;28:323–330, with permission, and ArkDB genome database developed by The Roslin Institute Bioinformatics Group (http://www.ri.bbsrc.ac.uk).
[b] a, saline agglutination; c, Coombs' test; d, dextran test; h, hemolytic test.
[c] − (negative) indicates presence of recessive null allele.
[d] Chromosome assignment made by author based on report of linkage of C and J systems by Andresen E, Baker LN. The C blood-group system in pigs and the defection and estimation of linkage between the C and J systems. Genetics 1964;49:379–386, with permission.

TABLE 114.3   Sheep Blood Groups

System	Map Location[a]	Blood Factors	Number of Alleles	Alleles[c]
EAA	6	a, b	3	−, a, b
EAB	10	a, b, c, d, e, f, g, h, i	>50[b]	−, a, ab, abc
EAC	20	a, b	4[b]	−, a, ab, b
EAD	Unknown	a, b	2	−, a
EAM	18	a, b, c	4	−, a, b, ac, c
EAR	Unknown	R, O	2	R, O
EAX	Unknown	X, Z	2	X, Z

[a] Map location was obtained from ArkDB genome database developed by The Roslin Institute Bioinformatics Group (http://www.ri.bbsrc.ac.uk)
[b] Number of alleles is based on internationally recognized factors. Additional factors with provisional designations have been identified that increase number to 100 EAB and 20 EAC alleles.
[c] − (negative) indicates presence of recessive null allele.

system. Blood groups in llamas and alpacas are detected by hemolytic tests.

APPLICATIONS OF BLOOD GROUPS

Animal Breeding

The major application of blood-group variation in cattle, pigs, sheep, and goats is associated with its use in parentage testing to verify accuracy of pedigree records for breed registries and in helping breeders solve problems of questionable paternity or maternity. The variability of blood groups, supplemented by electrophoretic tests that detect additional genetic variation in blood proteins, produce probabilities of exclusion of incorrect parentage of as much as 98%. Parentage testing is based on the principle of exclusion. The blood group or type that an animal possesses in any system is determined by a single pair of allelic genes, one transmitted by the sire and the other by the dam. Therefore, all factors found in any individual must also be present in one or both parents. Exceptions to this rule are grounds for illegitimacy and parentage exclusion. Accurate pedigree records are essential to many aspects of animal breeding related to planned breedings, genetic selection and estimation of heritabilities, and breeding values based on progeny testing.

Cattle breed registries throughout the world have rules requiring that bulls used in artificial insemination (AI) programs and embryo donor cows have blood types on record so that calves resulting from AI service or embryo transfer can be verified as to their parentage. Requirements vary from country to country and may, in some cases, involve testing of all animals submitted for registration.

Mandatory blood-typing programs for pigs, sheep and goats are virtually nonexistent in North America, and there has been little demand for parentage testing in these species in the United States and Canada. In contrast, several countries in Europe have active parentage testing programs for these species.

Blood groups have played a minor role in parentage testing of llamas and alpacas. Blood-typing tests for these animals are based on genetic variation of blood proteins. Parentage testing is required by llama and alpaca registries in the United States and Canada.

Blood groups in cattle, pigs, sheep, and goats have also been used for estimating genetic diversity within breeds and between breeds. Such studies provide useful information regarding structure of populations, historic development of breeds and effects of inbreeding. They also contribute to formulation of management programs for preservation of endangered breeds. Knowledge of genetic distances between breeds may also play a role in designing crossbreeding programs to maximize heterozygosity and heterosis.

Developments in molecular biology and DNA technologies during the past 10 years have provided alternative procedures to blood-typing tests for assaying genetic variation in domestic animals and for use in parentage testing or population studies. Among these procedures, DNA testing for microsatellite loci is presently the method of choice because of the availability of large number of markers with high degree of polymorphism.

Blood Transfusion

Clinically, knowledge of blood groups in these species has not affected conventional practice in transfusion. Matching of blood types for antigenic compatibility is not practical because of the high variability of blood groups between individuals. Availability of donors can also be limited. Blood transfusions in large animals are indicated for certain acute, life-threatening conditions and for plasma transfusion for failure of passive transfer. Single, unmatched whole-blood transfusions are generally safe in cattle, pigs, sheep, goats, and llamas. If repeated transfusions are required, a gross cross matching, involving testing the recipient's serum for antibodies against the donor's red cells (major) and testing of the donor's serum for antibodies against the recipient's red cells (minor), is recommended. When required, the specific antibodies engendered can be determined by testing the recipient's serum against a panel of red cells with known blood types.

In cattle, some vaccinations (e.g., for anaplasmosis), can stimulate production of antibodies against blood-group factors and cause neonatal isoerythrolysis (NI) of newborn calves after suckling of colostrum. Screening of sera from vaccinated cows for presence of blood-group antibodies before calving is recommended. Management of newborn calves at risk of developing NI requires prevention of maternal colostrum intake and replacement with stored colostrum obtained from non-sensitized cows.

REFERENCES

1. **Stormont C.** Current status of blood groups in cattle. Ann N Y Acad Sci 1962;97:251–268.
2. **Bell K.** The blood groups of domestic mammals. In: Agar NS, Board PG, eds. Red blood cells of domestic mammals. Amsterdam: Elsevier, 1983;133–164.
3. **DiStasio L.** Biochemical genetics. In: Piper L, Ruvinsky A, eds. The genetics of sheep. Wallingford, Oxon, UK: CAB International, 1997;133–148.
4. **Juneja RK, Vögeli P.** Biochemical genetics. In: Rothschild MF, Ruvinsky A, eds. The genetics of the pig. Wallingford, Oxon, UK: CAB International, 1998;105–134.
5. **Stormont C, Owen RD, Irwin MR.** The B and C systems of bovine blood groups. Genetics 1951;36:134–161.
6. **Stormont C.** Linked genes, pseudoalleles and blood groups. Am Nat 1955;89:105–116.
7. **Kappes SM, Bishop MD, Keele JW, et al.** Linkage of bovine erythrocyte antigen loci B, C, L, S, Z, R' and T' and the serum protein loci post-transferrin 2 (PTF-2), vitamin-D binding protein (Gc) and albumin (ALB) to DNA microsatellite markers. Anim Genet 1994;25:133–140.
8. **Rohrer GA, Vögeli P, Stranzinger G, et al.** Mapping 28 erythrocyte antigen, plasma protein and enzyme polymorphisms using an efficient genomic scan of the porcine genome. Anim Genet 1997;28:323–330.
9. **Nguyen TC.** Genetic systems of red cell blood groups in goats. Anim Genet 1990;21:233–245.
10. **Penedo MCT, Fowler ME, Bowling AT, et al.** Genetic variation in the blood of llamas, *Lama glama*, and alpacas, *Lama pacos*. Anim Genet 1988;19:267–276.
11. **Andresen E, Baker LN.** The C blood-group system in pigs and the detection and estimation of linkage between the C and J systems. Genetics 1964; 49:379–386.

CHAPTER 115

Granulocyte and Platelet Antigens

• MICHAEL A. SCOTT

Granulocyte and platelet antigens are the targets of antibodies in several clinically significant immune-mediated conditions (Table 115.1). Some of these conditions are well known in veterinary medicine, but others are better recognized in human medicine in which there is more extensive use of transfusion therapy and in which the human hemochorial placentation predisposes to neonatal neutropenic and thrombocytopenic disorders. In this chapter, the human model is used as a guide to understanding the contributions of granulocyte and platelet antigens to disease.

The identification and characterization of specific antigens involved in pathologic conditions generally begins with the recognition that antibodies are associated with a particular clinical disorder. The pathologic antibodies may be autoantibodies, alloantibodies, isoantibodies, or drug-induced antibodies. Autoantibodies are specifically reactive with normal self-antigens that are common to most individuals of a species. Alloantibodies are reactive with alloantigens, usually proteins, that are recognized as different by different individuals of the same species. Alloantigenic sites often result from inherited polymorphisms of the amino acid residues of a common protein. Isoantibodies, in the purist sense, react with nonpolymorphic epitopes that exist in all normal individuals of the species.[1] They usually occur after transfusion of an individual who has an inherited deficiency of an antigenic protein. The resulting isoantibodies are not specific for any of the allelic forms of the deficient protein, so they are not alloantibodies. Drug-induced antibodies occur with drug exposure. Some appear to be autoantibodies that bind to autoantigens in a drug-independent manner and persist long after drug cessation.[2] Most bind in a drug-dependent manner only in the presence of the causative drug. Drug-dependent binding may be Fab-mediated or Fc-mediated.

Once a pathogenic antibody is documented by specialized antibody assays,[3-7] its target antigen can be characterized. Several of the human granulocyte and platelet alloantigens have been defined to the level of nucleic acid polymorphisms of their genes, so the amino acid substitutions responsible for their antigenicity are known. Molecular allotyping techniques have shown that the genotypic and phenotypic frequencies of human platelet and granulocyte alloantigens vary considerably among ethnic groups, so species and breed differences in expression of alloantigens are likely in veterinary medicine.[8-10]

Human granulocyte and platelet antigens that are reactive with pathologic antibodies include protein, lipid, and carbohydrate molecules. Protein antigens are most important and best characterized. They may be cytosolic or exosolic, but it is the exosolic antigens that are responsible for most of the clinical conditions related to granulocyte and platelet antigens. The orientation, distribution density,[11] and tertiary (three-dimensional) structure[10,11] of these antigens appear to be important factors affecting their immunogenicity. Integrins tend to be polymorphic and alloimmunogenic.

GRANULOCYTE ANTIGENS

The granulocyte subset of leukocytes comprises the neutrophils, the eosinophils, and the basophils. Of these, neutrophils circulate at the greatest concentrations and appear to contribute most to immunologic conditions involving granulocyte antigens. The antigens found on human neutrophils have various tissue distribution patterns ranging from neutrophil-specific to widespread.[12] The latter include class I human leukocyte antigens[9] (HLA) and some blood group antigens.[9,12] Some antigens are common to a wide range of hemic cells,[9,12] and others are common to just the granulocytes.[12] Similar antigen distribution patterns are expected to exist in domestic mammals.

Many of the disease-associated human granulocyte antigens have not yet been identified, and none has been characterized in veterinary medicine. To date, three major immunogenic membrane antigens have been identified on human neutrophils: (1) FcγRIIIb, a low-affinity receptor for small immune complexes that is also on monocytes and some lymphocytes, (2) CR3 (CD11b/CD18, Mac-1), a β_2-integrin adhesion molecule that is also on monocytes and some lymphocytes and that mediates binding to endothelial cells and certain complement proteins, and (3) lymphocyte function-associated antigen (LFA)-1 (CD11a/CD18), a β_2-integrin on most

TABLE 115.1	Clinical Conditions Resulting from Antibodies to Granulocytes and Platelets[a]	
Granulocytes		**Platelets**
Autoimmune		Autoimmune
Primary immune-mediated neutropenia (autoimmune, idiopathic)		Primary immune-mediated thrombocytopenia (autoimmune, idiopathic)
Secondary immune-mediated neutropenia (e.g., with SLE)		Secondary immune-mediated thrombocytopenia (e.g., with SLE)
Chronic neutropenia of infancy/childhood		Transient neonatal thrombocytopenia secondary to maternal autoimmune thrombocytopenia
Transient neonatal neutropenia secondary to maternal autoimmune neutropenia		Alloimmune
Alloimmune		Neonatal alloimmune thrombocytopenia
Neonatal alloimmune neutropenia		Posttransfusion purpura
Transfusion reactions		Refractoriness to platelet transfusions
Febrile		Drug-induced
Pulmonary		Drug-induced, immune-mediated thrombocytopenia (drug-dependent or drug-independent antibodies)
Drug-induced		Isoimmune (rare)
Drug-induced, immune-mediated neutropenia (drug-dependent or drug-independent antibodies)		Refractoriness to platelet transfusions
Isoimmune (rare)		Neonatal isoimmune thrombocytopenia (potentially)
Neonatal isoimmune neutropenia		

[a] The categories are based on human diseases; nonhuman analogs have either been recognized or are likely to be recognized.

leukocytes that also mediates binding to endothelial cells.[9,11] Several alloantigens and autoantigens have been mapped to these proteins. Because these antigens are functional membrane proteins, antibody binding may affect cell functions.[13] The neutrophil-specific epitopes defined by human antibodies have not been identified on nonprimate neutrophils, but similar surface proteins have been identified in several species.[14–18] The epitopes recognized by monoclonal antibodies bear no necessary relation to the reactive epitopes of disease-associated pathologic antibodies.

Granulocyte Alloantigens

Most of the known human granulocyte antigens are alloantigens, often associated with FcγRIIIb. A few of them have been characterized to the nucleic acid level,[8,11] but their presence on granulocytes of veterinary species has not been assessed.

Alloantibodies induced by previous transfusion or pregnancy may target common or neutrophil-specific antigens and lead to febrile or pulmonary transfusion reactions.[9,19] Febrile reactions occur when a transfusion recipient has alloantibodies reactive with transfused leukocytes. Depleting blood of leukocytes before transfusing an immunized patient helps prevent further febrile reactions.[9] Transfusion-related lung injury usually occurs when antileukocyte antibodies are present in transfusions of plasma or whole blood from donors who have been alloimmunized by multiple pregnancies or transfusions.[12] Because of granulocyte and neutrophil-specific sites on antigens such as FcγRIIIb,[11] histocompatibility matching does not prevent these transfusion reactions. The incidence of antileukocyte antibodies and their contribution to transfusion reactions in dogs and other species is unknown.[20] Febrile reactions in dogs transfused with platelet concentrates has been weakly

associated with leukocyte contamination of the concentrates.[21]

Neonatal alloimmune neutropenia occurs because of maternal sensitization to paternal alloantigens on fetal neutrophils during pregnancy or parturition.[12] Alloantibodies may gain access to the fetus in utero, or the neonate may ingest and absorb them with intake of colostrum. Leukopenias associated with suspected antileukocyte antibodies have been reported in newborn pigs, calves, and foals.[22,23] Common antigens may be less pathogenic than neutrophil-specific antigens because the offending antibodies may have diluted effects as they react to multiple cell types instead of just to neutrophils.[12]

Granulocyte Autoantigens

Primary immune-mediated neutropenia (chronic idiopathic neutropenia) occurs when antineutrophil autoantibodies bind to autoepitopes and mediate premature neutrophil destruction.[13] Most granulocyte autoantibodies are panreactive with neutrophils of different alloantigenicity,[9,11] but reactivity to neutrophil-specific alloantigens has been reported.[24] Many human autoantigens are directed to nonpolymorphic sites on FcγRIIIb, whereas some target common antigens.[24] Autoantibodies reactive with antigens on myeloid precursors may result in pure white cell aplasia.[24,25] Chronic idiopathic neutropenias have rarely been described in veterinary medicine, but the steroid responsiveness of some suggests an immune-mediated and possibly autoimmune pathogenesis.[26,27]

Chronic neutropenia of infancy and childhood has not been described in veterinary medicine, but it is a common transient form of chronic idiopathic neutropenia in human infants.[12] Autoantibodies usually bind to neutrophil-specific epitopes, including some on alloantigens.[8] Autoimmune neutropenia, sometimes culminating in pancytopenia, can occur secondary to systemic lupus erythematosis, lymphoproliferative disorders, and infectious diseases.[12,24]

Granulocyte Isoantigens

Some human patients are absolutely or functionally deficient in FcγRIIIb.[9,28] In offspring of these patients, neonatal isoimmune neutropenia has occurred because of maternal isoimmunization by normal fetal FcγRIIIb. Transfusions could also lead to isoantibody production. Similar outcomes may occur with other neutrophil membrane protein deficiencies such as the CD11/CD18 complex deficiency reported in dogs and cattle that have leukocyte adhesion deficiency syndromes.[18]

Drug-Induced Granulocyte Antigens

Drug-induced neutropenias are usually the result of dose-dependent myelosuppression. However, drugs or their metabolites may cause neutropenia by inducing cell-mediated or antibody-mediated destruction of peripheral neutrophils or their marrow precursors.[24,25,29] The specific mechanisms and antigens involved are unknown, but in at least some cases, the drug's presence is important in maintaining the antigenic site for antibody binding to cells.[29] Removal of the offending drug typically prevents antibody binding and allows rapid recovery. White cell aplasia may occur when marrow precursors are targeted.[24,25] Several drugs have been implicated in causing myelosuppression in veterinary species, but immune-mediated mechanisms have not been proven.[30]

Serologic Detection Methods for Granulocyte Antigen-Antibody Interactions

No single assay can detect all granulocyte antigens.[8,13] Agglutination and immunofluorescence tests have been used most widely, but antigen capture methods have been evaluated more recently.[11] Immunofluorescence assays can be positive in granulocyte colony-stimulating factor (G-CSF)-treated human patients because G-CSF induces expression of FcγRI receptors that bind monomeric plasma IgG.[31] The use of G-CSF in other species may produce similar results. Only preliminary attempts have been made to detect pathogenic granulocyte antigen-antibody interactions in veterinary medicine.[6,32]

PLATELET ANTIGENS

The study of platelet immunogenicity has largely mirrored the study of platelet glycoproteins, the main targets of antiplatelet autoantibodies, alloantibodies, and drug-dependent antibodies. The major membrane glycoproteins that are also antibody targets belong to the integrin ($\alpha_x\beta_y$) and leucine-rich motif (glycoprotein [GP] Ib, IX, V) families.[1] $\alpha_{IIb}\beta_3$ is an activation-dependent receptor that mediates platelet aggregation by freely binding several adhesion molecules, including fibrinogen and von Willebrand's factor (vWf). Platelets from humans and animals[33] with Glanzmann's thrombasthenia either physically or functionally lack $\alpha_{IIb}\beta_3$ and cannot aggregate. $\alpha_2\beta_1$ is important as a collagen receptor, and inherited defects in $\alpha_2\beta_1$ also have functional consequences. GPIbIX binds vWF and is thought to be the primary mediator of platelet-vessel wall interactions under shear-stress conditions. Patients that have Bernard-Soulier syndrome are quantitatively or qualitatively deficient in GPIbIX (and V) and have defects in hemostasis.

Autoantibodies and alloantibodies to these functional membrane glycoproteins occasionally exacerbate hemorrhage either by activating platelets leading to more severe thrombocytopenia, or by causing functional impairments similar to those of inherited glycoprotein deficiencies.[1,34] Some autoantibodies have been shown to induce dysfunction without thrombocytopenia.[35,36] The frequency with which antiplatelet antibodies interfere with platelet function in dogs that have immune-mediated thrombocytopenia (IMT) is unknown, but one study suggests it may occur.[37] This may help explain hemorrhage in animals whose platelet concentrations are high enough to expect normal hemostasis.

As with granulocytes, the tissue specificity of platelet antigens varies from widespread to platelet-specific. Widespread antigens on human platelets include class I (but not class II) HLAs, and some of the major blood-group antigens that are present either intrinsically or as adsorbed antigens.[38] Other antigens are shared with leukocytes, endothelial cells, vascular smooth muscle cells, fibroblasts, and osteoclasts.[39] The presence of common antigenic molecules among cell types does not guarantee that the specific pathologic epitopes of these antigens are conserved, but some are. Antibodies to the Pl^A and Pen epitopes of the β_3 integrin (GPIIIa) on platelets and endothelial cells may exacerbate bleeding tendencies.[1] Evidence of shared antigenicity between canine endothelial cells and platelets exists.[40]

Platelet Alloantigens

Of the many platelet GPs, only the few discussed above seem polymorphic and immunogenic enough for consistent induction of alloantibody production.[10] Some of them are diallelic antigens, whereas all the human allotypes related to β_3 are mutations of the same region of the molecule and actually represent multiple epitopes of the same antigen.[10] The major platelet GPs are conserved among species,[33,41–44] and the human Pl^A1 and Pl^E1 epitopes have been reported in nonhuman species, including dogs.[33,45–47] However, their importance to alloimmune diseases in different species is unknown.

Neonatal alloimmune thrombocytopenia is caused by maternal sensitization to paternal alloantigens on fetal platelets. Thrombocytopenia may occur in the fetus or neonate after passive transfer of alloantibodies through the placenta or colostrum, but most of the offspring of mismatched human parents do not develop thrombocytopenia.[35] The Pl[A1] allotype is commonly involved in some human ethnic groups, but the responsible allotypes vary with ethnicity and may be rare and familial.[35] Neonatal alloimmune thrombocytopenia has been well described in pigs.[47,48] The participating antigens are unknown, but multiple platelet epitopes appear to be involved.[49] Antibodies to erythrocytes and leukocytes may be present concurrently, but they appear to differ in specificity.[23,48] Neonatal alloimmune thrombocytopenia was reported in a foal, and it may occur in mules.[50] The reactive epitopes were not identified.

Posttransfusion purpura is a poorly understood condition. It occurs 7 to 10 days after immunogenic platelet transfusions and results from antibody-mediated destruction of the transfused platelets as well as the recipient's own platelets, which lack the sensitizing antigen. Posttransfusion purpura has been described in dogs[51] and pigs,[52] but the conditions may not be the same as the human condition.

Platelet refractoriness occurs in patients receiving multiple platelet transfusions when they produce alloantibodies that mediate destruction of the transfused platelets. Common antigens are usually the cause of platelet refractoriness, but platelet-specific antigens can be contributory. Refractoriness to platelet transfusions has been reported in multiply transfused dogs; shortened life spans of transfused, but not autologous, platelets were documented.[21,51,53,54] Alloantibodies may exist in dogs that have never been pregnant or transfused.[53]

Platelet Autoantigens

Autoimmune thrombocytopenia is caused by autoantibodies that bind to platelet autoantigens and mediate their premature destruction.[55] The autoepitopes targeted in human primary IMT are usually public antigens.[56] Any transfused platelets may therefore be cleared quickly if there is a significant plasma antibody titer in the recipient. Multiple autoepitopes have been identified,[56] but the course, hemorrhagic tendency, and response to therapy of human primary IMT cannot currently be predicted by the autoepitopes involved.[1,35] Target epitopes are usually on GPs $\alpha_{IIb}\beta_3$, IbIX, $\alpha_2\beta_1$, or V, most of them being on the β_3 subunit of $\alpha_{IIb}\beta_3$. Some of the epitopes require the normal association of the cation-dependent $\alpha_{IIb}\beta_3$ complex, so ethylenediaminetetraacetic acid (EDTA) can dissociate the subunits and remove the reactive epitope.[35] Based on studies of monoclonal antibody binding to ovine and bovine $\alpha_{IIb}\beta_3$, cation-dependent epitopes also occur in at least some of our domestic species.[42]

IMT has frequently been diagnosed in dogs, and idiopathic thrombocytopenias in some horses and cats are probably immune-mediated.[57-62] Autoimmunity is often suspected but rarely proven. However, immunoprecipitation of canine samples have identified platelet membrane α_{IIb}, β_3, and GPIb as specific targets of antibodies in some dogs that have clinical diagnoses of primary IMT.[33,63,64] Thrombocytopenia suspected of being immune-mediated also frequently accompanies immune-mediated hemolytic anemia in dogs,[65,66] but it is unknown if specific antiplatelet antibodies are involved. The autoantigens targeted in IMT secondary to systemic autoimmune diseases may be different from those of primary IMT.[1]

Platelet Isoantigens

Isoantibodies have been produced in people with Glanzmann's thrombasthenia or Bernard–Soulier syndrome after transfusions with normal platelets. The antibodies may bind to α_{IIb}, β_3, the $\alpha_{IIb}\beta_3$ complex, or to GPIbIX.[38] GPIV deficiency has also led to isoimmunization.[38] Similar antibody production may occur in animals that have membrane GP deficiencies.[33]

Drug-Induced Platelet Antigens

Drugs can induce thrombocytopenia by immune and nonimmune mechanisms. Immune-mediated mechanisms have been documented for several drugs, and suspected with many more.[67] Some drugs or their metabolites appear to induce membrane neoepitopes that antibodies recognize in the presence but not in the absence of the specific drug or metabolite.[35,67] Several mechanisms have been postulated.[68] In people, quinine and quinidine induce such antibodies that bind to GPIbIX and $\alpha_{IIb}\beta_3$, often concurrently in the same patient.[68,69] Some drug-dependent antibodies require intact $\alpha_{IIb}\beta_3$ and will not bind after complex dissociation by EDTA.[70] Drugs may also induce autoantibodies that bind to platelets in a drug-independent manner long after the drug is gone.[67] In dogs, gold compounds, very high dose cefonizid and cefazedone, and trimethoprim/sulfonamides have been best implicated in causing drug-induced IMT.[3,32,71,72] Propylthiouracil may cause IMT in cats.[73]

Heparin-induced IMT is mostly the result of immune complex binding to platelet Fc receptors; platelet antigens are not involved.[68] Data are scarce, but platelets of pigs, sheep, goats, cattle, and nonhuman primates reportedly express Fc receptors, whereas platelets of rabbits, dogs, mice, and horses reportedly do not.[74-76] Heparin-induced IMT has not been recognized in veterinary medicine.

Platelet Cryptic Autoantigens

Human plasma sometimes contains antibodies that bind to platelets in an EDTA-dependent manner. EDTA appears to induce the expression of reactive cryptantigens, at least some of which are on $\alpha_{IIb}\beta_3$.[77,78] The presence of antibodies to these epitopes suggests the possibility that there are other means of exposing these epitopes in vivo and that they may be pathogenic or a reflection of immunologic activation.[1] EDTA has induced platelet agglutination in horses, pigs, and dogs, so similar cryptantigens likely exist in these species.[79–81] Formalin also induces the expression of hidden epitopes that are reactive with antibodies in some individuals.[77]

Platelet Glycolipid Autoantigens

Protein antigens have received much more attention, but acidic and neutral membrane glycolipids have also been identified as autoantigens in people that have IMT.[35] Platelet monogalactosylsulfatides have been implicated as cross-reactive autoepitopes with anti-DNA antibodies in people.[35]

Serologic Detection Methods for Platelet Antigen-Antibody Interactions

Platelet antibody assays have progressed from phase I (functional) assays to phase III assays that detect antibody binding to specific antigens.[7] Phase II assays for platelet surface-associated immunoglobulin have recently been developed for dogs.[3,4,64] As mentioned above, phase III immunoprecipitation studies have been done to characterize canine antiplatelet antibody specificities.[63,64] Immunoblotting studies are more difficult to interpret because reactive epitopes may be destroyed,[56] and many protein bands can be seen with sera from normal individuals.[82] These bands may be the result of autoantibodies to surface or cytosolic proteins unassociated with disease, or they may be the result of nonspecific immunoglobulin binding.

REFERENCES

1. **Kunicki TJ, Newman PJ.** The molecular immunology of human platelet proteins. Blood 1992;80:1386–1404.
2. **Aster RH.** The immunologic thrombocytopenias. In: Kunicki TJ, George JN, eds. Platelet immunobiology: molecular and clinical aspects. Philadephia: JB Lippincott, 1989;387–435.
3. **Lewis DC, Meyers KM, Callan MB, Bücheler J, Giger U.** Detection of platelet-bound and serum platelet-bindable antibodies for diagnosis of idiopathic thrombocytopenic purpura in dogs. J Am Vet Med Assoc 1995;206:47–52.
4. **Lewis DC, McVey DS, Shuman WS, Muller WB.** Development and characterization of a flow cytometric assay for detection of platelet-bound immunoglobulin G in dogs. Am J Vet Res 1995;56:1555–1558.
5. **Kristensen AT, Weiss DJ, Klausner JS, Laber J, Christie DJ.** Comparison of microscopic and flow cytometric detection of platelet antibody in dogs suspected of having immune-mediated thrombocytopenia. Am J Vet Res 1994;55:1111–1114.
6. **Jain NC, Vegad JL, Kono CS.** Methods for detection of immune-mediated neutropenia in horses, using antineutrophil serum of rabbit origin. Am J Vet Res 1990;51:1026–1031.
7. **Warner M, Kelton JG.** Laboratory investigation of immune thrombocytopenia. J Clin Pathol 1997;50:5–12.
8. **Hessner MJ, Curtis BR, Endean DJ, Aster RH.** Determination of neutrophil antigen gene frequencies in five ethnic groups by polymerase chain reaction with sequence-specific primers. Transfusion 1996;36:895–899.
9. **von dem Borne AEGKr.** Neutrophil alloantigens nature and clinical relevance. Vox Sang 1994;67:105–112.
10. **Newman PJ, Valentin N.** Human platelet alloantigens: recent findings, new perspectives. Thromb Haemost 1995;74:234–239.
11. **Bux J, Stein E-L, Bierling P, Fromont P, Clay M, Stroncek D, Santoso S.** Characterization of a new alloantigen (SH) on the human neutrophil Fcγ receptor IIIb. Blood 1997;89:1027–1034.
12. **Lalezari P.** Leukocyte antigens and antibodies. In: Hoffman R, Furie B, Shattil SJ, Benz EJ Jr, Cohen HJ, Silberstein LE, eds. Hematology: basic principles and practice. 2nd ed. New York: Churchill Livingstone, 1995; 1974–1980.
13. **Shastri KA, Logue GL.** Autoimmune neutropenia. Blood 1993;81:1984–1995.
14. **Horton MA, Fowler P, Simpson A, Onions D.** Monoclonal antibodies to

15. **Sweeney SE, Halloran PJ, Kim YB.** Identification of a unique porcine FcγRIIIAα molecular complex. Cellular Immunology 1996;172:92–99.
16. **Nagahata H, Higuchi H, Nochi H, Tamoto K, Noda H, Kociba GJ.** Enhanced expression of Fc receptors on neutrophils from calves with leukocyte adhesion deficiency. Microbiol Immunol 1995;39:703–708.
17. **Cox E, Mast J, MacHugh N, Schwenger B, Goddeeris BM.** Expression of β2 integrins on blood leukocytes of cows with or without bovine leukocyte adhesion deficiency. Vet Immuno Immunopathol 1997;58:249–263.
18. **Giger U, Boxer LA, Simpson PJ, Lucchesi BR, Todd RF III.** Deficiency of leukocyte surface glycoproteins Mo1, LFA-1, and Leu M5 in a dog with recurrent bacterial infections: an animal model. Blood 1987;69:1622–1630.
19. **Harrell K, Parrow J, Kristensen A.** Canine transfusion reactions. Part II. prevention and treatment. Compend Contin Educ Pract Vet 1997;February:193–200.
20. **Harrell K, Parrow J, Kristensen A.** Canine transfusion reactions. Part I. Causes and consequences. Compend Contin Educ Pract Vet 1997;February:181–190.
21. **Abrams-Ogg ACG, Kruth SA, Carter RF, Valli VE, Kamel-Reid S, Dubé ID.** Preparation and transfusion of canine platelet concentrates. Am J Vet Res 1993;54:635–642.
22. **Jain NC.** Immunohematology. In: Jain NC, editor. Essentials of veterinary hematology. Philadelphia: Lea & Febiger, 1993;381–408.
23. **Linklater KA, McTaggart HS, Imlah P.** Haemolytic disease of the newborn, thrombocytopenic purpura and neutropenia occurring concurrently in a litter of piglets. Br Vet J 1973;129:35–46.
24. **Coates TD, Baehner R.** Leukocytosis and leukopenia. In: Hoffman R, Benz EJ Jr, Shattil SJ, Furie B, Cohen HJ, Silberstein LE, eds. Hematology: basic principles and practice. 2nd ed. New York: Churchill Livingstone, 1995; 769–783.
25. **Marinone G, Roncoli B, Marinone MG Jr.** Pure white cell aplasia. Semin Hematol 1991;28:298–302.
26. **Maddison JE, Hoff B, Johnson RP.** Steroid responsive neutropenia in a dog. J Am Anim Hosp Assoc 1983;19:881–886.
27. **Swenson CL, Kociba GJ, Arnold P.** Chronic idiopathic neutropenia in a cat. J Vet Intern Med 1988;2:100–102.
28. **de Haas M, Kleijer M, van Zwieten R, Roos D, von dem Borne AEGKr.** Neutrophil FcγRIIIb deficiency, nature, and clinical consequences: a study of 21 individuals from 14 families. Blood 1995;86:2403–2413.
29. **Stroncek DF, Herr GP.** The chemical and immunoglobulin structural features necessary for reactions of quinine-dependent antibodies to neutrophils. Transfusion 1995;35:247–253.
30. **Jacobs G, Calvert C, Kaufman A.** Neutropenia and thrombocytopenia in three dogs treated with anticonvulsants. J Am Vet Med Assoc 1998; 212:681–684.
31. **Repp R, Valerius Th, Sendler A, Gramatzki M, Iro H, Kalden JR, Platzer E.** Neutrophils express the high affinity receptor for IgG (FcγRI, CD64) after in vivo application of recombinant human granulocyte colony-stimulating factor. Blood 1991;78:885–889.
32. **Bloom JC, Thiem PA, Sellers TS, Deldar A, Lewis HB.** Cephalosporin-induced immune cytopenia in the dog: demonstration of erythrocyte-, neutrophil-, and platelet-associated IgG following treatment with cefazedone. Am J Hematol 1988;28:71–78.
33. **Boudreaux MK, Kvan K, Dillon AR, Bourne C, Scott M, Schwartz KA, Toivio-Kinnucan M.** Type I Glanzmann's thrombasthenia in a great Pyrenees dog. Vet Pathol 1996;33:503–511.
34. **Deckmyn H, De Reys S.** Functional effects of human antiplatelet antibodies. Semin Thromb Hemost 1995;21:46–59.
35. **Kunicki TJ.** Human platelet antigens. In: Hoffman R, Benz EJ Jr, Shattil SJ, Furie B, Cohen HJ, Silberstein LE, eds. Hematology: basic principles and practice. 2nd ed. New York: Churchill Livingstone, 1995;1961–1973.
36. **George JN, Shattil SJ.** Acquired disorders of platelet function. In: Hoffman R, Benz EJ, Jr, Shattil SJ, Cohen HJ, Silberstein LE, Furie B, eds. Hematology: basic principles and practice. 2nd ed. New York: Churchill Livingstone, 1995;1926–1946.
37. **Kristensen AT, Weiss DJ, Klausner JS.** Platelet dysfunction associated with immune-mediated thrombocytopenia in dogs. J Vet Intern Med 1994; 8:323–327.
38. **Kunicki TJ.** Biochemistry of platelet-associated isoantigens and alloantigens. In: Kunicki TJ, George JN, eds. Platelet immunobiology: molecular and clinical aspects. Philadelphia: JB Lippincott, 1989;99–120.
39. **Shattil SJ.** Function and regulation of the β3 integrins in hemostasis and vascular biology. Thromb Haemost 1995;74:149–155.
40. **Morrison FS, Baldini MG.** Antigenic relationship between blood platelets and vascular endothelium. Blood 1969;33:46–56.
41. **Newman PJ.** Phylogeny and tissue distribution of platelet antigens. In: Kunicki TJ, George JN, eds. Platelet immunobiology: molecular and clinical aspects. Philadelphia: JB Lippincott, 1989;148–165.
42. **Mateo A, de la Lastra JP, Moreno A, Dusinsky R, Bilka F, Simon M, Horovska L, Llanes D.** Biochemical characterization of antigens detected with anti-platelet monoclonal antibodies. Vet Immuno Immunopathol 1996;52:363–370.

43. Raymond SL, Dodds J. Platelet membrane glycoproteins in normal dogs and dogs with hemostatic defects. J Lab Clin Med 1979;93:607–613.

44. Pintado CO, Friend M, Llanes D. Characterisation of a membrane receptor on ruminants and equine platelets and peripheral blood leukocytes similar to the human integrin receptor glycoprotein IIb/IIIa (CD41/61). Vet Immuno Immunopathol 1995;44:359–368.

45. Lane J, Brown M, Bernstein I, Wilcox PK, Slichter SJ, Nowinski RC. Serological and biochemical analysis of the PlA1 alloantigen of human platelets. Br J Haematol 1982;50:351–359.

46. Shulman NR, Marder VJ, Hiller MC, Collier EM. Platelet and leukocyte isoantigens and their antibodies: serologic, physiologic, and clinical studies. Prog Hematol 1964;4:222–304.

47. Jain NC. Immunohematology. In: Jain NC, ed. Schalm's veterinary hematology. 4th ed. Philadelphia: Lea & Febiger, 1986:990–1039.

48. Linklater KA. Iso-antibodies to red cell antigens in pigs' sera. 1. Iso-immunisation of pregnancy in sows. Animal Blood Groups and Biochemical Genetics 1971;2:201–214.

49. Lie H. The complexity of platelet antigens in pig. In: Xth European Conference on Animal Blood Groups and Biochemical Polymorphism Institut National De La Recherche Agronomique, Paris, 1966;181–184.

50. Buechner-Maxwell V, Scott M, Godber L, Kristensen A. Neonatal alloimmune thrombocytopenia in a quarter horse foal. J Vet Intern Med 1997;11:304–308.

51. Baldini M. Acute "ITP" in isoimmunized dogs. Ann N Y Acad Sci 1965;124:543–549.

52. Linklater KA. Post-transfusion purpura in a pig. Res Vet Sci 1977;22:257–258.

53. Slichter S, O'Donnell MR, Weiden PL, Storb R, Schroeder M-L. Canine platelet alloimmunization: the role of donor selection. Br J Haematol 1986;63:713–727.

54. Slichter S, Weiden PL, Kane PJ, Storb RF. Approaches to preventing or reversing platelet alloimmunization using animal models. Transfusion 1988;28:103–108.

55. George JN, Raskob GE. Idiopathic thrombocytopenic purpura: a concise summary of the pathophysiology and diagnosis in children and adults. Semin Hematol 1998;35:5–8.

56. Kiefel V, Santoso S, Mueller-Eckhardt C. Serological, biochemical, and molecular aspects of platelet autoantigens. Semin Hematol 1992;29:26–33.

57. Gaschen FP, Meyer BS, Harvey JW. Amegakaryocytic thrombocytopenia and immune-mediated haemolytic anaemia in a cat. Comp Haematol Int 1992;2:175–178.

58. Jordan HL, Grindem CB, Breitschwerdt EB. Thrombocytopenia in cats: a retrospective study of 41 cases. J Vet Intern Med 1993;7:261–265.

59. Peterson JL, Couto CG, Wellman ML. Hemostatic disorders in cats: a retrospective study and review of the literature. J Vet Intern Med 1995;9:298–303.

60. Lubas G, Ciattini F, Gavazza A. Immune-mediated thrombocytopenia and hemolytic anemia (Evan's syndrome) in a horse. Equine Pract 1997;19:27–32.

61. Morris DD, Whitlock RH. Relapsing idiopathic thrombocytopenia in a horse. Equine Vet J 1983;15:73–75.

62. Sockett DC, Traub-Dargatz J, Weiser MG. Immune-mediated hemolytic anemia and thrombocytopenia in a foal. J Am Vet Med Assoc 1987;190:308–310.

63. Lewis DC, Meyers KM. Studies of platelet-bound and serum platelet-bindable immunoglobulins in dogs with idiopathic thrombocytopenic purpura. Exp Hematol 1996;24:696–701.

64. Scott MA. Canine immune-mediated thrombocytopenia: assay development, a role for complement, and assessment in a toxicologic study. Michigan State University, PhD, 1995;451.

65. Klag AR, Giger U, Shofer FS. Idiopathic immune-mediated hemolytic anemia in dogs: 42 cases (1986–1990). J Am Vet Med Assoc 1993;202:783–788.

66. Jackson ML, Kruth SA. Immune-mediated hemolytic anemia and thrombocytopenia in the dog: a retrospective study of 55 cases diagnosed from 1969 through 1983 at the Western College of Veterinary Medicine. Can Vet J 1985;26:245–250.

67. Warkentin TE, Trimble MS, Kelton JG. Thrombocytopenia due to platelet destruction and hypersplenism. In: Hoffman R, Benz EJ Jr, Shattil SJ, Furie B, Cohen HJ, Silberstein LE, eds. Hematology: basic principles and practice. 2nd ed. New York: Churchill Livingstone, 1995;1889–1908.

68. Berndt MC, Chong BH, Andrews RK. Biochemistry of drug-dependent platelet autoantigens. In: Kunicki TJ, George JN, eds. Platelet immunobiology: molecular and clinical aspects. Philadelphia: JB Lippincott, 1989;132–147.

69. Visentin GP, Newman PJ, Aster RH. Characteristics of quinine- and quinidine-induced antibodies specific for platelet glycoproteins IIb and IIIa. Blood 1991;77:2668–2676.

70. Curtis BR, McFarland JG, Wu G-G, Visentin GP, Aster RH. Antibodies in sulfonamide-induced immune thrombocytopenia recognize calcium-dependent epitopes on the glycoprotein IIb/IIIa complex. Blood 1994;84:176–183.

71. Bloom JC, Blackmer SA, Bugelski PJ, Sowinski JM, Saunders LZ. Gold-induced immune thrombocytopenia in the dog. Vet Pathol 1985;22:492–499.

72. Sullivan PS, Arrington K, West R, McDonald TP. Thrombocytopenia associated with administration of trimethoprim/sulfadiazine in a dog. J Am Vet Med Assoc 1992;201:1741–1744.

73. Peterson ME, Hurvitz AI, Leib MS, Cavanagh PG, Dutton RE. Propylthiouracil-associated hemolytic anemia, thrombocytopenia, and antinuclear antibodies in cats with hyperthyroidism. J Am Vet Med Assoc 1984;184:806–808.

74. Siuha RK, Santos AV, Smith JW, Horsewood P, Andrew M, Kelton JG. Rabbit platelets do not express Fc receptors for IgG. Platelets 1992;3:35–39.

75. Rosenfeld SI, Anderson CL. Fc receptors of human platelets. In: Kunicki TJ, George JN, eds. Platelet immunobiology: molecular and clinical aspects. Philadelphia: JB Lippincott, 1989:337–353.

76. Nelson DS. Immune adherence. In: Dixon FJ, Humphrey JH, eds. Advances in immunology. New York: Academic Press, 1963;3:131–180.

77. von dem Borne AEGKr, Vos JJE, van der Lelie J, Bossers B, van Dalen CM. Clinical significance of positive platelet immunofluorescence test in thrombocytopenia. Br J Haematol 1986;64:767–776.

78. Casonato A, Bertomoro A, Pontara E, Dannhauser D, Lazzaro AR, Girolami A. EDTA dependent pseudothrombocytopenia caused by antibodies against the cytoadhesive receptor of platelet gpIIB-IIIA. J Clin Pathol 1994;47:625–630.

79. Tvedten HW. Artifacts: Case A-4. In: Tvedten HW, ed. Multi-species hematology Atlas Technicon H 1E system. Tarrytown: Miles, 1993:132–133.

80. Boudreaux MK. Platelets and coagulation; an update. Vet Clin North Am Small Anim Pract 1996;26:1065–1087.

81. Ragan HA. Platelet agglutination induced by ethylenediaminetetraacetic acid in blood samples from a miniature pig. Am J Vet Res 1972;33:2601–2603.

82. Reid DM, Jones CE, Vostal JG, Shulman NR. Western blot identification of platelet proteins that bind normal serum immunoglobulins. Characteristics of a 95-Kd reactive protein. Blood 1990;75:2194–2203.

CHAPTER 116

Major Histocompatibility Complex Antigens

• ANNE S. HALE and JOHN A. GERLACH

The major histocompatibility complex (MHC), a large region of associated genes, is the backbone of the mammalian immune system. Genes in this region are responsible for encoding proteins that control all aspects of antigen presentation and processing leading to disease resistance or immune tolerance. This region seems extremely polymorphic and highly conserved as a unit in all mammals, birds, fish, amphibians, and reptiles.[1] MHC is made up of three classes: I, II, and III. Class I MHC genes encode for surface glycoproteins or histocompatibility antigens found on all somatic cell surfaces. Responsible for presentation of endogenously derived peptides to the T-lymphocyte cell receptor (TCR), class I molecules mediate the destruction of virus and tumor through activation of CD8-positive, CD4-negative cytotoxic T cells and natural killer cells. Class II MHC genes encode for surface glycoproteins found on antigen-processing cells (APC) like B lymphocytes, dendritic cells, macrophages and epithelial cells. Class II molecules present exogenously derived peptides and mediate the activation of CD4-positive, CD8-negative T-helper cells, resulting in the secretion of specific cytokines leading cell mediated and humoral immune responses. Within the class II region of most MHC complexes lay genes that encode proteins responsible for endogenous antigen processing. For example, genes encoding subunits for the 20S proteasome (LMP2 and LMP7) are here. Proeasomes are responsible for intracellular peptide degradation.[2] These genes are inducible. Peptide transporter molecules (TAP1 and TAP2) move peptides derived by the 20S proteasome across the membrane of the endoplasmic reticulum for loading into class I molecules for presentation. TAP genes are also within the class II region. It is interesting that genes encoding antigen-processing and genes-presenting antigen to the immune system are linked in most species. The class III region of the MHC encodes for several complement factors (Bf, C2, C4), 21 hydroxylase (CYP21), tumor necrosis factor α and β (TNF α and β), and heat shock protein 70 (HSP70). Nomenclature for the MHC has included different names for different species with the lymphocyte antigen (LA) designation. Recent attempts at standardization have led to the suggestion of a new naming system reliant on the first letters of the genus and species. For example, dog LA (DLA) would be replaced with *MHCCafa*.[3] Several species would retain their old designation: H-2/mouse, HLA/human, RT-1/rat. This new system is frequently seen in the literature but has not been accepted by the entire scientific community; therefore, both nomenclatures are in use.

TYPING PARADIGMS

Typing paradigms to recognize and define the highly polymorphic MHC genes and gene products (antigen expressed on the cell surface) have undergone evolutions. Complement-mediated cell lysis with absorbed complement and sera derived from multiparous or immunized animals or man was one of the early, serologic methods used.[4] This assay is often referred to as the microlymphocytotoxicity assay. It was run in Terasaki microtiter plates and used microliter quantities of reagents. The sera used were often validated through international workshops under the auspices of the International Society of Animal Genetics. Examples of sera validation are cited under species-specific information later in this chapter.[5-9] Serologic typing can be used for both class I and class II antigen characterization.[4,10]

Cellular typing was first used to recognize class II antigen and is still useful for determining functionality for the plethora of class II antigens seen in most species. Cellular assays include the use of the mixed lymphocyte culture or reaction.[11] In brief, lymphocytes of two test subjects are mixed together in culture. The lymphocytes of one subject are treated with either chemicals or radiant energy to render them incapable of response and serve as stimulator for the other population of cells. If stimulated, the untreated cells undergo lymphoblastogenesis. The intensity of the response is proportional to the increase in the number of cells. A second form of cellular typing is termed primed lymphocyte testing.[12] The format of this testing is very similar to a mixed lymphocyte culture, with treated and untreated cells used, except it often employs well-characterized cell lines that are used as a reference base.

Molecular methods now dominate the MHC typing modalities.[13] Initially, these methods offered very crude estimates of the alleles present by the performance of restriction fragment length polymorphism (RFLP) testing, often using xenogeneic probes. For many species this is still the norm. Further refinement has brought forward methods based on amplification of a portion of a MHC gene (usually exon 2 for class II and exon 2 and 3 for class I molecules). The polymerase chain reaction (PCR) is most often used for this amplification.[14] Amplified fragments may be bound to a membrane and probed with sequence specific oligonucleotide probes (SSOP) that recognize the polymorphic position within the gene; this method is termed PCR-SSOP typing.[13,15] Fragments may also be digested with endonuclease and the resulting RFLP patterns used to recognize polymorphic variation within the region tested, this is termed PCR RFLP.[13,16] Secondary structure differences introduced by the sequence variation can be seen when the molecules migrate within a gel. Such structures can be single stranded or double stranded. Amplified fragments can also display secondary structure, and this characteristic is used to recognize variation seen in different MHC alleles. This type of testing, based on secondary structure, is termed single-strand conformation polymorphism (SSCP) typing or double-strand conformation polymorphism (DSCP) typing. When amplified products are used, the terms PCR SSCP or PCR DSCP are used.[13,17]

Specific alleles can also be specifically amplified with PCR in a testing protocol that allows for high-resolution typing.[13,18] Briefly, primer pairs are anchored in the polymorphic regions of specific alleles. This methodology may share one of the primers with other alleles but each allele has a unique set. This type of testing is often referred to as PCR SSP.

The most definitive type of MHC typing is sequenced-based typing.[13] This form of analysis allows for discrete allele assignments even in the presence of heterozygous alleles. One note of caution though, although the detection of alleles can be accomplished at the molecular level, there is no assurance that these molecules may be expressed.[19] This can lead to errors in expected outcomes of research protocols and transplantation results.

As a result of the numerous genomic mapping projects underway in many of the species, the identification of microsatellite markers within the MHC complex provides unique tools for haplotype studies within a family.[20] Microsatellite markers are short tandem repeats present in the genome. Primers flanking the tandem repeat are designed so that, when amplified, the product length variation depends on the number of repeats present. Because of the high degree of linkage disequilibrium or lack of recombination, the haplotype (full complement of MHC of one parental chromosome) can be followed throughout a family for pedigree, transplant, or disease association. Microsatellites may be used to track MHC alleles within a family but not outside the family or species.

Recent advances in molecular typing, described above, have allowed for definition of the MHC in nonhuman species. Knowledge of MHC "type" allows several clinical applications: paternity testing, disease resistance prediction and transplantation pairing. Paternity testing

has been used in man and animals for the purpose of defining shared alleles. Because of the high degree of polymorphism within the MHC, unique inheritance patterns can be used to predict the likelihood of unknown paternity. Study of the MHC in man and mouse have led to the association of MHC type with disease resistance, disease inheritance, and potential autoimmune disease. As a point of example, ankylosing spondylitis occurs in 96% of the Caucasians demonstrating a class I haplotype, HLA-B27. This association of ankylosing spondylitis is also seen in rats, mice, and primates carrying a B27-like haplotype.[21] Frequent association of MHC haplotype and virally mediated leukemia has been made. Species that demonstrate this association include the mouse, bovine, and rat.[1]

Transplantation in the human has relied on MHC typing for selection of donor-recipient pairs for over 25 years. Strong clinical evidence supports the theory that concise allelic matching minimizes the graft versus host disease seen in solid organ and bone marrow transplantation. With the advent of molecular typing techniques, nonhuman species may be evaluated for MHC type before transplantation in an attempt to maximize postgraft survival. The algorithm provided (Figure 116.1) is designed to offer a general means of selecting donor-recipient pairs for transplant in which MHC haplotype is used.[22]

The human MHC, often referred to as the HLA complex, is perhaps one of the most well-defined systems (Table 116.1). This characterization was initially performed by serologic and cellular techniques and over the past 10 years by molecular methods.[13] The need for definitive typing methods has pushed molecular typing to the forefront, employing allele-specific typing paradigms for all three classes of HLA genes. HLA-A, -B, and -C are traditional class I genes, present on most nucleated cells of man; nontraditional genes, HLA-E, -F, -G, -H, -J, and -K, are also present.[1] The class II regions have HLA-DR, -DQ and -DP genes. The numbers of DRβ genes present can vary, depending on which DRB gene is present. Within the class II region are the antigen-processing and transporter molecules, TAP and LMP. The class III region of man has the complement components Bf, C2, and C4. There are also genes in this class III region for HSPs and the 21-hydroxylase (CYP21) gene responsible for steroid metabolism. TNF genes are also present in the HLA class III region. There are numerous microsatellites in the HLA region suitable for haplotype assignment and disease association studies.[20]

The mouse MHC, H-2, has been extensively characterized by serologic, cellular, and molecular techniques.[23] Situated on chromosome 17, the H-2 is organized in a similar fashion to the human MHC. Mouse class I equivalents include H2-K, -D and -L. Class II is made up of H2-A and -E. Class III is found exactly patterning the human.[1] Many microsatellite markers have been characterized within the H-2. Strains of mice have been developed demonstrating H-2 disease associations. Examples of disease associations include leukemia and Gross virus infection.

The canine MHC (DLA) complex was characterized

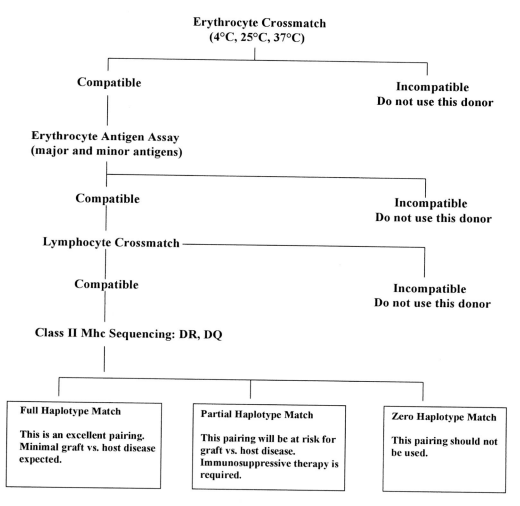

FIGURE 116.1 Donor-recipient pair selection in transplantation.

by both serologic and cellular assays and defined as having both class I and class II antigens present.[5,6] It was initially thought that DLA-A, -B, and -C were class I and that DLA-D was class II. It has been determined that DLA-B was actually a class II antigen. Class II antigens are expressed on nonstimulated canine T cells.[24] The class I and class II regions of DLA have been also characterized by molecular methods.[25,26] The class I genes present in the DLA class I region are DLA-A, -C, and -E. The DLA-D region of the dog has DR, DQ, and DP homologues as seen in man. DO and DN homologues are also seen as well as an LMP-2 gene. The dog also has a representative class III region associated with classes I and II. The class III region has C2, C4, CYP21, and TNF genes present.[27] There are numerous microsatellite markers associated with DLA class I and class II genes.[28,29]

The feline MHC, feline LA (FLA) complex could not be characterized until the advent of molecular typing. Cats do not readily form the postpartum antibody necessary for routine serologic identification. Until molecular characterizations were performed, the cat was considered uniquely monomorphic.[30] Class I, class II, and class III equivalents have been found and are polymorphic.

Cats have FLA-B, a class I homologue, and have FLA-DR, a class II molecule. Other class II equivalents, but as yet unconfirmed, are similar to HLA-DQ, H2-A, and H2-E.

The cattle MHC, bovine LA (BoLA), complex has been well characterized by both serologic and molecular methods.[8,9] Cattle have a BoLA-A and -B class I homologue and have BoLA-DR and -DQ class II equivalents. Cattle do not have a DP homologue but do have a third class II gene expressed, BoLA-DY. Cattle have the following class III genes linked to the complex, Bf, C4, CYP21, HSP70 and the blood group M. The BoLA system is well characterized by molecular typing methods and has been associated with the susceptibility and resistance to several pathogens.[1,31]

The ovine MHC, ovine LA (OLA) complex, has been primarily defined with molecular methods.[32] There are OLA-A and -B class I genes and OLA-DR and -DQ class II products. There is a DN homologue in sheep as well as a DM. Whether sheep have a third class II allele (-DP or -DY) is not yet determined. Class III gene products C4, CYP21, and TNF have also been defined. Sheep also have microsatellite markers associated with the OLA complex.[1,33]

TABLE 116.1   Characteristics of Animal MHC Systems

Species	Nomenclature	Class I	Class II	Class III	Unique Feature	Preferred Testing Modality
Human	HLA	A, B, C	DR, DQ, DP	C2, C4, TNF, HSP, CYP21		Molecular
Mice	H-2	K, D, L	A, E	Bf, C2, C4, M, TNF, HSP70		Molecular
Canine	DLA (Cafa)	A, C	DR, DQ, DP	C2, C4, CYP21, TNF		
Feline	FLA (Feca)	B	DR	C2, C4, HSP70, TNF	No DP	Molecular
Bovine	BoLA (Bota)	A, B	DR, DQ, DY	Bf, CR, CYP21, HSP70, M	No DP (DY)	Serologic or molecular
Ovine	OLA (Ovar)	A, B	DR, DQ	C4, CYP21, TNF		Molecular
Caprine	CLA (Cahi)	Unnamed	DR, DY	CYP21, C4, C2	Class I unnamed	Serologic or molecular
Equine	ELA (Eqca)	A	DR, DQ	C4		Molecular
Swine	SLA (Sudo)	A, B, C	DR, DQ	CYP21, Bf, TNF, C2, C4, HSP70	Class II on resting T cells	Molecular
Rhesus	RhLA (Mamu)	A, B				Molecular
Chimpanzee	ChLA (Patr)	A, B, C	DR, DQ, DP	C2, C4, TNF, HSP70, CYP21		Molecular
Rats	RT1	A	DR, DP	Bf, C2, C4, TNF, HSP70		Molecular
Rabbits	RLA (Orcu)	A	DR, DQ, DP	Not Linked		Molecular
Guinea Pig	GPLA (Capo)	A	DR	Bf, C2, C4, TNF, HSP70	No DP	Molecular
Chickens	B complex	F	L	Not Linked	Expression on RBC	Molecular
Reptilian	Species specific	Unnamed	Unnamed		Expression on RBC	Serologic or molecular
Amphibian	Species specific	A	DR			Molecular
Fish	Species specific	Present	Present			Molecular

The MHC complex of goats, caprine LA (CLA), is less well defined than other ruminants and food animals. There are class I genes present, but as yet it is not clear how many are present nor is clear nomenclature assigned. The class II region of the goat has DR and DY homologues present. The class III region contains CYP21, C2, C4, HSP, and TNF genes. To date, serologic, biochemical, and molecular methods are in use for typing and characterizing the goat MHC. Informative microsatellites are also present in the goat LA (GLA) complex.[1,34]

The horse MHC, equine LA (ELA) complex has been characterized by both serologic, cellular and, most recently, molecular methods.[7,35] The loci defined are ELA-A for class I and ELA-DR and -DQ for class II. There has not been a second class I loci defined, although it is suspected to be present. The C4 gene has been mapped to the ELA complex.[36]

The swine MHC, swine LA (SLA), complex is well characterized and very similar to that of man. There are three class I loci present, SLA-A, -B, and -C. SLA-DR and -DQ have also been documented. The class three region of the pig has homologues for CYP21, TNF, Bf, C2, C4, HSP70, and TNF. As with several other species, class II gene products are present on resting pig T lym-

phocytes.[37] Several microsatellites are present on swine chromosome 7, within SLA.[38]

Primate MHC is very similar to man.[21] Class I products are defined as A and B. Higher monkeys such as the chimpanzee also have a C loci. The class II products vary by Old World or New World variation with Old World monkeys demonstrating DR, DQ, and DP. New World monkeys have dropped some of these class II alleles.[39] Both serologic and molecular typing systems exist for class I and class II. Class III region in the primate has homologues for Bf, C2, C4, CYP21, and HSP70.[1]

The rat MHC, R-1, is most like the human. Homologues for class I loci A, class II loci DR, and DP have been identified. Class III molecules include Bf, C2, C4, CYP21, and HSP 70.[1]

The rabbit MHC, or rabbit LA (RLA), has been largely characterized by molecular means. RLA-A is a class I gene product. RLA-DR, RLA-DQ, and RLA-DP are class II gene products. Class III is not linked physically to the class I and II genes as in many other species.[1]

The guinea pig MHC, or guinea pig LA (GPLA), has class I, II, and III gene products. Class I products have been identified by serology, GPLA-A. A class II DR homologue has been defined by serology as well.[40,41] Class III molecules include Bf, C2, C4, TNF, and HSP70.

The chicken MHC, B complex, is unique in that it has Class I, II, III, and IV products present. Class I products are defined as F, whereas class II products are L. Unlike other MHC complexes reviewed, chicken class III products are not physically linked to the class I or the class II genetic region. Also unlike other species discussed, chicken class IV (B-G) products are expressed on erythrocytes.[1,42]

Reptilian MHC has been largely defined by serologic means. Evidence exists for both class I and class II homologues, but to date, these remain undefined and unnamed.[43]

Great interest has been shown in the amphibian MHC in an attempt to explain the great decline in world population over the past 10 years. Molecular methods have been established for evaluation of class I and class II genes. Class I in *Xenopus laevis* demonstrates *Xela A*.[44] Class II contains DR homologues.[1] Adults demonstrate class III homologues as well. Class I molecules are found on the red blood cell of the adult.[45] Interestingly, the immature phase of the amphibian does not demonstrate MHC molecules at all.

The MHC of fish has been studied for various reasons.[1,46] Driving forces are aimed at basic immunology, evolutionary biology, and improved commercial production. Fish have genes analogous to the class I and class II of other species. It is yet unclear exactly how many class I or class II genes are produced and which homologues are present.

Major histocompatibility genes defined through serologic and molecular means are the basis for antigen presentation and processing for the immune system. Polymorphism within this gene complex allows for species preservation through disease resistance and immune surveillance. The MHC is also responsible, in part, for disease association and autoimmune conditions. Through evaluation of this gene complex, clues to the evolutionary history of all species can be found.

REFERENCES

1. **Trowsdale J.** "Both man & bird & beast": comparative organization of Mhc genes. Immunogenetics 1995;41:1–17.
2. **Nonaka M, Namikawa-Yamada C, Sasaki M,** et al. Evolution of proteasome subunits Y and LMP2. J Immunol 1997;159(2):734–740.
3. **Klein J, Bontrop RE,** Dawkins RL, et al. Nomenclature for the major histocompatibility complexes of different species: a proposal. Immunogenetics 1990;31:217–219.
4. **McCloskey DJ, Brown J, Navarrete C.** Serological typing of HLA-A, -B and -C antigens. In: Hui KM, Bidwell JL, eds. Handbook of HLA typing techniques. Boca Raton: CRC Press, 1993;175–248.
5. **Deeg HJ, Raff RF, Grosse-Wilde H,** et al. Joint report of the third international workshop on canine immunogenetics I. Analysis of homozygous typing cells. Transplantation 1986;41:111–117.
6. **Bull RW, Vriesendorp HM, Cech R,** et al. Joint report of the third international workshop on canine immunogenetics. II. Analysis of the serological typing of cells. Transplantation 1987;43:154–161.
7. **Lazary S, Antczak DF, Bailey E,** et al. Joint report of the fifth international workshop in lymphocyte alloantigens of the horse, Baton Rouge, Louisiana, October 31–November 1, 1987. Anim Genet, 1987;19:447–456.
8. **Davies CJ, Joosten I, Bernoco D,** et al. Polymorphism of bovine MHC class I genes. Joint report of the fifth international bovine lymphocyte antigen (BoLA) workshop, Interlaken, Switzerland, August 1992. Eur J Immunogenet 1994;21:239A–258A.
9. **Davies CJ, Joosten I, Andersson L,** et al. Polymorphism of bovine MHC class II genes. Joint report of the fifth international bovine lymphocyte antigen (BoLA) workshop, Interlaken, Switzerland, August 1992. Eur J Immunogenet 1994;21:259B–289B.
10. **Brown J, McCloskey DJ, Navarrete C.** HLA-DR and -DQ serotyping. In:
11. Hui KM, Bidwell JL, eds. Handbook of HLA typing techniques. Boca Raton: CRC Press, 1993;249–308.
12. **Navarrete C, Brown J, McCloskey DJ,** et al. Definition of HLA-Dw determinants using homozygous typing cells and the mixed lymphocyte culture. In: Hui KM, Bidwell JL, eds. Handbook of HLA typing techniques. Boca Raton: CRC Press, 1993;309A–350A.
13. **Navarrete C, McCloskey DJ, Brown J.** Definition of HLA-Dw and HLA-DPw determinants by the primed lymphocyte test. In: Hui KM, Bidwell JL, eds. Handbook of HLA typing techniques. Boca Raton: CRC Press, 1993;351B–372B.
14. **Bunce M, Young NT, Welsh K.** Molecular HLA typing-the brave new world. Transplantation 1997;64:1505–1513.
15. **Saidi RK, Scharf S, Fallon F,** et al. Enzymatic amplification of beta-globin genomic sequences and restriction site analysis for diagnosis of sickle cell anemia. Science 1985;230:1350–1354.
16. **Tiercy JM, Grundschober C, Jeannet M,** et al. A comprehensive HL-DRB, -DQB and -DPB oligotyping procedure by hybridization with sequence specific oligonucleotide probes. In: Hui KM, Bidwell JL, eds. Handbook of HLA typing techniques. Boca Raton: CRC Press, 1993;117–148.
17. **Inoko H, Ota M.** PCR-RFLP. In: Hui KM, Ota M, eds. Handbook of HLA typing techniques. Boca Raton: CRC Press, 1993;9B–71B.
18. **Bidwell JL, Clay TM, Wood NAP,** et al. Rapid HLA-DR-Dw and DP matching by PCR fingerprinting and related DNA heteroduplex technologies. In: Hui KM, Bidwell JL, eds. Handbook of HLA typing techniques. Boca Raton: CRC Press, 1993;99B–116B.
19. **Olerup O, Zetterquist H.** HLA-DR typing by polymerase chain reaction amplification with sequence specific primers. In: Hui KM, Bidwell JL, eds. Handbook of HLA typing techniques. Boca Raton: CRC Press, 1993;149–174.
20. **Parham R.** Filling in the blanks. Tissue Antigens 1997;50:318–321.
21. **Foissac A, Crouau-Roy FA, Faure B,** et al. Microsatellites in the HLA region: on overview. Tissue Antigens 1997;49:197–214.
22. **Watkins DI.** The evolution of major histocompatibility class I genes in primates. Crit Rev Immunol 1995;15(1):1–29.
23. **Hale AS, Bull RW** "Compatibility Testing For Transplantation" in Proceedings of the 15th ACVIM Forum, 1997; 82–83.
24. **Klein J.** Biology of the mouse histocompatibility-2 complex. 1975; 8–15.
25. **Doxiadis IS, Krumbash K, Neffjes JJ,** et al. Biochemical evidence that the DLA-B locus codes for a class II determinant expressed on canine peripheral blood lymphocytes. Exp Clin Immunogenet 1989;6:642–651.
26. **Sarmiento UM, Storb R.** Characterization of class II alpha genes and DLA-D region allelic associations in the dog. Tissue Antigens 1988;32:224–234.
27. **Sarmiento UM, Storb R.** RFLP analysis of DLA class I genes in the dog. Tissue Antigens 1989;34:1548–63.
28. **Sarmiento UM.** The canine major histocompatibility complex: genetic structure and function of the Mhc of dogs. In: Shook LB, Lamont SJ, eds. The Mhc of domestic animal species. Boca Raton: CRC Press, 1996;177–186.
29. **Burnett RC, Francisco LV, DeRose SA,** et al. Identification and characterization of a highly polymorphic microsatellite marker within the canine Mhc class I region. Mamm Genome 1995;6:684–685.
30. **Wagner JL, Burnett RC, DeRose SA,** et al. Histocompatibility testing of dog families with highly polymorphic microsatellite markers. Transplantation 1996;62:876–877.
31. **Yuhki N, Winkler C, O'Brien SJ.** Mhc genes of the domestic cat. In: Srivastava, Ram, Tyle, eds. Immunogenetics of the major histocompatibility complex 1991;348–365.
32. **Lewin HA.** Genetic organization, polymorphism, and function of the bovine major histocompatibility complex. In: Shook LB, Lamont SJ, eds. The Mhc of domestic animal species. Boca Raton: CRC Press, 1996;65–98.
33. **Millot P.** The major histocompatibility complex of sheep (OLA) and two minor loci. Anim Genet 1978;9:115–121.
34. **Schweiger FW, Makkox J, Ballingall K,** et al. The ovine major histocompatibility complex. In: Shook LB, Lamont SJ, eds. The Mhc of domestic animal species. Boca Raton: CRC Press, 1996;121–176.
35. **Obexer-Ruff G, Joosten I, Schwaiger FW.** The caprine major histocompatibility complex. In: Shook LB, Lamont SJ, eds. The Mhc of domestic animal species. Boca Raton: CRC Press, 1996;99–119.
36. **Marti E, Szalai G, Antczak DF,** et al. The equine major histocompatibility complex. In: Shook LB, Lamont SJ, eds. The Mhc of domestic animal species. Boca Raton: CRC Press, 1996;245–267.
37. **Guerin G, Bertaud M, Chardon P,** et al. Molecular Genetic analysis of the major histocompatibility complex in an ELA type horse family. Anim Genet 1987;18:323–336.
38. **Schook LB, Rutherford MS, Lee JK,** et al. The swine major histocompatibility complex. In: Shook LB, Lamont SJ eds. The Mhc of domestic animal species. Boca Raton: CRC Press, 1996;213–244.
39. **Smith TP, Rohrer GA, Alexander LJ,** et al. Directed integration of the physical and genetic linkage maps of swine chromosome 7 reveals that the SLA spans the centromere. Genome Res 1995;5:259–271.
40. **Slierendregt BL, Otting N, Kenter M, Bontrop RE.** Allelic diversity at the Mhc-DP locus in rhesus macaques (Macaca mulatta). Immunogenetics 1995;41(1):29–37.

40. **Wilcox CE, Baker D, Butter C,** et al. Differential expression of guinea pig class II MHC antigens on vascular endothelial cells. Cell Immunol 1989;120:82–91.

41. **Steernberg PA, Jong WH, Geerse E,** et al. Major-histocompatibility-complex-class-II-positive cells and interleukin-2-dependent proliferation of immune T cells are required to reject carcinoma cells in the guinea pig. Cancer Immunol Immunother 1990;31:297–304.

42. **Kaufman JF, Lamont SJ.** The chicken major histocompatibility complex. In: Shook LB, Lamont SJ, eds. The Mhc of domestic animal species. Boca Raton: CRC Press, 1996;35–64.

43. **Farag MA, el Ridi R.** Functional markers of the major histocompatibility gene complex of snakes. Eur J Immunol 1990;20(9):2029–2033.

44. **Shum BP, Avila D, Pasquier LD,** et al. Isolation of a Classical MHC Class I cDNA from an Amphibian. J Immunol 1993;151(10):5376–5386.

45. **Kaufman JF, Skjoedt K, Salomonsen J.** The MHC molecules of nonmammalian vertebrates. Immunol Rev 1990;113:83–117.

46. **Oystein L, Grimholt U.** The major histocompatibility complex of fish: genetic structure and function of the Mhc of teleost species In: Shook LB, Lamont SJ, eds. The Mhc of domestic animal species. Boca Raton: CRC Press, 1996;17–29.

CHAPTER 117

Clinical Blood Typing and Crossmatching

• K. JANE WARDROP

Blood typing and crossmatching are techniques used in the selection of blood components before transfusion. When blood typing is performed, antisera or other reagents are used to identify selected red blood cell (RBC) antigens. In crossmatching, antibodies are detected by reacting donor sera and donor RBC with recipient sera and recipient RBC. The primary purpose of this pretransfusion testing is to ensure that the transfused RBC has optimal survival when transfused and does not cause harm to the recipient.

Pretransfusion testing in humans generally involves a type and screen procedure. This consists of an initial typing for ABO and Rh antigens and detection of patient antibody by use of commercially available reagent RBC-containing defined antigens. An indirect antiglobulin test (IAT) is used during this antibody screen. When no clinically significant antibodies are detected, an immediate spin crossmatch, in which serum is mixed with saline-suspended RBC and centrifuged immediately, can be performed to ensure ABO compatibility. If clinically significant antibodies are found, RBCs that lack the corresponding antigens are used, and an IAT crossmatchis performed. The IAT is best for detecting IgG antibodies. Use of a low-ionic-strength saline solution in the IAT further enhances its sensitivity. Recently, techniques with microplates, solid-phase systems, and microtubes, where antiglobulin reagent is contained within a matrix of sephadex or glass microbeads, have been developed.[1]

Blood typing and crossmatching can also be used before transfusion in most domestic animals. The development of veterinary blood banks for animals and an increased awareness of the benefits of transfusion have resulted in increased availability and use of blood products, especially whole blood, packed RBC, and plasma. Transfusions performed with untyped or uncrossmatched blood can sensitize recipients to future transfusions or can result in reactions that range from enhanced removal of the transfused RBC to death of the patient. Pretransfusion testing in veterinary clinical practice is often less complex than that performed in the human field, largely because of a lack of appropriate reagents.

BLOOD TYPING

Blood typing of most animal species is typically performed in commercial veterinary laboratories. A partial listing of these laboratories (regional veterinary diagnostic or clinical pathology laboratories may also offer these services and can be contacted) is provided:

1. Midwest Animal Blood Services, Inc. (dogs and cats)
   P.O. Box 626
   120 E. Main Street
   Stockbridge, Michigan 49285
   517-851-8244
2. Stormont Laboratories (dogs, cats, horses, and cattle)
   1237 East Beamer Street, Suite D
   Woodland, California 95695
   530-661-3078
3. Veterinary Genetics Laboratory (horses and cattle)
   University of California, Davis
   Davis, California 95616
   530-752-2211
4. Equine Blood Typing Research Laboratory (horses)
   University of Kentucky
   Department of Veterinary Science
   Lexington, Kentucky 40546
   606-257-3022

To perform blood typing, laboratories usually require the submission of either ethylenediamine tetra-acetic acid (EDTA) or acid citrate dextrose (ACD) whole blood. Serum may also be required for antibody testing. It is beyond the scope of this chapter to list in detail the RBC antigens found in the common domestic animal species, and the reader is referred to other chapters within this section. Canine RBC antigens are primarily identified by use of polyclonal antibodies generated through canine alloimmunization. DEA 1.1, an antigen capable of producing acute hemolytic reactions in the sensitized animal, can be identified with a monoclonal antibody.[2] This antibody is commonly used in canine blood-typing cards. Other RBC antigens may be present, however, lack of appropriate antisera prohibits or prevents their identification. For example, DEA 1.3 has recently been identified as an antigen capable of eliciting a hemolytic antibody response.[3] Typing sera is presently unavailable. Also DEA 6 and 8 are common antigens (DEA 6 is present in 99% of dogs; DEA 8 may be present in 40% of dogs) previously identified in dogs. Lack of available antisera prevents their identification by most typing laboratories. DEA typing for the dog varies, depending on the laboratory used, with some laboratories only typing for DEA 1.1, and others typing for DEA 1.1, 1.2, 3, 4, 5, and 7.

The one recognized blood-group system in the cat is the AB system. This system consists of three blood types, A, B, and AB. Type A is the most common blood type, occurring in >95% of domestic short-hair and long-hair cats in the United States. Type-B blood occurs in <5% of domestic short-hair and long-hair cats; however, the frequency of type A and B in cats varies with the breed of cat and the geographic location.[4,5] As an example, as much as 45% of Exotic and British short-hair cats and Cornish and Devon rex cats can have the B blood type. Type-AB cats are rare. Most laboratories type for both the A and B antigen in cats.

All type-B cats older than 3 months of age have high titers of anti-A antibodies. These antibodies act as strong hemolysins and hemagglutinins.[6] Type-B cats transfused with type-A RBC have a significant hemolytic transfusion reaction, and type-A or -AB kittens born to type-B queens are at risk of developing neonatal isoerythrolysis. Cats that have type-A blood have weak anti-B alloantibodies that produce a delayed transfusion reaction characterized by premature removal of transfused cells. Type-AB cats have no alloantibodies in their plasma.

Recently, typing of the dog and cat has been simplified by use of typing cards (DMS Laboratories, Inc., Farmington, NJ). These cards contain antisera or reagent that has been lyophilized onto the cards. The antisera is reconstituted with a diluent, and a drop of EDTA whole blood from the patient is added; the card is rocked for approximately 2 minutes. Agglutination indicates a positive response (Fig. 117.1). Controls are included to aid in reading the reactions. For the dog, cards are available that type for DEA 1.1. Cats that have type A, B, or AB can be identified with the feline blood-typing cards. The advantage of these cards lies in their speed and simplicity. False-positive DEA 1.1 reactions on the card assay have been noted.[7]

Blood typing in large animals is best performed by commercial veterinary laboratories, and blood typing cards are not available. Blood typing in large animals can be complex. For example, 34 different erythrocyte antigens from 7 blood groups have been identified in horses.[8] Cattle have at least 11 blood-group systems; sheep have 7.[8] This means that identification of a blood donor with identical alloantigen and antibody profiles is difficult, if not impossible. Compatibility testing in these species, however, can be used to help avoid severe transfusion reactions by identification of existing antibodies. Alloantigens Aa and Qa are the most immunogenic of the equine RBC antigens and are responsible for the majority of equine neonatal isoerythrolysis (NI)

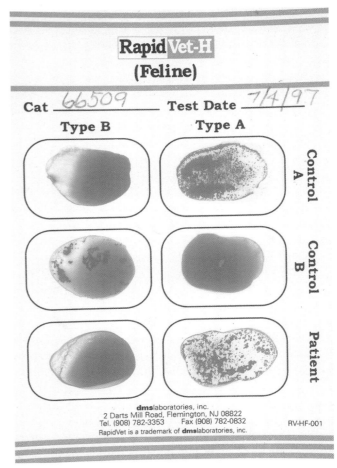

FIGURE 117.1 Example of a feline blood-typing card. The feline patient in this case is reacting with the anti-A reagent, indicating that the cat has type-A blood. Controls are included to aid in reading the reactions.

cases.[9,10] Mares that lack Aa and Qa are at risk of producing antibody to them on exposure. Mares known to be at risk, either because of blood type or because of previous foaling of an affected foal, can have sera tested for antibody before foaling.

CROSSMATCHING

Blood typing permits the identification of RBC antigens in a patient. It does not allow the detection of antibodies between a patient and a potential blood donor. In a clinical situation this is generally determined by crossmatching. Even in animals that have been blood typed, crossmatching should be considered to detect antibodies against RBC.

Crossmatching does have its limitations. A compatible crossmatch does not necessarily indicate that the donor and recipient have the same blood type, merely that antibodies against RBC cannot be detected. Also, the crossmatch technique may lack the appropriate sensitivity to detect some antibodies, thus it is possible to have a compatible crossmatch and still have increased removal of the transfused cells. A standard crossmatch does not detect platelet or granulocyte antibodies. It cannot predict some types of transfusion reactions, such as urticarial reactions. Nevertheless, crossmatching can be a useful technique and should be performed before transfusion. Ideally, crossmatching should be performed before all transfusions, however, where this is not possible, it should certainly be performed before those transfusions in which the recipient has a history of previous blood exposure. Crossmatching should always be performed before feline transfusions, regardless of the previous transfusion history, because of the presence of naturally occurring antibody in the cat and the serious consequences of transfusing type-A blood into a blood-type-B cat.

Crossmatching in large animals generally requires both a saline-agglutinating technique and a technique that can detect hemolysis. Agglutination tests can be performed by most veterinary practices; however, the hemolytic tests require the addition of exogenous complement, usually provided by rabbit or guinea pig serum.[11] This serum is diluted or absorbed first with RBCs of the species to be tested, to remove the natural heterolysins and heteroagglutinins present in the rabbit serum. Consequently, detection of hemolytic antibodies is often confined to the veterinary laboratory.

One crossmatching technique used in the identification of mare antibody in cases of suspected NI is the jaundiced foal agglutination test.[9,12] In this test, colostrum from the mare is reacted with RBCs from the foal. The colostrum can also be tested with potential donor blood. Serial dilutions (1:2 to 1:128) with saline of colostrum are made, and one drop of EDTA foal blood is added to 1 mL of the dilution. Blood is also added to a saline control tube that lacks colostrum. The tubes are centrifuged and judged for agglutination. Positive reactions at dilutions of 1:16 or greater are considered significant in horses.

The crossmatching procedure described in Table 117.1 is a saline-agglutination crossmatch commonly performed by many veterinary laboratories. Some laboratories also use an IAT in this procedure, adding species-specific Coombs' reagent after the initial RBC or sera reactions have been interpreted. Antisera-treated cells are washed in saline, the Coombs' reagent is added in an amount and dilution determined by the manufacturer, and the mixture is incubated. The mixture is then centrifuged, and the sample is checked for agglutination. A saline replacement technique is useful to detect rouleaux in species such as the horse and cat, in which rouleaux is common and can be erroneously identified as agglutination in the cross-match procedure. Steps in the saline replacement technique[13] are as follows:

1. Recentrifuge the serum or the RBC mixture when rouleaux formation is suspected.
2. Remove the serum.
3. Replace the serum with an equal volume of saline (two drops) and gently mix.
4. Centrifuge the saline or the RBC mixture at 1000 × g for 15 seconds.

TABLE 117.1 Crossmatching Procedure

1. Obtain an anticoagulated (EDTA) and/or non-anticoagulated specimen of blood from both patient and donor. The EDTA tube will serve as the source of RBC (antigen), and the non-anticoagulated tube will serve as the source of serum (antibody).
2. Centrifuge and separate plasma or serum from RBC.
3. Wash RBC by adding saline or phosphate buffered saline (PBS) to a small amount of packed RBC, mixing, and centrifuging. Decant the saline and repeat 3 times, filling the tubes with saline, mixing, centrifuging, and decanting.
4. After last wash, decant supernatant and resuspend cells with saline to give a 2–4% ("weak" tomato juice) suspension of RBC. The suspension may also be calculated; for example, 0.1 mL blood in 2.4 mL saline gives a 4% suspension.
5. Make the following mixtures by adding the indicated amount of the well-mixed RBC suspension and serum to 12 × 75 mm tubes:

Major crossmatch: 2 drops patient sera, 1 drop donor 2–4% RBC

Minor crossmatch: 2 drops donor sera, 1 drop patient 2–4% RBC

Include controls: 2 drops patient sera, 1 drop patient 2–4% RBC
2 drops donor sera, 1 drop donor 2–4% RBC

6. Incubate tubes 15–30 minutes at 37°C.
7. Centrifuge for 15 seconds (3400 rpm/1000 × g).
8. Read tubes:

Macroscopic—Examine tubes first for hemolysis. Then rotate tubes gently and observe cells coming off the red cell "button" in the bottom of the tube. In a compatible reaction, i.e., where there is no antigen–antibody reaction, the cells should float off freely, with no clumping/hemagglutination (compare to the control tubes). Rouleaux formation can be falsely interpreted as a reaction. If rouleaux is suspected, a saline replacement technique can be used. Proceed to the microscopic examination in those tubes with weak or no obvious reactions.

Microscopic—After tubes have been viewed macroscopically, place a drop of the cells/sera mixture on a slide, coverslip, and examine microscopically. The RBC should normally appear as individual cells, with no clumping or rouleaux formation.

---

5. Resuspend the saline or the RBC mixture and observe for agglutination. Rouleaux disperse when suspended in saline, whereas true agglutination remains.

Grading of reactions or antibody titration can also be performed.[14]

Blood typing and crossmatching are valuable techniques that must be considered before transfusion in all species. Although some testing should be performed in specialized veterinary laboratories, other tests, such as card blood typing and some crossmatching, can be performed in most clinical veterinary practices and provide information that aids in the safe selection of blood components.

REFERENCES

1. **Knight RC, de Silva M.** New technologies for red cell serology. Blood Rev 1996;10:101–110.
2. **Andrews GA, Chavey PS, Smith JE.** Production, characterization, and application of a murine monoclonal antibody to dog erythrocyte antigen 1.1. J Am Vet Med Assoc 1992;201:1549–1552.
3. **Symons M, Bell K.** Expansion of the canine A blood group system. Anim Genet 1991;22:227–235.
4. **Giger U, Kilrain CG, Filippich LJ, et al.** Frequencies of feline blood groups in the United Statesd. J Am Vet Med Assoc 1989;195:1230–1232.
5. **Giger U, Griot-Wenk M, Bucheler J, et al.** Geographical variation of the feline blood type frequencies in the United States. Feline Pract 1991;19:21–27.
6. **Bucheler J, Giger U.** Alloantibodies against A and B blood types in cats. Vet Immunol Immunopathol 1993;38:283–295.
7. **Moritz A, Widmann T, Hale AS.** Comparison of current typing techniques for evaluation of dog erythrocyte antigen 1.1. Proc 16th ACVIM Forum 1998;716.
8. **McClure JJ, Parish SM.** Diseases caused by allogeneic incompatibilities. In: Smith BP, ed. Large animal internal medicine. 2nd ed. St. Louis: Mosby Year Book, 1996;1862–1873.
9. **Stormont C.** Neonatal isoerythrolysis in domestic animals: a comparative review. Adv Vet Sci Comp Med 1975;19:23–45.
10. **Witham CL, Carlson GP, Bowling AT.** Neonatal isoerythrolysis in foals: management and prevention. Calif Vet 1984;11:21–23.
11. **Stormont C, Suzuki Y, Rhode EA.** Serology of horse blood groups. Cornell Vet 1964;54:439–452.
12. **McClure JJ, Parish SM.** Diseases caused by allogeneic incompatibilities. In: Smith BP, ed. Large animal internal medicine. St. Louis: Mosby-Year Book, 1996;1862–1873.
13. **Vengelen-Tyler V, ed.** Antibody detection and compatibility testing: saline replacement to demonstrate alloantibody in the presence of rouleaux. In: Technical manual, 12th edition. Bethesda, MD, American Association of Blood Banks, 1996, 636.
14. **Marsh WL.** Scoring of hemagglutination reactions. Transfusion 1972;12:352–353.

CHAPTER 118

Immune-Mediated Hemolytic Anemia

• MICHAEL J. DAY

DEFINITION

An immune-mediated hemolytic anemia (IMHA) arises when erythrocytes (or rarely bone marrow erythroid precursors) are destroyed by means of the mechanism of type II hypersensitivity, after the attachment of immunoglobulin to the cell membrane (Fig. 118.1). Antibody binding may activate the classical pathway of the complement system and result in deposition of complement components on the erythrocyte surface. If complement activation proceeds through the terminal pathway to the formation of transmembrane channels (membrane attack complexes), the red cell may be destroyed by osmotic lysis within the circulation (intravascular hemolysis). Alternatively, the surface immunoglobulin and complement may interact with immunoglobulin heavy chain (Fc) and complement receptors expressed by phagocytic cells (chiefly macrophages), resulting in damage to, or removal of, coated erythrocytes in extravascular sites such as the spleen or liver (extravascular hemolysis).

The terminology used to describe these effects must be used with care. An IMHA may be primary or secondary in nature. Secondary IMHA occurs when there is an underlying reason for the attachment of immunoglobulin to erythrocytes. For example, IMHA may occur as a secondary phenomenon in neoplastic disease (e.g., lymphoma, hemangiosarcoma) or when antibody has specificity for an infectious agent (e.g., *Haemobartonella felis*) or drug (e.g., penicillin) that is associated with the red blood cell (RBC) surface. In these latter cases, the erythrocyte destruction is due to bystander hemolysis as the causative antibody is not specific for the RBC itself.

By contrast, in primary idiopathic IMHA there is no underlying disease or evidence of recent drug administration, and the antibody is a true autoantibody with specificity for a self-antigen of the erythrocyte membrane. Only this form of disease is true autoimmune hemolytic anemia (AIHA), and the terms IMHA and AIHA should not be used interchangeably. AIHA may occur as a single clinical entity, may be recognized concurrently with autoimmune thrombocytopenia (AITP; the combined disease is Evans' syndrome), or may be part of the multisystemic autoimmune disease systemic lupus erythematosus (SLE). Rarely, the autoimmune response is directed against the bone marrow erythroid precursors, resulting in acquired pure red cell aplasia (PRCA).[1] In this disease, there may be autoantibodies that react with circulating erythrocytes in addition to the precursor population. In AIHA or acquired PRCA, erythrocyte-specific autoantibody is rarely found free in the circulation, as most is bound to RBC or precursors. The reactions to blood-group antigens (blood transfusion reactions, neonatal isoerythrolysis) and the uncommon cold agglutinin disease may be considered as forms of IMHA, but these disorders are not considered in this chapter.

IMHA is not an uncommon condition in veterinary species. In the dog, the majority of cases are primary AIHA, whereas in other species (particularly the cat and horse) secondary IMHA is the predominant form of immune-mediated hemolytic reaction. In this chapter, primary idiopathic AIHA of the dog, for which most information is available, is the predominant focus.

IMMUNOPATHOGENESIS OF AUTOIMMUNE HEMOLYTIC ANEMIA

The factors underlying the development of autoimmunity are discussed in detail in Chapter 121, Systemic Lupus Erythematosus. Briefly, the expression of any autoimmune disease requires that a combination of predisposing factors permits the development of an immunologic alteration that results in the observed autoimmune pathology. Such immunologic alterations have been experimentally investigated with murine models of AIHA. For example, AIHA may be induced in particular inbred strains of mice that are immunized with rat erythrocytes[2] or that are transgenic for high expression of interleukin (IL)-4,[3] or expression of an erythrocyte autoantibody.[4] IL-2 deficient mice, created by targeted disruption of the IL-2 gene, develop a lymphoproliferative syndrome with multisystemic autoimmunity, including Coombs' positive hemolytic anemia.[5] Mice of the New Zealand black (NZB) strain, spontaneously develop autoimmunity, including AIHA or an SLE-like disease characterized by immune complex glomerulonephritis and serum antinuclear antibody (ANA). The AIHA is mediated by CD4+ Th1 lymphocytes that are first activated in young

FIGURE 118.1 Pathogenesis of IMHA. IMHA may be primary AIHA, or secondary to a defined underlying cause. In AIHA, a series of predisposing factors interact to allow activation of self-reactive T and B lymphocytes and production of autoantibody specific for an antigen of the erythrocyte membrane. In secondary IMHA, the erythrocyte becomes an innocent bystander in an immune response that is directed toward the infectious agent or drug associated with the red cell membrane or that generates immune complexes that nonspecifically adsorb to the erythrocyte surface. In either case, the erythrocyte may be destroyed after complement fixation and formation of the membrane attack complex (intravascular hemolysis), or it may interact with phagocytic cells that express surface Fc and complement receptors. In this case the RBC may be entirely removed by erythrophagocytosis, or suffer partial loss of its cell membrane to form a spherocyte. These processes occur in the spleen or liver (extravascular hemolysis).

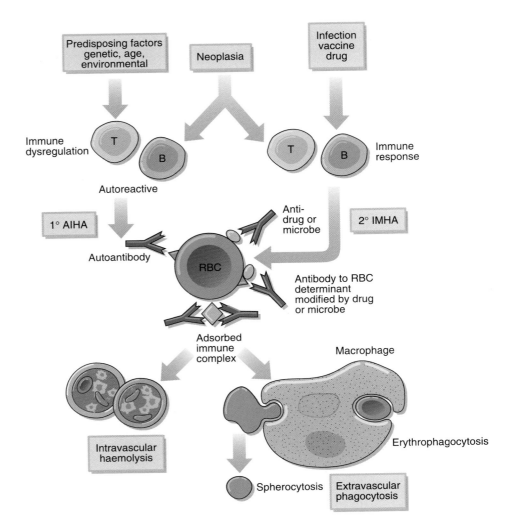

mice before the appearance of autoantibodies and anemia.[6] Nonobese diabetic (NOD) mice that fail to develop autoimmune diabetes, may develop Coombs' positive hemolytic anemia late in life.[7]

It is now believed that microbial infection is of particular importance in the induction of autoimmune diseases. Clinically normal individuals have circulating lymphocytes that are programmed to recognize self-antigens, but these cells are normally incapable of responding to autoantigens (self-tolerance). The altered immunoregulation that follows infection may permit loss of self-tolerance and the subsequent expression of autoimmune disease. For example, mice infected with a particular substrain of the lymphocytic choriomeningitis virus develop a transient AIHA. In this instance the anemia is not caused by antibodies that react with a shared epitope on the virus and RBC, but by true erythrocyte-specific autoantibodies.[8] The induction of this autoimmune response is thought to be caused by inappropriate activation of autoreactive T lymphocytes by virally derived peptides that are molecular mimics of erythrocyte-derived peptides. Such self-peptides would normally not be presented by the antigen-presenting

cells (APCs) of the immune system, to maintain the autoreactive T cells in a state of immunologic ignorance.

FACTORS PREDISPOSING TO AUTOIMMUNE HEMOLYTIC ANEMIA IN ANIMALS

Numerous factors predisposing to the development of AIHA are defined in the dog. A strong genetic influence is suggested by the greater prevalence of the disease in particular breeds (old English sheepdog, cocker spaniel, border collie, poodle, English springer spaniel, Irish setter) and within particular pedigrees.[9,10,11] Specific genetic associations have not been extensively defined, but one early study suggested association with genes of the major histocompatibility complex, and this area warrants further investigation.

Canine AIHA is generally a disease of middle age (6 to 8 years), and although there is no clear gender predisposition, the disease can be precipitated in bitches by whelping or estrous. Of current importance is the suggestion of an association between the development

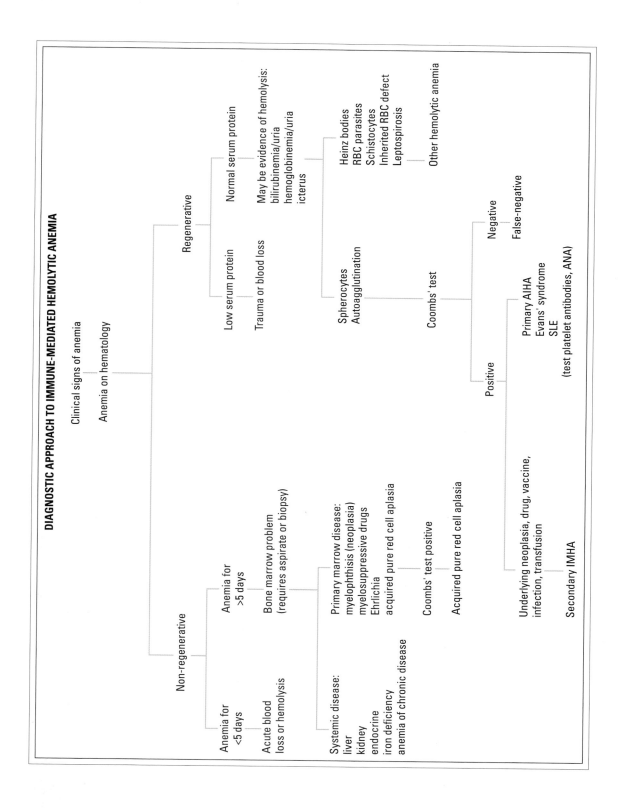

DIAGNOSTIC APPROACH TO IMMUNE-MEDIATED HEMOLYTIC ANEMIA

of canine AIHA and vaccination in the immediately preceding 4-week period. Anecdotal evidence for this association has been available for some time,[9] however a recent study by Duval and Giger[12] characterized two subgroups within a population of 58 dogs that had AIHA. One group (n = 15) had been vaccinated before disease onset, but the remaining dogs had not. A further difference between these two groups was the presence of serum ANA. None of the vaccine-associated AIHA cases had serum ANA, but 5 of 31 non-vaccine-associated cases were ANA positive, consistent with a primary, autoimmune pathogenesis. A similar epidemiologic survey was subsequently conducted in the United Kingdom. The data from 127,146 dogs were reviewed on a pet insurance company database. In this instance, there was no clear evidence that 41 dogs that had Coombs' positive AIHA or AITP had a greater prevalence of recent vaccination than 200 control dogs selected at random from the survey population.[13]

A seasonal incidence has been proposed for canine AIHA, although this is not consistent between different studies and may in fact be related to the prevalence of underlying infections, or timing of vaccinations[12,14] (Fig. 118.2).

Primary idiopathic AIHA is relatively less common in the cat, where most cases of IMHA are secondary to feline leukemia virus (FeLV) or *H. felis* (feline infectious anemia) infections.[15–17] Similarly, in the horse, IMHA is most frequently documented secondary to infection by equine infectious anemia virus or to administration of drugs such as penicillin[18] or trimethoprim-sulphonamide.[19]

IMMUNOPATHOGENESIS OF AUTOIMMUNE HEMOLYTIC ANEMIA IN THE DOG

A series of recent investigations has revealed many parallels between canine AIHA and the disease in human and experimental rodent models. The autoantibodies that characterize the canine disease are heterogeneous in their class and specificity, suggesting that a range of different underlying mechanisms may be involved in triggering the disease. Both immunoglobulin M (IgM) and immunoglobulin G (IgG) autoantibodies are found, and particular subclasses (IgG1 and IgG4) dominate the IgG response.[20] Significant quantities of immunoglobulin A (IgA) may also be associated with the erythrocyte membrane in AIHA, but the presence of this immunoglobulin is of questionable relevance. The specificity of the IgG autoantibodies has been characterized by means of eluting them from the surface of patient erythrocytes and incubating them with biotin-labeled normal canine RBC in the technique of immunoprecipitation.[21] The autoantibodies react with erythrocyte membrane glycophorins, the anion exchange molecule (band 3) and the cytoskeletal molecule spectrin (Fig. 118.3). Of note is the conserved specificity for band 3 that is found in murine models (in addition to glycophorin) of AIHA and in the

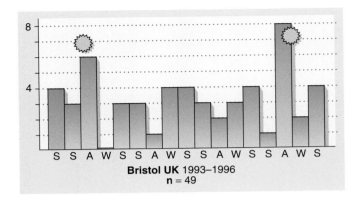

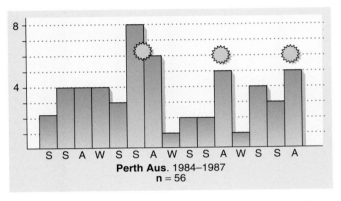

FIGURE 118.2 Seasonal distribution of cases of canine AIHA. Data are presented from the Northern (United Kingdom) and Southern (Australia) Hemispheres. The number of cases in each season (Spring, Summer, Autumn, Winter; SSAW) over a 3-year period are shown. Although there is a spread of cases, peaks (stars) are noted in some autumn periods and one Southern Hemisphere summer. Interpretation of such data is difficult but may reflect seasonal infections or annual cycles of administration of vaccines.

human disease (human patients also react to components of the Rhesus blood-group antigen system).

T-lymphocyte reactivity in canine AIHA has also been examined. Like other species, clinically normal dogs harbor erythrocyte-reactive lymphocytes that can be induced to proliferate in vitro when challenged with RBC-derived antigens. Such cells have a greater degree of reactivity when they are obtained from dogs recovered from AIHA (memory lymphocytes) or from normal dogs that are closely related to AIHA cases.[22] The latter observation suggests an immunologic mechanism for genetic susceptibility to AIHA in the dog. It is important to further investigate the fine specificity of such autoimmune responses, as this knowledge forms the basis for developing novel immunotherapeutic agents in future years.

CLINICAL PRESENTATION

There are two main clinical presentations of canine AIHA. That most commonly recognized has a chronic

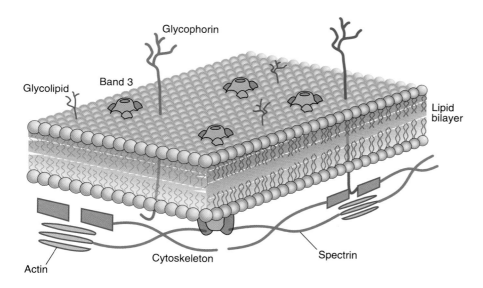

FIGURE 118.3 Schematic diagram of the erythrocyte membrane showing the major target autoantigens in canine AIHA: the glycophorins, the anion exchange molecule (band 3), and the cytoskeletal molecule spectrin. There is conservation of some of these autoantigens across species. Band 3 may be recognized in dogs and humans that have AIHA and is the target of the autoimmune response in some experimental mouse models of the disease.

onset (days to weeks) and is characterized by signs referable to anemia, erythrophagocytosis, and immunologic activity. These signs may include weakness, lethargy, exercise intolerance, anorexia, pyrexia, pallor of mucous membranes, tachypnea, tachycardia, hepatosplenomegaly, and lymphadenomegaly. Acute onset (one to two days) AIHA is less commonly recorded and is associated with severe intravascular hemolysis with jaundice, hemoglobinemia and hemoglobinuria, pyrexia and vomiting.

A proportion of dogs that have AIHA subsequently develop disseminated intravascular coagulation (DIC) or dyspnea caused by pulmonary thromboembolism.[23] Risk factors for development of these complications include hyperbilirubinemia, a negative Coombs' test, and the presence of indwelling catheters. These complications arise after the development of a hypercoagulable state that may be associated with the presence of an antiphospholipid antibody (misnamed the lupus anticoagulant) that enhances platelet aggregation and depresses regulation of the coagulation pathways.[24]

The range of clinical signs described for the dog is similar for cats that have AIHA, and as extravascular hemolysis is more common than intravascular, hemoglobinemia and hemoglobinuria are uncommon.[16,25]

DIAGNOSIS

AIHA diagnosis proceeds through a series of stages after the identification of compatible clinical history and presenting signs. An ethylenediamine tetra-acetic acid (EDTA) blood sample should be withdrawn for hematologic examination. This should be examined for the phenomenon of autoagglutination that may be observed by rotation of the collection tube or by placement of a drop of blood onto a microscope slide. Autoagglutination may only occur at 4°C, so blood should be refrigerated before making this assessment. True autoagglutination may be grossly distinguished from rouleaux formation

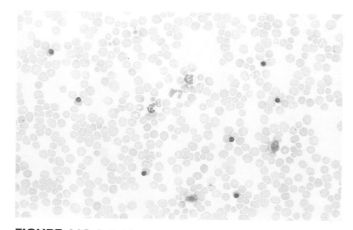

FIGURE 118.4 Leishman's stain. ×125. Blood smear from a dog that has AIHA, demonstrating the features of anisocytosis, polychromasia, and spherocytosis and the presence of nucleated erythrocytes.

by addition of an equal volume of saline to the drop of blood. Rouleaux is dispersed by this procedure, but agglutinates persist. One study previously reported the occurrence of cold autoagglutinins in normal dogs; but RBC suspensions were used, and the titers were weak.[26] It is often said that a positive slide autoagglutination test provides definitive evidence for AIHA and precludes the need for a Coombs' test. However, as described below, the Coombs' test can provide additional valuable information and should always be requested where possible.

Standard hematologic examination demonstrates the features of anemia. Canine AIHA is often a severe disease with a packed cell volume (PCV) of less than 20%. The anemia is generally regenerative (except for acquired PRCA), and reticulocytosis, polychromasia, anisocytosis and nucleated erythrocytes may be present (Fig. 118.4). Microscopic evidence of autoagglutination may be found, and the presence of spherocytosis is strongly suggestive of immune-mediated erythrocyte damage. AIHA is often accompanied by left shift neutrophilia that may reflect inflammatory cytokine production by activated macrophages, and the effect of these cytokines on hematopoiesis. Platelet numbers will be adequate in AIHA, but significant reduction in platelet count may indicate concurrent AITP or DIC.

In the presence of clinical and hematologic evidence for AIHA, the definitive diagnostic procedure is the Coombs' test (direct antiglobulin test, DAT) (Fig. 118.5). This test demonstrates the presence of erythrocyte-bound immunoglobulin or complement, but it does not distinguish between AIHA and secondary IMHA. The Coombs' test is performed with EDTA blood, and there is variation in the methodology used by different laboratories. A full Coombs' test is performed with a polyvalent Coombs' reagent (that recognizes IgG, IgM, and

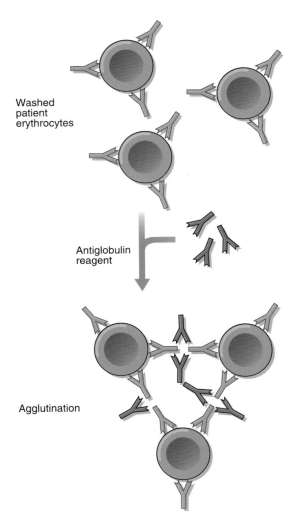

Washed patient erythrocytes

Antiglobulin reagent

Agglutination

FIGURE 118.5 Principle of the Coombs' test. A suspension of washed patient erythrocytes with membrane immunoglobulin or complement attached in vivo, are incubated with an antiglobulin reagent that cross-links these immunoreactants, forming a lattice that appears grossly as an agglutinate of red cells.

complement C3) specific for the species of the patient, but also with antisera specific for each of these immunoreactants alone. Each reagent should be fully titrated and mixed with a suspension of washed patient erythrocytes, and the test should be performed in duplicate at 4°C and 37°C (some laboratories also use room temperature). The performance of the test at temperatures other than 37°C is somewhat controversial, as nonpathologic cold antibodies may affect the results.[27] The read-out for the test is erythrocyte agglutination, and the titer of each positive reaction should be determined. The incidence of false-negative reactions is greatly reduced when the full test is performed in this manner. The results of the Coombs' test indicates the class of immunoglobulin bound to the erythrocytes, whether complement has been deposited, the titer of the reaction, and the optimum temperature reactivity of the antibody.

In general terms, two broad patterns of Coombs' reactivity are identified and these have some correlation with clinical presentation. The most commonly recorded pattern involves an IgG antibody that may be present with IgM or C3 and that reacts equally at 4°C and 37°C. This pattern often correlates with disease of chronic onset and is compatible with extravascular erythrocyte removal. Occasionally, a cold-reactive IgM antibody is identified that may fix complement and occurs in the absence of IgG. This pattern of Coombs' reactivity is more often associated with sample autoagglutination, intravascular hemolysis and acute onset, severe clinical disease. No clear association between the titer of RBC-bound antibody and disease severity exists, although low-titered reactions are more consistent with secondary IMHA than AIHA. Similarly, the presence of complement alone on the erythrocyte surface is most commonly associated with underlying disease.

Although the Coombs' test remains the gold standard for diagnosis of IMHA, other diagnostic tests are reported. The indirect Coombs' test (for detection of circulating autoantibody by incubation with normal erythrocytes) is not considered valid for use in veterinary species because of the low prevalence of non-cell-bound autoantibody. However, autoantibody may be eluted from the surface of patient RBC and bound back to normal erythrocytes as a further diagnostic procedure.[25] A cell-enzyme-linked immunosorbent assay (ELISA)-based method (direct enzyme-linked antiglobulin test [DELAT]) has been described, but is a time-consuming procedure and is largely used as a research tool.[28]

Other immunodiagnostic procedures may be used in canine AIHA. Many cases have significant serum titers of ANA, which may provide further evidence for a primary idiopathic autoimmune disease. In the presence of concurrent thrombocytopenia, tests for platelet autoantibody should be requested, although this is not routinely possible in many areas of the world. Adjunct immunodiagnostic tests such as determination of serum complement concentration (decreased levels of C3 or C4 may reflect deposition on erythrocyte membranes) or serum IgA concentration (IgA deficiency may be associated with canine autoimmunity) may be requested.

The diagnostic process is similar for feline IMHA.

Autoagglutination is more commonly documented in the feline disease and must be distinguished from rouleaux. Regeneration and spherocytosis are more problematic to define in the cat, and the Coombs' test must be interpreted carefully in this species as Coombs' positive anemia may occur with infection by *H. felis,* feline immunodeficiency virus, and feline coronavirus (feline infectious peritonitis [FIP]) as well as with a range of chronic inflammatory diseases. Cats are reported to have spontaneously arising, cold-reactive IgM antibodies at low titer,[17] so a full Coombs' test is essential.

TREATMENT

The first-line approach to therapy for canine AIHA involves the use of tapered immunosuppressive doses of glucocorticoids (e.g., prednisolone commencing at 2 to 4 mg/kg daily). In dogs that have severe, acute-onset intravascular hemolysis, or with acquired PRCA, or with anemia that is nonresponsive to glucocorticoid, the addition of cytotoxic agents (e.g., cyclophosphamide 50 mg/m² orally for the first 4 days of each week for 4 to 5 months only; azathioprine commencing at 2 mg/kg daily) to the regime is indicated. A recent study has questioned the efficacy of cyclophosphamide in therapy for AIHA.[29]

In severely anaemic dogs (PCV < 10%), supportive therapy in the form of matched whole blood or packed RBC transfusion may be required. The benefits of transfusion outweigh any possibility of enhancing hemolysis by providing greater antigenic load. Numerous other approaches to therapy are documented. The use of danazol (5 mg/kg orally twice daily) is controversial as recent studies have suggested that this drug may have little beneficial effect.[30] Cyclosporine (15 mg/kg orally per day) is efficacious in the therapy of AIHA but is costly. Similarly, the use of intravenous human gamma-globulin (0.5 to 1.5 g/kg given over 4 hours) to block macrophage Fc receptors or to bind circulating autoantibody, is of documented benefit but is an expensive undertaking.[31] No evidence exists that splenectomy (to remove a major site of extravascular hemolysis and autoantibody production) has any beneficial effect. In dogs that have acute, severe AIHA the use of prophylactic heparin treatment to prevent the complications of DIC or pulmonary thromboembolism is advocated.[32,33]

Immunosuppressive therapy (e.g., prednisolone 4 to 8 mg/kg daily) is also indicated for feline AIHA, although this is often combined with tetracycline to ensure treatment of underlying *H. felis* that may be difficult to diagnose on hematologic examination. Cytotoxic drugs may also be used for treatment of AIHA in the cat. Both cyclophosphamide and azathioprine are reported to be of benefit, but other therapies have not been evaluated in the cat.

MONITORING

Dogs that have chronic onset AIHA may make excellent recovery with appropriate supportive and immunosup-

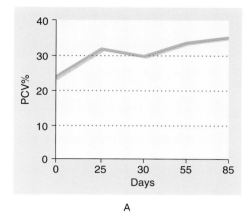

A

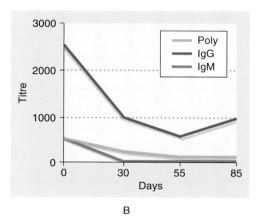

B

FIGURE 118.6 Serial monitoring of AIHA in a dog that has AIHA. The dog was treated with prednisolone at an initial dose of 2 mg/kg daily that was gradually tapered and withdrawn on day 76. Despite the rise and plateau in PCV, **A,** the dog remained Coombs' positive throughout the period of monitoring, **B.** Also in **B** serial titers obtained with polyvalent canine Coombs' reagent, anti-dog IgG and anti-dog IgM are shown. Data from **Day MJ.** Serial monitoring of clinical, haematological and immunological parameters in canine autoimmune haemolytic anemia. J Small Anim Pract 1996;37:523–534, with permission.

pressive therapy, but they remain at risk for disease relapse. There is often rapid clinical and hematologic response to therapy in such patients; however, serial monitoring of the Coombs' test has revealed striking persistence (for many months) of erythrocyte-bound autoantibody in many cases[34] (Fig. 118.6). Relapses may occur months or years after the initial episode and are often more severe, resulting in death. Alternatively, another manifestation of autoimmunity may surface in dogs recovered from AIHA, sometimes several years later. For example, a dog may present with AITP (and no anemia) subsequent to AIHA (without thrombocytopenia), but SLE and immune-mediated skin disease are also reported sequels. The mortality rate for dogs that have severe, acute-onset AIHA is greater than for the chronic form of disease.[35]

Therefore, recovery from AIHA necessitates regular

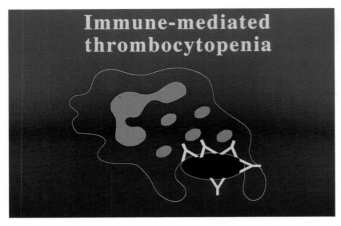

FIGURE 119.1 Pathogenesis of IMT. Antibodies (primarily IgG) bound to the surface of platelets result in accelerated platelet destruction by macrophages.

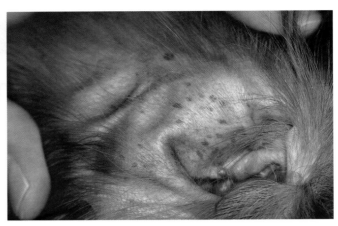

FIGURE 119.3 Petechial hemorrhages in the skin on the concave surface of the pinna of a dog that has primary IMT.

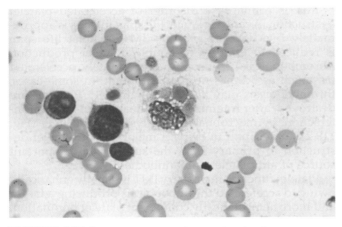

FIGURE 119.2 Splenic aspirate from a dog that has primary IMT and IMHA, showing a macrophage phagocytizing two platelets and a red cell. The other nucleated cells present are red-cell precursors.

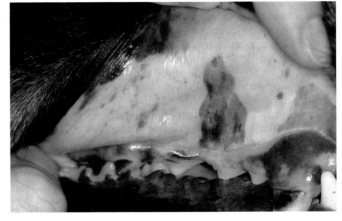

FIGURE 119.4 Petechial hemorrhages on the labial mucosa of a dog that has primary IMT.

Physical Examination Findings

Mucosal and cutaneous petechia, purpura, and ecchymoses, hyphema, retinal hemorrhages, melena, hematemesis, epistaxis, and mucous membrane pallor are frequent findings (Figs. 119.3 through 119.5).[20,22-24] Central nervous system or intraocular hemorrhage can lead to neurologic signs or blindness, respectively (Fig. 119.6). The degree of hemorrhage for any given platelet count is unpredictable. Dogs that have primary IMT may have less than 10,000 platelets/μL without evidence of hemorrhage. Fever, splenomegaly, hepatomegaly, and lymphadenopathy are uncommon in dogs with primary IMT.[20,22-24]

DIAGNOSIS

Complete Blood Count and Platelet Count

Dogs that have primary IMT usually have marked thrombocytopenia (<30,000 platelets per μL) on presen-

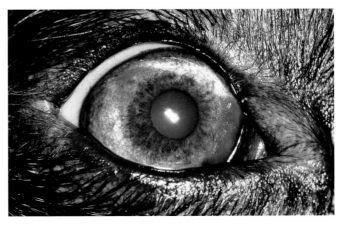

FIGURE 119.5 Iris petechia in a dog that has primary IMT.

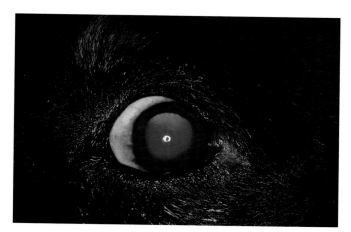

FIGURE 119.6 Hyphema in a dog that has primary IMT. Blindness can be the presenting complaint in dogs that have intraocular hemorrhage caused by thrombocytopenia.

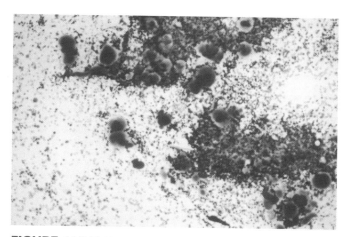

FIGURE 119.7 Bone marrow aspirate from a dog that has primary IMT (20× objective). Bone marrow is hypercellular with increased numbers of megakaryocytes, an appropriate thrombopoietic response to accelerated peripheral platelet destruction or use.

tation.[11,23-25] Examination of a peripheral blood smear is a reliable way to assess the presence of thrombocytopenia, although a platelet count is necessary to quantify its severity. Megathrombocytes (large, densely stained platelets suggestive of active thrombopoiesis) and microthrombocytes may be seen on blood smears from dogs that have IMT.[26]

Total and differential leukocyte counts are variable in dogs that have ITP. Neutrophilia with a left shift may be present owing to nonspecific bone marrow response to thrombocytopenia or anemia or to chemotactic activity of platelet activating factor or leukotrienes.[24,27] A stress leukogram may be evident.[23,27] Anemia, due to hemorrhage or concurrent IMHA, may be present, and may be regenerative or nonregenerative, depending on the time course of red-cell loss and the presence of immunologic targeting of red-cell precursors. IMHA is reported in approximately 20% of dogs that have primary IMT.[20,23,24]

Various criteria have been used to confirm a diagnosis of primary IMT in dogs, including the severity of thrombocytopenia, presence of microthrombocytosis, normal to increased numbers of megakaryocytes in bone marrow, detection of antiplatelet autoantibodies, increased platelet counts subsequent to administration of immunosuppressive doses of glucocorticoids, and exclusion of other causes for thrombocytopenia.

Severity of Thrombocytopenia

Although thrombocytopenia in dogs that have primary IMT is typically severe, thrombocytopenia associated with other diseases (e.g., disseminated intravascular coagulation [DIC], rickettsial infection) can also be marked.[28,29] The degree of thrombocytopenia cannot, alone, be considered a dependable diagnostic indicator of primary IMT.

Microthrombocytosis

Microthrombocytosis, the presence of a predominantly small population of platelets, is reported to be a specific indicator of primary IMT in dogs (specificity 95%) but is detected in less than 50% of cases.[25] Microthrombocytosis may result from preferential destruction of larger, more heavily IgG-sensitized platelets or from platelet fragmentation after immune injury. Although microthrombocytosis may increase diagnostic suspicion for IMT in dogs, it is unlikely to be helpful in differentiating primary from secondary causes of IMT.

Bone Marrow Evaluation

The value of bone marrow evaluation in dogs that have primary IMT is equivocal. Bone marrow disease is unlikely in the absence of leukopenia, nonregenerative anemia, or abnormal blood-cell morphology, and bone marrow evaluation is, therefore, not routinely indicated in dogs that have thrombocytopenia.[30,31] Finding normal to increased numbers of bone marrow megakaryocytes is indicative that thrombocytopenia is attributable to accelerated platelet destruction or use, but it is not specific for primary IMT (Fig. 119.7).[30] Furthermore, some dogs with primary IMT may have decreased numbers of bone marrow megakaryocytes caused by failure of bone marrow samples to provide a representative sample of bone marrow or caused by immunologic targeting of megakaryocytes.[24,27] One study reported that dogs that have primary IMT and decreased numbers of bone marrow megakaryocytes had a poorer prognosis.[24] Thrombocytopenia is not a contraindication to bone marrow aspiration or core biopsy, as severe hemorrhage is unusual, and can be readily controlled with local pressure.

Mean platelet volume (MPV) measurements can also be used to gauge the adequacy of platelet production.

Increased MPV is a sensitive and specific indicator of the adequacy of bone marrow response in dogs that have thrombocytopenia.[26]

Detection of Antiplatelet Autoantibodies

Various tests have been used to detect serum or plasma antibodies (usually IgG) that are capable of binding to platelets (platelet-bindable IgG) or that are bound to the dog's own megakaryocytes or platelets (platelet-bound IgG). None of these tests allow dogs that have primary IMT to be differentiated from dogs that have secondary IMT.

Platelet Factor 3 Test

The platelet factor 3 (PF3) test is based on the principle that normal canine platelets will be damaged by platelet-bindable IgG in the plasma sample being tested and release PF3, causing acceleration of the partial thromboplastin time (PTT).[32] Unfortunately, the PF3 test has variable sensitivity (from 28 to 80%) in dogs that have primary IMT, lacks specificity, and is of little diagnostic use in evaluating patients that have thrombocytopenia.[23,24,27,32]

Megakaryocyte Direct Immunofluorescence Test

The megakaryocyte direct immunofluorescence (MK-DIF) test detects IgG bound to megakaryocytes. The MK-DIF test also has variable sensitivity (from 30 to 80%) in dogs that have primary IMT.[20,27,33] A major disadvantage is that a bone marrow aspirate, which is otherwise not routinely necessary in patients that have thrombocytopenia, is required.

Detection of Platelet-Bound IgG

Detection of increased concentrations of platelet-bound IgG is extremely sensitive (approximately 90%) for primary IMT.[7] Because of the high sensitivity of tests for platelet-bound IgG, a diagnosis of primary IMT is unlikely if the test result is negative. A positive test for platelet-bound IgG in dogs that have thrombocytopenia implicates an immune pathogenesis for thrombocytopenia, but it is not specific for primary IMT. Positive tests for platelet-bound IgG have been reported in dogs with thrombocytopenia associated with SLE, *Ehrlichia canis* infection, dirofilariasis, sulfadiazine or trimethoprim administration, and cancer (lymphoproliferative disease and hemangiosarcoma).[7]

Detection of Platelet-Bindable IgG in Serum

Tests for platelet-bindable IgG are less sensitive (approximate sensitivity 60%) than tests for platelet-bound IgG, probably because most platelet-bindable IgG is already bound to platelets and little remains free in the circulation, but they may be helpful in those cases in which sufficient numbers of platelets cannot be isolated for testing. A positive test result for platelet-bindable IgG is not specific for primary IMT.[7,33]

Response to Glucocorticoid Therapy

The majority (approximately 70%) of dogs that have ITP have platelet counts of greater than 100,000 per μL within 7 days of initiating immunosuppressive glucocorticoid treatment.[12,20,24] However, because the principal action of glucocorticoids is to impair macrophage phagocytosis of antibody-sensitized platelets, primary and secondary IMTs may respond similarly.

Exclusion of Other Causes for Thrombocytopenia

Although patient signalment, history, clinical findings, and laboratory tests are helpful in increasing diagnostic suspicion, none are specific for primary IMT. A diagnosis of primary IMT is made, ultimately, by exclusion of other causes for thrombocytopenia. Absolute certainty of a diagnosis of ITP is unattainable. Other causes of thrombocytopenia must be excluded to reduce diagnostic uncertainty enough to permit optimal and timely treatment decisions. The degree to which other causes for thrombocytopenia must be or can be excluded varies with each patient and each client.

Splenomegaly

Thrombocytopenia caused by splenomegaly is mild (not less than 100,000 platelets/μL), which allows it to be easily distinguished from primary IMT.[33] Splenomegaly is unusual in dogs that have primary IMT.

Disseminated Intravascular Coagulation

Thrombocytopenia is a frequent finding in dogs that have DIC.[34] The absence of overt signs of illness in dogs that have thrombocytopenia makes DIC unlikely. Evaluation of a coagulation profile, including prothrombin time, PTT, fibrin degradation products, antithrombin III concentrations, and evaluation of a peripheral blood smear for schistocytes allow most cases of DIC to be diagnosed.

Hemolytic Uremic Syndrome

A disorder of platelet hyperaggregability with intravascular platelet thrombi and widespread tissue ischemia is called hemolytic uremic syndrome.[35,36] Clinical and laboratory findings in hemolytic uremic syndrome, including neurologic signs, renal failure, microangiopathic hemolytic anemia (schistocytosis), thrombocytopenia, and fever, make it distinguishable from primary IMT.

Anticoagulant Rodenticide Toxicity

Moderate to severe thrombocytopenia can occur in dogs that have hemorrhage subsequent to ingestion of anticoagulant rodenticide toxins.[37] Bleeding manifestations typical of a secondary hemostatic disorder and abnormal coagulation profiles allow differentiation from dogs that have primary IMT.

Neoplasia

Thrombocytopenia is frequently associated with neoplasia in dogs, particularly lymphoproliferative neoplasia and hemangiosarcoma,[5,38] but can occur with various solid neoplasms. Mechanisms for thrombocytopenia associated with neoplasia include DIC; splenic sequestration; myelophthisis; bone marrow suppression by chemotherapy, radiation therapy, or tumor-elaborated estrogens; and IMT. IMT is well documented in dogs that have lymphoproliferative and solid neoplasia and may precede the discovery of neoplasia.[5]

Systemic Lupus Erythematosus

IMT may be a component of SLE in dogs. Other clinical and laboratory manifestations of SLE, such as polyarthritis, dermatitis, polymyositis, glomerulonephritis, neutropenia, IMHA, lupus erythematosus cells, and antinuclear antibodies would permit a diagnosis of primary IMT to be excluded.[39]

Drug-Associated Immune-Mediated Thrombocytopenia

The gold salt auranofin, cephalosporins, and trimethoprim sulfonamide have been associated with IMT in dogs.[7,40,41] Any drug can potentially provoke IMT. Drug-induced IMT usually develops after weeks to months of therapy, resolves within 2 weeks of cessation of the drug, and does not recur and hence should be readily distinguishable from primary IMT.[4]

Infectious Disease

In North America, infectious diseases are reported to account for 20 to 60% of dogs that have thrombocytopenia.[10,11] Ehrlichiosis, Rocky Mountain spotted fever, and dirofilariasis are frequently diagnosed infectious causes of thrombocytopenia in dogs.[10,11] A decrease in platelet number or mild thrombocytopenia may occur subsequent to modified-live virus vaccination.[42,43] Immune-mediated platelet destruction may contribute to thrombocytopenia in dogs infected with *E. canis*, *Babesia canis*, *Dirofilaria immitis*, or distemper.[3,7,44]

Spurious Thrombocytopenia

Spurious thrombocytopenia is a consideration in dogs that have asymptomatic thrombocytopenia. Causes of spurious thrombocytopenia include platelet clumping caused by poor sampling technique, platelet activation by glass surfaces, ethylenediamine tetra-acetic acid (EDTA)-induced platelet clumping, and exclusion of large or small platelets caused by inappropriate machine settings or calibration.[30] Macrothrombocytosis in Cavalier King Charles spaniels can result in spurious throm-

bocytopenia.[45] Abnormal platelet counts should always be verified by examination of a peripheral blood smear.

Breed Differences

Normal Greyhounds, Shibas, and Cavalier King Charles spaniels may have lower platelet counts than those seen in other breeds of dogs.[46,47] Such breed differences must be remembered, so that these dogs are not erroneously classified as being thrombocytopenic.

TREATMENT

Supportive Care

Cage rest and minimization of trauma are important. Drugs and fluids should be administered enterally if feasible; the intravenous route is otherwise preferred.

Transfusion Therapy

Life-threatening hemorrhage is uncommon in dogs that have primary IMT.[23,24] Hypovolemia or anemia should be treated by administration of crystalloid or colloid solutions, packed red cells, or whole blood. Platelet transfusions in dogs that have IMT are rarely necessary, but they are indicated in dogs that have central nervous system hemorrhage (dogs that have severe thrombocytopenia and sudden onset of neurologic signs) to control bleeding until platelet numbers are able to be increased by other therapies. In this circumstance, transfusion of multiple units of platelets is necessary because transfused platelets are destroyed rapidly.[48] The inaccessibility of platelet components makes this therapy impractical for most veterinarians.

Glucocorticoids

Glucocorticoids are the initial therapy of choice for dogs that have primary IMT. The initial beneficial effect of glucocorticoids in dogs that have IMT is primarily inhibition of macrophage destruction of antibody-sensitized platelets.[49] Autoantibody production may also be impaired. Glucocorticoids also increase capillary resistance to hemorrhage, often reducing the severity of hemorrhage before platelet counts increase.[50] Glucocorticoids may also stimulate platelet production in some patients that have IMT.[51] Prednisolone or prednisone (2 mg/kg by mouth q12h) is used most frequently,[12,20,22–24] although some clinicians favor dexamethasone (0.1 to 0.6 mg/kg q24h).[21,24] The majority of dogs that have primary IMT attain platelet counts of 50,000 to 100,000/μL within 7 days of commencing glucocorticoid therapy.[12,20,24] Initial glucocorticoid therapy should ideally be continued until the platelet count normalizes (although this may not be achievable in some dogs) followed by dose tapering over weeks to months. Platelet counts should be monitored frequently, and glucocorticoid therapy and glucocorticoid tapering should continue as long as thrombocytopenia does not recur. In many cases, glucocorticoids cannot be discontinued once the disease is in remission.

Adjunctive Therapies

Various additional treatments, including cyclophosphamide, azathioprine, vincristine, splenectomy, danazol, cyclosporine, and human immunoglobulin, have been used in conjunction with glucocorticoids to treat dogs that have primary IMT. These treatments are generally reserved for dogs failing to respond to glucocorticoids, dogs that have recurrent disease, or dogs experiencing unacceptable glucocorticoid-induced adverse effects.

Vincristine

Vincristine administration to dogs that have primary IMT results in prompt (within one week) increases in platelet numbers.[52,53] Vincristine diminishes phagocytosis of platelets by macrophages caused by impaired microtubule assembly. To accentuate targeting of macrophages, vincristine can be incubated with homologous platelets in vitro (vincristine-loaded platelets) or infused intravenously for 6 to 8 hours to achieve in vivo platelet uptake.[53,54] Vincristine may also increase platelet counts by stimulating thrombopoiesis.[55] Vincristine's inhibitory effects on platelet function by means of disruption of platelet microtubules has not been shown to be clinically important.[55]

Cyclophosphamide

Cyclophosphamide is a frequently used treatment for dogs that have primary IMT. Cyclophosphamide is administered orally or intravenously, in conjunction with glucocorticoids, at a dose of 200 mg/m² weekly until an adequate response is attained. In humans who have primary IMT, an adequate response may take 1 to 16 weeks.[56] The efficacy of cyclophosphamide in dogs that have primary IMT is not documented.

Azathioprine

Azathioprine is administered (2 mg/kg per os) once daily initially and, once the desired clinical response is obtained, tapered in tandem with glucocorticoids to a maintenance dose of 0.5 to 1 mg/kg administered every 48 hours. An adequate response may take as long as 6 to 16 weeks.[57] The efficacy of azathioprine in dogs that have primary IMT is not documented.

Splenectomy

In dogs that have primary IMT, splenectomy is reserved for those dogs that fail to respond to or relapse after medical therapy. Rates of clinical disease remission in dogs that have primary IMT subsequent to splenectomy vary from 0% (0 of 4) to 80% (4 of 5), with a mean response rate of approximately 25%.[12,20,22,24]

Danazol

Danazol, a synthetic androgen with low capacity for masculinization, reduces the number of Fc receptors on macrophages and may act synergistically with glucocorticoids by displacing them from glucocorticoid-binding globulin. Documentation of danazol treatment of dogs that have primary IMT is limited. Two dogs that had primary IMT refractory to prednisone (1 mg/kg orally q12h) had greater than 100,000 platelets/µL within 1 to 2 weeks of starting danazol therapy (5 mg/kg orally q12h) in conjunction with prednisone.[58,59]

Cyclosporine

Experience with cyclosporine in dogs that have primary IMT is limited; there is one preliminary report of cyclosporine treatment of dogs that had primary IMT. Cyclosporine (15 to 30 mg/kg daily, to maintain trough blood concentrations of 400 to 600 ng/mL), in addition to other immunosuppressive therapies, was administered to 4 dogs that had ITP refractory to glucocorticoids. Three dogs achieved normal platelet counts after 3 to 5 weeks; one of these dogs died from systemic aspergillosis.[60] Others recommend a dose of 10 mg/kg q24h to maintain trough blood concentrations of 250 to 400 ng/mL.[61]

Human Immunoglobulin

Platelet count increases in humans who have primary IMT subsequent to intravenous administration of human immunoglobulin (IVIG) are more rapid than platelet responses to oral prednisone therapy, and IVIG is a frequently used emergency therapy in humans who have primary IMT.[62] Human IVIG binds to dog mononuclear cells and can modulate immune responses in dogs.[63] One dog that had IMHA and IMT had resolution of thrombocytopenia subsequent to IVIG therapy.[63]

Although the rationale for the use of vincristine, cyclophosphamide, azathioprine, splenectomy, danazol, cyclosporine, and IVIG in the treatment of dogs that have primary IMT may be valid, their proclaimed efficacy is based largely on subjective clinical impressions. Until appropriately controlled clinical trials test the efficacy and place of these treatments in the management of dogs with primary IMT, clinicians should use the therapies with which they have most experience.

Goals of Therapy

The goal of treatment in dogs with primary IMT is to withdraw all therapy while maintaining disease remission. This may not be attainable in all cases and some dogs require long-term immunosuppressive therapy to maintain remission.

PROGNOSIS

The majority (more than 70%) of dogs that have primary IMT, with or without concurrent IMHA, have platelet

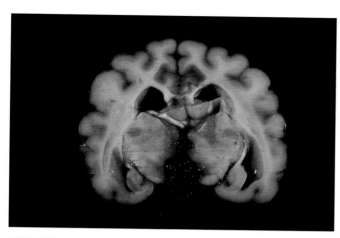

FIGURE 119.8 Intracranial hemorrhage, which caused rapid onset of altered mentation and seizures in this dog that has IMT, may occur with severe thrombocytopenia and is frequently fatal.

counts of greater than 50,000 to 100,000 platelets/μL subsequent to initial therapy (glucocorticoids alone or in conjunction with vincristine, cyclophosphamide, azathioprine, or fresh whole-blood or platelet transfusions).[12,20,24] Based on reported cases from referral hospitals, which may not be representative of cases seen by practitioners in the field, approximately 30% of dogs that have ITP die or are euthanatized during the initial episode of thrombocytopenia or because of disease recurrence (Fig. 119.8).[12,20,23,24] Approximately 40% of dogs have recurrence of clinical signs of primary IMT. The remaining dogs are either cured, have subclinical disease, or are lost to follow-up. The prognosis for dogs that have primary IMT and IMHA may be considerably worse than for dogs that have primary IMT only.[20]

REFERENCES

1. **Lewis DC, Meyers KM.** Canine idiopathic thrombocytopenic purpura—a review. J Vet Intern Med 1996;10:207–218.
2. **Mackin A.** Canine immune-mediated thrombocytopenia. Compend Cont Educ Pract Vet 1995;17:353–364.
3. **Axthelm MK, Krakowka S.** Canine distemper virus-induced thrombocytopenia. Am J Vet Res 1987;48:1269–1275.
4. **Chong BH.** Drug-induced immune thrombocytopenia. Platelets 1991;2:173–181.
5. **Helfand SC, Couto CG, Madewell BR.** Immune-mediated thrombocytopenia associated with solid tumors in dogs. J Am Anim Hosp Assoc 1985;21:787–794.
6. **Kristensen AT, Weiss DJ, Klausner JS, Laber J, Christie DJ.** Comparison of microscopic and flow cytometric detection of platelet antibody in dogs suspected of having immune-mediated thrombocytopenia. Am J Vet Res 1994;55:1111–1114.
7. **Lewis DC, Meyers KM, Callan MB,** et al. Detection of platelet-bound and serum platelet-bindable antibodies in the diagnosis of canine ITP. J Am Vet Med Assoc 1995;206:47–52.
9. **Lewis DC, Meyers KM.** Studies of platelet-bound and serum platelet-bindable immunoglobulins in dogs with idiopathic thrombocytopenic purpura. Exp Hematol 1996;24:696–701.
10. **Cockburn C, Troy GC.** A retrospective study of 62 cases of thrombocytopenia in the dog. Southwest Vet 1986;37:133–141.
11. **Grindem CB, Breitschwerdt EB, Corbett WT, Jans HE.** Epidemiologic survey of thrombocytopenia in dogs: A report on 987 cases. Vet Clin Pathol 1991;20:38–43.
12. **Jans HE, Armstrong PJ, Price GS.** Therapy of immune-mediated thrombocytopenia. A retrospective study of 15 dogs. J Vet Intern Med 1990;4:4–7.
13. **Jordan HL, Grindem CB, Breitschwerdt EB.** Thrombocytopenia in cats: a retrospective study of 41 cases. J Vet Intern Med 1993;7:261–265.
14. **Shulman NR, Jordan JV.** Platelet kinetics. In: Colman RW, Hirsh J, Marder VJ, Salzman EW, eds. Hemostasis and thrombosis, basic principles and clinical practice. Philadelphia: JB Lippincott, 1987;452–529.
15. **Ballem PJ, Segal AM, Stratton JR, Gernsheimer T, Adamson JW, Slichter SJ.** Mechanisms of thrombocytopenia in chronic autoimmune thrombocytopenic purpura. Evidence of both impaired platelet production and increased platelet clearance. J Clin Invest 1987;80:33–40.
16. **Joshi BC, Jain NC.** Experimental immunologic thrombocytopenia in dogs: a study of thrombocytopenia and megakaryocytopoiesis. Res Vet Sci 1977;22:11–17.
17. **McMillan R, Longmire RL, Yelenosky R, Donnell RL, Armstrong S.** Quantitation of platelet-binding IgG produced in vitro by spleens from patients with idiopathic thrombocytopenic purpura. N Engl J Med 1974;291:812–817.
18. **Harker LA, Slichter SJ.** The bleeding time as a screening test for evaluation of platelet function. N Engl J Med 1972;287:155–159.
19. **Kristensen AT, Weiss DJ, Klausner JS.** Platelet dysfunction associated with canine immune-mediated thrombocytopenia (ITP). J Vet Intern Med 1994;8:323–327.
20. **Jackson ML, Kruth SA.** Immune-mediated hemolytic anemia and thrombocytopenia in the dog: a retrospective study of 55 cases diagnosed from 1969 through 1983 at the Western College of Veterinary Medicine. Can Vet J 1985;26:245–250.
21. **Dodds WJ.** Immune-mediated diseases of the blood. Adv Vet Sci Comp Med 1983;27:163–196.
22. **Feldman BF, Handagama P, Lubberink AA.** Splenectomy as adjunctive therapy for immune-mediated thrombocytopenia and hemolytic anemia in the dog. J Am Vet Med Assoc 1985;187:617–619.
23. **Wilkins RJ, Hurvitz AL, Dodds WJ.** Immunologically mediated thrombocytopenia in the dog. J Am Vet Med Assoc 1973;163:277–282.
24. **Williams DA, Maggio-Price L.** Canine idiopathic thrombocytopenic purpura: clinical observation and long-term follow-up in 54 cases. J Am Vet Med Assoc 1984;185:660–663.
25. **Northern J, Tvedten HW.** Diagnosis of microthrombocytosis and immune-mediated thrombocytopenia in dogs with thrombocytopenia: 68 cases (1987–1989). J Am Vet Med Assoc 1992;200:368–372.
26. **Sullivan PS, Manning K, McDonald TP.** Association of mean platelet volume and bone marrow megakaryocytopoiesis in thrombocytopenic dogs: 60 cases (1984–1993). J Am Vet Med Assoc 1995;206:332–334.
27. **Joshi BC, Jain NC.** Detection of antiplatelet antibody in serum and on megakaryocytes of dogs with autoimmune thrombocytopenia. Am J Vet Res 1976;37:681–685.
28. **Harvey JW.** Ehrlichia platys infection (Infectious cyclic thrombocytopenia of dogs). In: Greene CE, ed. Infectious diseases of the dog and cat. Philadelphia: WB Saunders, 1990;415–418.
29. **Waddle JR, Littman MP.** A retrospective study of 27 cases of naturally occurring canine ehrlichiosis. J Am Anim Hosp Assoc 1988;24:615–620.
30. **Jain NC.** Essentials of veterinary hematology. Philadelphia: Lea and Febiger, 1993.
31. **Jones EC, Boyko WJ.** Diagnostic value of bone marrow examination in isolated thrombocytopenia. Am J Clin Pathol 1985;84:665–667.
32. **Jain NC, Kono CS.** The platelet factor-3 test for detection of canine antiplatelet antibody. Vet Clin Pathol 1970;9:10–14.
33. **Kristensen AT, Klausner JS, Weiss DJ, Laber J, Christie DJ.** Detection of antiplatelet antibody with a platelet immunofluorescence assay. J Vet Intern Med 1994;8:36–39.
34. **Feldman BF, Madewell BR, O'Neill S.** Disseminated intravascular coagulation: antithrombin, plasminogen, and coagulation abnormalities in 41 dogs. J Am Vet Med Assoc 1981;179:151–154.
35. **Hertzke DM, Cowan LA, Schoning P, Fenwick BW.** Glomerular ultrastructural lesions of idiopathic cutaneous and renal glomerular vasculopathy of greyhounds. Vet Pathol 1995;32:451–459.
36. **Holloway SA, Senior DF.** Hemolytic-uremic syndrome in dogs. J Vet Intern Med 1993;7:220–227.
37. **Lewis DC, Bruyette DS, Kellerman DL, Smith SA.** Thrombocytopenia in dogs subsequent to anticoagulant rodenticide-induced hemorrhage: 8 cases (1990–1995). J Am Anim Hosp Assoc 1997;33:417–422.
38. **Grindem CB, Breitschwerdt EB, Corbett WT, Page RL, Jans HE.** Thrombocytopenia associated with neoplasia in dogs. J Vet Intern Med 1994;8:400–405.
39. **Scott DW, Walton DK, Manning TO, Smith CA, Lewis RM.** Canine lupus erythematosus. I. Systemic lupus erythematosus. J Am Anim Hosp Assoc 1983;19:461–479.
40. **Bloom JC, Blackmer SA, Bugelski PJ,** et al. Gold-induced immune thrombocytopenia in the dog. Vet Pathol 1985;22:492–499.
41. **Bloom JC, Thiem PA, Sellers TS, Deldar A, Lewis HB.** Cephalosporin-induced immune cytopenia in the dog: demonstration of erythrocyte-, neutrophil-, and platelet-associated IgG following treatment with cefazedone. Am J Hematol 1988;28:71–78.
42. **McAnulty JF, Rudd RG.** Thrombocytopenia associated with vaccination of a dog with a modified-live paramyxovirus vaccine. J Am Vet Med Assoc 1985;186:1217–1219.
43. **Stokol T, Parry BW.** The effect of modified-live virus vaccination on von

Willebrand factor antigen concentrations and platelet counts in dogs. Vet Clin Pathol 1997;28:135–137.

44. **Waner T, Harrus S, Weiss DJ, Bark H, Keysary A.** Demonstration of serum antiplatelet antibodies in experimental acute canine ehrlichiosis. Vet Immunol Immunopath 1995;48:177–182.

45. **Brown S, Simpson KW, Baker S, Spagnoletti MA, Elwood CM.** Macrothrombocytosis in Cavalier King Charles Spaniels. Vet Rec 1994;135:281–283.

46. **Sullivan PS, Evans HL, McDonald TP.** Platelet concentration and hemoglobin function in Greyhounds. J Am Vet Med Assoc 1994;205:838–841.

47. **Eksell P, Haggstrom J, Kvart C, Karlsson A.** Thrombocytopenia in the cavalier King Charles Spaniel. J Small Anim Pract 1994;35:153–155.

48. **Carr JM, Kruskall MS, Kaye JA, Robinson SH.** Efficacy of platelet transfusions in immune thrombocytopenia. Am J Med 1986;80:1051–1054.

49. **Branehog I, Weinfeld A.** Platelet survival and platelet production in idiopathic thrombocytopenic purpura (ITP) before and during treatment with corticosteroids. Scand J Haematol 1974;12:69–79.

50. **Freund LA, Berild D, Hainau B.** Haemostatic effect of prednisolone in thrombocytopenia. Scand J Haematol 1983;31:485–487.

51. **Gernsheimer T, Stratton J, Ballem PJ, Slichter SJ.** Mechanisms of response to treatment in autoimmune thrombocytopenic purpura. N Engl J Med 1989;320:974–980.

52. **Greene CE, Scoggin J, Thomas JE, Barsanti JA.** Vincristine in the treatment of thrombocytopenia in five dogs. J Am Vet Med Assoc 1982;180:140–143.

53. **Helfand SC, Jain NC, Paul M.** Vincristine-loaded platelet therapy for idiopathic thrombocytopenia in a dog. J Am Vet Med Assoc 1984;185:224–226.

54. **Ahn YS, Harrington WJ, Mylvaganam R, Allen LM, Pall LM.** Slow infusion of vinca alkaloids in the treatment of idiopathic thrombocytopenic purpura. Ann Intern Med 1984;100:192–196.

55. **Mackin AJ, Allen DG, Johnstone IB.** Effects of vincristine sulfate and prednisone on platelet numbers and function in clinically normal dogs. Am J Vet Res 1995;56:100–108.

56. **Reiner A, Gernsheimer T, Slichter SJ.** Pulse cyclophosphamide therapy for refractory autoimmune thrombocytopenic purpura. Blood 1995;2:351–358.

57. **Quiquandon I, Fenaus P, Caulier MT, Pagniez D, Huart JJ, Bauters F.** Reevaluation of the role of azathioprine in the treatment of adult chronic idiopathic thrombocytopenic purpura: a report on 53 cases. Br J Haematol 1990;74:223–228.

58. **Bloom JC, Meunier LD, Thiem PA, Sellers TS.** Use of danazol for treatment of corticosteroid-resistant immune-mediated thrombocytopenia in a dog. J Am Vet Med Assoc 1989;194:76–77.

59. **Roseler BJ, Mason KV.** Use of danazol and corticosteroids for the treatment of immune-mediated thrombocytopaenia in a dog. Aust Vet Pract 1994;24:126–130.

60. **Cook AK, Bertoy EH, Gregory CR, Stewart AF.** Effect of oral cyclosporine (CS) in dogs with refractory immune-mediated anemia (IMA) or thrombocytopenia (ITP) [abstract]. J Vet Intern Med 1994;8:170.

61. **Vaden SL.** Cyclosporine. In: Bonagura JD, ed. Kirk's current veterinary therapy XII. Philadelphia: WB Saunders, 1995;73–77.

62. **Blanchette VS, Kirby MA, Turner C.** Role of intravenous immunoglobulin G in autoimmune hematologic disorders. Semin Hematol 1992;29:72–82.

63. **Scott-Moncrieff JC, Regan WJ, Glickman LT, DeNicola DB, Harrington D.** Treatment of nonregenerative anemia with human gamma-globulin in dogs. J Am Vet Med Assoc 1995;206:1895–1900.

CHAPTER 120

Immune-Mediated Neutropenia

• C. GUILLERMO COUTO

I mmune-mediated neutropenia (IMN) is relatively common in people.[1,2] Despite references to immune-mediated (or corticosteroid-responsive) neutropenia in animals being scarce in the literature,[3–7] in the author's experience it is fairly common in small animal patients. Although in most cases antibodies directed against neutrophils are difficult to demonstrate, the prompt and sustained response to corticosteroids or other immuno-suppressive drugs has led to the definition of this syndrome. In addition, a syndrome identical to the IMN seen in clinical patients can be induced by use of antineutrophil antibodies in cats.[8]

CLINICAL FEATURES

Although IMN is more common in dogs and cats, it also occurs in herbivores. The following discussion applies to all species, although it is primarily based on the syndrome as it occurs in dogs and cats.

Dogs and cats of any age or gender may present with either asymptomatic or symptomatic IMN. Most patients that have IMN are asymptomatic, although occasionally dogs (and, rarely, cats) with IMN in association with other immune-mediated cytopenias (i.e., anemia, thrombocytopenia, or both) present for evaluation of signs resulting from the latter (e.g., exercise intolerance, pallor, jaundice, and spontaneous bleeding).

Frequently IMN is diagnosed in a healthy dog or cat undergoing routine hematologic evaluation as part of an annual physical examination or before anesthesia. In this subset of patients, results of physical examination are normal, and the only abnormality detected is the cytopenia in the complete blood count (CBC).

Occasionally dogs that have IMN present for evaluation of fever or signs associated with infection. Persistent fever and malaise without other associated signs of infection are somewhat common in dogs that have IMN. Patients usually are referred for evaluation of fever of unknown origin (FUO) in association with neutropenia, since antibiotic therapy has failed to resolve the fever. Extensive clinical, clinicopathologic, and microbiologi-

cal evaluations do not reveal the presence of causal agents and, as discussed below, upon institution of immunosuppressive therapy, both the neutropenia and the fever resolve, only to reoccur after discontinuing the medication. This presentation is rare in cats.

Some dogs present for evaluation of neurologic signs, primarily nonlocalizable or spinal pain. In those patients, cerebrospinal fluid analysis usually reveals a suppurative nonseptic meningitis that resolves after instituting immunosuppressive therapy. Other dogs that have IMN have immune-mediated nonerosive polyarthritis, diagnosed by the presence of suppurative nonseptic joint cytology; these signs also resolve after immunosuppressive therapy. Felty's syndrome, a combination of neutropenia, erosive (i.e., rheumatoid) arthritis, and splenomegaly is rare in dogs. Occasionally, dogs that have IMN have other immune-mediated lesions, such as panniculitis or vasculitis.

A subset of dogs that have IMN present for evaluation of fever and signs of infection. In these dogs a septic focus can usually be found after thorough clinical and clinicopathologic evaluation. After evaluating the CBC and finding neutropenia and toxic changes in these leukocytes, it is usually assumed that the neutropenia is caused by an overwhelming bacterial infection. However, after the signs of infection resolve with appropriate antibiotic therapy, the neutropenia persists. In these patients, it is likely that the IMN predisposed the patient to a secondary bacterial infection. This form of presentation is also rare in cats.

CLINICOPATHOLOGIC FINDINGS

The CBC is helpful in diagnosing IMN. In most asymptomatic dogs and cats, severe neutropenia ($<500/\mu$L) is the only hematologic abnormality present; neutrophil counts of 100 to $200/\mu$L are common, and most cells do not have toxic changes (e.g., cytoplasmic basophilia, Döhle bodies). Moderate to marked lymphocytosis (i.e., 5000 to $9000/\mu$L) and mild thrombocytopenia (i.e., 100,000 to $130,000/\mu$L) are common in cats that have

IMN. Increases in the numbers of large granular lymphocytes are not common in either dogs or cats that have IMN. In symptomatic patients, the presence of immune-mediated hemolytic anemia, thrombocytopenia, or both, may result in additional changes in the CBC (e.g., regenerative anemia, thrombocytopenia, spherocytosis, autoagglutination). For additional information, please see corresponding chapters.

Dogs that present for evaluation of infection associated with IMN also have severe neutropenia, but toxic changes in the neutrophils are evident. Treatment with appropriate antibiotics results in resolution of the toxic changes, but the neutropenia remains unchanged.

Bone marrow aspiration in dogs or cats that have IMN typically reveals a hypercellular bone marrow with myeloid and megakaryocytic hyperplasia, although myeloid hypoplasia can also occur. The cytologic changes in most patients (i.e., myeloid hyperplasia with abundant bands but few mature neutrophils) suggest that the pathogenesis of the neutropenia is peripheral neutrophil destruction, rather than decreased production.

Although various tests to detect antineutrophil antibodies, including immunofluorescence, leukoagglutination, flow cytometry, and radioimmunoassays, among others, are used in people who have IMN and have been cursorily evaluated in animals, they are not reliable in a clinical setting.[2,9–11] In dogs that have anemia in association with neutropenia, a positive direct Coombs' test indirectly supports a diagnosis of immune-mediated cell destruction (i.e., there are antibodies on the red blood cells, so the neutropenia is also likely to be immune mediated). A positive antiplatelet antibody test in a dog that has thrombocytopenia and neutropenia may be interpreted in a similar fashion.

A positive antinuclear antibody (ANA) test in a dog that has neutropenia should be interpreted with caution, since this test can be positive in various disorders that are nonimmune in origin. Dogs that have Felty's syndrome may have positive rheumatoid factor (RF) tests.

Serologic evaluation for diseases associated with neutropenia should be conducted in dogs and cats that have severe neutropenia of undetermined origin. Ehrlichiosis in dogs and retroviral diseases in cats (i.e., feline leukemia virus and feline immunodeficiency virus infections) are important rule outs before instituting therapy for IMN. Polymerase chain reaction (PCR) for these infectious agents can also be used if the titer is negative but the index of suspicion is high.

Dogs that have neutropenia and fever or other clinical signs suggestive of infection should undergo thoracic radiography to detect an infectious pulmonary focus (e.g., abscess, pneumonia) and abdominal ultrasonography to detect hepatic (or less frequently, splenic) abscesses. Neutrophil scans can be performed by labeling allogeneic (i.e., normal canine donor) neutrophils with technetium 99; these neutrophils are then administered intravenously to the patient, who is then imaged with a gamma camera. Accumulation of labeled neutrophils in a site of hidden infection appears as a hot spot on the scan, suggesting a consumptive infectious neutropenia.

DIAGNOSIS

IMN is usually a diagnosis of exclusion. In the experience of the author, specific tests to detect antibodies on the surface of the neutrophils are not clinically reliable. The patient should undergo a thorough physical examination in search of a hidden infectious focus. This is probably more important in symptomatic dogs than in those that lack clinical signs, since it is unlikely than an asymptomatic dog or cat that has neutropenia has a clinically undetectable infection.

If there are changes in the CBC that support a regenerative cytopenia (i.e., polychromasia or reticulocytosis in association with anemia and thrombocytopenia), the most likely pathogenesis is peripheral destruction of both cell lines, and bone marrow evaluation may not be necessary. However, if there are no other cytopenias, or if the cytopenias are nonregenerative, a bone marrow specimen should be evaluated cytologically to rule out

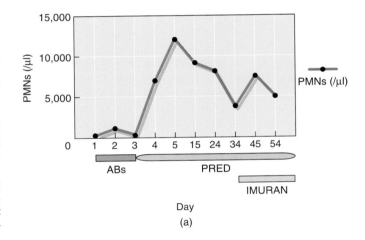

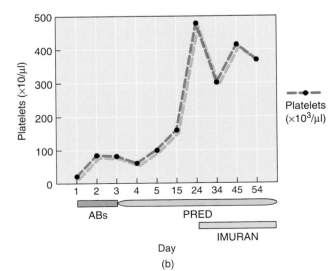

FIGURE 120.1 **A**—Changes in neutrophil counts in response to immunosuppressive therapy in an 8-year-old female Airedale Terrier. **B**—Changes in platelet counts in the same dog.

TABLE 120.1	Immunosuppressive Drugs Used to Treat Dogs and Cats That Have IMN[a]			
Drug	Dose	Interval	Species	Adverse Effects
Prednisone	2–4 mg/kg	q/24 h for 1 week; then q/48 hr	Dog	PU/PD; hepatopathy
Prednisone	4–8 mg/kg	q/24 h for 1 week; then q/48 hr	Cat	DM[b]
Azathioprine (Imuran)	50 mg/m^2	q/24 h; then q/48	Dog	myelosuppression
Cyclophosphamide (Cytoxan)	200–300 mg/m^2	q/2–3 weeks	Dog	myelosuppression, cystitis
Chlorambucil (Leukeran)	20 mg/m^2	q/2 weeks	Cat	myelosuppression?

[a] All drugs are administered orally.
[b] Diabetes mellitus.

other disorders. Disorders commonly associated with blood cytopenias in dogs include ehrlichiosis, bone marrow hypoplasia (drug induced or idiopathic), and leukemias; in cats, retroviral diseases and leukemias are the most common differential diagnoses. As discussed above, serologic evaluation (or PCR) for these diseases should be part of the routine evaluation of a neutropenic patient.

In asymptomatic neutropenic patients that have no toxic changes in the neutrophils, once infectious diseases and leukemia have been ruled out, an in-hospital therapeutic trial of immunosuppressive doses of corticosteroids is warranted. Before this, a 2- to 3-day course of bactericidal antibiotics (e.g., sulfa-trimethoprim or fluoroquinolones) is indicated to cover for hidden sources of bacterial infection. Dogs that have clinical signs associated with infection should be treated as discussed below before issuing a tentative diagnosis of IMN.

TREATMENT

Immunosuppressive drugs constitute the mainstay of therapy in dogs and cats with IMN. As discussed above, an in-hospital therapeutic trial of immunosuppressive doses of corticosteroids after 2 to 3 days on antibiotics is a sure way to retrospectively confirm a diagnosis. The antibiotics used are discussed below.

To this effect, the patients should be treated with 2 to 4 mg/kg/day of prednisone (dogs) or 4 to 8 mg/kg/day of prednisone (cats). Their rectal temperature should be monitored every 4 to 6 hours, and steroid therapy should be discontinued if fever develops; treatment should also be discontinued if the patient develops unexplained clinical signs while receiving steroids.

As a general rule, in dogs and cats that have IMN, neutrophil counts increase within 24 to 72 hours of instituting immunosuppressive therapy (Fig. 120.1). If the patient responds, the dose of corticosteroids is eventually tapered off to determine the lowest possible dose that maintains the neutrophil count above the target range (usually >1,500/μL in dogs and >1,000/μL in cats). Every-other-day corticosteroid therapy should be instituted after the first week of daily administration.

Other immunosuppressive drugs commonly used to treat IMN are listed in Table 120.1.

Other drugs can be used nonspecifically to stimulate neutrophil production in neutropenic dogs and cats. For example, lithium carbonate (10 mg/kg, orally, q/12 h) is effective in increasing neutrophil counts in dogs (but not in cats) that have chemotherapy-associated neutropenia in our clinic. The patient should receive the drug for 3 to 5 days, and trough serum lithium concentrations should be measured; the therapeutic range is between 0.8 and 1.5 mEq/L. Recently, human and canine recombinant granulocyte-colony stimulating factors (G-CSFs) have been evaluated in dogs that have chemotherapy-associated neutropenia, and their effects are similar to those of lithium when used at a dose of 5 μg/kg, subcutaneously q/24 h. However, the human-derived product (Neupogen) typically causes persistent neutropenia because of the development of antibodies against this human protein, that cross-react with the patient's own G-CSF.[12] Canine G-CSF is not commercially available. The role of lithium carbonate and G-CSFs in dogs and cats that have IMN is yet to be determined.

As discussed above, when antibiotics are indicated in dogs and cats that have neutropenia, bactericidal drugs should be chosen, since a functional neutrophil mass is needed to eliminate organisms after bacteriostatic antibiotic therapy. The antibiotics of choice used by the author for neutropenic asymptomatic dogs are either sulfa-trimethoprim (15 mg/kg, orally, q/12 h) or enrofloxacin (2.5 to 5 mg/kg, PO, q/12 h). Dogs and cats that have neutropenia and signs of infection or fever should be treated with a combination of intravenous bactericidal drugs. A combination of cephalothin, at a dose of 20 mg/kg intravenously q/8 h in combination with amikacin at a dose of 15 mg/kg intravenously q/24 h provides good results.

The long-term prognosis for dogs and cats that have IMN is good; however, approximately half of the patients need lifelong immunosuppressive therapy.

REFERENCES

1. **Dale DC.** Immune and idiopathic neutropenia. Curr Opin Hematol 1988;5:33–36.
2. **Chickering WR, Prasse KW.** Immune mediated neutropenia in man and animals: a review. Vet Clin Pathol 1981;10:6–16.

3. **Alexander JW, Jones JB, Michel RL.** Recurrent neutropenia in a Pomeranian: a case report. J Am Anim Hosp Assoc 1981;17:841–844.

4. **Maddison JE, Hoff B, Johnson RP.** Steroid responsive neutropenia in a dog. J Am Anim Hosp Assoc 1983;19:881–886.

5. **Gabbert NH.** Cyclic neutropenia in a feline leukemia-positive cat: A case report. J Am Anim Hosp Assoc 1984;20:343–348.

6. **Willard MD.** Corticosteroid-responsive leukopenia and neutropenia associated with FeLV infection in 2 cats. Mod Vet Pract 1985:719–722.

7. **Swenson CL, Kociba GJ, O'Keefe DA, et al.** Cyclic hematopoiesis associated with feline leukemia virus infection in two cats. J Am Vet Med Assoc 1987;191:93–96.

8. **Chickering WR, Brown J, Prasse KW, Dawe DL.** Effects of heterologous antineutrophil antibody in the cat. Am J Vet Res 1985;46:1815–1819.

9. **Lalezari P.** Neutrophil and platelet antibodies in immune neutropenia and thrombocytopenia. In: Rose NR, et al, eds. Manual of clinical laboratory immunology. 3rd ed. Washington, DC: American Society for Microbiology, 1986;630–634.

10. **Chickering WR, Prasse KW, Dawe DL.** Development and clinical application of methods for detection of antineutrophil antibodies in serum of the cat. Am J Vet Res 1985;46:1809–1814.

11. **Jain NC, Stott JL, Vegad JL, Dhawedkar RG.** Detection of anti-equine neutrophil antibodies by use of flow cytometry. Am J Vet Res 1991;52:1883–1890.

12. **Hammond WP, Csiba E, Canin A, et al.** Chronic neutropenia. A new canine model induced by human granulocyte colony-stimulating factor. J Clin Invest 1991;87:704–710.

CHAPTER 121

Systemic Lupus Erythematosus

• MICHAEL J. DAY

DEFINITION

In some individuals, an autoimmune response may involve multiple organ systems and present as polysystemic disease. The pathology of such conditions may be attributed to true autoantibody binding, immune complex deposition, or cell-mediated autoimmunity (types II to IV hypersensitivity mechanisms). There is a spectrum of such multisystems autoimmunity that includes conditions such as dermatomyositis, dermatouveitis, and the various vasculitides and polyarthritides, but the best defined entity is that of systemic lupus erythematosus (SLE). SLE is considered an uncommon disease of the dog and is rare in the cat and horse; thus, most information presented in this chapter derives from canine studies. In humans, this disorder is clearly defined by clinical and serologic criteria specified by the American Rheumatism Association.[1] Numerous diagnostic criteria have been proposed for SLE in veterinary species, the most universally accepted of which are that a patient should have at least two separate clinically and serologically defined manifestations of autoimmunity in addition to the presence of a high-titered serum antinuclear antibody (ANA). Occasional patients may have clinical and serologic features of polysystemic autoimmunity but lack serum ANA; by definition the disease is not SLE but is likely a related variant within the same spectrum. One further distinct SLE-like syndrome is the combination of immune-mediated polyarthropathy, serum ANA, and nonspecific illness that is documented in dogs of the German shepherd breed.[2]

AUTOIMMUNITY

SLE is a primary idiopathic autoimmune disease in which the immune system loses 'self-tolerance' toward autoantigens and mounts an inappropriate attack on target tissues. The machinery required to effect an autoimmune disease (e.g. autoreactive T and B lymphocytes) is always present within normal individuals but must be carefully regulated to maintain self-tolerance (Fig. 121.1). Such immunoregulatory mechanisms include: (1) deletion of autoreactive lymphocytes during intrathymic (T cell) or bone marrow (B cell) development ('clonal deletion') by inducing autoreactive cells to undergo programmed cell death (apoptosis); (2) deletion (by apoptosis) of autoreactive T lymphocytes following recognition of autoantigen after release from the thymus ('peripheral deletion'); (3) failure of antigen-presenting cells (APCs) to present autoantigens to autoreactive T cells ('immunologic ignorance'); (4) failure to deliver appropriate costimulatory signals to autoreactive T cells despite presentation of autoantigen by APC (anergy); and (5) active suppression of autoreactive T cells by other regulatory lymphoid populations. Expression of autoimmune disease therefore requires that self-tolerance be broken with activation of autoreactive lymphocytes. Although an abundance of theories explains how this may be achieved, current research suggests that microbial infection may provide the required immunologic disturbance by nonspecific activation of autoreactive clones by microbially derived substances such as 'superantigens', by binding to autoantigens to create 'bystander' damage or modifying self-antigens to create novel determinants, or by providing microbial peptides or epitopes that are 'molecular mimics' of self-peptides or antigens. These are presented by APC as part of the antimicrobial immune response but simultaneously bypass 'immunologic ignorance,' enabling activation of autoreactive clones.

The key interactions in induction of autoimmune disease are therefore between self-peptides, particular genetic forms of molecules of the major histocompatibility complex (MHC), and T cell receptors (Fig. 121.1). This trimolecular complex is the current focus of investigations into autoimmunity and research into development of immunotherapeutic means of treating these diseases.

PREDISPOSING FACTORS

As with all autoimmune diseases, SLE is a multifactorial disorder in which clinical expression relies on the presence of an optimum array of predisposing factors (Fig. 121.2). A number of such factors are recognized in human and companion animal SLE. The strongest risk factor for SLE is genetic background, and this association

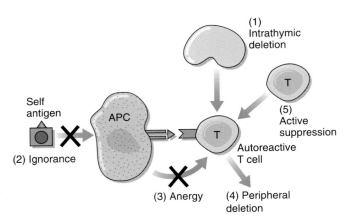

FIGURE 121.1 Maintenance of self-tolerance for autoreactive T lymphocytes. T lymphocytes expressing a T cell receptor (TCR) capable of recognizing self-peptide may be deleted during intrathymic development (1). Some autoreactive T cells are exported from the thymus and must be regulated to prevent autoimmune disease. These cells may fail to be activated because there is no presentation of self-peptide by MHC on antigen-presenting cell (APC) to engage the TCR [immunologic ignorance, (2)] or because no costimulatory signal is delivered by the APC despite antigen presentation [anergy, (3)]. Alternatively, when the autoreactive T cell recognizes self-peptide it may undergo apoptosis [peripheral deletion, (4)], or the T cell may be under the control of other regulatory lymphocytes [active suppression, (5)].

is well-defined in the dog where there are both breed (German shepherd dog, collie, Shetland sheepdog, English cocker spaniel) and familial associations. The disease is clearly inherited (but not by a simple mechanism), and experimental colonies of dogs with SLE have been established. In 1965, Lewis and Schwartz[3] established three inbred lines of dog from founder stock with SLE. These dogs developed serum ANA, and those kept long-term later developed clinical manifestations of SLE or other autoimmune diseases. Two further colonies have been reported in recent years, one in which disease was spontaneously arising[4] and a second in which the prevalence was enhanced by experimental matings.[5] Feline SLE occurs more frequently in purebred cats, particularly those with a Siamese or Persian background.[6]

The most powerful genetic associations with autoimmune diseases are with particular allelic variants of the polymorphic genes of the MHC, which encode the molecules involved in antigen presentation by APC. In human populations, there are well-established data that indicate the relative risk for development of specific autoimmune diseases if an individual carries particular combinations of MHC allotypes. Similar data are reported for canine SLE. In one of the colonies of dogs with SLE described above, disease expression was associated with the DLA (dog leukocyte antigen, the canine MHC) allele DLA A7, and a negative (or 'protective') association with DLA A1 and B5 was recorded.[5] Human SLE is also strongly associated with the presence of a null allele for the fourth component of complement (C4) and

with genetically determined insufficiency of various complement components. In a similar manner, dogs with SLE-like disease (immune-mediated polyarthritis, pyrexia, and ANA) are reported as having greater genetic expression of a specific complement C4 allotype.[7]

Numerous associations with microbial infection (particularly viral) have been suggested for human SLE, and viral infection has been proposed to underlie the canine disease, although no direct isolation of virus from canine tissues has been described. In early studies, blood lymphocytes taken from dogs with SLE were shown to express antigens that were cross-reactive with retroviral molecules, and cell-free extracts were able to transfer the serologic abnormalities of SLE from normal to affected dogs.[8] The feline viruses FeLV and FIV can induce disease in cats with similarity to SLE, and serum ANA may occur in the early stages of FeLV infection. However, the rare cases of feline SLE test negative for both viruses.[6]

Associations between IgA deficiency and autoimmune diseases (including SLE) and between IgA deficiency and serum ANA are well-documented in man and recognized in the dog.[9] Inefficient mucosal immune defenses may permit colonization by microbes that trigger the processes leading to loss of self-tolerance.

There may be geographic influence in expression of canine SLE. The disease is considered uncommon in Australia, Northern Europe, and the United States but is recognized not infrequently in Mediterranean countries. This may reflect an association with infections prevalent in these areas, such as leishmaniasis, in which there may be multiple immune-mediated pathologies.

Although there are strong hormonal influences on the expression of human SLE (predominantly female), such gender distribution is not clearly defined in the dog. Particular drugs have been able to induce SLE-like syndromes in both the dog (hydralazine)[10] and cat (propylthiouracil).[11]

IMMUNOPATHOGENESIS

The immunopathogenesis of SLE is complex and in any one individual case will reflect the particular self-antigens targeted for autoimmune attack. The disease may involve both humoral (autoantibody and immune complex) and cell-mediated immunologic effects (Fig. 121.2). A range of autoantibodies may be produced with specificity for autoantigens derived from erythrocytes, platelets, synovium, or endocrine tissue. The most significant autoantibodies are those which define the disease, the ANAs. These are specific for various constituents of the nucleus such as double- or single-stranded DNA, histones, and nonhistone proteins. ANA may be present in the serum of animals with any chronic inflammatory, infectious, or neoplastic disease, presumably as a consequence of cellular breakdown and exposure of nuclear material. However, in such situations the ANA is generally of low titer compared with the higher titers that characterize autoimmune disorders such as SLE.

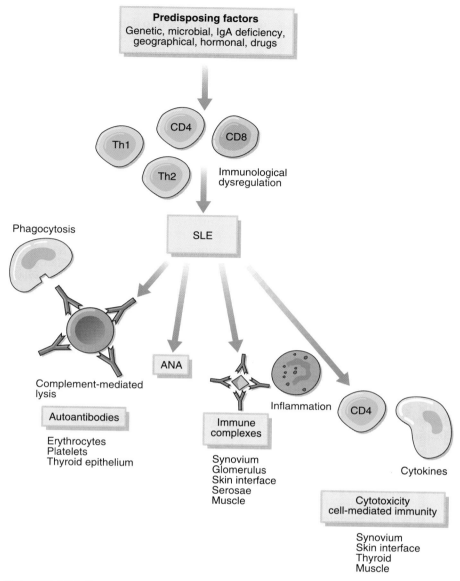

FIGURE 121.2 Pathogenesis of SLE. Initiation of disease involves a combination of predisposing factors that give rise to immunologic dysregulation, resulting in loss of self-tolerance. The multisystem pathology is caused by (1) antigen-specific autoantibodies, (2) immune complex deposition, and (3) cell-mediated immunity.

In human SLE there is much data on the clinical significance of individual specificities of ANAs, but these have only recently been investigated in the dog and no strong clinical associations are described.[12,13] Canine ANAs are heterogeneous and may be directed against components of the nucleosome (native DNA and histone proteins) or extractable nuclear antigens (Sm and ribonucleoprotein [RNP]). There are clear differences in the specificity of these antibodies in dogs compared with humans with SLE. In dogs, antibody directed against native DNA is far less commonly found, and there is a restricted pattern of reactivity against the various individual histone antigens. The lack of antibody specific for double-stranded DNA has generally been attributed to the presence of a nonspecific DNA binding protein in canine serum that interferes with the assay system. Recent studies, however, have shown that canine serum does not affect the binding of monoclonal antibody to DNA, confirming that the absence of canine native DNA antibody is a real phenomenon.[12] Canine ANAs also appear to have additional reactivities not found with human SLE sera (e.g., for the glycoprotein hnRNP G). In contrast, the pattern of reactivity to the Sm and RNP antigens is relatively conserved between the two species.[13] Antibodies to the proliferating cell nuclear antigen (PCNA) have also been described in dogs.

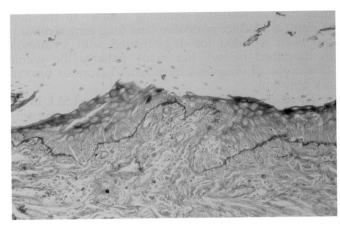

FIGURE 121.3 Interface band. Indirect immunoperoxidase staining, ×100. The 'lupus band test' aims to demonstrate the presence of immune complex deposition at the basement membrane zone (BMZ) of lesional skin with histopathologic evidence of interface dermatitis. This biopsy is taken from a dog with discoid lupus erythematosus and shows IgG deposition at the BMZ by an indirect immunoperoxidase technique.

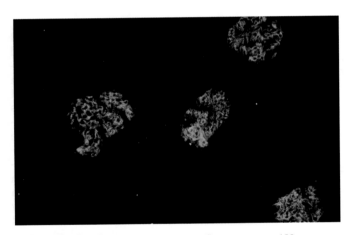

FIGURE 121.4 Glomeruli. Immunofluorescence, ×100. Deposition of immune complex within glomeruli may be demonstrated by immunohistochemistry. In this renal biopsy from a cat with protein-losing nephropathy, deposition of IgG has been demonstrated by indirect immunofluorescence.

strated by immunohistochemistry (Fig. 121.4), and electron microscopic examination may be performed to localize the level of deposition of glomerular immune complexes.

The definitive diagnostic procedure is detection of serum ANA that is most readily demonstrated by indirect immunofluorescence or immunoperoxidase tests using a substrate of nucleated cells (Fig. 121.5). Traditionally these have been frozen sections of rat liver, but cell lines propagated in culture (e.g., vero cells, human epithelial cells HEp-2) are increasingly used. There is debate as to the relative merits of these substrate cells and there is no universally accepted standard protocol

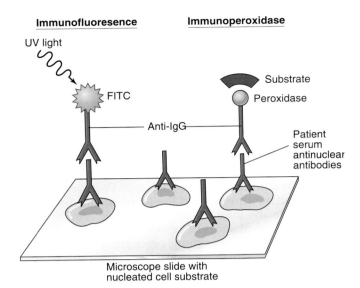

FIGURE 121.5 In the antinuclear antibody (ANA) test, patient serum is incubated with a substrate slide of nucleated cells (sections of rat liver or cell lines grown in culture). ANA bound to the nucleus are detected by the use of a secondary antibody specific for IgG of the patient species that has been conjugated to fluorescein isothiocyanate (FITC) or an enzyme (peroxidase). Positive nuclear staining is identified by the use of ultraviolet microscopy (immunofluorescence) or the addition of appropriate substrate and chromagen (immunoperoxidase). A range of serial dilutions of the serum sample are tested to obtain the titer of the reaction.

used by veterinary laboratories.[21,22] The result of an ANA test will be reported as a serum titer and pattern of nuclear staining. The most commonly observed patterns are speckled or homogenous staining (rim or nucleolar staining is less common), but there is no clear association between these patterns and the nature of clinical disease (Fig. 121.6). Interpretation of the titer must be made by the testing laboratory and a clinically significant titer distinguished from the low ANA titers that may be present in the serum of up to 10% of normal animals and animals with a wide range of nonimmune disease. A number of methods are used to assay antibody levels to the specific nuclear components detailed above (immunoprecipitation, ELISA, radioimmunoassay, western blotting), but again there are no clear associations between the presence of particular antibodies and clinical disease. These latter assays are rarely available outside the research setting. It should be noted that the ANA test has largely replaced the relatively insensitive lupus erythematosus (LE) cell test. In this test, heparinized or clotted blood is collected from the patient and mechanically disrupted so that free cell nuclei are obtained. LE cells are formed when the cell nuclei are exposed in vitro to ANA. The resultant opsonized nuclear material is phagocytized, and those cells containing the phagocytized material (LE cells) can be identified on blood smears (Fig. 121.7). LE cells can occasionally

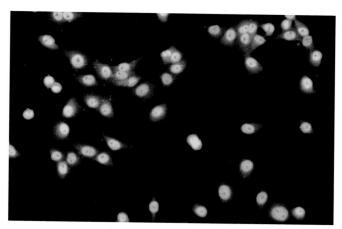

FIGURE 121.6 ANA. Immunofluorescence, ×50. Homogenous nuclear staining in a positive ANA test using the immunofluorescence method on a cell line substrate. Note the absence of nucleolar staining. The speckled and homogenous staining patterns are most commonly observed in veterinary species, but staining of the nuclear rim or nucleolus is occasionally reported.

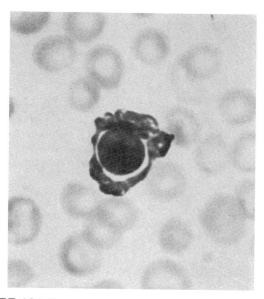

FIGURE 121.7 LE cell in clotted blood preparation from a dog with myopathy. Wright-Leishman stain, ×4000. (Reprinted with permission from Schalm and Ling, 1970; courtesy of *The California Veterinarian*).

be seen in vivo in joint fluid and when present are highly suggestive of SLE.

A range of other immunologic procedures are applicable to the diagnosis and monitoring of SLE but may be less readily available. Serum immune complex (circulating immune complex [CIC]) concentrations can be determined and will fall during clinical remission. Serum complement function (the CH_{50} test) or the concentration of specific complement components (C3 and C4)

can be measured. Reduced levels of complement in canine SLE are less likely to reflect inherited complement deficiency than utilization of complement in clearance of immune complexes. Complement levels will rise to normal during periods of remission or following therapy. Also, serum immunoglobulin concentrations, particularly those of IgG and IgA, can be measured.

THERAPY

The therapeutic approach to SLE will reflect the range of clinical manifestations present and should be tailored to each individual case. For example, specific supportive care may be necessary for renal disease (dietary management) or hemolytic anemia/thrombocytopenia (transfusion of packed red cells or platelet-rich plasma). The standard primary approach to therapy involves the use of tapered immunosuppressive doses of glucocorticoids that may be used in combination with other immunosuppressives such as cyclophosphamide or azathioprine.[15] One protocol using glucocorticoids in combination with the immunomodulatory drug levamisole is also reported.[23] Levamisole is administered at 3 to 7 mg/kg every 48 hours (a maximum dose of 150 mg/dog is used) together with prednisolone (1–2 mg/kg daily). The prednisolone is tapered and discontinued after 2 months, while levamisole is given continuously for 4 months and then stopped. If there is relapse of disease, levamisole is reinstituted for a further 4-month period.

Other reported therapeutic approaches include plasmapheresis (rarely available) in combination with glucocorticoids[24] or the use of cyclosporine to treat refractory disease. Feline SLE is also treated with glucocorticoids (prednisolone), and these may be used in combination with cyclophosphamide or chlorambucil.[6,18] It has been suggested that therapy should be more aggressive when the clinical presentation of feline SLE includes renal disease. Dexamethasone has been used in the treatment of equine SLE.[20]

Animals with SLE should be closely monitored throughout therapy and periodically during periods of remission. Appropriate parameters for monitoring include hematology, urinalysis, biochemistry, synovial fluid analysis, and serum ANA. The titer of this autoantibody may correlate with clinical severity and fall with clinical improvement, but the antibody may persist at lower titer during clinical remission.

REFERENCES

1. **Tan EM, Cohen AS, Fries JF, Masi AT, McShane DJ, Rothfield NF, Schaffer JG, Talal N, Winchester RJ.** The 1982 revised criteria for the classification of systemic lupus erythematosus. Arthritis Rheum 1982;25:1271–1277.
2. **Thoren-Tolling K, Ryden L.** Serum autoantibodies and clinical/pathological features in German shepherd dogs with a lupuslike syndrome. Acta Vet Scand 1991;32:15–26.
3. **Lewis RM, Schwartz RS.** Canine systemic lupus erythematosus: genetic analysis of an established breeding colony. J Exp Med 1971;134:417–438.
4. **Hubert B, Teichner M, Fournel C, Monier JC.** Spontaneous familial systemic lupus erythematosus in a canine breeding colony. J Comp Pathol 1988;98:81–89.

5. Teichner M, Krumbacher K, Doxiadis I, Doxiadis G, Fournel C, Rigal D, Monier JC, Gross-Wilde H. Systemic lupus erythematosus in dogs: association to the major histocompatibility complex class I antigen DLA-A7. Clin Immunol Immunopathol 1990;55:255–262.

6. Pedersen NC, Barlough JE. Systemic lupus erythematosus in the cat. Feline Practice 1991;19:5–13.

7. Day MJ, Kay PH, Clark WT, Shaw SE, Penhale WJ, Dawkins RL. Complement C4 allotype association with and serum C4 concentration in an autoimmune disease of the dog. Clin Immunol Immunopathol 1985;35:85–91.

8. Quimby FW, Gebert R, Datta S, Andre-Schwartz J, Tannenberg WJ, Lewis RM, Weinstein IB, Schwartz RS. Characterization of a retrovirus that cross-reacts serologically with canine and human systemic lupus erythematosus. Clin Immunol Immunopathol 1978;9:194–210.

9. Day MJ. Inheritance of serum autoantibody, reduced serum immunoglobulin A and autoimmune disease in a canine breeding colony. Vet Immunol Immunopathol 1996;53:207–219.

10. Balazs T, Robinson CJG, Balter N. Hydralazine-induced antinuclear antibodies in beagle dogs. Toxicol Appl Pharmacol 1981;57:452–456.

11. Aucoin DP, Peterson ME, Hurvitz AI, Drayer DE, Lahita RG, Quimby FW, Reidenberg MM. Propylthiouracil-induced immune-mediated disease in the cat. J Pharmacol Exp Ther 1985;234:13–18.

12. Monestier M, Novick KE, Karam ET, Chabanne L, Monier J-C, Rigal D. Autoantibodies to histone, DNA and nucleosome antigens in canine systemic lupus erythematosus. Clin Exp Immunol 1995;99:37–41.

13. Welin Henriksson E, Hansson H, Karlsson-Parra A, Pettersson I. Autoantibody profiles in canine ANA-positive sera investigated by immunoblot and ELISA. Vet Immunol Immunopathol 1998;61:157–170.

14. Chabanne L, Fournel C, Caux C, Bernaud J, Bonnefond C, Monier JC, Rigal D. Abnormalities of lymphocyte subsets in canine systemic lupus erythematosus. Autoimmunity 1995;22:1–8.

15. Bennett D. Immune-based non-erosive inflammatory joint disease of the dog. 1. Canine systemic lupus erythematosus. J Small Animal Pract 1987; 28:871–889.

16. Scott DW, Walton DK, Manning TO, Smith CA, Lewis RM. Canine lupus erythematosus. I. Systemic lupus erythematosus. JAAHA 1983;19:461–479.

17. Grindem CB, Johnson KH. Systemic lupus erythematosus: literature review and report of 42 new canine cases. JAAHA 1983;19:489–503.

18. Vitale CB, Ihrke PJ, Gross TL, Werner LL. Systemic lupus erythematosus in a cat: fulfilment of the American Rheumatism Association criteria with supportive skin histopathology. Vet Dermatol 1997;8:133–138.

19. Vrins A, Feldman B. Lupus-erythematosus-like syndrome in a horse. Equine Practice 1983;5:18–25.

20. Geor RJ, Clark EG, Haines DM, Napier PG. Systemic lupus erythematosus in a filly. JAVMA 1990;197:1489–1492.

21. Hansson H, Trowald-Wigh G, Karlsson-Parra A. Detection of antinuclear antibodies by indirect immunofluorescence in dog sera: comparison of rat liver tissue and human epithelial-2 cells as antigenic substrate. J Vet Intern Med 1996;10:199–203.

22. Bell SC, Hughes DE, Bennett D, Bari ASM, Kelly DF, Carter SD. Analysis and significance of anti-nuclear antibodies in dogs. Res Vet Sci 1997;62:83–84.

23. Fournel C, Chabanne L, Caux C, Faure JR, Rigal D, Magnol JP, Monier JC. Canine systemic lupus erythematosus. I: A study of 75 cases. Lupus 1992;1:133–139.

24. Matus RE, Scott RC, Saal S, Gordon BR, Hurvitz AI. Plasmapheresis-immunoadsorption for treatment of systemic lupus erythematosus in a dog. JAVMA 1983;182:499–502.

CHAPTER 122

Principles of Blood Collection and Processing[a]

• ANN SCHNEIDER

The advent of large-scale veterinary blood banks has made the practice of high-quality transfusion medicine possible. However, this is clearly dependent not just on component availability and appropriate use but also on the quality of the blood components. Strict adherence to collection, processing, and storage guidelines is the best way to achieve this quality.

This chapter details the currently accepted blend of human protocol and veterinary modifications where necessary for the collection, processing, and storage of blood components.

DONOR CONSIDERATIONS

Canine

Choosing donors carefully, when possible, greatly reduces the supplies wasted and the time spent drawing each unit. Although any dog more than 27 kg is able to donate 450 mL of blood as often as every three to four weeks without need for nutritional supplementation, the use of a 35- to 40-kg dog who is docile and of suitable body type (lean with a long neck, no excess skin folds, and a prominent jugular) will streamline the process.[1,2] The author has also had success drawing 225 mL units from donors 16 to 27 kg, although drawing nonstandard volumes necessitates careful planning (see Blood Collection Supplies).

Blood typing concerns are discussed elsewhere in this volume. All donors should receive a physical examination and hematocrit check before each donation. Periodic rechecks should be performed for both general health and endemic infectious diseases. This is for the protection of the recipient and the donor, and provides incentive for dog owners to become involved in the voluntary donor programs. Donors should also be maintained on

standard veterinary health protocol such as vaccination and heartworm prevention. Donors who have been transfused themselves or who have had a litter previously should be designated for red blood cell (RBC) unit production only, as the possibility of antibody levels to foreign RBC antigens is increased in these donors.

Feline

Feline donors should be indoor cats to minimize the risk of disease transmission. Donation volumes can be calculated based on *lean body weight;* recommendations range from 11 mL/kg to 15 mL/kg.[1,3,4] However, very large cats donating less than 11 mL/kg are less likely to have hypotension-related problems with the procedure and thus this situation is preferable. Donations may be taken as often as every 2 to 3 weeks if the hematocrit is acceptable.[3] Because cats are generally sedated for donation, personality is less of a concern than it is with canine donors. Previous litters and previous transfusions are not a concern for feline donors.

Initial screening should include blood type, general health, and infectious diseases. Infectious disease screening recommendations vary with institution, with region, and with the donor's environment and exposure to other cats and ectoparasites.[1,3,5]

Feline blood donors' diets should be nutritionally supplemented with iron based on the volume of blood drawn. Blood contains 0.5 mg iron per mL.[5] Based on an individual cat's donation volume and frequency, at least this amount should be replaced gradually with regular oral supplementation of ferrous sulfate.[3,5]

BLOOD COLLECTION PRINCIPLES

For optimal quality, blood is collected into a sterile, airtight system that is known as a closed system. Blood components made in a closed system are not exposed to air except when the needle is uncapped for insertion into the donor and when the component unit is entered

---

[a]Portions of this chapter are excerpted with the permission of the publisher from Schneider A. Blood components: collection, processing, and storage. In: Transfusion medicine. Philadelphia: WB Saunders, 1995;1245–1261.

with an administration set for transfusion. An open system is one with one or more additional sites of possible bacterial contamination, such as occurs when preparing for blood collection into syringes, ACD bottles, or bags to which anticoagulant is added after manufacture. An open system should be used only when a closed system is not available. The American Association of Blood Banks (AABB) advises that products stored in a refrigerator (1–6°C) that were collected into an open system be used within 24 hours and that platelet products stored at 20–24°C be used within 4 hours.[6] The shelf life of plasma from an open system is unaffected if it is frozen within 6 hours.[6] Despite the inconvenience, veterinary transfusion medicine should be subject to the same recommendations. Throughout the following sections, processing and storage will refer to closed systems unless otherwise specified.

BLOOD COLLECTION SUPPLIES

Commercial blood collection bags contain anticoagulant, and a sterile collection line with a needle (gauge 16 or 17) is attached to the bag. The bags are available as singles, doubles, triples, or quads, which indicate whether zero, one, two, or three empty satellite bags are attached via tubing to the primary bag. These satellite bags are used for the separation of components (see Separation Techniques).

Blood collection bags are available with a variety of anticoagulants and red blood cell nutrient solution additives. The anticoagulant is in the primary bag and, if present, the nutrient additive solution is in an attached satellite bag. After centrifugation and removal of plasma from the primary bag, the nutrient solution is added to the packed red blood cells (pRBCs) in the primary bag. When an additive is not used, a portion of the plasma must be left with the pRBCs for proper preparation of components (see Separation Techniques.) When an additive solution is to be used, complete removal of plasma from the pRBCs is possible.

Blood collection bags are available with anticoagulants CPDA-1, CPD, and CP2D. Bags with CPD contain the additive solutions Adsol (Baxter Healthcare Corporation, Fenwall Division, Deerfield, IL) or Optisol (Terumo Medical Corporation, Somerset, NJ). Bags with CP2D contain the additive solution Nutricel (Medsep Corporation, Covena, CA). Bags with CPDA-1 do not contain an additive solution.

Several different types of plastics are used in blood bag manufacture. Platelet products are most sensitive to these differences, which affect oxygen permeability and subsequently shelf life. Recommended bags for platelet products are CLX, PL-1240, and PL-732. These bags are actually inferior for pRBC storage but plasma storage is not affected.[7]

Canine

The standard commercially available blood collection bags are designed for the collection of 450 mL of blood. For the collection of amounts of blood less than 450 mL, the unwanted portion of the anticoagulant in the primary bag can be transferred before blood collection to an empty satellite bag; that bag is discarded after collection or separation. This technique allows collection of proportionately smaller units without excessive anticoagulant concentration. Bags are also now available for the collection of 225 mL units (Terumo Medical Corporation) with appropriate amounts of anticoagulant (CPD) and RBC preservative (Optisol).

Feline

Bags for collection of feline blood into a sterile system are not commercially available at present. Current open-system options include transfer of anticoagulant into an empty, sterile bag or set of bags and collection of blood into that bag via attached needle set (with or without suction), and transfer of anticoagulant into a syringe and collection of blood into the syringe via attached needle set. A closed system can be made in a fashion similar to that described for small-volume canine units, but *all* of the anticoagulant is transferred to a satellite bag that is then sealed. The anticoagulant remaining in the collection line is satisfactory for collection of a feline unit. However, the author finds the gauge and length of these needles to be prohibitively bulky when working with a feline jugular vein. The excessively large bags also cause the loss of a portion of the feline donation as a result of adherence to the bag.

If the blood is collected into a set of small sterile bags or into a syringe and then transferred to a set of small sterile bags (Pedi-Pak Pediatric Transfer Pack, National Hospital Specialties, Hackensack, NJ), components can be made. However, if an open system was used, the components are subject to the storage stipulations for any open system (see Blood Collection Principles.)

PREPARATION AND COLLECTION

Canine

A full blood unit contains 450 mL of blood, but 10% variation (405–495 mL) is acceptable. The specific gravity of whole blood is 1.053, so an ideal unit weighs 474 g and the acceptable range is 426–521 g.[6]

The jugular is the only site routinely used for blood collection. The author's choice position for the donor is in lateral recumbency on a table, with the head and neck placed on a pillow. If the donor is uncooperative in this position, sternal recumbency on a table, sitting on a table, sitting on the floor, or sternal recumbency on the floor are other options in order of decreasing desirability for the purposes of ease in restraint and rapidity of blood flow.

Once the donor is properly positioned and restrained, the hair over the desired site over the jugular is clipped and the site is surgically prepared. Further palpation of the jugular must be done above or below the prepared site to avoid contamination.

Blood can be collected into blood collection bags aided only by gravity and the donor's blood pressure, but the use of light suction quickens the pace and therefore facilitates the use of less cooperative donors. A technique devised by the Animal Blood Bank (Dixon, CA) is used by the author with excellent results.

The blood collection bag is hung from a hook inside a clear cylinder with a flat lid. The collection line with attached needle is brought through a notch between the cylinder and lid, and a hemostat is clamped on the line near the needle. A vacuum source is connected via tubing to an inlet in the chamber. The cylinder is placed on a scale, the scale is tared to zero, and the suction is adjusted to ≤5–7 inches of mercury for canine blood collection.[8] With one hand, the person who will draw the blood puts gentle pressure on the jugular below the prepared skin site, and the needle held in the other hand is inserted through the prepared site into the donor's jugular. When the hemostat is removed, blood flows into the collection line to the bag as the scale measures the grams of blood collected. When the desired amount has been obtained, pressure is released from the jugular below the venipuncture site, the hemostat is clamped on the line, and the needle is removed from the vein as the technician applies pressure over the site. If gravity alone is used to collect the blood, a third person should ideally be present to gently mix the blood with the anticoagulant, as this procedure is more prolonged.

During blood collection, the well-being of the donor should be constantly monitored. Mucous membrane color, pulse rate and strength, and respiratory rate are easily evaluated by the person drawing the blood. Donor attitude is also a useful indicator of potential problems. Any indication of donor compromise is cause for discontinuation of the collection.

Once the needle is removed from the donor, the blood in the line is stripped into the bag (Stripper/Sealer, Terumo Medical Corporation), the bag is gently mixed, and the line is sealed with aluminum clips or a thermal sealer. Alternatively, the line can be sealed without stripping the blood into the bag, and the blood in the line can then be used for testing.

Feline

Cats are routinely sedated for blood donation because of their often uncooperative nature during this procedure. Recommended protocols are discussed elsewhere.[1,3,5,9] Avoidance of hypotension is a major concern.

The sedated cat is positioned as desired (the author prefers lateral recumbency for the cat as well as for the dog) and the site over the jugular is prepared as described for the dog. If suction is being used, the procedure as described for the dog may be used, but using ≤3 inches of mercury has been suggested for use in the cat.[4] If a syringe is being used, only gentle suction is applied to avoid collapsing the vein or hemolyzing the blood.

Careful monitoring of the feline donor is essential because hypotension can be encountered despite all pre-cautions. Some institutions routinely give donors intravenous saline at a dose of 2 to 3 times the volume of blood drawn immediately after donation to avoid poor recovery.[3,5] Others only treat the donors if hypotension or symptoms of hypotension occur.

SEPARATION OPTIONS

Canine

Standard separation involves the preparation of plasma and pRBCs from whole blood (WB). This fresh plasma contains albumin, globulins, and maximum possible quantities of all coagulation factors, missing only the fraction that is unavoidably destroyed by collection and processing.[6,10] If this plasma is frozen within 8 hours of collection it is called fresh frozen plasma (FFP).[6] If the plasma is not frozen within 8 hours of collection, it can still be frozen and termed frozen plasma (FP). FP contains albumin, globulins, and adequate levels of the more stable factors, such as factors II, VII, IX, and X.[6,11]

Once frozen, FFP may be further processed into cryoprecipitate (cryo) and cryopoor plasma (cryoPP). According to studies of human cryo, cryo contains approximately 50% of factor VIII (VIII:C and von Willebrand's factor) and 20–40% of the fibrinogen from the original fresh plasma.[6]

Platelet products and pRBCs can also be made from WB if the blood is not refrigerated after drawing. These nonrefrigerated units must be made within 8 hours of collection.[6] Platelet-rich plasma (PRP) contains platelets, coagulation factors (although some of these rapidly deteriorate under the storage conditions for PRP), albumin, and immunoglobulins. PRP can be further processed into platelet concentrate (PC) and FFP if processed within 8 hours.

Feline

Feline blood, if collected into a set of sterile bags or transferred to a set of bags after collection (see Blood Collection Supplies), can be processed into components as described above. Limitations are incurred when the blood was collected into an open system, particularly with platelet products but also with pRBCs. Plasma storage, however, is unaffected. (See Principles of Blood Collection.)

SEPARATION TECHNIQUES

Canine

Standard: FFP or FP and pRBCs

Within 8 hours of collection, separation of WB into FFP and pRBCs must be complete, the plasma solidly frozen at −18°C, and the pRBCs chilled to 1–6°C.[6]

Standard separation of WB into pRBCs and plasma is begun by centrifugation of the set of blood collection bags in a refrigerated centrifuge at 5000 × g for 5 minutes.[6] The centrifugation time includes acceleration time but not deceleration time.

To transfer the plasma to a satellite bag, the segments of tubing connecting the primary bag to the satellite bags are clamped with hemostats. The seal in the tubing of the primary bag is broken and the bag is placed in a plasma extractor. One satellite bag is placed on a scale, and the scale is tared to zero. The plasma extractor gently squeezes the primary bag. The hemostat clamping the line between the primary bag and the bag on the scale is released, allowing plasma to flow into the satellite bag. The specific gravity of plasma is 1.023, so, for example, 120 mL of plasma weighs 123 g.[6] When the weight of the plasma in the satellite bag corresponds to the volume desired, the hemostat is clamped on the tubing and the plasma extractor is disengaged. The tubing at the top of the satellite bag will be used later to form samples for crossmatch procedures. Depending on the number of satellite bags in the set, plasma may be transferred entirely to one satellite bag or divided between one to three bags.

Bags containing CPDA-1 do not contain an additive solution. pRBCs in CPDA-1 must have a packed cell volume of 80% or less to have the full shelf life.[6] Therefore, a portion of the plasma must be left in the primary bag with the pRBCs. Bags containing CPD or CP2D have an attached satellite bag containing Adsol, Optisol, or Nutricel. All of the plasma can be removed from the pRBCs when using these systems, as the RBC additive solutions will provide the RBCs with the necessary fluid and nutrients.

Once the plasma has been removed to one or more satellite bags, the RBC nutrient solution, if available, is added to the pRBCs. The seal in the tubing to the additive bag is broken, and the solution is poured into the primary bag and gently mixed. If desired and if an additional empty satellite bag is available, half of the pRBCs can then be transferred to a separate bag.

The tubing attached to each component bag is sealed near its junction with the tubing segments of other bags. The plasma or pRBCs in the tubing should be saved for use in crossmatch procedures by making additional seals along the tubing and one adjacent to the bag, thus sequestering small samples in the tubing.

When the components are separated, each bag is labeled as to product, blood type, donor, dates of collection and expiration, and volume. Plasma units are placed into labeled cardboard plasma boxes (Baxter Healthcare Corporation). All components should be stored appropriately immediately after separation (see Storage).

Platelets

WB units to be used for the preparation of platelet products are stored at room temperature from the moment of collection and should be processed as soon as possible, but no longer than 8 hours from collection.[6]

Platelet processing is extremely sensitive to technique. For this reason, the AABB recommends establishing a protocol for each individual centrifuge by determining the platelet yield. This calculation and acceptable results are described elsewhere.[6] An acceptable starting protocol is to centrifuge at 2000 × g for 2.5 minutes at 20 to 24°C.[12] Alterations to this can be made based on results obtained with an individual centrifuge.

PRP is obtained by centrifuging a WB unit according to the established protocol just described. The PRP unit should be separated from the pRBCs immediately and the pRBCs should be refrigerated. PC and FFP can be made from PRP. The tubing between the PRP unit and an empty, attached satellite bag is temporarily obstructed by folding and securing with a rubber band. The two bags are centrifuged together at 5000 g for 5 minutes. Most of the supernatant plasma is transferred into the empty bag, leaving 35–70 mL of liquid in the original bag with the PC. The bags are separated and the plasma is stored as FFP if frozen within 8 hours of collection.[6] The PC is allowed to sit for 1 hour and then gently manipulated to resuspend the platelets.

Cryoprecipitate/Cryopoor Plasma

Cryo and cryoPP are made from already frozen FFP. When separating plasma from WB, if the unit is intended for further processing into cryo and cryoPP, the plasma is transferred into a satellite bag and an empty satellite bag is left attached via tubing. The tubing connecting the two is temporarily obstructed by folding and securing with a rubber band. The two bags are frozen together in a plasma box. After freezing, the unit is slowly thawed in a refrigerator at 1 to 6°C. When the unit reaches a slushy consistency, it is centrifuged at 5000 × g for 7 minutes and all but 10–15 mL of the liquid is transferred to the empty bag, leaving the precipitate and a small amount of fluid in the first bag. The bags are separated, and the liquid is labeled as cryoPP. The precipitate is labeled cryo, and both units are immediately refrozen.[6]

Feline

FFP and pRBCs can be made from feline WB if the blood is collected or transferred into a set of sterile bags. The WB is placed in one bag, and the tubing between this bag and an empty satellite bag is obstructed by folding and securing with a rubber band. If the bags being used are not designed to withstand centrifugation, they can still be centrifuged using a technique from the Eastern Veterinary Blood Bank. The bags are placed inside an empty standard blood bag whose top has been cut off. The bags are then bound to a bag of saline with rubber bands to keep the bags from collapsing. Centrifugation at 3000 × g for 10 minutes, which is contrary to the recommendations of the distributor of the bags, has been successful for separation in the author's experience.

STORAGE

RBC Products

Units of pRBCs should be stored at 1 to 6°C. Whereas a refrigerator with an alarm to indicate unsafe temperatures is ideal, minimally a thermometer stored in a container of fluid the volume of a small unit of pRBCs should be maintained and checked regularly. pRBC units should also be gently mixed twice weekly to maximize exposure to the preservative solution.[1,3]

RBC viability decreases with time. The AABB defines shelf life as the number of days after collection, assuming proper collection (closed system) and storage, at which 75% RBC viability is maintained. This viability is measured 24 hours after the transfusion is given.[6] Shelf life for canine pRBCs in a closed sytem of CPDA-1, CP2D and Nutricel, and CPD and Adsol is 20 days,[13] 35 days,[14] and 37 days,[15] respectively. A definitive shelf life for CPD and Optisol has not yet been researched using canine pRBCs. Human pRBCs in CPD and Optisol have a shelf life of 42 days;[6] however, it should be noted there can be significant differences between human and canine RBCs in different anticoagulants and preservatives.

Plasma Products

All plasma products should be stored at −18°C or lower. A freezer with an alarm to indicate unsafe temperatures is ideal. Known shelf lives are based on proper storage at this temperature. It may be logically assumed that shelf lives are shorter when plasma products are stored at warmer temperatures; if this is unavoidable, rapid turnover is recommended.

The shelf life of FFP is 1 year from collection.[6] The shelf life of FP is 5 years from collection.[6] After FFP has been stored for 1 year, it may be relabeled as FP and stored for 4 additional years.

The shelf life of cryo is 1 year from the date of collection, regardless of when during that year it was made from FFP.[13] CryoPP can be stored for a total of 5 years from the date of collection.[6]

Platelet Products

Platelet products are extremely sensitive to improper handling. PRP and PC have three requirements for maximal platelet survival and function: (1) storage at 20 to 24°C, (2) constant gentle agitation, and (3) storage in certain types of plastic bags (see Blood Collection Supplies). When collected into a closed system and under these specific conditions, the shelf life is 5 days.[11] If the unit was collected as an open system, shelf life is only 4 hours.[6]

QUALITY CONTROL

The best way to ensure high-quality blood components with maximal quantities of desired ingredients and minimal quantities of contaminants or deactivated ingredients is to precisely follow collection, processing, and storage protocol. Visual inspection before administration will help to identify units that were damaged in some way despite all efforts.

RBC Products

Units of pRBCs should not be removed from refrigeration needlessly. Each unit should be carefully evaluated as to color and texture. The presence of cloudy, purple, brown, or red supernatant, purplish red blood cell mass, clots, blood in the ports, or differences in color between the unit and the crossmatch tubing segments gives reason to suspect contamination.[6,16] If the unit was exposed to light such as through glass refrigerator doors, light-induced changes in bilirubin pigments may cause a greenish color.[11] If there was no light exposure, this color should cause concern.

Plasma Products

Properly prepared frozen plasma products may be rendered useless as a result of breakage or thawing. Storage of units in boxes will greatly reduce breakage but gentle handling is essential. Units should not be removed from the box until after thawing for administration, and inspection for cracks and leaks should occur at that time. Units with cracks or leaks should be discarded.

Thawing during storage may significantly reduce labile coagulation factors VIII:C, vWF, and XII.[10] Several techniques have been suggested to alert the staff that a unit was thawed after its original freezing: (1) Store the box initially laying flat in the freezer. After complete freezing, shift the box to sit on one end. Air bubbles present in the bag will move from the front edge to the upper edge of the bag if thawing occurs. The unit will also be thicker on the lower edge. (2) Place a rubber band around the unit before freezing, so that it makes an indentation in the bag. After complete freezing, cut the rubber band. If thawing occurs, the indentation left by the rubber band will be less obvious or will vanish. Units of FFP or cryo with evidence of thawing may have lost their labile factors.

Platelet Products

Proper preparation and handling as already described are the best ways to ensure an acceptable platelet yield and active platelets. Platelet units should not have grossly visible aggregates.[6]

CONCLUSION

Preparation of high-quality blood components requires great care and attention to detail. Lapses in proper protocol or storage mishaps may result in bacterial contamination, shortened shelf life, or decrease or absence of desired elements. Preparation of components must therefore only be attempted with proper equipment and a commitment to quality.

REFERENCES

1. **Brooks M.** Transfusion medicine, part I. In Proceedings of the American College of Veterinary Internal Medicine, Blacksburg, VA, 1990;8:77–80.
2. **Potkay S, Zinn RD.** Effect of collection interval, body weight, and season on the hemograms of canine blood donors. Lab Animal Sci 1969;19:192–197.
3. **Giger U.** Feline transfusion medicine. In: AE Hohenhaus, ed. Transfusion medicine (problems in veterinary medicine). Philadelphia: JB Lippincott, 1992;600–611.
4. **Kaufman PM.** Management of the feline blood donor. In: AE Hohenhaus, ed. Transfusion medicine (problems in veterinary medicine). Philadelphia: JB Lippincott, 1992;555–564.
5. **Cotter SM.** Blood Banking I: Collection and storage. In Proceedings of the American College of Veterinary Internal Medicine, Blacksburg, VA, 1988;6:45–47.
6. **Vengelen-Tyler V.** Technical manual, 12th ed. Bethesda, MD: American Association of Blood Banks, 1996.
7. **Schneider A.** Blood components: Collection, processing, and storage. In: AT Kristensen and BF Feldman, eds. Canine and feline transfusion medicine. Philadelphia: WB Saunders, 1995;1245–1261.
8. **Kaufman PM.** Transfusion supplies for dogs and cats. In: AE Hohenhaus, ed. Transfusion medicine (problems in veterinary medicine). Philadelphia: JB Lippincott, 1992;582–593.
9. **Bucheler J, Cotter SM.** Outpatient blood donor program. In: AE Hohenhaus, ed. Transfusion medicine (problems in veterinary medicine). Philadelphia: JB Lippincott, 1992;572–581.
10. **Anstall HR, Grove-Rasmussen M, Shaw RS.** Optimal conditions for storage of fresh frozen plasma. Transfusion 1961;1:87–93.
11. **Walker RH.** Technical manual, 11th ed. Bethesda, MD: American Association of Blood Banks, 1993.
12. **Clemmons RM, Bliss EL, Borsey-Lee MR, et al.** Platelet function, size and yield in whole blood and in platelet rich plasma prepared using different centrifugation force and time in domestic and food producing animals. Thromb Haemost 1983;50:838–843.
13. **Price GS, Armstrong PJ, McLeod DA, et al.** Evaluation of citrate-phosphate-dextrose-adenine as a storage medium for packed canine erythrocytes. J Vet Internal Med 1998;2:126–132.
14. **Wardrop KJ, Tucker RL, Mugnai, K.** Evaluation of canine red blood cells stored in a saline, adenine and glucose solution for 35 days. J Vet Internal Med 1997;11:5–8.
15. **Wardrop KJ, Owen TJ, Meyers KM.** Evaluation of an additive solution for preservation of canine red blood cells. J Vet Internal Med 1994;8:253–257.
16. **Kim DM, Brecher ME, Bland LA, et al.** Visual identification of bacterially contaminated red cells. Transfusion 1992;32:221–225.

CHAPTER 123

Red Blood Cell Transfusions in the Dog and Cat

• MARY BETH CALLAN

The term red blood cell (RBC) transfusion includes administration of packed red blood cells (pRBCs), fresh whole blood (FWB), or stored whole blood (SWB). The number of RBC transfusions administered to both dogs and cats has increased dramatically during the past 10 years[1,2] with the establishment of national commercial animal blood banks, as well as large donor programs at veterinary teaching hospitals. Concurrently, a move has occurred toward the more specific use of the pRBC component rather than FWB or SWB for initial treatment of anemia in the dog.[1,3] Such a change is a reflection of growing knowledge and expertise in veterinary transfusion medicine, which promotes the use of blood component therapy suited to a particular patient's needs, the benefits of which include more efficient use of blood and a decrease in potential adverse events associated with blood transfusion.

INDICATIONS

RBC transfusions are indicated in the treatment of anemia caused by hemorrhage, hemolysis, or ineffective erythropoiesis. Because oxygen is poorly soluble in plasma, nearly all oxygen contained in blood is carried by hemoglobin. Therefore, RBC transfusions increase the oxygen-carrying capacity of the anemic patient and, thus, treat or prevent inadequate delivery of oxygen to tissues, with consequent tissue hypoxia.[4] In two retrospective studies of RBC transfusions in dogs,[1,5] hemorrhage (acute or chronic) was the major cause of anemia in 70% of the dogs receiving RBC transfusions. In cats, the most common reason for RBC transfusion was ineffective erythropoiesis (46%), rather than hemorrhage or hemolysis.[2]

'Transfusion Trigger'

The decision to administer a RBC transfusion is usually based on measurement of the patient's packed cell volume (PCV), hematocrit (HCT), or hemoglobin (Hgb) concentration and, more importantly, on clinical evaluation of the patient. A 'transfusion trigger,' or threshold PCV below which a RBC transfusion is administered, has not been clearly defined in human or veterinary medicine. The concern regarding transmission of HIV and hepatitis C via blood transfusions has led to a significant decrease in the number of blood transfusions administered to humans in the United States during the past 15 years, as well as a lowering of the 'transfusion trigger' in a normovolemic anemic patient from an HCT of 30% and Hgb concentration of 10 g/dL to an HCT of 21% and Hgb concentration of 7 g/dL.[6] However, measurement of PCV alone is an inadequate determinant of the threshold for RBC transfusion because many additional factors (e.g., cardiac output and oxygen consumption) are involved in adequacy of tissue oxygenation. Also, in patients with hypovolemic anemia, the PCV is falsely elevated; as the total blood volume normalizes because of an increase in the plasma volume, the PCV decreases.[4] Animals with chronic anemia (e.g., anemia of chronic renal failure or iron deficiency anemia secondary to slow bleeding from an intestinal tumor) typically better cope with a lower PCV than do animals with an acute onset of anemia (e.g., an acute blood loss or hemolytic crisis) because of cardiovascular and other compensatory mechanisms. Because many factors can influence the need for a RBC transfusion, it is imperative that clinical judgement, not PCV, be the ultimate factor in the decision to administer RBCs to a patient. Tachycardia, poor pulse quality, pallor, lethargy, weakness, and decreased appetite are important clinical signs and symptoms that may indicate that a patient may be in need of additional oxygen-carrying support.

Whole Blood Versus pRBCs

Although administration of pRBCs is appropriate in the medical management of anemia resulting from any cause (i.e., hemorrhage, hemolysis, or ineffective erythropoiesis), whole blood (WB) transfusion may be considered in certain situations. By definition, FWB is blood that is less than 8 hours old from the time of collection and has not been refrigerated; therefore, FWB contains functional platelets, coagulation factors, and plasma proteins in addition to RBCs. Indications for FWB include anemia and a combined hemostatic disorder (e.g., DIC); anemia and thrombocytopenia or thrombopathia resulting in uncontrolled or life-threatening bleeding; and possibly massive transfusion (i.e., replacement of the patient's blood volume within a 24-hour period). SWB is more than 8 hours old; the length of storage depends on the anticoagulant/preservative solution used and varies from 48 hours for 3.8% sodium citrate (no preservative) to 4 weeks for CPD-A (citrate, phosphate, dextrose, and adenine). SWB contains plasma proteins and RBCs but not functional platelets or coagulation factors. A possible indication for SWB is anemia and hypoproteinemia (e.g., chronic gastrointestinal bleeding), although administration of pRBCs and, if there is a clinical need to increase the patient's oncotic pressure, a synthetic colloid or plasma (fresh or stored) would be appropriate. Given the loss of important blood components with storage, it is much more efficient to separate WB into pRBC and fresh frozen plasma than to store as WB.

As a result of the lack of a commercially available closed blood collection system for cats and the difficulty in preparing blood components from small WB units (typically 50 mL), anemic feline patients are more likely to receive FWB than pRBC.[2,7] However, the recent development of a closed blood collection system for cats will likely improve the quality of processing and storage of feline blood products.[7]

Fresh Versus Stored RBCs

Although storage of blood components allows for a readily available supply of RBCs for transfusion, it has been well-documented that RBCs develop a 'storage lesion' characterized by shape alterations, vesicle formation, and various biochemical alterations including decreased pH, ATP, and 2,3-diphosphoglycerate (DPG) concentrations, all of which ultimately affect RBC viability and function.[8] Addition of various preservative solutions containing dextrose, adenine, and phosphate—substrates for RBC energy metabolism—improve RBC posttransfusion viability.[8] A study of the effect of storage on canine pRBCs collected in citrate-phosphate-dextrose solution and resuspended in the additive solution Adsol (containing adenine, dextrose, saline, and mannitol) has documented a steady decrease in 2,3-DPG concentration (mean ± SD) from 15.2 ± 2.6 μmol/g Hgb on day 1 to 3.7 ± 1.9 μmol/g Hgb on day 44.[9] The reduction in RBC 2,3-DPG results in a decrease in the P_{50} value—the partial pressure of oxygen at which Hgb is 50% saturated with oxygen—of stored blood, thus increasing the Hgb-oxygen affinity and decreasing oxygen delivery to the tissues. Although a diminished release of oxygen to tissue from stored canine RBCs in comparison with fresh RBCs was demonstrated in an isolated hindlimb model in the dog,[10] a study comparing the effects of autologous

stored (21 days) red cells and freshly donated blood in restoring muscular tissue oxygenation after profound isovolemic hemodilution in dogs did not reveal a difference in tissue oxygenation between the two groups at comparable Hgb concentrations.[11] Regardless, the decrease in 2,3-DPG concentration in stored human and presumably other animal RBCs is a reversible change, with restoration of 2,3-DPG levels to 50% of normal within 7 to 24 hours posttransfusion.[8] Given the concern regarding possible impairment in oxygen delivery immediately postadministration of stored RBCs in comparison with fresh RBCs, the use of fresh RBCs (FWB or fresh pRBCs) has been recommended in certain clinical situations, e.g., a seriously ill and acutely anemic dog undergoing surgery. Such patients may also benefit from Oxyglobin®, a bovine Hgb solution with a low Hgb-O_2 affinity independent of 2,3-DPG. However, for the majority of dogs and cats in need of additional oxygen-carrying support, administration of stored RBCs is most appropriate. Decrease in erythrocyte 2,3-DPG concentration with storage is not an issue when transfusing cats because feline RBCs contain very low levels of 2,3-DPG and feline Hgb does not require 2,3-DPG for release of oxygen.

Red Blood Cell Transfusions in Immune-mediated Hemolytic Anemia

Although causes of anemia are discussed elsewhere in this text, a disease process that deserves mention with regard to RBC transfusion is immune-mediated hemolytic anemia (IMHA). IMHA is a disorder in which antibody bound to the surface of the RBC results in premature destruction of the patient's RBCs by macrophages. A widely held belief is that administration of RBCs to dogs with IMHA will "fuel the fire," or lead to accelerated destruction of RBCs and worsen the patient's overall condition. However, transfused RBCs are not more likely attacked by the autoantibodies than the patient's own cells. Furthermore, many dogs with IMHA are acutely and profoundly anemic (PCV <15%), which results in tissue hypoxia and failure, particularly when experiencing thromboembolic complications. During initial hospitalization, the reported mortality rate associated with IMHA is variable: 14%,[12] 29%,[13] and 41%.[14] In a retrospective study of RBC transfusions in dogs, IMHA accounted for 67% (29/43) of the dogs with hemolysis receiving RBC transfusions; 76% of the dogs with IMHA receiving RBC transfusions survived hospitalization.[1] In the study by Klag, 57% (24/42) of the dogs with IMHA received at least one blood transfusion, and no hemolytic transfusion reactions were observed.[13] Also, the incidence of mortality was not significantly different between dogs that received blood and those that did not, a remarkable finding given that the dogs receiving blood transfusions were more likely severely affected than those not receiving blood products.[13] RBC transfusions are, therefore, not contraindicated in patients with IMHA and are necessary in the successful medical management of many of these patients. Persistent autoagglutination precludes the ability to blood type the patient and perform a cross-match; therefore, it is safest to assume that the canine patient is DEA 1.1-negative and administer DEA 1.1-negative RBCs. However, because of the many canine blood types, the potential for RBC incompatibility reactions increases with repeated blood transfusions one week after the first transfusion.

ADDITIONAL BENEFITS OF RBC TRANSFUSIONS

RBC transfusions are an excellent source of iron, with 1 mL of blood containing 0.5 mg of iron, and thus are of benefit in the initial treatment of patients with severe iron-deficiency anemia. The iron in RBC transfusions is readily bioavailable, whereas oral absorption of iron is limited and continuous blood loss can worsen iron status. Alternatively, injectable iron may be used, but this is associated with pain and possibly anaphylaxis. Iron supplementation may have to be continued for months, and body iron stores may still remain marginal.

Enhanced hemostasis is an often overlooked benefit of RBC transfusions. A correlation between anemia and prolonged bleeding time has been reported in humans, and correction of the anemia results in shortening of the bleeding time.[15] The effect of HCT on the volume of blood shed during a bleeding time test can be dramatic: a reduction in HCT from 45 to 35% in normal, healthy humans resulted in a greater than two-fold increase in the volume of shed blood.[16] In human medicine, the clinical situation in which the hemostatic effect of RBCs is most apparent is chronic renal failure; administration of RBCs and erythropoietin to correct the anemia in uremic patients has resulted in improved platelet function, shortening of the bleeding time, and decreased frequency and severity of bleeding episodes.[17-19] One potential mechanism for RBCs leading to an improvement in primary hemostasis is the dispersion of platelets from the center of the blood vessel toward the endothelial cells of the vessel wall, facilitating the platelet-vessel adhesion.[15,17,19]

ADMINISTRATION

Careful attention to administration is essential to prevent damage of the blood product and harm to the patient. Prior to a RBC transfusion, blood typing and/or crossmatching should be performed to assure RBC compatibility. Segments of tubing from the donor blood bag may be used for the blood cross-match and for quality control and investigation of transfusion reactions. Storage of segments from the donor blood bag and the patient's serum/plasma at 1 to 6°C for 7 days following administration of an RBC product is recommended to aid in the laboratory investigation of adverse reactions noted after a blood transfusion has been completed.[20]

Canine pRBCs in a special RBC preservative solution such as Adsol can be administered directly, whereas other pRBC products should be diluted by adding 100 mL of saline to the blood bag, thus decreasing the viscosity of the donor blood. Concurrent administration of any drugs or fluids other than physiologic saline through the same catheter should be avoided to prevent blood coagulation and lysis of RBCs induced by contact with calcium-containing solutions and hypotonic solutions, respectively.

Warming of Blood

In the routine administration of RBC products to normovolemic anemic patients, refrigerated blood components do not require warming prior to transfusion; in fact, warming may accelerate the deterioration of stored RBCs and may permit rapid growth of contaminating microorganisms.[21] However, in patients that are hypothermic or receiving large volumes of blood, refrigerated RBC products should be prewarmed to temperatures between 22°C and 37°C immediately before transfusion to prevent exacerbation or development of hypothermia, the consequences of which may include cardiac arrhythmias and coagulopathies.[21] Blood units can be warmed by keeping the unit at room temperature for 30 minutes, placing the unit in a water bath not to exceed 37°C for 15 minutes, or running the tubing of the blood administration set through a warm water bath during the transfusion. In human medicine the most commonly used blood warmers are commercially available in-line warmers in which the IV tubing is immersed in water baths, with or without a countercurrent modification, or passed through dry heaters.[21] In the case of rapid RBC transfusion in humans, an admixture of warmed (70°C) isotonic saline with a unit of cold (4°C) pRBCs in a 1:1 dilution results in a diluted unit at 37°C without an adverse effect on osmotic fragility, plasma hemoglobin, or RBC survival in vivo.[21] Conventional microwave ovens and medical microwave warmers for thawing plasma are not designed for warming blood and can damage RBCs.[20] While it is typically unnecessary to warm blood for elective RBC transfusions at conventional rates, in situations requiring blood warming it is necessary to carefully monitor the temperature of the warming system to prevent RBC vesiculation and fragmentation, as well as hemolysis.

Blood Filters and Infusion Devices

RBC transfusions must be administered through a filter designed to remove clots and particles potentially harmful to the patient. Standard blood infusion sets have in-line filters with a pore size ranging from 170 to 260 μm that trap large cells, cellular debris, and coagulated proteins.[20] According to human blood banking standards, a filter may be used to administer two to four units of blood to a patient or for a maximum time limit of 4 hours; the combination of a high protein concentration at the filter surface and room temperature conditions promotes proliferation of any contaminating micro-organisms, and accumulated material slows the rate of flow.[20] Other blood filters with a pore size of 20 to 40 μm remove microaggregates composed of degenerating platelets, leukocytes, and fibrin strands that form in blood after 5 or more days of refrigerated storage, but a benefit to the routine use of microaggregate filters for low-volume transfusions has not been reported for humans.[20] Microaggregate filters are designed primarily for transfusion of RBCs, and a pediatric microaggregate blood filter with reduced dead space (Hemo-Nate Filter, Gesco International, San Antonio, TX) is particularly helpful in administering small volumes of blood to cats and small dogs. Special leukocyte reduction filters have recently received much attention in human blood banking because of the potential complications in transfusion recipients associated with residual white blood cells (WBCs) in cellular blood components, namely febrile nonhemolytic transfusion reactions, alloimmunization, transmission of infectious diseases, graft-versus-host disease, transfusion-related acute lung injury, and immunomodulation.[22] The frequency of adverse effects attributed to WBCs in blood products has not yet been well-documented in our veterinary patients. It remains to be seen if leukodepletion filters will be cost effective and play an important role in general RBC transfusions in dogs and cats.

In most instances the blood flow rate through an administration set by gravity alone is adequate to meet a patient's needs. Electromechanical infusion devices that deliver crystalloid or colloid solutions at a controlled rate have been evaluated for administration of blood. Depending on the pump design, many of the infusion devices may induce hemolysis, and some require special plastic disposables or tubing supplied by the manufacturer for use with blood.[20] In addition to pump design, the degree of hemolysis induced by mechanical pumps depends on the age of the blood (storage time), flow rates, and viscosity of the blood.[20,23] If considering the use of an infusion pump designed for crystalloid or colloid solutions to administer RBCs, the manufacturer should be consulted first. In the event that a blood flow rate greater than gravity can provide is needed, the rate may be increased by using an administration set with an in-line pump that the transfusionist squeezes by hand or by using a specially designed pressure bag that completely encases the blood unit and applies pressure evenly to the bag surface; pressures greater than 300 mm Hg may cause the seams of the blood bag to rupture or leak, necessitating close monitoring.[20] If blood is administered under pressure, large-bore catheters/needles are recommended for venous access to decrease hemolysis.

Route, Volume, and Rate of Transfusion

The intravenous route of administration is recommended for all RBC transfusions unless venous access cannot be obtained. Blood may be administered through peripheral (e.g., cephalic or saphenous) or central (e.g., jugular) vein catheters (16–22 gauge). Central lines are less positional and allow for the use of larger catheters and thereby more rapid transfusion in the case of hemorrhagic shock. However, peripheral veins may be preferred in animals with an increased bleeding tendency. The intraosseous route is an excellent alternative to the venous route because greater than 90% of donor RBCs enter the peripheral circulation within a few minutes of administration.[24] The intraperitoneal route of transfusion is no longer recommended because of the relatively slow and poor absorption of RBCs from the peritoneal cavity.

The volume of blood to be administered depends on the degree of anemia, the patient's clinical status, and the size of the animal. Similar to the transfusion trigger, a 'target PCV,' or the desired PCV posttransfusion, has not been clearly defined and is likely to vary depending on the patient's overall condition. It is typically not necessary to transfuse RBCs with the aim of restoring a normal PCV. Dogs and cats with chronic anemia may be cardiovascularly stable with a PCV of 20%, whereas those with an acute onset of anemia and ongoing blood loss or hemolysis may require transfusion to a higher PCV for stabilization. As a general guideline, administration of 2 mL/kg of WB will increase the patient's PCV by 1%, assuming that there is not ongoing hemorrhage or hemolysis. As an alternative to calculating the volume of donor blood required to reach a target PCV, one may administer an average volume of 10 mL/kg of pRBCs or 20 mL/kg of WB to a normovolemic dog and, if deemed necessary based on clinical evaluation of the patient posttransfusion, follow with additional blood. For practical purposes, most anemic cats will initially receive 1 unit of WB (typically 50 mL). If appropriately collected and stored, transfused compatible RBCs are expected to have a normal lifespan.[8,25]

The rate of blood administration depends on the patient's overall condition. In normovolemic anemic patients, the maximum rate of transfusion is 10–20 mL/kg/hr to avoid hypervolemia and pulmonary edema; hypovolemic anemic patients may tolerate replacement of their blood volume as quickly as the blood can be infused. In animals with cardiac failure, the infusion rate should not exceed 2–4 mL/kg/hr; pRBCs are preferable to WB in such cases where the transfusion volume tolerated by the patient may be a limiting factor in providing sufficient oxygen-carrying support. In all cases, including those in which the donor and recipient have been blood typed and/or crossmatched, the initial rate of transfusion should be slow (i.e., 2–3 mL during the first 5 minutes) while observing for any immediate adverse reactions. In general, a blood transfusion should be complete within 4 hours to ensure administration of functional blood components and to prevent growth of bacteria in the event of contamination.[20]

PATIENT MONITORING

Early recognition of transfusion reactions requires careful evaluation of the patient's attitude, vital signs, and perfusion (i.e., capillary refill time and pulse quality) before, during, and after a RBC transfusion. Measurement of PCV and total solids prior to and after (at least immediately and 24 hours after) transfusion and evaluation of the plasma and urine for the presence of Hgb is recommended. Any unexpected change in attitude, vital signs, or laboratory parameters may be indicative of an adverse reaction, in which case the RBC transfusion should be stopped immediately, the intravenous line left open with physiologic saline, and other supportive care provided as necessary (see Chapter 129 for a complete discussion of transfusion reactions).

It has been previously thought that equilibration of Hgb concentration after RBC transfusion in humans may take approximately 24 hours.[8] However, some recent studies in humans have provided data that Hgb and/or HCT measurements performed as early as 15 minutes posttransfusion reflect steady-state values in normovolemic patients not actively bleeding,[26] as well as in patients recovering from an acute bleeding episode.[27] Measurement of PCV in dogs and cats immediately posttransfusion and as clinically indicated during the following 24 hours is helpful in assessing ongoing blood loss or hemolysis.

Dogs and cats receiving RBC transfusions frequently have serious underlying diseases, reflected by a high mortality rate. In retrospective studies from two large institutions, the percentage of dogs receiving RBC transfusions and surviving hospitalization ranged from 47[5] to 61%[1]. However, the benefit of RBC transfusions in providing additional oxygen-carrying support to anemic dogs and cats is readily apparent. RBC transfusions can be lifesaving, provided that blood typing and crossmatching are performed to assure RBC compatibility and that donor blood is collected, stored, and administered according to blood banking guidelines.

REFERENCES

1. **Callan MB, Oakley DA, Shofer FS, Giger U.** Canine red blood cell transfusion practice. JAAHA 1996;32:303–311.
2. **Griot-Wenk ME, Giger U.** Feline transfusion medicine. In: AT Kristensen and BF Feldman, eds. Veterinary Clinics of North America, vol. 25. Philadelphia: WB Saunders, 1995.
3. **Stone E, Badner D, Cotter SM.** Trends in transfusion medicine in dogs at a veterinary school clinic: 315 cases (1986–1989). JAVMA 1992;200:1000–1004.
4. **Weiskopf RB.** Do we know when to transfuse red cells to treat acute anemia? Transfusion 1998;38:517–521.
5. **Kerl ME, Hohenhaus AE.** Packed red blood cell transfusions in dogs: 131 cases (1989). JAVMA 1993;202:1495–1499.
6. **Valeri CR, Crowley JP, Loscalzo J.** The red cell transfusion trigger: has a sin of commission become a sin of omission? Transfusion 1998;38:602–610.
7. **Springer T, Hatchett WL, Oakley DA, Niggemeier A, Giger U.** Feline blood storage and component therapy using a closed collection system. J Vet Intern Med 1998;12:248 (abstract).
8. **Mollison PL, Engelfriet CP, Contreras M.** Blood transfusion in clinical medicine, 9th ed. Oxford: Blackwell Scientific Publications, 1993;377–433.
9. **Wardrop KJ, Owen TJ, Meyers KM.** Evaluation of an additive solution for preservation of canine red blood cells. J Vet Intern Med 1994;8:253–257.
10. **Yhap EO, Wright CB, Popovic NA, Alix EC.** Decreased oxygen uptake with stored blood in the isolated hindlimb. J Appl Physiol 1975;38:882–885.
11. **Standl T, Horn P, Wilhelm S, Greim C, Freitag M, Freitag U, Sputtek A, Jacobs E, Schulte am Esch J.** Bovine haemoglobin is more potent than autologous red blood cells in restoring muscular tissue oxygenation after profound isovolaemic haemodilution in dogs. Can J Anaesth 1996;43:714–723.
12. **Day MJ.** Serial monitoring of clinical, haematological and immunological parameters in canine autoimmune haemolytic anaemia. J Small Animal Pract 1996;37:523–534.
13. **Klag AR, Giger U, Shofer FS.** Idiopathic immune-mediated hemolytic anemia in dogs: 42 cases (1986–1990). JAVMA 1993;202:783–788.
14. **Allyn ME, Troy GC.** Immune-mediated hemolytic anemia—a retrospective study: focus on treatment and mortality (1988–1996). J Vet Internal Med 1997;11:131 (abstract).
15. **Boneu B, Fernandez F.** The role of the hematocrit in bleeding. Trans Med Rev 1987;1:182–185.
16. **Crowley JP, Metzger JB, Valeri CR.** The volume of blood shed during the bleeding time correlates with the peripheral venous hematocrit. Am J Clin Pathol 1997;108:579–584.
17. **Livio M, Marchesi D, Remuzzi G, Gotti E, Mecca G, de Gaetano G.** Uraemic bleeding: role of anaemia and beneficial effect of red cell transfusions. Lancet 1982;2:1013–1015.
18. **Fernandez F, Goudable C, Sie P, Ton-That H, Durand D, Suc JM.** Low haematocrit and prolonged bleeding time in uraemic patients: effect of red cell transfusions. Br J Haematol 1985;59:139–148.
19. **van Geet C, Hauglustaine D, Verresen L, Vanrusselt M, Vermylen J.** Haemostatic effects of recombinant human erythropoietin in chronic haemodialysis patients. Thromb Haemost 1989;61:117–121.
20. **Vengelen-Tyler V, ed.** AABB technical manual. 12th ed. Bethesda, MD: American Association of Blood Banks, 1996.
21. **Iserson KV, Huestis DW.** Blood warming: current applications and techniques. Transfusion 1991;31:558–569.
22. **Bordin JO, Heddle NM, Blajchman MA.** Biologic effects of leukocytes present in transfused cellular blood products. Blood 1994;84:1703–1721.
23. **Stiles J, Raffe MR.** Hemolysis of canine fresh and stored blood associated with peristaltic pump infusion. Vet Emerg Crit Care 1991;1:50–53.
24. **Otto CM, Crowe DT.** Intraosseous resuscitation techniques and applications. In: RW Kirk and JD Bonagura, eds. Current veterinary therapy XI. Philadelphia: WB Saunders, 1992.
25. **Giger U, Bucheler J.** Transfusion of type-A and type-B blood to cats. JAVMA 1991;198:411–418.
26. **Wiesen AR, Hospenthal DR, Byrd JC, Glass KL, Howard RS, Diehl LF.** Equilibration of hemoglobin concentration after transfusion in medical inpatients not actively bleeding. Ann Intern Med 1994;121:278–280.
27. **Elizalde JI, Clemente J, Marin JL, Panes J, Aragon B, Mas A, Pique JM, Teres J.** Early changes in hemoglobin and hematocrit levels after packed red cell transfusion in patients with acute anemia. Transfusion 1997;37:573–576.

CHAPTER 124

Transfusion of Plasma and Plasma Derivatives

• MARJORY BROOKS

PLASMA CONSTITUENTS

Many proteins, carbohydrates, lipids, and electrolytes circulate in plasma, but the primary therapeutic constituents are hemostatic proteins, albumin, and immunoglobulins. The need for a single constituent predominates for most patients. Transfusion of plasma components, not whole blood (WB), is the most efficient and safest means for supplying the required protein. Recent advances in veterinary transfusion medicine have increased the availability of plasma and plasma derivatives, enabling their use in clinical practice.

Hemostatic Proteins

All of the clotting factors required for fibrin clot formation are present in plasma. Factors II, VII, IX, X, XI, and XII are serine protease enzymes, factors V and VIII are coagulation cofactors, and fibrinogen is the final substrate of the coagulation cascade reactions. The adhesive plasma glycoprotein, von Willebrand factor (vWF), is critical for platelet adhesion. Plasma anticoagulant factors include antithrombin and proteins C and S. Plasma also contains the fibrinolytic enzyme plasminogen and its regulatory proteins, tissue plasminogen activator, antiplasmin, and plasminogen activator inhibitor.

Albumin and Immunoglobulins

Albumin is the major oncotically active protein in plasma, present at a concentration of approximately 2 to 4 g/dL. Immunoglobulins circulate in canine and feline plasma at slightly lower concentration than albumin, with IgG representing the major class (up to 85%) and IgA and IgM comprising the remainder. Concentrated human albumin solutions (5–50 g/dL) and immunoglobulins (5–10 g/dL) are antigenic in animals, and the corresponding veterinary protein concentrates are not yet available.

PLASMA COMPONENTS

Centrifugation of WB separates heavier cellular elements from supernatant plasma. If centrifugation is performed within 4 to 6 hours of blood collection and blood has been maintained under refrigeration, then the supernatant retains the activity and concentration of all the plasma constituents in fresh WB. That supernatant can be immediately transfused as fresh plasma, but more frequently it is processed into components, such as fresh frozen plasma (FFP), frozen plasma (FP), cryoprecipitate, and cryosupernatant (Fig. 124.1). Optimum storage temperatures and maximum storage times for canine and feline components have not been determined. Current veterinary practice is adapted from techniques used for human plasma components.[1,2] All plasma products should be stored at or below temperatures of −20°C.

Fresh Frozen Plasma

FFP is separated from WB and frozen within 6 hours of collection. It contains equivalent amounts of all hemostatic proteins, albumin, and globulin as the plasma from which it was prepared. Stability of canine factor VIII and vWF was demonstrated in FFP after 10 months of storage at either −20°C or −70°C.[3] Pending additional studies, FFP should be transfused within 1 year of collection.

Frozen Plasma

Plasma that is separated from WB more than 6 hours after collection and then stored frozen is called frozen plasma (FP). This term also describes FFP that has been stored for more than 1 year. FP has low activity of the most labile coagulation factors (V and VIII) but is believed to retain activity of the vitamin-K-dependent factors (II, VII, IX, X) and albumin and immunoglobulin. FP is stored for up to 5 years.

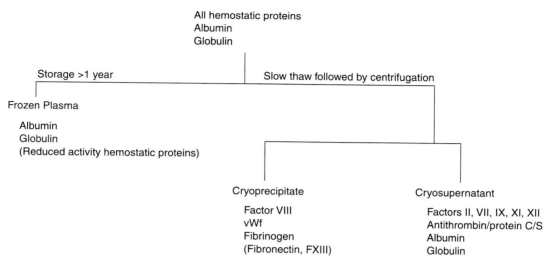

FIGURE 124.1 Composition of plasma products.

Cryoprecipitate

Cryoprecipitate is prepared by slowly thawing FFP at 1 to 6°C, and then centrifuging the partially thawed plasma to sediment the heavy, cold-insoluble proteins. The resultant cryoprecipitate contains factor VIII, vWF, fibrinogen, and fibronectin. The process of cryoprecipitation results in an average factor yield of approximately 50%, with reduction in volume to one-tenth that of the starting volume of FFP. Volume reduction is a major advantage of cryoprecipitate transfusion; therapeutic levels of factors are attained within minutes of a single intravenous bolus. Cryoprecipitate should be transfused within 1 year from the date of FFP collection.

Cryosupernatant

Cryosupernatant (cryosuper) or cryopoor plasma is the supernatant plasma remaining after production of cryoprecipitate. Cryosupernatant contains all clotting factors (except factor VIII and fibrinogen), anticoagulant and fibrinolytic factors, albumin, and immunoglobulins in a volume approximately equal to that of the starting FFP. Cryosuper should be transfused within 1 year for maximum factor activity, but transfusion for up to 5 years from the time of collection is believed to supply albumin, immunoglobulin, and some activity of vitamin-K-dependent factors.

INDICATIONS FOR PLASMA COMPONENT THERAPY

Plasma components are most often transfused to treat inherited and acquired hemostatic disorders and less frequently to supply albumin or immunoglobulin.[4] In each case, specific diagnosis enables selection of the optimum replacement product (Table 124.1). Diagnostic samples should be drawn before transfusion or at least 36 hours after transfusion to measure patients' endogenous plasma values. Cost and availability are additional factors to consider in designing specific treatment protocols.

Inherited Bleeding Disorders

Plasma components are transfused to control active hemorrhage or as preoperative prophylaxis. Appropriate transfusion of components often prevents red cell transfusion, thereby eliminating the risk of sensitization to red cell antigens.

von Willebrand disease (vWD) is the most common canine heritable bleeding disorder. The most clinically severe forms occur in dogs having no plasma vWF or a low concentration of vWF having an abnormal structure. Expression of milder forms of vWD is variable; some dogs experience repeated, spontaneous bleeding episodes and other dogs undergo surgery without complication. Clinical severity of vWD usually correlates with plasma vWF concentration, but history, in vivo bleeding time, breed, and concurrent disorders should all be considered when planning transfusion for individual dogs. Cryoprecipitate is the best product for treating or preventing hemorrhage in vWD-affected dogs. If cryoprecipitate is unavailable, FFP can be transfused to supply active vWF.[5]

Hemophilia is the most common inherited coagulation factor deficiency in dogs and cats. Hemophilia consists of two distinct forms: factor VIII deficiency (hemophilia A) and factor IX deficiency (hemophilia B). Both are X-linked recessive traits; therefore, hemizygous males express a bleeding tendency and heterozygous females are clinically normal. The transfusion require-

TABLE 124.1 Transfusion of Plasma and Plasma Components[a]

Product	Volume	Frequency	Indications
Fresh plasma Fresh frozen plasma	6–12 mL/kg	q8–12h	Inherited and acquired clotting factor deficiencies, vWD, DIC, hypoproteinemia, hypoglobulinemia
Frozen plasma	6–12 mL/kg	q8–12h	Hypoproteinemia, hypoglobulinemia
Cryoprecipitate	1 unit[b]/10 kg	q4–12h	Hemophilia (factor VIII deficiency), dysfibrinogenemia, hypofibrinogenemia, vWd
Cryosupernatant[c]	6–12 mL/kg	q8–12h	Hemophilia B (factor IX deficiency), inherited factor II, VII, X, XI deficiency, anticoagulant rodenticide toxicity, hypoproteinemia, hypoglobulinemia

[a]Transfuse plasma products at initial rate of 1–2 mL/min for all patients, maximum rate of 3–6 mL/min for adult dogs with normal cardiac function.
[b]One unit = cryoprecipitate prepared from 200 mL of FFP.
[c]Supernatant plasma remaining after cryoprecipitate preparation.

ments for hemophilia A and B differ. Cryoprecipitate is the best replacement therapy for hemophilia A. If cryoprecipitate is unavailable, then FFP can be used. Hemophilia B can be treated with either cryosupernatant or FFP. FP contains factor IX, but the biologic activity of factor IX after prolonged storage in animal plasma units is unknown.

Heritable deficiencies of other clotting factors (II, VII, X, XI, and fibrinogen) are less frequently identified in dogs and cats. Fibrinogen deficiency or dysfunction (dysfibrinogenemia) is best treated with transfusion of cryoprecipitate, or FFP if cryoprecipitate is unavailable. All of the other factor deficiencies can be treated with FFP or cryosupernatant.

Acquired Disorders

Acquired disorders are associated with simultaneous deficiencies of many factors, not with specific deficiency of a single factor. Acquired hemostatic defects are common and occur most frequently as a result of liver failure (production defect), vitamin K deficiency (activation defect), disseminated intravascular coagulation (consumption and localization defect), or severe, acute blood loss treated with crystalloid or colloid infusion (depletion/dilution defect).

Hepatic disorders most commonly associated with coagulopathy and therefore likely to benefit from transfusion include hepatic necrosis, cirrhosis, portosystemic shunt, and cholestasis. All of the procoagulant and anticoagulant factors, plasminogen, and albumin are synthesized in the liver, and transfusion with FFP will supply all of these proteins.

Vitamin K is required for a posttranslational modification of factors II, VII, IX, and X that enables these factors to participate in the coagulation cascade. Vitamin K deficiencies caused by anticoagulant rodenticide toxicity, biliary obstruction, and severe infiltrative bowel disease are most commonly associated with signs of coagulopathy. Transfusion (FFP or cryosuper) and vitamin K therapy are indicated to treat signs of hemorrhage in the respiratory tract or central nervous system.

Disseminated intravascular coagulation (DIC) is characterized by early systemic activation of coagulation, followed by secondary systemic fibrinolysis. The DIC process is always initiated by a primary disorder, most commonly sepsis, neoplasia, or vasculitis. Clinical signs of thrombosis, hemorrhage, or both may accompany DIC. Transfusion of FFP is indicated in the severe, hemorrhagic phase of DIC to replace hemostatic proteins. The thrombotic phase of DIC may be modulated by replacement of antithrombin and profibrinolytic factors through transfusion of cryosuper, a product that contains low concentration of procoagulant factors VIII and fibrinogen.

Circulatory shock caused by acute blood loss and then treated with crystalloid and/or colloid fluids may result in a secondary coagulopathy caused by depletion and dilution of factors. The best replacement product is FFP.

Hypoproteinemia caused by acute vasculitis, protein-losing nephropathies and enteropathies, hepatic failure or peritonitis, and hypoglobulinemia in neonates can be treated short-term with FFP, FP, or cryosuper transfusions. The benefit of replacement therapy is short lived. Specific and alternate treatment modalities must be administered concurrently for recovery.

GUIDELINES FOR TRANSFUSION OF PLASMA COMPONENTS

At present there are 4 commercial veterinary blood banks (Table 124.2) and additional university or regional blood banks that supply plasma products for in-house or local use. Because there are no accepted standards for unit size, potency, or processing techniques, veterinarians should contact their suppliers for details of quality assurance and quality control.

Plasma components are prepared in sterile plastic bags, and these bags are stored and shipped frozen in individual boxes. Plasma bags are brittle and must be handled carefully to prevent breakage. All FP products should be stored at temperatures of −20°C or lower,

TABLE 124.2	Veterinary Blood Banks[a]		
Blood Bank	**Location**	**Phone Number**	**Species**
Animal Blood Bank	CA	800-243-5759	Canine products
Eastern Veterinary Blood Bank	MD	800-949-3822	Canine products
Hemopet	CA	949-252-8455	Canine products
Midwest Animal Blood Services	MI	517-851-8244	Canine, feline products (and other species)

Information current July 1998.

and warmed to 37°C in a water bath or incubator immediately before administration. Unopened bags can be refrozen without significant loss of activity of labile factors,[6] but any product remaining in opened bags should be discarded if not transfused within 3 to 4 hours to prevent contamination.

Intravenous administration of plasma components is preferred, but intraosseous transfusion is an acceptable alternate route. Catheter sites should be aseptically prepared and components should be administered through blood filters. Plasma should never be mixed or allowed to come in contact with any fluid other than sterile, isotonic saline.

In the author's experience, routine treatment with corticosteroid or antihistamine is not required before plasma transfusion. The initial infusion rate should be 1 to 2 mL/min, with maintenance of this rate for cats, kittens, puppies, or recipients at risk for volume overload. The maximum infusion rate is 3 to 6 mL/min. Cryoprecipitates can be administered as a slow intravenous bolus over a period of 10 to 20 minutes.

The dose and frequency of transfusion varies for different products and different disease conditions (Table 124.1). In general, FFP, FP, and cryosupernatant are administered at 6 to 12 mL/kg, with maximum frequency of q8h. Cryoprecipitates are usually supplied in arbitrary 'units' based on the volume of FFP from which they were prepared. Each supplier must specify the volume to transfuse on the basis of recipients' body weight and disease process. High dose and short interval are most appropriate for initial transfusions, with reduction in volume and increase in interval as the patient responds. The high end of dosage range should be given as preoperative prophylaxis for animals having inherited bleeding disorders. The dose and frequency of postoperative transfusion depends on the severity of bleeding tendency. In general, animals affected with clinically severe vWD or clotting factor deficiencies should be transfused 4 to 6 hours postoperatively and then q8–12 h using the lower end of the dosage range for an additional 1 to 3 treatments. For most disease processes, plasma component transfusions are given for a period of 1 to 3 days.

PLASMA TRANSFUSION REACTIONS

Plasma component transfusions can be complicated by either immune or nonimmune adverse reactions.[7] Immune reactions are caused by a specific interaction between a constituent of the donor product and the recipient's immune system. Nonimmune reactions are caused by improper collection, processing, or administration techniques and are not specific to the donor–recipient pair. All plasma recipients should be observed during transfusion, and temperature, pulse, and respiration should be measured before and after transfusion. If there are any signs of discomfort or a change in clinical status during transfusion, the infusion should be immediately stopped and the product saved for analysis.

Clinical signs of immune reactions include fever, pruritus, urticaria, facial edema, erythema, pallor, dyspnea, and hypotension. These reactions may occur in response to a first transfusion or after many transfusions, usually within 15 to 30 minutes of initiating transfusion. The antigens or factors responsible for immune-mediated plasma reactions have not yet been identified in animals; however, cryoprecipitate rarely causes this complication. Treatment includes discontinuing transfusion and initiation of symptomatic or supportive care (Table 124.3). If needed, plasma from a different donor can be transfused after all signs have completely resolved.

Volume overload is the most common nonimmune transfusion reaction, caused by either too rapid a rate or too large a volume of transfusion. Clinical signs include emesis, vocalization, and dyspnea as a result of pulmonary edema. Cats, puppies, and cardiac-insufficient patients are most at risk for this complication. Transfusion of plasma products containing fibrin clot fragments, or precipitates formed by plasma contact with calcium or glucose-containing solutions, may cause signs of pulmonary edema, thrombosis, or DIC. Insufficient donor screening or contamination during processing or transfusion can result in transmission of infectious agents or sepsis in the recipient. More information on transfusion reactions is presented elsewhere in this section.

ALTERNATE AND ADJUNCT THERAPY

Supportive Care

Management practices can help to reduce transfusion requirements for animals having acquired and inherited bleeding disorders. Intravenous catheters are best placed in peripheral veins because catheterization of the jugular vein might cause perivascular hemorrhage and

TABLE 124.3	Management[a] of Plasma Transfusion Reactions	
Signs	**Differential Dx**	**Management/Treatment**
Fever	Immune response to platelet or WB antigens (donor or recipient antibodies)	Monitor Mild, transient: no treatment Severe, persistent: antipyretic, fluids If sepsis suspected: blood culture recipient; Gram stain/culture unit, intravenous fluid, antibiotic
Pruritus, urticaria, erythema, facial edema	Acute, hypersensitivity response to donor proteins (immunoglobulin, other plasma proteins)	Diphenhydramine (1.0–2.0 mg/kg) Dexamethasone (0.5 mg/kg) or Prednisone (1 mg/kg)
Pallor, hypotension, shock	Complement activation Vasoactive mediators in plasma product	Intravenous fluid (10–20 mL/kg) Dexamethasone sodium phosphate (1–2 mg/kg)
Dyspnea, emesis, cough (pulmonary edema)	Volume overload	Monitor Mild volume overload: resume transfusion at slower rate If severe signs: furosemide (2–5 mL/kg), O_2, ventilation, consider dopamine, hetastarch infusion
	Pulmonary microaggregates/increased pulmonary vascular permeability	

[a]The first step in any suspect reaction is to STOP transfusion (save unit for further evaluation).

interfere with respiration. The oral route of drug administration is preferred. Avoid intramuscular injections and invasive diagnostic procedures. Electrocautery, small vessel ligation, multilayer closure of incisions, and application of pressure wraps help to minimize hemorrhage from wounds. Topical tissue adhesive is useful for treating small cutaneous or mucosal wounds, provided hemorrhage is first controlled with direct pressure and tissues are dry. Cage confinement to limit activity is indicated during initial treatment periods. Do not administer drugs that might further impair hemostasis, including nonsteroidal anti-inflammatory drugs, sulfa drugs, and dextrans.

Drug Therapy

Drugs cannot replace the need for active hemostatic proteins. Human recombinant and plasma-derived clotting factor concentrates induce an antibody response when transfused in animals and are much more expensive than animal plasma products.

Desmopressin (DDAVP; 1 ug/kg SQ; ½ hr before surgery) has been described as preoperative prophylaxis for Doberman pinschers affected with vWD.[8] Close monitoring is indicated to determine duration and extent of response, and cryoprecipitate or FFP should be readily available if response to desmopressin is inadequate. Desmopressin is not indicated as treatment or prophylaxis for severe vWD or hemophilia.

Vitamin K deficiency is treated using vitamin K_1 (not vitamin K_3). A parenteral dose of vitamin K_1 (2.2 mg/kg SQ), followed by a dose of 1.1 mg/kg q12h is usually sufficient for initial therapy, with correction of coagulopathy seen within 1 to 2 days. Poisonings caused by ingestion of second-generation rodenticides can be treated using a tapering dosage schedule of oral vitamin K_1 (1.1 mg/kg q12h for 2 weeks; 1.1 mg/kg q24h for 2 weeks; 0.5 mg/kg q24h for 2 weeks).

Heparin may be useful in management of diseases associated with venous thrombosis, pulmonary thromboemboli, and the early or thrombotic phase of DIC. Safe and effective treatment regimens have not been documented in controlled veterinary trials. A frequently used heparin dose is 100 U/kg SQ q6–8h with monitoring to obtain a target prolongation of activated partial thromboplastin time to 1.5× pretreatment value.

Colloid administration (dextrans, hetastarch, oxypolygelatin) is useful for volume resuscitation. Hetastarch (up to 40 mL/kg/day), a high-molecular-weight colloid, is used to maintain intravascular oncotic pressure and minimize or eliminate the need for plasma transfusion in hypoproteinemic animals or in animals with inflammatory disease causing increased capillary permeability and hypovolemia. Infusion of a hemoglobin-based, oxygen-carrying solution (Oxyglobin; 30 mL/kg) may be useful to replace red cell and plasma transfusion requirements for animals with acute blood loss anemia.

The demand for plasma and plasma products has increased and will continue to increase as veterinarians gain experience in their use. The challenge now is for clinicians and researchers to develop controlled studies to optimize methods for plasma component production, clinical trials to determine safe and effective treatment protocols, and alternate therapies to ensure sufficient supply of plasma resources.

REFERENCES

1. **Mooney S.** Preparation of blood components. Problems in veterinary medicine. Trans Med 1992;4:594.
2. **Allain JP, Griedli H, Morgenthaler JJ, et al.** What are the critical factors in production and quality control of frozen plasma intended for direct transfu-

sion or for fractionation to provide medically needed labile coagulation factors? Vox Sanguinis 1983;44:246.

3. **Stokol T, Parry BW.** Stability of factor VIII and von Willebrand factor antigen concentration in the frozen state. Res Vet Sci 1995;59:156.

4. **Wardrop KJ.** Medical indications for plasma therapy. Proceedings of the 14th ACVIM forum. San Antonio, TX: 1996:31.

5. **Brooks M.** Emergency management of canine von Willebrand disease. Proceedings of the 14th ACVIM forum. San Antonio, TX: 1996:34.

6. **Stokol T, Parry BW.** Stability of von Willebrand factor and factor VIII in canine cryoprecipitate under various conditions of storage. Res Vet Sci 1995;59:152.

7. **Harreli KA, Kristensen AT.** Canine transfusion reactions and their management. Vet Clin North Am 1995;25:1333.

8. **Kraus KH, Turrentine MA, Jergens AE, et al.** Effect of desmopressin on bleeding time and plasma von Willebrand factor in Doberman pinscher dogs with von Willebrand disease. Vet Surg 1989;18:103.

CHAPTER 125

Platelet and Granulocyte Transfusions

• ANTHONY C.G. ABRAMS-OGG

PLATELET TRANSFUSION

Platelet transfusion is potentially indicated in the management of bleeding caused by thrombocytopenia and thrombocytopathia. Platelet transfusion has not been widely used in small animal medicine, and most reports concern experimental bone marrow transplantation. This reflects the reduced utility of platelet transfusion in immune-mediated thrombocytopenia (ITP), the restricted use of aggressive cytotoxic therapy for cancer, and the cost and historically poor prognosis of treating acute leukemia, aplastic anemia, and disseminated intravascular coagulation. However, with the use of more aggressive anticancer therapy and the increased willingness to treat complex hematologic disorders, there is an increasing need for platelet-rich blood products.

Donor Selection and Blood Donation

Blood donation is discussed in more detail elsewhere in this section. Donor blood type is important because platelet-rich products contain red blood cells. Donors should have platelet counts above 200,000/μL. If there is anticipated need for intensive platelet transfusion, such as occurs with bone marrow transplantation, vincristine (Oncovin, Eli Lilly and Co, Indianapolis, IN) at 0.02 mg/kg IV can be used to raise canine donor platelet counts. Platelet counts will rise by 35 to 45% 8 days postinjection.[1] Routine administration of vincristine to donors is not recommended because of the drug's potential for causing hematologic, gastrointestinal, and neurologic disorders and because this practice increases exposure of personnel to cytotoxic waste. Recombinant human interleukin-11 (Neumega, Genetics Institute, Cambridge, MA) can be used at 50 μg/kg SC daily for 7 to 14 days to increase canine donor platelet counts by the same increment as occurs with vincristine.[2] The drug's cost and formation of antibodies against it preclude its routine use.

Femoral artery or jugular vein collection may be used for dogs, with the latter using gravity or vacuum assistance. If platelet products are to be stored, a closed collection system should be used that includes the appropriate satellite bags and CPD or CPDA-1 as the anticoagulant-preservative solution. The collecting bag should be gently and continuously rocked during collection. If this is not possible during vacuum collection, the bag should be hung upside down in the vacuum chamber such that the blood is forced to pass through the anticoagulant-preservative solution. Glass vacuum bottles should not be used because glass inactivates platelets. Blood is preferably collected in less than 15 minutes, although blood collected over longer periods may still be adequate to prepare platelet-rich products.[3,4] Cat blood and small-volume dog donations may be collected with a 60-mL syringe containing the anticoagulant-preservative solution.

Platelet Products

Platelet-rich products include fresh whole blood (FWB), platelet-rich plasma (PRP), and platelet concentrate (PC). These products are prepared and stored at room temperature (20–24°C) because of the deleterious effects of chilling on platelets.[5-7] Platelet-rich products should be handled gently to minimize platelet activation, which impairs platelet viability (defined as posttransfusion circulation time).

FWB is whole blood less than 8 hours old. It contains a maximum number of functional platelets if kept at room temperature. If whole blood (WB) has been refrigerated (4°C), it is best used for platelet transfusion within 6 hours.[5-7] Platelets refrigerated for up to 24 hours have normal-to-increased immediate hemostatic efficacy, but markedly reduced viability after 6 to 8 hours. After 24 hours of refrigeration, viability is less than 10%; hemostatic efficacy is lost by 72 hours.

PRP is prepared by centrifugation of FWB. The FWB should rest at least 1 hour after collection to minimize platelet activation, and the bag should be gently massaged before centrifugation to resuspend platelets. Preparation of PRP from refrigerated WB is not recommended. If no other WB is available, refrigeration time should ideally be less than 6 hours and the PRP should not be stored. (Special techniques to prepare human platelet products from WB refrigerated for 1 to 5 days have been described, but are not standard procedure.[8]) Centrifugation to make PRP uses lighter gravitational forces than that used to separate red cells and plasma. This isolates most of the platelets in the plasma, with a higher concentration of platelets near the buffy coat. The plasma is expressed into a satellite bag, resulting in PRP. Stopping the expression when the red cell-plasma interface is 1 cm from the top of the bag will minimize leukocyte and red cell content of PRP while not sacrificing too many platelets.[3,9] One unit of WB (450 mL) yields one unit of PRP.

Percent platelet yield (platelets in PRP/platelets in WB × 100) and PRP platelet count vary with the donor, donor platelet count, blood volume being centrifuged, technician, centrifuge, and centrifugation protocol.[4,9] In a study comparing protocols to make PRP from small volumes of dog blood, protocols with shorter centrifugation times and higher gravitational forces had better yields than did protocols with longer times and lower forces.[10] A number of centrifugation protocols to make PRP for transfusion have been reported. Most current protocols use approximately 1000 × g for 4–6 min[3] (Callan B, Dodds J, personal communications) or 2000–2500 × g for 2.5 to 3 min[11,12] (Hale A, Thompson J, Wardrop J, personal communications). The centrifugation time is measured from the start of acceleration to the start of deceleration. The brake on the centrifuge should be turned to a low setting or turned off. Results with most protocols have not been reported. In the protocol used by the author (1000 × g for 4 min), average yield is approximately 80% (range 35–97%), resulting in a mean of 6×10^{10} platelets/unit (range of $3–10 \times 10^{10}$ platelets/unit).[3,9] A second centrifugation of the WB can be used to increase yield and is particularly useful with greyhounds, which have low normal platelet counts (Dodds J, personal communication). Good quality PRP will swirl intensely when agitated.

PC is prepared by centrifugation of PRP. A higher gravitational force is used than in preparing PRP, resulting in pelleting of nearly all the platelets. The platelet-poor plasma (PPP) is expressed, leaving 35 to 70 mL of plasma and the platelet pellet behind in the satellite bag. The resulting PC is left undisturbed for 60 to 90 minutes to promote disaggregation. Macroscopic leukocyte-platelet aggregates are dispersed and platelets are resuspended by gentle manual kneading and agitation. The PPP may be used as fresh or fresh frozen plasma (FFP). If PRP has been made using 1000 × g for 4 minutes, the typical centrifugation protocol to make PC is 2000 × g for 10 minutes. If PRP has been made using 2000–2500 × g for 2.5 to 3 minutes, the typical centrifugation protocol to make PC is 4000–5000 × g for 5 to 6 minutes. Most platelet loss occurs in PRP preparation, and the various centrifugation protocols to make PC from PRP are probably equivalent. One unit of PRP yields one unit of PC. Protocols for preparing human PC from WB by differential centrifugation are considered to be satisfactory if 75% of PC units contain more than 5.5×10^{10} platelets.[4] Units of PC can be pooled via transfer tubing. The pooled units are centrifuged at 570 × g for 15 minutes and PPP is expressed, leaving behind 8 to 10 mL per unit pooled (Wardrop J, personal communication).

Another method of preparing human PC by centrifugation uses a higher gravitational force to force platelets into the buffy coat.[13] The platelets are separated from the buffy coat by a second centrifugation. This method increases platelet yield per unit and may reduce platelet activation but has not been reported in dogs.

Plateletpheresis may also be used to prepare PC.[4] In a study using 10–24 kg beagles,[14] PC volume was 148–322 mL, platelet count was $1.26–2.95 \times 10^{11}$ platelets/PC, leukocyte concentration was $1–7 \times 10^7$/L, and red cell concentration was less than $1–2 \times 10^{10}$/L. Preparation time was 51 to 104 minutes. Donor platelet counts dropped to a median of 140,000/μL (minimum value 60,000/μL) by the end of the procedure, and returned to initial values after 4 days. Donor ionized calcium levels dropped during preparation, but clinical signs of hypocalcemia did not occur.

In contrast with dogs, cat PRP is best prepared using longer centrifugation times and lower gravitational forces.[10] In a protocol with documented utility in vivo,[15] FWB was transferred to 50-mL polypropylene tubes (small volume bags could also be used). Following a 30-minute sedimentation period, the tubes were centrifuged at 150 × g for 10 minutes and the PRP was aspirated. (Sedimentation alone has also been used to prepare cat PRP). The 60-mL collecting syringe is held vertically for 1 hour, at which time the PRP is expressed.) To make PC, PRP pooled from three units was centrifuged at 1100 × g for 10 minutes, and PPP was aspirated. The platelet pellet was left undisturbed for 60 minutes and then gently resuspended in 5 mL of PPP. Postfiltration yield was 60%.[15]

Vincristine-loaded platelets (VLP) are a unique platelet product used in the treatment of ITP. VLPs are produced by incubating platelets with vincristine. The platelets act as a drug carrier because they are rich in tubulin, which avidly binds vincristine. On transfusion to patients with ITP, the VLP are engulfed by the macrophages responsible for platelet destruction and release the drug intracellularly. The macrophages thus receive a higher dose of vincristine than is possible with bolus injection, maximizing cytotoxic effects in macrophages while minimizing cytotoxic effects in other cells. The cytotoxic effects inhibit macrophage function.[16]

In the first report in dogs,[16] 100 mL of PRP containing 2.5×10^{10} platelets were incubated with 3 mg vincristine for 1 hour at 37°C in the dark under continuous rotation. The PRP was centrifuged to produce a 35-mL volume PC, which was transfused over 30 minutes. The recipient was a dog with recurrent ITP refractory to therapy with prednisone and splenectomy. The dog showed prompt and sustained response. Similarly, seven dogs with acute refractory ITP given VLP showed prompt and sustained responses (unpublished observations). However, the apparent response to VLP may have been coincidental. In all cases dogs were receiving concurrent therapy, and the same dose of VLP was used to treat 9- to 30-kg dogs. The original protocol was extrapolated from human medicine, and there are no comparative data on the uptake of vincristine by human and dog platelets.

Storage

Recommendations allow room temperature storage of WB for 8 hours, PRP for 3 days, and PC for 5 days.[4] Bags approved for 5-day storage of human platelets are recommended for dog components.[3] Components are stored under continuous agitation; end-over-end, elliptical, and to-and-fro agitation are standard.[3,4] A tilting blood sample rocker could be used for short-term storage if other agitators are not available. Interruption of agitation of human PC (e.g., during shipment) for up to 24 hours has minimal effects on PC quality.[17] Indeed, manual agitation every 24 hours has been reported to be equivalent to continuous agitation.[17] It is likely, therefore, that the current practice of veterinary blood banks to ship fresh dog PRP without agitation does not impair platelet hemostatic properties.

During storage, physical and metabolic changes referred to as the storage lesion occur, which compromise platelet viability and function.[3,4] Optimal storage conditions for human PC to minimize the storage lesion have been the focus of continuous investigations.[3,4] Numerous tests have been used to evaluate platelet quality, including (in decreasing order of preference) correction of bleeding in thrombocytopenic and thrombocytopathic patients, viability, platelet morphology scoring, response to hypotonic stress, metabolic assessment, and aggregation.[3,9]

Few studies have investigated storage of dog and cat platelets. Dog PC was stored for 7 days with to-and-fro agitation while maintaining platelet numbers, metabolic activity, and pH above 6.0, a standard for human PC storage.[3] The author has similarly stored PRP for up to 7 days while maintaining acceptable pH and platelet counts (unpublished observations). Storage of cat PRP or PC for transfusion has not been reported.

Cryopreservation may be used to store dog PC for 6 months or longer. Platelets are cryopreserved using a cryoprotectant solution in approved plastic bags at a freezing rate of 1 to 3°C/min. In general, cryopreserved platelets have reduced function and viability compared with platelets stored at room temperature.[4] Dog platelets cryopreserved in 6% dimethyl sulfoxide were shown to be hemostatically effective in vivo[18] but severely damaged based on in vitro assessment.[3] The discordant results may reflect in part the poor predictive value of in vitro tests on in vivo function. Dog platelets cryopreserved in polyethylene glycol-dimethyl sulfoxide[19] were effective in controlling bleeding in basset hounds and otter hounds with thrombocytopathia and in dogs with ITP (Dodds J, personal communication).

Lyophilization has recently been reported for long-term storage of canine platelets[20] and for preparing infusible platelet membranes (a platelet transfusion substitute) using a proprietary freeze-thaw process.[21] Liposome-encapsulated platelet membrane fractions[22] and other platelet substitutes are being developed.

Transfusion

Platelet transfusion is most useful in thrombocytopenia caused by decreased platelet production, where transfused platelet lifespan is normal. It is clinically most rewarding when prompt marrow recovery is anticipated, e.g., following anticancer chemotherapy. Platelet transfusion is less beneficial in disseminated intravascular coagulation (increased platelet consumption) and splenomegaly (increased platelet sequestration), but should be given if the patient is bleeding. Platelet transfusion is least beneficial in ITP because transfused platelets may be rapidly destroyed. However, platelet transfusion should be considered in critical patients, as even a transient benefit may be life-saving. Platelet transfusion is of benefit in most cases of thrombocytopathia.

Platelet transfusions should be given using standard transfusion sets and 170-μm filters. Transfusion sets should be free of latex, which can bind platelets. Most infusion pumps will not damage platelets, but the manufacturer should be consulted in this regard.

The success of a platelet transfusion is judged by control of hemorrhage and by comparing the expected and measured 1-hour platelet increment.[9] If the transfusion was beneficial, active hemorrhage will be reduced. If bleeding is well-controlled, existing petechiae and ecchymoses will fade over 12 hours. The 1-hour platelet increment refers to the difference between recipient platelet counts before and 1 hour after transfusion. The expected 1-hour platelet count in the dog is calculated as follows:

Expected 1-hour platelet count ($\times 10^9$/L) =

$$\frac{\substack{\text{Platelet count pretransfusion} \\ (\times 10^9/\text{L}) + \text{unit platelet count} \\ (\times 10^9/\text{L}) \times \text{unit volume (L)} \times 0.51}}{\text{Recipient weight (kg)} \times 0.085 \,(\text{L}/\text{kg})}$$

where 0.085 $\times$ weight = estimated blood volume and 0.51 corrects for splenic sequestration of transfused platelets.[9,23]

If the measured platelet count is much below the expected count, there is accelerated platelet loss (destruction or consumption) or sequestration. If there is minimal platelet production but no accelerated platelet loss or sequestration, the recipient's platelet count should drop by 33% each day following transfusion. When interpreting the success of a platelet transfusion, it should be noted that platelet counts at low values are imprecise.

FWB is the only platelet-rich product available to many veterinary clinics. As a rule-of-thumb, a FWB transfusion of 10 mL/kg will raise the recipient's platelet count by approximately 10,000/μL and will stop critical hemorrhage if there is no ongoing platelet loss. (Transfusion of red cells may also reduce bleeding time in anemic patients independent from a transfused platelet effect.) The transfusion is given over 1 hour unless a slower rate is indicated.

Because large-volume transfusions are required to substantially raise platelet counts, polycythemia will result if FWB is used for chronic platelet support. Increased blood viscosity and altered rheology may be detrimental in septic animals (ideal PCV − 30%) or those at risk for thrombosis and ischemia. Phlebotomy at an initial volume of 20 mL/kg may be necessary. Repetitive red cell transfusions may also delay marrow recovery following irradiation.[9]

The initial dose for PRP or PC is one unit per 10 kg. If the units contain on average 6×10^{10} platelets, the 1-hour platelet increment should be 30,000 − 35,000/μL, if there is no ongoing platelet loss. PCs are transfused over 1 hour and PRP at 10 mL/kg/hr, unless a slower rate is indicated. PC is preferred for chronic support because hyperproteinemia may result from multiple PRP transfusions.

If a platelet-rich product is not available, the patient should be transfused with FFP (10 mL/kg) or cryoprecipitate (1 unit/10 kg). These products contain hemostatically functional platelet microparticles and have been beneficial in humans and dogs in treating bleeding caused by platelet disorders.[24]

Platelet transfusion may be cost prohibitive, especially in large dogs, and it may not be necessary to raise the platelet count by large increments. Critical hemorrhage can usually be prevented by transfusions to keep the platelet count above 10,000–15,000/μL. Transfusing when hemorrhage is detected will consume less blood products than prophylactic transfusion[4,9] but requires close patient monitoring and a readily available blood supply.

Transfusion Reactions

Transfusion reactions and their treatment are discussed in greater detail elsewhere in this section. Febrile transfusion reactions are the most common reaction to PC, and are more likely to occur when transfusing PC containing high numbers of leukocytes.[9,25] The reactions are usually not severe but do affect patient well-being and cannot be immediately distinguished from sepsis.

Platelet alloimmunization is a concern with repetitive transfusions and can be minimized by changing donors.[23] Repetitive transfusion from the same donor carries an 86% risk of alloimmunization following 2.4 ± 2.1 transfusions.[26] In contrast, with repetitive transfusions from multiple unrelated donors, the risk of alloimmunization to all donors is 60% after 14 ± 5 transfusions.[23] The alloimmunization can be abrogated by cyclosporine[27] but not by prednisone or cyclophosphamide.[26] Leukocyte depletion using special centrifugation bags or white cell filters may retard the onset of alloimmunization,[4,9] but these are expensive to use. Platelet crossmatching could theoretically be performed by a laboratory offering antiplatelet antibody tests for ITP, but the predictive value is not consistently high.[4] Other experimental modalities to reduce alloimmunization include ultraviolet irradiation[27] and use of platelet substitutes.

Transfusion-associated graft-versus-host disease may result from T lymphocytes present in blood products.[4] It has not been described in veterinary cases but has probably occurred. It is a concern when transfusing severely immunosuppressed patients, especially during bone marrow transplantation, where platelet-rich products (which contain leukocytes) should be irradiated with a minimum dose of 2500 cGy.[4]

Storage of PC at room temperature increases the risk of bacterial contamination.[4] Dog PRP and PC have been stored at room temperature without microbial growth,[3] but any veterinary blood bank should closely monitor such products microbiologically.

GRANULOCYTE TRANSFUSION

Granulocyte transfusion is potentially indicated in the treatment of neutropenic sepsis. Neutrophils have short circulation and tissue residence times. These times are even shorter during sepsis, such that transfused neutrophils are rapidly consumed. Nonetheless, a transient increase in neutrophil numbers to a critical level may permit survival in otherwise fatal sepsis.

Granulocyte concentrate (GC) is usually prepared by continuous-flow centrifugation leukapheresis.[28–30] Addition of synthetic colloid facilitates erythrocyte-leukocyte separation in humans and dogs but is not needed in horses, which have a rapid erythrocyte sedimentation rate.[31] Filtration leukapheresis has a higher yield but causes more cell damage and has fallen out of favor.[28–30] Granulocytes may also be obtained from single units of FWB.[32] Six-percent hetastarch (Hespan, DuPont Pharma, Wilmington, DE) is added in a 1 to 8 ratio to a unit of FWB. After a 1-hour sedimentation period, the plasma and buffy coat are expressed into a satellite bag, which is centrifuged at $5000 \times g$ for 5 minutes at room temperature. The plasma is then expressed, leaving the granulocytes in 20 mL of plasma.[32] Because of a rapid erythrocyte sedimentation rate, cat granulocytes could be obtained by sedimentation without synthetic colloid. Granulocytes may be stored at room temperature without agitation for 24 hours.[4] Exchange transfusion is an alternative means of providing granulocytes to neonates.[33]

Granulocyte transfusion was promoted in the 1970s and early 1980s. Usage then declined in humans because of expense, febrile reactions, controversial benefit, and newer antibiotics.[29] The recent availability of granulocyte colony-stimulating factor (Neupogen, Amgen, Thousand Oaks, CA) has paradoxically led to a resurgence of GC transfusion.[30] A major problem in GC preparation is the large volume of blood that must be processed to obtain sufficient neutrophils. This problem has been reduced by administration of granulocyte colony-stimulating factor to donors, which also improves transfused neutrophil lifespan.

Granulocyte transfusion is most useful in humans in the treatment of severe, prolonged neutropenia, where antibiotics alone cannot control sepsis, and in neonatal sepsis, where neutrophil reserve is limited and GC volume requirements are small. Transfusion is given on demand—prophylactic transfusion is of limited benefit.[34] Granulocyte crossmatching is necessary to minimize alloimmunization and decreased neutrophil survival resulting from incompatibility.[28–30] Irradiation of GC is recommended to minimize transfusion-associated graft-versus-host disease.[4]

Granulocyte transfusions in animals have been used primarily in experimental models of myelosuppression and neonatal sepsis.[28–30,35] They have been rarely used in clinical veterinary medicine. Granulocytes have been transfused to septic foals but details have not been reported.[36] FWB transfusion (20 mL/kg) is anecdotally beneficial in treating severe parvoviral infection in kittens.[37] Some of the benefit may be due to transfused neutrophils. Preparation of dog and cat GC for neonates is feasible in veterinary clinics but, like other aspects of small animal neonatology, is hampered by cost. The initial dose is 1×10^9 granulocytes/kg in a volume of 15 mL/kg once to twice daily. Assuming a donor neutrophil count of 4000/μL and a yield of 75%, approximately 175 mL of FWB will be needed to prepare a GC for a 0.5 kg pediatric recipient. The transfusion should be given through a standard 17-μm filter over 2 hours.

REFERENCES

1. **Mackin AJ, Allen DG, Johnstone IB.** Effects of vincristine and prednisone on platelet numbers and function in clinically normal dogs. Am J Vet Res 1995;56:100–107.
2. **Frank J, Abrams-Ogg A, O'Grady M, LaMarre J.** The mechanisms by which interleukin-11 causes plasma volume expansion in dogs [Abstract]. J Vet Intern Med 1998;12:239.
3. **Allyson K, Abrams-Ogg ACG, Johnstone IB.** Room temperature storage and cryopreservation of canine platelet concentrates. Am J Vet Res 1997;58:1338–1347.
4. **Vengelen-Tyler V, ed.** Technical manual, 12th ed. Bethesda, MD: American Association of Blood Banks, 1996.
5. **Vostal JG, Mondoro TH.** Liquid cold storage of platelets: A revitalized possible alternative for limiting bacterial contamination of platelet products. Transfus Med Rev 1997;11:286–295.
6. **Nolte I, Niemann C, Käufer-Weiss I, Bowry SK, Müller-Berghaus G.** Konservierung von Vollblut des Hundes für Transfusionszwecke in CPDA-1 Stabilisator beschicktem PVC-Beutel: Einfluß der Lagerung auf die Zahl, die Volumenverteilung und die Ultrastruktur der Thrombozyten. Berl Münch Tierärztl Wschr 1988;101:365–373.
7. **Nolte I, Mischke R.** Investigations of platelet aggregation and platelet counts from stored canine whole blood. Res Vet Sci 1995;58:190–192.
8. **Agranenko VA, Lisovskaya IL, Volkova RI.** Preparing platelet concentrates from banked blood stored for 1–5 days by using tetracycline antibiotics. Folia Haematol Int Mag Klin Morphol Blutforsch 1983;110:879–886.
9. **Abrams-Ogg ACG, Kruth S, Carter RF, Valli VE, Kamel-Reid S, Dubé ID.** Preparation and transfusion of canine platelet concentrates. Am J Vet Res 1993;54:635–642.
10. **Clemmons RM, Bliss EL, Dorsey-Lee MR, Sechord CL, Meyers KM.** Platelet function, size and yield in whole blood and in platelet-rich plasma prepared using differing centrifugation force and time in domestic and food-producing animals. Thromb Haemostas 1983;50:838–843.
11. **Mooney S.** Preparation of blood components. Problems Vet Med 1992; 4:594–599.
12. **Schneider A.** Blood components: collection, processing, and storage. Vet Clin North Am Small Animal Pract 1995;25:1245–1261.
13. **Fijnheer R, Pietersz RN, Korte de D.** Platelet activation during preparation of platelet concentrates: A comparison of the platelet-rich plasma and the buffy coat methods. Transfusion 1990;30:634–638.
14. **Adamik von A, Klein A, Mischke R.** Technische Aspekte bei der Gewin-
15. **Cowles BE, Meyers KM, Wardrop KJ, Menard M, Sylvester D.** Prolonged bleeding time of Chédiak-Higashi cats corrected by platelet transfusion. Thromb Haemostas 1992;67:708–712.
16. **Helfand SC, Jain NC, Paul M.** Vincristine-loaded platelet therapy for idiopathic thrombocytopenia in a dog. JAVMA 1984;185:224–226.
17. **Mitchell SG, Hawker RJ, Turner VS, Hesslewood SR, Harding LK.** Effect of agitation on the quality of platelet concentrates. Vox Sang 1994; 67: 160–165.
18. **Valeri CR, Feingold H, Melaragno J, Vecchione JJ.** Cryopreservation of dog platelets with dimethyl sulfoxide: therapeutic effectiveness of cryopreserved platelets in the treatment of thrombocytopenic dogs and the effect of platelet storage at −80°C. Cryobiology 1986;23:387–394.
19. **Raymond SL, Pert JH, Dodds WJ.** Evaluation of platelet cryopreservation techniques by isolated kidney perfusion. Transfusion 1975:15:219–225.
20. **Read M, Reddick RL, Bode AP, Bellinger DA, Nichols TC, Taylor K, Smith SV, McMahon DK, Griggs TR, Brinkhous KM.** Rehydrated lyophilized platelets: Potential for long-term storage of dried platelets for transfusion. Proc Natl Acad Sci USA 1995;92:391–401.
21. **Chao FC, Kim BK, Houranieh AM, Liang FH, Konrad MW, Swisher SN, Tulis JL.** Infusible platelet membrane microvesicles: A potential transfusion substitute for platelets. Transfusion 1996;36:536–542.
22. **Rybak ME, Renzulli LA.** A liposome based platelet substitute, the plateletsome, with hemostatic efficiency. Biomater Artif Cells Immobilization Biotechnol 1993;21:101–118.
23. **Slichter SJ, O'Donnell MR, Weiden PL, Torb R, Schroeder ML.** Canine platelet alloimmunization: The role of donor selection. Br J Haematol 1986;63:713–727.
24. **George JN, Pickett EB, Heinz R.** Platelet membrane microparticles in blood bank fresh frozen plasma and cryoprecipitate. Blood 1986;68:307–309.
25. **Heddle NM.** Febrile non-hemolytic transfusion reactions to platelets. Current Opinion Hematol 1995;2:478–483.
26. **Slichter SJ, Weiden PL, Kane PJ, Storb RF.** Approaches to preventing or reversing platelet alloimmunization using animal models. Transfusion 1988;28:103–108.
27. **Slichter SJ, Deeg HJ, Kennedy MS.** Prevention of platelet alloimmunization in dogs with cyclosporine and by UV-irradiation or cyclosporine-loading of donor platelets. Blood 1987;69:414–418.
28. **Weiss DJ.** White cells. In: SM Cotter, ed. Advances in veterinary science and comparative medicine, vol. 36: Comparative transfusion medicine. San Diego: Academic Press Inc, 1991;57–86.
29. **Strauss RG.** Therapeutic granulocyte transfusions in 1993 [Editorial]. Blood 1993;81:1675–1678.
30. **Dale DC, Liles WC, Price TH.** Renewed interest in granulocyte transfusion therapy [Annotation]. Br J Haematol 1997;98:497–501.
31. **Gordon BJ, Latimer KS, Murray CM, Moore JN.** Continuous-flow centrifugation hemapheresis in the horse. Am J Vet Res 1986;47:342–345.
32. **Rock G, Zurakowski S, Baxter A, Adams G.** Simple and rapid preparation of granulocytes for the treatment of neonatal septicemia. Transfusion 1984;24:510–512.
33. **Christensen RD, Anstall HB, Rothstein G.** Use of whole blood exchange transfusion to supply neutrophils to septic, neutropenic neonates. Transfusion 1982;22:504–506.
34. **Vamvakas EC, Pineda AA.** Determinants of the efficacy of prophylactic granulocyte transfusions: A meta-analysis. J Clin Apheresis 1997;12:74–81.
35. **Epstein RB, Zander AR.** Granulocyte transfusions in leukopenic dogs. In: TJ Greenwalt and GA Jamieson, eds. The granulocyte: Function and clinical utilization. New York: Alan R. Liss Inc, 1977;227–241.
36. **Cotter SM.** Clinical transfusion medicine. In: SM Cotter SM, ed. Advances in veterinary science and comparative medicine, vol. 36: Comparative transfusion medicine. San Diego: Academic Press Inc, 1991;187–223.
37. **Kowall NL.** Feline panleukopenia. In: RW Kirk, ed. Current veterinary therapy V small animal practice. Philadelphia: WB Saunders, 1974;957–959.

CHAPTER 126

Blood Transfusions in Large Animals

• DEBRA C. SELLON

W hole blood (WB) or blood component transfusions may be used as temporary lifesaving therapy for animals with a variety of serious hematologic abnormalities. This chapter will provide guidelines for selection of patients likely to benefit from transfusion therapy and practical instructions for collection, handling, and administration of blood products to large animals. The majority of the information will be specifically related to equine blood product therapy; however, a section devoted to ruminant transfusion medicine is included at the conclusion of this chapter.

INDICATIONS FOR BLOOD TRANSFUSIONS

WB transfusions are indicated in horses with anemia severe enough to impair tissue oxygenation. The most common clinical conditions treated with WB transfusion include hemorrhagic shock, coagulation disorders, hemolytic crises, and nonresponsive anemias. The decision for WB transfusion is usually based on a clinical assessment of the severity of the anemia, the rapidity of progression of the anemia, and the likelihood of adequate bone marrow regenerative responses in the patient. In horses, allogeneic, crossmatch-compatible erythrocytes survive less than 5 days after transfusion into the recipient.[1] Therefore, the oxygen delivery benefit of transfusion is transient and should be viewed as a temporary lifesaving measure designed to provide support until the erythropoietic response of the patient's bone marrow is effectively increasing red blood cell (RBC) numbers. Because multiple blood transfusions over a period of several weeks dramatically increase the risk of transfusion reaction, even with crossmatched donors a rapid and effective bone marrow response is essential for the long-term survival of the patient.

Often the source of the anemia and its regenerative nature are immediately apparent, as with acute severe hemorrhage or hemolysis in an otherwise healthy young horse. After acute hemorrhage, the severity of blood loss may be masked for 24 hours, pending fluid shifts in the body to restore circulating blood volume. In horses this situation is further complicated by transient increases in packed cell volume (PCV) as splenic erythrocyte reserves are mobilized. Serial monitoring of PCV is crucial. In horses with acute, severe blood loss approaching 20 to 30% of the total blood volume, transfusion is usually indicated regardless of the PCV. The blood transfusion may be administered concurrently or immediately following volume replacement therapy with other types of solutions. Most horses with a PCV of <12% and evidence of progressive hemorrhage or hemolysis, regardless of the nature or duration of the underlying problem, require a transfusion.

Severity of the anemia and its rapidity of progression can be difficult to assess in some horses. Acute internal hemorrhage, as with ruptured uterine arteries in brood mares, or chronic blood loss, as with gastrointestinal hemorrhage, can be more difficult to confirm or assess. The only change in equine peripheral blood after acute hemorrhage or hemolysis may be a slight anisocytosis that is quantitatively assessed through changes in red cell distribution width (RDW).[2-4] Accelerated bone marrow erythropoiesis is usually evident by 3 days after acute hemorrhage and is maximal by 7 days.[5] In most cases, serial monitoring of PCV is adequate to assess marrow responses. After experimental phlebotomy to mimic blood loss anemia in the horse, PCV increased 0.5 to 1% per day, more slowly than in other species.[6] Serial bone marrow aspirates may be evaluated if regenerative responses remain questionable after 3 to 5 days. A bone marrow myeloid : erythroid (M : E) ratio of <0.5 is indicative of erythrocyte regeneration (or myeloid suppression).[7] Reticulocyte counts in the bone marrow may also be used to assess regenerative responses in the horse. Normal equine bone marrow contains approximately 3% reticulocytes, but this may increase to >60% in response to severe blood loss.[7,8]

Plasma transfusions are indicated for treatment of failure of passive transfer in foals, restoration of plasma oncotic pressure in horses with severe hypoalbuminemia, replacement of essential coagulation factors, or replenishment of immunologic proteins. Plasma transfusions are recommended for most foals with a serum IgG concentration of <800 mg/dL. Plasma transfusions for replacement of albumin are recommended in horses with hypoalbuminemia and progressive peripheral pitting edema. Most horses with a total plasma protein of <3 g/dL or a serum albumin concentration of

<1.2 g/dL would benefit from plasma transfusion to improve plasma oncotic pressure and maintain vascular volume. Horses with endotoxemia, septicemia, and/or disseminated intravascular coagulation may benefit from fresh plasma transfusions. Horses with hereditary or acquired deficiencies in coagulative proteins will also benefit from fresh plasma transfusions or infusion of cryoprecipitates containing specific coagulation factors.

DONOR SELECTION AND MANAGEMENT

Selecting an appropriate blood donor horse is critical to the safety and efficacy of blood transfusion therapy. There is a high degree of blood group polymorphism among horses, with several blood group systems and factors resulting in as many as 400,000 possible blood types.[9] The very short half-life of transfused red cells in horses is probably the result of minor alloantigen incompatibilities that are not detected in routine crossmatching procedures. Because of the great diversity in alloantigens among horses, there is no such thing as a 'universal' equine donor, and clinicians must rationally choose the safest available alternative. Even though it is almost impossible to identify a perfect match between donor and recipient horses, careful selection of a donor will greatly decrease the risk of severe transfusion reactions.

Three approaches may be used in selection of a blood donor horse: (1) blood typing and regular alloantibody testing of potential donors; (2) crossmatching of potential donors with recipients immediately prior to transfusion; or (3) transfusion from an untyped, uncrossmatched donor with a low probability of prior exposure to blood products. In all cases, blood donors should be healthy adult horses that are recently seronegative for equine infectious anemia virus. Appropriate vaccination against common equine pathogens is highly recommended, especially for potential plasma donor horses.

Of the seven major blood groups currently recognized internationally in horses, alloantigens Aa of the A system and Qa of the Q system are the most immunogenic and the most likely to cause acute severe reactions following incompatible transfusions.[10,11] These alloantigens are extremely prevalent in most horse breeds.[12] Therefore, it is common for horses that are negative for Aa and Qa alloantigens to be exposed to these antigens through prior blood product transfusions, pregnancy,[13] or following immunization with an equine-origin biological[14] and develop serum alloantibodies that can be detrimental in the event of future blood transfusions.

Because of the severity of potential reactions to Aa and Qa alloantigens, the optimal equine blood donor should be negative for these antigens and their respective alloantibodies. Blood typing can be accomplished by sending samples of serum and blood anticoagulated with acid-citrate-dextrose (ACD) from potential donor horses to any of a number of laboratories experienced with equine blood typing (Table 126.1). Frequency of specific alloantigens varies between breeds of horses. In

TABLE 126.1	Veterinary Laboratories That Blood Type Horses[a]

Veterinary Genetics Laboratory
University of California
Davis, CA 95616
Phone: 530-752-2211

Stormont Laboratory, Inc.
1237 East Beamer Street, Suite D
Woodland, CA 95695
Phone: 530-661-3078

Dr. Melba Ketchum
Shelterwood Equine Laboratory, Inc.
Box 215
Carthage, TX 75633
Phone: 903-693-6424

Dr. Gus Cothran
Equine Blood-Typing Research Laboratory
Department of Veterinary Science
University of Kentucky
Lexington, KY 40546
Phone: 606-257-3777

[a]Serum and acid-citrate-dextrose anticoagulated blood are required by most laboratories. Contact the laboratory directly prior to submitting samples to confirm appropriate submission procedures.

general, Shetland ponies have a lower prevalence of both Aa and Qa than do most light breeds of horses.[12] Unfortunately, their small size makes them unsuitable as donors in most cases. Belgian draft horses, Standardbreds, and Quarter Horses have a lower frequency of Aa and Qa than do most other horses.[12] Routine testing of potential donor horses for serum alloantibodies should greatly decrease the risk of unexpected adverse transfusion reactions.

If previously blood-typed donor horses are not available, crossmatching can be performed to detect major incompatibilities between donor and recipient. In the major crossmatch procedure, washed erythrocytes from the potential donor horse are incubated with serum from the recipient and observed for gross or microscopic evidence of clumping. In the minor crossmatch procedure, washed erythrocytes from the recipient are similarly incubated with serum from the potential donor. Routine major and minor crossmatching most effectively demonstrates the presence of agglutinating alloantibodies. Hemolyzing alloantibodies are detected by adding exogenous complement to the reaction mixture. Agglutinating crossmatches are appropriate in an emergency situation as long as the clinician realizes that they may not accurately predict all severe transfusion reactions.

In the absence of previously blood-typed donor horses or a laboratory capable of performing equine crossmatches, a clinician may select a young, previously untransfused gelding as an unmatched donor. Mares that have been previously pregnant[13] or any horse that has received a transfusion of a blood product or has been immunized with an equine-origin biological[14] should be considered inappropriate as a blood donor. Ideally, the donor should be genetically similar to the recipient horse because alloantigen patterns tend to be similar among most light breeds of horses.[12] Because naturally occurring equine alloantibodies are uncommon and only weakly reactive, the first transfusion to a recipient is unlikely to result in a severe transfusion reaction unless the recipient horse has a prior history of receiving blood products or had an incompatible pregnancy. After the initial transfusion, alloantibodies can develop within a few days, and subsequent transfusions from the same or a different donor are increasingly hazardous even with prior blood typing and/or crossmatching.[1]

Selection of a plasma donor is similar to selection of WB donors. Several commercial plasma sources market equine plasma from Aa-, Qa-negative donors free of detectable alloantibodies. These plasma products can usually be administered without crossmatching to the recipient. If blood is collected without prior typing, the minor crossmatch (donor serum incubated with recipient RBCs) is most critical for plasma transfusions.

BLOOD COLLECTION TECHNIQUES

Blood for transfusion should be collected aseptically into sterile containers. An appropriate area over the donor's jugular vein is clipped and prepared with routine surgical scrub techniques. A large-gauge (10–14 gauge) intravenous catheter or needle attached to sterile tubing is inserted into the vein. The horse may be lightly sedated with xylazine, if necessary. Tubing may be attached to a variety of receptacles including commercially available blood collection bags or sterile glass containers. In general, plastic bags or glass jars specifically manufactured for blood collection are the best choice. Other types of plastic bags and glass containers may induce RBC lysis or activate complement and white blood cells. Glass containers for blood collection have the advantage of being able to establish and maintain a vacuum to speed the process of blood collection. However, the vacuum may induce more red cell lysis than gravity flow collection techniques. Tubing is flushed with anticoagulant solution prior to use, and appropriate anticoagulant should be present in the collection receptacle prior to blood collection.

The most frequently used anticoagulant for blood collection is a solution of ACD at a ratio of 1:9 with blood (100 mL ACD mixed with 900 mL blood). The citrate anticoagulates blood by chelating calcium and inhibiting calcium-dependent steps in blood coagulation. Dextrose provides an energy substrate for RBC glycolysis to prolong the life of harvested erythrocytes. Many commercially available blood collection bags are marketed with ACD already added to the bags. Alternatively, ACD may be purchased separately or prepared by mixing 11 g dextrose, 9.9 g sodium citrate, 3.3 g citric acid, and enough distilled water to total 300 mL.[15] The resulting solution is autoclaved or filter sterilized and stored at room temperature prior to use. This volume of ACD (300 mL) is sufficient to anticoagulate 3 liters of equine blood.

Heparin or sodium citrate solutions may be used as anticoagulants in an emergency situation where blood is to be used immediately after collection.[15] Heparin is used at 5 to 10 units per mL of blood. If large quantities of blood anticoagulated with heparin are administered, there is a risk that as the cumulative heparin dose approaches 50 to 100 units/kg, coagulative processes will be inhibited in the recipient, leading to inappropriate hemorrhage. This is most likely to occur with transfused quantities of >10–20 mL/kg.[16] Heparinized blood cannot be safely stored and should be used within two hours of collection. Sodium citrate may be used as a 2.5–4% solution (2.5–4 gm sodium citrate added to 100 mL distilled water). This stock solution is added at a rate of one part sodium citrate to nine parts blood.[17] If sodium citrate is used as an anticoagulant, the blood should be administered to the recipient horse within 2 to 3 hours of collection.

After adding anticoagulant as needed and attaching all tubing to appropriate blood receptacles, the donor's jugular vein is manually occluded distal to the needle or catheter. The receptacle is gently rotated at frequent intervals during the collection process to facilitate even mixing of anticoagulant and blood. The storage lifespan of equine RBCs has not been accurately assessed. In other species, WB anticoagulated with ACD may be stored at 4°C for up to 6 weeks. However, there are significant species-related differences in storage lifespan, and, in the absence of specific equine data, it is advisable to refrigerate the blood if there is more than 1 to 2 hours between collection and administration and to administer the blood to the recipient horse within a few days of collection.

For plasma collection, WB should be refrigerated after collection and sufficient time allowed for the RBCs to sediment (at least 2 hours). Alternatively, the blood can be centrifuged to rapidly pellet RBCs. After red cell sedimentation, the plasma is aseptically removed from the container by pouring, siphoning, or using a plasma extraction device.[15] Plasma can be frozen at −20°C for at least 1 year without loss of immunoglobulin content. There are many commercial sources of purified equine plasma harvested from healthy, immunized Aa- and Qa-negative alloantibody-negative donor horses. Commercial plasma is usually prepared by plasmapheresis under strict manufacturing conditions. It is often of superior quality with fewer contaminating red cell fragments than traditionally prepared plasma and can be safely administered without prior compatibility testing.

Adult horses have a blood volume of approximately 72 mL/kg, for a total blood volume of approximately 36 L in a 500-kg horse.[18] Most adult horses can safely donate 20 to 25% of their total blood volume (approximately 8–10 L for a 500-kg donor) every 30 days. If donor horses are bled regularly (monthly), they should receive supplemental dietary iron to maximize their bone marrow regenerative responses.

ADMINISTRATION OF BLOOD PRODUCTS

The quantity of WB or plasma to be administered depends on the size of the recipient, the nature and severity of the underlying problem (failure of passive transfer, blood loss, hypoproteinemia, etc.), the quantity of blood available, and the financial constraints of the client. In horses with severe anemia, the goal of transfusion is to provide the patient with sufficient oxygen-carrying capacity to maintain tissue oxygenation without eliminating the hypoxic stimulus necessary to elicit erythropoietin production in the kidneys. In most cases, replacement of 25 to 30% of the calculated loss in red cell mass or total blood volume is sufficient. Sample calculations are shown in Figure 126.1. In plasma transfusions to foals with failure of passive transfer, the goal is to provide sufficient immunoglobulin to increase plasma IgG concentrations to >800 mg/dL. A transfusion volume of 1–2 L plasma is sufficient for most 45- to 50-kg foals.

Example 1: A 450 kg horse has lost 40% of its blood volume from hemorrhage. Hemorrhage has now been controlled. Using a value of 72 mL/kg as the average blood volume for adult horses:

450 kg × 72 mL/kg = 32.4 L total blood volume

A loss of 40% of this total blood volume means a loss of 13 L of whole blood:

32.4 L × 40% loss = 13 L blood loss

With a goal of replacing 30% of the lost blood, replacement requirements can be calculated:

13 L × 30% = 3.9 L replacement estimate

Therefore, a transfusion of approximately 4 L of compatible whole blood should be sufficient. In this case, the remainder of the volume loss (9–10 L) should be replaced with isotonic electrolyte solutions.

Example 2: A 500 kg horse presents with severe hemolytic anemia (PCV 11%) that has occurred over 1 to 2 weeks.

Assuming an average adult horse PCV of 35%, approximate red cell loss can be calculated:

35% − 11%/35% = 69% total red cell mass has been lost

To replace 30% of this loss, calculate the replacement mass:

69% × 30% = 20.7% of total red cell mass should be replaced

To calculate the total blood volume in the horse:

500 kg × 72 mL/kg = 36 L total blood volume

Replacement volume can now be calculated:

36 L total blood volume × 20.7% to be replaced
  = 7.5 L replacement volume

Therefore, a transfusion of approximately 7–8 L of compatible whole blood would be appropriate. Alternatively, because this horse has lost only red cells and not plasma, a lesser volume of packed red blood cells may be administered.

FIGURE 126.1 Sample calculations of approximate transfusion volumes.

For treatment of hypoproteinemia, a total plasma or colloid transfusion volume of 10 to 20 mL/kg is recommended.

After warming the blood or plasma to body temperature (approximately 37°C), the transfusion should be administered through an intravenous administration set with an in-line filter to remove small clots, fibrin strands, and debris. Even when donors have been typed and/or crossmatches are compatible, the initial transfusion flow rate should be slow to assess for unexpected adverse reactions. A rate of 0.1 mL/kg for 10 to 20 minutes is appropriate. This would be approximately 50 mL in 10 minutes to a 500-kg horse, or 5 to 10 mL over 10 to 20 minutes for a 50-kg foal. During this time the recipient should be monitored for signs of adverse reactions as described below. If there are no adverse reactions at this initial flow rate, the remainder of the transfusion may be administered at rates of up to 20 mL/kg/hr. Slower flow rates are generally safer because transfusion reactions can be recognized before large volumes are administered. Slower infusion rates are also recommended for horses with suspected or confirmed endotoxemia. Rapid flow rates in normovolemic foals may induce iatrogenic volume overload. The recipient's vital signs and behavior should be monitored throughout the transfusion and the flow rate slowed or stopped if significant changes are observed.

ALTERNATIVES TO WB TRANSFUSION

There are few practical alternatives to WB transfusion in equine practice. In normovolemic, anemic horses, packed RBC transfusions may be administered instead of WB transfusions. This exposes the recipient to fewer foreign blood proteins. Preparation of packed RBCs requires sedimentation of WB from the donor and resuspension of the RBCs in a quantity of saline sufficient to permit transfusion. This is a labor-intensive and time-consuming process that is often not practical in emergency or field practice. Washed RBCs may be used if the donor horse is compatible with a major crossmatch (donor red cells incubated with recipient serum) but not a minor crossmatch. Washed RBCs from the dam are considered the transfusion of choice for foals with neonatal isoerythrolysis. Washing and resuspension of RBCs should be performed with 0.9% saline or similar calcium-free solutions to prevent interference with citrate-based anticoagulants. Donor erythrocytes should be washed three times to remove all plasma proteins. After resuspension in saline, centrifugation at 2000 rpm for 20 minutes is necessary to separate erythrocytes because they will not sediment adequately when suspended in saline.[19]

There has been much interest in blood substitutes in human and veterinary medicine in recent years. However, only one report of their use in horses is available in the veterinary literature.[20] Polymerized ultrapurified bovine hemoglobin was transfused into a Miniature Horse mare with severe estrus-associated ovarian hemorrhage. It was administered to this 75-kg mare at a total dose of 30 mL/kg and a rate of 600 mL/hr. A transient increase in pulmonary artery and central venous pressure was observed, with a concomitant decrease in cardiac output. The estimated half-life of the product was approximately 40.3 hours.[20]

Erythropoietin has been used to increase circulating RBC mass and indirectly improve athletic performance in horses. However, relatively high doses of recombinant human erythropoietin are required to produce changes in RBC count.[21] Repeated administration of recombinant human erythropoietin in horses can result in profound nonregenerative anemia secondary to anti-erythropoietin antibody production.[22,23] Erythropoietin administration to stimulate bone marrow erythropoiesis in horses is not recommended.

ADVERSE REACTIONS

Transfusion of blood or blood products has many inherent risks, including immediate or delayed reactions as a result of alloantigen incompatibility, hypersensitivity reaction to other blood or plasma proteins, hypocalcemia, inadvertent transmission of blood-borne infectious organisms, activation of complement in the recipient, infusion of bacterial- or endotoxin-contaminated blood, and allosensitization of the recipient. The most common clinical signs of a transfusion reaction are non-specific and include increases in heart and respiratory rate, dyspnea, fever, sweating, muscle fasciculations, piloerection, weakness, hypotension, diarrhea, and abdominal pain. Because it is often difficult to determine the exact cause of these clinical signs, it is advisable to immediately stop the transfusion and initiate therapy with isotonic crystalline fluids. In most cases this is sufficient to control the clinical signs.

Acute hemolytic reactions with hemoglobinemia and hemoglobinuria may occasionally occur if there are major alloantigen incompatibilities between donor and recipient. These are rare if donors are typed and/or appropriate crossmatching procedures are performed prior to transfusion. Hypersensitivity (allergic) reactions may range from acute anaphylaxis to urticaria. Sudden collapse with profound respiratory difficulty is characteristic of anaphylactic reactions and can be treated with 1:1000 epinephrine solution IM at 0.01 to 0.02 mL/kg (5–10 mL for a 450-kg horse). Intravenous fluids will improve peripheral circulation in hypotensive patients and help to maintain renal perfusion. Rapid-acting corticosteroids such as prednisolone sodium succinate are also indicated in treatment of acute anaphylactic reactions. Doses from 0.25 to 10 mg/kg IV have been recommended. Alternatively, dexamethasone sodium phosphate may be administered at 0.05 to 0.2 mg/kg IV. Nonsteroidal anti-inflammatory drugs may be beneficial in some horses.

Occasionally, a horse will develop symptomatic hypocalcemia while receiving blood product transfusions because of chelation of calcium by ACD or sodium citrate anticoagulants. These horses will develop signs of apprehension, weakness, muscle fasciculations, arrhyth-

mias, and collapse. Treatment should include discontinuation of the transfusion and administration of calcium gluconate.

All blood donor horses should have a recent negative test for serum antibodies to equine infectious anemia to prevent inadvertent transmission of the causative virus from donor to recipient.[24] Other blood-borne diseases that may be transmitted include *Ehrlichia equi* and *Babesia* spp. All blood donor horses should be healthy at the time of blood collection.

Improper handling of blood during collection and administration may result in contamination of the product with bacteria or bacterial products (e.g. endotoxin). This can result in severe septicemia and/or endotoxemia in the recipient with clinical signs of uncontrollable trembling, weakness, tachycardia, tachypnea, fever, hypotension, and collapse. The transfusion should immediately be discontinued and appropriate supportive care administered. The remaining blood or plasma can be cultured for evidence of gross bacterial contamination. A Gram stain may reveal bacteria in severe cases. Appropriate antibacterial therapy should be initiated. Nonsteroidal anti-inflammatory drugs may be useful in alleviating some of the hemodynamic consequences of endotoxemia. Strict aseptic technique and careful handling is essential throughout the process of blood collection and transfusion to prevent these types of reactions.

Because of the extreme alloantigen diversity among horses, a single blood product transfusion frequently results in allosensitization of the recipient.[11] This places the recipient horse at increased risk for adverse reactions to subsequent transfusions. It also makes that recipient significantly less desirable as a future blood donor. If the recipient is a mare, future foals are at increased risk for neonatal isoerythrolysis.

TRANSFUSION THERAPY IN RUMINANTS

Of the eleven blood groups that have been identified in cattle, the B and J groups have the greatest clinical relevance. The B group alone has over 60 different antigens. A similar degree of polymorphism is present in other ruminants (sheep and goats). The marked diversity of red cell alloantigens in ruminants makes it extremely difficult to identify donors that are closely matched to recipients. However, it is also highly unlikely that recipients will have clinically significant quantities of pre-existing alloantibodies, and transfusion reactions in ruminants are uncommon. From a practical clinical standpoint, almost any adult ruminant can be a donor for any recipient of the same species.

Occasionally, transfusion reactions may occur because of J antigen incompatibilities. The J antigen is not a true erythrocyte antigen but a soluble lipid that adsorbs to the surface of erythrocytes. Newborn cattle acquire this antigen within the first 6 months of life. The quantity of erythrocyte-associated J antigen varies between groups of cattle. Cattle with no J antigen may develop anti-J alloantibodies and experience transfusion reactions when transfused with blood from J-positive donors.[25] Cattle may also become sensitized to alloantigens by administration of vaccines derived from blood origin, such as some anaplasmosis and babesiosis vaccines. When used on breeding females these vaccines may sensitize the cow to some blood groups, especially in the A and F systems. If the blood types of the sire and the calf are positive for these types, and the cow has produced sufficient alloantibodies, an isoimmune hemolysis similar to neonatal isoerythrolysis of foals may occur.

The same general guidelines for collection, handling, storage, and administration of blood products apply for ruminants as described above for horses. Ruminant blood donors should be healthy adults that are negative for blood-borne parasites, including *Anaplasma marginale* and *Babesia* spp. Similar collection techniques and volumes are recommended for adult cattle as for adult horses. The safety and efficacy of long-term storage of ruminant WB has not been reported. Therefore, it is recommended that WB be transfused within 24 hours of collection. A blood administration set with in-line filter should be used for the transfusion.

REFERENCES

1. **Kallfelz FA, Whitlock RH, Schultz RD.** Survival of ^{59}Fe-labeled erythrocytes in cross-transfused equine blood. Am J Vet Res 1978;39:617–620.
2. **Radin MJ, Eubank MC, Weiser MG.** Electronic measurement of erythrocyte volume and volume heterogeneity in horses during erythrocyte regeneration associated with experimental anemias. Vet Pathol 1986;23:656–660.
3. **Easley JR.** Erythrogram and red cell distribution width of equidae with experimentally induced anaemia. Am J Vet Res 1985;46:2378–2384.
4. **Weiser G, Kohn C, Vachon A.** Erythrocyte volume distribution analysis and hematologic changes in two horses with immune-mediated hemolytic anemia. Vet Pathol 1983;20:424–433.
5. **Duncan JR, Prasse KW.** Veterinary laboratory medicine. Ames, IA: Iowa State University Press, 1977;3–29.
6. **Smith JE, Agar NS.** Studies on erythrocyte metabolism following acute blood loss in the horse. Equine Vet J 1976;8:34–37.
7. **Schalm OW.** Equine hematology: Part IV. Erythroid marrow cytology in response to anemia. Equine Practice 1980;2:35–40.
8. **Tablin F, Weiss L.** Equine bone marrow: A quantitative analysis of erythroid maturation. Anat Rec 1985;213:202–206.
9. **Stormont CJ.** Blood groups in animals. JAVMA 1982;181:1120–1124.
10. **Bailey E.** Prevalence of anti-red blood cell antibodies in the serum and colostrum of mares and its relationship to neonatal isoerythrolysis. Am J Vet Res 1982;43:1917–1921.
11. **Wong PL, Nickel LS, Bowling AT, et al.** Clinical survey of antibodies against red blood cells in horses after homologous blood transfusion. Am J Vet Res 1986;47:2566–2571.
12. **Suzuki Y.** Alloantibodies: The blood groups they define. Procedures from the First International Symposium. Equine Hematol 1975;1:34–41.
13. **Becht JL.** Neonatal isoerythrolysis in the foal: Part 1. Background, blood group antigens and pathogenesis. Comp Cont Ed Pract Vet 1983;5:S591–S598.
14. **Doll ER.** The influence of equine fetal tissue vaccine upon hemagglutination activity of mare serums: Its relation to hemolytic icterus of newborn foals. Cornell Vet 1952;42:495–505.
15. **Schmotzer WB, Riebold TW, Porter SL, et al.** Time-saving techniques for the collection, storage, and administration of equine blood and plasma. Vet Med 1985;89–94.
16. **Morris DD.** Blood transfusion. In: NE Robinson, ed. Current therapy in equine medicine. Philadelphia: WB Saunders, 1983;325–328.
17. **Becht JL, Gordon BJ.** Blood and plasma therapy. In: NE Robinson, ed. Current therapy in equine medicine, 2nd ed. Philadelphia: WB Saunders, 1987;317–322.
18. **Carlson GP, Rumbaugh GE, Harrold D.** Physiologic alterations in the horse produced by food and water deprivation during periods of high environmental temperatures. Am J Vet Res 1979;40:982–985.
19. **Williamson L.** Highlights of blood transfusions in horses. Comp Cont Ed Pract Vet 1993;15:267–269.
20. **Maxson AD, Giger U, Sweeney CR, et al.** Use of a bovine hemoglobin preparation in the treatment of cyclic ovarian hemorrhage in a miniature horse. JAVMA 1993;203:1308–1311.
21. **Jaussaud P, Audran M, Gareau RL, et al.** Kinetics and haematological effects of erythropoietin in horses. Vet Res 1994;25:568–573.
22. **Piercy RJ, Swardson CJ, Hinchcliff KW.** Erythroid hypoplasia and anemia following administration of recombinant human erythropoietin to two horses. JAVMA 1998;212:244–247.
23. **Woods PR, Campbell G, Cowell RL.** Nonregenerative anaemia associated with administration of recombinant human erythropoietin to a thoroughbred racehorse. Equine Vet J 1997;29:326–328.
24. **Sellon DC.** Equine infectious anemia. Vet Clin North Am Equine Pract 1993;9:321.
25. **Tizard IR.** Veterinary immunology: An introduction, 5th ed. Philadelphia: WB Saunders, 1996;359–367.

CHAPTER 127

Blood Transfusions in Exotic Species

• JAMES K. MORRISEY

The field of exotic animal medicine is rapidly growing and accumulating new information. The variety of species makes this field both exciting and frustrating for the clinician. Often, information is anecdotal or unknown. This holds true for transfusion medicine of exotic species as well. Blood groups are often unknown and controlled studies of transfusions and transfusion reactions may not exist for all species. Most research work has been done with birds and ferrets; therefore, much of the emphasis in this chapter will be on these species. Other species, such as rabbits and rodents, will be mentioned and the author's experiences added to supplement the available information.

AVIAN

Before beginning a discussion of transfusion medicine in avian species, there are some differences in the avian erythrocyte that should be discussed. Avian erythrocytes are oval and nucleated and considerably larger than mammalian erythrocytes. The avian red cell is typically 10 to 15 μm in length, depending on the species, whereas the typical mammalian erythrocyte is biconcave and 6 to 7 μm in diameter. The lifespan of the avian erythrocyte is 28 to 45 days, compared with that of the human erythrocyte, which lives nearly 110 days.[1] This shorter lifespan is thought to be a function of the increased metabolism and higher body temperature of birds. The avian erythrocyte can consume 7 to 10 times more oxygen at room temperature than can the mammalian erythrocyte.[2] Being nucleated, avian erythrocytes do not rely on anaerobic glycolysis for cellular energy as in mammalian cells but instead use aerobic metabolism of fat and protein.[3] Additionally, avian erythrocytes contain three types of hemoglobin and are capable of synthesizing hemoglobin in situ.[1]

Anemia

Total red blood cell (RBC) numbers in birds are affected by age, sex, environment, hormonal influences, and hypoxia.[1, 4] RBC numbers tend to be lower in young birds and females. Because the erythrocytes are larger, red cell numbers are lower in birds compared with mammals. The normal RBC count in birds ranges from 1.5 to 4.5×10^6 cells/μL.[5] The packed cell volume (PCV) for most species ranges from 35 to 55%.[6] A PCV less than 35% is considered an anemia. Reticulocytes can be measured as an indication of the response to an anemia. Normal reticulocyte counts in most species are 1 to 5% of the erythrocytes.[6] Although diffuse polychromasia is common in avian erythrocytes, an increased amount may still be used as an indication of regeneration.[7]

Anemia in birds is caused by many of the same mechanisms as in mammals, such as decreased production, increased destruction, or blood loss. Decreased production is often seen as an anemia of chronic inflammation. This type of anemia may be caused by chronic diseases of an infectious, metabolic, or neoplastic etiology. Birds develop this type of anemia more quickly than do mammals because of the shorter lifespan of the avian erythrocytes.[4] More avian erythrocytes are destroyed on a daily basis and thus alterations of erythroid production are seen earlier. Hemolytic anemias are less common in birds but can be caused by toxicities, hemoparasites, and septicemia. Immune-mediated anemias have not been reported in birds.

Hemorrhagic anemias are common in birds secondary to injuries. Healthy birds are remarkably adept at dealing with acute blood loss, and hemorrhagic shock rarely occurs. Studies in chickens have shown that after removal of 30% of the blood volume, the PCV returns to normal within 72 hours.[8] The removal of 60% of the blood volume in pigeons did not cause significant clinical effects and resulted in a return to normal PCV by day 7 without treatment.[9] This extraordinary response to hemorrhage in birds is thought to be the result of an increased capillary surface area within skeletal muscles, which allows rapid extravascular fluid resorption to maintain vascular volume. Birds also possess the ability to mobilize large numbers of immature RBCs, and there is an absence of the autonomic response to hemorrhage that contributes to irreversible shock.[10]

Indications

The decision to administer a transfusion is based on several factors: PCV, chronicity of anemia, cause and severity of anemia, possibility of further blood loss (by either hemorrhage or diagnostic purposes), and the ability of the patient to tolerate the stress associated with transfusion administration. Studies of acute blood loss in pigeons demonstrated that birds receiving intravenous fluids only had the best response to hemorrhage, as judged by PCV at 24 and 48 hours, when compared with birds receiving heterologous (different species) or homologous (same species) transfusions.[11] This might suggest that the best course of treatment for acute blood loss may be IV administration of a balanced crystalloid. A similar study in which 60% of the blood volume of pigeons was removed showed that the homologous transfusion of 30% of the blood volume ameliorated the effects of the anemia but both groups returned to a normal PCV by day 6.[9] In light of these conclusions, the effectiveness of a transfusion in acute hemorrhage in birds is debatable. The PCV should be determined and a homologous transfusion considered in patients showing clinical signs associated with anemia and a PCV less than 20%.[11,12]

Mild to moderate anemias of a chronic nature may not require transfusion if the patient is stable and will not require extensive hematologic testing (which will effectively worsen the anemia) or surgery. Cases of severe anemia (<15%) may benefit from a transfusion because the patient may be stabilized while diagnostic testing to determine the cause of the anemia is performed.

Blood Groups

Blood grouping is determined by chemical structures on the erythrocyte membrane called blood group antigens. For example, in man, antigens from the ABO blood group system result in four blood types: A (A antigen only), B (B antigen only), AB (both antigens), and O (neither antigen). Blood grouping has been studied in chickens in an attempt to identify gene markers associated with desirable traits and for pedigree purposes.[13] At least 28 different blood group antigens have been found to date in the chicken, many of which have more than 10 alleles for a single antigen.[14] Blood group antigens have also been studied in other species, including pheasants, quail, turkeys, guinea fowl, and ducks. There has been no work on blood grouping in psittacines and other pet species.

Compatibility and Donor Selection

Because of a lack of identified blood groups in most avian species, compatibility for transfusion is based on the use of major and minor crossmatches. A major crossmatch is performed by mixing donor RBCs with recipient plasma, and a minor crossmatch uses recipient cells and donor plasma. The appearance of agglutination or cell lysis indicates incompatibility.

For avian medicine, the donor should be of the same species for the most effective transfusions. Several studies have shown homologous transfusions to have a longer RBC survival time when compared with heterologous transfusions.[11,15,16] Recent work has shown that heterologous transfusions between members of the same genus may have similar survival times as homologous transfusions.[17,18] Therefore, the recommended donor is the same species or the same genus if that is not possible. Unlike mammals, a single transfusion between different species can be safe and efficacious.[19,20] When donors of the same genus or species are not available, a single transfusion can be given from a separate species. The half-life of heterologous transfusions may range from 12 hours to 3 days, whereas a homologous transfusion may have a half-life of 6 to 11 days.[15,16]

With the number of avian species presented to clinicians, keeping a large variety of blood donors is impractical. A feasible option for many practices is to have a list of client-owned, healthy birds of a variety of species to use as donors when necessary. These birds may be owned by individual clients or aviaries. Singly housed birds should be used when possible to avoid transmission of infectious diseases. All donor birds should be screened by performing yearly physical examinations, complete blood counts (CBCs), and biochemical profiles. Donors should also be screened at least once for infectious diseases that are pertinent to the species.

Blood Collection and Storage

The site of blood collection from the donor depends on the size and species of bird used and the amount of blood needed. In general, it is safe to withdraw approximately 10% of the blood volume, which is approximately 1% of the body weight. For example, a 500-g Amazon parrot can have 5 cc safely removed. For psittacines, ratites, and soft bills the right jugular vein is usually the most reliable and readily accessible site for blood collection. In waterfowl and gallinaceous birds, the medial metatarsal vein is easily identified on the medial aspect of the lower leg and can be used for blood collection (in addition to the jugular vein). The basilic or wing vein can be visualized as it crosses the proximal ulna and can be used in most species, especially pigeons and doves, but may be smaller and more fragile than other veins.

Blood may be collected into syringes containing an anticoagulant. Blood collection bags are not used routinely in avian medicine because of the small volume of blood collected in most instances. The anticoagulant of choice is sodium citrate, although heparin, acid-citrate-dextrose (ACD), citrate-phosphate-dextrose (CPD), or CPD with adenine (CPDA-1) can also be used. Sodium citrate is added to the syringe before collection of the sample at 0.1 cc of citrate per 0.9 cc of blood to be collected. A similar volume of ACD, CPD or CPDA-1 can be used. Care should be taken in transfusing smaller species or patients with hypocalcemia when using these media, because they act by binding calcium in the blood. Heparin can be used safely at 0.25 mL/10 mL of blood collected for avian transfusions.[4]

Blood is collected into a syringe using a butterfly

catheter or injection needle. A small amount of anticoagulant should be flushed through the needle to prevent clotting in the needle. The sample may then be administered to the recipient from the collection syringe or, for larger amounts, transferred into a pediatric transfusion bag. The author has used blood stored in ACD and citrate for 12 to 24 hours without apparent deleterious effects. Long-term storage of avian blood is not currently practiced. A recent study showed common mammalian storage media were inadequate for storage of avian whole blood because of the differences in erythrocyte metabolism.[21] Future work is necessary in this area in light of the importance of species-specific transfusions.

Transfusion Administration

The amount of blood administered will depend on several factors, including the degree of anemia, the size of the donor, and the stability of the recipient. As a guideline, the amount of blood transfused should be approximately 10 to 20% of the blood volume of the recipient, which is approximately 1 to 2% of the body weight. Transfusions may be given IV or IO (intraosseously) as a bolus or by constant rate infusion. The infusion method is less likely to cause circulatory overload but requires the placement of an in-dwelling IV or IO catheter. An additional advantage with an in-dwelling catheter is that it gives continued IV access for fluid and drug administration. In-dwelling IV catheters can be placed in the median metatarsal vein in larger birds (>300 g) or in the jugular vein in most birds. IO catheters are placed in the distal ulna or proximal tibiotarsus. The transfusion is given over 2 to 4 hours. A small animal blood filter can be used to remove clots or other large material from the transfusion.

The bolus method of transfusion delivery has the advantage of requiring only temporary venous access but can cause circulatory overload and may require longer handling time. In some patients it can be useful to use a butterfly catheter to obtain blood for analysis and then deliver a transfusion and other IV treatments using the same catheter. The transfusion should be given over 1 to 5 minutes if using the bolus therapy. The bolus may be given in the jugular, basilic, or median metatarsal vein. Boluses may also be given IO. The bolus should be delivered quickly enough to avoid overstressing the patient but slowly enough to prevent circulatory overload.

Transfusion Reactions

Transfusion reactions are caused by the incompatibility of donor red cells with host plasma. Transfusion reactions may result in hemolysis of the donor red cells, fever, urticaria, and anaphylaxis.[4] These signs may be difficult to assess in avian patients; therefore, death may be the only adverse sign associated with a transfusion in a bird. Reactions can be reduced by crossmatching

individuals before giving a transfusion. Transfusion reactions have been reported in birds given multiple heterologous transfusions.[19,20] These birds were given three transfusions at two-week intervals, resulting in the deaths of five of six birds. Pathology showed changes consistent with transfusion reactions such as hemoglobin casts in the renal tubules. Titers against heterologous RBCs lasted approximately 3 weeks in one group of birds studied. Regurgitation has also been seen and was thought to be a result of hypervolemia from administration of the transfusion too quickly or in too large a volume.

FERRETS

The domestic ferret (*Mustela putorius furo*) is a popular pet in Europe and the United States. In 1992, there were an estimated 1 million pet ferrets kept in the United States.[22] The ferret is similar to other companion mammals such as the dog and cat, and many aspects of transfusion medicine are similar and will be discussed only briefly.

Hematologic Characteristics

The PCV of the ferret is slightly higher than that of other companion mammals and has a range of 41 to 63%.[23,24] Consequently, RBC numbers are slightly higher, with a range of 7.30 to 12.18 $\times$ 10^6 cells/μL. There are no discernible blood types in the domestic ferret.[25] Attempts to demonstrate naturally or experimentally induced antierythrocyte antibodies in ferrets has been unsuccessful, even when using as many as six transfusions between the same animals. The absence of these isoantibodies suggests that there is little risk of transfusion reaction in ferrets and that crossmatching is not necessary. Clinically this seems to be the case, as there are no reported transfusion reactions in ferrets. Crossmatching is still advised, especially if a ferret is receiving multiple transfusions.

Anemia

The causes of anemia in the ferret are similar to that of other species. Blood loss may be caused by trauma, severe flea infestation, and gastrointestinal bleeding secondary to foreign bodies, gastric ulcers, and gastroenteritis. These conditions can result in severe hemorrhage that warrants a transfusion as a part of the supportive care regimen. Immune-mediated destruction of RBCs has not been reported in the ferret but should be considered in cases of anemia in which blood loss or decreased production cannot be identified.

Bone marrow suppression can occur in ferrets for a variety of reasons, including renal disease, neoplasia, hyperestrogenism, Aleutian disease, and as anemia of chronic inflammation. Ferrets are induced ovulators; therefore, hyperestrogenism can develop in female ferrets as a result of chronic estrus. Hyperadrenocorticism in ferrets can also result in hyperestrogenism (along with elevation of other reproductive hormones). The author has seen anemia in male and female ferrets as a result of adrenocortical disease.

Indications

The indications for transfusion in the ferret are similar to that of other companion mammals. The decision to perform a transfusion should be based on the PCV and the clinical status of the ferret. A transfusion should be considered in acute blood loss if the PCV falls below 18%. If the anemia has developed more gradually, a ferret may tolerate a PCV as low as 12% without the need for a transfusion.[23] The blood volume required for transfusion can be estimated using the following formula:

$$\text{mL of blood required} = BV_{recipient} \times [(\text{desired PCV} - \text{pretransfusion PCV})/PCV_{donor\ blood}]$$

BV is blood volume in mL and is calculated as 8% of the body weight in kilograms, multiplied by 1000 to convert liters to milliliters. A simpler method is to administer 10 to 20% of the recipient's blood volume in a single transfusion.

Donor Selection

Healthy male ferrets are suggested for blood donors because of their larger size and larger blood volume.[4,23] The donors should have yearly CBC and serum biochemistries performed if less than 3 years of age and every 6 months if over 3 years of age. Blood glucose levels should be measured every 3 months in ferrets over 3 years of age to detect early signs of insulinomas. Ferrets are susceptible to heartworm disease caused by *Dirofilaria immitis* and should be screened for the disease using both antigen and microfilaremia tests. Both tests are useful because there is typically a low number of adult worms, resulting in a higher likelihood of false-negatives for both testing methods. All donors should be vaccinated for canine distemper and rabies using approved vaccines.

Blood Collection

Blood for transfusion is typically collected in the donor ferret using isoflurane anesthesia or other sedation. Isoflurane anesthesia has been shown to decrease PCV, hemoglobin concentrations, and RBC numbers in ferrets as soon as 15 minutes after injection.[26] In light of this, blood should be collected as quickly as possible if using isoflurane anesthesia. The effects of other anesthetics have not been determined.

Blood for transfusion is best collected from the cranial vena cava or jugular vein using a small-gauge (25–23 gauge) butterfly catheter. Jugular venipuncture is simi-

lar to other species. The cranial vena cava cannot be palpated or visualized and is accessed at the thoracic inlet once the ferret is anesthetized. The needle is aimed toward the opposite back limb and inserted at the angle between the manubrium and first rib. Negative pressure is applied to the syringe once the skin has been punctured and advanced slowly until the vein is encountered.

The blood is collected into an appropriately sized syringe containing sodium citrate, ACD, CPD, or CPDA-1. If citrate is used, 0.1 mL of citrate is used for each 0.9 mL of blood collected. For ACD, 1 mL of ACD per 6 mL of blood is recommended.[4] Long-term storage of ferret blood is possible using typical mammalian storage media, but it is not currently practiced.

Administration

The blood can be administered by syringe pump or placed in a pediatric transfusion bag and administered by constant rate infusion. The blood should be administered over a 4- to 6-hour period. Pretreatment with short-acting corticosteroids has been advised[4] but is unwarranted.

The blood is administered into a peripheral or jugular catheter to the recipient ferret. Intravenous catheters can be placed in the cephalic and lateral saphenous veins. A small nick in the skin should be made using a 20-gauge needle before placing the catheter. A cutdown procedure may be required to place a jugular catheter. IO catheters can be placed in the proximal femur or tibial crest in small patients or in patients with vascular compromise. A small-animal blood filter should be used to prevent the transfusion of clots or other large particles.

Transfusion Reactions

Transfusion reactions have not been reported in ferrets, ostensibly because of the lack of detectable blood groups. Ferrets have received up to 13 separate transfusions from several different donors without apparent ill effects.[27] Signs of transfusion reactions should be similar to those for other mammals and include urticaria, fever, hemolysis of erythrocytes, and anaphylaxis.

RABBITS AND RODENTS

Little information is available concerning transfusion medicine in rabbits and rodents. Experimental work in this area has been performed in laboratory rabbits and rodents; however, the clinical relevance of such work is limited.

Rabbits

The normal PCV of the domestic rabbit is 30 to 50%.[5] The blood volume is approximately 57 mL/kg body weight.[28] Anemia can be caused by several conditions, including blood loss and decreased production. Significant blood loss can occur with trauma, with infectious diseases such as rabbit hemorrhagic disease, and with uterine diseases such as adenocarcinoma and endometriosis. Anemia of chronic inflammation is common in rabbits secondary to renal failure and other chronic disease conditions.

A transfusion should be considered in a rabbit with a PCV of less than 15%, especially if surgical treatment of the disease is indicated. The donor should be a large, healthy rabbit. The easiest vessel from which to collect blood is the central artery of the ear; however, severe damage to this artery could result in complete or partial loss of the pinna and owner consent to this is mandatory. Additional sites to collect blood include the jugular, lateral saphenous, or cephalic veins. Information on blood groups is not available; therefore, a major and minor crossmatch should be performed. The formula presented in ferrets for determining the optimum transfusion amount can be applied to rabbits. The transfusion should be collected in citrate, ACD, CPD, or CPDA-1 and used immediately. A blood filter should be used to prevent the transfusion of clots. The transfusion should be given over 4 to 6 hours.

Guinea Pigs and Chinchillas

The normal PCV for the guinea pig and chinchilla are 35 to 45% and 27 to 54%, respectively.[5] The blood volume for the guinea pig is 70 mL/kg. Blood loss can occur secondary to trauma and reproductive disease as in the rabbit. The author has seen a hemolytic anemia in a guinea pig secondary to a refeeding hypophosphatemia. Anemia of chronic inflammation is common in both species with renal disease and other chronic disorders.

A transfusion in either species should be considered when the PCV is below 15%. Blood should be collected from large, healthy donors that appear to be in good physical condition and have no abnormalities on CBC or serum chemical profiles. The amount of blood that can be safely removed in either species in unknown, but 10% of blood volume is unlikely to compromise the donor. The donor should be anesthetized and blood collected from the cranial vena cava (as described for the ferret) or jugular vein. The blood should be collected in citrate or ACD as described above. A major and minor crossmatch should be performed as there is little information regarding blood types in these species. The transfusion should be given as discussed for the ferret and rabbit.

GUIDELINES FOR NONDOMESTIC MAMMALS

Little information is available on transfusion medicine in many of the species that are seen commonly in zoologic and exotic animal medicine; however, there are several guidelines to follow when considering a transfusion in an unknown species. The need for a transfusion should be based on the normal PCV and blood volume for each animal. In general, a transfusion is warranted in acute blood loss of greater than 30% of an animal's blood volume or a 50% decrease in low normal PCV. An animal with a chronic anemia may tolerate a loss of 60% of blood volume before a transfusion is necessary. The clinical assessment of the animal is crucial. Signs of anemia are related to hypoxia and decreased viscosity of the blood and include tachypnea, tachycardia, cardiac murmurs, and lethargy. If the patient is tolerating an anemia, the risks and benefits of a transfusion must be considered. A healthy donor of the same species should always be used. A major and minor crossmatch will give some indication for transfusion reactions. Pretreatment of the recipient with ultra short-acting corticosteroids may be in order. The transfusion should be given slowly and the animal monitored continuously for signs of transfusion reaction.

REFERENCES

1. **Sturkie PD, Griminger P.** Body fluids: Blood. In: PD Sturkie, ed. Avian physiology. New York: Springer-Verlag, 1986;102–114.
2. **Lumeij JT.** A contribution to clinical investigative methods for birds with special reference to the racing pigeon, *Columbia livia domestica*. PhD Thesis. Utrecht: University of Utrecht, 1987;3–17.
3. **Hazelwood RL.** Carbohydrate metabolism. In: PD Sturkie, ed. Avian physiology. New York: Springer-Verlag, 1986;303–325.
4. **Hoefer HL.** Transfusions in exotic species. Probs Vet Med 1992;4:625–635.
5. **Carpenter JW, Mashima TY, Rupiper DJ.** Exotic animal formulary. Manhattan, KS: Greystone, 1996.
6. **Campbell TW.** Cytology. In: BW Ritchie, GJ Harrison, and LR Harrison, eds. Avian medicine: Principals and applications. Lake Worth: Wingers, 1994;199–222.
7. **Dein FJ.** Avian hematology: Erythrocytes and anemia. Proc Am Assoc Zoo Vet 1989;10–23.
8. **Ploucha JM, Scott JB, Ringer RK.** Vascular and hematologic effects of hemorrhage in the chicken. Am J Physiol 1981;240:H9–H17.
9. **Finnegan VM, Daniel GB, Ramsay EC.** Evaluation of whole blood transfusions in domestic pigeons (*Columba livia*). J Avian Med Surg 1997;11:7–14.
10. **Schindler SL, Gildersleeve RP, Thaxton JP, McRee DI.** Hematological response of hemorrhaged Japanese quail after blood volume replacement with saline. Comp Biochem Physiol 1987;87:933–945.
11. **Bos JH, Todd B, Tell LA, et al.** Treatment of anemic birds with iron dextran therapy, homologous and heterologous blood transfusions. Proc Annu Conf Assoc Avian Vet 1990;221–225.
12. **Quesenberry KE, Hillyer EV.** Supportive care and emergency therapy. In: BW Ritchie, GJ Harrison, and LR Harrison, eds. Avian medicine: principals and applications. Lake Worth: Wingers, 1994;382–398.
13. **Gilmour DG.** Blood groups. In: BM Freeman, ed. Physiology and biochemistry of the domestic fowl, vol 5. New York: Academic Press, 1988;4:263–273.
14. **Dietert MF, Taylor RL, Dietert RR.** Avian blood groups. Poultry Sci Rev 1992;4:87–105.
15. **Degernes LA, Crosier M, Harrison LD, et al.** Investigation of homologous and heterologous avian blood transfusions. Proc Assoc Avian Vet 1997;277–278.
16. **Sandmeier P, Stauber EH, Wardrop KJ, Washizuka A.** Survival of pigeon red blood cells after transfusion into selected raptors. JAVMA 1994;204:427–429.
17. **Degernes LA, Crosier ML, Harrison LD, et al.** Autologous, homologous, and heterologus red blood cell transfusions in cockatiel (*nymphicus hollandicus*). J Avian Med Surg 1999;13:2–9.
18. **Degernes LA, Harrison LD, Smith DW, et al.** Autologus, homologous, and heterologus red blood cell transfusions in conures of the genus *Aratinga*. J Avian Med Surg 1999;13:10–14.
19. **Altman RB.** Heterologous blood transfusions in avian species. Proc Am Assoc Zoo Vet 1982;7–8.
20. **Harrison GJ.** Experimental interspecies avian blood transfusions. Proc Am Assoc Zoo Vet 1977;118–119.
21. **Morrisey JK, Hohenhaus AE, Rosenthal KL, Giger U.** Comparison of three media for the storage of avian whole blood. Proc Assoc Avian Vet 1997;279–280.
22. **Carpenter JW, Harms CA, Harrenstein L.** Biology and medicine of the domestic ferret. J Small Exotic Animal Med 1994;2:151–162.
23. **Quesenberry KE.** Basic approach to veterinary care. In: EV Hillyer and KE Quesenberry, eds. Ferrets, rabbits and rodents. Philadelphia: WB Saunders, 1997;1:14–25.

24. **Fox JG.** Normal clinical and biological parameters. In: JG Fox, ed. Biology and diseases of ferrets. Philadelphia: Lea & Febiger, 1988;159–164.
25. **Manning DD, Bell JA.** Lack of detectable blood groups in domestic ferrets: Implications for transfusions. JAVMA 1990;197:84–86.
26. **Marini RP, Jackson LR, Esteves MI, et al.** Effect of isoflurane on hematologic variables in ferrets. Am J Vet Res 1994;55:1479–1482.
27. **Ryland LM.** Remission of estrus-associated anemia following ovariohysterectomy and multiple blood transfusions in a ferret. JAVMA 1981;178: 820–822.
28. **Jenkins JR.** Soft tissue surgery and dental procedures. In: EV Hillyer and KE Quesenberry, eds. Ferrets, rabbits and rodents. Philadelphia: WB Saunders, 1997;227–239.

CHAPTER 128

Autologous Transfusion

• TIMOTHY HACKETT

Veterinarians facing real and practical shortages of stored blood have used or considered autotransfusion during major surgery, in cases of anticoagulant rodenticide intoxication, trauma, and internal hemorrhage resulting from ruptured mass lesions. Autotransfusion is used to describe the return to the patient's own circulation of blood lost or removed as a result of surgery or internal hemorrhage. The term "autologous" refers to any blood derived from the same individual. An autologous transfusion is one in which the patient receives only his/her own blood. Autotransfusion has been used sporadically for more than a century. It has been an emergency treatment of sudden massive hemorrhage in the face of inadequate supplies of donor blood. Early canine autotransfusion studies were first reported in 1818. The first report of autotransfusion in man was in 1864, when 50 mL of blood from an amputated limb was autotransfused back into the patient. A report in the Lancet in 1874 suggested that recovery of postpartum hemorrhage was an overlooked source that could be used to great advantage.[1] Shortly after these reports, much more significant discoveries involving homologous transfusions were occurring. In 1900, Landsteiner discovered the ABO blood group. Then came the development of anticoagulants and preservatives, and by 1935 the first blood bank was established at the Mayo Clinic. Problems with blood availability and storage were addressed during World War II, when a great need for blood led to the development of widespread civilian blood banking.

The Korean and Vietnam wars placed high demands on banked blood supplies. Expanding surgical techniques, the use of open heart and advanced orthopaedic surgery, and improved emergency care further depleted banked blood reserves. Severe shortages of banked blood during the Vietnam War led to the development of autotransfusion equipment designed to salvage blood for reinfusion.[2] The early equipment used a suction tip with circulating anticoagulant, a reservoir, and a filter system. There were significant problems associated with poor blood quality, damaged cells, risk of infection, coagulopathies, and air embolism. Most of the early problems have been eliminated with newer equipment, but they may have limited the growth of autotransfusion practices. Techniques have improved and with the advent of human immunodeficiency virus, the increased incidence of hepatitis, a decreasing blood supply, and the rising cost of processing blood, there has been a renewed interest in autotransfusion.

ADVANTAGES OF AUTOLOGOUS TRANSFUSION

Autologous transfusion has several important advantages over homologous blood. In veterinary medicine the most important of these is the immediate availability of red blood cells (RBCs) in times of need and the conservation of limited banked blood. Autologous blood also eliminates the risk of blood-borne infections. Crossmatching is not a concern, yet while autologous blood is usually compatible, the use of autotransfusion does not eliminate the risk of transfusion reactions. Despite the fact that the blood given is the patient's own, transfusion reactions to autologous blood have been reported in man and include febrile nonhemolytic and allergic reactions.[3]

INDICATIONS AND CONTRAINDICATIONS FOR AUTOLOGOUS TRANSFUSION

Autologous transfusion is indicated when the alternative is death as a result of blood loss. This is particularly true when no other blood or hemoglobin replacement is available and the patient is showing signs of poor oxygen delivery. If more blood is required than is readily available, autologous blood can augment the supply. Occasionally, an owner may object to the use of homologous blood.

Autotransfusion is relatively contraindicated when the blood is contaminated with gastrointestinal contents or micro-organisms. With oncologic surgery or hemorrhage from intracavitary masses, malignant cells may be present and alternatives to autotransfusion should be explored. Contamination with amniotic fluid or drugs not intended for intravenous use are other potential contraindications for autotransfusion.

The risk of autotransfusion for some of the previously mentioned conditions must be weighed against the severity of hemorrhage and the need for immediate oxygen-carrying capacity. When whole blood, packed red cells, or cell-free hemoglobin products are available, autotransfusion should not be performed. If not, and the alternative is death as a result of hemorrhage, autotransfusion should be considered.

AUTOLOGOUS BLOOD COLLECTION

Blood collection for reinfusion should be performed in an aseptic, controlled manner. In emergency settings, blood may be collected into standard blood administration sets and reinfused to the patient through a micropore filter.[4] Specific autotransfusion equipment was developed by a military surgeon during the Vietnam War. The Klebenoff machine named for this surgeon was later modified and introduced commercially by Bentley Laboratories. The Bentley device was a simple suction, storage, and filtration device. A similar, inexpensive device has been described in the veterinary literature using a cardiotomy reservoir and readily available tubing materials.[5]

Problems associated with the Bentley system led to the development of centrifuge-based blood salvage devices. These devices separated whole blood for cell washing before returning the blood to the patient. As the red cell mass is separated from the plasma, contaminants and cellular debris are removed with a saline rinse solution. When the wash is complete, the cleaned RBCs are stored for later reinfusion to the patient. A unit of salvaged blood can be washed in a very short time, making these units practical for blood recovery in cases of surgical hemorrhage. Modern autotransfusion systems minimize contamination and provide the patient's own RBCs free of plasma and circulating mediators that may present more problems to critically ill patients. The Elmd-500 Portable Auto Transfusion System (Electromedics, Englewood, CO) is in use in veterinary patients at Colorado State University Veterinary Teaching Hospital. Although useful for intraoperative blood salvage, the equipment is expensive and requires additional manpower to operate. The cell washing system seems to be most useful for operative cases with anticipated yet controlled blood loss, as in the case of cardiopulmonary bypass.

Many other emergency cases requiring autotransfusion do have access to an automated cell salvage system. In these cases, one of two other methods may be employed. A passive canister collection system can be incorporated into a suction drainage system. A sterile collection bag is placed in the suction line of a standard underwater-seal continuous suction chest drainage system. The collected blood can then be examined for gross contamination, filtered, and quickly reinfused. A similar system is commonly used in people following thoracotomy. Chest tube drainage from the mediastinum is directed to a rigid canister containing two collection bags. The first contains a 170-micron filter to trap large clots and cellular debris. The blood passes into the second collection bag, which can then be removed from the canister, suspended, and the blood returned to the patient through smaller filters. Because the blood is sufficiently defibrinated, additional anticoagulants are not used.

The other method familiar to veterinary emergency clinicians is the direct aspiration and reinfusion of the patient's own blood.[6] This method involves the use of equipment available to any emergency veterinarian. Blood is aspirated from the chest or abdomen through a chest tube or percutaneous peritoneal dialysis catheter. The tube is connected to a standard blood bag collection system (Teruflex blood bag system, Terumo Corp, Tokyo, Japan) via a three-way stopcock. A large 35- to 60-mL syringe attached to the stopcock will facilitate aspiration. Blood is slowly aspirated into the syringe, then infused into the blood collection bag. When the bag is full or the cavity evacuated, the blood can be washed if time permits or immediately reinfused using a filtered blood administration set. If the blood is not washed with a centrifugation cell saver system, it should be filtered through a 40/150–micron dual screen filter (Fenwal Straight type blood set, Baxter Healthcare Corp., Deerfield, IL). This set is specifically designed for autotransfusion and has a smaller filter size to remove cell debris, aggregated platelets, leukocytes, and other particulates found in salvaged blood.[4]

PROBLEMS ASSOCIATED WITH AUTOLOGOUS TRANSFUSION

Autologous blood replacement is not equivalent to giving a patient a fresh unit of his/her own blood. Blood that has been in contact with the pleural or peritoneal surfaces for even 1 hour may become depleted of platelets, fibrin, and many essential clotting factors. The trauma of surgery, suction filtration, and reinfusion can lead to hemolysis. Free hemoglobin can cause acute renal tubular necrosis. Patients with pre-existing renal disease or hypovolemia should have urine output and renal perfusion closely monitored following autotransfusion.

Dilutional coagulopathies may be seen in patients receiving large amounts of autotransfused blood. Factor deficiencies and thrombocytopenia have already been mentioned. Additionally, these patients may be receiving large volumes of anticoagulant. The use of anticoagulants is controversial. If bleeding is fresh and ongoing, the addition of citrate-phosphate-dextrose (CPD) is probably indicated. If the patient is suffering from the effects of warfarin overdose, further anticoagulation is not justified. Multiple doses of CPD will worsen bleeding tendencies and can cause significant hypocalcemia. Serial tests of clotting function such as activated clotting time and partial thromboplastin time should be performed. Calcium levels should also be monitored closely. Replacement therapy with calcium gluconate is often necessary in small patients and in those patients receiving extremely large volumes of citrate-based anticoagulants.[3]

A consumptive coagulopathy and acute respiratory failure have been reported in people receiving autologous, salvaged blood. This complication has been termed salvaged blood syndrome and may be caused by the reinfusion of activated leukocytes and high concentrations of leukocyte elastase.[7,8]

One concern with autologous blood replacement is sepsis. Intracavitary blood is a potential media for the growth of micro-organisms. Although abdominal trauma can lead to possible fecal contamination, the use of intraoperative autologous transfusion in the presence of enteric contamination has been explored and in at least one study found to be safe if used in conjunction with parenteral antibiotics.[9]

Because abdominal mass lesions are a source of massive internal blood loss, the use of autologous blood salvage procedures may seem logical. However, there is concern over the possible systemic dissemination of malignant cells during autotransfusion. Viable tumor cells, which have demonstrated proliferation capacity and invasiveness, have been detected in the blood shed during human oncologic surgery.[10] Human clinical studies have failed to define any evidence for dissemination of tumor caused by autotransfusion in patients who underwent radical cystectomy for carcinoma of the bladder.[11] A similar study comparing recurrence and survival rates in groups of patients undergoing hepatectomy for hepatocellular carcinoma also found no difference between groups receiving autologous blood and homologous blood.[12] Similar studies in veterinary patients have not been done.

CONCLUSIONS

With the recent problems associated with blood-borne infections in people, preoperative autologous blood banking has gained popularity. Through the use of recombinant erythropoietin to stimulate RBC production, strict hemostasis, and the use of autologous-banked blood, the need for homologous donor blood units may decrease. The pre-need collection of autologous blood is commonly practiced for a variety of elective surgeries in humans. Because the risk of blood-borne infections in prescreened blood is less of a concern in our pet population, presurgical autologous blood collection is unlikely to become commonplace in veterinary medicine.

In veterinary medicine, the appropriate use of autologous blood replacement can provide immediate help when donor blood is unavailable. When collected in an aseptic manner and properly filtered, autologous blood can provide lifesaving oxygen-carrying capacity to critically ill patients.

REFERENCES

1. **Highmore W.** Overlooked source of blood supply for transfusion in postpartum hemorrhage. Lancet 1874;1:89.
2. **Purvis D.** Autotransfusion in the emergency patient. Vet Clin North Am Small Animal Pract 1995;25:1291–1304.
3. **Domen RE.** Adverse reactions associated with autologous blood transfusion: Evaluation and incidence at a large academic hospital. Transfusion 1998;38:296–300.
4. **Dodds WJ.** Autologous transfusion. Adv Vet Sci Comp Med 1991;36:239–256.
5. **Neibauer GW.** Autotransfusion for intraoperative blood salvage: A new technique. Comp Cont Ed Pract Vet 1991;13:1105.
6. **Crowe DT.** Autotransfusion in the trauma patient. Vet Clin North Am Small Animal Pract 1980;10:583.
7. **Bull BS, Bull MH.** The salvaged blood syndrome: A sequel to mechano-chemical activation of platelets and leukocytes? Blood Cells 1990;16:5–20.
8. **Harbison S, Chung S, Kucick B, Marino PL.** Leukocyte disruption and elastase release in autotransfused blood. Crit Care Med 1989;17:S42.
9. **Timberlake KA, McSwain NE.** Autotransfusion of blood contaminated by enteric contents: A potentially lifesaving measure in the massively hemorrhaging trauma patient? J Trauma 1988;28:855–857.
10. **Hansen E, Wolff N, Knuechel R, et al.** Tumor cells in blood shed from the surgical field. Arch Surg 1995;130:387–393.
11. **Hart OJ III, Klimberg IW, Wajsman Z, Baker J.** Intraoperative autotransfusion in radical cystectomy for carcinoma of the bladder. Surg Gynecol Obstet 1989;168:302–306.
12. **Fujimoto J, Okamoto E, Yamanaka N, et al.** Efficacy of autotransfusion in hepatectomy for hepatocellular carcinoma. Arch Surg 1993;128:1065–1069.

CHAPTER 129

Transfusion Reactions

• ANN E. HOHENHAUS

Although transfusions are frequently considered necessary and lifesaving therapy, they are not without risk of adverse effects. The term transfusion reactions is typically used to describe the consequences of transfusion, although a wide variety of adverse effects occur. Because each transfusion carries some risk of adverse effects, the veterinarian must consider both the therapeutic benefit of the transfusion and the risk of reaction prior to administration. Pretransfusion testing may eliminate some transfusion reactions, but because some adverse effects of transfusion are not predictable or preventable, each transfusion recipient must be monitored for adverse effects during and following the transfusion.

This chapter will classify the adverse effects of transfusion into four main categories: acute immunologic, acute nonimmunologic, delayed immunologic, and delayed nonimmunologic transfusion reactions. Acute reactions are those reactions occurring during or within hours of transfusion, and delayed reactions are those reactions occurring days to years later. The pathophysiologic mechanism of each type of transfusion reaction will be discussed and the clinical signs, diagnostic testing, management, and prevention strategies for each type of reaction will be outlined.

ACUTE TRANSFUSION REACTIONS—IMMUNOLOGIC

Several studies have reported fever without hemolysis as the most common acute immunologic reaction in veterinary patients.[1-3] Fever is defined as a >1°C increase in temperature over the pretransfusion value. Although the underlying mechanism is unknown in dogs and cats, febrile nonhemolytic transfusion reactions occur in multiply transfused human patients who have developed antibodies against donor leukocyte antigens. The incidence is approximately 2 to 3% of dogs transfused and less than 1% of cats.[1,3]

A febrile nonhemolytic transfusion reaction should be suspected in a dog or cat developing a fever during or 1 to 2 hours following a transfusion (Fig. 129.1). Fever associated with transfusion can also result from an acute hemolytic transfusion reaction, transfusion of blood con-

taminated with micro-organisms, or as a feature of an underlying disease process. Observation of hemoglobinemia when a packed cell volume (PCV) is measured, or hemoglobinuria during or immediately following a transfusion, suggests an acute hemolytic transfusion reaction. Brown discoloration of the unit of blood, the presence of gross hemolysis or clots, and identification of micro-organisms would suggest the fever is caused by transfusion of contaminated blood.

If the possibility of an acute hemolytic transfusion reaction or transfusion of contaminated blood is eliminated, a febrile, nonhemolytic transfusion reaction requires no immediate therapy other than antipyretic agents when the fever is high or the patient is uncomfortable. The fever is likely to recur with subsequent transfusions, and antipyretic agents may be given prior to transfusion. In humans, blood has been depleted of leukocytes prior to transfusion by special filters or washing.[4]

Transfusion of incompatible red blood cells (RBCs) results in an acute hemolytic reaction. Antibodies in the transfusion recipient's plasma form complexes with the transfused cells, triggering an inflammatory pathway similar if not identical to the systemic inflammatory response syndrome.[5] Acute hemolytic transfusion reactions are estimated to occur in 1:2000 canine transfusions and 1:6000 human transfusions.[3,6] The incidence of acute hemolytic transfusion reactions appears to be less than 1% in cats, but acute hemolytic transfusion reactions are more commonly reported in the cat than in the dog, probably as a result of naturally occurring antibodies present in the plasma of blood type B cats, which react against type A cells.[1,7-9]

The clinical signs of acute hemolytic transfusion reactions in dogs and cats differ. Cats of blood type B receiving type A blood exhibit signs of a transfusion reaction following administration of as little as 1 mL of blood.[10] The signs of administration of incompatible blood in cats include stretching, tachycardia, and tachypnea followed by bradycardia and apnea.[7] Hypotension and death may ensue. Abnormalities in laboratory tests result from hemolysis and include icterus, pigmenturia, positive direct Coombs' test, and a decreasing PCV.[8] Neither dogs nor cats have acute tubular necrosis associated with acute hemolytic transfusion reactions, as is seen in hu-

FEVER (> 1°C PRETRANSFUSION)

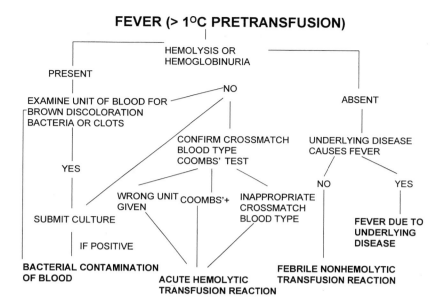

FIGURE 129.1 An algorithm for the diagnostic evaluation of a dog or cat with a transfusion-associated fever.

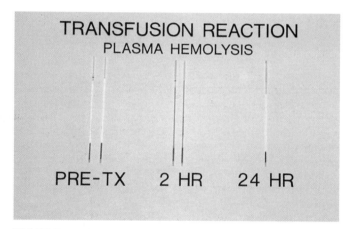

TRANSFUSION REACTION
PLASMA HEMOLYSIS

PRE-TX   2 HR   24 HR

FIGURE 129.2 Serial packed cell volumes (PCVs) from a dog experiencing an acute hemolytic transfusion reaction. Note the transition of plasma from clear to hemolyzed to icteric over 24 hours. As a consequence of the transfusion reaction, the PCV fell following the transfusion.

TABLE 129.1	Drugs Potentially Useful in the Management of Transfusion Complications

Antihistamines
   Diphenhydramine 1–2 mg/kg IM

Glucocorticoids
   For urticaria:
      Prednisone 0.1 mg/kg PO BID for 24–48 hours
   For shock:
      Methylprednisolone succinate 30 mg/kg, IV once
      Dexamethasone sodium phosphate 4–6 mg/kg, IV once

Pressor agent
   Dopamine 2–5 μg/kg/min constant rate infusion

Calcium supplementation
   Calcium gluconate 10% solution 50–150 mg/kg IV to effect
   Calcium chloride 10% solution 50–150 mg/kg, IV to effect
   Monitor heart rate, may cause bradycardia

Rapidly acting diuretic
   Furosemide 2–4 mg/kg, IV once

Rapidly acting venodilator
   Nitroglycerine paste (2%) 1/4 to 1 inch applied to skin, once
   Monitor blood pressure, may cause hypotension

mans.[6,11,12] Dogs receiving incompatible blood exhibit fever, tachypnea, salivation, urinations, and defecation as well as hemoglobinemia and hemoglobinuria (Fig. 129.2).[13] The Coombs' test is not always positive.

In any patient displaying signs of a hemolytic transfusion reaction, the transfusion should be immediately discontinued until the source of the reaction is identified (Fig. 129.1). Intravenous access should be maintained by infusion with a crystalloid solution. Cytokine-mediated hypotension may ensue; consequently, blood pressure and urine output should be monitored. Pressor agents such as dopamine and diuretics such as furosemide should be considered if blood pressure or urine output is low (Table 129.1). Evaluation of coagulation parameters in dogs and cats is reasonable because disseminated intravascular coagulation occurs following transfusion of incompatible blood in humans. The role of glucocorticoids has not been evaluated in this clinical situation, but their use has been recommended (Table 129.1).[3]

Prevention of acute hemolytic transfusion reactions is dependent on identification of compatible RBCs for transfusion. Both donor and recipient cats must be of the same blood type or accelerated clearance of transfused RBCs follows transfusion.[10] If blood typing is not possible prior to transfusion, a compatible crossmatch will indicate compatibility between donor and recipient but will not prevent sensitization of the recipient to future transfusions. Dogs differ from cats and man in that they do not appear to have any clinically important naturally occurring alloantibodies against RBCs. This means a crossmatch between two dogs never before transfused should be compatible, and an initial transfusion between two such dogs is not expected to cause an acute hemolytic transfusion reaction. If a second transfusion is given to a dog more than 4 days after the first, a crossmatch should be performed because antibodies against donor RBCs may form during that time. Dogs negative for dog erythrocyte antigen (DEA) 1.1 or untyped dogs should receive only DEA 1.1-negative blood to prevent formation of antibodies against DEA 1.1, which will result in a serious acute hemolytic transfusion reaction.

Urticaria or hives is a mild complication of transfusion that is attributed to antibodies against serum proteins (Fig. 129.3). The incidence of urticaria in canine and feline transfusions is less than 1%.[1-3] If urticaria occurs without other signs, the transfusion may be continued at a slower rate after administration of antihistamines (Table 129.1).

ACUTE TRANSFUSION REACTIONS—NONIMMUNOLOGIC

In dogs, vomiting in association with transfusion occurs approximately 1% of the time.[2,3] Rapid administration of blood or consumption of food prior or during transfusion is believed to be the cause. Vomiting typically resolves spontaneously and is easily prevented by withholding food and controlling the rate of administration of the transfusion. Vomiting has also been reported to be a common clinical sign in cats receiving bacterially contaminated blood.[14]

Blood, like any other fluid, can cause volume overload during transfusion if the cardiovascular status of the patient is not monitored during transfusion. It is expected to occur most often in patients with chronic or normovolemic anemia, pre-existing cardiac disease, and rapid transfusions. Treatment of volume overload consists of intravenous administration of a rapidly acting diuretic, rapid venodilation with nitroglycerine, and administration of oxygen in an oxygen cage, via a mask or nasal cannula (Table 129.1). Administration of the smallest volume of blood or component possible—for example, transfusion of packed RBCs instead of whole blood in cases of chronic anemia—is essential to decrease the risk of volume overload. Blood should be administered no faster than 1 mL/kg/hr.[15] If the planned volume cannot be administered in less than 4 hours, the blood should be split into two aliquots using sterile transfer packs to allow half the blood to be stored in the refrigerator while the other half is transfused.

Bacterial contamination of blood can occur at any point during the collection, processing, or storage of blood. RBCs are stored at 4°C in an attempt to inhibit bacterial growth, but certain bacteria can proliferate under these conditions. Platelets are stored at 24°C and have been most frequently associated with bacterial contamination.[16] Transfusion of blood containing high levels of endotoxin to humans results in a severe transfusion reaction consisting of fever, chills, nausea, and vomiting. Fatality is as high as 35%.[17] Cats receiving *Serratia marcescens*-contaminated whole blood most commonly developed vomiting or acute collapse. Fever was uncommon, occurring in only 1 of 14 cats receiving a contaminated transfusion.[14] If a contaminated transfusion is suspected, the patient's blood and the transfused blood should be cultured and broad-spectrum antibiotic therapy instituted based on the results of a Gram stain performed on a sample of blood from the bag (Fig. 129.1).

Preventing transfusion of contaminated blood is a multistep process.[15,17] Only completely healthy blood donors are eligible to donate. Blood must be collected with strict aseptic technique to prevent contamination by the donor's skin flora. Blood must be processed into components using closed multibag systems designed to prevent contamination and stored under conditions designed to limit bacterial proliferation. Finally, inspection of each unit of blood before transfusion for abnormal color or the presence of clots will help prevent administration of a contaminated unit (Fig. 129.4).

The presence of free hemoglobin in the blood bag or in the recipient's urine or plasma may be caused by bacterial contamination, an acute hemolytic transfusion reaction, or physical damage to the RBCs during collection, storage, or administration. As discussed above, transfusion of contaminated blood or an acute hemolytic transfusion reaction typically occurs with dramatic clinical signs. Transfusion of damaged RBCs is typically asymptomatic except for hemoglobinuria in the absence of worsening anemia.

Freezing, overheating, or excessive pressure from an infusion pump during transfusion can all result in physical trauma to RBCs and subsequent hemolysis. Addition of hypertonic (intravenous medications) or hypotonic

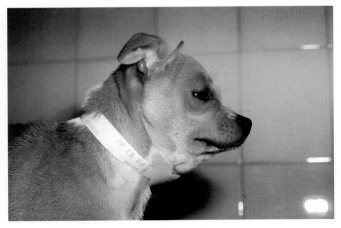

FIGURE 129.3 A urticarial reaction in a dog receiving plasma to treat rodenticide intoxication. Treatment with antihistamines and steroids induced resolution in 24 hours.

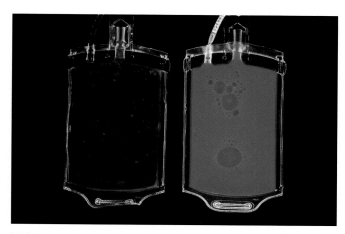

FIGURE 129.4 A unit of blood contaminated by bacterial and a normal unit. The contaminated blood on the left is an abnormal brown color and has visible clots. (Reprinted with permission from JAVMA 1997;210:795, with permission from the American Veterinary Medical Association, Schaumburg, IL.)

solutions (5% dextrose in water) to RBCs may also cause hemolysis. This complication can be prevented by storing blood under controlled conditions, never adding any solution except normal saline, and using only those pumps approved for use with blood products.[18]

Embolism with air occurs following transfusion of blood stored in glass bottles.[19] When the bottle is vented, air is introduced and if transfused may cause acute death. Glass bottles should not be used for the collection and storage of blood.

Although rarely performed in veterinary medicine, massive transfusion (transfusion of greater than 1 blood volume) may result in abnormalities of electrolytes, body temperature, and coagulation. Calcium is bound by citrate, a component of anticoagulant-preservative solutions, causing hypocalcemia and myocardial depression.[20] If hypocalcemia occurs, calcium chloride or calcium gluconate can be used to reverse the citrate effects (Table 129.1).[21] Potassium leaks from RBCs into the anticoagulant-preservative solution and in patients with pre-existing hyperkalemia or renal failure may exacerbate elevations in serum potassium. Transfusion of recently collected blood will help prevent this complication in patients at risk. Hypothermia, resulting from rapid infusion of refrigerated blood, will potentiate arrhythmias from hyperkalemia or hypocalcemia. Massive transfusion of stored blood, which is deficient in clotting factors, results in a dilutional coagulopathy.

Monitoring calcium, potassium, coagulation parameters, and body temperature during a massive transfusion is necessary to allow intervention before abnormalities become life-threatening. An electrocardiogram may be an adjunct to the measurement of serum electrolytes. Hypocalcemia is suspected when prolongation of the Q–T interval, depression of P and T waves, or ventricular arrhythmias are seen. The electrocardiogram is also useful to monitor for hyperkalemia. Decreased height of P waves, loss of P waves, or widening of the QRS

complex with large T waves are seen with hyperkalemia. If coagulation tests become prolonged, fresh frozen plasma can be administered to correct the deficiency of clotting factors.

DELAYED TRANSFUSION EFFECTS—IMMUNOLOGIC

The late effects of transfusion, such as posttransfusion purpura or delayed hemolytic transfusion reactions, occur as the result of an anamnestic immunologic response induced by a previous transfusion. The antibodies produced result in destruction of the transfused cells or platelets. Delayed hemolytic transfusion reactions, consisting of a falling hematocrit, icterus, fever, and a positive Coombs' test have not been well-documented in veterinary patients.[1,22] Posttransfusion purpura has recently been reported in a hemophiliac dog.[23] Thrombocytopenia and petechiation were subsequent to production of antibodies induced by previous transfusions and directed against the recipient's platelets. Optimal therapy for this disorder is unknown in veterinary patients, but corticosteroid administration may be beneficial. Delayed immunologic transfusion reactions cannot be predicted by performing a crossmatch.

DELAYED TRANSFUSION EFFECTS—NONIMMUNOLOGIC

Although extensive screening is typically performed on blood collected for transfusion, transmission of disease from donors to recipients is possible. In the cat, transmission of retroviruses (feline leukemia virus and feline immunodeficiency virus) and corona viruses is of the greatest concern. *Bartonella henselae* is an emerging disease in the cat that has been transmitted to other cats via transfusion.[24] Transmission of *Hemobartonella canis* and *Babesia canis* to canine transfusion recipients is a documented delayed complication of transfusion.[25,26] Theoretically, transmission of *Ehrlichia sp.*, *Borrelia burgdorferi*, and the microfilaria of *Dirofilaria immitis* is possible but has not been demonstrated. Screening of donors for infectious diseases potentially transmitted by transfusion is necessary to prevent this transfusion complication.

EVALUATION OF PATIENT EXPERIENCING A TRANSFUSION COMPLICATION

Monitoring a patient during a transfusion will allow early detection of complications. Baseline assessments of PCV, plasma, urine color, temperature, pulse, and respiratory rate should be made immediately prior to transfusion. Administration of a transfusion in an area of the hospital where the recipient can be continuously observed for signs such as restlessness, panting, vomiting, defecation, or collapse will assist in the identification of a transfusion reaction. The material provided in the cage to absorb urine should be white to facilitate recognition of hemoglobinuria. Before the transfusion is initiated, the information of the bag of blood should be checked against the crossmatch or blood type information in the medical record to ensure the correct unit of blood is being administered.[27] Because acute hemolytic reactions or signs resulting from transfusion of contaminated blood can occur following only 1 to 2 mL of blood, monitoring in the first half hour of the transfusion is critical.

If an adverse effect of transfusion is recognized, the transfusion must be discontinued immediately and the intravenous line maintained with an infusion of crystalloid solution while an assessment of the seriousness of the reaction is assessed. The PCV, plasma, urine color, temperature, pulse, and respiratory rate should be compared with baseline values. Hemoglobin in the plasma suggests an acute hemolytic transfusion reaction, bacterial contamination of blood, or physical damage to RBCs. A contaminated unit of blood may be identified several ways. Visual observation of the unit prior to transfusion may reveal a brown discoloration, hemolysis, or clots (Fig. 129.4). Samples of the blood remaining in the blood bag or tubing should be evaluated for hemolysis and Gram-stained for microscopic evaluation. If other signs of an acute hemolytic reaction or bacterial contamination are present, culture of the blood is necessary. Any intravenous solution administered concurrently with the transfusion or used to dilute packed RBCs is a potential source for contamination, and thus a Gram stain and culture are important. Blood from the recipient should also be cultured and submitted for Coombs' testing. A positive Coombs' test following transfusion in a patient with a negative Coombs' test prior to transfusion suggests an acute hemolytic reaction. The Coombs' test may be negative if all the transfused cells have been cleared from circulation when the sample is obtained. If an acute hemolytic transfusion reaction is suspected, the blood type and/or crossmatch should be repeated to eliminate laboratory error as the cause. In dogs or cats exhibiting respiratory distress during a transfusion, a central venous pressure measurement, thoracic auscultation, or thoracic radiographs help to identify patients with volume overload. If vomiting occurs in the absence of other clinical or laboratory abnormalities, the transfusion may be continued.

REFERENCES

1. **Henson MS, Kristensen AT, Armstrong PJ, et al.** Feline blood component therapy: Retrospective study of 246 transfusions. J Vet Intern Med 1994;8:169.
2. **Callan MB, Oakley DA, Shofer FS, et al.** Canine red blood cell transfusion practice. JAAHA 1996;32:303–311.
3. **Harrell K, Parrow J, Kristensen A.** Canine transfusion reactions. Part II. Prevention and treatment. Comp Cont Ed Small Animal Pract 1997;19:193–200.
4. **Rogers SE, Edmondson D, Goodrick MJ, et al.** Prestorage white cell reduction in saline-adenine-glucose-mannitol red cells by use of an integral filter: Evaluation of storage values and in vivo recovery. Transfusion 1995;35:727–733.
5. **Capon SM, Goldfinger D.** Acute hemolytic transfusion reaction, a paradigm of the systemic inflammatory response: New insights into pathophysiology and treatment. Transfusion 1995;35(6):513–520.
6. **Pineda AA, Brzica SM, Taswell HF.** Hemolytic transfusion reaction. Mayo Clin Proc 1978;53:378–390.
7. **Auer L, Bell K.** Blood transfusion reactions in the cat. JAVMA 1982;180:729–730.
8. **Giger U, Akol KG.** Acute hemolytic transfusion reaction in an Abyssinian cat with blood type B. J Vet Intern Med 1990;4:315–316.
9. **Wilkerson MJ, Wardrop KJ, Giger U, et al.** Two cat colonies with A and B blood types and a clinical transfusion reaction. Feline Pract 1991;19(2):22–27.
10. **Giger U, Bucheler J.** Transfusion of type-A and type-B blood to cats. J Vet Med Assoc 1991;198:411–418.
11. **Giger U, Gelens CJ, Callan MB, et al.** An acute hemolytic transfusion reaction caused by dog erythrocyte antigen 1.1 incompatibility in a previously sensitized dog. JAVMA 1995;206:1358–1362.
12. **Yuile CL, VanZandt TF, Ervin DM, et al.** Hemolytic reactions produced in dogs by transfusion of incompatible dog blood and plasma. Blood 1948;4:1232–1239.
13. **Young LE, Ervin DM, Yuile CL.** Hemolytic reactions produced in dogs by transfusion of incompatible dog blood and plasma. Blood 1948;4:1218–1231.
14. **Hohenhaus AE, Drusin LM, Garvey MS.** *Serratia marcescens* contamination of feline whole blood in a hospital blood bank. JAVMA 1997;210:794–798.
15. **Green CE.** Blood transfusion therapy: An updated overview. Proceedings of the American Animal Hospital Association's 49th Annual Meeting, 1982;187–189.
16. **Goldman M, Blajchman MA.** Blood product associated bacterial sepsis. Trans Med Rev 1991;5:73–83.
17. **Morduchowicz G, Pitlik SD, Huminer D, et al.** Transfusion reactions due to bacterial contamination of blood and blood products. Rev Infect Dis 1991;13:307–314.
18. **Stiles J, Raffe MR.** Hemolysis of canine fresh and stored blood associated with peristaltic pump infusion. Vet Emerg Crit Care 1991;1:50–53.
19. **Turnwald GH, Pichler ME.** Blood transfusion in dogs and cats. Part II. Administration, adverse effects, and component therapy. Compend Cont Educ Pract Vet 1985;7:115–126.
20. **Cooper N, Brazier JR, Huttenrott C, et al.** Myocardial depression following citrated blood transfusion. Arch Surg 1973;107:756–763.
21. **Cote CJ, Drop LJ, et al.** Calcium chloride versus calcium gluconate: Comparison of ionization and cardiovascular effects in children and dogs. Anesthesiology 1987;66:465–470.
22. **Kerl ME, Hohenhaus AE.** Packed red blood cell transfusions in dogs: 131 cases (1989). JAVMA 1993;202:1495–1499.
23. **Wardrop KJ, Lewis D, Marks S, et al.** Posttransfusion purpura in a dog with hemophilia A. J Vet Intern Med 1997;11:261–263.
24. **Kordick DL, Brietschwerdt EB.** Relapsing bacteremia after blood transmission of *Bartonella henselae* to cats. Am J Vet Res 1997;58:492–497.
25. **Lester SJ, Hume JB, Phipps B.** *Haemobartonella canis* infection following splenectomy and transfusion. Can Vet J 1995;36:444–445.
26. **Freeman MJ, Kirby BM, Panciera DL, et al.** Hypotensive shock syndrome associated with acute *Babesia canis* infection in a dog. JAVMA 1994;204;94–96.
27. **Sazama K.** Reports of 355 transfusion associated deaths: 1976–1985. Transfusion 1990;30:583–590.

CHAPTER 130

Hemapheresis

• GERALD S. POST

METHODOLOGY

The first cell separator was codeveloped by the NCI and IBM.[1] This began the era of therapeutic hemapheresis, which is defined as the process by which components thought to cause disease are removed from the blood.

Because of the availability of automated equipment to perform hemapheresis in human medicine, the use of manual techniques (whole blood exchange and component extraction/exchange) is usually reserved only for infants or special cases.[1] Manual techniques are often necessary in veterinary medicine because of the small blood volume of many of our patients (see the section on future applications in this chapter for more information). These manual techniques can be divided into two types. Whole blood exchange is the removal of some volume of blood and its replacement with a similar volume of donor blood. This procedure is rapid, inexpensive, and needs no special equipment. Because multiple units of compatible blood are needed for *one* exchange, transfusion reactions, cost, sodium or citrate overload (from anticoagulant), and disease transmission are problems. A second manual method involves the withdrawal of blood, which is then subjected to centrifugation and fractionation and the plasma or offending agent (buffy coat, red cells) being removed. The remaining normal components are reinfused with appropriate volume replacement. This technique is also inexpensive in terms of specialized equipment but is extremely labor-intensive and requires much manipulation of the blood.

Automated in-line blood cell separators have revolutionized hemapheresis. Some of the companies that manufacture in-line cell separators are COBE Lab., Fresenius, Haemonetics Co., Baxter-Fenwal Lab., Therakos, J. & J. Co., Asahi Medical Co., and Kuraray Co. Currently there are two techniques for automated cell separators: centrifugal and filtration/absorption methods. In centrifugal separation, whole blood is separated into its various components based on the separation coefficients of these components.[2] Intermittent and continuous separation devices are made. These machines can be utilized for various forms of apheresis. Plasmapheresis involves the removal and exchange of plasma. Cytapheresis involves the removal of specific cells; leukapheresis is the removal of leukocytes, plateletpheresis is the removal of platelets, and lymphoplasmapheresis involves the removal of lymphocytes and plasma.[2]

The second methodology in automated therapeutic apheresis involves the use of filter/membrane technology. In these types of machines, plasma is separated from cells using a low transmembrane pressure gradient (typically less than 50 mm Hg) across a microporous filter/membrane.[2] The size of the pores in the fibers of the filter or in the membrane determines the substance(s) removed, based on their molecular weight. Numerous filters are available commercially depending on the desired use. The companies that manufacture these filters include Travenol Lab., COBE Lab., Fresenius, Asahi Medical Co., Kuraray Co., Terumo, Organon Teknika, and Kawasumi Lab., Inc. These filters are typically made from cellulose, polypropylene, polyethylene alcohol, or polyvinyl alcohol.[2] Multiple filters can often be used in serial fashion to create a cascade filtration machine. The problem associated with this methodology is the increase in extracorporeal volume and the high incidence of filter clogging. Additional technologies utilized in filtration systems involve, but are not limited to, cryoprecipitation, dextran sulfate precipitation, thermofiltration, cryofiltration, and heparin acidification. One of the most selective apheresis techniques involves the use of adsorption methods. This involves the selective removal of molecules based on their adsorption to nonspecific or specific ligands. Examples of nonspecific adsorption filters are charcoal and heparin. Specific adsorption filters include anion exchange resins, tryptophan, DNA, staphylococcal protein A, and various specific monoclonal antibodies for specific antigen removal.[2]

Plasmapheresis

Current Uses in Veterinary Medicine

The use of plasmapheresis in veterinary medicine started in the late 1970s and early 1980s. Over the last 10 to 20 years many diseases have been treated with this modality. There are no reports that evaluate more than a few animals; therefore, larger clinical trials for each disease state are needed to determine the true efficacy of this modality in veterinary medicine.

Paraproteinemias and Hyperviscosity Syndrome

Paraproteinemias and hyperviscosity syndrome can be treated with plasmapheresis. This syndrome involves the abnormal production of a monoclonal gammopathy, usually involving IgA or IgM but occasionally involving IgG. Plasma viscosity is raised because of increased production of these paraproteins, and altered blood flow to many organs is resultant. Multiple myeloma and ehrlichiosis are the two most common diseases associated with paraproteinemia and hyperviscosity in veterinary medicine.[3-6] Lymphoma,[7] chronic lymphocytic leukemia,[8] macroglobulinemia,[9] and other inflammatory/infectious conditions[10,11] can cause paraproteinemias as well. The standard therapy for these various conditions, ranging from ehrlichiosis to multiple myeloma, involves the use of specific drug therapy. Cytotoxic chemotherapy is used in the various malignancies and antibiotic therapy is used in the treatment of infectious diseases. These drug therapies often have a substantial lag time between initiation of therapy and response. Plasmapheresis can be used to immediately lower the circulating levels of immunoglobulins in these disease states. Multiple dogs have been treated with between 1 and 3 plasmapheresis treatments for hyperviscosity syndrome, resulting in rapid improvement in clinical signs.[3,4] One cat with hyperviscosity syndrome treated with manual plasmapheresis is reported in the veterinary literature.[4]

Immune-mediated Diseases

Plasmapheresis has been used to treat immune-mediated diseases such as immune-mediated hemolytic anemia, immune-mediated thrombocytopenia, myasthenia gravis, systemic lupus erythematosus, and acute inflammatory polyradiculoneuropathy.

Immune-mediated hemolytic anemia (IMHA) involves the destruction of erythrocytes by antibodies directed against red cell antigens. Plasmapheresis can rapidly decrease the level of these circulating antibodies. There are only two dogs reported in the veterinary literature with a documented response to plasmapheresis for IMHA.[12] Because of the small sample size, it is therefore unknown what role, if any, plasmapheresis has in the management of veterinary patients with IMHA. Plasmapheresis for the rapid removal of antiplatelet antibodies has been advocated but also poorly described.[13]

Myasthenia gravis is caused by the production of antibodies directed against the acetylcholine receptors of skeletal muscles. A solitary dog with this disease treated with plasmapheresis is documented.[14]

Canine systemic lupus erythematosus (SLE) is an immune-mediated disorder characterized by immune complex deposition and the presence of antinuclear antibodies. Despite this simplistic view of this complex disorder, SLE can be a difficult diagnosis to establish.[15] Six dogs with SLE treated with plasmapheresis are de-

scribed in the literature.[15,16] Plasmapheresis is used to remove circulating immune complexes and autoantibodies. The dogs in these studies had clinical responses within 48 hours.[15,16] The use of immunosuppressive drugs in combination with the plasmapheresis is advocated in these reports to enhance and prolong the clinical response.[16] Leukapheresis was utilized in two of these dogs to further augment immunosuppression.[16] Plasmapheresis was unsuccessfully attempted in one dog with polyradiculoneuropathy.[13] This disease is characterized by an acute inflammatory cell infiltrate in the pericapillary area of the peripheral nerve tissue.[13]

Neoplastic Disorders

Plasmapheresis can be used to remove circulating immune complexes and other 'blocking' factors that are thought to contribute to the body's altered immune response to cancer.[17] There are three studies that evaluate the utility of plasmapheresis in various neoplastic conditions in dogs.[18-20] (See the section on ultrapheresis in this chapter for additional information.) One study reported a positive response to using an asparaginase-glutaminase reactor plasmapheresis system in dogs with lymphoma.[20] There are numerous articles pertaining to the use of staphylococcal protein A immunoadsorption in the treatment of feline leukemia.[21,22] This technique cleared the viremia, improved the FeLV-associated diseases, and induced a proliferative bone marrow response in a percentage of the affected cats.[21,22]

Plasmapheresis in Human Medicine with Possible Future Applications in Veterinary Medicine

An extensive review of the uses of plasmapheresis in human medicine is beyond the scope of this chapter; hundreds of diseases have been treated with plasmapheresis. I will attempt to highlight the major diseases treated with plasmapheresis in human medicine. An overview of the disease states for which therapeutic hemapheresis is an option, has been published.[23]

Plasmapheresis is listed as the standard of care for the following diseases (some which may have relevance to veterinary medicine): HIV-related polyneuropathy, HIV-related hyperviscosity, ABO incompatible bone marrow transplant, polycythemia vera, leukocytosis, thrombocytosis, sickle cell disease, cutaneous lymphoma, familial hypercholesterolemia, Guillain-Barré syndrome, inflammatory demyelinating polyneuropathy, myasthenia gravis, porphyria, hemochromatosis, cryoglobulinemia, Goodpasture's syndrome, and thrombotic thrombocytopenia.[23] Other disease states seen in veterinary medicine for which therapeutic apheresis is considered acceptable include systemic lupus erythematosus, pemphigus vulgaris, bullous pemphigoid, systemic vasculitis, paraproteinemia, multiple myeloma, hemolytic uremic syndrome, and progressive nephritis.[23] The diseases in veterinary medicine for which the use of plasmapheresis is of uncertain value, even in human medicine are: IMHA, aplastic anemia/red cell aplasia, cancer, immune-mediated thrombocytopenia, paraneoplastic syndromes (neurologic), polymyositis-dermatomyositis, and rheumatoid arthritis.[23]

The use of plasmapheresis in veterinary medicine is severely limited by the cost of the equipment and small size and blood volume of many of our veterinary patients. Equipment costs can be reduced by obtaining older equipment from human hospitals and by reusing filters.[24] Pediatricians also face the problem of small size and blood volume faced by veterinarians. There have been a number of recent articles describing techniques on how to circumvent these problems and safely and effectively use therapeutic apheresis in these small patients.[25-27] The use of continuous flow machines is recommended, as discontinuous flow machines cause intermittent hypovolemia and hypervolemia, which are poorly tolerated by small patients.[25] The pediatric literature suggests priming the machine with red cells when the extracorporeal circuit is 15% or greater than the patient's whole blood volume or when the patient is anemic or unstable.[25] (The extracorporeal circuit volume varies by manufacturer and model, but is generally between 125–300 mL.) The whole blood volume is calculated as 85 to 90 mL/kg for the dog and 65 to 75 mL/kg for the cat, which is in the range of 70 mL/kg for infants and children to 100 mL/kg for neonates.[25] Inlet flow rates also are often slow because of the smaller vascular access. It is therefore important to use cell separators that will flow at low rates.[25] In addition, inlet or replacement fluid rates in pediatrics are generally limited to 25 mL/min to limit the severity of potential side effects.[25] Anticoagulant-citrate-dextrose formula A (ACD-A) is the most widely used anticoagulant in apheresis, but citrate toxicity can occur.[25] The use of ACD-A in pediatrics (and possibly in veterinary medicine) has some limitations because of its calcium-binding effect.[25] Therefore, in addition to PT, PTT, and ACT measurements, ionized calcium is also monitored during and after apheresis.[25] Prevention of citrate toxicity may include the addition of 10% calcium gluconate to the replacement fluid, a decreased rate of citrate infusion, or calcium gluconate infusion.[25] The goal for pediatric anticoagulation is to maintain an ACT of 180 to 220 seconds during the procedure. Heparin can also be used as an anticoagulant for apheresis. The amount of heparin needed to maintain an ACT of 1.5 times normal and no clogging of the membranes/filters (if membrane or filter machines are used) is higher for dogs than for humans (G. Post, personal experience). A blood warmer is also more essential in small patients because a higher percentage of their blood volume is extracorporeal at any given time.

Numerous disease states may benefit from plasmapheresis. FIV-related neuropathy[28] may be similar in etiopathogenesis to HIV-related polyneuropathy and therefore possibly responsive to plasmapheresis. A specific form of plasmapheresis called photopheresis[29] is used to treat cutaneous lymphoma in people. This procedure involves the irradiation of the extracorporeal blood, usually after the administration of a photoreactive moiety such as psoralen.[30] This irradiation activates the psoralen, which then binds to, amongst others, DNA and causes interstrand cross-links and apoptosis.[31] This therapeutic option may be tried in cutaneous lymphoma of the dog or cat, for which no effective treatment exists. Familial hyperlipidemia of Schnauzers[32] and other dogs will be discussed later (under the section on lipidpheresis). Guillain-Barré syndrome, described in a few veterinary patients,[33,34] may benefit from plasmapheresis as it does in people based on the removal of the likely pathogenic IgM antiperipheral nerve myelin antibodies and the IgG antiganglioside antibodies.[35] Inflammatory demyelinating neuropathy, although infrequently described in the veterinary literature, may benefit from this treatment. Myasthenia gravis, a condition well described in both dogs[36,37] and cats[38,39] is another neurologic condition that may benefit from this treatment. Cryoglobulinemia has already been discussed. Thrombotic thrombocytopenia, a well-documented syndrome in people,[40] has some similarities to a vasculitic disease in Greyhounds[41] and certain cases of disseminated intravascular coagulation.[42] Plasmapheresis is often considered the standard of care for thrombotic thrombocytopenia in people[23,40] and may be useful for these related syndromes in veterinary medicine.

Other more common diseases in veterinary medicine for which plasmapheresis may be useful include refractory IMHA and immune-mediated thrombocytopenia. Even in human medicine there is insufficient evidence to establish the efficacy of this modality in these disease states, and thus further study is warranted.[23] Therapeutic plasmapheresis is used in these conditions for individuals for whom conventional therapy has failed.[23]

Tick-borne diseases are another common entity in our veterinary patients. To my knowledge, the only reported use of plasmapheresis for a tick-borne disease in veterinary medicine involves a dog with monoclonal gammopathy associated with *Ehrlichia canis*.[4] Interestingly, two cases of human babesiosis treated with therapeutic apheresis were recently reported.[43] Those veterinary patients with refractory babesiosis, ehrlichiosis, or other similar infectious disease may benefit from plasmapheresis even in the absence of a monoclonal gammopathy.

Leukapheresis

Leukapheresis is the removal of white blood cells from the circulation. The use of this modality in human medicine is reserved for certain leukemic patients[44] and as a technique to collect peripheral blood progenitor or stem cells for use in cancer patients receiving high-dose chemotherapy or radiation therapy.[45,46] To my knowledge, leukapheresis is not used clinically in veterinary medicine at the present time; however, a canine model for the collection of colony-forming units in peripheral blood using leukapheresis has been described.[47] As advances in veterinary oncology continue it is conceivable that leukapheresis, for the harvest of progenitor cells, could be utilized in conjunction with high-dose chemotherapy to treat certain canine and feline malignancies.

Plateletpheresis

Plateletpheresis is the removal of platelets from the circulation and is mainly utilized in human medicine to obtain platelets for transfusions.[48] These platelet transfusions are most commonly given to patients with severe thrombocytopenia as a result of chemotherapy, radiation therapy, bone marrow failure or aplastic anemia, or myelophthisis as a result of tumor infiltration.[48] As veterinary transfusion medicine continues its advances in the field of component therapy, it is likely that plateletpheresis will someday be utilized to treat similar conditions.

Lipoprotein and Lipid Apheresis

Low-density lipoprotein apheresis involves the removal of low-density lipoprotein (LDL) cholesterol via specific immunoadsorption columns.[49] Any posttreatment level of LDL cholesterol can be obtained because time of filtration is the limiting factor.[49] This procedure leads to an increase of high-density lipoproteins (HDL) in more than 50% of human patients.[49] A newer technique called lipidapheresis involves the removal of cholesterol and triglycerides from the plasma while retaining the apolipoproteins.[50] The utility of one or both of these techniques to treat coronary heart disease is still under investigation;[50] the treatment of familial hypercholesterolemia by LDL-apheresis is well-accepted.[23] In veterinary medicine, miniature Schnauzers and some other breeds have a familial hyperlipidemic syndrome.[32,51,52] The very low-density lipoproteins are elevated in these miniature Schnauzers, and chylomicronemia may or may not be present.[32] With modification of the immunoadsorption column, lipidapheresis may be a possible treatment for this disorder.

Ultrapheresis

Ultrapheresis is a term coined by Dr. M. Rigdon Lentz to describe a form of therapeutic apheresis in which molecules less than 100 kd are removed from the blood. This type of apheresis does not remove molecules greater than 150 kd; consequently, platelets, immunoglobulins, clotting factors, and cells are not removed. The moieties removed include shed receptors to IL-1, IL-2, IL-6, interferon gamma, and the shed receptor to TNF-α and TNF-β.[53]

Immunosuppression is a common finding in both people and animals with advanced malignancy. This immunosuppression has been ascribed to many factors, including shed tumor antigens, immunoglobulins, and cytokine inhibitors. By removing these immunosuppressive factors, an immunologic attack on the malignant cells is brought about. Both people[54] and dogs[55] with cancer have been treated with ultrapheresis, with demonstration of tumor regression in many cases. Currently, multiple human malignancies are undergoing clinical trials with this form of therapy, and further therapy is warranted in the veterinary field.

REFERENCES

1. **James L. Mac Pherson, Duke O. Kasprisin,** eds. Therapeutic hemapheresis. Boca Raton, FL: CRC Press Inc, 1985.
2. **Sawada K, Malchesky PS, Nose Y.** Available removal systems: State of the art. Curr Stud Hematol Blood Trans 1990;57:51–113.
3. **Matus RE, Leifer CE, Gordon BR, MacEwen EG, Hurvitz AI.** Plasmapheresis and chemotherapy of hyperviscosity syndrome associated with monoclonal gammopathy in the dog. JAVMA 1983;183:215–218.
4. **Forrester SD, Greco DS, Relford RL.** Serum hyperviscosity syndrome associated with multiple myeloma in two cats. JAVMA 1992;200:79–82.
5. **Matus RE, Leifer CE, Hurvitz AI.** Use of plasmapheresis and chemotherapy for treatment of monoclonal gammopathy associated with *Ehrlichia canis* infection in a dog. JAVMA 1987;190:1302–1304.
6. **Hribernik TN, Barta O, Gaunt SD, Boudreaux MK.** Serum hyperviscosity syndrome associated with IgG myeloma in a cat. JAVMA 1982;181:169–170.
7. **Williams DA, Goldschmidt MH.** Hyperviscosity syndrome with IgM monoclonal gammopathy and hepatic plasmacytoid lymphosarcoma in a cat. J Small Animal Pract 1982;23:311–323.
8. **MacEwen EG, Hurvitz AI, Hayes A.** Hyperviscosity syndrome associated with lymphocytic leukemia in three dogs. JAVMA 1977;170:1309–1312.
9. **Hurvitz AI, MacEwen EG, Middaugh CR, Litman GW.** Monoclonal cryoglobulinemia with macroglobulinemia in a dog. JAVMA 1977;170:511–513.
10. **Shelly SM, Scarlet-Kranz J, Blue JT.** Protein electrophoresis on effusions from cats as a diagnostic test for feline infectious peritonitis. JAAHA 1988;24:495.
11. **Wiedenkeller DE, Rosenberg MP.** Dysproteinemias. In: J August, ed. Consultations in feline medicine, 2nd ed. Philadelphia: WB Saunders, 1994:573.
12. **Matus RE, Schrader LA, Leifer CE, Gordon BR, Hurvitz AI.** Plasmapheresis as adjuvant therapy for autoimmune hemolytic anemia in two dogs. JAVMA 1985;186:691–693.
13. **Bartges JW.** Therapeutic plasmapheresis. Sem Vet Med Surg (Sm Animal) 1997;12:170–177.
14. **Bartges JW, Klausner JS, Bostwick EF, et al.** Clinical remission following plasmapheresis and corticosteroid treatment in a dog with acquired myasthenia gravis. JAVMA 1990;196:1276–1278.
15. **Matus RE, Scott RC, Saal S, Gordon BR, Hurvitz AI.** Plasmapheresis-immunoadsorption for treatment of systemic lupus erythematosus in a dog. JAVMA 1983;182:499–502.
16. **Matus RE, Gordon BR, Leifer CE, Saal S, Hurvitz AI.** Plasmapheresis in five dogs with systemic immune-mediated disease. JAVMA 1985;187:595–599.
17. **Nand S, Molokie R.** Therapeutic plasmapheresis and protein A immunoadsorption in malignancy: A brief review. J Clin Apheresis 1990;5:206–212.
18. **Klausner JS, Miller WJ, O'Brien TD, et al.** Effects of plasma treatment with purified protein A and *Staphylococcus aureus* Cowan I on spontaneous animal neoplasms. Cancer Res 1985;45:1263–1266.
19. **Gordon BR, Matus RE, Saal SD, et al.** Protein A independent tumoricidal responses following extracorporeal perfusion of plasma over *Staphylococcus aureus.* J Natl Cancer Inst 1983;70:1127–1131.
20. **Dennis MB Jr, Schmer G, Rastelli LN, Newman ML, Detter JC, Applebaum FR, Holcenberg JS.** Successful long-term use of a plasmapheresis reactor system in dogs with lymphoma. Trans Am Soc Artif Intern Organs 1983;744–748.
21. **Lafrado LJ, Mathes LE, Zack PM, Olsen RG.** Biological effects of staphylococcal protein A immunotherapy in cats with induced feline leukemia virus infection. Am J Vet Res 1990;51(3):482–486.
22. **Engelman RW, Tyler RD, Trang LQ, Liu WT, Good RA, Day NK.** Clinicopathologic responses in cats with feline leukemia virus-associated leukemia-lymphoma treated with staphylococcal protein A. Am J Pathol 1985;118:367–378.
23. **Strauss RG, Ciavarella D, Gilcher RO, Kasprisin DO, Kiprov DD, Klein HG, McLeod BC.** An overview of current management. J Clin Apheresis 193;8:189–194.
24. **Klinkmann H, Schmitt E, Falkenhagen D, Schmidt R, Osten B, Ahrenholtz P, Tessenow D.** Reuse of membrane plasma filters. In: Nose Y, Malchesky PS, Smith JW, Krakauer RS, et al, eds. Plasmapheresis. New York: Raven Press, 1983;107–112.
25. **Galacki DM.** An overview of therapeutic apheresis in pediatrics. J Clin Apheresis 1997;12:1–3.
26. **Kasprisin DO.** Techniques, indications and toxicity of therapeutic hemapheresis in children. J Clin Apheresis 1989;5:21–24.
27. **Kevy SV, Fosburg M.** Therapeutic apheresis in childhood. J Clin Apheresis 1990;5:87–90.
28. **Dow SW, Poss ML, Hoover EH.** Feline immunodeficiency virus: A neurotropic lentivirus. J Acquir Immune Defic Syndr 1990;3:658.
29. **Rook AH, Wolfe JT.** Role of extracorporeal photopheresis in the treatment of cutaneous t-cell lymphoma, autoimmune disease, and allograft rejection. J Clin Apheresis 1994;9:28–30.
30. **van Iperen HP, Brun BM, Cattieri S, Dell-Acqua F, Gasparro FP, Beijersbergen Henegouwen GM.** The lack of efficacy of 4,6,6'-trimethylangelicin to induce immune suppression in an animal model for photopheresis: A comparison with 8-MOP. Photochem Photobiol 1996;63:577–582.
31. **Yoo EK, Rook AH, Elenitsas R, Gasparro FP, Vowels BR.** Apoptosis induc-

tion of ultraviolet light A and photochemotherapy in cutaneous T-cell lymphoma: Relevance to mechanism of therapeutic action. J Invest Dermatol 1996;107:235–242.

32. **Whitney MS, Boon GD, Rebar AH, Story JA, Bottoms GD.** Ultracentrifugal and electrophoretic characteristics of the plasma lipoproteins of miniature Schnauzer dogs with idiopathic hyperproteinemia. J Vet Intern Med 1993;7:253–260.

33. **Cuddon PA.** Electrophysiologic assessment of acute polyradiculoneuropathy in dogs: Comparison with Guillain-Barré syndrome in people. J Vet Intern Med 1998;12:294–303.

34. **Northington JW, Brown MJ.** Acute idiopathic polyneuropathy. A Guillain-Barré-like syndrome in dogs. J Neurol Sci 1982;56:259–273.

35. **Weinstein R.** Is there a scientific rationale for therapeutic plasma exchange or intravenous immune globulin in the treatment of acute Guillain-Barré syndrome. J Clin Apheresis 1995;10:150–157.

36. **Miller LM, Lennon VA, Lambert EH, et al.** Congenital myasthenia gravis in thirteen smooth fox terriers. JAVMA 1983;182:694.

37. **Shelton GD.** Disorders of neuromuscular transmission Semin Vet Med Surg (Sm Animal) 1989;4:126.

38. **Cuddon PA.** Acquired immune-mediated myasthenia gravis in a cat. J Small Animal Pract 1989;30:511.

39. **O'Dair HA, Holt PE, Pearson GR, et al.** Acquired immune-mediated myasthenia gravis in a cat associated with a cystic thymus. J Small Animal Pract 1991;32:198.

40. **Elkins SL, Wilson PP Jr, Files JC, Morrison FS.** Thrombotic thrombocytopenic purpura: Evolution across 15 years. J Clin Apheresis 1996;11:173–175.

41. **Carpenter JL, Andelman NC, Moore FM, King NW Jr.** Idiopathic cutaneous and renal glomerular vasculopathy of Greyhounds. Vet Pathol 1988;25:401–407.

42. **Robbins SL, Cotran RS, Kumar V.** Pathologic basis of disease, 3rd ed. Philadelphia: WB Saunders, 1984;1048–1049.

43. **Evenson DI, Perry E, Kloster B, Hurley R, Stroncek DF.** Therapeutic apheresis for babesiosis. J Clin Apheresis 1998;13:32–36.

44. **Hale B.** Leukocytapheresis. In: Richard SA Tindall, ed. Therapeutic apheresis and plasma perfusion. New York: Alan R. Liss Inc, 1982;421–424.

45. **Keung Y, Cobos E, Dunn D, Park M, Dixon S, Wu, K, Park CH.** Determining factors for the outcome of peripheral blood progenitor cells harvests. J Clin Apheresis 1996;11:23–26.

46. **Murea S, Goldschmidt H, Hahn U, Pforsich M, Moos M, Haas R.** Successful collection and transplantation of peripheral blood stem cells in cancer patients using large-volume leukapheresis. J Clin Apheresis 1996;11:185–194.

47. **Kovacs P, Bruch C, Herbst EW, Friedner TM.** Collection of in vitro colony-forming units from dogs by repeated continuous flow leukapheresis. Acta Haemat 1978;60:172–180.

48. **Strauss RG.** Clinical perspectives of platelet transfusions: Defining the optimal dose. J Clin Apheresis 1995;10:124–127.

49. **Borberg H, Kadar J, Oette K.** The current status of low-density lipoprotein apheresis. Curr Stud Hematol Blood Transfus 1990;57:239–248.

50. **Cham BE, Kostner KM, Dwivedy AK, Shafey TM, Fang NX, Mahon MG, Iannuzzi CI, Colquhoun DM, Smith JL.** Lipid apheresis: An in vivo application of plasma delipidation with organic solvents resulting in acute transient reduction of circulating plasma lipids in animals. J Clin Apheresis 1995;10:61–69.

51. **Rogers WA, Donovan EF, Kociba GJ.** Idiopathic hyperlipoproteinemia in dogs. JAVMA 1975;166:1087–1091.

52. **Wada M, Minamisono T, Ehrhart LA, et al.** Familial hyperlipoproteinemia in beagles. Life Sci 1977;20:999–1008.

53. **Gatanaga T, Lentz R, Masunaka I, Tomich J, Jeffes EWB III, Baird M, Granger GA.** Identification of TNF-LT blocking factor(s) in the serum and ultrafiltrates of human cancer patients. Lymphokine Research 1990;9(2):225–229.

54. **Lentz MR.** Continuous whole blood ultrapheresis procedure in patients with metastatic cancer. J Bio Respir Modif 1989;8:511–27.

55. **Post GP, Mauldin GN, Lentz MR, Orentreich N.** The use of ultrapheresis in the treatment of canine malignancies. Proc Vet Cancer Soc 1997:10.

CHAPTER 131

Red Blood Cell Substitutes

• VIRGINIA T. RENTKO and TERRILYN A. SHARPE

Oxygen is poorly soluble in plasma; the plasma carries only 2% of the oxygen content of the blood. Hemoglobin transports the majority of oxygen in the blood. Mammalian hemoglobin is saturated with oxygen (97%) under ambient air conditions. Substitutes for the oxygen-carrying ability of blood have been in development for use in human medicine for over 50 years. The two major groups of red blood cell (RBC) substitutes are modified hemoglobin solutions and perfluorochemicals (PFC).

Solutions of hemoglobin seem a logical substitute for red cells. Survival of animals following total blood exchange with a hemoglobin-based oxygen-carrying (HBOC) solution was demonstrated in the 1930s by Amberson and more recently by Vlahakes.[1,2] Several hurdles have been overcome in the development of a clinically useful hemoglobin solution. First, outside of the RBC, tetrameric hemoglobin dissociates into two alpha-beta dimers (molecular weight 32 kd). These dimers readily pass through the renal glomeruli, resulting in rapid plasma clearance. Second, the oxygen affinity of hemoglobin in solution is greater than that of intracellular hemoglobin because of a loss of 2,3-DPG. Third, hemoglobin in solution has a high colloid osmotic pressure that limits the concentration able to be administered.

Bovine hemoglobin is preferable to other mammalian hemoglobins for use as an HBOC because unlike most hemoglobins it does not rely on 2,3-DPG to modulate oxygen uptake and release. In stored blood, the levels of 2,3-DPG naturally decrease, leading to a change in the oxygen-binding characteristic of canine hemoglobin. However, the oxygen binding of bovine hemoglobin is controlled by chloride, so changes in oxygen binding during storage are not seen. The molecular structure of bovine hemoglobin is similar to that of other mammalian hemoglobins. The amino acid sequence of hemoglobin is well-conserved across species.

PFCs are liquid organic compounds in which oxygen can dissolve. Their advantage is that they are formed from synthetic material that can be made in large quantities. However, compared with hemoglobin, PFCs have a lower capacity for carrying oxygen. High concentrations of oxygen (60–100%) must be administered with PFC infusions. One PFC, Fluosol-DA (20%) (Alpha Ther-apeutics Corporation, Los Angeles, CA) was FDA-approved for coronary artery angioplasty. It was subsequently withdrawn from the market because of poor utilization.

OXYGEN DELIVERY

Blood transfusions are considered life-saving owing to the oxygen-carrying ability of blood. The goal of administering blood is to improve systemic oxygen delivery. Oxygen delivery to tissues cannot be measured directly and therefore is represented by the following:

$$\text{oxygen delivery} = \text{cardiac output} \times \text{arterial oxygen content;}$$

$$\text{arterial oxygen content}^3 = \text{hemoglobin concentration} \times \text{\% saturation} \times 1.34$$

In anemic conditions, the decrease in arterial oxygen content is compensated by an increase in cardiac output to maintain oxygen delivery. Normally, oxygen delivery exceeds whole body oxygen requirements by four to fivefold. An additional compensatory mechanism is to increase oxygen extraction by the tissues. With severe anemia, the limits of these physiologic compensations are reached. Cardiac output and oxygen extraction can no longer compensate for the decrease in oxygen content. Oxygen consumption cannot be supported and tissues become hypoxic. Non–oxygen-carrying solutions such as crystalloids and synthetic colloids improve oxygen delivery via hemodilution, a resultant decrease in blood viscosity and an increase in cardiac output. Oxygen-carrying solutions (whole blood, packed red blood cells, and hemoglobin solutions) improve oxygen delivery by increasing arterial oxygen content, without associated cardiac work. An understanding of these physiologic mechanisms is key to establishing an optimal treatment plan for the anemic patient.

The clinical endpoints of oxygen delivery and signs of tissue hypoxia are not easily measured. Oxygen content of the blood can be directly measured in the laboratory but only indirectly assessed in a clinical setting. Clinically accessible parameters such as blood gases and pulse oximetry only indirectly reflect oxygen content.

Blood gas measurement of P_aO_2 (solubilized oxygen content in the plasma) aids in distinguishing hypoxemia due to hypoventilation, right to left stunting, ventilation-perfusion mismatching, and diffusion impairment, but it does not measure the majority of oxygen in the blood that is carried by hemoglobin. An anemic patient without a ventilatory disturbance maintains a normal P_aO_2. A second clinical assessment of oxygen-carrying requirements is pulse oximetry, which measures the arterial oxygen saturation of hemoglobin (in the red cell and plasma). Therefore, it reflects the oxygen content of the blood better than measurement of P_aO_2, but only reflects oxygen content indirectly. Because of the limitations with clinical measurements, clinical signs such as heart rate, blood pressure, pulse quality, mentation, and activity level are the most reliable indicators of improved oxygen delivery to tissues.

With the addition of hemoglobin to the plasma, oxygen transport is achieved by a fundamentally different mechanism than that performed by RBCs. Hemoglobin solutions are more efficient transporters of oxygen than are RBC suspensions.[4,5] Page et al.[5] investigated the oxygen transport function of RBC/hemoglobin solution mixtures in an in vitro model of an artificial capillary. Keeping the total hemoglobin concentration constant, the intracellular/extracellular hemoglobin ratio was varied. When a low concentration of hemoglobin solution was added to an RBC suspension, increased extraction of oxygen per gram of hemoglobin was seen compared with the red cell suspension alone. This increase in efficiency was attributed to an increase in the solubility of oxygen in the plasma, supporting the concept of hemoglobin solutions as therapeutics. Plasma hemoglobin facilitates diffusion of oxygen from red cells. This fact coupled with the low viscosity of the hemoglobin solution enables enhanced perfusion of tissues.

ASSESSING THE NEED FOR OXYGEN-CARRYING SUPPORT

A clinician's assessment of the severity of clinical signs and the hematocrit of an anemic animal form the basis on which a decision to transfuse is made. No controlled clinical studies examine the clinical consequences of anemia and transfusion practice in critically ill animals. The optimal lower limit to the transfusion trigger has not been established. A review of the literature in human patients suggests that improving oxygen delivery may decrease mortality in critically ill patients.[6] Historically, the transfusion trigger was called the '10/30 rule,' referring to a hemoglobin concentration of 10 g/dL or a packed cell volume (PCV) of 30%.[7] With the safety of human blood transfusions called into question in the mid-1980s, a limit of 8 g/dL hemoglobin was suggested by the Transfusion Practices Committee of the American Association of Blood Banks, and a limit of 7 g/dL hemoglobin was suggested by the NIH Consensus Conference of Perioperative Blood Transfusion. Currently, transfusions are administered at a much lower hemoglobin concentration to our veterinary patients. In fact, only

20% of small animal clinics perform transfusions regularly, despite the large number of anemic cases seen in practice.[8] The infrequency of administering blood likely reflects limited access to blood products. Veterinary practitioners have restricted access to blood components because of the constraints associated with availability of a sufficient number of compatible, disease-free donors. The technical limitations of blood typing, collecting, preparing, and storing blood components also restrict blood use. Because of the lack of compatible blood available to clinicians, dogs may not be transfused or may be placed at risk for a transfusion reaction from the use of unmatched blood. If blood or a suitable substitute were more readily available, transfusions would be administered earlier, before the anemia becomes too severe or life-threatening.

CHARACTERISTICS OF AN HBOC SOLUTION

One solution, Oxyglobin Solution (Biopure Corp., Cambridge, MA) is FDA-approved for use in dogs. Oxyglobin Solution [hemoglobin glutamer-200 (bovine)] is an ultrapurified, polymerized solution of bovine origin (13 g/dL) in a modified Ringer's lactate (Table 131.1). It has a physiologic pH (7.8) and osmolality (300 mOsm/kg). The viscosity is low (1.3 centipoise) comparable to that of crystalloid fluids (1.0 centipoise).

Oxyglobin is manufactured by stabilizing purified bovine hemoglobin. The purification process consists of various diafiltration, centrifugation, and chromatography steps designed to first isolate the RBCs from other blood cells and proteins, lysing the red cells to extract the hemoglobin. The purified hemoglobin is then chemically cross-linked to form stabilized tetramers and larger hemoglobin polymers (up to 500 kd) that are well-retained by the vascular system (plasma half-life 30–40 hours). Polymerization also allows for a physiologic concentration of hemoglobin (13 g/dL) with an acceptable oncotic pressure, 37 torr. After polymerization, less than 5% of

TABLE 131.1	Characteristics of a Hemoglobin-Based Oxygen-Carrying Solution[a]
Hemoglobin concentration	13 g/dL
P_{50}	38 torr
Osmolality	300 mOsm/kg
pH	7.8
Average molecular weight	200 kd
Methemoglobin	<10%
Colloid osmotic pressure	37 torr
Plasma half-life	30–40 hours[b]
Shelf life	2 years (room temperature)

[a] Oxyglobin Solution, Biopure Corp., Cambridge, MA
[b] (at 30 mL/kg), Dose-dependent

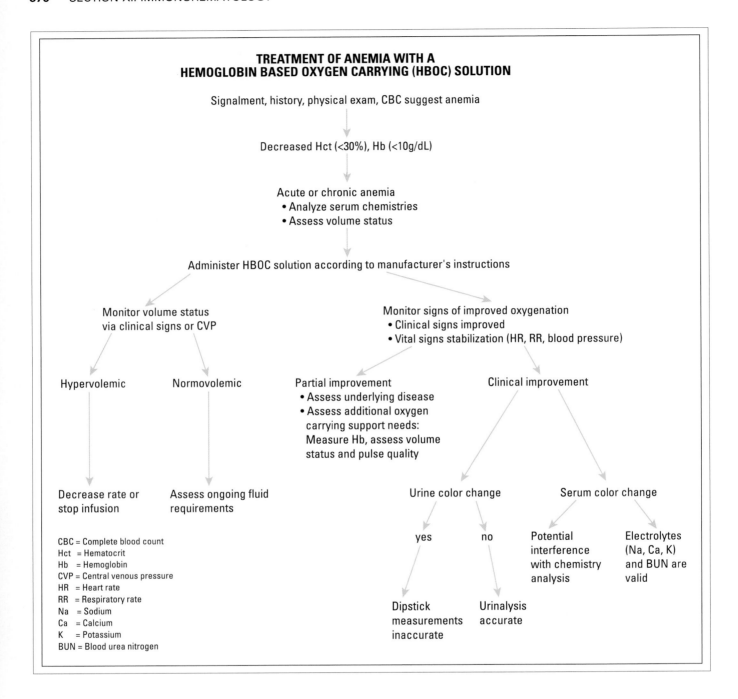

**TREATMENT OF ANEMIA WITH A
HEMOGLOBIN BASED OXYGEN CARRYING (HBOC) SOLUTION**

Signalment, history, physical exam, CBC suggest anemia

Decreased Hct (<30%), Hb (<10g/dL)

Acute or chronic anemia
• Analyze serum chemistries
• Assess volume status

Administer HBOC solution according to manufacturer's instructions

Monitor volume status
via clinical signs or CVP

Monitor signs of improved oxygenation
• Clinical signs improved
• Vital signs stabilization (HR, RR, blood pressure)

Hypervolemic   Normovolemic

Partial improvement
• Assess underlying disease
• Assess additional oxygen
  carrying support needs:
  Measure Hb, assess volume
  status and pulse quality

Clinical improvement

Decrease rate or
stop infusion

Assess ongoing fluid
requirements

Urine color change

Serum color change

CBC = Complete blood count
Hct = Hematocrit
Hb   = Hemoglobin
CVP = Central venous pressure
HR   = Heart rate
RR   = Respiratory rate
Na   = Sodium
Ca   = Calcium
K   = Potassium
BUN = Blood urea nitrogen

yes   no

Potential
interference
with chemistry
analysis

Electrolytes
(Na, Ca, K)
and BUN are
valid

Dipstick
measurements
inaccurate

Urinalysis
accurate

the hemoglobin remains as unstabilized tetramer. The product is stable at 2 to 30°C for up to 2 years. It has a P_{50} of 35 torr, higher than that of canine blood. The increased P_{50} allows oxygen to be onloaded and off-loaded in the tissues more easily than from canine hemoglobin.

MONITORING PATIENTS WITH HEMOGLOBIN IN THE PLASMA

The presence of a red pigment, hemoglobin, in the plasma causes changes in coloration of tissues and plasma, resulting in clinical signs and laboratory differences related to its use. One HBOC has been shown to be associated with a dose-dependent yellow-red discoloration of the skin, mucous membranes, and sclera. Following infusion, the plasma and total hemoglobin concentrations increase but the hematocrit may decrease related to hemodilution. An accurate estimate of the oxygen-carrying capacity of the blood is made using measurement of hemoglobin such that:

$$\text{Total hemoglobin} = \text{hemoglobin (RBC)} + \text{plasma hemoglobin}$$

Because of the presence of exogenous hemoglobin, hemoglobin concentration, mean corpuscular hemoglobin, and mean corpuscular hemoglobin concentration increase following infusion. Artifactual increases or decreases in serum chemistry tests occur because many chemistry tests use colorimetric methods.[9,10] The serum appears hemolyzed; however, the interferences are not those predicted based on hemolysis.

Electrolytes and BUN are valid in the presence of plasma hemoglobin. Coagulation tests, prothrombin, and activated partial thromboplastin time show interference with instruments using optical methods. No interference is seen using electromagnetic, mechanical, and light-scattering methods.[11] Accurate results are obtained for platelet counts and fibrin degradation products using the Thrombo-Wellco Test Kit (Murex®, Kent, England).

Urine may be transiently discolored as a result of excretion of a minor amount (<5%) of the smallest molecular component of the hemoglobin polymers. Evaluation of the urine sediment and specific gravity is not affected by the presence of hemoglobin in the urine. However, colorimetric measurements made using a dipstick (i.e., pH, glucose, ketones, and protein) are inaccurate while gross discoloration of the urine is present.

CLINICAL APPLICATIONS

An HBOC is potentially useful in three broad areas for the treatment of anemia related to the replacement of RBCs: (1) emergency use for hemodynamic stabilization; (2) surgical use; and (3) when blood is not available. Treatment of anemia is independent of its underlying cause. Diseases that may be treated using an oxygen-carrying solution are listed in Table 131.2. The treatment of anemia with an HBOC is illustrated in the algorithm.

A clinical trial using an HBOC was conducted in 64 client-owned dogs with moderate to severe anemia (PCV = 6–23%) resulting from hemolysis, blood loss, or ineffective erythropoiesis.[12] Dogs were either treated

TABLE 131.2 Anemic Indications for Oxygen-Carrying Solutions

Hemolysis	Blood Loss
Immune-mediated	Gastrointestinal
Toxic	Ulcers
Infectious	Parasitic
Ineffective Erythropoiesis	Neoplasia
	Infectious
Aplasia	Rodenticide toxicity
Infectious	Trauma
Toxic	Surgical blood loss
Metabolic	Neoplasia

TABLE 131.3 Theoretic Indications for Oxygen-Carrying Solutions

Hypovolemic shock

States of localized poor perfusion

Support for anesthetized patients

Adjunctive therapy with radiation or chemotherapy

with the HBOC or received supportive care with an option to receive the solution if their condition worsened. Plasma hemoglobin concentration significantly increased and the clinical signs associated with anemia (lethargy/depression, exercise intolerance, and increased heart rate) significantly improved in the HBOC-treated group relative to pretreatment. Treatment success, defined as the lack of need for additional oxygen-carrying support for 24 hours, was 95% in the HBOC-treated group compared with 32% in the control group.

The clinical field trial included dogs with anemia resulting from immune-mediated hemolytic anemia, gastrointestinal bleeding, trauma, surgery, rodenticide intoxication, red cell aplasia, and chronic renal failure. Because of the severity of the animals' illnesses and the design of the trial, it was difficult to ascertain if adverse events seen in the study were related to the administration of the HBOC or to the animal's underlying disease. The most common adverse effects and the incidence of the events seen in the trial included discolored mucous membranes (69%), sclera (56%), and urine (52%), increased central venous pressure (33%), vomiting (35%), and fever (17%).

Future clinical research may show oxygen-carrying solutions to have potential applications where RBCs may not be indicated (i.e., states of poor perfusion) (Table 131.3). As more clinical experience is gained with these solutions, new indications will be determined.

REFERENCES

1. Amberson WR, Flexman J, Stegyarde FR, Mulder AG, Tendler MJ, Pankratz DS, Lang EP. On the use of Ringer-Locke solutions containing hemoglobin as a substitute for normal blood in animals. J Cellular Comp Physiol 1934;5:359–382.
2. Vlahakes GJ, Lee R, Jacobs EE, LaRaia PJ, Austen WG. Hemodynamic effects and oxygen transport properties of a raw blood substitute in a model of massive blood replacement. J Thoracic Cardiovasc Surg 1990;100:379–388.
3. Nunn JF, Freeman J. Problems of oxygenation and oxygen transport during anaesthesia. Anaesthesia 1964;19:120–121.
4. Nair PK, Hellums JD, Olson JS. Prediction of oxygen transport rates in blood flowing in large capillaries. Microvasc Res 1989;38:269–285.
5. Page TC, Light WR, McKay CB, Hellums JD. Oxygen transport by erythrocyte/hemoglobin solution mixtures in an in vitro capillary as a model of hemoglobin-based oxygen carrier performance. Microvasc Res 1998;55(1):54–64.
6. Hebert PC, Wells G, Tweeddale M, Martin C, Marshall J, Pham BA, Blajchman M, Schweitzer I, Pagliarello G. Does transfusion practice affect mortality in critically ill patients? Am J Respir Crit Care Med 1997;155:1618–1623.
7. Welch HG, Meehan KR, Goodnough LT. Prudent strategies for elective red blood cell transfusion. Ann Intern Med 1992;116(5):393–402.
8. Howard A, Callan B, Sweeney M, Giger U. Transfusion practices and costs in dogs. JAVMA 1992;201(11):1697–1701.

was combined with rhG-CSF without recombinant human IL-6, the SCF led to an early increase in GM precursors in liquid cultures.[28] It appears that recombinant canine SCF has the ability to influence the survival and proliferation of various granulocyte-macrophage precursors.

Recombinant canine SCF possesses the unique ability to maintain the viability of progenitor cells for up to 5 weeks.[21] Therefore, SCF may be of value in vitro and may be effective when combined with other hemopoietic growth factors for reconstituting the bone marrow. SCF may provide a more rapid recovery from BMT and from diseases that result in aplasia of a number of different cell lines, especially the granulocytic cell lines.

CONCLUSION

Hemopoietic CSFs are potentially of great benefit for veterinary patients with a wide variety of diseases that result in bone marrow failure. These conditions include but are not limited to chemotherapy-induced bone marrow, aplasia, parvoviral enteritis, panleukopenia, estrogen toxicity, ehrlichiosis, anemia of chronic disease caused by CRF, and anemia caused by other disorders.

Currently, only recombinant human EPO, GM-CSF, and G-CSF are commercially available, and these cytokines should be used by the veterinarian with extreme caution because of the potential development of antibodies in their patients. Recombinant human EPO and G-CSF appear to work better than recombinant human GM-CSF and IL-3. It is anticipated that the recombinant canine growth factors will be commercially available in the future. Perhaps the greatest benefit associated with the use of hemopoietic growth factors is for those patients with profound neutropenia, such as those that receive chemotherapeutic agents. These growth factors have a great potential for improving quality of life and for reducing toxicity. The CSFs provide a tool that will allow safer exploration of increased anticancer dose intensity in settings where this approach may be beneficial. This may result in increased survival time and quality of life. Combinations of CSFs (e.g., IL-3 plus GM-CSF, or G-CSF plus GM-CSF) have the greatest potential for stimulating bone marrow function.

The newer cytokines are likely to be of great benefit in the future; however, further research is necessary to evaluate these hemopoietic growth factors. At a minimum, the serious toxicities associated with curative therapies will be less in the future. Some cancers that are incurable may be treatable with cures or increased survival times with the use of hemopoietic growth factors. In addition, the reduced quality of life associated with CRF will be substantially improved with the use of recombinant EPO.

REFERENCES

1. **Avalos BR, Broudy VC, Ceselski SK, et al.** Abnormal response to granulocyte colony-stimulating factor (G-CSF) in canine cyclic hemopoiesis is not caused by altered G-CSF receptor expression. Blood 1994;84(3):789–794.

2. **Bloomberg RM, Pook HA, Jacobs RM, et al.** Human recombinant erythropoietin therapy in a cat with chronic renal failure. Can Vet J 1992; 33(9):612–613.

3. **Ciekot PE, Ogilvie GK, Fettman MJ, et al.** Evaluation of GM-CSF, IL-3, and GM-CSF/IL-3 fusion protein (PIXY321) as multilineage-CSFs in the dog [Abstract]. Vet Cancer Soc Ann Meeting, Minneapolis, MN, 1991:41–43.

4. **Cowgill LD.** Clinical experience and use of recombinant human erythropoietin in uremic dogs and cats. Proceedings of the 9th ACVIM Forum, New Orleans, LA, 1991:147–149.

5. **Elmslie RE, Dow SW, Ogilvie GK.** Interleukins: Their biological properties and therapeutic potential. J Vet Intern Med 1991;5:283–293.

6. **Fulton R, Gasper PW, Ogilvie GK, et al.** Effect of recombinant human granulocyte colony-stimulating factor on hemopoiesis in normal cats. Exp Hematol 1991;19:759–767.

7. **Giger U.** Erythropoietin and its clinical use. Compend Cont Edu Pract Vet 1992;14(1):25–34.

8. **King LG, Giger U, Diserens D, et al.** Anemia of chronic renal failure in dogs. J Vet Intern Med 1992;6(5):264–270.

9. **Lothrop CD Jr, Warren DJ, Souza LM, et al.** Correction of canine cyclic hematopoiesis with recombinant human granulocyte colony-stimulating factor. Blood 1988;72:1324.

10. **Masunaga H, Uteda M, Sawai T, et al.** Effective administration of erythropoietin for renal anemia. Jap J Vet Sci 1989;51(4):783–788.

11. **Michu L, Callahan G, Allebban Z, Maddux JM, et al.** Effects of recombinant canine granulocyte colony-stimulating factor on white blood cell production in clinically normal and neutropenic dogs. JAVMA 1992;200(12):1957–1964.

12. **Ogilvie GK.** Hemopoietic growth factors: Revolution in oncology and hematology. Compend Cont Edu Pract Vet 1993;15:851–859.

13. **Ogilvie GK, Elmslie RE, Pearson F.** The use of a biological extract of *Serratia marcescens* to decrease myelosuppression associated with doxorubicin-induced myelosuppression in the dog. Am J Vet Res 1992;53:1787–1790.

14. **Ogilvie GK, Moore AS.** Hemopoietic growth factor support. In: Managing the veterinary cancer patient. Trenton, NJ: Veterinary Learning Systems, 1995:142–156.

15. **Ogilvie GK, Obradovich JE.** Hemopoietic growth factors: Clinical use and implications. In: Kirk RW, ed. Current veterinary therapy XI. Philadelphia: WB Saunders, 1992:466–470.

16. **Ogilvie GK, Obradovich JE, Cooper MF, et al.** The use of recombinant canine granulocyte colony-stimulating factor to decrease myelosuppression associated with the administration of mitoxantrone in the dog. J Vet Intern Med 1992;6:44–47.

17. **Obradovich JE, Ogilvie GL, Cooper MF, et al.** Effect of increasing dosages of canine recombinant granulocyte colony-stimulating factor on neutrophil counts in normal dogs. Proceedings of the 10th Annual Conference of the Veterinarian Cancer Society, Auburn, AL, 1990:5.

18. **Obradovich JE, Ogilvie GK.** Evaluation of recombinant canine granulocyte colony-stimulating factor as an inducer of granulopoiesis. J Vet Intern Med 1991;5:75–79.

19. **Obradovich JE, Ogilvie GK, Stadler-Morris S, et al.** Evaluation of canine recombinant granulocyte colony-stimulating factor in the cat. J Vet Intern Med 1993;7:65–69.

20. **Schumm M, Gunther W, Kolb HJ, et al.** Prevention of graft-versus-host disease in DLA-haplotype mismatched dogs and hemopoietic engraftment of CD6 depleted marrow with and without cG-CSF treatment after transplantation. Tissue Antigens 1994;43(3):170–178.

21. **Shull RM, Suggs SV, Langley KE, et al.** Canine stem cell factor (c-kit ligand) supports the survival of hemopoietic progenitors in long-term canine marrow culture. Exp Hematol 1992;20(9):1118–1124.

22. **Suda O, Iida Y, Yasuda T, et al.** Clinical effects of human erythropoietin on renal anaemia in cats. J Jap Vet Med Assoc 1993;46(1):51–53.

23. **Cowgill LD, James KM, Levy JK, Browne JK, Miller A, Lobingier, Egrie JC.** Use of recombinant human erythropoietin for management of anemia in dogs and cats with renal failure. JAVMA 1998;212 (4):521–528.

24. **Pechereau D, Martel P, Braun JP.** Plasma erythropoietin concentrations in dogs and cats: Reference values and changes with anaemia and/or chronic renal failure. Res Vet Sci 1997;62(2):185–188.

25. **Wolf RF, Peng J, Friese P, Gilmore LS, Burstein SA, Dale GL.** Erythropoietin administration increases production and reactivity of platelets in dogs. Thromb Haemost 1997;78(1):1505–1509.

26. **Bravo L, Legendre AM, Hahn KA, Rohrbach BW, Abraham T, Lothrop CD Jr.** Serum granulocyte colony-stimulating factor (G-CSF) and interleukin-1 (IL-1) concentrations after chemotherapy-induced neutropenia in normal and tumor-bearing dogs. Exp Hematol 1996;24(1):11–17.

27. **Henry CJ, Michael S, Buss MS, Lothrop CD Jr.** Veterinary uses of recombinant human granulocyte colony-stimulating factor. Part I. Oncology. Compend Cont Edu Pract Vet 1998;20(6):728–734.

28. **Schuening FG, von Kalle C, Kiem HP, Appelbaum FR, Deeg HJ, Pepe M, Gooley T, Graham TC, Hackman RC, Storb R.** Effect of recombinant canine stem cell factor, a c-kit ligand, on hematopoietic recovery after DLA-identical littermate marrow transplants in dogs. Exp Hematol 1997;25(12):1240–1245.

SECTION XII
Plasma Proteins
Kenita S. Rogers

CHAPTER 134

Overview of Plasma Proteins

• JENNIFER S. THOMAS

Plasma proteins consist of hundreds of proteins with a wide range of functions and structures (Table 134.1).[1] Based on protein electrophoresis, they are divided into albumin and into α, β, and γ globulins. Physiologic roles include: (1) providing a source of amino acids to the tissues; (2) maintaining colloidal oncotic pressure; (3) serving as a buffer to regulate acid-base status; (4) transporting a wide assortment of molecules or ions; (5) maintaining hemostasis; (6) regulating the inflammatory response; and (7) providing resistance to infection.[1,2] The liver synthesizes most of the plasma proteins, including albumin and the majority of the α- and β-globulins. Lymphoid organs are the primary sites of γ-globulin production.

The concentration of protein in the plasma reflects an equilibrium between intravascular and extravascular protein concentrations; however, the concentration of protein in the blood does not adequately predict total body stores of protein.[3] The half-life of plasma proteins is species-dependent and is, as a general rule, inversely proportional to animal size.[2] There is ongoing removal of plasma protein from circulation because of catabolism by the tissues, as well as loss into the gastrointestinal and urinary tracts.[1] This protein loss must be compensated for by dietary intake and production.

FACTORS AFFECTING PLASMA PROTEIN CONCENTRATION

Patient age must be taken into consideration when evaluating plasma protein concentration. At birth, both albumin and globulin concentrations are generally low. Following ingestion of colostrum, globulin concentrations increase as a result of absorption of immunoglobulins. Albumin and globulin production increases as the animal matures and reaches adulthood.[2] Total protein is generally higher in old animals because of slight decreases in albumin[1] and increases in α- and γ-globulins.[4]

Dietary requirements for maintenance of body protein vary according to species, age, and physiologic demands. In healthy adults, nitrogen balance is maintained so that dietary intake equals loss. Ruminants do not require protein in the diet. In other species, dietary re-

striction of protein may cause hypoproteinemia and hypoalbuminemia.[2,3] Globulin concentrations are usually not affected except in cases of extreme dietary protein restriction.[1] Decreased plasma protein may also occur in those patients whose nutritional requirements are not met as a result of malabsorption or maldigestion syndromes.[5] Young animals have greater nutritional demands compared with adult animals because of growth requirements. Nutritional demands increase in adult animals as a result of lactation, pregnancy, or recovery from tissue damage or injury.[1]

Although numerous hormones have dramatic effects on the quantity of tissue protein, hormonal alterations minimally affect plasma protein concentrations.[5] Hormonal effects on plasma protein may be difficult to predict because of opposing effects on albumin and globulins. For example, dogs with spontaneous hyperadrenocorticism may have increased total protein because of increased α-globulins despite simultaneously decreased albumin and γ-globulins.[6]

Plasma protein concentrations are affected by fluid balance and disease state. Dehydration causes loss of the fluid component of the blood and subsequent hyperproteinemia, although the absolute protein quantity in plasma does not increase. External hemorrhage causes loss of both blood cells and protein. Fluid is rapidly shifted from extravascular regions into the blood to maintain blood volume, causing a transient hypoproteinemia that will remain until plasma proteins can be replaced by induction of production. Both albumin and globulins tend to decrease equally with blood loss. Plasma protein levels often decrease during pregnancy and lactation.[2] Inflammatory disorders have significant effects on plasma protein. Protein uptake from plasma increases during tissue repair from injury, and tissue inflammation causes increased vascular permeability, leakage of proteins (primarily albumin) into the extravascular spaces, and a subsequent loss of protein from the vascular spaces.[1] With both stress and inflammation there is increased production of an assortment of globulins that migrate in the α and β fractions as part of the acute phase response.[7,8] Chronic inflammation or infection is associated with increased production of γ-globulins.[5]

TABLE 134.1   Function of Major Globulins and Causes of Alterations Reported in Animals

Protein	Function	Alteration: Common Associated Disorders
α-Globulins		
α_1-Fetoprotein	Unknown	Increase: hepatic neoplasia
α_1-Proteinase inhibitor	Protease inhibitor	Increase: Inflammation, hepatitis
		Decrease: cirrhosis
α_1-Acid glycoprotein	Immunoregulation	Increase: inflammation, tissue trauma, neoplasia, acute or chronic hepatitis
α_1-Antichymotrypsin	Enzyme inhibitor	Increase: inflammation
High-density lipoprotein (HDL)	Cholesterol transport	Increase: hypothyroidism
α_2-Macroglobulin	Protease inhibitor	Increase: inflammation, acute or chronic hepatitis
Ceruloplasmin	Copper transport	Increase: inflammation, tissue trauma
		Decrease: experimental copper deficiency
Haptoglobin	Bind dimeric hemoglobin immunoregulation	Increase: inflammation, tissue trauma, administration of corticosteroids, pregnancy/parturition
		Decrease: acute hemolysis, hematoma formation
Serum amyloid-A (SAA)	Immunoregulation Lipoprotein metabolism	Increase: inflammation, tissue trauma, parturition, familial amyloidosis in Abyssinians
β-Globulin		
Low-density lipoprotein (LDL)	Lipid transport	Increase: nephrotic syndrome, hypothyroidism, cholestatic liver disease
Transferrin	Transport iron	Increase: iron deficiency, chronic blood loss
		Decrease: Inflammation
Ferritin	Iron storage	Increase: inflammation, iron overload, acute hemolysis
		Decrease: iron deficiency, chronic blood loss
C-reactive protein	Modulate inflammatory response	Increase: Inflammation, tissue trauma, neoplasia, corticosteroid administration, parturition
Fibrinogen	Hemostasis Scaffold for tissue repair	Increase: inflammation, parturition/pregnancy
		Decrease: disseminated intravascular coagulation
Hemopexin	Bind heme	Decrease: hemolysis
Complement components (C3, C4), some immunoglobulins	Complement pathway factors	Increase: inflammation
γ-Globulin		
IgG, IgA, IgM	Immune defense	Increase: chronic infection, chronic inflammation, neoplasia, immune-mediated disorders, liver disease
		Decrease: failure of passive transport, acquired or inherited immunodeficiency syndromes

MEASUREMENT OF PLASMA PROTEINS

Plasma protein concentration can be quickly estimated on plasma (anticoagulated with EDTA or heparin) or serum using a refractometer. Serum values will be lower than plasma values primarily because of consumption of fibrinogen during clot formation. Because only a drop of fluid is required, the plasma remaining at the top of a microhematocrit tube following measurement of a packed cell volume can be used. Although the refractometer method is less sensitive than biochemical assays, it is adequate for routine determination of plasma or serum protein concentrations. Because the protein estimate is based on transmission of light, refractometers require clear, nonturbid fluid for accurate measurement; the presence of lipemia or severe hemoglobinemia or bilirubinemia will artificially increase the measured protein concentration.[1,5] Extremely high con-

centrations of glucose, urea, sodium, or chloride may also falsely increase the measured proteins.[9]

Fibrinogen concentrations can be easily estimated using a refractometer by comparing the protein in nonheated plasma with that in the same sample heated to 56 to 58°C for 3 minutes. Heating causes precipitation of fibrinogen, and the difference between the heated and nonheated sample is approximately equal to the fibrinogen concentration. The heat precipitation technique is not sensitive enough to detect the decreased fibrinogen concentrations associated with hemostatic disorders such as disseminated intravascular coagulopathy (DIC), and alternative methods to measure fibrinogen, such as a thrombin clotting time, are recommended.[9] Hyperfibrinogenemia is best interpreted by calculation of the plasma protein to fibrinogen ratio = [total plasma protein (g/dL) − fibrinogen (g/dL)]/fibrinogen (g/dL).[2] Ratios greater than 15 are found in normal animals or are consistent with dehydration. Ratios less than 10 indicate a selective increase in fibrinogen and are consistent with active inflammation. Ratios between 10 and 15 suggest selective increase in fibrinogen and are suspicious for inflammation.[10]

Total protein can be biochemically measured in serum or plasma (anticoagulated with heparin) using colorimetric methods and a spectrophotometer. Compared with the refractometer method, larger samples are required. Total protein concentrations are usually measured using a variation of the biuret method, which is based on the ability of proteins to bind to copper tartrate and form a colored complex. The intensity of color produced is proportional to the protein concentration. This method is accurate in protein ranges found in blood; however, it is not sensitive enough to pick up the low concentrations found in other body fluids such as cerebrospinal fluid.[1] Albumin concentrations are commonly measured using a method based on the ability of albumin to bind to bromcresol green and form a colored complex that can be measured. The avidity of binding between albumin and bromcresol green varies between species.[9] Globulin concentrations are not routinely measured but can be determined by subtracting the albumin concentration from the total protein concentration.

Protein electrophoresis is usually performed in patients with unexplained hyperglobulinemia or hypoglobulinemia. Individual globulins cannot be detected using protein electrophoresis; instead, globulins are divided into α, β, and γ fractions that can then be quantitated. The pattern of alterations in these fractions is rarely pathognomonic for a specific disease but can provide diagnostic information when interpreted in light of other clinical and laboratory findings. Immunoelectrophoresis can be used to qualitatively evaluate immunoglobulins.[2] If necessary, the quantity of individual proteins can be measured using spectrophotometric assays based on the biochemical activity of the protein or immunoassays such as radial immunodiffusion, latex agglutination, immunoturbidity, or enzyme-linked immunosorbent assays (ELISA).[7] Turbidimetric assays can be used to estimate the concentration of immunoglobulin in neonates to determine adequacy of passive transfer of colostrum.[2,9]

SPECIFIC TYPES OF PLASMA PROTEINS AND ASSOCIATED ALTERATIONS

Prealbumin

Prealbumin is produced by the liver and serves as a transport protein for thyroxine. It has been identified in the plasma of humans and some animals. In humans, the concentration of prealbumin decreases with malnutrition, surgery, trauma, and infections.[2] A protein similar to prealbumin is present in the blood of dogs. On protein electrophoresis, this protein migrates in the α_2-globulin region and concentrations remain within reference limits in dogs with hypothyroidism.[11] In horses, prealbumin concentration is negatively correlated with

albumin concentrations and the concentration increases following acute infection, laminitis, and neoplasia.[12]

Albumin

Albumin is the most abundant plasma protein, comprising approximately 35 to 50% of the protein in the blood of animals.[1] It provides a source of amino acids to the tissues, regulates colloid osmotic pressure, and binds to and transports a wide range of molecules and ions. The half-life of albumin is inversely related to animal size (e.g., 8.2 days in dogs, 16.5 days in cattle, and 19.4 days in horses).[2] Albumin concentrations increase with dehydration. Decreased albumin concentrations are best evaluated in conjunction with the albumin:globulin (A:G) ratio. Hypoalbuminemia in combination with normal to increased globulin concentrations (decreased A:G ratio) occurs secondary to selective loss of albumin (e.g., nephrotic syndrome or glomerulonephritis), sequestration into extravascular spaces (e.g., body cavity effusion, vasculopathy), or decreased production (e.g., hepatic failure, malnutrition, malabsorption, maldigestion, acute phase response associated with elevated globulin production). Hypoalbuminemia in conjunction with hypoglobulinemia (normal A:G ratio) suggests overhydration, acute blood loss, exudative lesions, or protein-losing enteropathy.[1,5,9]

Globulins: Acute Phase Proteins

Inflammation or tissue injury causes the release of pro-inflammatory cytokines (e.g., interleukin-1 [IL-1], interleukin-6 [IL-6], and tumor necrosis factor [TNF]), which alter the blood concentration of a variety of proteins (Table 134.2) that are produced primarily in the liver.[7] Proteins that decrease as part of the response are termed negative acute phase proteins, and include albumin[13,14] and transferrin.[1] Proteins that increase as part of the inflammatory response are termed positive acute phase proteins, and include C-reactive protein, α_1-acid glycoprotein (seromucoid, orosomucoid),

TABLE 134.2	Major Acute Phase Proteins Reported in Animals	
Positive Acute Phase Proteins	**Negative Acute Phase Proteins**
Fibrinogen	Albumin
Haptoglobin	Transferrin
C-reactive protein	
Ceruloplasmin	
Serum amyloid-A (SAA)	
α_1-Proteinase inhibitor	
α_1-Acid glycoprotein	
α_1-Antichymotrypsin	
α_2-Macroglobulin	
Ferritin	
Complement components	

α_1-proteinase inhibitor (α_1-antitrypsin), α_1-antichymotrypsin, serum amyloid A, ceruloplasmin, haptoglobin, α_2-macroglobulin, fibrinogen, and complement components.[2,10] Overall increases in these proteins are recognized by finding elevations in the α- and/or β-regions by serum protein electrophoresis. Increases in specific proteins are detected by biochemical assays or immunoassays. The concentration of these proteins is generally low to nondetectable in healthy animals, and elevations are used to diagnose and monitor inflammatory disease. The specific acute phase proteins that are increased and the time course for alterations in these proteins vary between species and according to the initiating disorder or underlying inflammatory disease process. As a general rule, some of the acute phase proteins (e.g., C-reactive protein) decrease rapidly once the underlying disorder is resolved, while others (e.g., fibrinogen) take days to weeks to return to baseline levels.[15]

Fibrinogen

Fibrinogen is a glycoprotein that is an integral component in hemostasis, providing a substrate for thrombin-mediated formation of fibrin, and in tissue repair, providing a matrix for migration of inflammatory cells, fibroblasts, and endothelial cells.[10] Fibrinogen elevations are detectable within 2 days of either turpentine injection[13] or administration of recombinant IL-1[16] in cattle. Fibrinogen levels increase with a variety of spontaneous inflammatory conditions in many species. It is commonly measured as part of a routine complete blood count in horses and cows because it may be a better indicator of inflammation in some situations than alterations in leukocyte counts.[9] In a retrospective study in 510 horses, fibrinogen levels were increased in 23.7% of 135 horses without evidence of an inflammatory leukogram. Of these, 25 and 72% had protein:fibrinogen ratios of <10 and 10 to 15, respectively.[10] However, many horses with inflammatory leukograms in this study did not have plasma protein:fibrinogen ratios suggestive of inflammatory disease, indicating that normal ratios may occur in some inflammatory processes. In dogs, fibrinogen measurement had similar sensitivity and specificity for detection of inflammation compared with measurement of leukocyte counts.[17]

Fibrinogen levels also increase with physiologic stress. In pregnant mares, fibrinogen levels begin to increase midgestation and peak 12 to 36 hours postpartum.[18] It is unclear whether fibrinogen levels increase secondary to elevated cortisol concentrations. Administration of a single dose of adrenocorticotropic hormone (ACTH) to healthy calves causes increased circulating concentrations of cortisol but has no significant effect on fibrinogen levels, whereas similar administration of ACTH to rabbits increases fibrinogen concentrations within 24 hours.[19] In contrast, administration of metyrapone to healthy calves inhibits endogenous production of cortisol and also significantly inhibits the hyperfibrinogenemia associated with surgical trauma.[20]

Hypofibrinogenemia occurs most commonly in DIC because of increased consumption. However, fibrinogen concentrations may be normal in cases of DIC associated with underlying inflammatory disease as a result of increased production associated with the acute phase response.[10]

C-Reactive Protein

C-reactive protein is involved in modulation of the inflammatory response. Proposed functions include: (1) opsonization of foreign organisms or damaged cells; (2) regulation of leukocyte and platelet activity; and (3) activation of the complement cascade.[21] C-reactive protein has been demonstrated to be an acute phase protein in dogs, horses, and pigs. It is present in low concentrations in healthy animals. Levels increase within 24 to 48 hours of experimentally induced inflammation (e.g., injection of turpentine or casein)[14,22-24] or surgery.[22,24-26] It is increased in a variety of spontaneous inflammatory disorders in dogs, including bacterial infections, acute and chronic ehrlichiosis, pyometra, polyarthritis, immune-mediated hemolytic anemia, glomerulonephritis, and enteritis.[7,22,27] The degree of elevation appears to correlate with severity of the inflammatory disease in some cases.[22] C-reactive protein is increased in horses with a variety of spontaneous inflammatory diseases, including pneumonitis, enteritis, and arthritis.[26]

Increased levels are also present in a significant percentage in dogs with neoplasia[22] or with a variety of diseases not generally associated with inflammation, including diabetes mellitus, hepatic failure, renal failure, and exocrine pancreatic insufficiency.[7,22] C-reactive protein increases in pigs following administration of ACTH or prednisolone without any underlying evidence of inflammatory disease,[28] suggesting that levels increase with physiologic stress. In pregnant mares, C-reactive protein increases at parturition.[24] Although C-reactive protein is present in the serum of cattle, it does not react as an acute phase protein.[29] Elevations do occur with lactation in healthy cows.[30]

Haptoglobin

Haptoglobin binds free hemoglobin in the plasma after which the complex is removed. Haptoglobin concentrations decrease in animals with hemolytic anemia[2] or with significant hematoma formation.[31] Intravenous injection of hemoglobin into normal cats causes disappearance of haptoglobin, which returns to normal within 48 hours.[32] Haptoglobin acts as a positive acute phase protein in numerous species, including cats, dogs, cattle, horses, sheep, and pigs. It may be involved in immunoregulation as indicated by an ability to inhibit lymphocyte blastogenesis.[33] Haptoglobin concentration in the blood elevates within 24 to 48 hours following surgery,[25,32,34-36] experimentally induced abscess formation (i.e., injection of turpentine),[7,13,23,32] or administration of recombinant IL-1[16] or endotoxin.[37] Levels increase following experimentally induced viral infections (including feline immunodeficiency virus or feline infectious peritonitis in cats, foot-and-mouth disease virus in cattle, and influenza virus in horses)[31,39,40] or bacterial infections (including *Corynebacterium pseudotuberculosis* in lambs, and *Pasteurella haemolytica* in calves).[37,38,41]

Haptoglobin concentrations are increased in a variety of spontaneous inflammatory diseases. Elevations occur in dogs with acute or chronic hepatitis, although levels decrease in dogs with terminal cirrhosis.[42] In dogs, measurement of haptoglobin is a more sensitive parameter of inflammation than is measurement of fibrinogen or leukocyte counts.[17] In cats, levels are elevated with naturally occurring feline infectious peritonitis and upper respiratory infections.[32] In cattle, increased haptoglobin occurs with mastitis, pneumonia, enteritis, peritonitis, endocarditis, abscesses, trauma, and endometritis.[43–45] Haptoglobin is lower in acute conditions than in chronic conditions.[43] In horses, elevations occur with enteritis, pneumonitis, shopping fever, cellulitis, colic, abortion, trauma, and rhabdomyolysis.[36,46]

Elevated haptoglobin concentrations also occur with some conditions not generally associated with inflammation or tissue damage. Haptoglobin increases in acute and chronic grass sickness in horses,[46] and concentrations are high in pregnant mares for 4 months prepartum and at parturition.[36] Levels increase in healthy cows at parturition,[47] in calves following the stress associated with transport,[33] and concentrations are elevated in cows with hepatic lipidosis,[48] possibly as a result of induction of haptoglobin production by hepatocytes in response to glucocorticoids or estradiol.[49] Haptoglobin peaks within 3 days of administration of prednisone in dogs[8] and following administration of dexamethasone to fasted cows.[50]

α_1-Acid Glycoprotein

α_1-Acid glycoprotein (AGP) may play a role in limiting the systemic immunologic response by inhibiting lymphocyte blastogenesis and antibody production.[51] Levels increase in response to tissue inflammation or injury in numerous species, including dogs, cats, horses, and cattle. Elevations are detected within 24 to 72 hours following experimentally induced inflammation (i.e., injection of turpentine),[13,14] surgery,[25,52] or administration of endotoxin[37] or recombinant IL-1.[16] Levels return to normal within 2 to 3 weeks. In dogs, elevated AGP occurs in acute and chronic ehrlichiosis[27] or hepatitis.[42] Levels are increased in dogs with a variety of neoplasms (lymphoma, carcinomas, sarcomas), and concentrations decrease following induction of clinical remission in patients with lymphoma.[53] In cats, AGP is increased with feline infectious peritonitis or feline immunodeficiency virus infection.[39] In cattle, levels of AGP increase with acute, subacute, and chronic inflammatory diseases[7] including infection with pasteurellosis,[37] traumatic pericarditis, arthritis, mastitis, pneumonia, mesenteric liponecrosis,[54] and hepatic abscesses.[51] Unlike haptoglobin, AGP does not increase following the stress of transportation in calves.[33] In pregnant mares, AGP concentrations increase 3 to 4 months prior to parturition. Elevated levels also are present in horses with grass sickness (a disorder generally not considered to be associated with inflammation) and with an assortment of spontaneous inflammatory diseases.[46] In one study in pigs, AGP did not consistently increase following induction of inflammation; however, preinduction concentrations of AGP were high and may have indicated underlying inflammatory disease.[23]

Ceruloplasmin

Ceruloplasmin transports copper and plays a role in iron metabolism.[2] Although less commonly measured than haptoglobin, ceruloplasmin has been identified as an acute phase protein in many species, including dogs, cats,[55] horses, and cows. Ceruloplasmin elevations are detectable 3 to 4 days following turpentine injection[7,13,56,57] and remain elevated for 2 to 4 weeks. Levels increase following endotoxin administration in cattle but not following *Pasteurella* infection.[37] Elevated levels are detectable 4 to 6 days following surgical trauma in dogs and horses[25,56] and may remain high for several weeks. Ceruloplasmin concentrations increase in some, but not all, spontaneous inflammatory diseases. In one study in horses, ceruloplasmin was not increased in patients with a variety of inflammatory diseases, whereas haptoglobin and AGP were significantly increased.[46] In contrast, levels were increased in significant numbers in foals with pneumonitis and enteritis and occasionally in foals with arthritis.[56] In dogs with a variety of spontaneous conditions, measurement of ceruloplasmin concentration was more sensitive than measurement of either fibrinogen or leukocyte counts but less sensitive than measurement of haptoglobin concentrations in detecting inflammatory disease.[17] Increased concentrations occur in some conditions not considered to be inflammatory in origin, including grass sickness[46] in horses. Ceruloplasmin concentrations decrease in cattle with experimentally induced copper deficiency.[58]

Serum Amyloid-A

The function of serum amyloid-A (SAA) is not clear but it may play a role in immunoregulation and clearance of high-density lipoproteins (HDL).[59] SAA increases four- to fortyfold within 24 hours of experimentally induced inflammation in horses, remaining high for 4 to 6 days, then decreasing to baseline levels by 2 to 4 weeks.[60] Levels rise rapidly following administration of endotoxin to cattle[59] or experimental inoculation of calves with *Pasteurella haemolytica*[61] or dogs with *Bordetella bronchiseptica*.[62] SAA is present in trace levels in healthy horses and peaks within 2 to 3 days following surgery.[63] Elevations in SAA occur in spontaneous inflammatory conditions, with levels being highest in acute conditions but remaining high in chronic conditions.[43] In cattle, SAA increases with pneumonia, enteritis, peritonitis, endocarditis, abscesses, trauma, and endometritis.[43] SAA is elevated in most horses with clinical evidence of inflammation[60] and in animals with herpesvirus infection, bacterial arthritis, strangles, enteritis, pneumonitis, cellulitis, and other miscellaneous infections.[63] SAA is significantly elevated in Abyssinian cats with familial amyloidosis and in non-Abyssinian cats hospitalized with a variety of illnesses.[64]

Elevations in SAA also occur in conditions not generally associated with inflammation. Levels peak within 1 to 3 days of parturition in healthy cows[65] and horses.[60] In healthy calves, SAA increases in animals subjected to physical stress, though the values remained within the normal range for adult cattle.[66] The cause for the elevation in this case is not clear. Administration of ACTH to healthy cows causes elevated cortisol concentrations without concurrent alterations in SAA concentrations.[67]

α_1-Proteinase Inhibitor (α_1-Antitrypsin)

α_1-Proteinase inhibitor is a serine protease inhibitor that modulates the inflammatory response by forming complexes with enzymes released from inflammatory cells.[68] Serum concentrations of α_1-proteinase inhibitor increase in the majority of dogs with acute or chronic hepatitis, although levels decrease in dogs with chronic progressive hepatitis or cirrhosis.[69] α_1-Proteinase inhibitor has been measured in animals to determine its diagnostic value for detecting inflammatory disease, but results have been mixed. α_1-Proteinase inhibitor is an unreliable indicator of inflammation in cows with mastitis,[44] whereas concentrations do increase following infection with *Pasteurella haemolytica*, administration of endotoxin,[37] or experimental turpentine injection.[13] Levels are not altered in hospitalized dogs with a variety of spontaneous diseases[68] or following surgical trauma.[25]

α_2-Macroglobulin

α_2-Macroglobulin acts as an acute phase protein in cattle infected with *Pasteurella* or administered endotoxin.[37] Elevations occur in horses with grass sickness, whereas levels are not detected in horses with an assortment of spontaneous inflammatory diseases[46] or with colic and endotoxemia.[70] Concentrations of α_2-macroglobulin increase in dogs with acute or chronic hepatitis.[42]

Ferritin

Ferritin consists of polypeptide chains surrounding an internal site for iron storage. Most of ferritin is located within the cytoplasm of cells; however, because ferritin is water-soluble, small amounts leak into the blood. Serum ferritin can be used to estimate body iron stores in dogs, cats, horses, and pigs.[15,55] Ferritin levels decrease with iron deficiency or chronic blood loss and increase in hemolytic anemia or iron overload.[15] Ferritin also acts as an acute phase protein. Levels increase following turpentine injection in ponies.[57] Concentrations are increased in horses with a variety of spontaneous inflammatory disorders, including pneumonia, guttural pouch infections, and lacerations.[71] Ferritin concentrations are high in humans with various neoplasms. Hyperferritinemia was documented in a dog with malignant histiocytosis.[72] Ferritin levels are not altered by administration of corticosteroids to horses.[73]

Transferrin

Transferrin is a plasma protein that binds iron for transport to the tissues. Transferrin can be measured immunologically, although it is more commonly estimated by measuring the total iron-binding capacity of the serum. Total iron-binding capacity increases with iron deficiency in most species with the exception of the dog.[15] Transferrin concentrations are also affected by inflammatory disease or tissue trauma. Transferrin tends to decrease following turpentine injection in ponies, although the decrease is not statistically significant.[57] Transferrin concentrations are decreased in horses with acute infections or laminitis.[74] Levels decrease in cattle with chronic inflammatory diseases but are normal in cattle with acute infections, ketosis, or following endotoxin administration.[75] Levels decrease in pigs experimentally infected with *Salmonella choleraesuis*.[76] Administration of corticosteroids to normal horses does not significantly alter serum transferrin concentrations.[73]

Other Globulins

α-Fetoprotein

α-Fetoprotein is a plasma protein that is normally present only in the fetus. In humans, levels increase with pregnancy, hepatic disease, and neoplasia.[77] Increased serum concentrations have been identified in a filly with hepatocellular carcinoma[78] and in the majority of dogs tested with cholangiocarcinoma, hepatocellular carcinoma, and hepatic lymphoma.[77]

Lipoprotein

Lipoproteins function in lipid transportation and consist of a core of triglyceride and cholesteryl esters surrounded by an outer covering of phospholipids, unesterified cholesterol, and apoproteins.[79] The four major classes of lipoproteins include HDL, low-density lipoprotein (LDL), very low-density lipoprotein (VLDL), and chylomicrons (CMs). CMs deliver dietary lipids from the intestine to the tissues and VLDLs carry triglycerides from the liver to extrahepatic tissues. LDLs transports cholesterol from the liver to extrahepatic tissues; HDLs deliver excess cholesterol from extrahepatic tissues to the liver.[80] HDL is the predominant lipoprotein in most mammals, including dogs, cats, horses, and ruminants.[79] The lipoprotein classes can be separated by electrophoresis and detected using a lipophilic stain.[80] HDL is in the α-globulin region, VLDL is in the pre-β region, LDL is in the β-globulin region, and CM stays at the site of sample application. Alterations in lipoproteins may occur with diabetes mellitus, hypothyroidism, pancreatitis, cholestatic liver disease, hyperadrenocorticism, and nephrotic syndrome.[80]

REFERENCES

1. **Kaneko JJ.** Clinical biochemistry of domestic animals, 4th ed. San Diego: Academic Press, 1989;142–165.
2. **Jain NC.** Essentials of veterinary hematology. Philadelphia: Lea & Febiger, 1993;349–380.

3. **Jahoor F, Bhattiprolu S, Del Rosario M, et al.** Chronic protein deficiency differentially affects the kinetics of plasma proteins in young pigs. J Nutr 1996;126:1489–1495.

4. **Batamuzi EK, Kristensen E, Jansen AL.** Serum protein electrophoresis: Potential test for use in geriatric companion animal health programmes. Zentralblatt Fur Veterinarmedizin 1996;43:501–508.

5. **Werner LL, Turnwald GH, Barta O.** Immunologic and plasma protein disorders. In: Willard MD, Tvedten H, Turnwald GH, eds. Small animal clinical diagnosis by laboratory methods, 2nd ed. Philadelphia: WB Saunders, 1994.

6. **van den Broek AHM, Lida J.** Serum protein electrophoresis in spontaneous canine hyperadrenocorticism. Res Vet Sci 1989;46:100–104.

7. **Eckersall PD.** Acute phase proteins as markers of inflammatory lesions. Comp Haematol Int 1995;5:93–97.

8. **Harvey JW, West CL.** Prednisone-induced increases in serum alpha-2-globulin and haptoglobin concentrations in dogs. Vet Pathol 1987;24:90–92.

9. **Duncan JR, Prasse KW, Mahaffey EA.** Veterinary laboratory medicine, 3rd ed. Ames, IA: Iowa State University Press, 1994;112–118.

10. **Andrews DA, Reagan WJ, DeNicola DB.** Plasma fibrinogen in recognizing equine inflammatory disease. Compend Cont Edu Pract Vet 1994;16:1349–1356.

11. **Larsson M, Petterson T.** Purification and partial characterization of thyroid hormone binding proteins in canine serum. Domest Animal Endocrinol 1987;4:215–229.

12. **Ek N.** Concentration of serum prealbumin (Pr) protein in sick horses and its correlation to blood leucocyte count and albumin content in serum. Acta Vet Scand 1980;21:482–497.

13. **Conner JG, Eckersall PD.** Bovine acute phase response following turpentine injection. Res Vet Sci 1988;44:82–88.

14. **Yamashita K, Fujinaga T, Miyamato T, et al.** Canine acute phase response: Relationship between serum cytokine activity and acute phase protein in dogs. J Vet Med Sci 1994;56:487–492.

15. **Smith JE.** Iron metabolism in dogs and cats. Compend Cont Edu Pract Vet 1992;14:39–43.

16. **Godsel DL, Baca-Estrada ME, Van Kessel AG, et al.** Regulation of bovine acute phase responses by recombinant interleukin-1 beta. Can J Vet Res 1995;59:249–255.

17. **Solter PF, Hoffman WE, Hungerford LL, et al.** Haptoglobin and ceruloplasmin as determinants of inflammation in dogs. Am J Vet Res 1991;52:1738–1742.

18. **Gentry PA, Feldman BF, O'Neill SL, et al.** Evaluation of the haemostatic profile in the pre- and postparturient mare, with particular focus on the perinatal period. Equine Vet J 1992;24:33–36.

19. **Gentry PA, Liptrap RM, Tremblay RR, et al.** Adrenocorticotrophic hormone fails to alter plasma fibrinogen and fibronectin values in calves but does so in rabbits. Vet Res Commun 1992;16:253–264.

20. **Fisher AD, Crowe MA, O'Nuallain EM, et al.** Effects of suppressing cortisol following castration of bull calves on adrenocorticotropic hormone, in vitro interferon-gamma production, leukocytes, acute-phase proteins, growth, and feed intake. J Animal Sci 1997;75:1899–1908.

21. **Cheryk LA, Haynes MA, Gentry PA.** Modulation of bovine platelet function by C-reactive protein. Vet Immunol Immunopathol 1996;52:27–36.

22. **Caspi D, Snel JJ, Batt RM, et al.** C-reactive protein in dogs. Am J Vet Res 1987;48:919–922.

23. **Eckersall PD, Saini PK, McComb C.** The acute phase response of acid soluble glycoprotein, alpha-1 acid glycoprotein, ceruloplasmin, haptoglobin and C-reactive protein in the pig. Vet Immunol Immunopathol 1995;51:377–385.

24. **Yamashita K, Fujinaga T, Okumura M, et al.** Serum C-reactive protein (CRP) in horses: The effect of aging, sex, delivery, and inflammations on its concentration. J Vet Med Sci 1991;53:1019–1024.

25. **Conner JG, Eckersall PD.** Acute phase response in the dog following surgical trauma. Res Vet Sci 1988;45:107–110.

26. **Takiguchi M, Fujinaga T, Naiki M, et al.** Isolation, characterization, and quantitative analysis of C-reactive protein from horses. Am J Vet Res 1990;51:1215–1220.

27. **Rikihisa Y, Yamamoto S, Kwak I, et al.** C-Reactive protein and α_1-acid glycoprotein levels in dogs infected with Ehrlichia canis. J Clin Micro 1994;32:912–917.

28. **Burger W, Ewald C, Fennert EM.** Increase in C-reactive protein in the serum of piglets (pCRP) following ACTH or corticosteroid administration. Zentralblatt Fur Veterinarmedizin 1998;45:1–6.

29. **Maudsley S, Rowe IF, de Beer FC, et al.** Identification and isolation of two pentraxins from bovine serum. Clin Exper Immunol 1987;67:662–673.

30. **Morimatsu M, Watanabe A, Yoshimatsu K, et al.** Elevation of bovine serum C-reactive protein and serum amyloid P component levels by lactation. J Dairy Res 1991;58:257–261.

31. **Kent JE, Goodall J.** Assessment of an immunoturbidimetric method for measuring equine serum haptoglobin concentrations. Equine Vet J 1991;23:59–66.

32. **Harvey JW, Gaskin JM.** Feline haptoglobin. Am J Vet Res 1978;39:549.

33. **Murata H, Miyamato T.** Bovine haptoglobin as a possible immunomodulator in the sera of transported calves. Br Vet J 1993;149:277–283.

34. **Eurell TE, Wilson DA, Baker GJ.** The effect of exploratory laparotomy on the serum and peritoneal haptoglobin concentrations of the pony. Can J Vet Res 1993;57:42–44.

35. **Morimatsu M, Sarikaputi M, Syuto B, et al.** Bovine haptoglobin: Single radial immunodiffusion assay of its polymeric forms and dramatic rise in acute-phase sera. Vet Immunol Immunopathol 1992;33:365–372.

36. **Taira T, Fujinaga T, Okumura M, et al.** Equine haptoglobin: isolation, characterization, and the effects of aging, delivery, and inflammation on its serum concentrations. J Vet Med Sci 1992;54:435–442.

37. **Conner JG, Eckersall PD, Wiseman RK, et al.** Acute phase response in calves following infection with Pasteurella haemolytica, Ostertagia ostertagi and endotoxin administration. Res Vet Sci 1989;47:203–207.

38. **Cheryk LA, Hooper-McGrevy KE, Gentry PA.** Alterations in bovine platelet function and acute-phase proteins induced by Pasteurella haemolytica A1. Can J Vet Res 1998;62:1–8.

39. **Duthie S, Eckersall PD, Addie DD, et al.** Value of alpha 1-acid glycoprotein in the diagnosis of feline infectious peritonitis. Vet Rec 1997;141:299–303.

40. **Hofner MC, Fosbery MW, Eckersall PD, et al.** Haptoglobin response of cattle infected with foot-and-mouth disease virus. Res Vet Sci 1994;57:125.

41. **Pépin M, Pardon P, Lantier F, et al.** Experimental Corynebacterium pseudotuberculosis infection in lambs: Kinetics of bacterial dissemination and inflammation. Vet Micro 1991;26:381–392.

42. **Sevelius E, Andersson M.** Serum protein electrophoresis as a prognostic marker of chronic liver disease in dogs. Vet Rec 1995;137:663–667.

43. **Alsemgeest SP, Kalsbeek HC, Wensing T, et al.** Concentrations of serum amyloid-A (SAA) and haptoglobin (HP) as parameters of inflammatory disease in cattle. Vet Quarterly 1994;16:21–23.

44. **Hirvonen J, Pyorala S, Jousimies-Somer H.** Acute phase response in heifers with experimentally induced mastitis. J Dairy Res 1996;63:351–360.

45. **Skinner JG, Brown RA, Roberts L.** Bovine haptoglobin responses in clinically defined field conditions. Vet Rec 1991;128:147–149.

46. **Milne EM, Doxey DL, Kent JE, et al.** Acute phase proteins in grass sickness (equine dysautonomia). Res Vet Sci 1992;50:272–278.

47. **Uchida E, Katoh N, Takahashi K.** Appearance of haptoglobin in serum from cows at parturition. J Vet Med Sci 1993;55:893–894.

48. **Nakagawa H, Yamamoto O, Oikawa S, et al.** Detection of serum haptoglobin by enzyme-linked immunosorbent assay in cows with fatty liver. Res Vet Sci 1997;62:137–141.

49. **Higuchi H, Katoh N, Miyamoto T, et al.** Dexamethasone-induced haptoglobin release by calf liver parenchymal cells. Am J Vet Res 1994;55:1080–1085.

50. **Yoshino K, Katoh N, Takahashi K, et al.** Possible involvement of protein kinase C with induction of haptoglobin in cows by treatment with dexamethasone and by starvation. Am J Vet Res 1993;54:689–694.

51. **Motoi Y, Itoh H, Tamura K, et al.** Correlation of serum concentration of α_1-acid glycoprotein with lymphocyte blastogenesis and development of experimentally induced or naturally acquired hepatic abscesses in cattle. Am J Vet Res 1992;53:574–579.

52. **Taira T, Fujinaga T, Tamura K, et al.** Isolation and characterization of alpha-1-acid glycoprotein from horses, and its evaluation as an acute-phase reactive protein in horses. Am J Vet Res 1992;53:961–965.

53. **Ogilivie GK, Walters LM, Greeley SG, et al.** Concentration of alpha-1-acid glycoprotein in dogs with malignant neoplasia. JAVMA 1993;203:1144–1146.

54. **Tamura K, Toshiroh Y, Itoh H, et al.** Isolation, characterization, and quantitative measurement of serum α_1-acid glycoprotein in cattle. Jpn J Vet Sci 1989;51:987–994.

55. **Andrews GA, Chavey PS, Smith JE.** Enzyme-linked immunosorbent assays to measure serum ferritin and the relationship between serum ferritin and nonheme iron stores in cats. Vet Pathol 1994;31:674–678.

56. **Okumura M, Fujinaga T, Yamashita K, et al.** Isolation, characterization, and quantitative analysis of ceruloplasmin from horses. Am J Vet Res 1991;52:1979–1985.

57. **Smith JE, Cipriano JE.** Inflammation-induced changes in serum iron analytes and ceruloplasmin of Shetland ponies. Vet Pathol 1987;24:354–356.

58. **Cerone SI, Sansinanea AS, Streitenberger SA, et al.** The effect of copper deficiency on the peripheral blood cells of cattle. Vet Res Commun 1988;22:47–57.

59. **Boosman R, Niewold TA, Mutsaers CWAAM, et al.** Serum amyloid A concentrations in cows given endotoxin as an acute-phase stimulant. Am J Vet Res 1989;50:1690–1694.

60. **Satoh M, Fujinaga T, Okumura M, et al.** Sandwich enzyme-linked immunosorbent assay for quantitative measurement of serum amyloid A protein in horses. Am J Vet Res 1995;56:1286–1291.

61. **Horadagoda A, Eckersall PD, Alsemgeest SP, et al.** Purification and quantitative measurement of bovine serum amyloid-A. Res Vet Sci 1993;55:317–325.

62. **Yomamoto S, Miyaji S, Ashida Y.** Preparation of anti-canine serum amyloid A (SAA) serum and purification of SAA from canine high-density lipoprotein. Vet Immunol Immunopathol 1994;41:41–53.

63. **Pepys MB, Baltz ML, Tennent GA, et al.** Serum amyloid A protein (SAA) in horses: Objective measurement of the acute phase response. Equine Vet J 1989;21:106–109.

64. **DiBartola SP, Reiter JA, Cornacoff JB, et al.** Serum amyloid A protein concentration measured by radial immunodiffusion in Abyssinian and non-Abyssinian cats. Am J Vet Res 1989;50:1414–1417.

65. **Alsemgeest SP, Taverne MAM, Boosman R, et al.** Peripartum acute-phase protein serum amyloid-A concentration in plasma of cows and fetuses. Am J Vet Res 1993;54:164–167.

66. **Alsemgeest SP, Lambooy IE, Wierenga HK.** Influence of physical stress on the plasma concentration of serum amyloid-A (SAA) and haptoglobin (Hp) in calves. Vet Quarterly 1995;17:9–12.

67. **van der Kolk JH, Alsemgeest SP, Wensing T, et al.** Failure of adrenocortico-trophic hormone to release serum amyloid A in cattle. Res Vet Sci 1992; 52:113–114.

68. **Hughes D, Elliott DA, Washabau RJ, et al.** Effects of age, sex, reproductive status, and hospitalization on serum alpha-1-antitrypsin concentration in dogs. Am J Vet Res 1995;56:568–572.

69. **Sevelius E, Andersson M, Jönsson L.** Hepatic accumulation of alpha-1-antitrypsin in chronic liver disease in the dog. J Comp Path 1994;111:401–412.

70. **Cote N, Trout DR, Hayes AM.** Evaluation of plasma alpha-2-macroglobulin and interactions with tumor necrosis factor-alpha in horses with endotoxe-mia signs. Can J Vet Res 1996;60:150–157.

71. **Smith JE, Cipriano JE, DeBowes R, et al.** Iron deficiency and pseudo-iron deficiency in hospitalized horses. JAVMA 1986;188:285–287.

72. **Newlands CE, Houston DM, Vaxconcelos DY.** Hyperferritinemia associ-ated with malignant histiocytosis in a dog. JAVMA 1994;205:849–851.

73. **Smith JE, DeBowes R, Cipriano JE.** Exogenous corticosteroids increase serum iron concentrations in mature horses and ponies. JAVMA 1986; 188:1296–1298.

74. **Ek N.** Concentration of serum transferrin in sick horses and its relationship to serum albumin content. Acta Vet Scand 1981;22:260–271.

75. **Moser M, Pfister H, Bruckmaier RM, et al.** Blood serum transferrin concen-tration in cattle in various physiological states, in veal cattle fed different amounts of iron, and in cattle affected by infectious and non-infectious diseases. Zentralblatt Fur Veterinarmedizin 1994;41:413–420.

76. **Kramer TT, Griffith RW, Saucke L.** Iron and transferrin in acute experimen-tal *Salmonella choleraesuis* infection in pigs. Am J Vet Res 1985;46:451–455.

77. **Lowseth LA, Gillett NA, Chang IY.** Detection of serum α-fetoprotein in dogs with hepatic tumors. JAVMA 1991;199:735–741.

78. **Roby KAW, Beech J, Bloom JC, et al.** Hepatocellular carcinoma associated with erythrocytosis and hypoglycemia in a yearling filly. JAVMA 1990;196:465–467.

79. **Bauer JE.** Comparative lipid and lipoprotein metabolism. Vet Clin Pathol 1996;25:49–56.

80. **Whitney MS.** Evaluation of hyperlipidemias in dogs and cats. Sem Vet Med Surg 1992;7:292–300.

CHAPTER 135

Protein Electrophoresis

• JENNIFER S. THOMAS

Serum protein electrophoresis is recommended when a patient has an unexplained hyperglobulinemia or hypoglobulinemia. Albumin will be separated and quantitated; however, individual globulins will not be identified using routine electrophoretic protocols. Instead, the globulins will be separated into α, β, and γ fractions, which contain groups of proteins with similar electrophoretic migration rates. The quantity of protein within each fraction is determined and compared with reference values for each species. The electrophoretic pattern provides information about relative increases and decreases of proteins, as well as information about the homogeneity of the proteins within a particular fraction. Patterns of alterations in these fractions are rarely pathognomonic for a particular disease but may provide useful diagnostic information when used in conjunction with other clinical and laboratory findings. If warranted, alterations in the concentrations of individual proteins can be determined using spectrophotometric assays based on the biological activity of that protein or immunoassays (e.g., radial immunodiffusion, turbidimetry, enzyme-linked immunosorbent assays [ELISA]).[1]

METHODOLOGY

Protein electrophoresis can be performed on either serum or plasma. Serum is generally preferred because the fibrinogen in plasma will often obscure the electrophoretogram in the β–γ region.[2] With electrophoresis, proteins are separated based on their migration rate in an electrical field. The rate of migration depends on the charge of the protein, the size of the protein, the strength of the electrical field, and the medium through which the proteins are migrating.[3] The rate of migration of the proteins will be affected by the pH and the ionic strength and composition of the buffer system used.[2,3] The standard buffer is barbital pH 8.6 at which the majority of plasma proteins will carry a negative charge.[3] The medium of choice for routine diagnostic purposes is either agarose[4,5] or cellulose

acetate[3] because each is relatively simple to use and provides accurate results. Other media that can be used include starch or polyacrylamide gel. By altering experimental conditions, proteins can often be separated into greater numbers of bands, which may be useful in a research setting.

Once electrophoresis is completed, the support medium is stained to visualize the protein bands (Fig. 135.1). Commonly used stains include Coomassie blue, Amido black, and Ponceau S.[2] Alternative stains specific for glycoproteins or lipids can also be used if improved visualization of only these types of proteins is desired.[6] The membranes can then be cleared and the intensity of the individual bands recorded using a densitometer. An electrophoretogram is generated and the area under the curve for each protein band is translated into a percentage of the total area. Multiplication of the total protein (as determined by biochemical assay) by the percentage of each of the fractions will yield the quantity of protein in each fraction. Narrow bands with high staining intensity such as albumin[7] or monoclonal proteins[8] may be underestimated using electrophoresis when compared with biochemical assays using spectrophotometric methods.

In an alkaline environment, most proteins will be negatively charged and will migrate from the point of application at the cathode region toward the anode.[3] Albumin is a relatively small protein with a strong negative charge and it migrates the farthest. The globulins consist of a heterogenous group of proteins that have a weaker negative charge. They migrate at a slower rate than albumin and are generally separated into α, β, and γ bands. The α-globulins migrate the furthest; the γ-globulins stay closest to the origin. The degree of migration of the albumin and globulin fractions varies between species.[6] In normal animals, each fraction is usually further divided into one or two zones. The actual number of zones will depend on both the animal species and laboratory conditions (e.g., medium, buffer characteristics, and voltage settings), so it is important that results be interpreted based on normals established for each reporting laboratory.[9]

ALTERATIONS IN ELECTROPHORETOGRAMS

Alteration in Albumin

Protein electrophoresis is rarely performed to evaluate a patient with hypoalbuminemia unless there is associated abnormalities in the serum globulins. Hypoalbuminemia can be readily detected on electrophoretograms and is best interpreted in conjunction with concomitant changes in globulin concentrations and the calculated albumin:globulin (A:G) ratio (Table 135.1). Hypoalbuminemia in conjunction with hypoglobulinemia (normal A:G ratio) occurs with blood loss, severe exudative skin disease, protein-losing enteropathy, or overhydration. Hypoalbuminemia in combination with normal to increased globulin concentrations (decreased A:G ratio) suggests decreased albumin production, selective loss of albumin, or sequestration of albumin into third body spaces.[3,7]

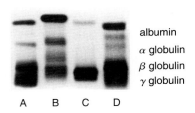

albumin
α globulin
β globulin
γ globulin

A   B   C   D

FIGURE 135.1 Serum protein electrophoresis using agarose gel and stained for protein (from Texas Veterinary Medical Diagnostic Laboratory, College Station, TX). Lane A is from a dog with coccidioidomycosis. Lane B is from a cat with feline infectious peritonitis. Lane C is from a dog with a multiple myeloma. Lane D is from a cow with pyelonephritis. Note the difference in the migration rate of the albumin band between the different species.

Overview of Globulins

The globulins consist of hundreds of proteins that perform a wide range of physiologic functions.[3] The division of globulins into α, β, and γ fractions is based solely on electrophoretic migration rates and is not determined by function. Many globulins are present in quantities too small to be detected by routine serum electrophoresis.[5] These proteins can only be detected by more sensitive biochemical assays or immunoassays. With certain types of diseases or disorders, the concentration of some of the globulins will significantly increase or decrease. If the magnitude of the change of these proteins is large enough, it will cause alterations that will be reflected in the serum protein electrophoresis profile.

Alterations in α-Globulins

Proteins that migrate in the α-globulin fraction include the acute phase proteins, high-density lipoprotein, and α_1-fetoprotein (Table 135.2). Increases in the α-globulin fraction occur commonly in animals secondary to tissue damage or inflammation as part of an acute phase response (Fig. 135.2). Cytokines (such as interleukin-1, interleukin-6, or tumor necrosis factor) released during an inflammatory reaction induce the release of a variety of proteins—termed positive acute phase proteins—primarily from the liver.[1] Many of these acute phase proteins help regulate the inflammatory reaction, remove products from damaged cells or byproducts of the inflammatory response, or modulate the immune response. Major acute phase proteins identified in animals in the α-globulin fraction include α_1-proteinase inhibitor (α_1-antitrypsin), α_1-acid glycoprotein (orosomucoid, seromucoid), serum amyloid-A, haptoglobin, ceruloplasmin, and α_2-macroglobulin.[6] Elevations in one

TABLE 135.1	Patterns of Alterations in Protein Electrophoretograms and Commonly Associated Disorders		
Zone Affected	**Change in Zone**	**A:G Ratio**	**Associated Disorder**
Albumin	Decrease	Decrease	Selective loss (e.g., protein-losing nephropathy)
			Decreased production (e.g., hepatic disease, malnutrition, maldigestion/malabsorption, acute phase response)
			Sequestration (e.g., body cavity effusion, vasculopathy)
	Decrease	Normal	Blood loss, exudative disorders (e.g., severe burns), protein-losing enteropathy
α-Globulin	Increase	Decrease	Inflammation (acute or chronic), neoplasia, nephrotic syndrome, hepatic disease, corticosteroid administration
β-Globulin	Increase	Decrease	Inflammation (acute or chronic), nephrotic syndrome, hepatic disease
γ-Globulin	Increase: polyclonal	Decrease	Systemic infections (e.g., bacterial, viral, fungal, rickettsial, parasitic), immune-mediated disorders, neoplasia, severe hepatic disease
	Increase: monoclonal	Decrease	Neoplasia (e.g., multiple myeloma, lymphoma), chronic infection (e.g., ehrlichiosis, feline infectious peritonitis virus, equine infectious anemia virus), chronic inflammation (e.g., pyoderma, plasmacytic gastroenterocolitis), idiopathic
	Decrease	Increase	Immunodeficiency (hereditary or acquired), failure of passive transfer

TABLE 135.2 Major Proteins in the Globulin Fractions

α-Globulin	β-Globulin	γ-Globulin
α_1-Fetoprotein	Low-density lipoprotein	IgG
α_1-Proteinase inhibitor[a]	Ferritin[a]	IgM
α_1-Acid glycoprotein[a]	C-reactive protein[a]	IgA
High-density lipoprotein	Fibrinogen[a]	IgE
α_2-Macroglobulin[a]	Transferrin[b]	
Ceruloplasmin[a]	Some immunoglobulins	
Haptoglobin[a]		
Serum amyloid-A[a]		

[a] Positive acute phase protein
[b] Negative acute phase protein

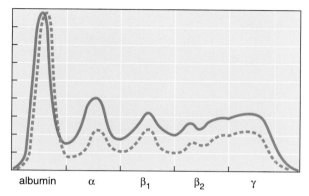

FIGURE 135.2 Electrophoretogram from a normal horse (dashed blue line) and a horse with bacterial discospondylitis (solid red line). This horse had a decreased A:G ratio and hyperglobulinemia composed of increased α-globulins with mildly increased β- and γ-globulins.

or more of these proteins may cause an increased α-globulin fraction on an electrophoretogram. In dogs, heightened α-globulin peaks have been associated with an assortment of spontaneous inflammatory diseases including chronic dermatitis, pyoderma, atopy, immune-mediated diseases, severe cutaneous burns, or parvovirus enteritis.[10–12] Increased α-globulin peaks have also been reported in dogs with various neoplasms,[10] in horses with diarrhea,[13] and in cattle with traumatic pericarditis.[14] Alterations in the α-globulins on an electrophoretogram occur rapidly and have been detected within 24 hours of experimental inoculation with feline infectious peritonitis (FIP) virus in cats.[15]

α-Globulin elevations also occur in disorders not associated with inflammation. Increased α-globulin fractions, caused primarily by elevated haptoglobin concentrations, have been detected 24 hours after administration of prednisone using serum electrophoresis in healthy dogs.[16] Increased α-globulin peaks also occur in dogs with spontaneous hyperadrenocorticism[17] or with diabetes mellitus.[18] Dogs with congenital or acquired renal failure have increased α-globulin peaks.[10] Nephrotic syndrome is associated with increased α-globulin peaks caused by elevated α_2-macroglobulin

and lipoprotein.[3] Hepatic disease (either acute or chronic) is associated with α-globulin elevations caused by increased concentrations of α_1-acid glycoprotein, α_1-antitrypsin, haptoglobin, and α_2-macroglobulin.[19] In vitro hemolysis of samples may cause an increased α_2-globulin peak as a result of the formation of haptoglobin-hemoglobin complexes.[20]

Decreased α-globulin peaks have been demonstrated using serum protein electrophoresis in dogs with end-stage hepatic cirrhosis. The decreases, which result from decreased α_1-antitrypsin and haptoglobin, are predictive of a poor prognosis.[19]

Alterations in β-Globulins

Proteins that migrate in the β-globulin fractions include acute phase proteins, low-density lipoprotein, transferrin, and some of the immunoglobulins (Table 135.2). Increases in β-globulins often occur in association with elevations in α-globulins as part of the acute phase response or with γ-globulins as part of a response to chronic inflammation or infection. Sometimes it may be difficult to separate the β- and γ-globulins on an electrophoretogram (Fig. 135.3). Acute phase proteins that migrate in the β fraction include C-reactive protein, ferritin, fibrinogen (which will be detected on plasma protein electrophoresis but not on serum electrophoresis), and transferrin.[3] Although transferrin is considered to be a negative acute phase protein that decreases with inflammation in most mammals,[3,6] transient elevations in transferrin have been detected using serum protein electrophoresis in cats with experimentally induced FIP.[15] Increased β-globulins as the only alteration are unusual but have been reported with nephrotic syndrome (increased low-density lipoprotein and transferrin), active hepatic disease (increased transferrin and hemopexin), or suppurative dermatitis (increased IgM or C3).[3] Occasionally, a monoclonal peak in the β fraction may occur in patients with multiple myeloma or

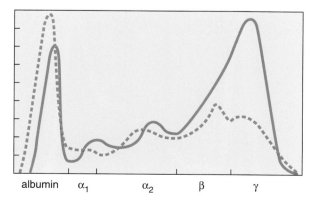

FIGURE 135.3 Electrophoretogram from a normal dog (dashed blue line) and a dog with chronic ehrlichiosis (solid red line). This dog had a decreased A:G ratio and hyperglobulinemia composed of increased β-γ-globulins with no detectable separation between the 2 fractions. The γ-globulin peak is polyclonal.

lymphoma.[3] An increased β-globulin peak occurs secondary to in vitro sample hemolysis as the result of the presence of free hemoglobin.[20]

Decreased β-globulin peaks have been detected using serum protein electrophoresis in dogs with hypoadrenocorticism[18] or with hyperadrenocorticism following mitotane therapy,[17] suggesting that decreased β-globulins may occur secondary to impaired production of adrenocortical hormones.

Alterations in γ-Globulins

The γ-globulin fraction in animals contains IgG, IgM, IgA, and IgE. Many immune responses in animals stimulate increased immunoglobulin concentrations too small to be detected by routine protein electrophoresis, even though elevated antibody titers will be detectable by more sensitive immunoassays.[6] When an elevation in the γ-globulin fraction is discernible on an electrophoretogram, the alteration is classified as either a polyclonal (Fig. 135.4) or a monoclonal (Fig. 135.5) gammopathy based on the width of the peak. A polyclonal peak will be broad-based, and a monoclonal peak will be narrow-based and as sharp as or sharper than the albumin peak.[3]

Polyclonal gammopathies result from increased production of a mixture of immunoglobulin types by multiple clones of plasma cells. Polyclonal increases occur secondary to chronic or severe infections (including infections with bacterial, fungal, viral, rickettsial, or parasitic organisms), neoplasia, or immune-mediated disorders.[3,7,21] Organisms that have a tendency to produce a marked polyclonal gammopathy include *Ehrlichia canis* in dogs, the viruses that cause FIP in cats and equine infectious anemia in horses.[22] Polyclonal gammopathies also occur in severe liver disease, possibly as a result of reduced clearance of foreign antigens from the intestine or autoantibody production secondary to the release of antigens from the liver into the systemic circulation.[19] Polyclonal elevations in the γ-globulins may occur as

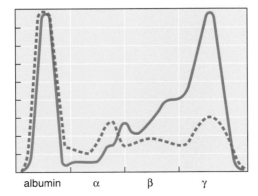

FIGURE 135.4 Electrophoretogram from a normal cat (dashed blue line) and a cat with systemic histoplasmosis (solid red line). This cat had a decreased A:G ratio and hyperglobulinemia composed of increased β-globulins and γ-globulins. The γ-globulin peak is polyclonal.

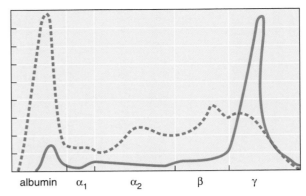

FIGURE 135.5 Electrophoretogram from a normal dog (dashed blue line) and a dog with multiple myeloma (solid red line). This dog had a decreased A:G ratio and hyperglobulinemia composed of increased γ-globulins. The γ-globulin peak is monoclonal.

animals age. Compared with young dogs, healthy geriatric dogs have significantly greater concentrations of γ-globulins, possibly because of a lifetime of exposure to foreign antigens.[10]

Monoclonal gammopathies are commonly associated with lymphoproliferative disorders such as lymphoma or multiple myeloma.[21] Less common causes include chronic infectious or inflammatory diseases. Some are considered idiopathic.[22] In dogs, monoclonal gammopathies have been reported secondary to ehrlichiosis,[23] chronic pyoderma,[24] and plasmacytic gastroenterocolitis.[25] Monoclonal gammopathies have been rarely reported in cats with FIP.[7] Biclonal peaks occasionally occur. A biclonal peak was documented in a cat with two discrete plasmacytomas in the liver[26] and in a dog with a multiple myeloma that produced two paraproteins that were dimers and trimers or tetramers of IgA.[27]

Decreases in the γ-globulin peak in conjunction with normal albumin concentrations occur in acquired or hereditary immunodeficiency syndromes, or in neonates with failure of passive transfer of colostrum.[3] The diagnosis of immunodeficiency should not be made based on serum protein electrophoresis alone. Documentation of decreased immunoglobulin concentrations using more sensitive immunoassays is needed. Decreased γ-globulin peaks may occur in association with decreased albumin concentrations as a result of loss of blood or plasma in protein-losing enteropathies[28] or in puppies with spontaneous parvovirus enteritis.[11] Dogs with spontaneous hyperadrenocorticism have decreased γ-globulin peaks, suggesting that chronic elevations in glucocorticoids may inhibit immunoglobulin production.[17]

REFERENCES

1. **Eckersall PD.** Acute phase proteins as markers of inflammatory lesions. Comp Haematol Int 1995;5:93–97.
2. **Tietz NW.** Fundamentals of clinical chemistry, 3rd ed. Philadelphia: WB Saunders, 1987;317–319.
3. **Kaneko JJ.** Serum proteins and the dysproteinemias. In: Clinical biochemistry of domestic animals, 4th ed. San Diego: Academic Press, 1989.
4. **Baker RJ, Valli.** Electrophoretic and immunoelectrophoretic analysis of feline serum proteins. Can J Vet Res 1988;52:308–314.

5. **Matthews AG.** Serum protein electrophoresis in horses and ponies. Equine Vet J 1982;14:322–324.
6. **Jain NC.** The plasma proteins, dysproteinemias, and immune deficiency disorders. In: Essentials of veterinary hematology. Philadelphia: Lea & Febiger, 1993.
7. **Werner LL, Turnwald GH, Barta O.** Immunologic and plasma protein disorders. In: Willard MD, Tvedten H, Turnwald GH, eds. Small animal clinical diagnosis by laboratory methods, 2nd ed. Philadelphia: WB Saunders, 1994.
8. **Chang CY, Fristche HA, Glassman AB, et al.** Underestimation of monoclonal proteins by agarose serum protein electrophoresis. Ann Clin Lab Sci 1997;27:123–129.
9. **Keay G.** Serum protein values from clinically normal cats and dogs determined by agarose gel electrophoresis. Res Vet Sci 1982;33:343–346.
10. **Batamuzi EK, Kristensen E, Jansen AL.** Serum protein electrophoresis: Potential test for use in geriatric companion animal health programmes. Zentralblatt Fur Veterinarmedizin 1996;43:501–508.
11. **van den Broek AHM.** Serum protein electrophoresis in canine parvovirus enteritis. Br Vet J 1990;146:255–259.
12. **Kern MR, Stockham SL, Coates JR.** Analysis of serum protein concentrations after severe thermal injury in a dog. Vet Clin Pathol 1992;21:19–22.
13. **Mair TS, Cripps PJ, Ricketts SW.** Diagnostic and prognostic value of serum protein electrophoresis in horses with chronic diarrhoea. Equine Vet J 1993;25:324–326.
14. **Yoshida Y.** Electrophoretic studies on serum proteins in cows with traumatic pericarditis. J Vet Med Sci 1991;53:5–11.
15. **Stoddart ME, Whicher JT, Harbour DA.** Cats inoculated with feline infectious peritonitis virus exhibit a biphasic acute phase plasma protein response. Vet Rec 1988;123:621–624.
16. **Harvey JW, West CL.** Prednisone-induced increases in serum alpha-2-globulin and haptoglobin concentrations in dogs. Vet Pathol 1987;24:90–92.
17. **van den Broek AHM, Lida J.** Serum protein electrophoresis in spontaneous canine hyperadrenocorticism. Res Vet Sci 1989;46:100–104.
18. **van den Broek AHM.** Serum protein electrophoresis in canine diabetes mellitus, hypothyroidism and hypoadrenocorticism. Br Vet J 1992;148:259–262.
19. **Sevelius E, Andersson M.** Serum protein electrophoresis as a prognostic marker of chronic liver disease in dogs. Vet Rec 1995;137:663–667.
20. **Amog VM, Bull RW, Michel RL.** Comparison of electrophoretograms of normal canine serum and plasma and of serum and plasma of hemolyzed specimens. Am J Vet Res 1977;38:387–390.
21. **Dorfman M, Dimski DS.** Paraproteinemias in small animal medicine. Compend Cont Edu Pract Vet 1992;14:621–631.
22. **Williams DA.** Gammopathies. Compend Cont Edu Pract Vet 1981;3:815–822.
23. **Breitschwerdt EB, Woody BJ, Zerbe CA, et al.** Monoclonal gammopathy associated with naturally occurring canine ehrlichiosis. J Vet Intern Med 1987;1:2–9.
24. **Burkhard MJ, Meyer DJ, Rosychuk RA, et al.** Monoclonal gammopathy in a dog with chronic pyoderma. J Vet Intern Med 1995;9:357–360.
25. **Diehl KJ, Lappin MR, Jones RL, et al.** Monoclonal gammopathy in a dog with plasmacytic gastroenterocolitis. JAVMA 1992;201:1233–1236.
26. **Larsen AE, Carpenter JL.** Hepatic plasmacytoma and bioclonal gammopathy in a cat. JAVMA 1994;205:708–710.
27. **Kato H, Momoi Y, Omori K, et al.** Gammopathy with two M-components in a dog with IgA-type multiple myeloma. Vet Immunol Immunopathol 1995;49:161–168.
28. **Finco DR, Duncan JR, Schall WD, et al.** Chronic enteric disease and hypoproteinemia in 9 dogs. JAVMA 1973;163:262–271.

CHAPTER 136

Immunoglobulins

- JAIME F. MODIANO

Immunoglobulins are major protein components of plasma, and some can be easily measured to provide clinically significant information. They are the prototypical members of a superfamily of proteins with canonical globular domains that also include T-cell antigen receptors and intercellular adhesion molecules.[1] Immunoglobulins are critical mediators of the humoral immune response to antigen, and in this context they are called antibodies. Over the course of evolution, vertebrates have developed various modes to generate a large repertoire of antibodies, yet there has been extensive conservation of the structural and functional features despite the appearance of substantial divergence in the sequence and genetic organization of these molecules.[2–4]

Immunoglobulin production is restricted to lymphoid cells of the B-cell lineage. Most immunoglobulins come from terminally differentiated plasma cells. Immunoglobulins are unique in their dichotomous function as membrane-bound and soluble proteins. Membrane-bound immunoglobulins (also called surface immunoglobulins) act as B-cell antigen receptors (BCR). Binding of antigen to the BCR initiates a cascade of signals that can alternatively lead to B-cell activation, differentiation, or anergy.[1] Binding of antigens by antibodies in the plasma enhances the clearance rate of these antigens and also promotes the activation of various components of the cellular immune response. The diseases and clinical syndromes observed in humans and animals with immunoglobulin deficiencies help to illustrate the critical roles of antibodies in supporting immune function and homeostasis.[5–7]

The significance of immunoglobulins in clinical medicine is not limited to their protective role in mediating host immunity. They are also important participants in the pathogenesis and progression of many immune-mediated disorders.[6,8] Moreover, the use of antibodies as tools for discovery and diagnosis has played a major role in many recent advances in medical knowledge and therapy (see Chapter 137, Immunoassays).

This chapter will review briefly the relationships between immunoglobulin structure and function, the genetic basis for generating antibody diversity, the role of antibodies in the adaptive immune response, their significance in immunopathology, and their importance in diagnostic laboratory medicine.

STRUCTURAL FEATURES OF IMMUNOGLOBULINS

The immunoglobulin molecule is comprised of two heavy (H) and two light (L) polypeptide chains, each having domains that are folded as β-sandwichlike structures.[9–12] The V-region domains of the L- and H-chains (VL-VH) form a region of the antibody known as the Fv, for 'fragment variable,' and the Fv portion maintains its antigen-binding properties even when separated from the remainder of the intact molecule. The Fab molecule, for 'antigen-binding fragment,' contains additional constant domains CL and CH1, but these do not appear to significantly influence antigen recognition.[13,14] The H- and L-chains are joined by disulfide bridges, and each H-L dimer is in turn assembled with another identical H-L dimer via an H-H disulfide bridge to generate the classical Y-shaped immunoglobulin molecule (Fig. 136.1). Hence, every basic antibody molecule has two antigen-binding sites.

The antigen-binding site on each VL-VH dimer consists of an area located near the top of the Fv and is formed by six polypeptide segments or 'complementarity determining region' (CDR) loops: three contributed by the L chain-L1, L2, and L3-and three from the H chain-H1, H2, H3.[13,15] The CDR loops are formed at the ends of the antiparallel β-strands of the polypeptide segments segments from each chain. The amino acid sequences of these CDR segments varies extensively from one antibody to another[16] and thus also bear the name of 'hypervariable regions.' X-ray diffraction studies of Fab and Fv crystals from over 50 different antibodies revealed that the six CDR loops are paramount to antigen recognition.[15,17] The affinity of most antigen-antibody interactions is on the order of $10^{-6} - 10^{-9}$ moles/L.

The function of antibodies in solution is predominantly related to their ability to bind antigens and mediate their removal. An antigen is essentially defined as any molecule that is 'not self.' The production of anti-

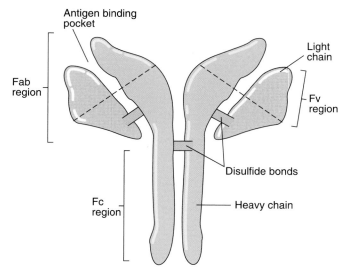

FIGURE 136.1 Schematic representation of an immunoglobulin. An IgG1 molecule is used to illustrate the basic arrangement of an immunoglobulin. Each molecule is composed of two heavy chain-light chain dimers joined by disulfide bonds. The Fv region consists of the variable domains that contain the antigen-binding pocket. The Fab region contains additional constant domains. The Fc region determines the immunoglobulin isotype. (Adapted from the space filling model of IgG1 available at http://www.umass.edu/microbio/rasmol, the RasMol World Wide Web site.)

bodies against self-molecules is prevented through the induction of tolerance and anergy (eliminating self-reactive B cells or suppressing their activation). Among the biologically relevant functions of immunoglobulins are neutralization, mediated through competitive binding or steric inhibition; agglutination; and opsonization, mediated by complement- or Fc-dependent removal.

The carboxy-terminal portion of the immunoglobulin molecule (Fc region) consists of class-specific sequences determined by the heavy chain. The fate of an immunoglobulin molecule to assemble into a transmembrane protein complexed noncovalently to the CD79 complex molecules (CD79a and CD79b, also called Igα and Igβ) to form a BCR, or to be secreted, is determined by alternative splicing of the heavy chain mRNA.

IMMUNOGLOBULIN ISOTYPES

Five distinct heavy chain genes (μ, δ, γ, α, and ϵ) are present in mammals. Heavy chain gene usage determines the immunoglobulin class or isotype (IgM, IgD, IgG, IgA, or IgE). IgM is the first antibody produced by all B cells. In solution, IgM assembles into a pentameric macromolecular complex (high-molecular-weight antibody) joined by a J chain (a polypeptide of ~15 KDa). The pentameric structure of IgM provides the molecule with 10 functional antigen-binding sites that increase its functional affinity (avidity); this multimeric structure also makes IgM exquisitely efficient at agglutination,

opsonization, and complement binding. IgD is found predominantly as a membrane-associated protein in immature B cells (and may not be used at all in some species).[7] IgG is the predominant form of immunoglobulin present in plasma and plays a major role in humoral defense mechanisms. It is usually present as monomers and can readily extravasate. IgG3 has a long hinge region similar to avian IgY, and may be the earliest form of mammalian IgG (see below). IgA is produced in lymphoid organs located at the mucosal interface of the gut, respiratory tract, urinary tract, and mammary gland, and it is largely responsible for providing a 'barrier' of defense against the large numbers of organisms found in these locations. IgA assembles into dimers that are joined by a J chain. These dimers are transported across the mucosal epithelial barrier by a large protein called the secretory component, which also protects the IgA molecules from digestion within the intestinal tract. IgE is predominantly associated with hypersensitivity. Its production is generally restricted to responses against parasitic nematodes and atopy. Among the different classes of antibodies, IgG and IgE are notable for their binding to specialized receptors (Fc receptors) on the surface of inflammatory cells. Fcγ receptors are present on the surface of monocytes and macrophages, neutrophils, and lymphocytes.[1,7] Fcε receptors are found on the surface of mast cells and basophils. IgE binds these Fc receptors, exposing its antigen-binding domain away from the cell. Cross-linking Fcε receptors on mast cells via the binding of antigen to IgE provides the signal for mast cell degranulation and release of histamine and other vasoactive substances that mediate type I hypersensitivity responses.

Isotype switching occurs following specific signals that are mediated by the microenvironment. The switch from IgM to IgG requires ligation of the BCR with antigen, as well as the ligation of a surface molecule called CD40 by the CD40 ligand (CD40L) present on the membrane of helper T cells. The functional significance of this interaction is underscored by the finding that the hyper-IgM immunodeficiency syndrome (where patients are unable to produce any isotype other than IgM) is mediated by a defect in the CD40L gene.[5,18] Switch signals also require the concerted action of various cytokines, with IL-4 leading to IgE production and IL-5 contributing significantly to IgA production.

ANTIBODY DIVERSITY

The origin of antibodies can be traced to a common vertebrate ancestor that lived before the divergence of cartilaginous fishes.[2,4,19] Although globular domain proteins may have initially developed as means of intercellular communication, the specific role of immunoglobulins in host defense has become indispensable for all vertebrates.[20] The ability of the immune response to discriminate self from nonself and to evolve in a time scale measured by cell divisions, rather than by generations of individuals, provided animals a survival advantage in the fight against microbial pathogens that reproduce and evolve on a scale lasting hours to days.[21] It is these properties that set the immune system apart from all other anatomic and functional systems in the body.

The first immunoglobulins to evolve were high-molecular-weight immunoglobulins similar to IgM. IgM-type immunoglobulins that are structurally and functionally similar are found in every species, from cartilaginous fishes to higher mammals.[4,22,23] A low-molecular-weight immunoglobulin called IgY may be the precursor to mammalian IgG (and IgE) and is present in amphibians, reptiles, and birds. IgY may have originated with the evolution of bony fishes.[4,23]

Different species have used various, nonmutually exclusive methods to diversify their antibody repertoire. These methods share the use of gene segments encoding variable (V) regions with the antigen-binding domains, diversity-generating (D) regions, joining (J) regions, and constant (C) regions that determine the class (or isotype) of the antibody (Fig. 136.2).[1,7] The recombinatorial processes in genomic DNA seen in primates and rodents have received the most attention,[24-26] but they are not used universally by all animals.[27] In humans and mice there is evidence of extensive duplication of V genes, with less so of D and J genes. Families of contiguous V genes are present in a single chromosome that are susceptible to rearrangement at the level of the germline DNA in developing B cells (Fig. 136.2).[26] A functional heavy (H) chain gene is generated by the transpo-

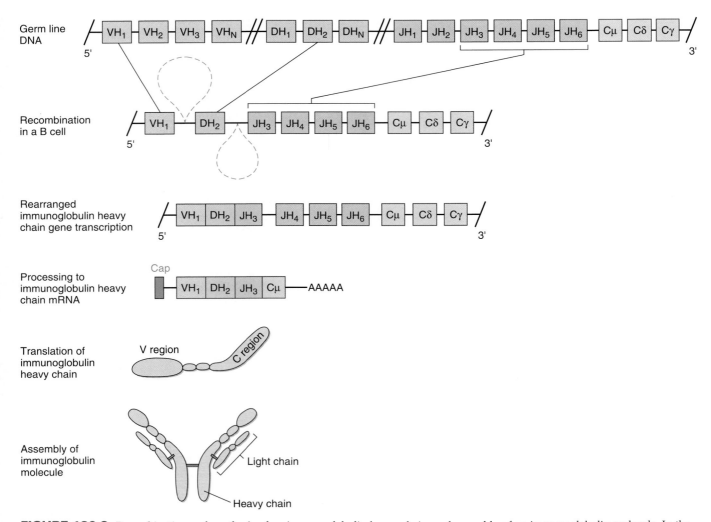

FIGURE 136.2 Recombination and synthesis of an immunoglobulin heavy chain, and assembly of an immunoglobulin molecule. In the germ-line DNA, families of contiguous V_H, D_H, and J_H genes are present in a single chromosome that are susceptible to rearrangement in developing B cells. Two rearrangement events must take place to produce a functional heavy chain gene. In this figure, the D_{H2} gene is joined to the J_{H3} gene, and the V_{H1} gene is joined to the rearranged DJ segment. The intervening DNA sequences are 'looped out' and deleted. The initial RNA transcript of the heavy chain gene begins upstream from the rearranged gene segments and ends beyond the heavy chain genes ($C\alpha$ and $C\varepsilon$ are not shown here). The rearranged VDJ genes are joined to the appropriate C-region gene by excision of the intervening sequence, and the transcript is capped and polyadenylated during processing to mRNA. This mRNA is then translated, and the heavy chain polypeptide dimerizes with a rearranged light chain polypeptide. Two heavy chain-light chain dimers are then joined to form a functional immunoglobulin molecule.

sition of a single D region to a location adjacent to a J_H region. A similar event follows that transposes a single V_H region to a location adjacent to the rearranged DJ segment. Similar events take place among the light chain genes, except that there are no D regions. Successful recombination leads to transcription and translation of the rearranged immunoglobulin gene. In humans, the estimated number of distinct specificities that can be generated from recombination of 50 V_H segments, 12 D segments, and 6 J_H segments (50 × 12 × 6) is 3600.[1] When the combination of these with as many as 200 kappa (κ) light chains and 150 lambda (λ) light chains is considered, the antibody repertoire increases to >1 × 10⁶ specificities. Additional diversity is generated by junctional diversification, that is, the fact that the joints between segments are 'imperfect' and allow for nucleotide deletions and insertions.[28,29] Somatic hypermutation is another mode that many animals use during secondary immune responses to increase antibody diversity, but it may be the mainstay of antibody diversification during primary responses in some species such as sheep.[27,30,31] Any human thus has the potential to generate ≥ 1 × 10⁹ distinct antibodies, apparently a sufficient number to survive in a hostile environment with countless pathogens. Similar recombinatorial processes are believed to occur in dogs, cats, and perhaps horses.

The genetic machinery that mediates these recombination events consists of various DNA excision and repair proteins such as recombinase and DNA protein kinase, and defects in any one of these will produce a severe combined immunodeficiency phenotype such as those characterized in humans,[5] mice,[32] and Arabian horses.[33]

Alternative methods to generate diversity at the level of the germ line have been shown to occur in other species. For example, cartilaginous fishes such as sharks rely on the presence of over 100 clusters of 'prerearranged' immunoglobulin gene segments, and antibodies generated through recombination events account for only a small proportion of the repertoires.[22] Birds, lagomorphs, and artiodactyls (cloven-hoofed mammals) appear to use gene conversion as a means to achieve diversity.[27,34] In this process, a 'master' pair of V and C genes is expressed in all B cells. Short segments of surrogate V genes (or pseudogenes) are copied to the master V gene (following an unknown inciting event), leading to the generation of new specificities.

ANTIBODIES IN ADAPTIVE IMMUNITY

Adaptive immunity refers to those responses mediated by lymphocytes that exhibit specificity and memory. Primary immune responses occur when a naive (previously unstimulated) B cell encounters antigen for the first time. These responses are frequently T-cell independent and are characterized by large amounts of IgM production. Secondary responses (also called memory or anamnestic responses) occur when memory B cells encounter antigen. These responses frequently require

T-cell help, and they are characterized by the production of IgG. Whereas it usually takes 5 to 7 days to mount a primary response, secondary responses appear faster (2 to 3 days) and are of greater magnitude as measured by antibody production. The apparent affinity of antibodies against a particular antigen also appears to increase during a secondary response. This is due to affinity maturation. During the course of a secondary response as reactive B cells proliferate, their DNA is subject to hypermutation in 'hotspots' found within the rearranged immunoglobulin V-region gene.[31] Thus, many of the clonal progeny will produce slightly different (mutant) antibodies from the parent B cell. The mutations are random, and may be neutral (have no effect on binding affinity), deleterious (reduce affinity), or beneficial (increase affinity). The expansion of those B cells bearing the mutant immunoglobulins with increased affinity will be favored during a secondary response because of the increased likelihood of extended interactions between the antigen and the BCR. The mechanisms that promote somatic hypermutation are incompletely understood, albeit it is clear that they are highly regulated.[30,31]

IMMUNOGLOBULIN IMMUNOPATHOLOGY

Heritable or acquired defects that interfere with immunoglobulin production can lead to immunodeficiency. Affected individuals show increased susceptibility to microbial pathogens and can succumb to infections by opportunistic or commensal agents.[5] Heritable defects that result in decreased levels of immunoglobulins include severe combined immunodeficiency, agammaglobulinemia, hyper-IgM syndrome, and selective deficiencies of IgM, IgG, or IgA.[5] The genetic lesions for many of these conditions have been identified in humans,[5] but relatively few have been characterized in domestic animals.[7]

Acquired conditions that interfere with immunoglobulin production and lead to immunodeficiency are seen frequently in domestic animals. Some of the more common causes include failure of passive transfer in newborns and infections with lymphotropic, immunosuppressive retroviruses. The reader is referred to recent textbooks in veterinary and comparative immunology for detailed discussions of animal immunodeficiencies.[7,23]

Excessive or inappropriate immunoglobulin production also can lead to pathologic conditions.[6,8] Type I or immediate hypersensitivity responses are mediated through the action of IgE on mast cells. Type II hypersensitivity responses and blood group incompatibilities are generally mediated by circulating IgG, as are type III hypersensitivity reactions and immune complex disease.

Autoimmune disorders wherein individuals mount antibody responses against self-antigens occur commonly. The event(s) that incites production of autoantibodies in most autoimmune diseases is unclear, but they all share in common a break in immune tolerance. Breaks in immune tolerance leading to autoimmune diseases may result from cross-reactivity between self and non-self antigens (molecular mimicry), exposure to hidden antigens, or defects in the regulatory mechanisms that dampen immune responses such as activation-induced apoptosis.[35] It is noteworthy that the mechanisms controlling B-cell tolerance are significantly less rigorous than those controlling T-cell tolerance. Autoimmunity can manifest as organ- or tissue-specific diseases, or it can cause systemic diseases. Table 136.1 lists some common immune-mediated diseases seen in domestic animals.

Hypergammaglobulinemias are another important manifestation of immunoglobulin immunopathology. Increased immunoglobulin production by many (polyclonal) or few (oligoclonal) B cells can result from a vigorous inflammatory response to infectious agents such as *Dirofilaria immitis* and *Ehrlichia canis*.[36-38] Conversely, B-cell tumors (lymphoma, leukemia) and plasma cell tumors (plasmacytoma, myeloma) are characterized by the production of a monoclonal immunoglobulin (paraprotein).[39] The paraneoplastic conditions caused by the elevated levels of immunoglobulin in these cases are significant determinants of prognosis and outcome.

DIAGNOSTIC APPLICATIONS

The measurement of immunoglobulins in plasma or serum has been the mainstay of serology in clinical laboratory medicine. An improved understanding of the biology of antibody production and of the biochemistry of antigen-antibody interactions has led to explosive advances in immunodiagnostics. New approaches to generate and manipulate antibodies in vitro promise to expand the applications of these molecules in clinical laboratory medicine and into the therapeutic arena.

TABLE 136.1 Some Common Antibody-Mediated Autoimmune Diseases Seen In Domestic Animals

Disease	Autoantigen
Hypothyroidism	Thyroglobulin
Pemphigus vulgaris	Desmoglein-3
Pemphigus foliaceous	? desmoglein-1
Bullous pemphigoid	Desmoplakin
Autoimmune nephritis	? glomerular basement membrane antigens
Immune-mediated hemolytic anemia	? glycophorins
Immune-mediated thrombocytopenia	? platelet/megakaryocyte membrane antigen
Myasthenia gravis	Acetylcholine receptor
Systemic lupus erythematosus	Nuclear proteins (? histones)
Rheumatoid arthritis	? IgG ? collagen

Adapted from Tizard IR. Veterinary immunology, 5th ed. Philadelphia: WB Saunders, 1996.

REFERENCES

1. Klein J, Horjesi V. Immunology, 2nd ed. London: Blackwell Science Ltd, 1997.
2. Hsu E. The variation in immunoglobulin heavy chain constant regions in evolution. Semin Immunol 1994;6:383–391.
3. Marchalonis JJ, Schluter SF. Evolution of variable and constant domains and joining segments of rearranging immunoglobulins. FASEB J 1989; 3:2469–2479.
4. Warr GW, Magor KE, Higgins DA. IgY: Clues to the origins of modern antibodies. Immunol Today 1995;16:392–398.
5. Rosen FS, Cooper MD, Wedgwood RJ. The primary immunodeficiencies. New Engl J Med 1995;333:431–440.
6. Sell S. Immunology, immunopathology and immunity, 5th ed. Stamford, CT: Appleton & Lange, 1996.
7. Tizard IR. Veterinary immunology, 5th ed. Philadelphia: WB Saunders, 1996.
8. Steinman L. Escape from "horror autotoxicus": Pathogenesis and treatment of autoimmune disease. Cell 1995;80:7–10.
9. Davies DR, Metzger H. Structural basis of antibody function. Ann Rev Immunol 1983;1:87–117.
10. Huber R. Structural basis for antigen-antibody recognition. Science 1986; 233:702–703.
11. Poljak RJ. X-ray diffraction studies of immunoglobulins. Adv Immunol 1975;21:1–33.
12. Poljak RJ, Amzel LM, Chen BL, Phizackerley RP, Saul F. Three-dimensional structure of the Fab fragment of a human immunoglobulin at 2.8 Å resolution. Proc Natl Acad Sci USA 1973;70:3305–3310.
13. Amit AG, Mariuzza RA, Phillips SE, Poljak RJ. Three-dimensional structure of an antigen-antibody complex at 2.8 Å resolution. Science 1986; 233:747–753.
14. Padlan EA. Anatomy of the antibody molecule. Molecular Immunol 1994;31:169–217.
15. Davies DR, Padlan EA, Sheriff S. Antibody-antigen complexes. Ann Rev Biochem 1990;59:439–473.
16. Kabat EA, Wu TT, Bilofsky H. Unusual distribution of amino acids in complementarity-determining (hypervariable) segments of heavy and light chains of immunoglobulins and their possible roles in specificity of antibody-combining sites. J Biol Chem 1977;252:6609–6616.
17. Bernstein FC, Koetzle TF, Williams EJB, Meyer EFJ, Kennard O, Shimanouchi T, Tasumi M. The protein data bank: A computer-based archival file for molecular structures. J Molecular Biol 1977;112:535–542.
18. Castigli E, Fuleihan R, Ramesh N, Tsitsikov E, Tsytsykova A, Geha RS. CD40 ligand/CD40 deficiency. Int Arch Allergy Immunol 1995; 107:37–39.
19. Pilstrom L. Immunology of fishes: Immunoglobulins. In: PP Pastoret, P Griebel, H Bazin, A Govaerts, eds. Handbook of vertebrate immunology. San Diego: Academic Press, 1998;15–23.
20. Stewart J. Immunoglobulins did not arise in evolution to fight infection. Immunol Today 1992;13:396–399.
21. Langman R. Comment on immunoglobulins did not arise in evolution to fight infection. Immunol Today 1992;13:396–397.
22. Litman GW. Sharks and the origins of vertebrate immunity. Sci Am 1996;275:67–71.
23. Pastoret PP, Griebel P, Bazin H, Govaerts A. Handbook of vertebrate immunology. San Diego: Academic Press, 1998.
24. Brack C, Hirama M, Lenhard-Schuller R, Tonegawa S. A complete immunoglobulin gene is created by somatic recombination. Cell 1978; 15:1–14.
25. Lewis S, Gifford A, Baltimore D. DNA elements are asymmetrically joined during the site-specific recombination of kappa immunoglobulin genes. Science 1985;228:677–685.
26. Tonegawa S. Somatic generation of antibody diversity. Nature 1983; 302:575–581.
27. Weill JC, Reynaud CA. Rearrangement/hypermutation/gene conversion: When, where and why? Immunol Today 1996;17:92–97.
28. Jeske DJ, Jarvis J, Milstein C, Capra JD. Junctional diversity is essential to antibody activity. J Immunol 1984;133:1090–1092.
29. Victor KD, Capra JD. An apparently common mechanism of generating antibody diversity: Length variation of the VL-JL junction. Molecular Immunol 1994;31:39–46.
30. Jolly CJ, Wagner SD, Rada C, Klix N, Milstein C, Neuberger MS. The targeting of somatic hypermutation. Semin Immunol 1996;8:159–168.
31. Neuberger MS, Milstein C. Somatic hypermutation. Curr Opin Immunol 1995;7:248–254.
32. Bosma M, Schuler W, Bosma G. The SCID mouse mutant. Curr Topics Immunol Microbiol 1988;137:197–202.
33. Wiler R, Leber R, Moore BB, VanDyk LF, Perryman LE, Meek K. Equine severe combined immunodeficiency: A defect in V(D)J recombination and DNA-dependent protein kinase activity. Proc Natl Acad Sci USA 1995;92:11485–11489.
34. Butler JE, Sun J, Kacskovics I, Brown WR, Navarro P. The VH and CH

immunoglobulin genes of swine: Implications for repertoire development. Vet Immunol Immunopathol 1996;54:7–17.

35. **Thompson CB.** Apoptosis in the pathogenesis and treatment of disease. Science 1995;267:1456–1462.

36. **Breitschwerdt EB, Woody BJ, Zerbe CA, De Buysscher EV, Barta O.** Monoclonal gammopathy associated with naturally occurring canine ehrlichiosis. J Vet Intern Med 1987;1:2–9.

37. **Drazner FH.** Renal amyloidosis and glomerulonephritis secondary to dirofilariasis. Canine Pract 1978;5:66–68.

38. **Michels GM, Boon GD, Jones BD, Puget B.** Hypergammaglobulinemia in a dog. JAVMA 1995;207:567–568.

39. **Thrall MA.** Lymphoproliferative disorders. Lymphocytic leukemia and plasma cell myeloma. Vet Clin North Am Small Animal Pract 1981; 11:321–347.

CHAPTER 137

Immunoassays

• JAIME F. MODIANO and MICHELLE G. RITT

The recognition of the functional differences between classes of immunoglobulins and the clinical significance of these differences spurred the development of various techniques to separate immunoglobulins in the early- to mid-20th century. Among the first techniques to be used for this purpose were agar gel immunodiffusion (AGID) and immunoelectrophoresis (IEP), both of which are still in use today. The development of a method to generate monoclonal antibodies in vitro[1] was perhaps the most significant event that propelled the development of reliable and cost-effective immunologic tests for clinical laboratory medicine. Further refinements in monoclonal antibody technology (especially the ability to produce antibodies in mass scale and the use of tracers that could be covalently linked to these antibodies) along with microassays, robotics, and sensitive, nonradiometric detection systems allowed for the development of radioimmunoassays (RIAs), enzyme-linked immunosorbent assays (ELISAs), and immunoblotting methods. These techniques are generally faster and easier to interpret than AGID and IEP.

This chapter will describe immunologically based, clinical laboratory methods that are presently used to measure antigens in plasma or serum. The antigens that can be measured by these techniques include 'self' molecules, such as hormones, vitamins, immunoglobulins, and other serum proteins; 'altered self' proteins, such as cancer-associated antigens; and 'foreign' proteins, including microbial antigens and vaccine antigens. There are various additional serologic tests that are used in veterinary clinical laboratories to detect antibodies against infectious organisms. These tests include agglutination, agglutination inhibition, complement fixation, immunofluorescence, and plaque assays, among others. The principles behind these tests and their applications have been reviewed elsewhere[2-4] and will not be considered here.

IMMUNOLOGIC ASSAYS USED TO MEASURE PLASMA PROTEINS

Immunodiffusion

The principle of immunodiffusion is based on the diffusion of molecules along concentration gradients, along with the properties of antigen-antibody interactions. The interaction between antigens and antibodies is determined partly by the bivalent (two binding sites) nature of antibodies and the presence of multiple epitopes on each antigen.[2-4] When either the antibody or the antigens are present in excess, small immune complexes are formed that can remain in solution. At optimal concentrations (equivalence), the antigen and the antibodies will form large complexes that precipitate out of solution (Fig. 137.1). These precipitates can be visualized within a translucent solid matrix such as an agar gel.

The Mancini technique, or radial immunodiffusion (RID), is used commonly to identify immunoglobulin isotypes in serum.[3-5] For RID, serum is placed into a well on a gel that is impregnated with antibodies against each specific immunoglobulin isotype (most commonly IgM, IgG, or IgA). The immunoglobulin in serum diffuses outwardly (radially) from the well and will precipitate with the antibody in the gel at the zone of equivalence (Fig. 137.2). The diameter of the precipitin ring is proportional to the concentration of immunoglobulin in the serum. Ouchterlony devised a clever modification of this technique whereby the presence of similar or cross-reactive antigens could be examined.[2-4,6] For this double immunodiffusion method, the unknown antigen, a known control antigen, and the known antibody are placed in wells at ~45° angles. If the antigens are dissimilar, only the positive control and the antibody will form a precipitate. If the antigens are similar but not identical, a 'spur' will be seen in the reaction (Fig. 137.3).

Immunoelectrophoresis

Electrophoresis describes the process of separating proteins in a gel using an electrochemical gradient. In IEP, protein detection relies on the precipitation of antigen-antibody complexes. The resultant 'bands' of precipitation represent the read-out of the test. In veterinary medicine, IEP is used predominantly to determine the isotype of paraproteins in monoclonal gammopathies. However, the development of more sensitive, specific, and reliable techniques that are less time-consuming and less laborious to perform is likely to make traditional IEP obsolete.

Several variations of immunoelectrophoretic tech-

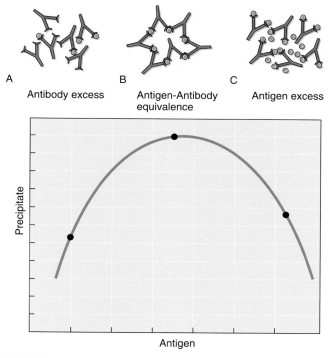

FIGURE 137.1 Precipitin reaction. The formation of insoluble complexes is a characteristic of antigen-antibody interactions when their concentrations are approximately equivalent. In this schematic representation, (**A**) little precipitate forms when antibodies are in excess. As the concentration of antigen increases, (**B**) so does precipitation due to the formation of a multivalent lattice and displacement of water molecules. This interaction is possible due to the presence of two binding sites on each antibody, and the presence of multiple epitopes on the antigen. Favorable conditions for the formation of a multivalent lattice diminsh (**C**) as the concentration of antigen exceeds the number of antibody binding sites.

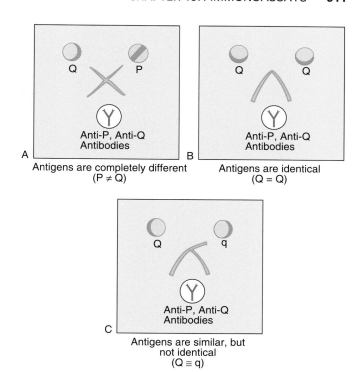

FIGURE 137.3 Double immunodiffusion. Cross-reactive antigens can be identified by the method of Ouchterlony. Antibodies against dissimilar antigens are placed in a well and allowed to diffuse towards antigens present in serum samples. In (**A**) the samples contain the distinct antigens 'P' and 'Q' recognized by the anti-P and anti-Q antibodies. The precipitates formed by these interactions are independent of each other and appear as a cross in the gel plate. In (**B**) both samples contain identical antigens represented by 'Q'. Precipitation will occur equally in both directions, thus the precipitin bands fuse without crossing. In (**C**) the samples contain similar, but not identical antigens represented by 'Q' and 'q'. While the similarity is sufficient to elicit a reaction with the anti-Q antibodies, precipitation will not occur equally in both directions because of different affinities of the antibody to 'Q' and 'q'. This leads to the formation of a spur, or a line of partial identity.

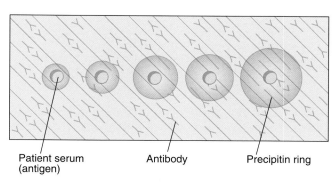

FIGURE 137.2 Radial immunodiffusion (RID). Serum is placed in wells within a gel that is impregnated with antibodies against the antigen to be measured. Serum proteins diffuse radially by osmosis. Precipitation occurs if the relevant antigen is present in the serum at concentrations that will create a zone of equivalence (see Fig. 137.1). The diameter of the precipitin ring is proportional to the concentration of antigen, and can be determined by generating standard curves.

niques were developed in the 1950s and refined over the years.[7] The most common types of IEP techniques include standard (zone) IEP, rocket IEP, counterimmunoelectrophoresis (CIE), and immunofixation.[2-4,6,7] The techniques differ from each other in the preparation of the immunochemical reaction. Standard or zone IEP involves the separation of serum proteins by charge. Once the electrophoresis is completed, antibody is placed in a trough alongside the zone of electrophoresis. Precipitation occurs if the antibody and a relevant antigen interact following diffusion through the gel matrix (Fig. 137.4A).

In rocket IEP, the gel is impregnated with antibody prior to electrophoretic separation. Different concentrations of antigen along the electrophoretic gradient create zones of diffusion that are cone- or rocket-shaped, hence the name (Fig. 137.4B). Although the quantitative estimates of immunoglobulin concentration provided by

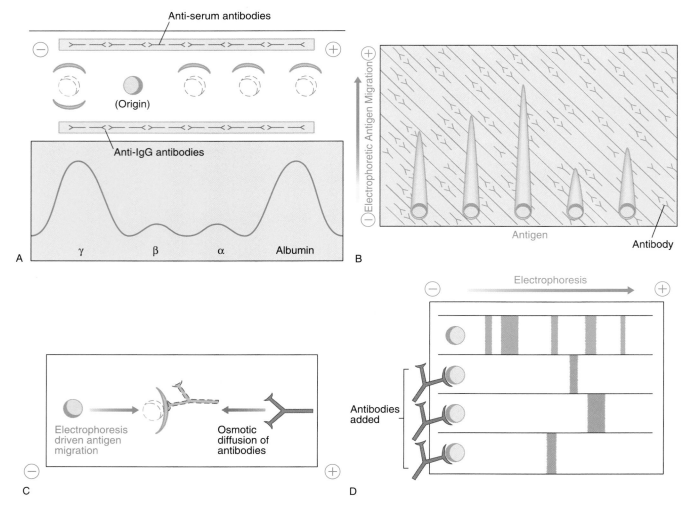

FIGURE 137.4 Immunoelectrophoresis (IEP). (**A**) In zone IEP, serum proteins are separated in a gel using an electrochemical gradient. Antibodies are then placed on troughs running parallel to the separated proteins. The separated serum proteins and the antibodies are allowed to diffuse into the gel, and precipitation will occur if the relevant antigens are present in the serum at concentrations that will create a zone of equivalence. In this schematic figure, anti-serum antibodies (containing antibodies against all major serum proteins) are used in the upper trough, and anti-IgG antibodies are used in the lower trough. Bands of precipitation are seen on top of each major serum component (albumin, alpha globulins, beta globulins, and gamma globulins) where the interactions with the anti-serum antibodies occur. However, a band of precipitation is only seen below the gamma globulin region that contains the serum IgG. (**B**) In rocket IEP, the serum proteins are separated electrophoretically through a gel that is impregnated with antibody. Precipitation occurs at the zones of equivalence for each sample. The height of the precipitation zone is proportional to the concentration of antigen. (**C**) In counterimmunoelectrophoresis (CIE), the antibody is allowed to diffuse towards the antigen during the electrophoretic separation. Precipitation will occur when the antibody and antigen concentrations reach a zone of equivalence. (**D**) For immunofixation, the antibodies are added directly to the lanes following electrophoretic separation and the precipitation reaction occurs at the spot where the antigen migrated.

rocket IEP are more accurate than those obtained by zone IEP, rocket IEP also is more expensive to run.

In CIE, a band of precipitation is formed where the antigen and antibody meet as they migrate in opposite directions through the gel. The pH of the buffer is identical to the isoelectric point of the antibody, thus allowing the antibody to diffuse along its concentration gradient unimpeded by the electric field that governs the migration of the antigen (Fig. 137.4C). CIE is commonly used in the diagnosis of autoimmune diseases such as systemic lupus erythematosus. Prediffusion of serum for 2 hours prior to separation improves the efficiency of CIE to identify autoantibodies.[8] Immunofixation utilizes the principle of electric separation of the antigen, but

unlike the other techniques described, antibody is added directly to each lane in the gel following electrophoresis.[6] In this case, the precipitins appear as straight bands within the lane (Fig. 137.4D).

Immunofixation is faster, easier to perform, and provides a more accurate estimate of immunoglobulin concentration than do IEP procedures.[6]

Radioimmunoassay

The development of a radiometric test to measure insulin in plasma[9] revolutionized the field of immunodiagnostics. RIAs are the mainstay of clinical endocrinology testing to detect and quantify protein and steroid hormones (insulin, ACTH, thyroid hormone, cortisol, progesterone, estradiol, testosterone, etc.) and vitamins such as cobalamin and folate.[3,10] RIAs are also prevalent in clinical pharmacology to measure blood levels of many drugs and drug metabolites such as digoxin.[11] RIAs are simple competitive-binding assays, where the target analyte in serum (competitor) is used to displace a known, radiolabeled standard (Fig. 137.5). After the reaction reaches equilibrium, the bound and unbound fraction are separated by precipitation, or by attaching the antibody to a solid phase. The concentration of the target molecule is proportional to the decrease in the concentration of the radioactive tracer.

A modification of the RIA called immunoradiometric assay (IRMA) uses a radiolabeled antibody in excess to bind the target molecule.[10] Because IRMAs rely on direct measurements and require fewer steps, they are more precise than RIAs. An important drawback of RIAs and IRMAs is the generation of radioactive waste materials

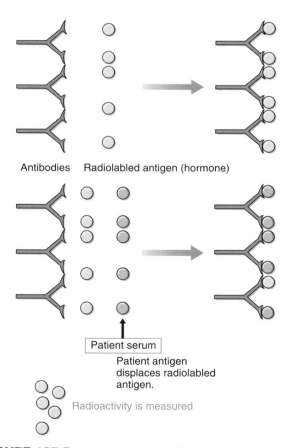

FIGURE 137.5 Radioimmunoassay (RIA). A simple competitive binding assay is the basis for RIA. Antibodies are incubated with a ligand that is a known radiolabeled standard (e.g., a hormone) in the presence of the patient's serum. Any hormone present in the serum will effectively compete for antibody binding sites and displace an equivalent concentration of the standard. Antigen-antibody complexes are removed from the reaction by precipitation or by attaching the antibody to a solid phase. The displaced standard can be quantified by measuring the radioactivity left in solution.

whose handling and disposal are hazardous and costly. Thus, most RIAs and IRMAs will likely be replaced by nonradiometric techniques in the near future.

Enzyme-Linked Immunosorbent Assay

The adaptation of enzyme conjugates that did not alter the binding properties of the antibody led to the development and widespread use of ELISA tests.[12] Horseradish peroxidase (HRP) and alkaline phosphatase (AP) are the two enzymes used most commonly in these conjugates, and various substrates are available for each of these enzymes that can produce reaction products of different colors.[2–4,10,12] These precipitates can be visualized without the aid of instrumentation to obtain qualitative answers. More importantly, they can provide accurate quantitative data when analyzed spectrophotometrically. Both HRP and AP also can catalyze reactions leading to photon emission (light), allowing for the development of chemiluminescent ELISA tests. These tests are several orders of magnitude more sensitive than their spectrophotometric counterparts and are likely to account for most of the test development in the coming years.[12]

ELISAs can be provided as kits with internal standards and controls. The reactions do not use or generate hazardous materials or byproducts, and they are extremely easy to perform. These advantages make them versatile enough to be used as screening tools at the cage-side, or in large-scale commercial laboratories. The principle of the ELISA is similar to that of the IRMA. When there is only one antibody against the antigen available, the antigen (serum) is attached to a solid phase (filter or microtiter plate). The labeled antibody is added to the matrix containing the antigen, followed by the addition of the substrate. The enzyme catalyzes the color (or chemiluminescent) reaction, providing results in a matter of minutes (Fig. 137.6A). If two antibodies with distinct specificities are available against the antigen, a 'capture' or 'sandwich' ELISA can be performed. For this test, the first (unlabeled) antibody is attached to the matrix or microtiter plate. The antigen is allowed to bind to this antibody, followed by the addition of the second (labeled) antibody. The antigen is thus 'captured' by the first antibody and 'sandwiched' between the two antibodies (Fig. 137.6B). The colorimetric or chemiluminescent reaction is then allowed to proceed by the addition of substrate, providing results within minutes. Capture ELISAs add specificity by reducing the likelihood of detecting cross-reactive proteins, as more than one epitope must be recognized in the antigen to generate a positive result. Another modification of the ELISA is a competitive ELISA, whereby a labeled substrate is used (much like a competitive RIA) and the presence of relevant antigens in serum is measured by displacement of the labeled standard.

Immunoblotting (Western Blotting)

Immunoblotting has been a powerful research tool, combining electrophoresis through a gel followed by trans-

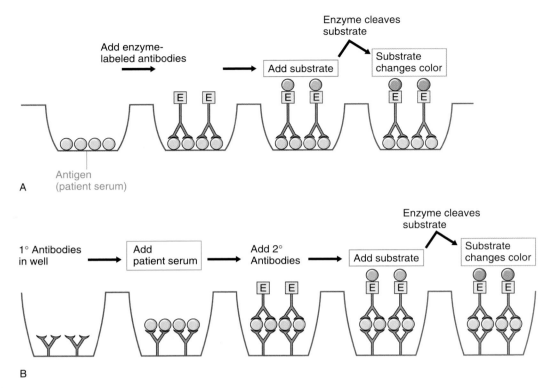

FIGURE 137.6 Enzyme-linked immunosorbent assay. In the standard ELISA (**A**), serum components are allowed to adhere to a surface such as a filter or a multiwell plate. Enzyme-conjugated antibodies are added to the filter or the plate, followed by a substrate. The enzyme catalyzes a reaction that causes a color change in the substrate. The color change can be appreciated visually, or quantified using a spectrophotometer. In the sandwich ELISA (**B**), an antibody is attached to the filter or plate before adding the serum. The unknown samples are then added, and the antigen is 'captured' by the primary antibody. A second, enzyme-conjugated antibody directed against a distinct epitope on that antigen is then added, followed by the substrate. The detection is as for the standard ELISA.

fer of the proteins to a solid matrix and detection of specific protein components by immunochemical reactions.[2–4,13] It is practically an extension of immunofixation and ELISA, and provides many of the advantages of both of these tests. The added electrophoresis step can improve the specificity of the test over ELISA by providing information on the mass (molecular weight) of the target. Although immunoblotting is no more difficult or labor-intensive than IEP or immunofixation, it is substantially more so than ELISAs; thus it remains primarily a tool of research. Its clinical applications are generally confined to confirm other diagnostic tests (e.g., the presence of anti-HIV antibody in humans or anti-FIV antibody in cats that have tested positive by ELISA).

To perform an immunoblot, the proteins are separated electrophoretically through a polyacrylamide gel, followed by electrochemical transfer to a filter made of nitrocellulose or synthetic fibers. Antibodies against specific antigens present in patient serum can be identified by incubating the serum with a blot containing standard antigens (e.g., extracts from an infectious agent such as FIV). This step is followed by a second incubation using a labeled secondary antibody directed against the patient's immunoglobulin for the immunochemical reaction (e.g., anti-cat immunoglobulin). The labeled antibody can be conjugated to a radioisotope (usually ^{125}I)

or an enzyme (HRP or AP). The detection step depends on the label and can include quantification of the radioactive isotope, a colorimetric reaction catalyzed by the enzyme, or a chemiluminescent reaction catalyzed by the enzyme (Fig. 137.7).

Although immunoblotting is not ideally suited for detection of serum components present in small quantities, many clinical applications are under development that use immunoblotting to detect the presence or absence of cellular proteins.[14–21]

CLINICAL APPLICATIONS IN VETERINARY MEDICINE

Immunodiffusion and IEP are useful methods to provide qualitative and quantitative estimates of immunoglobulins present in plasma. These tests were initially used to detect exposure to infectious organisms (based on an antibody responses), as well as to determine the isotypes of serum immunoglobulins in patients with monoclonal gammopathies based on serum protein electrophoresis. Additional applications are limited only by the availability of reagents (species-specific antibodies directed against clinically relevant targets). RID is still a common method to quantify immunoglobulins in vet-

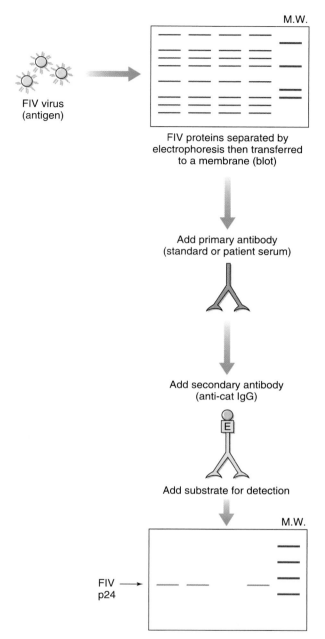

FIGURE 137.7 Immunoblotting. For clinical immunoblotting, antigens (e.g., FIV proteins) are separated by electrophoresis and transferred to a membrane (blot). Known standards (anti-FIV antibodies) and unknowns (patient serum) are added to individual lanes on the blot. Antibodies are allowed to react with antigens immobilized on the blot. An enzyme-conjugated secondary antibody directed against the serum immunoglobulins (e.g., anti-cat IgG) is then added followed by a substrate. The enzyme catalyzes a reaction that causes a color change (or light emission) in the substrate. The reaction can be appreciated visually, or quantified by autoradiography or densitometry.

erinary laboratories. AGID techniques to measure specific immunoglobulins also are used widely, and they include important assays such as the Coggin's test for equine infectious anemia virus (EIAV) and tests to measure titers against other viral and fungal pathogens. RIAs are available to measure steroid hormone and vitamins, but commercially important RIAs such as that used to measure canine thyroid hormone are likely to be replaced by chemiluminescent assays.

ELISA tests are becoming more commonplace and are likely to replace many immunoelectrophoretic and gel immunodiffusion tests soon. An ELISA test to measure EIAV antigen is available and has been shown to be superior to AGID (Coggin's test).[22] The cage-side ELISA tests used to measure FeLV antigen and anti-FIV antibody in cats and heartworm antigen in dogs are among the most commonly used immunoassays in veterinary medicine.[14] A modified ELISA to detect antibodies against *Dirofilaria immitis* in cats (feline heartworm test) has received approval by the USDA recently. ELISA tests also are available to diagnose other infectious diseases, such as Lyme disease and leishmaniasis.[23,24]

The simplicity of ELISA and chemiluminescent immunoassays make the widespread use of immunoblotting in clinical laboratories unlikely, except as a confirmatory test. An important application of immunoblots may be to distinguish natural exposure to microbial antigens from vaccine exposure. In these cases, it is important to demonstrate not only the presence of antibodies against particular organisms but also whether these antibodies were elicited by and react only to the vaccine antigen(s) or to other antigens on the microbe. For example, in one study of canine Lyme disease, serum from dogs with clinical signs of joint disease and positive antibody titers to *Borrelia burgdorferi* had antibodies against outer surface protein A (OspA), OspB, flagellin, and p39 as determined by immunoblotting. Conversely, vaccinated dogs with no clinical signs had antibodies against OspA and OspB, but not against flagellin and p39.[24]

Limitations

The limitations of each of the immunoassays described include availability of reagents and appropriate controls, the expertise required to perform and interpret the tests, and often the associated costs. The rapid progress in this field of clinical laboratory medicine precludes the provision of a complete list of immunoassays that are available in veterinary medicine. The use of the World Wide Web and other similar information media will simplify the search for updated immunoassays. Some useful sites at the time of publication include http://aginfo.snu.ac.kr/www/kvetcom.htm (a compilation of links to companies that manufacture or sell veterinary products) and http://netvet.wustl.edu/vetmed.htm (the World Wide Web Library of Veterinary Medicine, with extensive links to government and private organizations).

ADAPTATIONS OF REAGENTS FOR VETERINARY PATIENTS

The role of the immune system in myriad disease states has provided the impetus to develop diagnostic reagents to detect immunologically important cytokines. Many kits (mostly based on ELISA technology) are available to measure human and murine cytokines. However, in the experience of the authors and others, the usefulness of these kits to measure cytokines in other species has been limited.[25] It is imperative that the specificity and sensitivity of any immunoassay be confirmed using appropriate controls before they are adopted for use by commercial, research, or in-house laboratories.

It also is important to note that kits that work for one species may not necessarily work for other, even closely related species. Some of the cytokines that have been successfully measured in domestic animals using ELISA kits are tumor necrosis factor alpha (TNFα) in cats, horses, cows, and sheep[26–28]; interferon gamma (IFN-γ) in cows[29,30]; interleukin-1 (IL-1) and IL-2 in cows[30,31]; IL-8 in cows and dogs[32,33]; transforming growth factor beta (TGFβ) in dogs[34]; erythropoietin in dogs and cats[35]; and GM-CSF in sheep.[36] The use of polyclonal antibodies to measure cytokines by immunoblotting also has been reported.[17]

REFERENCES

1. **Kohler G, Milstein C.** Continuous cultures of fused cells secreting antibody of predefined specificity. Nature 1975;256:495–497.
2. **Klein J, Horejsi V.** Immunology, 2nd ed. London: Blackwell Science Ltd, 1977;422–441.
3. **Sell S.** Immunology, immunopathology and immunity, 5th ed. Stamford, CT: Appleton & Lange, 1996;108–118.
4. **Tizard IR.** Veterinary immunology, 5th ed. Philadelphia: WB Saunders, 1996;216–236.
5. **Reynolds HY, Johnson JS.** Quantitation of canine immunoglobulins. J Immunol 1970;105:689–703.
6. **Keren DK.** High-resolution electrophoresis and immunofixation, 2nd ed. Boston: Butterworth-Heinemann, 1994;171–209.
7. **Westermeier R.** Electrophoresis in practice, 2nd ed. Weinheim: VCH, 1997;13–15.
8. **Walravens MJ, Vanherrewegen H, Lacquet F, Godefridis G, Korevits G, Stevens E, Marien G, Molenberghs G.** Counterimmunoelectrophoresis with serum prediffusion: An improved method for the detection and identification of antibodies against extractable nuclear and cytoplasmic antigens. J Immunol Methods 1997;201:89–98.
9. **Yallow RS, Berson SA.** Immunoassay of endogenous plasma insulin in man. J Clin Invest 1960;39:1157–1175.
10. **Bennett BD, Wells DJ.** Endocrinology. In: Bishop ML, Duben-Engelkirk JL, Fody EP, eds. Clinical chemistry: Principles, procedures, correlations, 2nd ed. Philadelphia: JB Lippincott, 1992;319–352.
11. **Bittikofer JA.** Therapeutic drug monitoring. In: Bishop ML, Duben-Engelkirk JL, Fody EP, eds. Clinical chemistry: Principles, procedures, correlations, 2nd ed. Philadelphia: JB Lippincott, 1992;577–598.
12. **Gosling JP.** Enzyme immunoassay. In: Diamands EP and Christopoulos TK, eds. Immunoassay. San Diego: Academic Press, 1996;287–308.
13. **Renart J, Behrens MM, Fernandez-Renart M, Martinez JL.** Immunoblotting techniques. In: Diamands EP and Christopoulous TK, eds. Immunoassay. San Diego: Academic Press, 1996;537–554.
14. **Barr MC.** FIV, FeLV, and FIPV: Interpretation and misinterpretation of serological test results. Semin Vet Med Surg 1996;11:144–153.
15. **Cobb MA, Odedra R, Latif N, Dunn MJ.** Use of indirect immunofluorescence and Western blotting to assess the role of circulating antimyocardial antibodies in dogs with dilated cardiomyopathy. Res Vet Sci 1994;56:245–251.
16. **Cooley WA, Clark JK, Stack MJ.** Comparison of scrapie-associated fibril detection and Western immunoblotting for the diagnosis of natural ovine scrapie. J Comp Pathol 1998;118:41–49.
17. **Helfand SC, Modiano JF, Moore PF, Soergel SA, MacWilliams PS, Dubielzig RD, Hank JA, Gelfand EW, Sondel PM.** Functional interleukin-2 receptors are expressed on natural killer-like leukemic cells from a dog with cutaneous lymphoma. Blood 1995;86:636–645.
18. **Iqbal Z, Chaichanasiriwithaya W, Rikihisa Y.** Comparison of PCR with other tests for early diagnosis of canine ehrlichiosis. J Clin Microbiol 1994;32:1658–1662.
19. **Katz JB, Pedersen JC, Jenny AL, Taylor WD.** Assessment of Western immunoblotting for the confirmatory diagnosis of ovine scrapie and bovine spongiform encephalopathy (BSE). J Vet Diagn Invest 1992;4:447–449.
20. **McVey DS, Shuman WS.** Detection of antiplatelet immunoglobulin in thrombocytopenic dogs. Vet Immunol Immunopathol 1989;22:101–111.
21. **Peavy GM, Holland CJ, Dutta SK, Smith G, Moore A, Rich LJ, Lappin MR, Richter K.** Suspected ehrlichial infection in five cats from a household. JAVMA 1997;210:231–234.
22. **Lew AM, Thomas LM, Huntington PJ.** A comparison of ELISA, FAST-ELISA and gel diffusion tests for detecting antibody to equine infectious anaemia virus. Vet Microbiol 1993;34:1–5.
23. **Aisa MJ, Castillejo S, Gallego M, Fisa R, Riera MC, de Colmenares M, Torras S, Roura X, Sentis J, Portus M.** Diagnostic potential of Western blot analysis of sera from dogs with leishmaniasis in endemic areas and significance of the pattern. Am J Trop Med Hygiene 1998;58:154–159.
24. **Barthold SW, Levy SA, Fikrig E, Bockenstedt LK, Smith AL.** Serologic responses of dogs naturally exposed to or vaccinated against Borrelia burgdorferi infection. JAVMA 1995;207:1435–1440.
25. **Ahne W, Mayr A, Wiesner H.** Immunoreactive cytokines within primates. Zentralblatt Fur Veterinarmedizin 1996;43:607–611.
26. **Ellis JA, Godson D, Campos M, Sileghem M, Babiuk LA.** Capture immunoassay for ruminant tumor necrosis factor-alpha: Comparison with bioassay. Vet Immunol Immunopathol 1993;35:289–300.
27. **Lehmann R, Joller H, Haagmans BL, Lutz H.** Tumor necrosis factor alpha levels in cats experimentally infected with feline immunodeficiency virus: Effects of immunization and feline leukemia virus infection. Vet Immunol Immunopathol 1992;35:61–69.
28. **Su X, Morris DD, Crowe NA, Moore JN, Fischer KJ, McGraw RA.** Equine tumor necrosis factor alpha: Cloning and expression in Escherichia coli, generation of monoclonal antibodies, and development of a sensitive enzyme-linked immunosorbent assay. Hybridoma 1992;11:715–727.
29. **Billman-Jacobe H, Carrigan M, Cockram F, Corner LA, Gill IJ, Hill JF, Jessep T, Milner AR, Wood PR.** A comparison of the interferon gamma assay with the absorbed ELISA for the diagnosis of Johne's disease in cattle. Australian Vet 1992;69:25–28.
30. **Ng KH, Aldwell FE, Wedlock DN, Watson JD, Buddle BM.** Antigen-induced interferon-gamma and interleukin-2 responses of cattle inoculated with Mycobacterium bovis. Vet Immunol Immunopathol 1997;57:59–68.
31. **Goto M, Maruyama M, Kitadate K, Kirisawa R, Obata Y, Koiwa M, Iwai H.** Detection of interleukin-1 beta in sera and colostrum of dairy cattle and in sera of neonates. J Vet Med Sci 1997;59:437–441.
32. **Caswell JL, Middleton DM, Sorden SD, Gordon JR.** Expression of the neutrophil chemoattractant interleukin-8 in the lesions of bovine pneumonic pasteurellosis. Vet Pathol 1998;35:124–131.
33. **Mohamed A, Matsumoto Y, Yoshihara K, Watari T, Tsujimoto H, Hasegawa A, Onodera T, Hirota Y.** Establishment of a sandwich enzyme linked immunosorbent assay for canine interleukin-8. J Vet Med Sci 1997;59:39–41.
34. **Skaleric U, Kramar B, Petelin M, Pavlica Z, Wahl SM.** Changes in TGF-beta 1 levels in gingiva, crevicular fluid and serum associated with periodontal inflammation in humans and dogs. Eur J Oral Sci 1997;105:136–142.
35. **Pechereau D, Martel P, Braun JP.** Plasma erythropoietin concentrations in dogs and cats: Reference values and changes with anaemia and/or chronic renal failure. Res Vet Sci 1997;62:185–188.
36. **Entrican G, Deane D, MacLean M, Inglis L, Thomson J, McInnes C, Haig DM.** Development of a sandwich ELISA for ovine granulocyte/macrophage colony-stimulating factor. Vet Immunol Immunopathol 1996;50:105–115.

CHAPTER 138

Cerebrospinal Proteins

• JOAN R. COATES

Isolated evaluation of cerebrospinal fluid (CSF) protein is considered a poor tool for diagnosis of central nervous system (CNS) disorders; however, as an adjunct to clinical and laboratory data it provides information to support or refute a diagnosis of neurologic disease. Evaluation of CSF protein composition provides an in-depth approach toward the understanding of neurologic disorders. In addition, refined laboratory techniques may suggest other diagnostic and therapeutic options. Previous comprehensive literature reviews of humans[1-4] and domestic animals[5-11] have contributed to our understanding in the evolution of CSF protein evaluation.

SOURCES OF CSF PROTEIN

CSF protein is ultimately derived from plasma by ultra-filtration and secretory processes of the choroid plexus and active transport of compounds across the blood-brain barrier (BBB).[1] Approximately 80% of CSF protein is serum-derived. Serum proteins are largely excluded from CSF by the blood-CSF barrier, which consists of the interepithelial tight junctions of the choroid plexus and arachnoid mater.[12] Permeability of larger protein molecules into the brain parenchyma is determined by integrity of capillary endothelial tight junctions. Secondary lysosomes, known as the 'enzymatic barrier,' also contribute to the endothelial BBB and epithelial blood-CSF barriers.[12] Protein transport is bidirectional across the epithelial cells of the choroid plexus by transcytosis or by carrier-mediated mechanisms. Four properties govern concentration of serum proteins in the CSF: molecular radius, electrical charge, plasma concentration, and functional state of the blood-CSF barrier.[1] The most important determinant for protein transport from plasma into the CNS and CSF is the hydrodynamic radius of the protein molecule, not its molecular weight.[13] Proteins egress from the CNS into the venous sinus circulation via the arachnoid villi.

Although protein composition is primarily maintained by BBB function, the choroid plexus has a major role in de novo protein synthesis. Prealbumin, transferrin, and ceruloplasmin are synthesized by the brain and the choroid plexus epithelium.[14,15] Prealbumin (transthyretin) is also produced by the liver and functions as a carrier protein for thyroxine and vitamin A or retinol.[3] CSF transferrin consists of two isoforms that originate from CSF and serum.[3] The CSF isoform is produced by cerebral neuramidase modification of serum transferrin and represents a carbohydrate-deficient moiety of transferrin (tau protein, tau fraction). CSF transferrin is not present in serum or external secretions, making it useful as a means to detect CSF leakage in human patients (i.e., otorrhea and rhinorrhea).[16] Transferrin mRNA in the choroid plexus is species-specific. Large proportions of transferrin mRNA in total RNA have been demonstrated only in rats; smaller proportions were demonstrated in total RNA of mice, dogs, and rabbits.[17]

CNS-specific proteins, characterized by higher ratios in CSF than in plasma, constitute 1 to 2% of the total protein in normal CSF.[18] Such CSF-specific proteins include β_2-microglobulin, glial fibrillary acidic protein, myelin basic protein, P_2 protein, C-reactive protein, S-100 protein, neuron-specific enolase, and β- and γ-trace proteins.[3] Other CNS-specific proteins are released into the CSF in disease states. In humans, these proteins are utilized as markers or indicators for discriminating between infectious and noninfectious CNS inflammatory disorders and neoplasms.[3,4,18-20] Myelin basic protein and P_2 protein aid in evaluation of demyelinating diseases and CNS damage.[3,4] Myelin basic protein has been detected in the CSF of dogs affected with demyelinating canine distemper encephalomyelitis.[21] The significance of these CSF-specific proteins in domestic animals during normal and disease states remains to be determined.

METHODS FOR CSF TOTAL PROTEIN DETERMINATION

Several qualitative techniques assess excessive protein amounts in CSF. Nonspecific methods for determining excess in total protein in CSF are the foam test and urinary reagent strips. The foam test is performed by agitating the CSF sample; a positive test is the presence of foam remaining for 5 minutes or longer.[7] Urinary reagent strips ('dipstick' method) measure only the albumin content based on pH change of indicator dye (tetrabromol). Results are reliable below 30 mg/dL and above 100 mg/dL, but concentrations between 30 and 60 mg/dL may be read as negative.[22] Crude screening tests for globulins are the Nonne-Apelt (Ross-Jones) and Pandy's tests.[7,8] The Nonne-Apelt test involves the addition of CSF to an ammonium sulfate solution. The presence of globulin is detected by visual presence of a white to gray ring at the interface between the solution and CSF. Pandy's test is performed by mixing CSF and carbolic acid solution. Development of turbidity indicates the presence of globulin (graded 0–4).

Clinical laboratories quantify CSF total protein concentrations by utilizing turbidimetric, colorimetric, protein-dye binding, and automated assays.[2,3] Accurate interpretation requires understanding several principles: protein content in CSF is much lower as compared with serum; reagent reactions vary with different proteins (albumin and globulin); smaller quantities of CSF are available; and disparity exists between assay techniques.[3] Turbidimetric assays apply chemical precipitation techniques with trichloroacetic acid and sulfosalicylic acid reagents. Although relatively easy to perform, accurate protein determination is dependent on the albumin:globulin ratio (albumin produces four times more turbidity than does globulin) and ambient temperature.[23] Common colorimetric assays are referenced to the Lowry method.[24] Sensitivity is affected little by the albumin:globulin ratio; however, the assay is more labor-intensive. Protein-dye binding assays[25] using Coomassie Brilliant Blue G-250 are less time-consuming and require smaller amounts of CSF (25–100 μL). Automated techniques such as dry-slide methodology (*Vitros PROT Slide*) have become popular for colorimetric, quantitative measurements of CSF protein concentration and show similar results when compared with previously described reference methods.[26] Cerebrospinal fluid protein values in domestic animals must be interpreted in the context of species-specific reference values for that particular laboratory method.

TOTAL PROTEIN CONCENTRATION IN NORMAL CSF

Normal CSF total protein concentrations have been established for most domestic animal species (Table 138.1). Any value must be interpreted in light of age and sampling site variables. Gradients exist in the CNS for CSF protein content along the neuraxis.[27] Cerebellomedullary cisternal and ventricular fluids have lower protein concentrations than lumbar fluid. Caudorostral gradients of CSF protein concentration have been determined in dogs,[28–30] cats,[31] horses,[32–34] and humans.[4] Protein concentration in the lumbar region is higher because of slower fluid flow with relation to distance from the cranial fluid source and greater blood-CSF barrier permeability to proteins in the lumbar region.[27] Protein additions from adjacent nervous tissue also contribute to total protein content variations along the neuraxis. Albumin permeates the blood-CSF barrier at multiple sites along the neuraxis.[35] Globulin concentrations increase along the neuraxis.[4] Prealbumin concentration is decreased in lumbar fluid in comparison with cerebellomedullary cisternal fluid.[27] This change, in part, is due to its origination from the ventricular region and diffusion into nervous tissue across the linings of the subarachnoid space.

CSF protein concentrations and composition vary in young animals, probably as a result of increased permeability and immaturity of the blood-CSF barrier. Puppies at 4 weeks of age when compared at 10 weeks of age had significantly higher protein concentrations.[36] Studies describe age-related changes in protein composition in equine CSF.[37–39] Protein values of neonatal foals are initially elevated but approach adult reference values by 3 weeks of age.[37] High protein concentrations in CSF from the developing brain have been found in different species; the highest concentration appearing in the early stage of brain development, relates to the phase of brain maturation and not to the time of birth.[17,40,41]

Neurotransmitter metabolites have been evaluated in normal domestic animal species. Concentrations of dopamine (dihydroxyphenylacetic acid [DOPAC], homovanillic acid [HVA]) and serotonin metabolites (5-hydroxyindoleacetic acid [5-HIAA]) have been determined in dogs,[42] horses,[43] and cattle.[44] Gradients for neurotransmitter metabolites have been determined in the dog and horse. Rostrocaudal gradients (higher concentrations in the cerebellomedullary cistern site) exist for metabolites of serotonin (5-HIAA), DOPAC, and HVA in the dog.[29] Likewise, similar gradients have been established in the horse for 5-HIAA and HVA.[33]

Enzymes in CSF originate from neural tissue, serum, or cellular constituents.[4] Lactate dehydrogenase isoenzyme and creatine kinase activities have been evaluated in domestic animals. Enzyme activities have been assayed in the CSF of dogs,[45,46] cats,[47] horses,[32,39] cattle,[48] and llamas.[49] Creatine kinase activity in the CSF of horses with various neurologic disorders showed no association between the CSF red blood cell (RBC) count, CSF-nucleated cell count, CSF protein concentration, or serum creatine kinase activity and was determined to be an unreliable diagnostic indicator of disease.[50] However, one study in dogs with neurologic disease detected correlations between increased CSF creatine kinase activities and a poor disease prognosis.[51] Blood and epidural fat contamination have been implicated to cause falsely increased creatine kinase activity.[50,52] In conclusion, enzyme assay results in neurologic disorders are not sensitive or specific enough to warrant routine use in clinical practice.

CSF TOTAL PROTEIN IN DISEASE

Alterations in CSF protein concentrations are the most common and least specific of CSF alterations in disease and indicate presence of organic disease in the CNS or its membranes.[19] CSF pleocytosis and elevated protein

TABLE 138.1   Cerebrospinal Fluid Total Protein Concentration (mg/dL) in Reference to Species and Methodology

Dog	27 ± 4.2^a (23–35)[b] Sorjonen, 1987 Coomassie brilliant blue	29.9 ± 1.57 (23–38.5) Sorjonen, 1981 Micro-Lowry	CM 13.97 ± 4.54 (3–23) LS 28.68 ± 5.52 (18–44) Bailey, 1985 Coomassie brilliant blue	27.6 ± 1.1SE (15.5–42) Krakowka, 1981	27.5 (11–55) Fankhauser
Cat	18 ± 7 (6–36) Rand, 1990 Ponceau S	CM 27.0 ± 8.8 LS 44.0 ± 1.7 Hochwald, 1969 Biuret			
Horse	4–9 years CM 87 ± 17.0 (59–118) LS 93 ± 16 (65–124) Andrews, 1990 Coomassie brilliant blue	<10 days CM 82.8 ± 19.2 (56.7–115) LS 83.6 ± 16.1 (60.5–116) Andrews, 1994 Coomassie brilliant blue	<40 hours CM 138 ± 50 (70–210) Rossdale, 1982 Biuret	Adult CM 105 ± 38 (40–170) Rossdale, 1982 Biuret	0.75–15 years CM 37.23 ± 28.4 (5–100) Mayhew, 1977
Cow	LS 39.16 ± 3.39 (23.6–66.3) Welles, 1992 Coomassie brilliant blue				
Sheep	CM 27 ± 1SE Dziegielewska, 1980 Lowry				
Pig	CM 31 ± 3 Cavanagh, 1982 Lowry				
Llama	LS 43.1 ± 9.0 (31.2–66.8) Welles, 1994 Coomassie brilliant blue				

[a] Data are expressed as mean $\pm$ standard deviation.
[b] Data in parentheses indicate minimum-maximum values.

concentrations commonly coexist. Elevated protein concentrations without pleocytosis is referred to as protein-cytologic (albuminocytologic) dissociation. This condition occurs in viral infections and compressive and neoplastic processes.[9,53,54] Extreme protein elevation accompanied by entry of fibrinogen and clot formation is known as Froin's syndrome. Cerebrospinal fluid coagulation can be associated with inflammatory diseases, neoplasia, trauma, and CNS hemorrhage.[3] The highest CSF protein concentrations in dogs have been observed in purulent inflammatory diseases[55] and neoplasia.[53] Similarities exist for cattle,[56] horses,[10] and sheep.[57] Pathologic causes for CSF protein elevation include increased permeability of the blood-CSF barrier, decreased removal of protein via the arachnoid villi, obstruction of CSF circulation, and intrathecal synthesis of immunoglobulins.[53]

Increased protein concentration during CNS inflammation occurs from disruption of tight junctions between endothelial cells of venules and, to a lesser extent, meningeal or parenchymal vessels.[58] Additionally, any increase in cellular constituents or cellular disintegration will result in protein concentration elevation. Inflammation near the meninges or surface of the CNS is more likely to have marked CSF protein alterations than deep-seated parenchymal lesions. Inflammatory diseases in dogs commonly associated with elevated CSF protein concentrations include inflammatory canine distemper, other viral encephalitides, protozoal encephalitis, granulomatous meningoencephalomyelitis (GME), and steroid-responsive meningoencephalitis.[59] Elevated protein concentrations were determined in 71% of dogs with CNS inflammatory disease, and the highest values (>300 mg/dL) were determined for steroid-responsive meningitis-arteritis. Elevated protein concentrations in cats with inflammatory disease are most severe (200 mg/dL) in feline infectious peritonitis infections.[57] Infectious inflammatory disorders and parasitic diseases were common causes for severe CSF protein elevations in sheep,[60] cattle,[56] and horses.[10]

Blockage of spinal fluid pathways by focal disease processes may increase permeability and decrease absorption of proteins.[3] Focal destruction of nervous tissue causes secondary edema, ischemia, and necrosis that cause release of neural protein and transudation of serum proteins into the spinal fluid. CSF protein concentrations were highest in dogs with acute and severe compressive spinal cord lesions.[54] Cerebrospinal fluid alterations of dogs with intervertebral disc disease were identified in 85% of lumbar samples compared with 37% of cerebellomedullary cisternal samples (same dogs).[61] Increased protein concentration in lumbar CSF is most likely related to the predominant caudal flow of CSF from the brain to the terminal spinal cord. CSF total protein concentrations were not significantly elevated in horses with compressive spinal cord disease.[62]

CSF protein elevations from neoplastic processes occur as a result of tissue necrosis, focal blood-CSF barrier disruption, or local production of immunoglobulins. Secondary edema of nervous tissue and meninges causes protein transudation from perineural spaces into the spinal fluid. Both cerebellomedullary cisternal and lumbar CSF samples showed changes in protein concentration in dogs with intracranial disease.[54] The most common CSF abnormality in dogs with brain tumors was an increase in total protein content.[63] Choroid plexus papilloma had the highest mean total protein concentrations.[53]

CSF protein concentrations may be falsely elevated from blood contamination following subarachnoid hemorrhage or traumatic collection. Iatrogenic blood contamination of CSF samples usually occurs from puncture of meningeal or associated vertebral and spinal cord vessels. Problems with blood contamination are more frequently encountered in lumbar puncture than in cerebellomedullary cisternal puncture.[28,54] Correction factors accommodate for the effects of blood contamination on protein concentration and include the subtraction of 1 mg/dL protein from the total protein concentration per 700 RBCs in humans,[4] per 500 RBCs in dogs,[28] and per 100 RBCs in cats.[52] A formula[64] to more accurately represent the effects of blood contamination is as follows:

$$[\text{protein}]_{\text{corrected}} = [\text{protein}]_{\text{CSF}} - \frac{[\text{protein}]_{\text{blood}} \times \text{RBC}_{\text{CSF}}}{\text{RBC}_{\text{blood}}}$$

However, studies in clinically normal dogs and dogs confirmed with neurologic disease showed that low-level RBC contamination (RBC count $\leq 13,200/\mu\text{L}$) does not significantly alter CSF-nucleated cell count or protein concentration.[64,65] Furthermore, these correction formulas were shown to be unreliable.[64] Increased CSF white blood cell and protein concentrations is indicative of CNS disease even with moderate blood contamination.

Concentrations of neurotransmitter metabolites have been evaluated in neurologic disorders of domestic animals. Dopamine (HVA) and serotonin metabolites (5-HIAA) were evaluated in 12 Collie dogs administered ivermectin. Elevated CSF concentrations of both metabolites suggested an association between altered neurotransmission and the neurologic status in two dogs with ivermectin toxicosis.[66] γ-Aminobutyric acid, a major inhibitory neurotransmitter in the CNS and glutamate, an excitatory amino neurotransmitter in the brain have been clinically evaluated in epileptic dogs. Low γ-aminobutyric acid and high glutamate concentrations were determined in the CSF of epileptic dogs.[67,68] In addition, γ-aminobutyric acid and glutamate concentrations in CSF may serve as important markers for evaluating response to antiepileptic drugs.[67] Neurotransmitter metabolites also have been evaluated in the CSF of normal and narcoleptic dogs and horses.[69-71]

Decreased CSF protein concentrations are not commonly encountered. Potential causes documented in humans include removal of excessive quantities of CSF; CSF leakage from a dural tear secondary to trauma; benign intracranial hypertension; acute water intoxication associated with increased intracranial pressure; and hyperthyroidism (mechanism unknown).[2]

CSF PROTEIN FRACTIONATION

CSF protein composition can be further defined by semiquantitative electrophoretic techniques. Spinal fluid proteins are readily separated into specified zones by electrophoresis using paper, cellulose acetate, agarose, and polyacrylamide gel matrices on the basis of electrical charge and mobility.[3] Polyacrylamide gel and high-resolution electrophoresis on agarose gel offer more precise definition of protein composition, especially of the γ-globulin fraction.[72,73] High-resolution protein electrophoresis on agarose gel has been utilized for evaluation of equine CSF.[62] Polyacrylamide gel electrophoresis has higher resolution capacity than does agarose gel but gives electrophoretic patterns that are more difficult to interpret.[74] Isoelectric focusing, as another protein-separation method, involves separation of protein constituents on the basis of the isoelectric points via a pH gradient in the medium.[75,76] Although high-resolution protein electrophoresis on agarose may be the more conventional method, isoelectric focusing combined with silver staining techniques has the additional advantage of requiring smaller quantities of *unconcentrated* CSF.[77] Clinical utility of isoelectric focusing has increased the sensitivity of pattern definition in abnormal CSF samples.[78] More than 300 different proteins have been detected in the CSF of human patients by electrophoretic techniques.[3]

Zone electrophoresis was first developed as a clinical method by Kabat.[79] Major electrophoretic zones include prealbumin, albumin, α_1, α_2, β-, and γ-globulins.[4,11] Prealbumin (transthyretin) constitutes 5% of the total CSF protein. Albumin is considered the major band on CSF protein electrophoresis. The α_1-band primarily consists of α_1-antitrypsin. The α_2-region is not a dominant fraction because of relative decreases in large serum proteins such as α_2-macroglobulin and haptoglobin in normal

CSF. β-Globulins include two major components: transferrin and complement (C3). Other constituents of the β-fraction include β-lipoprotein, tau protein (modified transferrin), plasminogen, hemopexin, and β-trace protein. Serum-derived transferrin is detected within the β_1-region, and the modified CSF transferrin isoform migrates more cathodal in the β_2-region (τ region). γ-Globulins include the immunoglobulins and γ-trace protein. Electrophoretic patterns have been defined in normal dogs,[30,80] cats,[52] horses,[62,81,82] cattle,[48] and llamas[49] (Table 138.2).

Characterizations of Electrophoretic Patterns in CSF Dysproteinemia

Four patterns observed by electrophoretic techniques and used to classify CSF include intrathecal immunoglobulin production (increased IgG), intrathecal immunoglobulin production combined with BBB disturbance (increased IgG and albumin), BBB disturbance (increased albumin), and unaltered CSF.[30] Electrophoretic patterns in neurologic disorders of domestic animals have been described for dogs and horses. Dogs with spinal cord compression had a relative increase in the albumin fraction and cathodal dispersion of the α-globulin zone with relative decrease in the β- and γ-globulin fractions.[30] Furr described similar findings in horses and the additional presence of post-β peaks (τ-fraction).[62] Canine distemper viral (CDV) infections were electrophoretically characterized by a transient increase in CSF albumin concentration and a sustained increase in CSF γ-globulin concentration. Increases of γ-globulin concentration were more suggestive of the leukoencephalomyelopathy form of CDV.[62,83,84] Dogs with GME had increases in total albumin and in β- and γ-globulin zones resulting in β-γ bridging.[84] The electrophoretic pattern in dogs with neoplasms revealed an increase in the albumin, and α-, and β-globulin zones.[84] An increase in the γ-globulin zone was observed in neoplasms producing γ-globulins.[84]

Further qualitative evaluation of the γ-globulin zone using higher resolution electrophoretic techniques in humans has revealed discrete patterns of protein bands: monoclonal, polyclonal, and oligoclonal.[3,4] Oligoclonal IgG bands unique to CSF (not detectable on serum electrophoresis) provide additional evidence of an immune response within the CNS.[2,85] Although explanations are unclear, the presence of these bands may be the result of activation of certain clones of B lymphocytes and synthesis of specific populations of IgG. Oligoclonal bands are described in a variety of acute and chronic infections and noninfectious neurologic disorders; therefore, these findings lack specificity.[86,87] In humans, demonstration of oligoclonal bands is considered the single most reliable laboratory method for diagnosis of multiple sclerosis.[72,73]

CSF Albumin/Albumin Index

Albumin is the main protein constituent in CSF, comprising 50 to 70% of the total CSF proteins. Quantitative

techniques for albumin determination in CSF mainly applied to domestic animals include immunoelectrophoresis and agarose gel electrophoresis.[30,74,80,88] Because CSF albumin is serum-derived, determination of CSF albumin content may provide additional information when compared with determination of CSF total protein regarding the presence of BBB disruption.[89,90] The CSF/serum albumin ratio or quota is the most reliable variable to assess blood-CSF barrier integrity.[91]

CSF/serum albumin ratio

$$= \frac{\text{total protein}_{CSF}\,(\text{mg}/\text{dL}) \times \text{albumin}_{CSF}\,(\%)}{\text{Albumin}_{serum}\,(\text{g}/\text{dL}) \times 10}$$

$$= \frac{\text{Albumin}_{CSF}\,(\text{mg}/\text{dL})}{\text{Albumin}_{serum}\,(\text{g}/\text{dL}) \times 10}$$

Normal CSF/serum albumin ratio has been determined for the dog, horse, pig, and llama (Table 138.2). Serum albumin alterations may influence the overall increase in CSF albumin; however, the CSF/serum albumin ratio corrects for reduced serum albumin in patients with neurologic disease.[89] Albumin ratio is influenced by age and in humans is highest in neonates and in adults older than 40 years of age.[89] The albumin ratio was higher in neonatal foals than in adult horses.[38]

Increased ratios in dogs occur in traumatic collection procedures and in conditions associated with increased blood-CSF barrier permeability.[30,89,90] Dogs with compressive spinal cord disease had varying degrees of BBB disturbance, with mild to severe increases in the albumin ratio.[30,92] BBB disturbance with a marked to severe increase of the albumin quota was the predominate pattern in dogs with brain neoplasia.[92] Tumors located in proximity to the ventricular system or highly malignant tumors are more likely to produce evidence of BBB dysfunction. The albumin ratio varied in dogs with CDV infections.[84,92] BBB disturbance indicating severe endothelial damage was the predominant pattern in CSF of dogs with acute or subacute CDV infection. Increases in the albumin ratio and CSF albumin were greatest in dogs with GME.[92]

Immunoglobulins/IgG Index

Immunoglobulin levels in CSF are minimal and do not enter via the choroid plexus, in contrast to other proteins.[93] Increased CSF immunoglobulin values occur with BBB disturbance or local antibody synthesis.[85,91] During various CNS disorders, plasma cells and T lymphocytes locally synthesize immunoglobulins. Electrophoresis identifies γ-globulins as a heterogenous group that migrate in the 'γ' electrophoretic region. The major immunoglobulins (IgG, IgA, IgM, IgD, and IgE) in domestic animals are identified by immunochemical techniques such as rocket immunoelectrophoresis,[90] immunodiffusion,[88] single radial immunodiffusion[83,88] and enzyme-linked immunoadsorbent assay (ELISA).[94] IgG is considered the predominant CSF immunoglobulin. Concentrations of γ-globulin components have been evaluated in dogs.[49,88,90]

TABLE 138.2   Protein Constituents in the Cerebrospinal Fluid of Domestic Animals

	Dog-CM[30,88,93]	Cat-CM[47]	Horse (Adult)[34,81]		Foal (<10 Days)[38]		Cow-LS[48]	Pig[41]	Llama-LS[49]
CSF albumin mg/dL	37 ± 4.29 (31–44)	11 ± 15 (1–53)	CM	35.8 ± 9.7 (24.1–50.9)	CM	52.0 ± 8.6 (34–64)	15.747 ± 1.531SE (8.213–28.708)	13.0 ± 0.2SE	17.9 ± 4.45 (11.8–27.1)
			LS	37.8 ± 11.2 (24.4–56.4)	LS	53.8 ± 15.7 (37–92)			
Albumin quota	0.22 ± 0.05 (0.17–0.3)		CM	1.4 ± 0.4 (1.05–2.12)	CM	1.86 ± 0.29 (1.55–2.33)		0.23 ± 0.04SE	0.523 ± 0.114 (0.38–0.75)
			LS	1.5 ± 0.40 (0.92–2.35)	LS	1.85 ± 0.51 (1.39–2.88)			
α-Globulin %	28 ± 5.31 (24–31)	21 ± 11 (0–48)	α_1 LS	5.2 ± 0.9SE (2–11)			14.763 ± 1.108SE (9.775–24.332)		5.9 ± 1.45 (3.1–9.0)
			α_2 LS	6.7 ± 0.4SE (5–8)					
β-Globulin %	5 ± 5.31 (19–30)	57 ± 15 (37–91)	LS	5.8 ± 0.6SE (4–8)			3.789 ± 0.450SE (1.875–8.850)		12.5 ± 1.98 (9.4–16.8)
γ-Globulin %	7.75 ± 1.84 (6–9)	12 ± 7 (0–29)	LS	5.7 ± 0.8SE (3–9)			4.836 ± 0.442SE (2.457–8.850)		6.4 ± 2.5 (3.4–13.8)
CSF IgG mg/dL	17.45 ± 0.83 (14.0–21.1)	1.4 ± 1.7 (0–5.3)	CM	5.6 ± 1.4 (3.0–8.0)	CM	10.2 ± 5.5 (3.0–22)			
			LS	6.02 ± 2.1 (3.00–10.50)	LS	9.9 ± 5.7 (3.0–22.5)			
IgG index	0.38 ± 0.24 (0.15–0.9)	IgG-TP index 0.321 ± 0.210 (0.086–1.297)	CM	0.194 ± 0.046 (0.125–0.239)	CM	0.52 ± 0.28 (0.14–0.942)			
			LS	0.194 ± .05 (0.12–0.262)	LS	0.48 ± 0.27 (0.26–2.09)			
CSF IgM µg/mL	1.7 (0–5.8)								
CSF IgA µg/mL	0.08 (0–0.2)								

Data are expressed as mean ± std. dev.; Data in parentheses indicate min-max values; SE = standard error of mean; CM = cerebellomedullary cistern; LS = lumbosacral region.

The CSF/serum IgG ratio or CSF/serum IgG index has been suggested as an indicator of intrathecal IgG synthesis. The CSF/serum IgG ratio is less well-established. Because the ratio reflects both synthesis of IgG in the CNS and blood-CSF permeability, dual consideration of the IgG ratio and the albumin ratio (IgG index) is necessary to determine whether increased IgG concentrations are the result of intrathecal synthesis, BBB disruption, or both.[89] Albumin is a quantitative marker for blood-CSF barrier permeability and corrects for leakage of serum IgG into the CNS by incorporating a series of constants into the equation (CSF IgG index). The CSF IgG index is calculated using the quotient of the CSF/serum IgG ratio and the CSF/serum albumin ratio.[89] The equation factors out all sources of CSF IgG except de novo synthesis. Normal values for the CSF IgG index have been determined for dogs, cats, and horses (Table 138.2).

$$\text{CSF IgG index} = \frac{\text{IgG ratio}}{\text{Albumin ratio}} \quad \frac{\text{IgG}_{CSF}/\text{IgG}_{serum}}{\text{Alb}_{CSF}/\text{Alb}_{serum} \times 10}$$

The IgG index has been evaluated in neuroinflammatory disorders in dogs.[94–96] Intrathecal IgG synthesis was demonstrated in cases with chronic CDV, GME, steroid-responsive meningitis, and nonsuppurative encephalitis. Chronic CDV infections had the highest increases in the IgG index.

IgM and IgA indices are calculated in a similar manner. Intrathecal synthesis is most likely the source of excess IgA and IgM in CSF under normal or neuroinflammatory conditions.[97] In humans, IgA predominated in purulent meningitis and neurotuberculosis, and IgM predominated in tick-borne meningoencephalitis.[13] Diagnostic significance was independent of the disease stage, suggesting compartmental IgM and IgA response within the CNS. Significance of IgM and IgA in disease has been evaluated in dogs. Intrathecal IgM and IgA production were determined in dogs with distemper encephalitis, GME, and steroid-responsive meningitis.[95] High IgA concentrations in the CSF were more suggestive of steroid-responsive meningitis-arteritis than of other inflammatory disorders.[96,98]

REFERENCES

1. **Davson H, Welch K, Segal MB.** The proteins and other macromolecules of the CSF. In: H Davson, K Welch, MB Segal, eds. Physiology and pathophysiology of the cerebrospinal fluid. New York: Churchill Livingstone, 1987; 583–622.
2. **Krieg AF, Kjeldsberg CR.** Cerebrospinal fluid and other body fluids. In: JB Henry, ed. Clinical and diagnostic management: By laboratory methods, 18th ed. Philadelphia: WB Saunders, 1991;445–474.
3. **Kjeldsberg CR, Knight JA.** Cerebrospinal fluid. In: CR Kjeldsberg CR and JA Knight, eds. Body fluids: Laboratory examination of amniotic, cerebrospinal, seminal, serous and synovial fluids, 3rd ed. Hong Kong: American Society of Clinical Pathologists, 1993;65–157.
4. **Fishman RA.** Cerebrospinal fluid in diseases of the nervous system, 2nd ed. Philadelphia: WB Saunders, 1992.
5. **Fankhauser R.** The cerebrospinal fluid. In: JRM Innes and LZ Saunders, eds. Comparative neuropathology. New York: Academic Press, 1962;21–54.
6. **Feldman BF.** Cerebrospinal fluid. In: JJ Kaneko, ed. Clinical biochemistry of domestic animals, 4th ed. San Diego: Academic Press, 1989;835–865.
7. **Mayhew IG, Beal CR.** Techniques of analysis of cerebrospinal fluid. Vet Clin North Am Small Anim Pract 1980;10:155–176.
8. **Jamison EM, Lumsden JH.** Cerebrospinal fluid analysis in the dog: Methodology and interpretation. Semin Vet Med Surg (Small Animal) 1988;3: 122–132.
9. **Chrisman CL.** Cerebrospinal fluid analysis. Vet Clin North Am Small Animal Pract 1992;22:781–810.
10. **Green EM, Constantinescu GM, Kroll RA.** Equine cerebrospinal fluid: Physiologic principles and collection techniques. Comp Cont Edu Pract Vet 1992;14:229–238.
11. **Bailey CS, Vernau W.** Cerebrospinal fluid. In: JJ Kaneko, JW Harvey, ML Bruss, eds. Clinical biochemistry of domestic animals, 5th ed. San Diego: Academic Press, 1997;785–827.
12. **Broadwell RD, Banks WA.** A cell biological perspective for the transcytosis of peptides and proteins through the mammalian blood-brain fluid barriers. In: WM Pardridge, ed. The blood-brain barrier: Cellular and molecular biology. New York: Raven Press, 1993;165–199.
13. **Felgenhauer K, Schliep G, Rapic N.** Protein permeability of the blood-CSF barrier. Proteins Biol Fluids Proc Colloq 1976;23:481–487.
14. **Dickson PW, Alread AP, Marley PD.** High prealbumin and transferrin mRNA levels in the choroid plexus of rat brain. Biochem Biophys Res Commun 1985;127:890–895.
15. **Aldred AR, Grimes A, Schreeber G.** Rat ceruloplasmin. J Biol Chem 1987;262:2875–2878.
16. **Rouah E, Rogers BB, Buffone GJ.** Transferrin analysis by immunofixation as an aid in the diagnosis of cerebrospinal fluid otorrhea. Arch Pathol Lab Med 1987;111:756–757.
17. **Dziegielewska KM, Saunders NR.** The origins and functions of proteins in CSF in the developing brain. In: L Rakic, DJ Begley, H Davson, BV Zlokovic, eds. Peptides and amino acid transport mechanisms in the central nervous system. London: Macmillan, 1988;105–121.
18. **Watson MA, Scott MG.** Clinical utility of biochemical analysis of cerebrospinal fluid. Clin Chem 1995;41:343–360.
19. **Greenlee JE, Carroll KC.** Cerebrospinal fluid in CNS infections. In: WM Scheld, RJ Whitley, DT Durack, eds. Infections of the central nervous system, 2nd ed. Philadelphia: Lippincott-Raven, 1997;899–922.
20. **Mavligit GM, Stuckey SE, Cabanillas FF.** Diagnosis of leukemia or lymphoma in the central nervous system by beta$_2$-microglobulin determination. N Engl J Med 1980;303:718–722.
21. **Summers BA, Whitaker JN, Appel MJ.** Demyelinating canine distemper encephalomyelitis measurement of myelin basic protein in cerebrospinal fluid. J Neuroimmunol 1987;14:227–233.
22. **Jacobs RM, Cochrane SM, Lumsden JH, Norris AM.** Relationship of cerebrospinal fluid protein concentration determined by dye-binding and urinary dipstick methodologies. Can Vet J 1998;31:587–588.
23. **Schriever H, Gambino SR.** Protein turbidity produced by trichloracetic acid and sulfosalicylic acid at varying temperatures and varying ratios of albumin and globulin. Am J Clin Path 1975;44:667
24. **Lowry OH, Rosebrough NJ, Farr AL.** Protein measurement with the folin phenol reagent. J Biol Chem 1951;193:265–275.
25. **Bradford MM.** A rapid and sensitive method for the quantitation of microgram quantities of protein utilizing the principle of protein-dye binding. Anal Biochem 1976;72:248–254.
26. **Lott JA, Warren P.** Estimation of reference intervals for total protein in cerebrospinal fluid. Clin Chem 1989;35:1766–1770.
27. **Fishman RA, Ransohoff J, Osserman EF.** Factors influencing the concentration gradient of protein in cerebrospinal fluid. J Clin Invest 1958;37:1419–1428.
28. **Bailey CS, Higgins RJ.** Comparison of total white blood cell count and total protein of lumbar and cisternal cerebrospinal fluid of healthy dogs. Am J Vet Res 1985;46:1162–1165.
29. **Vaughn DM, Coleman E, Simpson ST, Whitmer WL, Satjawatcharaphong C.** A rostrocaudal gradient for neurotransmitter metabolites and a caudorostral gradient for protein in canine cerebrospinal fluid. Am J Vet Res 1988;49:2134–2137.
30. **Sorjonen DC.** Total protein, albumin quota, and electrophoretic patterns in cerebrospinal fluid of dogs with central nervous system disorders. Am J Vet Res 1987;48:301–305.
31. **Hochwald GM, Wallenstein MC, Matthews ES.** Exchange of proteins between blood and spinal arachnoid fluid. Am J Physiol 1969;217:348–353.
32. **Mayhew IG, Whitlock RH, Tasker JB.** Equine cerebrospinal fluid: Reference values of normal horses. Am J Vet Res 1977;38:1271–1274.
33. **Vaughn DM, Smyth GB.** Different gradients for neurotransmitter metabolites and protein in horse cerebrospinal fluid. Vet Res Commun 1989; 13:413–419.
34. **Andrews FM, Maddux JM, Faulk D.** Total protein, albumin quotient, IgG and IgG index determinations for horse cerebrospinal fluid. Prog Vet Neurol 1991;1:197–204.
35. **Fishman RA.** Exchange of albumin between plasma and cerebrospinal fluid. Am J Physiol 1953;175:96.
36. **Meeks JC, Christopher ML, Chrisman CL, Hopkins AL.** The maturation of canine cerebrospinal fluid. Proceedings of the 12th ACVIM Forum, 1994:1008.
37. **Furr MO, Bender H.** Cerebrospinal fluid variables in clinically normal foals from birth to 42 days of age. Am J Vet Res 1994;55:781–784.
38. **Andrews FM, Geiser DR, Sommardahl CS, Green EM, Provenza M.** Albumin quotient, IgG concentration, and IgG index determinations in cerebrospinal fluid of neonatal foals. Am J Vet Res 1994;55:741–745.

39. **Rossdale PD, Cash RSF, Leadon DP.** Biochemical constituents of cerebrospinal fluid in premature and full term foals. Equine Vet J 1982;14:134–138.

40. **Dziegielewska KM, Saunders NR.** The development of the blood-brain barrier: Proteins in fetal and neonatal CSF, their nature and origins. In: E Meisami and PJ Timiras, eds. Handbook of human growth and biological development. Boca Raton: CRC Press, 1987.

41. **Cavanagh ME, Cornelis ME, Dziegielewska KM, Luft AJ, Lai PCW, Lorscheider FL, Saunders NR.** Proteins in cerebrospinal fluid and plasma of fetal pigs during development. Dev Neurosci 1982;5:492–502.

42. **Vaughn DM, Coleman E, Simpson ST, Satjawatcharaphong C.** Analysis of neurotransmitter metabolite concentrations in canine cerebrospinal fluid. Am J Vet Res 1988;49:1302–1305.

43. **Vaughn DM, Smyth GB, Whitmer WL, Satjawatcharaphong C.** Analysis of equine cisterna magna cerebrospinal fluid for the presence of some monoamine neurotransmitters and transmitter metabolites. Vet Res Commun 1989;13:237–249.

44. **Ruckebusch M, Costes G.** Revue Med Vet 1988;139:1125–1131.

45. **Wilson JW, Wiltrout SK.** Cerebrospinal fluid creatine phosphokinase in the normal dog. Am J Vet Res 1976;37:1099–1100.

46. **Heavner JE, Colaianne J, Roper M.** Lactate dehydrogenase isoenzymes in blood and cerebrospinal fluid from healthy beagles. Am J Vet Res 1986;47:1772–1775.

47. **Rand JS, Parent J, Jacobs R, Johnson R.** Reference intervals for feline cerebrospinal fluid: Biochemical and serologic variables, IgG concentration, and electrophoretic fractionation. Am J Vet Res 1990;51:1049–1054.

48. **Welles EG, Tyler JW, Sorjonen DC, Whitley EM.** Composition and analysis of cerebrospinal fluid in clinically normal adult cattle. Am J Vet Res 1992;53:2050–2057.

49. **Welles EG, Pugh DG, Wenzel JGW, Sorjonen DC.** Composition of cerebrospinal fluid in healthy adult llamas. Am J Vet Res 1994;55:1075–1079.

50. **Jackson C, de Lahunta A, Divers T, Ainsworth D.** The diagnostic utility of cerebrospinal fluid creatine kinase activity in the horse. J Vet Intern Med 1996;10:246–251.

51. **Indrieri RJ, Holliday TA, Keen CL.** Critical evaluation of creatine phosphokinase in cerebrospinal fluid of dogs with neurologic disease. Am J Vet Res 1998;41:1299–1303.

52. **Rand JS, Parent J, Jacobs R, Percy D.** Reference intervals for feline cerebrospinal fluid: Cell counts and cytologic features. Am J Vet Res 1990;51:1044–1048.

53. **Bailey CS, Higgins RJ.** Characteristics of cerebrospinal fluid associated with canine granulomatous meningoencephalomyelitis: A retrospective study. JAVMA 1986;188:418–421.

54. **Thomson CE, Kornegay JN, Stevens JB.** Analysis of cerebrospinal fluid from the cerebellomedullary and lumbar cisterns of dogs with focal neurologic disease: 145 cases (1985–1987). JAVMA 1990;196:1841–1844.

55. **Scott PR, Will RG.** A report of Froin's syndrome in five ovine thoracolumbar epidural abscess cases. Br Vet J 1991;147:582–584.

56. **Tvedten HW.** Clinical pathology of bovine neurologic disease. Vet Clin North Am Food Animal Pract 1987;3:25–44.

57. **Scott PR.** Total protein and electrophoretic pattern of cerebrospinal fluid in sheep with some common neurological disorders. Cornell Vet 1993;83:199–204.

58. **Quagliarello VJ, Ma A, Stukenbrok H, Palade GE.** Ultrastructural localization of albumin transport across the cerebral microvasculature during experimental meningitis in the rat. J Exp Med 1991;175:657–672.

59. **Tipold A.** Diagnosis of inflammatory and infectious disease of the central nervous system in dogs: A retrospective study. J Vet Intern Med 1995;9:304–314.

60. **Scott PR.** Analysis of cerebrospinal fluid from field cases of some common ovine neurological diseases. Br Vet J 1998;148:15–22.

61. **Thomson CE, Kornegay JN, Stevens JB.** Canine intervertebral disc disease: Changes in the cerebrospinal fluid. J Small Animal Pract 1989;30:685–688.

62. **Furr M, Chickering WR, Robertson J.** High resolution protein electrophoresis of equine cerebrospinal fluid. Am J Vet Res 1997;58:939–941.

63. **Bailey CS, Higgins RJ.** Characteristics of cisternal cerebrospinal fluid associated with primary brain tumors in the dog: A retrospective study. JAVMA 1986;188:414–417.

64. **Wilson JW, Stevens JB.** Effects of blood contamination on cerebrospinal fluid analysis. JAVMA 1977;171:256–258.

65. **Hurtt AE, Smith MO.** Effects of iatrogenic blood contamination on results of cerebrospinal fluid analysis in clinically normal dogs and dogs with neurologic disease. JAVMA 1997;211:866–867.

66. **Vaughn DM, Simpson ST, Blagburn BL, Whitmer WL, Heddens-Mysinger R, Hendrix CM.** Determination of homovanillic acid, 5-hydroxyindoleacetic acid and pressure in the cerebrospinal fluid of Collie dogs following administration of ivermectin. Vet Res Commun 1989;13:47–55.

67. **Podell M, Hadjicontantinou M.** Cerebrospinal fluid γ-aminobutyric acid and glutamate values in dogs with epilepsy. Am J Vet Res 1997;58:451–456.

68. **Löscher W, Schwartz-Porsche D.** Low levels of γ-aminobutyric acid in cerebrospinal fluid of dogs with epilepsy. J Neurosci 1986;46:1322–1325.

69. **Faull K, Barchas J, Foutz A, Dement W, Holman R.** Monoamine metabolite concentrations in cerebrospinal fluid of normal and narcoleptic dogs. Brain Res 1982;242:137–143.

70. **Mefford IM, Baker TL, Boehme R, Foutz AS, Ciaranello RD, Barchas JD, Dement NC.** Narcolepsy: Biogenic amine deficits in an animal model. Science 1983;220:629–632.

71. **Lunn DP, Cuddon PA, Shaftoe S, Archer RM.** Familial occurrence of narcolepsy in miniature horses. Equine Vet J 1993;25:476

72. **Laterre EC, Callewaert A, Heremans JF, Sfaello Z.** Electrophoretic morphology of gamma globulins in cerebrospinal fluid of multiple sclerosis and other diseases of the nervous system. Neurology 1970;20:982–990.

73. **Link H, Muller R.** Immunoglobulins in multiple sclerosis and infections of the nervous system. Arch Neurol 1971;25:326–344.

74. **Takeoka T, Gotoh F, Furumi K, Mori K.** Polyacrylamide-gel disc electrophoresis of native cerebrospinal fluid proteins, with special reference to immunoglobulins and some clinical applications. J Neurol Sci 1976;29:213.

75. **Delmotte P.** Gel isoelectric focusing of cerebrospinal fluid proteins as a potential diagnostic tool. J Clin Chem Clin Biochem 1971;9:334.

76. **Nilsson K, Olsson JE.** Analysis for cerebrospinal fluid proteins by isoelectric focusing on polyacrylamide gel: Methodological aspects and normal values, with special reference to the alkaline region. Clin Chem 1978;24:1134–1139.

77. **Mehta PD, Mehta SP, Patrick BA.** Silver staining of unconcentrated cerebrospinal fluid in agarose gel (Panagel) electrophoresis. Clin Chem 1984;30:735–736.

78. **Link H, Kostulas V.** Utility of isoelectric focusing of cerebrospinal fluid and serum on agarose evaluated for neurological patients. Clin Chem 1983;29:810–815.

79. **Kabat EA, Glusman M, Knaub V.** Quantitative estimation of the albumin and gamma globulin in normal and pathologic cerebrospinal fluid by immunochemical methods. Am J Med 1948;4:653–662.

80. **Krakowka S, Fenner W, Miele JA.** Quantitative determination of serum origin cerebrospinal fluid protein in the dog. Am J Vet Res 1981;42:1975–1977.

81. **Kirk GR, Neate S, McClure RC, Hutcheson DP.** Electrophoretic pattern of cerebrospinal fluid. Am J Vet Res 1974;35:1263–1264.

82. **Kristenson F, Firth ER.** Analysis of serum protein and cerebrospinal fluid. Am J Vet Res 1977;38:1089–1092.

83. **Johnson GC, Fenner WR, Krakowka S.** Production of immunoglobulin G and increased antiviral antibody in cerebrospinal fluid of dogs with delayed–onset canine distemper viral encephalitis. J Neuroimmunol 1988;38:1089–1092.

84. **Sorjonen DC, Cox NR, Swango LJ.** Electrophoretic determination of albumin and gamma globulin concentrations in the cerebrospinal fluid of dogs with encephalomyelitis attributable to canine distemper virus infection: 13 cases (1980–1987). JAVMA 1989;195:977–980.

85. **Link H, Tibbling G.** Principles of albumin and IgG analysis in neurological disorders. II. Relation of the concentration of the proteins in serum and cerebrospinal fluid. Scand J Clin Lab Invest 1977;37:391–396.

86. **Chu AB, Sever JL, Madden DL, Iivanainen M, Leon M, Wallen N, Brooks BR, Lee YJ, Huoff S.** Oligoclonal IgG bands in cerebrospinal fluid in various neurological diseases. Ann Neurol 1983;13:434–439.

87. **Zeman A, McLean B, Keir G, Luxton R, Sharief M, Thompson E.** The significance of serum oligoclonal bands in neurological diseases. J Neurol Neurosurg Psychiatry. 1993;56:32–35.

88. **Sorjonen DC, Warren JN, Schultz RD.** Qualitative and quantitative determination of albumin, IgG, IgM and IgA in normal cerebrospinal fluid of dogs. J Am Animal Hosp Assoc 1981;17:833–839.

89. **Tibbling G, Link H, Ohman S.** Principles of albumin and IgG analyses in neurological disorders. I. Establishment of reference values. Scand J Clin Lab Invest 1977;37:385–390.

90. **Bichsel P, Vandevelde M, Vandevelde E, Affolter U, Pfister H.** Immunoelectrophoretic determination of albumin and IgG in serum and cerebrospinal fluid in dogs with neurologic diseases. Res Vet Sci 1984;37:101–107.

91. **Link H, Tibbling G.** Principles of albumin and IgG analyses in neurologic disorders. III. Evaluation of IgG synthesis within the central nervous system in multiple sclerosis. Scand J Clin Lab Invest 1977;37:397–401.

92. **Sorjonen DC, Golden DL, Levesque DC, Shores A, Moore MP.** Cerebrospinal fluid protein electrophoresis: A clinical evaluation of a previously reported diagnostic technique. Prog Vet Neurol 1991;2:261–267.

93. **Aleshire SL, Hajdu I, Bradley CA, Parl FF.** Choroid plexus as a barrier to immunoglobulin delivery into cerebrospinal fluid. J Neurosurg 1985;63:593–597.

94. **Tipold A, Pfister H, Vandevelde M.** Determination of the IgG index for the detection of intrathecal immunoglobulin synthesis in dogs using an ELISA. Res Vet Sci 1993;54:40–44.

95. **Tipold A, Pfister H, Zurbriggen A, Vandevelde M.** Intrathecal synthesis of major immunoglobulin classes in inflammatory diseases of the canine CNS. Vet Immunol Immunopathol 1994;42:149–159.

96. **Tipold A, Vandevelde M, Zurbriggen A.** Neuroimmunological studies in steroid–responsive meningitis-arteritis dogs. Res Vet Sci 1995;58:103–108.

97. **Woo AH, Cserr HF, Knopf PM.** Elevated cerebrospinal fluid IgA in humans and rats is not associated with secretory component. J Neuroimmunol 1993;44:129–136.

98. **Tipold A, Jaggy A.** Steroid-responsive meningitis-arteritis in dogs: Long-term study of 32 cases. J Small Animal Pract 1994;311–316.

CHAPTER 139

Bence-Jones Proteins

• LAURA I. BOONE

Immunoglobulin molecules produced by a population of cells originating from clonal expansion of a single plasma cell are called monoclonal proteins (M-proteins or myeloma proteins) or, alternatively, paraproteins. Unlike normal plasma cells, which produce complete immunoglobulins and small quantities of free light chains, these clonal cells can produce complete or incomplete immunoglobulins and free individualized, fragmented, or dimerized light chains.[1]

Unassociated light chains produced in excess by abnormal plasma cells are called Bence-Jones proteins. Approximately 20 kDa in molecular mass, they consist of two different structural domains, the constant and variable regions. Although one gene encodes the constant region, several gene segments are rearranged to form a variable region unique for each protein. Therefore, although these proteins share structural similarities, they often vary physicochemically as a result of unique properties of the variable regions.[2,3]

Because of their small size, serum Bence-Jones proteins filter through the glomerulus for metabolism by proximal tubular epithelial cells following receptor-mediated endocytosis. Paraproteinuria occurs if this receptor is saturated as a result of pronounced light chain proteinemia or increased protein filtration as a result of glomerular damage.[1,3]

METHODS OF DETECTION FOR URINARY BENCE-JONES PROTEINS

Because Bence-Jones proteins can be found in the serum or urine, screening for urinary light chains is indicated in patients with a serum monoclonal gammopathy. Routine evaluation procedures for proteinuria, specifically commercial dipsticks and the sulfosalicylic acid (SSA) test, are not satisfactory for accurate identification of Bence-Jones protein. Bence-Jones proteins are not detected by dipsticks, and although the SSA test semiquantitatively measures all proteins, it is not specific for urine light chains.[4,5] Classically, Bence-Jones proteins have been detected by heating the urine to 40 to 60°C, causing precipitation of most, but not all, monoclonal light chains. The precipitate disappears with further heating

to 100°C and reappears on cooling to 40 to 60°C. False-positives and negatives occur frequently, however, decreasing the usefulness of this test.[5,6]

Because of the unreliability of the above tests, more sensitive methods are required for detection of Bence-Jones proteins. Identification of light chain proteinuria begins with agarose or cellulose acetate electrophoresis of concentrated urine samples coupled with densitometric evaluation of protein bands.[4] Although 100–fold concentration of urine samples is adequate for moderate to high concentrations of light chains,[2] concentrating the samples 300- to 600-fold is recommended for low levels of proteinuria. Concentration of urine samples to this degree is accomplished by polyethylene glycol dialysis or reduced pressure extraction in collodium bags.[7] Paraproteins are represented as a peak in either the β or the γ region of the densitometric pattern from urine proteins separated with electrophoresis.[6]

Immunoelectrophoresis (IEP) or immunofixation electrophoresis (IFE) techniques using antisera against α-, γ-, and μ-heavy chains, and κ- and λ-light chains allow classification of the light chain and/or heavy chain component of the urine paraprotein.[4] For IEP, the anti-heavy or anti-light chain antisera is placed in a trough adjacent to proteins isolated by electrophoresis. Diffusion of the antibody and protein antigen results in precipitin arcs identifying the immunoglobulin chains of the paraprotein.[8] With IFE, the patient's urine is aliquoted into six lanes on an agarose gel for separation by electrophoresis. Once separated, protein bands in one lane are chemically fixed in the gel to provide a reference pattern. The remaining five lanes are treated with anti-heavy chain or anti-light chain antisera. If the appropriate heavy or light chain is present, an antigen-antibody complex will form, fixing the protein precipitate in the gel. Proteins not immobilized by this interaction are lost with washing. Following staining, fixed proteins are compared with the bands in the reference lane.[4] Bence-Jones proteins are identified as a precipitin band with anti-light chain antisera. Corresponding bands fixed in two lanes with anti-light and anti-heavy chain antisera indicate a monoclonal immunoglobulin (Fig. 139.1). Although both procedures are useful in identification of monoclonal gammopathies and Bence-

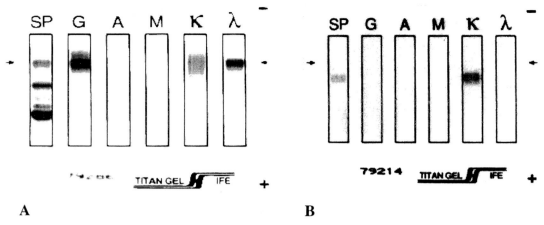

FIGURE 139.1 Immunofixation electrophoresis (IFE) gels from the urine of two human patients with serum monoclonal gammopathies. (SP: fixed protein reference lane; G: anti-γ heavy chain antisera; A: anti-α heavy chain antisera; M: anti-μ heavy chain antisera; κ: anti-κ light chain antisera; λ: anti-λ light chain antisera) (**A**) Single discrete precipitin bands in the γ heavy chain lane and the λ light chain lane indicate IgG-λ monoclonal immunoglobulin in the urine. Notice the broad diffuse band in the κ light chain lane, indicating polyclonal urinary κ light chains. (**B**) Single discrete precipitin band in the κ light chain lane indicates Bence-Jones proteinuria. (Courtesy of Helena Laboratories, Beaumont, TX)

proteinuria, IFE is the preferred method. Advantages of IFE over IEP include faster turnaround time, increased sensitivity, and easier interpretation of results.[9]

BENCE-JONES PROTEINURIA IN HUMANS

Bence-Jones proteinuria with or without a concomitant monoclonal gammopathy is a diagnostic feature for human plasma cell and lymphocytic disorders, including multiple myeloma, Waldenström's macroglobulinemia, and systemic amyloidosis. Classically, concomitant Bence-Jones proteinuria and serum monoclonal gammopathy has been a feature of multiple myeloma; however, in up to 20% of cases, Bence-Jones proteinuria alone is present at the time of diagnosis.[7] Significant Bence-Jones proteinuria is also present in approximately 55% of patients with Waldenström's macroglobulinemia, a relatively rare, slowly proliferating small-cell (plasmacytoid) lymphoma associated with monoclonal IgM production, infiltration of the bone marrow, and peripheral lymphocytosis.[10]

Multisystemic deposition of amyloid fibrils from light chains produced by a slowly proliferating monoclonal plasma cell population occurs in individuals with primary systemic amyloidosis (AL). Although serum monoclonal gammopathies are a consistent feature of AL, circulation of free light chains alone is rare. Bence-Jones proteinuria can be present in up to 67% of AL patients.[11]

The increased sensitivity of high-resolution agarose gel electrophoresis and IFE has improved detection of Bence-Jones proteinuria in 32% of patients with chronic lymphocytic leukemia, in 18% of patients with non-Hodgkin's lymphoma, and in 3 to 6% of patients with hairy cell leukemia. These conditions were previously identified as nonsecretory because the low level of light

chain proteinuria in these patients was undetectable by traditional electrophoresis.[7,12]

A monoclonal gammopathy and/or Bence-Jones proteinuria without evidence of plasmacytic neoplasia or lymphoproliferative disease is the diagnostic criteria for monoclonal gammopathy of undetermined significance. Although apparently disease-free at the time of diagnosis, these patients may develop a plasma cell dyscrasia or lymphoproliferative disease during long-term follow-up. Rarely, Bence-Jones proteinuria has been detected in apparently normal individuals without development of lymphoproliferative disease or plasma cell abnormalities during long-term follow-up.[7]

BENCE-JONES PROTEINS IN DOMESTIC SPECIES

Classically, Bence-Jones proteinuria has been one of four diagnostic criteria for multiple myeloma in domestic species. The remaining three criteria include serum monoclonal gammopathy (excluding IgM), radiographically evident osteolytic bone lesions, and marrow plasmacytosis, preferably with sheet or cluster formation.[13] In domestic species, either the heat precipitation test or urine electrophoresis has been used for identification of Bence-Jones proteinuria.

In the dog, multiple myeloma is almost always associated with a monoclonal gammopathy. Bence-Jones proteinuria occurs less commonly. In two retrospective studies of canine multiple myeloma, 31 to 40% of affected animals had positive heat precipitation tests, suggesting Bence-Jones proteinuria.[13,14] Bence-Jones proteinuria was detected in 33% of recently reported cases of IgA myeloma with heat precipitation[15,16] or IEP.[17] A similar incidence of paraproteinuria has been reported in recent cases of IgG myeloma.[18-20] Bence-Jones proteinuria has also been reported in 46% of dogs with chronic lymphocytic leukemia.[21] Although lymphoproliferative disease with excessive IgM production, similar to the human syndrome Waldenström's macroglobulinemia, has been reported in the dog,[22-24] Bence-Jones proteinuria has not been a feature of this disease.

Bence-Jones proteinuria with a concurrent serum monoclonal IgG gammopathy has rarely been reported in association with chronic infectious diseases in the dog.[25,26] Bence-Jones proteinuria was suggested by a monoclonal peak with urine electrophoresis in a dog with chronic pyoderma and a serum monoclonal IgG gammopathy.[25] Additionally, light chain proteinuria was suggested by urine immunoprecipitation in a dog with *Ehrlichia canis* and an IgG monoclonal gammopathy.[26] These cases suggest that light chain proteinuria in the dog is not limited to lymphoproliferative disease or plasma cell dyscrasias but may occur secondary to chronic antigenic stimulation. Surveillance of serum and urine in dogs with hyperglobulinemia using electrophoresis, IEP, and IFE techniques will help to identify monoclonal gammopathies and/or paraproteinuria with other causes of chronic antigenic stimulation.

Multiple myeloma with either monoclonal IgA or IgG gammopathies has been infrequently reported in the cat. In a retrospective study of feline cases of myeloma, 17% of affected animals had a positive heat precipitation test for Bence-Jones proteinuria.[13] Immunoelectrophoresis has been used to confirm Bence-Jones proteinuria in a cat with IgA myeloma[27] and in two cats with IgG myeloma.[28]

A cat with lymphoplasmacytic stomatitis and gingivitis also had a serum monoclonal gammopathy and urine M-protein spike in the β region.[29] This case suggests that other diseases with chronic antigenic stimulation should be considered as possible differential diagnoses for monoclonal gammopathies in the cat. Examination of serum and urine from hyperglobulinemic cats using electrophoresis, IEP, and IFE techniques may help to identify other nonneoplastic conditions associated with monoclonal gammopathies and/or paraproteinuria.

Serum monoclonal gammopathy was a consistent feature in a review of 10 published cases of equine multiple myeloma. Only one of five animals tested with the heat precipitation test was positive for paraproteinuria. Two of the four negative horses had a monoclonal spike in the urine electrophoresis pattern corresponding to a monoclonal peak in the serum.[30]

Monoclonal IgG gammopathy has been reported in a case of equine chronic lymphocytic leukemia. Concurrent Bence-Jones proteinuria was suggested by a positive heat precipitation test and demonstration of a monoclonal peak in the γ region by electrophoresis.[31] This would suggest that other equine lymphoproliferative disorders are associated with paraprotein production. Further evaluation of serum and urine from hyperglobulinemic horses using immunologic methods may identify other conditions with monoclonal gammopathies and/or paraproteinuria.

DETECTION OF BENCE-JONES PROTEINS IN DOMESTIC SPECIES

Although heat precipitation or electrophoresis has classically been used for Bence-Jones protein identification, serious drawbacks to these methods preclude their usefulness in detection of paraproteinuria in domestic species. Urinary M-proteins have been detected by electrophoresis or IEP despite a negative heat test (false-negative test) in human[5] and veterinary patients.[17,30] Positive heat tests without evidence of a urinary M-protein with IEP have also been reported in humans (false-positive test).[5] Because the incidence of false-positive heat tests in veterinary patients is unknown, positive precipitation tests should be confirmed with IFE or IEP. Additionally, because it is unclear whether other proteins may precipitate in the heat test, it is essential that antisera for κ- and λ-light chains confirm free light chains in heat-precipitated urine protein. Until free light chains can be demonstrated in heat-precipitated proteins, this test should be considered unreliable for Bence-Jones proteinuria detection in veterinary patients.

Urine free light chains are expected to appear as a discrete peak in the globulin region (β and γ region) of densitometric tracings from urine agarose electrophoresis samples (Fig. 139.2).[6,32] However, protein loss from concurrent glomerular disease can complicate evaluation of tracings from patients with suspected Bence-Jones proteinuria. One commonly interfering protein in the β region is transferrin.[4] Use of antitransferrin antisera in IEP or IFE procedures will help in differentiating transferrin from paraproteins in urine samples.

Incomplete or intact monoclonal immunoglobulins can also be lost with concurrent glomerular disease. Because of similar migration in the β or γ regions during electrophoresis,[6] these proteins can mimic or mask a urinary M-spike as a result of Bence-Jones proteins alone. IEP or IFE is required for definitive characterization of urinary paraproteins. Although antisera for human immunoglobulin isotypes is available, these products may not be adequate for IEP or IFE in veterinary

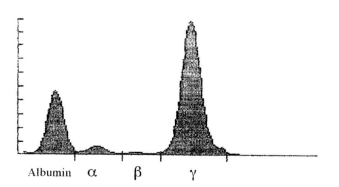

FIGURE 139.2 Representative urine protein electrophoresis from a dog with a serum monoclonal gammopathy. Notice the monoclonal spike in the γ region, which indicates a urinary paraprotein. (Courtesy of Texas Veterinary Medical Diagnostic Laboratory, College Station, TX)

patients because of the potential interspecies variability in immunoglobulins. For this reason, species-specific antisera against heavy and light chains should be used for these methods.

REFERENCES

1. **Picken MM, Shen S.** Immunoglobulin light chains and the kidney: An overview. Ultrastruct Pathol 1994;18:105–112.
2. **Levinson SS, Keren DF.** Free light chains of immunoglobulins: Clinical laboratory analysis. Clin Chem 1994;40(10):1869–1878.
3. **Sanders PW.** Pathogenesis and treatment of myeloma kidney. J Lab Clin Med 1994;124:484–488.
4. **Silverman LM, Christenson RH.** Amino acids and proteins. In: CA Burtis and ER Ashwood, eds. Tietz fundamentals of clinical chemistry, 4th ed. Philadelphia: WB Saunders, 1996.
5. **Kyle RA, Greipp PR.** The laboratory investigation of monoclonal gammopathies. Mayo Clin Proc 1978;53:719–739.
6. **Kyle RA.** The monoclonal gammopathies. Clin Chem 1994;40(11):2154–2161.
7. **Pascali E, Pezzoli A.** The clinical spectrum of pure Bence-Jones proteinuria: A study of 66 patients. Cancer 1988;62:2408–2415.
8. **Kricka LJ.** Principles of immunochemical techniques. In: CA Burtis CA and ER Ashwood, eds. Tietz fundamentals of clinical chemistry, 4th ed. Philadelphia: WB Saunders, 1996.
9. **Keren DF.** Immunofixation technique. In: High-resolution electrophoresis and immunofixation: Techniques and interpretation, 2nd ed. Boston: Butterworth-Heinemann, 1994.
10. **Dimopoulos MA, Alexanian R.** Waldenström's macroglobulinemia. Blood 1994;83(6):1452–1459.
11. **Kyle RA, Linos A, Beard CM, Linke RP, Gertz MA, O'Fallon M, Kurland LT.** Incidence and natural history of primary systemic amyloidosis in Olmsted County, Minnesota, 1950 through 1989. Blood 1992;79(7):1817–1822.
12. **Hansen DA, Robbins BA, Bylund DJ, Piro LD, Saven A, Ellison DJ.** Identification of monoclonal immunoglobulins and quantitative immunoglobulin abnormalities in hairy cell leukemia and chronic lymphocytic leukemia. Am J Clin Pathol 1994;102:580–585.
13. **MacEwen EG, Hurvitz AI.** Diagnosis and management of monoclonal gammopathies. Vet Clin North Am 1977;7(1):119–132.
14. **Matus RE, Leifer CE, MacEwen G, Hurvitz AI.** Prognostic factors for multiple myeloma in the dog. J Am Vet Assoc 1986;188(11):1288–1292.
15. **Day MJ, Penhale WJ, McKenna RP, Mills JN, Pass DA.** Two cases of IgA multiple myeloma in the dog. J Small Animal Pract 1987;28:147–156.
16. **Zinkl JG, LeCouteur RA, Davis DC, Saunders GK.** "Flaming" plasma cells in a dog with IgA multiple myeloma. Vet Clin Pathol 1983;12(3):15–19.
17. **Kirschner SE, Niyo Y, Hill BL, Betts DM.** Blindness in a dog with IgA-forming myeloma. JAVMA 1988;193(3):349–350.
18. **Campbell KL, Latimer KS.** Polysystemic manifestations of plasma cell myeloma in the dog: A case report and review. J Am Animal Hosp Assoc 1985;21:59–66.
19. **Couto CG, Ruehl W, Muir S.** Plasma cell leukemia and monoclonal (IgG) gammopathy in a dog. JAVMA 1984;184(1):90–92.
20. **Altman DH, Meyer DJ, Thompson JP, Bailey EA.** Canine IgG$_{2c}$ myeloma with mott and flame cells. J Am Animal Hosp Assoc 1991;27:419–423.
21. **Leifer CE, Matus RE.** Chronic lymphocytic leukemia in the dog: 22 cases (1974–1984). JAVMA 1986;189(2)214–217.
22. **Hurvitz AI, MacEwen EG, Middaugh CR, Litman GW.** Monoclonal cryoglobulinemia with macroglobulinemia in a dog. JAVMA 1977;170(5):511–513.
23. **Mejia EB, Carman S, Lumsden JH.** Macroglobulinemia in a dog. Can Vet J 1979;20:28–33.
24. **Hurvitz AI, Haskins SC, Fischer CA.** Macroglobulinemia with hyperviscosity syndrome in a dog. JAVMA 1970;157(4):455–460.
25. **Burkhard MJ, Meyer DJ, Rosychuk RA, O'Neil SP, Schultheiss PC.** Monoclonal gammopathy in a dog with chronic pyoderma. J Vet Intern Med 1995;9(5):357–360.
26. **Varela F, Font X, Valladares JE, Alberola J.** Thrombocytopathia and light-proteinuria in a dog naturally infected with *Ehrlichia canis*. J Vet Intern Med 1997;11(5):309–311.
27. **Yamada T, Shirota K, Matsuda M, Takahashi T, Ogata M, Nomura Y, Suzuki T, Yamamaoto H.** A case of feline IgA-monoclonal gammopathy associated with Bence-Jones proteinuria. Jpn J Vet Sci 1986;48(3):637–641.
28. **Forrester SD, Greco DS, Relford RL.** Serum hyperviscosity syndrome associated with multiple myeloma in two cats. JAVMA 1992;200(1):79–82.
29. **Lyon KF.** Feline lymphoplasmacytic stomatitis associated with monoclonal gammopathy and Bence-Jones proteinuria. J Vet Dent 1994;11(1):25–27.
30. **Edwards DF, Parker JW, Wilkinson JE, Helman RG.** Plasma cell myeloma in the horse. A case report and literature review. J Vet Intern Med 1993;7:169–176.
31. **Dascanio JJ, Zhang CH, Antczak DF, Blue JT, Simmons TR.** Differentiation of chronic lymphocytic leukemia in the horse: A report of two cases. J Vet Intern Med 1992;6:225–229.
32. **Lees GE, Willard MD, Green RA.** Urinary disorders. In: MD Willard, H Tvedten, GH Turnwald, eds. Small animal clinical diagnosis by laboratory methods, 2nd ed. Philadelphia: WB Saunders, 1994.

CHAPTER 140

Hyperviscosity Syndrome

• S. DRU FORRESTER and KENITA S. ROGERS

Hyperviscosity syndrome (HVS) is a group of clinical signs that occur with increased serum or whole blood viscosity. Although HVS may result from polycythemia, it usually occurs secondary to serum hyperviscosity. Serum viscosity is determined by the concentration, size, and shape of serum proteins. Hyperviscosity is most likely to occur with monoclonal elevations in IgM because it is the largest globulin (molecular weight of 900,000) and in IgA because it is capable of forming dimers. Even though IgG is relatively smaller (molecular weight of 160,000), monoclonal elevations of this immunoglobulin have been associated with HVS in dogs and cats.

Hyperviscosity syndrome in dogs and cats occurs with monoclonal hyperglobulinemia, most often as a result of increased γ-globulin concentrations and, rarely, as a result of increased β-globulin concentrations (Table 140.1).[1-23] Approximately 20 to 30% of dogs with monoclonal gammopathy have HVS, whereas HVS is rare in cats.[1-14,16-25] The most common cause of monoclonal hyperglobulinemia and HVS in dogs and cats is multiple myeloma (Fig. 140. 1).[2,4,8,9,12,13,16,17,20,21,23,25] In dogs with multiple myeloma and HVS, the immunoglobulin identified in 80% of cases is IgA.[1,4,8,16,17,20] In contrast, IgG is the monoclonal immunoglobulin most often present in cats with multiple myeloma and HVS.[2,12,13] Although neoplasia is the underlying disease in almost all cases with HVS, some dogs have developed HVS associated with ehrlichiosis and IgG monoclonal gammopathy.[3,5,7]

Hyperviscosity causes decreased blood flow to the tissues, which is often associated with clinical signs of ophthalmic, neurologic, cardiac, or coagulation abnormalities. Ophthalmic findings of HVS include blindness, decreased menace and pupillary light responses, corneal edema, aqueous flare, retinal detachments, retinal edema, multifocal retinal hemorrhages, dilated and tortuous retinal vessels, and secondary glaucoma (Fig. 140.2).[4,6,10,14,15,20,21] Neurologic abnormalities include depression, disorientation, seizures, cranial nerve deficits, and vestibular signs (e.g., head tilt, nystagmus, circling).[2,5,6,12] Signs of cardiac disease including tachycardia and gallop rhythm are present in some patients. Cardiac hypertrophy may result from the increased work of pumping hyperviscous blood, eventually resulting in congestive heart failure (Fig. 140.3). Coagula-

tion disturbances in patients with HVS tend be characterized by bleeding from mucous membrane surfaces and are most often manifested as epistaxis, gingival bleeding, melena, or prolonged hemorrhage from venipuncture sites.[1,3,4,14,16,20,22] Bleeding tendencies in patients with HVS probably result from platelet dysfunction but also may occur secondary to thrombocytopenia, which often exists in patients with HVS as a result of the underlying disease.

A tentative diagnosis of HVS is made after finding clinical signs of hyperviscosity in a patient with monoclonal gammopathy (see chapter 141 in this volume for diagnostic evaluation of patients with monoclonal gammopathy). Hyperviscosity is most often confirmed in veterinary patients by determining relative serum viscosity (i.e., time required for serum to flow through a tube compared with the time for water to flow through the same tube).[26-28] Relative serum viscosity in normal patients is <2.5; patients with clinical signs of HVS usually have values >5 and often >10.[1-4,11-22]

Treatment for patients with HVS includes chemotherapy for the underlying disease and plasmapheresis to control signs of HVS.[1-3,28] Plasmapheresis is the process of separating plasma and cells and returning the cells, resuspended in crystalloid solution, to the patient. Plasmapheresis decreases serum protein concentration, which subsequently lowers serum viscosity. Indications for plasmapheresis include uncontrolled hemorrhage, progressive vision loss, severe neurologic dysfunction,

TABLE 140.1	Diseases Associated with Hyperviscosity Syndrome in 52 Dogs and 7 Cats[1-13]	
Dogs	**Cats**
Multiple myeloma (n = 30)	Multiple myeloma (n = 4)
Lymphocytic leukemia (n = 11)	Lymphoma (n = 2)
Ehrlichiosis (n = 5)	Extramedullary plasmacytoma (n = 1)
Macroglobulinemia (n = 5)	
Extramedullary plasmacytoma (n = 1)	

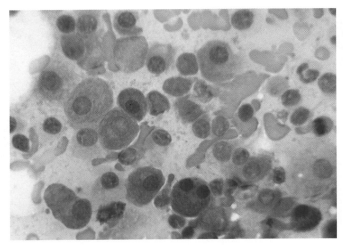

FIGURE 140.1 Bone marrow from a dog with multiple myeloma, a common cause of hyperviscosity syndrome. Note the presence of numerous plasma cells, some with multiple nuclei. (100×, Wright's stain)

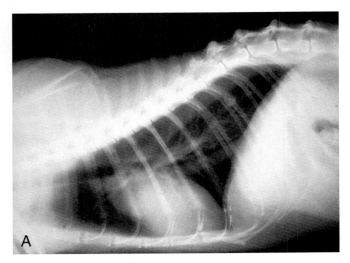

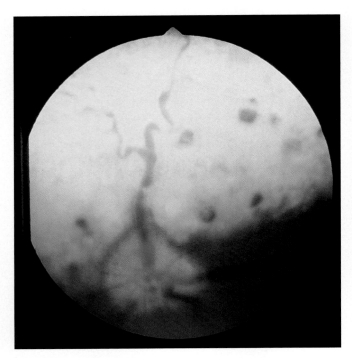

FIGURE 140.2 Retinal lesions in a cat with multiple myeloma and hyperviscosity syndrome. Note the presence of dilated and tortuous retinal vessels and multifocal retinal hemorrhages.

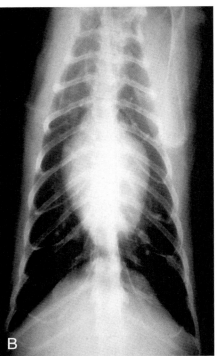

FIGURE 140.3 Lateral and ventrodorsal thoracic radiographs of a cat with multiple myeloma, hyperviscosity syndrome, and hypertrophic cardiomyopathy. There is generalized cardiomegaly with a valentine-shaped heart evident on the ventrodorsal view. There are osteolytic lesions in the dorsal spinous processes (T_{9-11}) and pedicles (T_{11-13}) of the thoracic vertebrae.

and uncontrollable cardiac failure. Continuous plasmapheresis is very effective for lowering serum viscosity but is not widely available for veterinary patients.[1,3] Intermittent plasma exchange has also been used successfully to lower serum protein and viscosity.[2,4,27] The volume of blood to be removed is calculated using a range of 10 to 15 mg/kg body weight.[27] The whole blood is collected in transfer packs with anticoagulant and centri-

fuged to separate plasma and cells. The plasma is removed and the cells are suspended in normal saline. The cells are administered intravenously to the patient. If the patient is severely anemic, a red blood cell transfusion is administered immediately after removal of whole blood for plasma exchange. The frequency of the procedure depends on the severity of clinical signs and response to other therapies. The goal is to decrease the serum viscosity to the point that clinical signs of HVS resolve. Although there may be an initial response to treatment, the overall prognosis for patients with HVS associated with neoplasia is grave. Patients with HVS and monoclonal gammopathy resulting from ehrlichiosis have a good prognosis after appropriate treatment.

REFERENCES

1. **Matus RE, Leifer CE, Gordon BR,** et al. Plasmapheresis and chemotherapy of hyperviscosity syndrome associated with monoclonal gammopathy in the dog. JAVMA 1983; 183:215–218.
2. **Forrester SD, Greco DS, Relford RL.** Serum hyperviscosity syndrome associated with multiple myeloma in two cats. JAVMA 1992;200:79–82.
3. **Matus RE, Leifer CE, Hurvitz AI.** Use of plasmapheresis and chemotherapy for treatment of monoclonal gammopathy associated with *Ehrlichia canis* infection in a dog. JAVMA 1987;190:1302–1304.
4. **Shull RM, Osborne CA, Barrett RE,** et al. Serum hyperviscosity syndrome associated with IgA multiple myeloma in two dogs. J Am Animal Hosp Assoc 1978;14:58–70.
5. **Hoskins JD, Barta O, Rothschmitt J.** Serum hyperviscosity syndrome associated with *Ehrlichia canis* infection in a dog. JAVMA 1983;183:1011–1012.
6. **Braund KG, Everett RM, Albert RA.** Neurologic manifestations of monoclonal IgM gammopathy associated with lymphocytic leukemia in a dog. JAVMA 1978;172:1407–1410.
7. **Breitschwerdt EB, Woody BJ, Zerbe CA,** et al. Monoclonal gammopathy associated with naturally occurring canine ehrlichiosis. J Vet Intern Med 1987;1:2–9.
8. **MacEwen EG, Hurvitz AI.** Diagnosis and management of monoclonal gammopathies. Vet Clin North Am Small Animal Pract 1977;7:119–132.
9. **Jackson MW, Helfand SC, Smedes SL,** et al. Primary IgG-secreting plasma cell tumor in the gastrointestinal tract of a dog. JAVMA 1994;204:404–406.
10. **Ward DA, McEntee MF, Weddle DL.** Orbital plasmacytoma in a cat. J Small Animal Pract 1997;38:576–578.
11. **Willard MD, Krehbiel JD, Schmidt GM,** et al. Serum and urine protein abnormalities associated with lymphocytic leukemia and glomerulonephritis in a dog. J Am Animal Hosp Assoc 1981;17:381–386.
12. **Hribernik TN, Barta O, Gaunt SD,** et al. Serum hyperviscosity syndrome associated with IgG myeloma in a cat. JAVMA 1982;181:169–170.
13. **Hawkins EC.** Immunoglobulin A myeloma in a cat with pleural effusion and serum hyperviscosity. JAVMA 1986;188:876–878.
14. **Williams DA, Goldschmidt MH.** Hyperviscosity syndrome with IgM monoclonal gammopathy and hepatic plasmacytoid lymphosarcoma in a cat. J Small Animal Pract 1982;23:311–323.
15. **Dust A, Norris AM, Valli VEO.** Cutaneous lymphosarcoma with IgG monoclonal gammopathy, serum hyperviscosity and hypercalcemia in a cat. Can Vet J 1982;23:235–239.
16. **Matus RE, Leifer CE, MacEwen EG,** et al. Prognostic factors for multiple myeloma in the dog. JAVMA 1986;188:1288–1292.
17. **Miller C, Fish MB, Danelski TF.** IgA multiple myeloma with multi-system manifestations in the dog: A case report. J Am Animal Hosp Assoc 1982;18:53–56.
18. **MacEwen EG, Hurvitz AI, Hayes A.** Hyperviscosity syndrome associated with lymphocytic leukemia in three dogs. JAVMA 1977;170:1309–1312.
19. **Leifer CE, Matus RE.** Chronic lymphocytic leukemia in the dog: 22 cases (1974–1984). JAVMA 1986;189:214–217.
20. **Center SA, Smith JF.** Ocular lesions in a dog with serum hyperviscosity secondary to an IgA myeloma. JAVMA 1982;181:811–814.
21. **Hendrix DVH, Gelatt KN, Smith PJ,** et al. Ophthalmic disease as the presenting complaint in five dogs with multiple myeloma. J Am Animal Hosp Assoc 1998;34:121–128.
22. **Hurvitz AI, Haskins SC, Fischer CA.** Macroglobulinemia with hyperviscosity syndrome in a dog. JAVMA 1970;157:455–460.
23. **Virella G, Slappendel RJ, Goudswaard J.** Multiple myeloma, IgA cryoglobulinemia and serum hyperviscosity in a dog. Int Arch Allergy Appl Immunol 1977;55:537–541.
24. **Drazner FH.** Multiple myeloma in the cat. Compend Cont Edu Pract Vet 1982;4:206–219.
25. **Mills JN, Eger CE, Robinson WF,** et al. A case of multiple myeloma in a cat. J Am Animal Hosp Assoc 1982;18:79–82.
26. **Wright DJ, Jenkins DE.** Simplified method for estimation of serum and plasma viscosity in multiple myeloma and related disorders. Blood 1970;36:516–522.
27. **Forrester SD, Relford RL.** Serum hyperviscosity syndrome: Its diagnosis and treatment. Vet Med 1992;87:48–54.
28. **Fahey JL, Barth WF, Solomon A.** Serum hyperviscosity syndrome. J Am Med Assoc 1965;192:120–123.

CHAPTER 141

Monoclonal Gammopathy

• KENITA S. ROGERS and S. DRU FORRESTER

Monoclonal gammopathy, or paraproteinemia, is identified as excessive production of immunoglobulin by clonal expansion of a single plasma cell. These proliferating cells synthesize abnormally large quantities of a homogeneous monoclonal immunoglobulin or a polypeptide subunit of the immunoglobulin (heavy or light chains).[1] These paraproteins are of a single immunoglobulin class and subclass and exhibit only one light chain type, either kappa or lambda.[2] Normal and neoplastic plasma cells can be adapted to high rates of synthesis and secretion of immunoglobulin. Gammopathies are classified as polyclonal or monoclonal on the basis of the relative spreading of the gamma-globulin zone on serum electrophoresis.[3] Polyclonal gammopathies are characteristic of benign plasma cell proliferation in response to persistent antigenic stimulation with chronic infectious or inflammatory diseases. Stimulation by an antigen normally results in a heterogenous population of differentiating B-cell clones. This diversity exists because most antigens have multiple sites to which the host responds.[1]

Monoclonal gammopathies are typically found in association with a variety of plasma cell and lymphoid dyscrasias. Immunoglobulins most often associated with plasma cell neoplasia in dogs and cats are IgG and IgA. More rarely, IgM or incomplete immunoglobulins are secreted. The specific syndrome associated with B-cell neoplasia is determined by the stage at which B-cell maturation is arrested.[1] For example, primary (Waldenstrom's) macroglobulinemia is a neoplasm of lymphocytes of intermediate differentiation that can synthesize and secrete IgM. Multiple myeloma is a tumor of more mature plasma cells, which typically secrete IgG or IgA. In addition to neoplasia, a variety of inflammatory or infectious diseases have been infrequently reported to develop monoclonal gammopathy, presumably as a sequelae of atypical benign clonal proliferation of plasma cells.

DIFFERENTIAL DIAGNOSIS

Although development of monoclonal gammopathy has been reported with both neoplastic and nonneoplastic disorders, the most common cause is multiple myeloma. Interesting clinical variants include primary macroglobulinemia, plasma cell leukemia, alpha chain disease, and nonsecretory myeloma. Two additional plasma cell disorders, extramedullary plasmacytoma and monoclonal gammopathy of undetermined significance, have an unclear relationship to myeloma. Two other diseases in the lymphoproliferative spectrum, malignant lymphoma and chronic lymphocytic leukemia (CLL), have also been reported to produce monoclonal gammopathy.[4-7] Occasionally, there will be clonal proliferation of plasma cells in infectious or inflammatory diseases. Reports in veterinary medicine are sparse, but monoclonal gammopathy has been reported in cats with feline infectious peritonitis and dogs with ehrlichiosis, chronic pyoderma, leishmaniasis, plasmacytic gastroenterocolitis, and amyloidosis.

Multiple myeloma is the most common cause of monoclonal gammopathy in small animal patients but remains an uncommon diagnosis.[7-9] Disease prevalence is less than 1% of all canine malignant tumors; it accounts for approximately 8% of canine hematopoietic tumors and less than 4% of primary bone tumors.[2,10] Myeloma is considered a rare tumor in the cat. Neoplastic proliferation typically occurs within the bone marrow, and patients subsequently develop diffuse systemic disease. In dogs, the excessively produced immunoglobulin is relatively equally distributed between IgG and IgA, whereas IgG appears to predominate in the small number of feline cases. There are also clinical reports of multiple myeloma resulting in monoclonal gammopathy in horses.[11-15] The clinical signs and laboratory abnormalities are similar to those reported in humans, dogs, and cats. Cryoglobulinemia, monoclonal proteins that form precipitates at less than 37°C, has been found in association with both canine multiple myeloma and macroglobulinemia.[7]

Primary macroglobulinemia is a proliferation of lymphoplasmacytoid cells intermediate between B lymphocytes and plasma cells in differentiation.[9] These tumors produce excessive quantities of IgM and are often associated with hyperviscosity syndrome (HVS) due to the structural size of this immunoglobulin class. Plasma cell leukemia is rare and is diagnosed by identifying circulating plasma cells from the bone marrow.[16] Alpha chain disease is a syndrome in which the neoplastic infiltrate is largely restricted to the small intestine and the circulating paraprotein is an IgA Fc fragment without an associated light chain. Typically, there is lymphoid or plasmacytoid intestinal infiltration. Heavy and light chain diseases have been rarely documented in dogs.[17-19] Nonsecretory myeloma is a variant of plasma cell neoplasia which does not result in production of monoclonal immunoglobulin and therefore lacks monoclonal gammopathy and Bence Jones proteinuria. It exhibits all other clinical features of myeloma but may require immunohistochemistry or electron microscopy for definitive diagnosis.[20,21]

Extramedullary plasmacytomas are generally considered to be benign tumors, but have occasionally been found in association with myeloma or lymphoma and have rarely been reported to metastasize.[22-28] These soft tissue tumors are composed of plasma cells at a location distant from the bone marrow and have been found in association with a monoclonal gammopathy. On some occasions, localized and systemic amyloid formation has been reported.[23-27,29-33] Common sites for extramedullary plasmacytomas are the feet, trunk, ears, mouth, and gastrointestinal tract. Although they are infrequently associated with circulating monoclonal gammopathy, demonstration of the monoclonal nature of the immunoglobulin produced locally is one of the diagnostic characteristics used to differentiate extramedullary plasmacytomas from an inflammatory plasma cell response. A rare biclonal gammopathy was identified in a cat with two hepatic extramedullary plasmacytomas.[34] One study suggested that simultaneous analysis of ploidy and relative $p62^{c\text{-}myc}$ oncoprotein concentrations can be used as an aid in assessment of malignant potential in canine plasma cell tumors.[35]

Monoclonal gammopathy of undetermined significance has been rarely reported in the dog.[36,37] It is an asymptomatic plasma cell dyscrasia characterized by paraproteinemia, but not associated with documented causes of monoclonal gammopathy. There are no apparent clinical signs of disease and it is most often an incidental finding that may be transient or remain constant for long periods. Bence Jones proteins may be present in the urine in small quantities. In humans, it occurs in approximately 0.15% of the general population. Long-term follow-up of this condition has shown that multiple myeloma develops in up to 16% of these patients, with an annual actuarial risk of 0.8%.[38] Diagnosis is by exclusion of all other causes of monoclonal gammopathy. Long-term follow-up is necessary to establish the benign nature of the gammopathy; the two identified canine cases were followed for 18 and 24 months.[36,37]

Other lymphoproliferative disorders have resulted in monoclonal gammopathy in both dogs and cats. Monoclonal gammopathy occurs in lymphoma patients if the phenotype of the neoplastic cells is a B cell capable of secreting immunoglobulin. Approximately 6% of canine lymphoma cases have monoclonal gammopathy.[2] Monoclonal gammopathy has been reported in a small number of cats with lymphoma, some of which were feline-leukemia-virus-positive or feline-immunodefi-

ciency-virus–positive.[39-41] CLL is a tumor of well-differentiated B lymphocytes. A monoclonal gammopathy can be identified in 68% of these dogs, and Bence Jones proteins in 40%[4]; CLL is a rare disorder in the cat.

Although neoplasia accounts for most cases of monoclonal gammopathy, several infectious diseases have also been reported to lead to this laboratory abnormality. Most infectious and inflammatory diseases result in antigenic stimulation that yields a polyclonal gammopathy, but under some circumstances, a monoclonal gammopathy can be identified. The infectious disease most commonly associated with monoclonal gammopathy in veterinary patients is canine ehrlichiosis.[42-46] All reported cases have been shown to have monoclonal IgG protein and frequently exhibit bone marrow plasmacytosis. The serum protein pattern has been variably characterized by a distinct narrow-base monoclonal spike, a broad-base monoclonal spike, or a monoclonal spike superimposed on a polyclonal gammopathy.[43] However, in some cases of canine ehrlichiosis, the apparent monoclonal spike is the result of polyclonal gammopathy consisting of one heavy chain class of IgG and at least four subclasses (IgG_{1-4}), rather than a true monoclonal gammopathy with a single heavy chain class, subclass, and light chain class.[47] In the absence of monospecific antisera, immunoelectrophoresis cannot reliably distinguish between polyclonal and monoclonal gammopathy if only isotype-specific heavy chain class antibody is used for reagents. In a recent report, serum electrophoresis suggested a monoclonal gammopathy in a dog with thrombocytopathia due to *Ehrlichia canis* infection, but heterogeneity of light chains in the urine suggested that the gammopathy was actually polyclonal.[48]

Because there are numerous similarities in the clinical, hematologic, and immunologic findings between multiple myeloma and ehrlichiosis, an *E. canis* titer should be performed in all dogs in which definitive evidence of myeloma, lymphoma, or macroglobulinemia is lacking or a diagnosis of monoclonal gammopathy of undetermined significance is contemplated.[43] Although in most cases the gammopathy will resolve with appropriate doxycycline or tetracycline therapy, plasmapheresis and chemotherapy have been used to treat the monoclonal gammopathy associated with this rickettsial disease.[43,44]

Other infectious or inflammatory diseases that have been associated with monoclonal gammopathy include feline infectious peritonitis, visceral leishmaniasis, chronic pyoderma, plasmacytic gastroenterocolitis, and Aleutian mink disease.[49-53] Monoclonal gammopathy in these cases has typically been due to excessive production of IgG. In rare circumstances, amyloidosis has been associated with monoclonal gammopathy.[54]

DIAGNOSTIC APPROACH

With the listed differential diagnoses in mind, evaluation of the patient with monoclonal gammopathy must define the underlying etiology and extent of organ involvement as well as determine the presence of associated abnormalities including HVS and hypercalcemia. The first diagnostic step is to recognize the presence of a hyperglobulinemia, which must still be identified as polyclonal or monoclonal gammopathy by serum electrophoresis. Serum electrophoresis should be performed if globulins are greater than or equal to 5 gm/dL or there is a high degree of suspicion for plasma cell neoplasia.[2] A sharp spike-like peak is considered monoclonal if its width is less than or equal to the serum albumin spike.[9] If electrophoresis identifies a monoclonal spike, immunoelectrophoresis can specifically identify the class of immunoglobulin that has been produced in excessive quantities in serum or urine specimens. Urine immunoelectrophoresis tends to be cumbersome due to the requirement of 24-hour urine collection to retrieve a specimen appropriate for concentration. Evaluation of urine for the presence of Bence Jones proteins can be a useful diagnostic test, but urine dipsticks are insensitive to this protein. A heat precipitation test is most often used to identify Bence Jones proteins, but urine electrophoresis remains the preferred method. The heat precipitation method is useful as a screening test, but fails to detect the proteins in some cases and may give false-positive results with renal insufficiency, connective tissue diseases, and certain malignancies.[9] Approximately 40% of dogs and 30% of cats with myeloma have Bence Jones proteinuria.[9]

The diagnostic evaluation for identification of the underlying etiology of monoclonal gammopathy will be dictated by the clinical signs exhibited. Clinical signs associated with paraproteinemia are secondary to neoplastic infiltration of specific organ systems, excessive production of paraproteins, or both of these processes. Dogs with multiple myeloma are more likely to experience paraneoplastic syndromes than patients with other malignancies.[55] Indeed, bone lesions, hypercalcemia, and anemia correlate directly with the total mass of myeloma cells.[38] However, regardless of the presenting clinical syndrome, all patients should be assessed with a complete blood count, platelet count, biochemical profile, and urinalysis.

Because multiple myeloma is the most common cause of monoclonal gammopathy, appropriate testing for this lymphoproliferative disorder is always indicated. For a diagnosis of myeloma to be confirmed, at least three of the following five criteria should be met: monoclonal gammopathy of IgG or IgA type, radiographic evidence of osteolytic bone lesions or diffuse osteoporosis, Bence Jones proteinuria, excessive numbers of plasma cells in the bone marrow, or histologic diagnosis of plasma cell tumor of soft tissues in a patient with concurrent bone marrow neoplasia.

A bone marrow examination by aspiration or biopsy is indicated in any case of monoclonal gammopathy because some cases of multiple myeloma, lymphoma, and CLL may be diagnosed definitively by this technique. The number of plasma cells found in the canine marrow should be less than 2% of the cellular population.[56] Collection of a diagnostic bone marrow specimen may require more than one attempt, because distribution of myeloma within the marrow cavity can be focal

and discrete. Diffuse infiltration of lymphocytoid plasma cells with cluster formation is a criterion for diagnosis in multiple myeloma, but possible sampling error and difficulty in determining malignancy in suspected cases with reactive marrow plasmacytosis must always be considered before making a definitive diagnosis.[7] Whereas sheets and clusters of plasma cells can be seen with myeloma, increased numbers of plasma cells scattered among normal bone marrow elements may be more supportive of a diagnosis of ehrlichiosis or other causes of chronic antigenic stimulation.[2] Myeloma plasma cells may be atypical in appearance or appear similar to normal plasma cells. Other indicated tests include assessment for the presence of Bence Jones proteins in the urine and evaluation for osteolytic bone lesions with a bone scan or radiographic surveys of the thorax, abdomen, pelvis, and spine. Many dogs with multiple myeloma have osteolysis or diffuse osteoporosis; this finding is uncommon in cats.[9]

The diagnosis of canine ehrlichiosis is considered in endemic portions of the country or in patients with an appropriate travel history, and is based on serology and response to doxycycline or tetracycline therapy. Any abnormal masses or enlarged lymph nodes in a patient with monoclonal gammopathy should be subjected to aspiration cytology or surgical biopsy. Abnormal fluid accumulations can be evaluated cytologically and electrophoresis can be performed, particularly in patients in which feline infectious peritonitis remains an important differential diagnosis. However, peritoneal and pleural effusion has been reported in a cat with IgA monoclonal gammopathy secondary to multiple myeloma.[57] A diagnosis of benign monoclonal gammopathy can be made only after elimination of all other possible diseases that can be associated with monoclonal gammopathy and evaluation of the stability of the paraprotein concentrations over time.[1]

Evaluation of the extent of organ involvement or associated abnormalities will also be based on presenting clinical signs. HVS should be suspected if coagulopathies, retinal hemorrhage, neurologic signs, or difficulty with blood withdrawal during venipuncture are noted.[55,58–63] Hyperviscosity is diagnosed by comparing the viscosity of the patient's serum to water. If hyperviscosity is diagnosed, it is most often associated with IgM and IgA paraproteinemia, but has also been recognized when large quantities of IgG are present.

Renal insufficiency is common in patients with monoclonal gammopathy, particularly myeloma patients. Mechanisms contributing to renal dysfunction include damage caused by light chain precipitation within renal tubular epithelium and tubular lumens, pyelonephritis, secondary amyloidosis or glomerulonephritis, dehydration, and hypercalcemia.[55,64] Hypercalcemia is identified in approximately 16% of dogs with myeloma and 20% of dogs with lymphoma.[8,65] In patients with monoclonal gammopathy secondary to myeloma, hypercalcemia has been associated with shorter median survival times.[8]

Bleeding disorders may occur as sequelae of thrombocytopenia, altered platelet function, interaction between paraproteins and coagulation factors, inhibitors of coagulation proteins, abnormal fibrin polymerization, HVS, and disseminated intravascular coagulation.[8,48,55,66,67] Approximately 66% of dogs with myeloma have radiographic evidence of bone involvement and nearly half of these have spinal involvement.[68] Increased osteoclast activity is believed to be the underlying mechanism.[55] The presence of extensive bony lesions adversely affects the prognosis in myeloma patients, with significantly shorter median survival times.[8]

THERAPY

Therapy for monoclonal gammopathy is dependent on the definitive diagnosis of the underlying disease condition as well as the severity of the accompanying clinical manifestations including hyperviscosity, renal failure, hypercalcemia, coagulopathies, and pathologic fracture. Treatment success can be judged by the decreasing size of the monoclonal spike (which is proportional to tumor burden in myeloma patients), amelioration of clinical signs, and resolution of Bence Jones proteinuria.[9] The most important premise of therapy is to treat the underlying disease process while providing supportive care for the frequent complications associated with these diseases. Indicated therapies may include chemotherapy (myeloma, macroglobulinemia, lymphoma, CLL), plasma exchange or plasmapheresis, transfusions, fluid therapy, antibiotics, and specific treatment of hypercalcemia. No therapy is recommended for monoclonal gammopathy of undetermined significance, but long-term follow-up is clearly warranted in these cases.

REFERENCES

1. **Dorfman M. Dimski DS.** Paraproteinemias in small animal medicine. Compend Cont Educ Pract Vet 1992;14:621–632.
2. **Thompson JP.** Immunologic diseases. In: Ettinger SJ, Feldman EC, eds. Textbook of veterinary internal medicine. 4th ed. Philadelphia: WB Saunders, 1995;2002–2029.
3. **Jain NC.** The plasma proteins, dysproteinemias, and immune deficiency disorders. In: Jain NC, ed. Schalm's veterinary hematology. 4th ed. Philadelphia: Lea & Febiger, 1986;940–989.
4. **Leifer CE, Matus RE.** Chronic lymphocytic leukemia in the dog: 22 cases (1974–1984). J Am Vet Med Assoc 1986;189:214–217.
5. **MacEwen EG, Hurvitz AI, Hayes A.** Hyperviscosity syndrome associated with lymphocytic leukemia in three dogs. J Am Vet Med Assoc 1977; 170:1309–1312.
6. **Kristensen AT, Klausner JS, Weiss DJ.** Spurious hyperphosphatemia in a dog with chronic lymphocytic leukemia and an IgM monoclonal gammopathy. Vet Clin Pathol 1991;20:45–48.
7. **Matus RE, Leifer CE.** Immunoglobulin-producing tumors. Vet Clin North Am Small Anim Pract 1985;15:741–753.
8. **Matus RE, Leifer CE, MacEwen EG, Hurvitz AI.** Prognostic factors for multiple myeloma. J Am Vet Med Assoc 1986;188:1288–1292.
9. **Hohenhaus AE.** Syndromes of hyperglobulinemia: diagnosis and therapy. In: Bonagura JD, ed. Current vaterinary therapy XII. Philadelphia: WB Saunders, 1995;523–530.
10. **Morrison WB.** Plasma cell neoplasms. In: Morrison WB, ed. Cancer in dogs and cats. Baltimore: Williams & Wilkins, 1998;697–704.
11. **Edwards DF, Parker JW, Wilkinson JE, Helman RG.** Plasma cell myeloma in the horse: a case report and literature review. J Vet Intern Med 1993;7:169–176.
12. **Mac Allister C, Qualls C, Tyler R, Root CR.** Multiple myeloma in a horse. J Am Vet Med Assoc 1987;191:337–339.
13. **Markel MD, Dorr TE.** Multiple myeloma in a horse. J Am Vet Med Assoc 1986;188:621–623.
14. **Henry M, Presse K, White S.** Hemorrhagic diathesis caused by multiple myeloma in a three-month-old foal. J Am Vet Med Assoc 1989;194:392–394.
15. **Geelen SNJ, Bernadine WE, Grinwis GCM, Kalsbeek HC.** Monoclonal gammopathy in Dutch warmblood mare. Vet Q 1997;19:29–32.
16. **Couto CG, Ruehl W, Muir S.** Plasma cell leukemia and monoclonal (IgG) gammopathy in a dog. J Am Vet Med Assoc 1984;185:90–92.
17. **Hoenig M.** Multiple myeloma associated with the heavy chains of immunoglobulin A in a dog. J Am Vet Med Assoc 1987;190:1191–1192.
18. **Gopegui RR, Espada Y, Vilafranca M, Cuadradas C, Fontcuberta E, Milla F, Roncales J, Ruzafa A.** Paraprotein-induced defective haemostasis in a dog with IgA (kappa-light chain) forming myeloma. Vet Clin Pathol 1994;23:70–71.
19. **Day MJ, Penhale WJ, McKenna RP, Mills JN, Pass DA.** Two cases of IgA multiple myeloma in the dog. J Small Anim Pract 1987;28:147–156.
20. **Marks SL, Moore PF, Taylor DW, Munn RJ.** Nonsecretory multiple myeloma in a dog: immunohistologic and ultrastructural observation. J Vet Intern Med 1995;9:50–54.
21. **MacEwen EG, Patnaik AK, Hurvitz AI, Bradley R, Claypoole TF, Withrow SJ, Erlandson RA, Lieberman PH.** Nonsecretory multiple myeloma in two dogs. J Am Vet Med Assoc 1984;184:1283–1286.
22. **Lester SJ, Mesfin GM.** A solitary plasmacytoma in a dog with progression to a disseminated myeloma. Can Vet J 1980;21:284–286.
23. **Rakich PM, Latimer KS, Weiss R, Steffens WL.** Mucocutaneous plasmacytomas in dogs: 75 cases (1980–1987). J Am Vet Med Assoc 1989;194:803–810.
24. **Carothers MA, Johnson GC, DiBartola, Liepnicks J, Benson MD.** Extramedullary plasmacytoma and immunoglobulin-associated amyloidosis in a cat. J Am Vet Med Assoc 1989;195:1593–1597.
25. **Mandel NS, Esplin DG.** A retroperitoneal extramedullary plasmacytoma in a cat with a monoclonal gammopathy. J Am Anim Hosp Assoc 1994;30:603–608.
26. **Trevor PB, Saunders GK, Waldron DR, Leib MS.** Metastatic extramedullary plasmacytoma of the colon and rectum in a dog. J Am Vet Med Assoc 1993;203:406–409.
27. **Jackson MW, Helfand SC, Smedes SL, Bradley GA, Schultz RD.** Primary IgG secreting plasma cell tumor in the gastrointestinal tract of a dog. J Am Vet Med Assoc 1994;204:404–406.
28. **Trigo FJ, Hargis AM.** Canine cutaneous plasmacytoma with regional lymph node metastasis. Vet Med 1983;78:1749–1751.
29. **Baer KE, Patnaik AK, Gilbertson SR, Hurvitz AI.** Cutaneous plasmacytomas in dogs: a morphologic and immunohistochemical study. Vet Pathol 1989;26:216–221.
30. **Clark GN, Berg J, Engler SJ, Bronson RT.** Extramedullary plasmacytomas in dogs: results of surgical excision in 131 cases. J Am Anim Hosp Assoc 1992;28:105–111.
31. **Rowland PH, Valentine BA, Stebbins KE, Smith CA.** Cutaneous plasmacytomas with amyloid in six dogs. Vet Pathol 1991;28:125–130.
32. **Geisel O, Stiglmair-Herb M, Linke RP.** Myeloma associated with immunoglobulin lambda-light chain derived amyloid in a dog. Vet Pathol 1990;27:374–376.
33. **MacEwen EG, Patnaik AK, Johnson GF, Hurvitz AI, Erlandson RA.** Extramedullary plasmacytoma of the gastrointestinal tract in two dogs. J Am Vet Med Assoc 1984;184:1396–1398.
34. **Larsen AE, Carpenter JL.** Hepatic plasmacytoma and biclonal gammopathy in a cat. J Am Vet Med Assoc 1994;205:708–710.
35. **Frazier KS, Hines ME, Hurvitz AI, Robinson PG, Herron AJ.** Analysis of DNA aneuploidy and c-myc oncoprotein content of canine plasma cell tumors using flow cytometry. Vet Pathol 1993;30:505–511.
36. **Dewhirst MW, Stamp GL, Hurvitz AI.** Idiopathic monoclonal (IgA) gammopathy on a dog. J Am Vet Med Assoc 1977;170:1313–1316.
37. **Hoenig M, O'Brien JA.** A benign hypergammaglobulinemia mimicking plasma cell myeloma. J Am Anim Hosp Assoc 1988;24:688–690.
38. **Bataille R, Harousseau JL.** Multiple myeloma. N Engl J Med 1997;336:1657–1662.
39. **Williams DA, Goldschmidt MH.** Hyperviscosity syndrome with IgM monoclonal gammopathy and hepatic plasmacytoid lymphosarcoma in a cat. J Small Anim Pract 1982;23:311–323.
40. **Rosenberg MP, Hohenhaus AE, Matus RE.** Monoclonal gammopathy and lymphoma in a cat infected with feline immunodeficiency virus. J Am Anim Hosp Assoc 1991;27:335–337.
41. **Dust A, Norris Am, Valli VEO.** Cutaneous lymphosarcoma with IgG monoclonal gammopathy, serum hyperviscosity and hypercalcemia in a cat. Can Vet J 1982;23:235–239.
42. **Hoskins JD, Barta O, Rothschmitt J.** Serum hyperviscosity syndrome associated with Ehrlichia canis infection in a dog. J Am Vet Med Assoc 1983;183:1011–1012.
43. **Breitschwerdt EB, Woody BJ, Zerbe CA, De Buysscher EV, Barta O.** Monoclonal gammopathy associated with naturally occurring canine ehrlichiosis. J Vet Intern Med 1987;1:2–9.
44. **Matus RE, Leifer CE, Hurvitz AI.** Use of plasmapheresis and chemotherapy for treatment of monoclonal gammopathy associated with Ehrlichia canis infection in a dog. J Am Vet Med Assoc 1987;190:1302–1304.
45. **Perille AL, Matus RE.** Canine ehrlichiosis in six dogs with persistently increased antibody titers. J Vet Intern Med 1991;5:195–198.
46. **Harrus S, Waner T, Avidar Y, Bogin E, Peh H, Bark H.** Serum protein alterations in canine ehrlichiosis. Vet Parasitol 1996;66:241–249.

47. **Michels GM, Boon GD, Jones BD, Puget B.** Hypergammaglobulinemia in a dog. J Am Vet Med Assoc 1995;207:567–570.

48. **Varela F, Font X, Valladares JE, Alberola J.** Thrombocytopathia and light-chain proteinuria in a dog naturally infected with *Ehrlichia canis*. J Vet Intern Med 1997;11:309–311.

49. **MacEwen EG, Hurvitz AI.** Diagnosis and management of monoclonal gammopathies. Vet Clin North Am Small Anim Pract 1977;7:119–132.

50. **Front A, Closa JM, Mascort J.** Monoclonal gammopathy in a dog with visceral leishmaniasis. J Vet Intern Med 1994;8:233–235.

51. **Burkhard MJ, Meyer DJ, Rosychuk RA, O'Neill SP, Schultheiss PC.** Monoclonal gammopathy in a dog with chronic pyoderma. J Vet Intern Med 1995;9:357–360.

52. **Diehl KJ, Lappin MR, Jones RL, Cayatte S.** Monoclonal gammopathy in a dog with plasmacytic gastroenteritis. J Am Vet Med Assoc 1992;201:1233–1236.

53. **Tizard IR.** B cells and their response to antigen. In: Tizard IR, ed. Veterinary immunology: an introduction. 5th ed. Philadelphia: WB Saunders, 1996, 121–140.

54. **Schwartzman RM.** Cutaneous amyloidosis associated with a monoclonal gammopathy in a dog. J Am Vet Med Assoc 1984;185:102–104.

55. **Hammer AS, Couto CG.** Complications of multiple myeloma. J Am Anim Hosp Assoc 1994;30:9–14.

56. **Tyler RD, Cowell RL, Meinkoth JH.** Bone marrow. In: Cowell RL, Tyler RD, Meinkoth JH, eds. Diagnostic cytology and hematology of the dog and cat. 2nd ed. St. Louis: Mosby, 1999, 284–304.

57. **Hawkins EC, Feldman BF, Blanchard PC.** Immunoglobulin A myeloma in a cat with pleural effusion and serum hyperviscosity. J Am Vet Med Assoc 1986;188;876–878.

58. **Forrester SD, Relford RL.** Serum hyperviscosity syndrome: its diagnosis and treatment. Vet Med 1992;87:48–54.

59. **Forrester SD, Greco DS, Relford RL.** Serum hyperviscosity syndrome associated with multiple myeloma in two cats. J Am Vet Med Assoc 1992;200:79–82.

60. **Hribernik TN, Barta O, Gaunt SD, Boudreaux MK.** Serum hyperviscosity syndrome associated with IgG myeloma in a cat. J Am Vet Med Assoc 1982;181:169–170.

61. **Shull RM, Osborne CA, Barrett RE, Schultz RD, Stevens JB, Hammer RF, Hurvitz AI.** Serum hyperviscosity syndrome associated with IgA multiple myeloma in two dogs. J Am Anim Hosp Assoc 1978;14:58–70.

62. **Kirschner SE, Niyo Y, Hill BL, Betts DM.** Blindness in a dog with IgA-forming myeloma. J Am Ved Med Assoc 1988;193:349–350.

63. **Center SA, Smith JF.** Ocular lesions in a dog with serum hyperviscosity secondary to an IgA myeloma. J Am Vet Med Assoc 1982;181:811–813.

64. **Campbell KL, Latimer KS.** Polysystemic manifestations of plasma cell myeloma in the dog: a case report and review. J Am Anim Hosp Assoc 1985;21:59–66.

65. **Rosenberg MP, Matus RE, Patnaik AK.** Prognostic factors in dogs with lymphoma and associated hypercalcemia. J Vet Intern Med 1991;5:268–271.

66. **Shepard VJ, Dodds-Laffin WJ, Laffin RJ.** Gamma A myeloma in a dog with defective hemostasis. J Am Vet Med Assoc 1972;160:1121–1127.

67. **Miller C, Fish MB, Danelski TF.** IgA multiple myeloma with multi-system manifestations in the dog: a case report. J Am Anim Hosp Assoc 1982;18:53–56.

68. **van Bree H, Pollet L, Cousement W, Van Der Stock J, Mattheeuws D.** Cervical cord compression as a neurologic complication in an IgG multiple myeloma in a dog. J Am Anim Hosp Assoc 1983;19:317–323.

CHAPTER 142

Hypoalbuminemia

• M.D. WILLARD

Finding hypoalbuminemia often helps the clinician quickly narrow the list of differential diagnoses to be considered in a given patient. Although found in all species, hypoalbuminemia tends to be more common in dogs than in cats. Severe hypoalbuminemia (i. e., serum albumin less than or equal to 2.0 gm/dL [normal, 2.5 to 4.4 gm/dL]) will be considered separately from mild hypoalbuminemia (i.e., serum albumin 2.1 to 2.5 gm/dL).

Hypoalbuminemia should be suspected whenever pitting edema or a low-protein, pure transudate (abdominal or pleural) is found. Failing to find such abnormal fluid accumulations does not lessen the likelihood of hypoalbuminemia; some pets have ascites when the serum albumin concentration is 1.5 gm/dL, whereas some will not have ascites even when the serum albumin is less than or equal to 1.0 gm/dL. Serum albumin should be less than or equal to 1.5 gm/dL to consider hypoalbuminemia as the sole cause of such effusions.

The first step after finding hypoalbuminemia is to eliminate artifact. Artifactual hypoalbuminemia is one of the more common serum chemistry profile problems encountered in veterinary medicine. Laboratories designed to evaluate human sera typically report canine serum samples as having serum albumin concentrations of less than 2.0 gm/dL, and sometimes less than 1.0 gm/dL, even if the true value is greater than 3.0 gm/dL. Newer chemistry analyzers are inconsistently affected by lipemia, hemolysis, and icterus, meaning that one cannot predict the effects of these variables without knowing the specifics of the particular system being used in the laboratory. Therefore, anytime the serum albumin concentration is unexpectedly low (even when using a laboratory dedicated to analyzing canine and feline samples), it should be redetermined on another serum sample.

There are four major considerations for severe hypoalbuminemia: decreased production due to hepatic insufficiency (HI), increased loss due to protein-losing nephropathy (PLN), protein-losing enteropathy (PLE) including gastric protein loss, or loss from cutaneous lesions or hemorrhage. Although some clinicians recommend evaluating the serum globulin concentration in conjunction with the serum albumin concentration to help determine the cause of hypoalbuminemia, the au-

thor discourages this approach. Although PLE often causes panhypoproteinemia, in contrast to PLN and HI (which often have a normal to increased serum globulin concentration), there are many exceptions. In addition, it is practical and relatively easy to diagnose HI and PLN definitively with specific laboratory testing (see below). If serum globulins are increased by any of several diseases (e.g., heartworm disease, Ehrlichiosis), the serum globulin concentration may remain in the normal range despite excessive loss into the alimentary tract. Furthermore, some hepatic diseases are associated with decreased serum globulin concentrations.[1]

Cutaneous loss is usually the easiest cause of hypoalbuminemia to diagnose, because there must be either major hemorrhage or severely inflamed lesions with large amounts of exuding serum. Examples of the latter include deep burns (fortunately rare in small animals) and tumors. These lesions are usually easy to diagnose in the examination room. Animals undergoing open abdominal drainage for peritonitis lose albumin but seldom become hypoalbuminemic.[2]

Protein-losing nephropathies due to glomerular disease are also easily diagnosed. Urinalysis typically reveals significant protein loss, but there are potential diagnostic pitfalls. If the urine is dilute (e.g., specific gravity less than 1.017), there may be substantial urinary protein loss with little or no protein detected by a urinary dipstick. High urine pH may be associated with false-positive protein readings on urine dipsticks. For questionable cases, a urine protein:creatinine ratio should be requested after the urine sediment has been examined. If the sediment is active (i.e., white blood cells, red blood cells, bacteria), the cause should be determined and resolved, because hemorrhage and inflammation can cause dramatically high ratios that disappear after resolution of the infection or hemorrhage. However, if the ratio is less than 0.5, urinary protein losses are not responsible for hypoalbuminemia even if the sediment is active. If the ratio is between 0.5 and 1 and the sediment is inactive, then it is not clear whether there is abnormal protein loss in the urine. If the ratio is greater than 1 despite an inactive sediment, then the pet is losing excessive amounts of protein into the urine.[3] Not all dogs with ratios greater than 1 will be hypoalbuminemic; ratios between 1 and 4 are variably associated with hypoalbuminemia. Most dogs with glomerular disease severe enough to cause severe hypoalbuminemia have ratios greater than 5. Many animals with PLN are not azotemic. Renal biopsy in animals with PLN is currently of questionable value, because until there is specific therapy for either amyloidosis or glomerulonephritis (the two main causes of PLN), the therapeutic approach is often the same with symptomatic treatment and attempts to eliminate the underlying cause. The prognosis tends to be worse for amyloidosis, but some patients with glomerulonephritis have similarly bad clinical courses. In general, dogs with renal amyloidosis tend to have higher protein: creatinine ratios than dogs with glomerulonephritis (i.e., greater than 20 versus 5 to 15, respectively).

After PLN and cutaneous losses are eliminated, HI is the next consideration. HI is not the same as hepatic disease. Hepatic disease must be so severe that function is lost before HI occurs. Classic causes of severe HI causing hypoalbuminemia include chronic hepatitis,[4] hepatic cirrhosis,[4] hepatic tumors,[5] and hepatic atrophy (especially due to congenital portosystemic shunts[1]), although inflammatory disease may also be responsible. If a pet is icteric due to hepatocellular disease or has major increases in alanine aminotransferase (ALT) (e.g., greater than 5 to 6 times normal), then it is reasonable to tentatively attribute hypoalbuminemia to HI (assuming that PLN has already been eliminated). However, if the ALT and serum albumin protein (SAP) are only modestly increased, then it may be uncertain whether hepatic disease is causing hypoalbuminemia. Furthermore, animals with HI due to cirrhosis, hepatic tumors, or hepatic atrophy may have normal ALT, SAP, and/or serum bilirubin.[1,4] Although decreased blood urea nitrogen (BUN) and hypoglycemia are classic signs in HI, they are missing in many HI patients with hypoalbuminemia. Postprandial bile acid determinations are usually the quickest and most reliable method of diagnosing HI.[6] There is seldom any benefit in measuring them in animals that are icteric from hepatobiliary disease. Postprandial bile acid concentrations greater than 80 to 100 μmol/L typically (but not invariably) reflect HI severe enough to cause hypoalbuminemia. Postprandial values greater than 20 but less than 80 μmol/L are typically associated with hepatic pathology, but the disease may not be severe enough to cause marked hypoalbuminemia. Preprandial bile acid determinations are often diagnostic of HI (especially in dogs), but postprandial values sometimes detect HI (especially congenital portosystemic shunt) that is missed by preprandial determinations. Serum bile acid concentrations cannot differentiate one hepatic disease from another; they are only used to identify HI. Ultimately, hepatic biopsy is indicated in most animals with hepatic parenchymal disease to determine the cause and severity of HI. If a congenital portosystemic shunt is suspected, abdominal ultrasonography is usually performed to attempt to distinguish intrahepatic from extrahepatic shunts. Abdominal imaging sometimes identifies hepatic disease quickly, with evidence such as marked microhepatia or hepatic masses.

After cutaneous losses, PLN, and HI have been eliminated by physical examination, urine protein: creatinine ratio, and postprandial bile acid concentrations, PLE becomes the next major consideration. PLE tends to be a diagnosis of exclusion but laboratory tests that definitively diagnose PLE, including fecal alpha 1-protease inhibitor,[7] are becoming more available. Even if the patient has "obvious" alimentary tract disease, urinalysis and postprandial bile acid determinations are reasonable diagnostic tests to perform to be sure there is not concurrent PLN or HI. Finally, many pets with PLE do not have vomiting or diarrhea; therefore, one cannot presumptively eliminate PLE based on history and physical examination.

If PLE exists, it is imperative to determine the cause. The most common causes in adult dogs are inflammatory bowel disease, alimentary lymphoma, intestinal lymphangiectasia, intestinal fungal infections (i.e., histoplasmosis and pythiosis), and hemorrhage due to ulceration/erosion. A patient may be bleeding into the gastrointestinal tract enough to cause hypoalbuminemia without having obviously bloody (i.e., melenic) stools. The most common causes in puppies are hookworms and chronic intussusception. The most common causes in cats are inflammatory bowel disease and alimentary lymphoma. Abdominal ultrasonography is usually a good first step in patients with PLE because lesions causing PLE may be diffuse or focal. Laparotomy may be preferred if ultrasonography reveals that there is a focal lesion out of reach of an endoscope, an intussusception, or that there is a localized mass lesion that could be resected. Otherwise, gastroduodenoscopy and colon-oileoscopy are usually diagnostic. Regardless of whether intestinal biopsy specimens are obtained endoscopically or surgically, multiple biopsies are indicated unless there is an obvious bleeding tumor or intussusception. Lymphangiectasia may be hard to detect, especially if the patient has been fasted or anorexic for more than 2 days. Feeding cream or corn oil the night before endoscopy or surgery may make it much easier to see the lesions and diagnostic histologic changes.[8]

Biopsies of the liver and intestine are usually the ultimate diagnostic tests for HI and PLE, respectively. Therefore, some clinicians perform a laparotomy as soon as PLN is eliminated (especially if ultrasonography and endoscopy are unavailable) in order to biopsy the liver and intestines. However, if ultrasonography and endoscopy are available, the diagnosis can usually be made with less trauma and risk to the patient.

Canine hypoadrenocorticism has also been associated with hypoalbuminemia.[9] The low albumin is often found after 1 to 3 days of fluid therapy, rather than on presentation when the patient is usually hemoconcentrated. The mechanism is unknown but may be due to PLE.

Finally, a patient may have more than one cause of hypoalbuminemia, PLN may be caused by a hepatic tumor or alimentary tract inflammation, which is also capable of causing hypoalbuminemia. In general, anorexia and/or cachexia by themselves are inadequate reasons for *severe* hypoalbuminemia. Although anorexia can obviously worsen hypoalbuminemia caused by HI

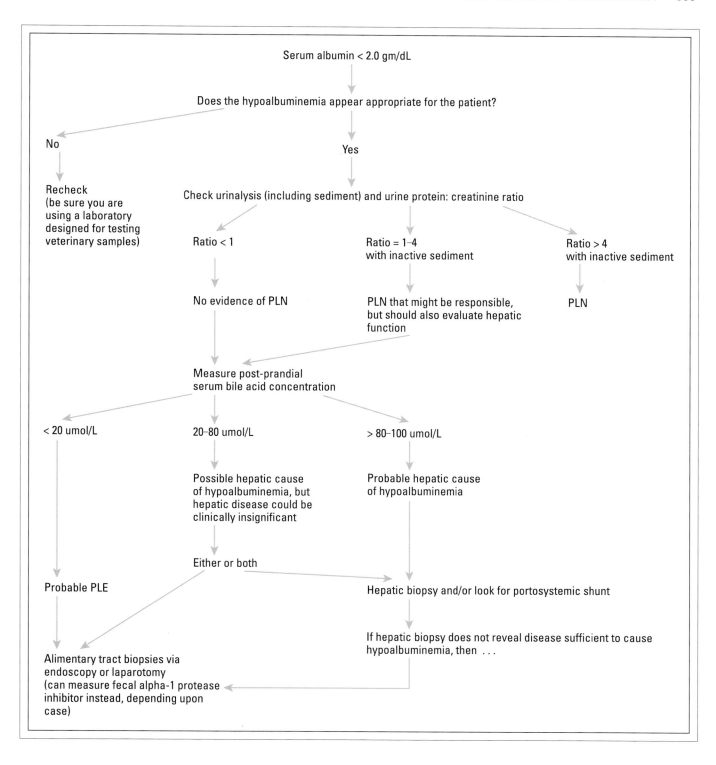

or PLE, it is generally unable to cause severe hypoalbuminemia by itself. If a cachectic and / or anorexic animal has severe hypoalbuminemia, these other causes need to be investigated.

Animals with mild hypoalbuminemia may have the same diseases that cause severe hypoalbuminemia. They may also have excessive fluid retention, which dilutes the serum albumin concentration. For example, a dog with ascites due to right-sided congestive heart failure or abdominal neoplasia may have low serum albumin detected on a chemistry profile. If there is repeated removal of abdominal effusion by paracentesis, this constitutes an additional loss of albumin as all effusions contain some albumin. The consequence will be a further lowering of the serum albumin concentration, which makes it that much easier for the effusion to recur due to progressively decreasing plasma oncotic pressure, regardless of its original cause. Reformation of the effusion then lowers the serum albumin concentration as still more albumin is drawn into the body cavity, creating a positive feedback loop. Severe accumulations of edema fluid might likewise sequester and dilute the serum albumin concentration. Severe vasculitis might cause substantial edema and subsequent albumin sequestration. However, edema and vasculitis appear to be rare causes of hypoalbuminemia.

Malabsorptive diseases and/or exocrine pancreatic insufficiency might cause hypoalbuminemia in some patients. However, it seems more likely that these patients have PLE due to the disease process causing the malabsorption or concurrent small intestinal bacterial problems. Compensatory decrease of serum albumin due to hyperglobulinemia has been mentioned in many texts, but little has been done to de-termine the importance of this phenomena in veterinary patients.

REFERENCES

1. **Center SA.** Hepatic vascular diseases. In: Strombeck's small animal gastroenterology. 3rd ed. Philadelphia. WB Saunders, 1996;802–846.
2. **Greenfield CL, Walshaw R.** Open peritoneal drainage for treatment of contaminated peritoneal cavity and septic peritonitis in dogs and cats: 24 cases (1980–1986). J Am Vet Med Assoc 1987;191:100–105.
3. **Lulich JP, Osborne CA.** Interpretation of urine protein-creatinine ratios in dogs with glomerular and nonglomerular disorders. Compend Cont Educ Pract Vet 1990;12:59–72.
4. **Center SA.** Chronic hepatitis, cirrhosis, breed-specific hepatopathies, copper storage hepatopathy, suppurative hepatitis, granulomatous hepatitis, and idiopathic hepatic fibrosis. In: Strombeck's small animal gastroenterology. 3rd ed. Philadelphia: WB Saunders, 1996;705–765.
5. **Strombeck DR, Guilford WG.** Hepatic neoplasms. In: Strombeck's small animal gastroenterology. 3rd ed. Philadelphia: WB Saunders, 1996; 847–859.
6. **Center SA.** Serum bile acids in companion animal medicine. Vet Clin North Am Small Anim Pract 1993;23:625–657.
7. **Melgarejo T, Williams DA, Tamayo A.** Fecal alpha 1-protease inhibitor for the diagnosis of canine protein-losing enteropathy (PLE). Proc Am Coll Vet Intern Med 1997; 15:45.
8. **Veldhuyzen Van Zanten SJO, Bartelsman JFWM, Tytgat GNJ.** Endoscopic diagnosis of primary intestinal lymphangiectasia using a high-fat meal. Endoscopy 1986;18:108–110.
9. **Langlais-Burgess L, Lumsden JH, Mackin A.** Concurrent hypoadrenocorticism and hypoalbuminemia in dogs: a retrospective study. J Am Anim Hosp Assoc 1995;31:307–311.

CHAPTER 143

Immunodeficiency Disorders

• DEBRA ZORAN

Mammalian immune defenses are composed of two primary components, the nonspecific (innate) and specific (acquired) immune systems. The nonspecific immune system is made up of phagocytic cells (such as neutrophils, monocytes, and macrophages) and the complement components, both of which are responsible for engulfment, digestion, or elimination of foreign substances. Alternatively, lymphocytes make up the specific immune system and are the only cells in the body capable of specifically recognizing antigenic determinants. Lymphocytes are subdivided into two functional groups: B cells, which are part of the humoral immune system, and T lymphocytes, which comprise the cell-mediated immune system. The interaction of antigen with the membrane-bound antibody on the surface of B cells triggers B-cell activation and development of effector cells which actively secrete antibody.[1] T lymphocytes recognize foreign protein antigens that are associated with major histocompatibility complex (MHC) molecules on the surfaces of antigen presenting cells or target cells.[2] Antigen recognition by T cells is the initiating stimulus for T-cell activation, which, depending on the type of T cell, leads to secretion of cytokines (e.g., interleukins), clonal proliferation, or the performance of regulatory or effector functions of T cells. A deficiency in either component of the immune system results in an increased susceptibility to infection, which is the hallmark of immunodeficiency disease. The severity, location, and type of infections observed will depend on the part of the immune system affected. For example, defects in B-cell numbers or function usually predispose the animal to increased susceptibility to bacterial infections, whereas animals with abnormal T-cell numbers or function have increased susceptibility to fungal, protozoal, and viral infections.[3] Because immunodeficiencies in the broadest sense involve all aspects of immunity, including the nonspecific response, this discussion will only be concerned with the specific immune response.

Immunodeficiency diseases can be classified as either primary (hereditary or congenital) or secondary (acquired) immunodeficiency disorders. Primary immune deficiency disorders are associated with severe, recurrent infections in neonatal animals and often result in death. Acquired immunodeficiency disorders are more common and occur secondary to a disease process, such as feline immunodeficiency virus, or result from neoplastic, metabolic, or nutritional causes that alter the immune system. The clinical picture (e. g., recurrent infections) is the same as in primary immunodeficiency disorders; however, secondary immune deficiencies may be transient if the inciting cause is corrected.

CLINICAL SIGNS AND DIAGNOSIS

There is a wide variation in the clinical presentation of animals with immune system disease. The classic clinical manifestation of immunodeficiency is increased susceptibility to infections and chronic or recurrent infections.[4] However, other signs of immunodeficiency include unexplained neonatal death, repeated infections affecting more than one animal in a litter, chronic infections that are unresponsive to appropriate antibiotic treatment, increased susceptibility to commensal or unusual pathogens, systemic illness following vaccination, or failure to respond to immunoprophylaxis.[5]

The initial diagnostic approach in animals with suspected immunodeficiency disease is to obtain a minimum database of historical, physical, and biochemical information, including a complete blood count, serum biochemical profile, urinalysis, and radiographs or ultrasound (if indicated). Other tests that may be considered include a serum protein electrophoresis, immunoglobulin (Ig) electrophoresis and radial immunodiffusion to determine Ig subtypes, lymphocyte counts and determination of T- and B-cell subsets, histopathology of lymphoid organs (thymus, spleen, and lymph nodes), intradermal skin testing (T-cell function), an in vitro evaluation of lymphocyte function (using phytohemagglutinin [PHA], pokeweed mitogen, or concanavalin A to evaluate B- or T-cell responses), and an evaluation of the response to vaccination.

Immunodeficiency disorders involving the humoral immune system are identified by determining individual Ig concentrations. The gold standard for quantification of Ig concentrations in serum is the serial radial immunodiffusion (SRID) assay, which is now commercially available. In addition to the SRID assay, the humoral immune system is evaluated by performing a lymphocyte count, separating B- and T-cell subsets (e.g.,

B cells can be identified by a monoclonal antibody test), evaluating B-cell function via in vitro blastogenesis assays (pokeweed mitogen), measuring the response to vaccination (e.g., determination of prevaccination and postvaccination titers), and evaluating the histopathologic structure of lymphoid organs. Finally, if the disease is suspected to be a primary immunodeficiency, all pertinent genetic information about the sire, dam, and other related animals should be obtained.

The cell-mediated immune system is more difficult to evaluate in the clinical setting. However, some of the basic tests are similar and include determination of T-cell numbers and subsets, evaluation of T-cell function via blastogenesis assays (PHA or concanavalin A) or intradermal skin testing, and histopathologic evaluation of lymphoid organs (e.g., thymus). T-cell subsets can be determined because T cells have different cell surface markers (antigen receptors) that determine their primary functions. For example, T lymphocytes are classified into functional groups: T-helper cells, T-suppressor cells, and cytotoxic T cells. T-helper cells are further divided into subsets of T-helper (Th)-1 and Th-2, which are the primary regulators of immune function.[6] Th-1 cells are generally involved with stimulation of nonspecific and cell-mediated immunity, whereas Th-2 cells stimulate humoral immunity.[7] In addition to T-cell subsets, one of the most important advances in the identification and analysis of T cells was the discovery of functionally distinct cell surface proteins that can be recognized by distinct monoclonal antibodies.[2] These surface markers have been identified by the stage of differentiation, lineage, or structural characteristics and divided into the so-called clusters of differentiation (CD) groups. T lymphocytes typically fall into either the CD4 (helper cells) or CD8 (cytotoxic) cluster designations; however, many other designations have been assigned and are beyond the scope of this review. CD antigens are important phenotypic markers of lymphocytes but have also been shown to be involved in cell-to-cell interactions, cell adhesion, and the transduction of cellular signals leading to lymphocyte activation.[2] Unfortunately, determination of T-cell subsets and in vitro blastogenesis assays are not available in all veterinary or reference laboratories, require a relatively large quantity of whole blood to perform the assay (10 to 20 ml), and are only an approximation of what is happening in vivo.

PRIMARY IMMUNODEFICIENCY DISORDERS

Severe Combined Immunodeficiency

Severe combined immunodeficiency (SCID) is the most severe of all primary immunodeficiencies because it involves both the humoral and cell-mediated components of the immune system (natural killer cells are unaffected). SCID has been observed in dogs, horses, and humans. In humans, there are many different genetic causes of SCID, and the mode of inheritance may be X-linked (most common) or autosomal recessive.[8] The genetic components in dogs have not been defined, but an X-linked form of SCID was identified in a family of Cardigan Welsh corgis.[9,10] Affected puppies had pyoderma, otitis externa, gastrointestinal disease, and respiratory infections that were typically bacterial in origin but unresponsive to antibiotics. Most of the pups were dead by 4 months of age, either from overwhelming bacterial infections or canine distemper (both naturally occurring and vaccine-induced). With the X-linked form of SCID, approximately half the males in a litter from a carrier female will be affected, and half of the female puppies will be carriers.[4] The characteristic laboratory findings are low to absent B- and T-cell numbers; low to absent concentrations of IgG, IgM, and IgA (some Ig crosses the placenta in pups); and nonfunctional T cells (no response to mitogens and no ability to support B-cell function).[9] The affected pups had a small thymus with lymphoid hypoplasia and extremely small to absent lymph nodes. In humans with SCID, the only successful treatment is bone marrow transplantation to reconstitute the patient with lymphoid stem cells. However, this is not technically practical in dogs.

SCID in horses was first recognized in Arabian foals in the 1970s.[11] SCID in Arabian foals is inherited as an autosomal recessive trait and is characterized by foals that appear normal at birth, but become increasingly susceptible to infections over the first two months of life as the circulating immunoglobulins that the foal acquired from colostrum gradually diminish.[12] These foals often die by 4 to 6 months of age due to overwhelming bacterial infections, viral infections such as adenovirus or coronavirus, or cryptosporidia or *Pneumocystis carinii* infections. The histologic findings in foals are similar to those found in dogs with SCID.

A presumptive diagnosis of SCID in foals can be made at birth by evaluation of a blood sample for (1) presence of severe lymphopenia (less than 1000 per μL), (2) absence of circulating IgM, (3) hypoplastic lymphoid tissues (e.g., spleen, thymus, lymph nodes), and (4) unaffected other white blood cell lines, either numerically or functionally.[13] Recently, genetic tests have been developed that identify horses and foals that carry the trait.[14] The absence of IgM is a useful screening tool because normal equine neonates begin to synthesize IgM at approximately 190 days of gestation.[15] Thus, a lack of IgM at birth is diagnostic for a primary immunodeficiency. Any IgM that the foal receives from the mare in the colostrum will have a very short half-life (days) compared to IgG (weeks to months). Therefore, if IgM is present at birth but the levels decrease to low or absent by day 21, this is diagnostic for a primary immunodeficiency. As in dogs, there is no practical treatment currently available, making SCID prevention of utmost importance.

Transient Hypogammaglobulinemia

This syndrome has been reported in horses[16] and cattle[17] and is characterized by the delayed onset of autologous production of Ig. There is a period between the decline of maternal, colostrally derived Ig and the development of autologous concentrations of Ig that results in the foal or calf being susceptible to infections. This syndrome is typically observed in neonates between 2 and 6 months of age. Diagnosis of this condition is made by finding low but not absent Ig levels, normal lymphocyte numbers, normal responses to immunization, and a normal cellular immune response (e.g., skin test).[13] Treatment of this condition is simply to prevent exposure of the neonate to pathogens and to control existing infections until normal Ig levels are attained. Plasma transfusions may be required in some cases with extremely low Ig concentrations or as adjunct therapy of severe infections.

Agammaglobulinemia

Agammaglobulinemia is a rare immune deficiency disorder but has been reported in Thoroughbreds, Standardbreds, and Quarter Horses.[18,19] In affected foals, there is a complete failure to produce Ig that affects all classes, low numbers of B lymphocytes, abnormal responses to immunization, but normal cell-mediated immune responses and T-cell numbers.[13] Clinical signs develop in foals at 2 to 4 weeks of age when passive (maternally derived) immunity starts to wane. The syndrome has only been reported in males to date and may represent an X-linked condition, but this remains to be proven. Because of the severity of the disease and lack of effective treatment, survival has not been reported beyond 18 months.

Miscellaneous Immune Deficiency Disorders

Primary immunodeficiency disorders of selected Ig's are rare and have only been reported in dogs and horses. A primary immunodeficiency involving aspects of both the cell-mediated and humoral immune responses has been documented in 10 Shar Pei dogs.[20] The dogs presented with recurrent infections or malignancies and were subsequently found to have abnormal IgM, IgA, and occasionally IgG concentrations as well as decreased T-cell response to pokeweed mitogen. The relatedness of these dogs and heritability of this condition were not established.

In 1997, Day et al.[21] reported a combined deficiency of IgG and IgA in a group of related Weimaraner dogs from the United Kingdom. These dogs presented with recurrent musculoskeletal, cutaneous, and gastrointestinal tract diseases that were first identified at 15 weeks of age and subsequently followed for 7 months. During that time, the dogs had waxing-waning neutrophilia and persistently low serum IgG and IgA levels. All the dogs died of secondary infections. On further examination, the dam and three other related dogs had reduced serum IgA levels; however, no mode of inheritance was determined.

A selective IgA deficiency has been reported in German Shepherd dogs[22] and Beagles,[23] but many other dog breeds such as Dachshunds, Dalmatians, Akitas, Chow Chows, Schnauzers, and West Highland White terriers may have IgA deficiency as well. The syndrome in German Shepherd dogs has been well documented, but the relatedness and specific genetic defects have not been determined. Affected dogs have chronic gastrointestinal disease (colitis), respiratory infections, and recurrent dermatopathies (recurrent otitis, allergies, pyoderma) that are poorly responsive to antibiotic therapy.[22]

IgM deficiencies have been reported in a dog[24] and in horses,[25] and are suspected but have not yet been documented in other species. The dog with IgM deficiency also had concurrent hypothyroidism, multiple cutaneous tumors, and impaired T-cell function, suggesting multiple metabolic and immune defects. Selective IgM deficiency has been reported in horses as a primary condition in foals[26] but also occurs concurrently with lymphosarcoma; thus, it is presumed to be a secondary immunodeficiency.[27] Affected horses have low or absent concentrations of IgM, normal concentrations of other Ig, normal cell-mediated immune function, and normal lymphocyte numbers. Horses with IgM deficiency can present in one of several ways: (1) severe, life-threatening infections in 8- to 10-month old foals; (2) chronic, recurrent, intermittent, but responsive infections and failure to thrive in animals up to 2 years of age; or (3) chronic debilitation in adult animals (2 to 5 years of age) often occurring in association with lymphosarcoma.[26,27] Diagnosis of this condition is relatively straightforward, because all tests of immune function are normal except for low or absent IgM levels. Many foals will be born with detectable IgM levels (obtained from colostrum) that gradually wane over time. The inheritance of this condition is not known, and there is no known treatment for this disease other than replacement therapy.

There are a few reported primary, selective immunodeficiencies involving T cells or T-cell function. One report described three related Irish wolfhounds with a history of chronic nasal discharge and respiratory disease.[28] The immunodeficiency syndrome was not completely characterized, but the dogs had decreased T-cell response to mitogens without other defects, suggesting a defect in cell-mediated immunity. Finally, T-cell deficiency was also identified in a flock of related Suffolk lambs, but this defect was not well characterized.[29]

SECONDARY IMMUNE DEFICIENCY DISORDERS

The immune system is a complex system whose function is influenced by both external and internal factors. The external factors that influence immune system function include diet (e.g., protein deficiency), drugs (e.g., steroids, chemotherapy agents), infectious agents (e.g., viral, protozoal, parasitic), stressors, and toxins. Internal factors that influence immune system function are frequently associated with the neuroendocrine system (e.g., catecholamines, glucocorticosteroids).[30] The end result is mild to moderate immunosuppression, which results in an increased susceptibility to infection as well as development of neoplastic diseases, autoimmune diseases, and allergies. The major causes of secondary immunodeficiency will be reviewed below.

Failure of Passive Transfer

Passive transfer of immunity from the dam to the neonate can occur transplacentally or by ingestion of colostrum. Both puppies and kittens receive a small amount of IgG (equivalent to approximately 10% of the maternal Ig level) transplacentally during gestation.[31] Thus, these neonates are not at a complete disadvantage if they do not receive colostrum within the first 6 to 12 hours postpartum. Nevertheless, maternal immunity received transplacentally wanes at an early age (3 to 6 weeks). Puppies and kittens that do not receive colostrum will be more susceptible to infections but will also be responsive to vaccination at an earlier age.

In horses, donkeys, cows, sheep, llamas, and pigs, there is no transfer of Ig across the placenta. Thus, failure of a newborn to suckle in the immediate postpartum period results in low to absent Ig levels and a high incidence of neonatal infections. The most common reasons for failure of the neonate to receive Ig, which is called failure of passive transfer (FPT), include a sick or injured neonate, injury or death of the dam, lack of adequate Ig production by the dam, failure of lactation or inadequate volume of colostrum due to premature letdown, failure of the neonate to nurse soon enough after birth, or failure of the neonate to absorb ingested colostrum.[32–34] This problem has been well documented in horses and cattle, with the incidence rate in horses estimated to be between 2.9 and 25%.[32] Dairy calves have a higher incidence of FPT than beef calves because of the greater selection for maternal ability with the beef breeds.[34] In foals, some IgM production begins while the neonate is in utero, but there is essentially no IgG, IgG (T), or IgA produced until after birth, and autologously produced Ig levels are not detectable until 2 to 3 weeks postpartum.[13] Foals that are immunodeficient because of FPT are particularly susceptible to omphalophlebitis, septic arthritis, and respiratory infections. Alternatively, calves that fail to receive colostrum have a high incidence of scours (diarrhea) and neonatal septicemia. The mortality rate of neonates with FPT is quite high unless early diagnosis and intervention occurs.[32–34]

There are several methods available for the diagnosis of FPT. However, the standard for diagnosis of FPT is measurement of serum Ig concentrations by SRID. The problem with SRID is that it requires 12 to 18 hours to perform the assay and thus is not a good "field" test. Several other assays continue to be used as predictors of FPT in neonates, including the zinc sulfate turbidity test, the sodium sulfite turbidity test, the latex agglutination test, serum protein electrophoresis, and serum refractometry (correlating Ig levels to a refractive index of serum protein). The zinc sulfate turbidity test is the oldest and most commonly used field screening test but it has a high false-positive rate.[35] The sodium sulfite turbidity test was recently shown to be the most sensitive (85%) and specific (87%) field test for early detection of FPT, with the serum refractometry test being a close second in assessing passive transfer.[35] Finally, the Ig levels in colostrum can be tested with SRID, or an estimate of colostrum quality (e.g., Ig content) can be made by determining its specific gravity. Normal equine colostrum will have an IgG concentration of greater than 3000 mg/dl and a specific gravity of greater than 1.060 (1.090 is ideal), whereas normal bovine, caprine, or ovine colostrum has IgG concentrations greater than 4500 mg/dL.[33,34,36]

The concentration of Ig in the foal, determined by SRID, that is considered adequate is variable but has been accepted to be greater than 800 mg IgG/dL.[36] In calves and llamas, the concentration should be greater than 1000 mg IgG/dL.[33,34] A concentration of less than 200 mg IgG/dL in all species is considered to be total FPT. Values in the 200 to 400 range suggest partial transfer, but if the neonate has an infection at the time the Ig concentration is measured, any value less than 800 mg/dL is abnormal.[13] Other tests of immunity—such as lymphocyte counts, tests of cellular immunity, response to vaccination, and determination of the presence of other Ig's (e.g., IgM)—are normal in animals with FPT.

Treatment of FPT is aimed at anticipation of the problem and correcting it before "gut closure" occurs (6 to 12 hours postpartum) and before the neonate is exposed to infectious agents that will cause illness. Once gut closure occurs, no further absorption of Ig will occur enterally. Ideally, colostrum of the same species should be given, but bovine colostrum has been successfully given to equine neonates (the half-life is less than 10 days).[13] If colostrum replacement is unavailable, plasma or commercial Ig products can be given. Because the Ig from plasma is not efficiently absorbed enterally, 6 to 9 L of plasma administered intravenously may be required to achieve adequate transfer.[13] Plasma administered at 20 to 40 ml per kg body weight will generally increase the serum IgG concentration by 200 to 300 mg/dL.[36] The ideal way to determine the adequacy of treatment is to measure serum Ig levels after transfusion.

Acquired Immunodeficiency Syndromes

Feline immunodeficiency virus (FIV) was first isolated in 1987 in a cat with a clinical syndrome similar to that caused by the human immunodeficiency virus.[37] FIV is a lentivirus of the retroviridae family and is endemic throughout most of the world.[38–40] The disease is transmitted through saliva or blood (T lymphocytes), and is most actively transmitted via deep puncture wounds obtained during fighting or from the queen to her kittens through milk. The virus is rarely transmitted via casual contact, venereal contact, or in utero because of the low level of viremia that occurs with this virus. FIV is primarily a disease of T lymphocytes (both CD4 and CD8 cells) but also infects macrophages and B cells in the later stages.[41] Cats with clinical diseases associated with FIV infection have lymphopenia, anemia, neutropenia, and hyperproteinemia along with a history of chronic illness.[42] In addition to the quantitative changes in lymphocytes, there are also functional immune deficits that develop. These changes include the loss of memory cells and functional memory, the loss of proliferative responses to mitogens, a decrease in cytokine production (e.g., interleukin 2), and an increase in B-cell activation resulting in polyclonal gammopathies.[43] Cats infected with the virus may survive for long periods (years) with the waxing and waning illnesses, but ultimately will die of chronic wasting diseases, neoplasia, or debilitating neurologic diseases that are the result of feline acquired immunodeficiency syndrome.

The diagnosis of FIV is based on the detection of antibody to the virus by a membrane-bound enzyme-linked immunosorbent assay (ELISA). The test is highly sensitive (100%) and specific (99.6%), but there will be instances in which a positive test result should be reevaluated (e.g., in a healthy adult cat with no signs of disease or in healthy kittens). In both these instances, the cat should be retested in 2 to 6 months, either with ELISA or Western immunoblot to confirm the result.[44] Although numerous antiviral therapies have been used in humans, most are not available, are extremely expensive, or are ineffective in cats with the disease. Thus, the care of an FIV-infected cat is primarily supportive. Many FIV-positive cats will have long asymptomatic (latent) periods (greater than 5 years) before the immunodeficiency syndrome develops.[45] If the cat is housed indoors to protect it from other cats and exposure to other diseases, many symptomatic cats will have prolonged periods of normal health between the periods of illness. There is no vaccine currently available for prevention of FIV, and the long-term prognosis remains guarded.

Miscellaneous Causes of Secondary Immunodeficiency Disorders

Acquired immunodeficiency disease is a common complication of many systemic diseases. These diseases have been better characterized in dogs and cats but are also recognized in horses and ruminants. The most common causes of secondary immune deficiencies in dogs and cats are viral diseases (e.g., canine distemper, canine parvovirus, feline panleukopenia virus, and feline leukemia virus), lymphoreticular neoplasms, treatment with chemotherapeutic agents or corticosteroids, severe protein malnutrition (dietary or anorexia induced), and parasitism (e.g., demodicosis, leishmaniasis, toxoplasmosis, trypanosomiasis).[46] In horses, candidiasis (an equine acquired immunodeficiency syndrome of unknown cause) and equine herpesvirus-1 infection are most often associated with secondary immune dysfunction. Cattle infected with the bovine immunodeficiency virus may develop immunodeficiency disorders, but the most common presentation is bovine leukemia.

REFERENCES

1. **Abbas AK, Lichtman AH, Pober JS.** Cells and tissues of the immune system. In: Cellular and molecular immunology. 2nd ed. Philadelphia: WB Saunders, 1994;14–30.
2. **Abbas AK, Lichtman AH, Pober JS.** Molecular basis of T cell antigen recognition and activation. In: Cellular and molecular immunology. 2nd ed. Philadelphia: WB Saunders, 1994;136–165.
3. **Rosen FS, Cooper MD, Wedgwood RJP.** The primary immunodeficiencies. N Engl J Med 1995;333:431–440.
4. **Felsburg PJ.** Primary immunodeficiencies. In: Bonagura JD, ed. Kirk's current veterinary therapy XII. Philadelphia: WB Saunders, 1995;448–456.
5. **Halliwell REW, Gorman NT.** Diseases associated with immunodeficiency. In: Veterinary clinical immunology. Philadelphia: WB Saunders, 1989;449–466.
6. **Kelso A.** Th-1 and Th-2 subsets: paradigms lost? Immunol Today 1995;16:374–379.
7. **Hnilica KA, Angarano DW.** Advances in immunology: role of T-helper lymphocyte subsets. Comp Cont Educ Pract Vet 1997;19:87–93.
8. **Noguchi M, Rosenblatt HM, Filipovich AH, Adelstein S, Modi WS, McBride OW, Leonard WJ.** Interleukin 2 gamma chain mutation results in X-linked severe combined immunodeficiency in humans. Cell 1993;73:147–157.
9. **Jezyk PF, Felsburg PJ, Haskins ME, Patterson DF.** X-linked severe combined immunodeficiency in the dog. Clin Immunol Immunopathol 1989;52:173–179.
10. **Pullen RP, Somberg RL, Felsburg PJ, Herthorn PS.** X-linked severe combined immunodeficiency in a family of Cardigan Welsh corgis. J Am Anim Hosp Assoc 1997;33:494–499.
11. **McGuire TC, Banks KL, Poppie MJ.** Combined immunodeficiency in horses: characterization of the lymphocytic defect. Clin Immunol Immunopathol 1975;3:555–559.
12. **Poppie MJ, McGuire TC.** Combined immunodeficiency in foals of Arabian breeding: evaluation of mode of inheritance and estimation of prevalence of affected foals and carrier mares and stallions. J Am Vet Med Assoc 1977;170:33–36.
13. **McClure JJ.** Diseases of the immune system. In: Kobluk CN, Ames TR, Geor R, eds. The horse: diseases and clinical management. Philadelphia: WB Saunders, 1995;1051–1063.
14. **Shin EK, Perryman LE, Meek K.** Evaluation of a test for identification of Arabian horses heterozygous for severe combined immunodeficiency trait. J Am Vet Med Assoc 1997;211:1268–1270.
15. **Jeffcott LB.** The transfer of passive immunity to the foal and its relation to immune status after birth. J Reprod Fertil 1975;23:727–730.
16. **McGuire TC, Poppie MJ, Banks KL.** Hypogammaglobulinemia predisposing to infections in foals. J Am Vet Med Assoc 1975;166:71–75.
17. **Vivrette SL, Smith BP.** Transient hypogammaglobulinemia in a Simmental heifer. J Vet Intern Med 1998;12:50–52.
18. **Banks KL, McGuire TC.** Absence of B lymphocytes in a horse with primary agammaglobulinemia. Clin Immunol Immunopathol 1976;5:282–287.
19. **Deem DA, Traver DS, Thacker HL.** Agammaglobulinemia in a horse. J Am Vet Med Assoc 1979;175:469–473.
20. **Rivas AL, Tintle L, Argentieri D, Kimball ES, Goodman MG, Anderson DW, Capefola RJ, Quimby FW.** A primary immunodeficiency syndrome in Shar Pei dogs. Clin Immunol Immunopathol 1995;74:243–251.
21. **Day MJ, Power C, Oleshko J, Rose M.** Low serum immunoglobulin concentrations in related Weimaraner dogs. J Small Anim Pract 1997;38:311–315.
22. **Magne ML.** Selective IgA deficiency in German Shepherd dogs. J Vet All Clin Immunol 1996;4:23–24.
23. **Glickman LT, Shofer FS, Payton AJ, Laster LL, Felsburg PJ.** Survey of serum IgA, IgG and IgM concentrations in a large beagle population in which IgA deficiency has been identified. Am J Vet Res 1988;49:1240–1245.
24. **Mill AB, Campbell KL.** Concurrent hypothyroidism, IgM deficiency, impaired T cell mitogen response, and multifocal cutaneous squamous papillomas in a dog. Canine Pract 1992;17:15–21.
25. **Weldon AD, Zhang C, Antczak DF, Rebhun WC.** Selective IgM deficiency and abnormal B cell response in a foal. J Am Vet Med Assoc 1992;201:1396–1398.
26. **Perryman LE, McGuire TC, Hilbert BJ.** Selective IgM deficiency in foals. J Am Vet Med Assoc 1977;170:212–217.
27. **Perryman LE, Wyatt CR, Magnuson NS.** Biochemical and functional characterization of lymphocytes from a horse with lymphosarcoma and IgM deficiency. Comp Immunol Microbiol Infect Dis 1984;7:53–58.
28. **Leisewitz AL, Spencer JA, Jacobson LS, Schroeder H.** Suspected primary immunodeficiency syndrome in three related Irish wolfhounds. J Small Anim Pract 1997;38:209–212.
29. **Zomborszky Z, Horn E, Tuboly S, Megyeri Z, Tilly P, Szabo C.** T cell deficiency in Suffolk lambs. Acta Vet Hung 1993;41:3–4.
30. **McEwen BS.** Protective and damaging effects of stress mediators. N Engl J Med 1998;338:171–179.
31. **Roth JA.** Immunosuppression and immunodeficiency. In: Bonagura JD, Kirk RW, eds. Kirk's current veterinary therapy, XI. Philadelphia: WB Saunders, 1992;560–563.
32. **Morris DD, Meirs DA, Merryman GS.** Passive transfer failure in horses: incidence and causative factors on a breeding farm. Am J Vet Res 1985;46:2294–2298.
33. **Smith BB.** Post partum care of the dam and neonate. In: Youngquist RS, ed. Current therapy in large animal theriogenology. Philadelphia: WB Saunders, 1997;822–824.

34. **Kersting K.** Post partum care of the cow and calf. In: Youngquist RS, ed. Current therapy in large animal theriogenology. Philadelphia: WB Saunders, 1997;324–329.
35. **Tyler JW, Hancock DD, Parish SM, Rea DE, Besser TE, Sanders SQ, Wilson LK.** Evaluation of 3 assays for failure of passive transfer in calves. J Vet Intern Med 1996;10:304–307.
36. **LeBlanc MM.** Immunologic considerations. In: Kotuba AM, Drummond WH, Kosch PC, eds. Equine clinical neonatology. Philadelphia: Lea & Febiger, 1990;275–294.
37. **Pedersen NC, Ho E, Brown ML, Yamamoto JK.** Isolation of a T-lymphotrophic virus from domestic cats with an immunodeficiency like syndrome. Science 1987;235:790–792.
38. **Ishida T, Washizu T, Toriyabe K, Motoyoshi S, Tomoda I, Pedersen NC.** Feline immunodeficiency virus infection in cats of Japan. J Am Vet Med Assoc 1989;194:221–225.
39. **Friend SLE, Birch CJ, Lording PM, Marshall JA, Studdert MJ.** Feline immunodeficiency virus: prevalence, disease association, and isolation. Aust Vet J 1990;67:237–243.
40. **Gruffydd-Jones TJ, Hopper CD, Harbour DA, Lutz H.** Serological evidence of feline immunodeficiency virus infection in UK cats from 1975-1976. Vet Rec 1988;123:569–570.
41. **English RV, Johnson CM.** In vivo lymphocyte tropism of feline immunodeficiency virus. J Virol 1993;67:5175–5179.
42. **Sparkes AH, Hopper CD, Millard WG, Gruffydd-Jones TJ, Harbour DA.** Feline immunodeficiency virus infection: clinicopathologic findings in 90 naturally occurring cases. J Vet Intern Med 1993;7:85–90.
43. **Siebelink KH, Chu H, Rimmelzwaan QF, Weijer K, van Herwijnen R, Knell P, Egberink HF, Bosch ML, Osterhaus AD.** Feline immunodeficiency virus infection in the cat as a model for HIV infection in man: FIV induced impairment of immune function. AIDS Res Hum Retroviruses 1990;6:1373–1379.
44. **English RV.** Feline immunodeficiency virus. In: Bonagura JD, ed. Kirk's current veterinary therapy XII. Philadelphia: WB Saunders, 1995;280–286.
45. **Shelton GH, Linenberger MC, Persik MT, Abkowitz JL.** Prospective hematologic and clinicopathologic study of asymptomatic cats with naturally occurring FIV infection. J Vet Intern Med 1995;9:133–140.
46. **Krakowa S.** Acquired immunodeficiency diseases. In: Bonagura JD, ed. Kirk's current veterinary therapy XII. Philadelphia: WB Saunders, 1995;453–456.

CHAPTER 144

Amyloidosis

• ROBERTA L. RELFORD

Amyloidosis is a diverse group of diseases that have in common the extracellular deposition of a protein that is composed of fibrils linked together in a beta-pleated sheet formation. This specific biophysical confirmation of the fibrils results in the protein being insoluble and resistant to proteolysis. The accumulation of amyloid protein in extracellular space compresses the adjacent cells and / or tissue. The normal tissue eventually atrophies or dies due to pressure or lack of blood supply, leading to dysfunction of certain tissues. The resultant disease conditions and associated clinical signs are extremely variable and dependent on the organ involved and the specific sites of amyloid deposition within the organ. Amyloidosis is a progressive disease that responds poorly to the limited treatment options that are available today.

Amyloid deposits are not composed of the same protein in each case, but all amyloid deposits have identical light and electron microscopic characteristics. The unique optical and staining characteristics of amyloid are due to the protein fibrils being linked together in the beta-pleated sheet formation.[1-3] The beta-pleated sheet formation occurs by polymerization of repeated peptides from an entire protein or protein segment. When viewed by electron microscopy, the major component of amyloid appears as nonbranching fibrils of variable length with a diameter of 7 to 10 nm.[2] X-ray crystallography has shown that the fibrils are aligned and stacked in a repeating pattern to create the beta-pleated sheet formation. Amyloid deposits can be derived from at least 15 different proteins called amyloid precursor proteins. However, only six amyloid precursor proteins have been documented in the pathogenesis of amyloidosis in domestic animals. The formation of amyloid deposits involves different mechanisms for each precursor protein.

Regardless of the major protein component of the amyloid, two other components are consistently found on transmission electron microscopy. One minor component is a group of pentagonal-shaped structures known as P-components that constitute 10% of the deposit. Amyloid P-component is derived from circulating serum amyloid P-component and has strong homology to C-reactive protein, which is an acute phase protein in the mouse but not other species.[4] Its role in the pathogenesis of amyloidosis is unknown. The final component of amyloid is sulfated glycosaminoglycan. It is thought to have an effect on the precursor protein leading to its conformational change into the beta-pleated sheet formation.

DIAGNOSIS

Screening for amyloid can be done on gross tissue by applying an iodine solution to the cut surface of an organ. When rinsed with sulfuric acid, amyloid will turn blue violet, similar to the reaction seen with starch. This reaction led to the use of the term "amyloid," because it means "starch-like." It has since been discovered that the glycoprotein, amyloid P-component, is responsible for the reaction with iodine in all amyloid deposits.

Further identification of amyloid is aided by the fact that all types of amyloid deposits, regardless of the associated precursor protein, have identical light and electron microscopic characteristics. The characteristic staining properties are due to the binding of the stain to the beta-pleated sheet fibrils and not due to reaction with the amino acid components of the amyloid protein. When stained with hematoxylin and eosin and viewed under routine light microscopy, amyloid appears as an eosinophilic homogenous to fibrillar extracellular substance. The amyloid deposits must be distinguished from other similar-appearing extracellular substances such as collagen, fibrin, and immune deposits.

Histochemical staining techniques used to identify amyloid include Congo red, Thioflavin-T or S, and toludine-blue. Other stains, such as blue crystal violet and periodic acid-Schiff, will stain amyloid but are not specific.[1] Congo red stain is used most commonly and stains amyloid an orange-red when viewed under routine light microscopy. If viewed under polarized light, the amyloid is birefringent and has a characteristic apple-green color. Congo red stain works best if the tissue has been preserved in formalin, whereas it may lose its affinity if other fixatives are used. Thioflavin-T or S, when applied to amyloid and viewed under ultraviolet light, will exhibit a yellow-green fluorescence. Thioflavin-T seems to stain amyloid from cats more consistently.[5] Toluidine-blue-stained amyloid will impart a reddish

Current veterinary therapy XI. 11th ed. Philadelphia: WB Saunders, 1992;59–62.

4. **Pepys MB, Baltz ML.** Acute phase proteins with special reference to C-reactive protein and related proteins (pentaxins) and serum amyloid A protein. Adv Immunol 1983;34:141–212.

5. **Guilford WG, Center SA, Strombeck DR, Williams DA, Meyer DJ.** Strombeck's small animal gastroenterology. 3rd ed. Philadelphia: WB Saunders, 1996.

6. **Libbey CA, Skinner M, Cohen AS.** Use of abdominal fat tissue aspirate in the diagnosis of systemic amyloidosis. Arch Intern Med 1983;143:1549–1552.

7. **Glenner GG.** Amyloid deposits and amyloidosis: the beta fibrilloses. N Engl J Med 1980;302:1283–1292, 1333–1343.

8. **Carothers MA.** Extramedullary plasmacytoma and immunoglobulin-associated amyloidosis in a cat. J Am Vet Med Assoc 1989;195:1593–1597.

9. **Giesel O, Stiglmair-Herm M, Linke RP.** Myeloma associated with immunoglobulin lambda-light chain derived amyloid in a dog. Vet Pathol 1990;27:374–376.

10. **Schwartzman RM.** Cutaneous amyloidosis associated with a monoclonal gammopathy in a dog. J Am Vet Med Assoc 1984;185:102–104.

11. **van Andel ACJ, Gruys E, Kroneman J.** Amyloid in the horse: a report of nine cases. Equine Vet J 1988;20:277–285.

12. **Sherwood BF, Lemay JC, Castellanos RA.** Blastomycosis with secondary amyloidosis in the dog. J Am Vet Med Assoc 1967;150:1377–1381.

13. **Grindem CB, Johnson KH.** Amyloidosis in a case of canine systemic lupus erythematosus. J Comp Pathol 1984;94:569–573.

14. **Cheville NF.** Amyloidosis associated with cyclic neutropenia in the dog. Blood 1968;31:111–114.

15. **Winkelmann J, Veltmann E, Trautwein G.** Amyloidosis in chronic erysipelas polyarthritis in pigs. DTW 1979;86:131–138.

16. **Rings DM, Garry FB.** Amyloidosis associated with paratuberculosis in a sheep. Compend Cont Educ Pract Vet 1988;10:381–385.

17. **Hoffman JS, Benditt EP.** Changes in high density lipoprotein content following endotoxin administration in the mouse. J Biol Chem 1982;257:10510–10517.

18. **Hoffman JS, Benditt EP.** Plasma clearance kinetics of the amyloid-related high density lipoprotein apoprotein, serum amyloid protein (ApoSAA), in the mouse. J Clin Invest 1983;71:926–934.

19. **DiBartola SP, Tarr MJ, Parker AT, Powers JD.** Clinicopathologic findings in dogs with renal amyloidosis: 59 cases (1976–1986). J Am Vet Med Assoc 1989;195:358–364.

20. **Kasper CA, Fretz PB.** Nasal amyloidosis: a case report and review. Equine Pract 1994;16:25–30.

21. **Stone MJ.** Amyloidosis: a final common pathway for protein deposition in tissues. Blood 1990;75:531–545.

22. **Chew DJ, DiBartola SP, Boyce JT.** Renal amyloidosis in related Abyssimian cats. J Am Vet Med Assoc 1982;181:139–142.

23. **Boyce JT, DiBartola SP, Chew DJ.** Familial renal amyloidosis in Abyssinian cats. Vet Pathol 1984;21:33–38.

24. **Zuber RM.** Systemic amyloidosis in Oriental and Siamese cats. Aust Vet Pract 1993;23:66.

25. **Biller DS, DiBartola SP.** Familial renal disease in cats. In: Kirk RW, ed. Current veterinary therapy XII. 12th ed. Philadelphia: WB Saunders, 1995.

26. **Bowles MH, Mosier DA.** Renal amyloidosis in a family of beagles. J Am Vet Med Assoc 1992;201:569–574.

27. **Mason NJ, Day MJ.** Renal amyloidosis in related English foxhounds. J Small Anim Pract 1996;37:255–260.

28. **DiBartola SP, Tarr MJ, Webb DM, Giger U.** Familial renal amyloidosis in Chinese Shar Pei dogs. J Am Vet Med Assoc 1990;197:483–487.

29. **Zuber RM.** Amyloidosis in Oriental shorthair cats. In: August JR, ed. Consultations in feline internal medicine. 3rd ed. Philadelphia: WB Saunders, 1997.

30. **Loeven KO.** Hepatic amyloidosis in two Chinese Shar Pei dogs. J Am Vet Med Assoc 1994;204:1212–1216.

31. **Cummings BJ, Head E, Ruehl W, Milgram NW, Cotman CW.** The canine as an animal model of human aging and dementia. Neurobiol Aging 1996;17:259–268.

32. **Russell MJ, Bobik M, White RG, Hou Y, Benjamin SA, Geddes JW.** Age-specific onset of beta-amyloid in beagle brains. Neurobiol Aging 1996;17:269–273.

33. **Roertgen KE, Lund EM, O'Brien TD, Westermark P, Hayden DW, Johnson KH.** Apolipoprotein AI derived pulmonary vascular amyloid in aged dogs. Am J Pathol 1995;147:1311–1317.

34. **Tekirian TL, Cole GM, Russell MJ, Yang F, Wekstein DR, Patel E, Snowdon DA, Markesbery WR, Geddes JW.** Caboxy terminal of beta amyloid deposits in aged human, canine, and polar bear brains. Neurobiol Aging 1996;17:249–257.

35. **Roertgen KE, Parisi JW, Clark HB, Barnes DL, O'Brien TD, Johnson KH.** A beta associated cerebral angiopathy and senile plaques with neurofibrillary tangles and cerebral hemorrhage in an aged wolverine. Neurobiol Aging 1996;17:243–247.

36. **Ruehl WW, Bruyette DS, DePaoli A, Cotman CW, Head E, Milgram NW, Cummings BJ.** Canine cognitive dysfunction as a model for human age-related cognitive decline, dementia and Alzheimer's disease: clinical presentation, cognitive testing, pathology and response to 1-deprenyl therapy. Prog Brain Res 1995;106:217–225.

37. **Uchida K, Nakayama H, Goto N.** Pathological studies on cerebral amyloid angiopathy, senile plaques and amyloid deposition in visceral organs in aged dogs. J Vet Med Sci 1991;53:1037–1042.

38. **Tani Y, Uchida K, Uetsuka K, Nakamura S, Nakayama H, Goto N, Doi K.** Amyloid deposits in the gastrointestinal tract of aging dogs. Vet Pathol 1997;34:415–420.

39. **Yoshino T, Uchida K, Tateyama S, Yamaguchi R, Nakayama H, Goto N.** A retrospective study of canine senile plaques and cerebral amyloid angiopathy. Vet Pathol 1996;33:230–234.

40. **Uchida K, Tani Y, Uetsuka K, Nakayama H, Goto N.** Immunohistochemical studies on canine cerebral amyloid angiopathy and senile plaques. J Vet Med Sci 1992;54:659–667.

41. **Cummings BJ, Head E, Afagh AJ, Milgram NW, Cotman CW.** Beta amyloid accumulation correlates with cognitive dysfunction in the aged canine. Neurobiol Learn Mem 1996;66:11–23.

42. **Breuer W, Geisel RP, Linke RP, Hermanns W.** Light microscopic, ultrastructural, and immunohistochemical examinations of two calcifying epithelial odontogenic tumors (CEOT) in a dog and a cat. Vet Pathol 1994;31:415–420.

43. **Rowland PH, Valentine BA, Stebbins KE, Smith CA.** Cutaneous plasmacytomas with amyloid in six dogs. Vet Pathol 1991;28:125–130.

44. **O'Brien TD, Norton F, Turner TM, Johnson KH.** Pancreatic endocrine tumor in a cat: clinical, pathological, and immunohistochemical evaluation, J Am Anim Hosp Assoc 1990;26:453–457.

45. **O'Brien TD, Butler PC, Westermark P, Johnson KH.** Islet amyloid polypeptide: a review of its biology and potential roles in the pathogenesis of diabetes mellitus. Vet Pathol 1993;30:317–332.

46. **O'Brien TD, Wagner JD, Litwak KN, Carlson CS, Cefalu WT, Jordan K, Johnson KH, Butler PC.** Islet amyloid and islet amyloid polypeptide in cynomolgus macaques (Macaca fascicularis): an animal model of human non-insulin-dependent diabetes mellitus. Vet Pathol 1996;33:479–485.

47. **Lutz TA, Rand JS.** A review of new developments in type 2 diabetes in human beings and cats. Br Vet J 1993;149:527–536.

48. **Yano BL, Hayden DW, Johnson KH.** Feline insular amyloid: association with diabetes mellitus. Vet Pathol 1981;18:621–627.

49. **Johnson KH, Hayden DW, O'Brien TD, Westermark P.** Spontaneous diabetes mellitus-islet amyloid complex in adult cats. Am J Pathol 1986;125:416–419.

50. **Struble AL. Nelson RW.** Non-insulin-dependent diabetes mellitus in cats and humans. Compend Cont Educ Pract Vet 1997;19:935–945.

51. **Rowland PH, Linke RP.** Immunohistochemical characterization of lambda light-chain-derived amyloid in one feline and five canine plasma cell tumors. Vet Pathol 1994;31:390–393.

52. **O'Brien TD, Hayden DW, O'Leary TP, Caywood DD, Johnson KH.** Canine pancreatic endocrine tumors: immunohistochemical analysis of hormone content and amyloid. Vet Pathol 1987;24:308–314.

53. **Shaw DP, Gunson DE, Evans LH.** Nasal amyloidosis in four horses. Vet Pathol 1987;24:183–185.

54. **DiBartola SP, Tarr MJ, Benson MD.** Tissue distribution of amyloid deposits in Abyssinian cats with familial amyloidosis. J Comp Pathol 1986;96:387–398.

55. **Spyridakis L, Brown S, Barsanti JA, Hardie EM, Carlton B.** Amyloidosis in a dog: treatment with dimethylsulfoxide. J. Am Vet Med Assoc 1986;189:690–691.

56. **Cowgill LD.** Diseases of the kidney In: Ettinger SJ, ed. Textbook of veterinary internal medicine. 2nd ed. Philadelphia: WB Saunders, 1983.

57. **Gruys E, Sijens RJ, Biewenga WJ.** Dubious effect of dimethylsulfoxide (DMSO) therapy on amyloid deposits and amyloidosis. Vet Res Commun 1981;5:21–32.

recognized. Some primary immunodeficiencies have been well defined (Table 145.2), whereas for others only a breed predilection to particular infections suggests a genetic basis. Similarly, breed predispositions have been recognized for certain hematologic immune-mediated disorders and hematopoietic cancers without knowing the molecular basis. These disorders are covered elsewhere.

should not be used for breeding. If carriers are used because of other highly desirable traits, they should only be bred to clear (homozygous normal) animals in order to prevent the breeding of affected animals, and all offspring need to be tested before their use for breeding. Three comprehensive lists of hereditary erythrocyte, immune, and bleeding disorders follow (Tables 145.1 to 145.3).

CHAPTER 146

Cyclic Hemopoiesis

• GLENN P. NIEMEYER and CLINTON D. LOTHROP, JR

Hemopoiesis is a remarkable process whereby pluripotent stem cells self-renew, proliferate, and differentiate into eight distinct blood cell lineages.[1] The bone marrow is the principal source of blood cell formation in normal adults, although lymphocytes undergo maturation in peripheral lymphoid organs. Bone marrow contains cells at all stages of hemopoietic cell development and includes the most primitive precursors as well as maturing hemopoietic cells. Blood-forming tissues are divided into hemopoietic progenitor cells (including stem cells), multiprogenitor and committed progenitor cells, and a microenvironment composed of endothelium and reticular cells that form a three-dimensional network throughout the hematopoietic spaces (Fig. 146.1). The microenvironment provides a substratum, growth factors, and nutrients necessary for normal hemopoiesis. The turnover of cells in the hemopoietic system of an adult human is approximately 1 trillion cells a day, including 200 billion erythrocytes and 70 billion polymorphonuclear leukocytes, because most mature blood cells have a limited lifespan.

The process in which a hemopoietic stem cell either self-renews or differentiates into the various hemopoietic lineages is currently undefined (Fig. 146.2). It is not clear whether hemopoietic cell fate decisions occur through stochastic mechanisms or are the result of signals mediated through specific receptor ligand interactions.[2] A major goal of contemporary experimental hematology has been to define the complex network of positive and negative regulatory signals generated by the interaction of growth factors with their receptors.[3]

HEMOPOIETIC GROWTH FACTORS

Hemopoietic growth factors can be divided into three groups: (1) factors affecting specific cellular lineages at later stages of the maturation process (e.g., erythropoietin, granulocyte-colony-stimulating factor [CSF], thrombopoietin, monocyte-CSF), (2) intermediate-acting factors that support proliferation of multipotential progenitors after they have exited G_0 of the cell cycle (e.g., interleukin-3 [IL-3], granulocyte/monocyte CSF), and (3) early factors that alter the kinetics of cell-cycle

dormant primitive stem cells[4] (stem cell factor, flt-3 ligand, IL-1, IL-6). Late-acting factors, such as granulocyte-colony-stimulating factor (G-CSF) and thrombopoietin, also have synergistic activity with early-acting factors to activate quiescent stem cells into the cell cycle. In addition to the above classification, many hemopoietic growth factors have multiple isoforms. In many instances, the predominant isoform is a transmembrane protein that is biologically active when expressed on the cell surface. Membrane-bound growth factors have activities distinct from soluble growth factors. Soluble factors reach hematopoietic cells via the bloodstream and tend to act on more differentiated cells affecting their growth and maturation. The soluble growth factors have been the subject of extensive studies, and clinical use of G-CSF and erythropoietin (Epo) is already commonplace in medical practice.[5-7] Recombinant human G-CSF and Epo can be used to treat neutropenia and anemia in dogs and cats, but there is a risk for development of neutralizing antibodies with chronic administration. The interaction between membrane-bound growth factors and their cognizant receptor is an important mechanism for the regulatory interactions occurring between progenitor cells and the microenvironment. Membrane-bound growth factors may function in part as adhesion molecules. Other important differences between membrane-bound growth factors and soluble growth factors are that membrane-bound growth factors induce (1) more intrinsic receptor kinase activity, (2) decreased downregulation of cell-surface receptor expression, (3) increased receptor stability, and (4) sustained activation of important cellular signal transduction components.[8] Membrane-bound growth factors act synergistically with other similar factors, leading to cellular differentiation and thus rendering the cells subject to the effect of soluble, late-acting factors.[9]

Defining hemopoietic regulatory pathways has proven difficult due to certain inherent features of the hemopoietic growth factor network. First, a characteristic feature of a given group of growth factors is their functional redundancy. Second, in addition to their effect on progenitor cells, hemopoietic growth factors also modulate the effector function of differentiated cells. Third, combinations of growth factors can interact

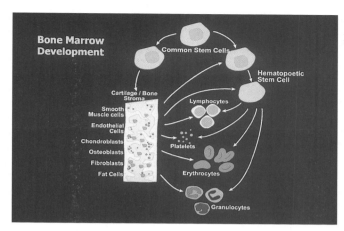

FIGURE 146.1 Bone marrow is composed of a three dimensional network of mesenchymal and hemopoietic precursor cells.

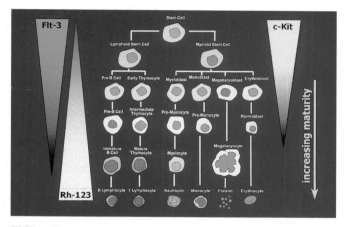

FIGURE 146.2 Hemopoietic stem cells give rise to multiple cell lineages. Some of the receptors known to be expressed on early hemopoietic progenitor cells are shown. Decreased staining of progenitor cells with Rh-123, a fluorescent vital dye, is due to expression of p-glycoprotein.

synergistically to produce a greater biologic effect than would be predicted from the additive effect of the individual factors. Fourth, many of the effects of the growth factors observed both in vitro and in vivo do not represent direct effects of the factors on progenitor cells; rather, they represent indirect effects mediated by other factors produced in response to the first factor.[10] Biochemical and molecular biology techniques are providing insight into these complex interactions.

RECEPTORS

The receptors for many of the cytokines and growth factors involved in hemopoiesis have been defined at the molecular level. The receptor structure provides a basis for the functional redundancy present in the hemo-

poietic growth factor network. Molecular analysis of cytokine receptors has shown that many cytokines have both low- and high-affinity receptors and functional receptors consist of more than one subunit. It is also apparent that receptors for cytokines with similar functions share a common subunit that is essential for signal transduction. The sharing of common subunits provides an explanation for why different cytokines may exhibit similar effects on the same target cell. Furthermore, because cytokines may have more than one type of receptor, a cytokine may elicit multiple effects depending on the cell and type of the receptor expressed.[11] Exactly how cell-surface receptors are coupled to intracellular signaling pathways and how each signaling pathway is coupled to diverse cellular function is not completely understood.

REGULATORY MECHANISMS

The regulatory mechanisms that induce a pluripotent stem cell to proliferate and differentiate along a single lineage or hemopoietic pathway are as yet undefined, even though the concept of a common pluripotent stem cell that can give rise to all the lineages of the hemopoietic system was first proposed a century ago by Arthur Pappenheim. The difficulties in characterizing the hemopoietic stem cell as well as defining regulatory mechanisms involved in the process of hemopoiesis can be attributed to the relatively low frequency of stem cells. Pluripotent hemopoietic stem cells are extremely rare and represent approximately 0.01% of bone marrow cells, which makes it difficult to obtain stem cells in sufficient quantity and purity for analysis.

Cyclic hemopoiesis (CH) is an unusual genetic disease of the pluripotent stem cell that disrupts normal steady-state hemopoiesis and results in an on/off production of blood cells. CH is inherited as an autosomal recessive trait in dogs, and both autosomal recessive and autosomal incomplete dominant forms have been described in humans. CH is always linked to a diluted coat color (Fig. 146.3), hence the acronym "lethal Gray

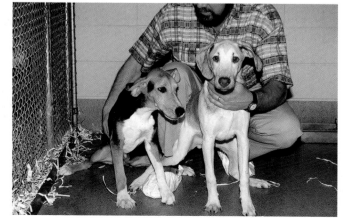

FIGURE 146.3 Normal and cyclic hemopoietic littermates. Cyclic hemopoiesis is always linked to a diluted or gray coat color.

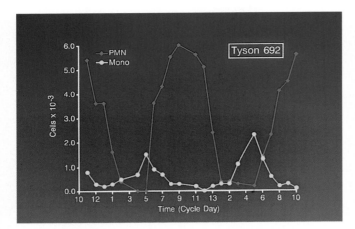

FIGURE 146.4 Cyclic neutropenia is the hallmark of canine cyclic hemopoiesis. Monocytes also cycle with a 12 to 14 day periodicity but out of phase with the neutrophil cycles.

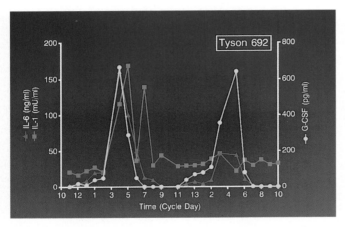

FIGURE 146.5 Serum levels of the hemopoietic growth factors IL-1 and IL-6 and G-CSF cycle concurrently with the periods of neutropenia and monocytosis.

Clinical symptoms in dogs and human patients with CH include gingivitis, lymphadenopathy, excessive bleeding, pneumonia, diarrhea, subcutaneous abscesses, and intermittent lameness. Dogs and humans with CH often die of overwhelming infections; however, in a controlled laboratory setting, most dogs die of hepatic and renal amyloidosis. Systemic amyloidosis has also been reported in human cyclic neutropenia.[24] The systemic amyloidosis was initially theorized to be secondary to repeated inflammation associated with recurrent infections during periods of neutropenia.[25] However, laboratory animals largely free of intercurrent infections also die of systemic amyloidosis. It is now known that systemic amyloidosis in CH dogs is the result of the inherent cyclic activation of the acute phase response mechanism by cytokines produced during periods of monocytosis (Fig. 146.6). The coordinated peaks of G-CSF, IL-1, and IL-6 in serum from CH dogs occur during the monocytosis phase of the dog's cycle. These cytokines are not normally detectable in serum from any species. Acute phase proteins that have been shown to cycle in CH dogs include amyloid A protein, fibrinogen, von Willebrand's factor, and undefined alpha-2 globulins. The peak activities of the acute phase proteins are also always associated with periods of monocytosis.[25] In addition to the activation of the acute phase response, IL-1 and IL-6 produced by activated monocytes and macrophages at periods of monocytosis stimulate the neuroendocrine axis, leading to cyclic production of corticotropin and cortisol.[26] Cortisol may then serve to downregulate IL-1 and IL-6 production, because glucocorticoid negative response elements are found in the promoters of the IL-1 and IL-6 genes. Although the exact genetic lesion that causes CH in dogs is not known, these findings provide a molecular explanation for many of the clinical and cellular phenomena that are associated with CH. The CH dog model is a paradigm of

Collie disease." Dogs heterozygous for the CH trait have normal coat color and do not have hemopoietic cycles. The hallmark of CH is the cyclic neutropenia that occurs at 14-day and 21-day intervals in dogs and humans, respectively[12-14] (Fig. 146.4). In CH, monocytes, platelets, and reticulocytes also cycle with the same periodicity but out of phase with neutrophils. However, unlike neutrophils, monocytes, platelets, and reticulocytes cycle from normal to above normal levels. The hemopoietic growth factors erythropoietin, thrombopoietin, G-CSF, IL-1, and IL-6 also fluctuate in a cyclic manner in CH dogs[15-19] (Fig. 146.5). Morphologic examination of bone marrow cells and committed progenitor assays have shown an alternating erythroid-myeloid pattern that precedes changes in the circulating blood cells, suggesting a bone marrow origin of the hemopoietic cycles.[20,21] CH has been induced and cured by bone marrow transplantation, which strongly suggests that CH is a disease of the pluripotent stem cell.[22,23]

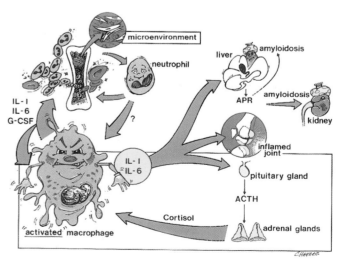

FIGURE 146.6 Chronic recurrent activation of the acute phase response by monocyte-derived cytokines results in systemic amyloidosis in cyclic hemopoietic dogs.

hormonal cross-talk between the hemopoietic, immune, and endocrine systems.

Several in vivo and in vitro studies have shown that hemopoietic progenitor cells from CH dogs have decreased responsiveness to multiple hemopoietic growth factors.[6,27-29] Recombinant G-CSF is effective at reducing the neutropenic nadir associated with CH in both humans and dogs. In CH dogs, pharmacologic but not physiologic doses of recombinant human or canine G-CSF can eliminate the cyclical oscillations of neutrophils associated with the disease. Avalos et al.[30] reported decreased in vitro colony formation in CH dogs in response to G-CSF. In that study, bone marrow mononuclear cells from CH dogs required sevenfold higher G-CSF concentrations than normal dog cells to achieve half-maximal colony growth. We have also characterized the in vitro responsiveness of myeloid progenitor cells from normal and CH dogs to multiple recombinant canine hemopoietic growth factors (Niemeyer et al, submitted 2000). Bone marrow mononuclear cells from normal and CH dogs responded similarly to G-CSF and granulocyte-macrophage-colony stimulating factor (GM-CSF). These data differ from that reported by Avalos et al. and others in that we did not observe a significant difference in half-maximal colony production by normal and CH dogs in response to G-CSF or GM-CSF. This discrepancy may be explained by different methods used to generate maximal colony production in the two laboratories. We also characterized the responsiveness of bone marrow progenitor cells to stem cell factor (SCF), an early-acting hemopoietic growth factor. Bone marrow mononuclear cells from CH dogs had a significantly decreased response to SCF compared with normal dogs.

In another study, Dale et al.[31] reported on the efficacy of SCF in the treatment of canine CH. The characteristic neutrophil nadirs were less severe and regular oscillations of other blood lineages became less distinct following recombinant canine SCF administration to CH dogs. The in vitro colony formation data, the observation that CH dogs have cutaneous mast cell deficiency, and CH dog coat color dilution suggest that an abnormality in *c-kit* or *c-kit* signaling may play a role in the pathogenesis of CH in dogs. However, this has not yet been definitively demonstrated.

Cyclic hemopoietic dogs also have qualitative platelet function defects due to dense granule storage pool disease (SPD) that results in decreased stores of serotonin and Ca^{2+}.[32] In addition to SPD, platelets from CH dogs have defective platelet aggregation to multiple platelet agonists such as collagen, platelet activating factor, and thrombin. Administration of G-CSF to CH dogs corrects hemopoietic cycles but does not correct the qualitative platelet defects, suggesting that the platelet defects are not 2° to the hemopoietic cycles. The relationship of the platelet defects to the hemopoietic cycles is not known, but it is possible that there are common defects in second messenger signaling molecules crucial to platelet and pluripotent stem cells.

In summary, CH is an unusual hemopoietic stem cell disease of undetermined cause that dampens steady-state hemopoiesis and unmasks the inherent cyclic na-

ture of blood cell production. Although not definitely proven, CH most likely results from abnormal signal transduction in response to a hemopoietic growth factor(s) such as SCF. Understanding the molecular basis for CH will provide insight into key regulatory steps and the basic mechanism of steady-state hemopoiesis, which may lead to improved understanding of bone marrow aplasias, leukemias, and interactions of the hematopoietic, endocrine, and immune systems.

REFERENCES

1. **Uchida N.** Heterogenicity of hematopoietic stem cells. Curr Opin Immunol 1993;5:177.
2. **Goldsmith MA, Mikami A, You Y, Liu KD, Thomas L, Pharr P, Longmore GD.** Absence of cytokine receptor-dependent specificity in red blood cell differentiation in vivo. Proc Natl Acad Sci USA 1998;95:7006.
3. **Socolovsky M, Lodish HF, Daley GQ.** Control of hematopoietic differentiation: lack of specificity in signaling by cytokine receptors. Proc Natl Acad Sci USA 1998;95:6573.
4. **Ogawa M.** Differentiation and proliferation of hematopoietic stem cells. Blood 1993;81:2844.
5. **Moore MA.** The clinical use of colony stimulating factors. Annu Rev Immunol 1991;9:159.
6. **Hammond WP 4th, Price TH, Souza LM, Dale DC.** Treatment of cyclic neutropenia with granulocyte colony-stimulating factor. N Engl J Med 1989;320:1306.
7. **Yano M, Iwama A, Nishio H, Suda J, Takada G, Suda T.** Expression and function of murine receptor tyrosine kinases, TIE and TEK, in hematopoietic stem cells. Blood 1997;89:4317.
8. **Kapur R, Majumdar M, Xiao X, McAndrews-Hill M, Schindler K, Williams DA.** Signaling through the interaction of membrane-restricted stem cell factor and c-kit receptor tyrosine kinase: genetic evidence for a differential role in erythropoiesis. Blood 1998;91:879.
9. **Slanicka Krieger M, Nissen C, Manz CY, Tokosoz D, Lyman SD, Wodnar-Filipowicz A.** The membrane-bound isoform of stem cell factor synergizes with soluble flt-3 ligand in supporting early hematopoietic cells in long-term cultures of normal and aplastic anemia bone marrow. Exp Hematol 1998;26:365.
10. **Kishimoto T, Taga T, Akira S.** Cytokine signal transduction. Cell 1994;76:253.
11. **Miyajima A, Mui AL, Ogorochi T, Sakamaki K.** Receptors for granulocyte-macrophage colony-stimulating factor, interleukin-3, and interleukin-5. Blood 1993;82:1960.
12. **Lund JE, Padgett GA, Ott RL.** Cyclic neutropenia in grey collie dogs. Blood 1967;29:452.
13. **Dale DC, Hammond WP 4th.** Cyclic neutropenia: a clinical review. Blood Rev 1988;2:178.
14. **Wright DG, Dale DC, Fauci AS, Wolff SM.** Human cyclic neutropenia: clinical review and long-term follow-up of patients. Medicine (Baltimore) 1981;60:1.
15. **Adamson JW, Dale DC, Elin RJ.** Hematopoiesis in the grey collie dog. Studies of the regulation of erythropoiesis. J Clin Invest 1974;54:965.
16. **McDonald TP, Clift R, Jones JB.** Canine cyclic hematopoiesis: platelet size and thrombopoietin level in relation to platelet count (39561). Proc Soc Exp Biol Med 1976;153:424-428.
17. **Dale DC, Brown CH, Carbone P, Wolff SM.** Cyclic urinary leukopoietic activity in grey collie dogs. Science 1971;173:152.
18. **Yang TJ, Jones JB, Jones ES, Lange RD.** Serum colony-stimulating activity of dogs with cyclic neutropenia. Blood 1974;44:41.
19. **Warren DJ, Maniatis M, Moore MAS, Pratt HL, Jones JB, Lothrop CD Jr.** Cyclic production of granulocyte-colony stimulating factor in cyclic hematopoietic dogs. Hematopoiesis 1990;273:252.
20. **Machado EA, Jones JB, Aggio MC, Chernoff AL, Maxwell PA, Lange RD.** Ultrastructural changes of bone marrow in canine cyclic hematopoiesis (CH dog). Virchows Arch 1981;390:93–108.
21. **Scott R, Dale D, Rosenthal A, Wolff S.** Cyclic neutropenia in grey collie dogs. Ultrastructural evidence for abnormal neutrophil granulopoiesis. Lab Invest 1973;28:514–525.
22. **Dale DC, Graw RD.** Transplantation of allogenic bone marrow in canine cyclic neutropenia. Science 1974;183:83.
23. **Jones JB, Yang TJ, Dale JB, Lange RD.** Canine cyclic hematopoiesis: marrow transplantation between littermates. Br J Haematol 1975;30:215.
24. **Lange RD, Crowder CG, Cruz P, Hawkinson SW, Lozzio CB, Machado E, Painter P, Terry W, Jones JB.** Cyclic neutropenia. A tale of two brothers and their family. Am J Pediatr Hematol Oncol 1981;3:127.

25. **Machado EA, Gregory RS, Jones JB, Lange RD.** The cyclic hematopoietic dog: a model for spontaneous secondary amyloidosis. A morphologic study. Am J Pathol 1978;92:23.

26. **Lothrop CD Jr, Coulson PA, Nolan HL, Cole B, Jones JB, Sanders WL.** Cyclic hormonogenesis in grey collie dogs: interactions of hematopoietic and endocrine systems. Endocrinology 1987;120:1027.

27. **Hammond WP, Chatta GS, Andres RG, Dale DC.** Abnormal responsiveness of granulocyte-committed progenitor cells in cyclic neutropenia. Blood 1992;79:2536.

28. **Lothrop CD Jr, Warren DJ, Souza LM, Jones JB, Moore MA.** Correction of canine cyclic hematopoiesis with recombinant human granulocyte colony-stimulating factor. Blood 1988;72:1324.

29. **Hammond WP, Boone TC, Donahue RE, Souza LM, Dale DC.** A comparison of treatment of canine cyclic hematopoiesis with recombinant human granulocyte-macrophage colony-stimulating factor (GM-CSF), G-CSF interleukin-3, and canine G-CSF. Blood 1990;76:523.

30. **Avalos BR, Broudy VC, Ceselski SK, Druker BJ, Griffin JD, Hammond WP.** Abnormal response to granulocyte colony-stimulating factor (G-CSF) in canine cyclic hematopoiesis is not caused by altered G-CSF receptor expression. Blood 1994;84:789.

31. **Dale DC, Rodger E, Cebon J, Ramesh N, Hammond WP, Zsebo KM.** Long-term treatment of canine cyclic hematopoiesis with recombinant canine stem cell factor. Blood 1995;85:74.

32. **Lothrop CD, Candler RV, Pratt HL, Uso IM, Jones JB, Carroll RC.** Characterization of platelet function in cyclic hematopoietic dogs. Exp Hematol 1991;19:916–922.

CHAPTER 147

Hematology of Selective Intestinal Cobalamin Malabsorption

• JOHN C. FYFE

Investigation of inherited selective intestinal cobalamin (vitamin B_{12}) malabsorption in giant schnauzers confirmed that cobalamin is an essential vitamin for good nutrition in dogs and that gastrointestinal cobalamin absorption occurs in dogs via a route mediated by intrinsic factor and an intestinal receptor.[1-3] Investigation of this group of dogs also allowed description of the canine hematologic responses specific to cobalamin deficiency and allowed determination of the earliest and most reliable diagnostic indicators of cobalamin deficiency in dogs. All animal species must obtain exogenous cobalamin by gastrointestinal absorption of the vitamin either produced by microorganisms within the gastrointestinal tract (i.e., ruminants) or liberated by digestion of foodstuffs of animal, and ultimately, microbial origin.[4] There are comparative differences in cobalamin-dependent metabolism and in gastrointestinal cobalamin absorption. Therefore, the signs and biochemical indications of cobalamin deficiency and the clinical situations in which one can expect cobalamin malabsorption differ somewhat among species.

The coenzyme forms of the dietary vitamin are essential cofactors for the activity of two enzymes of intermediary metabolism in mammals, methylmalonyl-CoA mutase and methionine synthase (Fig. 147.1).[5] Reduced activity of these two enzymes causes the biochemical signatures of cobalamin deficiency, methylmalonic acidemia/uria and homocysteinemia, respectively. In addition, low activity of the latter enzyme creates a "metabolic trap" of 5-methyl tetrahydrofolate and deprives the enzymes of purine and pyrimidine synthesis of essential folate derived cofactors.[6] Thereby, cobalamin deficiency indirectly inhibits nucleic acid synthesis; thus, the tissues that are most affected are those in which cells divide most rapidly. In the adult animal these include hematopoietic tissue, testes, and intestinal epithelium but involve most tissues in a developing fetus or rapidly growing newborn.

Inhibition of nuclear maturation during hematopoiesis leads to the hematologic hallmarks of cobalamin deficiency, nonregenerative anemia and neutropenia with megaloblastosis of erythroid and myeloid precursor cells in bone marrow, and release of macrocytic erythrocytes and hypersegmented neutrophils.[7] Although the presence of macrocytic erythrocytes in peripheral blood is a feature common to cobalamin deficiency in many species, macrocytosis—as defined by an increase in mean corpuscular volume (MCV)—is not observed in most species other than humans and nonhuman primates. The presence of many abnormally small and distorted erythrocytes counters the large forms in MCV during the dyserythropoiesis of canine cobalamin deficiency.

The resistance to macrocytic changes in the erythron of dogs is not only seen in cobalamin deficiency. Young adult beagles were studied in toxicity trials of azidothymidine (AZT), an anti-human immunodeficiency virus (HIV) drug well known to cause macrocytic anemia in humans by inhibiting thymidine triphosphate formation and nucleic acid synthesis (K. Ayers, Burroughs Wellcome, personal communication 1991). In 6 weeks of the study with AZT dosages up to 160 mg/kg/day, there was no change in MCV in treated dogs. However, the red cell distribution widths (RDWs) increased from 13.0 ± 0.2 to 16.1 ± 2.2 at all dosages by the fourth week, and red blood cell (RBC) counts dropped to just below normal ($5.4 \times 10^6/\mu L$) at higher dosages by the fifth week. There were also significant effects on leukocytes and platelets.

CLINICAL ABNORMALITIES IN CANINE COBALAMIN DEFICIENCY

Selective intestinal cobalamin malabsorption described in giant schnauzers is an autosomal recessive disorder caused by failure to express the receptor for intrinsic factor-cobalamin complex, now called cubilin, on the apical brush border membrane of small intestinal and renal tubule epithelial cells.[3] This disorder is the canine homologue of Imerslund-Gräsbeck syndrome in humans. Affected dogs fail to absorb dietary cobalamin, and all clinical abnormalities are attributable to the ensuing cobalamin deficiency.[2] Inherited cobalamin malab-

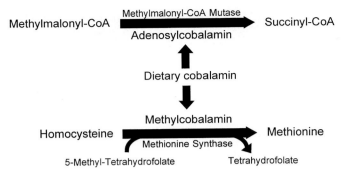

FIGURE 147.1 Cobalamin-dependent metabolism. Cobalamin absorbed from the gastrointestinal tract and delivered to tissues is converted to coenzyme forms essential for the enzymatic activities of methylmalonyl-CoA mutase and methionine synthase. Cobalamin deficiency leads to reduced activity of both enzymes and increased serum concentrations of methylmalonic acid and homocysteine.

sorption has also been reported in a family of border collies.[8] Single cases of apparent congenital cobalamin malabsorption have been investigated in a beagle[8a] and in a cat (JC Fyfe, unpublished data 1988). It has not been determined whether the border collies or these sporadic cases had defects of cubilin expression or of some other gene product involved in cobalamin absorption and transport.

The signs of cobalamin deficiency developing in the neonatal period are somewhat different from the signs of cobalamin deficiency that develops in adulthood. The most apparent effect of cobalamin deficiency in the young is growth failure. In puppies affected with selective cobalamin malabsorption, inappetence and failure to thrive begin variably between 8 and 12 weeks of age. While linear growth velocity is maintained almost normally, weight gain is suppressed, with loss of previously attained body condition by 15 weeks of age. Weight gains plateau between 12 and 20 weeks of age. Untreated dogs may die suddenly at 5 to 6 months of age or later. Some affected dogs have had mildly elevated serum alanine aminotransferase activity and centrolobular degeneration of hepatocytes. Some have exhibited transient mild hyperammonemia or seizures. Along with growth stunting, these signs may mimic those of portocaval shunt. Cobalamin-deficient kittens also exhibit growth failure[9] and may exhibit signs of hepatic dysfunction.[10]

Complete blood counts reveal dyserythropoiesis and dysgranulopoiesis. Absolute neutropenia (1.7 to $3.6 \times 10^3/\mu L$) develops in affected puppies between 8 and 16 weeks of age, followed by development of nonregenerative, normochromic, normocytic anemia (hematocrit, 27 to 31%; 3.9 to 4.5×10^6 RBC/μL; 3.7 to 5.6×10^4 reticulocytes/μL; MCV, 65 to 68 fL; mean corpuscular hemoglobin concentration, 32.8 to 33.9 g/dL) by 20 to 22 weeks of age. The RDW is elevated with statistical significance in affected dogs (14.7 ± 0.1) by this age when compared with age-matched normal dogs (13.3 ± 0.7; n = 3/group; $P < 0.05$). Accordingly,

examination of blood smears reveals moderate to severe anisocytosis and poikilocytosis, many small RBCs, some large ovalocytes (elliptocytes), and occasional megaloblasts (Fig. 147.2). The latter are macrocytes with fully hemoglobinized cytoplasm that retain an immature nucleus. Careful examination also reveals occasional large, hypersegmented neutrophils and some giant platelets.

Although platelet counts remain normal, platelet

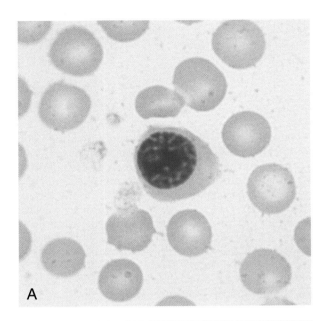

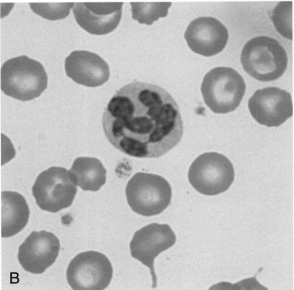

FIGURE 147.2 Peripheral blood smears from cobalamin-deficient dogs. Erythrocytes in both panels demonstrate anisocytosis and poikilocytosis. The nucleated cell in **A** is a megaloblast exhibiting nuclear/cytoplasmic asynchrony, an immature nucleus in fully hemoglobinized cytoplasm. The nucleated cell in **B** is a neutrophil exhibiting six to seven nuclear lobations, indicative of slowed development of granulocytic cells. This smear was made when the neutrophil count was 3870/μL.

counts of affected dogs are significantly increased (470 ± 90 vs. $275 \pm 35 \times 10^3/\mu L$; n = 3/group; $P < 0.05$) and mean platelet volumes are significantly decreased (7.4 ± 0.2 vs. 9.4 ± 0.8 fL; n = 3/group; $P < 0.02$) when compared with age-matched normal controls. Although these data indicate that cobalamin deficiency causes detectable dysthrombocytopoiesis by 5 to 6 months of age in affected dogs, the abnormalities are too subtle to be diagnostically useful in a clinical setting.

Examination of bone marrow aspirates reveals hypersegmented neutrophils, large band forms, and some giant metamyelocytes (Fig. 147.3). Erythroid precursors may be reduced in number, and total cellularity of the marrow decreased or normal. Erythroid dysplasia is evident as nuclear to cytoplasm asynchrony, abnormal nuclear chromatin, and some nuclear lobation.

There is complete resolution of hematologic, biochemical, and growth abnormalities in affected puppies on treatment with parenteral, but not oral, cyanocobalamin. A megadose of cyanocobalamin (1 mg, once) administered parenterally is sufficient to maintain an affected dog in complete remission for more than 1 month, even during periods of greater requirements such as gestation, lactation, and rapid postnatal growth. Normal 12-week-old puppies are in the steepest part of their growth curves. In affected puppies, serum cobalamin concentrations were undetectable at 7 weeks, and growth failure became evident variably between 8 and 12 weeks. Parenteral cyanocobalamin (2.5 μg but not 0.5 μg) begun at 12 weeks of age and given daily was sufficient to return each puppy to a normal rate of growth within 1 week. Ten days of treatment with 5 μg/day prevented relapse for up to 4 weeks. Each of three affected puppies with onset of growth failure between 6 and 7 weeks of age that were treated once

with 1 mg of parenteral cyanocobalamin maintained a normal rate of growth for the following 10 weeks.

The rapidity of responses to parenteral cobalamin treatment varies in cobalamin-deficient dogs. Appetite returns within 12 to 48 hours, and weight gain ensues immediately thereafter. Reticulocytosis begins 3 to 4 days after parenteral treatment and may last for 10 to 14 days. Total white blood cell and neutrophil counts increase rapidly and are within normal range within 10 days. Urinary methylmalonic acid excretion drops to within normal limits within 1 week. Serum methylmalonic acid concentrations drop equally soon after treatment, but serum total homocysteine concentrations may not be within normal limits for 2 weeks.

Adult dogs may become cobalamin-deficient without exhibiting recognizable clinical signs. In an adult affected dog from which parenteral cobalamin treatment was withheld for 6 months, the onset of cobalamin deficiency was clinically occult. Inappetence was not readily apparent, although appetite notably increased on parenteral cobalamin replacement. No hematologic abnormalities were noted. In another small study, an adult dog was maintained on a cobalamin-deficient diet for 5 years (CA Hall, personal communication, 1987). At 10 months, the experimental dog was excreting methylmalonic acid in urine, and its serum cobalamin concentration was 14% that of the control dog maintained on a normal canine diet. At the end of the study, the cobalamin content of most tissues of the depleted dog was 4 to 12% the content of control dog tissues. Exceptions were thyroid (21%) and brain (23%). Serum cobalamin was 6% of the control. Despite the cobalamin depletion of the experimental dog, the MCV was 67 fL and RBC count was $5.6 \times 10^6/\mu L$, neither value outside the limits of normal.

CLINICAL DIAGNOSIS OF COBALAMIN DEFICIENCY

Serum cobalamin concentration has proven to be the earliest and most convenient indicator of cobalamin deficiency in dogs. By 4 weeks of age, serum cobalamin concentrations are subnormal in puppies affected with selective cobalamin malabsorption. Puppies obtain the vitamin transplacentally during fetal life.[11] By comparing serum cobalamin concentrations of affected puppies and their normal littermates, developing cobalamin deficiency is evident as early as 2 weeks of age, indicating that their defect of cobalamin absorption is present at or soon after birth. Serum concentrations of methylmalonic acid and total homocysteine become significantly elevated by 6 weeks, but serum methionine concentrations are not significantly reduced until approximately 16 weeks of age.

In adult affected dogs from which monthly parenteral cobalamin treatment is withheld, serum cobalamin concentrations fall below normal within 2 weeks. Serum methylmalonic acid concentrations rise above normal within 4 weeks, but serum total homocysteine concentrations do not rise above the normal range for 17 to 18 weeks. Thus, in adult dogs and in growing puppies,

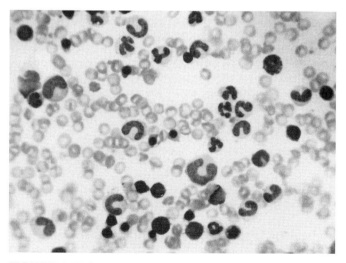

FIGURE 147.3 Bone marrow aspirate of a cobalamin-deficient dog. This bone marrow aspirate was prepared from the dog exhibiting the peripheral smear shown in Figure 147.2B. Cells of the erythropoietic series are underrepresented, and giant metamyelocytes and band neutrophils are evident.

the serum cobalamin concentration is the earliest indicator of cobalamin malabsorption and developing deficiency of the vitamin. Elevation of serum or urine methylmalonic acid indicates cobalamin deficiency at the tissue level, and the additional finding of elevated serum total homocysteine indicates long-standing deficiency with reduced activity of both cobalamin-dependent enzymes.

Experience with clinical cases of congenital and adult-onset cobalamin malabsorption in cats suggests that the serum cobalamin concentration is the earliest indicator of cobalamin deficiency in this species as well. Whereas cats with low serum cobalamin exhibit methylmalonic acidemia/-uria, they have not exhibited elevated serum homocysteine concentrations or homocystinuria. One such cat was found to have a serum betaine concentration of 1400 μM, 7- to 14-fold higher than serum betaine concentrations in cobalamin-deficient dogs and 25-fold higher than found in cobalamin-deficient humans.[12] High betaine concentrations in cats may allow homocysteine methylation in the absence of cobalamin-dependent methionine synthase activity.

Newly absorbed cobalamin in transit to target tissues is bound to the specific transport protein, trans-cobalamin-II (TC-II).[13] In both dogs and cats, nearly all serum cobalamin is bound to TC-II, and interruption of cobalamin absorption is quickly reflected in reduced serum cobalamin concentrations.[14] This is in contrast to the situation in humans, in which 75 to 90% of plasma cobalamin is bound to haptocorrin (a nonspecific cobalamin-binding protein) and in which cobalamin malabsorption may be long standing and tissue deficiency of the vitamin severe before serum cobalamin concentrations fall below the normal range.[13] Accordingly, studies of cobalamin turnover indicate a biologic half-life of the vitamin of 50 to 100 days in dogs compared with 330 to 400 days in humans.[11,15] It is likely that cats are more like dogs than humans in this respect.

GASTROINTESTINAL COBALAMIN ABSORPTION

Cobalamin is a complex organometallic compound containing a cobalt atom; thus, cobalamin deficiency due to reduced rumenal production of the vitamin may occur in ruminants grazing cobalt-deficient pastures. Although nonruminant diets vary widely in cobalamin content, the most common cause of cobalamin deficiency is gastrointestinal cobalamin malabsorption, either as selective cobalamin malabsorption or as part of a disorder causing intestinal malabsorption of other nutrients as well.[16]

Ingested cobalamin freed from foodstuffs by digestion is bound initially by a nonspecific corrin-binding glycoprotein, haptocorrin (HC or transcobalamin-I), found in salivary, gastric, pancreatic, and biliary secretions (Fig. 147.4).[17] When subjected to proteolysis and the rising pH of intestinal chyme, both caused by pancreatic secretions, HC releases cobalamin and the vitamin binds

to intrinsic factor (IF), a 50 kDa glycoprotein that still bears the moniker given it by William Castle in 1929.

IF is a highly specific cobalamin-binding protein that does not bind the many naturally occurring cobalamin analogs. IF is produced by the gastric mucosa in humans and rats, but dogs secrete intrinsic factor from pancreatic duct cells and the gastric mucosa[18,19]; intrinsic factor production in the domestic cat is entirely pancreatic.[20] A specific receptor on the apical membrane of epithelial cells in the distal small intestine mediates endocytosis of the cobalamin-IF complex. The intestinal receptor, previously designated IFCR, was recently dubbed cubilin due to its unusual structure composed of 8 tandem EGF domains followed by 27 tandem CUB domains.[21] After endocytosis, IF is degraded in lysosomes, and cobalamin is delivered to the portal plasma bound to the transport protein TC-II.[22]

There is a large flux of enterohepatic recirculation of cobalamin, up to 10-fold the daily dietary requirement, with cobalamin bound to HC secreted in bile, transfer of the vitamin to IF, and subsequent reabsorption in the distal small intestine.[23] This is suggested to be a means of eliminating altered cobalamin compounds, which are inhibitory to the enzymes of cobalamin-dependent metabolism, by exposing them again to the structural discrimination of IF-binding. Cobalamin excretion in bile has been demonstrated in dogs.[24]

Cubilin mRNA is expressed in the distal half of the canine small intestine, with peak expression in the distal quarter.[25] This correlates well with in vivo studies localizing the site of absorption of orally administered cobalamin to the distal ileum of dogs.[26,27] Cubilin is more restricted in cat intestine; the receptor activity is found only in the distal third of the small intestine, and peak expression is restricted to the distal sixth.[28] Again, this correlates with the site of absorption of orally administered cobalamin determined experimentally in cats.[20]

The intestinal epithelial receptor for the IF-cobalamin complex was recently shown to be identical to the receptor designated gp280 in studies of rat yolk sac and renal proximal tubule epithelium.[29] Genetic evidence stemming from studies of canine selective intestinal cobalamin malabsorption indicates that the intestinal and renal receptors are products of the same gene.[3] In the kidney, it appears to function as a salvage receptor of several proteins filtered by the glomerulus. Cloning of cubilin cDNAs of rats, humans, and dogs indicates that the receptor is a 460 kDa glycoprotein that is highly conserved among the three species data.[21,30,31]

DIAGNOSIS OF COBALAMIN MALABSORPTION

Cobalamin malabsorption can be considered a cobalamin wasting disorder because it interrupts absorption of the larger proportion of cobalamin undergoing enterohepatic recirculation as well as dietary cobalamin (Fig. 147.4). Due to the complexity of mechanisms involved in cobalamin absorption, cobalamin malabsorption may accompany a wide variety of acquired gastro-

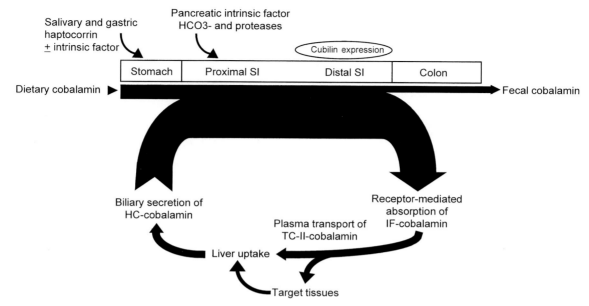

FIGURE 147.4 Gastrointestinal cobalamin absorption and transport. Dietary cobalamin is transferred from haptocorrin to intrinsic factor in the proximal small intestine (SI), and the intrinsic factor-cobalamin complex is absorbed in the distal small intestine. Absorption is mediated by the specific IF-cobalamin receptor, cubilin. Interruption of cobalamin absorption causes rapid cobalamin wasting because a large daily flux of cobalamin undergoes enterohepatic recirculation.

intestinal disorders in addition to the hereditary forms. These may variously affect the production of cobalamin binding proteins, the transfer of cobalamin from HC to IF in the proximal small intestine, and the binding of the IF-cobalamin complex to cubilin in the distal small intestine. Failure anywhere along the gastrointestinal absorptive pathway results in cobalamin deficiency, characteristic metabolic abnormalities, and, when sufficiently prolonged, dyshematopoiesis.

Cobalamin absorption may be demonstrated directly by means of oral administration of radiolabeled cobalamin and collection of feces, urine, and/or serum samples.[32] In all such tests, the patient is fed a physiologic dose of radioactive cobalamin, and the ability to absorb is determined by measuring radioactivity in the stool, urine, blood, liver, or whole body. Such a test was developed to evaluate cobalamin absorption in normal controls and dogs with selective intestinal cobalamin malabsorption.[2] Under the conditions used, normal control dogs absorbed approximately one-third of the administered dose, with kinetics identical to those described in similarly tested humans[33]; there was no detectable cobalamin absorption in affected dogs.[2]

Canine cobalamin absorption can be determined directly in this way because the radiotracer allows the detection of newly absorbed cobalamin within the relatively large pool of cobalamin already in circulation, but the radioactive excretory products present regulatory and contamination problems. A promising alternative approach that does not use radioactive material is to document cobalamin wasting. This has been used in cats with small intestinal disease causing cobalamin deficiency and in a cat with congenital cobalamin malab-

sorption (KW Simpson, JC Fyfe, unpublished data, 2000). Serum cobalamin concentrations were measured at weekly intervals after parenteral administration of a 1-mg megadose of the vitamin. Cobalamin wasting was inferred when serum cobalamin concentrations dropped from supranormal levels to subnormal within 4 weeks, a rate of decline not seen in normal control cats. In cats with acquired conditions, specific treatment led to reduced cobalamin wasting and, by inference, restored cobalamin absorption. As indicated previously, similar kinetics of cobalamin wasting occur in dogs with selective cobalamin malabsorption, suggesting that cobalamin wasting determination may be clinically useful in dogs as well.

REFERENCES

1. **Fyfe JC, Jezyk PF, Giger U, Patterson DF.** Inherited selective malabsorption of vitamin B_{12} in giant schnauzers. J Am Anim Hosp Assoc 1989;25:533–539.
2. **Fyfe JC, Giger U, Hall CA, Jezyk PF, Klumpp SA, Levine JS, Patterson DF.** Inherited selective intestinal cobalamin malabsorption and cobalamin deficiency in dogs. Pediatr Res 1991;29:24–31.
3. **Fyfe JC, Ramanujam KS, Ramaswamy K, Patterson DF, Seetharam B.** Defective brush-border expression of intrinsic factor-cobalamin receptor in canine inherited intestinal malabsorption. J Biol Chem 1991;266:4489–4494.
4. **Beck WS.** Biological and medical aspects of vitamin B_{12}. In: Dolphin D, ed. B_{12} biochemistry and medicine. New York: John Wiley & Sons, 1982;2.
5. **Allen RH, Stabler SP, Savage DG, Lindenbaum J.** Metabolic abnormalities in cobalamin (vitamin B_{12}) and folate deficiency. FASEB J 1993;7:1344–1353.
6. **Scott J, Weir D.** Folate/vitamin B_{12} inter-relationships. Essays Biochem 1994;28:63–72.
7. **Babior BM.** The megaloblastic anemias. In: Williams WJ, Beutler E, Erslev AJ, Lichtman MA, eds. Hematology. 4th ed. New York: McGraw-Hill 1990.
8. **Outerbridge CA, Myers SL, Giger U.** Hereditary cobalamin deficiency in border collie dogs. J Vet Intern Med 1996;10:169.
8a. **Fordyce HH, Callan MB, Giger U.** Persistent cobalamin deficiency causing failure to thrive in a juvenile beagle. JSAP, 2000, in press.
9. **Keesling PT, Morris JG.** Vitamin B_{12} deficiency in the cat. J Anim Sci 1975;41:317.

10. **Vaden SL, Wood PA, Ledley FD, Cornwell PE, Miller RT, Page R.** Cobalamin deficiency associated with methylmalonic acidemia in a cat. J Am Vet Med Assoc 1992;200:1101–1103.

11. **Luhby AL, Cooperman JM, Donnenfeld AM.** Placental transfer and biological half-life of radioactive vit. B_{12} in the dog. Proc Soc Exp Biol Med 1959;100:214–217.

12. **Allen RH, Stabler SP, Lindenbaum J.** Serum betaine, N,N-dimethylglycine and N-methylglycine levels in patients with cobalamin and folate deficiency and related inborn errors of metabolism. Metabolism 1993;42:1448–1460.

13. **Hall CA.** Transcobalamins I and II as natural transport proteins of vitamin B_{12}. J Clin Invest 1975;56:1125–1131.

14. **Linnell JC, Collings L, Down MC, England JM.** Distribution of endogenous cobalamin between the transcobalamins in various mammals. Clin Sci 1979;57:139–144.

15. **Schloesser LL, Deshpande P, Schilling RF.** Biologic turnover rate of cyanocobalamin (vitamin B_{12}) in human liver. Arch Intern Med 1958;101:306–309.

16. **Sullivan LW.** Vitamin B_{12} metabolism and megaloblastic anemia. Semin Hematol 1970;7:6–22.

17. **Allen RH, Seetharam B, Allen NC, Podell E, Alpers DH.** Correction of cobalamin malabsorption in pancreatic insufficiency with a cobalamin analogue that binds with high affinity to R protein but not to intrinsic factor: *in vivo* evidence that a failure to partially degrade R protein is responsible for cobalamin malabsorption in pancreatic insufficiency. J Clin Invest 1978;61:1628–1634.

18. **Batt RM, Horadagoda NU, McLean L, Morton DB, Simpson KW.** Identification and characterization of a pancreatic intrinsic factor in the dog. Am J Physiol 1989;256:G517–G523.

19. **Simpson KW, Alpers DH, De Wille J, Swanson P, Farmer S, Sherding RG.** Cellular localization and hormonal regulation of pancreatic intrinsic factor secretion in dogs. Am J Physiol 1993;265:G178–G188.

20. **Fyfe JC.** Feline intrinsic factor (IF) is pancreatic in origin and mediates ileal cobalamin (Cbl) absorption. J Vet Intern Med 1993;7:133.

21. **Moestrup SK, Kozyraki R, Kristiansen M, Kaysen JH, Rasmussen HH, Brault D, Pontillon F, Goda FO, Christensen EI, Hammond TG, Verroust PJ.** The intrinsic factor-vitamin B_{12} receptor and target of teratogenic antibodies is a megalin-binding peripheral membrane protein with homology to developmental proteins. J Biol Chem 1998;273:5235–5242.

22. **Rappazzo ME, Hall CA.** Cyanocobalamin transport proteins in canine plasma. Am J Physiol 1972;222:202–206.

23. **Kanazawa S, Herbert V.** Mechanism of enterohepatic circulation of vitamin B_{12}: movement of vitamin B_{12} from bile R-binder to intrinsic factor due to the action of pancreatic trypsin. Trans Assoc Am Physicians 1983;96:336–343.

24. **Willigan DA, Cronkite EP, Meyer LM, Noto SL.** 1958 Biliary excretion of Co^{60} labeled vitamin B_{12} in dogs. Proc Soc Exp Biol Med 1958;99:81–84.

25. **Xu D, Fyfe JC.** Determination of longitudinal intrinsic factor-cobalamin receptor expression in dog intestine. Proc 8th Annu Phi Zeta Res Day, East Lansing, Michigan, 1998.

26. **Drapanas T, Williams JS, McDonald JC, Heyden W, Bow T, Spencer RP.** Role of the ileum in the absorption of vitamin B_{12} and intrinsic factor (NF). JAMA 1963;184:337–341.

27. **Marcoullis G, Rothenberg SP.** Intrinsic factor-mediated intestinal absorption of cobalamin in the dog. Am J Physiol 1981;241:G294–G299.

28. **Stolt LB, Fyfe JC.** Localization of proteins that mediate gastrointestinal cobalamin absorption in cats and dogs. Proc 6th Annu Phi Zeta Res Day, East Lansing, Michigan, 1995.

29. **Seetharam B, Christensen EI, Moestrup SK, Hammond TG, Verroust PJ.** Identification of rat yolk sac target protein of teratogenic antibodies, gp280, as intrinsic factor-cobalamin receptor. J Clin Invest 1997;99:2317–2322.

30. **Kozyraki R, Kristiansen M, Silahtaroglu A, Hansen C, Jacobsen C, Tommerup N, Verroust PJ, Moestrup SK.** The human intrinsic factor-vitamin B_{12} receptor, *cubilin*: molecular characterization and chromosomal mapping of the gene to 10p within the autosomal recessive megaloblastic anemia (MGA1) region. Blood 1998;91:3593–3600.

31. **Xu D, Kozyraki R, Newman TC, Fyfe JC.** Genetic evidence of an accessory protein activity required specifically for cubilin brush-border expression and intrinsic factor-cobalamin absorption. Blood 1999;94:3604–3606.

32. **Herbert V.** Detection of malabsorption of vitamin B_{12} due to gastric or intestinal dysfunction. Semin Nucl Med 1972;2:220–234.

33. **Arkun SN, Miller IF, Meyers LM.** Vitamin B_{12} absorption test. Acta Haematol 1969;41:341–348.

CHAPTER 148

Chédiak-Higashi Syndrome

• KENNETH M. MEYERS

Chédiak-Higashi syndrome (CHS) is an inherited disease that is transmitted as an autosomal recessive trait. It has been described in humans; Hereford, Brangus, and Japanese Black cattle; Aleutian mink; beige (bg) mice; Persian cats; blue and silver foxes; beige rats; and an albino killer whale.[1,2] A partial oculocutaneous albinism, recurrent pyogenic infections, and a bleeding tendency characterize the syndrome (Fig. 148.1). Children, but not animals, with CHS often enter an accelerated phase of the disease characterized by fever, lymphoadenopathy, hepatosplenomegaly, and pancytopenia with widespread lymphohistiocytic organ infiltration.[3] The accelerated phase may occur shortly after birth or may be delayed for years and is usually fatal. There is an increased morbidity and mortality in animals with CHS.[4]

CLINICAL SIGNS AND DIAGNOSIS

Diagnosis of CHS is based on the presence of hypopigmentation of the skin, hair, and eyes; enlarged or giant granules in granule-forming cells; and a platelet storage pool disease. The most consistent diagnostic pathologic feature in humans is the presence of giant eosinophilic, peroxidase-positive granules in peripheral leukocytes (Fig. 148.2). In some species, such as cats,[5] the enlarged granules in neutrophils are only lightly eosinophilic; in others, such as mice and rats, the enlarged granules are more prominent in cells other than neutrophils.[6,7]

Early prenatal diagnosis of CHS is possible based on the presence of enlarged granules. Most prenatal diagnoses of CHS have been made through cytologic examination of fetal blood cells with or without fetal tissue. Cultured amniotic fluid cells and chorionic villus cells have also been used for diagnostic purposes.[8]

Hypopigmentation

The pigmentary dilution in animals is seen as a lightened hair coat and lightened irises. In animals, the pigmentary dilution leads to unusual coat colors that are sought by the fur industry. The degree of hypopigmentation in humans is variable.

The enlarged melanin granules may have a regular shape or they may be complex. They can be observed in peripheral areas of the hair shaft under microscopic examination.[5] The presence of a few large melanin granules rather than a dispersed population of normal-sized granules contributes significantly to the pigmentary dilution in a manner that is analogous to the mechanism used by amphibians to change color. Amphibian skin becomes lighter when melanin granules aggregate and darker when melanin granules disperse. In addition, the enlarged granules have a paucity of some melanin-forming enzymes, such as tyrosinase.[9]

CHS has an associated photophobia, and tapetal areas are not apparent on ophthalmoscopic examination.[10] The tapetal defect in CHS cats is associated with a degeneration of tapetal rods, found within tapetal cells, when the kittens are between 2 and 4 weeks of age.

Increased Susceptibility to Pyogenic Infections

Humans and animals with CHS have an increased susceptibility to bacterial infections, which is associated with multiple defects in the host defense system. There is neutropenia that is due, in part, to impaired release of mature neutrophils from the bone marrow.[3] The intracellular killing of phagocytized bacteria by CHS granulocytes is inhibited.[11] The number of phagocytes at the site of bacterial invasion is likely to be limited due to a defective chemotactic response.[12] Natural killer (NK)[13] cells and cytotoxic lymphocytes (CTL)[14] have enlarged granules, and the cytotoxic function of these cells is significantly impaired in bg mice and human patients with CHS.

Bleeding Diathesis

The bleeding tendency in CHS is due to platelet storage pool deficiency (SPD).[1] Template bleeding times are prolonged, whereas platelet counts and coagulation times are normal. Collagen-induced platelet aggregation in vitro is markedly depressed, especially at low agonist concentrations (Fig. 148.3). Platelet serotonin and secre-

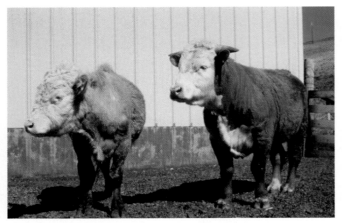

FIGURE 148.1 Two Hereford bulls with CHS. Hypopigmentation is apparent. The bull on the right was 2 years old; the bull on the left was 7 years old and exhibits marked wasting. There is a steady deterioration in CHS cattle due to chronic respiratory and other infections. The older bull died of subdermal bleeding complications following trauma.

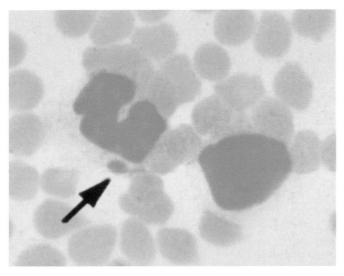

FIGURE 148.2 The arrow points to an enlarged granule in a monocyte from a CHS mink. There may be more than one granule per cell, and they can be as large as 2.5 μm in diameter (original magnification, 1000×).

mine (5HT).[16,17] The release of platelet agonists from activated platelets initiates a positive-feedback process, which enables platelet-to-platelet aggregates to plug the perforated blood vessel. CHS platelets, which have a virtual absence of dense granules and their stored platelet agonists, lack this feedback pathway.

Similar Disorders

Other syndromes have been described in animals (the fawn-hooded rat[18] and 14 strains of mice[19]) and people in which there is a pigmentary dilution and a platelet SPD. The triad of oculocutaneous albinism, a bleeding diathesis that is due to a platelet SPD, and pigmented macrophages characterizes the Hermansky-Pudlak syndrome (HPS).[20] Ceroid is present in large amounts in macrophages and accumulates in the lungs, bladder, and oral mucosa. The pale ear pigmented mouse (ep/ep) is an animal model for HPS.[21] The gene responsible for HPS has been identified in humans and the ep mouse.[21] The gene is located on chromosome 19 in mice and on human chromosome 10q24q25. Similar to CHS,

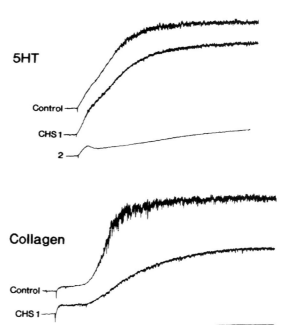

FIGURE 148.3 Aggregometer tracing of platelets from a normal cat and two cats with CHS in response to serotonin (5HT) (12.5 μM) and collagen (25 ug/mL). The bar represents 0.25 minutes. The impaired aggregation response was more pronounced in platelets from CHS cat 2 than in platelets from CHS cat 1. Feline platelets form the platelet agonist thromboxane (Tx) A2 in response to an agonist, such as 5HT and collagen, and they are sensitive to TxA2. The degree of platelet impairment in SPD platelets from animals like the cat is dependent not only on the loss of dense granule agonists, but also on the amount of TxA2 formed. In this case, the platelet SPD of the two CHS cats was the same, but platelets from CHS cat 1 formed three times more TxA2 than did platelets from CHS cat 2.

table adenosine triphosphate (ATP) and adenosine diphosphate (ADP) are virtually absent, as are ultrastructurally identifiable dense granules.

The most prominent ultrastructural feature of platelets is the presence of a large number of granules.[15] Platelets contain four granule types, alpha granules, lysosomes, microperoxisomes, and dense granules (Fig. 148.4). Alpha granules and lysosomes contain proteins and acid hydrolases, respectively. Dense granules (also known as amine storage organelles, very dense granules, dense bodies, and bull's-eye granules) store a high (molar) concentration of the platelet agonists adenosine diphosphate (ADP) and serotonin or 5-hydroxytrypta-

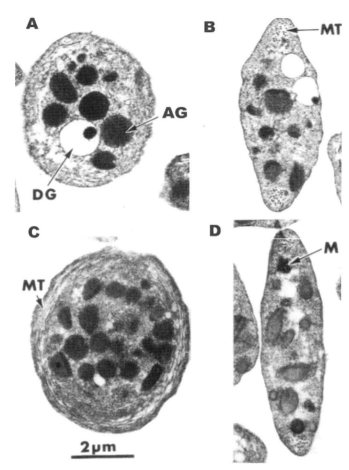

FIGURE 148.4 Platelets from normal (**A, B**) and CHS (**C, D**) cattle fixed with glutaraldehyde followed by osmium tetroxide postfixation. Dense granules (DG) are seen in normal but not CHS platelets. *AG,* alpha granules; *M,* microtubules; *Mito,* mitochondria.

the degree of hypopigmentation differs among HPS patients. These differences among patients and the large number of mutations that result in both a pigment abnormality and a platelet-dense granule abnormality point out that multiple factors are involved in the formation of granules and that platelet-dense granules and melanosomes have several processes in common.

CELLULAR DEFECTS

Enlarged Granules

Enlarged granules have been observed in most granule-forming cells including renal tubules and fibroblasts (Fig. 148.2). The enlarged granules have been so closely associated with lysosomes that CHS is generally considered a lysosomal disease. Where there is more than one granule type within a cell, the granule with lysosomal-like properties is the primary granule affected.[22] For example, neutrophils have azurophilic, specific, and gelatinase granules. Azurophilic granules are lysosomal-like

granules. They contain acid hydrolases and myeloperoxidase, which provides the term peroxidase-positive granules. Giant granules are derived from azurophilic granules, and the peroxidase-negative granules are not major participants in the formation of giant granules. Melanosomes, which are not lysosomes but are enlarged in CHS, have lysosomal-like properties and contain hydrolytic enzymes and lysosomal-associated membrane proteins.

Within a species, not all cells have the same phenotypic expression of the CHS defect. Although massive giant granules are observed in nearly all leukocytes from human CHS patients, giant granules are seldom seen in human CHS platelets.[16]

Within a given cell line there are differences in expression of the CHS trait as species lines are crossed. Enlarged giant granules have not been identified in platelets and megakaryocytes (MKs) from CHS cattle, mink, and cats.[15] Conversely, enlarged granules have been identified in human CHS platelets and mice MK.[15,16]

The enlarged granules in many CHS cells are not secreted appropriately, and the granule secretory defect has clinical significance. The enlarged melanosomes are not efficiently transferred from melanocytes into keratinocytes.[9] This may further limit granule dispersion and enhance the pigmentary dilution seen in CHS. The ineffective bactericidal activity of phagocytes is attributed to impaired phago-lysosome fusion, whereas the defective cytolytic function is related to an inability of NK cells and CTL to exocytose their lytic granules.[14]

Although the pathophysiology of the CHS trait is beginning to be described, several steps need clarification. Substances to be digested within lysosomes are received from endosomes containing endocytosed material or proteins from the *trans* Golgi network, from autophagosomes containing cell organelles, or from phagosomes containing phagocytosed material. There are two defined populations of endosomes vesicles, early and late endosomes. Early endosomes may make a transition into late endosomes by a granule fusion process that is dependent on normal microtubule function. Late endosomes also receive vesicles from the *trans* Golgi network. Late endosomes make a transition into lysosomes by a process that involves granule fusion. In CHS there is a severe misdirection of vesicles from the *trans* Golgi network and/or early endosomes into late endosomes.[23] As a consequence, the transported enzyme may not be incorporated into the target granule but may be secreted to the exterior.[9] This may lead to a deficiency of microbicidal/cytotoxic proteins in host defense cells[3] and a reduction of tyrosinase in melanocytes.[9] The enlarged granules in CHS are lysosomes and not early or late endosomes.[23] The relationship between the sorting defect and enlarged lysosomal granules has not yet been described.

Cellular Defects Other Than Enlarged Granules

Cytoskeletal abnormalities and impaired cyclic nucleotide metabolism have been described in neutrophils from some humans[24] and animals[25] with CHS. Although these abnormalities may be present and contribute to the bactericidal defect in CHS, they do not represent the basic defect in CHS. They are not seen in all CHS neutrophils[24] or in other cells.[1,26]

In a syndrome that is characterized by the presence of enlarged granules in granule-forming cells, platelets represent an unusual expression of the gene. There is a virtual absence of dense granules in CHS animal platelets and most CHS human patients (Fig. 148.4).[1,15] Enlarged platelet alpha granules and lysosomes have not been observed in CHS cats, mink, and Hereford cattle. They are rarely observed in platelets from human CHS patients or in CHS foxes or MKs from bg mice. Platelet-dense granules accumulate and store nucleotides, divalent cations, and amines. Most of the adenine nucleotides contained in dense granules are synthesized by MKs. Within MKs, granules having the typical appearance of dense granules cannot be identified, but granules that are the precursors to platelet-dense granules are observed. Once platelets are in circulation, they acquire 5HT that is released from enterochromaffin cells into plasma. Serotonin is stored within dense granules as a nucleotide-bivalent cation macromolecular complex[17] that can be demonstrated by transmission electron microscopy. In cattle there is a dense eccentrically located core that appears attached to the luminal side of the membrane (Fig. 148.4). The remaining contents of the dense granule have a clear, empty appearance. The virtual absence of platelet-dense granules appears to be due to a granule-forming defect in MKs where the precursor to the platelet-dense granule is not formed.

GENE ABNORMALITY

The CHS gene has been identified.[27-29] The *beige* gene in mice, which is located on chromosome 13, and the human CHS gene (also termed lysosomal trafficking regulator or LYST) have been cloned and sequenced. The mouse *beige* and the human CHS are homologous. A 5-kilobase deletion has been described in *beige*. Three gene defects have been identified in human CHS patients, a nonsense and two frame shift mutations. Genetic and cellular complementation studies suggest that the defective gene in CHS mink is homologous to in that in humans and mice.[30]

The function of the Beige/CHS protein or LYST is unknown. Based on sequence analysis, the CHS protein contains transmembrane association regions.[29] The modular architecture of BG/CHS is similar to the yeast protein kinase VPS15, which is involved with vacuolar protein sorting.[29] In cellular immunolocalization studies, the Beige protein was not membrane associated but colocalized with microtubules.[23]

TREATMENT

Temporary improvement has been achieved in some[31] but not all[32] human CHS patents through the use of ascorbic acid. Other temporary treatments include steroids, cytotoxic and chemotherapeutic agents[32,33] (vincristine and colchicine, etoposide and methotrexate), or splenectomy.[34] Platelet transfusions may provide short-term correction of the bleeding diathesis.[35] Neutrophil function of CHS cats is temporarily improved with recombinant granulocyte-colony-stimulating factor[36] or interleukin-2[37] treatment. Long-term correction of the platelet, granulocytic, and cytotoxic T-cell abnormalities is provided by bone marrow transplantation.[38,39] Drugs that affect platelet function, such as cyclooxygenase inhibitors, are contraindicated.

REFERENCES

1. **Meyers KM, Menard M.** Platelet storage pool deficiency. In: Meyers KM, Barnes CD, eds. The platelet amine storage granule. Ann Arbor: CRC Press, 1992.
2. **Ogawa H, Tu C-H, Kagamizono H, Soki K, Inoue Y, Akatsuka H, Nagata S-I, Wada T, Ikeya M, Makimura S, Uchida K, Yamaguchi R, Otsuka H.** Clinical, morphological, and biochemical characteristics of Chediak-Higashi syndrome in fifty-six Japanese Black cattle. Am J Vet Res 1997;58:1221–1226.
3. **Blume RS, Wolff SM.** The Chediak-Higashi syndrome: studies in four patients and a review of the literature. Medicine 1972;51:247–263.
4. **Windhorst DB, Padgett G.** The Chediak-Higashi syndrome and the homologous trait in animals. J Invest Dermatol 1973;60:529–537.
5. **Prieur DJ, Collier LL, Bryan GM, Meyers KM.** The diagnosis of feline Chediak-Higashi syndrome. Feline Pract 1979;9:26–32.
6. **Ozaki K, Maeda H, Nishikawa T, Nishimura M, Narama I.** Chediak-Higashi syndrome in rats: light and electron microscopical characterization of abnormal granules in beige rats. J Comp Pathol 1994;110:369–379.
7. **Oliver C, Essner E.** Distribution of anomalous lysosomes in the beige mouse: a homologue of Chediak-Higashi syndrome. J Histochem Cytochem 1973;21:218–228.
8. **Diukman R, Tanigawara S, Cowan M, Golbus M.** Prenatal diagnosis of Chediak-Higashi syndrome. Prenat Diagn 1992;12:877–885.
9. **Zhao H, Boissy Y, Abdel-Malek Z, King R, Nordlund J, Boissy R.** On the analysis of the pathophysiology of Chediak-Higashi syndrome: defects expressed by cultured melanocytes. Lab Invest 1994;71:25–34.
10. **Collier LL, King EJ, Prieur DJ.** Tapetal degeneration in cats with Chediak-Higashi syndrome. Curr Eye Res 1985;4:767–773.
11. **Renshaw HW, Davis WC, Fudenberg HH, Padgett GA.** Leukocyte dysfunction in the bovine homologue of the Chediak-Higashi syndrome of humans. Infect Immun 1974;10:928–937.
12. **Colgan SP, Blancquaert AB, Thrall MA, Bruyninckx WJ.** Defective *in vitro* motility of polymorphonuclear leukocytes of homozygote and heterozygote Chediak-Higashi cats. Vet Immunol Immunopathol 1992;31:205–227.
13. **Roder J, Duwe A.** The beige mutation in the mouse selectively impairs natural killer cell function. Nature 1979;278:451–453.
14. **Baetz K, Isaaz S, Griffiths G.** Loss of cytotoxic T lymphocyte function in Chediak-Higashi syndrome arises from a secretory defect that prevents lytic granule exocytosis. J Immunol 1995;154:6122–6131.
15. **Ménard M, Meyers K.** Ultrastructure of dense granule precursor development in megakaryocytes. In: Meyers KM, Barnes CD, eds. The platelet amine storage granule. Ann Arbor: CRC Press, 1992.
16. **White JG.** The dense bodies of human platelets. In: Meyers KM, Barnes CD, eds. The platelet amine storage granule. Ann Arbor: CRC Press, 1992.
17. **Holmsen H, Ugurbil K.** Nuclear magnetic resonance studies of amine and nucleotide storage mechanisms in platelet dense granules. In: Meyers KM, Barnes CD, eds. The platelet amine storage granule. Ann Arbor: CRC Press, 1992.
18. **Tschopp TB, Zucker MB.** Hereditary defect in platelet function in rats. Blood 1972;40:217–226.
19. **Swank RT, Reddington M, Novak EK.** Inherited prolonged bleeding time and platelet storage pool deficiency in subtle gray (SUT) mouse. Lab Anim Sci 1996;46:56–60.
20. **Gahl WA, Brantly M, Kaiser-Kupfer MI, Iwata F, Hazelwood S, Shotelersuk V, Duffy LF, Kuehl EM, Troendle J, Bernardini I.** Genetic defects and clinical characteristics of patients with a form of oculocutaneous albinism (Hermansky-Pudlak syndrome). N Engl J Med 1998;338:1258–1264.
21. **Gardner JM, Wildenberg SC, Keiper NM, Novak EK, Rusiniak ME, Swank RT, Puri N, Finger JN, Hagiwara N, Lehman AL, Gales TL, Bayer ME, King RA, Brilliant MH.** The mouse pale ear (ep) mutation is the homologue of human Hermansky-Pudlak syndrome. Proc Natl Acad Sci USA 1997;94:9238–9243.
22. **Kjeldsen L, Calafat J, Borregaard N.** Giant granules of neutrophils in Chediak-Higashi syndrome are derived from azurophil granules but not from specific and gelatinase granules. J Leukoc Biol 1998;64:72–77.
23. **Faigle W, Raposo G, Tenza D, Pinet V, Vogt AB, Kropshofer H, Fischer**

A, de Saint-Basile G, Amigorena S. Deficient peptide loading and MHC class II endosomal sorting in a human genetic immunodeficiency disease: the Chediak-Higashi syndrome. J Cell Biol 1998;141:1121–1134.

24. **Pryzwansky KB, Schliwa M, Boxer LA.** Microtubule organization of un-stimulated and stimulated adherent human neutrophils in Chediak-Higashi syndrome. Blood 1985;66:1398–1403.

25. **Oliver JM.** Impaired microtubule assembly correctable by cyclic GMP and cholinergic agonists in the Chediak-Higashi syndrome. Am J Pathol 1976;85:395–418.

26. **Perou CM, Kaplan J.** Chediak-Higashi syndrome is not due to a defect in microtubule-based lysosomal mobility. J Cell Sci 1993;106:99–107.

27. **Perou CM, Moore KJ, Nagle DL, Misumi DJ, Woolf EA, McGrail SH, Holmgren L, Brody TH, Dussault BJ Jr, Monroe CA, Duyk GM, Pryor RJ, Li L, Justice MJ, Kaplan J.** Identification of the murine beige gene by YAC complementation and positional cloning. Nat Genet 1996;13:303–308.

28. **Barbosa MDFS, Nguyen QA, Tchernev VT, Ashley JA, Detter JC, Blaydes SM, Brandt SJ, Chotai D, Hodgman C, Solari CE, Lovett M, Kingsmore SF.** Identification of the homologous beige and Chediak-Higashi syndrome genes. Nature 1996;382:262–265.

29. **Nagle DL, Karim MA, Woolf EA, Holmgren L, Bork P, Misumi DJ, McGrail SH, Dussault BJ Jr, Perou CM, Boissy RE, Duyk GM, Spritz RA, Moore KJ.** Identification and mutation analysis of the complete gene for Chediak-Higashi syndrome. Nat Genet 1996;14:307–311.

30. **Perou CM, Justice MJ, Pryor RJ, Kaplan J.** Complementation of the beige mutation in cultured cells by episomally replicating murine yeast artificial chromosomes. Proc Natl Acad Sci USA 1996;93:5905–5909.

31. **Boxer LA, Watanabe AM, Rister M, Besch HR, Allen J, Baehner RL.** Correc-tion of leukocyte function in Chediak-Higashi syndrome by ascorbate. N Engl J Med 1976;259:1041–1045.

32. **Saitoh H, Komiyama A, Norose N, Morosawa H, Akabane T.** Development of the accelerated phase during ascorbic acid therapy in Chediak-Higashi syndrome and efficacy of colchicine on its management. Br J Haematol 1981;48:79–84.

33. **Bejaoui M, Veber F, Girault D, Gaud C, Blanche S, Griscelli C, Fisher A.** Phase accélérée de la maladie de Chediak-Higashi. Arch Fr Pediatr 1989; 46:733–736.

34. **Harfi HA, Malik SA.** Chediak-Higashi syndrome: clinical, hematologic, and immunologic improvement after splenectomy. Ann Allergy 1992;69:147–149.

35. **Cowles BE, Meyers KM, Wardrop KJ, Menard M, Sylvester D.** Transfusion of normal feline platelets corrects the bleeding time in cats with the Chediak-Higashi syndrome. Thromb Haemost 1992;67:708–712.

36. **Colgan SP, Gasper PW, Thrall MA, Boone TC, Blancquaert AMB, Bruyninckx WJ.** Neutrophil function in normal and Chediak-Higashi syndrome cats following administration of recombinant canine granulocyte colony-stimulating factor. Exp Hematol 1992;20:1229–1234.

37. **Holcombe RF.** Interleukin-2-induced cytotoxicity of Chediak-Higashi lym-phocytes. Acta Haematol 1992;87:45–48.

38. **Colgan SP, Hull-Thrall MA, Gasper PW, Gould DH, rose BJ, Fulton R, Blanquaert AMB, Bruyninckx WJ.** Restoration of neutrophil and platelet function in feline Chediak-Higashi syndrome by bone marrow transplanta-tion. Bone Marrow Transplant 1991;7:365–374.

39. **Haddad E, Le Deist F, Blanche S, Benkerrou M, Rohrlich P, Vilmer E, Griscelli C, Fisher A.** Treatment of Chediak-Higashi syndrome by allogenic bone marrow transplantation: report of 10 cases. Blood 1995;85:3328–3333.

CHAPTER 149

Pelger-Huët Anomaly

• KENNETH S. LATIMER

Pelger-Huët (P-H) anomaly is generally a benign congenital anomaly of leukocytes characterized by nuclear hyposegmentation of granulocytes with the retention of a coarse, mature chromatin pattern.[1] Alterations in granulocyte morphology are especially noticeable in the neutrophil series where band cells and metamyelocytes predominate in the stained blood smear. Nuclear morphology is variable and may be round, oval, dumb-bell-shaped, peanut-shaped, band, or bilobate. The latter nuclear shape often consists of two rounded lobes of chromatin connected by a thin filament. This is referred to as the spectacle or "pince-nez" form, resembling eyeglasses that pinch the bridge of the nose to remain in place.[2] Barr bodies or sex chromatin bodies, typical of neutrophil nuclei of females, are not observed or are exceedingly rare.[3] The overall impression derived from examination of the stained blood smear is that of a degenerative left shift (neutrophil bands and less mature forms outnumber segmenters) without toxic changes of neutrophils.

Eosinophils and basophils have similar nuclear hyposegmentation. More detailed studies also have documented nuclear hypolobulation of both monocytes and megakaryocytes.[4] P-H anomaly, therefore, is a natural reflection of the interrelated development of granulocytes, monocytes, and megakaryocytes. Examination of Romanowsky-stained bone marrow smears reveals a normal maturation sequence with the exception of nuclear hyposegmentation. Furthermore, observations of the congenital nature of the anomaly have included transfer of P-H anomaly by bone marrow transplantation[5] and presence of the anomaly in identical triplets.[6]

P-H anomaly occasionally is a serendipitous laboratory finding in a healthy individual. More often, however, the anomaly is encountered in ill patients in whom it may be misdiagnosed as chronic infection, preleukemic syndrome, or a drug-induced change in granulocyte morphology.[1] Diagnosis of P-H anomaly, however, requires the exclusion of possible causes of acquired nuclear hyposegmentation of granulocytes (pseudo-Pelger-Huët anomaly) such as chronic bacterial and viral infections, drug administration, and developing neoplasia.

HISTORICAL BACKGROUND

Karl Pelger, a Dutch physician specializing in tuberculosis, first reported the unique appearance of neutrophils with nuclear hyposegmentation and a mature, coarse chromatin pattern in the blood of a woman with tuberculosis in 1928.[7] Subsequently, he reported similar hematologic findings in a second tuberculosis patient in 1931, leading to an association between these unique hematologic findings and severe tuberculosis with a poor clinical prognosis.[8] In the same year, G. J. Huët, a Dutch pediatrician, examined a young girl for suspected tuberculosis. Tuberculosis could not be documented despite the presence of nuclear hyposegmentation of neutrophils as previously described by Pelger. A detailed medical history, however, indicated that this girl was the niece of Pelger's first patient. Subsequent hematologic study of family members revealed that the unique neutrophil morphology was inherited as an autosomal dominant trait.[9] Other familial descriptions of this new anomaly subsequently were reported. In the interim, professional debate ensued on the proper name for this hematologic syndrome. Schilling ultimately proposed that this hereditary hematologic syndrome should be called Pelger-Huët anomaly.[10]

Following the initial description and study of P-H anomaly in humans, the anomaly was subsequently identified in rabbits in 1938.[11] The anomaly was not reported in another species for approximately three decades, until it was observed simultaneously in a German shepherd dog in Eastern Europe and in a red bone hound in the United States in 1965.[12,13] Subsequently, P-H anomaly was first reported in cats from the United States in 1981.[14]

AFFECTED SPECIES AND INCIDENCE

P-H anomaly has been described in humans,[2] rabbits,[15] dogs,[1] and cats.[14,16,17] The anomaly has been reported or observed in both mongrel[18] and purebred dogs, including the Australian cattle dog (blue heeler)[1]; Australian shepherd[1,19,20]; Basenji[21-23]; border collie[4]; Boston terrier[1]; cocker spaniel[24]; black and tan, blue tick, and red bone coonhounds[1,13,25]; German shepherd dog[12]; English-American (Walker) foxhounds[4,26]; and Samoyed.[4,27] The anomaly has only been described in eight domestic shorthair cats.[14,16,17] To date, congenital P-H anomaly has not been observed in large animals. Although P-H anomaly reportedly has been observed in reptiles,[14,19,28,29] these species, as well as amphibians, fish, and birds, normally have hyposegmented granulocyte nuclei in health. The appearance of the granulocytes mimics P-H anomaly, but distinct nuclear segmentation of granulocytes is not the norm as occurs in mammalian blood smears.

Most studies of the incidence of P-H anomaly have focused on humans. The overall incidence of P-H anomaly generally is low, but increased incidence of the anomaly may be associated with familial intermarriage or geographic clustering of populations in isolated locales. In humans, the incidence of the anomaly ranges from 1:320 in Advasi, India[30] to 1:43,000 in Spokane, Washington.[31] On the average, the incidence of the anomaly more closely approximates 1:6000 to 1:8000 in the general population. Based on the largest survey performed,[32] the incidence of P-H anomaly in rabbits exceeds 1:1786. In dogs, the incidence of P-H anomaly in the general hospital population exceeds approximately 1:10,000.[13] However, the incidence of the anomaly is higher in certain canine breeds because of line breeding and inbreeding. Recently, a large prospective study of P-H anomaly in Australian shepherds indicated a 9.8% incidence of the anomaly, especially in dogs from the west coast of the United States.[20] The incidence of P-H anomaly in cats is unknown, but probably is rare compared with that reported for dogs.

PHENOTYPIC EXPRESSION IN HEALTH AND INHERITANCE PATTERN

Heterozygous Phenotype

When P-H anomaly is encountered in clinical practice, it is usually in the heterozygous form. This form of the anomaly presents as a persistent left shift with a preponderance of band neutrophils and younger forms in the stained blood smear. The chromatin pattern is coarse and mature. Although the morphologic change is most apparent within neutrophils (Figs. 149.1 and 149.2), it is also present in eosinophils and basophils (Figs. 149.3 and 149.4).

Homozygous Phenotype

The homozygous form of P-H anomaly is rare. In this form of the anomaly, granulocytes have round to oval nuclei with an exceedingly coarse or "chunky" chromatin pattern (Fig. 149.5). The homozygous form of P-H anomaly was originally observed and studied in rabbits.[15] Homozygotes (super-Pelgers) were observed less

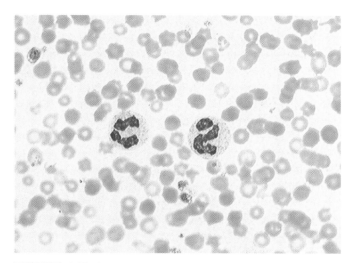

FIGURE 149.1 Blood smear from a cat (Wright-Leishman stain). Neutrophils with a normal phenotype exhibit distinct nuclear lobulation.

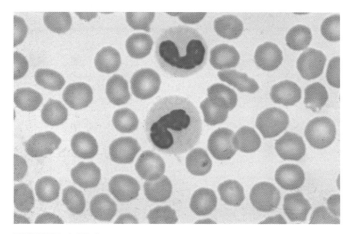

FIGURE 149.2 Blood smear from a cat with heterozygous P-H anomaly (Wright-Leishman stain). Neutrophils have band-shaped nuclei with a coarse, mature chromatin pattern.

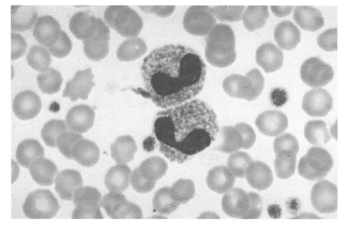

FIGURE 149.3 Blood smear from a cat with heterozygous P-H anomaly (Wright-Leishman stain). Eosinophil metamyelocytes have a coarse, mature chromatin pattern.

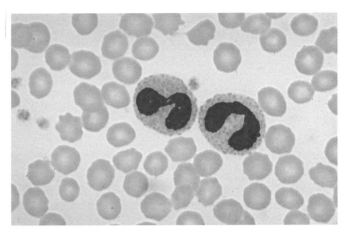

FIGURE 149.4 Blood smear from a cat with heterozygous P-H anomaly (Wright-Leishman stain). Basophils exhibit nuclear hyposegmentation with a coarse, mature chromatin pattern.

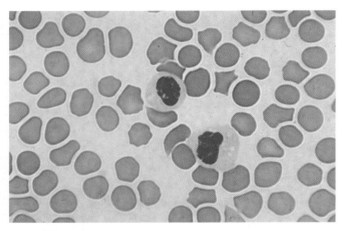

FIGURE 149.5 Blood smear from a cat with homozygous P-H anomaly (Wright-Leishman stain). Neutrophils have round to oval nuclei with an extremely condensed or "chunky" chromatin pattern.

frequently than expected, indicating that this form of the anomaly was lethal in utero. The few homozygous rabbits that were carried to term were usually stillborn or died within the first months of life. These individuals were also smaller and less vigorous than their heterozygous counterparts. Only 2 of 39 homozygous rabbits survived to adulthood,[15] and most of these had skeletal abnormalities related to chondrodysplasia.[15,33] Subsequently, homozygous P-H anomaly has been reported in 11 persons, but without skeletal deformity.[34–43] One individual was 94 years old when he was initially referred for hematologic study, indicating that humans with the homozygous form of P-H anomaly may have a prolonged lifespan.[39] The homozygous form of P-H anomaly also has been observed in one stillborn kitten with chondrodysplasia[17] but has not been observed in dogs.

Initial hematologic investigations in humans and rabbits indicated that P-H anomaly was inherited as a sim-

ple Mendelian autosomal dominant characteristic with almost 100% penetrance.[2,15] Presumptive evidence for a similar pattern of autosomal dominant transmittance also exists in dogs[25,26] and cats.[16] Despite the general acceptance of autosomal dominant transmittance of P-H anomaly, evidence in humans also suggests rare transmittance as an autosomal recessive trait.[44] For instance, two children with P-H anomaly were the progeny of parents with a normal leukocyte phenotype.[45,46] This observation suggests that P-H anomaly may not always exhibit 100% penetrance, a new mutation occurred, or the children were illegitimate. Recently, a large study of P-H anomaly in Australian shepherds has demonstrated autosomal dominant transmittance with incomplete penetrance.[20] Incomplete penetrance may allow the anomaly to skip generations where the typical leukocyte phenotype is not expressed (e.g., P-H progeny from patients with a normal leukocyte phenotype). Further studies will be required to determine if P-H anomaly is inherited in this manner in other dog breeds and to determine the mode of inheritance in cats.

Shift in Phenotypic Expression in Disease

The appearance of P-H cells in the blood may change somewhat in disease states. With severe bacterial infection, the "left shift" may intensify as nuclear morphology appears more immature and may occasionally mimic the homozygous form of P-H anomaly.[47] In dogs and cats with P-H anomaly, severe bacterial infection may be associated with toxic changes (basophilia, vacuolation, and/or Döhle bodies) of the neutrophil cytoplasm. Although the chromatin pattern should appear less mature in left shifts associated with bacterial infection, this may be difficult to confirm in stained blood smears from dogs or cats with the anomaly. If the intensified left shift results in a homozygous phenocopy, granulocyte morphology will revert to the heterozygous phenotype with successful treatment of the infection. Homozygous phenocopies of P-H anomaly also have been produced experimentally by administration of colchicine to rabbits with the heterozygous form of P-H anomaly.[48] Leukocyte morphology returned to the heterozygous phenotype when drug administration ceased.

Despite the presence of P-H anomaly, human P-H neutrophils may become hypersegmented with vitamin B_{12} or folate deficiency.[49,50] Affected neutrophils often have three to five nuclear lobes and appear more "normal." Following successful treatment of the megaloblastic anemia, the hypersegmented neutrophils revert to the heterozygous phenotype with typical nuclear hyposegmentation.

ULTRASTRUCTURAL, CYTOCHEMICAL, AND CYTOGENETIC STUDIES

One of the earliest ultrastructural studies of human P-H neutrophils reported nuclear hyposegmentation with occasional nuclear appendices and bridges. Subjectively, the number of cytoplasmic granules appeared decreased, but the size of the secondary granules was markedly increased.[51] The nuclear bridges may have represented filaments connecting nuclear lobes in cells with a pince-nez appearance. Furthermore, the change in granule number and size was not evaluated critically. More recent ultrastructural studies of P-H granulocytes from humans[52] and dogs[4,26] have reported nuclear hyposegmentation, occasional nuclear clefts, coarse heterochromatin, and normal cytoplasmic granules. These latter ultrastructural studies indicate that only nuclear changes exist in P-H cells, which is consistent with light microscopic observations.

Cytochemical staining has been performed on P-H granulocytes from both human and canine patients.[4,42,52,53] Stain applications have included Sudan black B, naphthol ASD chloroacetate esterase, peroxidase, alkaline and acid phosphatase, alpha-naphthyl acetate esterase, and periodic acid-Schiff reaction. Abnormalities in cytochemical staining have not been detected for either species. Collectively, these observations indicate that P-H neutrophils have adequate granules and granule constituents for bactericidal activity.

Limited cytogenetic studies of human patients with P-H anomaly have been performed.[52,54,55] In most instances, the karyotype has been normal; however, chromosomal abnormalities have been observed in a few individuals and within some families. The relationship of these abnormalities to either P-H anomaly or the population at large has not been determined. Similar studies have not been performed in animals.

CELL FUNCTION STUDIES

Controversy has existed since the 1930s whether P-H patients are predisposed to infection or other maladies.[56] Most clinical observations of human P-H patients fail to mention an increased incidence of clinical infection[31,57]; however, one report suggested an increased incidence of localized infections including appendicitis, meningitis, and pulmonary tuberculosis.[58] Another family was reported to have recurrent abdominal pain and fever similar to familial Mediterranean fever.[59] Personal experience with P-H dogs and cats indicates that these individuals are not clinically predisposed to infection. Although fewer weaned puppies have been reported from foxhound bitches with P-H anomaly,[26] it is unknown whether these dams were experienced or inexperienced at parenting. Thus, P-H anomaly generally is unassociated with an increased incidence of infection from a clinical viewpoint.

Early studies of P-H cell function have been controversial in both humans and dogs. In humans, neutrophil random and chemotactic movement has been reported as defective[60-62] or normal.[55-63] The larger, more recent studies have shown that P-H and control neutrophils exhibit comparable movement when tested in vitro.[55,63] In dogs, neutrophil chemotaxis was reported as defective (using in vivo skin chambers)[26] or normal (using

in vitro modified Boyden chambers).[21] Each study only examined one dog with P-H anomaly, and test methods differed. In a more recent report, five unrelated dogs with P-H anomaly were studied. Abnormalities in neutrophil movement were not discerned when measured by the skin window, migration under agarose, or modified Boyden chamber techniques.[64]

Various biochemical assays such as nitroblue tetrazolium (NBT) dye reduction, hexose monophosphate shunt activity, superoxide generation, chemiluminescence, and protein iodination suggest that P-H neutrophils are metabolically active and have adequate constituents for bactericidal activity.[52,55,61,63] The ultimate expression of bactericidal potential is the ability of human and canine P-H neutrophils to rapidly phagocytose and kill both bacteria and yeasts.[37,42,46,53,55,61,63,64] Reports of decreased phagocytic or bactericidal activity of P-H neutrophils are infrequent.[56,60]

Studies of immune function in humans and dogs with P-H anomaly reveal normal responses to T- and B-cell mitogens, normal antibody responses to thymus-dependent and thymus-independent antigens, and adequate immunoglobulin concentrations in serum.[55,61,64] Decreased lymphoblast transformation to T- and B-cell mitogens and retarded antibody response to immunization with sheep erythrocytes have been reported in foxhounds.[26] The case for immunodeficiency in these dogs is very weak, however, because marked variability of the lymphoblast transformation data obscures interpretation, the antibody titer to sheep erythrocytes reached control values by 28 days, and it is unclear if more than one P-H dog was tested for immune function. In summary, there is no basis to support immunodeficiency in either humans or dogs with P-H anomaly.

P-H granulocytes have been used as a biologic marker to estimate neutrophil circulating half-life (T½) in people.[65] Donor blood from people with P-H anomaly was transfused into compatible ABO and Rh typed recipients. The disappearance of transfused P-H neutrophils from the circulation over a 6- to 8-hour period indirectly reflected the circulating T½ of these cells. The neutrophil circulating T½ determined using P-H anomaly as a biologic marker was similar to the neutrophil circulating T½ determined by radioisotope studies.[65] A similar transfusion experiment also was performed in a dog.[66] Blood was obtained from a red bone hound with P-H anomaly and transfused into a normal Walker hound recipient. The recipient was of A-negative blood type, but the donor was not typed nor was compatibility crossmatching performed. The circulating T½ for neutrophils was 4.8 hours, which is shorter than the normal canine neutrophil circulating T½ of 5.6 hours, as determined by DFP[32] labeling studies.[1] The circulating T½ for canine eosinophils was slightly less than 30 minutes.[66] In contrast, the normal circulating T½ for human eosinophils is much longer, ranging from 2 to 12 hours. Based on this single transfusion experiment, the circulating T½ for "normal" canine eosinophils repeatedly has been quoted as 30 minutes. However, this value probably significantly underestimates the real circulating eosinophils T½ in dogs. Potential sources of error in the circu-

CHAPTER 150

X-Linked Severe Combined Immunodeficiency

• PAULA S. HENTHORN and PETER J. FELSBURG

Severe combined immunodeficiency (SCID) describes a group of heterogeneous genetic diseases characterized by defects in both humoral and cell-mediated immune responses that usually result in infantile death.[1] Clinically different forms have been described in both humans and animals, and molecular defects responsible for several types of SCID have been identified in recent years.[2-4] Forms of SCID exhibiting autosomal recessive inheritance include adenosine deaminase deficiency, purine nucleoside phosphorylase deficiency, and jak-3 deficiency in humans as well as protein kinase-C catalytic subunit deficiency in Arabian foals (see Chapter 151). However, the X-linked recessive form of SCID (XSCID) is the most common form in humans[5] and has also been well-characterized in the dog.[6-10]

HUMAN XSCID AND THE COMMON GAMMA CHAIN

XSCID in boys was first described in 1963[11] and is characterized by failure to thrive, susceptibility to a wide range of infectious agents including opportunistic pathogens, absence of a thymic shadow on thoracic radiographs, lack of palpable peripheral lymph nodes, and lack of a T lymphocyte mitogenic response.[12] Patients may have near normal serum concentrations of circulating immunoglobulin M (IgM) but low or absent IgG and IgA concentrations. Most patients have normal to increased numbers of circulating B lymphocytes, while percentages of blood T lymphocytes are variably low. XSCID is lethal in humans by 2 years of age unless treated by bone marrow transplantation.[13,14]

The gene responsible for XSCID has been identified as the third or gamma chain of the interleukin-2 (IL-2) receptor.[15] (The IL-2 receptor is composed of three distinct polypeptide chains, α, β, and λ[18].) This initial finding was somewhat of a puzzle, because mice lacking the cytokine IL-2 do not exhibit a severe immunodeficient phenotype.[16,17] However, the findings that the IL-2 receptor gamma chain is also a component of additional cytokine receptors—including the receptors for IL-4, IL-7, IL-9, and IL-15—made the understanding of the

severity of XSCID in the face of the IL-2 receptor (IL-2R) defect more complete.[18-20] Because of its involvement in multiple cytokine receptor, the IL-2 receptor gamma chain has come to be referred to as the common gamma chain, or γc. Hundreds of different mutations have been identified in the γc gene in human XSCID patients (see http://www.nhgri.nih.gov/DIR/LGT/SCID/IL2RGbase.html and references therein).

The placement of the XSCID/γc gene on the X chromosome has allowed particular insights into the involvement of this protein in the ontogeny of various hemopoietic cell lineages. Early in development in females, one of the two X chromosomes (referred to as the paternal or maternal X-chromosome, based on which parent it was inherited from) becomes inactive, with little or no gene expression from that chromosome. This process is known as lyonization. In general, whether the paternal X or the maternal X is inactivated is a random event. X inactivation is also stable, such that all the daughter cells of a cell have the same inactive X chromosome. In any tissue, there is generally a 1:1 ratio of cells with an inactive paternal X to cells with an inactive maternal X chromosome. However, if one of the X chromosomes, for example the maternally derived X chromosome, carries a mutation in an X-linked gene that is important or necessary in the growth or survival of that cell type, that 1:1 ratio will be skewed. Instead, there will be a preponderance of cells that contain the paternal X chromosome as the active X, the chromosome that contains the normal copy of the important gene. Human carrier females of XSCID, while demonstrating completely normal immune function, show skewed X chromosome inactivation patterns in T cells, mature B cells, and natural killer cells, reflecting the loss of cells with the X-linked SCID mutation on the active X chromosome in these cell lineages.[21-24]

CANINE XSCID

Clinical Features

Canine XSCID is characterized clinically by growth retardation and increased susceptibility to bacterial and viral infections in young pups.[6] Generally, pups appear normal at birth and for several weeks thereafter, during the time when they are presumably protected from overwhelming infection by maternal antibodies. Pups then begin to lag behind their normal littermates in size and weight, and infections begin to become apparent. The most prominent infections vary from individual to individual but include a wide range of opportunistic organisms that rarely are responsible for disease in normal animals. Bacterial infections, including pyoderma, otitis externa, and cystitis, are common. Diarrhea secondary to gastrointestinal infections with various parasites (Giardia, Coccidia, Campylobacter, Cryptosporidium) is also seen. Vaccination with modified-live virus distemper-hepatitis vaccine causes these diseases in XSCID pups. Affected pups lack palpable peripheral lymph nodes, and no thymus shadow is visible on thoracic radiographs. Antibiotic therapy is not effective in clearing infections. Pups experience recurrent infections and die or are euthanized by 5 to 6 months of age.

XSCID pups are variably lymphopenic, with normal or increased percentages of B cells, and usually decreased percentages of T cells.[9] Serum immunoglobulin levels can be diagnostically helpful, but must be compared with age-matched or littermate controls. Affected pups have normal IgM levels, undetectable IgA after 2 weeks of age, and low IgG levels, particularly as the pups age. Lymphocytes show a severely reduced response to mitogen stimulation (PHA—phytohemaglutinin, ConA—conconavalin A, PWM—poke weed mitogen) compared with lymphocytes from normal littermates. The most specific test for XSCID that can be performed antemortem is an assay to determine if lymphocytes can bind IL-2, using human recombinant IL-2 labeled with phycoerythrin and flow cytometry.[25] Nearly 100% of lymphocytes from normal dogs bind IL-2, whereas only a few percent of XSCID lymphocytes bind IL-2.[8]

Postmortem Findings

Thymuses from XSCID pups are often less than 10% of the size (by weight) of normal age-matched controls and are usually obscured by adipose tissue.[7] The thymocyte numbers can vary considerably, ranging from 40- to 1300-fold reduction compared to normal. Thymuses from XSCID dogs fall into three histologic patterns that differ in the presence of Hassall's corpuscles and corticomedullary demarcation. Descriptions of thymuses can range from simple dysplasia with varying numbers of lymphocytes, no corticomedullary demarcations, and no Hassall's corpuscles to relatively normal-looking thymuses with well-defined corticomedullary demarcation and numerous Hassall's corpuscles with extremely small lobules and lack of lymphocytes in the subcapsular cortical region.[7] In general, the thymuses of young pups (less than 4 weeks) are simply dysplastic.

Generally, most lymph nodes are not grossly identifiable on postmortem examination. The rare lymph nodes that are found (mesenteric and hepatic have been seen) are disorganized and contain few small lympho-

cytes but do contain large blast-like cells in the cortical areas.[6]

Further Immunologic Findings

The major problem in XSCID appears to be the defect in T-cell development. In the thymus, thymocyte development is followed by the study of cell-surface marker expression, including CD3, CD4, and CD8. Early thymocytes progress from triple negative for these three markers to positive for CD3; this is referred to as double negative (DN or CD4−, CD8−). (The cells remain positive for CD3 throughout T-cell development.) In a proliferation dependent step, the cells acquire both CD4 and CD8 to become double positive (DP). In a subsequent proliferation independent step, they lose either the CD4 or the CD8 marker to become single positive (SP). The mature SP cells exit to the periphery. The proportions of thymocytes that are DN, DP, and SP are altered in thymuses of XSCID dogs compared with normal dog thymuses.[8] There is an increased percentage of DN thymocytes and a reduced percentage of DP thymocytes. The percentage of SP thymocytes is normal. These data indicate that there is a partial block during the proliferation-dependent DN to DP transition. As in human XSCID, canine carriers of XSCID show nonrandom X-inactivation in T lymphocytes and thymocytes.[26]

Molecular Basis of Canine XSCID

Not unexpectedly, XSCID in dogs is also caused by mutations in the γc gene.[27,28] The normal γc polypeptide is 373 amino acids in length and is 84% and 71% identical to the human and mouse protein sequences, respectively.[27] The protein has several evolutionarily conserved potential functional domains, including the amino terminal signal protein used in targeting the protein to the cell surface, the conserved extracellular cysteine residues, the WSXWS motif found in members of the cytokine receptor family,[29] a membrane-spanning region, and an Src homology region (Fig. 150.1). This Src homology region at the carboxyl terminus of the protein interacts with a protein kinase in the cell to initiate the cascade of signals necessary for cell activation. Basset hounds have a four base pair deletion in the signal peptide region of the γc gene, causing a shift in the translation reading frame and premature truncation of the γc protein during its synthesis. The mutant polypeptide would be only 21 amino acids in length compared with its normal counterpart and is clearly nonfunctional.[27] The mutation in the Cardigan Welsh Corgi dogs is a single nucleotide insertion that also causes a shift in the translation reading frame and premature truncation of the γc protein at amino acid 196, eliminating the transmembrane domain and portion of the molecule that initiates signal transduction.[28] Again, this is a protein that could not be anchored stably in the cell membrane and could not perform its normal functions.

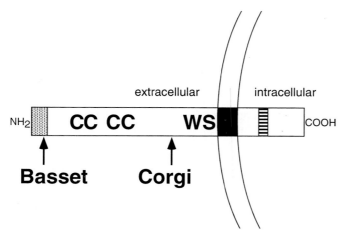

FIGURE 150.1 Representation of the γc polypeptide chain in the cell membrane. The black area represents the transmembrane domain; the shaded area is the signal peptide, which is cleaved off before the protein reaches the cell membrane; and the dashed area is the Src region necessary for signal transduction. Arrows point to the locations of the mutations found in Basset hounds and Cardigan Welsh Corgis. C, conserved cystine residues; WS, conserved WSXWS motif.

Treatment of XSCID

Bone marrow transplantation is the only treatment for XSCID in humans, although gene therapy is a promising future therapy. In humans with XSCID, rates of bone marrow transplantation success range from 50% to nearly 100%, depending on factors such as the availability of a donor matched at the major histocompatibility genes (referred to as HLA in humans and as DLA in dogs) or the use of pretransplant cytoablative treatment.[2,14,30–32] Bone marrow transplantation for XSCID has been performed in dogs in an experimental setting. Several XSCID dogs that have received both normal and carrier bone marrow without cytoablative therapy have completely engrafted donor T cells, have partially engrafted donor B cells, and can be maintained in a conventional environment.[33] However, the methodology is not identical to that used in human transplants, and a large proportion of successfully engrafted dogs develop cutaneous papillomas within 1 year of transplant. Thus, susceptibility to papillomas may reflect a lack of engraftment of some γc-dependent cell lineage, probably in the skin, that participates in the immune response to this virus.[10]

Genetic Considerations

In the veterinary setting, there is no treatment for XSCID, but an understanding of the inheritance and genetic basis for the disease allows the incidence of XSCID to be controlled in future generations.

X-Linked Recessive Inheritance

XSCID is a lethal X-linked recessive disease, and there are some unique properties of this mode of inheritance

that warrant discussion. Carriers of XSCID are phenotypically normal because, while they have one copy of the γc gene that cannot produce the normal protein, they still have one copy of the gene that can produce the normal protein. Because males only have one X chromosome, males that have an X chromosome with a mutant copy of the γc gene are affected (they have no normal copy of the γc gene to provide the normal γc protein). Carrier females do not have to mate with other carriers to produce affected pups. On average, half the male offspring of a carrier female are affected and half the female offspring are carriers. A carrier female will not necessarily produce any affected offspring, but can still pass the disease to future generations through her carrier female offspring.

A genetic disease begins with a mutation, or mistake, in the DNA of a gene. Mutations can be caused by environmental insult (chemicals, radiation) or by a rare mistake in the cell's normal metabolism. The mutation in the gene of interest must have occurred sometime in the past, in the germ line of an ancestor of the affected animal. The mutation could have occurred any number of generations back, and by chance no affected males were produced or none were recognized as having the disease in intervening generations. Alternatively, it could have occurred in the egg or sperm that gave rise to the affected animal. Because only one mutant copy of an X-linked gene must be present to produce the disease in a male animal, X-linked diseases are often discovered within just a few generations of the original mutation event that gave rise to the disease.

As a consequence of these features of X-linked inheritance, X-linked diseases can appear to be sporadic with no family history of the disease. If there is a family history, including instances when multiple littermates are infected, it may be possible to trace the mutant gene back to the animal in which the mutation occurred, which may only be a few generations back (see below).

Incidence of Canine XSCID

Canine XSCID was first recognized in a litter of Basset hounds in 1978.[6] Repeat breedings and additional breeding studies performed in a colony established from the mother of the original litter confirmed that the disease was X-linked. XSCID in Basset hounds has not been reported since. XSCID was again recognized in 1993 in closely related Cardigan Welsh Corgi dogs.[34] The pedigree of this family was consistent with X-linked inheritance, and the diagnosis of XSCID was confirmed with DNA studies identifying a γc gene mutation in the studied affected male dog and related obligate carrier females (see molecular defect above).[28] DNA analysis established that the γc mutation was present in the grandmother of the affected dog but not in her parents, indicating that only her female offspring were at risk of being carriers of the disease. Subsequent genetic testing was used to identify carrier females so they could be removed from the breeding population, and this prevented the spread of the disease.

Because it is believed that controlled breeding and random chance have prevented the spread of XSCID among the Corgi and Basset populations, XSCID is no more likely to occur in these two breeds than in any other breed. New cases of XSCID can occur in any breed and will likely be the result of different mutations in the canine γc gene.

REFERENCES

1. **Rosen FS, Cooper MD, Wedgwood RJ.** The primary immunodeficiencies. N Engl J Med 1995;333:431–440.
2. **Fischer A, Malissen B.** Natural and engineered disorders of lymphocyte development. Science 1998;280:237–243.
3. **Shin EK, Perryman LE, Meek K.** A kinase-negative mutation of DNA-PK(CS) in equine SCID results in defective coding and signal joint formation. J Immunol 1997;158:3565–3569.
4. **Fischer A, Cavazzana-Calvo M, de Saint Basile G, di Santo JP, Hivroz C, Rieux-Laucat F, Le Deist F.** Naturally occurring primary deficiencies of the immune system. Annu Rev Immunol 1997;15:93–124.
5. **Conley ME, Buckley RH, Hong R, Guerra-Hanson C, Roifman CM, Brochstein JA, Pahwa S, Puck JM.** X-linked severe combined immunodeficiency: diagnosis in males with sporadic severe combined immunodeficiency and clarification of clinical findings. J Clin Invest 1990;85:1548–1554.
6. **Jezyk PF, Felsburg PJ, Haskins ME, Patterson DF.** X-linked severe combined immunodeficiency in the dog. Clin Immunol Immunopathol 1989; 52:173–189.
7. **Snyder PW, Kazacos EA, Felsburg PJ.** Histologic characterization of the thymus in canine X-linked severe combined immunodeficiency. Immunol Immunopathol 1993;67:55–67.
8. **Somberg RL, Robinson JP, Felsburg PJ.** T lymphocyte development and function in dogs with X-linked severe combined immunodeficiency. J Immunol 1994;153:4006–4015.
9. **Somberg RL, Tipold A, Hartnett BJ, Moore PF, Henthorn PS.** Postnatal development of T cells in dogs with X-linked severe combined immunodeficiency. J Immunol 1996;156:1431–1435.
10. **Felsburg PJ, Somberg RL, Hartnett BJ, Henthorn PS, Carding SR.** Canine X-linked severe combined immunodeficiency. A model for investigating the requirement for the common gamma chain (gamma c) in human lymphocyte development and function. Immunol Res 1998;17:63–73.
11. **Gitlin D, Craig JM.** The thymus and other lymphoid tissues in congenital agammaglobulinemia. I. Thymic alymphoplasia and lymphocytic hypoplasia and their relation to infection. Pediatrics 1963;32:517–530.
12. **Shim EK, Perrymann OE, Meek K.** A kinase-negative mutation of DNA-PK(CS) in equine SCID results in defective coding and signal joint formation. J Immunol 1997;158:3454–3549.
13. **Conley ME.** X-linked severe combined immunodeficiency. Clin Immunol Immunopathol 1991;61:S94–S99.
14. **Fischer A, Landais P, Friedrich W, Morgan G, Gerritsen B, Fasth A, Porta F, Griscelli C, Goldman SF, Levinsky R.** European experience of bone-marrow transplantation for severe combined immunodeficiency. Lancet 1990;336:850–854.
15. **Noguchi M, Huafang Y, Rosenblatt HM, Filipovich AH, Adelstein S, Modi WS, McBride OW, Leonard WJ.** Interleukin-2 receptor g chain mutation results in X-linked severe combined immunodeficiency in humans. Cell 1993;73:147–157.
16. **Sadlack B, Merz H, Schorle H, Schimpl A, Feller AC.** Ulcerative colitis-like disease in mice with a disrupted interleukin-2 gene. Cell 1993;75:253–261.
17. **Schorle H, Holtschke T, Hunig T, Schimpl A, Horak I.** Development and function of T cells in mice rendered interleukin-2 deficient by gene targeting. Nature 1991;352:621–624.
18. **Sugamura K, Asao H, Kondo M, Tanaka N, Ishii N, Ohbo K, Nakamura M.** The interleukin-2 receptor gamma chain: its role in the multiple cytokine receptor complexes and T cell development in XSCID. Annu Rev Immunol 1996;14:179–205.
19. **Leonard WJ.** Dysfunctional cytokine receptor signaling in severe combined immunodeficiency. J Invest Med 1996;44:304–311.
20. **Leonard WJ.** The molecular basis of X-linked severe combined immunodeficiency: defective cytokine receptor signaling. Annu Rev Med 1996; 47:229–239.
21. **Puck JM, Nussbaum RL, Conley ME.** Carrier detection in X-linked severe combined immunodeficiency based on patterns of X chromosome inactivation. J Clin Invest 1987;79:1395–1400.
22. **Conley ME, Lavoie A, Briggs C, Brown P, Guerra C, Puck JM.** Nonrandom X chromosome inactivation in B cells from carriers of X chromosome-linked severe combined immunodeficiency. Proc Natl Acad Sci USA 1988;85:3090–3094.
23. **Puck JM, Stewart CC, Nussbaum RL.** Maximum-likelihood analysis of human T-cell X chromosome inactivation patterns: normal women versus carriers of X-linked severe combined immunodeficiency. Am J Hum Genet 1992;50:742–748.
24. **Wengler GS, Allen RC, Parolini O, Smith H, Conley ME.** Nonrandom X chromosome inactivation in natural killer cells from obligate carriers of X-linked severe combined immunodeficiency. J Immunol 1993;150:700–704.
25. **Somberg RL, Robinson JP, Felsburg PJ.** Detection of canine interleukin-2 receptors by flow cytometry. Vet Immunol Immunopathol 1992;33:17–24.
26. **Deschenes SM, Puck JM, Dutra AS, Somberg RL, Felsburg PJ, Henthorn PS.** Comparative mapping of canine and human proximal Xq and genetic analysis of canine X-linked severe combined immunodeficiency. Genomics 1994;23:62–68.
27. **Henthorn PS, Somberg RL, Fimiani VM, Puck JM, Patterson DF.** IL-2R gamma gene microdeletion demonstrates that canine X-linked severe combined immunodeficiency is a homologue of the human disease. Genomics 1994;23:69–74.
28. **Somberg RL, Pullen RP, Casal ML, Patterson DF, Felsburg PJ, Henthorn PS.** A single nucleotide insertion in the canine interleukin-2 receptor gamma chain results in X-linked severe combined immunodeficiency disease. Vet Immunol Immunopathol 1995;47:203–213.
29. **Bazan JF.** Structural design and molecular evolution of a cytokine receptor superfamily. Proc Natl Acad Sci USA 1990;87:6934–6938.
30. **Buckley RH, Schiff SE, Schiff RI, Roberts JL, Markert ML, Peters W, Williams LW, Ward FE.** Haploidentical bone marrow stem cell transplantation in human severe combined immunodeficiency. Semin Hematol 1993; 30:92–101.
31. **van Leeuwen JE, van Tol MJ, Joosten AM, Schellekens PT, van den Bergh RL, Oudeman-Gruber NJ, van der Weijden-Ragas CP, Gerritsen EJ, et al.** Relationship between patterns of engraftment in peripheral blood and immune reconstitution after allogeneic bone marrow transplantation for (severe) combined immunodeficiency. Blood 1994;84:3936–3947.
32. **Dror Y, Gallagher R, Wara DW, Colombe BW, Merino A, Cowan MJ.** Immune reconstitution in severe combined immunodeficiency disease after lectin-treated, T-cell-depleted haplocompatible bone marrow transplantation. Blood 1993;81:2021–2030.
33. **Felsburg PJ, Somberg RL, Hartnett BJ, Suter SF, Henthorn PS, Moore PF, Weinberg KI, Ochs HD.** Full immunologic reconstitution following nonconditioned bone marrow transplantation for canine X-linked severe combined immunodeficiency. Blood 1997;90:3214–3221.
34. **Pullen RP, Somberg RL, Felsburg PJ, Henthorn PS.** X-linked severe combined immunodeficiency in a family of Cardigan Welsh corgis. J Am Anim Hosp Assoc 1997;33:494–499.

CHAPTER 151

Severe Combined Immunodeficiency in Arabian Foals

• LANCE E. PERRYMAN

MOLECULAR BASIS OF DISEASE

Severe combined immunodeficiency (SCID), a uniformly fatal inherited disease of Arabian foals, was first reported in 1973.[1] The disorder is inherited as an autosomal recessive trait and appears to be limited to foals in which both dam and sire are descendants of Arabian horses.[2-4] Affected foals have been reported in the United States, Australia, Canada, and Great Britain.[1,5-7]

SCID foals appear normal at birth but cannot generate antigen-specific immune responses.[8,9] Affected foals lack mature T and B lymphocytes, which accounts for the lymphopenia and hypoplasia of lymphoid organs characteristic of this disorder.[10-13] Failure to produce mature lymphocytes is explained by a mutation in the gene encoding the catalytic subunit of DNA-dependent protein kinase (DNA-PK).[14] DNA-PK is required to carry out V(D)J recombination, the gene rearrangement process that provides for expression of antigen receptors on B and T lymphocytes.[15] In the absence of these gene rearrangement events, B lymphocytes do not produce immunoglobulins or express immunoglobulin M (IgM) on the cell surface. Likewise, the inability to rearrange T-cell receptor genes results in failure to express antigen-specific receptors on the surface of T lymphocytes. Progenitors of B and T lymphocytes that are unable to complete the maturation process are eliminated, resulting in the paucity of lymphocytes observed in SCID foals.

SCID foals lack DNA-PK activity because of a defect in the catalytic subunit (DNA-PK$_{CS}$) of the enzyme.[14,16] Equine DNA-PK$_{CS}$ has a molecular mass of approximately 350 kD and contains 4127 amino acids. Sequence analysis of the gene encoding DNA-PK$_{CS}$ revealed a five base pair deletion in SCID foals. The deletion causes a frame shift mutation at codon 3155 and formation of a premature stop codon at amino acid position 3160. The resulting 967 amino acid deletion eliminates the protein kinase active sites and renders the enzyme functionally inactive. The gene encoding DNA-PK$_{CS}$ is located on equine chromosome 9.[17]

SCID also occurs in mice, humans, and dogs.[9,18,19] Mutations in DNA-PK$_{CS}$ are the basis for SCID in Arabian horses and mice, but the site of the mutation differs in these two species.[20] As of 1998, characterized mutations in humans and dogs with SCID involved other enzymes and receptor proteins, but not DNA-PK$_{CS}$. Basset hounds and Cardigan Welsh Corgis with canine X-linked SCID have distinct mutations in the gene encoding the gamma chain of the receptor common to interleukin-2 (IL-2) and other cytokines (see Chapter 150).

CLINICAL FEATURES

The typical foal with SCID appears normal at birth and remains free of infections and grows well for 3 to 8 weeks if it received colostrum. Initial signs usually involve the respiratory tract, consisting of mucopurulent nasal and ocular discharge and abnormal respiratory sounds. These initial signs of bacterial infection often respond to antimicrobial therapy. With time, respiratory infections increase in severity and frequency and respond poorly to therapy. Affected foals lose condition and inevitably die, usually between 2 and 4 months of age.

Equine adenovirus is the most common and important pathogen in SCID foals.[21,22] Infection usually starts in the upper respiratory tract but occasionally begins within intestinal epithelial cells.[21] Adenovirus spreads to bronchiolar epithelial, renal epithelial, and pancreatic duct epithelial cells. Pancreatic changes are profound in SCID foals infected with adenovirus. There is marked reduction in pancreatic exocrine tissue and substantial increase in fibrous connective tissue. These changes may contribute to growth reduction and loss of condition in SCID foals.

Pneumocystis carinii, an opportunistic pathogen commonly found in immunodeficient patients, contributes to the decline of pulmonary function in several foals with SCID.[22] Several bacteria, most notably *Rhodococcus equi,* are cultured from pulmonary and extrapulmonary lesions of SCID foals.

Some SCID foals become infected with *Cryptosporidium parvum* and develop severe, life-threatening diarrhea. This may occur prior to, or concomitant with, respiratory disease and dramatically shortens the time from onset of initial infection to death.[23,24]

Equine herpes viruses are rarely described as the cause of serious infections in SCID foals. The presence of natural killer (NK) cells and NK cell activity in SCID foals may explain this observation.[25,26]

The age at onset of infections is determined by the amount of protective antibodies absorbed from maternal colostrum and the degree to which affected foals are isolated from other horses. The length of the clinical course also depends on these factors as well as the intensity of antimicrobial and supportive therapy. Death is inevitable by 5 months. With increased awareness of the disease and availability of definitive diagnostic criteria, most SCID foals are humanely euthanized early in the clinical course.

DIAGNOSIS

The clinical signs of SCID are not readily distinguishable from those in foals with selective IgM deficiency or failure to absorb adequate maternal immunoglobulins from colostrum.[27] Before 1997, a definitive diagnosis of SCID required demonstration of (1) profound lymphopenia (less than 1000 lymphocytes/μL blood), (2) absence of IgM in serum, and (3) hypoplasia of thymus and spleen. A tentative diagnosis of SCID was made in living foals by analyzing blood for IgM concentration and absolute lymphocyte counts. However, the diagnosis could not be confirmed until spleen and other lymphoid tissues were examined histologically. Thus, a definitive diagnosis could not be established until after the foal died, but owners were often reluctant to authorize euthanasia without assurance that the disease was untreatable. This resulted in prolonged physical discomfort to the foal, extra cost, and anxiety to owners struggling to manage multiple infections in foals for which successful treatment was impossible. Anxiety was also heightened by the realization that SCID is a genetic disorder inherited as an autosomal recessive trait. Definitive diagnosis of SCID in a foal identifies both dam and sire as heterozygotes for the SCID trait. Before 1997, the heterozygote status could only be determined by progeny testing. Furthermore, designation of mares and stallions as heterozygotes for the SCID trait could not be verified by molecular analysis until recently.

Definitive molecular criteria for diagnosis of SCID in Arabian foals were published in 1997.[14] The mutation responsible for SCID is a five base pair deletion in the gene encoding the catalytic subunit of DNA-PK. Knowledge of the defect and the sequence of nucleotides surrounding the critical sight allows definitive evaluation of the DNA-PK$_{CS}$ genotype in horses of any age. The critical region of DNA is amplified by polymerase chain reaction and evaluated by Southern blots using a nucleotide probe complimentary to the normal gene sequence and a DNA probe complimentary to the SCID mutant gene sequence. Amplified DNA from SCID foals hybridizes only to the DNA probe complimentary to the SCID mutant gene sequence. In contrast, amplified DNA from

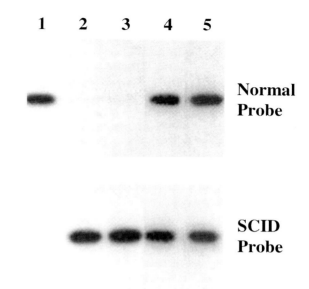

FIGURE 151.1 Southern blot analysis for the normal and SCID mutant sequence of DNA-PK$_{CS}$. **Lane 1:** normal foal control; **lane 2:** SCID foal control; **lane 3:** foal homozygous for the mutant SCID gene sequence; **lane 4:** sire of SCID foal shown in lane 3; **lane 5:** dam of SCID foal shown in lane 3.

genotypically normal foals hybridizes only to the probe complimentary to the normal gene sequence. Of particular significance is the observation that amplified DNA from horses heterozygous for the SCID trait hybridizes with both probes (Fig. 151.1).[14,28] Thus, definitive genotype information can be obtained from Arabian horses of any age and well before the expected time of onset of infectious diseases in immunodeficient foals. Diagnostic service is available from VetGen, Inc. (www.vetgen.com).

TREATMENT

The disorder is uniformly fatal. The complete inability to generate antigen-specific immune responses renders the affected foal incapable of preventing and recovering from infections through immune mechanisms. Onset of fatal infections can be delayed but not prevented by transfusion of plasma as a source of antibodies. Once infections occur, the clinical course can be prolonged but not resolved by treatment with antimicrobial agents. Eventually, SCID foals acquire infections for which antimicrobial agents are ineffective. Death is inevitable, usually between 2 and 4 months of age. SCID foals do not survive past 5 months of age when maintained under standard equine husbandry conditions.

SCID in a single foal was corrected by transplantation of histocompatible bone marrow cells from a full sibling donor.[29,30] Neither radiation nor chemotherapy was used to prepare the recipient foal. Lymphocyte counts increased within 2 weeks of transplantation. Although a full year was required for normalization of immune functions, the foal developed ability to respond to vaccine antigens and resist infections while pastured and stabled with other horses. The horse survived 5 years after transplantation before dying of an intestinal disorder unrelated to SCID or bone marrow transplantation. This experiment demonstrated that lymphoid precursor cells with the normal gene sequence for DNA-PK$_{CS}$ are able to differentiate to functional, mature T and B lymphocytes within the microenvironment of the bone marrow, thymus, and peripheral lymphoid organs of SCID foals. However, bone marrow transplantation is not a realistic solution to management of SCID. The procedure requires a histocompatible donor and is both technically demanding and prohibitively expensive. Even though the reconstituted foal was immunocompetent, it remained homozygous for the SCID trait and would transmit the mutant DNA-PK$_{CS}$ gene to all offspring. Therefore, reconstituted foals would be unsuitable for breeding purposes.

CONTROL OF THE DEFECT IN THE ARABIAN HORSE POPULATION

The solution to SCID in Arabian horses is to avoid the production of affected foals. SCID foals can only be produced when both the sire and dam are heterozygous for the mutant DNA-PK$_{CS}$ gene. Therefore, mares and stallions should be tested and classified as homozygous normal or heterozygous for the SCID gene. Once this information is known, breeding programs are structured to ensure that heterozygous stallions are never mated to heterozygous mares. Implementation of this strategy would curtail the production of SCID foals.

The second goal should be to encourage preferential use of homozygous normal horses in breeding programs. In the interim, continued use of known heterozygous horses can be done effectively under controlled conditions. For example, the owner of an otherwise highly desirable SCID heterozygous stallion could selectively breed him to genotypically normal mares. The foals could be tested anytime after birth to determine genotype. The breeding of a heterozygous stallion to homozygous normal mares is expected to yield equal numbers of heterozygous and homozygous normal foals.[31] The homozygous normal foals could be selected for future breeding programs. The heterozygous colts could be gelded, and all heterozygous offspring used for nonreproductive activities for which Arabian horses are well suited.

The incidence of SCID in the Arabian horse population is unknown as of 1998. Surveys in the 1970s suggested SCID occurred in more than 2% of Arabian foals examined.[3] The availability of definitive molecular criteria and the testing of large numbers of Arabian horses will result in more accurate and contemporary estimates of SCID incidence and heterozygote frequency in the Arabian horse population. More importantly, the ability to test mares and stallions before breeding makes it possible to eliminate the production of SCID foals and

to reduce the SCID gene frequency while preserving the desirable genetic traits of horses that are heterozygous for the SCID trait. This is a striking example of the benefits derived from defining the molecular basis of a disease. Understanding the molecular basis facilitates effective diseases control while preserving the goals of the industry affected by the disease.

REFERENCES

1. **McGuire TC, Poppie MJ.** Hypogammaglobulinemia and thymic hypoplasia in horses: a primary combined immunodeficiency disorder. Infect Immun 1973;8:272–277.
2. **Thompson DB, Studdert MJ, Beilharz RG, Littlejohns IR.** Inheritance of a lethal immunodeficiency disease of Arabian foals. Aust Vet J 1975;51:109–113.
3. **Poppie MJ, McGuire TC.** Combined immunodeficiency in foals of Arabian breeding: evaluation of mode of inheritance and estimation of prevalence of affected foals and carrier mares and stallions. J Am Vet Med Assoc 1977;170:31–33.
4. **Perryman LE, Torbeck RL.** Combined immunodeficiency of Arabian horses: confirmation of autosomal recessive mode of inheritance. J Am Vet Med Assoc 1980;176:1250–1251.
5. **Studdert MJ.** Primary, severe, combined immunodeficiency disease of Arabian foals. Aust Vet J 1978;54:411–417.
6. **Clark EG, Turner AS, Boysen BG, Rouse BT.** Listeriosis in an Arabian foal with combined immunodeficiency. J Am Vet Med Assoc 1978;172:363–366.
7. **Whitwell KE.** Combined immunodeficiency in Arab foals. Vet Rec 1978; 103:568.
8. **McGuire TC, Poppie MJ, Banks KL.** Combined (B- and T-lymphocyte) immunodeficiency: a fatal genetic disease in Arabian foals. J Am Vet Med Assoc 1974;164:70–76.
9. **Felsburg PJ, Somberg RL, Perryman LE.** Domestic animal models of severe combined immunodeficiency: canine X-linked severe combined immunodeficiency and severe combined immunodeficiency in horses. Immunodef Rev 1992;3:277–303.
10. **McGuire TC, Banks KL, Poppie MJ.** Combined immunodeficiency in horses: characterization of the lymphocyte defect. Clin Immunol Immunopathol 1975;3:555–566.
11. **Wyatt CR, Magnuson NS, Perryman LE.** Defective thymocyte maturation in horses with severe combined immunodeficiency. J Immunol 1987; 139:4072–4076.
12. **McGuire TC, Perryman LE, Davis WC.** Analysis of serum and lymphocyte surface IgM of normal and immunodeficient horses with monoclonal antibodies. Am J Vet Res 1983;44:1284–1288.
13. **McGuire TC, Banks KL, Davis WC.** Alterations of the thymus and other lymphoid tissue in young horses with combined immunodeficiency. Am J Pathol 1976;84:39–54.
14. **Shin EK, Perryman LE, Meek K.** A kinase negative mutation of DNA-PK$_{CS}$ in equine SCID results in defective coding and signal joint formation. J Immunol 1997;158:3565–3569.
15. **Weaver DT.** V(D)J recombination and double-strand break repair. Adv Immunol 1995;58:29–85.
16. **Wiler R, Leber R, Moore BB, VanDyk LE, Perryman LE, Meek K.** Equine severe combined immunodeficiency: a defect in V(D)J recombination and DNA-dependent protein kinase activity. Proc Natl Acad Sci USA 1995;92:11485–11489.
17. **Bailey E, Reid RC, Skow LC, Mathiason K, Lear TL, McGuire TC.** Linkage of the gene for equine combined immunodeficiency disease to microsatellite markers HTG8 and HTG4: synteny and FISH mapping to ECA9. Anim Genet 1997;28:268–273.
18. **Bosma GC, Custer RP, Bosma MJ.** A severe combined immunodeficiency mutation in the mouse. Nature 1983;301:527–530.
19. **Rosen FS, Cooper MD, Wedgwood RJP.** The primary immunodeficiencies. N Engl J Med 1995;333:431–440.
20. **Leber R, Wiler R, Perryman LE, Meek KD.** Equine SCID: mechanistic analysis and comparison to murine SCID. Vet Immunol Immunopathol 1998;65:1–9.
21. **McChesney AE, England JJ, Whiteman CE, Adcock JL, Rich LJ, Chow TL.** Experimental transmission of equine adenovirus in Arabian and non-Arabian foals. Am J Vet Res 1974;35:1015–1023.
22. **Perryman LE, McGuire TC, Crawford TB.** Maintenance of foals with combined immunodeficiency: causes and control of secondary infections. Am J Vet Res 1978;39:1161–1167.
23. **Snyder SP, England JJ, McChesney AE.** Cryptosporidiosis in immunodeficient Arabian foals. Vet Pathol 1978;15:12–17.
24. **Bjorneby JM, Leach DR, Perryman LE.** Persistent cryptosporidiosis in horses with severe combined immunodeficiency. Infect Immun 1991; 59:3823–3826.
25. **Magnuson NS, Perryman LE, Wyatt CR, Mason PH, Talmadge JE.** Large

granular lymphocytes from SCID horses develop potent cytotoxic activity after treatment with human recombinant interleukin 2. J Immunol 1987;139:61–67.

26. **Lunn DP, McClure JT, Schobert CS, Holmes MA.** Abnormal patterns of equine leucocyte differentiation antigen expression in severe combined immunodeficiency foals suggests the phenotype of normal equine natural killer cells. Immunology 1995;84:495–499.

27. **Perryman LE, McGuire TC.** Evaluation for immune system failures in horses and ponies. J Am Vet Med Assoc 1980;176:1374–1377.

28. **Shin EK, Perryman LE, Meek K.** Evaluation of a test for identification of Arabian horses heterozygous for the severe combined immunodeficiency trait. J Am Vet Med Assoc 1997;211:1268–1270.

29. **Bue CM, Davis WC, Magnuson NS, Mottironi VD, Ochs HD, Wyatt CR, Perryman LE.** Correction of equine severe combined immunodeficiency by bone marrow transplantation. Transplantation 1986;42:14–19.

30. **Perryman LE, Bue CM, Magnuson NS, Mottironi VD, Ochs HD, Wyatt CR.** Immunologic reconstitution of foals with combined immunodeficiency. Vet Immunol Immunopathol 1987;17:495–508.

31. **Damjanov I.** Developmental and genetic diseases. In: Rubin E, Farber JL, eds. Pathology. Philadelphia: JB Lippincott, 1988;196–249.

CHAPTER 152

IgA Deficiency

• PETER FELSBURG

THE MUCOSAL IMMUNE SYSTEM

The mucosal surfaces are a major site of antigenic exposure because they are in direct contact with the external environment. The secretions that are associated with the various mucosal surfaces form a unique immunologic mechanism involved in host defense—the mucosal immune system. The organ systems involved in the mucosal immune system include the gastrointestinal tract, respiratory tract, urogenital tract, salivary glands, lacrimal glands, mammary glands, and the skin.

There are both immune and nonimmune defense mechanisms functioning to protect these mucosal surfaces from infection. The nonimmunologic host protective mechanisms of the mucosal organs relate to the physical properties of the individual organs. For example, the skin acts as a physical barrier to potential pathogens. The skin also has a dense and stable resident bacterial flora whose composition is regulated by a number of factors such as desquamation, desiccation, and a relatively low pH. If any of these physical factors is altered, the composition of the skin flora is disturbed, its protective properties reduced, and colonization of pathogens may occur. The resident flora of the gastrointestinal tract is essential not only for the control of potential pathogens but also for digestion. If the natural flora of the intestine is altered (e.g., antibiotic therapy), the overgrowth of potential pathogens may occur. The flushing action of saliva and intestinal motility are also important physical factors in preventing colonization of pathogens. The mucociliary tree of the upper respiratory tract is an important physical factor in regulating colonization of the respiratory tract with potential pathogens. The flushing action of the urogenital system and mammary glands is important in limiting bacterial growth in these organs.

The primary immune effector molecule of the mucosal immune system is a special form of immunoglobulin A (IgA) called secretory IgA (sIgA). Serum IgA is primarily composed of a single IgA molecule, whereas IgA found in secretions consists of a dimer of IgA, two molecules bound together by a molecule called the J (joining) chain, surrounded by another molecule referred to as secretory component. IgA represents the product of two cell types, submucosal plasma cells, such as those in the lamina propria of the intestinal tract, and epithelial cells that line the mucosal surfaces. The submucosal plasma cells synthesize IgA and the J chain. The J chain forms disulfide bonds with two monomeric IgA molecules to form a dimeric IgA molecule within the plasma cell. The dimeric IgA molecule is secreted into the lamina propria. The epithelial cells that line the mucosal surfaces produce a protein called secretory component (SC) that localizes to the basal surface of the epithelial cell. The SC binds to the J chain of the dimeric IgA molecule and transports it across the epithelial cell and releases it into the secretions that coat the mucosal surfaces. The SC also protects the sIgA molecule from digestion by proteolytic enzymes found in the various secretions of the organs comprising the mucosal immune system. In the skin, IgA is found in the apocrine sweat glands, suggesting that it functions as a cutaneous secretory immunoglobulin. SC can also transport any locally produced IgM across the epithelial lining because IgM also contains a J chain that is responsible for the formation of the pentameric IgM molecule.

Because sIgA is found in the secretions covering the mucosal surfaces, it provides the first line of defense against infectious disease agents, primarily toxins, bacteria, and viruses. sIgA is capable of neutralizing toxins before they bind to their cell receptors. The antibacterial activity of sIgA is related to its ability to bind antigenic determinants on the bacteria, thereby inhibiting adherence and colonization of the bacteria. sIgA also binds to viruses to prevent adherence. If the virus cannot adhere to the epithelial surface, infection is prevented. sIgA has also been shown to inhibit absorption of macromolecular antigens such as potential allergens. In summary, the interaction of sIgA with the various nonimmunologic defense mechanisms is important in preventing infection of mucosal organs.

A deficiency of IgA results in the failure to mount a local immune response to bacteria and viruses and predisposes the individual to infections. IgA-deficient individuals also have an increased absorption of antigens, predisposing them to the potential development of allergies and autoimmune disease. IgA deficiency has only been documented in humans and dogs.

IgA DEFICIENCY IN HUMANS

IgA deficiency (IgAD) is the most common primary immunodeficiency in humans.[1] The prevalence, based on screening large populations of "healthy" adult blood donors, is approximately 1/600 in Western populations. IgAD is actually a heterogeneous group of diseases consisting of two main types: severe IgAD, defined as undetectable IgA, and partial IgAD, defined as low IgA (less than 2 standard deviations of the mean for age-matched normal individuals). A further complication of IgAD is that it may be transient, particularly in pediatric patients. The importance of the transience of IgAD has recently been addressed by long-term follow-up studies of both pediatric and adult IgAD patients. In pediatric patients, IgA will normalize by adulthood (15 years of age) in approximately 8% of severe IgAD patients and approximately 50% of partial IgAD patients. Thus, it appears that in pediatric patients severe IgAD is usually persistent, whereas partial IgAD is often transient, probably representing delayed maturation of IgA production. In a 20-year follow-up study of "healthy" adult blood donors diagnosed as having severe IgAD (mean age at diagnosis, 24 years), severe IgAD remained in 78% of patients and converted to partial IgAD in 21% (remaining partial IgAD during the study).[2] Therefore, primary IgAD appears to be permanent in adults.

Although individuals with IgAD are often asymptomatic, reduced levels of IgA predispose to a variety of diseases including upper respiratory infections, skin infections, neurologic problems, allergies, and autoimmune disease. In fact, symptomatic IgAD accounts for 10 to 15% of all cases of clinically important primary immunodeficiencies. Approximately 50% of symptomatic IgAD patients present with recurrent infections, particularly of the upper respiratory tract. Approximately 7% of IgAD patients have recurrent or chronic skin infections. Surprisingly, chronic gastrointestinal tract infections are rare, probably due to compensatory mechanisms operating in the gastrointestinal tract. The exception is an increased incidence of *Giardia* in IgAD patients. Atopic disease has been reported to occur in 21 to 45% of symptomatic IgAD patients. Up to 60% of atopic IgAD patients have a history of nonspecific dermatitis or eczema. The frequency of autoimmune disease in symptomatic IgAD patients ranges from 7 to 36%, with rheumatoid arthritis and systemic lupus erythematosus being the most frequently associated with IgAD.[3] Autoantibodies in the absence of overt clinical autoimmune disease are frequently present in IgAD patients. Rheumatoid factor is present in 13 to 30% of IgAD patients, and anti-DNA antibodies are present in 11 to 22% of IgAD patients. Anti-IgA antibodies have been found in approximately 25 to 50% of individuals with IgAD. It is unclear whether these antibodies play a role in the pathogenesis of IgAD; however, they are more common in patients who have other autoantibodies (80%) than in patients with no other autoantibodies (20%).

The question remains why so many IgAD patients are asymptomatic at the time of diagnosis. A recently completed 20-year follow-up study of "healthy" adult blood donors diagnosed with IgAD has shown that these individuals had significantly more respiratory infections than did "normal" individuals.[4] In addition, this study showed that individuals with IgAD who are healthy as young adults had a risk of developing various autoimmune diseases in middle age, particularly rheumatoid arthritis and systemic lupus erythematosus. There are two possible explanations why some IgAD patients do not experience problems with recurrent or chronic infections. First, increased local production and passage of secretory IgM (sIgM) into mucosal secretions may compensate in some individuals who lack IgA. sIgM is significantly elevated in secretions of IgAD individuals without any increased susceptibility to infection; however, those individuals with IgAD and frequent infections do not show increased sIgM. A second reason for the discrepancy is that approximately 50% of IgAD adults also have either an IgG2 and/or IgG4 subclass deficiency. These individuals appear to have more serious problems with infections than those with isolated IgAD.

Although the familial aggregation of IgAD suggests a genetic basis for IgAD, the mode of inheritance is unknown. Hypothesized patterns of inheritance include autosomal recessive, autosomal dominant with low penetrance, multifactorial, and polygenic. There are associations with certain human leukocyte antigen (HLA) types. There is a higher association of IgAD relating mother to child than father to child.

IgA DEFICIENCY IN THE DOG

The initial descriptions of IgAD in the dog were in the beagle and Shar pei.[5,6] The most common clinical problems in dogs with IgAD include recurrent upper respiratory infections due to *Bordetella bronchiseptica* and canine parainfluenza virus, otitis, staphylococcal dermatitis, and atopic dermatitis. The infections associated with IgAD in the dog begin within the first few months of life but are usually not life-threatening. Several dogs have experienced convulsive episodes. During a 5-year study of dogs with chronic skin disease, 40 were identified with IgAD.[7] Breeds represented in this study included Shar peis, German shepherds, cocker spaniels, Doberman pinschers, miniature schnauzers, miniature pinchers, Akitas, and isolated cases in a Yorkshire terrier, Welsh corgi, Newfoundland, West Highland white terrier, Keeshound, Irish setter, Wheaton terrier, and Old English sheepdog. The two major clinical presentations were atopy with secondary staphylococcal pyoderma (14 dogs) and chronic or recurrent staphylococcal pyoderma (12 dogs). IgAD has also been associated with disseminated aspergillosis, particularly in German shepherds.[8] The relationship of IgAD and any potential IgG subclass deficiency has not been evaluated in dogs.

In a 1-year prospective study of beagle puppies diagnosed with IgAD, the incidence of upper respiratory disease was 2.4 times greater in the IgAD dogs than in age-matched dogs with normal IgA concentrations. In addition, the IgAD dogs were three times more likely to be infected with *Giardia* than were dogs with normal IgA concentrations.[9]

Screening of large populations of "healthy" adult dogs has demonstrated that IgAD is present in clinically normal adult dogs and can take the form of either severe or partial IgAD. Determination of serum IgA concentrations in 829 clinically normal adult beagles revealed the presence of IgAD in approximately 9% of the dogs, 1% with severe IgAD and 8% with partial IgAD.[9] IgAD diagnosed in these healthy adult dogs appears to be persistent, similar to the observations in humans. In a 2-year study of 5 severe IgAD and 15 partial IgAD healthy adult beagles, all 5 of the dogs with severe IgAD remained severely IgA-deficient and 12 of 15 dogs with partial IgAD remained partially IgA-deficient. Six of these dogs developed nonspecific dermatitis during the study period, with 50% of these dogs having positive skin tests for several environmental antigens. Thirty-two percent of dogs developed rheumatoid factor in the absence of overt clinical rheumatoid arthritis. Anti-IgA antibodies were found in 30% of the IgAD dogs. Partial IgAD has been reported to occur in up to 75% of clinically normal adult Shar pei dogs.[6] A relative IgAD has been reported in "healthy" adult German shepherd dogs.[10] This observation was based on comparing the mean IgA values of 13 adult German shepherd dogs and comparing their values with those of 13 adult mongrels and 14 adult Irish setters. A major problem was that the mean IgA values for the German shepherds in the study, although approximately half of the other two groups, were the same as previously published mean IgA concentrations for normal adult mongrels and purebred dogs; the mean values for the mongrels and Irish setters were twice as high as the previously published normal values. Therefore, whether "relative" IgA deficiency exists in the German shepherd remains questionable.

Although the mode of inheritance of IgAD in the dog remains unknown, epidemiologic studies have shown that puppies born to clinically healthy IgAD dams are at much higher risk of developing upper respiratory infections than puppies born to dams with normal concentrations of IgA.[11] In addition, an experimental breeding of an IgAD dam and IgAD sire resulted in a litter of five puppies. At 3 months of age, four of five puppies had undetectable IgA; at 1 year of age, one dog still had severe IgAD and two dogs had partial IgAD. All three IgAD dogs experienced recurrent upper respiratory infections during the 1-year study.[9] The infections occurred despite vaccination with a *B. bronchiseptica* and canine parainfluenza intranasal vaccine. The severe IgAD dog also experienced chronic dermatitis and several episodes of seizures.

DIAGNOSIS OF IgAD

The diagnosis of IgAD, both in humans and dogs, is based on the quantitation of serum IgA. An important consideration in the diagnosis of IgAD is the age of the dog.[12] Levels of serum IgA are low in all puppies. By 3 to 4 months of age, serum IgA levels have increased to

TABLE 152.1 Example of Transient IgA Deficiency in the Dog

Immunoglobulin (mg/dL)	Age (months)				
	3	6	9	12	18
IgA[a]	<10	<10	<10	22	125
IgG	850	1350	1600	1825	1950
IgM	110	140	180	165	200

[a]At 3 months of age, IgA values in normal dogs are 26 ± 9 mg/dL. Normal adult values IgA range between 30 to 50 mg/dL.

levels at which normal and IgAD dogs can be differentiated. Unlike IgM and IgG, serum IgA concentrations do not reach normal adult levels until 12 to 18 months of age. It is imperative to evaluate a young, potentially IgAD dog with values for age-matched normal dogs and not compare pediatric values with the published normal values for adult dogs. Another important consideration is the transient nature of IgAD, especially in pediatric patients. Approximately 20% of dogs diagnosed with IgAD before 1 year of age will revert to normal IgA levels between 12 to 18 months of age; however, approximately 90% of dogs diagnosed with IgAD after 1 year of age will remain IgAD.[9] An example of transient IgA deficiency is illustrated in Table 152.1.

MANAGEMENT OF IgAD

Treatment of IgAD patients is limited to symptomatic treatment of the various infections, allergies, and/or autoimmune diseases. No specific immunotherapy exists for the treatment of IgAD itself. Immune globulin is contraindicated, because many IgAD patients may possess or produce anti-IgA antibodies that could result in serious anaphylactic reactions. In addition, it would not replace sIgA, which is the cause of IgAD.

REFERENCES

1. **Burrows PD, Cooper MD.** IgA deficiency. Adv Immunol 1997;65:245–276.
2. **Koskinen S, Tolo H, Hirvonen M, Koistinen J.** Long-term persistence of selective IgA deficiency in healthy adults. J Clin Immunol 1994;14:116–119.
3. **Liblau RS, Bach JF.** Selective IgA deficiency and autoimmunity. Int Arch Allergy Immunol 1992;99:16–27.
4. **Koskinen S.** Long-term follow-up of health in blood donors with primary IgA deficiency. J Clin Immunol 1996;16:165–170.
5. **Felsburg PJ, Glickman LT, Jezyk PF.** Selective IgA deficiency in the dog. Clin Immunol Immunopathol 1985;36:297–305.
6. **Moroff SD, Hurvitz AI, Peterson ME, Saunders L, Noone K.** IgA deficiency in Shar-pei dogs. Vet Immunol Immunopathol 1986;13:181–188.
7. **Campbell KL, Felsburg PJ.** IgA deficiency and skin disorders. In: Kirk RW, ed. Current veterinary therapy, XI. Philadelphia: WB Saunders, 1992;528–531.
8. **Day MJ, Penhale WJ, Eger CE, Shaw SE, Kabay MJ, Robinson WF, Huxtable CRR, Mills JN, Wyburn RS.** Disseminated aspergillosis in dogs. Aust Vet J 1986;63:55–59.
9. **Felsburg PJ, HogenEsch H, Shofer F, Kirkpatrick CE, Glickman LT.** Clinical epidemiologic and immunologic characteristics of canine selective IgA deficiency. Adv Exp Med Biol 1987;216B:1461–1470.
10. **Whitbread TJ, Batt RM, Garthwaire G.** Relative deficiency of serum IgA in German shepherd dogs: a breed abnormality. Res Vet Sci 1984;37:350–352.
11. **Shofer FS, Glickman LT, Payton AJ, Laster LL, Felsburg PJ.** Influence of parental serum immunoglobulins on morbidity and mortality of Beagles and their offspring. Am J Vet Res 1990;51:239–244.
12. **Glickman LT, Shofer FS, Payton AJ, Laster LL, Felsburg PJ.** Survey of serum IgA, IgG, and IgM concentrations in a large Beagle population in which IgA deficiency had been identified. Am J Vet Res 1988;49:1240–1245.

CHAPTER 153

Leukocyte Adhesion Deficiency

• MARCUS E. KEHRLI, JR, MARK R. ACKERMANN, ROBERT O. GILBERT, and DALE E. SHUSTER

MOLECULAR BASIS OF DISEASE

Leukocyte adhesion deficiency (LAD) in dogs,[1] humans,[2] and cattle[3,4] is a fatal primary immunodeficiency first reported as a granulocytopathy syndrome in Irish Setters in 1975. In all three species, LAD is inherited as an autosomal recessive trait and is characterized by persistent progressive neutrophilia in patients suffering from severe recurrent bacterial and mycotic infections. These patients suffer from a failure to form pus and, in all three species, the condition is a heritable deficiency of leukocyte surface glycoproteins associated with cell adherence and egress into tissues.[5-9] Leukocytes of patients with LAD have a deficiency or total lack of a family of structurally and functionally related glycoproteins called the β_2-integrins. Failure to express functional β_2-integrins is responsible for the inability of neutrophils to leave the bloodstream efficiently in response to chemotactic signals from tissues. Because neutrophils do not reach sites of infection, the organisms inducing the inflammatory response persist and recruitment signals from the tissues continue to stimulate neutrophil production and release from the bone marrow. Hence, a failure of neutrophil egress from blood combined with increased bone marrow output results in a striking and persistent leukocytosis characterized primarily as a neutrophilia.

The β_2-integrins include Mac-1, LFA-1, and p150,95[10] which are expressed primarily on leukocytes. These molecules are now termed CD11/CD18 by the World Health Organization.[11] Each of these molecules contains an α and a β subunit, noncovalently associated in an $\alpha_1\beta_1$ structure. The heterodimers share an identical β subunit (CD18) and are distinguished by their α subunits designated CD11a, CD11b, and CD11c for LFA-1α, Mac-1α, and p150,95α, respectively. A fourth member of the β_2-integrin family, CD11d, has also been described.[12-16] Mac-1 (CD11b/CD18) is also known as complement receptor 3 (CR3) and binds the opsonin C3bi and intercellular adhesion molecule-1 (ICAM-1; CD54) on endothelial cells. In vivo, Mac-1 mediates tight adherence of neutrophils to activated postcapillary venule endothelial cells that express ICAM-1; the selectin family of adhesion molecules mediates initial tethering to and rolling adherence of leukocytes across nonactivated endothelial cells.[17,18] The primary adhesion molecule family that neutrophils express is the β_2-integrins, whereas lymphocytes and monocytes express significant levels of other adhesion molecule families. These other adhesion molecule families provide a functionally redundant capacity for egress into tissues, thus allowing lymphocytes and monocytes to leave the bloodstream to combat infection and provide immune surveillance.

More than a dozen distinct mutations of the gene encoding the common β subunit (CD18) have been identified as the basis for LAD in human patients.[19-23] Each of these mutations results in an allele that fails to produce a functional protein. In cattle, only one CD18 allele has been found that encodes for a defective protein, and a single defective CD18 allele in Irish Setters has been documented.

Although the molecular basis for LAD was first reported in humans and predicted in dogs,[9] far more affected cattle have been identified. This is because using a few bulls to breed large numbers of cows is greatly facilitated by the management practice of artificial insemination. Studies leading to the molecular definition of bovine LAD (BLAD) identified neutrophils from a calf apparently affected by LAD that were deficient in the expression of the α-subunit of the Mac-1 β_2-integrin heterodimer.[8] Flow cytometric analysis of neutrophils from the sire and dam of this proband using a monoclonal antibody (mAb) specific for canine CD18 indicated the proband's parents expressed 65 to 70% of apparently normal levels of CD18 on neutrophils of other cattle.[8] Based on the apparent deficiency of the Mac-1 β_2-integrin heterodimer on neutrophils of the proband and the reduced expression of all β_2-integrins on all leukocytes in the parents of the proband, it was predicted that the defective allele was that of CD18, the common β-subunit shared among the leukocyte integrins. Eventually, the cDNA sequence of a normal bovine CD18 allele from a healthy Holstein calf was determined.[24] The 2833 nucleotide bovine CD18 sequence coded for a protein with 769 amino acids. Compared to human and murine sequences, the deduced amino acid sequences were greater than 80% identical among the three species. Amino acids 96-389 (95% identity) were very highly conserved when compared to the human sequence, a region where several mutations of the human CD18 sequence were found to cause LAD. These interspecies conserved regions identify portions of the CD18 molecule which presumably are functionally important for neutrophil egress.

The sequence of the defective allele for bovine CD18 was initially determined in two Holstein calves (10 and 14 months of age) with signs of BLAD. Northern blot analysis revealed that transcript (mRNA) from the defective CD18 allele was present at normal levels and of expected size in BLAD calves, ruling out genetic defects that block transcription or cause large deletions. mRNA was isolated from these BLAD calves and used to generate cDNA for sequencing of the bovine CD18 alleles present in BLAD cattle.[25] Comparing the cDNA sequence for CD18 in a BLAD calf with the normal sequence revealed a point mutation (adenine→guanine) resulting in a substitution of glycine for an aspartic acid at position 128 (referred to as the D128G allele) of the protein sequence for CD18. This mutation occurs near the center of 26 consecutive amino acids that are identical in normal bovine, human, and murine CD18 and lies within the larger extracellular region (aa 96-389) that is highly conserved across integrin β subunits.[22,24-26] Another mutation detected in the sequence from BLAD calves replaced a cytosine at nucleotide 775 with thymine; however, the mutation at nucleotide 775 was silent, as it did not alter the deduced amino acid sequence. Several retrospective and prospective case studies indicated the presence of only one allele in Holstein cattle which causes BLAD.[7,27-29] Although the first published reports of LAD in a veterinary species were on canine LAD (CLAD),[9] the mutation in the genetic code has only recently been determined.

In Irish setters, the presence of a single missense mutation (a G to C transversion at nucleotide 107 of the cDNA sequence) has been demonstrated responsible for causing a serine where a cysteine substitution at position 36 of the amino acid sequence.[29a] Using retroviral vectors expressing the normal (C36) or defective allele (C36S) for canine CD18, these authors elegantly demonstrated this mutation causes a failure to express detectable β_2-integrins on human LAD B-cells. The normal canine allele was able to resurrect β_2-integrin expression on these cells. This cysteine residue is conserved across all species in which alleles for CD18 have been sequenced. Moreover, this cysteine is conserved among all mammalian integrins sequenced [β_1(CD29), β_2(CD18) and β_3(CD61)]. This cysteine presumably forms a critical intrachain disulfide bond in the extracellular region of the CD18 protein. An oligonucleotide ligation assay (OLA) utilizing genomic DNA was developed as a screening method for detecting canine carriers of this eventually lethal autosomal recessive genetic disease.[29a] Results from screening a population of 208 Irish setters in the United Kingdom identified 19 carrier dogs (a 9% carrier rate). This genetic disease has not been reported in other breeds and OLA testing of 48 dogs representing 12 other

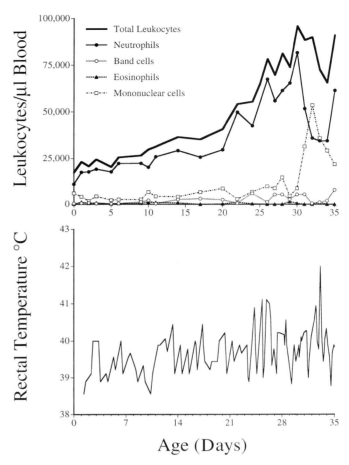

FIGURE 153.1 Leukogram and rectal temperature of a BLAD calf from birth to death. A persistent progressive neutrophilia accompanied by recurrent febrile episodes is a hallmark feature of BLAD.

breeds failed to detect the defective C36S CD18 allele.[29a] The absence of this defective allele in other breeds suggests that, as with BLAD, the defective CD18 allele likely arose after divergence of the Irish setter and Holstein breeds from the other breeds in each species.

CLINICAL FEATURES

LAD in all species is clinically characterized by recurrent soft tissue infections, severely impaired pus formation, persistent leukocytosis (primarily neutrophilia) (Fig 153.1), and abnormalities of various adhesion-dependent functions of leukocytes in vitro. Typically, animals reaching ages greater than 6 months will present with a history of respiratory disease and diarrhea, exhibit periodontal gingivitis with gingival recession (Fig. 153.2) and tooth loss, and will achieve ~60% of normal weight and ~80% of expected stature. Oral ulcers are common in all species and are refractory to treatment. BLAD calves will likely present with a persistent and pronounced mature neutrophilia of greater than 40,000 neutrophils/μL blood, compared with a normal level of less than 4000 neutrophils/μL. Neutrophils from BLAD calves will express less than 2% of normal level of β_2 integrins by flow cytometry; although not good for heterozygote detection, flow cytometry can provide an extremely rapid diagnosis of affecteds.

The original bovine granulocytopathy syndrome was described as a disease of young Holstein cattle characterized by recurrent pneumonia, ulcerative and granulomatous stomatitis, enteritis with bacterial overgrowth, periodontitis, delayed wound healing, persistent neutrophilia, and death at an early age.[3,4,7,8] For some time clinicians in North America had recognized a condition colloquially known as "leukemoid response of calves" that now is thought to have represented BLAD calves. Most of these calves exhibited stunted growth and a persistent, progressive neutrophilia (often exceeding 100,000/μL) and a less dramatic lymphocytosis.[3,4,7,8,30] The concomitant increase in lymphocytes and monocytes is presumably due to increased bone marrow production of leukocytes in response to recurrent infectious episodes. The stunting of growth in these immunologically compromised patients is presumably due to several factors: (1) continuous recurrent disease inducing inflammatory cytokine release and catabolic processes in response to normal microbial flora and pathogens, (2) periodontal gingivitis and tooth loss impairing normal feed consumption, and (3) elevated basal metabolic rates associated with recurrent febrile episodes.

At birth, BLAD calves will appear healthy and have leukocyte counts within the normal range for newborns. However, within 1 week calves may exhibit a leukocytosis of more than 34,000 cells/μL. These calves may only have a mild fever (e.g., 39.6°C) if examined closely. A

hallmark feature of BLAD is that analysis of subsequent blood samples obtained over the next several weeks will reveal a chronic progressive neutrophilia, which will eventually be greater than 85% neutrophils and exceed 100,000 leukocytes/μL. In vitro assessment of isolated blood neutrophils will reveal selected functional abnormalities. These calves will die prematurely, following persistent fever and chronic diarrhea, despite administration of antibiotics.

β_2-integrin deficiency in Holstein calves is analogous to severe LAD phenotypes seen in humans. Neutrophils in LAD patients are unable to adhere to the endothelial lining of postcapillary venules, thus interrupting egression of neutrophils into infected tissues. Calves with BLAD die prematurely as a result of the failure of neutrophils to extravasate into infected tissues, as is the case with most untreated human LAD patients. Moreover, severe generalized prepubertal periodontitis, similar to that seen in cattle with LAD, has been reported in children with LAD.[30,31] Often, the infections in LAD patients are the result of otherwise normal flora for immunologically competent individuals. A second form of LAD (Type II) has been reported in human patients who lack fucosylated glycoconjugates.[32,33] These glycoconjugates include the selectin ligand, sialyl LewisX, and various fucosylated blood group antigens.

The severe clinicopathologic consequences of CD11/CD18 deficiency in people as well as dogs and cattle reflect the diverse contributions of the β_2-integrins to leukocyte adherence reactions of importance in inflammation and host defense. The severity of neutrophil function abnormalities and clinical complications among humans with LAD is directly related to the degree of glycoprotein deficiency. Human patients with the severe phenotype (expressing less than 1% of normal $\alpha\beta$ complexes on cell surfaces) are susceptible to life-threatening infectious complications in infancy, whereas patients with moderate deficiency (expressing 3 to 10% of normal amounts) develop less severe complications and generally survive into adulthood.[34] Studies of their neutrophils in vitro indicate less severe functional impairment than has been observed among subjects with the severe phenotype.[34] Cattle and dogs with LAD have a moderately severe phenotype because affected animals express ~2% of normal amounts of CD18 protein on neutrophil surfaces. It is clear that LAD is a lethal genetic condition for homozygous animals; because environmental hygiene conditions for dogs and cattle are more challenging than for humans, the likelihood of premature death is greatly increased versus human LAD patients. It is likely that BLAD calves would be the first to die if a disease outbreak due to a recognized pathogen would occur on a farm. It is also possible that BLAD calves may die as a result of disease caused by normal flora.[35] Clinical and research experience with BLAD patients predicts the majority of these calves would die before 1 year of age. It is possible, however, for some of the animals to live past 2 years of age, but they are severely stunted in growth (~50% of expected body weight) and suffer from the various infectious conditions of the skin (including severe ringworm) and gas-

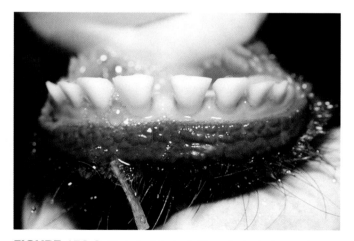

FIGURE 153.2 Periodontal gingivitis and gingival recession evident in a 14-month-old Holstein bull. Leukocyte counts in this bull ranged between 35,000 and 75,000 over a nearly 3-year life span. This bull was one of the healthiest BLAD animals ever studied over a 7-year period during which BLAD animals were maintained at the National Animal Disease Center-USDA-ARS. This bull was humanely euthanized after 2000 U of semen were collected.

trointestinal and respiratory tracts. Of the older survivors, a striking periodontal gingivitis with marked recession of the gingiva may be the most obvious clinical sign.

Histologically, capillaries, sinusoids, and blood vessels throughout the body contain numerous neutrophils although a few neutrophils are present subjacent to ulcerated lesions of mucosal surfaces. Large crescents of numerous neutrophils often circumscribe splenic periarteriolar lymphocytic sheaths, and increased myeloid/erythroid ratios are present in the bone marrow. Neutrophils have also been noted in the lung of some calves with BLAD. Lymph nodes range from hyperplastic, in some reports, to diffuse, hypocellularity with necrosis of secondary follicles.[4,8]

IMMUNOLOGIC ASSESSMENTS OF BLAD CALVES

Neutrophils from LAD patients fail to adhere to postcapillary venule endothelial cells in a β_2-integrin–dependent manner. This is significant in that this precludes the efficient egress of neutrophils into tissues to combat pathogens and normal flora in tissues and on mucosal surfaces. Lymphocytes and monocytes from LAD patients also fail to express β_2-integrins and fail to adhere in a β_2-integrin–dependent manner. However, as mentioned above, these leukocytes express other adhesion molecules that are not affected by the β_2-integrin deficiency and thus provide a redundant adhesion mechanism for lymphocytes and monocytes to adhere tightly to endothelial cells for egress.

The presence or absence of β_2-integrin molecules has been demonstrated on the surface of neutrophils, monocytes, and lymphocytes from normal or BLAD calves using specific monoclonal antibodies and flow cytometry,[25,36] or by colloidal gold immunolabeling and scanning electron microscopy in backscatter mode.[37] Surface expression of CD18, CD11a, and CD11b evaluated by flow cytometry detected CD11a and CD11b expression at 6% and 10% of norm values. Analyses of numerous BLAD patients have found CD18 to be expressed at ~2% of normal levels for resting and platelet activating factor (PAF)-stimulated neutrophils. Curiously, resting neutrophil L-selectin expression in BLAD patients is markedly reduced compared to controls.[30] The low levels of L-selectin in BLAD patients may be a reflection of chronic immunological activation resulting from subclinical infections. Similar findings from canine LAD patients have been reported.[9,38]

Neutrophils from BLAD patients have several functional deficits consistent with deficient expression of CD11/CD18 glycoproteins. In vitro assessments have identified abnormalities of motile, phagocytic, and oxidative functions of neutrophils which appear to mediate inflammatory deficits in vivo.[3,4,7,8,39] Diminished phagocytosis-associated oxidative and secretory functions during ingestion of C3bi opsonized zymosan by neutrophils of BLAD patients are consistent with a deficiency of the Mac-1α subunit that contains the CR3 epitope

reactive with C3bi deposited on zymosan particles.[6,34] Adherence and surface CD18 levels on neutrophils from normal cattle increase following stimulation with PAF.[30] These responses are not observed with neutrophils from BLAD patients. PAF-enhanced neutrophil adherence from normal cattle can be inhibited by treating control neutrophils with anti-CD18 mAb, but this mAb is without effect when incubated with neutrophils from BLAD patients.

DIAGNOSIS

The clinical hallmarks of LAD include recurrent infections accompanied by a persistent progressive neutrophilia that fails to return to normal leukocyte numbers and fever (Fig. 153.1). These infections may affect the respiratory or enteric tracts or both. Older animals also may suffer from severe ringworm or papilloma warts. The periodontal gingivitis with gingival recession (Fig. 153.2) and subsequent tooth loss are nearly pathognomonic when combined with the striking neutrophilia. Supportive laboratory analysis of CD18 expression by flow cytometry can provide an extremely rapid confirmatory diagnosis (Fig. 153.3).

On the basis of the two point mutations within the D128G allele encoding the bovine CD18 responsible for BLAD, a rapid DNA-based diagnostic test was developed.[25] A DNA-polymerase chain reaction (PCR)-restriction fragment length polymorphism (RFLP) technique was developed around the locus of the mutation. This mutation is used to identify unequivocally the genotype of cattle at the CD18 locus. Testing is performed with genomic DNA. Several commercial laboratories conduct the DNA-PCR-RFLP test for BLAD. This test has been

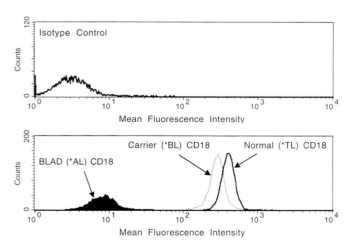

FIGURE 153.3 Flow cytometric analysis of CD18 expression on neutrophils of cattle. **Upper panel:** background fluorescence of neutrophils labeled with an irrelevant isotype control mAb. **Lower panel:** expression of CD18 on neutrophils from homozygous normal cattle (*TL), heterozygous carriers (*BL), and a homozygous BLAD calf (*AL). Neutrophils were stained with saturating amounts of mAb specific for CD18.

licensed to Immgen Inc., College Station, Texas, and the Bovine Blood Typing Laboratory of Canada, Saskatoon, Saskatchewan. All testing in the United States is co-ordinated through and recorded with the Holstein Association of America (802-254-4551). Several hundred Holstein bovine LAD cases have been confirmed by DNA-PCR-RFLP to be homozygous for the D128G mutation.[25,27–29,40] Many of these cases (dating back to 1977) were found using formalin-fixed tissues from cattle suspected to have bovine granulocytopathy syndrome. All evidence to date indicates that all BLAD patients worldwide represent a homozygous genotype for a single mutant allele of CD18 (D128G).

TREATMENT

No effective treatments exist for LAD in cattle or dogs. Human patients with LAD may undergo successful bone marrow transplantation from histocompatible donors. Because the β_2-integrins are involved in cell:cell adhesion between cytotoxic T cells and foreign target cells, the rejection of donor cells is not as efficient. An attempt at bone marrow transplantation from a nonhistocompatible calf into a 3-year-old BLAD heifer was unsuccessful (ME Kehrli and JL Burton, unpublished data, 1993). Leukocyte transfusions (greater than 10^{10} total isolated leukocytes) from nonhistocompatible donors were also attempted with BLAD patients exhibiting dramatically elevated leukocyte counts (greater than 125,000 leukocytes/μL). During the hours following transfusion, no evidence of leukocytes expressing normal levels of CD18 was found by flow cytometric analysis of more than 100,000 circulating leukocytes from the recipient. It is possible that leukocyte transfusions resulted in virtually immediate migration of donor cells into tissues, especially because the recipients exhibited clinical improvement as assessed by a reduction in leukocyte count and fever. Leukochimeric, nonidentical twins have been observed in which one twin's true genotype is a homozygous affected BLAD animal and the other twin's genotype is a heterozygote or homozygous normal for CD18 expression (ME Kehrli, unpublished data, 1995; P. Healy, New South Wales, Australia, unpublished data, 1994). Leukochimerism in these animals is a result of the anastomosis of the chorioallantoic membranes between nonidentical twins that allows the exchange of bone marrow stem cells between each fetus. In effect, this results in a natural bone marrow transplant in utero before full immunologic competence develops and a stable transplant results. Each of these sets of twins were born with roughly equal proportions of distinct populations of CD18$^+$ and CD18$^-$ leukocytes in their circulation; within a few months, the proportion of CD18$^-$ leukocytes reached as high as 85 to 90% of the circulating leukocytes. With as few as 10% CD18$^+$ circulating leukocytes, these patients experienced apparently normal health and growth, suggesting that only minimal success is necessary with bone marrow transplantation to achieve a healthy outcome in CD18-deficient patients.

Because expression of CD18 is restricted to cells derived from bone marrow, LAD has been a target for somatic gene therapy using ex vivo infection of bone marrow stem cells. Successful in vitro correction of CD18 expression in human lymphocytes has been achieved by gene therapy.[41] Transplantation of syngeneic murine stem cells infected with a retrovirus containing human CD18 expressed human CD18 on 17 to 36% of circulating granulocytes at 2 weeks after transplantation in mice.[42]

CONTROL OF THE DEFECT IN CATTLE

BLAD has an inheritance pattern of an autosomal recessive trait.[7] Testing of bulls and cows mated for the purpose of producing future sires used in artificial insemination throughout the world was initiated in 1991. BLAD was an especially serious condition within the Holstein breed because some of the most prominent sires were heterozygous for the D128G allele. Osborndale Ivanhoe, Penstate Ivanhoe Star, Carlin-M Ivanhoe Bell, and Thonyma Secret are some of the elite sires of the breed diagnosed as carriers of this allele on the basis of DNA testing. Cattle that have been tested for this genetic condition and found free of the defective allele are designated *TL; carrier animals are designated *BL. To date, tens of thousands of cattle around the world have been genotyped for the CD18 locus. From January 1991 to January 1996, the BLAD carrier rate averaged 12.5% among the semiannual summary rankings of the top 100 Holstein bulls in the United States. The BLAD carrier rate among these bulls peaked at 17% in 1991 and again during the summer of 1994. However, as a result of the DNA-PCR-RFLP test, the number of young *BL bulls entering artificial insemination service has been virtually zero since 1993.[43] Since 1994, the carrier rate among artifical insemination bulls has been steadily declining, and it is estimated that after 1998 virtually no carriers will be ranked among the top 100 genetic merit bulls. Results from this testing have provided the necessary information to phase out the use of carrier bulls designated *BL by 1998 without any significant loss of the existing gene pool necessary for high-quality milk production.[43] The frequency of *BL cows in 1991 was ~8%, and this frequency undoubtedly continued to rise through the mid-1990s as the generations of replacement heifers from the numerous *BL bulls came into milk production.

It is certain that a small proportion of calfhood deaths in this breed were, in fact, attributed to infectious complications of BLAD. Assuming random mating and a carrier rate for the D128G allele of 13.5% among bulls and 8% among cows, not more than 1.1% of all random matings would be between carrier animals. Of these matings, only 25% would result in homozygous affected BLAD progeny; therefore, only 0.27% of all random matings would result in an affected BLAD calf. With 9.7 million dairy cows in the United States in the early 1990s, this predicted about 26,000 BLAD calves born each year. Worldwide, this number may have approached 100,000 calves per year. The extensive use of artificial insemination in the dairy industry allows for relatively few bulls to sire most of the progeny; this also allows rapid elimination of autosomal recessive diseases if bulls with such undesirable traits are eliminated. Although the heterozygotic condition has not been completely studied with regard to effects on health, at this time it appears that there are no detrimental effects on cattle carrying the defective allele. A slight favorable advantage has been reported for carrier cows to have a reduced clinical mastitis incidence.[44]

Due to the existence in dizygotic bovine twins of the leukochimeric condition, it is important to identify even slight aberrations in DNA polymorphism assays. The potential risk of false genotyping of cattle and the expense to breeders emphasizes the importance of this issue. Reports of leukochimerism warrant against the exclusive use of blood samples for DNA typing when twinning is properly documented.[45] Breed associations have determined it is important to eliminate the presence of genetic lethal conditions from populations of animals. The dairy cattle industry affords the most striking example of how rapidly the use of DNA-PCR technologies can be applied with minimal negative impact on the available finite gene pool. Previous efforts to screen for a genetic defect in Australian Holstein cattle were the first to use DNA-PCR technology (typically DNA extracted from blood).[46] Testing of animals for citrullinemia using blood leukocyte DNA led to the false genotyping of a few animals that were not originally known to be twins. Apparently, a certain percentage of live births (~1 in 1500 animals) involve a calf with a twin that died in utero and was resorbed during gestation or was never observed in the placental membranes (P Healy, personal communication, 1992). These unidentified twins pose a potential delay to breed associations who desire to eliminate genetic defects quickly through DNA testing methods. A similar lack of a known twin has recently been reported in a parentage dispute involving a mare who was excluded as a parent based on blood-derived DNA.[47]

Limitations of applying DNA-PCR for genotype identification include financial and technical errors. If 1499 of 1500 births are accurately recorded as twin or single births, then a test performed on blood-derived DNA would be 99.93% accurate. This level of accuracy should be acceptable, provided twinning is documented and it offers the cattle industry the ability to test the DNA of calves shortly after birth, thus saving considerable expense associated with performing skin biopsies or waiting until semen is available from bulls that need to be tested. For cows, only an alternative source of DNA (such as skin) is a satisfactory solution to the potential leukochimerism condition causing a false genotype. Testing of the most influential Holstein sires and any sire's descendent from a known carrier through the use of semen would be prudent. Matings between known carriers should be avoided unless a deliberate effort to identify homozygotically normal embryos or fetuses is made. This type of mating might result in valuable progeny but would be achieved only through considerable expense and effort.

REFERENCES

1. **Renshaw HW, et al.** Canine granulocytopathy syndrome: neutrophil dysfunction in a dog with recurrent infections. J Am Vet Med Assoc 1975;166:443–447.
2. **Crowley CA, et al.** An inherited abnormality of neutrophil adhesion: its genetic transmission and its association with a missing protein. N Engl J Med 1980;302:1163–1168.
3. **Hagemoser WA, et al.** Granulocytopathy in a Holstein heifer. J Am Vet Med Assoc 1983;183:1093–1094.
4. **Nagahata H, et al.** Bovine granulocytopathy syndrome: neutrophil dysfunction in Holstein Friesian calves. J Vet Med Ser A 1987;34:445–451.
5. **Dana N, et al.** Deficiencies of a surface membrane glycoprotein (Mo1) in man. J Clin Invest 1984;73:153–159.
6. **Anderson DC, et al.** Abnormalities of polymorphonuclear leukocyte function associated with a heritable deficiency of high molecular weight surface glycoproteins (GP138): common relationship to diminished cell adherence. J Clin Invest 1984;74:536–551.
7. **Takahashi K, et al.** Bovine granulocytopathy syndrome of Holstein-Friesian calves and heifers. Jpn J Vet Sci 1987;49:733–736.
8. **Kehrli ME Jr, et al.** Molecular definition of the bovine granulocytopathy syndrome: identification of deficiency of the Mac-1 (CD11b/CD18) glycoprotein. Am J Vet Res 1990;51:1826–1836.
9. **Giger U, et al.** Deficiency of leukocyte surface glycoproteins Mo1, LFA-1, and Leu M5 in a dog with recurrent bacterial infections: an animal model. Blood 1987;69:1622–1630.
10. **Sanchez-Madrid F, et al.** A human leukocyte differentiation antigen family with distinct α-subunits and a common β-subunit: the lymphocyte function-associated antigen (LFA-1), the C3bi complement receptor (OKM1/Mac-1), and the p150,95 molecule. J Exp Med 1983;158:1785–1803.
11. **Reinherz EL.** Human myeloid and hematopoietic cells In: Reinherz EL, et al. eds. Leukocyte typing II. New York: Springer-Verlag, 1986;124–129.
12. **Danilenko DM, et al.** A novel canine leukointegrin, $\alpha_d\beta_2$, is expressed by specific macrophage subpopulations in tissue and a minor CD8+ lymphocyte subpopulation in peripheral blood. J Immunol 1995;155:35–44.
13. **Van der Vieren M, et al.** A novel leukointegrin, $\alpha_d\beta_2$, binds preferentially to ICAM-3. Immunity 1995;3:683–690.
14. **el-Gabalawy H, et al.** Synovial distribution of alpha d/CD18, a novel leukointegrin. Comparison with other integrins and their ligands. Arthritis Rheum 1996;39:1913–1921.
15. **Rabb H, et al.** The leukointegrin $\alpha d/\beta_2$ ($\alpha d/CD18$): specific changes in surface expression in patients on hemodialysis. Cell Adhes Commun 1998;6:13–20.
16. **Shelley CS, et al.** Mapping of the human CD11c (ITGAX) and CD11d (ITGAD) genes demonstrates that they are arranged in tandem separated by no more than 11.5 kb. Genomics 1998;49:334–336.
17. **Kishimoto TK, et al.** Neutrophil Mac-1 and MEL-14 adhesion proteins inversely regulated by chemotactic factors. Science 1989;245:1238–1241.
18. **Ley K, Tedder TF.** Leukocyte interactions with vascular endothelium. J Immunol 1995;155:525–528.
19. **Kishimoto TK, et al.** Heterogenous mutations in the β subunit common to the LFA-1, Mac-1, and p150,95 glycoproteins cause leukocyte adhesion deficiency. Cell 1987;50:193–202.
20. **Marlin SD, et al.** LFA-1 immunodeficiency disease: definition of the genetic defect and chromosomal mapping of alpha and beta subunits by complementation in hybrid cells. J Exp Med 1986;164:855–867.
21. **Dana N, et al.** Leukocytes from four patients with complete or partial LeuCAM deficiency contain the common beta-subunit precursor and beta-subunit messenger RNA. J Clin Invest 1987;79:1010–1015.
22. **Kishimoto TK, et al.** Leukocyte adhesion deficiency: aberrant splicing of a conserved integrin sequence causes a moderate deficiency phenotype. J Biol Chem 1989;264:3588–3595.
23. **Hibbs ML, et al.** Transfection of cells from patients with leukocyte adhesion deficiency with an integrin β subunit (CD18) restore lymphocyte function-associated antigen-1 expression and function. J Clin Invest 1990;85:674–681.
24. **Shuster DE, et al.** Sequence of the bovine CD18-encoding cDNA: comparison with the human and murine glycoproteins. Gene 1992;114:267–271.
25. **Shuster DE, et al.** Identification and prevalence of a genetic defect that causes leukocyte adhesion deficiency in Holstein cattle. Proc Natl Acad Sci USA 1992;89:9225–9229.
26. **Wilson RW, et al.** Nucleotide sequence of the cDNA from the mouse leukocyte adhesion protein CD18. Nucleic Acids Res 1989;17:5397.
27. **Stöber M, et al.** Bovine leukocyte adhesion deficiency (BLAD = Hagemoser-Takahashi-Syndrome): clinical, patho-anatomical and -histological findings. DTW 1991;98:443–448.
28. **Gilbert RO, et al.** Clinical manifestations of leukocyte adhesion deficiency in cattle: 14 cases (1977–1991). J Am Vet Med Assoc 1993;202:445–449.
29. **Lienau A, et al.** Bovine leukocyte adhesion deficiency: clinical picture and differential diagnosis. DTW 1994;101:405–406.
29a. **Kijas JM, Bauer TR Jr, Gafvert S, Marklund S, Trowald-Wigh G, Johannisson A, Hedhammar A, Binns M, Juneja RK, Hickstein DD, Andersson L.** A missense mutation in the β-2 integrin gene (ITGB2) causes canine leukocyte adhesion deficiency. Genomics 1999;61:101–107.

30. **Kehrli ME Jr, et al.** Clinical and immunological features associated with bovine leukocyte adhesion deficiency In: Lipsky PE, et al., eds. Structure, function, and regulation of molecules involved in leukocyte adhesion. New York: Springer-Verlag, 1993;314–327.

31. **Waldrop TC, et al.** Periodontal manifestations of the heritable Mac-1, LFA-1, deficiency syndrome. Clinical, histopathologic and molecular characteristics. J Periodontol 1987;58:400–416.

32. **Maly P, et al.** The alpha(1,3)fucosyltransferase Fuc-TVII controls leukocyte trafficking through an essential role in L-, E-, and P-selectin ligand biosynthesis. Cell 1996;86:643–653.

33. **Karsan A, et al.** Leukocyte adhesion deficiency type II is a generalized defect of de novo GDP-fucose biosynthesis. Endothelial cell fucosylation is not required for neutrophil rolling on human nonlymphoid endothelium. J Clin Invest 1998;101:2438–2445.

34. **Anderson DC, et al.** The severe and moderate phenotypes of heritable Mac-1, LFA-1 deficiency: their quantitative definition and relation to leukocyte dysfunction and clinical features. J Infect Dis 1985;152:668–689.

35. **Ackermann MR, et al.** Alimentary and respiratory tract lesions in eight medically fragile Holstein cattle with bovine leukocyte adhesion deficiency (BLAD). Vet Pathol 1996;33:273–281.

36. **Rutten VP, et al.** Identification of monoclonal antibodies with specificity to α- or β-chains of β_2-integrins using peripheral blood leucocytes of normal and bovine leukocyte adhesion deficient (BLAD) cattle. Vet Immunol Immunopathol 1996;52:341–345.

37. **Ackermann MR, et al.** Identification of β_2 integrins in bovine neutrophils by scanning electron microscopy in the backscatter mode and transmission electron microscopy. Vet Pathol 1993;30:296–298.

38. **Trowald-Wigh G, et al.** Leucocyte adhesion protein deficiency in Irish setter dogs. Vet Immunol Immunopathol 1992;32:261–280.

39. **Nagahata H, et al.** Bovine leukocyte adhesion deficiency: neutrophil function and pathological analysis. Am J Vet Res 1994;55:40–48.

40. **Agerholm JS, et al.** Bovine leukocyte adhesion deficiency in Danish Holstein-Friesian cattle. II. Patho-anatomical description of affected calves. Acta Vet Scand 1993;34:237–243.

41. **Wilson JM, et al.** Correction of CD18 deficient lymphocytes by retrovirus mediated gene transfer. Science 1990;248:1413–1416.

42. **Wilson RW, et al.** Expression of human CD18 in murine granulocytes and improved efficiency for infection of deficient human lymphoblasts. Hum Gene Ther 1993;4:25–34.

43. **Powell RL, et al.** Relationship of bovine leukocyte adhesion deficiency with genetic merit for performance traits. J Dairy Sci 1996;79:895–899.

44. **Kelm SC, et al.** Genetic association between parameters of innate immunity and measures of mastitis in periparturient Holstein cattle. J Dairy Sci 1997;80:1767–1775.

45. **Ryncarz RE, et al.** Recognition of leukochimerism during genotyping for bovine leukocyte adhesion deficiency (BLAD) by polymerase chain reaction amplified DNA extracted from blood. J Vet Diagn Invest 1995;7:569–572.

46. **Dennis JA, et al.** Molecular definition of bovine argininosuccinate synthetase deficiency. Proc Natl Acad Sci USA 1989;86:7947–7951.

47. **Bowling AT, et al.** Silent blood chimaerism in a mare confirmed by DNA marker analysis of hair bulbs. Anim Genet 1993;24:323–324.

CHAPTER 154

The Porphyrias and the Porphyrinurias

• J. JERRY KANEKO

Diseases associated with the accumulation of porphyrin compounds in cells, tissues, and in all body fluids are classified as porphyrias and porphyrinurias. The porphyrias are those inherited enzyme defects of the metabolic pathway leading to synthesis of porphyrins and their metal complexes, the hemoglobins and other heme proteins. The porphyrinurias are those acquired defects of the same pathway due to chemical and metal toxicities.[1] The heme proteins are found widespread in nature, as would be expected of compounds so closely associated with the fundamental metabolic processes. The photosynthetic pigment of plants, chlorophyll, is a magnesium-porphyrin. The heme proteins of animals include hemoglobins, myoglobins, and heme enzymes such as catalase, peroxidase, and cytochromes. As such, the heme compounds are vital to the capture and delivery of oxygen to the tissues and to the subsequent generation of chemical energy to sustain life. The normal sequence of events and the enzymes involved in the synthesis of the porphyrins have been described in detail in Chapter 23 ("Hemoglobin Synthesis and Destruction"). This chapter will focus on porphyrias, those hereditary forms, in which the toxic porphyrin compounds accumulate amid failures to synthesize the precise porphyrin structures required for their incorporation into functional heme proteins.

Depending on the fundamental biochemical defect, the porphyrias are further classified by the major tissue of origin, the erythropoietic system, or the liver. Thus, the two major porphyrias are the erythropoietic and hepatic porphyrias. There are other systems of classification of the porphyrias, and although there is general agreement on the erythropoietic forms, there is still some confusion about the classification of the hepatic forms.[2] A useful system of classification is given in Table 154.1.

PORPHYRIN SYNTHESIS, THE PORPHYRIAS, AND THE PORPHYRINURIAS

The biochemical pathway for the synthesis of porphyrins and the heme of hemoglobin are now well known[1]

(see Chapter 23) and are outlined in Figure 154.1. The nomenclature of the enzymes involved and deficiencies are given in Table 154.1, and their numbers correspond to the numbered steps given in Figure 154.1.

The first step in the pathway of porphyrin synthesis requires vitamin B_6 as a cofactor for δ-aminolevulinic synthetase (ALA-syn); this is the underlying deficiency in pyridoxine responsive anemia but has not been recognized as hereditary enzyme deficiency. ALA-dehydrase (ALA-D) may be deficient or inhibited by a toxin such as lead. This is also seen in the incorporation of iron into protoporphyrin IX by ferrochelatase (FER-Ch), where its deficiency is the cause of congenital erythropoietic protoporphyria (CEP) of cattle and humans. FER-Ch inhibition is a major toxic effect of lead, particularly in dogs and children.

The synthesis of porphyrins and heme can occur only in respiring cells with a full complement of mitochondrial and cytosolic enzymes. The Krebs cycle is an aerobic cycle, so oxygen would be required to supply the succinyl-CoA. The predominant tissues that synthesize heme are the bone marrow for hemoglobin and the liver for the heme enzymes. As would be expected, these are the two tissues that are central to the pathogenesis of the porphyrias and the porphyrinurias.

DIAGNOSIS OF PORPHYRIAS

Clinically, the detection of porphyrins is based on their reddish-brown color, their characteristic red fluorescence when exposed to ultraviolet (UV) light, and the lesions of photosensitivity due to the photosensitizing nature of the porphyrin compounds. Because they are present in all body cells, tissues, and fluids, the porphyrins stain all tissues. This is particularly noticeable in the reddish-orange staining of the teeth and dentine, hence the name "Pink Tooth" is colloquially used for congenital erythropoietic porphyria. In well-vascularized tissues (e.g., mucous membranes) a muddy color is readily detected. Porphyrins in body fluids are readily excreted in the urine, in all excreta, and in saliva, sweat, tears, and mucous secretions. The reddish-orange discoloration of the urine is readily visible and is often

TABLE 154.1   Classification of the Porphyrias

No. in Figure 154.1	Porphyria Type	Inheritance	Enzyme Deficiency Abbreviation	Enzyme Deficiency Full Name
Erythropoietic porphyrias				
4.	Congenital erythropoietic porphyria (CEP)	AR Cattle	UROgenIII-Cosyn	Uroporphyrinogen III cosynthase (cosynthetase)
8.	Erythropoietic protoporphyria (EPP)	AD Siamese Swine	FER-Ch	Ferrochelatase; heme synthase (synthetase)
Hepatic porphyrias				
2.	ALA-D deficiency porphyria	AR	ALA-D	Delta-aminolevulinate dehydrase (dehydratase); porbobilinogen synthase
3.	Acute intermittant porphyria	AD	UROgenI-Syn	Uroporphyrinogen I synthase (synthetase); porphobilinogen deaminase (PBG-D)
5.	Porphyria cutanea tarda	AD	UROgen-D	Uroporphyrinogen decarboxylase
5.	Hepatoerythropoietic porphyria	AR	UROgen-D	Uroporphyrinogen decarboxylase
6.	Harderoporphyria	AR	COPROgenIII-Ox	Coproporphyringen III oxidase
6.	Hereditary coproporphyria	AD	COPROgenIII-Ox	Coproporphyringen III oxidase
7.	Variegate porphyria	AD	PROTOgen-Ox	Protoporphyrinogen oxidase

From Kaneko JJ. Porphyrins and the porphyrias. In: Kaneko JJ, Harvey JW, Bruss ML, eds. Clinical biochemistry of domestic animals. 5th ed. San Diego: Academic Press, 1997.
A, autosomal; *R*, recessive; *D*, dominant; *U*, unknown.

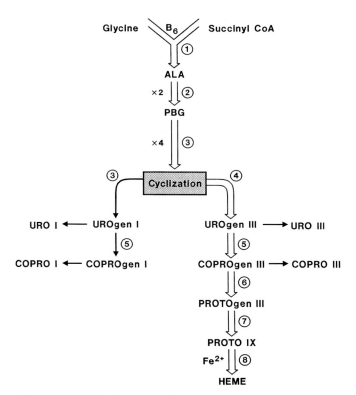

FIGURE 154.1 Alternate pathways for porphyrin synthesis. Normally, enzymes 3 and 4 function together in a coordinated manner to form heme. In the absence of enzyme 4, the alternate and terminal pathway to form the type I isomers is taken. The circled numbers correspond to the enzymes listed in Table 154.1. From Kaneko JJ. Porphyrins and the porphyrias. In: Kaneko JJ, Harvey JW, Bruss ML, eds. Clinical biochemistry of domestic animals. 5th ed. San Diego: Academic Press, 1997, with permission.

the presenting complaint. When UV light of the Soret band (405 nm) or a Wood's lamp is shined on the teeth or urine, an intense reddish fluorescence is seen. This is virtually pathognomonic of porphyria, but this red fluorescence should not be confused with the yellow-green fluorescence of the tetracycline drugs. The third major clinical observation is the photodermatitis that is evident on the light-colored areas of the skin. This may be accompanied by light sensitivity of the eyes. When exposed to UV light, the porphyrins in the skin are excited by absorption of the UV light energy and raised to an unstable, higher-level energy state. The excitation energy is then emitted when the unstable excited molecule returns to its ground state. The excitation energy can be emitted as fluorescence or transferred to molecular oxygen to form singlet oxygen. Singlet oxygen is a powerful oxidant for many forms of biologically important compounds, including the peroxidation of membrane lipids, membrane and cellular proteins, and cell organelles. Peroxidation is the primary event in the photosensitivity and photodermatitis seen in the porphyrias.[3]

The principal method now used for the detection of porphyrins in biologic materials in the clinical laboratory is also based on the characteristic red fluorescence observed when acidic solutions of the porphyrins are exposed to UV light. Fluorescence does not differentiate the uroporphyrins from the coproporphyrins, so these are separated on the basis of their solubilities in organic solvents before exposure. Various screening and chemical procedures are described in detail for urine, fecal and blood porphyrins, as well as for urinary porphobilinogen.[1]

ERYTHROPOIETIC PORPHYRIAS

Bovine Congenital Erythropoietic Porphyria

The most characteristic finding in bovine congenital erythropoietic porphyria (CEP) is a reddish brown discoloration of the teeth and bones. The disease is seen primarily in Holsteins, with a few cases in Shorthorns and Jamaican cattle. Bovine CEP is inherited as an autosomal recessive trait. The condition is present at birth, and severely affected calves must be protected from sunlight if they are to survive.

Although the predominant signs of teeth and urine discoloration and the photosensitization of the severely affected animal are readily apparent, they may vary widely depending on the degree of enzyme deficiency, age, time of year, proportion of whitish hair coat, and exposure to sunlight. The urinary excretion of the porphyrins and, therefore, urine color may vary widely.

Normally, free porphyrins are found in very low concentrations in cells, tissues, and body fluids. Thus, the finding of porphyrins in any detectable amounts is always noteworthy. In urine, porphyrin excretion varies over extremely wide limits, ranging from uroporphyrins between 6.3 and 3900 μg/dL (0.076 to 46.96 μmol/l) and coproporphyrins between 2.1 and 8300 μg/dL (0.032 to 126.74 μmol/l). At concentrations of 100 μg/dL (1.53 μmol/l) or more, a reddish discoloration is discernible in the urine. At 1000 μg/dL (15.27 μmol/l) or more, an intense red fluorescence of the urine is readily observed when examined with a Wood's lamp. The principal porphyrins excreted are URO I and COPRO I, and the amount of each appearing in the urine is also variable.

Bovine fecal porphyrins may be derived from two sources: the bile and chlorophyll of the food. The porphyrins derived from chlorophyll are excluded by the usual analytical method. Essentially, the only porphyrin found in the bile and feces of CEP cattle is COPRO I, and its concentration varies over wide limits. Fecal coproporphyrin varies between 1.9 and 11,800 μg/g (0.003 to 18.0 μmol/g) and biliary coproporphyrin between 320 and 13,600 μg/dL (4.88 to 207.67 μmol/l). Only small amounts of COPRO III have been observed in feces.

Only traces of free porphyrins are normally present in the plasma and in erythrocytes. In bovine CEP, plasma variable amounts of URO I (1 to 27 μg/dL; 0.012 to 0.33 μmol/l) and COPRO I (4.2 to 25 μg/dL; 0.064 to 0.38 μmol/l) are seen. A striking difference as compared to the human disease is the high level of free PROTO IX in the erythrocytes of the CEP cow. Excess PROTO IX is commonly found in iron deficiency, hemolytic anemia, and lead poisoning. In iron deficiency, PROTO IX accumulates because of failure to form hemoglobin. Similarly, PROTO IX accumulates in lead poisoning due to inhibition of FER-Ch and a subsequent inability to insert iron into hemoglobin.

The hematologic picture in CEP is one of a responsive hemolytic anemia with the degree of response directly related to the severity of the anemia. The anemia in mild cases of bovine CEP is normocytic; in the more severe cases, it is macrocytic accompanied by reticulocytosis, polychromasia, anisocytosis, basophilic stippling, and an increase in nucleated erythrocytes. There is a markedly decreased M:E ratio, indicating a strong erythroid hyperplasia.

The presence of porphyrins in the nucleated erythrocytes is clearly evident by examination of unfixed and unstained bone marrow smears with a fluorescent microscope. These fluorescent cells have been called fluorocytes. The fluorescence is seen only in morphologically abnormal nucleated erythrocytes that contain abnormal nuclear inclusions.

The hematology of newborn CEP calves is strikingly different from that of older CEP calves and cows.[4] There is an intense erythrogenic response in the neonatal CEP calf which persists for the first 3 weeks of life. Nucleated erythrocyte counts during the first 24 hours of life ranged from 5000 to 63,500/μL. Reticulocyte counts were lower than expected (6.4%) and increased to a peak of only 12.5% at 4 days of age. The persistent reticulocytosis is thought to be due to a delay in maturation of the reticulocytes.[5,6]

Erythrocyte life span is shortened in bovine and human CEP and is inversely correlated with erythrocyte coproporphyrin concentration.[7] The shortest erythrocyte survival time of 27 days (normal, 150 days) was associated with the highest erythrocytic coproporphyrin concentration. The porphyrins, through their lipid solubility, are presumed to damage the erythrocyte membrane, thereby leading to hemolysis. In vivo ^{59}Fe metabolic studies were compatible with a hemolytic type of anemia and ineffective erythropoiesis (i.e., intramedullary erythroid phagocytosis).[8] Plasma iron turnover and transfer rates, erythrocyte iron uptake, and organ uptakes were increased as expected in a hemolytic process.

A biochemical defect in the bovine CEP reticulocyte in vitro was expressed as an increase in porphyrin synthesis, a marked decrease in heme synthesis, and a delay in the maturation time of the reticulocyte.[5] The half-life for the maturation of the reticulocyte was 50 hours compared with a normal value of 3 to 10 hours. This delay in reticulocyte maturation is thought to be the direct result of the defect in heme synthesis, because the rate of heme synthesis controls the rate of maturation of the reticulocyte. This means that reticulocyte survival time is inversely proportional to the degree of anemia.

A similar delay in the maturation of the metarubricyte to the reticulocyte was observed in the bone marrow cells of CEP cows,[6] but there was no effect on the earlier nucleated erythrocytes. Therefore, the more mature erythrocytic cells are the cells most noticeably affected by the high porphyrin content. This is not surprising because heme and hemoglobin synthesis are most active in the later stages of erythrocytic cell development. Ultimately, the accumulation of porphyrins in these cells, whether in bone marrow or in blood, induces hemolysis. On exposure of surface capillaries to sunlight, photohemolysis of the type observed in erythropoietic protoporphyria further aggravates the hemolysis.

In summary, excess porphyrin in the mature and developing erythrocytes induces their hemolysis in the circulation or in the bone marrow with a corresponding shortening of erythrocyte life span. In addition, the decrease in heme synthesis induces an increase in the survival time of the reticulocyte by inhibiting the maturation of the developing erythrocytes, which further aggravates the anemia. This biochemical defect in heme synthesis is morphologically expressed in the fluorocytes and in the evidence of erythrogenic response in the blood and bone marrow, the degree of which is directly related to the severity of the enzymatic defect of the porphyria.

The activity of uroporphyrinogen III cosynthase (UROgenIII-Cosyn) is considerably less in homozygous CEP cattle as compared to normals,[9] and the heterozygotes have UROgenIII-Cosyn activities intermediate between porphyric and normal animals.[10] Similarly, low UROgenIII-Cosyn activity is found in human CEP. The genetic aspects of all forms of hereditary porphyrias have been reviewed.[11]

Normally in heme synthesis, the combined action of uroporphyrinogen I synthase (UROgenI-Syn) and UROgenIII-Cosyn catalyzes the formation of the normal type III porphyrin isomer, UROgenIII, which ultimately leads to heme formation. In a deficiency of UROgenIII-Cosyn, the type I isomers, UROgenI and COPROgenI are formed, the amounts of which are governed by the relative activities of these enzymes. The type I isomers that are formed cannot be converted into a PROTOgenI, so there is no Type I heme. This is because coproporphyrinogen III oxidase (COPROgenIII-Ox) is absolutely specific only for the Type III isomer and there is no specific coproporphyrinogen I oxidase. The UROgenI and COPROgenI isomers are readily oxidized to their corresponding free and toxic uroporphyrins and coproporphyrins. These oxidized free porphyrins accumulate in the erythropoietic tissues, developing erythrocytic cells, and mature erythrocytes where they induce the hemolysis characteristic of CEP.

Total deficiency of UROgenIII-Cosyn is obviously incompatible with life, so surviving patients with CEP have only a partial deficiency of UROgenIII-Cosyn. The central theme for the metabolic basis for bovine CEP is the genetically controlled deficiency of UROgenIII-Cosyn with the accumulation of the resultant type I porphyrins. These type I porphyrins are the ultimate cause of the clinical and pathophysiologic manifestations of the failure in the heme synthetic pathway in CEP.

Bovine Erythropoietic Protoporphyria

The fundamental enzymatic defect in bovine erythropoietic protoporphyria (EPP) is a generalized deficiency of FER-Ch with a resulting accumulation of PROTO IX. EPP is well recognized in humans, in whom it is inherited as an autosomal dominant trait.[11] Patients do not have the major signs of CEP such as anemia, porphyrinuria, or discolored teeth. Photosensitivity of the skin is the only clinical manifestation of the disease and is associated with a high plasma protoporphyrin concentration. In the laboratory, the most striking findings are the high concentrations of PROTO IX in the erythrocytes and feces.[12]

In cattle, EPP has a pattern of recessive inheritance in contrast to humans and may be sex related, because to date it has only been seen in females. The photosensitivity also seems to diminish in adult life.

Porphyria of Swine

Porphyria in swine is inherited as a dominant trait. Except for very severe cases, there appears to be little or no effect on the general health of the pig. Photosensitivity is not seen, even in the white pigs. The predominant feature in the affected pig is a characteristic reddish discoloration and pink fluorescence of the teeth. Porphyrin deposition in the teeth of the newborn is virtually pathognomonic of porphyria in swine. The porphyrins are principally URO I.

The urine of the affected pig is discolored only in more severely affected cases. The 24-hour urinary excretion of uroporphyrins ranged between 100 and 10,000 μg and for coproporphyrin, only 50 μg. These were both the type I isomers. Porphobilinogen (PBG) is absent in the urine. Close similarities in this pattern of porphyrin excretion to that found in bovine CEP are apparent, but the localization of the defect in erythropoiesis has not been established; however, no affected animals are available for study.

Porphyria of Cats

There are at least two forms of porphyria described in cats. Excessive accumulation of URO I, COPRO I, and PROTO IX were observed in the erythrocytes, urine, feces, and tissues in a family of porphyric Siamese cats.[13] These cats had photosensitivity, severe anemia, and severe renal disease. It was concluded that the principal defect in these cats was a deficiency of UROgenIII-Cosyn similar to CEP of humans and cows. The other cases of porphyria were seen in domestic cats and had a similar discoloration of the teeth which fluoresced under UV light. Their urine was also discolored due to the presence of uroporphyrin, coproporphyrin, and porphobilinogen but there was no evidence of anemia or photosensitization. The porphyria appeared to be inherited as an autosomal dominant trait.

PHYSIOLOGIC PORPHYRIAS

All fox squirrels (*Sciurus niger*) have red bones due to the accumulation of URO I and COPRO I.[14] Fox squirrel porphyria resembles CEP of humans, cows, and cats by having a deficiency of UROgenIII-Cosyn, the accumulation of type I porphyrins in the urine and feces, as well as discolored bones, teeth, and tissues which fluoresce upon exposure to UV light. There is increased erythropoiesis but no apparent hemolytic anemia, no photosensitivity, or any other deleterious effects of the porphyrins. These relatively benign effects are most likely due to the animal's thick hair coats and nocturnal living habits. It is interesting that an enzyme deficiency with serious health effects in other species should have evolved as a "normal" characteristic in the fox squirrel. This is understandable when one appreciates that CEP cattle always kept indoors and protected from sunlight thrive and reproduce normally.

The UROgenIII-Cosyn deficiency is found only in the fox squirrel and not in the closely related gray squirrel (*Sciurus carolinensis*). Urine porphyrin excretion in the fox squirrel is 10-fold greater than in the gray squirrel and is significantly increased when erythropoiesis is stimulated by bleeding. The UROgenIII-Cosyn of fox squirrel erythrocytes is very heat-sensitive; this may indicate that its' CEP is additionally due to an increased lability of the enzyme.

Porphyrins accumulate in the feathers of certain brightly colored birds (e.g., Touracos) and certain lower animals and microorganisms, but this appears to be a normal phenomenon.

HEPATIC PORPHYRIAS

This group of porphyrias has been seen only in humans, in whom they are the most common group of porphyrias. The salient features of important members of this group of porphyrias are summarized in Table 154.1. As the name of this group implies, the predominant site of the metabolic defect is localized in the liver, and the group is further subdivided on the basis of their principal clinical manifestations. Specific enzyme deficiencies have been identified for all forms of hepatic porphyrias (Table 154.1).

δ-Amino-Levulinic Acid Dehydratase Porphyria

This rare hepatic form of porphyria, called ALA-D porphyria (ADP), has a marked deficiency of the enzyme ALA-D.[15] It is inherited as an autosomal recessive trait and is characterized by neurologic signs without skin photosensitivity.

Acute Intermittent Porphyria

Acute intermittent porphyria (AIP), a deficiency of UROgenI-Syn, is the major autosomal dominant form of hepatic porphyria seen in humans and is characterized by acute abdominal attacks and neurologic signs, but no photosensitivity. Most patients are asymptomatic unless some form of aggravating factor induces an attack, such as exposure to barbiturates, sulfonamides, estrogens, and alcohol. The disease occurs more commonly in women than in men. The principal urinary finding is the excretion of large amounts of ALA and PBG.

Porphyria Cutanea Tarda

Porphyria cutanea tarda (PCT) is caused by a deficiency of uroporphyrinogen decarboxylase (UROgen-D) and presents as both a sporadic and familial form. The sporadic form is the acquired form of PCT and is the most common of all forms of human porphyria. The familial form is inherited as an autosomal dominant trait. As the name implies, the characteristic clinical signs of PCT are the photosensitive lesions of the skin. The disease occurs in mid- to late-adult life, and common precipitating causes of this disease are alcohol and estrogens. In the hereditary form, there is a decrease in hepatic and erythrocytic UROgen-D activity.[16]

Hepatoerythropoietic Porphyria

Hepatoerythropoietic porphyria (HEP) is a form that clinically resembles CEP but there is a marked deficiency of UROgen-D, as in PCT. It is thought to be the homozygous form of familial PCT. HEP is characterized by a very severe photosensitivity but there is no liver involvement.

HARDEROPORPHYRIA

This is a form of porphyria in which the propionate group on the A ring is converted to a vinyl group, whereas the normal next step of B ring conversion is somehow disrupted. There is a deficiency of COPROgenIII-Ox, but the mechanism explaining why the groups on both rings are not oxidized is unknown.

Hereditary Coproporphyria

Hereditary coproporphyria (HCP) is clinically similar to PCT with a mild cutaneous photosensitivity; it may also have neurologic signs as in AIP. Like AIP, HCP is commonly precipitated by drugs. As in harderoporphyria, COPROgenIII-Ox is the deficient enzyme.

Variegate Porphyria

The signs of variegate porphyria (VP) are generally more variable than the other forms, but in most cases acute abdominal attacks and photosensitivity are seen. VP is most common among the South African white population. VP is inherited as an autosomal dominant trait. There is a deficiency of PROTOgenIII-Ox that can be observed in cultured fibroblasts and leukocytes of VP patients.

REFERENCES

1. **Kaneko JJ.** Porphyrins and the porphyrias. In: Kaneko JJ, Harvey JW, Bruss ML, eds. Clinical biochemistry of domestic animals. 5th ed. San Diego: Academic Press, 1997.
2. **Kappas A, Sassa S, Galbraith RA, Nordmann Y.** The porphyrias. In: Scriver CR, Beaudet AL, Sly WS Valle D, eds. The metabolic and molecular bases of inherited disease. 7th ed. New York: McGraw-Hill, 1995;2.

3. **Poh-Fitzpatrick MB.** Pathogenesis and treatment photocutaneous manifestations of the porphyrias. Semin Liver Dis 1982;2:164–176.
4. **Kaneko JJ, Mills R.** Erythrocyte enzyme activity, ion concentration, osmotic fragility, and glutathione stabity in bovine erythropoietic porphyria and its carrier state. Am J Vet Res 1969;30:1805–1810.
5. **Smith JJ, Kaneko JJ.** Rate of heme and porphyrin synthesis by bovine porphyric reticulocytes in vitro. Am J Vet Res 1966;27:931–940.
6. **Rudolph WG, Kaneko JJ.** Kinetics of erythroid bone marrow cells of normal and porphyric calves in vitro. Acta Haematol 1971;45:330–335.
7. **Kaneko JJ, Zinkl JG, Keeton KS.** Erythrocyte porphyrin and erythrocyte survival in bovine erythropoietic porphyria. Am J Vet Res 1971;32:1981–1985.
8. **Kaneko JJ, Mattheeuws DRG.** Iron metabolism in normal and porphyric calves. Am J Vet Res 1966;27:923–929.
9. **Levin EY.** Uroporphryinogen 3 cosynthetase activity in bovine erythropoietic porphyria. Science 1968;161:907–908.
10. **Romeo G, Glenn BC, Levin EY.** Uroporphryrinogen 3 cosynthetase in asymptomatic carriers of congenital erythropoietic porphyria. Biochem Genet 1970;4:719–726.
11. **Romeo G.** Enzymatic defects of hereditary porphyrias: an explanation of dominance at the molecular level. Hum Genet 1977;39:261–276.
12. **Ruth GR, Schwartz S, Stephenson B.** Bovine protoporphyria: first nonhuman model of this hereditary photosensitizing disease. Science 1977;198:199–201.
13. **Giddens WE Jr, Labbe RF, Swango LJ, Padgett GA.** Feline congenital erythropoietic porphyria associated with severe anemia and renal disease. Am J Pathol 1975;80:367–386.
14. **Flyger V, Levin EY.** Animal model: normal porphyria of fox squirrels (Sciurus niger). Am J Pathol 1977;87:269–272.
15. **Brandt A, Doss M.** Hereditary porphobilinogensynthase deficiency in humans associated with acute hepatic porphyria. Hum Genet 1981;58:194–197.
16. **Pimstone NR.** Porphyria cutanea tarda. Semin Liver Dis 1982;11:132–142.

CHAPTER 155

Hereditary Methemoglobinemia

• J.W. HARVEY

Hemoglobin is a protein consisting of four polypeptide globin chains, each of which contains a heme prosthetic group within a hydrophobic pocket. Heme is composed of a tetrapyrrole with a central iron molecule that must be maintained in the ferrous (+2) state to reversibly bind oxygen. Methemoglobin differs from hemoglobin only in that the iron moiety of heme groups has been oxidized to the ferric (+3) state and it is no longer able to bind oxygen.

ENDOGENOUS METHEMOGLOBIN FORMATION

Approximately 3% of hemoglobin is oxidized to methemoglobin each day.[1] This formation results from spontaneous autoxidation of oxyhemoglobin and probably also secondarily to oxidants produced in normal metabolic reactions. Although the iron moiety of deoxyhemoglobin is in the ferrous state, in oxyhemoglobin it exists in (or near) the ferric state, with an electron being transferred to the O_2 molecule to give a bound superoxide (O_2^-) ion.[2] During deoxygenation, the electron returns to the iron moiety, O_2 is released, and deoxyhemoglobin (Hb^{2+}) is formed. Autoxidation of oxyhemoglobin to methemoglobin (Hb^{3+}) with the release of O_2^- occurs when the bound O_2^- is replaced by a nucleophile, such as Cl^-, as shown below.[3]

$Hb^{3+} \cdot O_2^- \rightarrow Hb^{2+} + O_2$ \hspace{1cm} Deoxygenation

$Hb^{3+} \cdot O_2^- + Cl^- \rightarrow Hb^{3+} \cdot Cl^- + O_2^-$ \hspace{0.5cm} Autoxidation

METHEMOGLOBIN REDUCTION

Methemoglobin usually accounts for less than 1% of total hemoglobin, because the formed methemoglobin is continuously reduced back to hemoglobin, primarily by the enzyme NADH-methemoglobin reductase (cytochrome-b_5 reductase, EC 1.6.2.2). In the reaction, ferricytochrome b_5 is first reduced enzymatically with NADH; then the resulting ferrocytochrome b_5 reduces methemoglobin nonenzymatically to hemoglobin.[4]

Erythrocytes contain another enzyme, NADPH dehydrogenase (NADPH methemoglobin reductase, NADPH diaphorase, NADPH flavin reductase, EC 1.6.99.1), that is capable of methemoglobin reduction when appropriate electron carriers are present. In addition to redox dyes, such as methylene blue, various flavins may function as substrates for reduction by NADPH. The contribution of this enzyme to methemoglobin reduction is believed to be negligible, at least in human erythrocytes, because erythrocyte flavin concentrations are normally low.[5]

Erythrocytes from most species use primarily glucose for energy to generate NADH for the reduction of methemoglobin.[4] Horse erythrocytes utilize lactate better than glucose to generate NADH by the lactate dehydrogenase reaction. Because lactate is present in blood and easily diffuses into erythrocytes, it may be an important substrate of methemoglobin reduction in vivo. Erythrocytes from adult pigs cannot reduce methemoglobin with glucose as the substrate because they lack a membrane glucose transporter, but they can reduce methemoglobin using either lactate or inosine for energy.[4,6]

Methylene blue is used to treat toxic methemoglobinemia because it causes methemoglobin to be reduced faster than occurs by the relatively slow methemoglobin reductase reaction. Methylene blue is reduced to leukomethylene blue by the NADPH-dependent diaphorase discussed earlier and leukomethylene blue reacts spontaneously with methemoglobin, reducing it to hemoglobin and regenerating methylene blue.[4] Other drugs such as ascorbate and N-acetylcysteine may promote methemoglobin reduction at slow rates in some species.[7] N-acetylcysteine is the drug of choice in the treatment of acetaminophen toxicity in cats, which results in both methemoglobinemia and Heinz body hemolytic anemia, but it appears to be more beneficial in preventing oxidant injury than in correcting it.[8]

METHEMOGLOBINEMIA

Causes

Methemoglobinemia results from either increased production of methemoglobin by oxidants or decreased reduction of methemoglobin associated with a deficiency in the erythrocyte methemoglobin reductase enzyme. Experimental studies indicate that many drugs can produce methemoglobinemia in animals. Significant methemoglobinemia has been associated with clinical cases of benzocaine, acetaminophen, and phenazopyridine toxicities in cats and/or dogs; nitrite toxicity in cattle; copper toxicity in sheep; and red maple toxicity in horses.[4]

Clinical Signs

Methemoglobinemia (approximately 20% or greater) results in cyanotic-appearing mucous membranes that may be difficult to recognize in heavily pigmented animals. Both low blood oxygen tension and methemoglobinemia can result in cyanotic-appearing mucous membranes and dark-colored blood samples. Hypoxemia is documented by measuring low pO_2 and/or low oxygen saturation by pulse oximetry of an arterial blood sample. Methemoglobinemia is suspected when arterial blood appears dark even in the face of normal or increased pO_2. Animals with slight to moderate methemoglobinemia may exhibit decreased exercise tolerance. Lethargy, ataxia, and stupor, resulting from hypoxia, do not become apparent until methemoglobin content exceeds 50%, with a coma-like state and death ensuing after it reaches 80%, based on experimental studies in animals.[4]

Laboratory Findings

Methemoglobinemia may not be recognized in venous blood samples, because the brownish color of methemoglobin is not readily apparent when mixed with large amounts of the deoxyhemoglobin that normally accounts for the dark, bluish color of venous blood. When deoxyhemoglobin binds oxygen to form oxyhemoglobin, it becomes bright red; consequently, the brownish coloration of methemoglobin becomes more apparent in oxygenated samples. A simple spot test provides a rapid way to oxygenate a venous blood sample and determine if clinically significant levels of methemoglobin are present. One drop of blood from the patient is placed on a piece of absorbent white paper and a drop of normal control blood is placed next to it. If the methemoglobin content is 10% or greater, the patient's blood will have a noticeably brown coloration compared with a bright red color of the control blood. Accurate determination of methemoglobin content requires that blood be submitted to a laboratory that has this test available.[9]

Differential Diagnosis

Animals with methemoglobin reductase deficiency exhibit little or no clinical signs of disease. Consequently, the recent onset of clinical signs of toxicosis such as anorexia, vomiting, diarrhea, depression, rapid heart rate, rapid respiratory rate, ataxia, stupor, hemoglobinuria, and/or subcutaneous edema in an animal with cyanotic-appearing tongue and mucous membranes suggest that toxic methemoglobinemia is present. With the exception of nitrite, chemicals that produce methemoglobinemia also produce hemolytic anemia.[4] Consequently, the concomitant occurrence of a hemolytic anemia and methemoglobinemia strongly suggests that a toxic methemoglobinemia is present.

HEREDITARY METHEMOGLOBINEMIA IN HUMANS

Types of inherited methemoglobinemia reported in humans include methemoglobin reductase deficiency, a deficiency of the cytochrome b_5 cofactor, and certain hemoglobinopathies.[2] A single gene is responsible for the formation of the cytochrome-b_5 reductase enzyme in many tissues.[10] In addition to its role in methemoglobin reduction in erythrocytes, a bound form of the enzyme functions in other tissues in the elongation and saturation of fatty acids, cholesterol biosynthesis, and cytochrome P-450–mediated drug metabolism.[11] Some methemoglobin-reductase–deficient humans exhibit only methemoglobinemia, whereas others have mental retardation and other neurologic defects in addition to methemoglobinemia. These different syndromes occur because different defects (base changes) occur in the gene. Defects that result in minimal functional enzyme activity in many tissues can cause methemoglobinemia and neurologic defects. Defects that result in the production of a functional but unstable enzyme may only result in methemoglobinemia. Mature erythrocytes cannot synthesize proteins. Consequently, during the erythrocyte life span of about 4 months in the circulation, the activity of an unstable enzyme decreases to the point that methemoglobin reduction can no longer be maintained. The enzyme deficiency is not as severe in other cell types because they can synthesize replacement enzymes and many turn over faster than erythrocytes.[10]

METHEMOGLOBIN REDUCTASE DEFICIENCY IN DOGS AND CATS

Persistent methemoglobinemia associated with erythrocyte methemoglobin reductase deficiency has been recognized in Chihuahua, Borzoi, English Setter, terrier-mix, Cockapoo, Poodle, Corgi, Pomeranian, Toy American Eskimo, Cocker-Toy American Eskimo, and Pit Bull-mix dogs (JW Harvey, unpublished studies, 1997)[1,12–14] and in domestic shorthair cats (JW Harvey, unpublished studies, 1997).[7,15] The deficiency is presumed to be an inherited autosomal recessive disorder, as it is in humans, but detailed family studies have not been reported. Intermediate (low % normal) activity was measured in erythrocytes from an offspring of the mating of an affected and a normal Pomeranian dog (see Case Study 1 at the end of this book), and two littermate Pit Bull-mix dogs were both found to have this deficiency (JW Harvey, unpublished studies, 1997), supporting the likelihood that it is an inherited disorder in dogs. Similarly, erythrocytes from two littermate cats were devoid of enzyme activity, with a third littermate having approximately 40% of normal methemoglobin reductase activity, suggesting an autosomal recessive mode of inheritance in cats.[7]

Clinical Signs

Affected animals have cyanotic-appearing mucous membranes and may exhibit lethargy or exercise intoler-

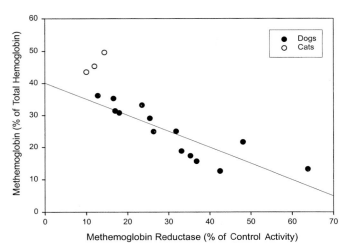

FIGURE 155.1 Comparison of the methemoglobin content in blood (percent of total hemoglobin that is methemoglobin) to the erythrocyte methemoglobin reductase enzyme activity (expressed as a percent of control activity) for methemoglobin-reductase–deficient animals assayed by the author. Linear regression analysis was used to determine the line of best fit for the dogs with an R value of 0.859 and $P < 0.001$.

ance at times, but frequently have no clinical signs of disease. In several cases, methemoglobinemia was recognized for the first time during routine surgery when mucous membranes and blood remained dark even when animals were given supplemental oxygen.

Laboratory Findings

Venous blood samples remain dark with a brownish tinge, rather than turning bright red, when exposed to air (see the methemoglobin spot test above). When assayed spectrophotometrically,[9] methemoglobin content in deficient dogs varies from 13 to 41%. The methemoglobin content in five deficient domestic shorthair cats varied from 44 to 52%. The hematocrit is usually normal in deficient dogs but was slightly to moderately increased in four of five deficient cats, secondary to the chronic methemoglobinemia and resultant decreased blood oxygen content. A definitive diagnosis is made by measuring erythrocyte methemoglobin reductase enzyme activity.[16] Because the test is time-consuming and requires special supplies and training of technologists, prior arrangements must be made with a laboratory before blood samples are submitted. Anticoagulated blood should be refrigerated and sent on wet ice (not frozen) to the laboratory so that the assay can be done within a day of sample collection. One or more samples from normal animals should be sent along with the patient's sample to be used as controls.

There is a significant indirect relationship between erythrocyte enzyme activity and methemoglobin content in deficient dogs (Fig. 155.1). Contrary to what might be expected based on enzyme activity alone, car-

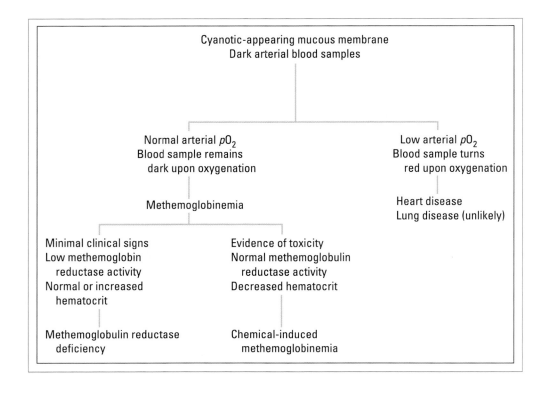

rier animals with about 50% of normal enzyme activity do not have methemoglobinemia. This can be explained if the abnormal enzyme present in deficient erythrocytes is unstable, as has been demonstrated in methemoglobin reductase deficient humans (see previous discussion).[10] Dog erythrocytes normally have a life span of approximately 100 days in the circulation and presumably the life span of deficient dogs is normal, as it is in methemoglobin reductase deficient humans.[4] If the defective enzyme is unstable, then methemoglobin reductase activity decreases substantially as the erythrocytes age, with the old erythrocytes having minimal or no activity and high methemoglobin content. In carrier animals, 50% of the enzyme present within erythrocytes is stable, providing enough activity to reduce the methemoglobin formed, even in old erythrocytes.

Therapy

Animals with methemoglobin reductase deficiency have normal life expectancy. Treatment is not needed, although veterinarians may wish to give a single intravenous injection of methylene blue (1 mg/kg) 1 hour before a deficient animal is anesthetized for surgery. Most of the methemoglobin will be converted to hemoglobin, providing an increased amount of hemoglobin that is capable of binding oxygen.

Riboflavin treatment has resulted in decreased methemoglobin content in some enzyme-deficient humans but had no effect when given to deficient dogs.[1] N-acetylcysteine and ascorbic acid treatments resulted in moderate reductions in methemoglobin content in deficient cats.[7] Because of the existing methemoglobinemia, exposure to oxidative drugs should be avoided in deficient animals.

FAMILIAL METHEMOGLOBINEMIA AND HEMOLYTIC ANEMIA IN HORSES

Methemoglobinemia and mild to moderate hemolytic anemia have been reported in a trotter mare and her dam.[17] The animals were examined because of poor performance. Reduced glutathione (GSH) values were about 50% of normal, and glutathione reductase activities were 25 to 50% that of normal erythrocytes. The glutathione reductase deficiency was not considered to be the result of riboflavin deficiency. It is unclear how these abnormalities are related to the pathogenesis of this disorder. In the absence of exogenous oxidants, the deficiencies do not seem severe enough to account for the hematologic abnormalities. No abnormal hemoglobin types were present, and glucose-6-phosphate dehydrogenase, glutathione peroxidase, and methemoglobin reductase activities were normal.

A horse with laboratory findings similar to those described above has recently been discovered.[18] This mustang of unknown parentage has persistent methemoglobinemia with eccentrocytes in blood. The hematocrit varied from normal to slightly decreased. Erythrocyte GSH is low and glutathione reductase activity is zero, unless flavin adenine dinucleotide (FAD) is added to the assay. In addition, methemoglobin reductase activity is less than half-normal. Studies underway suggest that there is a defect in converting flavin mononucleotide (FMN) to FAD within the erythrocytes. Both glutathione reductase and methemoglobin reductase are reportedly FAD containing enzymes. Consequently, a defect in FAD production may account for the low activities measured for each enzyme.

REFERENCES

1. **Harvey JW, King RR, Berry CR, Blue JT.** Methaemoglobin reductase deficiency in dogs. Comp Haematol Int 1991;1:55–59.
2. **Mansouri A, Lurie AA.** Methemoglobinemia. Am J Hematol 1993;42:7–12.
3. **Wallace WJ, Maxwell JC, Caughey WS.** The mechanisms of hemoglobin autoxidation evidence for proton-assisted nucleophilic displacement of superoxide by anions. Biochem Biophys Res Commun 1974;57:1104–1110.
4. **Harvey JW.** The erythrocyte: physiology, metabolism and biochemical disorders. In: Kaneko JJ, Harvey JW, Bruss ML, eds. Clinical biochemistry of domestic animals. 5th ed. San Diego: Academic Press, 1997;157–203.
5. **Hultquist DE, Xu F, Quandt KS, Shlafer M, Mack CP, Till GO, Seekamp A, Betz AL, Ennis SR.** Evidence that NADPH-dependent methemoglobin reductase and administered riboflavin protect tissues from oxidative injury. Am J Hematol 1993;42:13–18.
6. **Sartorelli P, Paltrinieri S, Agnes F, Baglioni T.** Role of inosine in prevention of methaemoglobinaemia in the pig: in vitro studies. Zentralbl Veterinarmed [A] 1996;43:489–493.
7. **Giger U, Wang P, Boyden M.** Familial methemoglobin reductase deficiency in domestic shorthair cats. Fel Pract Suppl 1999;31:14.
8. **Harvey JW.** Methemoglobinemia and Heinz-body hemolytic anemia. In: Bonagura JD, ed. Kirk's current veterinary therapy XII. Small animal practice. Philadelphia: WB Saunders, 1995;443–446.
9. **Christopher MM, Harvey JW.** Specialized hematology tests. Semin Vet Med Surg Small Anim 1992;7:301–310.
10. **Nagai T, Shirabe K, Yubisui T, Takeshita M.** Analysis of mutant NADH-cytochrome b_5 reductase: apparent "type III" methemoglobinemia can be explained as type I with an unstable reductase. Blood 1993;81:808–814.
11. **Shirabe K, Yubisui T, Borgese N, Tang C, Hultquist DE, Takeshita M.** Enzymatic instability of NADH-cytochrome b_5 reductase as a cause of hereditary methemoglobinemia type I (red cell type). J Biol Chem 1992;267:20416–20421.
12. **Harvey JW, Ling GV, Kaneko JJ.** Methemoglobin reductase deficiency in a dog. J Am Vet Med Assoc 1974;164:1030–1033.
13. **Letchworth GJ, Bentinck-Smith J, Bolton GR, Wootton JF, Family L.** Cyanosis and methemoglobinemia in two dogs due to NADH methemoglobin reductase deficiency. J Am Anim Hosp Assoc 1977;13:75–79.
14. **Atkins CE, Kaneko JJ, Congdon LL.** Methemoglobin reductase deficiency and methemoglobinemia in a dog. J Am Anim Hosp Assoc 1981;17:829–832.
15. **Harvey JW, Dahl M, High ME.** Methemoglobin reductase deficiency in a cat. J Am Vet Med Assoc 1994;205:1290–1291.
16. **Beutler E.** Red cell metabolism: a manual of biochemical methods. 3rd ed. Orlando: Grune & Stratton, 1984.
17. **Dixon PM, McPherson EA.** Familial methaemoglobinaemia and haemolytic anaemia in the horse associated with decreased erythrocytic glutathione reductase and glutathione. Equine Vet J 1977;9:198–201.
18. **Harvey JW, Stockham SL, Johnson PJ, Scott MA.** Methemoglobinemia and eccentrocytosis in a horse with erythrocyte flavin adenine dinucleotide (FAD) deficiency (abstract). Proc Int Soc Anim Clin Biochem 2000; in press.

CHAPTER 156

Red Blood Cell Membrane Defects

• MUTSUMI INABA

Red blood cells must be very durable and flexible to undergo marked deformation under high shear stress condition so that they can survive during repeated passages through the microcirculation. These important properties are determined by three major elements of their membranes: a lipid bilayer, integral or transmembrane proteins, and a membrane skeletal network (Fig. 156.1). A lipid bilayer provides a permeability barrier between the cytosol and the external environment. Major constituents of the membrane skeleton mechanically support the plasma membrane and are organized into a lattice-like meshwork that is linked with both integral membrane components and cytoskeletal elements. Some of the transmembrane proteins embedded within the lipid bilayer ensure selective permeability to maintain red cell homeostasis. Accelerated destruction of red cells (hemolytic anemia) may occur when these properties of the red cell membrane are affected or deficient by some genetic defects. This chapter reviews the current progress in the investigation of inherited red cell membrane disorders in animals.

HEMOLYTIC ANEMIAS CAUSED BY HEREDITARY RED CELL MEMBRANE DISORDERS

The membrane protein-protein and protein-lipid interactions are the critical determinants of red cell morphology and mechanical stability, as evidenced by the numerous hereditary red cell disorders in humans attributed to mutations of the membrane.[1,2] These interactions are divided into two categories (Fig. 156.1): (1) vertical interactions involving the band 3-ankyrin-spectrin and glycophorin C-protein 4.1-spectrin binding, which attach the spectrin-actin network to the plasma membrane and stabilize the lipid bilayer, and (2) horizontal interactions involving spectrin dimer-dimer association (tetramer formation), and contact of the distal ends of spectrin with F-actin by the aid of protein 4.1 and adducin within the junctional complex.

HEREDITARY SPHEROCYTOSIS

The cardinal features of hereditary spherocytosis (HS) are hemolytic anemia of varying severity, spherocytosis, increased red cell osmotic fragility, and splenomegaly. Pathophysiology of HS involves two major factors: intrinsic membrane defect, and selective sequestration of HS cells in the normal spleen. Hence, anemia can be corrected by splenectomy in human HS patients. Typical forms of HS need to be distinguished from other hemolytic anemias manifesting moderate to small numbers of spherocytes, such as autoimmune hemolytic anemia by Coombs' test as well as unstable hemoglobin and oxidative damage by Heinz body screening. HS is now considered to be a disorder of vertical interactions of the membrane proteins, although the primary molecular defects are heterogeneous including deficiencies or dysfunctions of spectrin, ankyrin, band 3, and protein 4.2. Consequently, the lipid bilayer is destabilized, leading to membrane and surface area loss, and spherocyte formation.[2]

Hereditary Band 3 Deficiency in Cattle (Band 3^Bov.Yamagata)

Hereditary band 3 deficiency in Japanese black cattle (band 3^Bov.Yamagata) is associated with HS and is inherited by an autosomal dominant trait. Homozygous affected animals totally lack band 3 due to a nonsense mutation Arg664 → Stop (R664X)[3] (Koshino et al., submitted) and show mild to moderate, chronic hemolytic anemia (hematocrit, 25 to 35%); slight acidosis; and growth retardation. The mechanisms resulting in a lack of the band 3 protein may involve selective reduction of the mutant band 3 mRNA and rapid breakdown of the mutant protein during translocation to the plasma membrane. Carrier cattle heterozygous for R664X mutation also have abnormal red cell morphology and impaired anion transport activity due to partial deficiency of red cell band 3 (about 30%). However, spherocytosis in heterozygotes is mild, and the hemolysis is well compensated. Genotypes for R664X mutation are easily determined using genomic DNA as the template by polymerase chain reaction-restriction fragment length polymorphism (PCR-RFLP) or PCR-single strand conformation polymorphism (PCR-SSCP) techniques. The ancestral origin of this genetic defect has not yet been identified.

Band 3 (anion exchanger 1, AE1) is the most abundant transmembrane protein in mammalian red blood cells.

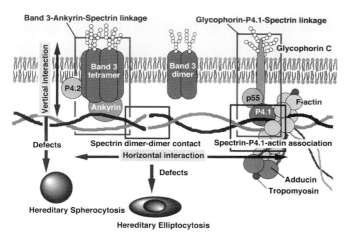

FIGURE 156.1 A schematic diagram illustrating structural and functional organization of red cell membrane proteins. Membrane protein-protein associations are divided into two categories: (1) vertical interactions involving band 3-ankyrin-spectrin linkage and glycophorin C-protein 4.1 (P4.1)-spectrin linkage, and (2) horizontal interactions involving the spectrin heterodimer contact (tetramer formation) and association of spectrin tetramer at the distal ends with F-actin at the junctional complex consisting of actin, P4.1, and adducin. In general, a defect of vertical interactions leads to hereditary spherocytosis, whereas a defect of horizontal interactions causes hereditary elliptocytosis and pyropoikilocytosis.

Band 3 has two putative functions[4–6]: (1) it mediates a rapid Cl^-/HCO_3^- exchange across the plasma membrane to increase five-fold the capacity of the blood to carry CO_2 from tissues to the lungs and maintains blood acid-base homeostasis together with the renal band 3 function; and (2) it may also participate in maintaining mechanical properties of red blood cell membranes by forming the band 3-ankyrin-spectrin complex. Various mutations leading to disorders and partial deficiency of red cell band 3 associated with abnormal red cell morphology (spherocytosis and ovalocytosis) have been reported in humans,[2,5,7,8] but none of them exhibited complete lack of the protein or its function.

The most surprising finding, therefore, is that cattle with total lack of band 3 survived to and thrived in adulthood. They suffered from extremely severe hemolytic anemia shortly after birth and exhibited jaundice and splenomegaly. The mortality rate is high during this period, particularly in the first week after birth. Once they overcome this neonatal crisis, jaundice subsides and hemolysis becomes modest. Until 1998, a half dozen homozygous affected cattle older than 3 years of age living in good condition have been found. One of three affected females had two normal parturitions. The studies on bovine hereditary band 3 deficiency have demonstrated the importance of band 3 in red cell morphology and homeostasis.

Red blood cells from homozygotes of band $3^{Bov.Yamagata}$ are also deficient in spectrin, ankyrin, actin (by 20–50%), and protein 4.2, resulting in a distorted and disrupted membrane skeletal network (Fig. 156.2). Their red cell membranes are extremely unstable and demonstrate the

spontaneous loss of surface area by invagination, vesiculation, extrusion of microvesicles, and fragmentation, thereby leading to the formation of spherocytes with irregular contours, gouging, and pitting (Fig. 156.3). Red cells from homozygous and heterozygous cattle constantly show considerably increased osmotic fragility with 50% hemolysis at 0.75% and 0.65 to 0.70% NaCl, respectively (normal, 0.45 to 0.55% NaCl), demonstrating that the surface area/volume ratios of red cells from both homozygotes and heterozygotes are remarkably reduced due to the mechanical instability of their red cell membranes (Fig. 156.4). Despite these severe changes, the affected animals show no reticulocytosis and no noticeable intravascular hemolysis. However, the protein 4.1a/4.1b ratio, which is a good marker of red cell aging,[9–11] is remarkably reduced and paralleled by increased erythropoiesis. These findings demonstrate the functional importance of band 3-ankyrin-spectrin association in maintaining mechanical stability of the membrane[12] but not in assembly of the membrane skeletal architecture; they also indicate that accelerated and continual destruction of red cells occur in homozygous cattle and also in heterozygotes with less severity.

Total deficiency of band 3 also results in defective Cl^-/HCO_3^- exchange. The Cl^- influx into the red cells from homozygotes requires approximately 2 hours to reach transmembranous equilibrium even at 37°C. Band 3 deficiency causes mild acidosis with decreases in the

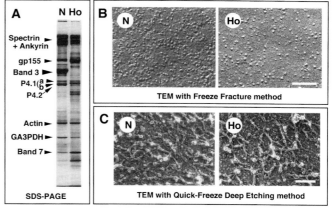

FIGURE 156.2 Abnormal red cell membrane structures in bovine band 3 deficiency (band $3^{Bov.Yamagata}$). **(A)** SDS-PAGE profiles of red cell membrane proteins from the normal (N) and the homozygote for R664X mutation (Ho). Note that spectrin (+ankyrin) and actin levels are markedly reduced compared to protein 4.1. Protein 4.2 is almost missing. A 66-kDa protein only found in the homozygote was albumin (Fig. 156.3). gp155 indicates a transmembrane protein characteristic to ruminant red cells.[65] **(B)** Markedly reduced number of intramembrane particles of normal (N) and the homozygous cells (Ho) on electron micrographs by the freeze fracture method. **(C)** Disrupted membrane skeletal network in the band-3–deficient red cells visualized by the quick-freeze deep etching method. The membrane skeletons in the band-3–deficient cells (Ho) are totally disrupted and distorted with filaments of uneven length and width compared with the well-organized normal red cells (N). Scale bars = 0.1 μm.

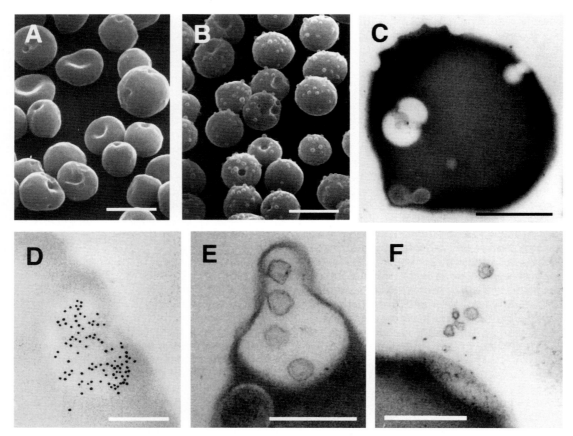

FIGURE 156.3 Morphologic anomaly in bovine band 3 deficiency. Scanning (A, B) and transmission (C–F) electron miographs of red cells from a homozygous animal of band 3[Bov.Yamagata]. **A:** The proband red cells look like potatoes and greatly vary in size, principally being spherocytic and stomatocytic with irregular contours. **B:** When blood is allowed to stand for several hours at ambient temperature, numerous small globules on the surface are observed. **C–F:** Marked endocytosis-like invagination, exocytosis-like projections, fusion of vesicles inside the cell, and extrusion of microvesicles. The vesicle in the cytoplasm contained plasma proteins as judged by immunoelectron micrography using anti-bovine albumin antibodies (D). Scale bars = 5 μm (A and B), 1 μm (C), and 0.2 μm (D–F).

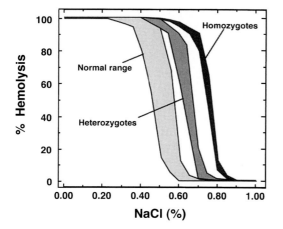

FIGURE 156.4 Increased red cell osmotic fragility in bovine band 3 deficiency. The osmotic fragility test was done by the standard method.[66] Data for normal cattle (n = 15) as well as homozygotes (n = 4) and heterozygotes (n = 8) of band 3 deficiency.

HCO_3^- concentration and total CO_2 in the blood. However, these values remain in the normal range. As CO_2 in blood rarely reaches saturation, it is suggested that the additional CO_2 carrying capacity facilitated by band 3 is probably not as critical as has been believed previously,[4,5] except under high stress conditions such as vigorous exercise or high altitude.

Transgenic mice with complete band 3 deficiency have similar red blood cell features.[13,14] These studies demonstrate that band 3 indeed contributes to red cell membrane organization, CO_2 transport, and acid-base homeostasis.

Several mutations that affect components of the erythrocyte membrane skeleton have also been reported in mice.[15,16] These include spectrin deficiencies in house[17,18] and deer mice[19] as well as ankyrin deficiency in nb mice[16] with moderate to life-threatening hemolytic anemia and fragile short-lived spherocytes.

HEREDITARY ELLIPTOCYTOSIS

The principal lesion of human hereditary elliptocytosis (HE) involves heterogeneous defects in horizontal membrane protein interactions (Fig. 156.1), such as abnormal spectrin structure affecting the spectrin heterodimer contacts and deficiency or dysfunction of protein 4.1.[2] Common HE is morphologically characterized by elliptocytes and rod-shaped cells in some patients. Aberrant disruption of the horizontal interactions results in fragmentation of red blood cells, leading to hereditary pyropoikilocytosis (HPP). Ovalocytosis, spherocytic HE, is a rare condition in which both round oval cells lacking central concavity and spherocytes are present on the blood film. It is likely that elliptocytes and poikilocytes are permanently stabilized in their abnormal shape. The weakened horizontal connections facilitate reorganization of skeleton, which follows axial deformation of cells by a prolonged shear stress.[2] Although cameline red cells are elliptocytic by nature, the molecular basis and physiologic importance of this unique feature remains unknown.

Hereditary Protein 4.1 Deficiency in Dogs (HE in Dogs)

Canine HE was discovered by Smith et al.[20] The proband exhibited elliptocytosis, membrane fragmentation, microcytosis, and poikilocytosis without anemia (Fig. 156.5). Red cell mechanical stability was markedly decreased, and osmotic fragility was remarkably increased. The proband red cell membranes were deficient in protein 4.1 (4.1a and 4.1b). The parents of the proband had decreased amounts (approximately 50% of normal) of protein 4.1 and some elliptocytes.

Protein 4.1 forms a tertiary complex with spectrin and actin within the junctional complex. This spectrin-actin binding region was mapped to the 10-kDa domain[21] containing amino acid sequences encoded by a 21-amino acid alternative exon and a 59-amino acid constitutive exon.[22] Immunoblotting of erythrocyte membrane proteins from the proband showed the presence of a small amount of 76-kDa polypeptide lacking the 21 amino acid segment and a very faint band of normal protein 4.1. RT-PCR analysis and sequencing of cloned reticulocyte protein 4.1 cDNA consistently showed that mRNA with a deletion of the alternative exon encoding 21 amino acid peptide was the predominant form with only a small quantity of normal mRNA. Therefore, the functional defect in the HE dog is likely due to the combined influences of two factors: a quantitative deficiency of protein 4.1 and a failure to activate efficiently expression of an alternatively spliced exon encoding 21 amino acids in the spectrin-actin binding region during erythropoiesis.[23] The primary cause leading to inefficient erythroid-specific alternative splicing has not been defined.

HEREDITARY STOMATOCYTOSIS

Stomatocytes are uniconcave or bowl-shaped red cells in suspension but have a slit-like appearance, an artifact on dried blood films (Fig. 156.6). Overhydrated hereditary stomatocytosis (HSt) (hydrocytosis) is a heterogeneous group of disorders in humans characterized by moderate to severe hemolytic anemia with stomatocytes, an elevated mean corpuscular volume, and a reduced mean corpuscular hemoglobin concentration. The principal lesion involves a remarkable increase of Na^+ influx into cells, resulting in a marked increase of intracellular Na^+ and water content and a corresponding decrease of K^+.[24,25] The molecular basis of this permeability defect is unknown. Human HSt (hydrocytosis) is often but not necessarily associated with absence of a specific membrane protein.[26,27] A possible defect of a 31-kDa integral membrane protein 7.2b (stomatin), which may function in the regulation of cation transport and stretch- or pressure-sensitive system, in HSt remains to be proven.[2]

HSt in Dogs and Cats

Stomatocytosis is recognized in dogs and cats with undefined etiologies. All disorders appear to be transmitted as autosomal recessive traits.

HSt in Miniature Schnauzers

Stomatocytosis inherited by autosomal recessive trait has been reported in miniature schnauzers (Fig. 156.6A) without clinical signs of disease.[28,29] HSt in schnauzers is characterized by macrocytosis, relatively high packed cell volume, remarkably decreased mean corpuscular hemoglobin concentration, and increased osmotic fragility. Red cell survival is only slightly shortened. Affected miniature schnauzers are of normal stature.

HSt in Chondrodysplastic Alaskan Malamute Dwarf Dogs

In Alaskan malamutes, chondrodysplasia (short-limbed dwarfism) occurs along with stomatocytosis[30,31] (Fig.

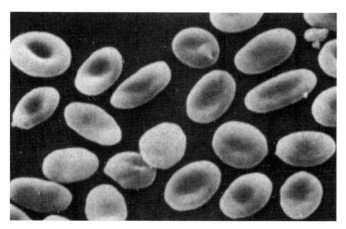

FIGURE 156.5 Scanning electron micrograph of red cells from the proband with HE. The proband red cells reveal biconcave elliptocytes. (From Smith JE, Moore K, Arens M, Rinderknecht GA, Ledet A. Hereditary elliptocytosis with protein band 4.1 deficiency in the dog. Blood 1983;61:373–377 with permission.) Scale bar = 5 μm.

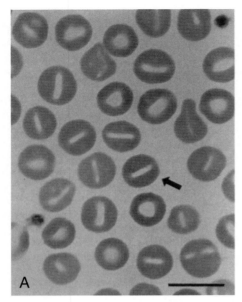
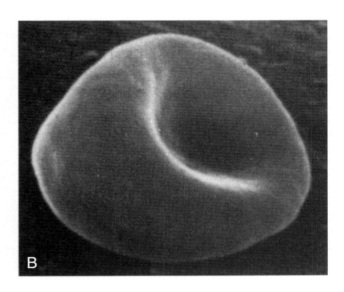

FIGURE 156.6 Red cell morphology of canine HSt (hydrocytosis). **(A)** Numerous stomatocytes with a slit-like appearance are present on the Wright-Giemsa–stained blood smear from a miniature schnauzer. A representative stomatocyte is indicated by the arrow. (From Brown DE, Weiser MG, Thrall MA, Giger U, Just CA. Erythrocyte indices and volume distribution in a dog with stomatocytosis. Vet Pathol 1994;31:247–250 with permission.) **(B)** Scanning electron micrograph of a typical stomatocyte from an affected Alaskan malamute. (From Pinkerton PH, Fletch SM, Brueckner PJ, Miller DR. Hereditary stomatocytosis with hemolytic anemia in the dog. Blood 1974;44:557–567 with permission.) Scale bar = 10 μm.

156.6B). The affected malamutes have macrocytosis, decreased mean corpuscular hemoglobin concentration, increased osmotic fragility, shortened red cell survival, reticulocytosis, erythroid hyperplasia, and increased iron turnover.[32] Although heterozygous carriers have minor changes in their red cells, they have a normal red cell life span and no dwarfism. Red cell Na concentration and water content are increased in affected dogs.

The pathogenesis of stomatocyte formation in malamutes and schnauzers is attributed to an increase in monovalent cation and, consequently, increased water content of red cells as is reported in human HSt. However, the exact nature of membrane defects leading to the changes in red cell indices in these breeds is obscure.

Familial Stomatocytosis–Hypertrophic Gastritis in Dogs

Familial stomatocytosis-hypertrophic gastritis is a multiorgan disease with hemolytic anemia, HSt, and hypertrophic gastritis described in the Drentse partrijshond breed.[33,34] The main clinical signs are diarrhea, jaundice, and ataxia and paresis of the pelvic limbs. Pathologic findings involve hypertrophic gastritis, progressive liver disease, renal cysts in aged subjects, and polyneuropathy.[33]

Red cells from affected dogs show increased osmotic fragility. In contrast to malamutes and schnauzers with stomatocytosis, red cells from affected partrijshonds have normal mean corpuscular volume, slightly increased cell water with basically normal content, and fluxes of Na and K, suggesting a different mechanism for stomatocyte formation.[34] Affected dogs have normal red cell membrane protein profile, but a decrease of phosphatidylcholine with altered fatty acid composition and simultaneous increase of sphingomyelin in both red cells and plasma. It is suggested that this polysystemic disease is a disorder of lipid metabolism in which defective membrane function and red cell shape change are induced by abnormal phospholipid composition of the plasma. This is supported by a shortened half life of red cells from normal dogs after transfusion into dogs with this syndrome. Stomatocytic shape change may be attributed to membrane surface loss, presumably due to abnormal phospholipid composition of the bilayer. The exact relation between anomaly in phospholipid and hypertrophic gastritis and the primary cause of this syndrome are unknown.

Hemolytic Anemia With Increased Red Cell Osmotic Fragility in Cats

A hereditary red cell defect is suspected in Abyssinian and Somali cats with Coombs' negative hemolytic anemia.[35] The affected cats exhibited recurrent anemia (hematocrit, 15 to 25%); severe splenomegaly with extramedullary hemopoiesis, hemosiderosis, congestion, and lymphoid hyperplasia; weight loss; macrocytosis; and a few stomatocytes. The anemia was variably regenerative. The osmotic fragility of their red cells was markedly increased. Splenectomy partially corrected the anemia and prevented hemolytic crises, but long-term survival remains unknown.

DIAGNOSTIC APPROACHES TO RED CELL MEMBRANE DEFECTS

Genetic aberrations of red cell membranes described above are feasibly surveyed by evaluating red cell morphology, osmotic fragility, and red cell parameters. The osmotic fragility test is a simplified means to estimate the surface area/volume ratio of red cells. It is most valuable in the diagnosis of HS but is also useful in evaluation of most forms of HE and overhydrated HSt (hydrocytosis). Several laboratory tests, such as Coombs' test and Heinz body screening, may be required to eliminate a possibility that hemolytic anemia and abnormal red cell shapes result from extrinsic factors. As exemplified for bovine HS in Figure 156.2A, SDS-PAGE analysis followed by some immunochemical, biochemical, and biophysical techniques often provides insights into primary defects of membrane skeletal and integral proteins resulting in HS, HE, and HPP.

MEMBRANE TRANSPORT DEFECTS

Deficiency and dysfunction of membrane transport systems may affect red cell homeostasis. Particularly, defects in transport of amino acids involved in glutathione metabolism have been reported to generate hemolytic anemia when red cells are exposed to extrinsic factors including oxidants.

Amino Acid Transport Deficiency in Animals

Red cell glutathione deficiency, inherited as an autosomal recessive trait, occurs in Finnish Landrace sheep.[36] Affected animals are not anemic but have shortened red cell life span.[37] This is possibly caused by increased oxidant sensitivity as exemplified by Heinz bodies. Affected sheep are more likely to become anemic after the administration of oxidants in vivo.[38] Red cells from the affected animals are defective in the transport system for various amino acids including cysteine.[39,40] Consequently, cysteine uptake and glutathione synthesis are limited, and glutathione concentrations in red cells are decreased to approximately 30% of normal. The transport deficiency appears to develop during reticulocyte maturation.[41]

A similar defect of amino acid transport is found in about 30% of thoroughbred horses[42] but seems to cause no clinical signs. The lesion appears to result in increased amino acid levels and glutathione deficiency in some cases.

High Membrane Na,K-ATPase Activity in Dogs

Although canine reticulocytes have a considerable amount of membrane Na,K-ATPase (Na/K-pump) activity, its activity is rapidly lost during maturation into mature red cells.[43] Proteolytic degradation[44] and extrusion of vesicles (exosomes)[45] are likely involved in this process. As a consequence, dogs usually have red cells with low K$^+$ and high Na$^+$ concentrations (LK red cells).[46] However, some Japanese Shiba and mongrel dogs have HK red cells with high K$^+$ and low Na$^+$ concentrations, because the Na,K-ATPase protein and its activity are retained in mature red cells.[44,47,48] This HK phenotype representing immaturity of erythroid precursor cells[49,50] is inherited in an autosomal recessive manner and has also been found in Japanese Akita[51] and several breeds of Korean dogs.[52] Although dogs with HK red cells are not anemic, their red cells have shortened life spans,[49] increased osmotic fragility, increased mean corpuscular volume, and normal mean corpuscular hemoglobin values, suggesting an increase in cell water.[47] Molecular basis for red cell HK and LK phenotypes is unknown. Due to the leak of K$^+$ from red cells, blood from HK dogs may cause pseudohyperkalemia in vitro after storage or on delaying plasma or serum separation.[51] Thus, care should be taken, particularly when stored blood from HK dogs is used for transfusion.

Canine red cells possess a high-affinity Na$^+$-dependent transport system for glutamate and aspartate[53,54] which resembles the kinetic and pharmacologic properties of the transporter in the brain.[55,56] The increased concentration gradients of Na$^+$ and K$^+$ across the membrane produced by the presence of Na,K-ATPase with high activity accelerates transport of glutamate and aspartate into HK red cells.[54] The concentration of reduced glutathione is increased 5 to 7 times that of normal because the feedback inhibition of gamma glutamylcysteine synthetase by glutathione is released by glutamate accumulated in these cells at about 90 times that in normal cells.[57] Some variant dogs of HK phenotype that lacks the increase of red cell glutathione have been reported,[58,59] suggesting that several independent mutations have emerged in these breeds.[56]

The accumulation of glutathione in the canine HK cells only provides improved protection against oxidative damage induced by acetylphenylhydrazine, but these erythrocytes are more susceptible to oxidative damage induced by 4-aminophenyl disulfide,[60] onions,[61,62] and sodium n-propylthiosulfate,[63] one of the hemolytic thiosulfate compounds isolated from onions.[64] The increased glutathione concentration accelerates the generation of superoxide through its redox reaction with the aromatic disulfide,[60] but the exact mechanism by which HK red cells are more sensitive to the thiosulfates remains to be clarified.

ACKNOWLEDGMENTS

The author thanks Dr. Ken-ichiro Ono (University of Tokyo) for his enthusiastic support and discussion during the preparation of this manuscript. This work was supported by Grants-in-Aid (No. 07456140, 09460145, and 10556071) from the Ministry of Education, Science, Sports, and Culture of Japan.

REFERENCES

1. **Palek J, Sahr KE.** Mutations of the red blood cell membrane proteins: from clinical evaluation to detection of the underlying genetic defect. Blood 1992;80:308–330.
2. **Palek J, Jarolim P.** Hereditary spherocytosis, elliptocytosis, and related disorders. In: Beutler E, Lichtman MA, Coller BS, Kipps TJ, eds. Williams hematology. 5th ed. New York: McGraw-Hill, 1995;536–557.
3. **Inaba M, Yawata A, Koshino I, Sato K, Takeuchi M, Takakuwa Y, Manno S, Yawata Y, Kanzaki A, Sakai J, Ban A, Ono K, Maede Y.** Defective anion transport and marked spherocytosis with membrane instability caused by hereditary total deficiency of red cell band 3 in cattle due to a nonsense mutation. J Clin Invest 1996;97:1804–1817.
4. **Jay DG, Cantley L.** Structural aspects of the red cell anion exchanger protein. Annu Rev Biochem 1986;55:511–538.
5. **Tanner MJA.** Molecular and cellular biology of the erythrocyte anion exchanger (AE1). Semin Hematol 1993;30:34–57.
6. **Jay DG.** Role of band 3 in homeostasis and cell shape. Cell 1996;86:853–854.
7. **Jenkins PB, Abou-Alfa GK, Dhermy D, Bursaux E, Feo C, Scarpa AL, Lux SE, Garbarz M, Forget BG, Gallagher PG.** A nonsense mutation in the erythrocyte band 3 gene associated with decreased mRNA accumulation in a kindred with dominant hereditary spherocytosis. J Clin Invest 1996;97:373–380.
8. **Jarolim P, Murray JL, Rubin HL, Taylor WM, Prchal JT, Ballas SK, Snyder LM, Chrobak L, Melrose WD, Brabec V, Palek J.** Charaterization of 13 novel band 3 gene defects in hereditary spherocytosis with band 3 deficiency. Blood 1996;88:4366–4374.
9. **Inaba M, Gupta KC, Kuwabara M, Takahashi T, Benz EJ Jr, Maede Y.** Deamidation of human erythrocyte protein 4.1: possible role in aging. Blood 1992;79:3355–3361.
10. **Inaba M, Maede Y.** The critical role of aspargine 502 in post-translational alteration of protein 4.1. Comp Biochem Physiol 1992;103B:523–526.
11. **Inaba M, Maede Y.** Correlation between protein 4.1a/4.1b ratio and erythrocyte life span. Biochim Biophys Acta 1988;944:256–264.
12. **Low PS, Willardson BM, Mohandas N, Rossi M, Shohet S.** Contribution of the band 3-ankyrin interaction to erythrocyte membrane mechanical stability. Blood 1991;77:1581–1586.
13. **Peters LL, Shivdasani RA, Liu S-C, Hanspal M, John KM, Gonzalez JM, Brugnara C, Gwynn B, Mohandas N, Alper SL, Orkin SH, Lux SE.** Anion exchanger 1 (band 3) is required to prevent erythrocyte membrane surface loss but not to form the membrane skeleton. Cell 1996;86:917–927.
14. **Southgate CD, Chishti AH, Mitchell B, Yi SJ, Palek J.** Targeted disruption of the murine erythroid band 3 gene results in spherocytosis and severe haemolytic anaemia despite a normal membrane skeleton. Nat Genet 1996;14:227–230.
15. **Birkenmeier CS, McFarland-Starr EC, Barker JE.** Chromosomal location of three spectrin genes: relationship to the inherited hemolytic anemias of mouse and man. Proc Natl Acad Sci USA 1988;85:8121–8125.
16. **White RA, Birkenmeier CS, Lux SE, Barker JE.** Ankyrin and the hemolytic anemia mutation, nb, map to mouse chromosome 8: Presence of nb allele is associated with a truncated erythrocyte ankyrin. Proc Natl Acad Sci USA 1990;87:3117–3121.
17. **Greenquist AC, Shohet SB, Bernstein SE.** Marked reduction of spectrin in hereditary spherocytosis in the common house mouse. Blood 1978;51:1149–1155.
18. **Lux SE.** Spectrin-actin membrane skeleton of normal and abnormal red blood cells. Semin Hematol 1979;6:121–51.
19. **Shohet SB.** Reconstitution of spectrin-deficient spherocytic mouse erythrocyte membranes. J Clin Invest 1979;64:483–494.
20. **Smith JE, Moore K, Arens M, Rinderknecht GA, Ledet A.** Hereditary elliptocytosis with protein band 4.1 deficiency in the dog. Blood 1983;61:373–377.
21. **Correas I, Leto TL, Speicher DW, Marchesi VT.** Identification of the functional site of erythroid protein 4.1 involved in spectrin-actin associations. J Biol Chem 1986;261:3310–3315.
22. **Conboy JG, Chan JY, Chasis JA, Kan WY, Mohandas N.** Tissue- and development-specific alternative RNA splicing regulates expression of multiple isoforms of erythroid membrane protein 4.1. J Biol Chem 1991;266:8273–8280.
23. **Conboy JG, Shitamoto R, Parra M, Winardi R, Kabra A, Smith J, Mohandas N.** Hereditary elliptocytosis due to both qualitative and quantitative defects in membrane skeletal protein 4.1. Blood 1991;78:2438–2443.
24. **Zarkowsky HS, Oski FA, Shaafi R, Shohet SB, Nathan DG.** Congenital hemolytic anemia with high sodium, low potassium red cells. I. Studies of membrane permeability. N Engl J Med 1968;278:573–581.
25. **Mentzer WC, Smith WB, Goldstone J, Shohet SB.** Hereditary stomatocytosis: membrane and metabolism studies. Blood 1975;46:659–669.
26. **Lande WM, Thiemann PVW, Mentzer WC.** Missing band 7 protein in two patients with high Na, low K erythrocytes. J Clin Invest 1982;70:1273–1280.
27. **Eber SW, Lande WM, Iarocci TA, Mentzer WC, Hohn P, Wiley JS, Schroter W.** Hereditary stomatocytosis consistent association with an integral membrane protein deficiency. Br J Haematol 1989;72:452–455.
28. **Giger U, Amador A, Meyers–Wallen V, Patterson DF.** Stomatocytosis in miniature schnauzers. Am Coll Vet Intern Med Proc 1988;754.
29. **Brown DE, Weiser MG, Thrall MA, Giger U, Just CA.** Erythrocyte indices and volume distribution in a dog with stomatocytosis. Vet Pathol 1994;31:247–250.
30. **Fletch SM, Smart ME, Pennock PW, Subden RE.** Clinical and pathologic features of chondrodysplasia (dwarfism) in the Alaskan malamutes. J Am Vet Med Assoc 1973;162:357–361.
31. **Fletch SM, Pinkerton PH.** Animal model for human disease: inherited hemolytic anemia with stomatocytosis in the Alaskan Malamute dog. Am J Pathol 1973;71:477–480.
32. **Pinkerton PH, Fletch SM, Brueckner PJ, Miller DR.** Hereditary stomatocytosis with hemolytic anemia in the dog. Blood 1974;44:557–567.
33. **Slappendel RJ, van der Gaag I, van Nes JJ, van den Ingh TS, Happe RP.** Familial stomatocytosis–hypertrophic gastritis (FSHG), a newly recognized disease in the dog (Drentse partrijshond). Vet Q 1991;13:30–40.
34. **Slappendel RJ, Renooij W, de Bruijne JJ.** Normal cations and abnormal membrane lipids in the red blood cells of dogs with familial stomatocytosis–hypertrophic gastritis. Blood 1994;84:904–909.
35. **Kohn B, Hohenhaus A, Giger U.** Hemolytic anemia caused by increased osmotic fragility of erythrocytes in cats. Proc Annu Vet Forum 1996;760.
36. **Tucker EM, Kilgour L.** An inherited glutathione deficiency and a concomitant reduction in potassium concentration in sheep red cells. Experientia 1970;26:203–204.
37. **Tucker EM.** A shortened life span of sheep red cells with a glutathione deficiency. Res Vet Sci 1974;16:19–22.
38. **Tucker EM, Young JD, Crowley C.** Red cell glutathione deficiency: clinical and biochemical investigations using sheep as an experimental model system. Br J Haematol 1981;48:403–415.
39. **Young JD, Ellory JC, Tucker EM.** Amino acid transport defect in glutathione-deficient sheep erythrocytes. Nature 1975;254:156–157.
40. **Young JD, Ellory JC, Tucker EM.** Amino acid transport in normal and glutathione-deficient sheep erythrocytes. Biochem J 1976;154:43–48.
41. **Tucker EM, Young JD.** Biochemical changes during reticulocyte maturation in culture. A comparison of genetically different sheep erythrocytes. Biochem J 1980;192:33–39.
42. **Fincham DA, Young JD, Mason DK, Collins EA, Snow DH.** Breed and species comparison of amino acid transport variation in equine erythrocytes. Res Vet Sci 1985;38:346–351.
43. **Maede Y, Inaba M.** (Na,K)-ATPase and ouabain binding in reticulocytes from dogs with high K and low K erythrocytes and their changes during maturation. J Biol Chem 1985;260:3337–3343.
44. **Inaba M, Maede Y.** Na,K-ATPase in dog red cells. Immunological identification and maturation-associated degradation by the proteolytic system. J Biol Chem 1986;261:16099–16105.
45. **Johnstone RM, Adam M, Hammond JR, Orr L, Turbide C.** Vesicle formation during reticulocyte maturation. Association of plasma membrane activities with released vesicles (exosomes). J Biol Chem 1987;262:9412–9420.
46. **Parker JC.** Solute and water transport in dog and cat red blood cells. In: Ellory JC, Lew VL, eds. Membrane transport in red cells. London: Academic Press, 1977;427–465.
47. **Maede Y, Inaba M, Taniguchi N.** Increase of Na-K-ATPase activity, glutamate, and aspartate uptake in dog erythrocytes associated with hereditary high accumulation of GSH, glutamate, glutamine, and aspartate. Blood 1983;61:493–499.
48. **Maede Y, Amano Y, Nishida A, Murase T, Sasaki A, Inaba M.** Hereditary high-potassium erythrocytes with high Na,K-ATPase activity in Japanese Shiba dogs. Res Vet Sci 1990;50:123–125.
49. **Maede Y, Inaba M.** Energy metabolism in canine erythrocytes associated with inherited high Na$^+$- and K$^+$-stimulated adenosine phosphatase activity. Am J Vet Res 1987;48:114–118.
50. **Inaba M, Maede Y.** Inherited persistence of immature type pyruvate kinase and hexokinase isozymes in dog erythrocytes. Comp Biochem Physiol 1989;92B:151–156.
51. **Degen M.** Pseudohyperkalemia in akitas. J Am Vet Med Assoc 1987;190:541–543.
52. **Fujise H, Higa K, Nakayama T, Wada K, Ochiai H, Tanabe Y.** Incidence of dogs possessing red blood cells with high K in Japan and East Asia. J Vet Med Sci 1997;59:495–497.
53. **Ellory JC, Jones SEM, Preston RL, Young JD.** A high-affinity sodium-dependent transport system for glutamate in dog red cells. J Physiol 1981;320:79.
54. **Inaba M, Maede Y.** Increase of Na$^+$ gradient-dependent L-glutamate and L-aspartate transport in high K$^+$ dog erythrocytes associated with high activity of (Na$^+$,K$^+$)-ATPase. J Biol Chem 1984;259:312–317.
55. **Sato K, Inaba M, Maede Y.** Characterization of Na$^+$-dependent L-glutamate transport in canine erythrocytes. Biochim Biophys Acta 1994;1195:211–217.
56. **Sato K, Inaba M, Suwa Y, Matsuu A, Hikasa Y, Ono K, Kagota K.** Inherited defects of sodium-dependent glutamate transport mediated by glutamate/aspartate transporter in canine red cells due to a decreased level of transporter protein expression. J Biol Chem 2000;275:6620–6627.
57. **Maede Y, Kasai N, Taniguchi N.** Hereditary high concentration of glutathi-

one in canine erythrocytes associated with high accumulation of glutamate, glutamine, and aspartate. Blood 1982;59:883–889.

58. **Fujise H, Mori M, Ogawa E, Maede Y.** Variant of canine erythrocytes with high potassium content and lack of glutathione accumulation. Am J Vet Res 1993;54:602–606.

59. **Fujise H, Hishiyama N, Ochiai H.** Heredity of red blood cells with high K and low glutathione (HK/LG) and high K and high glutathione (HK/HG) in a family of Japanese Shiba dogs. Exp Anim 1997;46:41–46.

60. **Maede Y, Kuwabara M, Sasaki A, Inaba M, Hiraoka W.** Elevated glutathione accelerates oxidative damage to erythrocytes produced by aromatic disulfide. Blood 1989;73:312–317.

61. **Maede Y.** High concentration of blood glutathione in dogs with acute hemolytic anemia. Jpn J Vet Sci 1977;39:187–189.

62. **Yamato O, Maede Y.** Susceptibility to onion-induced hemolysis in dogs with hereditary high erythrocyte reduced glutathione and potassium concentrations. Am J Vet Res 1992;53:134–137.

63. **Yamato O, Hayashi M, Yamasaki M, Maede Y.** Induction of onion-induced haemolytic anaemia in dogs with sodium n-propylthiosulfate. Vet Rec 1998;142:216–219.

64. **Yamato O, Yoshihara T, Ichihara A, Maede Y.** Novel Heinz body hemolysis factors in onion (Allium cepa). Biosci Biotechnol Biochem 1994; 58:221–222.

65. **Inaba M, Maede Y.** A new major transmembrane glycoprotein, gp155, in goat erythrocytes. Isolation and characterization of its association to cytoskeleton through binding with band 3-ankyrin complex. J Biol Chem 1988;263:17763–17771.

66. **Beutler E.** Osmotic fragility. In: Williams WJ, Beutler E, Erslev AJ, Lichtman MA, eds. Hematology. 4th ed. New York: McGraw-Hill, 1990;1726–1728.

CHAPTER 157

Erythrocyte Phosphofructokinase and Pyruvate Kinase Deficiencies

• URS GIGER

Because erythrocytes lack mitochondria, their energy is solely generated by anaerobic glycolysis, also known as Embden-Meyerhof pathway (see Chapter 21, "Erythrocyte Metabolism").[1] Metabolism of one molecule of glucose to two molecules of lactate leads to the net production of two molecules of adenosine triphosphate (ATP) (Fig. 157.1). The rate of glycolysis depends on the need for ATP of erythrocytes to maintain the shape, deformability, membrane transport, and metabolic functions such as phosphorylation and synthesis of purines, pyrimidines, and glutathione. More than a dozen enzymes are involved in glycolysis and the two ancillary pathways, unique to erythrocytes, the hexose-monophosphate and Rapoport-Luebering shunt. Some of these enzymes exist in different isoforms allowing for cell and tissue specific expression and regulation. The key regulatory enzyme of anaerobic glycolysis is phosphofructokinase (PFK). Whereas ATP is the most important inhibitor of PFK activity, inorganic phosphate, adenosine monophosphate (AMP), and adenosine diphosphate (ADP) act in stimulatory fashions. In addition, glucose-1,6-biphosphate and fructose-2,6-biphosphate are activators. Under maximally activating conditions for PFK, an enzyme distal in glycolysis—pyruvate kinase (PK)—becomes rate-limiting. Therefore, it is not surprising that a deficiency of either PFK or PK activity will lead to erythrocytic malfunction and premature destruction, thereby causing hemolytic anemia. Although both erythroenzymopathies impair the same metabolic pathway, their clinical presentations are distinctly different. Subsequently, both erythroenzymopathies will be reviewed separately, and contrasting features between the two disorders as well as human patients and affected animals will be highlighted.

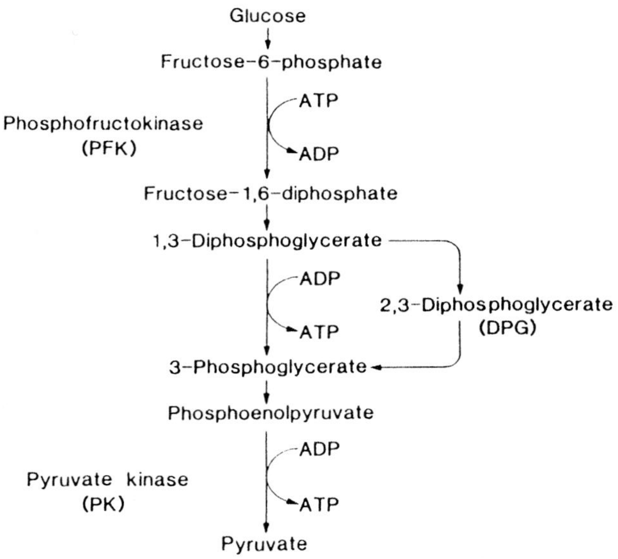

PFK DEFICIENCY

PFK (EC 2.7.1.11) catalyzes the regulatory phosphorylation step of fructose-6-phosphate to fructose-1,6-biphosphate. There are three isoforms of PFK, referred to as muscle (M-PFK), liver (L-PFK), and platelet (P-PFK) forms, that are encoded by three different genes.[2,3] The active PFK enzyme is a homo- or heterotetramer composed of one or more isoforms, each of these combinations providing unique enzyme kinetic properties. Their expression is cell and tissue specific and developmentally regulated. Skeletal muscle contains exclusively M-PFK homotetramers.[4] Human erythrocytes express equal amounts of M-PFK and L-PFK, whereas in canine erythrocytes the M-PFK isoform predominates in a ratio of 86:14 over P-PFK.[2-4] Furthermore, during myogenesis[5] and erythropoiesis as well as postnatal development,[6] the isoform composition in these cells changes from L-PFK to M-PFK and P-PFK. Deficiency of M-PFK has been associated with hemolysis and myopathy in humans and dogs, whereas in two Holstein calves PFK

FIGURE 157.1 Embden-Meyerhof (anaerobic glycolytic) pathway and Rapoport-Luebering shunt in erythrocytes (simplified). *ATP*, adenosine triphosphate; *ADP*, adenosine diphosphate.[13]

deficiency apparently did not cause any hematologic abnormalities[7] and will, therefore, not be discussed here.

PFK Deficiency in Humans

M-PFK deficiency, also known as Tarui-Layzer syndrome, is a rare genetic disorder in humans characterized by metabolic myopathy and a well-compensated hemolytic disorder.[8,9] PFK-deficient humans exhibit exercise intolerance, muscle weakness, and muscle cramping on exertion. Because of the residual half-normal PFK activity in affected erythrocytes, contributed by L-PFK isozymes and lack of alkaline fragility of human erythrocytes, overt clinical signs of hemolysis occur extremely rarely. In fact, human patients are overcompensating their hemolytic component and developing a mild erythrocytosis, because PFK-deficient erythrocytes do not readily release oxygen from hemoglobin. The ensuing tissue hypoxia accelerates erythropoiesis. A few mutations in the M-PFK gene have been described in human patients.[10]

Canine PFK Deficiency

Canine M-PFK deficiency was first described as a common autosomal recessive trait in English springer spaniels.[11–13] Molecular genetic studies revealed a non-sense mutation in the last exon of the M-PFK gene ($\Delta2228G{\rightarrow}A$).[14,15] The resulting change from a tryptophane to stop codon causes a truncation of the M-PFK protein by 40 amino acids, leading to rapid degradation and complete deficiency of the M-PFK enzyme.[15,16] Affected dogs are, therefore, completely lacking PFK activity in muscle and have 8 to 22% of control PFK activity in erythrocytes due to residual P-PFK and L-PFK expression (other tissues appear less affected as they express higher levels of other PFK isoforms).[2,6,17,18] The metabolic block at the PFK step results in a deficiency of ATP and 2,3-diphosphoglycerate (DPG) in erythrocytes as well as no lactate production and accumulation of sugar phosphates and glycogen in muscle; hence, the term glycogenosis or glycogen storage disease type VII.[12,17,19,20]

In erythroenzymopathies, the mechanism of accelerated lysis is generally not known but is assumed to be caused by energy depletion.[8] In dogs, the compensated hemolytic disorder with PFK deficiency, as seen in human patients, is accentuated by life-threatening hemolytic crises. A unique mechanism has been documented to be responsible for intravascular lysis, namely an increased alkaline-induced hemolysis.[11,13] Although incompletely understood, canine erythrocytes are more alkaline fragile than cells from other species.[21,22] As canine erythrocytes lyse at pH 7.6, canine blood left in open tubes on the bench is known to result in considerable hemolysis. In vivo, the intracellular pH of erythrocytes is determined by organic phosphate and chloride anions. Because PFK-deficient erythrocytes have markedly decreased DPG concentrations of approximately one-third of normal, chloride ions are moving in and increase the erythrocytic pH.[11,19,20] Thus, PFK-deficient erythrocytes

start lysing at a pH near 7.4 (Fig. 157.2). Consequently, even minor systemic alkalemia can induce intravascular hemolysis. Alkalemia is associated with any form of hyperventilation, and because dogs control their body temperature by panting and often bark, such situations occur readily.[11,13]

The low DPG content of PFK-deficient erythrocytes has another major effect, as the oxygen affinity of canine hemoglobin is DPG-dependent (Fig. 157.3). The hemoglobin-oxygen affinity of PFK-deficient erythrocytes is, therefore, significantly increased; this is reflected by a left shift of the hemoglobin-oxygen dissociation curve.[11,12] The relative tissue hypoxia impairs, for instance, muscle and other tissue metabolism and stimulates renal erythropoietin synthesis and erythropoiesis. Therefore, aside from the occasional hemolytic crises, the chronic hemolytic disorder is fully compensated with a robust regenerative response even at normal hematocrit.

Sporadic intravascular hemolytic crises associated with pigmenturia, anemia, and/or jaundice are the hallmark findings of PFK deficiency in dogs.[11,13,23] These episodes are induced by hyperventilation-associated events such as excessive panting and barking, strenuous exercise, and high environmental temperatures. Thus, guests or a new pet at home, a visit to the veterinarian, kenneling, and training for field trialing have precipitated hemolysis. These crises can be first observed at a few months of age, although some animals may not experience any problems until several years of age, or they are completely missed until the owner looks for them. During these episodes, which generally last one to several days, affected animals have pale to icteric mucous membranes; are lethargic, inappetent, and often febrile; and splenomegaly may be noted. Pigmenturia is characterized by hemoglobinuria during crises, whereas hyperbilirubinuria is persistently strong. The anemia may become life-threatening with hematocrits as low as 5%, but is always macrocytic, hypochromic, and strongly regenerative with corrected and absolute reticulocyte counts of greater than 4% and greater than $200,000/\mu L$, respectively. The apparent half-life of chromium-labeled PFK-deficient erythrocytes is only 16 days compared with 20 to 28 days for normal canine cells. Beside polychromasia, marked anisocytosis and normoblastosis (but no poikilocytosis) are observed on microscopic examination of a blood smear. Leukocytosis and hyperglobulinemia may also be present. The plasma may be discolored because of hemoglobinemia and hyperbilirubinuria due to hemolysis, although some hepatopathy may also exist. Transient hyperkalemia is due to lysis of high potassium containing reticulocytes and young erythrocytes.[3]

Less commonly, PFK-deficient dogs may develop muscle signs on exertion.[17,24–27] In fact, muscle cramping in one of the limbs even after mild exercise is the most dramatic presentation.[24] Affected dogs may suddenly refuse to run and have high serum creatine kinase activity. The mechanism of muscle contractures in metabolic myopathies is still not understood.[9] Despite a complete lack of PFK activity in muscle, clinical signs of myopathy

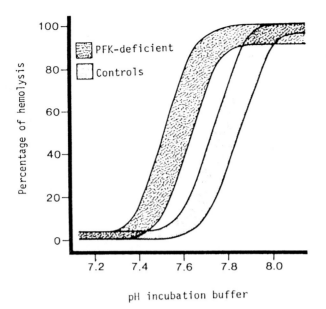

FIGURE 157.2 Alkaline fragility of erythrocytes from PFK-deficient and control dogs incubated at various pH values for 1 hour at 37°C. Shaded areas represent observed range of lysis. Erythrocytes from PK-deficient dogs behave like controls.[13]

are generally mild, presumably due to the high oxidative rate of canine skeletal muscle.[28] Nevertheless, impairments in oxidative and anaerobic muscle metabolism have been demonstrated experimentally.[25,26] Clinically affected dogs may only show mild exercise intolerance and intermittent muscle wasting. They train and perform poorly as field trial dogs. The serum creatine kinase activity is normal to slightly increased. PFK-deficient skeletal muscle accumulates slightly more glycogen and occasionally amylopectin.[17,27]

PFK deficiency is an autosomal recessive trait[12] and occurs commonly in the English springer spaniel breed.[29,30] Since the first description in 1985,[11] more than 100 cases have been documented, but the gene frequency remains at 2% despite extensive screening over the past decade.[30] Most of them are field trial rather than conformational (bench, show) springers from the United States, but affected springers were also found in Denmark and Britain. Based on extensive pedigree analyses, a common ancestor goes back to least the 1960s, if not earlier. PFK deficiency has also been reported in an American cocker spaniel and mixed-breed dogs.[31] Because they all had the same disease-causing DNA mutation, these animals must be related. In fact, the PFK-deficient Cocker with a six-generation pedigree was bred in a kennel that also had English springer spaniels, and one of the parents of an affected mixed-breed dog resembled a springer spaniel. Thus, related breeds may have the same disease-causing mutation; however, PFK deficiency in other breeds and species is likely due to another mutation in the PFK gene.

PFK deficiency may be suspected based on signalment, family history, typical clinical signs, and suggestive laboratory test abnormalities. However, a definitive diagnosis requires proof of the PFK mutation or reduced erythrocytic PFK enzyme activity. A simple polymerase chain reaction (PCR)-based DNA test accurately identifies PFK-deficient dogs (homozygotes, affected; two mutant alleles) and carriers (heterozygotes; one mutant and normal allele) in the English springer spaniel and related breeds.[14,29,30] EDTA-anticoagulated blood, but also a drop of blood dried on a special filter paper, a buccal swab with a special brush, and semen are suitable sources for DNA extraction and PCR testing. Whereas the PCR test is simple and permits a diagnosis from the first day of life, the PFK enzyme activity test is cumbersome and not accurate until 2 months of age. Normal and affected neonatal dogs express large quantities of L-PFK in erythrocytes.[6] Because the PCR-based test is mutation-specific, the measurement of PFK enzyme activity may be indicated in other breeds and species in which the same disease is suspected. It is recommended to screen with the PCR-based PFK test for English springer spaniels that have suspicious clinical signs and are used for breeding; testing should take place before training for field trialing.

PFK-deficient dogs may have a normal life expectancy if crises-inducing situations are avoided.[13] Dogs experiencing a hemolytic crisis are provided with supportive care including transfusions, if needed. Fever and excessive panting or barking should be avoided. Diamox (a carbonic anhydrase inhibitor) may acidify the blood, and aspirin and dipyrone may counter the fever accompanying hemolysis, thereby preventing further intravascular lysis during an acute crisis; however, these drugs have not been proven effective in clinical practice. Despite massive intravascular hemolysis, hemoprotein-induced acute nephropathy has not been observed. Nevertheless, hemolytic dogs should be well hydrated, but blood transfusions are only rarely needed. Affected dogs recover from these crises within days, which may be misinterpreted as a successful therapeutic response of a presumptive immune-mediated hemolytic disease. A proper diagnosis will alleviate unnecessary exposure to harmful immunotherapeutic agents. Finally, experimental bone marrow transplantation can successfully correct the hematologic abnormalities and oxygenation of muscle.[32]

PK DEFICIENCY

PK (EC 2.7.1.40) catalyzes the ATP-generating conversion of phosphoenolpyruvate to pyruvate and is, therefore, an important regulator in the terminal glycolytic pathway. There are two different genes coding by alternative splicing a total of four developmentally dependent and tissue-specific PK isoforms.[33-35] The PKLR gene encodes the red blood cell (R-PK) and liver (L-PK) isoenzymes, whereas the other (PKM) gene generates the muscle (M_1-PK) and M_2-PK isoform. R-PK is expressed almost exclusively in mature erythrocytes and has a different first exon, making the amino-terminal sequence longer when compared to that of L-PK. In contrast, erythroid precursors express M_2-PK and switch to R-PK isoforms during differentiation to mature red blood cells.[36] Erythrocytic PK deficiency causing hemolytic anemia has been described in humans, dogs, cats, and mice.[37,38]

PK Deficiency in Humans

PK deficiency is the most prevalent hereditary nonspherocytic hemolytic anemia caused by a glycolytic enzymopathy.[8,39] Many mutations in the PKLR gene have been found to cause R-PK deficiency; some of them are common in certain ethnic (Amish) and geographic regions.[10,40] Most of the patients, however, are compound heterozygotes. Clinical signs in PK-deficient humans are very variable, ranging from a mild compensated hemolytic disorder to severely anemic patients who become transfusion-dependent, develop iron overload, and die during early childhood. Splenectomy is helpful in some human patients.[8,39]

PK Deficiency in Dogs

In 1971, erythrocyte PK deficiency was first recognized in Basenji dogs.[41,42] It served as the classic example of an inborn error of metabolism in veterinary medicine, although the biochemical derangements turned out to be more complex, making a diagnosis more difficult. R-PK deficiency appears to occur most commonly in Basenjis[41-42] but has also been reported in Beagles,[44-46] West Highland white[47,48] and Cairn terriers,[49] miniature Poodles,[11] a Dachshund,[4] Chihuahua, Pug, and American Eskimo Toy dogs.[1,11] In Basenjis, a single base pair deletion in exon 5 of the R-PK gene has been identified causing a frameshift and severe truncation of the protein.[50,51] In contrast, a six base insertion ambiguously positioned at 3'-end of exon 10 in the R-PK sequence was found in West Highland white terriers.[48] This insertion results in the in-frame addition of two amino acids, threonine and lysine, and is likely also the causative mutation in Cairn terriers,[49] a related breed. In the other breeds a disease-causing mutation has not yet been identified. In the Beagle, the disease-causing mutation is likely in exon 1, which has not yet been sequenced from dogs, as the rest of the R-PK cDNA sequence is normal. Despite the varied mutations in R-PK, the biochemical changes and clinicopathologic manifestations of PK deficiency in any of the reported canine breeds appear identical.

The R-PK deficiency in erythrocytes of affected dogs can be demonstrated by agarose gel electrophoresis, immunoblotting, and immunoprecipitation studies.[43] However, all affected dogs express M_2-PK in erythrocytes, which increases total erythrocyte PK activity of affected dogs and is therefore misleading. For instance, miniature Poodles with nonspherocytic anemia and osteosclerosis may well have had R-PK deficiency,[52] despite high erythrocyte PK activity in vitro. M_2-PK expression is rarely observed in human patients. This M_2-PK isozyme, which is normally present in erythroid precur-

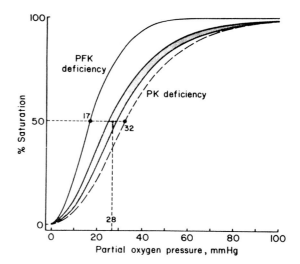

FIGURE 157.3 Hemoglobin-oxygen dissociation curves of PFK-deficient and PK-deficient canine erythrocytes.[11] Shaded area represents normal range.

sor cells but not mature erythrocytes, appears to be heat-labile and dysfunctional in vivo, because affected erythrocytes show a severe metabolic block at the PK step.[43] In addition to the accumulation of proximal glycolytic metabolites in erythrocytes, the DPG content is also increased. The resulting right shift of the hemoglobin-oxygen dissociation curve allows for improved oxygen delivery, thereby ameliorating the clinical signs of severe anemia in PK-deficient dogs (Fig. 157.3).

PK-deficient dogs present at a few months to a few years of age because of intermittent weakness and exercise intolerance. They appear to adapt well to the anemia, presumably due to the favorable tissue oxygenation despite severe anemia; in fact, pale mucous membranes during routine health checks may be the first sign. The hematocrit ranges between 12 and 26%; the anemia is highly regenerative, with reticulocyte counts reaching 90%, and is macrocytic-hypochromic. Echinocytes have been documented.[42] The erythrocyte half-life is 5.8 days in PK-deficient Basenjis compared with 19 to 28 days in normal dogs.[43] Hepatosplenomegaly may also be noted. Affected dogs die of anemia or hepatic failure between 1 and 5 years of age. Interestingly, all PK-deficient dogs develop a progressive myelofibrosis and osteosclerosis that remain unexplained and do not occur in other species with PK deficiency.[41-49] The osteosclerosis may be discovered by radiography of long bones at 1 year of age and completely obstructs the marrow cavities by 3 years.

A diagnosis of PK deficiency is strongly suggested by the concurrent occurrence of a highly regenerative severe anemia and osteosclerosis in a dog younger than 5 years of age. PCR-based PK tests are available for the Basenji[50,51] and West Highland white[48] (and likely Cairn) terrier breeds. These DNA tests are accurate to detect affected and carrier dogs in these breeds. However, because they are mutation-specific, they cannot be used for other breeds. In other breeds, cumbersome PK enzyme activity assays with agarose gel electrophoresis or immunologic methods specific for R-PK are required. PK carriers do not express M-PK and, therefore, have intermediate erythrocytic PK activity. Unfortunately, the PK activity assays are not very accurate in detecting carriers, as the carrier and normal range overlap.[43] PK deficiency has most commonly been reported in the Basenji breed, but the PK mutation frequency remains unknown in all canine breeds.

Affected dogs are managed symptomatically in clinical practice. Bone marrow transplantation, performed experimentally,[53] corrects the hemolytic anemia and halts the osteosclerosis. Splenectomy has not been shown to be effective in slowing the degree of hemolysis.

PK Deficiency in Cats

In the 1990s, erythrocytic PK was identified and characterized in the Abyssinian, Somali, and domestic shorthair cats.[54,55] A 13 base pair deletion at the 3'-end of exon 5 in the R-PK cDNA but not the genomic sequence is caused by a splicing defect and results in a severe reduction in erythrocytic PK enzyme activity. There is no anomalous M_2-PK expression in erythrocytes and no osteosclerosis in cats, which are observed in all PK-deficient dogs. Affected cats have chronic intermittent hemolytic anemia that might be first recognized between a few months of age to advanced age. The anemia is intermittent, mild to moderate, slightly macrocytic-hypochromic, and generally slightly to strongly regenerative. Splenectomy appears to reduce the severity of the hemolytic crises. PK deficiency is common in the two related breeds, Abyssinian and Somali, and the same mutation has also been identified in a domestic cat.

REFERENCES

1. **Harvey JW.** The erythrocyte—physiology, metabolism, and biochemical disorders. In: Kaneko JJ, Harvey JW, Bruss ML, eds. Clinical biochemistry of domestic animals. 5th ed. San Diego: Academic Press, 1997;157–203.
2. **Vora S, Giger U, Turchen S, Harvey JW.** Characterization of the enzymatic lesion in inherited phosphofructokinase deficiency in the dog: an animal analogue of human glycogen storage disease type VII. Proc Natl Acad Sci USA 1985;82:8109–8113.
3. **Giger U, Harvey JW, Yamaguchi RA, McNulty PK, Chiapella A, Beutler E.** Inherited phosphofructokinase deficiency in dogs with hyperventilation-induced hemolysis: increased in vitro and in vivo alkaline fragility of erythrocytes. Blood 1985;65:345–351.
4. **Mhaskar Y, Harvey JW, Dunaway GA.** Developmental changes of 6-phosphofructo-1-kinase subunit levels in erythrocytes from normal dogs and dogs affected by glycogen storage disease type VII. Comp Biochem Physiol 1992;101:303–307.
5. **Gekakis N, Gehnrich SC, Sul HS.** Phosphofructokinase isozyme expression during myoblast differentiation. J Biol Chem 1989;264:3658–3661.
6. **Harvey JW, Reddy GR.** Postnatal hematologic development in phosphofructokinase-deficient dogs. Blood 1989;74:2556–2561.
7. **Valberg SJ, Mickelson JR, DiMauro S.** Nonlysosomal glycogenoses in horses and cattle. Muscle Nerve 1998;7(Suppl):S89.
8. **Glader BE, Lukens JN.** Hereditary hemolytic anemias associated with abnormalities of erythrocyte glycolysis. In: Lee GR, et al., eds. Wintrobe's clinical hematology. 10th ed. Baltimore: Williams & Wilkins, 1160–1175.
9. **Rowland LP, DiMauro S, Layzer RB.** Phosphofructokinase deficiency. In: Engel A, Banker BQ, eds. Myology. New York: McGraw-Hill, 1986;1603–1617.
10. **Miwa S, Fujii H.** Molecular basis of erythroenzymopathies associated with hereditary hemolytic anemia. Tabulation of mutant enzymes. Am J Hematol 1996;51:122–128.
11. **Giger U.** Hereditary erythrocyte disorders. In: Bouagura JD. Kirk's Current Veterinary Therapy XIII 2000;414–420.
12. **Giger U, Reilly M, Asakura T, Baldwin CJ, Harvey JW.** Autosomal recessive inherited phosphofructokinase deficiency in English springer spaniels. Anim Genet 1986;17:15–23.
13. **Giger U, Harvey JW.** Hemolysis caused by phosphofructokinase deficiency in English springer spaniels: seven cases (1983-86). J Am Vet Med Assoc 1987;191:453–459.
14. **Smith BF, Henthorn PS, Rajpurohit Y, Stedman H, Wolfe JH, Patterson DF, Giger U.** A cDNA coding canine muscle type phosphofructokinase. Gene 1996;168:275–276.
15. **Smith BF, Stedman H, Rajpurohit Y, Henthorn PS, Wolfe JH, Patterson DF, Giger U.** The molecular basis of canine muscle-type phosphofructokinase deficiency. J Biol Chem 1996;271:20070–20074.
16. **Mhaskar Y, Giger U, Dunaway GA.** Presence of truncated M-type subunit and altered kinetic properties of 6-phosphofructo-1-kinase isozymes in canine brain affected by glycogen storage disease type VII. Enzyme 1991;45:137–144.
17. **Giger U, Kelly AM, Teno PS.** Biochemical studies of canine muscle phosphofructokinase deficiency. Enzyme 1988;40:25–29.
18. **Harvey JW, Pate MG, Mhaskar Y, Dunaway GA.** Characterization of phosphofructokinase-deficient canine erythrocytes. J Inherit Metab Dis 1992;15:747–759.
19. **Harvey JW, Sussman WA, Pate MG.** Effect of 2,3-diphosphoglycerate concentration on the alkaline fragility of phosphofructokinase-deficient canine erythrocytes. Comp Biochem Physiol [B] 1988;89:105–109.
20. **Giger U, Teno P, Reilly MP, Asakura T, McLaughlin AC.** Phosphofructokinase-deficient canine erythrocytes studied in vitro. Blood 1986;68:35a.
21. **Waddell WJ.** Lysis of dog erythrocytes in mildly alkaline isotonic media. Am J Physiol 1956;186:339–342.
22. **Iampietro PF, Burr MJ, Fiorica V, McKenzie JM, Higgins EA.** pH-dependent lysis of canine erythrocytes. J Appl Physiol 1967;23:505–510.
23. **Harvey JW, Smith JE.** Comp Hematol Int 1994;4:70–74.
24. **Giger U, Argov Z, Schnall M, Bank W, Chance B.** Metabolic myopathy in canine muscle-type phosphofructokinase deficiency studies by P-NMR. Muscle Nerve 1988;11:1260–1265.
25. **Brechue WF, et al.** Metabolic and work capacity of skeletal muscle of PFK-deficient dogs studied in situ. J Appl Physiol 1994;77:2456–2567.
26. **McCully K, Chance B, Giger U.** In vivo determination of altered hemoglobin saturation in dogs with M-type phosphofructokinase deficiency. Muscle Nerve 1999;22:621–627.
27. **Harvey JW, Calderwood-Mays MB, Gropp KE, Denaro FJ.** Polysaccharide storage myopathy in canine phosphofructokinase deficiency (Type VII glycogen storage disease). Vet Pathol 1990;27:1–8.
28. **Snow DH.** No classical type IIB fibres in dog skeletal muscle. Histochem 1982;75:53–65.
29. **Giger U, Smith BF, Rajpurohit Y.** PCR-based screening test for phosphofructokinase (PFK) deficiency: a common inherited disease in English springer spaniels. J Vet Intern Med 1995;9:187.
30. **Giger U, Kimmel A, Overley DB, Schwartz L, Smith BS, Rajpurohit Y.** Frequency of phosphofructokinase deficiency in English springer spaniels: A longitudinal and randomized survey. J Vet Intern Medicine 2000, in press.
31. **Giger U, Smith BF, Woods CB, Patterson DF, Stedman H.** Inherited phosphofructokinase deficiency in the American Cocker spaniel. J Am Vet Med Assoc 1992;201:1569–1571.
32. **Giger U, Smith BF, Griot-Wenk M, Rajpurohit Y, McCully K, Haskins ME, Stedman H.** The molecular basis of canine muscle phosphofructokinase deficiency is a point mutation. Blood 1991;78:365a.
33. **Imamura K, Tanaka T.** Multimolecular forms of pyruvate kinase from rat and other mammalian tissues. J Biochem 1972;71:1043–1051.
34. **Noguchi T, Inoue H, Tanaka T.** The M1 and M2-type isozymes of rat pyruvate kinase are produced from the same gene by alternative RNA splicing. J Biol Chem 1986;261:13807–13812.
35. **Noguchi T, Yamada K, Inoue H, Matsuda T, Tanaka T.** The L and R-type isozymes of rat pyruvate kinase are produced from a single gene by the use of different promoters. J Biol Chem 1987;262:14366–14371.
36. **Max-Audit I, Kechemir D, Mitjavila MJ, Vainchenker W, Rotten D, Rosa R.** Pyruvate kinase synthesis and degradation by normal and pathologic cells during erythroid maturation. Blood 1988;72:1039–1043.
37. **Kanno H, Morimoto M, Fujii H, Tsujimura T, Asai H, Noguchi T, Kitamura Y, Miwa S.** Primary structure of murine red blood cell-type pyruvate kinase (PK) and molecular characterization of PK deficiency identified in the CBA strain. Blood 1995;86:3205–3209.
38. **Morimoto M, Kanno H, Asai H, Tsujimura T, Fujii H, Moriyama Y, Kasugai T, Hirono A, Ohba Y, Miwa S, Kitamura Y.** Pyruvate kinase deficiency of mice associated with non-spherocytic hemolytic anemia and cure of the anemia by marrow transplantation without host irradiation. Blood 1995;86:4323–4328.
39. **Tanaka KR, Paglia DE.** Pyruvate kinase and other enzymopathies of the erythrocyte. In: Scriver CR, Beaudet AL, Sly WS, Valle D, eds. The metabolic and molecular basis of inherited disease. 7th ed. New York: McGraw-Hill, 1995;3488–3493.
40. **Demina A, Varughese KI, Barbot J, Forman L, Beutler E.** Six previously undescribed pyruvate kinase mutations causing enzyme deficiency. Blood 1998;92:647–652.

41. **Searcy GP, Miller DR, Tasker JB.** Congenital hemolytic anemia in the Basenji dog due to erythrocyte pyruvate kinase deficiency. Can J Comp Med Vet Sci 1971;35:67–70.
42. **Searcy GP, Tasker JB, Miller DR.** Animal model: pyruvate kinase deficiency in dogs. Am J Pathol 1979;94:689–692.
43. **Giger U, Noble NA.** Inherited erythrocyte pyruvate kinase deficiency in Basenji dogs. J Am Vet Med Assoc 1991;198:1755–1761.
44. **Harvey JW, Kaneko JJ, Hudson EB.** Erythrocyte pyruvate kinase deficiency in a Beagle dog. Vet Clin Pathol 1977;6:13–17.
45. **Prasse KW, Crouser D, Beutler E.** Pyruvate kinase deficiency with terminal myelofibrosis and osteosclerosis in a Beagle. J Am Vet Med Assoc 1975;166:117–1175.
46. **Giger U, Mason GD, Wang P.** Inherited erythrocyte pyruvate kinase deficiency in a Beagle. Vet Clin Pathol 1991;20:83–86.
47. **Chapman BL, Giger U.** Inherited erythrocyte pyruvate kinase deficiency in the West Highland White terrier. J Small Anim Pract 1990;31:610–616.
48. **Skelly B, Wallace M, Rajpurohit Y, Wang P, Giger U.** Identification of a 6 base pair insertion in West Highland White Terriers with erythrocyte pyruvate kinase deficiency. Am J Vet Res 1999;60:1169–1172.
49. **Schaer M, Harvey JW, Calderwood-Mays M, Giger U.** Pyruvate kinase deficiency causing hemolytic anemia with secondary hemochromatosis in a Cairn terrier. J Am Anim Hosp Assoc 1992;28:233–239.
50. **Whitney KM, Goodman S, Bailey E, Lothrop CE.** The molecular basis of canine pyruvate kinase deficiency. Exp Hematol 1994;22:866–874.
51. **Whitney KM, Lothrop CD.** Genetic test for pyruvate kinase deficiency in Basenjis. J Am Vet Med Assoc 1995;207:918–921.
52. **Randolph JF, Center SA, Kalfelz FA, et al.** Familial non-spherocytic hemolytic anemia in poodles. Am J Vet Res 1986;47:687–695.
53. **Weiden PL, Hackman RC, Deeg HJ, Storb R.** Long-term survival and reversal of iron overload after marrow transplantation in dogs with congenital hemolytic anemia. Blood 1981;57:66–70.
54. **Ford S, Giger U, Duesberg C, Beutler E, Wang P.** Inherited erythrocyte pyruvate kinase (PK) deficiency causing hemolytic anemia in an Abyssinian cat. J Vet Intern Med 1992;6:123.
55. **Giger U, Rajpurohit Y, Wang P, Ford S, Kohn B, Patterson DF, Beutler E, Henthorn PS.** Molecular basis of erythrocyte pyruvate kinase (R-PK) deficiency in cats. Blood 1997;90(Suppl):5b.

CHAPTER 158

Hemophilia A and B

• PETER MANSELL

HEMOPHILIA A

Hemophilia A is the most common inherited coagulopathy in domestic animals. The disease has been most widely documented in dogs, having been diagnosed in a large number of breeds, most notably the German Shepherd. The disease has also been reported in several other domestic species including cats,[1] horses,[2] and cattle.[3]

Hemophilia A is caused by a lack of functional factor VIII. The activation of factor X by a complex of activated factor IX, phospholipid, and calcium is markedly accelerated in the presence of activated factor VIII. Consequently, activated factor VIII helps to promote the rapid stabilization of the primary hemostatic plug by fibrin. When factor VIII is lacking, the speed of formation and also the strength of the hemostatic plug is compromised, and the plug is liable to breakdown, allowing recurrent or persistent hemorrhage from the site of vessel damage. Although factor VIII circulates in close association with von Willebrand factor (vWF), the two molecules are distinct. Association with the vWF molecule protects the circulating factor VIII molecule, and factor VIII activity may be decreased in individuals with some types of von Willebrand's disease, although this is more pronounced in humans than in domestic animal species.[4]

The factor VIII gene in humans is located near the tip of the X chromosome. The gene that codes for factor VIII has been sequenced.[5] It spans 186 kb with 26 coding exons, resulting in the production of a protein of 2351 amino acids. A wide variety of defects of the gene, both of base substitutions and either large or small deletions, have been identified and characterized in human hemophiliacs.[6] Many of these sites of point mutations contain the CpG dinucleotide. These defects result in either the failure of synthesis of factor VIII or the synthesis of dysfunctional factor VIII that is unable to fulfill its role in secondary hemostasis. Despite considerable efforts, attempts to identify the defects responsible for the disease in other species have not been as successful.[7,8]

As is the case in humans, hemophilia A in animals is an X-chromosomal recessive inherited disease. Consequently, there is a single allele of the gene in males and two copies in females. One of the alleles of the factor VIII gene in females is lost by the random inactivation of one of the two X chromosomes in female cells. Males may carry either a normal or a defective copy of the gene and so may be either normal or affected. Females may be homozygous normal, heterozygous (carriers), or extremely rarely homozygous affected animals. Although homozygous affected females have been reported, they are rare because they must inherit a defective gene from both parents (i.e., the father would have had to be affected). New mutations, in which the defect appears in families without a history of the disease, do occur and may be responsible for a substantial proportion of cases of the disease in humans.

Clinical Signs

The clinical severity of hemophilia A is dependent on both the magnitude of the deficiency of factor VIII and the exposure of the animal to trauma that may institute a hemorrhagic episode. Mildly affected animals, with factor VIII activities of 5% or above, do not tend to bleed spontaneously and may be able to maintain adequate hemostasis for most of the time. Moderately affected animals, with factor VIII activities of 2 to 5%, take longer to achieve hemostasis and are more likely to suffer serious sequelae to minor trauma. Severely affected animals, with less than 2% of normal factor VIII activity, may be prone to apparently spontaneous hemorrhagic episodes in which no trauma can be identified.

The consequences of a hemorrhagic episode depends largely on the site of the hemorrhage and the extent to which bleeding continues before hemostasis is achieved. Intramuscular and intraarticular hemorrhage that results in lameness is the most common manifestation of the disease in dogs. Subcutaneous hematomas and excessive bleeding from surgical sites are also commonly seen. The occurrence of large hematomas in the scrotum following castration is often the first recognized sign of the disease in dogs. Intramuscular, intracranial, and subdural bleeding may have serious sequelae due to subsequent pressure on nervous tissues. Clinical signs are not common in young puppies although there is no evidence of transplacental transfer of factor VIII from the dam. Puppies may or may not bleed excessively after minor surgical procedures, and bleeding from the gums at the loss of the deciduous teeth is often only noted retrospectively once a diagnosis has been made. Heterozygous carrier females generally do not exhibit clinical signs, but homozygous affected females may be more severely affected than males.[9]

Diagnosis

A diagnosis of hemophilia A should be considered in an animal with a prolonged activated partial thromboplastin time (APTT) and a normal prothrombin time (PT). There is only poor correlation between the degree of prolongation of the APTT and the activity of factor VIII in the plasma, and measurement of the APTT alone is not sufficient to establish the diagnosis. The definitive diagnosis of hemophilia A requires the demonstration of a deficiency of factor VIII by specific assay. One stage assay methods that detect the formation of a clot by the physical detection of fibrin strands, or by measuring the increase of the optical density of the test plasma, are easily amenable to automation and provide repeatable results. Factor VIII activity may also be below normal values in some cases of von Willebrand's disease.

There is no recognized international standard of factor VIII activity in animal plasma. The activity of factor VIII differs substantially between species, and this should be considered both in the selection of assay reagents and in the interpretation of assay results. Functional assay of factor VIII requires a substrate plasma that provides all other coagulation factors in adequate amounts so that factor VIII, which is supplied by the test plasma, is the only rate-limiting component. Factor VIII deficient plasma of human origin is suitable for use in the assay of canine factor VIII because the activity of the other coagulation factors is sufficient. However, normal canine plasma has five to eight times the factor VIII activity of human plasma. When interpreting factor VIII assays, it is wise to use species-specific plasma as the standard. There is a wide range of factor VIII activities in normal animals (60 to 160 U/dL), and it is common practice to use pooled plasma from at least 10 normal animals of the same species as the test plasma as a nominal 100 U/dL standard. Even animals with only mild hemophilia usually have a factor VIII activity of 5 to 40 U/dL, which is substantially below the normal range, and distinction of these animals is generally not difficult.

The lack of any transplacental transfer of factor VIII in dogs allows a correct diagnosis of hemophilia in young puppies, although the factor VIII activity of normal puppies may be marginally lower than that of adults.[10] Similarly, collection of blood samples from dogs that are under the influence of acepromazine or xylazine sedation and thiopentone anesthesia is satisfactory for subsequent factor VIII assay.[11] Factor VIII activity is reasonably stable in separated plasma that is stored for 24 to 48 hours at temperatures less than 20°C.[12] Careful venepuncture is critical for the correct interpretation of laboratory results. Factor VIII activity may be slightly elevated immediately after a clinical hemorrhagic episode.

Detection

Detection of carrier (heterozygous) females can be done by using a variety of methods based on evidence of mutation following analysis of DNA, pedigree information, or plasma. Analysis of DNA has the potential to provide definitive results and can be used in human medicine in those cases in which DNA analysis of related individuals provides sufficient information to trace the inheritance of the mutated gene.

In animals, pedigree analysis can draw information from either the anterior pedigree (ancestors) or the posterior pedigree (offspring). Determination of a female's anterior pedigree allows the calculation of a probability of the female being heterozygous for the trait, based on the principles of simple Mendelian inheritance. In some specific cases this information alone may be sufficient to establish a female to be a carrier (e.g., if the female is the daughter of a confirmed hemophiliac). Posterior pedigree information can only provide a likelihood ratio that the female is a carrier; a female may be proved to be a carrier using this method (if, for example, she produces hemophilic offspring), but the testing of offspring per se can never prove a female to be homozygous normal. Nevertheless, as the number of proven normal offspring increases without the detection of a hemophiliac, the odds of the maternal female being a carrier diminish (a female that has produced five normal male offspring without producing any hemophilic offspring has less than a 5% chance of being a carrier herself). The probability and likelihood ratio may be combined to provide a pedigree-based probability that the female is a carrier. In the absence of disease in an animal's pedigree, the possibility of the occurrence of a new mutation should be considered. The male offspring of an affected male are normal, as long as the offspring's dam is normal.

Numerous attempts have been made to discriminate between normal and carrier bitches using coagulation studies, with variable success. The APTT of carrier bitches is not prolonged. The reported accuracy of carrier detection in bitches on the basis of factor VIII activity, alone or in combination with vWF assay, varies among authors.[13–15] The factor VIII activity of carrier bitches is generally 30 to 60 U/dL, which is less than that of normal bitches, but many heterozygous females have factor VIII activities within the range of normality (60 to 160 U/dL).

Therapy

Basic therapy of hemophilic animals consists of simple nursing care so that the animal's own hemostatic mechanisms have a chance of stemming any hemorrhage. Bandaging, compression, local cautery and vessel ligation, and restriction of movement may be sufficient to allow healing, although treatment may need to be prolonged. It is preferable for exogenous factor VIII to be given, so that hemostasis is achieved more rapidly and reliably. Elective surgery should be avoided, although surgical procedures are feasible provided that the animal's own hemostasis is supplemented by the provision of exogenous factor VIII before, during, and after the procedure.

In cases in which blood loss has been extensive, the transfusion of fresh whole blood, or fresh frozen plasma and packed red blood cells, may be necessary. Fresh or fresh frozen plasma may be transfused (6 to 10 mL/kg) to provide factor VIII in a smaller volume. Plasma cryoprecipitate contains concentrations of factor VIII about 10 times higher than that of plasma and allows an even smaller volume of infusion to be used. If not available commercially, plasma cryoprecipitate is not difficult to prepare from whole plasma.[16] In addition to having a low factor VIII activity relative to many animal species, human factor VIII (either purified from donations or of recombinant DNA origin) is generally in high demand for the treatment of human cases and is unlikely to be readily available for veterinary use. Ideally, sufficient exogenous factor VIII would be transfused to return the patient's plasma factor VIII activity to normality; however, good therapeutic effects can generally be achieved by raising the plasma factor VIII activity to 15 to 30 U/dL. The use of factor VIII, especially from other species, may also result in the induction of factor VIII inhibitors.[17,18] Treatment of individuals with factor VIII inhibitors often requires the transfusion of very high doses of exogenous factor VIII or the use of alternative therapies.

The use of ancillary treatments, such as Desamino-D-arginine vasopressin (DDAVP) or fibrinolytic inhibitors, has not been critically assessed for clinical efficacy in the treatment of hemophilia A in animals. DDAVP has proved to be of some use in the treatment of human cases of hemophilia A, by promoting the release of sufficient factor VIII from hepatocytes into the circulation to promote hemostasis.[19] However, the use of DDAVP does not produce an increase of factor VIII activity of sufficient magnitude, duration, or reliability in hemophilic dogs to be of any great clinical value.[20] In humans with inhibitors, prothrombin complex concentrates or recombinant factor VIIa have been used as alternatives to exogenous factor VIII.

Gene therapy offers the potential of ongoing therapy of hemophiliacs, without relying on the repeated infusion of exogenous factor VIII. The latter carries the disadvantages of inconvenience, cost, and risk of contamination. Hemophilia A is a promising candidate for this approach because only a relatively small increase in factor VIII activity would be necessary to prevent clinical signs. Several difficulties have been noted. Factor VIII undergoes substantial posttranslational modifications that are necessary for full biologic activity. Introduction of a functional gene coding for factor VIII into appropriate target tissues has also proved difficult.[21] The size of the gene that codes for factor VIII presents difficulties in the choice of a vector of sufficient capacity. Complete correction of canine hemophilia A using gene therapy

techniques has been reported[22] using an adenoviral vector carrying human factor VIII cDNA; however, the therapeutic effect was only transient. Improvements in gene vectors and the development of methods that result in the sustained expression of the factor VIII gene in patients are still required but are now realistic goals.

HEMOPHILIA B

Hemophilia B (Christmas disease) is due to an absolute or functional deficiency of factor IX. Once it has been activated by activated factor XI, factor IX forms a complex with factor VIII, calcium, and phospholipid which rapidly activates factor X by enzymatic cleavage. Deficiency of factor IX results in slower activation of factor X, which subsequently results in poor stabilization of the platelet plug by fibrin, such that the plug is weakened and prone to disintegration. The gene that codes for factor IX in humans is located at the tip of the long arm of the X chromosome. The gene consists of 34 kb, arranged as eight exons coding for a protein of 415 amino acids. A base substitution mutation[23] and a mutation involving deletion and transition of the factor IX gene have both been described in animals.[24]

Clinical Signs

The inheritance and clinical signs of hemophilia B are similar to those of hemophilia A. The genes for factor VIII and factor IX are both located on the X chromosome, and both diseases are inherited as a recessive X-chromosomal trait, occurring predominantly in males. The clinical signs relate to an inability to form a stable hemostatic plug rapidly after rupture of blood vessels, with prolonged or inappropriate bleeding from localized sites of damage. The severity of clinical signs seen in hemophilia B is related to the size and activity of the affected animals, being more severe in larger, more active animals.

In both diseases, the APTT is prolonged and the PT is within normal limits. To differentiate between the two diseases, specific factor assays are required to identify the deficient factor. An APTT with the addition of plasma or serum may allow differentiation. The prolonged APTT of both hemophilia A and B can be corrected by the addition of normal fresh plasma. In contrast, the addition of normal fresh serum (which contains factor IX but not factor VIII) corrects the prolonged APTT of hemophilia B but not that of hemophilia A.

Detection

Hemophilia B has been reported in a variety of breeds of dogs and cats.[25] In contrast to the range of factor VIII activities seen in animals with hemophilia A, most animals with hemophilia B have quite low factor IX activities (5 U/dL or less), and heterozygous carriers have factor IX activities of 40 to 60 U/dL, less than the lower end of the normal range (60 U/dL), making identification of these animals somewhat more reliable.

Abnormal hemorrhage is not uncommon in human carriers of the disease. Detection of carriers by DNA analysis is possible only in those breeds or families in which the mutation has been characterized.

Therapy

Therapeutic correction of the factor IX deficiency can be attained by the transfusion of whole blood or plasma. Cryoprecipitate does not contain factor IX. Ancillary therapies such as confinement, bandaging, and possibly local cautery, all of which assist in the maintenance of the unstable platelet plug, are beneficial. Surgery should be avoided if possible; when this is not the case, supplementation of the patient's own hemostatic mechanisms by transfusion of exogenous factor IX in blood or plasma before and during the procedure is indicated.

Hemophilia B has a number of characteristics that make it a promising candidate for gene therapy—the factor IX gene is relatively small, and only small amounts of factor IX need be expressed in the patient for there to be a clinical improvement. In addition, expression of the gene does not need to be localized in any particular tissue. The introduction of functional genes encoding for factor IX using viral vectors has been successfully achieved in dogs with hemophilia B and, although the therapeutic effect was short-lived, an effect was detectable for several months.[26] Diminution or cessation of the clinical effect may be due to immune-mediated inactivation of cells expressing the transferred factor IX gene. Nonviral methods of introducing the factor IX gene into cells, utilizing the ability of some cells to take in conjugates by endocytosis, have been investigated by several researchers.[21]

REFERENCES

1. **Littlewood JD.** Haemophilia A (factor VIII deficiency) in the cat. J Small Anim Pract 1986;27:541–546.
2. **Henninger RW.** Hemophilia A in two related Quarter horse colts. J Am Vet Med Assoc 1988;193:91–94.
3. **Healy PJ, Sewell CA, Exner T, Morton AG, Adams BS.** Haemophilia in Hereford cattle: factor VIII deficiency. Aust Vet J 1984;61:132–133.
4. **Weiss HJ, Sussman II, Hoyer LW.** Stabilization of factor VIII in plasma by the von Willebrand factor: studies in posttransfusion and dissociated factor VIII and in patients with von Willebrand's disease. J Clin Invest 1977;60:390–404.
5. **Gitschier J, Wood WI, Goralka TM, Wion KL, Chen EY, Eaton DE, Vehar GA, Capon DJ, Lawn RM.** Characterization of the human factor VIII gene. Nature 1984;312:326–330.
6. **Antonarakis SE.** Molecular genetics of coagulation factor VIII gene and hemophilia A. Thromb Haemost 1995;74:322–328.
7. **Clark P.** Studies on the molecular biology of the factor VIII gene in normal and haemophilic dogs, with special reference to German shepherd dogs in Australia. PhD thesis, 1997, University of Melbourne, Australia.
8. **Clark P, Bowden DK, Parry BW.** Studies to detect carriers of haemophilia A in German shepherd dogs using diagnostic DNA polymorphisms in the human factor VIII gene. Vet J 1997;153:71–74.
9. **Pijnappels MIM, Briet E, van der Zwet GT, Huisden R, van Tilburg NH, Eulderink F.** Evaluation of the cuticle bleeding time in canine haemophilia A. Thromb Haemost 1986;55:70–73.
10. **Mansell PD, Parry BW.** Changes in factor VIII activity and von Willebrand factor antigen concentration with age in dogs. Br Vet J 1992;148:329–337.
11. **Mansell PD, Parry BW.** Effect of acepromazine, xylazine and thiopentone on factor VIII activity and von Willebrand factor antigen concentration in dogs. Aust Vet J 1992;69:187–190.
12. **Mansell PD, Parry BW.** Stability of canine factor VIII activity and von Willebrand factor antigen concentration in vitro. Res Vet Sci 1991;51:313–316.
13. **Fogh JM.** A study of hemophilia A in German shepherd dogs in Denmark. Vet Clin North Am Small Anim Pract 1988;18:245–254.
14. **Littlewood JD.** Inherited bleeding disorders of dogs and cats. J Small Anim Pract 1989;30:140–143.
15. **Mansell PD, Parry BW, Anderson GA.** Detection of canine carriers of haemophilia A using factor VIII activity and von Willebrand factor antigen concentration. Prev Vet Med 1993;16:133–139.
16. **Herschgold EJ, Pool JG, Pappenhagen AR.** The potent antihemophilic globulin concentrate derived from a cold insoluble fraction of human plasma: characterization and further data on preparation and clinical trial. J Lab Clin Med 1965;67:23–32.
17. **Strauss SH, Merler E.** Characterization and properties of an inhibitor of factor VIII in the plasma of patients with hemophilia A following repeated transfusions. Blood 1967;30:137–150.
18. **Giles AR, Tinlin A, Hoogendoorn H, Greenwood P, Greenwood R.** Development of factor VIII:c antibody in dogs with haemophilia A (factor VIII:c deficiency). Blood 1984;63:451–456.
19. **Mannucci PM.** Desmopressin: a nontransfusional form of treatment for congenital and acquired bleeding disorders. Blood 1988;72:1449–1455.
20. **Mansell PD, Parry BW.** Changes of factor VIII: coagulant activity and von Willebrand factor concentration following injection of DDAVP in dogs with mild hemophilia A. J Vet Int Med 1991;5:191–194.
21. **Fallaux FJ, Hoeben RC, Briet E.** State and prospects of gene therapy for the hemophilias. Thromb Haemost 1995;74:263–273.
22. **Connelly S, Mount J, Mauser A, Gardner JM, Kaleko M, McClelland A, Lothrop CD Jr.** Complete short-term correction of canine hemophilia A by in vivo gene therapy. Blood 1996;88:3846–3853.
23. **Evans JP, Brinkhous KM, Brayer GD, Reisner HM, High KA.** Canine hemophilia B resulting from a point mutation with unusual consequences. Proc Natl Acad Sci USA 1989;86:10095–10099.
24. **Mauser AE, Whitlark J, Whitney KM, Lothrop CD.** A deletion mutation causes hemophilia B in Lhasa apso dogs. Blood 1996;88:3451–3455.
25. **Maggio-Price L, Dodds WJ.** Factor IX deficiency (hemophilia B) in a family of British shorthair cats. J Am Vet Med Assoc 1993;203:1702–1704.
26. **Kay MA, Landen CN, Rothenberg SR, Taylor LA, Leland F, Wiehle S, Fang B, Bellinger D, Finegold M, Thompson AR, et al.** In vivo hepatic gene therapy: complete albeit transient correction of factor IX deficiency in hemophilia B dogs. Proc Natl Acad Sci USA 1994;91:2353–2357.

CHAPTER 159

Other Hereditary Coagulopathies

• W. JEAN DODS

Hemorrhagic diseases have been recognized and studied in humans and animals for more than 40 years. Today, reliable and useful animal models exist for nearly all the inherited and acquired hemostatic and thrombotic disorders, and much is known about their clinical, diagnostic, and therapeutic management.[1-8] Hemophilia A and B as well as factor XI deficiency are covered in separate chapters (Chapters 158 and 160, respectively). von Willebrand disease is the most common bleeding disorder and is discussed in Chapter 72.

Diagnostic Evaluation of Bleeding Disorders

Medical history typically includes information about the current bleeding problem, previous bleeding problems, family history, environmental influences, and drugs.[2-5] Animals with hereditary bleeding disorders often show signs at a young age, although adult onset does not exclude a mild hereditary bleeding tendency. Excessive hemorrhage occurs after minor trauma. Knowledge of the patient's present and past bleeding episodes often provides the key to diagnosis because bleeding problems, especially when internal, can mimic a variety of other disease states. Physical examination focuses on the location, severity, and nature of the bleeding (whether the hemorrhage is superficial or deep).

Laboratory Diagnosis of Bleeding Disorders

Screening tests used routinely for diagnosis of bleeding disorders include the following: toenail or buccal mucosal bleeding time, platelet count, prothrombin time (PT), activated partial thromboplastin time (APTT), fibrinogen concentration, d-dimer or other tests for fibrinogen-fibrin degradation products, and von Willebrand factor (vWF).[2-5] Because the PT and APTT tests are designed primarily for screening purposes, they are relatively insensitive to minor abnormalities and thus may fail to identify patients with only mild bleeding tendencies. If a defect is not found on screening but the history strongly suggests a hemorrhagic problem, more specialized coagulation tests should be considered.

Therapy of Bleeding Disorders

Control of the physiologic and physical environment to promote hemostasis, tissue repair, and prevention of recurrence are important adjuncts to management and treatment of bleeding disorders. Drugs known to interfere with hemostasis are contraindicated for patients with moderate to severe hemostatic defects because they impair platelet function and further compromise the stability of the hemostatic plug.[2-5] These include aspirin, promazine tranquilizers, phenylbutazone, nitrofurans, potentiated sulfonamides, glycosaminoglycans, penicillins, phenothiazines, antihistamines, local anesthetics, estrogens, antiinflammatory drugs, plasma expanders such as dextran and hydroxyethyl starch, and live virus vaccines.[4,5]

Adequate replacement therapy with the correct blood component is essential for the control of moderate or severe hemostatic defects.[2-8]

Until recently, most veterinarians have used random (untyped) blood donors, because typing sera for determining animal blood groups were not commercially available. Today, blood typing can be obtained through the larger veterinary diagnostic laboratories, and commercial card-typing systems for the canine DEA 1.1 antigen and feline A and B antigens have been developed.

Veterinarians can also purchase blood from the handful of private commercial or university-based blood banks recently established for dogs, cats, and horses. Alternatively, practitioners may keep DEA 1-negative dog donors in their hospital to provide fresh blood for emergency use to treat patients in need of repeated transfusions. However, whole blood is no longer the treatment of choice for most veterinary transfusions.[2-8] Processing freshly collected blood into several clinically useful components is more cost-effective, efficient, and safer. For hereditary coagulopathies other than factor VIII and fibrinogen deficiency, fresh-frozen plasma or supernatants from plasma cryoprecipitates are most appropriate. Treatment of vWD is discussed in Chapter 72.

FIBRINOGEN (FACTOR I) DEFICIENCY

Fibrinogen is a complex glycoprotein, the substrate for thrombin, and the precursor of fibrin. The human and bovine protein have a molecular mass of 340 kDa and a dimeric structure composed of three pairs of peptide chains ($A\alpha$,$B\beta$,γ) joined by disulfide bonds.[9] Most vertebrate fibrinogens share a similar structure.[1] Following the action of thrombin on fibrinogen, two major fibrinopeptides (A and B) are released from the amino termini of the α and β chains, respectively. The remaining fibrin monomers are then polymerized to form insoluble, cross-linked fibrin by the interaction of fibrin-stabilizing factor (factor XIII) and Ca^{2+}.[10]

Fibrinogen is an important cofactor that mediates platelet aggregation responses, as platelets contain relatively large amounts of fibrinogen. It has a half-life of approximately 36 hours.[1-3]

Fibrinogen is apparently synthesized by hepatic parenchymal cells as a heterogeneous group of molecules, which may explain the large number of abnormal or dysfibrinogens known to occur as inherited disorders, in the fetus, or with underlying disease (especially of the liver).[5] The α chain is especially heterogeneous and has been shown to vary in size during evolutionary development.[1]

Inheritance

Hereditary fibrinogen deficiencies are autosomal incompletely dominant or recessive traits.[1,5,11]

Incidence

Hereditary fibrinogen defects have been recognized in humans, goats, and dogs.[1-4] These can be caused by a complete lack of fibrinogen (afibrinogenemia), reduced fibrinogen (hypofibrinogenemia), or an abnormal fibrinogen (dysfibrinogenemia). Caprine afibrinogenemia was recognized in the Netherlands in a large family of Saanen dairy goats.[11]

Clinical Signs

The defect in dairy goats was characterized by a severe hemorrhagic diathesis in newborn and young kids, incompletely dominant inheritance, umbilical bleeding, recurrent hemarthroses, and bleeding into subcutaneous tissues and from mucous membranes. Fibrinogen was undetectable by bioassays and immunoassays. Heterozygotes had hypofibrinogenemia.[11]

Canine hypofibrinogenemia was recognized in a family of Bernese mountain dogs from Europe.[2,4,5] Both biologic and immunologic assays of fibrinogen were decreased. The propositus died of a severe hemorrhagic crisis. Related dogs appeared to be heterozygous for the trait. Inherited dysfibrinogenemia has been studied in an inbred borzoi family, and hypofibrinogenemia has been diagnosed in the Lhasa apso, vizsla, and collie.

These disorders usually are expressed as a mild bleeding tendency exacerbated by stress events, trauma, or surgery.[2-4]

Diagnosis

Quantitative or qualitative fibrinogen disorders result in a complete failure of plasma or whole blood to clot in any coagulation test or when thrombin is added, and plasma does not form a precipitate when heated to 56°C or treated with 25% ammonium sulfate. Thus, the PT and APTT are very prolonged or never clot, and fibrinogen levels are either very or moderately reduced.[1-5] Some abnormalities of platelet function, such as prolonged bleeding time and abnormal clot retraction, may also occur. Although biologic assays of fibrinogen are abnormal, the presence of fibrinogen is usually detected immunologically.[1-5]

Therapy

The treatment of choice for severe fibrinogen defects is plasma cryoprecipitate, although in typical clinical settings fresh-frozen plasma is usually given for cost and availability reasons.[2,4,8]

PROTHROMBIN (FACTOR II) DEFICIENCY

Prothrombin is an α-globulin glycoprotein of 71.6 kDa and 8.2% carbohydrate.[9] Prothrombin is converted the active enzyme, thrombin, by the action of a complex mixture of plasma or tissue thromboplastins and metal ions. Prothrombin is synthesized by the liver, and its reported half-life varies from 10 to 60 hours, with an average of ~36 hours. Both the synthesis and release of prothrombin require vitamin K. Vitamin K is also a known requirement for four other clotting factors—factors VII, IX, X, and protein C.[12,13]

Inheritance

Inherited prothrombin deficiency states (hypo- or dysprothrombinemia) are autosomal traits.[1-3]

Incidence

These are rare disorders in humans and animals. Canine hypoprothrombinemia is the only inherited prothrombin defect recognized to date in animals and has been reported in the boxer, otterhound, and English cocker spaniel.[2,4,5]

Clinical Signs

Both hypo- and dysprothrombinemia are recognized as clinical entities in humans and produce mild to moderately severe bleeding problems. Two generations of an affected family of boxers have been studied.[2-4] The defect was characterized by epistaxis and umbilical bleeding in newborn puppies and mild mucosal surface bleeding in young adults. Although the disease appeared at first to resemble dysprothrombinemia with reduced prothrombin activity and normal antigen, additional studies pointed to a metabolic or kinetic problem in turnover of all the vitamin K-dependent clotting factors. These dogs were also warfarin-sensitive and had a considerably delayed warfarin turnover time.

Diagnosis

Prothrombin defects are characterized by prolonged PT and APTT.[2,4,5]

Therapy

Because prothrombin complex clotting factor concentrates are not available for veterinary use, affected animals are given transfusions of fresh-frozen plasma or the supernatant from plasma cryoprecipitates.[2,4,8]

FACTOR VII DEFICIENCY

Factor VII is a single-chain glycoprotein that functions primarily in the extrinsic pathway of coagulation.[9,14,15] Factor VII has the most rapid turnover rate of any coagulation factor, with a half-life of 2 to 7 hours.[2,5] It is synthesized by the liver and secreted into the blood as a zymogen with a molecular weight of approximately 50 kDa.[12,13] Factor VII is the second component, along with tissue factor, that rapidly accelerates coagulation via the extrinsic pathway. Calcium ions are required, and the reaction proceeds by activating factor IX to factor IXa and factor X to factor Xa. The extrinsic system needs only factors VII, X, V, prothrombin, and fibrinogen to form fibrin.[16]

Recent studies with murine factor VII cDNA determined that the translated protein has high sequence homology to that of human, rabbit, rhesus monkey, canine, and bovine factor VII.[13] There is significant sequence similarity in the amino termini of factor VII, prothrombin, factor IX, factor X, and protein C. Despite structural similarities to the other vitamin K-dependent proteins, factor VII differs significantly in its metabolic behavior.

Inheritance

Factor VII deficiency is inherited as an autosomal trait with incomplete (or variable) penetrance.[14,15]

Incidence

To date, this disorder has only been reported in dogs and humans. It is recognized most often in large breeding colonies of beagles.[14,15] The high incidence in this breed probably reflects its widespread use in biomedical research. Factor VII deficiency has also been described in Alaskan malamute, boxer, bulldog, miniature schnauzer, and mixed-breed dogs.[4] The defect is usually discovered fortuitously during routine hematologic screening for drug testing, research, or clinical workup.[15]

Clinical Signs

Canine factor VII deficiency is a mild disease typically expressed by easy bruising and a predisposition to demodicosis, presumably because the animal's defective extrinsic clotting provides an ideal, moist environment for mange mites.[4,14]

Diagnosis

Affected homozygotes are detected by the presence of a prolonged PT, normal APTT and Stypven (Russell's viper venom) time, and reduced factor VII activity (less than 15% and usually below 5%).[1,2-5,15] Heterozygotes are difficult to identify with PT alone, because it is only slightly elevated or falls within the upper end of normal range; factor VII levels are typically 15 to 65%.[4,5,15] Factor VII antigen levels can also be measured.[2,15]

Therapy

Transfusion therapy is usually not required for factor VII-deficient dogs, but if bleeding is severe, treatment is the same as for prothrombin defects.[4,8]

FACTOR X DEFICIENCY

Factor X is activated by the action of factor IXa, phospholipid, and Ca^{2+}; the reaction is accelerated by tissue factor (extrinsic system) and factor VIII (intrinsic system). The factor Xa so formed activates factor V.[9] Factor X is a dimeric α-globulin of about 59 kDa in plasma and 36 kDa in serum, is synthesized by the liver in the presence of vitamin K, and is secreted into the plasma as a precursor to a serine protease. The half-life is 20 to 40 hours.

Inheritance

Factor X deficiency is inherited as an autosomal trait with incomplete (or variable) penetrance.[2,4]

Incidence

A rare coagulation disorder, factor X deficiency was first described in humans in the mid-1950s.[1] Some 20 years later, it was recognized in a family of American cocker spaniels.[17] Most of the original affected stock was screened for the trait and removed from the breeding

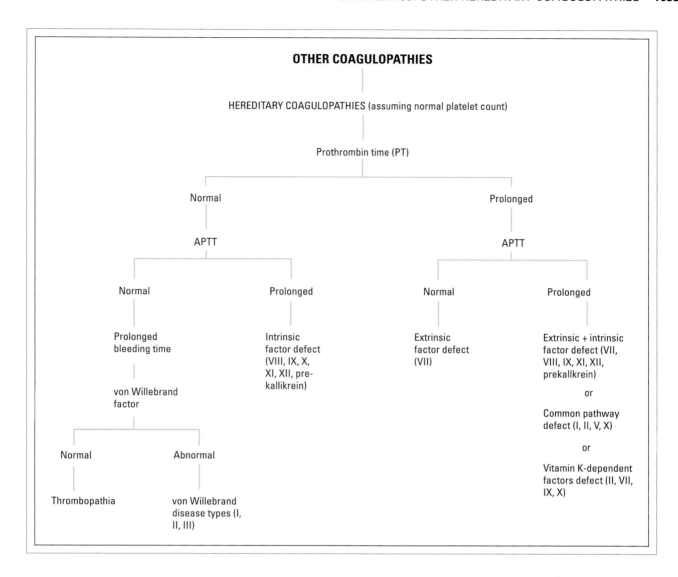

pool. Since then, factor X deficiency has been diagnosed occasionally in mongrel dogs and recently in the Jack Russell terrier.[18]

Clinical Signs

Dogs classified as homozygotes or strongly penetrant heterozygotes have very low to moderately low levels of factor X (less than 5 to 30%). This is expressed clinically in affected adults as a mild to moderately severe mucosal surface bleeding disease, whereas weakly penetrant heterozygotes (30 to 70% factor X) are usually asymptomatic.[17,18] Severely affected dogs with less than 10% factor X usually are stillborn or die as neonates from internal bleeding; this situation mimics the "fading puppy syndrome." Exceptions were an affected mongrel puppy with 6% factor X that lived for nearly 1 year before experiencing a fatal bleeding episode, and the propositus of the Jack Russell terrier family with 3 to 13% factor X that experienced excessive bleeding at tail

docking, during eruption of permanent dentition, and several days after ovariohysterectomy.[18] Three siblings of this female died of unknown cause during the perinatal period and may also have been affected. Complete absence of factor X is thought to be a lethal mutation because of its central role in coagulation.[1]

Diagnosis

Clinically affected individuals have mild to moderately prolonged PT, APTT, and Stypven time as well as low factor X levels (see above). In heterozygotes, screening tests may be at the upper end of normal ranges or slightly prolonged, and factor X levels are partially reduced.[2,4] Chromogenic substrate assays are also available for quantitating factor X levels.[2]

Therapy

Fresh-frozen plasma transfusions are given to treat factor X deficiency.[4,18]

VITAMIN K-DEPENDENT COAGULATION FACTOR DEFICIENCY

Combined deficiency of all vitamin K-dependent coagulation factors (II, VII, IX, and X) has occasionally been reported in humans and was thoroughly investigated in a family of Devon Rex cats.[19,20] A defective vitamin K-dependent carboxylase was identified which had decreased affinity for both vitamin K hydroquinone and propeptide.[20]

Inheritance

The feline disorder appears to be inherited as an autosomal recessive trait.[19]

Incidence

This type of disorder is rare. The incidence in the Devon Rex breed is unknown. Relatives of the affected kittens were identified; they had significantly reduced vitamin K-dependent coagulation factors but were clinically asymptomatic.[19,20] The disorder has been observed in Australia, the United States, and Great Britain.

Clinical Signs

Bleeding episodes in affected kittens were severe or fatal and included hematomas, hemarthroses, as well as intrathoracic and intraabdominal hemorrhages.[19]

Diagnosis

Affected cats (clinically affected or asymptomatic relatives) have significantly prolonged PT and APTT as well as very low levels of factors II, VII, IX, and X.[19,20]

Therapy

Treatment with oral and parenteral vitamin K_1 normalizes the defect.[19,20]

FACTOR XI (PTA) DEFICIENCY

Details about factor XI and its deficiency states[21-23] are reviewed in another section (see Chapter 160).

FACTOR XII (HAGEMAN FACTOR) DEFICIENCY

Hageman factor is an α-globulin involved in the initial stage of clotting through a surface-mediated or "contact activation" process. Factor XII is a single-chain sialoglycoprotein of 80 kDa which is activated by contact with biologic tissues, other than intact endothelium, and most foreign surfaces.[1,5,9] It is present in plasma as a precursor to a serine protease. Hageman factor is synthesized by the liver, and the half-life is 52 to 60 hours.[3]

The functions of activated factor XII include the conversion of plasma kininogens to kallikrein, enhancement of vascular permeability, activation of fibrinolysis, initiation of the Schwartzman reaction, activation of the extrinsic coagulation pathway, interaction with the Fletcher (prekallikrein) and Fitzgerald (high-molecular-weight kininogen [HMWK]) factors in surface-mediated reactions, and mediation of inflammatory and complement (C1-esterase) reactions.[9]

Inheritance

Factor XII deficiency is inherited as an autosomal recessive trait.[1-5,24-27]

Incidence

Hageman trait is an asymptomatic coagulation factor deficiency recognized in humans, dogs, and cats; it is a relatively common random finding in domestic cats.[1,24-27] Affected dog breeds include miniature poodle, standard poodle, German shorthair pointer, and shar pei.[4] The absence of detectable biologic or immunologic factor XII is also a normal phenomenon of a variety of other vertebrates and invertebrates, such as certain marine mammals (whales, dolphins), birds (common domestic fowl and waterfowl), reptiles, and possibly fish.[1-3]

Clinical Signs

Factor XII-deficient individuals do not exhibit a bleeding tendency, unless hemostasis is otherwise compromised.[4,26]

Diagnosis

The first feline case was discovered fortuitously because of prolonged screening tests of intrinsic clotting.[24] It had less than 5% factor XII and died without progeny. The second case, discovered similarly, had less than 1% factor XII and provided several generations of progeny.[25] Affected homozygous individuals have significantly prolonged APTT, recalcification times, and whole blood clotting times in glass tubes as well as very low factor XII activity; the PT is normal.[2,4,5,24-27] Heterozygotes have approximately 50% factor XII activity.[27]

Therapy

Treatment is usually not required.

PREKALLIKREIN (FLETCHER FACTOR) DEFICIENCY

Plasma prekallikrein is a 79.5 kDa γ-globulin glycoprotein that is synthesized in the liver and secreted into plasma, where nearly 75% circulates as a complex with factor XI and HMWK. The conversion of plasma prekallikrein to kallikrein is catalyzed by factor XIIa.[9,28–30] In a reciprocal response, prekallikrein stimulates the conversion of factor XII to XIIa by 50- to 100-fold; HMWK augments the reaction as well and releases the vasoactive peptide bradykinin.[27,30] Interaction of prekallikrein with factor XII also converts plasminogen to plasmin, thereby stimulating fibrinolysis; activates the alternative pathway of complement; and promotes neutrophil and monocyte chemotaxis.[30]

Inheritance

Human prekallikrein deficiency is inherited as an autosomal recessive trait and appears to have similar inheritance in miniature and Belgian horses.[29,30]

Incidence

Fletcher trait has been described in humans, dogs, and miniature and Belgian horses.[27–30] The incidence in Belgian horses is unknown but warrants investigation, as several horses closely related to the affected horse and two full siblings also had low or very low Fletcher factor activity.[30]

Clinical Signs

Although most affected humans do not experience abnormal bleeding, some have had excessive bleeding after tonsillectomy or tooth extraction and epistaxis.[30] Affected dogs have been admitted for diagnostic workup after recurrent gastrointestinal hemorrhage and hematuria,[27,28] and the propositus in the Belgian horse family had significant bleeding after castration.[30]

Diagnosis

Affected individuals have very long APTT (with particulate activators rather than ellagic acid), normal PT, and very low prekallikrein levels (typically less than 2.5%).[27–30] As ellagic acid activates factor XII directly, thereby bypassing the augmentation provided by prekallikrein, use of this reagent in the APTT assay makes it insensitive to prekallikrein deficiency.[27,30] Presumed heterozygous Belgian horses had variably reduced levels of prekallikrein (12.5 to 64%).[30]

Therapy

For clinically affected individuals, fresh-frozen plasma is the treatment of choice.[30]

COAGULOPATHIES NOT YET RECOGNIZED IN ANIMALS

Other human coagulopathies include factors V and XIII (fibrin stabilizing factor [FSF]) deficiencies, both rare autosomal traits. The former produces a moderate to severe bleeding diathesis, prolonged APTT and PT, and very low factor V activity.[5,9] Factor XIII-deficient patients have poor wound healing, bruise easily, and bleed at delivery or after minor surgery, especially dental extractions. FSF-deficient clots dissolve within 24 hours when placed in 5 M urea or 1% monochloroacetic acid.[10]

Another defect not recognized in animals is HMWK deficiency, although several nonmammalian species normally lack this activity. HMWK activity is detectable in primate, dog, and whale plasmas; is very low in rabbit and cattle plasmas; and is apparently absent when measured with conventional assays in fowl, reptilian, and amphibian plasmas.[1]

REFERENCES

1. **Lewis JH.** Comparative hemostasis in vertebrates. Plenum Press, 1996.
2. **Feldman BF, ed.** Hemostasis. Vet Clin North Am Small Anim Pract 1988;18.
3. **Dodds WJ.** Hemostasis. In: Kaneko JJ, ed. Clinical biochemistry of domestic animals. 4th ed. San Diego: Academic Press, 1989;274–315.
4. **Dodds WJ.** Bleeding disorders. In: Morgan RV, ed. Handbook of small animal practice. 2nd ed. New York: Churchill Livingstone, 1992;765–777.
5. **Dodds WJ.** Hemostasis. In: Kaneko JJ, Harvey JW, Bruss ML, eds. Clinical biochemistry of domestic animals. 5th ed. San Diego: Academic Press, 1997:241–283.
6. **Cotter SM, ed.** Comparative transfusion medicine. Adv Vet Sci Comp Med 1991;36.
7. **Hohenhaus AE, ed.** Transfusion medicine. Probl Vet Med 1992;4:555–670.
8. **Kristensen AT, Feldman BF, eds.** Canine and feline transfusion medicine. Vet Clin North Am Sm Anim Pract 1995;25:1231–1490.
9. **Davie EW.** Biochemical and molecular aspects of the coagulation cascade. Thromb Haemost 1995;74:1–6.
10. **Lopaciuk S, McDonagh RP, McDonagh J.** Comparative studies on blood coagulation factor XIII. Proc Soc Exp Biol Med 1978;158:68–72.
11. **Breukink HJ, Hart HC, Arkel C, Velden NA, Watering CC.** Congenital afibrinogenemia in goats. Zentralbl Vet Med [A]. 1972;19:661–678.
12. **Suttie JW.** Synthesis of vitamin K-dependent proteins. FASEB J 1993; 7:445–452.
13. **Idusogie E, Rosen E, Geng J-P, Carmeliet P, Collen D, Castellino FJ.** Characterization of a cDNA encoding murine coagulation factor VII. Thromb Haemost 1996;75:481–487.
14. **Spurling NW, Peacock R, Pilling T.** The clinical aspects of canine factor VII deficiency including some case histories. J Small Anim Pract 1974; 15:229–235.
15. **Spurling NW.** Hereditary blood coagulation factor VII deficiency in the beagle: immunological characterization of the defect. Comp Biochem Physiol 1986;83A:755–760.
16. **Kitchen S, Preston FE.** Factor VII clotting assays: influence of thromboplastin. Thromb Haemost 1994;71:720–723.
17. **Dodds WJ.** Canine factor X (Stuart-Prower factor) deficiency. J Lab Clin Med 1973:82:560–566.
18. **Cook AK, Werner LL, O'Neill SL, Brooks M, Feldman BF.** Factor X deficiency in a Jack Russell terrier. Vet Clin Pathol 1993;22:68–71.
19. **Maddison JE, Watson ADJ, Eade IG, Exner T.** Vitamin K-dependent multifactor coagulopathy in Devon rex cats. J Am Vet Med Assoc 1990;197:1495–1497.
20. **Soute BAM, Ulrich MMW, Watson ADJ, Maddison JE, Ebberink RHM, Vermeer C.** Congenital deficiency of all vitamin K-dependent blood coagulation factors due to a defective vitamin K-dependent carboxylase in Devon rex cats. Thromb Haemost 1992;68:521–525.
21. **Dodds WJ, Kull JE.** Canine factor XI (PTA) deficiency. J Lab Clin Med 1971:78:746–752.
22. **Knowler C, Giger U, Dodds WJ, Brooks M.** Factor XI deficiency in Kerry blue terriers. J Am Vet Med Assoc 1994;205:1557–1561.
23. **Gentry PA, Ross ML.** Coagulation factor XI deficiency in Holstein cattle: expression and distribution of factor XI activity. Can J Vet Res 1993; 57:242–247.

24. **Green RA, White F.** Feline factor XII (Hageman) deficiency. Am J Vet Res 1977;38:893–895.
25. **Kier AB, Bresnahan JF, White FJ, Wagner JE.** The inheritance pattern of factor XII (Hageman) deficiency in domestic cats. Can J Comp Med 1980;44:309–314.
26. **Peterson JL, Couto CG, Wellman ML.** Hemostatic disorders in cats: a retrospective study and review of the literature. J Vet Intern Med 1995;9:298–303.
27. **Otto CM, Dodds WJ, Greene CE.** Factor XII and partial prekallikrein defi-

ciencies in a dog with recurrent gastrointestinal hemorrhage. J Am Vet Med Assoc 1991;198:129–131.
28. **Chinn DR, Dodds WJ, Selcer BA.** Prekallikrein deficiency in a dog. J Am Vet Med Assoc 1986;188:69–71.
29. **Turrentine MA, Sculley PW, Green EM, Johnson GS.** Prekallikrein deficiency in a family of miniature horses. Am J Vet Res 1986;47:2464–2467.
30. **Geor RJ, Jackson ML, Lewis KM, Fretz PB.** Prekallikrein deficiency in a family of Belgian horses. J Am Vet Med Assoc 1990;197:741–745.

CHAPTER 160

Factor XI Deficiency

• PATRICIA A. GENTRY

Hereditary factor XI (FXI) deficiency in cattle, dogs, and humans is associated with a hemorrhagic diathesis that differs from that observed in classic hemophilia.[1-6] Spontaneous bleeding is rare, and hemorrhagic episodes generally occur following surgery or trauma. Bleeding occurs most frequently in tissues in which a fibrin clot is susceptible to premature degradation because of high endogenous fibrinolytic activity. The delayed bleeding response in individuals with reduced levels of FXI activity is due to the dual role of FXI in regulating coagulation. Although FXI is not involved in the initiation of coagulation after vascular injury, it is essential for maintaining the process until wound healing has occurred. It does this by catalyzing the biochemical pathway that sustains thrombin generation and hence fibrin formation, and by the downregulation of the activation of the fibrinolytic system which prevents premature fibrin degradation (Fig. 160.1).

CHARACTERISTICS OF FXI

FXI is a glycoprotein synthesized in the liver.[1] Normal plasma FXI levels have been estimated to be 3 to 6 μg/mL in humans and approximately 2 μg/mL in cattle. The protein has been purified to homogeneity from human, bovine, porcine, rabbit, and murine plasmas. With the exception of the rabbit, FXI circulates in plasma as a dimeric molecule consisting of two identical subunits linked by a disulfide bond. Although the complete amino acid sequence has only been determined for human FXI, analysis of partial amino acid sequences reveals close homology among human, bovine, and murine FXI sequences. The estimated molecular weight of bovine FXI is 113 to 124 kDa, which is smaller than the 140 to 175 kDa for human FXI and the 160 kDa for murine FXI. These molecular weight differences are likely due to posttranslational modification of the various types of FXI molecules which result in differences in carbohydrate content. During the conversion of FXI to its activated state, factor XIa (FXIa), each FXI subunit is cleaved at a single site to yield two identical peptides, each containing a catalytic site and linked by disulfide bonds. FXIa consists of a C-terminal trypsin-like cata-

lytic light chain and an N-terminal noncatalytic heavy chain composed of four repeated amino acid sequences called "apple" domains that are designated as A_1 through A_4 (Fig. 160.2). The A_4 domain not only provides the binding site for the primary activator of FXI, namely activated FXII (FXIIa), but it is also required for the molecular dimerization that is essential for the expression of a biologically functional protein.[7] The A_3 domain contains the binding site for both factor IX (FIX), which is the major plasma substrate for FXIa, and for activated platelets. The A_1 domain contains the binding site for high-molecular-weight kininogen (HK), a FXI cofactor, and for thrombin.[1] In plasma, FXI and HK circulate in an equimolar complex.[7]

The gene coding for human FXI is located on chromosome 4, is 23 kb long, and contains 15 exons and 14 introns.[8] The bovine gene for FXI is located on chromosome 27.[9] The bovine and human nucleotide sequences for exons 13, 14, and 15 exhibit 90%, 83%, and 86% homology, respectively. The bovine amino acid sequences, deduced from the nucleotide sequences, for both the active site serine region and for the seven cystine residue sequence that forms the intramolecule disulfide bonds in the FXI protein are similar to those of the human protein.[9] Preliminary evidence indicated that the mutation responsible for FXI deficiency in cattle is not associated with either exon 14 or exon 15, which code for the active site region of the protein. Subsequently, the elucidation of the complete sequence of the bovine FXI gene revealed that the mutation is due to an insertion in exon 12.

ROLES OF FXI IN HEMOSTASIS

Thrombin Generation

In the vascular system, there are two interrelated pathways that generate thrombin, the key enzyme in thrombus formation. The tissue factor, or extrinsic pathway involves the expression of the transmembrane protein tissue factor (TF) on the surface of perturbed endothelial cells which is the trigger for thrombin generation. Circulating factor VII (FVII) binds to TF, forming an active TF-FVII complex that initiates the conversion of pro-

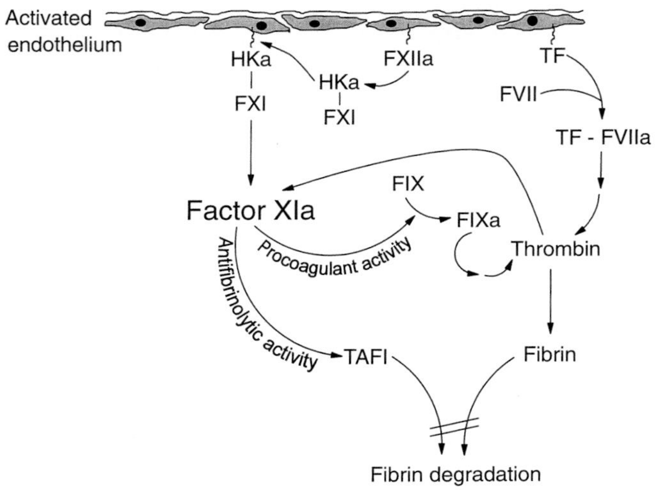

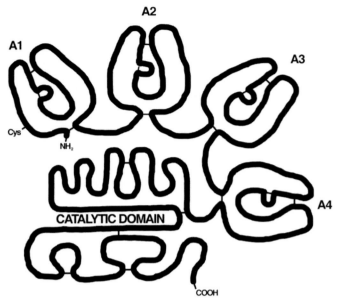

FIGURE 160.1 An outline of the participation of factor XI (FXI) in hemostasis as a procoagulant factor in thrombin generation and as antifibrinolytic agent through activation of thrombin activated fibrinolysis inhibitor (TAFI). The factor XI zymogen, which circulates in complex with high-molecular-weight kininogen (HK), is converted to its activated form (FXIa) by the surface-mediated interactions of activated factor XII (FXIIa) and activated HK (HKa). FXIa initiates thrombin generation by activation of factor IX (FIX). Factor XIa is also generated by the first few thrombin molecules formed by the action of the transiently active tissue factor (TF) pathway in a positive feedback reaction. FXIa is also essential for TAFI formation. TAFI functions to prevent the premature degradation of the fibrin clot at sites of vascular damage.

FIGURE 160.2 A schematic illustration of the structure of the factor XI (FXI) molecule illustrating the catalytic domain and the disulfide bond (-) structure. The four apple domains are shown as A1, A2, A3, and A4. The A1 domain contains the binding site for high-molecular-weight kininogen (HK). The A3 domain contains the binding site for factor IX, the substrate for activated FXI. The A2 domain is also associated with FIX activation. The A4 domain contains the binding site for activated FXII, a physiologic activator of FXI.

thrombin to thrombin through the activation of factor X (FX). However, this is only a transient pathway of thrombin formation because it is rapidly terminated by the action of a circulating inhibitor, tissue factor pathway inhibitor (TFPI). Thrombin generation is sustained at sites of trauma by the formation of FXIa on the negatively charged membranes of activated endothelial cells, platelets, or neutrophils through the interaction of FXI and other components of the contact activation pathway (Fig. 160.3).[7,10]

Activation of FXI

The primary physiologic activators of FXI in plasma are activated factor XII (FXIIa) and thrombin generated by the TF-FVII pathway (Fig. 160.1). The formation of FXIIa is triggered, at a site of vascular damage or inflammation, when the inactive zymogen comes into contact with a negatively charged surface and undergoes a conformation change resulting in its autoactivation.[7,10] A few molecules of FXIIa appear to be sufficient to convert the HK cofactor to a modified form, HKa, which exhibits increased surface binding affinity. Because the majority of plasma FXI circulates as bimolecular complexes with HK, the increased binding of HKa brings large amounts of FXI to the charged surface in proximity to FXIIa, causing it to be readily converted to FXIa (Fig. 160.1). The clinical observation that animals and humans con-

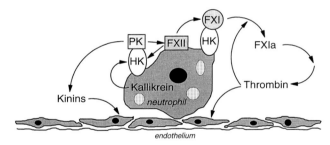

FIGURE 160.3 Diagrammatic representation of the assembly of the contact phase system and the generation of activated factor XI (FXIa) on the surface of an activated neutrophil. Both the high-molecular-weight kininogen-FXI (HK-FXI) and HK-prekallikrein (HK-PK) complexes and factor XII (FXII) can bind to the surface of activated neutrophils. The activation of HK-PK complex induces both local kinin formation and the activation of FXII, which in turn causes feedback activation of the HK-PK complex and the activation of the HK-FXI complex. The activated FXI (FXIa) initiates thrombin formation.

genitally deficient in either FXII or HK rarely bleed illustrates the importance of thrombin activation of FXI in maintaining hemostasis. Indeed, FXI activation by thrombin is the only mechanism that exists in reptiles, birds, and some marine mammals in which the absence of biologic or immunologic FXII is a normal phenomenon.[2]

Actions of Activated FXI

In plasma, even small amounts of FXIa are sufficient to induce thrombin formation. The procoagulant substrate for FXIa is FIX. The interaction between FXIa and FIX is facilitated by (1) the ability of FIX to adhere to the membrane of activated cells at specific sites in proximity to the already adherent FXIa, and (2) FIX binding to the heavy chain of FXIa. Both of these interactions render the FIX molecule accessible to cleavage by FXIa in a reaction that only requires calcium as a cofactor.[1,10] FIXa then functions to generate thrombin through the activation of FX in a reaction that requires FVIIIa, phospholipid, and calcium as cofactors.

In addition to the positive feedback activation of FXI, thrombin has multiple roles at a site of vascular lesion. These include the conversion of fibrinogen to fibrin and the activation of thrombin-activated fibrinolysis inhibitor (TAFI). The formation of TAFI during fibrin clot formation is dependent on adequate amounts of FXIa being present.[11] TAFI is similar to plasma procarboxypeptidase, also known as plasminogen-binding protein, and functions to attenuate fibrin degradation and hence prevents the dissolution of a thrombus until tissue repair has occurred. Hence, FXI has a unique role in the regulation of hemostasis because it can function both as a procoagulant and an antifibrinolytic factor (Fig. 160.1).

Modulation of FXI Activity

FXIa is inhibited by the same group of circulating inhibitors known to modulate other hemostatic serine proteases. These inhibitors include α_1-antitrypsin (α_1AT), C1-inhibitor, antithrombin (AT), and α_1-antiplasmin (α_1AP). Until recently $\alpha 1$AT was considered to be the main FXIa inhibitor in plasma. However, in vivo studies with both rabbits and chimpanzees have confirmed that C1-inhibitor is the major circulating FXIa inhibitor.[12] For example, in the primate model, 68% of infused FXIa was found to complex with the C1-inhibitor compared to 10% with α_1AT, 9% with AT, and 13% with α_1-AP. Further, the clearance half-life of the FXIa-α_1AT complex was 349 minutes compared with 95 to 104 minutes for the other FXIa-inhibitor complexes.

FXI LEVELS IN PLASMA

In veterinary medicine, plasma FXI levels are determined in a functional coagulation assay that is a modification of the routine coagulation screening assay, the activated partial thromboplastin time (APTT). The APTT assay will discriminate between FXI homozygous deficient and normal animals but is not sensitive enough to detect the heterozygous condition. The modified APTT assay involves mixing test plasma with plasma from an animal deficient in FXI and measuring the extent to which the test plasma sample can correct the clotting time of the FXI-deficient plasma relative to the correction produced by a pooled plasma prepared from multiple normal donors of the same species. For example, the concentration of FXI activity in the pooled donor plasma is designated as 100%, and a patient would be deemed to have an FXI activity 25% of normal if its plasma shortens the PTT of FXI-deficient plasma (0%) only 25% as well as that observed when pooled normal plasma is added.

In cattle, dogs, and humans the sex of the animal does not affect normal plasma FXI levels. Newborn calves exhibit plasma FXI activity at $74 \pm 3\%$ of adult values, but this rises to 100% within 72 hours. In contrast, in humans, adult plasma FXI levels are not reached until 2 to 6 months of age.[1] In dogs and cattle, circulating levels of FXI remain unchanged throughout pregnancy and parturition, whereas a 30 to 50% decline in FXI activity occurs in human females toward the end of pregnancy.[1,13]

OCCURRENCE AND EXPRESSION OF FXI DEFICIENCY

FXI deficiency is the most common hereditary coagulation disorder in cattle but is relatively rare in other domestic animals. It has been identified in three breeds of dogs (English springer Spaniels, Kerry blue terriers, and great Pyrenees) and in two breeds of cattle (North American Holstein and Japanese Black cattle).[2–6] Through worldwide exportation of Holstein semen, FXI deficiency is known to have been introduced into cattle herds in England, Australia, New Zealand, and the Netherlands. The majority of cases of FXI deficiency reported in the human population are in families of Jewish origin.[1,14] There are similarities in the clinical expression of this disorder in all species, with hemorrhagic episodes being more likely to occur in homozygous deficient animals that have essentially no circulating FXI activity than in mildly deficient heterozygous animals that have variable amounts of plasma FXI activity.[1,3,5,15] In Canadian Holstein cattle, the mean ($\pm$ standard deviation) plasma FXI activity was determined to be $2 \pm 2\%$ for 48 homozygous deficient animals, $38 \pm 10\%$ for 92 heterozygous animals, and $94 \pm 21\%$ for 316 normal animals.[3] These values for the homozygous and heterozygous animals are somewhat lower than the values of $4 \pm 3\%$ and $57 \pm 10\%$ reported for the FXI-deficient homozygous and FXI heterozygous human population, while the range of values for the normal population is similar.[15] In Japanese Black cattle, the mean plasma FXI activity for five homozygous animals was reported to be $6.2 \pm 2.0\%$ of normal on the basis of the efficiency with which the bovine plasma corrected human FXI-deficient plasma.[16] However, human FXI-deficient plasma is less sensitive in detecting reduced FXI activity in bovine plasma than bovine FXI-deficient plasma.

Although only a small number of FXI affected dogs have been studied, the values reported in the Spaniel and Kerry blue families are similar: in homozygous deficient dogs the range of plasma FXI activity is 2.5 to 11% of normal, while the range in heterozygous dogs is 23 to 46%.[5,6] Inherited FXI deficiency has not been reported in other domestic animals. Reduced plasma FXI activity appeared to be the cause of epistaxis in a cat. However, in this case, the depression of functional activity to less than 5% of normal was determined to be due to an acquired circulating FXI inhibitor rather than to impaired FXI synthesis.[17]

The hemorrhagic clinical symptoms associated with FXI deficiency in animals and humans are generally mild but can be catastrophic after surgery or severe trauma. Bleeding is generally not observed until 12 to 14 hours postsurgery and may be delayed up to 4 days. In Holstein cattle, as in humans, the incidence and severity of hemorrhagic episodes are variable. Although the majority of fatal bleeding episodes in Holstein cattle occur in FXI homozygous deficient animals, mild hemorrhage at castration has been noted in both homozygous and heterozygous bull calves. In contrast, an FXI homozygous Holstein cow underwent caesarian surgery uneventfully. Preliminary reports suggest that the risk of hemorrhage may be higher in Japanese Black cattle than in Holsteins.[16]

In FXI-deficient dogs, transfusions of fresh-frozen plasma can return the APTT and plasma FXI activity values to within reference range limits, although multiple transfusions may be needed to stop hemorrhage.[5] Transfusion of fresh whole blood also controlled the epistaxis that occurred in a cat with an acquired inhibitor to FXI.[17]

In all species, FXI deficiency appears to be transmitted as an autosomal recessive trait.[1,2,15,18] In both the cattle and human populations, the observation that there is a parallel reduction in the plasma levels of plasma FXI coagulant activity and FXI antigen suggests that the disorder is caused by a lack of expression of the FXI protein rather than the synthesis of a nonfunctional protein.[19,20] This conclusion is compatible with the gene mutation that results in expression of a shortened, inactive protein. In a mouse model, in which disruption of the FXI gene rendered the mice FXI deficient, the coagulation profile and bleeding tendencies were similar to those reported in cattle and humans.[21]

When the prevalence of FXI deficiency was first evaluated in Canadian Holsteins, the gene frequency for the heterozygous condition was estimated to be between 7 and 16%, which was similar to the value of 13.4% reported for the human population.[15,18] After more than a decade of screening plasma from Holstein bulls for FXI activity levels and using the results to eliminate heterozygous sires from breeding programs, the incidence of heterozygotes in Canadian Holsteins is now estimated to be less than 3%.[3] All Canadian Holstein semen used for export is obtained from bulls that have tested normal for FXI deficiency. The incidence of FXI heterozygous cattle will be further reduced when molecular technology is available for routine screening. The importance of eliminating FXI deficiency from the Holstein population is that although cattle with the disorder exhibit only infrequent hemorrhagic episodes, the reproductive performance of clinically asymptomatic FXI heterozygous cows is impaired.[22] Consequently, the disorder has

potential economic significance for the dairy industry. Reproductive problems related to menorrhagia, threatened miscarriages, and postpartum hemorrhage have also been reported in FXI-deficient human females.[1]

ASSOCIATION OF FXI WITH INFLAMMATORY RESPONSE

Although not observed in the human FXI-deficient population, cattle homozygous for FXI deficiency are more susceptible to secondary health problems such as mastitis, chronic pneumonia, and chronic dermatitis than their normal herd mates; this may be related to altered neutrophil function.[3,23] Neutrophils isolated from FXI homozygous cattle appear to be more susceptible to spontaneous activation, and exhibit an increased respiratory burst in response to mild stimulation with either C3b or C5a complement fractions, compared to neutrophils isolated from normal herd mates (Table 160.1). The neutrophil can serve as a circulating platform for the activation of the FXIIa-kallikrein cascade of the contact activation system in part because both HK-FXI and HK-prekallikrein (HK-PK) complexes, as well as FXII, can bind to the cell surface (Fig. 160.3). In normal animals, both FXI and prekallikrein compete as substrates for FXIIa.[10] Hence, when the FXI protein is absent, it is possible that higher than normal amounts of kallikrein can be formed. Kallikrein is not only chemotactic for neutrophils and stimulates them to undergo the respiratory burst and degranulation, but it also induces the generation of bradykinin, a potent vasodilator.[10] These reactions can produce increased vascular permeability that may contribute (at least in part) to the appearance of blood in the colostrum, which is consistently observed in cows that are either homozygous or heterozygous for FXI deficiency. It has yet to be determined whether an association between decreased plasma FXI and in-

TABLE 160.1	Comparison of Superoxide Anion Production (nmol) Between Unstimulated and Stimulated Neutrophils Isolated from Factor XI-Deficient Cows (FXI Neutrophils) and Normal Cows (Normal Neutrophils)

Assay Conditions	Normal Neutrophils (mean ± SEM)	FXI Neutrophils (mean ± SEM)
Unstimulated	0.5 ± 0.2	0.9 ± 0.2
Zymogen activated serum	3.5 ± 0.4	5.7 ± 1.2
Opsonized zymogen particles	12.7 ± 3.6	22.2 ± 2.2
12-myristate 13-acetate	37.2 ± 2.9	52.8 ± 2.3

The mean ± standard error values (SEM) were calculated from results of duplicate samples of neutrophils obtained from eight normal cows and from five FXI-deficient cows. Superoxide production was determined by the ability of neutrophil released to reduce cytochrome C as described in Liptrap RM, Gentry PA, Ross ML, Cummings E. Preliminary findings of altered follicular activity in Holstein cows with coagulation factor XI deficiency. Vet Res Commun 1995;19:463–471.

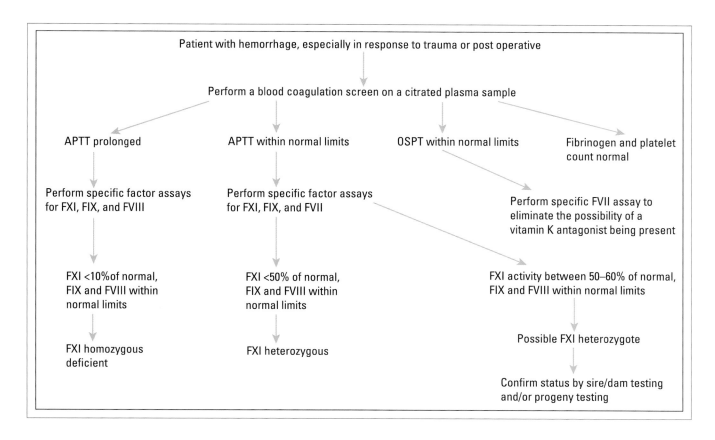

creased kallikrein production was responsible for the spontaneous hemorrhage into mammary tissue that led to the discovery of FXI deficiency in a British dairy herd.[24]

FXI deficiency in Kerry Blue terriers is associated with the development of lipoma-like skin tumors that frequently require surgical removal. Postoperative bleeding is observed in these animals.

REFERENCES

1. **Kitchens CS.** Factor XI: a review of its biochemistry and deficiency. Semin Thromb Hemost 1991;17:55–72.
2. **Dodds WJ.** Hemostasis. In: Kaneko JJ, Harvey JW, Bruss ML, eds. Clinical biochemistry of domestic animals. 5th ed. New York: Academic Press, 1997;241.
3. **Gentry PA, Ross ML.** Coagulation factor XI deficiency in Holstein cattle. Can J Vet Res 1995;58:242–247.
4. **Kociba GJ, Ratnoff OD, Loeb WF, Wall RL, Heider LE.** Bovine plasma thromboplastin antecedent (factor XI) deficiency. J Lab Clin Med 1969;74:37–41.
5. **Knowler C, Giger U, Dodds WJ, Brooks M.** Factor XI deficiency in Kerry blue terriers. J Am Vet Med Assoc 1994;205:1557–1561.
6. **Dodds WJ, Kull JE.** Canine factor XI (plasma thromboplastin antecedent) deficiency. J Lab Clin Med 1971;78:746–752.
7. **DeLa Cadena RA, Wachtfogel YT, Colman RW.** Contact activation pathway: inflammation and coagulation. In: Colman RW, Hirsh H, Marder VJ, Salzman EW, eds. Hemostasis and thrombosis: basic principles and clinical practice. 3rd ed. Philadelphia: JB Lippincott, 1994;219.
8. **Tuddenham EGD, Cooper DN.** The molecular genetics of haemostasis and its inherited disorders. Oxford: Oxford University Press, 1994;212.
9. **Robinson JL, Beever JE, Leeuw ND, Lewin HA, Gillings M, Dennis JA, Healy PJ.** Characterization of the 3′ end of the gene for bovine factor XI. J Dairy Sci 1998;81:539-543.
10. **Wachtfogel YT, DeLaCadena RA, Colman RW.** Structural biology, cellular
11. **Minnema MC, Friederich PW, Levi M, vondem Borne, PAKR, Mosnier LO, Meijers JCM, Biemond BJ, Hack CE, Bouma BN, tenCate H.** Enhancement of rabbit jugular vein thrombolysis by neutralization of Factor XI. J Clin Invest 1998;101:10–14.
12. **Wuillemin WA, Hack CE, Bleeker WK, Biemond BJ, Levi M, tenCate H.** Inactivation of factor XIa in vivo: studies in chimpanzees and humans. Thromb Haemost 1996;76:549–555.
13. **Gentry PA, Liptrap RM.** Comparative hemostatic protein alterations accompanying pregnancy and parturition. Can J Physiol Pharmacol 1988;66:671–678.
14. **Bolton-Maggs PHB, Patterson DA, Wensely RT, Tuddenham EGD.** Definition of the bleeding tendency in factor XI-deficient kindreds—a clinical and laboratory study. Thromb Haemost 1995;73:194–202.
15. **Bolon-Maggs PHB, Wan-Yin BY, McCraw AH, Slack J, Kernoff PBA.** Inheritance and bleeding in factor XI deficiency. Br J Haematol 1988; 69:521–528.
16. **Ogawa H, Iga Y.** Factor XI deficiency in Japanese black cattle. Proc Congr Int Soc Anim Clin Biochem 1998;24.
17. **Feldman BF, Soares CJ, Kitchell BE, Brown CC, O'Neill S.** Hemorrhage in a cat caused by inhibition of factor XI (plasma thromboplastin antecedent). J Am Vet Med Assoc 1993;182:589–591.
18. **Gentry PA, Black WD.** Prevalence and inheritance of factor XI (plasma thromboplastin antecedent) deficiency in cattle. J Dairy Sci 1980;63:616–620.
19. **Gentry PA.** The relationship between factor XI coagulant and factor XI antigenic activity in cattle. Can J Comp Med 1984;48:58–62.
20. **Ragni MV, Sinha D, Seaman F, Lewis JH, Spero JA, Walsh PN.** Comparison of bleeding tendency, factor XI coagulant activity, and factor XI antigen in 25 factor XI-deficient kindreds. Blood 1985;65:719–724.
21. **Gailani D, Lasky NM, Broze GJ.** A murine model of factor XI deficiency. Blood Coagul Fibrinolysis 1997;8:134–144.
22. **Liptrap RM, Gentry PA, Ross ML, Cummings E.** Preliminary findings of altered follicular activity in Holstein cows with coagulation factor XI deficiency. Vet Res Commun 1995;19:463–471.
23. **Coomber BL, Galligan CL, Gentry PA.** Comparison of in vivo function of neutrophils from cattle deficient in plasma factor XI activity and from normal animals. Vet Immunol Immunopathol 1997;58:121–131.
24. **Brush PJ, Anderson PH, Gunning RF.** Identification of factor XI deficiency in Holstein-Friesian cattle in Britain. Vet Rec 1978;121:14–17.

CHAPTER 161

Thrombopathias

• JAMES L. CATALFAMO and W. JEAN DODDS

NORMAL PLATELET FUNCTION

Effective diagnosis and clinical management of bleeding diatheses caused by thrombopathia, or platelet dysfunction, requires an understanding of the dynamics of normal platelet function. Platelets are derived from megakaryocytes, which are localized primarily to bone marrow but can also be found in other organs including the lungs.[1,2] Large numbers of these anucleated cell fragments circulate in the vascular compartment as quiescent, discrete, nonadhesive, smooth discs.

When a blood vessel is injured, platelets are rapidly transformed into adhesive spiny spheres capable of attaching to and spreading on damage-exposed matrix components of the subendothelium. The high shear conditions often encountered at sites of vascular trauma require the binding of von Willebrand factor (vWF) to platelet integrin receptors and to specific sites on fibrillar collagen for platelet adhesion to occur. Surface binding events initiate cell signaling pathways which mediate secretion from platelet storage organelles of adenine nucleotides, divalent cations, and serotonin along with anchor proteins including fibrinogen, vWF, fibronectin, and p-selectin.[3] The secreted substances accumulate locally and serve to recruit additional platelets to the injury site, where they anchor to each other to form larger order aggregates. In contrast to cats and most other species, canine platelets lack a secretable pool of vWF.[4] The in vivo significance of this species difference in adhesion and aggregation events has not been determined.

As recruited platelet numbers increase, large order platelet aggregates accumulate and bridge the zone of vascular damage to form a hemostatic plug. The initial hemostatic plug through the action of thrombin on fibrinogen is strengthened and stabilized by the generation of a platelet-fibrin meshwork. This provides a framework for trapping additional platelets and red blood cells (RBCs). Platelets have a highly organized cytoskeleton that regulates anchor protein function.[5] Contraction of cytoskeletal proteins linked to platelet integrin receptors for fibrin(ogen) serves to consolidate the growing clot and its subsequent retraction.

The ability of the normally quiescent platelet to respond within nanoseconds to injury-induced stimuli is central to its role in maintaining vascular integrity. This rapid response is initiated by the interaction of specific ligands with receptors embedded in the platelet membrane surface (Fig. 161.1). Multiple classes of receptors capable of binding the same ligand have recently been reported.[6,7] They apparently expand the extent and repertoire of platelet responses a specific ligand may signal. Species differences in response to platelet stimuli may reflect potential differences in the membrane distribution of receptor subclasses for a specific ligand. The endoperoxides prostacyclin (PGI_2), PGE_2, and PGD_2, which are synthesized by endothelial cells and released into the vascular space, serve as antagonist ligands that react with their respective platelet receptors to dampen platelet reactivity.[8] PGI_2 inhibits platelet reactivity by elevating intraplatelet cyclic adenosine monophosphate (cAMP) and decreasing free ionized calcium and inositol phosphate formation.[9] Endothelium-derived nitric oxide can also reduce platelet responsiveness by raising the level of intracellular cyclic guanosine monophosphate (GMP).[10]

Platelet integrin and non-integrin glycoprotein receptors play a critical role in adhesion (platelet-subendothelial matrix interactions) and aggregation (platelet-platelet association) events.[11] Integrin receptors are composed of alpha and beta subunits. The $\alpha_{IIb}\beta_3$ complex ($GPII_b$-III_a) is the most abundant platelet integrin and functions as the activation-dependent receptor for fibrinogen, fibronectin, and vWF.[12] The binding of fibrinogen to this receptor is essential for normal platelet aggregation.[13] Platelet adhesion and aggregation at high shear rates depend on vWF binding to $\alpha_{IIb}\beta_3$.[14] Platelet adhesion to collagen is supported by its binding to the integrin receptor $\alpha^2\beta_1$ (GPI_aII_a).[15] This receptor is also involved in signaling collagen-induced platelet activation.[16]

Platelets also intimately network with the coagulation system[17] and provide a phospholipid membrane surface for assembly of coagulation protein complexes on activated platelets. This serves to accelerate rates of clot formation dramatically at sites of vascular injury.

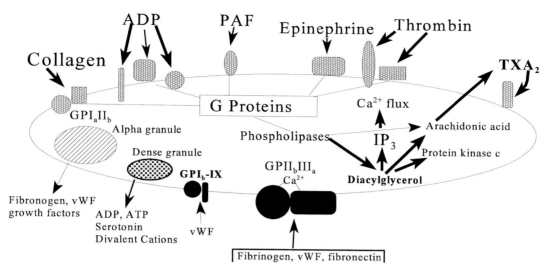

FIGURE 161.1 Platelet cell surface receptors and their role in initiating "outside in" and "inside out" cell signaling. Multiple receptors for a specific ligand may initiate different signaling events. Ligand binding activates phospholipase C via coupled G proteins to generate IP_3 and diacylglycerol (DAG) as well as mobilize ionized calcium from platelet storage sites. Ca^{2+} also activates phospholipase A_2 to release arachidonic acid, which is converted to thromboxane A_2. Thromboxane is released and activates other platelets via its surface receptor. DAG stimulates protein kinase C to phosphorylate intraplatelet proteins critical for platelet function, including dense and alpha granule release. Changes in the phosphorylation state or conformation of the cytoplasmic domains of adhesion receptors enhances binding of the anchor proteins fibrinogen and vWF. vWF binds to GPI_b-IX and under high shear to $GPII_b$-III_a to support platelet adhesion to damaged subendothelium. Platelet aggregation is mediated by bound fibrinogen bridging $GPII_b$-III_a receptors on adjacent platelets. Release of dense granule constituents serves to amplify platelet reactivity. Elevation of intraplatelet cAMP blocks ionized calcium mobilization and phosphoinositide hydrolysis; nitric oxide derived from the endothelium dampens platelet reactivity by increasing the level of cyclic GMP. (Adapted from Brooks, Catalfamo. Platelet dysfunction. In: Bounagura JD, ed. Kirk's current veterinary therapy XIII. Philadelphia: WB Saunders Co. 2000;443, Figure 1.)

CLINICAL SIGNS OF THROMBOPATHIA

Signs characteristic of platelet dysfunction include bleeding from mucosal surfaces. The patient may present with gingival hemorrhage, epistaxis, melena, or hematuria; cutaneous ecchymoses; and prolonged or excessive bleeding at sites of surgery or trauma. In contrast, pinpoint hemorrhages or petechiae are more commonly seen in thrombocytopenic patients. These signs are not unique to platelet dysfunction and may be similar to those seen in other disorders of primary hemostasis including von Willebrand disease (vWD).

The most obvious findings on initial examination are frequently signs of acute or chronic blood loss anemia. Effective diagnosis of an underlying defect of platelet function requires that the clinician suspect a bleeding diathesis and implement a diagnostic plan to evaluate hemostasis.

DIAGNOSTIC EVALUATION

The initial approach to evaluation of bleeding should focus on distinguishing blood loss caused by injury to blood vessels from a systemic bleeding disorder. Thorough history and physical examination, in some cases including ancillary diagnostic procedures (radiography, ultrasonography, endoscopy), is usually sufficient to locate the source and underlying cause of hemorrhage

from large vessels. A history of repeated episodes of hemorrhage, bleeding at multiple sites, and concurrent disease known to affect hemostasis suggests the presence of a systemic bleeding diathesis. Systematic evaluation of preliminary screening tests of hemostasis should then be performed to rule out the more common bleeding disorders before pursuing detailed studies of platelet function.

Thrombocytopenia and coagulation factor deficiencies are the most common bleeding diatheses in domestic animals. Platelet estimate from a blood smear and/or platelet count and coagulation screening tests (activated partial thromboplastin time [APTT], prothrombin time [PT], fibrinogen) are therefore performed as the first step in evaluating any patient suspected of having a bleeding disorder. Determination of plasma vWF concentration provides a rapid screening test for vWD. This defect of primary hemostasis is clinically indistinguishable from platelet dysfunction and should be ruled out before pursuing platelet function studies.

Complete drug history and metabolic profile are included in the preliminary evaluation to identify disease processes likely to impair platelet function and to direct therapy. Platelet dysfunction commonly accompanies disseminated intravascular coagulation (DIC). Tests to define or characterize DIC and fibrinolytic defects (fibrin degradation products and d-dimer titers) as well as hypercoagulable states (antithrombin III level) complete the initial laboratory screening process. An in vivo assessment of primary hemostasis is performed by measuring buccal mucosa bleeding time (BMBT).[18] The finding of long bleeding time, normal platelet count, and normal vWF concentration is compatible with either acquired or inherited platelet dysfunction. The clinical severity of bleeding caused by platelet dysfunction, however, may not always correlate with the degree of prolongation of bleeding time.

LABORATORY TESTS TO EVALUATE PLATELET FUNCTION

Platelet response and specific platelet defects are characterized by performing a series of in vitro tests to evaluate platelet function and structure (Table 161.1). Test procedures must be adapted and validated to accommodate species-specific differences. Accurate measurement of platelet function in aggregation and release studies requires that samples be analyzed within 3 hours of collection to ensure viability of patient platelets. This necessitates patient referral to the clinic or veterinary teaching hospital where testing is performed.

Platelet aggregation in response to different agonist compounds is measured by detecting changes in light transmission of platelet-rich plasma (PRP) samples or changes in electrical impedance of whole blood samples. Whole blood aggregation studies use small sample volumes and are simple to perform, features useful for detecting dysfunction in patients having acquired disorders secondary to disease or drug administration. Ag-

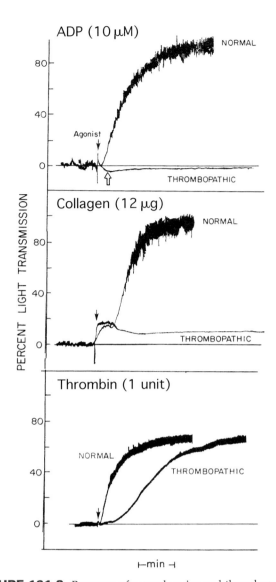

FIGURE 161.2 Response of normal canine and thrombopathic Basset hound platelets to platelet agonists. Percent platelet aggregation expressed as a function of increasing light transmission. Fifty microliters of agonist (↓) was added to a siliconized reaction cuvette containing 0.45 mL of citrated platelet-rich plasma (300,000 platelets/μL) at 37° C and stirred at 850 rpm. The open arrow indicates shape change response. Note the failure of thrombopathic platelets to aggregate in response to ADP and collagen. Thrombin elicits a rate-impaired aggregation response with normal maximal extent. The shape change response of thrombopathic Basset hound platelets is normal.

gregation studies using PRP and the turbidimetric technique are more difficult to perform but provide more detailed information for characterizing and defining platelet response in patients with inherited platelet function defects (Fig. 161.2).

In this method, a beam of light is passed through a heated (37°C) reaction cuvette containing a fixed number of stirred platelets suspended in PRP. Most of the incident light is scattered back to the light source; however,

TABLE 161.1	Laboratory Test to Identify and Characterize Platelet Dysfunction	
Specific Platelet Test	**Platelet Defect Identified**
Dilute whole blood clot retraction	Absent or abnormal GPII$_b$/III$_a$ receptors
Aperture closure time	Abnormal platelet adhesion or aggregation
Platelet aggregation studies: ADP, collagen, arachidonate, other agonists	Abnormal shape change Abnormal signal recognition Abnormal signal pathways Abnormal inter platelet adhesion Abnormal secretion response
Platelet secretion studies: serotonin, ATP, ADP, adenine nucleotide ratios	Abnormal uptake, storage, metabolism, or release of dense granule constituents
Platelet membrane glycoprotein analysis: GPI$_b$, GPII$_b$, GPIII$_a$	Abnormal adhesion receptors
Platelet ultrastructure (electron microscopy)	Abnormalities in the ultrastructural organization of the platelet including the presence or absence of specific platelet storage organelles

a small fraction of incident light passes through the suspension of platelets to the photo detector, which then transmits the signal to an output devise (chart recorder or digital image). A second cuvette containing platelet poor plasma (PPP) serves as the reference cuvette and represents 100% light transmittance (aggregation). The baseline transmittance (0% aggregation) is generally measured for 1 minute before agonist addition. If the platelets have been isolated in an unactivated state, the baseline transmittance signal will oscillate due to the light-scattering properties of disc-shaped particles when stirred in suspension. Agonist addition to the cuvette will induce a rapid change if platelets change shape from disc to sphere. This change is recorded as a decrease in light transmittance (spherical particles in contrast to discs pack together very efficiently and block more light). As the platelets begin to form aggregates, light transmission increases until it reaches a maximal plateau. The rate and maximal extent of platelet aggregation can then be calculated. Adenosine triphosphate (ATP) secretion from platelet dense granules can be monitored and quantified simultaneously with aggregation. An aggregometer capable of measuring a luminescence signal is required. Luciferin-luciferase reagent is added to the aggregation reaction cuvette prior to agonist. The luminescence signal (rate and maximal extent) generated by agonist-induced secretion of platelet dense granule ATP is recorded. An ATP standard is used to calibrate the luminescence signal.

The impedance method is generally performed using whole blood samples diluted in saline or buffer. Platelet aggregation is detected by measuring the electrical impedance between electrodes immersed in the sample. The electrodes must become coated with a monolayer of platelets before a stable base line is established. On addition of an agonist, platelets will form aggregates that gradually accumulate on the electrodes and thereby increase the impedance between them. The aggregation response is reported as a change in ohms (rate and maximal extent). The impedance method requires longer assay times (up to 15 minutes to reach maximal aggregation) than the optical method. The method is very sensitive to small changes in aggregation. High doses of agonist, therefore, may "mask" abnormal platelet function.

Evaluation of platelet function using the impedance or optical methods does not simulate the hemodynamic conditions of platelet adhesion and aggregation encountered at a vascular lesion. A new platelet function analyzer (PFA-100, Dade Berhing Inc., Miami, FL), which was designed based on work described by Kratzer and Born,[19] uses a small volume of citrated whole blood (0.8 mL) to evaluate the ability of platelets to support primary hemostasis under high shear stress. The anticoagulated blood is aspirated through a capillary under microprocessor-controlled conditions that simulate hemodynamic flow. The blood then passes through an aperture in a membrane coated with collagen and either epinephrine or adenosine diphosphate (ADP). The platelets adhere and aggregate at the aperture until blood flow stops. The results are reported in seconds as closure time. The ability of this system to detect rapidly

(within 5 minutes) defects in primary hemostasis in canines was evaluated (Table 161.2). These preliminary data suggest that the technique has the potential to identify abnormal primary hemostasis in dogs. Dogs diagnosed with Basset hound thrombopathia, Otterhound thrombasthenia, Type 2 vWD, and Type 3 vWD had infinite closure times (longer than 300 seconds for the instrument) for both epinephrine/collagen and ADP/collagen. When purified canine vWF was added to the blood of a dog with type 3 vWD, the closure time became finite for the ADP/collagen cartridge at 10% vWF and corrected at 30%. The epinephrine/collagen cartridge had a finite closure time at 30% vWF and at 50% was within normal reference range.

Platelet function testing is most effective when used to identify animals with severe phenotypes. Obligate carriers and relatives that exhibit mild functional abnormalities can also be identified using this approach. However, function testing is limited by its low test specificity for inherited versus acquired defects. This limitation is heightened for those defects with variable penetrance. Results obtained from platelet function analysis can be used to advise breeders on optimal strategies to control the defect within the population. Future development and utilization of molecular diagnostic techniques for control and elimination of inherited platelet defects will require identification of causative genetic lesions in candidate genes linked to expression of each defect. The genes for human $GPII_b$ and $GPIII_a$ have been sequenced, and causative mutations have been identified in patients with Glanzmann thrombasthenia.[20] Similar progress in dogs and cats will be seen for molecular diagnosis of Glanzmann variants and the other inherited platelet defects.

TABLE 161.2 PFA-100 Closure Times for Dogs with Defective Primary Hemostasis

Defect	Mean Closure Time (seconds)	
	Epinephrine/ Collagen	ADP/ Collagen
Normal dog (n = 5)	95 ± 6	68 ± 4
Adhesion receptor (II_bIII_a) Otterhound Glanzmann variant (n = 2)	>300	>300
Signaling defect (cAMP) Basset hound thrombopathia (n = 4)	>300	>300
Type 1 vWD (n = 2)	>300	143, 192
Type 2 vWD (n = 2)	>300	>300
Type 3 vWD (n = 3)	>300	>300
Type 3 vWD + vWF	94	86
Normal canine reference range (n = 20)	68–184	47–119

vWD, von Willebrand disease; *vWF*, von Willebrand factor.

INHERITED THROMBOPATHIAS

Inherited disorders of platelet function can be classified broadly into disorders of platelet membrane glycoproteins,[21,22] defects involving platelet storage granules,[23–26] and defects of intracellular signaling.[27–29] Inherited platelet defects are rare and are often breed-specific. Features of well-characterized inherited thrombopathias in domestic animals are summarized in Table 161.3.

Adhesion Receptor Defects

Thrombasthenic thrombopathia is a variant of human Glanzmann's thrombasthenia recognized in dogs. The original reports of this autosomally inherited defect in Otterhounds provided evidence that a variable proportion of their circulating platelets shared morphologic features with those of Bernard-Soulier syndrome, including circulating giant platelets. During the 1970s and mid-1980s an aggressive selective breeding program, which used the simple clot retraction assay for screening, dramatically reduced the incidence of this defect in the breed. However, by the late 1980s a variant form of the original platelet function defect was identified in several animals related by common ancestry to the original breeding stock. This variant is the defect now encountered in Otterhounds.

In contrast to individuals originally studied, platelets from these Otterhounds lack evidence of a combined defect. In fact, their mean platelet volumes are well within the normal reference range. The functional and biochemical features exhibited by platelets from affected Otterhounds are characteristic of human type I Glanzmann's thrombasthenia. Thrombasthenic Otterhound platelets fail to aggregate in response to physiologic stimuli (ADP, collagen, thrombin, arachidonic acid) and do not support clot retraction. The functional abnormalities are due to the absence or marked reduction in the activation-dependent integrin adhesion receptor shared by fibrinogen and vWF. There are approximately 40,000 to 50,000 copies of this receptor on the platelet surface, and its presence is also required for shear rate-dependent adhesion and aggregation mediated by vWF. α_{IIb} and β_3 integrins are not detected in thrombasthenic platelet membranes analyzed by electrophoretic or flow cytometry techniques using antibodies specific for α_{IIb} and β_3 or their Ca^{2+}-dependent complexes. These findings are similar to those reported for thrombasthenia reported in Great Pyrenees. Both defects appear to be homologues of Type I Glanzmann's thrombasthenia in humans. The Otterhound variant, more commonly

---

TABLE 161.3   Inherited Platelet Thrombopathias in Domestic Animals

Type Defect	Species (Breed)	Features	Reference No.
Adhesion receptor	Dog (Otterhound)	Abnormal platelet adhesion; absent or trace aggregation to most stimuli; abnormal clot retraction; absent or reduced GPII$_b$-III$_a$ complex	21
	Dog (Great Pyrenees)		22
Storage pool	Dog (American cocker spaniel)	Normal number dense granules; abnormal storage and secretion ADP; abnormal platelet aggregation to ADP and collagen; normal clot retraction	23
	Cat (Persian)	Associated with Chédiak-Higashi syndrome; reduced number dense granules; failure to secrete ADP and serotonin; abnormal platelet aggregation; normal clot retraction	24
Signal	Dog (Basset hound)	Abnormal platelet adhesion; absent or trace platelet aggregation in response to most stimuli; normal clot retraction, normal levels GPII$_b$-III$_a$ complex; abnormal phosphodiesterase activity, elevated cAMP	27
	Dog (Spitz)	Abnormal platelet adhesion; absent or trace platelet aggregation in response to most stimuli; normal clot retraction, normal levels GPII$_b$-III$_a$ complex; abnormal signaling pathway	28
	Cow (Simmental)	Absent platelet aggregation in response to most stimuli; abnormal clot retraction, normal GPII$_b$-II$_a$ complex, delayed binding of adhesion proteins, abnormal signaling pathway	29
Combined signal and storage pool	Dog (Grey collie)	Associated with cyclic neutropenia and primitive stem cell disorder; normal platelet aggregation to ADP, partially impaired for other stimuli; defective uptake and storage of serotonin; abnormal platelet protein phosphorylation	25
	Cow (Japanese black)	Associated with Chédiak-Higashi syndrome; reduced number dense granules; decreased serotonin, adenine nucleotides, and Mg^{2+}; abnormal platelet aggregation to collagen, impaired Ca^{2+} mobilization	26

ADP, adenosine diphosphate; *cAMP*, cyclic adenosine monophosphate.

called thrombasthenic thrombopathia, should be renamed Otterhound thrombasthenia.

Storage Pool Defects

The secretion of adenine nucleotides, serotonin, and divalent cations from platelet dense (δ) granules and adhesion proteins from alpha (α) granules is essential for normal platelet function. Most platelet secretion defects are acquired secondary to drug administration. Inherited abnormalities are rare and may be expressed as an isolated defect, as reported for the δ-storage pool defect in American cocker spaniels,[23] or associated with Chédiak-Higashi syndrome, as observed in Persian cats.[24] The defect reported in cats is due to a reduced number of dense granules and is inherited as an autosomal recessive trait. The bleeding diathesis varies from mild to severe. Platelets from affected cats fail to secrete serotonin and ADP and exhibit abnormal platelet aggregation with normal clot retraction. Similar defects have been reported in fawn-hooded rats, Aleutian mink, Hereford cattle, and beige mice.

The defect in the American cocker spaniel is a unique δ-storage pool defect that resembles human platelet δ-storage pool disease.[23] It is inherited as an autosomal recessive trait. Dense granules in platelets from affected dogs are normal in number and appearance. Most but not all affected individuals have a prolonged bleeding time. Clot retraction and serotonin uptake are normal. Platelets from affected dogs exhibit variably abnormal aggregation responses to ADP and collagen. Dense granule ATP content is normal; this is in marked contrast to ADP, which ranges from 10 to 30% of normal. This reduction results in an elevated ATP:ADP ratio (8.3 versus 1.9 for normal dogs) and is considered diagnostic for δ-storage pool disease. Dogs with this platelet storage pool defect serve as important animal models for understanding mechanisms of adenine nucleotide storage in δ granules. Studies using the model are likely to lead to elucidation and characterization of proteins involved in platelet ADP transport.

Signaling Defects

Defective platelet signal pathways have been implicated in thrombopathias reported in Basset hounds, Spitz dogs, and Simmental cattle. Basset hound thrombopathia is a unique autosomally inherited defect.[27] Variable penetrance and expression of the trait have made it difficult to establish the precise mode of genetic transmission despite the analysis of platelet function in more than 300 Basset hounds. Breeding studies suggested that the defect may be transmitted as an autosomal recessive trait. However, the existence of large numbers of dogs with intermediate function raised the possibility of an autosomal dominant mode of genetic transmission. Identification of a candidate gene specific for the defect and subsequent molecular genetic analysis of animals difficult to classify on the basis of their platelet function phenotype should establish the genotypes. This will help clarify the mode of genetic transmission for this defect.

Functional abnormalities in Basset hound thrombopathia are associated with impaired cyclic AMP metabolism and abnormal platelet phosphodiesterase activity (PDE). Elevation of basal levels of cyclic AMP in thrombopathic platelets interferes with cell signaling events critical to adhesion receptor function. This results in abnormal platelet aggregation in response to most agonists. In vitro shear-rate–dependent platelet adhesion and aggregation stimulated by epinephrine/collagen and ADP/collagen are also abnormal. Platelet shape change, clot retraction, and concentrations of membrane adhesion receptors (including $\alpha_{IIb}\beta_3$) are normal. Platelet content of adenine nucleotides, serotonin, and anchor molecules stored in alpha granules, including fibrinogen, are normal. However, signaling events leading to agonist-induced release of dense granule constituents are abnormal. Agonist-induced ionized calcium flux (mobilization from intraplatelet stores and extracellular transport) is normal. Turnover of inositol phosphates, including IP_3, is enhanced in thrombopathic Basset hound platelets. Animals affected with this defect serve as valuable animal models for elucidation of signaling events pivotal to adhesion receptor function and identification of proteins involved in regulation of platelet cyclic nucleotide metabolism. The defect reported in a Spitz is similar in clinical, functional, and biochemical features; however, the molecular basis for the defect may differ from that reported for thrombopathic Bassets.[28]

Thrombopathia in Simmental cattle is characterized by an absent or micro aggregation response to ADP, collagen, and the calcium ionophore A23187. Mobilization of ionized calcium and myosin-light chain phosphorylation are normal. Normal numbers of $\alpha_{IIb}\beta_3$ receptors are present on platelets of affected individuals. Although binding of fibrinogen to its $\alpha_{IIb}\beta_3$ receptor complex occurs, the rate of activated fibrinogen receptor expression is significantly delayed. The bleeding diathesis observed in this defect is attributed to delayed binding of adhesion receptor molecules. The molecular basis for the abnormal signaling remains to be established and has been attributed to possible abnormalities in events that regulate platelet cytoskeletal interaction with cytoplasmic domains of α_{IIb} and β_3 integrins and its assembly into a functional complex.[29]

Combined Signal and Storage Pool Defects

The combined defect identified in the Grey collie is found in association with cyclic neutropenia and primitive cell disorder. Platelets from these dogs aggregate normally in response to ADP and exhibit variable reactivity to other agonists including collagen. The uptake and dense granule storage of serotonin is abnormal. The defect in signaling has been attributed to abnormal platelet protein phosphorylation and is associated with reduced phospholipase C activity.[25]

5. **Morrison S, Uchida N, Weissman I.** The biology of hematopoietic stem cells. Annu Rev Cell Dev Biol 1995;11:35–71.

6. **Orlic D, Bodine D.** What defines a pluripotent hematopoietic stem cell (PHSC): will the real PHSC please stand up. Blood 1994;84:3991–3994.

7. **McSweeney PA, Rouleau KA, Storb R, Bolles L, Wallace PM, Beauchamp M, Krizanac- Bengez L, Moore P, Sale G, Sandmaier B, de Revel T, Appelbaum FR, Nash RA.** Canine CD34: cloning of the cDNA and evaluation of an antiserum to recombinant protein. Blood 1996;88:1192–2003.

8. **Shull RM, Hastings NE, Selcer RR, Jones JB, Smith JR, Cullen WC, Constantopoulos G.** Bone marrow transplantation in canine mucopolysaccharidosis I. Effects within the central nervous system. J Clin Invest 1987;79:435–443.

9. **O'Brien JS, Storb R, Raff RF, Harding J, Appelbaum F, Morimoto S, Kishimoto Y, Graham T, Ahern-Rindell A, O'Brien SL.** Bone marrow transplantation in canine GM1 gangliosidosis. Clin Genet 1990;38:274–280.

10. **Taylor RM, Farrow BR, Stewart GJ.** Amelioration of clinical disease following bone marrow transplantation in fucosidase-deficient dogs. Am J Med Genet 1992;42:628–632.

11. **Deeg HJ, Shulman HM, Albrechtsen D, Graham TC, Storb R, Koppang N.** Batten's disease: failure of allogeneic bone marrow transplantation to arrest disease progression in a canine model. Clin Genet 1990;37:264–270.

12. **Weiden PL, Storb R, Graham TC, Schroeder ML.** Severe hereditary haemolytic anemia in dogs treated by marrow transplantation. Br J Haematol 1976;33:357–362.

13. **Felsburg PJ, Somberg RL, Hartnett BJ, Suter SF, Henthron PS, Moore PF, Weinberg KI, Ochs HD.** Full immunologic reconstitution following nonconditioned bone marrow transplantation for canine X-linked severe combined immunodeficiency. Blood 1997;90:3214–3221.

14. **Kwok WW, Schuening F, Stead RB, Miller AD.** Retroviral transfer of genes into canine hemopoietic progenitor cells in culture: a model for human gene therapy. Proc Natl Acad Sci USA 1986;83:4552–4555.

15. **Eglitis MA, Kantoff PW, Jolly JD, Jones JB, Anderson WF, Lothrop CD Jr.** Gene transfer into hematopoietic progenitor cells from normal and cyclic hematopoietic dogs using retroviral vectors. Blood 1988;71:717–722.

16. **Al-Lebban ZS, Henry JM, Jones JB, Eglitis MA, Anderson WF, Lothrop CD Jr.** Increased efficiency of gene transfer with retroviral vectors in neonatal hematopoietic progenitor cells. Exp Hematol 1990;18:180–184.

17. **Stead RB, Kwok WW, Storb R, Miller AD.** Canine model for gene therapy: inefficient gene expression in dogs reconstituted with autologous marrow infected with retroviral vectors. Blood 1988;71:742–747.

18. **Schuening FG, Kawahara K, Miller AD, To R, Goehle S, Stewart D, Mullally K, Fisher L, Graham TC, Appelbaum FR, et al.** Retrovirus-mediated gene transduction into long-term repopulating marrow cells of dogs. Blood 1991;78:2568–2576.

19. **Schuening FG, Storb R, Stead RB, Goehle S, Nash R, Miller AD.** Improved retroviral transfer of genes into canine hematopoietic progenitor cells kept in long-term marrow culture. Blood 1989;74:152–155.

20. **Carter RF, Abrams-Ogg AC, Dick JE, Kruth SA, Valli VE, Kamel-Reid S, Dube ID.** Autologous transplantation of canine long-term marrow culture cells genetically marked by retroviral vectors. Blood 1992;79:356–364.

21. **Bienzle D, Abrams-Ogg AC, Kruth SA, Acland-Snow J, Carter RF, Dick JE, Jacobs RM, Kamel-Reid S, Dube ID.** Gene transfer into hematopoietic stem cells: long-term maintenance of in vitro activated progenitors without marrow ablation. Proc Natl Acad Sci USA 1994;91:350–354.

22. **Barquinero J, Kiem HP, von Kalle C, Darovsky B, Goehle S, Graham T, Siedel K, Strob R, Schuening FG.** Myelosuppressive conditioning improves autologous engraftment of genetically marked hematopoietic repopulating cells in dogs. Blood 1995;85:1195–1201.

23. **Hurwitz DR, Kirchgesser M, Merrill W, Galanopoulos T, McGrath CA, Emami S, Hansen M, Cherington V, Appel JM, Bizinkauskas CB, Brackmann HH, Levine PH, Greenberger JS.** Systemic delivery of human growth hormone or human factor IX in dogs by reintroduced genetically modified autologous bone marrow stromal cells. Hum Gene Ther 1997;8:137–156.

24. **Foley R, Ellis R, Walker I, Wan Y, Carter R, Boyle M, Braciak T, Addison C, Graham F, Gauldie J.** Intramarrow cytokine gene transfer by adenoviral vectors in dogs. Hum Gene Ther 1997;8:545–553.

25. **Ferrara ML, Occhiodoro T, Fuller M, Hawthorne WJ, Teutsch S, Tucker VE, Hopwood JJ, Stewart GJ, Anson DS.** Canine fucosidosis: a model for retroviral gene transfer into haematopoietic stem cells. Neuromuscul Disord 1997;7:361–366.

26. **Shull R, Lu X, Dube I, Lutzko C, Kruth S, Abrams-Ogg A, Kiem H, Goehle S, Schuening F, Millan C, Carter R.** Humoral immune response limits gene therapy in canine MPS I. Blood 1996;88:377–379.

SECTION XIV
Specific Species—Appropriate Hematology
Stephen A. Smith

CHAPTER 163

Normal Hematology of the Dog

• JAMES H. MEINKOTH and KENNETH D. CLINKENBEARD

ERYTHROCYTES

Morphology

The canine erythrocyte is a biconcave disc, approximately 7 μm in diameter. The biconcave shape is more pronounced in the dog than in other domestic animals, giving their red cells a clearly visible central pallor (Fig. 163.1) when viewed in the monolayer of well-made blood smears. This prominent central pallor, which normally encompasses approximately the central one-third to one-half of the diameter of the cell, makes recognition of spherocytes possible in this species. Central pallor may be lost at the edges of a smear, where shear forces distort normal morphology.

Canine erythrocytes normally display only mild anisocytosis and poikilocytosis. Echinocyte formation may be an artifact related to smear preparation (i.e., crenation) but has also been reported in certain disease states.[1] Clear, refractile areas (artifacts) within red cells may be seen if the blood smear is not adequately dried before staining.

When blood smears are stained with Romanowsky stains, such are Wright's stain, polychromatophilic (blue staining) cells may be seen occasionally, but these normally comprise less than 1% of the cells (Fig. 163.2). These represent erythrocytes recently released from the bone marrow and are recognized as reticulocytes when blood is stained with certain supravital stains, such as new methylene blue. Canine reticulocytes are mostly of the aggregate type, containing one or more large, distinct clumps of blue staining material (Fig. 163.3). In dogs, polychromasia noted on Romanowsky-stained smears correlates well with reticulocytosis,[2] although accurate, reproducible evaluation of polychromasia requires more microscopy experience.

Rare nucleated red cells and Howell-Jolly bodies can be seen in blood smears from normal dogs (Fig. 163.2). Nucleated red cells may be more numerous in newborn pups, but numbers decrease rapidly within the first week of life and reach adult levels by approximately 1 to 2 months of age.[3,4] Low numbers (1 to 10 per slide) of hemoglobin (Hgb) crystals have been reported in blood smears of clinically normal dogs younger than 3 months of age.[5] Hgb crystals are square to rectangular structures that stain similar to, or slightly darker than, Hgb and often deform the red cell that contains them.

Quantitative Parameters

Table 163.1 provides typical reference ranges for erythrocyte parameters of adult dogs. Reference ranges are designed to include values found in the majority (typically 90 to 95%) of "normal" animals. Reference ranges may vary according to the population used to collect the data and the definition of "normal." Many published reference ranges for canine hematologic values are derived from research animals and represent a single breed raised under confinement conditions. Such ranges may be narrower than would be applicable to a general patient population in which breed, age, and environmental variables are present. Alternatively, reference ranges that are derived from pound dogs or "clinically healthy" animals brought to a veterinary clinic may be inappropriately wide because of subclinical disease, nutritional status, and physiologic or environmental influences (e.g., fear associated with being in a strange environment and phlebotomy). Common, clinically significant sources of variability are discussed later.

Hgb, Hematocrit, and RBC Count

All three of these measurements of red cell mass are interrelated and, in the absence of significant alterations of red cell size and Hgb concentration, tend to parallel each other. Hematocrit (Hct) is the most easily measured by the practitioner and is most frequently used.

The red cell mass of neonatal animals varies significantly from adults (Table 163.2). At birth, Hgb, Hct, and RBC are near normal but decline rapidly over about the first 2 months of life. After this values start to increase, generally reaching adult levels by approximately 6 months to 1 year of age.[4,6,7] The magnitude of the drop is clinically significant, with packed cell volume (PCV) values reaching a nadir in the high 20s to low 30s.[3]

Some authors have found a gender affect on red cell mass. One study of beagles showed that males had a slightly higher Hgb concentration than females (16 g/dL versus 15.6 g/dL).[8] The magnitude of this

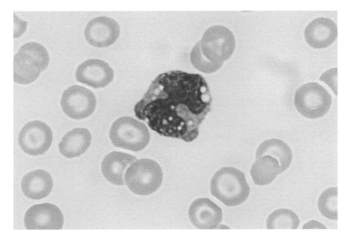

FIGURE 163.1 Vacuolated canine monocyte. Numerous erythrocytes in the background demonstrate distinct central pallor. (Wright-Giemsa, 250 × original magnification. Photo courtesy of Oklahoma State University Clinical Pathology Teaching Files.)

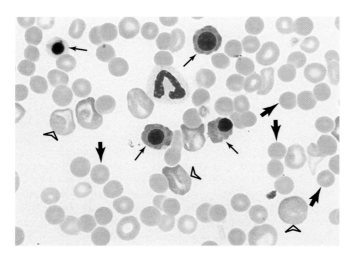

FIGURE 163.2 Blood smear from a dog with an immune-mediated hemolytic anemia. Many large, polychromatophilic erythrocytes are present (arrowheads). Four nucleated red cells (rubricytes and metarubricytes) are also present (thin arrows). Many of the mature erythrocytes are spherocytes (thick arrows). (Wright-Giemsa stain, 250X × original magnification. Photo courtesy of Oklahoma State University Clinical Pathology Teaching Files.)

Mean Corpuscular Volume (MCV), Mean Corpuscular Hemoglobin (MCH), and MCH Concentration (MCHC)

These red cell indices characterize the size and hemoglobinization of the red cell population. In the dog, fetal red cells are larger than those of adults. The MCV of newborn pups is 95 to 100 fL, but rapid replacement of fetal erythrocytes following birth brings this value to adult levels by 2 to 3 months.[3] Breed variations of erythrocyte size have been reported. Some lines of toy and miniature poodles have an inherited macrocytosis with abnormal erythropoiesis.[12,13] These animals have RBC

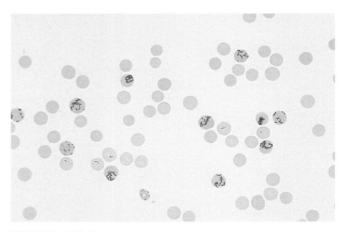

FIGURE 163.3 Canine reticulocytes. Most canine reticulocytes have large aggregates of blue staining precipitate. (new methylene blue stain, 250 × original magnification. Photo courtesy of Oklahoma State University Clinical Pathology Teaching Files.)

TABLE 163.1	Hematologic Reference Ranges for Normal Dogs
Erythrocytes ($\times 10^6$)	5.5–8.5
Hemoglobin (g/dL)	12.0–18.0
PCV (%)	37–55
MCV (fL)	60–77
MCHC (%)	32–36
Reticulocytes (%)	0.0–1.5
Leukocytes/μL	6000–17,000
Neutrophils	3000–11,500
Bands	0–300
Lymphocytes	1000–4800
Monocytes	150–1350
Eosinophil	100–1250
Basophils	Rare
Platelets/μL	200,000–500,000
Mean platelet volume (fL)	6.7–11.1[a]
	3.9–6.1[b]

Data from Jain NC. Schalm's veterinary hematology. 4th ed. Philadelphia: Lea & Febiger, 1986;103–125.
[a] Data from Meyer DJ, Harvey JW. Veterinary laboratory medicine. 2nd ed. Philadelphia: WB Saunders, 1998;345.
[b] Data from Willard MD, Tvedten H, Turnwald GH. Small animal clinical diagnosis by laboratory methods. 2nd ed. Philadelphia: WB Saunders, 1994;359.

change is not likely to be clinically significant as all values are well within the standard reference ranges for adult dogs. Pregnant females have significant changes during gestation. In one study, the PCV of pregnant dogs fell from a baseline of 53% to 32% at term.[6] Numerous studies have shown that Greyhound dogs generally have somewhat higher values related to red cell mass than other dogs.[9-11]

TABLE 163.2	Blood Values in Normal Beagles to 2 Months of Age[a]				
	Age				
	0–3 Days	**14–17 Days**	**28–31 Days**	**40–45 Days**	**56–59 Days**
Number of dogs	46	46	48	44	42
RBC ($\times 10^6$)	4.8 ± 0.8	3.5 ± 0.3	3.9 ± 0.4	4.1 ± 0.4	4.7 ± 0.4
Hemoglobin (g/dL)	15.8 ± 2.9	9.9 ± 1.1	9.6 ± 0.9	9.2 ± 0.7	10.3 ± 0.9
PCV (%)	46.3 ± 8.5	28.7 ± 2.9	28.4 ± 2.5	28.3 ± 2.3	31.4 ± 2.4
MCV (fL)	94.2 ± 5.9	81.5 ± 3.3	71.7 ± 3.5	68.2 ± 2.6	65.8 ± 2.3
MCH (pg)	32.7 ± 1.8	28.0 ± 2.0	24.3 ± 1.6	22.4 ± 1.0	21.8 ± 1.2
MCHC (%)	34.6 ± 1.4	34.3 ± 1.6	33.5 ± 1.4	32.4 ± 1.7	32.6 ± 1.8
nRBC/100 WBC	7.2 ± 6.7	2.4 ± 3.8	1.1 ± 1.5	0.6 ± 0.9	0.1 ± 0.4
Reticulocytes (%)	6.5	6.7	5.8	4.5	3.6
WBC/µL	16,800 ± 5,700	13,600 ± 4,400	13,900 ± 3,300	15,300 ± 3,700	15,700 ± 4,400
Absolute number of WBC/µL					
Band neutrophils	600 ± 500	200 ± 200	100 ± 200	200 ± 200	300 ± 300
Segmented neutrophils	9,200 ± 6,600	6,900 ± 3,100	6,800 ± 2,000	7,400 ± 2,400	8,500 ± 2,900
Lymphocytes	3,700 ± 2,300	4,900 ± 1,700	5,400 ± 1,600	6,100 ± 1,900	5,000 ± 1,500
Monocytes	1,400 ± 1,300	1,100 ± 600	1,100 ± 600	1,300 ± 600	1,400 ± 700
Eosinophils	400 ± 400	500 ± 500	400 ± 400	300 ± 300	400 ± 400
Platelets/µL[b]	302,000	290,000	287,000	321,000	411,000
M:E ratio[b]	1.6:1	1.7:1	1.7:1	1.8:1	1.4:1

[a] Data from Shifrine M, et al. Hematologic changes to 60 days of age in clinically normal Beagles. Lab Anim Sci 1973;23:894–898.
[b] Data from Earl FL, et al. The hemogram and bone marrow profile of normal neonatal, and weanling Beagle dogs. Lab Anim Sci 1973;23:690–695. Values were approximated for various age groups shown here; 5 males and 5 females were studied in each group.

counts that are below standard reference ranges, but due to the large size of the red cells and increased Hgb content, their PCV and Hgb are normal. The reported MCV of affected animals ranges from 84.5 to 106.7 fL (compared with 60 to 77 fL in unaffected animals). Japanese Akita dogs have microcytic red cells with an MCV ranging from 55 to 65 fL. Similarly, Japanese Shiba dogs have microcytic erythrocytes.

Reticulocytes

Reticulocytes are released from the canine marrow in a cyclic manner, with a periodicity of approximately 14 days.[14] Adult dogs generally have less than 1.0 % reticulocytes in peripheral blood. Neonatal animals have significantly higher reticulocyte counts, a manifestation of increased erythropoiesis needed to keep up with a rapidly expanding vascular volume. Reticulocyte counts up to approximately 10% can be seen in dogs during the first 2 months of life.[4,15] This number decreases to adult levels by approximately 5 to 6 months of age.

LEUKOCYTES

Normal Morphology

Neutrophils are the most abundant leukocyte in the peripheral blood of normal dogs. The mature neutrophil has an elongated nucleus that contains several distinct lobules separated by constricted areas (Fig. 163.4). These constricted areas are usually simply narrowing of the nuclear material, but may form thin filamentous structures. The nucleus stains dark purple and has a clumped chromatin pattern consisting of many areas of densely staining heterochromatin. Cytoplasm is generally clear to slightly eosinophilic. Neutrophil granules in the dog are generally indiscernible but may be faintly eosinophilic. Immature or band neutrophils may be present in low numbers in normal animals. These cells contain elongated nuclei that lack the distinct lobulation of the mature cell. The nucleus should have generally parallel sides, lacking any discrete nuclear constrictions (Fig. 163.4). The nuclear chromatin of a band cell is generally less condensed and lighter staining than that of a mature cell. Cytoplasm is similar to that of mature neutrophils.

Lymphocytes in the peripheral blood vary in size, with small lymphocytes being most abundant

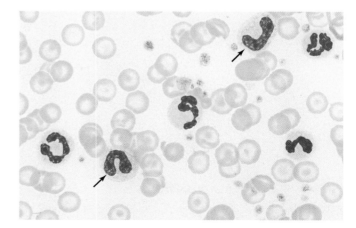

FIGURE 163.4 Four segmented neutrophils and two band neutrophils. Band neutrophils (arrows) lack any distinct nuclear constrictions and have lighter staining nuclear chromatin. (Wright-Giemsa stain, 250 × original magnification. Photo courtesy of Oklahoma State University Clinical Pathology Teaching Files.)

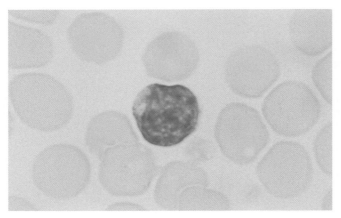

FIGURE 163.5 Small, mature lymphocyte. A small rim of cytoplasm is visible on only one side of the nucleus. (Wright-Giemsa stain, 250 × original magnification. Photo courtesy of Oklahoma State University Clinical Pathology Teaching Files.)

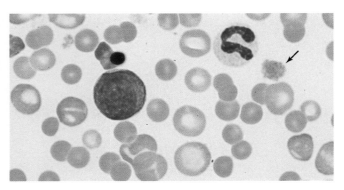

FIGURE 163.7 Blood smear from a dog with immune-mediated hemolytic anemia. A neutrophil, hematogone, and significantly reactive lymphocyte are present. The reactive lymphocyte is enlarged and contains an increased amount of intensely basophilic cytoplasm. An enlarged platelet is also present (arrow). Polychromatophilic erythrocytes and spherocytes are present as in Figure 163-2. (Wright-Giemsa stain, 250 × original magnification. Photo courtesy of Oklahoma State University Clinical Pathology Teaching Files.)

(Fig. 163.5). Small lymphocytes have densely staining nuclei that range from generally round with a flattened side to oval to slightly indented. Nuclear chromatin is densely clumped. Small lymphocytes have only scant amounts of cytoplasm which is pale blue. The cytoplasm is often only a thin rim or crescent that cannot be seen completely encircling the nucleus. Medium-sized lymphocytes occur in blood smears from normal dogs and have more abundant cytoplasm that may completely encircle the nucleus (Fig. 163.6). The nuclei stain lighter and the chromatin appears less dense. Medium-sized lymphocytes in peripheral blood may approach the size of neutrophils. Occasionally, lymphocytes will contain

several small red to azurophilic cytoplasmic granules. These granules are often confined to a small cluster near one side of the nucleus. Reactive lymphocytes (Fig. 163.7) can be seen in blood smears from dogs responding to an antigenic stimulation. Reactive lymphocytes may be larger and have increased amounts of intensely basophilic cytoplasm. Rarely, they may take on a morphology similar to mature plasma cells, with an eccentric nucleus and a perinuclear clear area.

Monocytes are larger than neutrophils (Fig. 163.8). Monocyte nuclei are extremely variable and may be round, multilobulated, band-shaped, or S-shaped (Figs. 163.1 and 163.8). Those that are band-shaped generally have rounded, knob-shaped ends that differenti-

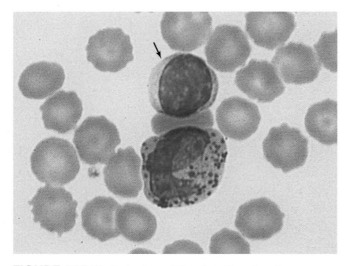

FIGURE 163.6 Canine basophil and medium lymphocyte. Canine basophils have a segmented nucleus and sparse granules. The lymphocyte (arrow) is slightly larger than a small lymphocyte and contains more abundant cytoplasm. (Wright-Giemsa stain, 250 × original magnification. Photo courtesy Oklahoma State University Clinical Pathology Teaching Files.)

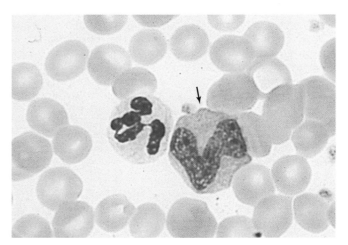

FIGURE 163.8 Neutrophil and monocyte. The monocyte (arrow) is larger than the neutrophil and contains a wider nucleus. This monocyte does not contain cytoplasmic vacuoles. (Wright-Giemsa stain, 250 × original magnification. Photo courtesy of Oklahoma State University Clinical Pathology Teaching Files.)

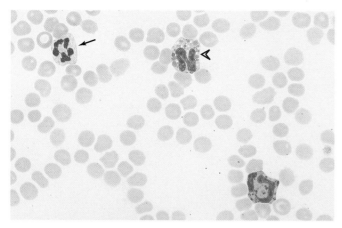

FIGURE 163.9 Blood smear from a dog showing a neutrophil (arrow), eosinophil (arrowhead), and basophil. The eosinophil has variably sized granules and a few distinct vacuoles. Canine basophils are sparsely granulated. (Wright-Giemsa stain, 250 × original magnification. Photo courtesy of Oklahoma State University Clinical Pathology Teaching Files.)

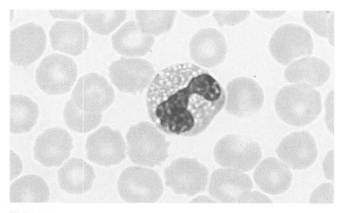

FIGURE 163.10 Vacuolated eosinophil from an adult Greyhound. (Wright-Giemsa stain, 250 × original magnification. Photo courtesy of Oklahoma State University Clinical Pathology Teaching Files.)

ate them from band neutrophils. The nuclear chromatin is less condensed than that of the mature neutrophil. Cytoplasm is moderate to abundant and grey-blue to deeply basophilic. Canine monocytes may have variable numbers of clear, distinct-walled cytoplasmic vacuoles. Occasionally, faint, dust-like azurophilic granules can be seen evenly spread throughout the blue cytoplasm.

Eosinophils can usually be found in low numbers on blood smears from healthy dogs. Eosinophils are slightly larger than neutrophils (Fig. 163.9). Their most characteristic feature is the presence of prominent eosinophilic granules. In dogs, the number and size of these granules is greatly variable. Size of the granules within a single cell may also be variable. Occasionally, an eosinophil may contain only one or two extremely large granules which could be mistaken for an inclusion body or parasite. Cytoplasm between the granules is lightly basophilic and may contain a few clear vacuoles. Eosinophil nuclei are less lobulated than those of neutrophils, usually having only two or three lobes. Eosinophils of adult Greyhounds are unique in that they contain numerous clear vacuoles and often lack distinct granules (Fig. 163.10).[16] Eosinophils of Greyhound pups contain granules, although these are a dull slate color rather than orange as in other species.

Basophils are rare in blood smears from normal dogs (Fig. 163.9). Basophils are larger than neutrophils and have a more elongated, convoluted nucleus. Compared to other species, canine basophils contain only scattered, small, purple to pink-purple cytoplasmic granules. The basophils' cytoplasm is blue-grey to slightly purple.

Quantitative Parameters

Reference ranges for leukocyte parameters of adult dogs are given in Table 163.1. As noted previously, reference ranges will be affected by the population from which they are derived. This could potentially have a greater effect on leukocyte parameters than on those of other cell lines, because animals not in controlled environments have greater exposure to a variety of antigens. Diurnal and seasonal variations have been reported in leukocyte counts, although the fluctuations are relatively minor and do not exceed the limits of standard reference ranges.[17,18] In some areas, animals may have higher eosinophil counts in certain seasons due to environmental allergens and parasite load. In addition, short-term alterations in leukocyte numbers may occur as part of epinephrine- or corticosteroid-induced responses in animals that are not conditioned to blood collection (see Chapter 55, Interpretation of Canine Leukocyte Responses).

Fluctuations in total white blood cell and neutrophil counts have been noted in Beagles during the first 2 months of life; however, with a few exceptions, values generally remained within the reference intervals listed in Table 163.2.[3] In one study, newborn animals (0 to 3 days) had band neutrophil counts that were slightly outside the adult reference range, indicating a left shift. Occasionally, metamyelocytes were seen during this period without any other evidence of disease. Band neutrophils decreased to within reference limits by 7 to 10 days of life. Lymphocyte counts are significantly higher in young dogs. Dogs younger than 6 months of age typically have lymphocyte counts of at least 2000/μL, with some as high as 10,000/μL.[3] After maturity, there is little change in hematologic parameters. Studies have found no significant trends in white cell counts of dogs from 1.5 to 14 years of age.[19,20] During pregnancy, total leukocyte counts may increase to levels that are slightly above reference ranges (~19,000/μL) near parturition. Leukocyte counts decrease into reference range during lactation but may not return to baseline values until the pups are weaned.[6]

PLATELETS

Morphology

Canine platelets appear as small, oval to round structures on blood smears (Fig. 163.11). Canine platelets are generally one-fourth to one-half the size of erythrocytes, but some platelets are larger than a red cell. They have clear to light grey cytoplasm and numerous small pink to purple granules. The granules may be dispersed throughout the platelet or aggregated into a central cluster. Occasionally, platelets become partially activated and have a spider-like appearance with small cytoplasmic pseudopodia. Alternatively, activated platelets may form small clumps or an agglutinated mass. Such large masses of platelets generally get pulled out to the feathered edge of a blood smear (Fig. 163.12).

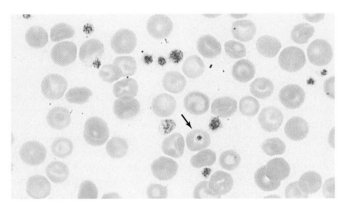

FIGURE 163.11 Canine platelets. One platelet overlies a red cell (arrow) mimicking an intraerythrocytic structure. (Wright-Giemsa stain, 250 × original magnification. Photo courtesy of Oklahoma State University Clinical Pathology Teaching Files.)

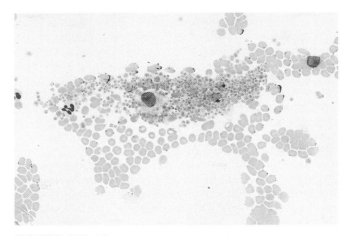

FIGURE 163.12 Large clump of platelets at the feathered edge of a blood smear. (Wright-Giemsa stain, 250 × original magnification. Photo courtesy of Oklahoma State University Clinical Pathology Teaching Files.)

TABLE 163.3	Differential Cell Counts from Bone Marrow Samples of Normal Dogs
Cell Type	**Mean ± SD**
Myeloid series	
Myeloblasts	0.9 ± 0.2
Progranulocytes	2.1 ± 0.4
Neutrophilic myelocytes	6.3 ± 1.0
Neutrophilic metamyelocytes	7.9 ± 2.1
Neutrophilic bands	11.3 ± 2.2
Neutrophils	23.5 ± 1.3
Eosinophilic myelocytes	0.6 ± 0.2
Eosinophilic metamyelocytes	0.7 ± 0.3
Eosinophilic bands	1.2 ± 0.4
Eosinophils	0.8 ± 0.5
Basophils	0.02 ± 0.04
Total myeloid series	55.32
Erythroid series	
Rubriblasts, prorubricytes	6.5 ± 0.5
Rubricytes, metarubricytes	27.6 ± 4.4
Total erythroid series	34.1
Myeloid/erythroid ratio	1.7 ± 0.4
Lymphocytes	8.2 ± 2.7
Plasma cells	0.7 ± 0.3
Mitotic figures	1.4 ± 0.3
Macrophages	0.4 ± 0.2

Adapted from Melveger BA, Earl FL, Van Loon ED. Sternal bone marrow biopsy in the dog. Lab Anim Care 1969;19:866–868.

Normal Parameters

Normal parameters for platelets in adult dogs are listed in Table 163.1. Platelet counts between 200,000 and 500,000/μL are considered normal. Low platelet counts have been noted in seemingly healthy racing Greyhounds.[21] The average platelet count from 36 Greyhounds in one study was 154 (±43) × 10^3/μL.

Mean platelet volumes (MPV) from colony-raised Beagles have been reported to be 8.5 (±0.53) fL.[22] Reference ranges can vary significantly among analyzers (Table 163.1).

BONE MARROW

The morphology of canine hemopoietic cells found in bone marrow aspirates has been reviewed.[23] The relative proportions of hematopoietic cells found in samples of bone marrow from normal dogs is given in Table 163.3.[24] The myeloid:erythroid (M:E) ratio of canine marrow is generally reported as being between 1.0:1 and 2.0:1. In one study, normal males had a significantly higher M:E ratio than females, some ranging as high as 2.9:1.[25] Comparison of marrow samples collected from various anatomic sites has shown that the percentages of various cellular elements is fairly uniform.[25,26] Also, repeated sampling of bone marrow from the same anatomic location seems to have little effect on differential cell counts.[27,28] Neonatal dogs have a significantly increased percentage of lymphocytes in bone marrow samples compared with adults.[15] In one study, mean lymphocyte percentages peaked at 54.7% by 21 days of age, decreasing to 17.6% by 56 days. Bone marrow samples from normal adult dogs generally have less than 10% lymphocytes.[29,30]

REFERENCES

1. **Weiss DJ, Kristenson A, Papenfuss N, McClay CB.** Quantitative evaluation of echinocytes in the dog. Vet Clin Pathol 1990;19:114–118.
2. **Laber J, Perman V, Stevens JB.** Polychromasia or reticulocytes: an assessment of the dog. J Am Anim Hosp Assoc 1974;10:399–406.
3. **Shifrine M, Munn SL, Rosenblatt LS, Bulgin MS, Wilson FD.** Hematologic changes to 60 days of age in clinically normal beagles. Lab Anim Sci 1973;23:894–898.
4. **Ewing G, Schalm OW, Smith RS.** Hematologic values of normal basenji dogs. J Am Vet Med Assoc 1972;161:1661–1664.
5. **Lund JE.** Hemoglobin crystals in canine blood. Am J Vet Res 1974;35:575–577.
6. **Anderson AC, Gee W.** Normal blood values in the beagle. Vet Med 1958;53:135–156.
7. **Bulgin MS, Munn SL, Gee W.** Hematologic changes to 4 ½ years of age in clinically normal beagles. J Am Vet Med Assoc 1970;157:1064–1070.
8. **Michaelson SM, Scheer K, Gilt S.** The blood of the normal beagle. J Am Vet Med Assoc 1966;148:532–534.
9. **Doxey DL.** Cellular changes in the blood as an aid to diagnosis. J Small Anim Pract 1966;7:77–89.
10. **Porter JA, Canaday WR.** Hematologic values in mongrel and greyhound dogs being screened for research use. J Am Vet Med Assoc 1971;159:1603–1606.
11. **Lassen D, Craig AM, Blythe LL.** Effects of racing on hematologic and serum biochemical values in greyhounds. J Am Vet Med Assoc 1986;188:1299–1303.
12. **Schalm OW.** Erythrocyte macrocytosis in miniature and toy poodles. Canine Pract 1976;3:55–57.
13. **Canfield PJ, Watson ADJ.** Investigations of bone marrow dyscrasia in a poodle with macrocytosis. J Comp Pathol 1989;101:270–278.
14. **Morley A, Stohlman F.** Erythropoiesis in the dog: the periodic nature of the steady state. Science 1969;165:1025–1027.
15. **Earl FL, Melveger BE, Wilson RL.** The hemogram and bone marrow profile of normal neonatal and weanling beagle dogs. Lab Anim Sci 1973;23:690–695.
16. **Jones RF, Paris R.** The greyhound eosinophil. J Small Anim Pract 1963;4(Suppl):29–33.
17. **Lilliehöök I.** Diurnal variation of canine blood leukocyte counts. Vet Clin Pathol 1997;26:113–117.
18. **Tsessarskaya TP, Burkovskaya TE.** Seasonal variation in the blood leukocyte count in dogs. Bull Exp Biol Med 1976;82:1465–1467.
19. **Lowseth LA, Gillett NA, Gerlach RF, Muggenburg BA.** The effects of aging on hematology and serum chemistry values in the beagle dog. Vet Clin Pathol 1990;19:13–19.
20. **Doughery JH, Rosenblatt LS.** Changes in the hemogram of the beagle with age. J Gerontol 1965;20:131–138.
21. **Sullivan PS, Evans HL, McDonald TP.** Platelet concentration and hemoglobin function in greyhounds. J Am Vet Med Assoc 1994;205:838–841.
22. **Waner T, Yuval D, Nyska A.** Electronic measurement of canine mean platelet volume. Vet Clin Pathol 1989;18:84–86.
23. **Harvey JW.** Canine bone marrow: normal hematopoiesis, biopsy techniques, and cell identification and evaluation. Compend Cont Educ Pract Vet 1984;6:909–925.
24. **Melveger BA, Earl FL, Van Loon ED.** Sternal bone marrow biopsy in the dog. Lab Anim Care 1969;19:866–868.
25. **Penny RHC, Carlisle CH.** The bone marrow of the dog: a comparative study of biopsy material obtained from the iliac crest, rib and sternum. J Small Anim Pract 1970;11:727–734.
26. **Rekers PE, Coulter M.** A hematological and histological study of the bone marrow and peripheral blood of the adult dog. Am J Med Sci 1948;216:643–655.
27. **Jain NC.** Schalm's veterinary hematology. 4th ed. Philadelphia: Lea & Febiger; 1986;103–125.
28. **Mitema ES.** Cytologic response of dogs to weekly bone marrow collections. Vet Med 1985;80:37–38.

CHAPTER 164

Normal Hematology of the Cat

• KENNETH D. CLINKENBEARD and JAMES H. MEINKOTH

ematologic references ranges are available from both research colonies and randomly sampled healthy cats.[1,2] These reference ranges show satisfactory agreement for the means of most values with the widest variation occurring in the white blood cell (WBC) count.[1] Sources of variation of hematologic values in cats are attributed to site of venipuncture, patient anxiety associated with sample collection, ratio of anticoagulant to blood, time of analysis after collection, and method and instrumentation used for analysis. In addition, age, sex, nutritional status, and husbandry as well as presence of pregnancy, anesthesia, or pharmacologic treatment can affect the measured hematologic values. The effect of most of these factors on hematologic values are not peculiar to the cat, but are common for all domestic species.

Means for hemoglobin (Hb) concentration, WBC, and absolute neutrophil and lymphocyte counts are statistically higher for samples collected from the jugular or cephalic veins versus the ear margin veins.[3] These differences are small enough (less than 10% of the reference range) that they are of no practical importance for interpretation in most cases. Clumping of feline platelets has the potential to affect data from hematologic analyzers. Collection of samples during anesthesia with agents that cause splenic sequestration, such as ketamine, acepromazine, barbiturates, or halothane, has the potential for lowering the red blood cell (RBC) count, Hb, and packed cell volume (PCV) compared with those values for the unanesthetized patient. The PCV nadirs for ketamine anesthesia can be $\approx$15 PCV units less than preanesthetic values.[4] Although there is no published data for cats, anesthetic agents that cause splenic contraction, such as ether or nitrous oxide, may increase the RBC, Hb, and PCV compared with preanesthetic values.

Several sets of reference normal values are available for kittens; however, many of the values in these sets are sufficiently divergent (i.e., it is difficult to determine which reference ranges are valid for diagnostic purposes).[5] The agreement among reference values for adult cats is better, particularly for the means. The ranges for the WBC and absolute neutrophil counts vary the most; this is likely caused by varying degrees of physiologic leukocytosis present in various groups of normal cats. The normal hematologic values for adult cats are presented in Table 164.1.[2]

ERYTHROCYTES

Feline RBCs typically lack discernible pale centers on blood smears and exhibit moderate anisocytosis (Fig. 164.1). At birth, the fetal RBCs are large (mean corpuscular volume [MCV], $\approx$90 fL), and the RBC, Hb, and PCV are low. The nadirs of means for RBC and PCV can be as low as $4.8 \times 10^6/\mu L$ and 26%, respectively.[6] Fetal RBCs are replaced by 1 to 4 months of age, resulting in the values for RBC, Hb, PCV, and MCV reaching those for the adult during this time. Male cats have slightly higher RBC, Hb, and PCV values than females. Queens can exhibit a mild normocytic, normochromic anemia with an average decrease of 8 PCV units during the last third of pregnancy; this resolves by 1 week postparturition.[7]

Moderate rouleau can be observed on blood smears from normal cats, and 0 to 1% of RBCs can contain Howell-Jolly bodies (Figs. 164.1 and 164.3). Low numbers of Heinz bodies (less than 5% of RBCs) can be found on blood smears of some healthy, nonanemic cats.[8] Reticulocytes in cats are classified as aggregate (type III or markedly aggregated reticulation) and punctate (type I or II or slight focal reticulation) (Fig. 164.2). In nonanemic cats, aggregated reticulocytes comprise less than 0.4% of RBCs, but the percentage of punctate reticulocytes is variable and can range as high as 10.8%.[9] Polychromatophilic RBCs are typically macrocytic, stain gray-blue with Wright's stain (Fig. 164.3), and constitute less than 0.5% of RBCs in nonanemic cats.

Cats have two natural blood types designated A and B. The prevalence of type A is much higher in most populations than type B. Sera of either type A or type B cats can contain isoantibodies to the opposite blood type, but only anti-A isoantibodies in type B cats are highly agglutinating and hemolytic; anti-B isoantibodies in type A cats are typically nonagglutinating and nonhemolytic.[10]

LEUKOCYTES

The WBC and differential counts in cats are more variable than those for dogs. This may be caused in part by a higher percentage of leukocytes in the marginated pool

TABLE 164.1 Hematologic Reference Range for Cats[a]

Data	Range	UC Davis Values[b]
Erythrogram		
Erythrocytes ($\times 10^6/\mu$L)	5.0–10.0	6.0–10.2
Hemoglobin (g/dL)	8.0–15.0	9.0–15.1
PCV (%)	24.0–45.0	29.0–48.0
MCV (fL)	39.0–55.0	41.5–52.5
MCHC (%)	31.0–35.0	30.0–33.5
Reticulocytes[c] (%)		
Aggregate	0–0.4	
Punctate	1.4–10.8	
RBC diameter (μm)	5.5–6.3	
Erythrocytes lifespan (days)	66–78	
Other data		
Platelet count ($\times 10^5/\mu$L)	3–8	200,000–600,000
MPV (fL)	12–17[d]	
Plasma proteins (g/dL)	6.0–8.0	6.8–8.3
Fibrinogen (g/dL)	0.05–0.30	
Leukogram		
Leukocytes (μL)	5500–19,500	5000–15,000
Band neutrophils	0–300	Rare
Segmented neutrophils	2500–12,500	2500–11,300
Lymphocytes	1500–7000	1400–8100
Monocytes	0–850	0–800
Eosinophils	0–1500	0–1500
Basophils	Rare	Rare

[a] Data adapted from Jain NC. The cat: normal hematology with comments on response to disease. In: Schalm's veterinary hematology. 4th ed. Philadelphia: Lea & Febiger, 1986;126–139.
[b] Recently determined values from the University of California, Davis, Veterinary Medical Teaching Hospital.
[c] Cramer DV, Lewis RM. Reticulocyte response in the cat. J Am Vet Med Assoc 1972;160:61–67.
[d] For nonaggregated platelets. Zelmanovic D, Hetherington EJ. Automated analysis of feline platelets in whole blood, including platelet count, mean platelet volume, and activation state. Vet Clin Pathol 1998;27:2–9.

Eosinophils typically are slightly larger than neutrophils and have segmented nuclei, which are often bilobulated with condensed chromatin, and the cytoplasm has abundant, small, uniform-sized, rod-shaped, pale orange staining granules (Figs. 164.1 and 164.4). Basophils are similar in size to eosinophils and have segmented nuclei with condensed chromatin and abundant, small, uniform-sized, round-shaped, pale lavender to pink to orange staining cytoplasmic granules (Fig. 164.5). A few less-mature dark purple granules may be observed occasionally in feline basophils. Lymphocytes are smaller than neutrophils, have rounded nuclei often with a flat side, condensed chromatin that appears smudged and

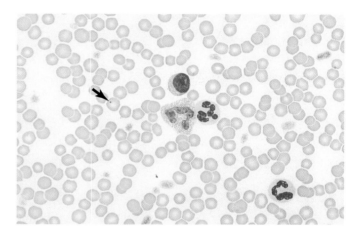

FIGURE 164.1 Feline RBCs exhibit moderate anisocytosis. Pale centers are frequently not readily discernible. A Howell-Jolly body (small arrow), two segmented neutrophils, a lymphocyte, an eosinophil, and both round and elongated platelets are present. (Wright-Giemsa stain, 250×. Courtesy of the Oklahoma State University, College of Veterinary Medicine Teaching Files.)

(estimated to be 70%[11]) than in other domestic species. Increased blood flow caused by anxiety shifts leukocytes from the marginated pool to the circulating pool, resulting in higher and more variable WBC and differential counts. Hematology analyzers with an automated differential leukocyte count feature provide accurate differential counts for feline neutrophils and lymphocytes, but not for monocytes, eosinophils, or basophils.[12] At birth, the WBC and differential counts are typically within the adult reference range. For kittens between 3 and 4 months of age, the WBC may increase to $\approx 23 \times 10^3/\mu$L and be composed of $\approx$50% segmented neutrophils and $\approx$50% lymphocytes.[5,6] The WBC declines to adult normal range for cats at 5 to 6 months of age.

The morphology of feline neutrophils is similar to that of other domestic species with segmented nuclei with condensed chromatin and nonstaining cytoplasm (Figs. 164.1, 164.3, and 164.4). Neutrophils from apparently healthy cats can contain a few Döhle bodies. Bar bodies or "drumstick" protrusions of the nucleus can be present in 4 to 11% of neutrophils of female cats.[13]

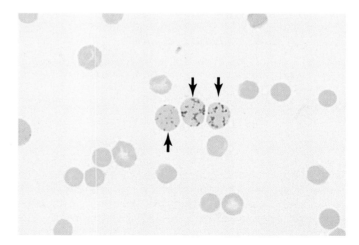

FIGURE 164.2 Two feline aggregate reticulocytes with markedly aggregated reticulation (top arrows) and one punctate reticulocyte with slight focal reticulation (bottom arrow) are present. (New methylene blue, 250×. Courtesy of the Oklahoma State University, College of Veterinary Medicine Teaching Files.)

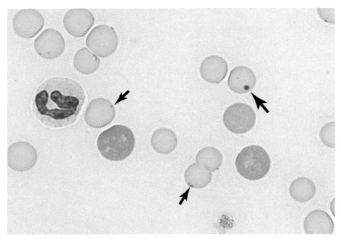

FIGURE 164.3 Macrocytic gray-blue polychromatophilic RBCs and normal feline RBCs are present. A single Howell Jolly body (large arrow) is seen in contrast to many rod-shaped, peripherally located *Hemobartonella felis* organisms (small arrows). A few platelets and a segmented neutrophil are also shown. (Wright-Giemsa stain, 250×. Courtesy of the Oklahoma State University, College of Veterinary Medicine Teaching Files.)

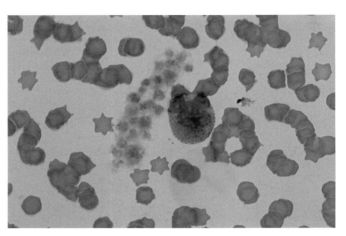

FIGURE 164.5 A feline basophil with lavender, round, intracytoplasmic granules. Platelet clump and rouleau are also present. (Wright-Giemsa stain, 1000×. Courtesy of the Oklahoma State University, College of Veterinary Medicine Teaching Files.)

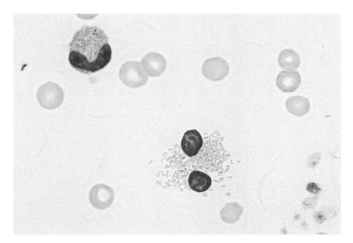

FIGURE 164.4 A ruptured eosinophil demonstrates the rod-shaped pale orange cytoplasmic granules of feline eosinophils. An intact eosinophil is also present. (Wright-Giemsa stain, 250×. Courtesy of the Oklahoma State University, College of Veterinary Medicine Teaching Files.)

lacks discernible nucleoli, and has scant basophilic cytoplasm that often appears to extend only one-third of the way around the nucleus (Fig. 164.6). Some lymphocytes can have a few small red-staining "azurophilic" cytoplasmic granules (Fig. 164.7). Monocytes are larger than neutrophils; have rounded, strap-, bi-, or tri-lobulated or ameboid-shaped nuclei with reticulated chromatin pattern; and abundant lightly basophilic to gray cytoplasm with a few to several clear variable-sized cytoplasmic vacuoles (Fig. 164.8).

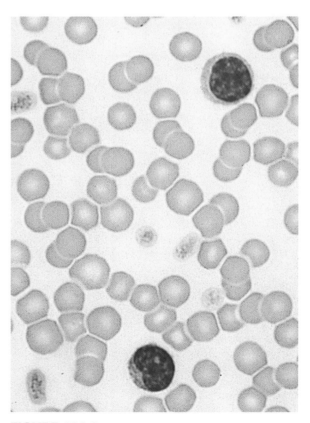

FIGURE 164.6 Two lymphocytes and round and elongated platelets are present. (Wright-Giemsa stain, 250×. Courtesy of the Oklahoma State University, College of Veterinary Medicine Teaching Files.)

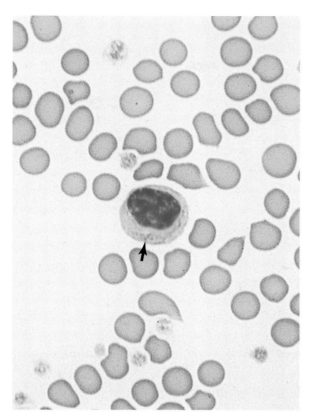

FIGURE 164.7 A lymphocyte containing small azurophilic intracytoplasmic granules (arrow). (Wright-Giemsa stain, 250×. Courtesy of the Oklahoma State University, College of Veterinary Medicine Teaching Files.)

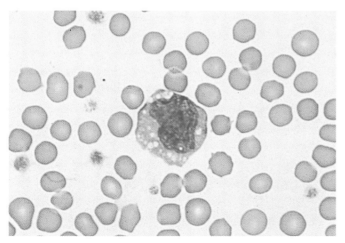

FIGURE 164.8 A monocyte with numerous cytoplasmic vacuoles. (Wright-Giemsa stain, 250×. Courtesy of the Oklahoma State University, College of Veterinary Medicine Teaching Files.)

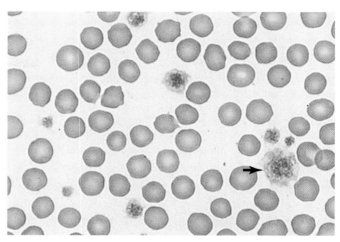

FIGURE 164.9 A megaplatelet (arrow) and normal-sized platelets. (Wright-Giemsa stain, 250×. Courtesy of the Oklahoma State University, College of Veterinary Medicine Teaching Files.)

TABLE 164.2	Bone Marrow Reference Range for Cats
	%
Erythroid series	
Rubriblast	0.17 ± 0.29
Prorubricyte	1.00 ± 0.54
Basophilic rubricyte	4.02 ± 1.56
Polychromatophilic rubricyte	17.57 ± 4.48
Metarubricyte	5.54 ± 3.15
Mitotic rubricyte	0.43 ± 0.24
Total erythrocytic cells	28.74 ± 4.64
Granulocytic series	
Myeloblast	0.08 ± 0.16
Promyelocyte	1.74 ± 1.04
Myelocyte, neutrophilic	4.31 ± 2.49
Myelocyte, eosinophilic	0.60 ± 0.42
Myelocyte, basophilic	0.11 ± 0.11
Metamyelocyte, neutrophilic	10.06 ± 3.20
Metamyelocyte, eosinophilic	0.54 ± 0.39
Metamyelocyte, basophilic	0.03 ± 0.07
Band, neutrophilic	14.4 ± 1.30
Band, eosinophilic	0.49 ± 0.40
Band, basophilic	0.0
Neutrophil	12.86 ± 4.85
Eosinophil	0.60 ± 0.20
Basophil	0.0
Total granulocytic cells	45.86 ± 3.78
Myeloid:erythroid ratio	1.63 ± 0.35:1
Other cell types	
Hematogones	0.83 ± 0.75
Lymphocytes	16.13 ± 2.92
Plasma cells	0.80 ± 0.60
Monocytes	0.77 ± 0.51
Mitotic cells	0.20 ± 0.26
Macrophages	0.06 ± 0.10
Unclassified cells	0.49 ± 0.28
Degenerated cells	6.31 ± 3.32
Total other cells	25.40 ± 4.75

Data adapted from Jain NC. The cat: normal hematology with comments on response to disease. In: Schalm's veterinary hematology. 4th ed. Philadelphia: Lea & Febiger, 1986;126–139.

PLATELETS

Feline platelets have morphology similar to other domestic animals, except occasional elongated forms or macrocytic (shift or megaplatelets) may be encountered on blood smears (Figs. 164.1, 164.6, and 164.9). Anxiety associated with blood collection in cats can cause splenic contraction and a sudden increase in circulating platelets. Feline platelets are prone to clumping after blood collection.

PLASMA PROTEINS

At birth, kittens are normoalbuminemic but hypogammaglobulinemic. Following assimilation of colostrum, the globulin concentration increases but may not reach the adult normal range until 4 to 6 months of age. The globulin concentration can continue to increase with age, so that total protein concentrations of up to 8.5 g/dL can be observed in some normal old-age cats.[2]

BONE MARROW

Published myeloid:erythroid (M:E) ratios for cats vary from 1.4:1 to 3.5:1.[1,2] Means and standard deviations from 500-cell differential counts on bone marrows from 7 normal cats is compiled in Table 164.2.[2] Aspirin and chloramphenicol can cause marrow hypoplasia in cats.

REFERENCES

1. **Gilmore CE, Gilmore VH, Jones TC.** Bone marrow and peripheral blood of cats: techniques and normal values. Pathol Vet 1964;1:18–40.
2. **Jain NC.** The cat: normal hematology with comments on response to disease. In: Schalm's veterinary hematology. 4th ed. Philadelphia: Lea & Febiger, 1986;126–139.
3. **Jacobsen JOG, Jensen AL.** Comparison of haematological analyses of blood taken from the cephalic and marginal ear veins in cats. J Small Anim Pract 1998;39:94–95.
4. **Frankel T, Hawkey CM.** Haematological changes during sedation in cats. Vet Rec 1980;107:512–513.
5. **Clinkenbeard KD, Cowell RL, Meinkoth JH, Decker L.** The hematopoietic system. In: Hoskins J, ed. Veterinary pediatrics, dogs and cats from birth to six months. 2nd ed. Philadelphia: WB Saunders (in press).
6. **Anderson L, Wilson R, Hay D.** Haematological values in normal cats from four weeks to one year of age. Res Vet Sci 1971;579–583.
7. **Berman E.** Hemogram of the cat during pregnancy and lactation and after lactation. Am J Vet Res 1974;35:457–460.
8. **Jain NC.** Demonstration of Heinz bodies in erythrocytes of the cat. Bull Am Soc Vet Clin Pathol 1973;2:13.
9. **Cramer DV, Lewis RM.** Reticulocyte response in the cat. J Am Vet Med Assoc 1972;160:61–67.
10. **Wilkerson MJ, Meyers KM, Wardrop KJ.** Anti-A isoagglutinins in two blood type B cats are IgG and IgM. Vet Clin Pathol 1991;20:10–14.
11. **Prasse KW, Kaeberle ML, Ramsey FK.** Blood neutrophil granulocyte kinetics in cats. Am J Vet Res 1973;34:1021–1025.
12. **Tvedten H, Korcal D.** Automated differential leukocyte counts in horses, cattle, and cats using the Technicon H-1E system. Vet Clin Pathol 1996;25:14–22.
13. **Loughman WD, Frye FL, Condon TB.** XY/XXY bone marrow mosaicism in three male tricolor cats. Am J Vet Res 1970;31:307–314.

CHAPTER 165

Normal Hematology of the Horse

• JOHN W. KRAMER

Reviews of equine hematology have been published,[1-3] and specifics of the neonate[4-6] and the equine athlete[7] have also been reported elsewhere.

The common domestic equi (horses, donkeys, and their hybrid the mule) have a few subtle hematologic differences.[2] Two basic types of horses and many breeds have developed. Horses of Arabian ancestry are called "hot-blooded" and include Arab, Thoroughbred, Standardbred, and Quarterhorse breeds. "Cold-blooded" horses are the draft stocks and pony. The hematologic difference is a slightly greater resting hematocrit in hot-blooded horses than in cold blooded ones (Tables 165.1 and 165.2). Other hematologic differences are not evident, and observations from ponies and horses are frequently interchanged in research projects. Reference values for ponies, donkeys, and other equi have been assembled.[2]

Automation and computerization has enhanced blood cell counting, but the major causes for variation in reference ranges remain age and emotional status of the sampled subjects. Quantification and identification of white blood cells is rapidly changing from counting nucleated cells remaining after hemolysis to cytochemical and immunocytochemical cell counting technology in which small populations of circulating blood cells can be detected and isolated.

ERYTHROCYTES

The horse's discocytic, biconcave erythrocytes have a width of about 5 to 6 μm, a mean corpuscular volume (MCV) of 44 to 52 fL, red cell distribution width (RDW) of 14 to 25%, and life span of about 140 to 155 days. Equine RDW range is greater than the range of other species. Equine reticulocytes mature completely to red blood cells (RBCs) in the bone marrow. Acceleration of equine erythropoieses appears to be slower than in many other species. Although only a relatively few polychromatophilic reticulocytes enter peripheral blood in anemia the young RBCs released can be sufficient to produce an MCV macrocytosis.[8] An anemia with a packed cell volume (PCV) of less than 25% may require more than 1 week before an accelerated bone marrow response exceeds the MCV reference range.[9]

Normal equine blood has a rapid erythrocyte sedimentation rate as the result of rouleaux formation. The reason for the rouleaux is poorly understood but hyperfibrinogenemia, unknown plasma proteins, and erythrocyte membrane factors are contributors.[10,11] Equine RBCs rapid sedimentation makes it essential to mix equine blood samples thoroughly before an aliquot is removed.

Mammalian erythropoietins are closely conserved but there is sufficient heterogeneity in the equine erythropoietin to believe that human recombinant erythropoietin is antigenic in the horse and its ability to stimulate erythropoiesis in the horse is questionable.[12-14]

Erythrocyte Metabolism

Animal erythrocyte metabolism has been reviewed by Harvey,[15] and intracellular metabolite concentrations and enzymes summarized. Erythrocyte glucose consumption of about 0.6 μmol/hr/mL of RBCs is less than that of humans, dogs, and goats but about equal to that of cattle and sheep.[15] An energy-dependent, Na^+/K^+ membrane pump maintains a high intraerythrocytic K^+ concentration (120 mEq/L) and low Na^+ concentration (10 mEq/L) in the horse.[16] Prolonged room temperature storage of a blood sample consumes the plasma glucose required for the Na^+/K^+ membrane pump, allowing the intracellular K^+ to leak into the plasma and produce a pseudohyperkalemia before hemolysis becomes visually evident.

Diuretic therapy and general electrolyte depletion are associated with echinocyte formation.[17-19] Eccentrocytosis are associated with familial, erythrocytic G6PDH deficiency.[20]

Two hemoglobins types are expressed in the same individual horse as the result of two alpha chain hemoglobin variants. Donkeys have another hemoglobin type, and the mule expresses all three hemoglobins of its parents.[21-23] Donkeys and horses have sufficient erythrocytic, antigenic surface differences that neonatal, isoimmune hemolytic anemia occurs in the neonatal mule.[24,25]

Mare to fetal gradient is maintained with the help of

a lower fetal erythrocytic 2-3-diphosphoglycerate concentration.[22] Although fetal erythrocytes maintain a low 2-3-diphosphoglycerate concentration, the oxygen debt of exercise dos not result in the increased 2-3-diphosphoglycerate concentration in trained exercised horses.[26]

Methemoglobin formation and the resulting Heinz bodies are seen in horses treated with oxidative drugs and drugs with oxidative products such as anthelminthic phenothiazine. Low methemoglobin concentrations are normal in erythrocytes. The oxidized ferric iron of methemoglobin is reduced to its O^2 carrying ferrous iron of hemoglobin by the enzyme NADH methemoglobin reductase. This methemoglobin reduction process is adequate at the normally low equine RBC concentrations, but at high methemoglobin concentrations reduction is slower than observed in some other species.[14]

Dynamics of the Erythron

The clinical measurement of the peripheral blood is an insensitive indicator of the size of the horse's erythron.

Apprehension- and excitement-induced epinephrine release results in splenic contraction injecting massive numbers of erythrocytes into the peripheral blood. Splenic contraction can cause as much as a 40% increase in PCV, masking the effects of training and the clinical evaluation of hemorrhage.[1,7,27] In cases of colic, the patient's PCV may increase from a resting, quiescent 40% to 75% PCV in a matter of minutes with no apparent change in hydration or movement in water compartments. Although the resulting polycythemia increases the bloods total oxygen carrying capacity, it is at the cost of increasing blood viscosity and cardiac load.[27] In colic cases, the PCV has become an intuitive prognosticator—the higher the PCV, the poorer the prognosis.

LEUKOCYTES

Neutrophils

Staging of the maturation of the neutrophil is based on the progressive nuclear lobulation as the result of

TABLE 165.1 Normal Blood Ranges for the Horse

	Hot-Blooded Breeds (Based on 147 Clinically Normal Horses)	Cold-Blooded Breeds (Collected from the Literature)
Erythrocytic series		
Erythrocytes ($\times 10^6/\mu L$)	6.8–12.9	5.5–9.5
Hemoglobin (g/dL)	11.0–19	8.0–14.0
PCV (%)	32–53	24.00–44.0
MCV (fL)	37.0–58.5 (37.0–58.0)[a]	—
MCH (pg)	12.3–19.9 (10.0–20.0)[a]	—
MCHC (%)	31.0–38.6 (31.0–36.0)[a]	—
RBC diameter (μm)	5.0–6.0	—
RDW (%)	24–27	—
Leukocytic series		
Total leukocytes/μL	5400–14,300	6000–12,000
Neutrophil (band)	0–100 (0–100)	—
Neutrophil (seg)	2260–8580	—
Lymphocyte	1500–7700	—
Monocyte	0–1000	—
Eosinophil	0–1000	—
Basophil	0–290	—
Percentage distribution		
Neutrophil (band)	0–8	0–2
Neutrophil (seg)	22–72	35–75
Lymphocyte	17–68	2–10
Monocyte	0–14	2–12
Eosinophil	0–10	0–3
Basophil	0–4	—
Other data		
Plasma proteins (g/dL)	5.8–8.7	—
Fibrinogen (g/dL)	0.1–0.4	—
Thrombocytes ($\times 10^3$)	1.0–3.5	—
Erythrocyte life span (days)	140–150	—
Myeloid:erythroid ratio	0.5–1.5:1.0	—

Adapted from Jain NC. Schalm's veterinary hematology. 4th ed. Philadelphia: Lea & Febiger, 1986;141.
[a] Parentheses contain recently determined values from the University of California, Davis, Veterinary Medical Teaching Hospital.

TABLE 165.2 Normal Blood Values of Thoroughbred and Quarter Horse Foals of Both Sexes (mean ± 1 SD)[a]					
	1st Day	**2–7 Days (Average 5)**	**8–14 Days (Average 9)**	**21–30 Days (Average 28)**	**1–3 Months (Average 51 days)**
Number of foals	34	16	15	8	14
RBC ($\times 10^6/\mu$L)	10.5 ± 1.4	9.5 ± 0.8	9.0 ± 0.8	11.2 ± 1.3	11.9 ± 1.3
Hb (g/dL)	14.2 ± 1.3	12.7 ± 0.9	11.8 ± 1.2	13.1 ± 1.1	13.4 ± 1.6
PCV (%)	41.7 ± 3.6	37.1 ± 2.8	34.9 ± 3.7	37.8 ± 3.3	38.3 ± 4.1
MCV (fL)	40.1 ± 3.8	39.2 ± 2.8	39.1 ± 2.2	34.2 ± 0.4	32.4 ± 1.9
MCH (pg)	13.6 ± 1.2	13.4 ± 1.0	13.1 ± 0.8	11.8 ± 0.8	11.2 ± 0.6
MCHC (%)	33.9 ± 1.6	43.2 ± 1.2	33.6 ± 0.9	34.5 ± 1.0	34.9 ± 1.2
Plasma proteins (g/dL)	6.2 ± 0.9 (32)	6.3 ± 0.5	6.1 ± 0.6	6.2 ± 0.4	6.4 ± 0.4
Fibrinogen (mg/dL)	270 ± 60 (15)	330 ± 130 (6)	300 ± 50 (9)	400 (5)	460 ± 70 (10)
Total leukocytes/μL	9602 ± 3372	9300 ± 2346	9483 ± 2196	9688 ± 1940	10,893 ± 2977
Band neutrophil	138 ± 198	29 ± 37	48 ± 125	19 ± 33	10 ± 28
Neutrophil (seg)	6824 ± 2757	6448 ± 2128	6338 ± 1849	5501 ± 1346	5315 ± 2437
Lymphocyte	2192 ± 891	2420 ± 739	2633 ± 933	3823 ± 863	5086 ± 1419
Monocyte	414 ± 373	308 ± 172	302 ± 124	266 ± 192	348 ± 175
Eosinophil	0	30 ± 34	21 ± 38	48 ± 53	115 ± 88
Basophil	14 ± 78	41 ± 44	29 ± 50	11 ± 29	12 ± 26
Leukocytes (%)					
Band neutrophil	1.5 ± 1.8	0.3 ± 0.4	0.5 ± 1.1	0.2 ± 0.3	0.1 ± 0.3
Segmented neutrophil	68.9 ± 10.7	68.2 ± 9.4	66.2 ± 9.0	56.8 ± 7.4	46.9 ± 12.1
Lymphocyte	25.1 ± 10.3	27.0 ± 9.8	28.5 ± 9.4	39.6 ± 6.5	48.5 ± 11.5
Monocyte	3.9 ± 2.9	3.4 ± 1.9	3.3 ± 1.5	2.6 ± 2.0	3.3 ± 1.8
Eosinophil	0	0.3 ± 0.4	0.2 ± 0.4	0.4 ± 0.5	1.0 ± 0.8
Basophil	0.02 ± 0.08	0.4 ± 0.4	0.3 ± 0.5	0.1 ± 0.3	0.1 ± 0.3
N:L	2.8:1	2.5:1	2.3:1	1.4:1.0	1.1:1

Adapted from Jain NC. Schalm's veterinary hematology. 4th ed. Philadelphia: Lea & Febiger, 1986.
[a] Numbers in parentheses indicate number of foals when less than total for series.

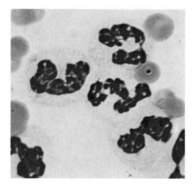

FIGURE 165.1 Three mature equine neutrophils in a row and one band neutrophil on the left.

chromatin condensation. Bertram's[28] review of domestic animal neutrophils includes the horse. Horses are less inclined to respond with a marked left shift of neutrophils than are some other species, such as the dog. If equine neutrophil maturation is to be used as an indicator of inflammation and a prognosticator, care must be taken to note subtle population shifts in the granulocytic series. Two transitional stages are recognized between the metamyelocyte and segmented neutrophil, the band and hyposegmented neutrophil. Hyposegmentation is the earliest indicator of a shift of the bone marrow's neutrophil storage pool out into peripheral blood and an accerated regenerative response (Fig. 165.1).

Hypersegmented neutrophils multiple fine filamentous bridging of nuclear lobules is indicative of aging of neutrophils. Although common to extravascular effusions, hypersegmented neutrophils are not normal in the peripheral blood. They become evident in peripheral blood when endogenous hyperadrenocorticism of stress and therapeutic steroids inhibit the neutrophils from leaving the vascular space.

The equine neutrophil's clear cytoplasm contains peroxidase-positive azurophilic, primary granules, and peroxidase-negative secondary granules. They occupy as much as 11% of the cytoplasmic space. The secondary granule is the most common granule. Ultrastructurally, primary and secondary granules are round to ellipsoidal with a crystal structure along the primary granule's axis.[28] Inflammatory disorders result in an increased intensity of staining of neutrophil's cytoplasmic granules, "toxic granulation." This intense staining is the result of a sulfated mucoid substance retained in the granules of bone marrow and peripheral blood neutrophils.[28]

Recombinant canine granulocyte-colony stimulating factor can accelerate neutrophil release and production.[29] Its long-term antigenic effects are unclear. A familial myeloid and megakaryocytic hypoplasia disorder has been reported in horses, but its mechanism is not understood.[30]

Bacterial endotoxins are neutrophil chemoattractants that produce marked degenerative left shifts and panleukopenia. Equine neutrophils are slower to respond

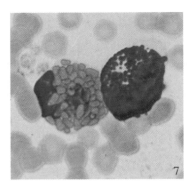

FIGURE 165.2 An equine eosinophil and basophil.

to some attractants, but the equine neutrophil is an appropriate model for chemoattractants-receptor research.[31–33] Cytochemical immunocytochemical staining reveals a range of enzymes and substrates in the horse's neutrophiles ultrastructure.[1,2,14,28] Immunocytochemical cell surface antigen serve to add to the specificity of neutrophils characterization[34] and parental testing.[35]

EOSINOPHILS

Eosinophils contain, large, eosinophilic, cytoplasm granules that may engorge the cytoplasm and mask the lobulated nucleus. Maturation of the lobulated nucleus seldom progresses to fine filamentation (Fig. 165.2).

BASOPHILS

As in other species, equine basophils are sparse in blood except in instances of eosinophiles. Its numerous, small, intensely basophilic granules may mask the incompletely segmented nucleus (Fig. 165.2).

LYMPHOCYTES

Lymphocytes comprise approximately 50% of the total white blood cell population. The T- and B-cell subsets of lymphocytes are separable by their cell surface markers[34] but inseparable with Wright's staining. As many as 5% of the lymphocytes may contain small, Wright's stained magenta, cytoplasmic granules.

Neonatal foals begin life with as few as $1000/\mu$L or less lymphocytes, but in a matter of a few month this increases to as many as 4000 to $5000/\mu$L (Table 165.2).[4,6] A physiologic lymphocytosis in excited, apprehensive, and fractious horses can result in rapid increase in lymphocyte concentration to $9000/\mu$L or more.[1] Once calmed, the horse's lymphocytosis returns to the reference range of normal horses.

MONOCYTES

The nucleus of the equine monocyte is typically large, broad, and indented with a lacy chromatin pattern. Cytoplasm is gray and granular, with small azurophilic granules and a few clear vacuoles.

THROMBOCYTES

Equine platelet concentrations are some of the lowest reported for mammals. A comparative review of platelets including the horse is available.[36] The platelet's azurophilic granules are so small they are difficult to see with an oil immersion lens. Giant platelet forms and pseudopodia are associated with recent proliferation from megakaryocytes. The platelet's ultrastructure reveals a smooth surface similar the human platelets, but their organelles to respond to different aggregating agents.[34]

Idiopathic thrombocytopenia similar to EDTA-associated pseudothrombocytopenias of humans has been reported in a horse.[37] Platelets are not aggregated on the stained slide, but the use of heparin as the anticoagulant rather than EDTA results in appreciably greater platelet counts.

PHYSIOLOGIC LEUKOCYTOSIS

Vigorously exercised and fractious horses frequently have hyperglycemia, polycythemia, and neutrophilia and occasionally lymphocytosis, which return to their reference ranges when the horse is calmed. This rapid, dramatic alteration is the result of the intravascular distribution of granulocytes and lymphocytes. Endogenous and therapeutic corticosteroids in horses produce an apparent neutrophilia, lymphopenia, and eosinopenia for various lengths of time with no change in erythrocyte, platelet, or monocyte counts.[1] Endogenous epinephrine and steroids are frequently simultaneously increased in exercised and stressed horses. If steroid release of exercise or stress[37] is imposed on a horse that already has an inflammatory neutrophilia with a regenerative left shift, the magnitude of the neutrophilia can be amplified, complicating the interpretation of the blood cell count.

BONE MARROW

The limited release of reticulocytosis into peripheral blood in regenerative anemias negates the use of a reticulocyte count as an indicator of accelerated erythropoiesis. Although a limited macrocytosis does increase the MCV in regenerative anemias, other indicators of accelerated erythropoiesis are sought. The horse's bone marrow, myeloid to erythroid ratio (M:E), macrophage activity, and bone marrow polychromatophilic, reticulocyte to normochromic erythrocyte ratio are used collectively to evaluate acceleration of erythropoiesis. The iliac crest, ribs and sternum are sources of bone marrow (see Chapter 3). Descriptions of the horse's bone marrow cytology have been published (Table 165.3). The M:E ratio ranges from 0.5 to 2.4. This large range limits the M:E's sensitivity as an indicator of accelerated erythropoiesis. Bone marrow proportions of polychromatophilic reticulocytes to normochromic erythrocytes is approximately 5%. A proportional increase in bone marrow reticulocytes can be accredited to accelerated erythropoiesis. However, bone marrow specimens are frequently heavily contaminated with reticulocyte-free, peripheral blood. This contamination serves to lower the observed bone marrow reticulocyte count. Increased bone marrow macrophage activity can subjectively be used as an indicator of accelerated erythrophagocytosis. Increased nucleophagocytosis, erythrophagocytosis, bilirubin, and iron pigments are indicators of accelerated erythropoiesis. Collectively, the MCV, macrophage activity, proportional reticulocyte numbers, and M:E are used to detect accelerated erythropoiesis.

NEONATES

Critical hematological evaluation of the foal and yearling require age-related reference values.[4-6] Foal erythron, lymphocyte, and fibrinogen concentrations are initially lower and serum iron higher than adult values; they achieve adult values at different times. Mean erythrocyte volume is relatively high in the neonate, decreasing during the first 4 months of life. They increase to the values of mature horses by 1 year of age. These changes are accompanied by proportional changes in the MCH.[1]

Neonatal hyperbilirubinemia is common[5] as the result of delayed fetal development of the hepatic bilirubin conjugation process. Unless age-related values for foals are used, the foal's lower-than-adult normal hematocrit and icterus can be interpreted incorrectly to be neonatal isoerythrolysis. Neonatal fibrinogen reference ranges are lower than those of adult horses,[4-6] but haptoglobin concentrations are similar to those of adult horse values.

Passive colostral immunoglobulin transfer to the neonate foal increases serum protein concentration from a presuckling value of 3 to 5 g/dl to 6 g/dl in the first 24 hours of life. This increase in the foal's serum globulin concentration is measured with a simple enzyme-linked immunosorbent assay (ELISA) test procedure. Along with the mare's colostral antibodies goes the absorption of colostral γ glutamyltransferase (GGT). However, the colostral GGT transfer from the mare to the foal is too

---

TABLE 165.3   Cellular Composition of the Bone Marrow of Horses

Cell Type	Archer (1954) (12 horses)		Calhoun (1954) (7 horses)		Tschudi et al. (1976) (15 horses)		Franken et al. (1982a) (24 horses)	
	Range (%)	Mean (%)	Range (%)	Mean (%)	Range (%)	Mean (%)	Range (%)	Mean (%)
Myeloblast	0–0.7	0.2	—	—	0.3–2.0	1.2	0–5.0	1.0
Promyelocyte	0.1–1.0	0.5	0.0–5.0	1.8	0.0–3.0	1.3	0.5–3.5	1.7
Myelocytes								
Neutrophilic	11.1–28.6	17.9	26.2–56.0	38.1	1.0–5.0	3.3	1.0–7.5	3.2
Eosinophilic	0.7–2.4	1.4	0.4–3.6	2.3	0.0–0.3	0.1	—	—
Metamyelocytes								
Neutrophilic	17.9–29.4	17.9–29.4	17.9–29.4	17.9–29.4	17.9–29.4	17.9–29.4	17.9–29.4	17.9–29.4
Eosinophilic	1.1–7.0	3.5	—	—	0.0–0.3	0.1	—	—
Basophilic	1.1–5.4	1.0	—	—	0.0–0.3	0.1	—	—
Band neutrophils	—	—	—	—	—	—	6.0–26.5	15.7
Mature granulocytes								
Neutrophils	7.8–25.3	14.7	1.8–20.2	13.3	11.0–30.0	20.4	3.0–16.5	8.4
Eosinophils	0.5–6.0	2.6	0.2–1.2	0.6	0.0–0.6	0.2	0.0–5.0	1.8
Basophils	0.0–0.3	0.1	0.0–0.6	0.6	0.0–0.5	0.1	0.0–1.0	0.3
Total myeloid series		63.7		56.7		34.5		37.9
Rubriblast	0.0–0.9	0.3	0.4–3.4	1.6	0.6–4.0	2.2	0.0–2.0	0.7
Prorubricyte	0.2–4.4	1.9	—	—	2.0–9.0	5.8	1.0–9.5	3.6
Rubricyte	2.2–13.0	6.3	8.0–32.0	20.9	10.0–23.0	16.2	14.5–44.0	28.2
Metarubricyte	4.2–39.2	17.6	5.0–24.2	13.7	25.0–45.0	34.9	14.0–36.0	23.2
Total erythroid series		26.2		34.7		60.5		55.9
Monocyte	—	—	1.2–4.8	2.7	0.0–2.0	0.8	0.0–1.0	0.2
Lymphocyte	2.5–20.9	9.7	2.0–5.6	3.9	1.0–6.0	3.8	1.5–8.5	3.8
Plasma cell	0.0–1.7	0.5	0.0–0.8	0.6	0.0–2.0	0.7	0.0–2.0	0.6
Megakaryocyte	—	—	—	—	—	—	—	—
Mitotic figures	—	—	—	—	—	—	—	—
Myeloid:erythroid ratio	1.1–10.2:1	2.4:1	0.9–3.8:1	1.6:1	0.3–0.9:1	0.6:1	0.5–0.9:1	0.7:1

From Jain NC. Schalm's veterinary hematology. 4th ed. Philadelphia: Lea & Febiger, 1986.

low to be a sensitive indicator of the transfer of protective levels of immunoglobulin.

REFERENCES

1. **Jain NC.** Schalm's veterinary hematology. 4th ed. Philadelphia: Lea & Febiger, 1986;140.
2. **Archer RK, Jefcott LB.** Comparative clinical hematology. 1st ed. Oxford: Blackwell Scientific, 1977;161.
3. **Lassen, ED, Swardson CJ.** Hematology and hemostasis in the horse normal functions and common abnormalities. Vet Clin North Am Equine Pract 1995;11:351–389.
4. **Harvey JW, Asquith RL, McNulty PK, Kivipelto J, Bauer JE.** Hematology of foals up to one year old. Equine Vet J 1984;16:347–353.
5. **Bauer JE, Harvey JW, Asquith RL, et al.** Clinical chemistry reference values of foals during the first year of life. Equine Vet J 1984;16:361–363.
6. **Becht JL, Semrad SD.** Hematology, blood typing, and immunology of the neonatal foal. Vet Clin North Am Equine Pract 1985;1:91–116.
7. **Rose RJ, Hodgson DR.** Hematology and biochemistry. In: Hodgson DR, Rose RJ, eds. The athletic horse: principles and practices of equine sports medicine. 1st ed. Philadelphia: WB Saunders, 1994;63.
8. **Tablin F, Weiss L.** Equine bone marrow: a quantitative analysis of erythroid maturation. Anat Rec 1985;213:202–206.
9. **Weiser G, Kohn C, Vachon A.** Erythrocyte volume distribution analysis and hematological changes in two horses with immune-mediated hemolytic anemia. Vet Pathol 1983;20:424–433.
10. **Allen BV.** Relationships between the erythrocyte sedimentation rate, plasma proteins and viscosity, and leucocyte counts in thoroughbred racehorses. Vet Rec 1988;122:329–332.
11. **Baskurt OK, Farley RA, Meiselman HJ.** Erythrocyte aggregation tendency and cellular properties in horses, human, and rat: a comparative study. Am J Physiol 1997;273:H2604–H2612.
12. **Wen D, Boissel JP, Tracy TE, Gruninger RH, et al.** Erythropoietin structure-function relationships: high degree of sequence homology among mammals. Blood 1993;83:1507–1516.
13. **Jaussaud P, Audran M, Gareau RL, Souillard A, Chavaneh L.** Kinetics and hematological effects of erythropoietin in horses. Vet Res 1994;25:568–573.
14. **Piercy RJ, Swaedson CJ, Hinchcliff KW.** Erythroid hypoplasia and anemia following administration of recombinant human erythropoietin to two horses. J Am Vet Med Assoc 1998;212:244–247.
15. **Harvey JW.** The erythrocyte: physiology, metabolism, and biochemical disorders. In: Kaneko JJ, Harvey JW, Bruss ML, eds. Clinical biochemistry of domestic animals. 5th ed. San Diego: Academic Press, 1998.
16. **Contreras A, Martinez R, Dives R, Marusic ET.** An unusual pattern of Na$^+$ and K$^+$ movements across the horse erythrocyte membrane. Biochem Biophys Acta 1986;856:388–391.
17. **Geor RJ, Weiss DJ.** Drugs affecting the hematologic system of the performance horse. Vet Clin North Am Equine Pract 1993;9:649–667.
18. **Boucher JH, Ferguson EW, Wilhelmsen CL, et al.** Erythrocyte alterations endurance exercise in horses. J Appl Physiol 1981;51:131–134.
19. **Geor RJ, Lund EM, Weiss DJ.** Echinocytosis in horses: 54 cases (1990). J Am Vet Med Assoc 1993;202:976–980.
20. **Stockham SL, Harvey JW, Kinden DA.** Equine glucose-6-phosphate dehydrogenase deficiency. 1995;31:518–527.
21. **Kitchen H, Brett I.** Embryonic and fetal hemoglobin in animals. Ann N Y Acad Sci 1974;241:653–671.
22. **Kitchen H, Bun HF.** Ontogeny of equine hemoglobins. J Reprod Fertil Suppl 1975;23:595–598.
23. **Mazur G, Braunitzer G.** The sequence of hemoglobins from an Asiatic wild ass and a mountain zebra. Hoppe Seylers Z Physiol Chem 1982;363;59–71.
24. **McClure JJ, Koch C, Traub-Dargatz J.** Characterization of a red blood cell antigen in donkeys and mules associated with neonatal isoerythrolysis. Anim Genet 1994;25:119–120.
25. **Traub Dargatz JL, McClure JJ, Koch C, et al.** Neonatal isoerythrolysis in a mule foal. J Am Vet Med Assoc 1995;206:67–70.
26. **Stull CL, Lawrence LM.** The effect of exercise and conditioning on equine red blood cell characteristics. J Equine Vet Sci 1986;6:170–174.
27. **Persson SGB.** On blood volume and working capacity in horses. Acta Physiol Scand 1967;(Suppl 19):5–35.
28. **Bertram TA.** Neutrophilic leukocytes structure and function in domestic animals. Adv Vet Sci Comp Med 1985;30:91–129.
29. **Zinkl JG, Madigan JE, Fridman DM, et al.** Haematological, bone marrow and clinical chemical changes in neonatal foals given recombinant granulocytic-stimulating factor. Equine Vet J 1994;26:313–328.
30. **Kohn CW, Swardson C, Provost P, et al.** Myeloid and megakaryocytic hypoplasia in related standardbreds. J Vet Intern Med 1995;9:315–323.
31. **Zinkl JG, Brown PD.** Chemotaxis of horse polymorphonuclear leukocytes to N-formyl–L leucyl-L-phenylalanine. Am J Vet Res 1982;43:613–616.
32. **Marr KA, Foster AP, Lees P, et al.** Effect of antigen challenge on the activation of peripheral blood neutrophils from horses with chronic obstructive pulmonary disease. Res Vet Sci 1997;62:253–260.
33. **Benbarek H, Deby Dupont G, Caudron I, et al.** Failure of lipopolysaccharides to directly trigger the chemiluminescence response of isolated equine polymorphonuclear leukocytes. Vet Res Commun 1997;21:477–82.
34. **Equine leukocyte antigens II. Lunn DP, Holmes MA, Antczak DF, eds.** Vet Immunol Immunopathol 1998;62:99–183.
35. **Bowling AT, Eggleston Stott ML, et al.** Validation of microsatellite markers for routine horse parentage testing. Anim Genet 1997;28:247–252.
36. **Meyer KM.** Pathobiology of animal platelets. Adv Vet Sci Comp Med 1985;30:131–165.
37. **Hinchcliff KW, Kociba GJ, Mitten LA.** Diagnosis of EDTA-dependent pseudothrombocytopenia in a horse. J Am Vet Med Assoc 1993;203:1715–1716.
38. **Calson GP.** Hematology and body fluids in the equine athlete: a review. In: Gillespie, Robinson, eds. Equine exercise physiology. 2nd ed. ICEEP Publications, 1987;393–425.

CHAPTER 166

Normal Hematology of Cattle, Sheep, and Goats

• JOHN W. KRAMER

GENERAL PHYSIOLOGIC AND ENVIRONMENTAL INFLUENCES

Exercise and emotional state are variables to be considered when establishing reference values in domestic ruminants. Despite the range and sensitivity of technology used, cattle, sheep, and goat blood reference values are uniformly broad (Tables 166.1–166.3).[1-3] Domesticated, cattle, sheep, and goats may have little or no direct physical contact with humans; therefore, when sampling occurs, the animals must be physically restrained and become emotionally upset. Reports of reference values seldom include such variables as exact age, emotional state, history, form of restraint, ambient temperature, state of hydration, or parasite burdens.

The numerous reference values for domestic cattle, sheep, and goats have been reported and reveal few hematologic breed differences. Breed differences have been reported for beef cattle, who have greater red blood cell (RBC) values than dairy cattle breeds, as well as sheep with different hemoglobins and goats with differing cell shapes. Care must be taken to use reference values that include similar environmental conditions and seasons as well as physiologic variables observed in the experimental population.

Lactating cows have consistently lower white blood cell (WBC), RBC, and plasma protein values than do nonlactating cows.[1] Some reports fail to recognize lactation as a physiologic process and use as their point of reference the general bovine population, including bulls, steers, calves, and nonlactating cows. Bulls have appreciably greater RBC counts than cows. As with growing maturing animals, appropriate reference values must be used to correct for physiologic variables.

Seasonal, environmental changes influence blood values. In all species, differing oxygen tensions of altitudes alter the erythron. The greater the altitude, the lower the O_2 tension and the higher the erythron reference ranges. Some Western American beef cattle experience two 5000-foot elevation changes a year that result in a packed cell volume (PCV) change of 10 to 15%. In the spring they are moved from low winter pastures to high spring and summer pastures and then back down again in the autumn. Seasonal parasite burdens also alter the complete blood cell (CBC) count.

ERYTHROCYTES

Morphology

The adult bovine's biconcave erythrocytes have a width of 5 to 6 μm and a relatively long life span of approximately 130 days (Table 166.1).[4] Anisocytosis of a slight to moderate degree characterizes the normal bovine erythrocyte. Central pallor in healthy cattle RBCs is unusual, and in disease a punched-out bowl shape uniconcavity is seen. Acanthocytosis is not unusual in blood smears from apparently healthy calves. The acanthocytes are not uniformly distributed on the slide, suggesting that their formation may be inherent to their RBC and a technical artifact. Rouleau formation is unusual in normal cattle RBCs, and the sedimentation rate is slow. Inflammatory hyperfibrinogenemia enhances rouleau formation and sedimentation. Because of the RBCs' small size and dispersion, a large amount of intercellular space is trapped in the hematocrit column.

Ovine RBCs also have an appreciably broad range (Table 166.2). This breadth may reflect the range in elevations at which sheep are raised. Caprine RBC is discoid, but the Angora breed frequently has a high percentage of fusiform RBCs (Fig. 166.1).[5] The fusiform configuration is the result of hemoglobin polymerization but is not associated with any of the species electrophoretically defined hemoglobins.

Polychromasia and reticulocytes are generally absent from the blood of normal adult cattle, sheep, and goats. When severe anemia occurs, reticulocytosis slowly appears in peripheral blood with macrocytosis, polychromasia, and basophilic stippled RBCs signaling accelerated erythropoiesis. Basophilic stippling in ruminants is common to accelerated erythropoiesis. The stippling is best demonstrated with rapidly dried, freshly made, unfixed smears of EDTA-preserved blood stained with Wright's-Giemsa stain.

TABLE 166.1   Normal Blood Values for Cattle

	Range	Mean
Erythrocytic series		
Erythrocytes ($\times10^6/\mu$L)	5.0–10.0	7.0
Hemoglobin (g/dL)	8.0–15.0	11.0
PCV (%)	24–46	35
MCV (fL)	40–60	52
MCH (pg)	11.0–17.0	14.0
MCHC (%)	30–36	32.7
RBC diameter (μm)	4.0–8.0	5.8
Miscellaneous data		
Plasma proteins (g/dL)	7.0–8.5	
Fibrinogen (mg/dL)	300–700	
Thrombocytes ($\times10^3$)	1100–800	500
RBC life span (days)	160	
Myeloid:erythroid ratio	0.3–1.9	0.7–1.0
Leukocytic series		
Total leukocytes/μL	4000–12,000	8000
Neutrophil (band)	0–120	20
Neutrophil (seg)	600–4000	2000
Lymphocyte	2500–7500	4500
Monocyte	25–840	400
Eosinophil	0–2400	700
Basophil	0–200	50
Percentage distribution		
Neutrophil (band)	0–2	0.5
Neutrophil (seg)	15–45	28
Lymphocyte	45–75	58
Monocyte	2–7	4.0
Eosinophil	0–20	9.0
Basophil	0–2	0.5

Summarized literature data from Jain NC. Schlam's veterinary hematology. 4th ed. Philadelphia: Lea & Febiger, 1986.

Hemoglobins

Studies of hemoglobin's tetrameric peptides, α and β chains, are the foundation of population and molecular genetics. Ruminant hemoglobins are of particular interest because of the large amount of polymorphism, which occurs between species, breeds, and within the individual as it develops from embryo to adult.[6] The polymorphism is greatest in the β chain. As in many other species, ruminants have two hemoglobin types. Embryonal type (HbE) to maintain a dam to in utero O_2 gradient, and adult type (HbA) for the ex utero environment. Transition from HbE to HbA begins in utero and may not be complete until months after birth. Like humans, cattle, sheep, and goats have a third hemoglobin, fetal hemoglobin (HbF), which replaces HbE in utero. As gestation progresses to the paranatal period, bovine HbF is gradually replaced by HbA. As the prenatal RBCs live out their lives, HbF-containing cells give way to HbA-containing RBCs.

Sheep and goats have a unique fourth hemoglobin type, HbC. The HbC replaces HbF at birth; within a few months, HbA replaces it. Although HbC and HbA have the same O_2 affinities at arterial pO_2, HbC's O_2 affinity is lower than HbA in the hypercapnic, hypoxic peripheral environment.[7] A unique feature of HbC and HbA of sheep and goats that is absent in HbE or HbF is the ability to switch HbC and HbA on and off by erythropoietin.[8]

All goats studied have HbC, but only sheep with HbA phenotypes A (α_2, β_2^A) or AB (α_2 $\beta_2^{A,B}$) express HbC, which makes up 15 to 30% of their total hemoglobin. Sheep with HbA phenotype B (α_2, β_2^B) do not express HbC.[1] By 30 days of a lamb's life, nearly all of the HbC is displaced by HbA. Kids, however, express the HbC for as long as 60 postnatal days, by which time the switch to HbA is complete.

Erythrocyte Metabolism

The metabolism of domestic animals' erythrocytes has recently been reviewed by Harvey.[9] Glucose consumption by bovine and ovine RBCs are similar at 0.6 and 0.7 μmol/hr/mL of RBCs, but caprine RBCs consumption rate is about 3 times greater at 1.9 μmol/hr/mL of RBCs.

An energy-dependent membrane pump maintains high intraerythrocytic/plasma ratios in many species. Most cattle, sheep, and goats have low Na^+ and K^+

TABLE 166.2   Normal Blood Values for Sheep

	Range	Mean
Erythrocytic series		
Erythrocytes ($\times10^6/\mu$L)	9–15	12.0
Hemoglobin (g/dL)	9–15	11.5
PCV (%)	27–45	35
MCV (fL)	28–40	34
MCH (pg)	8–12	10.0
MCHC (%)	31–34	32.5
RBC diameter (μm)	3.2–6.0	4.5
Miscellaneous data		
Plasma proteins (g/dL)	6.0–7.5	
Fibrinogen (mg/dL)	100–500	
Thrombocytes ($\times10^3$)	1100–800	500
RBC life span (days)	140–150	
Myeloid:erythroid ratio	0.77–1.7	1.1
Leukocytic series		
Total leukocytes/μL	4000–12,000	8000
Neutrophil (band)	Rare	—
Neutrophil (seg)	700–6000	2400
Lymphocyte	2000–9000	5000
Monocyte	0–750	200
Eosinophil	0–1000	400
Basophil	0–300	50
Percentage distribution		
Neutrophil (band)	Rare	—
Neutrophil (seg)	10–50	30.0
Lymphocyte	40–75	62
Monocyte	0–6	2.5
Eosinophil	0–10	5.0
Basophil	0–3	0.5

Summarized literature data from Jain NC. Schlam's veterinary hematology. 4th ed. Philadelphia: Lea & Febiger, 1986.

TABLE 166.3	Normal Blood Values for Goats	
	Range	Mean
Erythrocytic series		
Erythrocytes ($\times 10^6/\mu$L)	8.0–18.0	13.0
Hemoglobin (g/dL)	8.0–12.0	10.0
PCV (%)	22–38	28
MCV (fL)	16–25	19.5
MCH (pg)	5.2–8.0	6.5
MCHC (%)	30–36	33
RBC diameter (μm)	2.5–3.9	3.2
Miscellaneous data		
Plasma proteins (g/dL)	6.0–7.5	
Fibrinogen (mg/dL)	100–400	
Thrombocytes ($\times 10^3$)	300–600	450
RBC life span (days)	125	
Myeloid:erythroid ratio	0.7	
Leukocytic series		
Total leukocytes/μL	4000–13,000	9000
Neutrophil (band)	Rare	
Neutrophil (seg)	1200–7200	3250
Lymphocyte	2000–9000	5000
Monocyte	0–550	250
Eosinophil	50–650	450
Basophil	0–120	50
Percentage distribution		
Neutrophil (band)	Rare	
Neutrophil (seg)	30–48	36.0
Lymphocyte	50–70	56.0
Monocyte	0–4	2.5
Eosinophil	1–8	5.0
Basophil	0–1	0.5

Summarized literature data from Jain NC. Schlam's veterinary hematology. 4th ed. Philadelphia: Lea & Febiger, 1986.

intraerythrocytic to plasma gradients. Some cattle, sheep, and goats with specific autosomal recessive phenotypes have a high intraerythrocytic K^+ gradient associated with blood groups.[9]

Ferrous iron of oxyhemoglobins (OxHb) is constantly undergoing oxidation to ferric iron of methemoglobin (MetHb) by intracellular metabolic products.[10] Erythrocytes normally contain a low concentration of MetHb that is cyclically reduced back to OxHb by the intraerythrocytic antioxidant system's enzyme, NADH methemoglobin reductase. When the quantity of MetHb reaches a certain point, polymerization occurs and the precipitate Heinz body becomes associated with the cell membrane. Heinz bodies result in both intravascular and extravascular hemolysis and its sequela hemoglobinuria.

Erythrocytic 2,3 diphosphoglycerate (2,3 DPG) accumulation modifies some species Hb but not bovine, sheep, or goat. Ruminant feti and neonates have greater amounts of erythrocytic 2,3 DPG than adults, which have relatively low amounts of erythrocytic 2,3 DPG. However, unlike many other species, 2,3 DPG is not bound to ruminant HbF and HbA. Cattle, sheep, and goat HbFs have sufficient inherent oxygen affinity to maintain fetal pO_2.

The copper and zinc metalloenzyme superoxide dismutase was originally identified in cattle. Although dietary copper and zinc deficiencies can be characterized by reduced erythrocytic superoxide dismutase activity, its value as an in vivo antioxidant is unknown.

Another erythrocyte metalloenzyme of clinical diagnostic significance is selenium-containing glutathione peroxidase (GPX). There is a direct correlation between metal deficiency and enzyme activity.[11] Although erythrocytic GPX is directly related to a muscle disorder in ruminants, white muscle disease, it is inconsistently accompanied by methemoglobinemia. Hemolytic anemia is not a routinely reported clinical feature of selenium

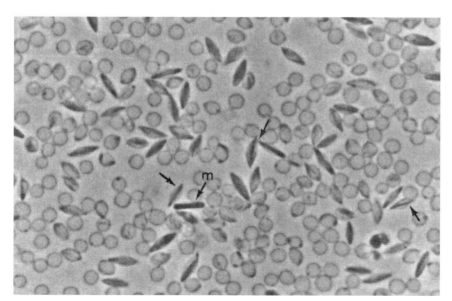

FIGURE 166.1 Blood film stained with new methylene blue. Partially lysed fusiform erythrocytes containing a dense bar of polymerized hemoglobin (arrows) can be seen among spheroidal erythrocytic ghosts. A matchstick form (m) with a dense hemoglobin rod is also present. Many spheroidal ghost cells contain one or two granules representing precipitated hemoglobin ($\times$425). (Reprinted with permission from Jain NC, Kono CS. Fusiform erythrocytes resembling sickle cell in Angora goats: light and electron microscopic observations. Res Vet Sci 1977;22:169.)

deficiency in ruminants. Heinz bodies in selenium-deficient Florida cattle is reported to be resolved by selenium treatment.[9,12] Whether the cause of the MetHb was selenium is not clear.

The various hemoglobin types and erythrocyte metabolism of cattle, sheep, and goats do not appear to make theses species' erythrocytes any more susceptible to oxidation than those of other species. Cattle have intermediate amounts of the erythrocytic pentose phosphate pathway's limiting enzyme activity, glucose phosphate dehydrogenase, and sheep and goats have appreciably less than other domestic species.[9] On occasion a ruminant's diet and microflora combination can prove to be a determinant. When plants containing large amounts of nitrates or fertilizer nitrates are eaten, the microflora reduce the nitrate to nitrite, which when absorbed oxidizes OxHb to MetHb without Heinz body formation. Sulfoxide-containing kale and other *Brassica* sp. are converted by rumen microflora to an oxidant that, when absorbed, produces Heinz body, hemolytic anemia. MetHb with and without Heinz body formation and hemoglobinuria are associated with consumption of onions and rye grass as well as copper deficiency, toxicosis, and hypophosphatemia.[13,14]

Erythrocyte Development

Erythropoietin (EPO) control of erythropoieses is well established, and a recombinant commercial human EPO is available. Because of EPO's highly conserved structure across species lines, sheep are the subject of experimental studies of EPO's control of erythropoiesis.[15] A unique feature of EPO is its direct control of the HbA to HbC shift.[8]

During gestation and at birth, the hemoglobins types change and the erythrons size increases. At birth about 60 to 90% of the neonatal calf's Hb is HbF and 9% of the RBCs reticulocytes. Fetal calves' RBCs are less fragile and larger than the adult bovine's RBCs. In early gestation, the bovine fetal RBCs have a mean corpuscular volume (MCV) of approximately 95 fL, but by birth it has decreased to about 46 fL. From birth to about 8 to 12 weeks of age, the MCV continues to decrease to approximately 37 fL as the population of HbF RBCs are replaced by RBCs containing HbA. There is a trend in cattle for the size of the erythron to decline between 6 months to about 2 years of age.

Veal calves raised solely on a diet of milk or milk replacer have lower erythron values than conventionally raised calves as the result of milk's low iron content.[2] Although veal calves have lower erythron values than conventionally reared calves, they do not have clinical signs of anemia.

Hemoglobinuria occurs in young water-deprived calves with hypertonic plasm and microcytic, hypertonic RBCs.[2,14] When dehydrated calves are allowed to drink water freely, their plasma become hypotonic within minutes. In this hypotonic matrix, the hypertonic RBCs rapidly absorb water and hemolyze before their RBC membrane can accommodate the change.[16]

There is a direct relationship between daily, abient temperature changes and hemoglobin concentration. As temperature rises, blood hemoglobin concentration increases. This fluctuation is considered to be an expression of water hypervolemia during the warmest part of the day.

LEUKOCYTES

Care must be taken in determining the significance of changes in WBCs absolute differential cell counts. Total WBC counts by electronic clinical counters have a reproducibility error of less than 1%. However, when the electronic cell count is combined with the poorly reproducible 100 differential hand cell count to calculate the absolute WBC counts, the reproducibility of minor cell type counts is poor.[17,18] This poor reproducibility of differential cell counts limits the clinical, interpretive value of absolute monocyte, eosinophile, and basophile counts. Electronic cell counting enhances the reproducibility of differential cell counts only to a minor degree.

Cell sorting by immune cell surface markers has improved specificity and sensitivity of cell counting.[19] The B lymphocytes paracrine dependency on the T lymphocytes is an example of the dynamic natural history of the cell. Specific cell subset profiles, blood and organ distribution, and cytokines are the current subjects of clinical diagnostics and prognostics research and development and may one day supplement or replace the conventional leukogram.[20–22]

Aging results in WBC changes (Table 166.4). In the first few weeks of life, neutrophils are the dominant WBC in calves, kids, and lambs. By about 2 weeks of age, the lymphocyte has become the dominant WBC, with a neutrophil to lymphocyte ratio of 0.5 in calves and lambs and 0.6 in kids. As bovine adults age, the concentration of neutrophils and lymphocytes decrease but lymphocytes continue to be the dominant cell.

Pregnancy causes minor changes in RBC and WBC concentrations. At birth, endogenous corticosteroids response of excitement and stress produces neutrophilia and lymphopenia.[1,2] The magnitude of steroid-induced neutrophilia is not as great in cattle, sheep, and goats as is reported in dogs, cats, and horses.

Neutrophils

Cattle, sheep, and goats have a smaller granulocyte bone marrow reserve than many other species, as indicated by their myeloid to erythroid ratio of about 0.5.[1,23] This small granulocyte reserve is seen in peripheral blood as a neutropenia in the early granulopoietic response to suppurative inflammatory disorders. Once the granulopoiesis is accelerated, a regenerative neutrophilia develops.[1]

Many domestic species have two types of cytoplasmic granules, secondary and primary granules, but cattle, sheep, and goats have third a granule, which gives the bovine neutrophil its eosinophilic cytoplasm.[23] In cattle,

TABLE 166.4   Absolute Leukocyte Blood Values for Female Jersey Cattle (N × 10⁻³)

Age	No. of Cattle	Total Leukocytes	Band Neutrophils	Segmented Neutrophils	Lymphocytes	Monocytes	Eosinophils	Basophils
1–6 mo	16	8.8 ± 2.5	<0.1	3.0 ± 1.8	4.7 ± 1.3	0.7 ± 0.5	0.2 ± 0.5	<0.1
6–12 mo	10	7.8 ± 1.8	0	0.8 ± 0.5	6.3 ± 1.5	0.6 ± 0.2	<0.1	0
1–2 yr	14	9.0 ± 2.5	0	2.4 ± 1.4	5.9 ± 1.6	0.4 ± 0.2	0.5 ± 0.4	<0.1
2–3 yr	31	9.4 ± 7.8	<0.1	2.2 ± 0.9	5.3 ± 1.2	0.5 ± 0.2	1.3 ± 1.0	<0.1
3–4 yr	28	7.7 ± 1.9	0	4.6 ± 1.1	4.6 ± 1.1	0.3 ± 0.2	0.9 ± 0.7	<0.1
4–6 yr	29	7.5 ± 1.1	<0.1	1.8 ± 0.7	4.0 ± 0.9	0.5 ± 0.2	1.2 ± 0.7	<0.1
>6 yr	21	7.7 ± 2.5	<0.1	1.8 ± 0.9	4.4 ± 2.1	0.4 ± 0.2	1.3 ± 0.7	<0.1

Adapted with modifications from Jain NC. Schlam's veterinary hematology. 4th ed. Philadelphia: Lea & Febiger, 1986.

this third neutrophil granule is larger than the primary and secondary granules and occupies twice the cytoplasmic space as they do in sheep and other domestic species. The bovine's large neutrophil granules have more antimicrobial activity than the cytoplasmic granules of nonruminant species. In sheep these large granules occupy less space and the cytoplasm is more of a granular eosinophilic texture (Figs. 166.2, 166.3, 166.4).

Cytochemical and immunocytochemical staining reveals a range of enzymes and substrates in ruminant neutrophils[1,9] (Fig. 166.6). Lysozyme, an enzyme common to many species, is not found in the neutrophils of cattle, sheep, or goats. Immunocytochemical cell membrane antigens serve to add to the specificity of neutrophil characterization.

Eosinophils

The ruminant's eosinophil's band to bilobed nucleus is surrounded by numerous, small, uniformly round, intensely stained red, refractile, cytoplasmic granules in sparse basophilic cytoplasm (Fig. 166.2 [4]). Ovine eosinophil granules are unique in containing a crystal ultrastructure, which is sometimes seen with the light microscope as a dark nevus in the granule (Figs. 166.4B, 166.5).

Parasite-free calves to tend to double their eosinophil values from 6 months of age to adulthood. As in other animals, parasites and their larvae can produce eosinophilia. Seasonal parasite infestations are reflected in seasonal eosinophilia. An example is the eosinophilia of subcutaneous migration of ox warble larva in the spring which produces transit marked eosinophilia in cattle free of intestinal nematodes. Eosinophilia has been associated with milk autoantibodies in dairy cows.[24]

Basophils

The basophil of sheep, cattle, and goats is a sparse cell of the same size as the eosinophil, with electron-dense, numerous, small, intensely blue-staining granules sometimes masking the nucleus. Basophils occurring at such low concentrations are not reliably quantified by the 100-cell differential cell method (Figs. 166.2 [5] and 166.3).

Lymphocytes

As in most species, the ruminant neonate begins life with fewer lymphocytes than granulocytes. In a matter of months, their concentration doubles and by 3 months of age they make up 70 to 80% of the total WBC (Tables 166.1–166.3). After a few years, a slow decline of lymphocytes occurs. The age-related fluctuations in lymphocyte concentration exemplify the need for age-related reference values, but its effect on the T- and B-cell subsets is not clear.[1,25]

Bovine lymphocytes are 8 to 15 μm in diameter and are described in three sizes.[1,2] Small lymphocytes have a small, round nucleus containing a densely staining chromatin pattern elliptically located in a small volume of clear to gray-blue cytoplasm. The sparsity of the cytoplasm and density of the chromatin suggest that the small lymphocyte may be metabolically dormant or at the least less active than the other two forms of lymphocytes. In comparison to small lymphocytes, the medium lymphocytes have larger, round to indented-shaped nuclei in which the same amount of chromatin is spread over a greater area, revealing lighter staining parachromatin adjoining areas of condensed chromatin. The cytoplasmic volume of medium lymphocytes is also greater than that seen in the small lymphocyte and encircles the eccentrically placed nucleus. Large lymphocytes have an even larger, lighter staining nucleus and more cytoplasm than the medium-sized lymphocyte. This large lymphocyte has a round or indented or deeply cleaved centrally placed nucleus. These lymphocytes are frequently confused with the monocytes and are sometimes called transitional lymphocytes. Like monocytes, large lymphocyte's cytoplasm stains blue to gray and sometimes contains small clear vacuoles. Unlike the monocyte, the lymphocyte's nucleus does become bilobed and the two cell's cytochemical and immunocytochemical staining are different. Variable shapes, sizes, and numbers of magenta cytoplasmic granules are frequently seen in a focal arrangement in the lymphocytes of cattle, sheep, and goats and may serve to identify the large bovine lymphocyte. Agranular large lymphocytes and monocytes are ultrastructurally inseparable, and cytochemical and immunocytochemical staining are needed to separate these two cell types. Chromatin cen-

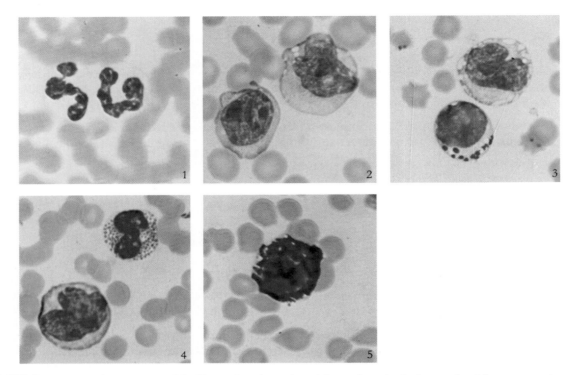

FIGURE 166.2 (1) Mature bovine neutrophils. The rouleau formation of the erythrocytes is abnormal and is a response to an inflammatory disease. (2) A bovine lymphocyte (cell with round nucleus) and a monocyte. (3) A bovine monocyte and a lymphocyte with azurophilic cytoplasmic granules. (4) A bovine eosinophil containing distinct reddish granules and a monocyte. From the same blood as 1. (5) A bovine basophil. Intensely stained metachromatic cytoplasmic granules usually mask the nucleus in basophils.

ters, nucleolar rings, and nucleoli are seen with a low frequency in Wright's-stained normal bovine lymphocytes, and caution must be taken in using these features as evidence of neoplasia.

Lymphocytes of sheep and goats do not have unique features. They are most commonly of the small and medium size, and confusion with monocytes is less of a problem than it is in cattle. Their sparse lymphocyte cytoplasm is blue to gray, and the variably sized and shaped magenta granules are frequently seen in a large proportion of lymphocytes present but with unknown significance (Figs. 166.3 and 166.4).

The subsets of ruminant leukocytes and their cytokines are active subjects of study. Cell sorting technology allows for the identification of subsets of lymphocytes beyond the T and B cells and their natural history.[22] Some subsets have a predilection for various anatomic sites, and disease states result in altered peripheral blood subset profiles.[21,26,27]

Monocytes

The ruminant monocyte is a round to convoluted-shaped cell from 13 to 19 μm in diameter. It has a large indented to bilobed nucleus containing a diffuse chromatin pattern in a gray cytoplasm containing fine, small, indistinct, magenta to eosinophilic granules. Vacuoles

are common and more irregular in shape than those seen in some large lymphocytes (Figs. 166.2 [4], 166.3, and 166.4D).

PLATELETS

Ruminant platelets in Wright's-stained peripheral blood are distributed singly and in aggregates with variable size and shape with azurophilic granules. Cytoplasmic projections are rare. Normal circulating survival time is thought to be about 10 days. Giant platelet forms and pseudopodia are associated with recent proliferation from megakaryocytes. The ultrastructure of the bovine platelets consists of extensive invaginations of surface membrane.[27,28]

BONE MARROW

Care must be taken when interpreting bone marrow aspirates. Clones of hemopoietic cell types are randomly distributed through the marrow, and the quantification is a relative expression and not as concentration per unit volume. Extensive studies of the bovine bone marrow in embryos, calves, and adults have been reported. The single most remarkable feature of bovine

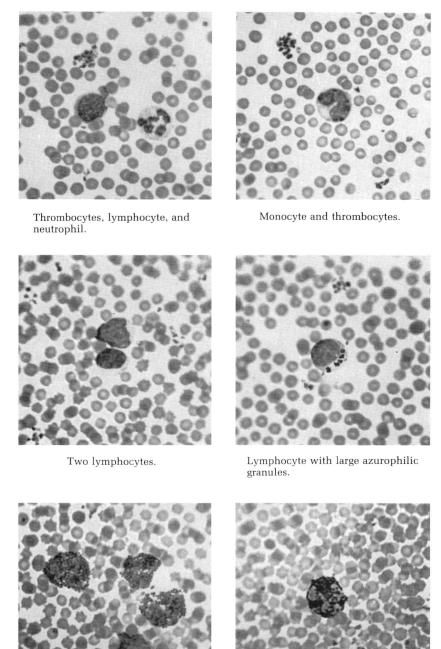

FIGURE 166.3 Ovine blood cells (original magnification, ×600).

Thrombocytes, lymphocyte, and neutrophil.

Monocyte and thrombocytes.

Two lymphocytes.

Lymphocyte with large azurophilic granules.

Three eosinophils and one lymphocyte.

Basophil.

bone marrow is the myeloid:erythroid (M:E) ratio of 0.5 to 0.6. A similar M:E ratio is reported in goats, but in sheep the ratio is about 1. The low bovine bone marrow M:E correlates with the low neutrophil concentration in their peripheral blood and the rapid rate at which they are depleted and a degenerative left shift occurs in an inflammation. The iliac crest and ribs are sources of bone marrow. Increased bone marrow macrophage activity is subjectively used to detect accelerated erythrophagocytosis. Increased nucleophagocytosis, erythrophagocytosis, bilirubin, and iron pigments are indicators of accelerated erythropoiesis.

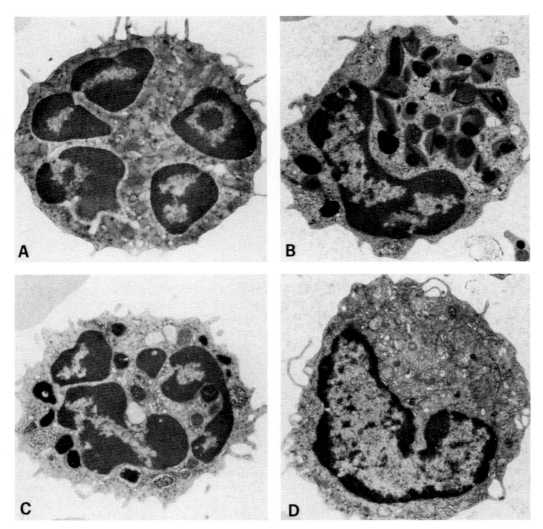

FIGURE 166.4 An ovine neutrophil **(A)**, eosinophil **(B)**, basophil **(C)**, and monocyte **(D)** prepared from the buffy coat of peripheral blood. The neutrophil **(A)** has a multilobed nucleus, and its cytoplasm is filled with larger, electron-dense primary granules and smaller, less-dense specific granules. Few other cellular organelles are seen (×14,000). The eosinophil **(B)** of the sheep is characterized by pleomorphic granules that contain crystalloid rods and membranous whorls. Cellular organelles are sparse (×12,000). The basophil **(C)** also contains a diverse population of cytoplasmic granules. Maturation of granules proceeds from lightly to densely stippled structures (×13,000). The cytoplasm of the monocyte **(D)** has granules, vesicles, and abundant ribosomes. Rough endoplasmic reticulum, mitochondria, and Golgi bodies are prominent (×13,000). (Photographs courtesy of Dr. Kurt H. Albertine and Dr. Norman C. Staub.)

PLASMA PROTEINS

The color of bovine plasma ranges from very yellow to colorless depending on the quantity of dietary plant chromogens. Summer green feed results in the deepest yellow, and winter dry fodder the lightest. This is in contrast to the plasma of sheep and goats, which is colorless independent of dietary chromogens.

Presuckled, neonatal ruminant plasma proteins are predominately albumin, hepatic origin alpha globulins, and very limited immunoglobulin. In the first day of life, dynamic changes occur in ruminant plasma proteins. Having suckled, colostral water and immunoglobulins are quickly absorbed through the rapidly closing gut wall into plasma. Total body water increases, lowering the plasma albumin concentration, and colostral immunoglobulins, and enzymes, GGT and AP, increase to their maximum by 48 hours. Total serum protein concentration in presuckled calves increases from about 4 g/dL to as much as 7 g/dL. There is an empiric, direct relationship between the amount of total plasma protein in the postsuckled calf and frequency of early calfhood diseases. This relationship is so well established in the veal calf industry that veal calf buyers will frequently only accept calves with greater than 5 g/dL of plasma protein.

Panhyperproteinemia is common to dehydration and when severe may rise to 10 g/dL. At this level hypervis-

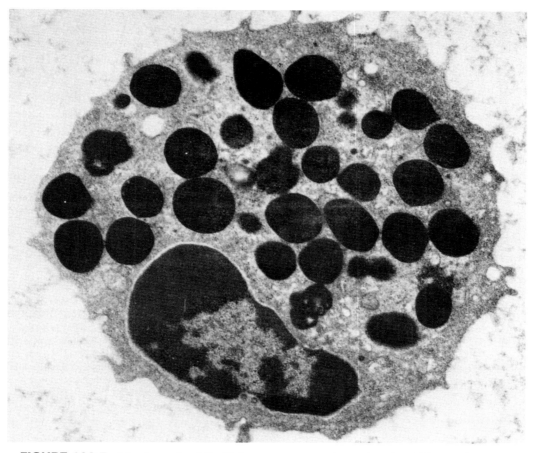

FIGURE 166.5 A bovine eosinophil with homogenous, round granules of variable sizes (×13,500).

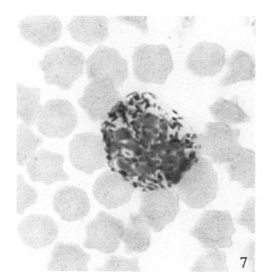

FIGURE 166.6 Sudan black B-positive granules in a bovine neutrophil. Sudanophilia in neutrophils generally parallels their peroxidase activity. Stained by the method of Sheehan and Storey.[31]

cosity can be of concern. Hyper-γ-globulinemia is common to inflammatory disorders and associated with hyperfibrinogenemia.

Plasma fibrinogen and haptoglobin are acute phase hepatic proteins. Fibrinogen has been a popular indicator of occult inflammatory disorders in ruminants for some time, and haptoglobin only recently has common into use. As a rule, the greater the magnitude of their increase, the greater the magnitude of inflammation. Some individuals regard hyperfibrinogenemia to be as good as or better than neutrophiles as an indicator of occult inflammation. Although fibrinogen haptoglobins are acute phase proteins which can increase appreciably in plasma in a single day at the onset of suppurative inflammations, they may remain elevated for as long as the inflammation is present.

Plasma fibrinogen is low (160 ± 130 mg/dL) to undetectable in neonatal calves. By 3 to 16 weeks of life it has risen to adult values of 300 to 700 mg/dL.[1] Independent of a calf's low baseline value, inflammation can still elicit a hyperfibrinogenemia of the magnitude seen in adult cattle with inflammatory diseases. Dehydration increases the plasma protein concentration, including fibrinogen. Compensation for dehydration in adult cattle can be determined by a ratio of plasma protein to fibrinogen. A ratio of less than 10:1, and more precisely 8:1, is indicative of an absolute increase in fibrinogen. An inherent problem with using the ratio is that hyperimmunoglobulinemia of inflammation may distort the ratio and present clinical chemistry profile dehydration in a subject not clinically dehydrated.

The efficacy of haptoglobins as an indicator of inflammation has been established, but because of greater ease in measurement and reported clinical use, fibrinogen is a more established diagnostic procedure.[29,30] With the recognition of structural conservation between species, simpler immunologic assays being developed may change haptoglobins status.

REFERENCES

1. **Jain NC.** Schalm's veterinary hematology. 4th ed. Philadelphia: Lea & Febiger, 1986:178, 208, 225.
2. **Archer RK, Jefcott LB.** Comparative clinical hematology. 1st ed. Oxford: Blackwell Scientific, 1977:215, 305.
3. **Mbassa GK, Poulsen JS.** The comparative hematology of cross-bred and indigenous east African goats of Tanzania and breeds reared in Denmark. Vet Res Commun 1992;16:221–229.
4. **Vacha J.** Red cell life span. In: Ager NS, Boards PG, eds. Red blood cells of domestic mammals. Amsterdam: Elsevier, 1983;67–132.
5. **Jain NC, Kono CS.** Fusiform erythrocytes resembling sickle cells in Angora goats: light and electron microscopic observations. Vet Sci 1977;22:169–180.
6. **Kitchen H, Brett I.** Embryonic and fetal Hb in animals. Ann N Y Acad Sci 1974;241:653–671.
7. **Winslow RM, Swenberg ML, Benson J, Perrella M, Benzzi L.** Gas exchange properties of goat hemoglobins A and C. J Biol Chem 1989;264:4812–4817.
8. **Barker JE, Pierce JE, Nienhuis AW.** Hemoglobin switching in sheep: a comparison of the erythropoietin-induced switch to HbC and the fetal to adult hemoglobin switch. Blood 1980;56:488–494.
9. **Harvey JW.** The erythrocyte: physiology, metabolism, and biochemical disorders. In: Kaneko JJ, Harvey JW, Bruss ML, eds. Clinical biochemistry of domestic animals. 5th ed. San Diego: Academic Press, 1998;157.
10. **Ohno H, Nomura M, Watanabe K.** A possible mechanism of Heinz body hemolytic anemia induced by DQ-2511, a new gastroprokinetic drug, in dogs. Fund Appl Toxicol 1996;32:269–277.
11. **Kramer JW, Hoffman WE.** Clinical enzymology. In: Kaneko JJ, Harvey JW, Bruss ML, eds. Clinical biochemistry of domestic animals. 5th ed. San Diego: Academic Press, 1998;303.
12. **Maas J, Parish SM, Hodgson DR, Valberg SJ.** Nutritional myopathies. In: Smith B, ed. Large animal internal medicine. 2nd ed. St. Louis: Mosby, 1996;1513.
13. **Carlson GP.** Heinz body hemolytic anemia. In: Smith B, ed. Large animal internal medicine. 2nd ed. St. Louis: Mosby, 1996;1227.
14. **Ogawa E, Kobayashi K, Yoshiura N, Mukai J.** Hemolytic anemia and red blood cell metabolic disorder attributable to low phosphorus intake in cows. Am J Vet Res 1989;50:388–392.
15. **Wen D, Boissel JP, Tracy TE, Gruninger RH, et al.** Erythropoietin structure-function relationships: high degree of sequence homology among mammals. Blood 1993;83:1507–1516.
16. **Shimizu Y, Naito Y, Murakami D.** The experimental study on the mechanism of hemolysis on paroxysmal hemoglobinuria in calves due to excessive water intake. Jpn J Vet Res 1979;19:583–592.
17. **Kjeldsberg CR.** Principles of hematologic examination. In: Lee GR, Bithell TC, Foerster J, Athens JW, Lukens JN, eds. Wintrobe's clinical hematology. 9th ed. Philadelphia: Lea & Febiger, 1993;7.
18. Leukocyte differential counting, HIO-T, tentative standard. Villanova, Pennsylvania, National Committee for Laboratory Standards. 1984;4:257.
19. **Naessens J, Hobkins J, eds.** 3rd workshop on ruminant leukocyte antigens. Vet Immunol Immunopathol 1996;52:213–472.
20. **Davis WC, Hamilton MJ.** Comparison of the unique characteristics of the immune system in different species of mammals. Vet Immunol Immunopathol 1998;63:7–13.
21. **Stone DM, McElwain, Davis WC.** Enhanced B-lymphocyte expression of IL-2Rα associated with T lymphocytosis in BLV-infected persistently lymphocytic cows. Leukemia 1994;8:1057–1061.
22. **Jolly PE, Gangopadhyay A, Chen S, et al.** Changes in the leukocyte phenotype profile of goats infected with caprine arthritis encephalitis virus. Vet Immunol Immunopathol 1997;56:97–106.
23. **Bertram TA.** Neutrophilic leukocytes structure and function in domestic animals. Adv Vet Sci Comp Med 1985;30:91–129.
24. **Campbell SG.** Milk allergy and autoallergy disease of cattle. Cornell Vet 1970;60:684.
25. **Bendixen HJ.** Bovine enzootic leukosis. Adv Vet Sci Comp Med 1965;10:129–203.
26. **Cullor JS, Tyler JW.** Mammary gland health and disorder. In: Smith B, ed. Large animal internal medicine. 2nd ed. St. Louis: Mosby, 1996;1177.
27. **Meyers KM.** Pathobiology of animal platelets. Adv Vet Sci Comp Med 1985;30:131–165.
28. **M'enard M, Meyers KM.** Storage pool deficiency in cattle with the Chédiak-Higashi syndrome results from an absence of dense granule precursors in their megakaryocytes. Blood 1988;72:1726–1734.
29. **McNair J, Kennedy DG, Bryson DG, Reilly GA, McDowell SW, Mackie DP.** Evaluation of a competitive immunoassay for the detection of bovine haptoglobin. Res Vet Sci 1997;63:145–149.
30. **Katnik I, Pupek M, Stefaniak T.** Cross reactivities among some mammalian haptoglobins studied by a monoclonal antibody. Comp Biochem Physiol [B] Biochem Mol Biol 1998;119:335–340.
31. **Sheehan JL, Ishmael DR.** Acute lymphocytic leukemia with atypical cytochemical features. Am J Clin Pathol 1975;63:415–420.

CHAPTER 167

Normal Blood Values of the Water Buffalo (*Bubalus bubalis*)

• JAWAHAR LAL VEGAD

Table 167.1 presents selected data from the literature on hematology of water buffaloes, and additional details can be found in references cited. Various blood values obtained for 50 clinically normal, lactating Indian Murrah water buffaloes are presented in Table 167.2.[1]

Prominent features in the normal hemogram of water buffaloes include an average size mean corpuscular volume (MCV) of the erythrocytes similar to that in cattle, low icterus index, pronounced erythrocyte sedimentation rate (ESR), absence of reticulocytes, and predominance of lymphocytes over neutrophils. Morphologic features of erythrocytes, leukocytes, and platelets are similar to those in cattle. A brief description of blood cells as seen in 50 Indian Murrah water buffaloes is presented.

Erythrocytes usually exhibit slight to marked rouleaux formation, slight anisocytosis, and uniform staining. Individual erythrocytes, however, appear as slightly biconcave discs with distinct or indistinct central pallor. Biconcave discocytic morphology of the erythrocytes is clearly visible in scanning electron microscopy (Fig. 167.1). Polychromasia is absent, as are reticulocytes in the new methylene blue-stained films. Howell-Jolly bodies are rare.

Platelets are abundant and usually distributed in small to large clumps. Individual platelets are pleomorphic, round to elongated, measure about a quarter to half the size of any erythrocyte, and contain small but distinct azurophilic granules.

Small, medium, and large lymphocytes are present in varying numbers. However, usually only one type predominates in an individual animal. Their nuclei are characteristically round or oval, with an occasional slight indentation, and contain coarsely granular and/or plaqued chromatin. The cytoplasm stains pale to dark blue. Some lymphocytes contain a few azurophilic granules (0.5 to 2 μm). Rarely, binucleated lymphocytes, lymphocytes with nucleated rings, and lymphocytes with few cytoplasmic vacuoles are observed.

Monocytes are usually larger than lymphocytes. Their nuclei are amoeboid in shape and contain finely granular, "lacy," or "stringy" and sometimes plaqued chromatin. The cytoplasm stains moderately blue and appears grainy or foamy and vacuolated. Rarely, a few fine azurophilic granules may be observed in the cytoplasm.

Neutrophils usually have coiled, multilobed, and sometimes monolobed nuclei and pale to slightly pink, fine, indistinct cytoplasmic granules. The multilobed nuclei have two to four lobes with plaqued chromatin, a few clear areas of euchromatin, and an irregular outline. The monolobed nuclei exhibit one or two shallow constrictions, slight membrane roughness, and relatively less chromatin condensation than multilobed neutrophils. Band cells are rare and have, in comparison, a smooth nuclear outline without constrictions.

Eosinophils contain small, uniformly round, bright pink granules almost filling the clear or pale cytoplasm. Their nuclei are usually smaller and less lobulated than those of neutrophils.

Basophils contain numerous large, dark purple granules that almost mask the nuclear lobes.

Hematologic examination carried out on buffalo fetuses of 3 to 10 months gestation revealed that red blood cells (RBCs), hemoglobin (Hb), packed cell volume (PCV), and white blood cells (WBCs) increased with age.[2] Reticulocytes were present in significant numbers at 3 to 4 months, after which their number decreased and were absent by the ninth month. Lymphocytes increased gradually until 6 months, when a sharp increase occurred. Neutrophils decreased between 3 and 10 months. Eosinophils, basophils, and monocytes were not seen before 5 months.

Hematologic changes with age have been studied in Indian Murrah water buffaloes from birth to 28 days of life[3] (Table 167.1). The RBC count decreased on day 1 and fluctuated up to 28 days. Hb and PCV values were higher at birth than in adults and decreased on day 28. The differential leukocyte count consisted of 60% neutrophils and 39.7% lymphocytes at birth and changed to 32.2% and 66.4%, respectively, by day 28. Monocytes and eosinophils increased during the 28-day period but were still below 1%. Similar studies were performed on Egyptian buffalo calves from birth to 6 months of age.[4] Lymphocytes increased from birth to a

TABLE 167.1 Selected Published Hematologic Values of Water Buffaloes (*Bubalus bubalis*)

Source	Species	Number, Age, Sex	RBC (×10⁶/μL)	Hb (g/dL)	PCV (%)	WBC (×10³/μL)	Neutrophils	Lymphocytes	Monocytes	Eosinophils	Basophils
Hafez and Anwar (1954)[a]	Egyptian water buffaloes	20 females	6.8	11.0–15.2 (13.0)	38–52 (44.3)	6.7	36.0	51.0	8.0	5.0	1.0
Thangaraj et al. (1979)[b]	Indian water buffaloes	Birth	8.07 ± 1.22	20.66 ± 2.18	50.9 ± 6.88	9.09 ± 2.56	60.0	39.7	0.08	0	—
		1 day	6.50 ± 2.0	—	—	7.30 ± 2.24	—	—	—	—	—
		28 days	—	17.31 ± 1.3	43.46 ± 4.43	8.39 ± 1.65	32.15	66.4	0.77	0.62	—
Murthy (1980)[a]	Indian water buffaloes	192 (4–8 yr)	5.7 ± 0.1	10.3 ± 0.2	37.9 ± 0.5	9.1 ± 0.1	24.1 ± 1.0	67.9 ± 12	—	4.4 ± 0.1	—
Patil et al. (1992 a,b)[a]	Indian water buffaloes	18 females	6.77 ± 0.08	11.81 ± 0.15	30.58 ± 0.25	7.96 ± 0.29	31.45 ± 0.78	63.33 ± 0.55	3.52 ± 0.22	1.99 ± 0.14	0.08 ± 0.00
Sulong et al. (1980)[c]	Malaysian swamp buffaloes	50 (2–4 yr)	8.8	13.4	39.2	10.7	35.2	54.2	3.7	6.6	0.3

[a] See Suggested Readings.
[b] See Reference 3.
[c] See Reference 9.

TABLE 167.2	Hematologic Values in 50 Clinically Normal, Lactating Indian Murrah Buffaloes		
Parameter	**Range**	**Mean**	**Standard Deviation**
RBC ($\times 10^6/\mu$L)	5.07–8.27	6.54	0.77
Hb (g/dL)	9–13.5	11.1	0.96
PCV (%)	26–34	31.0	2.0
MCV (fL)	40.6–55.2	48.2	4.60
MCHC (%)	30.5–38.5	35.2	2.34
MCH (pg)	13.5–20.5	17.10	1.85
Icterus index (units)	2–5	2	1.25
ESR (mm at 1 hr)	17–69	53	12.30
Plasma protein (g/dL)	6–9	7.8	0.70
Fibrinogen (g/dL)	0.2–0.8	0.37	0.20
Reticulocytes (%)	0	0	0
WBC (number/μL)	6250–13,050	9676	1789
Bands	0–106	18	40
Neutrophils	1285–6893	3257	1262
Lymphocytes	2554–9637	5065	1595
Monocytes	63–1349	584	301
Eosinophils	170–1471	592	452
Basophils	0–326	131	98
WBC, percentages			
Bands	0–1	0.2	0.34
Neutrophils	13–54	32.9	8.74
Lymphocytes	26–75	52.7	12.0
Monocytes	1–11.5	5.9	2.63
Eosinophils	2–14.0	6.9	4.64
Basophils	0–3.5	1.4	1.02

Modified from Jain NC, Vegad JL, Jain NK, et al. Haematological studies on normal lactating Indian water buffaloes. Res Vet Sci 1981;32:52.

peak at 4 months, while eosinophils were usually below 1% until 4 months, when they were nearly absent. In six Indian buffalo calves, plasma fibrinogen concentration was lower (0.53 g/dL) at 2 weeks of age than at 6 months of age (0.82 g/dL), and it was positively correlated with ESR and negatively correlated with PCV.[5]

Important age-related changes in the hemogram of Indian Murrah water buffaloes include a slight decline in PCV by 3 months of age, followed by a gradual increase to adult levels after 24 months. The ESR increases gradually and is highest in adults; similarly, whole blood viscosity increases with age. The neutrophil : lymphocyte ratio decreases gradually from birth to 2 to 4 years of age because of reduction in neutrophil numbers and a corresponding increase in lymphocytes.[6]

Water buffaloes, like horses, do not show significant reticulocytosis during recovery from acute blood loss anemia. Their leukocyte responses to corticosteroid and endotoxin administration[7] are generally similar to those of cattle.[8] Stress-related changes in differential leukocyte counts, similar to those in cattle, occur at parturition.

Malaysian swamp buffaloes were found to have higher RBC, Hb, PCV, and WBC values than river buffaloes and cattle.[9] Similar hematologic values were reported for mature Australian swamp buffaloes.[10] RBC, Hb, and PCV values were lower in spray-cooled or wallowing Indian water buffaloes than in those at normal environmental temperature.[11] Seasonal changes in blood values and serum proteins have been reported.[12,13] A significant correlation was found between red cell glutathione peroxidase activity and plasma selenium in 89 Egyptian water buffaloes.[14]

The American bison (*Bison bison*), or buffalo, shows some age-related variations in blood values.[15] Calves have higher red cell values and a leukogram typical of cattle in that lymphocytes exceed neutrophils. However, adults have higher numbers of neutrophils and eosinophils and lower lymphocyte numbers.

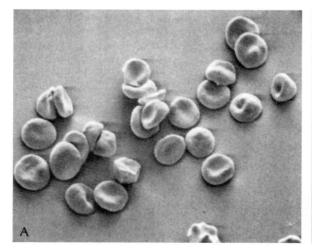
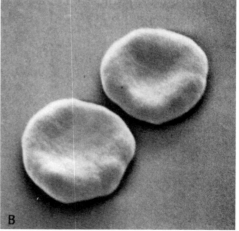

FIGURE 167.1 Scanning electron photomicrographs of buffalo blood depicting discocytic erythrocytes with typical concave surface and two erythrocytes with narrow concavity. **A,** ×1800; **B,** ×4000. (Reprinted with permission from Jain NC, et al. Haematological studies on normal lactating Indian water buffaloes. Res Vet Sci 1982;32:52.)

REFERENCES

1. **Jain NC, Vegad JL, Jain NK, Shrivastava AB.** Haematological studies on normal lactating Indian water buffaloes. Res Vet Sci 1981;32:52–56.
2. **El-Naggar MA, Ibrahim H, Serur BH.** Haematological parameters of buffalo foetus. Assiut Vet Med J 1982;9:167–169.
3. **Thangaraj TM, Seshagiri VN, Krishnan AR, Venkataswami V.** Haematological changes in neonate of *Bubalus bubalis*. Indian J Dairy Sci 1979;32:240–242.
4. **Karram MH, El-Amrousi SA, Raghib MF, Amer AA.** Studies on the red and white blood cells of buffalo calves from birth up to 6 months age. J Egypt Vet Med Assoc 1981;39:133–141.
5. **Nangia OP, Garg SL.** Age-related changes in plasma fibrinogen and related parameters in buffalo-calves. Indian J Anim Sci 1982;52:1024–1027.
6. **Sharma MC, Pathak NN, Verma RP, Hung NN, Cu NV, Lien NH, An DT, Mai HV, Vuc NV.** Normal haematology of Murrah buffaloes of various ages in the agroclimatic conditions in Viet Nam. Indian Vet J 1985;62:383–386.
7. **Jain NC, Vegad JL, Shrivastava AB, Jain NK, Garg UK, Kolte GN.** Haematological changes in buffalo calves inoculated with *Escherichia coli* endotoxin and corticosteroids. Res Vet Sci 1989;47:305–308.
8. **Jain NC, Lasmanis J.** Leucocytic changes in cows given intravenous injection of *Escherichia coli* endotoxin. Res Vet Sci 1978;24:386–387.
9. **Sulong A, Hilmi M, Jainudeen MR.** Haematology of the Malaysian swamp buffalo (*Bubalus bubalis*). Pertanika 1980;3:66–70 (Vet Bull 1981;51:688).
10. **Canfield PJ, Best FG, Fairburn AJ, Purdie J, Gilham M.** Normal haematological and biochemical values for the swamp Buffalo (*Bubalus bubalis*) in Australia. Aust Vet J 1984;61:89–93.
11. **Bahga GS, Gangwar PC, Srivastava RK, Dhigra DP.** Effect of spray cooling and wallowing on blood composition in buffaloes during summer. Indian J Dairy Sci 1980;33:294–298.
12. **Anwar M, Chaudhri AQ.** Haematology of buffalo during summer and winter. Pakistan Vet J 1984;4:5–6.
13. **Salem IA.** Seasonal variations in some body reactions and blood constituents in lactating buffaloes and Friesian cows with reference to acclimatization. J Egypt Vet Med Assoc 1980;40:63–72.
14. **Gazia N, Wegger I.** Glutathione peroxidase and selenium in blood from Egyptian water buffaloes. Acta Vet Scand 1980;21:137–139.
15. **Sikarskie JG, Schillhorn van Veen TW, van Selm G, Kock MD.** Comparative blood characteristics of ranched and free-ranging American bison (Bison). Am J Vet Res 1990;51:955–957.

SUGGESTED READINGS

Hafez ESE, Anwar A. Normal haematological values in the buffalo. Nature 1954;174:611–612.

Hafez AM, Ibrahim H, Gomaa A, Farrag AA, Salem IA. Enzymatic and haematological studies on buffaloes at periparturient periods. Assiut Vet Med J 1983;11:173–175.

Jain NC. Essentials of veterinary hematology. Philadelphia: Lea & Febiger, 1993.

Kohli RN, Singh S, Singh M. Studies on erythrocyte sedimentation rate in buffaloes. I. Evaluation of various techniques. Indian Vet J 1975;52:915–918.

Kumar R, Jindal R, Rattan PJS. Haematological investigations in buffaloes from birth to sexual maturity. Indian Vet J 1990;67:311–314.

Kumar R, Sharma TP, Rattan PJS. Haematological studies during estrogen cycle in Murrah buffalo heifers. Indian Vet J 1992;69:894–897.

Malik JK, Chand N, Singh RV, Singh PP, Bahga HS, Sud SC. Haematology of male buffalo calves. Indian Vet J 1974;51:95–99.

Moustafa IH, Soliman MK, Naser H. Some peculiarities of buffaloes blood. Vet Med J 1963;10:263–269.

Murthy TS. A note on certain cellular constituents of blood in buffaloes. Livestock Adviser, Bangalore, India 1980;5:44–45 (Vet Bull 1981;51:368).

Oshiro S, Shinjo A, Takahashi H, Koja Z. Comparative studies on the blood composition of water buffaloes, cattle and goats. Sci Bull College Agri, Univ Ryukyus, Okinawa, 1978;25:383–387 (Abstr Vet Bull 1979;49:985).

Patil MD, Talvelkar BA, Joshi VG, Deshmukh BT. Haematological studies in Murrah buffaloes. Indian Vet J 1992a;69:661–663.

Patil MD, Talvelkar BA, Joshi VG, Deshmukh BT. Haematological studies in Murrah buffaloes: TLC, DLC and micrometry of leucocytes. Indian Vet J 1992b;69:760–761.

Satija KC, Rajpal S, Pandey R, Sharma VK. Electrophoresis of buffalo (*Bos bubalis*) serum proteins including immunoglobulins. Infect Immun 1979;24:567–570.

Umesh KR, Reddy V, Chandra S, Rao AS, Reddy CE, Reddy VS, Reddy GVN. Studies on certain blood constituents of rural buffaloes during cyclic and post-partum periods. Indian Vet J 1995;72:469–471.

Vihan VS, Joshi BP, Rai P. A note on electrophoretic pattern of serum proteins in some disease conditions among buffaloes. Indian J Anim Sci 1973;43:546–549.

Vogel J, Vogel L. Some haematological indices of the buffalo (*Bubalus bubalis*). Veterinaria (Rio de Janeiro) 1967;20:166–169.

CHAPTER 168

Normal Hematology of the Pig

• CATHERINE E. THORN

Routine hematology is not often performed in pigs. The low intrinsic value of individual animals, difficulty in collecting blood, and wide ranges reported for many hematologic parameters reduce the utility of the complete blood count in swine. For more detailed information on porcine hematology and hematopoietic organs, the reader is referred to other reviews.[1-4] An extensive collection of photographs of porcine blood and bone marrow cells may be found in Sanderson and Phillips.[5]

EDTA anticoagulant and a Romanowsky type stain are preferred for optimal cytologic evaluation. Because porcine red cell is relatively fragile, excess turbulence or improper handling of the sample often results in hemolysis. Routine hemogram values, except the differential count, are stable at 20°C or 4°C for 36 hours,[6] whereas the white cell differential count becomes less reliable within 12 hours after collection.[6] Automated counting of leukocyte subsets[7] and reticulocytes[8] has been reported.

REFERENCE INTERVALS

Many reference intervals for porcine blood have been published.[3,5,9-11] Although most published intervals are comparable, the range for most elements of porcine blood are quite wide (Table 168.1). Variability may be due to sex, breed, growth rate, diet, age, stage of gestation or lactation, feeding method, management practices, or season.[10,12,13] Interpretation of porcine hematology data requires consideration of these factors.

ERYTHROCYTES

Porcine red cells have an average diameter of 6.0 μm (Fig. 168.1). Spiny crenation is common, and the cells tend to form rouleaux in health. Central pallor is not visible in every cell. Anisocytosis is seen in adults but is more prominent in young pigs. Blood from young pigs often contains many large polychromatic cells, nucleated red cells, and Howell-Jolly bodies.

The pig erythrocyte is highly susceptible to hemolysis by hypotonic saline. Porcine red cells display a bimodal pattern, with adult cells and fetal populations being more resistant to lysis than red cells from weaned pigs. Osmotic resistance is temperature-, pH-, and time-dependent[14,15] but not influenced by sex or breed.[16] The sedimentation rate of pig erythrocytes is faster than that of other domestic animals[1,17] and is subject to daily fluctuations.[18]

LEUKOCYTES

The mature neutrophil is 12 to 15 μm in diameter. It has an irregular nuclear membrane and moderately coarse chromatin with well-defined lobes. The cytoplasm stains a pale pink or blue and contains few pink granules. Band neutrophils have a U-shaped nucleus but are otherwise similar to the mature form (Fig. 168.2). Band cells may be present in the healthy animal. Metamyelocytes have a less mature chromatin pattern, and nuclear shape may vary from kidney-bean–shaped to a ring form with no lobation. The cytoplasm is pale blue. Eosinophil nuclei are poorly segmented and may appear immature (Fig. 168.3). The cytoplasmic granules are round to oval, stain a pale orange, and tend to fill the cytoplasm. The basophil nucleus stains lavender and has a smooth chromatin pattern (Fig. 168.4). The cytoplasmic granules of the basophil are coccoid to dumbell-shaped and stain similarly to or more intensely than the nucleus.

Small lymphocytes are 7 to 10 μm in diameter (Fig. 168.5), have a round to oval nucleus with a condensed chromatin pattern, and a small rim of pale blue cytoplasm. Large lymphocytes are 11 to 15 μm in diameter (Fig. 168.3). The chromatin pattern is slightly coarse and does not stain as intensely as the small lymphocyte. The cytoplasm stains pale blue. Large lymphocytes may contain low numbers of round to oblong azurophilic granules usually located at the margin of the cell. Many circulating lymphocytes are referred to as "null cells" based on lack of expression of cell surface antigens. Some T cells possess both CD4 and CD8 surface markers, and the CD4:CD8 ratio is about 0.6.[19]

Monocytes are 14 to 18 μm in diameter and have

TABLE 168.1 Normal Blood Values for the Pig

Erythrocytic Series	Range	Average	Leukocytic Series	Range	Average
Erythrocytes ($\times 10^6/\mu$L)	5.0–8.0	6.5	Leukocytes/μL	11,000–22,000	16,000
Hemoglobin (g/dL)	10.0–16.0	13.0	Percentage distribution		
PCV (%)	32–50	42.0	Neutrophil (band)	0–4	1.0
MCV (fL)	50–68	60	Neutrophil (mature)	28–47	37.0
MCH (pg)	17.0–21	19.0	Lymphocyte	39–62	53.0
MCHC (%)	30.0–34.0	32.0	Monocyte	2–10	5.0
Reticulocytes (%)	0.0–1.0	0.4	Eosinophil	0.5–11	3.5
ESR (mm in 1 hr)	Variable		Basophil	0–2	0.5
RBC diameter (μm)	4.0–8.0	6.0			
RBC life span (days)	86 $\pm$ 11.5		Other Data		
Resistance to hypotonic saline (%)			Thrombocytes ($\times 10^5/\mu$L)	5.2 $\pm$ 1.95	
Min.		0.70	Icterus index (units)	<5	
Max.		0.45	Plasma protein (g/dL)	6.0–8.0	
Myeloid:erythroid ratio	1.77 $\pm$ 0.52:1 (Lahey et al., 1952)		Fibrinogen (g/dL)	0.1–0.5	

a convoluted nucleus with lacy chromatin, often with localized condensation (Fig. 168.6). The abundant blue-grey cytoplasm may contain granules or vacuoles. Some monocytes may be difficult to distinguish from a large lymphocyte or immature neutrophil.[18]

PLATELETS

Porcine platelets are morphologically similar to those of other domestic species (Fig. 168.4). They are variable in shape and are generally small, 1 to 3 μm in diameter, with a mean volume of 6.9 to 8.9 fL.[11] Platelets are anucleate and have deeply staining purple cytoplasmic granules. Platelets are often found in variable-sized clumps.

BONE MARROW

Bone marrow samples are rarely evaluated in pigs. Myeloid to erythroid ratios of 1.77–2:1 have been reported.[4,5]

PLASMA PROTEIN

Plasma protein concentration in adult pigs is about 7 to 8 g/dL.[20] Fibrinogen concentration, an indicator of inflammation, in adults is 0.1 to 0.5 g/dL. The measurement of acute phase proteins is increasingly being used for identification of acute inflammation. C-reactive protein is regarded as the major acute phase protein in the pig.[21]

COAGULATION

Coagulation of pig blood not collected into anticoagulant is rapid.[2] Coagulation parameters, tests for bleeding time, and platelet function in pigs have been described but are seldom used.[18,22,23]

INFLUENCE OF AGE

Blood values for newborn and young piglets have been published.[4,5,24] Table 168.2 depicts the changes in the red and white cell parameters of piglets farrowed and kept on concrete for 10 days, then transferred outside to soil.

Many red cell changes take place after birth. Within a few days of age, red cell number and hemoglobin concentration drop 30 to 38% after expansion of plasma volume.[25] Cell size increases soon after birth, decreases to its smallest volume at 2 to 6 months of age, and then increases again to adult size. In suckling pigs, reticulocyte counts of 3 to 8% and nucleated red cell counts of 5% are common. These decrease as the pig matures. Polychromasia, Howell-Jolly bodies, crenation, rouleaux, and poikilocytes are often seen in the blood of young pigs. Red cell count and hemoglobin concentration increase to reach adult levels at about 5 months of age.

The white blood cell (WBC) count is high at birth. Total leukocyte count decreases shortly after birth, then increases at about the fifth week of life. Actual cell numbers are quite variable. At birth, neutrophils represent about 65 to 70% of the leukocytes and lymphocytes account for about 20%. In the first week, neutrophils and lymphocytes are in equal amounts; by 10 days of age, lymphocytes outnumber neutrophils. The ingestion of colostrum and age at weaning affect erythrocyte and leukocyte numbers as well as cell dynamics.[26,27] By 6 months, the neutrophil:lymphocyte ratio is about 1:2.

Platelet numbers appear to be age-dependent, but reported trends are inconsistent.[22,24] The concentration of plasma protein before and after the ingestion of

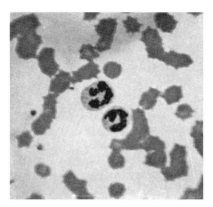

FIGURE 168.1 Erythrocytes and segmented neutrophils.

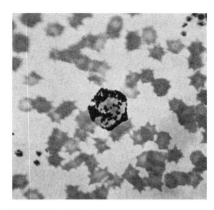

FIGURE 168.4 Basophil and platelets.

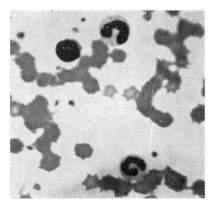

FIGURE 168.2 Small lymphocyte and two band neutrophils.

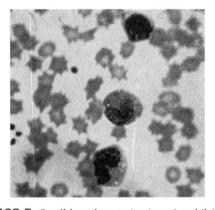

FIGURE 168.5 Small lymphocyte (top), eosinophil (middle), and monocyte (bottom).

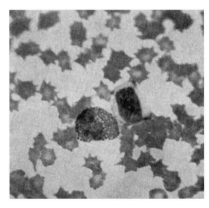

FIGURE 168.3 Eosinophil and large lymphocyte.

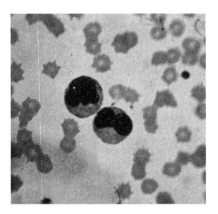

FIGURE 168.6 Monocytes.

colostrum is about 2.2 g/dL and 5.5 g/dL, respectively. It slowly increases during the first year of life to 7 to 8 g/dL.[20] In healthy pigs 2 to 3 months of age, plasma fibrinogen concentration ranges from 0.2 to 0.4 g/dL.

The rapid growth rate of young pigs places a large demand on iron requirements. Milk alone cannot meet this requirement. Unless a supplemental source of iron is provided, the pigs develop a severe microcytic, normocytic to hypochromic anemia. Serum ferritin and total iron binding capacity become reduced.[28] Early contact with soil[29] or intramuscular injection of iron dextran is recommended.[2] Spontaneous recovery occurs around the fifth week of life, when the pigs start to derive nutrients from other sources. The effect of low iron on leukocyte counts is variable.[30,31]

TABLE 168.2 Influence of Age and Husbandry on the Hematology of Young Duroc-Jersey Pigs. Ranges and Means for a Single Litter of 5 Males and 4 Females. Pigs Kept on Concrete Until 10 Days of Age and Then Placed on Soil[a]

Age (days)	Value	Wt. (lb)	RBC (×10^6/μL)	Hb (g/dL)	PCV (%)	MCV (fL)	MCHC (%)	MCH (pg)	Retic. (%)	Nuc. RBC/100 WBC	Sed. Rate (1 hr)	WBC (×10^3/μL)[b]	Differential Leukocyte Count (%)					
													Band	Neutrophil	Lymphocyte	Monocyte	Eosinophil	Basophil
1	Min.	1.7	4.3	8.4	27.0	57	28.9	18.0	4.5	0.5	0	7.6	1.0	64.5	16.0	0.5	0	0
	Max.	3.3	6.4	12.3	42.5	71	31.3	21.0	10.0	4.0	4	15.3	7.0	75.5	31.0	7.5	2.0	1.0
	Ave.	2.4	5.3	10.5	35	67	30.5	20	6.7	2	2	11.5	3.6	71	20	4.7	0.9	0.2
3	Min.	2.4	3.3	7.8	26.5	70	29.1	21.0	6.9	7	2	6.3	1.0	38.0	23.5	6.0	0	0
	Max.	4.0	5.2	11.0	36.5	81	30.3	24.0	16.6	57	12	13.4	5.5	61.5	54.0	9.5	1.5	0
	Ave.	3.2	4.5	9.8	33	73	29.5	22	12.0	17	5	9.4	3.3	51	37.6	6.8	0.8	0
6	Min.	3.5	3.4	6.4	22.0	60	26.4	17.0	4.5	5	12	7.4	1.0	33.0	32.5	2.0	0	0
	Max.	5.0	4.7	9.4	31.0	74	30.9	23.0	13.0	54	33	10.5	3.3	60.5	55	10.5	1.0	0
	Ave.	4.5	4.0	8.0	26.7	67	29.1	20	7.7	14	22.6	8.2	2	45.4	45.3	4.9	0.3	0
10	Min.	5.2	2.1	4.2	15.0	62	29.0	19.0	6.0	3	1	5.6	0	8.0	36.5	1.0	0	0
	Max.	7.1	4.3	8.7	20.0	78	31.0	24.0	12.0	30	35	19.1	2.0	51.0	82.0	10.0	0.5	0.5
	Ave.	6.4	3.5	7.0	24	68	29.6	20	10	11	12	10.9	1	27	64	7	0.1	0.05
20	Min.	8.5	4.4	9.0	35.5	70	26.0	19.0	9.0	1	0	6.2	0	13.5	55.0	2.0	0	0
	Max.	11.5	5.3	11.2	40.5	82	29.0	23.0	13.0	25	1	10.5	3.5	39.5	82.0	7.0	2.0	0.5
	Ave.	10.5	4.9	10.2	37	76	27.6	21	10.6	11.5	0	7.7	1.4	25.7	66.8	4.3	0.8	0.05
36	Min.	—	5.9	11.3	37.0	62	28.0	18.8	1.6	0	0	12.7	0	28.0	40.0	3.0	3.5	0
	Max.	—	6.8	13.3	44.0	68	32.0	20.0	6.8	1	2	20.9	5.0	43.0	68.0	10.5	14.0	1.5
	Ave.	—	6.2	12.1	39.7	64	30.5	19.4	3.0	0.5	0.5	16.3	1.8	33	52	6	7	0.5

[a] These data were developed in cooperation with Dr. Otto Straub.
[b] Corrected for nucleated red cells.

TABLE 168.3 The Hematology of Duroc-Jersey Swine as Influenced by Age, Sex, Castration, Pregnancy, and Parturition[a]

Classification	No.	Value	RBC (×10^6/μL)	Hb (g/dL)	PCV (%)	MCV (fL)	MCHC (%)	Sed. Rate (1 hr)	WBC (×10^3/μL)	Myelocyte	Metamyelocyte	Band	Neutrophil	Lymphocyte	Monocyte	Eosinophil	Basophil
Both sexes 3½ to 4 months	10	Min.	6.4	11.5	38	53	28	0	18.9	—	—	1.0	17	46	1.0	0.5	0.0
		Max.	8.0	13.3	44	61	31	6	33.8	—	—	3.0	42	77	8.0	8.5	1.5
		Ave.	7.1	12.0	40	57	30	2.6	26.9	0.0	0.0	2.0	27	63	5.0	2.5	0.5
Castrated males 3 to 6 months	16	Min.	6.0	9.8	31	54	28	0	11.1	—	—	0.5	17	44	2.0	0.0	0.0
		Max.	8.0	13.0	44	68	32	25	28.3	—	—	4.5	45	73	10.0	10.0	1.0
		Ave.	7.0	11.7	39	59	30	5	19.5	0.0	0.0	2.0	29	60	6.0	2.5	0.5
Males 6 to 12 months	9	Min.	6.3	11.5	37	55	29.5	1	13.4	—	—	0.0	30	51	4.0	0.5	0.0
		Max.	8.6	13.5	44	68	33	14	25.3	—	—	2.5	41	61	9.0	4.5	1.0
		Ave.	7.0	12.4	41	59	31	5	18.9	0.0	0.0	1.5	33	57	6.0	2.2	0.3
Males 1 year and older	8	Min.	5.8	12.8	41	62	30	0.5	10.0	—	—	0.0	11	36	5.0	2.0	0.0
		Max.	7.5	15.3	50	72	33	31	17.4	—	—	2.0	49	76	12.0	5.5	3.0
		Ave.	6.7	14.1	45	66	31	13	13.3	0.0	0.0	0.6	32	55	8.0	3.5	0.9
Females 6 to 12 months; not pregnant	10	Min.	5.4	10.4	36	53	30	5	14.5	—	—	0.5	19	53	3.5	0.0	0.0
		Max.	7.9	13.8	46	67	34	27	21.6	—	—	3.5	37	67	10.5	5.5	2.0
		Ave.	7.0	12.9	41	59	32	15	15.3	0.0	0.0	1.2	33	57	5.5	2.7	0.6
Females 1 year and over; not pregnant	9	Min.	4.7	9.6	31	56	30	24	11.6	—	—	0.0	28	38	0.0	0.5	0.0
		Max.	7.7	14.3	48	69	33	55	21.0	—	—	2.0	42	61	9.0	10.0	1.5
		Ave.	6.0	12.1	38	64	31	26	16.4	0.0	0.0	0.7	36	54	5.0	4.0	0.3
Females 1 year and over; pregnant 3 to 8 weeks	20	Min.	5.6	11.5	37	58	30	1	11.3	—	—	0.0	31	39	2.5	1.0	0.0
		Max.	8.0	14.7	48	68	32	30	22.3	—	—	2.5	48	61	11.0	12.0	2.0
		Ave.	6.4	13.3	43	63	31	7	16.3	0.0	0.0	1.0	37	51	6.0	4.0	1.0
Females 1 year and over; pregnant 2½ to 3½ months	38	Min.	5.1	11.2	35	59	29	3	9.8	—	—	0.0	23	30	0.5	0.0	0.0
		Max.	8.0	15.3	50	69	33	53	20.9	—	0.5	4.5	58	68	12.0	9.0	2.0
		Ave.	6.4	12.8	42	65	31	20	14.4	0.0	0.1	1.1	35	55	5.0	3.0	0.8
Females 2 weeks or less before parturition	14	Min.	4.9	11.0	34	63	30	0	11.5	—	—	0.0	25	34	1.5	0.0	0.0
		Max.	6.3	14.5	46	75	33	47	21.9	—	—	3.5	55	57	9.0	2.5	1.5
		Ave.	5.7	12.6	40	70	31.6	21	15.6	0.0	0.0	1.7	39	52	6.0	0.7	0.6
Females 1 to 6 hours postpartum	5	Min.	4.9	11.2	35	57	31	21	15.1	—	—	0.0	43	17	0.5	0.5	0.0
		Max.	6.5	12.8	42	73	32	45	19.2	—	1.0	5.5	67	48	9.0	11.5	0.0
		Ave.	5.7	12.1	38	66	31.8	33	17.3	0.0	0.2	2.8	52	33	5.0	7.0	0.0
Females 10 to 24 hours postpartum	8	Min.	4.5	10.0	30	57	31	10	7.0	0.0	0.0	0.0	8	34	2.5	1.0	0.0
		Max.	7.3	14.5	46	70	33	54	17.2	4.0	6.0	42.0	45	72	11.0	6.0	1.5
		Ave.	5.8	12.0	37	63	32	47	10.3	0.5	1.8	10.0	30	46	7.0	4.0	0.7
Females 2 to 10 days postpartum	13	Min.	4.5	9.8	30	59	31	0	7.8	—	—	0.0	4	29	2.5	0.5	0.0
		Max.	6.9	15.1	47	71	34	28	21.0	—	—	7.5	58	57	30.0	9.5	3.0
		Ave.	5.5	12.7	39	66	32	12	15.0	0.0	0.0	3.0	43	40	9.0	4.0	1.0
Females 15 to 49 days postpartum	10	Min.	2.4	5.1	15	61	29	3	8.8	—	—	0.5	36	31	2.0	2.0	0.0
		Max.	6.0	12.3	42	79	35	55	24.4	—	3.0	14.0	59	52	11.5	10.0	3.5
		Ave.	4.9	10.4	32	66	32	35	18.7	0.0	0.6	4.0	46	37	6.0	5.0	1.4

[a] These data were developed in cooperation with Dr. Otto Straub.

INFLUENCE OF BREED/SEX

There is no consistent significant influence of gender on hematologic parameters. Observed differences were not considered biologically important.[13,32-34] Breed differences in values have been reported.[12,34-36]

INFLUENCE OF PREGNANCY/ PARTURITION/LACTATION

Hematologic changes occur with pregnancy, parturition, and lactation (Table 168.3). Approximately 2 weeks before parturition, red cell parameters in the sow decrease and continue to do so until the end of lactation. Reticulocytes may be seen during this period. Total white cell number decreases during gestation, and anemia during pregnancy in sows has been documented.[37,38] Neutrophilia with a left shift and lymphopenia often occur at parturition. Within 24 hours of farrowing the neutrophil:lymphocyte ratio reverses.[39]

The influences of treatment with recombinant porcine somatotrophin,[40] growth hormone-releasing factor, and thyrotropin-releasing factor on sow blood during lactation have been reported.[41]

EFFECT OF STRESS

In swine, sampling stress is the largest source of hematologic variation.[42] The stress response develops within 2 minutes, rapidly affecting the leukogram.[10] The total leukocyte and neutrophil count can increase by two- to three-fold, resulting in a stress leukogram with significant elevations also seen in hemoglobin concentration, hematocrit, and erythrocyte sedimentation rate.[43] The effect of sedation on hematologic values is unpredictable; thus, sedation is not recommended for blood collection.[11]

EFFECT OF DISEASE

Hematologic changes associated with various inflammatory processes in swine have been examined.[32,44,45] Increased erythrocyte sedimentation rates as well as decreased hematocrit and hemoglobin concentrations were reported. Interpretation of these data is questionable.[11] Evaluation of a blood smear with a differential count may be a better indicator of an inflammatory process than total cell counts.[2]

THE FETAL PIG

A number of studies have reported the hematologic characteristics of fetal pigs.[38,46,47] Nucleated red cells are present in the fetal circulation at 30 days gestation. Red cell number and hemoglobin concentration increase with age as nucleated red cells decrease. Red cell size decreases during gestation.[38,46] Reticulocyte percent is maximal (6.5%) mid gestation but decreases to 1% by birth. Total WBC number increases throughout embryonic life, consisting mostly of neutrophils. Serum protein concentration is 2 to 3 g/dl throughout gestation, with no sex or breed differences reported.

MINIATURE SWINE

Miniature pigs are an important animal model in biomedical research[48,49] and are recently popular as pets.[50] Hematologic parameters of many breeds of miniature pigs have been characterized,[51-54] with similar characteristics and cell morphology as larger domestic swine. There was no effect on red or white cell parameters with regard to sex,[51,54,55] but breed differences have been reported.[56] Age-related changes in miniature pigs are comparable to those in domestic swine.[51,55,56] Adult values are attained at about 9 months of age.

REFERENCES

1. **Pond WG, Houpt KA.** Body fluids, hematology, and immunology. In: The biology of the pig. Ithaca: Cornell University Press, 1978;244–276.
2. **Friendship RM, Henry SC.** Cardiovascular system, hematology, and clinical chemistry. In: Leman AD, Straw BE, Mengeling WL, et al., eds. Diseases of swine. 7th ed. Ames: Iowa State University Press, 1992;3–11.
3. **Sims LD.** Blood. In: Sims LD, Glastonbury JRW, eds. Pathology of the pig: a diagnostic guide. Victoria, Australia: The Pig Research and Development Corporation and Agriculture, 1996;165–174.
4. **Jain NC.** The pig: normal hematology with comments on response to disease. In: Veterinary hematology. 4th ed. Philadelphia: Lea & Febiger, 1986; 240–255.
5. **Sanderson JH, Phillips CE.** Pigs. In: An atlas of laboratory animal haematology. New York: Oxford University Press, 1981;432–469.
6. **Fontaine M, Hamelin N, Martineau GP.** Effect of time, storage conditions and mailing on the stability of porcine blood values. Med Vet Quebec 1987;17:15–21.
7. **Wang F-I, Williams TJ, El-Awar FY, Pang VF, Hahn EC.** Characterization of porcine peripheral blood leukocytes by light-scattering flow cytometry. Can J Vet Res 1987;51:421–427.
8. **Fuchs A, Eder H.** Enumeration and maturation distribution of reticulocytes of six animal species. J Vet Med Series A 1991;38:749–754.
9. **Friendship RM, Lumsden JH, McMillan I, Wilson MR.** Hematology and biochemistry reference values for Ontario swine. Can J Comp Med 1984;48:390–393.
10. **Dubreuil P, Farmer C, Couture Y, Petitclerc D.** Hematological and biochemical changes following an acute stress in control and somatostatin-immunized pigs. Can J Anim Sci 1993;73:241–252.
11. **Evans RJ.** Porcine haematology: reference ranges and the clinical value of haematological examination in the pig. Pig J 1994;32:52–57.
12. **Yeh SH, Tai JJL, Chang HL, Lee CJ.** Blood profile of Lanyu pigs in Taiwan. J of Taiwan Livest Res 1994;27:187–195.
13. **Elbers ARW, Counotte GHM, Tielen MJM.** Haematological and clinico-chemical blood profiles in slaughter pigs. Vet Quart 1992;14:57–62.
14. **Oyewale JO.** Changes in osmotic resistance of erythrocytes of cattle, pigs, rats and rabbits during variation in temperature and pH. J Vet Med A 1992;39:98–104.
15. **Oyewale JO.** Effect of storage on the osmotic fragility of mammalian erythrocytes. J Vet Med A 1993;40:258–264.
16. **Makinde MO.** Osmotic fragility of erythrocytes in two breeds of swine. Anim Technol 1986;37:73–76.
17. **Weng X, Clouter G, Pibarot P, Durand LG.** Comparison and simulation of different levels of erythrocyte aggregation with pig, horse, sheep, calf and normal human blood. Biorheology 1996;33:4–5, 365–377.
18. **Imlah P, McTaggart HS.** Heamatology of the pig. In: Archer RK, Jeffcott LB, eds. Comparative clinical haematology. Oxford: Blackwell Scientific, 1977;271–303.
19. **Roth JA.** Immune system. In: Leman AD, Straw BE, Mengeling WL, et al., eds. Diseases of swine. 7th ed. Ames: Iowa State University Press, 1992;21–39.
20. **Miller ER, et al.** Swine hematology from birth to maturity I. Serum proteins J Anim Sci 1961;20:31.
21. **Eckersall PD, Saini PK, McComb C.** The acute phase response of acid soluble glycoprotein, alpha(1)-acid glycoprotein, ceruloplasmin, haptoglo-

bin and C-reactive protein, in the pig. Vet Immunol Immunopathol 1996; 51:377–385.

22. **Blecher TE, Gunstone MJ.** Fibrinolysis, coagulation and haematological findings in normal large White/Wessex cross pigs. Br Vet J 1969;125:74–81.

23. **Bowie EJW, Owen CA Jr, Zollman PE, Thompson JH Jr, Fass DN.** Tests of hemostasis in swine: normal values and values in pigs affected with von Willebrand's disease. Am J Vet Res 1973;34:1405–1407.

24. **Olowookoron MO, Makinde MO.** Thrombocytes, clotting time, haemoglobin value and packed cell volume in Nigerian piglets during the first four weeks of life. J Vet Med A 1980;27:508.

25. **Miller ER, et al.** Swine hematology from birth to maturity II. Erythrocyte population, size and hemoglobin concentration. J Anim Sci 1961;20:890–897.

26. **Vellenga L, Wensing T, Breukink HJ, Hagens FH.** Effects of irradiated sow colostrum on some biochemical and haematological measurements in newborn piglets. Res Vet Sci 1986;41:316–318.

27. **Gajecki M, Przala F, Zdunczyk E, Bakula T, Milosz Z, Rodziewicz M.** Variations in the blood cells and serum protein fractions of piglets weaned at different ages. Zeszyty Naukowe Akademii Rolniczo Technicznej Olsztynie Weterynaria 1984;15:173–183.

28. **Smith JE, Moore K, Boyington D, et al.** Serum ferritin and total iron-binding capacity to estimate iron storage in pigs. Vet Pathol 1984;21:597–600.

29. **Kernkamp HCH.** Soil, iron, copper and iron in the prevention and treatment of anemia in suckling pigs. J Am Vet Med Assoc 1935;87:37.

30. **Gainer JH, Guarnieri J, Das NK.** Neutropenia and anemia in the iron deficient baby pig. Calif Vet 1984;39:18–20, 41.

31. **Svetina A, Andreansky T, Jerovick I, Antoncic M.** Hematology and some blood chemical values in postnatal anemia of the pig. Veterinarski Arch 1994;64:4–6, 77–87.

32. **Odink J, Smeets JFM, Visser IJR, Sandman H, Snijders JMA.** Hematological and clinicochemical profiles of healthy swine and swine with inflammatory processes. J Anim Sci 1990;68:163–170.

33. **Makinde MO, Majok AA.** Biochemical and haematological values in abattoir pigs with and without subclinical lesions. Onderstepoort J Vet Res 1996;63:11–14.

34. **Egbunike GN, Akusu MO.** Breed and sex influences on porcine haematological picture under hot and humid climatic conditions. Vet Res Commun 1983;6:103–109.

35. **Falkenberg H, Micklich D, Matthes HD, Mohring H.** Reference blood values in different breeds of pigs in relation to indoor or outdoor keeping. Arch Tierzucht 1996;39:153–168.

36. **Kaneko H, Saito Y, Honjo A.** Growth and blood properties of primary SPF piglets. Jpn J Swine Sci 1987;24:212–217.

37. **Nachreiner RF, Ginther OJ.** Gestational and periparturient periods of sows: serum chemical and hematologic changes during gestation. Am J Vet Res 1972;33:2215–2219.

38. **Dungan LJ, Weist DB, Fyfe DA, Smith AC, Swindle MM.** Normal hematology, serology, and serum protein electrophoresis values in fetal Yucatan miniature swine. Lab Anim Sci 1995;45:285–289.

39. **Nachreiner RF, Ginther OJ.** Gestational and periparturient periods of sows:

serum chemical, hematologic and clinical changes during the periparturient period. Am J Vet Res 1972;33:2233–2238.

40. **Smith VG, Leman AD, Seaman WJ, VanRavenswaay F.** Pig weaning weight and changes in hematology and blood chemistry of sows injected with recombinant porcine somatotropin during lactation. J Anim Sci 1991;69:3501–3510.

41. **Dubreuil P, Pelletier G, Petitclerc D, Lapierre H, Couture Y, Gaudreau P. Morrisset J, Barzeau P.** Influence of growth hormone-releasing factor and/or thyrotropin-releasing factor on sow blood components, milk composition and piglet performance. Can J Anim Sci 1990;70:821–832.

42. **Dubreuil P, Couture Y, Tremblay A, Martineau GP.** Effects of experimenters and different blood sampling techniques on blood metabolite values in growing pigs. Can J Vet Res 1990;54:379–383.

43. **Elbers ARW, Visser IJR, Odink J, Smeets JFM.** Changes in haematological and clinicochemical profiles in blood of apparently healthy slaughter pigs, collected at the farm and at slaughter, in relation to the severity of pathological-anatomical lesions. Vet Quart 1991;13:1–9.

44. **Visser IJR, Odink J, Smeets JFM, Aarts PAMM, Elbers ARW, Alsemgeest SPM, Gruys E.** Relationship between pathological findings and values of haematological and blood-chemistry variables in apparently healthy finishing pigs at slaughter. J Vet Med B 1992;39:123–131.

45. **Smeets JFM, Odink J, Visser IJR, Schoen ED, Snijders JMA.** Haematology and blood-chemistry for predicting abscesses and other abnormalities in slaughtered pigs. Vet Quart 1990;12:146–151.

46. **Waddill DG, Ullrey DE, Miller ER, et al.** Blood cell populations and serum protein concentrations in the fetal pig. J Anim Sci 1962;21:583.

47. **Brooks CC, Davis JW.** Changes in hematology of the perinatal pig. J Anim Sci 1969;28:517.

48. **Panepinto LM, Tumbleson ME.** Miniature swine breeds used worldwide in research. In: Schook LB, ed. Advances in swine in biomedical research. New York: Plenum Press, 1996;2:681–691.

49. **Tumbleson ME,** ed. Advances in swine biomedical research. Conf Proc Univ Maryland, 1995;1, 2.

50. **Braun WF Jr, Casteel SW.** Potbellied pigs. Miniature porcine pets. Vet Clin North Am 1993;23:1149–1177.

51. **Parsons AH, Wells RE.** Hematologic values of the Yucatan miniature pig. Vet Clin Pathol 1989;18:90–92.

52. **McClellan RO, Vost G, et al.** Age-related changes in hematological and serum biochemical parameters in miniature swine. In: Bustad LK, et al., eds. Swine in biomedical research. Richland: Pacific Northwest Laboratories, 1966;597–610.

53. **Tumbleson ME, Middleton CC, Tinsley OW, Hutcheson DP.** Serum biochemic and hematologic parameters of Hormel miniature swine from four to nine months of age. Lab Anim Care 1969;19:345–351.

54. **Radin MJ, Weiser MG, Fettman MJ.** Hematologic and serum biochemical values for Yucatan miniature swine. Lab Anim Sci 1986;36:425–427.

55. **Oldigs B, Schmidt FW, Douwes F.** Blood and serum values for Gottingen miniature swine IV. Endogenous and exogenous factors affecting erythrocytes and granulocytes. J Vet Med A 1984;31:46–58.

56. **Ellegaard l, Jorgensen KD, Klastrup S, Hanesen AK, Svendsen O.** Haematologic and clinical chemical values in 3 and 6 months old Gottingen minipigs. Scand J Lab Anim Sci 1995;22:239–248.

CHAPTER 169

Hematology of the Ferret (*Mustela putorius furo*)

• DAVID M. MOORE

BLOOD COLLECTION

Several reviews[1,2] have described a number of methods for collection of blood from ferrets, including toenail clipping (yielding less than 0.5 mL of blood), retroorbital sinus blood collection (safely yielding 1 to 3 mL of blood in ferrets weighing 100 to 300 g and 5 to 10 mL of blood from adults[3]), cardiac puncture,[4] caudal arterial puncture in the tail, and jugular venipuncture.[5] Chronic jugular catheterization for repeated blood sampling has also been described.[6,7]

The total blood volume of the ferret is estimated to be between 5 and 7% of body weight, with a total blood volume in adult males of approximately 60 ml and approximately 40 mL in adult females.[8] Terminal blood collection (exsanguination) from the abdominal aorta in anesthetized ferrets will yield approximately 3% of body weight in blood.[9]

MORPHOLOGY AND NUMBERS OF PERIPHERAL BLOOD CELLS

Reported hematologic values for the ferret (*Mustela putorius furo*) are provided in Tables 169.1 and 169.2. Additional reported values for ferrets can be found in the literature.[10,11]

Erythrocytes

The mean diameters (in μm) reported for erythrocytes of ferrets were found to be 5.94 in males (range, 4.6 to 7.7) and 6.32 in females (range, 4.6 to 7.7).[9] Hematocrit and red blood cell (RBC) values for ferrets were found to be higher than indices for dogs and cats.[8] Thornton et al.[9] observed the range of reticulocytes in albino ferrets to be 1 to 12% (mean, 4%) in males and 2 to 14% (mean, 5.3%) in females. Howell-Jolly bodies were seen in about 5% of both male and female ferrets but were not observed in large numbers in those animals.[9]

Thrombocytes

The mean diameters (in μm) reported for platelets of ferrets were found to be 1.7 in males (range, 1.5 to 2.3) and 1.73 in females (range, 1.5 to 2.3).[9] Kawasaki[12] provided normal ranges of circulating platelets from ferrets seen in his practice, 297 to 730 $\times$ 10^3/mm^3 (mean, 453 $\times$ 10^3/mm^3), and a range suggested by his colleagues, 350 to 550 $\times$ 10^3/mm^3 (mean, 400 $\times$ 10^3/mm^3). Thornton et al.[9] observed the following platelet levels in adult albino ferrets: 297 to 730 $\times$ 10^3/mm^3 (mean, 453 $\times$ 10^3/mm^3) in males, and 310 to 910 $\times$ 10^3/mm^3 (mean, 545 $\times$ 10^3/mm^3) in females. Besch-Williford[13] presented a reference range of platelets as 245 to 910 $\times$ 10^3/mm^3, with a mean of 650 $\times$ 10^3/mm^3 in Fitch ferrets and a range of 453 to 545 $\times$ 10^3/mm^3 in albino ferrets. Female ferrets develop thrombocytopenia during estrus.[14] In females (jills) with severe anemia associated with hyperestrogenism, platelet counts may be less than or equal to 20 $\times$ 10^3/mm^3.[12]

Leukocytes

Neutrophils are the predominant leukocyte observed when performing differential counts. The mean diameter of neutrophils was reported as 11.2 μm in males (range, 10 to 13.1 μm) and 9.6 μm in females (range, 9.2 to 10.0 μm).[9] The cytoplasm of ferret neutrophils contains polychromatic granules. The mean diameter of small lymphocytes was reported as 7.7 μm in males (range, 6.2 to 9.2) and 8.7 μm in females (range, 7.7 to 10.0); the mean diameter of large lymphocytes was reported as 11.1 μm in males (range, 9.2 to 13.1) and 11.9 μm in females.[9] Eosinophils (mean diameter 12.7 μm in males, 12.6 μm in females) have either a one or two lobed nucleus.[9] The nucleus of basophils is segmented, and their mean diameter was reported as 13.5 μm in males and 13.8 μm in females.[9] Monocyte diameters were in the range of 12 to 18 μm, and almost all of those cells were found to be vacuolated.[9]

TABLE 169.1   Referenced Erythrocyte Parameters in the Ferret (*Mustela putorius furo*)

Reference	Breed/Type	Gender	RBC (×10⁶/mm³) Mean	RBC (×10⁶/mm³) Range	PCV (%) Mean	PCV (%) Range	Hb (g/dl) Mean	Hb (g/dl) Range	MCV (μ^3) Mean	MCV (μ^3) Range	MCH ($\mu\mu$g) Mean	MCH ($\mu\mu$g) Range	MCHC (%) Mean	MCHC (%) Range
16	NS	NS	9.98	—	—	35–51	12.8	—	—	—	—	—	—	—
9	Albino	M	10.23	7.3–12.18	55.4	44–61	17.8	16.3–18.2	—	—	—	—	—	—
	Albino	F	8.11	6.77–9.76	49.2	42–55	16.2	14.8–17.4	—	—	—	—	—	—
17	Fitch	M	—	—	43.4	36–50	14.3	12–16.3	—	—	—	—	—	—
	Fitch	F	—	—	48.4	47–51	15.9	15.2–17.4	—	—	—	—	—	—
14	Fitch	F (in estrus)	5.99 ± 2.02	1.81–9.06	36 ± 12	13–53	12.1 ± 3.9	4.4–17.7	61.0 ± 6.14	48.4–71.8	20.5 ± 1.39	18.8–24.3	33.8 ± 3.24	29.2–42.3
	Fitch	F (ovariectomized)	8.52 ± 0.44	8.07–8.77	45 ± 3	42–47	15.8 ± 1.0	14.6–16.4	53.4 ± 3.8	51.4–54.9	18.7 ± 1.1	18.2–19.3	35.2 ± 0.9	34.9–35.7
13	NS	NS (adult)	—	6.77–12.18	—	36–61	—	12.0–18.2	—	—	—	—	—	—
	Fitch	NS (adult)	—	6.5–8.7	—	43.4–48.4	—	14.3–15.9	—	—	—	—	—	—
	Albino	NS (adult)	—	8.11–10.23	—	49.2–55.4	—	16.2–17.8	—	—	—	—	—	—
18[a]	NS	M	—	9.64–9.69	—	49.4–49.8	—	16.7–16.8	51.4	—	17.3	—	—	33.7–33.8
	NS	F	—	9.3–9.34	—	48.4–48.8	—	16.2–16.3	—	52.1–52.2	17.5	—	—	33.4–33.5
18[b]	NS	NS	—	3.6–10.0	—	30–55	—	—	—	—	—	—	—	—
8	Fitch	M	11.3	10.1–13.2	53.1	48–59	16.9	15.4–18.5	47.1	42.6–51.0	15	13.7–16.0	32	30.3–34.9
8[a]	NS	M (10 wk)	6.4 ± 0.6	5.5–7.4	32.9 ± 1.9	29.3–36.8	11.8 ± 0.8	10.4–13.6	51.3 ± 1.8	47.8–54.8	18.3 ± 0.6	17.5–19.1	35.7 ± 0.6	34.7–37.0
		F (10 wk)	6.1 ± 0.7	5–7	32.1 ± 2.7	27.0–34.8	11.5 ± 1.0	9.6–12.5	52.0 ± 1.9	49.6–54.5	18.9 ± 0.7	17.8–19.6	35.7 ± 0.7	34.8–36.9
		M (12 wk)	6.4 ± 0.8	4.8–7.8	33.4 ± 2.3	30.9–38.1	12.0 ± 0.8	11.0–13.7	51.4 ± 1.6	49.0–53.6	18.9 ± 1.7	17.4–22.8	35.9 ± 0.5	34.7–36.7
		F (12 wk)	6.4 ± 0.7	5.7–7.8	34.1 ± 2.5	31.3–38.5	12.2 ± 0.9	11.2–13.8	52.5 ± 3.4	48.8–57.6	19.1 ± 1.0	17.7–20.4	35.8 ± 0.5	35.3–37.0
		M (14–16 wk)	8.2 ± 0.9	6.2–9.2	39.1 ± 4.0	29.8–43.2	14.3 ± 1.0	12.7–15.9	47.8 ± 2.4	44.9–53.6	17.6 ± 1.3	16.4–20.6	36.9 ± 2.2	35.1–42.6
		M (adult)	9.1 ± 0.9	7.1–10.2	42.3 ± 3.7	33.6–47.2	15.5 ± 1.3	12.0–16.9	46.6 ± 1.9	44.1–52.5	17.1 ± 0.8	16.5–19.7	37.0 ± 2.0	—
		F (nonestrus)	8.2 ± 0.6	7.5–9.3	39.1 ± 2.6	35.6–44.7	14.5 ± 1.0	12.9–15.9	48.4 ± 3.0	44.4–53.7	17.6 ± 1.0	16.4–19.4	37.0 ± 2.0	35.1–42.2
		F (in estrus)	8.3 ± 0.5	7.5–9.3	38.8 ± 2.5	34.6–43.3	13.4 ± 0.9	11.9–15.0	46.8 ± 1.3	45.2–48.7	16.2 ± 0.3	15.8–16.8	34.5 ± 0.6	33.2–35.3

[a] Data supplied by Marshall Farms.
[b] Reference data supplied by the University of Miami Avian Diagnostic Lab.
NS, not specified.

TABLE 169.2 Referenced Leukocyte Parameters in the Ferret (*Mustela putorius furo*)

Reference	Breed/Type	Gender	WBC (×10³/mm³) Mean	WBC (×10³/mm³) Range	Neutrophils (%) Mean	Neutrophils (%) Range	Lymphocytes (%) Mean	Lymphocytes (%) Range	Eosinophils (%) Mean	Eosinophils (%) Range	Basophils (%) Mean	Basophils (%) Range	Monocytes (%) Mean	Monocytes (%) Range
16	NS	NS	—	9–13	65	—	35	—	0	—	0	—	0	—
9	Albino	M	9.7	4.4–19.1	57	11–82	35.6	12–54	2.4	0–7	0.1	0–2	4.4	0–9
	Albino	F	10.5	4.0–18.2	59.5	43–84	33.4	12–50	2.6	0–5	0.2	0–1	4.4	2–8
17	Fitch	M	11.3	7.7–15.4	40.1	24–78	49.7	28–69	2.3	0–7	0.7	0–2.7	6.6	3.4–8.2
	Fitch	F	5.9	2.5–8.6	31.1	12–41	58	25–95	3.6	1–9	0.8	0–2.9	4.5	1.7–6.3
14	Fitch	F (in estrus)	3.84 ± 1.72	1.82–5.83	—	18.8–53.5	—	60.7–83.9	—	0–2.5	—	0–0.74	—	0–2.52
	Fitch	F (ovariectomized)	7.07 ± 1.42	5.98–8.1	—	21.6–44.5	—	53.7–57.5	—	2.3–4.0	—	0.2–1.1	—	0.5–1.3
13	NS	NS (adult)	—	2.5–19.1	—	11–84	—	12–95	—	1–9	—	0–3	—	0–9.1
	Fitch	NS (adult)	—	5.9–11.3	—	31.1–40.1	—	49.7–58.0	—	2.3–3.6	—	0.7–0.8	—	4.5–6.6
	Albino	NS (adult)	—	9.7–10.5	—	57.0–59.5	—	33.4–35.6	—	2.4–2.6	—	0.1–0.2	—	4.4–4.6
12	NS	NS	—	2.8–8.0	—	—	35	—	—	—	—	—	—	—
18[a]	NS	M	—	8.9–9.2	—	47–48	—	46–48	—	3.0–3.5	—	0–0.49	—	1.0–1.19
	NS	F	—	7.0–7.6	—	49–50	45	—	—	3.0–3.3	—	0–0.34	—	1.0–1.12
18[b]	NS	NS	—	3.3–15.9	—	9.0–54	—	34–85	—	0–10	—	0–3	—	0–8
8	Fitch	M	6.2	1.7–11.9	—	24–72	—	26–73	—	0–3	—	—	—	1–4
8[a]	NS	M (10 wk)	8.0 ± 2.1	5.3–12.0	32.7 ± 5.3	24.3–45.1	54.8 ± 5.9	42.2–64.3	4.4 ± 1.1	2.7–6.1	0.1 ± 0.1	0–0.2	2.8 ± 0.8	1.7–4.3
		F (10 wk)	9.2 ± 2.0	6.7–12.6	28.6 ± 4.9	20.6–76.6	60.0 ± 6.4	52.4–68.2	4.2 ± 1.8	2.1–6.9	0.1 ± 0.0	0–0.1	2.5 ± 1.0	1.4–4.1
		M (12 wk)	8.4 ± 2.0	5.3–11.7	43.3 ± 14.2	24.3–68.3	46.1 ± 14.1	22.1–62.8	4.4 ± 0.9	3.3–5.8	0.1 ± 0.3	0–1.3	2.1 ± 1.1	0.7–4.7
		F (12 wk)	6.7 ± 1.2	5.8–9.8	27.9 ± 3.7	21.7–32.4	61.8 ± 3.5	57.8–67.0	3.7 ± 1.0	2.2–5.7	0.1 ± 0.1	0–0.3	2.0 ± 0.3	1.5–2.4
		M (14–16 wk)	9.5 ± 3.7	—	37.5 ± 8.9	27.9–58.2	50.9 ± 9.0	30.1–60.6	5.4 ± 1.3	3.6–8.2	0.1 ± 0.1	0–0.2	1.7 ± 0.5	1.1–2.9
		M (adult)	8.4 ± 2.5	4.9–13.8	41.5 ± 15.4	24.0–76.6	47.4 ± 15.3	14.7–66.6	5.6 ± 1.5	1.9–8.5	0.1 ± 0.1	0–0.3	1.7 ± 1.0	0.7–5.0
		F (nonestrus)	7.2 ± 2.3	5.1–12.6	57.7 ± 6.8	48.8–71.0	33.3 ± 6.1	22.7–43.3	4.3 ± 2.1	2.3–8.5	0	0–0.1	1.8 ± 0.7	1.0–3.0
		F (in estrus)	5.7 ± 1.5	5.2–8.2	43.2 ± 9.4	33.1–60.9	48.2 ± 9.6	32.9–59.1	3.1 ± 1.2	1.6–5.6	0	0–0.1	1.6 ± 0.5	1.1–2.7

[a]Data supplied by Marshall Farms.
[b]Reference data supplied by the University of Miami Avian Diagnostic Lab.
NS, not specified.

TABLE 169.3	Observed Coagulation Values in Ferrets	
Parameter	**Mean ± SD**	**Reference**
Clotting time (sec)	120 ± 0.5	19
Prothrombin time (sec)	15.7 ± 0.4	9
	10.3 ± 0.1	19
Activated partial thrombo-plastin time (sec)	18.4 ± 1.4	19

BONE MARROW CYTOLOGY

In normal ferrets, the myeloid : erythroid (M:E) ratio was found to be 3.4 ± 1.1:1.0.[14] Hypoplasia of the bone marrow in ferrets is usually instigated by prolonged exposure to estrogens[15] and is associated with prolonged estrus in females.[14] Severely affected jills had a depletion of both erythroid and granulocytic precursors, with almost a total absence of megakaryocytes.[14]

OTHER HEMATOLOGIC VALUES

The erythrocyte sedimentation rate in ferrets was reported as 1 to 3 mm/hr.[16] Because of the almost negligible erythrocyte sedimentation rate in ferrets, blood for packed cell volume (PCV) determinations must be spun for 20% longer than samples from other species.[9] Observed coagulation values for ferrets are presented in Table 169.3.

REFERENCES

1. **Moody KD.** Laboratory management of the ferret for biomedical research. Lab Anim Sci 1985;35:272–279.
2. **Otto G, Rosenblad WD, Fox JG.** Practical venipuncture techniques for the ferret. Lab Anim 1993;27:26–29.
3. **Fox JG, Hewes K, Niemi SM.** Retro-orbital technique for blood collection from the ferret. Lab Anim Sci 1984;34:198–199.
4. **Buckland M.** A guide to laboratory animal technology. London: William Heinemann, 1971.
5. **Bleakley SP.** Simple technique for bleeding ferrets (*Mustela putorius furo*). Lab Anim 1980;14:59–60.
6. **Messina JE, Sylvina TJ, Hotaling LC, Goad ME, Fox JG.** A simple technique for chronic jugular catheterization in ferrets. Lab Anim Sci 1988;38:89–90.
7. **Florczyk AP, Schurig JE.** A technique for chronic jugular catheterization in the ferret. Pharmacol Biochem Behav 1981;14:255–257.
8. **Fox JG.** Biology and diseases of the ferret. 2nd ed. Baltimore: Williams & Wilkins, 1998.
9. **Thornton PC, Wright PA, Sacra PJ, Goodier TE.** The ferret, *Mustela putorius furo*, as a new species in toxicology. Lab Anim 1979;13:119–124.
10. **Carpenter JW, Hill EF.** Hematological values for the Siberian ferret. J Zoo Anim Med 1979;10:126.
11. **Fox JG, Hotaling L, Ackerman BP, Hewes K.** Serum chemistry and hematology reference values in the ferret (*Mustela putorius furo*). Lab Anim Sci 1986;36:583.
12. **Kawasaki TA.** Normal parameters and laboratory interpretation of disease states in the domestic ferret. Semin Avian Exotic Pet Med 1994;3:40.
13. **Besch-Williford CE.** Biology and medicine of the ferret. In: Harkness JE, ed. Exotic pet medicine. Vet Clin North Am Small Anim Pract 1987;17:1155–1183.
14. **Sherrill A, Gorham J.** Bone marrow hypoplasia associated with estrus in ferrets. Lab Anim Sci 1985;35:280–286.
15. **Ryland LM, Gorham KR.** The ferret and its diseases. J Am Vet Med Assoc 1978;173:1154–1158.
16. **Willis LS, Barrow MV.** The ferret (*Mustela putorius furo* L.) as a laboratory animal. Lab Anim Sci 1971;21:712–716.
17. **Lee EJ, Moore WE, Fryer HC, Minocha HC.** Haematological and serum chemistry profiles of ferrets (*Mustela putorius furo*). Lab Anim 1982;16:133–137.
18. **Johnson-Delaney CA.** Exotic companion medicine handbook. Lake Worth, FL: Wingers Publishing, 1996.
19. **Lewis JH.** Comparative hemostasis in vertebrates. New York: Plenum Press, 1996.

CHAPTER 170

Hematology of Rabbits

• DAVID M. MOORE

BLOOD COLLECTION

Blood is usually collected from the marginal ear veins of rabbits. The rabbit can be restrained in a commercial rabbit restrainer, a zippered cat bag (commonly available at most veterinary clinics), or by securely wrapping it in a large towel. The fur covering the marginal ear vein is plucked, which aids in visualization and dilation of the vessel. By warming the ear with a warm wash cloth, warming it next to an incandescent light bulb, and/or stroking the central artery from the base to the tip of the ear, dilation of the vein will be enhanced. Pretreatment with acetylpromazine, a tranquilizer (0.25 mL, injected subcutaneously), will also result in dilation of peripheral veins including the marginal ear vein. A 23- to 25-gauge needle can be used when collecting blood from the vein. The vacuum from a Vacutainer tube would likely collapse the vessel, and similarly, attempting rapid withdrawal with a syringe may also collapse the vessel and prevent the free flow of blood. Slow, steady pressure should be used when drawing blood with a syringe. Blood can be collected as it flows from the hub of a needle inserted in the marginal ear vein. A peristaltic pump,[1] or an Erlenmeyer flask to which a vacuum is applied using a vacuum pump, may also be used to facilitate blood collection from the marginal ear vein. When using the flask, the fur over the vessel is plucked, the vessel is pricked with a sterile lancet, and the ear is inserted into the flask. A rubber stopper on the outlet port of the flask is inserted into an appropriately sized centrifugation tube for collection of nonsterile blood. Although the central artery of the ear can be used for blood collection, it should be used with caution, because formation of a hematoma is a potential sequela to the procedure.

Alternate blood collection sites include the jugular vein, the lateral saphenous vein, and direct cardiac puncture (in an anesthetized animal). An 18-gauge or larger hypodermic needle, between 1.5 to 2 inches in length, attached to tubing from a human blood collection set, can be inserted in the third left intercostal space, about 4 mm lateral to the sternum, until it penetrates the heart and blood is seen flowing into the tube. Cardiac blood collection is usually reserved for terminal exsanguination procedures, and should not be used for clinical patients, because it can result in myocardial damage, hemothorax, pericardial tamponade, or death. Generally, collection of blood from the jugular veins also requires sedation or slight anesthesia (i.e., gas anesthesia administered with a nose cone).

The total blood volume in rabbits was estimated to be between 4.5 and 8.1% of total body weight,[2,3] or approximately 53.8 ± 5.2 mL/kg.[4] However, Jain[5] cautioned against introducing inaccuracies by expressing blood volume on the basis of actual body weight, and instead suggested that blood volume be correlated with lean body weight or body surface area. The recommended maximum volume of blood that can be collected safely during one bleeding is 7.7 mL/kg of body weight.[6]

MORPHOLOGY AND INDICES OF PERIPHERAL BLOOD CELLS

Reported hematologic values for the New Zealand white (NZW) rabbit (*Oryctolagus cuniculus*) are provided in Tables 170.1 and 170.2. Hematologic values reported for some other breeds or species of rabbits are provided in Tables 170.3 and 170.4. An excellent discussion of the sources of variation found in hematologic values was provided by McLaughlin and Fish.[7]

Erythrocytes

The rabbit erythrocyte is a biconcave disk whose average diameter ranges between 6.7 and 6.9 μm,[5] with the average thickness of approximately 2.15 to 2.4 μm.[8,9] There is a marked anisocytosis of the erythrocytes of rabbits, with microcytes of one-quarter the diameter of normal cells sometimes in evidence. Schermer[9] described the appearance of numerous thorn apple forms in blood smears as characteristic of rabbit blood, and observed that polychromasia was found in 1 to 2% of erythrocytes. Reticulocytes accounted for 1 to 7% of the total number of erythrocytes in adult animals and were determined to be, on average, $2 \pm 0.5\%$ in males and $3 \pm 0.5\%$ in females.[9] One- to two-month-old NZW rabbits were found to have reticulocyte counts of $7.4 \pm 4.7\%$, with a 50% reduction in those counts occurring during the third

TABLE 170.1 Referenced Erythrocyte Parameters of the New Zealand White (NZW) Rabbit (*Oryctolagus cuniculus*)

Reference	Gender	RBC (×10⁶/mm³) Mean	RBC (×10⁶/mm³) Range	PCV (%) Mean	PCV (%) Range	Hb (g/dl) Mean	Hb (g/dl) Range	MCV (μ³) Mean	MCV (μ³) Range	MCH (μμg) Mean	MCH (μμg) Range	MCHC (%) Mean	MCHC (%) Range
9	NS	5.25	4–6.4	—	—	12.4	8.4–15.5	—	—	—	—	—	—
36	NS	6.2	—	39	—	13.4	—	60	—	23	—	35	—
37	M/F (adult)	—	5.11–7.94	—	37–50	—	9.8–17.4	—	57.8–65.4	—	17.1–23.5	—	28.7–37
13	NS (1 yr)	7.73 ± 0.78	—	49.08 ± 3.98	—	15.97 ± 1.3	—	63.62 ± 2.47	—	20.7 ± 1.07	—	32.52 ± 1.04	—
	NS (adult)	7.79 ± 0.51	—	47.58 ± 2.89	—	15.95 ± 1.18	—	61.08 ± 2.45	—	20.48 ± 1.1	—	33.54 ± 1.2	—
6	M	6.7 ± 0.62	5.46–7.94	41.5 ± 4.25	33–50	13.9 ± 1.75	10.4–17.4	62.5 ± 2.0	58.5–66.5	20.7 ± 1.0	18.7–22.7	33.5 ± 1.85	33–50
	F	6.31 ± 0.6	5.11–6.51	32.2 ± 4.4	31.0–48.6	12.8 ± 1.5	9.8–15.8	63.1 ± 1.92	57.8–65.4	20.3 ± 1.6	17.1–23.5	32.2 ± 1.74	28.7–35.7
14	M (3 mo)	5.3 ± 0.4	—	34 ± 2	—	11.2 ± 0.7	—	65 ± 3	—	21 ± 1	—	33 ± 1	—
	F (3 mo)	5.4 ± 0.6	—	36 ± 3	—	11.7 ± 1	—	67 ± 4	—	22 ± 1	—	33 ± 1	—
26	NS	—	4–7	—	30–50	—	8–15	—	—	—	—	—	—
5	M (1–2 mo)	5.64 ± 0.49	—	40.5 ± 2.4	—	11.8 ± 0.8	—	72.2 ± 5.1	—	21 ± 1.3	—	28.4 ± 4.2	—
	F (1–2 mo)	5.5 ± 0.62	—	40.3 ± 2.2	—	11.5 ± 0.8	—	73.9 ± 6.4	—	21.1 ± 1.6	—	28.5 ± 0.9	—
	M (3 mo)	6.24 ± 0.24	—	42.5 ± 1.6	—	13.4 ± 0.5	—	68.1 ± 1.9	—	21.5 ± 0.6	—	31.4 ± 0.9	—
	F (3 mo)	6.02 ± 0.23	—	41.4 ± 2.5	—	12.6 ± 0.7	—	68.7 ± 2.5	—	20.9 ± 0.8	—	30.4 ± 1	—
	M (4–6 mo)	6.34 ± 0.39	—	43.3 ± 2.6	—	13.9 ± 1.1	—	68.2 ± 4.1	—	21.9 ± 1.5	—	32 ± 1.2	—
	F (4–6 mo)	6.32 ± 0.43	—	43.0 ± 2.3	—	13.5 ± 0.9	—	68.2 ± 3.0	—	21.4 ± 1.2	—	31.4 ± 1.1	—
	M (7–12 mo)	6.03 ± 0.3	—	42.4 ± 1.6	—	13.7 ± 0.6	—	70.9 ± 2.3	—	22.7 ± 0.8	—	32 ± 8	—
	F (7–12 mo)	5.95 ± 0.43	—	41.7 ± 3.2	—	13.1 ± 1.0	—	70.2 ± 3.1	—	22.1 ± 1.1	—	31.4 ± 1.2	—
	M (1–2 yr)	6.34 ± 0.7	—	42.7 ± 1.8	—	13.2 ± 1.0	—	67.9 ± 5.6	—	21 ± 1.1	—	31 ± 1.8	—
	F (1–2 yr)	5.96 ± 0.54	—	40.8 ± 3.5	—	12.7 ± 1.3	—	68.5 ± 2.7	—	21.4 ± 1	—	31.3 ± 1.4	—
15	M (n = 98)	6.75 ± 0.53	—	40.4 ± 3.05	—	13.7 ± 1.0	—	59.9 ± 2.78	—	20.4 ± 0.97	—	34.0 ± 0.52	—
	F (n = 98)	6.22 ± 0.48	—	37.8 ± 2.31	—	12.8 ± 0.78	—	60.9 ± 2.4	—	20.8 ± 0.93	—	34.1 ± 0.61	—
12	F (2.9–4.4 kg)	5.7 ± 0.4	—	36 ± 3	—	12.1 ± 1.0	—	62 ± 1	—	21	—	34	—
16	NS (4–7 mo)	6.0 ± 0.6	3.7–7.5	38 ± 3.1	26.7–47.2	12.8 ± 1.0	8.9–15.5	63.7 ± 3.1	58–79.6	21.4 ± 1.3	19.2–29.5	33.6 ± 0.6	31.1–37
17	M	6.4 ± 0.4	—	43 ± 2	—	14 ± 0.6	—	65 ± 4	—	21 ± 1	—	32.5 ± 0.4	—
	F	6.0 ± 0.6	—	39 ± 2	—	12.7 ± 0.6	—	66 ± 2	—	22 ± 1	—	32.8 ± 0.3	—
18	NS	—	4–7.2	—	36–48	—	10.0–15.5	—	—	—	—	—	—
19	NS	—	4–7	—	36–48	—	10.0–15.5	—	—	—	—	—	—
20	NS	—	5.1–7.9	—	33–50	—	10.0–17.4	—	57.8–66.5	—	17.1–23.5	—	29–37

NS, not specified.

TABLE 170.2 Referenced Leukocyte Parameters in the New Zealand White (NZW) Rabbit (*Oryctolagus cuniculus*)

Reference	Gender	WBC (×10³/mm³) Mean	WBC (×10³/mm³) Range	Neutrophils (%) Mean	Neutrophils (%) Range	Lymphocytes (%) Mean	Lymphocytes (%) Range	Eosinophils (%) Mean	Eosinophils (%) Range	Basophils (%) Mean	Basophils (%) Range	Monocytes (%) Mean	Monocytes (%) Range
9	NS	8	5.2–12	—	8–50	—	20–90	—	1–3	—	0.5–30	—	1–4
36	NS	8.1	—	32	—	63	—	1.3	—	2.4	—	4.1	—
37	NS	—	5.2–12.5	—	36.4–54	—	28–52.1	—	0.5–3.5	—	2.4–7.5	—	4.0–13.4
13	NS (1 yr)	4.91 ± 2.19	—	—	—	54.2 ± 11.6	—	4.5 ± 3.6	—	—	—	6.3 ± 3.5	—
	NS (adult)	7.46 ± 3.15	—	—	—	42.7 ± 19.8	—	2.2 ± 2.0	—	—	—	4.3 ± 3.0	—
6	M	9.0 ± 1.75	5.5–12.5	46 ± 4	38–54	39 ± 5.5	28–50	2 ± 0.75	0.5–3.5	5 ± 1.25	2.5–7.5	8 ± 2	4–12
	F	7.9 ± 1.35	5.2–10.6	43.4 ± 3.5	36.4–50.4	41.8 ± 5.15	31.5–52.1	2 ± 0.6	0.8–3.2	4.3 ± 0.95	2.4–6.2	9 ± 2.2	6.6–13.4
14	M (3 mo)	9.7 ± 3.3	—	30	—	60	—	1	—	3.1	—	3.1	—
	F (3 mo)	7.7 ± 2.2	—	25	—	64	—	0	—	3.9	—	5.5	—
26	NS	—	6–12	—	20–60	—	20–50	—	0–5	—	0–1	—	1–10
5	M (1–2 mo)	5.99 ± 1.98	—	34.7 ± 11.7	—	57.7 ± 13.1	—	0.8 ± 0.6	—	2.0 ± 1.7	—	5.5 ± 7.0	—
	F (1–2 mo)	5.38 ± 1.85	—	31.9 ± 12.2	—	61.1 ± 12.5	—	0.9 ± 0.9	—	2.3 ± 2.2	—	3.7 ± 2.6	—
	M (3 mo)	8.45 ± 1.34	—	28.9 ± 8.4	—	65.7 ± 9.2	—	1.6 ± 0.8	—	0.8 ± 0.6	—	5.6 ± 7.5	—
	F (3 mo)	9.1 ± 3.54	—	28.8 ± 10	—	67.5 ± 10.3	—	0.9 ± 0.8	—	1.5 ± 0.8	—	1.4 ± 0.9	—
	M (4–6 mo)	7.71 ± 1.08	—	27.6 ± 10.4	—	68.5 ± 11.1	—	0.8 ± 0.8	—	1.4 ± 1.3	—	1.7 ± 1.4	—
	F (4–6 mo)	7.69 ± 1.6	—	28.9 ± 10.4	—	63.9 ± 10.4	—	1.5 ± 0.9	—	2.5 ± 1.8	—	2.7 ± 2.3	—
	M (7–12 mo)	8.99 ± 1.75	—	27.9 ± 8	—	62 ± 16.9	—	0.8 ± 0.7	—	3.0 ± 2.6	—	2.5 ± 2.4	—
	F (7–12 mo)	7.69 ± 1.8	—	30 ± 9.7	—	62.8 ± 11.8	—	1.2 ± 1.1	—	2.4 ± 2.0	—	3.6 ± 2.6	—
	M (1–2 yr)	10.0 ± 2.85	—	47 ± 5.9	—	44.5 ± 7	—	1.5 ± 1	—	2.3 ± 2.3	—	4.9 ± 4.5	—
	F (1–2 yr)	9.72 ± 3.3	—	44.7 ± 14.6	—	45.6 ± 14.4	—	2.0 ± 1.6	—	3.3 ± 2.2	—	4.8 ± 2.5	—
15	M (2–7 mo)	9.5 ± 2.07	—	32 ± 10.95	—	62 ± 13.2	—	1 ± 0.8	—	2 ± 1.7	—	1 ± 1.4	—
	F (2–7 mo)	8.4 ± 2.24	—	34 ± 10.7	—	61 ± 11.3	—	1 ± 1.3	—	3 ± 1.8	—	1 ± 1.1	—
12	F (2.9–4.4 kg)	8.1 ± 2.7	—	32 ± 15	—	68 ± 15	—	—	—	—	—	—	—
16	NS	9.2 ± 2.2	5.2–16.5	—	—	—	—	—	—	—	—	—	—
17	M (1–2 yr)	6.8 ± 1.2	—	26 ± 7	—	58 ± 8	—	0.5 ± 0.4	—	3.2 ± 0.8	—	6.0 ± 2.4	—
	F (1–2 yr)	5.6 ± 0.9	—	35 ± 3	—	47 ± 7	—	1.2 ± 0.8	—	5.0 ± 2.5	—	6.6 ± 2.4	—
18	NS	—	7.5–13.5	—	20–35	—	55–80	—	0–4	—	2–10	—	1–4
19	NS	—	9–11	—	20–75	—	30–85	—	0–4	—	2–7	—	1–4
20	NS	—	5.2–12.5	—	20–75	—	30–85	—	1–4	—	1–7	—	1–4

NS, not specified.

TABLE 170.3 Referenced Erythrocyte Parameters for Some Other Rabbit Breeds/Species

Reference	Breed/Species	Gender	RBC (×10⁶/mm³) Mean	RBC (×10⁶/mm³) Range	PCV (%) Mean	PCV (%) Range	Hb (g/dl) Mean	Hb (g/dl) Range	MCV (μ³) Mean	MCV (μ³) Range	MCH (μμg) Mean	MCH (μμg) Range	MCHC (%) Mean	MCHC (%) Range
38	Dutch Belted *L. europaeus*	M	5.45 ± 0.13	—	41.18 ± 0.71	—	13.98 ± 0.25	—	—	—	—	—	—	—
		F	5.3 ± 0.14	—	41.79 ± 0.91	—	14.21 ± 0.35	—	—	—	—	—	—	—
6	Dutch Belted *L. europaeus*	NS	—	4.8–6.3	—	34.8–48.9	—	12.2–16.3	—	62.7–88.1	—	22.0–29.4	—	28.5–38.1
6	Polish White *L. europaeus*	NS	—	4.6–6.32	—	36.7–43.5	—	11.9–16.3	—	67.7–80.3	—	22.0–30.1	—	29.7–40.6
39	Jack Rabbit *L. californicus*	NS	—	6.59–8.56	—	42–53	—	13.7–17.5	—	57.6–70	—	18.1–23.1	—	28.8–36.8
6	Jack Rabbit *L. californicus*	NS (1 yr)	—	6.17–9.29	—	41.2–57	—	13.4–18.6	—	58.7–68.6	—	18.6–22.8	—	30.4–34.6
		NS (adult)	—	6.77–8.81	—	41.8–53.4	—	13.6–18.3	—	56.2–66	—	18.3–22.7	—	31.1–35.9
5	Jack Rabbit *L. californicus*	NS (<1 yr)	7.73 ± 0.78	—	49.08 ± 3.98	—	15.97 ± 1.3	—	63.62 ± 2.47	—	20.7 ± 1.07	—	32.52 ± 1.04	—
		NS (adult)	7.79 ± 0.51	—	47.58 ± 2.89	—	15.98 ± 1.18	—	61.08 ± 2.45	—	20.48 ± 1.1	—	33.54 ± 1.2	—
40	Cottontail (*Sylvalagus floridanus*)	NS (autumn)	—	—	34	—	—	—	—	—	—	—	—	—
		NS (winter)	—	—	45	44–54	—	—	—	—	—	—	—	—
		NS (spring)	—	—	42	31–46	—	—	—	—	—	—	—	—
		NS (summer)	—	—	40	31–47	—	—	—	—	—	—	—	—
41	Cottontail (*Sylvalagus floridanus*)	NS	—	—	37.2 ± 6.7	18–49	—	—	—	—	—	—	—	—

NS, not specified.

TABLE 170.4   Referenced Leukocyte Parameters for Some Other Rabbit Breeds/Species

Reference	Breed/Species	Gender	WBC (×10³/mm³) Mean	WBC (×10³/mm³) Range	Neutrophils (%) Mean	Neutrophils (%) Range	Lymphocytes (%) Mean	Lymphocytes (%) Range	Eosinophils (%) Mean	Eosinophils (%) Range	Basophils (%) Mean	Basophils (%) Range	Monocytes (%) Mean	Monocytes (%) Range
38	Dutch Belted L. europaeus	M	7.14 ± 0.74	—	36.29 ± 2.94	—	58.47 ± 2.79	—	2.0 ± 0.57	—	1.35 ± 0.43	—	2.47 ± 0.4	—
		F	7.01 ± 0.48	—	23.42 ± 2.51	—	71.53 ± 3.01	—	0.89 ± 0.2	—	1.74 ± 0.58	—	2.37 ± 0.43	—
6	Dutch Belted L. europaeus	NS	—	4–13	—	30–50	—	28.5–52.5	—	0.5–5.0	—	2–8	—	2–16
6	Polish White L. europaeus	NS	—	7.45–13.3	—	16.4–49.9	—	73–90.0	—	0.13–1.63	—	1.13–3.63	—	0.73–3.25
39	Jack Rabbit L. californicus	NS	—	2.2–14.7	—	13.0–81.5	—	25–83	—	0–8	—	0–1.5	—	2–10
6	Jack Rabbit L. californicus	NS (1 yr)	—	2.7–7.1	—	11.8–57.4	—	31.0–77.4	—	0.9–8.1	—	0–1	—	2.8–9.8
		NS (adult)	—	3.31–10.8	—	11.4–71.8	—	22.9–81.3	—	0.2–4.2	—	0–0.9	—	1.3–7.3
5	Jack Rabbit L. californicus	NS (<1 yr)	4.91 ± 2.2	—	34.6 ± 11.4	—	54.2 ± 11.6	—	4.5 ± 3.6	—	0.4 ± 0.6	—	6.3 ± 3.5	—
		NS (adult)	7.46 ± 3.15	—	50.4 ± 21.4	—	42.7 ± 19.8	—	2.2 ± 2.0	—	0.4 ± 0.5	—	4.3 ± 3.0	—
40	Cottontail (Sylvalagus floridanus)	NS (autumn)	—	—	51	—	43.5	—	1	0–9.5	1.5	—	1.5	—
		NS (winter)	—	—	28.5	21–45.5	62.5	48–71.5	1	1–1.5	1.5	0.5–2.5	2	1–2.5
		NS (spring)	—	—	48	47–69.5	43	25.5–45.5	0.5	0–1	2	1.0–2.5	2	1.5–3.5
		NS (summer)	—	—	43	5–67	53	29–94	0	0–1	0.75	0–3	2.7	1.0–5.5

NS, not specified.

month of life and a subsequent smaller decrease to $3.0 \pm 1.3\%$ in adult rabbits.[5] Reticulocyte counts were found to increase following repeated blood collections.[10]

The life span of rabbit erythrocytes was estimated to range between 45 to 70 days,[5] with an average life span of 57 days and a predicted random destruction rate of 0.5% per day.[11] Erythrocyte counts are low in newborn rabbits, whereas mean corpuscular volume (MCV) and mean corpuscular hemoglobin (MCH) values are higher than observed in adults.[12] Erythrocyte numbers and hemoglobin concentrations are slightly higher in male rabbits than in females (Table 170.1). Higher values for red blood cells (RBCs), hemoglobin (Hb), and packed cell volume (PCV) were seen in wild jackrabbits (Table 170.3), while that species has somewhat smaller erythrocytes.

Thrombocytes

Rabbit platelets appear as small clusters of azurophilic granules surrounded by pale blue cytoplasm. Observed ranges of numbers of circulating platelets have been reported in several references: 126 to $1000 \times 10^3/\text{mm}^3$;[9] 270 to $628 \times 10^3/\text{mm}^3$;[13] 304 to $656 \times 10^3/\text{mm}^3$ in males, and 270 to $630 \times 10^3/\text{mm}^3$ in females;[6] 322 to $734 \times 10^3/\text{mm}^3$ in males, and 248 to $438 \times 10^3/\text{mm}^3$ in females;[14] 197 to $385 \times 10^3/\text{mm}^3$ in males, and 249 to $449 \times 10^3/\text{mm}^3$ in females;[5] 369 to $629 \times 10^3/\text{mm}^3$ in males, and 384 to $556 \times 10^3/\text{mm}^3$ in females;[15] 112 to $795 \times 10^3/\text{mm}^3$;[16] 110 to $206 \times 10^3/\text{mm}^3$;[17] 200 to $1000 \times 10^3/\text{mm}^3$;[18] 250 to $270 \times 10^3/\text{mm}^3$;[19] and 250 to $650 \times 10^3/\text{mm}^3$.[20]

Leukocytes

The leukocyte count in rabbits may vary with rhythmic diurnal fluctuations, nutritional variation, and differences in age, gender, and breed; in addition, the differential count in a normal rabbit may be observed to fluctuate considerably when evaluated over 1 month.[6] Total leukocyte counts were lowest in newborn and juvenile rabbits, reaching adult levels after 12 months of age (Table 170.2). The neutrophil:lymphocyte ratio (expressed as %) at 2 months of age was found to be 33:60 and changed to 45:45 after 12 months of age.[5]

The rabbit heterophil (neutrophil) has been referred to as a pseudoeosinophil. The rabbit heterophil is approximately 10 to 15 μm in diameter.[14] Its polymorphic nucleus is stained a light purple with a light blue nuclear membrane. The nucleus is surrounded by a diffusely pink cytoplasm, which contains small acidophilic-specific granules and a variable number of large reddish granules. The nucleus of the rabbit lymphocyte is round, pyknotic, and surrounded by a narrow band of blue-staining cytoplasm, which may occasionally contain azurophilic granules in larger lymphocytes. Both small and large forms of lymphocytes may be observed. The rabbit monocyte is a large cell (15 to 18 μm in diameter) with an ameboid nuclear pattern (lobulated, horseshoe-shaped, or bean shaped) and diffuse and lightly stained

nuclear chromatin, with the nucleus surrounded by blue cytoplasm that may contain a few vacuoles.[14] The rabbit eosinophil is larger than the heterophil (12 to 16 μm diameter) and has a nucleus that is bilobed or horseshoe-shaped. Its intensely acidophilic cytoplasmic granules are more numerous within the cytoplasm and are three to four times the size of the granules observed in the heterophil. In contrast to other common laboratory animals, the basophil of the rabbit is regularly found in circulating blood in small to modest numbers.[5] Circulating basophil numbers were found to be inversely proportional to the number of tissue mast cells.[5] The nucleus of the rabbit basophil stains a light purple color, and its cytoplasm is packed with purple to black metachromic granules.

A rare dominant hereditary condition in humans and rabbits, referred to as the Pelger-Huët nuclear anomaly, is characterized by a lack of segmentation of the nuclei of leukocytes, primarily neutrophils, and secondary complications such as severe skeletal deformities and an increase in mortality rates.[21] Peripheral blood will be observed to contain neutrophils with round, single, or minimally segmented nuclei. The occasional observation of a few circulating Pelger cells may occur in otherwise normal rabbits and appears not to be genetic in origin.[7]

BONE MARROW CYTOLOGY

Bone marrow samples may be obtained from an anesthetized rabbit from three possible sites: the wing of the

---

TABLE 170.5   Differential Cell Distribution in the Bone Marrow of Normal Rabbits[24]

Erythrocyte series	
Rubriblast	0.2%
Prorubricyte	0.6%
Basophilic rubricyte	5.5%
Polychrom rubricyte	18.9%
Metarubricyte	16.7%
Total erythroid cells	41.9%
Other cells	
Lymphocyte	12.6%
Monocyte	1.6%
Plasma cell	0.2%
RE cell	1.0%
Other	0.3%
Granulocytic series	
Myeloblast	0.7%
Progranulocyte	0.6%
Myelocytes	3.1%
Metamyelocytes	7.4%
Band Pseudoeosinophils	23.2%
Segmenter Pseudoeosinophils	5.3%
Basophil	0.7%
Eosinophil	1.4%
Total granulocytic cells	42.4%

M:E = 1.01:1.0

TABLE 170.6 Observed Blood Coagulation Values in Rabbits

Parameter	Mean ± SD	Reference
Bleeding time (min)	1.4 ± 0.3	27
	2.1 ± 0.5	28
	1.9 ± 0.8	29
	5.4 ± 1.2	30
	4.6 ± 0.5	31
	3.87 ± 0.41	32
Clotting time (min)	4.3 ± 0.6	27
	4.0 ± 0.4	31
	4.0 ± 1.7	32
Prothrombin time (sec)	7.5 ± 1.5	32
	7.5 ± 0.3	33
Activated partial thrombo-plastin time (sec)	32.8 ± 4.5	32
	(19.5–22.5)	34
	(15.7–42.7)	35

ilium of the pelvis,[22] the proximal end of the femur, or the proximal end of the humerus. An 18-gauge Rosenthal pediatric biopsy needle can be used for bone marrow collection from the humerus and femur.[23] The appearance of most cells and the maturation sequence in rabbit bone marrow is similar to that in humans and other mammals.[7] Sanderson and Phillips[14] provided an excellent series of color photomicrographs of rabbit bone marrow. The myeloid to erythroid (M:E) ratio of rabbit bone marrow is approximately 1:1.[14,24] The M:E ratio in rabbits from birth to 5 months of age was reported as follows: 0.72:1 at birth, 0.19:1 at 1 week, 1.09:1 at 4 weeks, 0.61:1 at 2 months, 0.81:1 at 3 months, 1.42:1 at 4 months, and 0.89:1 at 5 months.[25]

Table 170.5 provides the differential percentages of cells found within the bone marrow of normal rabbits.

OTHER HEMATOLOGIC VALUES

Reported coagulation values for NZW rabbits are provided in Table 170.6.

The sedimentation rate for blood from rabbits was reported as follows: for male rabbits, 2.0 ± 0.5 mm/hr (range, 1 to 3 mm/hr); for female rabbits, 1.75 ± 0.4 mm/hr (range, 0.95 to 2.55 mm/hr);[6] and 2 to 4 mm/hr.[26]

REFERENCES

1. **Stickrod G, Ebaugh T, Garnett C.** Use of mini-peristaltic pump for collection of blood from rabbits. Lab Anim Sci 1981;31:87–88.
2. **Weisbroth SH, Flatt RE, Kraus AL.** The biology of the laboratory rabbit. New York: Academic Press, 1974.
3. **Kaplan HM, Timmons EH.** The rabbit: a model for the principles of mammalian physiology and surgery. New York: Academic Press, 1979.
4. **Prince H.** Blood volume in the pregnant rabbit. Q J Exp Physiol 1982;67:87.
5. **Jain NC.** Schalm's veterinary hematology. Philadelphia: Lea & Febiger, 1986.
6. **Mitruka BJ, Rawnsley HM.** Clinical biochemical and hematological reference values in normal experimental animals and normal humans. 2nd ed. New York: Masson, 1981.
7. **McLaughlin RM, Fish RE.** Clinical biochemistry and hematology. In: Manning PJ, et al., eds. The biology of the laboratory rabbit. San Diego, Academic Press, 1994.

8. **Hawkey CM, Dennett TB.** Color atlas of comparative veterinary hematology. Ames, IA: Iowa State University Press, 1989.
9. **Schermer S.** The blood morphology of laboratory animals. Philadelphia: FA Davis, 1967.
10. **Balin A, Koren G, Hasu M, Zipursky A.** Evaluation of a new method for the prevention of neonatal anemia. Pediatr Res 1989;25:274–275.
11. **Vacha J.** Red cell life-span. In: Agar NS, Boards PG, eds. Red blood cells of domestic animals. Amsterdam: Elsevier, 1983.
12. **Bartolotti A, Castelli D, Bonati M.** Hematology and serum chemistry of adult, pregnant, and newborn New Zealand rabbits (Oryctolagus cuniculus). Lab Anim Sci 1989;39:437–439.
13. **Loeb WF, Bannerman RM, Rininger BF, Johnson AJ.** Hematologic disorders. In: Benirschke KE, et al., eds. Pathology of laboratory animals. New York: Springer-Verlag, 1978;1.
14. **Sanderson JH, Phillips CE.** An atlas of laboratory animal hematology. Oxford: Oxford University Press, 1981.
15. **Wolford ST, Schroer RA, Gohs FX, Gallo PP, Brodeck M, Falk HB, Ruhren R.** Reference range data base for serum chemistry and hematology values in laboratory animals. J Toxicol Environ Health 1986;18:161–188.
16. **Hewitt CD, Hewitt CD, Innes DJ, Savory J, Wills MR.** Normal biochemical and hematological values in New Zealand white rabbits. Clin Chem 1989;35:1777–1779.
17. **Kabata J, Gratwohl A, Tichelli A, John L, Speck B.** Hematologic values of New Zealand white rabbits determined by automated flow cytometry. Lab Anim Sci 1991;41:613–619.
18. **Harkness JE, Wagner JE.** The biology and medicine of rabbits and rodents. 4th ed. Baltimore: Williams & Wilkins, 1995.
19. **Johnson-Delaney CA.** Exotic companion medicine handbook. Lake Worth, FL: Wingers Publishing, 1996.
20. **Hillyer EV, Quesenberry KE.** Ferrets, rabbits, and rodents—clinical medicine and surgery. Philadelphia: WB Saunders, 1997.
21. **Pelger S.** Nuclear anomaly of leucocytes. In: Undritz E, ed. Fol Ham Schweiz Med Wsch 1943;67:249.
22. **Wilson P.** Bone marrow biopsy in the rabbit. Lab Anim 1971;5:203–206.
23. **Horan PK, Muirhead KA, Gorton S, Irons RD.** Aseptic aspiration of rabbit bone marrow and enrichment for cycling Cells. Lab Anim Sci 1980;30:76–79.
24. **Dikovinova NV.** The absolute number of cells in the bone marrow and myelograms of normal rabbits. Bull Exp Biol Med 1957;44:1129.
25. **Sabin FR, et al.** Changes in the bone marrow and blood cells of developing rabbits. J Exp Med 1936;64:97.
26. **Wallach JD, Boever WJ.** Diseases of exotic animals—medical and surgical management. Philadelphia: WB Saunders, 1983.
27. **Livio M, Vigano G, Morigi M, Ubiali A, Galbusera M, Remuzzi G.** Role of platelet-activating factor in primary hemostasis. Am J Physiol 1988;254:H1218–1223.
28. **Vaughan DE, Declerck PJ, DeMol M, Collen D.** Recombinant plasminogen activator inhibitor—ru1 reverses the bleeding tendency associated with combined administration of tissue-type plasminogen activator and aspirin in rabbits. J Clin Invest 1989;84:586–591.
29. **Johnstone MT, Andrews T, Ware JA, Rudd MA, George D, Weinstein M, Loscalzo J.** Bleeding time prolongation with streptokinase and its reduction with l-desamino-8-d-arginine vasopressin. Circulation 1990;82:2142–2151.
30. **Ali BH.** The effect of ivermectin on some haematological indices in rabbits—influences of vitamin K treatment. Clin Exp Pharmacol Physiol 1990;17:735–738.
31. **Klokkevold PR, Lew DS, Ellis DG, Bertolami CN.** Effect of chitosan on lingual hemostasis in rabbits. J Oral Maxilofac Surg 1991;49:858–863.
32. **Lewis JH.** Comparative hemostasis in vertebrates. New York: Plenum Press, 1996.
33. **Lee MJ, Clement JG.** Effects of soman poisoning on hematology and coagulation parameters and serum biochemistry in rabbits. Mil Med 1990;155:244–249.
34. **Gentry PA.** The effect of administration of a single dose of T-2 toxin on blood coagulation in the rabbit. Can J Comp Med 1982;46:414–419.
35. **Meier P, Gygax P.** A comparison of different reagents for the activated partial prothromboplastin time in rabbit and rat plasma. Thromb Res 1990;59:883–886.
36. **Melby EC Jr, Altman NH.** Handbook of laboratory animal science. Cleveland: CRC Press, 1976.
37. **Mitruka BJ, Rawnsley HM.** Clinical biochemical and hematological reference values in normal experimental animals and normal humans. 1st ed. New York: Masson Publishing, 1977.
38. **Laird CW, Fox RR, Mitchell BP, Blau EM, Schultz HS.** Effect of strain and age on some hematological parameters in the rabbit. Am J Physiol 1970;218:1613–1617.
39. **Fetters MD.** Hematology of the black-tailed jack rabbit (Lepus californicus). Lab Anim Sci 1972;22:546–548.
40. **Jacobson HA, Kirkpatrick RL, Burkhart HE, Davis JW.** Hematologic comparisons of shot and live trapped cottontail rabbits. J Wildl Dis 1978;14:82–88.
41. **Lepitzki DAW, Woolf A.** Hematology and serum chemistry of cottontail rabbits of southern Illinois. J Wildl Dis 1991;27:643–649.

CHAPTER 171

Hematology of the Guinea Pig (*Cavia porcellus*)

• DAVID M. MOORE

BLOOD COLLECTION

Blood collection from pet guinea pigs is a balancing act—weighing the interests of the patient and client, determining the volume of blood needed for analysis, and selecting a vessel or method that will supply the required quantity without threatening the animal's well-being. Minimal quantities of blood can be obtained in a single microhematocrit tube from the metatarsal veins, ear veins, saphenous veins, or toenails of nonanesthetized guinea pigs, after the vessels are pricked with either a sterile lancet or a sterile hypodermic needle (23- to 27-gauge), or the toenails can be cut to the "quick" with nail clippers. Somewhat larger samples can be obtained from the saphenous veins of the hind limbs by first anesthetizing the guinea pig, then inserting a sterile hypodermic needle into the vessel, and then collecting the blood as it drips from the hub of the needle. In research laboratories, blood collection methods that yield significantly larger volumes of blood include cardiac or vena cava punctures (both are generally used as a terminal procedure in anesthetized cavies), venipuncture of the jugular vein, catheterization of the lateral saphenous vein[1,2], or collection from the retroorbital plexus in anesthetized animals (as described in Chapter 189 "Hematology of the Rat").

The blood volume of the adult guinea pig is approximately 69 to 75 ml/kg of body weight,[3] and approximately 7 to 10% of the blood volume (0.5 to 0.7 ml/100 g of body weight) can be withdrawn safely in a single collection from a healthy, nonanemic guinea pig.[4]

MORPHOLOGY AND INDICES OF PERIPHERAL BLOOD CELLS

Reported hematologic values for the guinea pig (*Cavia porcellus*) are provided in Tables 171.1 and 171.2.

Erythrocytes

Guinea pig erythrocytes are moderately anisocytotic, with a diameter ranging between 6.6 and 7.9 μm,[5] al-though microcytes, when present, may be only 3.5 μm in diameter. The guinea pig erythrocyte is the largest red blood cell (RBC) compared with other common laboratory animal species.[6] Polychromatic erythrocytes may total about 25% of circulating erythrocytes in neonates, 4.5% in juveniles, and 1.5% in adult cavies.[5,7] The erythrocytic indices in guinea pigs (i.e., erythrocyte count, hemoglobin, and packed cell volume [Table 171.1]), are relatively low when compared with the values observed in other laboratory rodent species.[8]

Thrombocytes

Guinea pig platelets have an irregular oval shape (2 to 3 μm in length), and the periphery of the cytoplasm is pale in comparison to a more intensely stained inner zone.[5] Observed ranges of numbers of circulating platelets have been reported in several references: 120 to 132 × 10³/mm³;[5] 161 to 368 × 10³/mm³;[9] 530 ± 149 × 10³/mm³;[10] 250 to 850 × 10³/mm³;[3] 250 to 850 × 10³/mm³;[11] and 260 to 740 × 10³/mm³.[4]

Leukocytes

Guinea pig neutrophils are approximately 10 to 12 μm in diameter, have a pyknotic, segmented nucleus (with up to five or more segments), and eosinophilic granules within its cytoplasm, causing some to refer to it as a pseudoeosinophil. A "drumstick" sex chromatin lobe may be present on the nuclei of neutrophils in female guinea pigs. Cavy eosinophils are larger than neutrophils (about 10 to 15 μm in diameter), have a less segmented but somewhat indented nucleus with a lesser degree of pyknosis, and thick, round bright red granules that almost completely fill the cytoplasm.[5] Basophils are rarely found, are about the same size as neutrophils or somewhat larger, have a lobulated homogeneously purple-stained nucleus, and their cytoplasm is closely packed with round violet granules of varying size.[5] Lymphocytes are the predominant leukocyte (Table 171.2), and the small lymphocytes, which are in greater num-

TABLE 171.1 Referenced Erythrocyte Parameters for the Guinea Pig (*Cavia porcellus*)

Reference	Gender	RBC (×10⁶/mm³) Mean	RBC (×10⁶/mm³) Range	PCV (%) Mean	PCV (%) Range	Hb (g/dL) Mean	Hb (g/dL) Range	MCV (μ^3) Mean	MCV (μ^3) Range	MCH ($\mu\mu g$) Mean	MCH ($\mu\mu g$) Range	MCHC (%) Mean	MCHC (%) Range
5	NS	5.37	4.62–6.48	—	—	15.3	11.2–16.1	—	—	—	—	—	—
20	NS	5.4	—	43	—	13.4	—	81	—	25	—	30	—
9	M/F	—	5.49–8.69	—	37.5–44.2	—	11.4–13.5	—	54.6–62	—	16.5–18.8	—	26.1–34.
21	F	5.4	—	43	—	13.4	—	81	—	25	—	30	—
10	NS	4.92 ± 0.54	—	41.2 ± 3.6	—	12.4 ± 1.3	—	84.1 ± 4.5	—	—	—	30.1 ± 1.2	—
22	NS	—	5–8	—	32–50	—	10–16	—	50–68	—	16–22	—	30–34
16	NS	—	5–8	—	32–50	—	10–16	—	50–67	—	—	—	30–34
23	M (n = 110)	5.6 ± 0.62	4.36–6.84	42 ± 2.5	37–47	14.4 ± 1.38	11.6–17.2	77 ± 3	71–83	25.7 ± 0.75	24.2–27.2	34.3 ± 2.28	29.7–38.
	F (n = 95)	4.75 ± 1.2	3.35–6.15	45.4 ± 2.25	40.9–49.9	14.2 ± 1.42	11.4–17	91 ± 2.45	86.1–95.9	25.7 ± 0.8	23.1–26.3	31.3 ± 1.55	28.2–34.
17	NS	—	4–7	—	35–45	—	11–17	—	—	—	—	—	—
6	M (2–30 d)	4.67 ± 0.65	—	38.3 ± 4.5	—	11.63 ± 1.5	—	82.4 ± 4.0	—	—	—	29.7 ± 1.4	—
	F (2–30 d)	4.58 ± 0.52	—	42.9 ± 2.9	—	11.07 ± 1.2	—	82.1 ± 4.6	—	—	—	29.5 ± 1.1	—
	M (31–60 d)	5.18 ± 0.47	—	42.9 ± 2.9	—	13.06 ± 1.0	—	82.9 ± 3.9	—	—	—	30.3 ± 0.9	—
	F (31–60 d)	5.19 ± 0.4	—	43.5 ± 3.1	—	13.3 ± 0.8	—	84.0 ± 4.7	—	—	—	30.7 ± 1.0	—
	M (63–90 d)	5.64 ± 0.38	—	46.3 ± 2.3	—	14.04 ± 0.9	—	82.2 ± 2.7	—	—	—	30.3 ± 1.2	—
	F (63–90 d)	5.52 ± 0.35	—	46.2 ± 2.8	—	14.2 ± 0.9	—	83.7 ± 1.9	—	—	—	30.8 ± 1.6	—
	M (4–6 mo)	5.81 ± 0.62	—	45.1 ± 4.5	—	14.07 ± 1.0	—	77.7 ± 3.8	—	—	—	31.2 ± 1.2	—
	F (4–6 mo)	5.27 ± 0.49	—	44.1 ± 3.8	—	13.55 ± 1.4	—	83.7 ± 3.1	—	—	—	30.7 ± 1.0	—
	M (7–12 mo)	5.55 ± 0.51	—	44.0 ± 3.7	—	13.9 ± 1.4	—	79.4 ± 3.7	—	—	—	31.6 ± 1.1	—
	F (7–12 mo)	4.87 ± 0.24	—	41.2 ± 2.4	—	12.4 ± 0.7	—	84.6 ± 3.0	—	—	—	30.1 ± 0.9	—
	M (13–28 mo)	5.37 ± 0.46	—	43.9 ± 3.7	—	13.56 ± 1.1	—	81.8 ± 3.5	—	—	—	30.9 ± 1.4	—
	F (13–28 mo)	4.67 ± 0.39	—	39.8 ± 2.6	—	11.76 ± 0.8	—	85.4 ± 4.5	—	—	—	29.6 ± 0.8	—
3	NS	—	4.5–7.0	—	37–48	—	11–15	—	—	—	—	—	—
11	NS	—	4.5–7.0	—	37–48	—	11–15	—	—	—	—	—	—
4	NS	—	3.2–8.0	—	32–50	—	10–17.2	—	71–96	—	23–27	—	26–39

NS, not specified.

TABLE 171.2 Referenced Leukocyte Parameters for the Guinea Pig (Cavia porcellus)

Reference	Gender	WBC (×10³/mm³) Mean	WBC (×10³/mm³) Range	Neutrophils (%) Mean	Neutrophils (%) Range	Lymphocytes (%) Mean	Lymphocytes (%) Range	Eosinophils (%) Mean	Eosinophils (%) Range	Basophils (%) Mean	Basophils (%) Range	Monocytes (%) Mean	Monocytes (%) Range
5	NS	9	3.2–15	—	18–35	—	55–75	—	1–5	—	0–3	—	3–12
20	NS	9.9	—	38	—	55	—	3.5	—	0.3	—	2.7	—
9	M/F	—	7.8–20.7	—	21.7–47.7	—	41.3–68.5	—	2.1–7.8	—	0.6–2.7	—	2.46–5.8
21	F	9.9	—	—	28–34	—	39–72	—	1–5	—	0–3	—	3–12
10	NS	11.2 ± 2.85	—	—	—	—	—	—	—	—	—	—	—
22	NS	—	11–22	—	28–47	—	39–52	—	0–11	—	0–2	—	2–10
16	NS	—	10–14	—	28–47	—	39–60	—	1–11	—	0–2	—	2–10
23	M (n = 84)	11.5 ± 3	5.5–17.5	42 ± 7	28–56	49 ± 6.75	40–62.5	4.0 ± 1.5	1–7	0.7 ± 0.5	0–1.7	4.3 ± 0.5	3.3–5.3
	F (n = 80)	10.8 ± 2.8	5.2–16.4	31.1 ± 5.4	20.3–41.9	63.4 ± 8.5	46.4–80.4	3.5 ± 1.75	0–7	0.2 ± 0.3	0–0.8	1.8 ± 0.4	1.0–2.6
17	NS	—	7–14	—	20–60	—	30–80	—	0–5	—	0–1	—	2–20
6	M (2–30 d)	3.73 ± 0.94	—	27.9 ± 10.8	—	70.7 ± 11.7	—	2.2 ± 2.1	—	0.22 ± 0.48	—	21. ± 1.9	—
	F (2–30 d)	4.09 ± 1.0	—	21.2 ± 6.4	—	74.9 ± 7.7	—	1.9 ± 1.7	—	0.13 ± 0.4	—	1.4 ± 1.4	—
	M (31–60 d)	5.52 ± 1.8	—	29.0 ± 10.7	—	66.2 ± 13.6	—	1.0 ± 0.8	—	0.13 ± 0.28	—	2.1 ± 1.5	—
	F (31–60 d)	7.04 ± 2.01	—	25.8 ± 11.7	—	71.5 ± 12.5	—	1.0 ± 0.8	—	0.08 ± 0.21	—	1.6 ± 1.5	—
	M (63–90 d)	5.94 ± 1.2	—	31.9 ± 10.7	—	65.9 ± 10.6	—	0.6 ± 0.6	—	0.19 ± 0.39	—	1.3 ± 1.1	—
	F (63–90 d)	7.98 ± 2.3	—	26.3 ± 7.1	—	70.5 ± 7.1	—	1.4 ± 1.2	—	0.1 ± 0.2	—	1.7 ± 2.0	—
	M (4–6 mo)	9.58 ± 3.17	—	20.8 ± 6.1	—	75.3 ± 6.7	—	1.2 ± 1.0	—	0.19 ± 0.24	—	1.9 ± 1.4	—
	F (4–6 mo)	10.24 ± 1.87	—	24.3 ± 11.3	—	71.3 ± 11.9	—	2.0 ± 1.8	—	0.31 ± 0.47	—	2.2 ± 1.6	—
	M (7–12 mo)	11.5 ± 2.0	—	23.2 ± 5.1	—	71.4 ± 4.0	—	2.6 ± 4.5	—	0	—	2.8 ± 1.4	—
	F (7–12 mo)	10.93 ± 3.2	—	23.5 ± 11.0	—	71.4 ± 11.3	—	2.3 ± 2.5	—	0.08 ± 0.18	—	2.7 ± 2.2	—
	M (13–28 mo)	13.53 ± 2.5	—	30.3 ± 15.7	—	64.8 ± 16.1	—	2.1 ± 2.4	—	0.18 ± 0.24	—	2.7 ± 1.6	—
	F (13–28 mo)	9.88 ± 2.1	—	24.7 ± 10.6	—	69.4 ± 13.2	—	2.3 ± 2.1	—	0.22 ± 0.29	—	3.4 ± 3.6	—
3	NS	—	7–18	—	28–44	—	39–72	—	1–5	—	0–3	—	3–12
11	NS	—	7–18	—	28–44	—	39–72	—	1–5	—	0–3	—	3–12
4	NS	—	5.5–17.5	—	22–48	—	39–72	—	0–7	—	0–2.7	—	1–10

NS, not specified.

1109

TABLE 171.3	Observed Coagulation Values in Guinea Pigs	
Parameter	Mean (± SD)	Reference
Bleeding time (min)		
Foreleg	4	18
Hindleg	4.5	18
Paw	3.5	18
Clotting time (min)	3 (±0.7)	18
Prothrombin time (sec)	17.6	19
	26 (±2.5)	18
Activated partial thrombo-plastin time (sec)	16.8 (range 13.0–22.9)	19
	28.7 (±3.8)	18

bers than the large lymphocyte forms, are not much larger than the erythrocytes. The small lymphocytes of cavies have a round, pyknotic nucleus surrounded by a narrow band of cytoplasm. The large lymphocytes are almost twice as large, with a less pyknotic, more oval-shaped nucleus and a brighter, broader zone of cytoplasm that may contain small to large azurophilic granules.[5] Guinea pig monocytes are usually larger than the large lymphocytes, have an oval nucleus with a loosely webbed chromatin structure, and have a grey-blue cytoplasm that is darker than the cytoplasm observed in large lymphocytes.

Occasional Foa-Kurloff cells (KC cells), which are unique to the guinea pig, may be observed in the circulation, accounting for up to 3 to 4% of the differential leukocyte count.[6,8] There is no significant difference in numbers of observed KC in males and females after 2 to 3 months of age.[6] The Kurloff cell is a specialized mononuclear leukocyte that contains an intracytoplasmic inclusion body consisting of a mucopolysaccharide. Whereas these cells may be found in blood vessels and in the thymus gland, their highest density shifts from the lungs and red pulp of the spleen to the thymus and placenta under estrogen stimulation and pregnancy.[12] The exact origin and function of these cells is unknown, although it has been speculated that they may function as killer cells in the general circulation or as protectors of fetal antigen in the placenta.[13,14]

BONE MARROW CYTOLOGY

Bone marrow is perhaps best obtained from the proximal end of the femur in guinea pigs. The myeloid to erythroid (M:E) ratio was estimated to be between 1.2 and 1.6:1.0.[15]

OTHER HEMATOLOGIC VALUES

The sedimentation rate for blood from guinea pigs was reported as follows: 2.3 to 8.1 mm/hr;[9] 1 to 14 mm/hr;[16] 2 to 4 mm/hr;[17] and 1.1 to 14 mm/hr.[4] Observed coagulation values for guinea pigs are presented in Table 171.3.

REFERENCES

1. **Desjardins C.** Indwelling vascular cannulas for remote blood sampling, infusion, and long-term instrumentation of small laboratory animals. In: Gay WI, ed. Methods of animal experimentation. Orlando: Academic Press, 1986.
2. **Nau R, Schunck O.** Cannulation of the lateral saphenous vein–a rapid method to gain access to the venous circulation in anesthetized guinea pigs. Lab Anim 1993;27:23–25.
3. **Harkness JE, Wagner JE.** The biology and medicine of rabbits and rodents, 4th ed. Baltimore: Williams & Wilkins, 1995.
4. **Hillyer EV, Quesenberry KE, Donnelly TM.** Biology, husbandry, and clinical techniques (of guinea pigs and chinchillas). In: Hillyer EV, Quesenberry KE, eds. Ferrets, rabbits, and rodents clinical medicine and surgery. Philadelphia: WB Saunders, 1996.
5. **Schermer S.** The blood morphology of laboratory animals. Philadelphia: FA Davis, 1967.
6. **Jain NC.** Schalm's veterinary hematology. 4th ed. Philadelphia: Lea & Febiger, 1986.
7. **Albritton AB.** Standard values in blood. Philadelphia: WB Saunders, 1958.
8. **Manning PJ, Wagner JE, Harkness JE.** Biology and diseases of guinea pigs. In: Fox JG, et al., eds. Laboratory animal medicine. Orlando: Academic Press, 1984.
9. **Mitruka BJ, Rawnsley HM.** Clinical biochemical and hematological reference values in normal experimental animals and normal humans. 1st ed. New York: Masson, 1977.
10. **Benirschke K, Garner FM, Jones TC, eds.** Pathology of laboratory animals. New York: Springer-Verlag, 1978;1.
11. **Johnson-Delaney CA.** Exotic companion medicine handbook. Lake Worth, FL: Wingers Publishing, 1996.
12. **Izard J, Barrellier MT, Quillec M.** The Kurloff cell–its differentiation in the blood and lymphatic system. Cell Tissue Res 1976;173:237–259.
13. **Marshall AHE, Swettenham KV, Vernon-Roberts B, Revell PA.** Studies on the function of the Kurloff cell. Int Arch Allergy Appl Immunol 1971;40:137–152.
14. **Eremin O, Wilson AB, Coombs RR, Ashby J, Plumb D.** Antibody-dependent cellular cytotoxicity in the guinea pig. Cell Immunol 1980;55:312–327.
15. **Epstein RD, Tompkins EH.** A comparison of techniques for the differential counting of bone marrow cells (guinea pig). Am J Med Sci 1943;206:249.
16. **Coles EH.** Veterinary clinical pathology. Philadelphia: WB Saunders, 1980.
17. **Wallach JD, Boever WJ.** Diseases of exotic animals–medical and surgical management. Philadelphia: WB Saunders, 1983.
18. **Lewis JH.** Comparative hemostasis in vertebrates. New York: Plenum Press, 1996.
19. **Kaspareit J, Messow C, Edel J.** Blood coagulation studies in guinea pigs (Cavia porcellus). Lab Anim 1988;22:206–211.
20. **Melby EC, Altman NH.** Handbook of laboratory animal science. Cleveland: CRC Press, 1976.
21. **Quillec M, Debout C, Izard J.** Red cell and white cell counts in adult female guinea pigs. Pathol Biol 1977;25:443–446.
22. **Benjamin MM.** Outline of veterinary pathology. Ames, IA: Iowa State University Press, 1978.
23. **Mitruka BJ, Rawnsley HM.** Clinical biochemical and hematological reference values in normal experimental animals and normal humans. 2nd ed. New York: Masson, 1981.

CHAPTER 172

Hematology of the Mongolian Gerbil (*Meriones unguiculatus*)

• DAVID M. MOORE

BLOOD COLLECTION

The gerbil's blood volume is approximately 7.7 ml/100 g of body weight, and thus approximately 0.8 ml of blood can be collected safely during one withdrawal without adversely affecting the animal's well-being.[1] In research laboratories, blood is usually collected from anesthetized gerbils from the retroorbital venous plexus or by cardiac puncture (both procedures are described in Chapter 189 "Hematology of the Rat"). Less invasive procedures, which yield significantly lower volumes of blood, involve filling a single microhematocrit tube with blood obtained from a cut toenail or from the saphenous vein following puncture with a sterile lancet or hypodermic needle. Analysis of blood samples obtained from the tail vein or heart demonstrated almost identical results for packed cell volume (PCV), hemoglobin (Hb), and erythrocyte numbers, whereas samples obtained from the tail vein had higher leukocyte counts associated with a greater concentration of lymphocytes.[2] Lipemic plasma, prevalent in both sexes and at all ages, with a more pronounced lipemia in males 13 months of age or older, was attributed to addition of sunflower seeds to the diet.[2]

MORPHOLOGY AND NUMBERS OF PERIPHERAL BLOOD CELLS

Reported hematologic values for the Mongolian gerbil (*Meriones unguiculatus*) are provided in Tables 172.1 and 172.2. A significant sexual dimorphism exists with respect to erythrocyte indices (i.e., mean corpuscular volume [MCV], Hb, hematocrit [HCT], and mean corpuscular hemoglobin concentration [MCHC]), total leukocyte count, and absolute numbers of circulating lymphocytes,[3] with higher values for the erythrocyte indices reported in adult male gerbils.[4]

Erythrocytes

An erythrocytic macrocytosis, panleukocytosis, and erythrocyte counts lower than in adults are observed

in neonatal gerbils, but these parameters approximate adult values by about 8 weeks of age.[4] Reticulocytes in the peripheral blood may be observed at a frequency of between 21 and 54/1000 red blood cells (RBCs).[1] Basophilic stippling of erythrocytes was observed in 40% of the cells of fetal and newborn gerbils, but declined in incidence until 20 weeks of age to a level of 5.4 ± 2.4% seen in adult gerbils.[5] A range of 5 to 40 basophilic particles, of approximately 0.3 μm in diameter, may be present in the stippled erythrocytes.[2] Erythrocytes with diffuse basophilic staining, when present, are usually larger than the erythrocytes. Erythrocytes with basophilic stippling may be relatively immature erythrocytes that still possess remnants of cytoplasmic ribonucleoprotein.[5] Normochromic stippled erythrocytes are as large or slightly larger than mature erythrocytes, but are smaller than the diffusely stained basophilic erythrocytes. The presence of stippled erythrocytes should not be confused with the intracellular organism Haemobartonella sp. Polychromatophilic RBCs are found with almost equal frequency in male and female gerbils, with 17/1000 RBCs in males and 16.8/1000 RBCs in females.[3] The presence of stippled red cells and reticulocytes at levels higher than observed in most other domestic rodent species may be a result of the relatively brief life span of erythrocytes in gerbils, noted as 9 to 10 days, which necessitates a continuous hyperactive state of erythropoiesis.[1,2]

Thrombocytes

Platelet counts for gerbils are similar to those found in rats.[2] Observed ranges of numbers of circulating platelets have been reported in several references: 638 × 10^3/mm^3;[6] 400 to 600 × 10^3/mm^3;[4] and 400 to 600 × 10^3/mm^3.[7] A comparison of platelet counts by age and gender is provided in Table 172.3.

Leukocytes

The ratio of lymphocytes to neutrophils averages 6.1:1 in male gerbils and 3.2:1 in females.[8] The total leukocyte

TABLE 172.1 Referenced Erythrocyte Parameters of the Mongolian Gerbil (*Meriones unguiculatus*)

Reference	Gender	RBC (×10⁶/μL) Mean ± SD	RBC (×10⁶/μL) Range	PCV (%) Mean	PCV (%) Range	Hb (g/dL) Mean	Hb (g/dL) Range	MCH Mean μμg	MCH Range μμg	MCV Mean (μ³)	MCV Range (μ³)	MCHC Mean %	MCHC Range %
2	M (2 mo.)	8.1	7.0–8.9	47	41–51	13.9	12.1–15.4	—	—	—	—	—	—
	M (7 mo.)	8.3	7.8–8.9	47	44–50	14.4	13.4–15.6	—	—	—	—	—	—
	M (13 mo.)	8.1	7.1–8.6	46	42–49	15.2	13.1–17.9	—	—	—	—	—	—
	F (2 mo.)	7.7	7.3–8.2	45	42–47	13	12.1–13.8	—	—	—	—	—	—
	F (7 mo.)	8.7	7.6–9.9	46	43–50	13.7	12.4–15.2	—	—	—	—	—	—
	F (13 mo.)	8.6	8.0–9.4	47	43–50	14.4	13.1–16.9	—	—	—	—	—	—
14	—	—	7–8	—	37–47	—	14–16	—	—	—	—	—	—
8	ns	8.849 ± 0.509	7.87–9.97	—	—	—	—	17.49 ± 1.089	16.13–19.40	54.46 ± 3.72	46.64–60.04	32.14 ± 0.71	30.64–33.33
	M	—	—	49.25 ± 2.03	46–52	15.88 ± 0.57	15.2–16.8	—	—	—	—	—	—
	F	—	—	46.80 ± 1.4	44–48	15.00 ± 0.39	14.4–15.6	—	—	—	—	—	—
3	M	—	—	47.5 ± 0.978	44–49	14.75 ± 0.44	13.8–16.2	—	—	—	—	—	—
	F	—	—	45.8 ± 1.32	43–49	14.14 ± 0.51	13.5–14.8	—	—	—	—	—	—
11	M (3 mo.)	8.9	—	47.4	—	15.9	—	17.1	—	54.5	—	32.4	—
13	ns	—	7.87–9.97	—	46–52	—	15.2–16.8	—	16.1–19.4	—	46.6–60	—	30.6–33.3
12	ns	—	7–8	—	35–45	—	14–16	—	16.3–19.40	—	46.64–60.04	—	30.64–33.33
6	ns	8.5	7.0–10	48	41–52	15	12.1–16.9	—	—	—	—	—	—
4	ns	8.5	7–10	—	35–50	—	10–17	—	—	—	—	—	—
1	ns	—	8–9	—	43–49	—	12.6–16.2	—	—	—	—	—	—
7	ns	8.5	7–10	48	41–52	15	12.6–16.2	—	—	—	—	—	—

TABLE 172.2 Referenced Leukocyte Parameters of the Mongolian Gerbil (*Meriones unguiculatus*)

Reference	Gender	WBC (×10³/μL) Mean ± SD	WBC (×10³/μL) Range	Neutrophils (%) Mean ± SD	Neutrophils (%) Range	Lymphocytes (%) Mean ± SD	Lymphocytes (%) Range	Monocytes (%) Mean ± SD	Monocytes (%) Range	Eosinophils (%) Mean (± SD)	Eosinophils (%) Range	Basophils (%) Mean (± SD)	Basophils (%) Range
2	M (2 mo.)	9.8	4.7–15.0	19.3	14.8–38	75.5	68–76.7	3	2.1–3.3	2	0–2.5	0.7	0–1.3
	M (7 mo.)	11.2	5.1–15.9	14.2	9.8–16.3	83	80.5–86.2	2.7	0–3.2	0.9	0–1.9	0.53	0–1.2
	M (13 mo.)	9.1	4.3–12.3	18.7	9.3–23.6	75.8	68–76.8	3.3	0–6.5	1.1	0–1.6	0.88	0–1.6
	F (2 mo.)	8.3	4.5–15.4	20.5	17.8–38.3	74.7	68.9–76	2.4	2.2–5.8	1.2	0–1.8	0.84	0–1.3
	F (7 mo.)	9.9	4.7–16.7	16.2	6.4–22.8	79.8	78.4–85.1	2	0–4.2	1	0–2.4	0.6	0–1.2
	F (13 mo.)	9.5	5.6–12.8	21	10.7–25.8	74.8	58.9–78.1	3.1	1.7–6.2	1	0–2.3	0.42	0–0.8
8	M	13.532 ± 5.85	6.506–21.600	13.9 ± 6.75	2–23	84.8 ± 7.90	73–97	—	—	—	—	—	—
	F	8.696 ± 0.415	7.509–10.900	23.4 ± 12.23	7–41	74.8 ± 12.36	58–92	—	—	—	—	—	—
	ns	—	—	—	—	—	—	0.3	0–3	1.1	0–4	0.05	0–1
3	M	12.1 ± 1.99	8.64–15.4	20.2	7.8–33.5	78.2	—	0.8	—	1.2	—	1.5	—
	F	9.65 ± 1.72	7.34–14.6	26.2	17.1–35.7	72.8	—	1.4	—	1.36	—	1.1	—
11	M (3 mo.)	12.4	—	15.6	—	80.6	—	0.2	—	1.1	—	0.7	—
13	ns	—	6.51–21.6	—	2–23	—	73–97	—	0–3	—	0–4	—	0–1
12	ns	—	7.5–10.9	22	7–41	75	—	—	0–4	—	0–3	—	0–1
6	ns	11	4.3–21.6	19	3–41	78	32–97	3	0–9	1	0–4	0.6	0–2
4	ns	—	4.3–22	—	2–41	—	58–98	—	0–3	—	0–4	—	0–1
1	ns	—	7–15	—	5–34	—	60–95	—	0–3	—	0–4	—	0–3
7	ns	11	4.3–21.6	29.9	5–34	73.5	60–95	—	0–3	—	0–4	—	0–1

			Platelets ($\times 10^3$/mm³)	Platelets ($\times 10^3$/mm³)
TABLE 172.3		**Platelet Counts in Mongolian Gerbils[2]**		
Age	No.	Gender	Mean	Range
2 mo	3	M	557.66	543–575
2 mo	3	F	794.16	767.5–830
7 mo	3	M	608.36	540–668.8
7 mo	3	F	669.60	603.8–720
13 mo	3	M	609.17	432–710
13 mo	3	F	590.67	540–632

count in gerbils is closer to that of the mouse than the hamster.[9] Reported normal leukocyte values for Mongolian gerbils are provided in Table 172.2.

BONE MARROW CYTOLOGY

The myeloid to erythroid (M:E) ratio in the bone marrow of gerbils was reported to be 1.6 ± 0.75:1, with an observed range of 0.6 to 3.6:1.[10] One laboratory calculated the mean percentages of selected bone marrow cells as follows: neutrophils, 38.5%; normoblasts, 26.8%; plasma cells, 2.0%; eosinophils, 1.9%; and basophils, 0.2%.[11] Basophilic stippling was seen in 26.1 ± 7.6% of erythrocytes in bone marrow.[5] Lymphocytes in marrow samples accounted for about 8.4 ± 4.2% of cells observed, with a range between 1.4 and 20.1%.[10] Ring heterophils are seen in gerbil marrow, similar to those observed in rats

and mice.[10] The bone marrow of adult gerbils contains a higher proportion of stippled red cells than is observed in the circulating blood.[5]

OTHER HEMATOLOGIC VALUES

The sedimentation rate (mm/hr) for normal gerbil blood was reported as 0 to 2 mm/hr.[12]

REFERENCES

1. **Harkness JE, Wagner JE.** The biology and medicine of rabbits and rodents. 4th ed. Baltimore: Williams & Wilkins, 1995.
2. **Ruhren R.** Normal values for hemoglobin concentration and cellular elements in the blood of Mongolian gerbils. Lab Anim Care 1965;15:313–320.
3. **Dillon WG, Glomski GA.** The Mongolian gerbil: qualitative and quantitative aspects of the cellular blood picture. Lab Anim 1975;9:283–287.
4. **Wagner JE, Farrar PL.** Husbandry and medicine of small rodents. Vet Clin North Am Small Anim Pract 1987;17:1061–1087.
5. **Smith RA, Termer EA, Glomski CA.** Erythrocyte basophilic stippling in the Mongolian gerbil. Lab Anim 1976;10:379.
6. **Clark JD.** Biology and diseases of other rodents. In: Fox JG, Cohen BJ, Loew FM, eds. Laboratory animal medicine. Orlando: Academic Press, 1984;192.
7. **Johnson-Delaney CA.** Exotic companion medicine handbook. Lake Worth, FL: Wingers Publishing, 1996.
8. **Mays A Jr.** Baseline hematological and blood biochemical parameters of the Mongolian gerbil (*Meriones unguiculatus*). Lab Anim Care 1969;19:838–842.
9. **Handler AH, Magalini SI, Pav D.** Oncogenic studies on the Mongolian gerbil. Cancer Res 1966;26:844–847.
10. **Weeks AM, Glomski CA.** Cytology of the bone marrow in the Mongolian gerbil. Lab Anim 1978;12:195.
11. **Robinson DG.** Physiological parameters and selected general data. Gerbil Dig 1979;6:1.
12. **Wallach JD, Boever WJ.** Diseases of exotic animals–medical and surgical management. Philadelphia: WB Saunders, 1983.
13. **Mitruka BM, Rawnsley HM.** Clinical biochemical and hematological reference values in normal experimental animals and normal humans. New York: Masson, 1981;413.
14. **Loew FM.** The management and diseases of gerbils. In: Current veterinary therapy. Philadelphia: WB Saunders, 1968;3416–418.

CHAPTER 173

Hematology of the Syrian (Golden) Hamster (*Mesocricetus auratus*)

• DAVID M. MOORE

BLOOD COLLECTION

Blood is collected from laboratory hamsters either from the retroorbital venous plexus or by cardiac puncture while the animals are anesthetized (these procedures are described in Chapter 189 "Hematology of the Rat"). Alternate blood collection methods for research of pet hamsters include use of a microhematocrit tube to obtain blood from a clipped toenail or from the saphenous vein following puncture with a sterile lancet or hypodermic needle. The blood volume in a hamster is between 65 and 80 mL/kg of body weight (of which approximately 1 to 1.5 mL can be withdrawn safely during a single collection).[1,2]

MORPHOLOGY AND NUMBERS OF PERIPHERAL BLOOD CELLS

Reported hematologic values for the Syrian hamster (*Mesocricetus auratus*) are provided in Tables 173.1 and 173.2. Additional published hematologic reference values can be found in the literature (Table 173.3).[3–6]

Erythrocytes

Hamster erythrocytes are biconcave, have an average diameter of 6 μm (range, 5 to 7 μm), and a small proportion of the red blood cells (RBCs) may show polychromasia. Nucleated erythrocyte levels may be as high as 10 to 30% in newborn hamsters, whereas levels of those cells in adults is usually less than or equal to 2%.[2,7] Reported ranges of reticulocyte numbers include 2.0 to 12.5%[8] and 0.4 to 2.8%.[9] The hematocrit and hemoglobin levels in neonates increase until about 8 to 9 weeks of age.[7] Elevated hemoglobin levels are observed in 2- to 3-week-old hamsters and in animals that are anorexic or have been starved.[10] The number of circulating erythrocytes declined by 25 to 30% following castration of male hamsters,[11] and testosterone administration was shown to restore erythrocyte levels to normal in castrates.[1] Erythrocyte counts and hemoglobin concentrations are higher in hibernating animals, with the mean number of erythrocytes increasing from 7.7 × 10^6/mm^3 to approximately 8.2 × 10^6/mm^3, and hemoglobin increasing from a mean value of 13.5 g/dL to approximately 16.7 g/dL.[9] RBC senescence was delayed and erythrocyte destruction was virtually absent during hibernation, with an observed increase in erythrocyte life span up to 160 days,[12] as compared with the normal erythrocyte life span of 60 to 70 days in nonhibernating hamsters.[13]

Thrombocytes

Platelets appear to be amorphous veils of a grey-blue ground substance with violet granulation.[9] Observed ranges of numbers of circulating platelets have been reported in several references: 336 to 587 × 10^3/mm^3;[9] 247 to 372 × 10^3/mm^3;[7] 300 to 573 × 10^3/mm^3;[10] 200 to 590 × 10^3/mm^3;[14] 200 to 500 × 10^3/mm^3;[2] 200 to 500 × 10^3/mm^3;[15] and 297 to 439 × 10^3/mm^3.[16] Platelet counts were found to be reduced during hibernation.[17]

Leukocytes

Hamster neutrophils, also referred to as heterophils, have annular lobulated pyknotic nuclei and contain acidophilic cytoplasmic granules of round or rod shapes. Neutrophils may be either segmented or unsegmented and generally have a diameter between 10 and 12 μm. Two classes of lymphocytes, small and large (with the small form in greater prevalence), comprise between 60 and 80% of all circulating white blood cells. The nucleus of the hamster lymphocyte is round, pyknotic to the point that it almost seems granulated, and is seldom indented.[9] A narrow band of blue-staining cytoplasm surrounds the nucleus of the lymphocyte and may occasionally contain azure granules. Occasionally, the band of cytoplasm of some lymphocytes may be reduced to

TABLE 173.1   Referenced Erythrocyte Parameters of the Syrian (Golden) Hamster (*Mesocricetus auratus*)

Reference	Gender	RBC (×10⁶/mm³) Mean	RBC (×10⁶/mm³) Range	PCV (%) Mean	PCV (%) Range	Hb (g/dL) Mean	Hb (g/dL) Range	MCV (μ^3) Mean	MCV (μ^3) Range	MCH ($\mu\mu$g) Mean	MCH ($\mu\mu$g) Range	MCHC (%) Mean	MCHC (%) Range
9	NS	7	6–9	—	—	14.88	—	—	—	—	—	—	—
7	NS	7.5 ± 2.4	—	52.5 ± 2.3	—	16.8 ± 1.2	—	71.2 ± 3.2	—	—	—	—	—
3	NS (n = 23)	6.8 ± 0.3	—	—	—	16.0 ± 0.3	—	73.9 ± 3.0	—	—	—	31.6 ± 2.1	—
4	NS	7.2	—	46	—	14.8	—	64	—	21	—	32	—
5	NS	7.5 ± 2.4	—	52.5 ± 2.3	—	16.8 ± 1.2	—	71.2 ± 3.19	—	22.3 ± 1.27	—	32.0 ± 2.23	27.8–37.4
18	M/F	—	3.96–10.3	—	32.9–58.8	—	13.1–19.2	—	64.0–77.6	—	19.9–25.8	—	—
10	M (n = 84)	7.5 ± 1.40	4.7–10.3	52.5 ± 2.3	47.9–57.1	16.8 ± 1.2	14.4–19.2	70.0 ± 3.19	64.8–77.6	22.4 ± 1.27	19.9–24.9	32.0 ± 2.23	27.5–36.5
	F (n = 80)	6.96 ± 1.50	3.96–9.96	49.0 ± 4.9	39.2–58.8	16.0 ± 1.45	13.1–18.9	70.0 ± 3.0	64.0–76.0	23.0 ± 1.4	20.2–25.8	32.6 ± 2.4	27.8–37.4
6	NS	—	7–8	—	45–49.8	—	16.6–18.6	—	—	—	—	—	—
14	NS	8	4–10	—	36–59	—	9.7–19	—	—	—	—	—	—
2	NS	—	6–10	—	36–55	—	10–16	—	—	—	—	—	—
15	NS	—	5–10	—	36–55	—	10–16	—	—	—	—	—	—
16	NS (n = 6)	7.1 ± 0.2	—	42 ± 1.9	—	15.2 ± 0.6	—	59 ± 1.0	—	21 ± 0.8	—	36 ± 0.8	—

NS, not specified.

TABLE 173.2 Referenced Leukocyte Parameters of the Syrian (Golden) Hamster (*Mesocricetus auratus*)

Reference	Gender	WBC ($\times 10^3$/mm^3) Mean	WBC ($\times 10^3$/mm^3) Range	Neutrophils (%) Mean	Neutrophils (%) Range	Lymphocytes (%) Mean	Lymphocytes (%) Range	Eosinophils (%) Mean	Eosinophils (%) Range	Basophils (%) Mean	Basophils (%) Range	Monocytes (%) Mean	Monocytes (%) Range
9	NS	6.2	3.4–7.6	—	3–43	—	50–96	—	0–2	—	0	—	0–1
7	NS	7.62 ± 1.3	—	29.9 ± 8.0	—	73.5 ± 9.4	—	1.1 ± 0.0	—	0	—	2.5 ± 0.8	—
4	NS	6.3	—	27	—	68	—	1.1	—	0	—	2.9	—
5	NS	7.62 ± 1.3	—	21.9 ± 5.5	—	73.5 ± 9.4	—	1.1 ± 0.02	—	—	—	2.5 ± 0.8	—
18	M/F	—	5.02–10.6	—	17.1–35.2	—	50.9–92.3	—	0.22–1.54	—	0–5	—	0.4–4.4
10	M (n = 84)	7.62 ± 1.3	5.02–10.2	22.1 ± 2.5	17.1–27.1	73.5 ± 9.4	54.7–92.3	0.9 ± 0.32	0.26–1.54	1.0 ± 2.0	0–5	2.5 ± 0.8	0.9–4.1
10	F (n = 80)	8.56 ± 1.54	6.48–10.6	29.0 ± 3.12	22.8–35.2	67.9 ± 8.52	50.9–84.9	0.7 ± 0.24	0.22–1.18	0.5 ± 0.7	0–2.1	2.4 ± 1.0	0.4–4.4
6	NS	—	5–23	—	10–50	—	50–70	—	0–5	—	0–1	—	0–10
14	NS	—	3–15	—	10–43	—	50–95	—	0–4.5	—	0–1	—	0–3
2	NS	—	3–11	—	10–42	—	50–95	—	0–4.5	—	0–1	—	0–3
15	NS	—	6.3–8.9	—	10–42	—	50–95	—	0–4.5	—	0–1	—	0–3
16	NS	4.7 ± 0.8	—	24 ± 9	—	74 ± 9	—	0	—	0	—	2 ± 1	—

NS, not specified.

TABLE 173.3   Referenced Ranges of Hematologic Values for Other Hamster Species

Parameter		European Hamster		Chinese Hamster
		Ref. 17	Ref. 9	Ref. 19
RBC	($\times 10^6/mm^3$)	6.04–9.10	6.4–8.8	4.4–9.10
PCV	(mL%)	44–49		36.5–47.7
Hemoglobin	(g/dL)	13.4–15.5	12.4–15.9	10.7–14.1
MCV	(μ^3)	58.7–71.4		53.6–65.2
MCH	($\mu\mu$g)	18.6–22.5		15.5–19.1
MCHC	(%)	26.4–32.5		27–32
WBC	($\times 10^3/mm^3$)	3.4–7.6		2.7–9.6
Neutrophils	(%)	3.5–41.6		14.8–23.6
Lymphocytes	(%)	50–95		68.1–84.8
Eosinophils	(%)	0.0–2.1		0.3–3.1
Basophils	(%)	0.0–0.2		0.0–0.5
Monocytes	(%)	0.0–1.0		0.0–2.4

TABLE 173.4   Bone Marrow Contituents in Hamsters[8]

Erythrocyte Series

Rubriblast	0.14%
Prorubricyte	1.94%
Basophilic rubricyte	9.34%
Polychrom rubricyte	22.10%
Metarubricyte	2.39%
Total erythroid cells	36.18%

Other cells

Lymphocyte	0.04%
Monocyte	0.07%
Plasma cell	0.47%
RE cell	1.91%
Other	0.03%

Granulocytic Series

Myeloblast	1.22%
Promyelocyte	3.03%
Myelocyte (neut)	13.72%
Myelocyte (eos)	0.29%
Metamyelocyte (neut)	29.59%
Metamyelocyte (eos)	0.55%
Metamyelocyte (bas)	0.05%
Neutrophil	12.69%
Eosinophil	0.20%
Basophil	0.10%
Total granulocytic cells	61.41%

M:E = 1.696:1.0

the extent that the cells may be mistaken as basophils, although basophils are rarely observed. The morphology of eosinophils, basophils, and monocytes is similar to that of other rodents. Eosinophils are relatively rare and may not be observed in some animals. Eosinophils have an annular nucleus, sometimes slightly twisted,

which fills the periphery of the cell as a wide pyknotic band, surrounded by a narrow zone of cytoplasm.[9] The closely packed cytoplasmic granules in the eosinophils of hamsters are shaped like short rods, in contrast to the more rounded granules observed in rats and mice. Monocytes are the largest cells observed in hamster blood and are characterized as having a large, swollen, indented, or trilobulate nucleus and a delicately reticulated grey-blue cytoplasm.[9]

A diurnal variation in the numbers and types of leukocytes can be observed in the hamster. It has been reported that leukocyte levels increase to a range of 8 to $10 \times 10^3/\mu L$ of blood at night when the nocturnal animal is most active, peaking in the early morning around 12×10^3 leukocytes/μL, and with an increase of neutrophils rather than lymphocytes.[9] Because most clinical and research manipulations of hamsters occur during daylight hours when the animals would typically be asleep, the implications of diurnal variation on hematologic indices should be considered when interpreting results.

White blood cell counts decline during hibernation to approximately 2500 cells/μL in Syrian hamsters[18] and to approximately 1000 cells/μL in European hamsters,[17] with an observed neutrophil to lymphocyte ratio of 45%:45%. Following awakening from hibernation, a pronounced leukocytosis can be observed (i.e., a range of 10,000 to 20,000 leukocytes/μL, and an average of 13,600 cells/μL), with a predominant neutrophilia, totalling 70 to 90% of the cells counted.[9]

BONE MARROW CYTOLOGY

The cellular constituents of the bone marrow of hamsters are quite similar to that observed in rats and mice. Reports differ widely as to the myeloid to erythroid (M:E) ratio in normal bone marrow, with Desai[7] reporting the M:E ratio as 8 to 10:1, and Trincao et al.[8] reporting a much lower ratio of 1.7:1. The results of the latter study are presented in Table 173.4.

Myeloblasts are commonly observed in the bone mar-

TABLE 173.5   Observed Coagulation Values in Hamsters

Parameter	Mean ± SD	Reference
Bleeding time (sec)	109 ± 19	7
Clotting time (sec)	143 ± 50	7
	60	9
	180 ± 42	16
Prothrombin time (sec)	10.5 ± 0.2	7
	9.0 ± 0.8	12
	14.8 ± 1.0	20
(Males)	9.9 ± 1.2	21
(Females)	9.3 ± 1.8	21
Partial thromboplastin time (sec)	22.2 ± 2.1	16
	24.4 ± 2.7	20

row of hamsters and have a large swollen nucleus, which may contain one or two nuclear bodies, and are surrounded by a narrow basophilic band of cytoplasm. Myelocytes, each with a large swollen nucleus, have a brighter appearing cytoplasm that may occasionally contain a few violet granules. Giant cells may be numerous, plasma cells are occasionally observed, and distinct lymphocytes or monocytes seldom are seen.[9]

OTHER HEMATOLOGIC VALUES

Reported coagulation values for Syrian hamsters are provided in Table 173.5. The sedimentation rate (mm/hr) for normal hamster blood was reported by a number of authors: 0.5 mm at 60 minutes, and 0.7 mm at 120 minutes;[9] 0.3 to 0.96 mm/hr;[18] and 0.32 to 0.96 mm/hr (mean, 0.64 ± 0.16 mm/hr) for males, and 0.30 to 0.70 mm/hr (mean, 0.50 ± 0.10 mm/hr) for females.[18]

REFERENCES

1. **Jain NC.** Schalm's veterinary hematology. 4th ed. Philadelphia: Lea & Febiger, 1986.
2. **Harkness JE, Wagner JE.** The biology and medicine of rabbits and rodents. 4th ed. Baltimore: Williams & Wilkins, 1995.
3. **Bannon PD, Friedell GH.** Values for plasma constituents in normal and tumor bearing Golden hamsters. Lab Anim Care 1966;16:417–420.
4. **Myerstein N, Cassuto Y.** Haematological changes in heat-acclimated golden hamsters. Br J Haematol 1970;18:417–423.
5. **Tomson FN, Wardrop KJ.** Clinical chemistry and hematology. In: Van Hoosier GL, McPherson CW, eds. Laboratory hamsters. Orlando: Academic Press, 1987.
6. **Wallach JD, Boever WJ.** Diseases of exotic animals—medical and surgical management. Philadelphia: WB Saunders, 1983.
7. **Desai RG.** Hematology and microcirculation. In: Hoffman RA, et al., eds. The golden hamster—its biology and use in medical research. Ames: Iowa State University Press, 1968:185–191.
8. **Trincao C, et al.** Blood and bone marrow of the golden hamster. Anais Inst Med Trop 1949;6:41.
9. **Schermer S.** The blood morphology of laboratory animals. Philadelphia: FA Davis, 1967.
10. **Mitruka BJ, Rawnsley HM.** Clinical biochemical and hematological reference values in normal experimental animals and normal humans. 2nd ed. New York: Masson, 1981.
11. **Stewart OM, et al.** Hematological findings in the golden hamster. J Exp Med 1944;80:189.
12. **Brock MA.** Production and life span of erythrocytes during hibernation in the golden hamster. Am J Physiol 1960;198:1181.
13. **Rigby PG, et al.** Erythrocyte survival in hamsters using intraperitoneal $Na_2Cr^{51}O_4$. Proc Soc Exp Biol Med 1961;106:313.
14. **Wagner JE, Farrar PL.** Husbandry and medicine of small rodents. Vet Clin North Am Small Anim Pract 1987;17:1061–1087.
15. **Johnson-Delaney CA.** Exotic companion medicine handbook. Lake Worth, FL: Wingers Publishing, 1996.
16. **Lewis JH.** Comparative hemostasis in vertebrates. New York: Plenum Press, 1996.
17. **Reznik G, Reznik-Schuller H, Emminger A, Mohr U.** Comparative studies of blood from hibernating and nonhibernating European hamsters (Cricetus cricetus L.). Lab Anim Sci 1975;25:210–215.
18. **Mitruka BJ, Rawnsley HM.** Clinical biochemical and hematological reference values in normal experimental animals and normal humans. 1st ed. New York: Masson, 1977.
19. **Moore W.** Hemogram of the Chinese hamster. Am J Vet Res 1966;27:608.
20. **Dodds WJ, Raymond SL, Moynihan AC, McMartin DN.** Spontaneous atrial thrombosis in aged Syrian hamsters. II. hemostasis. Thromb Haemost 1977;38:457–464.
21. **Dent NJ.** The use of the Syrian hamster to establish its clinical chemistry and hematology Profile Clin Toxicol 1977;18:321–323.

CHAPTER 174

Hematology of Fish

• TERRY C. HRUBEC and STEPHEN A. SMITH

A number of factors make diagnostic hematology more challenging in fish species than in mammals. First, a review of the literature provides inconsistencies concerning the nomenclature, cellular differentiation, maturation, and function of fish blood cells. Second, cell counts must be determined manually, because the nucleated erythrocytes and the overlap in leukocyte size prevent the use of automated methods. Third, the number of fish species and their diversity in morphologic form and ecologic function makes generalizations about fishes impossible. The generic term "fish" includes primitive jawless vertebrates and vertebrates with cartilaginous skeletons as well as more advanced species having bony skeletons. This chapter limits its scope to bony fishes (Class Osteichthyes) as these fishes are more closely related to other bony vertebrates and have certain similarities in blood cell morphology and function.

Study in the field of fish hematology has spanned the past 100 years;[1-3] however, the literature is often conflicting and incorrect. Significant advances to develop hematology as a diagnostic tool for fishes have only occurred in the past 15 years, mainly due to new information concerning the function and maturation of blood cells, the standardization of hematologic techniques, and the physiologic response to disease.

HEMATOLOGIC METHODS

Hematologic techniques used for mammals are generally applicable for fishes with slight modification. Most fishes respond adversely to being handled. Anesthesia before bleeding is recommended to decrease hematologic changes due to the stress of restraint. Hematologic changes due to hypoxia during anesthesia can be minimized by rapidly anesthetizing and bleeding the fish. A number of anesthetic agents have been used with fishes. Buffered MS-222 (tricaine methanesulfonate; Sigma Chemical, St. Louis, MO) at 100 to 200 mg/L is the most widely accepted. Unbuffered MS-222 should not be used because it decreases the pH of the anesthetic solution and causes significant physiologic changes in the fish. The anesthetic solution should be aerated and of sufficient concentration to induce stage 2 anesthesia (loss of equilibrium) within 30 seconds and stage 3 anesthesia within 1 minute. The fish is bled before respiratory depression induces significant hypoxia.

Collecting a Blood Sample

Fishes can be bled from a number of sites. However, the caudal tail vessels are used most frequently. Some investigators believe that this technique contaminates the blood with tissue fluid and prefer the cuvarian duct (a vessel within the oral cavity) or bleeding directly from the heart. However, cardiac puncture is highly traumatic, and the cuvarian duct can only be sampled in large fish. Collecting blood from a severed tail is not recommended as it causes tissue fluid contamination of the blood sample and is lethal for the fish. Blood should only be used for clinical evaluation if the sample is obtained with a "clean stick" (e.g., the vessels are located immediately, and negative pressure is applied to the syringe only after the needle is in the vessels).

Fish blood hemolyses easily, and best results are obtained with a 1- or 3-mL syringe. If a larger sample is required, a Vacutainer system can be used. Blood should be transferred immediately to a blood tube containing anticoagulant to minimize clotting. Pediatric tubes (0.5 mL) are an ideal size for most fishes. The choice of anticoagulant between heparin and EDTA for preservation of cellular morphology is species-specific. Salmonid and cyprinid blood cells retain morphology best with heparin, whereas catfish, bass, and tilapia cells preserve best in EDTA. Occasionally with stressed fish, blood will clot even in the presence of an anticoagulant. Clots may not be visible in the tube, but thrombocytes appear clumped in the hemacytometer and on smears, preventing accurate enumeration of thrombocytes and leukocytes. Use of a different anticoagulant may prevent thrombocyte clumping.

Determination of Cell Counts

One of the greatest problems with diagnostic hematology in fishes is the reliability of the complete blood count (CBC). Inaccuracies can occur because the cells must be counted manually with a hemacytometer. Sources of error associated with manual counting are incorrectly diluting and mixing the blood, incorrectly charging the hemacytometer, and incorrectly identifying and miscounting cells. Misidentification occurs because distinguishing leukocytes from thrombocytes or lysed erythrocytes is frequently difficult. As thrombocytes activate, they become round and appear similar to lymphocytes (Fig. 174.1). Erythrocytes can lyse in the blood diluent and the nucleus will take up the stain in a manner similar to a leukocyte. With practice, one can distinguish lysed erythrocytes from leukocytes; however, for many species, it is impossible to distinguish leukocytes from thrombocytes on the hemacytometer. Leukocytes and thrombocytes are more accurately distinguished during the differential count on a stained blood smear.

The following procedure is time-consuming but provides the greatest accuracy for a CBC in fishes. A blood diluent that differentially stains erythrocytes and leukocytes is required for counting cells on a hemocytometer. Natt-Herricks diluent[4] or Rees-Ecker diluent both work well with most fish species. Depending on the number of cells in the blood, a 1:100 or 1:200 dilution of blood to filtered diluent is used to stain the cells for about 4 minutes before charging the hemacytometer.

As in mammals, erythrocytes are counted in five of the secondary squares on the center primary square. The raw count, multiplied by 5000 for a 1:100 dilution or by 10,000 for a 1:200 dilution, will give the number of erythrocytes per microliter of blood. As the leukocyte count is much higher in fishes than in mammals, leukocytes and thrombocytes are counted only in the four corner primary squares. The raw count multiplied by

250 for a 1:100 dilution and by 500 for a 1:200 dilution will give the number of cells per microliter of blood. This method gives a combined total count for leukocytes and thrombocytes. Thrombocytes are then enumerated during the differential count on a stained blood smear.

Differential counts are determined from blood smears made with anticoagulated blood and stained with a Romanowsky stain (Wright's/Giemsa/Leishman). Direct smears made without anticoagulant will exhibit thrombocyte clumping and should be avoided. The quality of the smear will affect the quality and reliability of the cell counts. It is best to become familiar with the blood cells found in each species before beginning the differential. It is also good practice to scan each slide before the differential count to check the quality of the smear. In a region of the slide where a monolayer of cells is present, count leukocytes and thrombocytes until 200 leukocytes are enumerated. In other words, count all cell types except erythrocytes until the sum of the lymphocytes, monocytes, and various granulocytes equals 200, regardless of the number of thrombocytes counted. As thrombocytes frequently make up greater than 50% of the cells, total counts greater than 400 are common. The percentage of thrombocytes is then subtracted from the combined leukocyte-thrombocyte count determined on the hemacytometer. This gives the total leukocyte count and the thrombocyte count. The percentage of each leukocyte type is multiplied by the combined leukocyte-thrombocyte count to give the absolute number of each cell type.

If mild thrombocyte clumping prevents accurate enumeration of a combined leukocyte-thrombocyte count on the hemacytometer, an estimate of the combined count can be determined using the ratio of leukocytes-plus-thrombocytes to erythrocytes on the blood smear. The estimate is only reliable when thrombocyte clumping is minimal and thrombocytes can be counted accurately on a good-quality blood smear. The number of erythrocytes and leukocytes-plus-thrombocytes are counted in a monolayer of evenly distributed cells until a total of 2000 cells are counted (approximately 8 to 10 fields). The ratio of leukocytes-plus-thrombocytes to erythrocytes is multiplied by the erythrocyte count determined on the hemacytometer to give the combined leukocyte-thrombocyte count. Whenever possible, the counts should be made directly on the hemacytometer, because direct counts are more accurate than estimates.

Hemoglobin

Hemoglobin is determined using the standard cyanomethemoglobin method. However, because the erythrocytes are nucleated, nuclear contents are released into the test solution during cell lysis, causing a flocculent precipitate to affect test results. Samples should be centrifuged to pellet this precipitate before measuring the absorbance.

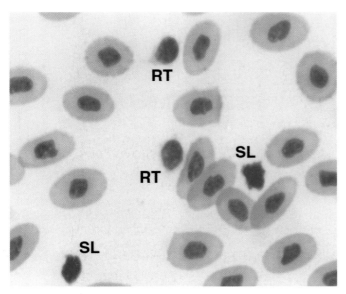

FIGURE 174.1 Hybrid striped bass. Reactive thrombocytes (RT) and small lymphocytes (SL).

BLOOD CELL MORPHOLOGY

The blood cells present in the peripheral blood of fishes vary with the species but include the following: erythrocytes, thrombocytes, lymphocytes, monocytes, neutrophils, heterophils, eosinophils, basophils, and immature forms.[2,3,5] Most cells appear to have similar functions in fishes as they do in mammals. All photomicrographs were taken at the same magnification; note the relative size of each cell type among the different species.

Fish erythrocytes, unlike mammalian erythrocytes, are nucleated and are the most numerous cells in the blood. Smaller and slightly basophilic reticulocytes may also be present. The developing erythrocyte continues to increase in size and hemoglobin content with time, resulting in higher mean corpuscular volume (MCV), mean corpuscular hemoglobin (MCH), and MCH concentration (MCHC) in older cells.[6] Erythrocyte counts may vary with different environmental and water quality conditions, although these changes are not well characterized.[7-9] Erythrocyte counts may decrease with disease,[9,10] but it is unclear whether the decrease is due to changes in red cell number or simply a change in the hydration status of the fish.

The thrombocyte is the cell type responsible for coagulation of blood (Figs. 174.1 and 174.2). Their shape is variable, depending on their activation state, and changes from spiked or oval to round as the cell becomes activated during clotting. In anticoagulated blood, the nucleus may segment or remain oval. Ultrastructurally, the cells are similar to mammalian platelets, with an interconnecting canalicular system and cytoplasmic granules.[11]

Fish lymphocytes are usually designated as small or large, although true functional differences between the

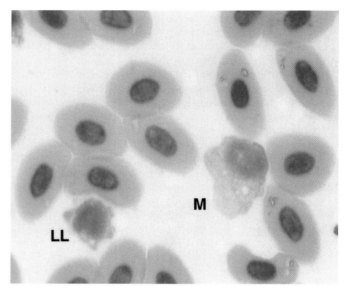

FIGURE 174.3 Goldfish. Monocyte (M) and large lymphocyte (LL).

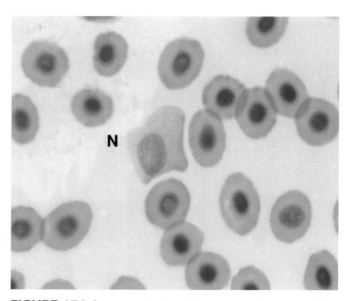

FIGURE 174.4 Channel catfish. Neutrophil, oval nucleus (N).

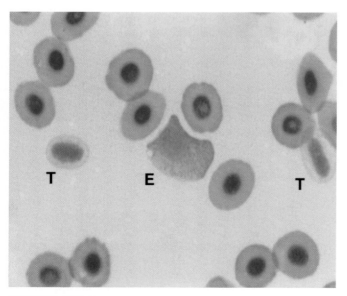

FIGURE 174.2 Channel catfish. Eosinophil (E) and thrombocytes (T).

sizes have not been documented (Figs. 174.1 and 174.3). As in mammals, there are T, B, and nonspecific cytotoxic lymphocytes.[12,13]

Neutrophils (often mistakenly referred to as heterophils) are one of the largest circulating cells in the blood (Figs. 174.4 and 174.5). Granules are not observed with light microscopy, but the cytoplasm may have a grainy appearance. In most species, the nucleus is open and usually oval to kidney-bean–shaped, but in some species the nucleus may be lobulated or segmented.

Heterophils have been described for a number of fish species. Heterophils are the same size or slightly smaller

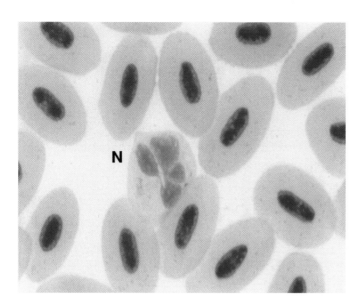

FIGURE 174.5 Rainbow trout. Neutrophil, segmented nucleus (N).

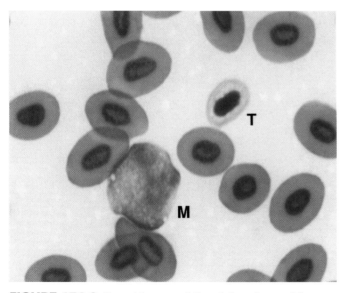

FIGURE 174.6 Pacu. Monocyte (M) and thrombocyte (T).

than neutrophils with pale eosinophilic to lavender granules. In the literature, it is often difficult to tell whether a cell is truly heterophilic or whether the cell is being called a heterophil under the mistaken belief that nonmammalian species have heterophils in place of neutrophils. Fishes usually have either neutrophils or heterophils, although some species have both. Functional differences between fish neutrophils and heterophils have not been determined.

Eosinophils and basophils are described for some species. Eosinophils are the same size or slightly smaller than neutrophils, with eosinophilic granules in the cytoplasm (Fig. 174.2). Eosinophils function in parasite kill-

ing and phagocytosis. Little is known about basophil morphology and function, but it is thought to be similar to basophils in mammals.

Monocytes are round, with the nucleus varying from round to horseshoe-shaped (Figs. 174.3 and 174.6). The cytoplasm stains a deep blue and is often vacuolated. As in mammals, monocytes circulate through the blood, migrate into the tissues, and become macrophages. Monocytes and macrophages are the primary phagocytic cell in fishes.[2,14]

The hemopoietic tissues in fishes are primarily the anterior kidney (pronephros) and the spleen. All the cellular elements in the blood are produced in these organs. The primary site of erythropoiesis is usually the anterior kidney with secondary sites in the spleen, although the spleen may be the primary site in some species.[15] The spleen is also the site for lymphopoiesis. Thrombocytes, monocytes, neutrophils, eosinophils, and basophils are produced in the anterior kidney.[16] Blood cells are produced in the hemopoietic tissues, but significant maturation occurs in circulation.

Blood coagulation in fishes is not well studied but appears to be similar to mammalian coagulation. Substances that are vasoactive or aggregate platelets in mammals have a similar function in fishes. The blood coagulation cascade contains both intrinsic and extrinsic pathways.[3,17] Stress causes thrombocytosis and a decrease in clotting time.[18]

BLOOD VALUES

Previously, the main focus of piscine hematology has been to determine the effects of toxicants and changes in environmental conditions on the blood analytes. These hematologic changes were almost never correlated with reference intervals and only rarely correlated with documented pathologic changes or disease. Hematologic changes due to stress are fairly well characterized in fishes, but other responses are not as well documented. This lack of knowledge has prevented the use of fish hematology for diagnostic purposes. The packed cell volume (PCV), hemoglobin, and erythrocyte numbers are frequently determined, but erythrocyte indices, leukocyte number, and differential counts are determined only occasionally. Hematologic values for a number of common fish species are given in Table 174.1.

In general, the hematocrit ranges from 20 to 45%, with more active species of fish usually having higher PCV values. The hematocrit can increase artifactually from splenic contraction and from erythrocyte swelling.[19] Changes in the hematocrit have been noted with seasonal variation.[8,9] However, other studies have demonstrated no change in the hematocrit at different temperatures.[7,20]

Hemoglobin concentrations are low compared to mammals, being 5 to 10 g/dL. As with the PCV, more active fishes generally have higher hemoglobin values. Although the hemoglobin and erythrocyte indices have been determined in a number of studies, not enough is known about anemia in fishes to utilize the data fully.

TABLE 174.1 Comparison of Hematologic Values Determined for Various Fish Species[a]

Species	No.	PCV (%)	Hb (g/dL)	MCV (fL)	MCH (pg)	MCHC (g/dL)	RBC (10^6/μL)	Reference
M. saxatilis X M. chrysops[b]	50	23–47	8–12	81–106	19.6–26.4	22–30	3.66–4.96	22
Oncorhyncus mykiss[b]	200	24–43	5.3–9.5	—	—	21.9–24.1		23
Oncorhyncus mykiss[b]	122	21–44	1.5–7.7	192–420	14.4–70.0	5.6–24.4	0.77–1.67	24
Tilapia[b]	40	27–37	7.0–9.8	115–183	28.3–42.3	22–29	1.91–2.83	25
Chanos chanos[b]	283	22–48	5–15	133–302	20.9–47.2	11–38	1.70–4.00	26
Morone saxatilis	31	48	9.1	—	—	—	3.79	27
Morone saxatilis	18	34–55	6.2–10.9	155	31.3	20.5	2.0–4.2	28
Carassius auratus	60	38–40	9.7–10.6	241–245	63–66	26	1.6–1.8	29
Cyprinus carpio	103	28	7.1	—	—	—	1.54	30
Ictalurus punctatus	35	40	—	—	—	—	2.44	31
Salmo salar	20	44–49	8.9–10.4	441–553	94–106	19.4–21.7	0.85–1.1	32
Salvelinus fontinalis	74	36.6	8.0	—	—	—	1.34	30
Oncorhyncus aquabonita	12	44–52	—	—	—	—	1.19–1.20	33
Sarotherodon melano-theron	40	31–34	7.3–9.0	203–228	54	24–26	1.37–1.69	34
Pleuronectes americanus	~20	17–26	4.2–6.0	90–126	25–33	—	1.7–2.6	35
Pleuronectes americanus	~20	21–28	2.8–6.4	101–126	15–26	—	1.8–2.5	9
Colossoma brachypomum	29	25	—	—	—	—	1.68	36

Species	No.	WBC (#/μL)	Lymphocyte (#/μL)	Neut/Hetero (#/μL)	Monocyte (#/μL)	Eosinophil (#/μL)	Thrombocyte (#/μL)	Reference
M. saxatilis X M. chrysops[b]	50	32600–115100	22500–115100	400–3500	1500–7500	0–400	30700–74100	22
Tilapia[b]	40	21600–154700	6800–136400	600–9900	400–4300	35–1600	25100–85200	25
Chanos chanos[b]	195	17500–92500	51–68%	3–7%	4–9%	—	12–32%	26
Crassius auratus	55	10100–14700	9540–13660	—	—	—	30000–46100	37
Ictalurus punctatus	35	164000	89900	5200	500	0	68400	31
Oncorhyncus aquabonita	5	21000	18799	1582	588	—	135000–310000	33
Sarotherodon melano-theron	40	61900–62900	10.9–11.6%	3.1–3.8%	3.6–4.2%	—	80.5–82.3%	34
Pleuronectes americanus	~20	88000–282000	38700–154540	2470–26630	—	—	36480–115500	35
Colossoms brachypomum	22	33500	21028	3183	1242	209	—	36

[a]Unless denoted as a reference interval, all values are means; a range indicates that means were determined for groups of fish based on sex, blood collection method, time of year, etc.
[b]The range given is a true reference interval.

The MCV, which on average ranges from 150 to 350 fL, is an effective way to determine the size of red cells. Active fish with higher oxygen demands tend to have smaller erythrocytes and consequently lower MCV. The MCH varies considerably due to the size variation in circulating erythrocytes and runs between 30 and 100 pg. The MCHC ranges from 18 to 30% and is lower in fishes than in mammals due to the space-occupying erythrocyte nucleus.

Erythrocyte numbers are usually lower than in mammals and range from 1 to 5×10^6/μL. Erythrocyte counts vary with the need for oxygen. Ice fish and thin larval fish often have no discernible erythrocytes, being able to absorb sufficient oxygen from the water directly into the plasma. Sedentary fish have values closer to 1×10^6, whereas active pelagic fish often have counts greater than 5×10^6/μL.

Leukocyte numbers are variable but generally range from 30,000 to 150,000 cells/μL. In most species, lymphocytes are the most abundant leukocyte present, followed by monocytes or neutrophils, and then eosino-phils. Basophils, when present, are only occasionally seen. Stress causes leukopenia characterized by lymphopenia and neutrophilia.[21] The leukocytic response to suboptimal temperatures is characterized by leukopenia, lymphopenia, and monocytopenia.[20] Changes with specific diseases are not well documented; however, Chinook salmon with bacterial kidney disease increased leukocyte counts to levels above controls after 16 days.[10]

REFERENCES

1. **Blaxhall PC.** The haematological assessment of the health of freshwater fish: a review of selected literature. J Fish Biol 1972;4:593–604.
2. **Ellis AE.** The leukocytes of fish: a review. J Fish Biol 1977;11:453–491.
3. **Fange R.** Fish blood cells. In: Hoar WS, Randall DJ, Farrel AP, eds. Fish physiology. The cardiovascular system. San Diego: Academic Press, 1992; 12(B):1–54.
4. **Natt MP, Herrick CA.** A new blood diluent for counting erythrocytes and leucocytes of the chicken. Poultry Sci 1952;31:735–738.
5. **Zinkl JG, Cox WT, Kono CS.** Morphology and cytochemistry of leukocytes and thrombocytes of six species of fish. Comp Hematol Int 1991;1:87–195.
6. **Speckner W, Schindler JF, Albers C.** Age-dependent changes in volume and hemoglobin content of erythrocytes in the carp (Cyprinus carpio L.). J Exp Biol 1989;141:133–149.
7. **Fourie FLR, Hattingh J.** A seasonal study of the hematology of carp (Cypri-

nus carpio) from a locality in the Transvaal, South Africa. Zool Africa 1976;11:75–80.

8. **Lane HC.,** Progressive changes in hematology and tissue water of sexually mature trout, *Salmo gairdneri* Richardson during the autumn and winter. J Fish Biol 1979;15:425–436.

9. **Mahoney JB, McNulty JK.** Disease associated changes and normal seasonal hematological variation in winter flounder in the Hudson-Raritan estuary. Trans Am Fish Soc 1992;121:261–268.

10. **Iwama GK, Greer GL, Randall DJ.** Changes in selected haemotological parameters in juvenile Chinook salmon subjected to a bacterial challenge and a toxicant. J Fish Biol 1986;28:563–572.

11. **Ferguson HW.** The ultrastructure of plaice (Pleuronectes platessa) leucocytes. J Fish Biol 1976;8:139–142.

12. **Clem LW, Miller NW, Bly JE.** Evolution of lymphocyte subpopulations, their interactions, and temperature sensitivities. In: Cohen N, Warr GW, eds. The phylogeny of immune functions. Boca Raton, FL: CRC Press, 1991;191–213.

13. **Evans DL, Jaso-Friedmann L.** Nonspecific cytotoxic cells as effectors of immunity in fish. Ann Rev Fish Dis 1992;2:109–121.

14. **Blazer VS.** Piscine macrophage function and nutritional influences: a review. J Aquat Anim Health 1991;3:77–86.

15. **Glomski CA, Tamburlin J, Chainani M.** The phylogenetic odyssey of the erythrocyte. III. Fish, the lower vertebrate experience. Histol Histopathol 1992;7:501–528.

16. **Pica A, Taglialatela R, Ferrandino I, Della Corte F.** The blood cells and the haemopoiesis of *Diplodus sargus* L: haematological values, cytochemistry and leukocytes' response to vaccine stimulation. Eur J Histochem 1996;40:57–66.

17. **VanVliet KJ, Smit GL, Pieterse JJ, Schoonbee HJ, van Vuren JHJ.** Thromb-elastographic diagnosis of blood coagulation in two freshwater fish species. Comp Biochem Physiol 1985;82A:19–21.

18. **Casillas E, Smith LS.** Effect of stress on blood coagulation and hematology in rainbow trout (*Salmo gairdneri*). J Fish Biol 1977;10:481–491.

19. **Heath AG.** Water pollution and fish physiology. Boca Raton, FL: CRC Press, 1987.

20. **Hrubec TC, Robertson JL, Smith SA.** Effects of temperature on hematologic and serum biochemical profiles of hybrid striped bass (*Morone chrysops X Morone saxatillis*). Am J Vet Res 1997;58:126–130.

21. **Ellsaesser CF, Clem LW.** Hematological and immunological changes in channel catfish stressed by handling and transport. J Fish Biol 1986;28:511–521.

22. **Hrubec TC, Smith SA, Robertson JL, Feldman B, Veit HP, Libey GS,** **Tinker MK.** Comparison of hematologic reference intervals between culture system and type of hybrid striped bass. Am J Vet Res 1996;57:618–623.

23. **Wedemeyer GA, Nelson NC.** Statistical methods for estimating normal blood chemistry ranges and variances in rainbow trout (*Salmo gairdneri*), Shasta stain. J Fish Res Board Can 1975;32:551–554.

24. **Miller WR, Hendricks AC, Cairns J.** Normal ranges for diagnostically important hematological and blood chemistry characteristics of rainbow trout (*Salmo gairdneri*). Can J Fish Aquat Sci 1983;40:420–425.

25. **Hrubec TC, Cardinale JL, Smith SA.** Hematology and plasma chemistry reference intervals for cultured Tilapia (*Oreochromis* hybrid). Vet Clin Path 2000;29.

26. **Ram-Bhaskar BR, Srinivasa-Rao KS.** Influence of environmental variables on hematology, and compendium of normal hematological ranges of milk-fish, *Chanos chanos* (Forskal) in brackish culture. Aquaculture 1989;83:123–136.

27. **Westin DT.** Serum and blood from adult striped bass, *Morone saxatillis*. Estuaries 1978;1:126–128.

28. **Lochmiller RL, Weichman JD, Zale AV.** Hematological assessment of temperature and oxygen stress in a reservoir population of striped bass (*Morone saxatillis*). Comp Biochem Physiol 1989;93A:535–541.

29. **Burton CB, Murray SA.** Effects of density on goldfish blood: I. hematology. Comp Biochem Physiol 1979;62A:555–558.

30. **Houston AH, DeWilde MA.** Some observations upon the relationship of microhaematocrit values to haemoglobin concentrations and erythrocyte numbers in the carp *Cyprinus carpio* L. and brook trout *Salvelinus fontinalis* (Mitchill). J Fish Biol 1972;4:109–115.

31. **Grizzle JM, Rogers WA.** Anatomy and histology of the channel catfish. Opelika, AL: Craftmaster Printers, 1976;18.

32. **Sandnes K, Lie O, Waagbo R.** Normal ranges of some blood chemistry parameters in adult farmed Atlantic salmon *Salmo salar*. J Fish Biol 1988;32:129–136.

33. **Hunn JB, Wiedmeyer RH, Greer IE, Grady AW.** Blood chemistry of laboratory-reared golden trout. J Aquat Anim Health 1992;4:218–221.

34. **LeaMaster RL, Brock JA, Fugioka RS, Nakamura RM.** Hematologic and blood chemistry values for *Sarotherodon melanotheron* and a red hybrid tilapia in freshwater and seawater. Comp Biochem Physiol 1990;97A:525–529.

35. **Bridges DW, Cech JJ Jr, Pedro DN.** Seasonal hematological changes in winter flounder. *Pseudopleuronectes americanus*. Trans Am Fish Soc 1976;105:596–600.

36. **Tocidlowski ME, Leubart GA, Stoskopf MK.** Hematologic study of the red pacu (*Colossoma brachypornum*). Vet Clin Pathol 1997;26:119–125.

37. **Murray SA, Burton CB.** Effects of density on goldfish blood: II. cell morphology. Comp Biochem Physiol 1979;62A:559–562.

CHAPTER 175

Normal Hematology of Reptiles

• DOUGLAS R. MADER

Considering the variety among exotic veterinary patients, evaluation of the hemogram can be difficult and requires substantial training and experience. The morphology of the cells often varies considerably between animal groups (e.g., birds, reptiles) and between species within a group (e.g., iguanas, chameleons). Unless the clinical laboratory examining and interpreting the blood smear is thoroughly familiar with the normals for each species, it is extremely difficult to evaluate either normal or abnormal samples from clinical cases and often leads to erroneous results. Thus, veterinary practices that concentrate on exotic species will benefit immensely from having in-house laboratory support. A veterinary technician specifically trained in reading hematology slides can provide consistency, reliability, and rapid turn-around of results. A technician skilled at reading exotic hemograms is a valuable asset and practically a necessity in any nondomestic practice.

SAMPLE COLLECTION

Obtaining samples for hematology and clinical chemistry in reptiles is not difficult; as with anything, it is readily accomplished with practice. Venipuncture techniques such as toenail and tail tip clips are antiquated and, with the state of knowledge in today's exotic marketplace, should be considered inappropriate.

Standard sampling techniques such as cardiocentesis and jugular, axillary, femoral, buccal, and tail vein venipuncture can all be used, depending on the type of patient being sampled and the experience of the practitioner. Each technique has its advantages and limitations; with practice and experience, practitioners will develop proficiency in the different methods. Comprehensive descriptions of these techniques are beyond the scope of this chapter and are well described in the reptile literature.[1] A brief review is in order, however, for the purposes of this discussion.

In snakes, either tail vein (especially in crotalids) or cardiocentesis are the best techniques for collecting blood. The author has routinely used cardiocentesis for snake patients and, after sampling literally thousands of animals, has never had a problem.

Ventral coccygeal tail vein venipuncture is the preferred collection site in lizards. Some practitioners prefer axillary sampling. However, caution must be practiced due to extensive perivascular lymph networks that may dilute the collected sample.

In chelonians, either right jugular vein bleeding or collection of blood from either the axillary or femoral plexus can be used. The former is the preferred method in gentle animals.

Small crocodilians can be bled much the same as lizards. Larger crocodilians can be sampled from the supravertebral or dorsal occipital sinus, a point just caudal to the base of the skull directly over the top of the cervical spinal column.

SAMPLE SIZE AND HANDLING

Blood volumes in reptiles vary from 5 to 8% of total body weight.[1] Of this amount, up to 10% of the patient's total blood volume can be collected safely for analysis. As a rough approximation, the sample size should never be larger than one-half percent of the animal's total body weight. For example, in a 450-g iguana, one can safely remove 2.25 cc of blood. This is more than required by even the most antiquated autoanalyzers.

The standard capillary tube holds 70 μl. This means that the volume of a single capillary tube is the maximum amount of blood that one would want to take from any patient weighing a minimum of 14 g. Although this is a small sample, enough blood is available to yield some valuable diagnostic information.

The total (plasma) protein (using a heparinized capillary tube), packed cell volume (PCV), and icterus index are all readily measured from a single capillary tube. Microscopic analysis of the blood-filled capillary tube may reveal microfilaria, and after centrifugation, will also give an estimated buffy coat size. A thin blood smear can be made, and an estimated white blood cell (WBC) count with a differential can be performed, and the red cells can be evaluated for any abnormalities or hemoparasites. An important observation here is the morphology of the leukocytes (specifically, degranulation or toxic changes). After the cells have been centrifuged, the remaining plasma can be used for a limited number of specific chemistries.

With very small patients, only a single drop of blood may be all that can be collected safely. A thin, well-prepared blood smear will always be valuable as a diagnostic aide.

Blood smears for staining should always be prepared from fresh, non-anticoagulated whole blood directly from the patient.[2] EDTA anticoagulant may cause the blood in some species of reptiles to lyse. This is most commonly seen in chelonians.[2] Heparin anticoagulated blood does not stain well, causing a bluish tinge in the erythrocytes as well as clumping of thrombocytes and leukocytes.[2]

Only lithium heparin should be used as an anticoagulant. Potassium heparin can be used, but the plasma chemistry values (specifically the electrolytes) may not be accurate. Blood can be collected in heparinized capillary tubes, heparinized microtainers, or heparinized plasma separator tubes. The preferred method varies among clinical laboratories, so it is wise to check with the laboratory before samples are collected. Every laboratory also has their own method of preference for blood smear preparation. Again, check with the laboratory to see if the preference is for coverslip or slide-on-slide method.

EVALUATING THE HEMOGRAM

A thorough hematologic analysis provides information on a patient's health status and includes evaluation of the erythrocytes, leukocytes, and thrombocytes in the peripheral blood.

Erythrocytes

The erythron is included in the calculation of the PCV, the total red blood cell (RBC) count, and hemoglobin. As practitioners learn more about exotic species, it is becoming more apparent how little is really known about these parameters.

In mammalian medicine, a calculated erythrocyte mass—called the hematocrit (HCT)—can be calculated by electronic cell counters rather than using a PCV. These cell counters have limitations, specifically, the necessity to be adjustable to accommodate erythrocyte size. Because reptilian cells are larger than mammalian cells, the calculated values may not accurately reflect the actual red cell mass.

The PCV is a simple, rapid, and inexpensive test to estimate red cell mass. A microhematocrit capillary tube is used. The sample must be centrifuged for a minimum of 5 minutes at $12,000 \times g$.[2] If the centrifugation is insufficient in speed or time, the erythrocytes will not pack, trapping plasma between the cells, and will result in a spuriously elevated PCV reading. When properly performed, the precision of the microhematocrit method in mammals is $\pm 1\%$.[3]

Calculation of the total RBC can be done either manu-

ally or by an electronic particle counter. Detailed descriptions of these techniques are described in the mammalian literature.

Most private clinics cannot afford the expense of electronic counters. The two most common manual methods, using either the Unopette System 5877 (Becton-Dickinson, Rutherford, NJ) or Natt and Herrick's solution, require the use of a hemocytometer.[2] There is an inherent error when using these latter two methods of approximately 20%.[3] A well-spun microhematocrit tube is the most cost-effective, reliable method for RBC screening in clinical practice.

"Normal" values for reptiles are difficult to come by and when found must be interpreted with some equivocation. Normals published by one laboratory may vary from those published by another source due to many factors. Nonstandardized methodology is perhaps the biggest variable. Nonetheless, some selected "normal" hematologic parameters for reptiles are shown in Table 175.1.

The RBC of an individual animal will vary with season, ambient temperature, sex (males have a higher RBC than females in some species), and nutritional status. Prehibernation animals will have a higher RBC than posthibernation animals.[4-8]

Reptiles have lower numbers of circulating erythrocytes than birds or mammals.[5] There is an inverse relationship between the size of the erythrocyte and the total number of circulating cells.[5] As mean corpuscular volume (MCV) decreases (turtles > snakes > lizards), the total number of circulating RBCs increases (lizards > snakes > turtles).[5,6]

The average life spans for the dog and cat erythrocyte are 68 and 115 days, respectively,[3] compared to 600 to 800 days in reptiles. It is suspected that this long turnover rate is due to the slower metabolic rate of reptiles compared to mammals.[4,5]

There are several types of stains that can be used for evaluating reptilian cells. Diff Quik (American Scientific Products, McGraw Park, IL) is one of the more commonly used stains in clinical practice. Most of the descriptions in the literature are based on Wright's

TABLE 175.1	Generalized Selected Normal Hematologic Parameters for Reptilian Patients—Iguanas, Snakes, and Turtles		
Parameter	**Iguana**	**Snake**	**Turtle**
PCV	22–35	26–42	23–35
RBC	1.4–6.0	0.5–2.5	0.5–1.5
WBC	3–8	5–10	3–8
HET	50–80	40–70	40–60
LC	20–50	30–60	40–60
MONO	0–1	0–1	0–1
BASO	0–1	0–1	0–1
EOS	0–1	0–1	0–1
AZ	0–4	0–4	0–4
TP	3.3–5.5	3.3–5.5	3.3–5.5

Courtesy of ANTECH Diagnostics.

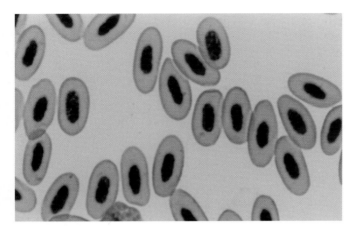

FIGURE 175.1 Reptilian erythrocytes are ellipsoidal with centrally positioned nuclei (Wright's Giemsa). (Photo courtesy of Dr. Jim Klaassen, ANTECH Diagnostics.)

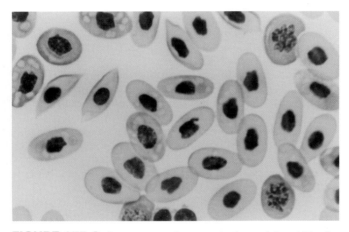

FIGURE 175.2 Immature erythrocytes in the peripheral blood of a turtle. These cells are smaller than mature erythrocytes and are round with large nuclei and basophilic cytoplasm (Wright's Giemsa). (Photo courtesy of Dr. Jim Klaassen, ANTECH Diagnostics.)

stain; however, Giemsa, Wright's-Giemsa, Wright's-Leishman's, and others can be used.[2]

Reptilian erythrocytes are ellipsoidal with a centrally positioned nuclei (Fig. 175.1). The cytoplasm stains orange-pink and is homogeneous in texture. The nuclear clumping within the mature nucleus becomes more condensed as the cell ages.[2]

Reptiles in stages of flux (such as in growth, ecdysis, and regenerative anemia) will often have immature erythrocytes in their peripheral blood. These cells are smaller than mature erythrocytes and are round with large nuclei and basophilic cytoplasm (Fig. 175.2).

Polychromasia, or the extent thereof, is a good indication of a responsive anemia. Reticulocyte counts can be done but are generally not needed. Standard stains may be used which show stained aggregates of reticulum encircling the nucleus.[2] Mitotic nuclei, binucleation, and

other nuclear abnormalities are found in patients with regenerative anemias, inflammatory diseases, and during the posthibernation period.[9] Likewise, mild anisocytosis, polychromasia, and poikilocytosis are not uncommon in normal animals but may be exaggerated in disease (Fig. 175.3).

Hemoglobin concentrations can be determined using the same techniques used in mammalian laboratories. The normal reported ranges for reptilian hemoglobin concentration is between 6 and 12 gm/dl.[5]

Thrombocytes

The reptilian thrombocyte is polymorphic. Commonly found in aggregates, these cells have characteristics and functions similar to the mammalian platelet. Although their nuclei are usually ellipsoid, polymorphic nuclei have been associated with inflammatory disease.[9] They also play a role in blood clotting, thrombus formation, and wound healing.[5]

Thrombocytes are readily ruptured during the making of the blood smear.[10] If undamaged, the thrombocyte appears ellipsoidal to fusiform in shape with a centrally placed nucleus (Fig. 175.4). The smooth nucleus is basophilic, surrounded by a clear cytoplasm, occasionally punctuated with azurophilic granules.[2] When activated, the cytoplasm shows vacuolization.

Normal thrombocyte numbers vary between groups and with environmental changes. Normal ranges are between 25 and 350 thrombocytes per 100 leukocytes.[5]

Leukocytes

The leukogram includes calculation of the total leukocyte count, determination of the differential leukocyte count, and evaluation of the overall cellular morphology. As with erythrocytes, manual methods for determination of total leukocyte, or WBC, counts are commonly

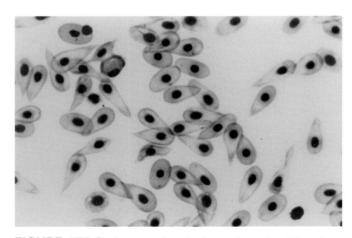

FIGURE 175.3 Anisocytosis, polychromasia, and poikilocosis are not uncommon in normal animals but may be exaggerated in disease, as shown in this tortoise (Wright's Giemsa). (Photo courtesy of Dr. Jim Klaassen, ANTECH Diagnostics.)

used. The nuclei in the erythrocytes and thrombocytes interfere with the electronic cell counters when trying to determine the total WBC count.

The most common manual methods include the direct count using Natt-Herrick's solution and a semidirect count using phloxine B solution (Eosinophil Unopette 5877, Becton-Dickinson). Detailed descriptions of these techniques are described elsewhere.[2]

Limitations of these manual methods include the difficulty in distinguishing small lymphocytes from thrombocytes while using the Natt and Herrick's solution, and an increased margin of error in species with low heterophil numbers when using the Unopette system.[2] In addition, although neither of these techniques are difficult, they do require training and practice for consistent results, and the procedure is somewhat labor-intensive.

An alternate method of determining total WBC is the "estimate." Using a well-prepared blood smear, the total number of leukocytes are counted under 40× magnification in each field for 10 fields. The average is taken and multiplied by 1000 for an estimated count (M. Kurian, ANTECH Diagnostics, personal communication). For instance, if the average number of leukocytes per 10 fields is 5.5, then the estimated WBC would be 5500/μl. The main obstacle for obtaining accurate estimates is having a properly prepared blood film. Clotted, streaky, or smears that are not monolayer can all lead to spurious results.

Heterophils

The heterophil is a cell unique to reptiles, fish, birds, and some mammals, such as the rabbit. It is also the cell that makes interpreting the leukogram so difficult. The heterophil varies in morphology between groups, between genera, and between species.

Functionally, the reptilian heterophil is similar to the mammalian neutrophil. This cell responds to tissue inflammation and infection, their primary function being

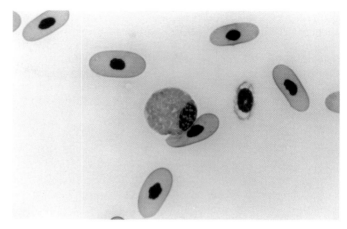

FIGURE 175.5 Heterophils distinguishing needle-like intracytoplasmic granules are a reddish-orange, as seen in this tortoise (Wright's Giemsa). (Photo courtesy of Dr. Jim Klaassen, ANTECH Diagnostics.)

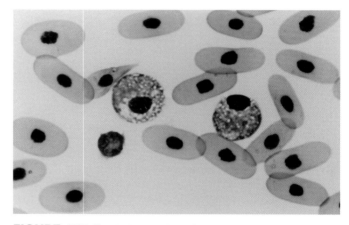

FIGURE 175.6 The heterophils of crocodilians have larger granules, although they are fewer in number than the numerous, smaller granules seen in lizards and snakes (Wright's Giemsa). (Photo courtesy of Dr. Jim Klaassen, ANTECH Diagnostics.)

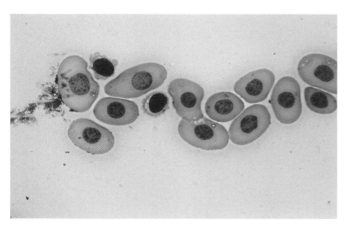

FIGURE 175.4 Thrombocytes appear ellipsoidal to fusiform in shape with a centrally placed nucleus (Wright's Giemsa). (Photo courtesy of Dr. Jim Klaassen, ANTECH Diagnostics.)

phagocytosis.[5,6] In health, this cell accounts for 30 to 45% of the total leukocyte count.[4] An increase in circulating heterophils indicates a response to inflammatory disease (infectious or injury). Stress, neoplasia, and myeloid leukemia have also been reported to cause heterophilia.[2]

With a Romanowsky stain, the heterophil's distinguishing needle-like intracytoplasmic granules are reddish-orange (Fig. 175.5). Crocodilians have larger granules, although they are fewer in numbers than the numerous, smaller granules seen in the lizards and snakes (Figure 175.6).[4] In chelonians, the granules are so numerous that they tend to displace the nucleus off to the side of the cell. The nucleus is light blue on staining[4] and may appear lobed in some species of lizards.[2]

Immature heterophils are not uncommonly seen in peripheral blood. Their presence usually indicates extensive demand of mature heterophils, such as in severe infection. In addition, the presence of abnormal appearing heterophils is an indication of infectious or inflammatory disease. Toxic cells have increased cytoplasmic vacuolization and basophilia.[2] The granules stain dark blue to purple and may take on abnormal shapes. Degranulation or excessive lobation in nonlobed species are additional indications of toxic changes to the heterophils in response to disease (Fig. 175.7).

Eosinophils

The reptilian eosinophil is as distinctive as the mammalian eosinophil. These large, round cells are peroxidase-positive and have bead-like or spherical, eosinophilic cytoplasmic granules.[5] The eosinophilic granules of some species, such as the iguana, may stain blue with Romanowsky's stain (Fig. 175.8A, B).[9] The nucleus may be simple or lobed and is usually eccentric.[4] Eosinophil size varies with species. Snakes have the largest cells, turtles and crocodilians have intermediate-sized cells, and lizards have the smallest eosinophils.[8]

Eosinophils numbers vary from 7 to 20% in normal, healthy reptile blood[2,4] but also vary with the seasons, being lowest during the summer and highest during hibernation.[2] Eosinophilia is also influenced by parasitic stimuli and other antigenic stimuli. In Chelonia, eosinophils participate in the immune response and will phagocytize immune complexes.[11]

Basophils

The basophil, like the eosinophil, is a readily recognizable cell, just as it is in mammalian hematology. These small cells have dark purple staining metachromatic granules with an slightly eccentric to centrally placed nonlobed nucleus (Fig. 175.9). The nucleus is often obscured by the darkly stained granules.[2,4]

Reptilian basophils appear to have similar function

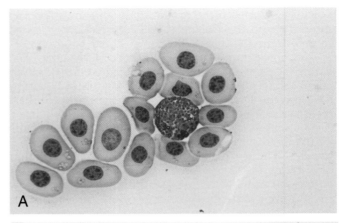

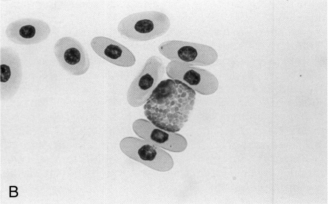

FIGURE 175.8 (**A**) Snake eosinophil stained with Wright's Giemsa. (Photo courtesy of Dr. Jim Klaassen, ANTECH Diagnostics.) (**B**) Tortoise eosinophil stained with Diff Quick. (Photo courtesy of Dr. Tom Boyer.) Note the bluish granules in the tortoise cell.

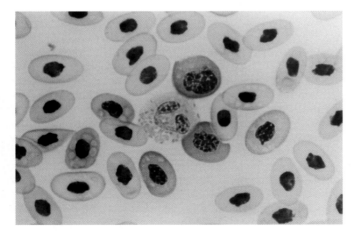

FIGURE 175.7 Degranulation or excessive lobation in nonlobed species are additional indications of toxic changes to the heterophils in response to disease (iguana, Wright's Giemsa). (Photo courtesy of Dr. Jim Klaassen, ANTECH Diagnostics.)

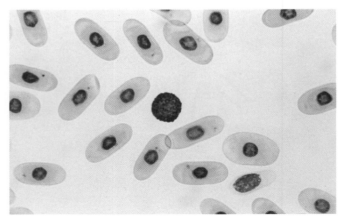

FIGURE 175.9 The basophil has dark purple staining metachromatic granules with a slightly eccentric to centrally placed nonlobed nucleus (Wright's Giemsa). (Photo courtesy of Dr. Tom Boyer.)

to mammalian basophils, being involved with the processing of surface immunoglobulins and histamine release.[5,12,13] Basophilia may also occur with the presence of blood parasites.[5]

Unlike most other leukocytes, there does not appear to be a seasonal variation in numbers of circulating basophils.[8] Normal ranges vary from 0 to 40% depending on the species.[2] Turtles have higher numbers of circulating basophils than other reptilian species, in some cases upward of 50 to 60%. There does not appear to be any pathology associated with these high numbers.

Lymphocytes

The reptilian lymphocyte is similar in appearance to those found in the blood of mammals. There are both small (5 to 10 μm) and large (15 μm) lymphocytes. These mononuclear cells may be round or found wrapped around other cells in the blood smear.[2] The basophilic cytoplasm is scant and may contain azurophilic granules. The small lymphocytes are frequently confused with thrombocytes when reading the differential (Fig. 175.10).

The lymphocytes originate from the thymus, bone marrow, spleen, and other lymphopoietic tissue.[2] There appears to be more than simple T- and B-cell diversity.[5] The B cells are responsible for producing certain immunoglobulins, and the T cells moderate the immune response.[2]

As with most other reptilian cells, there is a seasonal influence on the circulating numbers of lymphocytes in peripheral blood, in which the numbers are lowest during the cooler winter or hibernating months and highest during the warmer months.[5,6] This suggests that the animal's immune response would likewise be less during the colder months and augmented during the warmer time of the year.

For most reptiles, lymphocytes are the most prevalent

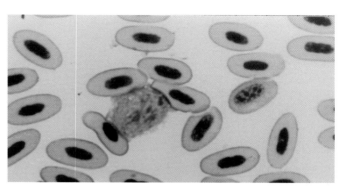

FIGURE 175.11 Monocytes have fine to moderately granular blue-gray cytoplasm, with or without vacuoles, and a ''U''-shaped or curved nucleus of granular chromatin (iguana, Wright's Giemsa). (Photo courtesy of Dr. Jim Klaassen, ANTECH Diagnostics.)

circulating cell and can be as high as 80% in some species.[5] Lymphocyte numbers are lower in males and also in starvation.[2] A lymphocytosis can occur with inflammation, wound healing, viral diseases, and certain parasitic infections.[2]

Plasma Cells

The reptilian plasma cell is similar in shape, morphology, and staining qualities to the mammalian plasma cell[4] but is rare in peripheral blood.[2] These cells have a deep staining basophilic cytoplasm with a prominent perinuclear halo that encompasses approximately one-third of the eccentric nucleus.[9,10,14] The nucleus has a dense perinuclear chromatin and chromatin clumping.[2]

The plasmacyte count in healthy reptiles is 0.2 to 0.5% or less but may increase in the presence of infection or other inflammatory conditions.[4]

Monocytes and Azurophils

The reptilian monocyte is similar in appearance to its mammalian counterpart. It is the largest cell in the normal leukogram, consisting of fine to moderately granular blue-gray cytoplasm, with or without vacuoles, and a ''U''-shaped or curved nucleus of granular chromatin (Fig. 175.11).[2,4] Monocytes with azurophilic appearance to the cytoplasm are often referred to as azurophils (Fig. 175.12).[2]

Regular, normal-appearing monocytes are not found with abundance, usually ranging less than 10% of the WBC. Snakes, on the other hand, will normally have azurophilic monocytes ranging from 15 to 20%.

Like the basophil, the monocyte shows little seasonal variation.[6] The monocyte and azurophilic monocyte counts will increase with antigenic stimulation and infectious disease. The monocytes also play an active role in granuloma and giant cell formation.[2]

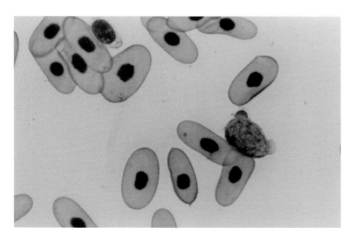

FIGURE 175.10 The small lymphocytes are frequently confused with thrombocytes when reading the differential (thrombocyte near the top of the figure) (tortoise, Wright's Giemsa). (Photo courtesy of Dr. Jim Klaassen, ANTECH Diagnostics.)

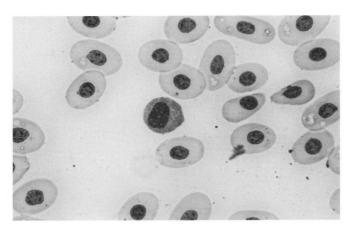

FIGURE 175.12 Monocytes with azurophilic appearance to the cytoplasm are often referred to as azurophils. These cells are often associated with inflammatory processes (iguana, Wright's Giemsa). (Photo courtesy of Dr. Jim Klaassen, ANTECH Diagnostics).

CONCLUSION

Although there are many values that have been published as "normal" over the years, clinicians must use these numbers cautiously. There are many factors that influence the hemogram of reptilian patients: age, sex, season, environmental conditions, and health status. In addition, variables such as laboratory techniques and sample handling can also affect the quality and reliability of results.

Ideally, veterinary practices that see a substantial number of exotic patients (reptiles, birds, and small mammals) would benefit from performing routine hematology in-house. Rapid turn-around of results and reproducibility are two obvious benefits.

It is critical to acquire a thorough history and perform a proper physical examination when collecting laboratory samples. When comparing results of follow-up samples, it is important to know if the samples were taken from a patient that had been housed at dramatically different temperatures.

Substantially more research has to be performed and documented before veterinarians can reliably use published normals when monitoring a patient's status. This does not mean that hematology has minimal value in clinical cases. Quite the contrary. Following changes in PCV, WBC and differential counts will help a clinician monitor progress and the effects of therapy. The key to ensuring the value of the hemogram is consistency in sampling and laboratory methodologies.

REFERENCES

1. **Jacobson ER.** Blood collection techniques in reptiles: laboratory investigations. In: Fowler ME, ed. Zoo and wild animal medicine: current therapy 3. Philadelphia: WB Saunders, 1993;144–152.
2. **Campbell TW.** Clinical pathology. In: Mader DR, ed. Reptile medicine and surgery. Philadelphia: WB Saunders, 1996;248–257.
3. **Coles EH.** Veterinary clinical pathology. Philadelphia: WB Saunders, 1986; 10–42.
4. **Frye FL.** Hematology as applied to clinical reptile medicine. In: Frye FL, ed. Biomedical and surgical aspects of captive reptile husbandry. 2nd ed. Melbourne, FL: Kreiger, 1991;1:209–277.
5. **Sypek J, Borysenko M.** Reptiles. In: Rowley AF, Ratcliffe NA, eds. Vertebrate blood cells. Cambridge: Cambridge University Press, 1988;211–256.
6. **Duguy R.** Numbers of blood cells and their variations. In: Gans C, Parsons TC, eds. Biology of the reptilia. San Diego: Academic Press, 1970;3:93–109.
7. **Mussachia XJ, Sievers ML.** Effects of induced cold torpor on blood of Chrysemys picta. Am J Physiol 1956;187:99.
8. **Saint Girons MC.** Morphology of the circulating blood cell. In: Gans C, Parsons TC, eds. Biology of the reptilia. San Diego: Academic Press, 1970; 3:73–91.
9. **Hawkey CM, Dennett TB.** Color atlas of comparative veterinary hematology. London: Wolfe Medical Publications, 1989;9:192.
10. **Campbell TW.** Avian hematology and cytology. Ames, IA: Iowa State University Press, 1988;3–17.
11. **Mead KF, Borysenko M.** Surface immunoglobulins on granular and agranular leukocytes in the thymus and spleen of the snapping turtle, Chyledra serpentina. Dev Comp Immunol 1984;8:109.
12. **Mead KF, Borysenko M, Findlay SR.** Naturally abundant basophils in the snapping turtle, Chyledra serpentina, possesses surface antibody with reaginic function. J Immunol 1983;130:334.
13. **Sypek JP, Borysenko M, Findlay SR.** Anti-immunoglobulin histamine release from naturally abundant basophils in the snapping turtle, Chyledra serpentina. Dev Comp Immunol 1984;8:358.
14. **Campbell TW.** Hematology of exotic animals. Comp Cont Ed Pract Vet 1991;13:95.

CHAPTER 176

Hematology of Nonhuman Primates

• DAVID M. MOORE

BLOOD COLLECTION

Blood may be collected from nonhuman primates (NHP) from a number of venipuncture sites depending on the size of the animal, the method of restraint, and the sample volume required. The cephalic vein of the forearm, the saphenous vein on the caudal aspect of the hindlimb, the femoral vein located in the femoral triangle, the jugular vein, and small samples can be obtained using a sterile lancet to puncture the marginal ear vein, a finger, or a heel. The blood volume in NHP was reported to be 7.35 to 9.02% of total body weight.[1]

In most instances, anesthesia is used for restraint before blood collection in NHP. Blood samples obtained from anesthetized and unanesthetized/physically restrained NHP had comparable hematocrit values up to 10 minutes after administration of ketamine hydrochloride, with a decrease in hematocrit noted 20 minutes after administration of ketamine anesthesia.[2] However, a subsequent comparative study found no change in erythrocyte counts over a 40-minute period following ketamine administration.[3] Markedly lower neutrophil numbers were observed in NHP chemically restrained with ketamine.[2,3] In physically restrained monkeys, with little or no conditioning to restraint, an "alarm reaction" leukogram can be observed, manifested as an elevated total white blood cell (WBC) count and altered differential leukocyte counts.[4] Although chemical restraint may negate the alarm reaction, appropriate training and conditioning of NHP may be more desirable in many circumstances. An excellent review article is available that describes and lists references for successful regimens for training NHP to cooperate during blood collection without the need for tranquilization or anesthetization.[5]

MORPHOLOGY AND INDICES OF PERIPHERAL BLOOD CELLS

Reported hematologic values for a number of NHP species are provided in Tables 176.1 through 176.10. Additional publications provide valuable hematologic reference data: for the rhesus monkey[6]; for rhesus macaques from birth to 2 years of age[7]; for rhesus macaques from birth to adulthood according to age, gender, and gravidity[8]; for normal baboons[9,10]; for normal chimpanzees[10]; for capuchin monkeys[11]; for the owl monkey[12]; for prosimian species including lemurs and galagos[1,13,14]; and for a variety of Old World and New World NHP species[1,15–23].

The morphology of peripheral blood cells is similar across the numerous species of NHPs,[24] and it was reported that there are no significant differences in cell counts between species, with the exception of thrombocyte counts.[1]

Erythrocytes

NHP erythrocytes are biconcave and have an average diameter of 7.1 to 7.5 μm (range, 3.5 to 8.5 μm).[24] A small number of polychromatic red blood cells (RBCs) are always found in NHP peripheral blood,[1] and reticulocyte counts are usually low in adults (0.3 to 0.7%).[24] The mean life span of the NHP RBC is 85 days (range, 52 to 128 days).[17] An alternate tagging technique found a range of erythrocyte life span for the rhesus monkey of 86 to 105 days (mean, 99.9 $\pm$ 1.0 days).[25]

Erythrocyte counts are slightly higher in NHP males than those observed in females, and hemoglobin concentration levels are also much lower in females.

Thrombocytes

The morphology of thrombocytes in NHP species is similar to that observed in other species, with amorphous pale-blue ground substance and pronounced violet granulation. Statistically significant differences in numbers of thrombocytes across NHP species have been observed, with the lowest mean value in chimpanzees, capuchin monkeys, and "long tailed" species (221 to 239 $\times$ 10^3/mm^3), and the highest mean values observed in baboons and rhesus macaques (356 $\times$ 10^3/mm^3 and 508 $\times$ 10^3/mm^3, respectively).[24] Mean platelet counts for the rhesus macaque (*Macaca mulatta*) have been reported as: 454 $\pm$ 104 $\times$ 10^3/mm^3;[26] 560 $\pm$ 174 $\times$ 10^3/mm^3;[27] and 417 $\pm$ 114.7 $\times$ 10^3/mm^3.[17] Mean platelet counts for the stumptailed macaque (*M. arctoides*) were found to be 353 $\pm$ 93.9 $\times$ 10^3/mm^3.[28] For chimpanzees, the number

TABLE 176.1   Referenced Erythrocyte Values for Several Species of New World Nonhuman Primates

Reference	Species	RBC ($\times 10^6$/mm³) Mean or [Range]	PCV (%) Mean or [Range]	Hb (g/dl) Mean or [Range]	MCV (μ^3) Mean	MCH ($\mu\mu$g) Mean or [Range]	MCHC (%) Mean or [Range]
	Howler monkey						
37	*Alouatta villosa* (female)	3.9 ± 0.7	36.8 ± 6.7	11.7 ± 1.8	97.7 ± 12.7	29.7 ± 1.4	31.4 ± 5.5
	A villosa (male)	3.8 ± 0.7	37.0 ± 5.8	11.2 ± 1.7	97.6 ± 5.3	29.8 ± 0.9	30.5 ± 1.7
1	*A. villosa*	[2.89–4.65]	[29–44]	[8.6–13.8]	[76.9–117.0]	[22.7–36.9]	[23.7–37.8]
	Owl monkey						
12	*Aotus trivirgatus*	5.17 ± 0.84	42.0 ± 5.4	14.3 ± 1.1	82.4 ± 11.9	26.9 ± 3.1	34.1 ± 3.1
1	*A. trivirgatus*	[3.50–7.74]	[32.5–51.6]	[11.9–16.0]	[57.8–91.8]	[21.7–29.5]	[28.6–39.4]
38	*A. vociferans*	6.4 ± 0.5	52.2 ± 3.7	17.1 ± 1.3	81.3 ± 4.1	26.6 ± 1.6	32.8 ± 0.6
		[5.6–7.4]	[44.0–57.8]	[14.0–18.9]	[72–90]	[22.7–30.3]	[31.0–33.8]
	Spider monkey						
1	*Ateles fusiceps*	[1.97–4.22]	[17–48]	[5.0–12.5]	[54.8–154.0]	[16.1–40.3]	[15.4–38.5]
	Ateles geoffroyi	3.68–4.98	[44–50]	[13.0–15.1]	[98–117]	[28.8–34.9]	[27.0–39.8]
37	*Ateles geoffroyi*	4.2 ± 0.6	40.5 ± 4.9	12.4 ± 1.7	97.0 ± 2.4	30.0 ± 0.4	31.0 ± 0.8
	Marmoset/tamarin						
39	*Callithrix jacchus*	6.7 ± 0.68	48.0 ± 3.5	15.5 ± 1.3	—	—	—
16	*Callithrix jacchus*	6.9	48	15.5	69	22	32
40	*Callithrix jacchus*	6.86	45	15.1	67	22	34
41	*Leontopithecus rosalia*	5.7	—	—	—	—	—
	L. rosalia (males)	—	—	15.4 ± 1.6	—	—	—
	L. rosalia (females)	—	—	14.8 ± 1.3	—	—	—
1	*Sanguinus geoffroyi*	[5.47–8.68]	[34–62]	[10.6–18.7]	[48.0–87.6]	[15.0–26.5]	[22.3–40.9]
42	*Sanguinus labiatus*	6.95	52	17	74	25	33
1	*Sanguinus mystax*	[4.7–7.7]	[35.3–60.7]	[8.7–19.6]	—	[18.3–29.9]	[26.1–35.1]
40	*Sanguinus oedipus*	6.59	45	15.5	69	23	34
	Capuchin monkey						
37	*Cebus capuchinus* (male)	4.92 ± 0.72	47.0 ± 6.7	14.4 ± 1.8	96.7 ± 1.8	29.7 ± 1.7	30.9 ± 2.2
1	*Cebus capuchinus*	[4.15–6.68]	[40–63]	[12.4–19.8]	[70–117]	[21.6–37.3]	[24.2–39.1]
11	*Cebus* sp. (female adult)	6.0 ± 0.6	49 ± 4	17 ± 1	79 ± 4	27 ± 2	34 ± 2
	Cebus sp. (at birth)	5.0 ± 0.5	55 ± 4	19 ± 1	105 ± 4	37 ± 3	36 ± 3
	Cebus sp. (1 month)	4.0 ± 0.5	39 ± 6	13 ± 1	97 ± 11	31 ± 3	32 ± 4
	Cebus sp. (2 months)	5.0 ± 0.4	43 ± 3	14 ± 1	89 ± 7	29 ± 2	32 ± 2
	Cebus sp. (4 months)	6.0 ± 0.4	46 ± 3	15 ± 1	83 ± 5	27 ± 2	32 ± 2
	Cebus sp. (12 months)	6.0 ± 0.4	47 ± 3	16 ± 1	79 ± 5	26 ± 2	33 ± 2
	Squirrel monkey						
43	*Saimiri sciureus* (at birth)	6.0 ± 0.7	55 ± 6	18 ± 2	89 ± 6	29 ± 3	33 ± 2
	S. sciureus (1 month)	5.0 ± 0.5	34 ± 3	11 ± 1	72 ± 4	23 ± 1	32 ± 2
	S. sciureus (2 months)	6.0 ± 0.5	38 ± 3	12 ± 1	66 ± 5	21 ± 2	32 ± 2
	S. sciureus (4 months)	7.0 ± 0.6	42 ± 3	13 ± 1	63 ± 5	20 ± 2	33 ± 2
	S. sciureus (12 months)	7.0 ± 0.6	43 ± 3	14 ± 1	62 ± 3	20 ± 1	33 ± 2
	S. sciureus (24 months)	7.0 ± 0.5	44 ± 3	14 ± 1	60 ± 3	20 ± 1	33 ± 2
1	*Saimiri sciureus*	[5.9–9.4]	[30.5–43.6]	[9.3–16.1]	[39–60]	[12.2–21.0]	[24.8–44.2]
44	*Saimiri sciureus*	7.26	—	14.25 ± 0.11	—	—	—

of platelets were found to be 272 ± 231 × 10^3/mm³ (range, 41 to 503 × 10^3/mm³) in males, and 273 ± 146 × 10^3/mm³ (range, 127 to 419 × 10^3/mm³) in females.[10]

Leukocytes

Total leukocyte counts are usually observed within a range of 6 to 16 × 10^3/μL of blood.[1] The WBC counts in infants were more variable than in adults, but mean values achieved adult levels by 12 weeks of age.[7] The neutrophil:lymphocyte ratio (in %) at birth was observed to be 72.4:22.7 and by 8 weeks of age was comparable to the adult ratio of 22.6:70.4.[7] The typical NHP neutrophil is a large round cell (12 to 14 μm diameter) with a pyknotic, twisted, or segmented nucleus (with up to 10 to 12 segments, although it commonly presents with 5 to 6 lobes) whose cytoplasm contains closely packed delicate pink, rod-shaped granules.[24] A "drumstick" chromatin lobe may be observed in female NHP and was found in 1.6% of 500 neutrophils in female rhesus macaques.[29] Stab neutrophils may be observed at a low frequency (0 to 2%). In contrast to other mamma-

TABLE 176.2   Referenced Leukocyte Values for Several Species of New World Nonhuman Primates

Reference	Species	WBC (×10³/mm³) Mean or [Range]	Neutrophils (%) Mean or [Range]	Lymphocytes (%) Mean or [Range]	Eosinophils (%) Mean or [Range]	Basophils (%) Mean or [Range]	Monocytes (%) Mean or [Range]
	Howler monkey						
37	*Alouatta villosa* (female)	11.9 ± 5.5	63.0 ± 18.9	34.5 ± 19.3	0.1 ± 0.4	0.4 ± 0.5	1.8 ± 1.3
	Alouatta villosa (male)	13.2 ± 5.0	60.3 ± 6.4	37.3 ± 6.1	0.3 ± 0.5	0	2.3 ± 1.0
1	*Alouatta villosa*	[7.2–22.9]	[51–64]	[32–49]	[0–2]	[0–1]	[0–3]
	Owl monkey						
12	*Aotus trivirgatus*	12.7 ± 4.7	55.4 ± 7.6	35.5 ± 18.3	9.5 ± 9.2	<0.1	—
1	*Aotus trivirgatus*	[3.2–28.5]	[13–91]	[5–80]	[0–37]	[0–1]	—
38	*A. vociferans*	8.8 ± 3.8	29	63	18	1	3
	Spider monkey						
1	*Ateles fusiceps*	[4.3–18.5]	[46–82]	[13–54]	[0–4]	[0–2]	0–3
	Ateles geoffroyi	[7.3–13.5]	—	[50.0–76.1]	[0–3]	[0–1]	0–6
37	*Ateles geoffroyi*	13.0 ± 4.5	39.0 ± 8.0	59 ± 8	1 ± 1	0	1 ± 1
	Marmoset/tamarin						
39	*Callithrix jacchus*	10.0 ± 2.7	37.4 ± 14.7	59.9 ± 14.7	0.9 ± 0.9	0.2 ± 0.3	1.6 ± 1.1
16	*Callithrix jacchus*	7.3	55	43	0.5	1.3	0.4
40	*Callithrix jacchus*	12.8	28	67	0.6	0.3	2.1
41	*Leontopithecus rosalia*	7.13 ± 2.8	62 ± 35.2	30.4 ± 16.0	4.2 ± 5.6	1.1 ± 2.0	2.2 ± 2.5
1	*Sanguinus geoffroyi*	[7.3–24.6]	[30–90]	[9–66]	[0–2]	[0–6]	[0–2]
42	*Sanguinus labiatus*	11.9	42	54	0.9	0.7	2.8
1	*Sanguinus mystax*	[7.7–20.8]	—	—	—	—	—
1	*Sanguinus nigricollis*	[6.8–20.8]	[4.0–72.5]	[20.5–91.0]	[0.0–11.5]	[0.0–7.5]	[0–11]
40	*Sanguinus oedipus*	12.6	43	49	1.2	0.1	5
1	*Sanguinus oedipus*	[7.3–24.6]	[30–90]	[9–66]	[0–2]	[0.0–7.5]	[0–11]
	Capuchin monkey						
37	*Cebus capuchinus*	16.0 ± 8.4	55.6 ± 6.6	40.9 ± 6.7	1.6 ± 2.2	0	1.8 ± 1.1
1	*Cebus capuchinus*	[6.3–34.3]	[40–70]	[25–55]	[0–5]	[0–1]	[0–4]
11	*Cebus* sp. (female adult)	8 ± 3	—	—	—	—	—
	Cebus sp. (at birth)	8 ± 2	62	33	<1	<1	4
	Cebus sp. (1 month)	7 ± 3	30	60	4	<1	6
	Cebus sp. (2 months)	8 ± 3	26	70	3	<1	3
	Cebus sp. (4 months)	10 ± 4	18	76	4	<1	4
	Cebus sp. (12 months)	8 ± 3	30	62	4	0	4
	Squirrel monkey						
43	*Saimiri sciureus* (at birth)	13	77	13	3	1	6
	S. sciureus (1 month)	6	40	53	4	<1	3
	S. sciureus (2 months)	8	40	54	2	<1	4
	S. sciureus (4 months)	8	31	62	4	<1	2
	S. sciureus (12 months)	8	30	63	2	<1	4
1	*Saimiri sciureus*	[4.6–11.7]	[22.5–80.0]	[20–68]	0–10	0–1	1–6
44	*Saimiri sciureus* (males)	8.0 ± 0.4	34.8 ± 2.1	58.0 ± 2.1	—	—	3.5 ± 0.5

TABLE 176.3   Referenced Erythrocyte Values for a Few Species of Old World Nonhuman Primates

Reference	Species	RBC (×10⁶/mm³) Mean or [Range]	PCV (%) Mean or [Range]	Hb (g/dl) Mean or [Range]	MCV (μ³) Mean or [Range]	MCH (μμg) Mean or [Range]	MCHC (%) Mean or [Range]
	African green monkey						
1	*Cercopithecus aethiops*	[4.34–6.34]	[35–44]	[10.8–13.2]	[70–96]	[23.4–28.6]	[27–34]
	Mangabey						
13	*Cercocebus* sp. (male)	4.72	38	11.7	80.5	24.8	30.8
	Cercocebus sp. (female)	6.15	46	14	74.8	22.8	30.4
	Silver leaf-eating monkey						
1	*Presbytis cristatus*	[4.0–7.6]	[40.4–51.6]	[9.7–12.9]	[69.7–89.0]	[16.7–22.2]	[21.1–28.0]

TABLE 176.4   Referenced Leukocyte Values for a Few Species of Old World Nonhuman Primates

Reference	Species	WBC (×10³/mm³) Mean or [Range]	Neutrophils (%) Mean or [Range]	Lymphocytes (%) Mean or [Range]	Eosinophils (%) Mean or [Range]	Basophils (%) Mean or [Range]	Monocytes (%) Mean or [Range]
1	African Green Monkey *Cercopithecus aethiops*	[9.7–17.0]	[20–61]	[32–75]	[0–11]	[0–1]	[0–2]
13	Mangabey *Cercocebus* sp. (male) *Cercocebus* sp. (female)	5.3 8.9	32 25	62 67	2 1	1	4 6
1	Silver leaf-eating monkey *Presbytis cristatus*	[5.5–15.9]	[22–81]	[15–63]	[0–8]	[0–3.5]	[0–6]

lian species, eosinophils of NHP are somewhat harder to distinguish from neutrophils. Both are of equivalent size, but the eosinophil can be identified using the following criteria: the granules of the eosinophil are almost twice as large and more rounded than those in neutrophils, have a brighter yellow-red color, and may be superimposed on the nucleus; the cytoplasm in eosinophils is a slightly darker grey-blue; and the nucleus of the eosinophil is not as pyknotic or segmented, and its shape may appear as a horseshoe, annular, or S-forms with up to three segments.[24] Eosinophil counts may be found in a range of 0 to 8% of total leukocyte count. Basophils may be as large or slightly larger than neutrophils, with dull grey cytoplasm closely packed with dull grey rods and additional pale violet to dark purple, round or rod-like granules of varying sizes. The nuclear outline is sharply defined and is only rarely obscured by cytoplasmic granules. The nucleus of basophils may be horseshoe-shaped or annular and fills most of the cell. Basophils may account for between 0 and 2% of total leukocyte counts. Lymphocytes are the predominant leukocyte in NHP blood, accounting for between 25 and 91% of total leukocyte counts. Small, medium, and large lymphocyte forms may be observed, accounting for 5 to 6%, 80 to 85%, and 10 to 12% of total lymphocyte numbers, respectively.[30] The small lymphocytes are larger than erythrocytes, have a basophilic staining cytoplasm, and a round, occasionally depress nucleus that can appear lumpy and pyknotic. The large lymphocyte is only slightly larger than the small lymphocyte, its cytoplasm and nucleus appear lighter in color, and the cytoplasm may contain delicate azurophilic granules. Monocytes in NHP are larger than the lymphocytes and may appear in two forms. The first type of monocyte has a broader band of cytoplasm than is observed in the lymphocytes, with a mottled grey-blue color with a foamy appearance or with discrete vacuoles. The second type of monocyte, a transitional form, has a large oval nucleus devoid of depressions, and its cytoplasm appears darker adjacent to the nucleus and often shows a delicate pale reddish granulation. Monocyte counts range form 0 to 4% of total leukocyte counts.

Total leukocyte counts are slightly higher in female NHP than those observed in males.

BONE MARROW CYTOLOGY

Bone marrow constituents were found to be similar when sampled from three separate sites—sternum, ribs, and femur.[24] Bone marrow can also be aspirated aseptically from the ischial tuberosity in rhesus macaques. Neutrophil myelocytes are the predominant cell type observed and have basophilic or lighter staining cytoplasm containing a round or oval nucleus (which may contain a nucleolus). Reported mean values were found to be $39.12 \pm 4.67\%$ for the nucleated erythrocytic cells, $53.04 \pm 4.13\%$ for the granulocytic series, and a myeloid:erythroid (M:E) ratio of $1.36 \pm 0.26{:}1.0$.[31,32] In another study the M:E ratios for several sample sites were evaluated: sternum, 1.37:1.0; vertebra, 1.36:1.0; rib, 1.28:1.0; femur, 1.11:1.0; and tibia, 0.92:1.0.[33] The cellular composition of bone marrow from adult baboons was described by Berchelman and Kalter[34] and had an average M:E ratio of 1.79:1.0 (range, 1.26 to 2.86:1.0).

OTHER HEMATOLOGIC VALUES

Reported coagulation values for a few species of NHP are provided in Table 176.11. Coagulation values in NHP are similar to those reported for humans.[35]

The erythrocyte sedimentation rate (ESR) (mm/hr) for normal rhesus macaque blood was reported by a number of authors and summarized by Schermer[24]: 1.5 to 3.5 mm at 60 minutes; 2.1 to 9.2 mm at 120 minutes; and 17.6 to 56.7 mm at 24 hours. The ESR in female rhesus macaques was found to accelerate around 120 days of gestation and continued to increase until parturition, followed by a rapid decline after delivery.[36] The mean ESR for adult male rhesus macaques was reported as 2.12 ± 0.28 mm/hr (range, 1.56 to 2.68 mm/hr); for adult rhesus females, the mean was 4.08 ± 0.36 mm/hr (range, 3.36 to 4.80 mm/hr).[1]

TABLE 176.5   Referenced Erythrocyte Values for Several Species of Macaques

Reference	Species	RBC (×10⁶/mm³) Mean or [Range]	PCV (%) Mean or [Range]	Hb (g/dl) Mean or [Range]	MCV (μ³) Mean or [Range]	MCH (μμg) Mean or [Range]	MCHC (%) Mean or [Range]
	Stumptail macaque						
18	*Macaca arctoides*	4.86 ± 0.41 [4.2–5.6]	37.8 ± 3.1 [30–43]	12.7 ± 1.11 [10.5–14.7]	77.7 ± 4.7 [71–88]	26.2 ± 2.8 [23–30]	33.7 ± 1.2 [31–36]
28	*M. arctoides* (males)	5.1 ± 0.34 [4.6–5.4]	39.8 ± 2.8 [36–43]	13.36 ± 0.77 [11.3–14.7]	78.0 ± 4.6 [71–88]	26.4 ± 4.6 [24–28]	33.9 ± 1.3 [32–36]
	M. arctoides (females)	4.76 ± 0.39 [4.2–5.6]	37.0 ± 3.0 [30–43]	12.38 ± 1.09 [10.5–14.1]	77.7 ± 4.8 [71–88]	26.1 ± 1.7 [23–30]	33.6 ± 1.2 [31–35]
	M. arctoides (M/F)	4.86 ± 0.41 [4.2–5.6]	37.8 ± 3.1 [30–43]	12.68 ± 1.11 [10.5–14.7]	77.7 ± 4.7 [71–88]	26.2 ± 2.8 [23–30]	33.7 ± 1.2 [31–36]
45	*M. arctoides* (males)	— —	39.32 ± 5.85 [14–47]	12.17 ± 1.20 [6.9–14.9]	— —	— —	— —
	M. arctoides (females)	— —	40.04 ± 5.20 [24–56]	12.02 ± 1.41 [6.3–19.2]	— —	— —	— —
1	*M. arctoides*	[4.4–5.9]	[36–43]	[11.3–14.7]	[70–88]	[20–30]	[28–38]
46	*M. arctoides* (males)	4.8 ± 0.28 [4.3–5.2]	36.2 ± 2.5 [32.6–39.2]	12.1 ± 0.84 [10.8–13.3]	75.3 ± 2.1 [71–77]	25.3 ± 0.6 [24.0–25.8]	33.4 ± 0.4 [32.9–33.9]
17	*M. speciosa* (arctoides)	4.7 ± 0.8	37.2 ± 5.1	12.1 ± 1.4	79.8 ± 4.6	25.9 ± 1.5	32.2 ± 1.5
1	*M. speciosa* (arctoides)	[3.1–6.3]	[32.5–42.3]	[9.3–14.9]	[70.6–89.0]	[22.9–28.9]	[29.2–35.2]
	Formosan rock macaque						
47	*Macaca cyclopis*	5.12 ± 0.66 [3.80–6.44]	38.9 ± 2.7 [33.5–44.3]	13.9 ± 0.9 [12.1–15.7]	— [71–88]	— [23–30]	— [31–36]
1	*M. cyclopis*						
	Cynomologous macaque						
1	*M. irus* (*fascicularis*)	—	[34.6–45.0]	[9.3–13.7]	[61.1–71.5]	[17.0–19.4]	[25.8–31.4]
	M. fascicularis	[3.9–7.1]	[38–50]	[11.6–14.5]	[69.1–90.0]	[21.1–26.4]	[26.4–33.0]
46	*M. fascicularis* (males)	5.8 ± 0.47 [5.0–6.7]	35.3 ± 2.2 [31.2–40.0]	11.7 ± 0.68 [10.5–13.3]	62.2 ± 3.4 [55–69]	20.1 ± 1.3 [17.4–22.1]	33.3 ± 1.5 [29.4–35.5]
48	*M. fascicularis* (males)	6.56 ± 0.53 [5.9–8.0]	38 ± 3 [34–46]	12 ± 1 [10–14]	59 ± 4 [51–67]	18 ± 1 [16–21]	31 ± 1 [28–34]
	M. fascicularis (females)	6.00 ± 0.59 [4.66–6.91]	36 ± 3 [30–42]	11 ± 1 [9–14]	60 ± 4 [51–69]	19 ± 1 [15–22]	31 ± 1 [29–33]
	Rhesus macaque						
6	*Macaca mulatta*	5.02 ± 0.55 [3.56–6.95]	39.60 ± 3.61 [26–48]	12.9 ± 1.81 [8.8–16.5]	79.48 ± 7.48 [58.1–116.9]	25.93 ± 2.89 [18.5–36.6]	32.63 ± 2.11 [25.6–40.2]
17	*M. mulatta*	5.6 ± 0.6	42.1 ± 3.2	12.3 ± 1.1	76.0 ± 6.5	22.0 ± 2.4	29.1 ± 2.0
1	*M. mulatta*	[3.1–8.6]	[32–50]	[9.0–16.5]	[58.4–104.0]	[18.0–35.4]	[24.8–39.0]
18	*M. mulatta*	4.48 ± 0.63	40.3 ± 3.5	12.5 ± 1.5	91.5 ± 11.7	28.2 ± 2.7	31.0 ± 2.7
50	*M. mulatta*	5.7 ± 0.6	44.0 ± 3.3	13.9 ± 1.1	78.0 ± 5.7	25.0 ± 1.9	32.0 ± 0.9
27	*M. mulatta* (females, <3 yrs)	5.57 ± 0.55	40.9 ± 3.0	13.4 ± 1.1	73	24	32.9
	M. mulatta (males, <3 yrs)	5.70 ± 0.59	41.9 ± 2.6	14.1 ± 0.9	74	25	33.6
	M. mulatta (females, >3 yrs)	5.60 ± 0.57	41.1 ± 2.8	13.5 ± 1.0	74	24	33
	M. mulatta (males, >3 yrs)	5.85 ± 0.62	42.1 ± 2.8	13.8 ± 1.0	72	24	32.8
	Pigtail macaque						
17	*Macaca nemistrina*	5.95 ± 0.34	42.5 ± 1.0	13.1 ± 0.9	71.5 ± 6.0	22.1 ± 2.0	31.0 ± 1.5
51	*M. nemistrina* (males)	— —	35.7 ± 3.5 [32–45]	11.32 ± 1.2 [9.2–13.2]	— —	— —	31.8 ± 2.5 [27.8–37.1]
	M. nemistrina (females)	— —	37.2 ± 3.7 [28–48]	11.53 ± 1.1 [9.2–14.4]	— —	— —	31.0 ± 2.0 [26.1–40.3]
1	*M. nemistrina*	[4.1–7.45]	[38–46]	[11.7–15.7]	[63.3–79.7]	[17.5–28.1]	[27.9–37.4]
	Bonnet macaque						
1	*M. radiata*	[3.17–4.80]	[34–48]	[10.6–14.8]	[85–120]	[26.5–37.0]	[25.8–36.1]

TABLE 176.6   Referenced Leukocyte Values for Several Species of Macaques

Reference	Species	WBC (×10³/mm³) Mean or [Range]	Neutrophils (%) Mean or [Range]	Lymphocytes (%) Mean or [Range]	Eosinophils (%) Mean or [Range]	MCH ($\mu\mu$g) Mean or [Range]	Monocytes (%) Mean or [Range]
	Stumptail macaque						
18	*Macaca arctoides*	9.28 ± 2.19 [5.2–14.9]	38.2 ± 18.3 [11–88]	54.1 ± 17.4 [12–79]	7.5 ± 6.3 [0–22]	0.2 ± 0.4 [0–1]	0.4 ± 0.7 [0–2]
28	*M. arctoides* (males)	9.33 ± 2.8 [5.2–14.9]	44.7 ± 18.3 [17–74]	46.5 ± 17.6 [13–73]	8.1 ± 5.4 [2–17]	0.18 ± 0.32 [0–1]	0.55 ± 0.84 [0–2]
	M. arctoides (females)	9.26 ± 1.94 [5.7–13.9]	35.3 ± 18.1 [11–88]	57.4 ± 16.5 [12–79]	7.3 ± 6.8 [0–22]	0.16 ± 0.41 [0–1]	0.28 ± 0.60 [0–2]
	M. arctoides (M/F)	9.28 ± 2.19 [5.2–14.9]	38.2 ± 18.3 [11–88]	54.1 ± 17.4 [12–79]	7.5 ± 6.3 [0–22]	0.17 ± 0.38 [0–1]	0.36 ± 0.68 [0–2]
45	*M. arctoides* (males)	14.69 ± 5.46 [3.9–37.8]	28.28 ± 15.2 [1–82]	67.35 ± 15.20 [29–98]	3.63 ± 3.50 [0–31]	0.2 ± 0.6 [0–5]	0.54 ± 1.39 [0–11]
	M. arctoides (females)	14.13 ± 5.05 [5.2–36.6]	31.42 ± 15.2 [4–88]	61.87 ± 16.91 [11–93]	5.15 ± 5.24 [0–40]	0.22 ± 0.57 [0–3]	0.52 ± 1.56 [0–12]
1	*M. arctoides*	[5.2–14.9]	[17–74]	[22–79]	[2–17]	[0–1]	[0–2]
46	*M. arctoides* (males)	9.3 ± 3.2 [4.7–18.5]	48 ± 13 [25–71]	45 ± 11 [27–63]	5.2 ± 3.9 [1–21]	— —	1.7 ± 1.3 [0–4]
17	*M. speciosa (arctoides)*	19.6 ± 6.0 [7.6–31.6]	39.5 ± 17.0 [22.5–56.5]	47.5 ± 15.0 [32.5–62.5]	10.0 ± 8.5 [1.5–18.5]	0.4 ± 0.7 [0–1]	2.5 ± 1.5 [1–4]
1	*M. speciosa (arctoides)*						
	Formosan rock macaque						
47	*Macaca cyclopis*	10.3 ± 4.1 [6.2–14.4]	49.56 ± 17.4 [32.2–67.0]	47.46 ± 17.15 [30.3–64.6]	1.44 ± 2.22 [0.0–3.6]	0.78 ± 0.87 [0.0–1.65]	0.62 ± 1.05 [0.0–1.67]
1	*M. cyclopis*						
	Cynomologous macaque						
1	*M. irus (fascicularis)*	[4.3–21.1]	[25–79]	[16–68]	[0–6]	[0.0–1.5]	[1–5]
	M. fascicularis	[8.15–21.3]	[13.8–81.0]	[35–83]	[0–11]	[0–1]	[1–1]
46	*M. fascicularis* (males)	9.8 ± 5.4 [5.4–21.2]	59 ± 17 [36–86]	35 ± 14 [12–55]	2.7 ± 1.6 [0–5]	— —	3.6 ± 1.3 [2–5]
	Rhesus macaque						
49	*Macaca mulatta* (males)	10.3 ± 2.8	32.9 ± 1.4	58.0 ± 1.4	4.1 ± 0.3	0.4 ± 0.06	4.2 ± 0.2
	M. mulatta (females)	10.3 ± 3.1	38.7 ± 1.4	52.1 ± 1.3	5.4 ± 0.4	0.5 ± 0.08	3.2 ± 0.3
17	*M. mulatta*	10.1 ± 3.6	40 ± 17	55.0 ± 16.5	3.5 ± 3.0	0.3 ± 0.5	1.1 ± 1.6
6	*M. mulatta*	8.17 ± 3.25 [2.5–26.7]	37.3 ± 9.5 [5–88]	58.8 ± 15.0 [8–92]	2.56 ± 2.65 [0–14]	0.2 ± 0.54 0–6	2.15 ± 2.21 [0–11]
1	*M. mulatta*	[4.6–21.6]	[14–71]	[23–95]	[0–16]	[0–4]	[0–8]
14	*M. mulatta*	11.5 ± 4.3	22.7 ± 11.1	68.7 ± 11.9	5.0 ± 5.3	0.2 ± 0.6	3.9 ± 2.8
50	*M. mulatta*	10.7 ± 3.8	41 ± 12	53 ± 12	4.0 ± 2.1	0	1.0 ± 1.3
27	*M. mulatta* (females, <3 yrs)	8.5 ± 3.18	37.0 ± 15.3	57.8 ± 14.3	—	—	—
	M. mulatta (males, <3 yrs)	7.88 ± 2.35	32.5 ± 13.5	63.8 ± 13.3	—	—	—
	M. mulatta (females, >3 yrs)	7.57 ± 2.37	38.7 ± 13.0	56.7 ± 12.3	—	—	—
	M. mulatta (males, >3 yrs)	8.2 ± 3.21	34.5 ± 14.3	61.3 ± 14.3	—	—	—
	Pigtail macaque						
17	*Macaca nemistrina*	11.5 ± 2.8	41.5 ± 17.0	52.5 ± 17.5	3.5 ± 5.0	0.1 ± 0.3	2.5 ± 1.5
51	*M. nemistrina* (males)	11.8 ± 3.7 [5.0–19.2]	50.53 ± 15.6 [14–90]	41.39 ± 14.7 [7–77]	2.19 ± 2.67 [0–16]	0.36 ± 0.55 [0–3]	4.15 ± 3.22 [0–19]
1	*M. nemistrina*	[5.3–13.1]	[23–58]	[37–69]	[0–8]	[0–1]	[0–4]
	Bonnet macaque						
1	*M. radiata*	[12.0–13.7]	[44–76]	[36–73]	[1.7–2.5]	—	[0–2]

TABLE 176.7   Referenced Erythrocyte Values for Several Species of Baboons

Reference	Species	RBC (×10⁶/mm³) Mean or [Range]	PCV (%) Mean or [Range]	Hb (g/dl) Mean or [Range]	MCV (μ^3) Mean or [Range]	MCH ($\mu\mu$g) Mean or [Range]	MCHC (%) Mean or [Range]
10	*Papio* sp. (M, single housed)	5.05 ± 0.64 [4.41–5.69]	39.0 ± 4.5 [34.5–43.5]	12.9 ± 1.5 [11.4–14.4]	76.9 ± 5.2 [71.7–82.1]	25.4 ± 1.7 [23.7–27.1]	33.1 ± 1.5 [31.6–34.6]
	Papio sp. (F, single housed)	4.86 ± 0.59 [4.27–5.45]	37.4 ± 5.0 [32.4–42.4]	12.3 ± 1.7 [10.6–14.0]	77.1 ± 6.3 [70.8–83.4]	25.3 ± 1.9 [23.4–27.2]	32.8 ± 1.1 [31.7–33.9]
	Papio sp. (M, gang housed)	4.99 ± 0.80 [4.19–5.79]	39.3 ± 5.6 [33.7–44.9]	12.9 ± 2.0 [10.9–14.9]	78.9 ± 6.6 [72.3–85.5]	25.9 ± 2.4 [23.5–28.3]	32.8 ± 1.1 [31.7–33.9]
	Papio sp. (F, gang housed)	4.82 ± 0.75 [4.07–5.57]	37.7 ± 5.2 [32.5–42.9]	12.2 ± 1.9 [10.3–14.1]	78.4 ± 4.8 [73.6–83.2]	25.3 ± 1.8 [23.5–27.1]	32.3 ± 1.4 [30.9–33.7]
50	*Papio* sp.	4.5 ± 0.5	36.0 ± 3.8	11.4 ± 1.2	80.0 ± 2.5	26.0 ± 0.5	32.0 ± 1.3
17	*Papio doguera (anubis)* (M/F)	4.45 ± 0.5	35.8 ± 8.7	11.8 ± 1.6	80.4	26.5	32
51	*P. anubis*	— —	35.6 ± 4.4 [24.5–49.0]	11.98 ± 1.6 [7.5–18.2]	— —	— —	33.5 ± 2.5 [22.5–43.3]
1	*Papio cynocephalus anubis*	—	[24.5–49.0]	[7.5–18.2]	—	—	[25.9–43.3]
	P.c. cynocephalus	[4.42–5.03]	[41–44]	[12.5–13.9]	[87.8–97.0]	—	[27.9–33.9]
	P. doguera (anubis)	[3.45–5.45]	[18.4–53.2]	[8.6–15.0]	[71.6–88.4]	[23.9–29.1]	[28.8–35.2]
52	*P.c. anubis* (males)	5.39 ± 0.49	41.8 ± 3.6	12.9 ± 0.9	77.8 ± 5.1	23.9 ± 1.5	30.8 ± 1.3
	P.c. cynocephalus (males)	5.97 ± 0.49	44.3 ± 4.0	13.8 ± 1.4	74.4 ± 4.1	23.6 ± 1.5	31.0 ± 1.7
34	*Papio cynocephalus* (M/F)	4.65 [4.42–5.03]	43 [41–44]	13.3 [12.5–13.9]	92.4 —	— —	30.9 —
1	*Papio hamadryas*	[3.87–6.07]	[35–49]	[11.4–14.7]	[69–88]	—	—
18	*P. hamadryas*	5.22 ± 0.38	41.3 ± 3.0	13.1 ± 0.72	76.9 ± 4.4	—	—
1	*Papio ursimus*	[4.49–6.34]	[30–43]	[7.6–14.0]	[53.4–83.0]	[14.0–25.8]	[20.8–38.3]

TABLE 176.8   Referenced Leukocyte Values for Several Species of Baboons

Reference	Species	WBC (×10³/mm³) Mean or [Range]	Neutrophils (%) Mean or [Range]	Lymphocytes (%) Mean or [Range]	Eosinophils (%) Mean or [range]	Basophils (%) Mean or [Range]	Monocytes (%) Mean or [Range]
9	*Papio* sp. (males)	10.9 ± 4.0	54 ± 20	42 ± 20	2.0 ± 1.7	0.1 ± 0.3	1.0 ± 1.2
	Papio sp. (females)	10.8 ± 3.0	64 ± 21	33 ± 19	1.0 ± 0.9	0.1 ± 0.3	1.0 ± 1.1
	Papio sp. (juveniles)	7.6 ± 2.7	44 ± 13	53 ± 13	1.6 ± 1.9	0.1 ± 0.2	1.6 ± 1.9
10	*Papio* sp. (M, single housed)	9.2 ± 6.1 [3.1–15.3]	62 ± 24 [38–86]	35 ± 24 [11–59]	1 ± 2 [0–3]	0 [0]	2 ± 3 [0–5]
	Papio sp. (F, single housed)	10.0 ± 5.5 [4.5–15.5]	61 ± 29 [32–90]	36 ± 30 [6–66]	1 ± 2 [0–3]	0 [0]	2 ± 3 [0–5]
	Papio sp. (M, gang housed)	8.1 ± 4.8 [3.3–12.9]	49 ± 35 [14–84]	48 ± 34 [14–82]	1 ± 2 [0–3]	0 ± 1 [0–1]	2 ± 3 [0–5]
	Papio sp. (F, gang housed)	10.1 ± 6.9 [3.2–17.0]	48 ± 39 [9–87]	49 ± 39 [10–88]	1 ± 3 [0–4]	0 ± 1 [0–1]	2 ± 3 [0–5]
50	*Papio* sp.	7.9 ± 2.6	44 ± 13	46 ± 13	2 ± 1	1 ± 1	7.0 ± 3.9
17	*Papio doguera (anubis)*	14.1 ± 2.3	60.5 ± 17.0	36.0 ± 15.5	1.5 ± 2.0	0.4 ± 0.7	1.5 ± 1.5
51	*P. anubis*	9.6 ± 3.2 [3.9–20.4]	51.0 ± 18.7 [8–93]	42.7 ± 17.9 [2–86]	3.01 ± 3.24 [0–25]	0.37 ± 0.66 [0–5]	2.82 ± 2.32 [0–13]
1	*Papio cynocephalus anubis*	[3.9–20.4]	[8–93]	[2–86]	[0–25]	[0–5]	[0–13]
	P.c. cynocephalus	[4.1–12.3]	[24–71]	[25–73]	[1–5]	[0–1]	[1–4]
	p. doguera (anubis)	[9.5–18.7]	[26.5–94.5]	[20.5–51.5]	[1–10]	[0.4–0.7]	[0.0–1.5]
52	*P.c. anubis* (males)	9.9 ± 4.06	—	—	—	—	—
	P.c. cynocephalus (males)	8.7 ± 2.33	—	—	—	—	—
34	*Papio cynocephalus*	7.1 [4.1–12.3]	51 [24–71]	45 [25–73]	3 [1–5]	1 [0–1]	2 [1–4]
1	*Papio hamadryas*	[4.9–15.4]	[21–68]	[21–74]	[0–16]	[0–3]	[0–9]
18	*P. hamadryas*	7.7 ± 2.4	44.5 ± 12.8	45.7 ± 12.8	6.6 ± 4.3	0.3 ± 0.6	2.9 ± 2.7
1	*Papio ursimus*	[4.75–17.1]	[27–73]	[26–59]	[1–4]	[0.0–0.5]	[0.0–5.8]

TABLE 176.9   Referenced Erythrocyte Values for Several Species of Great Apes

Reference	Species	RBC (×10⁶/mm³) Mean or [Range]	PCV (%) Mean or [Range]	Hb (g/dl) Mean or [Range]	MCV (μ^3) Mean or [Range]	MCH ($\mu\mu$g) Mean or [Range]	MCHC (%) Mean or [Range]
	Gorilla						
53	*Gorilla gorilla*	4.21 ± 0.34	40.4 ± 2.4	12.1 ± 0.74	95.4 ± 6.9	28.8 ± 2.1	30.2 ± 1.5
13	*Gorilla gorilla* (male)	5.34	43	13.1	80.5	24.5	30.5
	Chimpanzee						
54	*Pan troglodytes*	5.59 ± 0.46	41.4 ± 2.7	13.5 ± 0.95	74.3 ± 4.5	24.2 ± 1.3	32.6 ± 1.1
17	*P. troglodytes* (M/F adults)	4.6 ± 0.6	39.7 ± 5.0	12.5 ± 1.5	86.0 ± 8.2	27.2 ± 2.7	31.2 ± 2.2
55	*P. troglodytes* (Males, all ages)	5.19 ± 0.60 [3.05–6.23]	45.18 ± 5.48 [29–58]	14.44 ± 1.99 [7.9–18.9]	87.43 ± 7.08 [64.9–101.8]	27.86 ± 2.39 [20.3–33.5]	32.01 ± 1.63 [28.2–35.0]
	P. troglodytes (Females, all ages)	4.85 ± 0.39 [4.27–5.76]	42.64 ± 3.14 [32–49]	13.49 ± 1.15 [10.3–16.4]	88.18 ± 6.49 [70.0–109.1]	27.88 ± 2.18 [22–35]	31.67 ± 1.82 [27–36]
56	*P. troglodytes* (Males, 14–180 mo.)	5.34 ± 0.49	42.4 ± 3.7	13.6 ± 1.4	79.6 ± 5.54	25.4 ± 2.0	32.1 ± 2.1
	P. troglodytes (Females, 14–180 mo.)	5.37 ± 0.58	42.8 ± 3.4	13.9 ± 1.3	80.1 ± 5.57	26.0 ± 2.4	32.5 ± 2.2
57	*P. troglodytes* (M/F, 8–63 kg)	4.86 ± 0.72 [3.3–7.1]	38.32 ± 5.47 [26–52]	12.05 ± 1.88 [7.8–17.4]	75.28 ± 8.49 [55.46–95.15]	24.83 ± 2.48 [19.85–29.98]	31.28 ± 2.49 [26.92–40.00]
58	*P. troglodytes*	5.1 ± 0.6	—	13.0 ± 1.5	—	—	—
10	*P. troglodytes* (males)	5.44 ± 1.15 [4.29–6.59]	44.2 ± 7.7 [36.5–51.9]	14.5 ± 2.5 [12–17]	81.4 ± 8.9 [72.5–90.3]	26.7 ± 3.1 [23.6–29.8]	32.8 ± 1.0 [31.8–33.8]
	P. troglodytes (females)	5.02 ± 0.93 [4.09–5.95]	41.0 ± 6.3 [34.7–47.3]	13.4 ± 2.3 [11.1–15.7]	81.9 ± 8.0 [73.9–89.9]	26.7 ± 2.5 [24.2–29.2]	32.6 ± 1.1 [31.5–33.7]
50	*Pan troglodytes*	4.8 ± 0.3	39.0 ± 2.6	12.6 ± 0.9	82.0 ± 3.6	26.0 ± 0.9	33.0 ± 1.3
13	*Pan* sp. (female)	5.08	44	13.8	86.6	27.1	31.3
	Pan sp. (male)	5.46	45	15	82.4	27.4	33.3
	Orangutan						
59	*Pongo pygmaeus*	4.36 ± 0.63	37.9 ± 3.6	11.8 ± 1.27	86.8 ± 12.3	27.3 ± 3.2	31.0 ± 1.9
13	*P. pygmaeus* (neonatal male)	5.95	46	16.3	77.3	27.3	35.4
	P. pygmaeus (adult male)	5.7	44	14.3	76.4	24.8	32.5

TABLE 176.10   Referenced Leukocyte Values for Several Species of Great Apes

Reference	Species	WBC (×10³/mm³) Mean or [Range]	Neutrophils (%) Mean or [Range]	Lymphocytes (%) Mean or [Range]	Eosinophils (%) Mean or [Range]	Basophils (%) Mean or [Range]	Monocytes (%) Mean or [Range]
	Gorilla						
53	*Gorilla gorilla*	9.5 ± 4.1	63.8 ± 15.1	29.8 ± 13.6	2.6 ± 2.5	0.2 ± 0.4	3.2 ± 2.2
13	*Gorilla gorilla* (male)	5.6	84	24	2	—	10
	Chimpanzee						
54	*Pan troglodytes*	12.5 ± 5.1	52.0 ± 14.6	43 ± 14	2.6 ± 3.2	0.2 ± 0.5	1.1 ± 1.2
17	*Pan troglodytes* (M/F adults)	12.5 ± 5.1	63.0 ± 16.5	33.0 ± 15.5	2.5 ± 3.0	0.2 ± 0.5	1.1 ± 1.0
55	*P. troglodytes* (Males, all ages)	11.85 ± 5.00 [4.8–31.1]	64.5 ± 15.95 [26–91]	30.21 ± 15.88 [4–69]	2.24 ± 2.83 [0–17]	0.24 ± 0.56 [0–3]	2.21 ± 1.72 [0–7]
	P. troglodytes (Females, all ages)	13.64 ± 5.80 [5.5–50.3]	64.45 ± 19.48 [13–94]	30.43 ± 17.98 [4–67]	2.00 ± 2.61 [0–12]	0.20 ± 0.47 [0–3]	1.81 ± 1.70 [0–10]
56	*P. troglodytes* (Males, 14–180 mo.)	12.0 ± 4.8	42.3 ± 14.4	50.1 ± 13.4	3.6 ± 4.2	0.2 ± 0.4	1.5 ± 2.6
	P. troglodytes (Females, 14–180 mo.)	12.1 ± 4.3	41.8 ± 14.4	53.0 ± 14.3	2.7 ± 2.7	0.2 ± 0.4	0.9 ± 2.1
57	*P. troglodytes* (M/F, 8–63 kg)	10.13 ± 4.08 [4.33–20.18]	— —	— —	— —	— —	— —
10	*P. troglodytes* (males)	11.0 ± 7.6 [3.4–18.6]	46 ± 35 [11–81]	47 ± 32 [15–79]	4 ± 9 [0–13]	1 ± 4 [0–5]	2 ± 3 [0–5]
	P. troglodytes (females)	13.6 ± 8.6 [5.0–22.2]	44 ± 33 [11–77]	50 ± 31 [19–81]	3 ± 6 [0–9]	0 ± 2 [0–2]	2 ± 3 [0–5]
50	*Pan troglodytes*	13.3 ± 4.8	61 ± 17	35 ± 17	1.0 ± 0.9	0	2.0 ± 1.5
13	*Pan* sp. (female)	7	44.5	51	1.5	0.5	2.5
	Pan sp. (male)	9.7	49	26	1	—	4
	Orangutan						
59	*Pongo pygmaeus*	11.3 ± 5.2	51.3 ± 16.5	43 ± 16	2.9 ± 2.7	0.1 ± 0.4	2.6 ± 2.3
13	*P. pygmaeus* (neonatal male)	8.7	50	45	—	—	5
	P. pygmaeus (adult male)	9.3	67.5	26.5	1	0.5	4.5

TABLE 176.11   Observed Coagulation Values in Selected Nonhuman Primate Species

Parameter	Species	Mean ± SD	Reference
Bleeding time (sec)	*Papio* sp.	313 ± 139 (150–618)	50
Clotting time (sec)	*Macaca mulatta*	78 ± 46	24
	Macaca mulatta	11 ± 1.9	50
	Pan troglodytes	3.0 ± 1.1	50
	Papio sp.	21.0 ± 3.6	50
	Papio sp. (males)	32.5 ± 1.7	60
	Papio sp. (females)	31.0 ± 2.1	60
	Papio sp. (juveniles)	33.5 ± 2.1	60
Prothrombin time (sec)	*Macaca mulatta*	11.5 ± 1.4	50
	Macaca mulatta	12.0 ± 0.3	61
	Macaca nemistrina	12.6 ± 0.3	61
	Pan troglodytes (males)	11.7 ± 1.5	10
	Pan troglodytes (females)	11.8 ± 1.5	10
	Pan troglodytes	15.9 ± 1.4	50
	Papio sp. (males)	13.1 ± 1.4	10
	Papio sp. (females)	12.9 ± 1.0	10
	Papio sp.	12.1 ± 0.5	50
	Papio sp. (males)	13.0 ± 0.7	60
	Papio sp. (females)	12.5 ± 0.9	60
	Papio sp. (juveniles)	12.5 ± 0.4	60
	Saimiri sciureus	15.86 ± 1.13	61
Partial thromboplastin time (sec)	*Aotus trivirgatus* (M/F)	19.6 ± 1.8	62
	Aotus trivirgatus (females)	19.4 ± 1.9	62
	Aotus trivirgatus (males)	19.7 ± 1.8	62
	Aotus trivirgatus (<2 yrs)	20.6 ± 1.0	62
	Aotus trivirgatus (>2 yrs)	19.3 ± 1.9	62
	Macaca mulatta	35.5 ± 2.9	50
	Macaca mulatta (males)	94 ± 10	63
	Macaca mulatta (females)	98 ± 11	63
	Pan troglodytes (males)	21.1 ± 3.4	10
	Pan troglodytes (females)	20.9 ± 3.2	10
	Pan troglodytes	22.0 ± 1.8	50
	Papio sp. (males)	34.0 ± 5.4	10
	Papio sp. (females)	31.1 ± 4.2	10
	Papio sp.	33.1 ± 4.1	50
	Papio sp. (males)	32.5 ± 1.7	60
	Papio sp. (females)	31.0 ± 2.1	60
	Papio sp. (juveniles)	33.5 ± 2.1	60

REFERENCES

1. **Mitruka BJ, Rawnsley HM.** Clinical biochemical and hematological reference values in normal experimental animals and normal humans. 2nd ed. New York: Masson, 1981.
2. **Loomis MR, Henrickson RV, Anderson JH.** Effects of ketamine hydrochloride on the hemogram of rhesus monkeys (*Macaca mulata*). Lab Anim Sci 1980;30:851–853.
3. **Porter WP.** Hematologic and other effects of ketamine and ketamine-acepromazine in rhesus monkeys (*Macaca mulatta*). Lab Anim Sci 1982;32:373–375.
4. **Ives M, Dack GM.** "Alarm reaction" and normal blood picture in *Macaca mulatta*. J Lab Clin Med 1956;47:723.
5. **Reinhardt V.** Training nonhuman primates to cooperate during blood collection—a review. Lab Primate Newslett 1997;36:1.
6. **McClure HM.** Hematologic, blood chemistry, and cerebrospinal fluid data for the rhesus monkey. In: Bourne GH, ed. The rhesus monkey. New York: Academic Press, 1975.
7. **Martin DP, McGowan MJ, Loeb WF.** Age related changes of hematologic values in infant Macaca mulatta. Lab Anim Sci 1973;23:194–200.
8. **Buchl SJ, Howard B.** Hematologic and serum biochemical and electrolyte values in clinically normal domestically bred rhesus monkeys (Macaca mulatta) according to age, sex, and gravidity. Lab Anim Sci 1997;47:528–533.
9. **Hack CA, Gleiser CA.** Hematologic and serum chemical reference values for adult and juvenile baboons (*Papio* sp.). Lab Anim Sci 1982;32:502–505.
10. **Hainsey BM, Hubbard GB, Leland MM, Brasky KM.** Clinical parameters of normal baboons (*Papio* species) and chimpanzees (pan troglodytes). Lab Anim Sci 1993;43:236–243.
11. **Samonds KW, Hegsted DM.** Hematological development of the cebus monkey (*Cebus albifrons* and *apella*). Folia Primatol 1974;22:72–79.
12. **Wellde BT, Johnson AJ, Williams JS, Langbehn HR, Sadun EH.** Hematologic, biochemical, parasitologic parameters of the night monkey (*Aotus trivirgatus*). Lab Anim Sci 1971;21:575–580.
13. **Jain NC.** Schalm's veterinary hematology. 4th ed. Philadelphia: Lea & Febiger, 1986.
14. **Loeb WF, Bannerman RM, Rininger BF, Johnson AJ.** Hematologic disorders. In: Benirschke K, et al., eds. Pathology of laboratory animals. New York: Springer-Verlag, 1978;1.
15. **Caminiti B.** Biology of the platelets of nonhuman primates—a bibliography 1965–1980. Seattle: University of Washington Primate Information Center, 1980.
16. **Hawkey CM.** Comparative mammalian haematology. London: William Heinemann Medical Books, 1975.
17. **Huser HJ.** Atlas of comparative primate hematology. New York: Academic Press, 1970.
18. **Loeb W.** Clinical pathology. In: Fowler ME, ed. Zoo and wild animal medicine. Philadelphia: WB Saunders, 1986.
19. **Morrow AC, Terry MW.** Hematologic values for nonhuman primates tabulated from the literature—I. erythrocytes. Seattle: University of Washington Primate Information Center, 1970.
20. **Morrow AC, Terry MW.** Hematologic values for nonhuman primates tabu-

lated from the literature—II. Total leukocytes and differential counts. Seattle: University of Washington Primate Information Center, 1970.

21. **Vogin EE, Oser F.** Comparative blood values in several species of nonhuman primates. Lab Anim Sci 1971;21:937–941.
22. **Hawkey CM, et al.** Clinical hematology of the common marmoset (*Callithrix jacchus*). Am J Primatol 1982;3:179.
23. **Porter JA Jr.** Hematology of the night monkey (*Aotus trivirgatus*). Lab Anim Sci 1969;19:470.
24. **Schermer S.** The blood morphology of laboratory animals. Philadelphia: FA Davis, 1967.
25. **Kreier JP, et al.** Erythrocyte life span and label elution in monkeys (*Macaca mulatta*) and cats (*Felis catus*) determined with chromium-51 and diisopropyl fluorophosphate-32. Am J Vet Res 1970;31:1429.
26. **Melville GS Jr, et al.** Hematology of the *Macaca mulatta* monkey. Lab Anim Care 1967;17:189.
27. **Stanley RE, Cramer MB.** Hematologic values of the monkey (*Macaca mulatta*). Am J Vet Res 1968;29:1041.
28. **Vondruska JF.** Certain hematologic and blood chemical values in adult stumptailed macaques (*Macaca arctoides*). Lab Anim Care 1970;20:97.
29. **Chiarelli B, Barberis L.** Drumsticks in the leukocytes of primates. Experientia 1964;20:679.
30. **Hall BE.** The morphology of the cellular elements of the blood of the rhesus monkey, *Macacus rhesus*. Folia Haematol 1929;38:30.
31. **Switzer JW.** Bone marrow composition in the adult rhesus monkey (*Macaca mulatta*). J Am Vet Med Assoc 1967;151:823.
32. **Switzer JW.** A new technique for sampling bone marrow in the monkey. Lab Anim Care 1967;17:255.
33. **Stasney J, Higgin GM.** The bone marrow of the monkey (*Macacus rhesus*). Anat Rec 1936;67:219.
34. **Berchelman ML, Kalter SS.** Hematology. In: Kalter SS, ed. Primates in medicine. Basel: Karger, 1973;8.
35. **April M, Keith JC Jr.** Cardiovascular and lymphoreticular systems. In: Bennett BT, et al., eds. Nonhuman primates in biomedical research—diseases. San Diego: Academic Press, 1998.
36. **Allen JR, Siegfried LM.** Hematologic alterations in pregnant rhesus monkeys. Lab Anim Care 1966;16:465.
37. **Porter JA Jr.** Hematologic values of the black spider monkey (*Ateles geoffroyi*), white-face monkey (*Cebus capuchinus*), and black howler monkey (*Alouatta villosa*). Lab Anim Sci 1971;21:426.
38. **Malaga CA, et al.** Hematologic values of the wild-caught karyotype V owl monkey (*Aotus vociferans*). Lab Anim Sci 1995;45:574.
39. **Eccleston E.** Normal haematological values in rats, mice, and marmosets. In: Archer RK, Jeffcoat LB. Comparative clinical haematology. Oxford: Blackwell Scientific, 1977.
40. **Richter CB.** Part C—biology and diseases of callitrichidae. In: Fox JG, et al., eds. Laboratory animal medicine. Orlando: Academic Press, 1984.
41. **Bush M, et al.** Hematologic values of captive golden lion tamarins (*Leontopi-*

thecus rosalia)—variations with sex, age and health status. Lab Anim Sci 1982;32:294.
42. **Wadsworth PF, et al.** Hematological, coagulation and blood chemistry data in red-bellied tamarins (*Sanguinus labiatus*). Lab Anim 1982;16:327.
43. **Ausman LM, et al.** Hematologic development of the infant squirrel monkey (*Saimiri sciureus*). Folia Primatol 1976;26:292.
44. **Kakoma I, et al.** Distribution, characteristics and relationships between hematologic variables of healthy Bolivian squirrel monkeys. Lab Anim Sci 1987;37:352.
45. **Oser F, et al.** Blood values in stumptailed macaques (*Macaca arctoides*) under laboratory conditions. Lab Anim Care 1970;20:462.
46. **Verlangieri AJ, et al.** Normal serum biochemical, hematological, and EKG parameters in anesthetized adult male *Macaca fascicularis* and *Macaca arctoides*. Lab Anim Sci 1985;35:63.
47. **Taylor JF, et al.** Baseline blood determinations of the Taiwan macaque (*Macaca cyclopis*). Lab Anim Sci 1073;23:582.
48. **Giulietti M, et al.** Reference blood values of iron metabolism in cynomologous macaques. Lab Anim Sci 1991;41:606.
49. **Valerio DA, et al.** *Macaca mulatta*—management of a laboratory breeding colony. New York: Academic Press, 1969.
50. **Lewis JH.** Comparative hemostasis in vertebrates. New York: Plenum Press, 1996.
51. **Dillingham LA, et al.** A comparison of the hemograms of *Macaca mulatta*, *Macaca nemestrina*, and *Papio anubis*. Folia Primatol 1971;14:241.
52. **Newson J, Davies JDG.** Hematology of laboratory baboons in Kenya. J Med Primatol 1974;3:95.
53. **McClure HM, et al.** Hematologic and blood chemistry data for the gorilla (*Gorilla gorilla*). Folia Primatol 1972;18:300.
54. **DiGiacomo RF, et al.** The progression and evaluation of hematologic and serum biochemical values in the chimpanzee. J Med Primatol 1975;4:188.
55. **McClure HM, et al.** Hematologic and blood chemistry data for the chimpanzee (*Pan troglodytes*). Folia Primatol 1972;18:444.
56. **Hodson H, et al.** Baseline blood values of the chimpanzee. I. The relationship of age and sex and hematological values. Folia Primatol 1967;7:1.
57. **Burns KF, et al.** Compendium of normal blood values for baboons, chimpanzees, and marmosets. Am J Clin Pathol 1967;48:484.
58. **Vie JC, et al.** Megaloblastic anemia in a handreared chimpanzee. Lab Anim Sci 1989;39:613.
59. **McClure HM, et al.** Hematologic and blood chemistry data for the orangutan (*Pongo pygmaeus*). Folia Primatol 1972;18:284.
60. **Kelly CA, Gleiser CA.** Selected coagulation reference values for adult and juvenile baboons. Lab Anim Sci 1986;36:173.
61. **Seaman AJ, Malinow MR.** Blood clotting in nonhuman primates. Lab Anim Care 1968;18:80.
62. **Mrema JEK, et al.** Activated partial thromboplastin time of owl monkey (*Aotus trivirgatus*) plasma. Lab Anim Sci 1984;34:295.
63. **Schiffer SP, et al.** Activated coagulation time for rhesus monkeys (*Macaca mulata*). Lab Anim Sci 1984;34:191.

CHAPTER 177

Laboratory Techniques for Avian Hematology

• F. WILLIAM PIERSON

Automated complete blood counts using laser flow cytometry have only recently become valuable in avian species due to the presence of nucleated red blood cells and thrombocytes.[1] Therefore, the use of hand counting methods for the generation of avian hemograms is still standard practice in many laboratories. Because techniques for avian blood collection and hemogram interpretation have been addressed elsewhere, this chapter is limited to enumeration methods.

PACKED CELL VOLUME

Determination of packed cell volume (PCV) in birds is essentially the same as that for other species. Blood can be collected into standard (75 mm) heparinized microhematocrit tubes via transcutaneous puncture of a superficial vein (i.e., the ulnar or medial metatarsal vein) or from the hub of a needle. With smaller birds, 22 mm of blood in a standard microhematocrit is sufficient.[2] Alternatively, nonheparinized tubes may be used when blood has been collected and treated with ethylenediamine tetraacetate (EDTA). Tubes should be centrifuged at $12,000 \times g$ for 5 minutes and read on a standard microhematocrit graphic reader.[3]

TOTAL RED BLOOD CELL COUNT

The total red blood cell (TRBC) count can be determined automatically or manually. Sodium citrate appears to be the best anticoagulant for automated flow cytometric analysis,[1] as EDTA has a tendency to cause hemolysis in some species of birds.[4] More commonly, manual enumeration is performed using the method of Natt and Herrick[5] or the Unopette (5850) system (Bectin-Dickenson, Rutherford, NJ).

According to the Natt and Herrick method, fresh whole blood or blood containing EDTA is drawn into a standard blood dilution pipette to the 0.5 mark, followed by methyl violet 2B diluent (Table 177.1) to the 101 mark. This gives a final dilution 1:200. The pipette is then briefly agitated, blotted, and the counting chamber of a Neubauer hemacytometer (improved ruling) charged. After a few minutes to allow settling, the red cell count may be determined under high-dry magnification ($40\times$ objective). Erythrocytes appearing in the center and four corner squares are counted and the total multiplied by 1×10^4 to give the TRBC count per microliter.[1]

The Unopette 5850 system designed for mammalian erythrocytes works equally as well for avian species.[4,6] Briefly, blood is drawn into the Unopette and mixed. The hemocytometer is then charged. As with the method of Natt and Herrick, erythrocytes appearing in the center and four corner squares are counted, totaled, and multiplied by 1×10^4 to give the TRBC count per microliter.

HEMOGLOBIN CONCENTRATION AND MEAN CORPUSCULAR VALUES

Methods and formulae for determining the hemoglobin concentration, mean corpuscular volume (MCV), mean corpuscular hemoglobin (MCH), and MCH concentration (MCHC) are identical to those used for mammalian species. However, in the case of avian hemoglobin determinations, samples must be centrifuged at $1000 \times g$ for 10 minutes following red cell lysis to remove nuclei and other cellular debris adequately.[4]

DIFFERENTIAL WHITE BLOOD CELL COUNT

Difficulty is encountered with automated leukocyte determinations because of the presence of nucleated red blood cells and thrombocytes. Therefore, manual techniques are required.

Differential white blood cell counts require the preparation of stained blood smears. Whole blood or blood treated with EDTA may be used. The standard two-

TABLE 177.1	Natt and Herrick (Methyl Violet 2B) Diluent[5]
NaCl	3.88 g
Na_2SO_4	2.50 g
$Na_2HPO_4 \cdot 12H_2O$	2.91 g
KH_2PO_4	0.25 g
Formalin (37%)	7.50 ml
Methyl violet 2B	0.10 g

In the order listed, the above ingredients are dissolved and brought to volume with distilled water in a 1000 ml volumetric flask. The solution is allowed to sit overnight and then filtered through no. 2 Whatman paper. The final pH should be 7.3.

slide wedge technique for making blood smears has a tendency to produce a significant number of "smudge cells" with avian blood.[4] Therefore, the use of a slide and coverglass method[7] is preferred in most laboratories. Briefly, a drop of blood is placed on a precleaned microscope slide. While the slide is held between the fingers, a rectangular coverglass (22 mm × 60 mm) is placed on top of the blood. As the blood begins to spread, the coverslip is gently slipped off the microscope slide in a horizontal fashion. After air drying, commonly available stains such as Wright's, Giemsa, or Wright's/Giemsa may be used to prepare slides for examination either automatically or manually. Quick stains like Diff-Quik are also useful but have a tendency to damage some cell types and understain immature erythrocytes.[4] Differential counting methods are as described for mammalian species. Avian cellular morphology and leukogram interpretation are addressed in Chapter 60.

TOTAL WHITE BLOOD CELL COUNT

Two methods for manual total white blood cell (TWBC) determination have found wide acceptance in laboratories that process clinical avian samples.

The Natt and Herrick[5] method is a direct TWBC determination and differs from that previously described for TRBC counts only in the enumeration step. For the TWBC count, leukocytes (dark to light blue) appearing in the nine large squares of an improved Neubauer hemocytometer are totaled. The TWBC count is then calculated using the following corrected, simplified formula:

TWBC/μl = (number of leukocytes in 9 squares) × 220

The eosinophil Unopette 5877 technique[6,8] is an indi-

rect method for determination of TWBC. Briefly, whole blood (25 μl) is drawn into the pipette provided and mixed with the diluent (phloxine B). Both chambers of a Neubauer hemocytometer (improved ruling) are then charged. This should be done within 5 minutes of mixing to prevent staining of erythrocytes. The hemocytometer is then allowed to sit for at least 3 to 5 minutes in a humidified environment to permit settling. Those cells that appear granular, red-orange (heterophils and eosinophils), and are found within the nine large squares of both chambers should be counted. Before calculating the TWBC, a differential WBC count must be performed. The following corrected, simplified formula can then be used to calculate the TWBC count:

$$TWBC/\mu l = \frac{(number\ of\ cells\ in\ 18\ squares)}{(\%\ heterophils + eosinophils)} \times 1760$$

TOTAL THROMBOCYTE COUNT

An estimate of thrombocyte numbers may be obtained using blood smears prepared as described for the differential white blood cell count.[6] Normally, there should be 2 to 3 thrombocytes (10 to 15 per 1000 erythrocytes) per microscope field when a monolayer is viewed with the 100× objective under oil immersion. If the PCV is within the range of 40 to 50%, an estimate of total thrombocyte count (TTC) can be determined using the following simplified formula:

$$Estimated\ TTC/\mu l = $$
(number of thrombocytes in 5 fields) × 3500

If the PCV is outside the 40 to 50% range, then the estimated TTC must be corrected by multiplying it by the decimal percent deviation (e.g., observed PCV/normal PCV).

REFERENCES

1. **Fudge AM.** Avian clinical pathology–hematology and chemistry. In: Altman RB, Club SL, Dorrenstein GM, Quesenberry K, eds. Avian medicine and surgery. Philadelphia: WB Saunders, 1997;142–157.
2. **Leonard JL.** Clinical laboratory examinations. In: Petrak ML, ed. Diseases of caged and aviary birds. Philadelphia: Lea & Febiger, 1982;269–303.
3. **Cohen RR.** Anticoagulation, centrifugation time, and sample replicate number in microhematocrit method for avian blood. Poult Sci 1967;46:214–218.
4. **Dein FJ.** Hematology. In: Clinical avian medicine and surgery. Philadelphia: WB Saunders, 1984;174–191.
5. **Natt MP, Herrick CA.** A new blood diluent for counting erythrocytes and leucocytes of the chicken. Poult Sci 1952;31:735–738.
6. **Campbell TW.** Avian hematology and cytology. 2nd ed. Ames, IA: Iowa State University Press, 1995;3–19.
7. **Beacon DN.** Differential blood counts. J Lab Clin Med 1928;13:366–369.
8. **Costello RT.** A Unopette technique for eosinophil counts. Am J Clin Pathol 1970;54:249–250.

CHAPTER 178

Normal Avian Hematology: Chicken and Turkey

• DENISE I. BOUNOUS and NANCY L. STEDMAN

There are approximately 8600 species of birds representing 27 orders compared to 4500 species of mammals representing 18 orders. Birds recently have been moved into the class Reptilia and now are considered likely descendents from theropod dinosaurs (i.e., *Deinonychus* and *Velociraptor*).[1] Unique features of avian anatomy and physiology, including some relevant to hematology, have evolved to enable these modern dinosaurs to fly, whereas some features, like uricotelism and nucleated erythrocytes and thrombocytes, are retained. Progress in avian hematology largely is based on only a few domesticated species, (i.e., chicken, turkey, duck, pigeon). Effects of season, age, gender, and reproduction are mostly unknown but are beginning to be explored as our knowledge increases.

BLOOD COLLECTION

Several sites for blood collection have been described in the avian species. As in other birds, collection sites and techniques are partially dictated by the size, and hence age, of the chickens or turkeys.

The right jugular vein is the practical site for venipuncture in small chicks (i.e., those weighting less than 100 g). The right jugular vein is more superficial than the left, sits within a featherless tract, and is easily visualized. One person can carry out collection from this site in small chicks. A convenient technique is to hold the bird in the left hand, with the head between the second and third fingers and the neck outstretched. The thumb can be used to hold off the vein at the thoracic inlet. Hematoma formation is usually minimal at this site.

Cardiac puncture also can be performed in all sizes of chickens and in poults without assistance. By supporting the bird in dorsal recumbency against the left arm while holding it by the legs with the left hand, the right hand can be used to identify the ventral floor of thoracic inlet and insert the needle. In small birds, this site can be dangerous and use may be limited to situations where euthanization follows blood collection.

The cutaneous ulnar or brachial veins (i.e., the "wing veins") are superficial and easily visualized; therefore, they are commonly used in poultry. Unfortunately, the largest and most powerful muscle in the avian body, the flight muscles, are attached to the wings, and sudden flapping can result in vein laceration with significant hemorrhage and hematoma formation. Therefore, this technique generally requires an assistant.

The medial metatarsal vein is analogous to the caudal tibial vein and runs along the medial aspect of the tarsometatarsus. It is easily accessed for venipuncture in chickens or turkeys 300 g and larger, and hematoma formation is usually minimal in this area.

Bone marrow can be aspirated from the dorsal ulnar process on the dorsal aspect of the distal ulna or the tibial crest. The tibial crest is similar to its mammalian counterpart and probably easier to aspirate. The sternum can also be used, but in older chickens the marrow in this flat bone is largely replaced by fat. As an adaptation for flight, significant pneumatization occurs in many flat bones, including the sternum, and also in the humerus. These sites should be avoided for bone marrow aspiration.

A common rule of thumb is to limit blood collection to no more than 10% of the bird's blood volume. Blood volume as a percentage of body weight averages 7%. A convenient calculation is to draw 1% of the body weight (i.e., 1 mL from a 100-g chick). Birds are more tolerant to blood loss than mammals because rapid volume replacement occurs by resorption of tissue fluids. Ducks and pigeons are even more tolerant, likely through baroreceptor reflexes. Carotid sinus baroreceptors are not present in chickens.[2]

CELL COUNTS AND STAINING

Ideally, a smear should be made immediately after collection from blood containing no anticoagulant. Heparin can induce cellular and staining artifacts. The two-slide pushing technique or the two cover glass method can be used. The coverglass method may result in less cellular disruption or smudge cells (usually erythrocytes). Either

Wright's or Diff-Quik (American Scientific Products, McGraw Park, IL) stains can be used for staining avian blood smears; the authors prefer Wright's stain.

Total leukocyte counts may be performed using the eosinophil Unopette 5877 (Becton-Dickinson, Rutherford, NJ) or with Natt-Herrick's solution. The total leukocyte count is calculated using the following formula for counts performed using the eosinophil Unopette system:

Total WBC/μL

$$= \frac{\text{Number of cells stained in both sides of chamber} \times 1.1 \times 16 \times 100}{\text{percentage of granulocytes}}$$

If quantitative methods are unavailable, an estimated count can be determined from a well-made smear by averaging the number of leukocytes per high-power field for at least ten fields and multiplying by 2000. However, this method must be viewed as an estimate and may be useful only in cases of severe leukopenia or leukocytosis.

Total erythrocyte counts can be performed using an erythrocyte Unopette (Becton-Dickinson) system or an automated cell counter. Leukocytes and the nucleated erythrocytes will be counted together on automated impedance counters. Numbers of leukocytes are normally too low to make a significant impact on total erythrocyte numbers. Packed cell volume (PCV) may be obtained by the microhematocrit method. Hemoglobin concentration can be measured as for mammalian species, but it requires centrifugation to remove free erythrocyte nuclei following cell lysis. Thus, mean corpuscular volume (MCV), mean corpuscular hemoglobin (MCH), and MCH concentration (MCHC) can be calculated for avian species.[3]

A percentage of reticulocytes can be estimated using new methylene blue (NMB) staining method. Residual cytoplasmic RNA stains basophilic with NMB. A reticulocyte count of approximately 3% could be present in normal chickens. Higher percentages in the presence of anemia would indicate a regenerative response.

Thrombocyte quantitation is extremely difficult, and most methods result in an estimation at best. In some instances, thrombocytes are reported only as normal, increased, or decreased. Each oil immersion field observed when performing the differential count normally should have one or two thrombocytes.

HEMOPOIESIS

In chickens, embryonal mesenchyme gives rise to "blood islands" in the dorsal aorta and yolk sac that are detectable at 24 hours incubation. Avian erythrocytes arise from the endothelium of these blood islands. Thrombocytes are believed to arise similarly, but from a distinct mononuclear progenitor cell line other than megakaryocytic. Thus erythropoiesis, and probably thrombopoiesis, is intrasinusoidal or intravascular, whereas other cell lineages develop outside these vascu-

lar spaces.[4] Only erythrocytes, thrombocytes, and their precursors usually are found in the circulating blood of the chicken embryo, with the presence of leukocyte precursors being much less common. Most leukocytes and their precursors are retained in their hemopoietic compartments until shortly before hatch. Bone marrow, yolk sac, and spleen are the major sites of hemopoiesis, with the exception of lymphopoiesis, which occurs in the thymus and bursa. The yolk sac, which is rudimentary in mammals, is the primordial hemopoietic organ in the avian embryo and has its own limited hemopoietic stem cell population. The spleen is a significant hemopoietic organ in the avian embryo where granulopoiesis predominates.[5] Around the time of hatching, the spleen shifts to a lymphopoietic organ. Small islands of hemopoiesis, particularly around vascular spaces, also may be detected in virtually any tissue of the avian embryo, such as aorta, heart, pharynx, cranial nerves, spinal ganglia, subcutis, muscles, gonads, pancreas, and kidney.

After hatch, the bone marrow, particularly in long bones and vertebrae, is the major site of hemopoiesis in birds. Additional foci of hemopoiesis can occur in virtually any site, with the liver being most commonly involved.[6] Under the influence of estrogen, marrow spaces of long bones in maturing hens accumulate numerous spicules of woven bone, known as medullary bone, but this accumulation does not replace marrow elements.

The ultrastructural anatomy of embryonic and adult bone marrow in chickens is different from that of mammals.[4,7] Capillary branches from marrow arterioles empty into medullary sinuses. Unlike capillaries, these sinuses are lined by endothelium without a basement membrane. The endothelium is continuous with numerous intercellular junctions between immature erythrocytes and endothelial cells. This adherence to the endothelium is thought to play a role in preventing immature erythrocytes from entering the circulation and in regulating erythropoiesis. Thrombocyte precursors have not definitively been identified in avian bone marrow, presumably due to their fragility and subsequent loss during processing, but they also are believed to occur in the intravascular sinuses. Early thrombocyte precursors may be indistinguishable from erythrocyte precursors. Stem cells observed migrating through endothelium between intravascular and extravascular sinuses likely represent migration of the pluripotent stem cell to the extravascular sinus. Maturing granulocytes also migrate through the endothelium and may undergo final maturation intravascularly. Monocytogenesis is not apparent in avian marrow, and early monocyte precursors are likely indistinguishable from early granulocyte precursors. Macrophages are not prominent in avian bone marrow.

HEMOPOIETIC GROWTH FACTORS

There is limited knowledge of avian cytokines, with the vast majority of the work performed in chickens.[8,9]

TABLE 178.1 Hemopoietic Growth Factors of Chickens[8,9]

Cytokine	Source	Target	Activity
Erythropoietic stimulating factor	Serum of anemic chickens	CFU-E	Proliferation
IL-1	Chicken macrophage	T lymphocyte	Comitogen
IL-2	T lymphocytes	T lymphocytes	Proliferation
IL-8	Chicken fibroblasts	Heterophils	Chemotaxis
cMGF (myelomonocytic growth factor)	HD-11 (a chicken macrophage cell line), chicken serum	Myeloblasts, marrow	Colony formation
Lymphocyte inhibitory factor (MIF)	Chicken lymphocytes	Lymphocytes	Inhibits migration
Thrombocyte inhibitory factor	Chicken lymphocytes	Thrombocytes	Inhibits migration
Thrombocyte colony stimulating factor	Chicken spleen conditioned medium	Late thrombocyte precursors	Colony formation
Tumor necrosis factor-α	Chicken macrophage	Various	Cytolysis

TABLE 178.2 The Erythrocyte Maturation Sequence[29-31]

Cell Maturation Stage	Description
Rubriblast	Large cell, central round nuclei, granular chromatin, prominent nucleoli, very basophilic cytoplasm with mitochondrial spaces
Prorubricyte	Nucleoli and mitochondrial spaces inapparent
Basophilic rubricyte	Clumped chromatin pattern, very basophilic cytoplasm
Early polychromatic rubricyte	Cytoplasm becoming grayish, indicating hemoglobin production, chromatin more clumped, smaller nucleus
Late polychromatic rubricyte	More grayish to eosinophilic cytoplasm, clumped chromatin, small round nucleus
Polychromatic erythrocyte	Similar to mature erythrocytes but slightly larger with a more basophilic cytoplasm; should be 1–5% of circulating erythrocytes
Mature erythrocyte	Homogeneous eosinophilic cytoplasm, oval cell with central oval nucleus and condensed chromatin pattern

Current information regarding hemopoietic growth factors of chickens is shown in Table 178.1. In general, there is little to no cross-species effect of cytokines between chickens and mammalian species. The effect of cytokines isolated from chickens on cells from other avian species is not known.

ERYTHROCYTES

Erythrocyte precursors in the bone marrow are round cells that become oval as they mature. The maturation of erythrocytes is described in Table 178.2. Mature chicken and turkey erythrocytes found in the peripheral blood are large elliptical cells approximately $12 \times 6\ \mu$m. They have a homogeneous eosinophilic cytoplasm and a central round to oval nucleus with a condensed chromatin pattern. Because erythropoiesis is intravascular, occasional rubricytes rarely can be found in peripheral blood in healthy avian patients (Fig. 178.1). The percentage of reticulocytes seen in the peripheral blood of normal chickens and turkeys is somewhat higher than in most mammalian species. Polychromasia is more prominent in younger birds, but typically does not exceed 5%. Common artifactual abnormalities in erythrocyte morphology include cytoplasmic refractile vacuoles, smudge

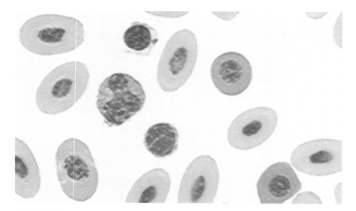

FIGURE 178.1 Thrombocyte with cytoplasmic azurophilic granule at one pole, two rubricytes, small lymphocyte, monocyte. Cells are identified in a clockwise manner.

cells, and various morphologies induced by stretching cells while preparing the smear, such as spindling, bilobed nuclei, and erythroplastids (anucleate fragments of erythrocyte cytoplasm).

Avian erythrocytes function similarly to mammalian erythrocytes with some notable biochemical differences.

TABLE 178.3   The Granulocytic Series Maturation Sequence[29–31]

Cell Maturation Stage	Description
Myeloblast	Large, round cell with rim of lightly basophilic cytoplasm around a large nucleus with a delicate chromatin pattern and nucleoli
Promyelocyte	Light blue cytoplasm, eccentric nucleus with delicate chromatin pattern, primary granules in cytoplasm are orange spheres, heterophil and basophil promyelocytes also have magenta granules and rings (smaller in basophil promyelocyte)
Myelocyte	Smaller, more condensed nucleus, contain less than half the definitive number of specific or secondary granules and still retain magenta granules and rings (except eosinophil myelocytes)
Metamyelocyte	Smaller, slightly indented nucleus, more than half the number of definitive granules
Band	Similar to mature cell without nuclear lobes; nucleus is elongate to U-shaped, rare to see bands in circulation in avian blood, usually see mature granulocytes only
Mature heterophil	Round cell with no cytoplasmic coloration, eosinophilic rod-shaped cytoplasmic granules with a distinct refractile central body, 2 to 3 lobbed nucleus with coarse chromatin often partially obscured by granules
Mature eosinophil	Round, similar to heterophil but granules more brightly eosinophilic (more arginine) and without central refractile body, cytoplasm usually pale blue
Mature basophil	Round cell with a round central nucleus, deeply basophilic cytoplasmic granules that may partially obscure the nucleus and dissolve or coalesce in alcohol solubilized stains like Wright's

The structure of avian hemoglobin, however, is similar to mammals. 2-3-bisphosphoglycerate is present only in chicken embryonal erythrocytes and disappears shortly after hatch. Myoinositol readily is taken up by erythrocyte precursors and converted to inositol pentaphosphate (IP5). IP5 and adenosine triphosphate (ATP) concentrations increase rapidly after hatch, with corresponding decreases in blood oxygen affinity due to IP5 binding to hemoglobin. The highest concentration of IP5 is in the mature erythrocyte, and this concentration does not change for the life of the cell regardless of requirements for oxygen.[10] Various degrees of IP5 binding result in a wide range of hemoglobin oxygen affinity among species. However, pH is a more important regulator of oxygen affinity. Decreasing pH results in decreasing oxygen affinity (Bohr effect), presumably linked to IP5 binding.[11] Carbon dioxide (CO_2) has a minimal effect on oxygen affinity because the efficient respiratory system of avian species is thought to maintain a very constant blood CO_2 level. Formation of bicarbonate from CO_2 and hydrogen ion release indirectly may regulate oxygen affinity.

GRANULOCYTIC CELLS

Granulocytes in the peripheral blood of chickens and turkeys include heterophils, eosinophils, and basophils. These cells arise from a common precursor in the bone marrow. Maturation of granulocytes is described in Table 178.3.

Heterophils

The heterophil is the predominant granulocyte in chickens and turkeys. The mature heterophil is a round cell approximately 13 μm in diameter. The cytoplasm is colorless with reddish-orange, rod-shaped cytoplasmic granules that often partially obscure the nucleus

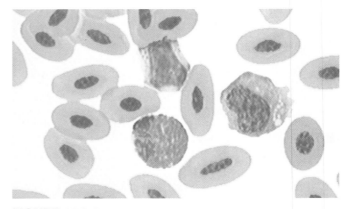

FIGURE 178.2 Medium lymphocyte with intracytoplasmic granules to left of nucleus, monocyte, and heterophil from a wild turkey. Cells are identified in a clockwise manner.

(Figs. 178.2 and 178.3). The nucleus has two to three lobes and a coarse chromatin pattern. Heterophil function parallels mammalian neutrophil function. However, differences in granule contents and response to some stimuli have been identified. Heterophils lack myeloperoxidase and alkaline phosphatase. Chicken and turkey heterophils, unlike neutrophils, do not respond to stimulation by formyl-methionyl-leucyl-phenylalanine (FMLP), and they only produce low amounts of detectable oxygen radicals.[12,13] Chicken heterophil bactericidal capabilities are similar to human and canine neutrophils, but phagocytosis capability and oxidant production are less than human and canine neutrophils.[12] Heterophil phagocytosis and killing are inefficient in post hatched chicks. In turkeys, heterophil functional maturity is reached by 14 to 21 days after hatch.[14] Cationic peptides with bactericidal capabilities (defensins) are found in chicken and turkey heterophils.[15] The largest (primary) granules contain lysozyme

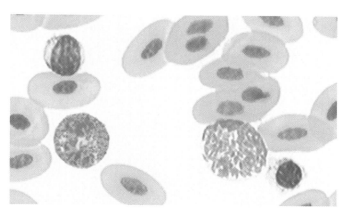

FIGURE 178.3 Lymphocyte, heterophil, thrombocyte, and eosinophil of a domestic chicken. Cells are identified in a clockwise manner.

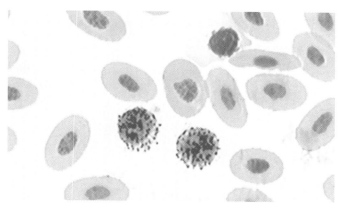

FIGURE 178.4 Thrombocyte and two basophils from a domestic chicken. Cells are identified in a clockwise manner.

and several cationic proteins, which are first detectable in the promyelocyte stage adjacent to the Golgi.

Eosinophils

These cells are round to irregularly shaped and are approximately 12 μm in diameter. They have a lobed nucleus and light blue cytoplasm with eosinophilic round to oval granules that stain brighter than those of heterophils do and lack the central body (Fig. 178.3). Immature heterophils have round granules and could be confused with eosinophils. Cytochemical stains can distinguish between the two types. Eosinophils are positive for peroxidase and acid phosphatase activity and Sudan black B, while heterophils are negative.[16] Eosinophils may participate in delayed type hypersensitivity reactions in birds,[17] but their importance in parasite immunity has not been established.

Basophils

Basophils are round cells approximately 12 μm in diameter with a round, central, light blue nucleus that is frequently partially obscured by the deeply basophilic cytoplasmic granules (Fig. 178.4). These granules may dissolve or coalesce in Wright's stains. Basophils are one of the first leukocytes to enter tissue as part of the early inflammatory response in birds.[18]

MONOCYTES

Chicken and turkey monocytes usually are the largest leukocytes (approximately 14 μm in diameter) on a peripheral blood smear and must be differentiated from large lymphocytes (Figs. 178.1 and 178.2). Monocytes are round cells with usually abundant blue-gray granular cytoplasm that can be vacuolated and contain a dusting of fine azurophilic granules. Their nuclei can be pleo-

morphic, ranging from round to oval to indented. Because of their varied appearances, monocytes can be the most difficult leukocyte to differentiate. Therefore, it is important to be consistent in their classification from lymphocytes when performing a leukocyte differential.

Chicken and turkey monocytes are similar to the mammalian cells. Monocytes from turkeys and chickens are capable of oxidative activity, as well as phagocytosis and killing (as in mammalian species); chicken monocytes also produce reactive nitrogen intermediates.[19] As with chicken heterophils, the degree of measured oxidant production of monocytes may be less than in mammalian species or produced via a different pathway.[20] Heterophils from chickens and turkeys have greater phagocytosis and killing activities than do monocytes.[21] The role of avian monocytes in antitumor and antimicrobial immunity is not well defined. Because birds are uricotelic, there is no de novo synthesis of L-arginine as in the mammalian urea cycle, and this amino acid is required in birds for the production of these intermediates. The monocyte maturation series is described in Table 178.4.

LYMPHOCYTES

Lymphocytes are the predominant leukocyte in the peripheral blood of chickens and turkeys. Both small and medium lymphocytes normally occur. The small lymphocytes are round with a round nucleus, clumped chromatin, high nuclear:cytoplasmic (N:C) ratio, and a rim or small amount of basophilic cytoplasm (Figs. 178.1 and 178.3). Occasionally the cytoplasm of small lymphocytes may only be seen as cytoplasmic projections, and they may be confused with thrombocytes. Thrombocytes can be distinguished by their clear cytoplasm. Medium lymphocytes have more abundant and sometimes more pale basophilic cytoplasm. They often "mold" around adjacent cells. Lymphocytes may have nuclear indentation, and sometimes larger lymphocytes may have more an-

TABLE 178.4 The Monocyte Maturation Sequence[29-31]	
Cell Maturation Stage	Description
Monoblast	A poorly defined cell, probably indistinguishable from the myeloblast
Early promonocyte	Large cells with abundant, clear blue cytoplasm, round nucleus, reticular chromatin
Late promonocyte	Round, eccentric nucleus with granular basophilic cytoplasm, sparse eosinophilic granules
Mature monocyte	Large and irregular with a round to bilobed nucleus, fine chromatin pattern, abundant blue-gray granular cytoplasm, and occasional cytoplasmic vacuoles and/or fine dust-like eosinophilic granules

gular nuclei or nuclei with a flattened side. Medium to large lymphocytes must be distinguished from monocytes. Monocytes have slightly more basophilic cytoplasm and sometimes fine eosinophilic granules (Figs. 178.1 and 178.2).

Reactive lymphocytes can be seen in peripheral blood. Cell size is increased and the cytoplasm is deeply basophilic, sometimes with a clear perinuclear area (Golgi). Plasma cells may only rarely be found in peripheral blood. Reactive lymphocytes are differentiated from plasma cells by their central nucleus. Reactive lymphocytes may also resemble rubricytes; however, rubricytes have a lower N:C ratio and are typically seen in peripheral blood with polychromatophilic erythrocytes in regenerative responses. The presence of eosinophilic (azurophilic) granules in peripheral blood lymphocytes is rare, and its significance is unknown (Fig. 178.2). It is possible that these cells could represent natural killer (NK) cells, but NK cells have yet to be identified definitively in the peripheral blood of chickens or turkeys. These cells are readily distinguished from monocytes, because lymphocyte azurophilic granules are larger and more intensely staining than the dust-like granules of monocytes.

Lymphocyte stem cells colonize the thymus and bursa of Fabricius (for which the B lymphocyte is named) at approximately 10 to 15 days embryonization in chickens. The thymus reaches maximum size around 16 weeks of age, the bursa reaches maximum size around 4 to 12 weeks of age, and then slowly regress.[22] The bursa is completely regressed by sexual maturity, and the thymus is completely regressed soon after sexual maturity in chickens. Variable numbers of periarteriolar lymphocytes have been described in avian bone marrow, usually increasing with age. In the authors' experience lymphocytes in the bone marrow of healthy chickens are infrequent.

THROMBOCYTES

Chicken and turkey thrombocytes are round to slightly oval cells with a round nucleus in the center of a clear cytoplasm. Small lymphocytes may resemble thrombocytes but can be differentiated by the blue-staining cytoplasm of lymphocytes. Thrombocytes stain positively with the periodic acid-Schiff and Grimelius staining methods.[23] Frequently one or more distinct small granules are present at the poles of the thrombocyte (Fig. 178.1). Thrombocytes can readily phagocytose colloidal carbon and may have a phagocytic role as well as a hemostatic role.[24] A C3b-like receptor and analogs to mammalian platelet glycoproteins IIb and IIIa have been identified in chicken thrombocytes.[25] Nuclear retention in avian thrombocytes may result in continued ability of the mature cell to synthesize proteins. Unlike mammalian platelets, chicken thrombocytes have been shown to be capable of synthesizing new molecules in vitro.[25] Similar to mammalian platelets, avian thrombocytes have fibrinogen receptors that localize when thrombocytes are activated, facilitating thrombocyte aggregation.[26] The thrombocytic maturation series is described in Table 178.5.

NORMAL REFERENCE INTERVALS FOR CHICKENS AND TURKEYS

Total erythrocyte numbers are approximately 3 million per microliter, or a PCV of 25 to 42%. Chicks typically have a lower PCV (as low as 24%) that increases with age. The MCV has been reported in the range of 90 to 140 fL.[3] Chicks tend to have fewer, larger erythrocytes. Hemoglobin concentrations of chickens and turkeys have been reported from 8.6 to 15.2 gm/dL.[2] Variation in erythrocyte parameters may reflect different lines of chickens and turkeys and different methods of determination. Erythrocyte life span is 28 to 35 days in chickens.[2]

Early data showed PCV to be lower in heavy-type (30.1% to 30.9%) than in leghorn type (31.9% to 33.9%) chickens.[27] More recent hematology data of chickens are shown in Tables 178.6, 178.7, and 178.8. Mean hematocrits from specific pathogen-free leghorn chicks of 5 to 42 days of age ranged from 32.7 to 36.7%, respectively.[28]

Limited hematologic data are available for domestic turkeys (Table 178.9), and that available is similar to reference intervals for 4-month-old wild turkeys (Table 178.10). As in chickens, studies have shown that differences exist in hematologic parameters of closed genetic lines and different commercial lines of turkeys.[29] Large body birds bred for meat production had lower lymphocyte counts, higher heterophil counts, and higher total erythrocyte counts than lines bred for egg production.

TABLE 178.5   The Thrombocyte Maturation Sequence[30-32]

Cell Maturation Stage	Description
Thromboblast	Large, ameboid cells with a rim of very basophilic cytoplasm around a large nucleus with punctate chromatin (chromatin is not coarse as in the rubriblast), nucleolus not always apparent, some clear vacuoles within cytoplasm
Early immature thrombocyte	Slightly lower N:C than thromboblast, more cytoplasmic vacuoles evident; chromatin becomes clumped
Mid immature thrombocyte	Oval, pale blue vacuolated cytoplasm, occasional eosinophilic granules, very clumped chromatin
Late immature thrombocyte	Oval, smaller than an erythrocyte, pale blue cytoplasm with much cytoplasmic clearing, eosinophilic granules at one pole of the cell
Thrombocyte	Round to slightly oval, smaller than an erythrocyte, high N:C ratio, dense clumped chromatin, and clear cytoplasm occasionally with sparse distinct eosinophilic granules

TABLE 178.6   Hematologic Values for the Chicken (*Gallus gallus domesticus*)[3]

Parameter	Interval
Erythrocytes/μL	2,500,000–3,500,000
Hemoglobin (g/dL)	7–13
PCV %	22–35
MCV (fL)	90–140
MCH (pg)	33–47
MCHC (%)	26–35
Reticulocytes (%)	0–0.6
Leukocytes/μL	12,000–30,000
Heterophil (band)	Rare
Heterophil	3000–6000
Lymphocyte	7000–17,500
Monocyte	150–2000
Eosinophil	0–1000
Basophil	Rare

TABLE 178.7   Reference Intervals for Leukocytes From Healthy 22- to 24-Week-Old Male Broiler-Type Chickens (N = 89)

Cell Type	Reference Interval
Leukocytes/μL	7940–24,280
Heterophils	1703–9746
Lymphocytes	2639–10,294
Monocytes	544–4123
Eosinophils	0–346
Basophils	382–2499

From DI Bounous, J Wilson, unpublished data, University of Georgia, 1995.

TABLE 178.8   Leukocyte Values From 10-Day-Old Broiler Breeder Chicks (N = 10)[33]

Cell Type	Values
Leukocytes/μL	25.19 ± 5.01
Heterophils	7.19 ± 3.39
Lymphocytes	13.86 ± 1.58
Monocytes	1.94 ± 1.01
Eosinophils	0.64 ± 0.92
Basophils	1.56 ± 0.25

TABLE 178.9   Hematologic Values for 3-Week-Old Domestic Turkeys (N = 24)[34]

Parameter	Value
Hemoglobin	9.14 gm/dL
Hematocrit	30.8%
MCV	164 μm
MCH	42.6 pg
MCHC	29.6%

TABLE 178.10   Reference Intervals for Healthy Wild Turkey Poults (*Meleagris gallopova* subspecies *silvestris*) (N = 48)[35]

Parameter	Reference Interval
PCV %	30–41.5
Leukocytes/μL	13,917–46,609
Heterophils	4046–24,231
Lymphocytes	4156–31,138
Monocytes	0–3756
Eosinophils	0–420
Basophils	23–2039

REFERENCES

1. **Forster CA, Sampson SD, Chiappe LM, Krause DW.** The Theropod ancestry of birds: new evidence from the late cretaceous of Madagascar. Science 1998;279:1915–1919.
2. **Sturkie PD.** Body fluids: blood. In: Sturkie PD, ed. Avian physiology. New York: Springer-Verlag, 1986;102–120.
3. **Zinkl JG.** Avian hematology. In: Jain NC, ed. Schalm's veterinary hematology. 4th ed. Philadelphia: Lea & Febiger, 1986;256–273.
4. **Campbell F.** Fine structure of the bone marrow of the chicken and pigeon. J Morphol 1967;123:405–440.
5. **Nicolas-Bolnet C, Yassine F, Cormier F, Dieterlien-Lievre F.** Developmental kinetics of hematopoietic progenitors in the avian spleen Exp Cell Res 1991;16:294–301.
6. **Barnes HJ.** Hemic system. In: Ridell C, ed. Avian histopathology. 2nd ed. Kennett Square, PA: American Association of Avian Pathologists, 1996;1–16.
7. **Sorrell JM, Weiss L.** Intercellular junctions in the hematopoietic compartments of embryonal chicken bone marrow. Am J Anat 1982;164:57–66.
8. **Klasing KC.** Avian leukocytic cytokines. Poult Sci 1994;73:1035–1043.
9. **Sharma JM.** Avian immunology. In: Pastoret P-P, ed. Handbook of vertebrate immunology. Bath, England: Academic Press, 1998;73–137.
10. **Isaacks RE, Lai LL, Kim CY, Goldman PH, Kim HD.** Studies on avian erythrocyte metabolism. XVII. Kinetics and transport properties of myo-inositol in chicken reticulocytes. Arch Biochem Biophys 1989;274:564–573.
11. **Isaacks R, Goldman P, Kim C.** Studies on avian erythrocyte metabolism XIV. Effect of carbon dioxide and pH on P50 in chickens. Am J Physiol 1986;250:R260–R266.
12. **Brooks RL, Bounous DI, Andreasen CB.** Functional comparison of avian heterophils with human and canine neutrophils. Comp Haem Int 1996;6:153–159.
13. **Kogut MH, Holtzapple C, Lowry VK, Stanker LH.** Functional responses of neonatal chicken and turkey heterophils following stimulation by inflammatory agonists. Am J Vet Res 1998;59:1404–1408.
14. **Lowry VK, Genovese KJ, Bowen LL, Kogut MH.** Ontogeny of the phagocytic and bactericidal activities of turkey heterophils and their potentiation by *Salmonella enteriditis* immune lymphokines. FEMS Immunol Med Microbiol 1997;19:95–100.
15. **Evans EW, Beach GG, Wunderlich J, Harmon BG.** Isolation of microbial peptides from avian heterophils. J Leuk Biol 1995;56:661–665.
16. **Andreasen CB, Latimer KS.** Cytochemical staining characteristics of chicken heterophils and eosinophils. Vet Clin Pathol 1990;19:51–54.
17. **Maxwell MH.** Histochemical identification of tissue eosinophils in the inflammatory response of the fowl (*Gallus domesticus*). Res Vet Sci 1984;37:7–11.
18. **Katiyar AK, Vegrad JL, Awadhiya RP.** Pathology of inflammatory-reparative response in punched wounds of the chicken skin. Avian Pathol 1992;21:471–480.
19. **Sung YJ, Hotchkiss JH, Austic RE, Dietert RR.** L-arginine dependent production of a reactive nitrogen intermediate by macrophages of a uricotelic species. J Leukoc Biol 1991;50:49–56.
20. **Van Nerom A, Desmidt M, Ducatelle R, Haesebrouck F.** Lucigenin- and luminol-enhanced chemiluminescence in turkey monocytes. J Biolumin Chemilumin 1997;12:207–214.
21. **Stabler JG, McCormick TW, Powell KC, Kogut MH.** Avian heterophils and monocytes: phagocytic and bactericidal activities against Salmonella enteritidis. Vet Microbiol 1994;38:293–305.
22. **Pope CR.** Lymphoid system. In: Ridell C, ed. Avian histopathology avian histopathology. 2nd ed. Kennett Square, PA: American Association of Avian Pathologists, 1996;17–44.
23. **Swayne DE, Stockham SL, Johnson GS.** Cytochemical properties of chicken blood cells resembling both thrombocytes and lymphocytes. Vet Clin Pathol 1996;15:17–24.
24. **Grecci R, Saliba AM, Mariano M.** Morphologic changes, surface receptors, and phagocytic potential of fowl mononuclear phagocytes and thrombocytes *in vivo* and *in vitro.* J Pathol 1980;130:23–31.
25. **Kunicki T, Newman PJ.** Synthesis of analogs of human platelet membrane glycoprotein IIb-IIIa complex by chicken peripheral blood thrombocytes. Proc Natl Acad Sci USA 1985;82:7319–7323.
26. **O'Toole ET, Hantgan RR, Lewis JC.** Location of fibrinogen during aggregation of avian thrombocytes. Exp Mol Pathol 1994;61:175–190.
27. **Washburn KW, Guill RA.** Comparison of hematology between leghorn-type and heavy type production stocks. Poult Sci 1971;51:946–950.
28. **Bounous DI, Goodwin MA, Brooks RL, Lamichhane CM, Campagnoli RP, Brown J, Snyder DB.** Immunosuppression and intracellular calcium signaling in splenocytes from chicks infected with chicken anemia virus, C1-isolate. Avian Dis 1995;39:135–140.
29. **Bayyari GR, Huff WE, Rath NC, Balog JM, Newberry LA, Villines JD, Skeeles JK, Anthony NB, Nestor KE.** Effect of the genetic selection of turkeys for increased body weight and egg production on immune and physiologic responses. Poult Sci 1997;76:289–296.
30. **Campbell TW.** Hematology. In: Ritchie BW, Harrison GJ, Harrison LR, eds. Avian medicine: principles and applications. Lake Worth: Wingers Publishing, 1994;176–198.
31. **Campbell TW.** Avian hematology and cytology. 2nd ed. Ames, IA: Iowa State University Press, 1995;3–34.
32. **Lucas AM, Jamroz C.** Atlas of avian hematology. Agricultural monograph 25.271. Washington, DC: United States Department of Agriculture, 1961.
33. **Bartholomew A, Latshaw D, Swayne DE.** Changes in blood chemistry, hematology, and histology caused by a selenium / vitamin E deficiency and recovery in chicks. Biol Trace Elem Res 1998;62:7–16.
34. **Kubena LF, Edrington TS, Kamps-Holtzapple C, Harvey RB, Elissalde MH, Rottinghaus GE.** Effects of feeding fumonisin B₁ present in Fusarium moniliforme culture material and aflatoxin singly and in combination to turkey poults. Poult Sci 1995;74:1295–1303.
35. **Bounous DI, Wyatt RF, Quist CF.** Normal hematologic and serum biochemical and K. E. intervals for juvenile wild turkeys (*Meleagris gallopova* subspecies *silvestris*) J Wildl Dis 2000, in press.

SUGGESTED READINGS

Glick B. Immunophysiology. In: Sturkie PD, ed. Avian physiology. New York: Springer-Verlag, 1986;87–101.

MacRae EK, Powell RE. Cytochemical reaction for cationic proteins as a marker of primary granules during development in chicken heterophils. Histochemistry 1979;60:295–308.

Samarut J, Bouabelli M. In vitro development of CFU-E and BFU-E in cultures of embryonic and post embryonic hematopoietic cells. J Cell Physiol 1980;105:553–563.

CHAPTER 179

Normal Hematology of Psittacines

• TERRY W. CAMPBELL

The blood of psittacine birds contains nucleated erythrocytes, nucleated thrombocytes, heterophils, eosinophils, basophils, lymphocytes, and monocytes. The blood of various species of psittacine birds is similar in many respects and exhibits only minor differences. Normal hematologic values for psittacine birds determined by different laboratories can vary significantly. This variation is caused by differences in blood sampling and analytic techniques. Other factors that influence the hematologic results include age, gender, anesthesia, nutrition, environmental conditions, physiologic status, and genetic factors (species) of psittacine birds used to establish normal blood values.

HEMATOLOGIC EXAMINATION

Blood from psittacine birds for hematologic examination is commonly collected by venipuncture of the jugular, medial metatarsal, basilic, or brachial veins. Ethylene-diamine-tetraacetic acid (EDTA) is the anticoagulant of choice for avian hematology because it allows proper staining of the cells and does not tend to clump leukocytes.[1–3] Lithium heparin has the advantage of providing anticoagulated blood for hematology and plasma for blood chemistry evaluations. However, heparinized blood may result in improper staining of cells resulting in erroneous leukocyte counts and poor cellular morphology in stained blood films.[1–3] Heparin also causes clumping of leukocytes and thrombocytes and resultant inaccurate cell counts. Blood films can be made using a variety of techniques; with proper attention to technique, cell disruption is minimized while maintaining good cellular distribution with monolayered areas for examination.[1,4–7]

The laboratory evaluation of psittacine blood involves the same routine procedures used for mammalian hematology with a few modifications. Hemoglobin concentration is determined by the cyanmethemoglobin method with one modification: the free nuclei from lysed erythrocytes must be removed by centrifugation of the cyanmethemoglobin reagent-blood mixture before obtaining the optical density value to avoid an overestimation of the hemoglobin concentration.

The presence of nucleated erythrocytes and thrombocytes in avian blood interferes with automated methods for counting white blood cells. Also, the size of erythrocytes is similar to the size of many of the leukocytes; thrombocytes and small lymphocytes are also similar in size. Therefore, direct and semidirect manual methods for obtaining total leukocyte concentrations in birds have been developed.[8–12] Accurate interpretation of leukocyte counts, especially when determined by the semidirect method, is dependent on accurate identification and differentiation of leukocytes in the stained blood film.

The thrombocyte concentration of most psittacine species studied ranges between 20,000 and 30,000 per mm^3 of blood, or 10 to 15 thrombocytes per 1000 erythrocytes.[1,13] An actual thrombocyte concentration is difficult to determine because thrombocytes tend to clump. Therefore, their concentration is often reported as normal, increased, or decreased based on estimates from peripheral blood films. Approximately one to five thrombocytes can be seen in a monolayer 1000× (oil immersion) field in a blood film from a normal bird, unless thrombocytes clump excessively on preparation.

ERYTHROCYTES

Mature psittacine erythrocytes are elliptical with an elliptical, centrally positioned nucleus. Nuclear chromatin is uniformly clumped and becomes increasingly condensed with cellular age. In Wright's stained blood films, the nucleus stains purple while the cytoplasm appears orange-pink with a uniform texture. Mature psittacine erythrocytes vary in size depending on the species; in most species, erythrocyte shape is relatively uniform. Polychromatophilic erythrocytes occur in low numbers (usually less than 5% of erythrocytes) in the peripheral blood of most normal birds. Determination of reticulocyte concentration can be made by staining erythrocytes with a vital stain, such as new methylene blue.[1,3]

Atypical erythrocytes are occasionally present in the peripheral blood of normal birds and may represent artifacts associated with blood film preparation; when observed in significant numbers, they indicate disorders affecting avian erythrocytes. The degree of polychromasia and reticulocytosis and the presence of immature erythrocytes in the peripheral blood aid in the assessment of red blood cell regeneration. The presence of a large number of hypochromatic erythrocytes is indicative of an erythrocyte disorder, such as iron deficiency and iron sequestration with infectious diseases.

A slight variation in the size of erythrocytes is considered normal for psittacine birds. A greater degree of anisocytosis is usually observed in birds with regenerative anemia and associated with polychromasia. Likewise, minor deviations from the normal shape of psittacine erythrocytes are considered normal in the peripheral blood of birds. However, marked poikilocytosis may indicate erythrocytic dysgenesis. Round erythrocytes with oval nuclei are occasionally found in the blood films of anemic birds and suggest a dysmaturation of the cell cytoplasm and nucleus, which may be a result of accelerated erythropoiesis.

Anucleated erythrocytes (erythroplastids) or cytoplasmic fragments are occasionally found in normal avian blood films. Mitotic activity associated with erythrocytes in blood films suggests a marked regenerative response or erythrocytic dyscrasia. Binucleate erythrocytes rarely occur in blood films of normal birds; however, the presence of large numbers of binucleated erythrocytes plus other features of red blood cell dyscrasia is suggestive of neoplastic, viral, or genetic disease.[14]

LEUKOCYTES

Leukocytes in normal psittacine birds are released into the peripheral circulation only when mature. The leukocytes in the peripheral blood film include lymphocytes, monocytes, and granulocytes. The granulocytes are classified as heterophils, eosinophils, and basophils.

Heterophils are the most abundant leukocyte in the peripheral blood of most psittacine birds in most studies, whereas lymphocytes are the most abundant in others (Tables 179.1 and 179.2). This may be a reflection of the variation associated with differences in the interpretation of the leukocyte differential among laboratories. The cytoplasm of normal mature heterophils appears colorless and contains eosinophilic granules (dark orange to brown red) with Romanowsky stains. The cytoplasmic granules are typically elongate (rod or spiculated-shaped) but may appear oval to round in some species. Heterophil granules frequently have a distinct central body that appears refractile and usually hide the partially lobed nucleus. Most psittacine eosinophils are the same size as heterophils but have round, strongly eosinophilic cytoplasmic granules. In general, eosinophil granules stain more intensely than heterophil granules. The cytoplasmic granules of eosinophils lack the central refractile body seen in many avian heterophils. The cytoplasm of eosinophils stains clear blue in contrast to the colorless cytoplasm of normal mature heterophils. The nucleus of eosinophils is lobed and usually stains darker than heterophil nuclei. The cyto-

plasmic granules of psittacine eosinophils stained with Romanowsky stains vary in appearance; granules may appear large, swollen, and round and may appear colorless or stain pale blue.

Basophils of psittacine birds contain deeply metachromic granules that often obscure the nucleus. The nucleus is usually nonlobed, causing the basophils to resemble mammalian mast cells.

Monocytes in peripheral blood films of psittacine birds are typically the largest leukocyte and resemble their mammalian counterparts.

As mentioned previously, some studies indicate lymphocytes are the most abundant leukocyte in the peripheral blood of normal psittacine birds, while most suggest heterophils are the most abundant leukocyte. This variation may be associated with differences in the interpretation of the leukocyte differential among laboratories. Lymphocytes of psittacine birds resemble mammalian lymphocytes. The lymphocyte cytoplasm usually appears homogenous and weakly basophilic (pale blue) and lacks vacuoles and granules. Cytoplasmic features are important when differentiating small lymphocytes from thrombocytes. The latter have clear, colorless cytoplasm that often appears vacuolated with a few distinct specific granules. Occasionally, cells in blood films of birds have features of both thrombocytes and lymphocytes. These intermediate cells have small, round to oval nuclei with coarsely clumped chromatin and moderately abundant blue-tinged cytoplasm that lacks vacuoles and granules. Cytochemical properties indicate these cells to be lymphocytes.[15] Occasionally, lymphocytes may contain distinct azurophilic granules or irregular cytoplasmic projections.

Abnormal appearing heterophils in blood films include both immature and toxic heterophils.[1,6,7] Immature heterophils have increased cytoplasmic basophilia, nonsegmented nuclei, and immature cytoplasmic granules when compared with normal mature heterophils. Immature heterophils most frequently encountered in the blood are myelocytes and metamyelocytes. Abnormal psittacine lymphocytes are classified as reactive or blast-transformed lymphocytes. Plasma cells can also be found in the peripheral blood of psittacine birds.

THROMBOCYTES

Thrombocytes are nucleated cells found in the peripheral blood of psittacine birds. Mature thrombocytes tend to be oval cells with a round to oval nucleus that contains densely clumped chromatin. The nucleus is more rounded than an erythrocyte nucleus, and thrombocytes have a high nucleus to cytoplasm (N:C) ratio. Normal mature thrombocytes have a colorless to pale gray cytoplasm that often has a reticulated appearance. Thrombocytes frequently contain one or more distinct eosinophilic granules usually located in one area of the cytoplasm. Thrombocytes aggregated in clumps show degranulation of specific granules, cellular degeneration, and nuclear pyknosis.

Avian thrombocytes are derived from mononuclear precursors in the bone marrow, and occasionally imma-

TABLE 179.1   Hematology Values for Selected Juvenile Hand-Raised Psittacine Birds [Mean ± Standard Deviation and Range]

	Cockatoos (*Cacatua* sp.)[a]	Macaws (*Ara* sp.)[b]	Eclectus parrot[c]
RBC [$\times 10^6/\mu$L]	2.53 ± 0.63 [1.5–4.0]	2.9 ± 0.8 [1.5–4.5]	2.69 ± 0.67 [1.5–4.0]
PCV [%]	39.7 ± 9.0 [25–59]	41.7 ± 8.4 [25–55]	43.8 ± 8.4 [26–58]
Hb [g/dL]	11.4 ± 2.9 [6.5–17.0]	12.3 ± 3.3 [7–17]	12.46 ± 3.01 [6.5–18]
MCV [fL]	160 ± 23 [210–215]	149 ± 24.7 [112–200]	166 ± 26 [125–215]
MCHC [g/dL]	27.2 ± 6.1 [24–33]	28.7 ± 2.9 [22.5–35.0]	27.7 ± 5.0 [23–32]
WBC [$\times 10^3/\mu$L]	12.9 ± 6.3 [5.5–25.0]	19.2 ± 6.9 [7–30]	13.7 ± 6.3 [5.5–25.0]
Band heterophils [%]	1.3 ± 2.3 [0–7]	0.6 ± 1.7 [0–5]	0.5 ± 1.5 [0–5]
[$\times 10^3/\mu$L]	0.16 ± 0.33 [0–1.4]	0.11 ± 0.31 [0–1.0]	0.07 ± 0.22 [0–1.0]
Heterophils [%]	50.8 ± 11.7 [27–74]	55.3 ± 10 [37–75]	53.9 ± 11.4 [35–75]
[$\times 10^3/\mu$L]	6.5 ± 4.5 [2.0–18.0]	10.1 ± 5.8 [3.0–20.0]	7.7 ± 4.8 [4.4–17.0]
Lymphocytes [%]	41.2 ± 11.9 [17–65]	39.0 ± 10 [20–60]	39.5 ± 11.5 [20–65]
[$\times 10^3/\mu$L]	4.9 ± 2.5 [1.8–10.0]	6.8 ± 3.2 [3.0–13.0]	5.1 ± 2.0 [2.5–10.0]
Monocytes [%]	5.8 ± 3.4 [0–12]	4.4 ± 2.9 [1–10]	5.0 ± 2.7 [1–11]
[$\times 10^3/\mu$L]	0.69 ± 0.53 [0–2.0]	0.75 ± 0.55 [0.2–14.0]	0.64 ± 0.43 [0–2.0]
Eosinophils [%]	0	0 ± 0.2 [0–1]	0.1 ± 0.3 [0–1]
[$\times 10^3/\mu$L]	0	0.05 ± 0.04 [0–0.28]	0 ± 0.4 [0–0.3]
Basophils [%]	0.9 ± 1.1 [0–4]	0.5 ± 1.0 [0–3]	1.1 ± 1.0 [0–3]
[$\times 10^3/\mu$L]	0.1 ± 0.14 [0–0.5]	0.09 ± 0.18 [0–0.6]	0.15 ± 0.17 [0–0.5]

[a] Modified from Clubb SL, et al. Hematologic and serum biochemical reference intervals in juvenile cockatoos. J Assoc Avian Vet 1991;5:16–26.
[b] Modified from Clubb SL, et al. Hematologic and serum biochemical reference intervals in juvenile macaws [*Ara* sp]. J Assoc Avian Vet 1991;5:154–162.
[c] Modified from Clubb SL, et al. Hematologic and serum biochemical reference intervals in juvenile eclectus parrots [*Eclectus roratus*]. J Assoc Avian Vet 1991;4:218–225.

ture thrombocytes are present in the peripheral blood of normal birds. They are larger, round to oval cells with round to oval nuclei and basophilic cytoplasm compared with mature thrombocytes. The mid-immature and late-immature thrombocytes are most commonly seen when immature cells are present.

HEMOPOIETIC FEATURES

The normal myeloid:erythroid (M:E) ratio of psittacine birds is presumed to be 1.0 : 1.0. Increased erythropoiesis is indicated by an increase in polychromasia (reticulocytes) in the blood and bone marrow films. A significant increase in erythropoiesis would reveal a decrease in the M:E ratio with a normal heterophil concentration in the peripheral blood. An anemic psittacine bird with a normal peripheral blood heterophil concentration, little or no polychromasia, and an increased M:E ratio has a decrease in erythropoiesis. Erythroid dysplasia in the peripheral blood film and a marked decrease in the M:E ratio in the bone marrow indicate a myelodysplastic disorder with erythroid predominance. Increased granulopoiesis is usually indicated by a peripheral heterophilia and an increased bone marrow M:E ratio. A decrease in peripheral blood heterophil concentration and bone marrow M:E ratio indicates a decrease in granulopoiesis. Myeloid leukemia exhibits increased numbers of myeloid blast cells in the peripheral blood and bone marrow M:E ratios.

HEMATOLOGIC RESPONSES

The packed cell volume (PCV) is the quickest and most practical method for evaluating the red cell mass of psittacine birds. The normal PCV of many species of psittacine birds ranges between 35 and 55%. Therefore, a PCV less than 35% suggests anemia and a PCV greater than 55% suggests dehydration or erythrocytosis (polycythemia). The latter condition can be differentiated by the total serum protein; increased total protein indicates dehydration, while normal or low total protein supports erythrocytosis.

Typically, polychromatic erythrocytes make up 5% or less of the erythrocyte population in blood films from normal birds. The degree of erythrocyte polychromasia and reticulocytosis is an indication of the degree of erythrogenesis. Other evidence of active erythropoiesis is the presence of binucleate immature erythrocytes and an increase in the number of normal immature erythrocytes in the peripheral blood. However, in cases of nonanemic birds, these cells indicate abnormal erythropoiesis. Immature erythrocytes may also suggest early release from the hematopoietic tissue following anoxic insult or toxicity.

The causes of anemia in psittacine birds include blood loss (hemorrhagic anemia), increased red cell destruction (hemolytic anemia), and decreased red cell production (depression anemia). The most common causes of hemorrhagic anemia in psittacine birds include traumatic injury and hemorrhagic lesions of internal organs, such as ulcerated neoplasms and gastric ulcerations. Heavy infestation with blood-sucking ectoparasites or gastrointestinal parasites and coagulopathies associated with toxicities or severe liver disease are less common causes of blood loss anemia in psittacine birds.[16–19] Hemolytic anemia can result from parasitemias, septicemia, and toxicities. Although rare, immune-mediated anemia may result in hemolysis with red cell agglutination present in the blood film.[3,20] A nonregenerative,

TABLE 179.2 Hematology Values for Selected Juvenile Captive Psittacine Birds [Mean ± Standard Deviation and Range]

	White Cockatoo (Cacatua alba)	Red Lory (Eos bornea)	Blue-fronted Amazon (Amazona aestiva)	Orange-winged Amazon (Amazona amazonica)	Scarlet Macaw (Ara macao)	Green-winged Macaw (Ara chloroptera)	Military Macaw (Ara militaris)	Blue and Gold Macaw (Ara ararauna)	Patagonian Conure (Cyanoliseu spatagonus)	African Grey Parrot (Psittacus erithacus)
RBC [×10⁶/µL]	2.98 ± 0.19 [2.75–3.2]	3.17 ± 0.49 [2.62–4.72]	2.92 ± 0.55 [2.11–3.53]	3.08 ± 0.20 [2.81–3.32]	3.07 ± 0.43 [2.29–3.67]	3.20 ± 0.38 [2.65–4.05]	3.44 ± 0.59 [2.72–5.16]	3.24 ± 0.50 [2.11–4.10]	3.54 ± 0.32 [3.16–4.09]	3.47 ± 0.41 [2.96–4.03]
PCV [%]	44.8 ± 4.4 [37.0–48.0]	48.8 ± 3.2 [44.0–54.0]	50.6 ± 6.2 [43.5–58.0]	48.4 ± 2.2 [46.0–51.0]	47.4 ± 4.4 [40.0–54.0]	46.1 ± 3.8 [39.0–54.0]	47.1 ± 4.3 [37.0–54.5]	44.6 ± 4.6 [31.5–51.8]	47.6 ± 3.1 [45.0–52.0]	46.4 ± 5.3 [32.0–54.0]
Hb [g/dL]	15.7 ± 1.9 [13.9–18.4]	16.0 ± 1.4 [14.2–18.7]	17.3 ± 0.9 [16.0–18.4]	16.3 ± 0.8 [15.5–17.5]	16.4 ± 2.2 [13.1–19.9]	13.6 ± 2.8 [9.6–18.7]	15.6 ± 2.3 [11.1–19.6]	14.4 ± 1.2 [11.7–17.0]	15.0 ± 0.8 [14.3–16.2]	15.4 ± 3.4 [10.7–21.7]
MCV [fL]	150.7 ± 14.3 [132–171]	155.9 ± 13.7 [111–172]	180.0 ± 19.7 [163–209]	157.6 ± 5.9 [151–166]	151.6 ± 10.7 [135–169]	145.0 ± 13.9 [116–177]	137.0 ± 16.0 [106–173]	141.0 ± 21.4 [102–199]	134.6 ± 7.1 [127–146]	137.7 ± 17.1 [106–166]
MCHC [g/dL]	33.5 ± 4.0 [30.0–39.2]	32.9 ± 1.0 [31.2–35.6]	34.3 ± 2.6 [31.7–37.8]	33.7 ± 1.5 [32.1–36.0]	34.4 ± 2.2 [29.7–37.3]	29.6 ± 4.6 [21.9–34.9]	33.5 ± 2.5 [33.9–40.7]	32.7 ± 3.4 [28.1–43.5]	31.6 ± 0.5 [30.9–32.3]	32.2 ± 5.4 [24.8–43.4]
WBC [×10³/µL]	6.7 ± 7.5 [1.3–18.7]	3.3 ± 2.2 [0.8–9.0]	6.5 ± 2.4 [4.7–11.0]	6.1 ± 3.8 [1.2–10.1]	9.8 ± 4.5 [4.7–22.0]	16.9 ± 8.9 [3.8–30.0]	9.5 ± 4.5 [13.7–18.0]	16.6 ± 9.0 [1.7–36.0]	5.8 ± 2.1 [2.5–8.7]	9.0 ± 3.6 [29.4–83.0]
Heterophils [%]	45.1 ± 28.5 [17.6–83.0]	55.2 ± 17.4 [25.6–79.2]	30.7 ± 15.0 [12.4–46.6]	36.2 ± 7.2 [21.9–40.7]	39.9 ± 13.0 [26.0–67.0]	32.2 ± 13.4 [14.0–62.0]	41.5 ± 15.4 [12.0–62.5]	37.2 ± 18.3 [12.8–60.0]	40.7 ± 13.7 [23.5–62.7]	60.8 ± 20.6 [29.4–83.0]
Lymphocytes [%]	52.7 ± 27.5 [15.0–80.3]	41.7 ± 16.6 [18.7–70.1]	67.0 ± 14.2 [52.4–83.5]	63.4 ± 7.0 [55.8–73.2]	55.1 ± 11.4 [36.0–68.2]	34.0 ± 13.8 [35.0–84.2]	55.3 ± 14.5 [43.3–80.0]	60.0 ± 17.6 [35.5–84.4]	54.3 ± 10.7 [34.7–65.8]	35.5 ± 20.9 [15.5–67.7]
Monocytes [%]	1.8 ± 1.6 [0.0–3.7]	1.4 ± 1.2 [0.0–4.5]	1.7 ± 0.9 [1.0–3.1]	3.5 ± 1.5 [2.0–5.0]	3.4 ± 2.4 [0.0–8.1]	2.1 ± 2.2 [0.0–8.3]	2.4 ± 2.4 [0.0–8.0]	1.3 ± 0.8 [0.0–2.0]	0.9 ± 1.1 [0.0–2.5]	2.8 ± 2.0 [1.0–6.0]
Eosinophils [%]	0.2 ± 0.4 [0.0–1.0]	1.5 ± 1.5 [0.0–4.6]	0.3 ± 0.5 [0.0–1.0]	1.0 ± 2.2 [0.0–5.0]	1.2 ± 1.4 [0.0–4.0]	0.5 ± 0.9 [0.0–3.0]	0.3 ± 0.7 [0.2–2.1]	0.7 ± 0.8 [0.0–2.0]	0.2 ± 0.4 [0.0–1.1]	1.0 ± 1.2 [0.0–2.8]
Basophils [%]	0.2 ± 0.4 [0.0–1.0]	0.2 ± 0.4 [0.0–1.2]	0.2 ± 0.5 [0.0–1.0]	0.3 ± 0.7 [0.0–1.7]	0.4 ± 0.7 [0.0–2.0]	0.3 ± 0.5 [0.0–1.7]	0.2 ± 0.4 [0.0–1.2]	0.3 ± 0.6 [0.0–1.2]	0.0	0.0

Adapted from Polo FJ, Peinado VI, Viscor G, Palomeque J. Hematologic and plasma chemistry values in captive psittacine birds. Avian Dis 1998;42:523–535.

normocytic, normochromic anemia is indicative of decreased erythropoiesis (depression anemia), which can develop rapidly in birds with inflammatory diseases, especially those involving infectious agents. Psittacine birds appear to develop anemias due to lack of erythropoiesis more quickly than do mammals, perhaps due to the relatively short avian erythrocyte half-life compared to mammalian erythrocytes.[21,22] Disorders frequently associated with depression anemia in psittacine birds include tuberculosis, aspergillosis, chlamydiosis, chronic hepatic or renal disease, hypothyroidism, neoplasia, and other chronic inflammatory diseases.[16]

Hypochromasia can be seen with iron deficiency, chronic inflammatory diseases, and lead toxicosis.[3,21] Hypochromasia is also associated with nutritional deficiencies, especially iron deficiency anemia. Hypochromatic erythrocytes frequently appear in blood films from birds with chronic inflammatory diseases, presumably related to iron sequestration as part of the bird's defense against infectious agents. In such cases, hypochromatic cells are often observed in blood films before the red cell indices (mean corpuscular hemoglobin [MCH] and MCH concentration [MCHC]) suggest hypochromasia.

Erythrocytosis (polycythemia) is rarely reported in psittacine birds.[23] The conditions associated with polycythemia in mammals most likely cause the same condition in birds.

Avian leukograms often vary widely among normal psittacines of the same species. Because birds often become excited when handled, the blood collection process usually results in a physiologic leukocytosis resulting in an increase in the concentration of heterophils and lymphocytes in the peripheral blood. Normal total leukocyte reference intervals obtained from psittacine birds are generally broad; thus, leukogram values of birds must differ greatly from normal reference intervals to have diagnostic significance (Tables 179.1 and 179.2).

The general causes of leukocytosis in psittacine birds include inflammation, toxicities, hemorrhage into the coelomic cavity, rapidly growing neoplasms, and leukemia. A leukocyte differential aids in the assessment of a leukocytosis. A heterophilia is usually present when leukocytosis is caused by inflammation. Because heterophils actively participate in inflammatory lesions, the magnitude of heterophilia is dependent on the severity of the inflammation and its etiology.[24,25] Leukocytosis and heterophilia can be associated with inflammation in response to localized or systemic infections caused by a spectrum of infectious agents and noninfectious etiologies. Marked leukocytosis and heterophilia are often associated with diseases produced by common psittacine pathogens, such as *Chlamydia, Mycobacterium,* and *Aspergillus.* Slight to moderate leukocytosis and lymphopenia can occur with excess endogenous or exogenous glucocorticoids (stress leukogram).

Heterophil morphology appears more important in the prediction of the outcome of the disease than the magnitude of the heterophil count. Increased numbers of immature heterophils usually result from excessive peripheral utilization of mature heterophils with deple-

tion of the mature storage pool in the hematopoietic tissue, indicating a severe inflammatory response, especially when associated with leukopenia.[26] Toxic heterophils are associated with severe systemic illness such as septicemia, viremia, chlamydiosis, mycotic infections, and severe tissue necrosis. The degree of heterophil toxicity usually indicates the severity of the bird's condition.

Leukopenia is associated with either consumption of peripheral leukocytes or decreased production. Leukopenias associated with heteropenias can occur with severe bacterial infections or certain viral diseases (e.g., Pacheco's parrot disease).[27,28] Leukopenia and heteropenia with the presence of immature heterophils suggest exhaustion of the mature heterophil storage pool because of excessive peripheral demand for heterophils as seen with severe inflammation. Leukopenia, heteropenia, immature heterophils, and toxic heterophils indicate a degenerative response. Degenerative responses and depletion are differentiated by the presence of toxic heterophils or by following the decreasing leukocyte count with serial leukograms. Lymphocytosis or the presence of many reactive lymphocytes is suggestive of antigenic stimulation associated with infectious diseases. Lymphocytosis can also occur with lymphocytic leukemia. In some cases of lymphocytic leukemia, immature lymphocytes may be present in the blood film. A marked lymphocytosis in which the majority of lymphocytes appear as small mature lymphocytes with scalloped cytoplasmic margins has also been associated with lymphoid neoplasia.[1,29,30] Lymphopenia can occur with glucocorticosteroid excess. Immunosuppressive drugs may also cause lymphopenia.

Monocytes exhibit phagocytic activity and migrate into tissues to become macrophages involved in inflammation and destruction of invading organisms; therefore, a monocytosis is often associated with infectious diseases caused by organisms that typically cause granulomatous inflammation, such as *Mycobacterium, Chlamydia,* and fungi. Chronic bacterial granulomas and massive tissue necrosis may also result in monocytosis.

Because the exact functions of avian eosinophils are not known, it is difficult to interpret the cause of peripheral eosinophilias in psittacine birds. Although this avian granulocyte was given the name "eosinophil," avian eosinophils may behave differently from mammalian eosinophils.[31,32] Despite the limited knowledge of the function of avian eosinophils, peripheral eosinophilias in psittacines can be interpreted loosely as responses to parasitism or exposure to foreign antigens (hypersensitivity response). Eosinopenia may be difficult to document in psittacine birds. If present, it would be expected to be associated with a stress response or glucocorticosteroid administration.

Basophilia is rare in psittacine birds. The function of avian basophils is not known but presumed to be similar to mammalian basophils and mast cells, because their cytoplasmic granules contain histamine and they appear to participate in acute inflammatory and Type IV hypersensitivity reactions.[13,33–35] Basophils appear to participate in the initial phase of acute inflammation in birds;

however, this is usually not reflected as basophilia in the leukogram.[36] Peripheral basophilia may suggest early inflammation or an immediate hypersensitivity reaction in psittacine birds.

Avian thrombocytes may participate in removing foreign materials from the blood.[37] The presence of immature thrombocytes usually indicates a regenerative response to excessive utilization of thrombocytes. Young psittacine birds tend to have relatively higher numbers of circulating thrombocytes than adult birds.[33]

Thrombocytopenia is a result of either decreased bone marrow production or excessive peripheral utilization or destruction. Decreased thrombocyte concentration is often associated with severe septicemia and possibly diffuse intravascular coagulation.

BLOOD PARASITES

Protozoan parasites, especially *Hemoproteus* sp., and microfilaria of filarial nematodes are commonly found as incidental findings in blood films from wild-caught psittacine birds.

REFERENCES

1. **Campbell TW.** Avian hematology and cytology. Ames, IA: Iowa State University Press, 1988.
2. **Dein FJ.** Hematology. In: Harrison GJ, Harrison LR, eds. Clinical avian medicine and surgery. Philadelphia: WB Saunders, 1986;174–191.
3. **Hawkey CM, Dennett TB.** Color atlas of comparative veterinary hematology. London: Wolfe Medical Publications, 1989.
4. **Davidson I, Henry JB.** Todd-Sanford clinical diagnosis by laboratory methods. 15th ed. Philadelphia: WB Saunders, 1974.
5. **Dein FJ.** Laboratory manual of avian hematology. East Northport, NY: Association of Avian Veterinarians, 1984.
6. **Coles EH.** Veterinary clinical pathology. 4th ed. Philadelphia: WB Saunders, 1986;53–54.
7. **Schalm OW, Jain NC, Carroll EJ.** Veterinary hematology. 3rd ed. Philadelphia: Lea & Febiger, 1975;21.
8. **Costello RT.** A Unopette for eosinophil counts. Am J Clin Pathol 1970;54:249.
9. **Robertson GW, Maxwell MH.** Modified staining techniques for avian blood cells. Br Poult Sci 1990;31:881–886.
10. **Zinkl JG.** Avian hematology. In: Jain CJ, ed. Schalm's veterinary hematology. Philadelphia: Lea & Febiger, 1986;261–262.
11. **Joseph V, Wagner D, Stouli J, Palagi-Lynn L.** Toluidine blue stain for avian WBC count. J Assoc Avian Vet 1989;3:191, 229.
12. **Dein FJ, Wilson BA, Fischer MT.** Avian leucocyte counting using the hemocytometer. J Zoo Wildl Med 1994;25:432–437.
13. **Fox AJ, Solomon JB.** Chicken non-lymphoid leukocytes. In: Rose LN, Payne LN, Freeman MB, eds. Avian immunology. Edinburgh:, Poultry Science, 1981;135–166.
14. **Romagnano A, Barnes HJ, Perkins P, Guy JS, Flammer K.** Binucleate erythrocytes and erythrocytic dysplasia in a cockatiel. Proc Assoc Avian Vet 1994;83–86.
15. **Swayne DE, Stockman SL, Johnson GS.** Cytochemical properties of chicken blood cells resembling both thrombocytes and lymphocytes. Vet Clin Pathol 1986;15:17–24.
16. **Gaskin JM.** Psittacine viral diseases: a perspective. J ZooWildl Med 1989; 20:249–264.
17. **Jacobson ER, Hines SA, Quesenberry K, Mladinich C, Davis RB, Kollias GV, Olsen J.** Epornitic of papova-like virus-associated disease in a psittacine nursery. J Am Vet Med Assoc 1984;185:1337–1341.
18. **Lothrop C, Harrison GJ, Schultz D, Utteridge T.** Miscellaneous diseases. In: Harrison GJ, Harrison LR, eds. Clinical avian medicine and surgery. Philadelphia: WB Saunders, 1988; 525–536.
19. **Wainright PO, Pritchard NG, Fletcher OJ, Davis RB, Clubb S.** Identification of viruses from Amazon parrots with a hemorrhagic syndrome and a chronic respiratory disease. First Int Conf Zool Avian Med 1987;15–19.
20. **Rupiper DJ, Read, DH.** Hemochromatosis in a Hawk-head parrot [Deroptyus accipitrinus]. J Avian Med Surg 1996;10:24–27.
21. **Campbell TW, Dein FJ.** Avian hematology, the basics. Vet Clin North Am Small Anim Pract 1984;14:223–248.
22. **Sturkie PD.** Blood: physical characteristics, formed elements, hemoglobin, and coagulation. In: Sturkie PD, ed. Avian physiology. New York: Springer-Verlag, 1976;53–75.
23. **Taylor M.** Polycythemia in the blue and gold macaw—a case report of three cases. Proc First Int Conf Zool Avian Med 1987;95–104.
24. **Topp RC, Carlson HC.** Studies on avian heterophils, II: histochemistry. Avian Dis 1972;16:369–373.
25. **Topp RC, Carlson HC.** Studies on avian heterophils, III: phagocytic properties. Avian Dis 1972;16:374–380.
26. **Tangredi BP.** Heterophilia and left shift with fatal diseases in four psittacine birds. J Zoo Anim Med 1981;12:13–16.
27. **Rosskopf WJ, Woerpel RW.** Chronic endocrine disorder associated with inclusion body hepatitis in a Sulfur-crested Cockatoo. J Am Vet Med Assoc 1981;179:1273–1276.
28. **Olson C.** Avian hematology. In: Biester HE, Swarte LH, eds. Diseases of poultry. 5th ed. Ames, IA: Iowa State University Press, 1965;100–119.
29. **Campbell TW.** Lymphoid leukosis in an Amazon parrot—a case report. Proc Assoc Avian Vet 1984;229–234.
30. **Purchase GH, Burmester BD.** Leukosis/sarcoma group. In: Hofstad MS, ed. Diseases of poultry. Ames, IA: Iowa State University Press, 1978;418–468.
31. **Maxwell MH, Burns RB.** Experimental stimulation of eosinophil production in the domestic fowl. Res Vet Sci 1986;41:114–123.
32. **Maxwell MH.** Attempted induction of an avian eosinophilia using various agents. Res Vet Sci 1980;29:293–297.
33. **Dieterien-Lievre F.** Birds. In: Rawley AF, Ratcliffe NA, eds. Vertebrate blood cells. Cambridge: Cambridge University Press,988;257–336.
34. **Hodges RD.** The histology of the fowl. London: Academic Press, 1974.
35. **Carlson HC, Allen JR.** The acute inflammatory reaction in chicken skin: blood cellular response. Avian Dis 1969;14:817–833.
36. **Montali RJ.** Comparative pathology of inflammation in the higher vertebrates [reptiles, birds, and mammals]. J Comp Pathol 1988;99:1–26.
37. **Grecchi R, Saliba AM, Mariano M.** Morphological changes, surface receptors and phagocytic potential of fowl mononuclear phagocytes and thrombocytes in vivo and in vitro. J Pathol 1980;130:23–31.

CHAPTER 180

Normal Hematology of Waterfowl

• TERRY W. CAMPBELL

Hematology is part of the clinical data used to assess the health of waterfowl, such as ducks and geese. Age, sex, and seasonal differences may occur and create variations in the hemogram of healthy waterfowl. Changes in the hemogram may also occur during migration, reproduction, molting, and maturation. Normal hematologic values determined by different laboratories can vary significantly. This variation is caused by differences in blood sampling and analytic techniques. Other factors that influence the hematologic results include anesthesia, nutrition, environmental conditions, physiologic status, and genetic factors (species) of birds used to establish normal blood values.

HEMATOLOGIC EXAMINATION

Blood for hematologic examination is commonly collected by venipuncture of the jugular, medial metatarsal, basilic, or brachial veins using ethylenediaminetetraacetic acid (EDTA) as the anticoagulant. Laboratory evaluation of the hemogram of waterfowl involves assessment of erythrocytes, leukocytes, and thrombocytes using the same routine procedures described for other birds.

ERYTHROCYTES

Seasonal variations, age, and species affect the erythrocyte parameters such as packed cell volume (PCV), total erythrocyte count (TRBC), hemoglobin (Hb) concentration, mean corpuscular hemoglobin concentration (MCHC), and mean corpuscular volume (MCV) of normal waterfowl (Table 180.1).] In general, the variation in the erythrocyte parameters between male and female ducks and geese are not statistically significant and may reflect seasonal variation.[1] Averages for PCV, Hb, TRBC, and MCHC are higher in females than males of various species of ducks in the prenesting period.[2] In general, averages for PCV, Hb, TRBC, and MCHC tend to be higher in the winter and prenesting period in adult ducks and geese of either gender than during the postnesting period and fall.[3] Midmigration ducks have

slightly lower erythrocyte counts than wintering ducks.[4] The postnesting MCV averages for these birds tend to be higher than the winter or prenesting periods.[3] The differences in adult ducks most likely reflect hormonal and nutritional changes caused by alterations in the photoperiod and migration.

Age differences are recognized as a cause of variation in the hemogram of healthy ducks and geese. Four- to ten-week-old ducklings have lower PCV and slightly higher total protein values than most adult ducks.[4] The difference between ducklings and adult ducks probably reflects the high metabolic rate associated with rapid growth and the consumption of a higher protein and carbohydrate diet.

Significant differences occur between species of waterfowl. For example, mallard ducks (*Anas platyrhynchos*), a dabbling duck, have higher average PCV and TRBC values during the winter and prenesting period compared with diving ducks.[3] Diving ducks have higher MCV values during the winter and prenesting period and higher PCV, Hb, and MCHC values during the postnesting period when compared with those of mallard ducks.[3] Ducks tend to have higher TRBC values than geese do during the winter, but geese have higher MCV and Hb values.[3]

Anemia occurs with hemolysis, hemorrhage, and decreased red blood cell production. A nonregenerative, normocytic, normochromic anemia is indicative of decreased erythropoiesis (depression anemia), which can develop rapidly in birds with inflammatory diseases, especially those involving infectious agents. Erythrocytosis occurs commonly with hemoconcentration associated with dehydration and rarely polycythemia.

LEUKOCYTES

Leukocytes in the peripheral blood film of waterfowl are the same as other birds which include lymphocytes, monocytes, and granulocytes. The granulocytes are classified as heterophils, eosinophils, and basophils. Lymphocytes are the most abundant leukocyte of most healthy adult ducks and geese, representing between 60 and 70% of the leukocyte differential (Table 180.1). The

TABLE 180.1   Selected Hematology Data for Normal Ducks and Geese

	American Black Duck[a]	Wood Duck[b]	Canada Goose[c] January	Canada Goose[c] June	Snow Goose[d]	Mallard Duck[e] January	Mallard Duck[e] June
RBC [× 10⁶/uL]	2.78 ± 0.22	2.79 ± 0.22	2.67 ± 0.3	2.18 ± 0.3	2.25	3.35 ± 0.3	2.01 ± 0.4
PCV [%]	40.24 ± 4.21	45.54 ± 3.41	51 ± 3.1	46 ± 3.5	46	49 ± 2.5	39 ± 5.1
Hb [g/dL]	12.96 ± 1.36	14.95 ± 1.22	16.2 ± 1.0	14.0 ± 1.2	14.0	15.6 ± 0.8	11.4 ± 1.6
MCV [fL]	144.68 ± 9.96	164.24 ± 14.43	193.3 ± 16.6	210.1 ± 19.4	204	148.4 ± 13.7	199.6 ± 27.7
MCHC [g/dL]	32.23 ± 1.16	32.99 ± 3.7	31.6 ± 0.1	30.7 ± 1.4	30.4	31.6 ± 0.2	29.2 ± 2.0
WBC [× 10³/uL]	19.7 ± 6.60	25.58 ± 5.72	20.4–21.8		20.1 ± 4.71	23.4–24.8	
Heterophils [× 10³/uL]	4.86 ± 1.37	8.45 ± 2.59	39%		7.0	38% ± 1.5	29% ± 1.4
Lymphocytes [× 10³/uL]	13.03 ± 1.53	13.28 ± 1.77	46%		12.3	54% ± 1.6	66% ± 1.4
Monocytes [× 10³/uL]	1.46 ± 0.99	1.05 ± 0.68	6.0%		0.2	3.6% ± 0.3	2.5% ± 0.3
Eosinophils [× 10³/uL]	0.22 ± 0.16	0.51 ± 0.06	2.0%		0.5	0.4% ± 0.1	0.2% ± 0.17
Basophils [× 10³/uL]	0.16 ± 0.15	0.41 ± 0.23	7.0%		0.1	3.6% ± 0.3	2.2% ± 0.3

[a]Mean ± standard deviation. Mulley RC. Haematology and blood chemistry of the Black duck [*Anas superciliosa*]. J Wildl Dis 1979;15:437–441.
[b]Mean ± standard deviation. Mulley RC. Haematology of the wood duck. *Chenonetta jubata.* J Wildl Dis 1980;16:271–273.
[c]Mean ± standard error. Erythrocyte data from Shave HJ, Howard V. A hematologic survey of captive waterfowl. J Wildl Dis 1976;12:195–201. Leukocyte data from Wallach JD, Boever WJ. Diseases of exotic animals. Philadelphia: WB Saunders, 1983;837.
[d]Mean values from Williams JI, Traines DO. A hematological study of snow, blue, and Canada geese. J Wildl Dis 1971;7:258.
[e]Mean ± standard error. Erythrocyte data from Shave HJ, Howard V. A hematologic survey of captive waterfowl. J Wildl Dis 1976;12:195–201. Relative distribution of leukocytes from Fairbrother A, O'Loughlin D. Differential white blood cell values of the mallard [*Anas platyrhynchos*] across different ages and reproductive states. J Wildl Dis 1990;26:78–82. Total leukocyte count from Wallach JD, Boever WJ. Diseases of exotic animals. Philadelphia: WB Saunders, 1983;837.

heterophil is the next most frequently observed leukocyte found in the blood of ducks and geese, representing an average of 35% of leukocytes. Ducklings and goslings younger than 60 days of age have lower relative lymphocyte counts and higher relative heterophil counts compared with adult ducks and geese.[5] The percentage of heterophils in the peripheral blood of ducks decreases during molting of the flight feathers (remige molt).[6] There is no significant difference in the heterophil to lymphocyte ratio between genders or with the state of reproduction (pre–egg-laying, egg-laying, incubation, molting, and post–egg-laying).[5]

The general causes of a leukocytosis in waterfowl include inflammation, toxicities, and hemorrhage into the coelomic cavity. Heterophilia is usually present when leukocytosis is caused by inflammation. The magnitude of heterophilia is dependent on the severity of the inflammation and its etiology. Increased numbers of immature heterophils usually result from excessive peripheral utilization of mature heterophils with depletion of the mature storage pool in the hematopoietic tissue. Toxic heterophils commonly occur with severe systemic illness associated with infectious agents and severe tissue necrosis. Leukopenia is associated with either consumption of peripheral leukocytes or decreased production. Lymphocytosis may occur with antigenic stimulation. Lymphopenia can occur with glucocorticosteroid excess. Because the exact functions of avian eosinophils are not known, it is difficult to interpret the cause of peripheral eosinophilias in waterfowl.

Abnormal appearing heterophils in blood films include both immature and toxic heterophils. Immature heterophils are rarely present in the peripheral blood of normal ducks and geese, and their presence usually indicates excessive peripheral utilization of mature heterophils and depletion of the mature storage pool in the hematopoietic tissue. The presence of immature heterophils in the blood film indicates a severe inflammatory response, especially when associated with leukopenia. Toxic heterophils are associated with severe systemic illness (i.e., septicemia, viremia, bacterial and mycotic infections, and severe tissue necrosis). Abnormal lymphocytes are classified as reactive or blast-transformed lymphocytes.

THROMBOCYTES

Thrombocytes of ducks and geese resemble those of other birds. Age, reproductive status, and health of the bird affect thrombocyte numbers in the peripheral blood. Young ducklings and goslings have a lower thrombocyte concentration compared with adult birds. The number of thrombocytes in the peripheral blood begins to increase at 5 days of age and reaches adult concentrations at 18 days of age.[5] Female ducks exhibit a decrease in the thrombocyte concentration during the incubation, molting, and postreproduction periods.[5]

Thrombocytopenia is a result of either decreased bone marrow production or excessive peripheral utilization or destruction Decreased thrombocyte numbers are often associated with severe septicemias and possibly diffuse intravascular coagulation (DIC).

BLOOD PARASITES

Common blood parasites of ducks and geese include species of *Hemoproteus, Leukocytozoon, Plasmodium,* and microfilaria of onchocercid helminths. *Leukocytozoon simondi* is a major factor in the high mortality rates of young waterfowl in some areas.[7]

REFERENCES

1. **Mulley RC.** Haematology and blood chemistry of the black duck (*Anas superciliosa*). J Wildl Dis 1979;15:437–441.
2. **Mulley RC.** Haematology of the wood duck, *Chenonetta jubata.* J Wildl Dis 1980;16:271–273.
3. **Shave HJ, Howard V.** A hematologic survey of captive waterfowl. J Wildl Dis 1976;12:195–201.
4. **Kocan RM, Pitts SM.** Blood values of the canvasback duck by age, sex, and season. J Wildl Dis 1976;12:341–346.
5. **Fairbrother A, O'Loughlin D.** Differential white blood cell values of the mallard (*Anas platyrhynchos*) across different ages and reproductive states. J Wildl Dis 1990;26:78–82.
6. **Driver EA.** Haematological and blood chemical values of mallard, *Anas platyrhynchos* platyrhynchos, drakes before, during, and after remige molt. J Wildl Dis 1981;17:413–421.
7. **Bennett GF, Blandin W, Huesmann HW, Campbell AG.** Hematozoa of the Anatidae of the Atlantic flyway. I. Massachusetts. J Wildl Dis 1974;10:442–451.

CHAPTER 181

Normal Hematology of Marine Mammals

• THOMAS H. REIDARSON, DEBORAH DUFFIELD, and JAMES McBAIN

Years of routine clinical tests on marine mammals have provided considerable data on hematology of these creatures. Statistical analyses for many of these parameters have been reported on killer whales (*Orcinus orca*), beluga whales (*Delphinapterus leucas*), captive and free-ranging bottlenose dolphins (*Tursiops truncatus*), and manatees (*Trichechus manatus latirostris*)[1-11] as well as a large collection of data for many other cetacean and pinniped species in the "Handbook of Marine Mammal Medicine."[12]

The source of animals for normal values typically consists of "clinically normal" individuals. For the purpose of this chapter, normal is defined by having a normal appearance (with respect to body weight, condition, and behavior), not being pregnant, and not receiving any medication for at least 2 weeks. For wild individuals, samples were drawn after humane capture; for individuals from oceanaria, samples were drawn either after humane capture or in an unrestrained trained fashion.

For cetaceans, blood samples were drawn from the ventral fluke vasculature. Pinnipeds were manually restrained, and blood was drawn from either the caudal gluteal vasculature (for otarids) or the extradural sinus (for phocids).[13] Manatees were manually restrained, and blood was drawn from the inter radial-ulnar vasculature.[11] Twenty-eight free-ranging polar bears, 26 subadults and 2 adults, were anesthetized using telazol, and blood was drawn from jugular veins. Finally, northern and southern sea otters were manually restrained, and blood was drawn from either the femoral or popliteal vein.[14]

For all animals, blood collection tubes with ethylenediamine tetraacetate (EDTA) as an anticoagulant were used for complete blood count (CBC) determinations. On filling, the tubes were gently rocked and then immediately analyzed (except for the free-ranging Sarasota bottlenose dolphins, for whom tubes were immediately refrigerated in an ice chest and analyzed within 24 hours of sampling). For protein and fibrinogen determinations, blood was drawn into tubes containing thrombin or citrate, respectively. For protein, once clot retraction had begun, serum tubes were centrifuged at 2500 RPM for 5 minutes. For fibrinogen, citrated blood was also spun at 2500 RPM for 5 minutes. Serum and plasma were analyzed within 1 hour of sampling (the Sarasota dolphins were analyzed within 24 hours of sampling).

Ranges were calculated as ±2 standard deviations around the means. We offer the following observation for the clinical interpretation of these normal values and ranges. Having several years of cumulative data for individuals over time for SeaWorld bottlenose dolphins and killer whales, it was possible to evaluate where individual animals fit in the overall species range. Based on these comparisons, it was very clear that the normal values for individual animals occupy a tightly described subsection of the overall species range. This cautions the need, when dealing with long-term maintenance of these species, to establish norms for individuals from which to track health changes from normal status. In dealing with free-ranging or rehabilitation of animals, this approach is not practical, and the normal means and ranges presented in these tables offer the best measure of the distribution of normal values in each of these species. Statistical analyses for age and sex differences for the SeaWorld bottlenose dolphins and killer whales were done using a General Linear Model, MANOVA, (SPSS, version 8).

Table 181.1 contains normal hematology values from eight different cetacean species (including data from free-ranging Sarasota bottlenose dolphins). The free-ranging Sarasota Bay dolphins data were provided by H. Rhinehart, J. Sweeney, F. Townsend, and R. Wells. Hematology values include all age groups and both sexes. All cetacean data (other than the Sarasota bottlenose dolphins) were obtained from long-term records of animals maintained by SeaWorld. Significant differences include increased mean corpuscular volume (MCV) for beluga whales and elevated erythrocyte sedimentation rates (ESRs) for pilot whales and false killer whales. Table 181.2 compares age differences in free-ranging versus captive bottlenose dolphins. Only statistically different values are noted (Student's t test $P < 0.05$). For free-ranging bottlenose dolphins these included platelet numbers, lymphocyte and eosinophil numbers, and globulins, whereas for captive bottlenose dolphins these values included MCV, platelet numbers, lymphocyte numbers, ESR, and globulins. The only statistically significant sex difference was lymphocyte numbers in captive bottlenose dolphins, in which

TABLE 181.1A   Normal Hematology and Proteins From Commerson's Dolphins, Common Dolphins, Beluga Whales, and Pilot Whales[a]

Parameter	Commerson's Dolphins (*Cephalorhynchus commersoni*) (n = 10; sample n = 250)		Common Dolphins (*Delphinus delphis*) (n = 2; sample n = 42)		Beluga Whales (*Delphinapterus leucas*) (n = 16; sample n = 260)		Pilot Whales (*Globicephala macrorhynchus*) (n = 2; sample n = 74)	
	Range[b]	Mean ± SD	Range[c]	Mean ± SD	Range[b]	Mean ± SD	Range[c]	Mean ± SD
RBC (10⁶/mm³)	4.2–5.6	4.9 ± 0.4	4.6–4.9	4.7 ± 0.2	3.6–4.0	3.8 ± 0.1	3.3–3.7	3.5 ± 0.1
Hb (g/dL)	15.1–18.7	16.9 ± 0.9	16.1–19.4	17.9 ± 1.4	18.7–21.4	20.1 ± 0.7	15.1–16	15.5 ± 0.1
HCT (%)	44–52	48 ± 2	46–55	50 ± 4	51–59	55 ± 2	43–45	44 ± 1
MCV (fl)	93–105	99 ± 3	100–114	107 ± 7	160–183	172 ± 6	123–129	126 ± 3
MCH (pg)	33–37	35 ± 1	35–40	38 ± 3	59–67	63 ± 2	43–46	44 ± 1
MCHC (g/dL)	34–36	35 ± 0.4	34–36	35 ± 1	35–39	37 ± 1	34–36	35 ± 1
Thrombocytes (10³/μL)	109–261	185 ± 38	55–100	80 ± 28	64–148	106 ± 21	70–90	85 ± 7
Reticulocytes (%)	0.9–2.1	1.5 ± 0.3	0.8–1.4	1 ± 0.1	0.2–1.0	0.6 ± 0.2	0.7–1.2	1.0 ± 0.1
nRBC	0–1.2	0.2 ± 0.5	0	0	0–1	0.5 ± 0.4	0	0
ESR (@ 60 min)	0	0	0	0	0–9	3 ± 3	16–52	32 ± 16
Leukocytes/μL	3620–8160	5890 ± 1140	4570–4900	4780 ± 110	5320–9560	7440 ± 1060	4720–6500	5550 ± 640
Neutrophil (band)	0	0	0	0	0	0	0	0
Neutrophil (mature)	1150–3250	2330 ± 590	2590–4150	3210 ± 230	2580–5520	4050 ± 740	2830–4220	3460 ± 110
Lymphocyte	1260–2420	1850 ± 300	380–850	540 ± 110	1100–4150	2310 ± 920	570–2080	1310 ± 735
Monocyte	150–270	210 ± 30	120–350	220 ± 85	220–780	500 ± 140	160–510	360 ± 20
Eosinophil	690–2200	1450 ± 380	620–1280	950 ± 70	90–640	340 ± 150	220–910	560 ± 230
Basophil	0	0	0	0	0	0	0	0
Plasma proteins (g/dL)	5.6–6.7	6.2 ± 0.3	6.3–7.3	6.8 ± 0.2	5.9–7.1	6.5 ± 0.3	5.3–6.0	5.6 ± 0.2
Albumin (g/dL)	3.6–3.8	3.7 ± 0.1	3.9–4.7	4.3 ± 0.3	4.0–4.8	4.4 ± 0.2	2.9–3.3	3.1 ± 0.2
Globulin (g/dL)	1.9–3.1	2.5 ± 0.3	1.8–3.0	2.4 ± 0.5	1.7–2.7	2.2 ± 0.3	2.2–3.0	2.6 ± 0.2
Fibrinogen (g/dL)	108–270	175 ± 50	NT	NT	64–139	102 ± 19	280–445	332 ± 32

[a]Data contributed by SeaWorld.
[b]Because n = 2, ranges are 25–75% quartiles around median value of combined data.
[c]If ± SD exceeds observed high or low value, we reported the high or low observed value.
NT, not tested.

case females had greater numbers (not included in Table 181.2).

Table 181.3 is a compilation of normal hematology values for seven species of pinnipeds. These values represent a compilation of data from L. Dunn, F. Gulland, and SeaWorld. As with cetaceans, these values include all age groups and both sexes. The only remarkable differences include increased MCV, mean corpuscular hemoglobin (MCH), and MCH concentration (MCHC) for northern elephant seals.

Table 181.4 is an age grouping compilation of normal hematology from free-ranging harbor seals (*Phoca vitulina*), northern elephant seals (*Mirounga angustirostris*), and California sea lions (*Zalophus californianus*) stranded in Northern California, treated for various illnesses, and released by The Marine Mammal Center in Sausalito, California, from 1992 to the present (contributed by F. Gulland). In all cases, blood samples were drawn immediately before release after individuals were deemed normal.

Table 181.5 contains three other marine mammal species, Florida manatee (*Trichechus manatus latirostris;* con-

tributed by G. Bossart and D. Odell), polar bears (*Ursus maritimus;* contributed by M. Cattet and N. Caulkett), and captive and wild sea otters (*Enhydra lutris;* contributed by T. Williams). The predominant segmented nucleated cell type of the Florida manatee contains small, pleomorphic, rod to round, eosinophilic cytoplasmic granules. Thus, this cell is termed a heterophil or heterophilic granulocyte; however, recent evidence has shown this cell to be related biochemically to the neutrophil.[11] For polar bears, MCH values were the greatest for all marine mammals. Other values are expected to change throughout the year due to variation in intravascular water content. Cattet and Caulkett (personal communication) have found mean total protein and mean hematocrit to vary from 6.8 mg/dl and 42.4% (n = 19) in spring (when polar bears are feeding) to 7.8 mg/dl and 52.6% (n = 20) during the summer (when polar bears begin prolonged fasting). Values obtained during fall, at the end of prolonged fasting, are similar to those obtained during spring. Correlation between total protein and hematocrit is highly significant at all times of the year (Pearson correlation r = 0.51, $P < 0.001$, n = 93).

TABLE 181.1B   Normal Hematology and Proteins from Pacific White Sided Dolphins, Killer Whales, False Killer Whales, and Bottlenose Dolphins

Parameter	Pacific White Sided Dolphins[a,c] (*Lagenorhynchus obliquidens*) (n = 10; sample n = 400) Range	Mean ± SD	Killer Whales[a,c] (*Orcinus orca*) (n = 18; sample n = 1334) Range	Mean ± SD	False Killer Whales[a,c] (*Pseudorca crassidens*) (n = 6; sample n = 83) Range	Mean ± SD	Free-Ranging Bottlenose Dolphins[b,d] (*Tursiops truncatus*) (n = 96; sample n = 96) Range	Mean ± SD	Captive Bottlenose Dolphins[a,c] (*Tursiops truncatus*) (n = 119; sample n = 1202) Range	Mean ± SD
RBC (10^6/mm³)	5.2–6.0	5.6 ± 0.2	3.4–4.2	3.8 ± 0.2	3.1–4.7	3.9 ± 0.4	3–4.1	3.6 ± 0.2	3.0–4.0	3.4 ± 0.3
Hb (g/dL)	17.0–20.6	18.8 ± 0.9	13.5–15.9	14.7 ± 0.6	13.3–18.1	15.7 ± 1.2	12.4–15.4	14.1 ± 0.7	12.6–15.8	14.2 ± 0.8
HCT (%)	48–56	52 ± 2	39–46	42 ± 2	39–51	45 ± 3	37–47	42 ± 2.4	36–46	41 ± 2.3
MCV (fl)	90–98	94 ± 2	103–117	111 ± 4	106–124	115 ± 4.5	106–134	120 ± 6.2	108–136	122 ± 7
MCH (pg)	33–35	34 ± 0.6	36–42	39 ± 1.5	36–44	40 ± 2	35–44	40 ± 2.1	37–47	42 ± 2.3
MCHC (g/dL)	34–36	35 ± 0.3	34–36	35 ± 0.6	33–37	35 ± 1	30–35	33 ± 1	32–38	35 ± 1.5
Thrombocytes (10^3/mm³)	78–162	120 ± 21	98–228	163 ± 35	58–154	106 ± 24	92–238	165 ± 34	58–178	117 ± 30
Reticulocytes (%)	0.8–2.3	1.5 ± 0.4	0.5–2.5	1.5 ± 0.5	0–3.7	1.4 ± 1.2	NT	NT	0.3–3.5	1.8 ± 0.8
nRBC	0–0.7	0.1 ± 0.3	0	0	0–1	0.2 ± 0.4	0	0	0–3	0.8 ± 1.3
ESR (@ 60 min)	0	0	0–2	0.5 ± 1	3–29	15 ± 7	NT	NT	0–30	11 ± 10
Leukocytes/µL	2530–6930	4730 ± 1100	3760–7890	5830 ± 1120	4450–9350	6650 ± 1350	5900–13700	9500 ± 1840	4480–9080	6770 ± 1150
Neutrophil (band)	0	0	0	0	0	0	0	0	98–522	310 ± 106
Neutrophil (mature)	1250–3730	2490 ± 620	2380–6060	4220 ± 990	2280–5040	3660 ± 690	2450–6850	4477 ± 937	2460–5980	4200 ± 880
Lymphocyte	390–1390	800 ± 300	520–1850	1180 ± 330	990–2490	1570 ± 460	310–3810	1750 ± 728	420–2500	1460 ± 520
Monocyte	80–240	160 ± 40	140–420	280 ± 70	120–400	260 ± 70	80–640	284 ± 141	110–430	270 ± 80
Eosinophil	720–1910	1190 ± 360	8–160	82 ± 40	410–1540	920 ± 310	1070–5340	2882 ± 1059	130–1510	820 ± 350
Basophil	0	0	0	0	0	0		13 ± 10	0	0
Plasma proteins (g/dL)	5.7–6.9	6.3 ± 0.3	5.5–6.6	6.1 ± 0.3	5.8–6.6	6.2 ± 0.2	6.3–8.7	7.5 ± 0.6	5.6–7.6	6.6 ± 0.5
Albumin (g/dL)	3.0–3.8	3.4 ± 0.2	3.0–3.7	3.3 ± 0.2	3.4–3.8	3.6 ± 0.1	2.8–3.7	3.3 ± 0.2	4.2–5.4	4.8 ± 0.3
Globulin (g/dL)	2.4–3.4	2.9 ± 0.3	2.0–3.4	2.7 ± 0.4	1.7–3.3	2.5 ± 0.4	3.0–5.5	4.2 ± 0.6	1.0–2.6	1.8 ± 0.4
Fibrinogen (g/dL)	147–333	213 ± 60	192–346	269 ± 38	176–340	259 ± 56	NT	NT	140–410	275 ± 68

[a] Data contributed by SeaWorld.
[b] Data contributed for Sarasota Bay free-ranging dolphins by H. Rhinehart, J. Sweeney, F. Townsend, and R. Wells.
[c] If ± SD exceeds observed high or low value, we reported the high or low observed value.
[d] Ranges were calculated as ±2 standard deviations around the means.
NT, not tested.

TABLE 181.2 **Normal Hematology and Proteins with Age-Related Differences from Free-Ranging and Captive Atlantic Bottlenose Dolphins (*Tursiops truncatus*)**

Parameter	Free-Ranging Atlantic Bottlenose Dolphins[a,c] (*Tursiops truncatus*) (n = 30; sample n = 96)		Captive Bottlenose Dolphins[b,d] (*Tursiops truncatus*) (n = 119; sample n = 1202)	
	Range	Mean ± SD	Range	Mean ± SD
RBC (10⁶/mm³)	3.0–4.0	3.4 ± 0.2	3.0–4.0	3.6 ± 0.3
<10 year	ND	ND	ND	ND
>10 year	ND	ND	ND	ND
Hb (g/dL)	12.6–15.4	14.1 ± 0.7	12.6–15.8	14.2 ± 0.8
<10 year	ND	ND	ND	ND
>10 year	ND	ND	ND	ND
HCT (%)	37–47	42 ± 2.4	36–46	41 ± 2.3
<10 year	ND	ND	ND	ND
>10 year	ND	ND	ND	ND
MCV (fL)	106–134	120 ± 6.2	108–136	122 ± 7
<10 year	ND	ND	107–133	120 ± 6.6
>10 year	ND	ND	111–137	124 ± 6.7
MCH (pg)	35–44	40 ± 2.1	37–47	42 ± 2.3
<10 year	ND	ND	ND	ND
>10 year	ND	ND	ND	ND
MCHC (g/dL)	30–35	33 ± 1.1	32–38	35 ± 1.5
<10 year	ND	ND	ND	ND
>10 year	ND	ND	ND	ND
Thrombocytes (10³/mm³)	92–238	165 ± 34	58–178	118 ± 30
<10 year	109–228	175 ± 32	76–184	130 ± 27
>10 year	100–238	157 ± 37	50–154	102 ± 26
Reticulocytes (%)	NT	NT	0.3–3.5	1.9 ± 0.8
<10 year	NT	NT	ND	ND
>10 year	NT	NT	ND	ND
nRBC	0	0	0–3	1 ± 1.3
<10 year	0	0	ND	ND
>10 year	0	0	ND	ND
ESR (@ 60 min)	NT	NT	0–31	12 ± 10
<10 year	NT	NT	0–27	9 ± 9
>10 year	NT	NT	0–32	14 ± 9
Leukocytes/μL	5900–13700	9500 ± 1840	4480–9080	6780 ± 1150
<10 year	ND	ND	ND	ND
>10 year	ND	ND	ND	ND
Neutrophil (band)	0	0	284–696	490 ± 106
<10 year	ND	ND	ND	ND
>10 year	ND	ND	ND	ND
Neutrophil (mature)	2450–6850	4477 ± 937	2460–5980	4220 ± 880
<10 year	ND	ND	ND	ND
>10 year	ND	ND	ND	ND
Lymphocyte	310–3810	1750 ± 728	430–2510	1470 ± 520
<10 year	340–3670	2103 ± 790	880–2460	1730 ± 425
>10 year	940–2410	1375 ± 460	310–1890	1100 ± 395
Monocyte	80–640	284 ± 141	110–430	270 ± 80
<10 year	ND	ND	ND	ND
>10 year	ND	ND	ND	ND

continued

TABLE 181.2   Normal Hematology and Proteins with Age-Related Differences from Free-Ranging and Captive Atlantic Bottlenose Dolphins (*Tursiops truncatus*)   (*continued*)

Parameter	Free-Ranging Atlantic Bottlenose Dolphins[a,c] (*Tursiops truncatus*) (n = 30; sample n = 96)		Captive Bottlenose Dolphins[b,d] (*Tursiops truncatus*) (n = 119; sample n = 1202)	
	Range	Mean ± SD	Range	Mean ± SD
Eosinophil	1070–5340	2882 ± 1059	140–1510	830 ± 347
<10 year	1070–4585	2504 ± 843	ND	ND
>10 year	1150–4240	2995 ± 1100	ND	ND
Basophil	0–50	13 ± 10	0	0
<10 year	ND	ND	ND	ND
>10 year	ND	ND	ND	ND
Plasma proteins (g/dL)	6.3–8.7	7.5 ± 0.6	5.6–7.6	6.6 ± 0.5
<10 year	ND	ND	ND	ND
>10 year	ND	ND	ND	ND
Albumin (g/dL)	2.8–3.7	3.3 ± 0.2	4.2–5.4	4.8 ± 0.3
<10 year	ND	ND	ND	ND
>10 year	ND	ND	ND	ND
Globulin (g/dL)	3.0–5.5	4.2 ± 0.6	1.0–2.6	1.8 ± 0.4
<10 year	3.2–5.3	4.0 ± 0.5	1.0–2.2	1.6 ± 0.3
>10 year	3.0–5.5	4.3 ± 0.6	1.4–2.6	2.0 ± 0.3
Fibrinogen (g/dL)	NT	NT	142–412	277 ± 68
<10 year	NT	NT	ND	ND
>10 year	NT	NT	ND	ND

[a]Data contributed for Sarasota Bay free-ranging bottlenose dolphins by H. Rhinehart, J. Sweeney, F. Townsend, and R. Wells.
[b]Data contributed by SeaWorld.
[c]Ranges were calculated as ±2 standard deviations around the means.
[d]If ± SD exceeds observed high or low value, we reported the high or low observed value.
ND, no difference; *NT,* not tested.

TABLE 181.3A   Normal Hematology and Proteins from Captive Northern Fur Seals, Steller's Sea Lions, Northern Elephant Seals, and Harp Seals

Parameter	Northern Fur Seals[a,c] (*Callorhinus ursinus*) (n = 17; sample n = 123)		Steller's Sea Lions[a,c] (*Eumetopias jubata*) (n = 5; sample n = 41)		Northern Elephant Seals[b,d] (*Mirounga angustirostris*) (n = 149; sample n = 149)		Harp Seals[a,c] (*Pagophilus groenlandicus*) (n = 12; sample n = 139)	
	Range	Mean ± SD	Range	Mean ± SD	Range	Mean ± SD	Range	Mean ± SD
RBC (10^6/mm³)	4.4–5.8	5.1 ± 0.4	4.1–5.2	4.5 ± 0.3	2.0–2.9	2.5 ± 0.3	4.2–5.3	4.6 ± 0.3
Hb (g/dL)	15.1–18.9	16.2 ± 2.4	15–19	16.4 ± 1	17.3–24.9	21.0 ± 1.9	18.5–24.8	21.3 ± 1.8
HCT (%)	42–53	46.4 ± 3.3	42–49	45 ± 2.5	38–55	46 ± 4	45–63	53 ± 3.9
MCV (fL)	92–102	96 ± 3.1	96–111	103 ± 3.9	170–199	185 ± 7	97–125	115 ± 8.5
MCH (pg)	31.7–36	34 ± 1.2	33–39	36 ± 2	70–102	85 ± 9	39–49	45 ± 2.8
MCHC (g/dL)	32–38	35 ± 2.6	32–36	35 ± 1.4	40–53	46 ± 3.5	36–44	40 ± 2.1
Thrombocytes (10^3/µL)	320–698	428 ± 155	196–489	243 ± 128	120–754	437 ± 160	159–755	500 ± 211
Reticulocytes (%)	0	0	NT	NT	NT	NT	NT	NT
nRBC	0	0	0	0	0	0	0–4	0
ESR (@ 60 min)	NT	NT	NT	NT	NT	NT	NT	NT
Leukocytes/µL	3400–11500	6300 ± 2100	4700–10200	7100 ± 1840	9840–28600	19300 ± 4720	8600–15030	11800 ± 1720
Neutrophil (band)	0–264	39 ± 50	0–264	26 ± 62	0–517	517 ± 43	0–328	52 ± 88
Neutrophil (mature)	2173–7738	3213 ± 950	2420–8568	4454 ± 1608	4970–21890	13430 ± 4230	4386–9512	6367 ± 1973
Lymphocyte	534–3960	1701 ± 968	584–2886	1351 ± 785	510–6170	3430 ± 1460	1440–3608	2024 ± 663
Monocyte	92–1221	693 ± 422	134–876	552 ± 195	0–2750	1360 ± 690	310–1376	758 ± 332
Eosinophil	0–1700	693 ± 540	0–378	69 ± 128	0–960	230 ± 360	453–2460	1422 ± 629
Basophil	0–240	18 ± 42	0	0	0	0	0	0
Plasma proteins (g/dL)	6.3–7.6	6.9 ± 0.3	7.8–8.8	8.2 ± 0.3	5.4–8.6	6.9 ± 0.8	6.3–7.4	6.8 ± 0.3
Albumin (g/dL)	2.5–3.5	3.0 ± 0.3	3.7–4.2	3.9 ± 0.2	2.6–4.2	3.4 ± 0.4	3.2–3.5	3.4 ± 0.1
Globulin (g/dL)	3.7–4.5	4.0 ± 0.2	3.7–5.0	4.2 ± 0.3	2.0–5.2	3.5 ± 0.8	3.0–4.7	3.5 ± 0.5

[a]Data contributed by L. Dunn.
[b]Data contributed by F. Gulland.
[c]Ranges specified by contributor.
[d]If ± SD exceeds observed high or low value, we reported the high or low observed value.
NT, not tested.

TABLE 181.3B   Normal Hematology and Proteins from Harbor Seals, Gray Seals, and California Sea Lions

Parameter	Harbor Seals[a,c] (*Phoca vitulina*) (n = 24; sample n = 37)		Gray Seals[b,d] (*Halichoerus grypus*) (n = 9; sample n = 36)		California Sea Lions[a,c] (*Zalophus californianus*) (n = 26; sample n = 54)	
	Range	Mean ± SD	Range	Mean ± SD	Range	Mean ± SD
RBC (10^6/mm³)	4.7–5.1	5.0 ± 0.2	3.5–4.9	4.2 ± 0.3	4.2–4.9	4.6 ± 0.3
Hb (g/dL)	19.4–20.8	20.6 ± 0.8	16.4–20	17.6 ± 1.8	15.7–19.3	17.7 ± 1.9
HCT (%)	54–59	58 ± 2	43–52	48 ± 3	47–56	50 ± 3
MCV (fL)	111–119	117 ± 3	104–129	110 ± 9	108–112	109 ± 5
MCH (pg)	39–43	41 ± 2	40–47	43 ± 2.3	36–43	39 ± 2
MCHC (g/dL)	35–37	35 ± 1	35–43	37 ± 3.3	34–37	36 ± 1
Thrombocytes (10^3/µL)	285–355	314 ± 78	244–519	378 ± 102	218–390	280 ± 50
Reticulocytes (%)	0.3–0.5	0.4 ± 0.2	NT	NT	0.2–0.5	0.4 ± 0.2
nRBC	0	0	0	0	0	0
ESR (@ 60 min)	3.0–11	5 ± 5	NT	NT	8.0–38	26 ± 14
Leukocytes/µL	7100–8900	8020 ± 610	6800–13600	9900 ± 2700	4700–6100	5490 ± 2270
Neutrophil (band)	0–157	27 ± 30	0–360	43 ± 88	0	0
Neutrophil (mature)	4690–6490	5410 ± 1410	4278–9559	6594 ± 1579	2690–3800	3260 ± 980
Lymphocyte	1620–2450	1770 ± 510	1666–3872	2726 ± 620	1060–2040	1550 ± 450
Monocyte	520–910	610 ± 290	192–1599	725 ± 333	200–440	320 ± 90
Eosinophil	100–490	210 ± 160	0–994	448 ± 321	100–490	350 ± 150
Basophil	0	0	0–396	30 ± 59	0	0
Plasma proteins (g/dL)	7.7–8.2	7.8 ± 0.3	7.8–9	8.3 ± 0.4	6.8–7.4	7.1 ± 0.2
Albumin (g/dL)	2.6–3.0	2.9 ± 0.2	3.3–4.2	3.6 ± 0.3	3.3–3.0	3.1 ± 0.2
Globulin (g/dL)	4.4–5.3	4.9 ± 0.3	3.9–5.4	4.7 ± 0.4	3.6–4.1	4.0 ± 0.5
Fibrinogen (g/dL)	146–234	189 ± 43	NT	NT	156–316	235 ± 67

[a]Data contributed by SeaWorld.
[b]Data contributed by L. Dunn.
[q]If ± SD exceeds observed high or low value we reported the high or low observed value.
[d]Ranges specified by contributor.
NT, not tested.

TABLE 181.4   Normal Hematology and Proteins from Wild Harbor Seals, Northern Elephant Seals, and California Sea Lions

Parameter	No.	Harbor Seals[a,b] (*Phoca vitulina*) Range	Mean ± SD	No.	Northern Elephant Seals[a,b] (*Mirounga angustirostris*) Range	Mean ± SD	No.	California Sea Lions[a,b] (*Zalophus californianus*) Range	Mean ± SD
RBC (10^6/mm^3)									
Pup	27	4.0–5.7	4.9 ± 0.6	126	1.8–2.9	2.5 ± 0.2	86	3.5–4.8	4.1 ± 0.3
Yearling	36	3.6–4.9	4.3 ± 0.3	23	1.8–2.8	2.4 ± 0.3	58	2.9–4.8	3.9 ± 0.5
Adult	0	NT	NT	0	NT	NT	13	3.6–5.0	4.2 ± 0.4
Hb (g/dL)									
Pup	27	14.5–22.5	18.4 ± 3.2	126	17.6–23.9	20.8 ± 1.6	86	12.2–16.9	14.7 ± 1.3
Yearling	36	15–19.6	17.2 ± 1.5	23	17.3–27.3	22.6 ± 2.6	58	11.2–16.7	14.2 ± 2
Adult	0	NT	NT	0	NT	NT	13	14.3–18.9	16.0 ± 2
HCT (%)									
Pup	27	42–62	52 ± 8	126	38–54	46 ± 4	86	36–53	44 ± 6
Yearling	36	37–56	46 ± 5	23	32–60	47 ± 6	58	28–56	41 ± 6
Adult	0	NT	NT	0	NT	NT	13	40–54	46 ± 5
MCV (fL)									
Pup	27	91–118	106 ± 10	126	170–197	184 ± 7	86	93–128	105 ± 13
Yearling	36	94–122	108 ± 9	23	175–201	192 ± 8	58	89–123	106 ± 9
Adult	0	NT	NT	0	NT	NT	13	100–115	110 ± 8
MCH (pg)									
Pup	27	32–45	37 ± 4	126	70–96	83 ± 6.5	86	32–38	36 ± 2
Yearling	36	37–45	40 ± 3	23	80–121	96 ± 12	58	32–41	37 ± 2
Adult	0	NT	NT	0	NT	NT	13	35–41	38 ± 2
MCHC (g/dL)									
Pup	27	33–38	35 ± 1.5	126	40–51	45 ± 3	86	30–38	34 ± 2
Yearling	36	33–41	38 ± 2.5	23	43–60	50 ± 5	58	30–39	35 ± 3
Adult	0	NT	NT	0	NT	NT	13	33–36	35 ± 1
Thrombocytes (10^3/μL)									
Pup	27	494–1079	702 ± 149	126	171–661	455 ± 124	86	211–689	450 ± 119
Yearling	36	404–999	720 ± 185	23	208–702	389 ± 136	58	192–708	431 ± 138
Adult	0	NT	NT	0	NT	NT	13	153–673	398 ± 137
Reticulocytes (%)									
Pup	27	NT	NT	126	NT	NT	86	NT	NT
Yearling	36	NT	NT	23	NT	NT	58	NT	NT
Adult	0	NT	NT	0	NT	NT	13	NT	NT
nRBC									
Pup	27	NT	NT	126	NT	NT	86	NT	NT
Yearling	36	NT	NT	23	NT	NT	58	NT	NT
Adult	0	NT	NT	0	NT	NT	13	NT	NT
ESR (@ 60 min)									
Pup	27	NT	NT	126	NT	NT	86	NT	NT
Yearling	36	NT	NT	23	NT	NT	58	NT	NT
Adult	0	NT	NT	0	NT	NT	13	NT	NT
Leukocytes/μL									
Pup	27	6800–15600	12700 ± 3550	126	11200–28600	19800 ± 4610	86	9200–23800	16500 ± 3910
Yearling	36	6300–16600	12000 ± 3770	23	7830–24600	16200 ± 4200	58	9410–22800	16600 ± 3410
Adult	0	NT	NT	0	NT	NT	13	9400–15800	13300 ± 2890
Neutrophil (band)									
Pup	27	0–770	260 ± 260	126	0–1580	470 ± 393	86	0–380	260 ± 230
Yearling	36	0–340	90 ± 125	23	0–1260	70 ± 100	58	0–680	230 ± 230
Adult	0	NT	NT	0	NT	NT	13	0–580	170 ± 20
Neutrophil (mature)									
Pup	27	3200–11590	9230 ± 3450	126	6190–22170	13800 ± 4183	86	4580–20660	11380 ± 1350
Yearling	36	3600–12790	7920 ± 2760	23	4270–15830	11450 ± 4000	58	5140–16680	10490 ± 3225
Adult	0	NT	NT	0	NT	NT	13	3760–13310	8790 ± 3080

continued

TABLE 181.4   Normal Hematology and Proteins from Wild Harbor Seals, Northern Elephant Seals, and California Sea Lions (*continued*)

Parameter	Harbor Seals[a,b] (*Phoca vitulina*)			Northern Elephant Seals[a,b] (*Mirounga angustirostris*)			California Sea Lions[a,b] (*Zalophus californianus*)		
	No.	Range	Mean ± SD	No.	Range	Mean ± SD	No.	Range	Mean ± SD
Lymphocyte									
Pup	27	700–2040	1400 ± 870	126	1150–6170	3630 ± 1550	86	430–8820	3400 ± 1480
Yearling	36	1040–3700	2250 ± 730	23	430–3920	2390 ± 1430	58	1180–6380	3780 ± 1300
Adult	0	NT	NT	0	NT	NT	13	1070–5640	3040 ± 1300
Monocyte									
Pup	27	0–1830	890 ± 510	126	0–2800	1380 ± 709	86	0–2400	740 ± 450
Yearling	36	0–2450	1110 ± 670	23	170–2380	1260 ± 604	58	0–1600	730 ± 440
Adult	0	NT	NT	0	NT	NT	13	0–1480	660 ± 480
Eosinophil									
Pup	27	0–140	30 ± 50	126	0–810	190 ± 306	86	0–240	660 ± 490
Yearling	36	0–1440	450 ± 490	23	0–1540	410 ± 567	58	0–1470	650 ± 410
Adult	0	NT	NT	0	NT	NT	13	300–1800	670 ± 560
Basophil									
Pup	27	0	0	126	0	0	86	0	0
Yearling	36	0	0	23	0	0	58	0	0
Adult	0	NT	NT	0	NT	NT	13	0	0
Plasma proteins (g/dL)									
Pup	27	5.2–7.6	6.2 ± 0.8	126	5.4–8.2	7.6 ± 1.0	86	7.0–10.9	8.9 ± 1.0
Yearling	36	6.6–8.2	7.7 ± 0.7	23	6.3–9.6	7.9 ± 1.1	58	7.7–11.4	9.4 ± 1.0
Adult	0	NT	NT	0	NT	NT	13	8.2–10.9	9.3 ± 0.7
Albumin (g/dL)									
Pup	27	2.1–4.1	3.2 ± 0.8	126	2.7–4.2	3.4 ± 0.4	86	2.4–4.3	3.4 ± 0.5
Yearling	36	2.7–3.9	3.2 ± 0.5	23	2.5–4.1	3.3 ± 0.4	58	2.7–4.5	3.6 ± 0.5
Adult	0	NT	NT	0	NT	NT	13	2.9–3.9	3.2 ± 0.3
Globulin (g/dL)									
Pup	27	1.7–5.1	3.0 ± 1.1	126	2.0–4.8	3.4 ± 0.7	86	3.4–7.6	5.5 ± 1.0
Yearling	36	2.4–6.5	4.5 ± 1.0	23	2.8–6.2	4.3 ± 1.0	58	3.7–8.1	5.8 ± 1.2
Adult	0	NT	NT	0	NT	NT	13	4.2–8.2	5.1 ± 0.7
Fibrinogen (g/dL)									
Pup	27	NT	NT	180	NT	NT	86	NT	NT
Yearling	36	NT	NT	30	NT	NT	58	NT	NT
Adult	0	NT	NT	0	NT	NT	13	NT	NT

[a]Data contributed by F. Gulland.
[b]If ± SD exceeds observed high or low value, we reported the high or low observed value.
NT, not tested.

TABLE 181.5 Normal Hematology and Proteins from Florida Manatees, Polar Bears, and Sea Otters

Parameter	Florida Manatee[a,d] (Trichechus manatus latirostris) Range	Mean ± SD	Polar Bears[b,e] (Ursus maritimus) Range	Mean ± SD	Sea Otters (Enhydra lutris)[c,e] Pups (n = 21; sample n = 21) Range	Mean ± SD	Captive adults (n = 43; sample n = 43) Range	Mean ± SD	Wild adults (n = 123; sample n = 123) Range	Mean ± SD
RBC (10^6/mm^3)	2.4–3.4	2.8 ± 0.1	5.4–8.2	6.2 ± 0.6	2.5–4.6	3.6 ± 0.5	4.6–6.0	5.3 ± 0.3	4.3–5.7	5.0 ± 0.3
Hb (g/dL)	9.8–13.2	11.6 ± 0.5	12.9–17.5	14.6 ± 1.1	6.1–17.7	11.9 ± 2.9	15.6–22.2	18.9 ± 1.6	15.1–21.2	18.4 ± 1.6
HCT (%)	30–40	35 ± 1	36.1–53.3	41.4 ± 3.8	23–51	37 ± 7	46–62	54 ± 3.9	48–64	56 ± 3.9
MCV (fL)	122–149	128 ± 2	62.4–72.5	66.2 ± 1.9	82–114	98 ± 8	92–120	106 ± 6.8	95–123	109 ± 6.8
MCH (pg)	38–46	41 ± 1	21.2–25.6	23.4 ± 0.8	24–42	33 ± 4.3	30–42	36 ± 3.2	30–42	36 ± 3.2
MCHC (g/dL)	30–33	31 ± 1	328–370	354 ± 10	28–38	33 ± 2.5	29–43	36 ± 3.6	30–42	33 ± 3.6
Thrombocytes (10^3/μL)	195–412	283 ± 54	60–1083	317 ± 179	NT	NT	NT	NT	NT	NT
Reticulocytes (%)	0–4	0	0	0	NT	NT	NT	NT	NT	NT
nRBC	0	0	0	0	NT	NT	NT	NT	0–3.0	0.12 ± 1.5
ESR (@ 60 min)	7.0–85	34 ± 7	NT	NT	NT	NT	NT	NT	NT	NT
Leukocytes/μL	4000–11800	8640 ± 1930	3300–10800	5700 ± 1900	1100–14440	4770 ± 4833	4300–15160	9730 ± 2714	3670–14530	9100 ± 2714
Neutrophil (band)	0	0	100–300	200 ± 90	0	0	0	0	0	0
Neutrophil (mature)	960–5990	4300 ± 370	1800–4900	3000 ± 1010	2150–10160	2980 ± 3590	1530–10350	5940 ± 2205	1240–10060	5650 ± 2205
Lymphocyte	960–8590	3810 ± 1400	600–1700	1000 ± 340	1000–4330	1480 ± 1427	1600–5320	3460 ± 931	1050–4780	2915 ± 931
Monocyte	0–1020	270 ± 175	300–1120	300 ± 590	0–1880	210 ± 837	0–1080	230 ± 425	0–1100	255 ± 425
Eosinophil	0	0	40–440	190 ± 110	0–930	80 ± 427	0–1020	270 ± 373	0–1160	415 ± 373
Basophil	0	0	0–130	40 ± 50	0	0	0	0	0	0
Plasma proteins (g/dL)	6.2–8.6	7.4 ± 0.4	6.5–9.1	7.4 ± 0.8	3.3–7.5	5.4 ± 1	6.0–8.2	7.1 ± 0.6	5.9–8.1	7.0 ± 0.6
Albumin (g/dL)	3.6–5.9	4.4 ± 0.3	3.7–5.2	4.5 ± 0.4	1.3–3.5	2.4 ± 0.5	2.8–4.0	3.4 ± 0.3	2.4–3.5	3.0 ± 0.3
Globulin (g/dL)	2.6–2.7	3.2 ± 0.5	2.3–4.2	3.0 ± 0.6	1.0–5.0	3.0 ± 1.0	2.7–4.7	3.7 ± 0.5	3.1–5.0	4.0 ± 0.5

[a] Data contributed by G. Bossart and D. Odell.
[b] Data contributed by M. Cattet and N. Caulkett.
[c] Data contributed by T. Williams.
[d] Ranges are 25–75% quartiles around median value of combined data.
[e] Ranges specified by contributor.
NT, not tested.

ACKNOWLEDGMENTS

The authors are grateful to the following contributors: Greg Bossart, DVM, PhD; Marc R.L. Cattet, DVM, Msc; Nigel A. Caulkett, DVM, MVetSc; Larry Dunn, DVM; Frances Gulland, DVM, PhD; Daniel Odell, PhD; Howard Rhinehart; Jay Sweeney, VMD; Forrest Townsend, DVM; Randall Wells, PhD; and Thomas Williams, DVM.

REFERENCES

1. **Ridgway SH.** Homeostasis in the aquatic environment. In: Ridgway SH, ed. Mammals of the sea, biology and medicine. Springfield, IL: Charles C. Thomas, 1972;605.

2. **Cornell LH.** Hematology and clinical chemistry values in the killer whale, Orcinus orca. J Wildl Dis 1983;19:259–264.

3. **Wallach JD, Boever WJ.** Cetaceans and sirenians. In: Diseases of exotic animals: medical and surgical management. Philadelphia: WB Saunders, 1983;687–725.

4. **Medway W, Geraci JR.** Clinical pathology of marine mammals. In: Fowler ME, ed. Zoo and wild animal medicine. 2nd ed. Philadelphia: WB Saunders, 1986;791–798.

5. **ISIS.** Average physiological values. Apple Valley, MN: ISIS and the AAZV, 1987.

6. **Cornell LH, Duffield DA, Joseph BE, Stark B.** Hematology and serum chemistry values in beluga (*Delphinapterus leucas*). J Wildl Dis 1988;224:220–224.

7. **Asper ED, Cornell LH, Duffield DA, Odell DK, Joseph BE, Stark BI, Perry CA.** Hematology and serum chemistry values in bottlenose dolphins. In: Leatherwood S, Reeves RR, eds. The bottlenose dolphin. San Diego: Academic Press, 1990;479–485.

8. **Rhinehart H, Wells RS, Townsend FI, Sweeney JC, Caspter DR.** Blood profiles of free-ranging bottlenose dolphins from the central west coast of Florida. Contract report to National Marine Fisheries Service, Southeast Fisheries Center, Miami, FL. Contract no. 40-WCNF-003060, 1991.

9. **Wells RS.** The role of long-term study of a bottlenose dolphin community. In: Pryor K, Norris KS, eds. Dolphin societies: discoveries and puzzles. Berkeley: University of California Press, 1991;199–225.

10. **Rhinehart HL, Wells RS, Townsend FI, Sweeney JC, Casper DR.** Blood profiles of free-ranging bottlenose dolphins from the central west coast of Florida: 1991–92. Contract report to National Marine Fisheries Service, Southeast Fisheries Center, Miami, FL. Contract no. 50-WCNF-706083, 1992.

11. **Walsh MT, Bossart GD.** Manatee medicine. In: Zoo and wild animal medicine: current therapy. Philadelphia: WB Saunders, 1998;507–516.

12. **Bossart GD, Dierauf LA.** Marine mammal clinical laboratory medicine. In: Dierauf LA, ed. Handbook of marine mammal medicine: health, disease, and rehabilitation. Boca Raton, FL: CRC Press, 1990;1–52.

13. **Dierauf L.** Marine mammal clinical laboratory medicine. In: Dierauf LA, ed. Handbook of marine mammal medicine: health, disease, and rehabilitation. Boca Raton, FL: CRC Press, 1990;553–590.

14. **Williams TM, Davis RW.** Emergency care and rehabilitation of oiled sea otters: a guide for oil spills involving fur-bearing marine mammals. Fairbanks: University of Alaska Press, 1995;48.

CHAPTER 182

Normal Hematology of Elasmobranchs

• MICHAEL K. STOSKOPF

The taxonomic radiation of the more than 500 species of extant elasmobranchs includes a wide variety of adaptations to different ecologic niches, so variation in hematologic parameters among the various families and genera of cartilaginous fishes should be expected. Unfortunately, the blood constituents of relatively few elasmobranch species have been investigated, and much of the published basic research has been conducted on species that are not commonly displayed or managed in captivity. Almost no work has been published correlating changes in hematologic parameters to the presence of disease in elasmobranchs.

Elasmobranchs have nucleated erythrocytes and circulating blast cells, and mitotic figures are commonly believed to be related to the erythrocytic series, although detailed studies to confirm this are not available (Table 182.1). All principal leukocyte types are found in elasmobranch blood (Table 182.2).[1,2] Detailed electron microscopy and some cytochemistry studies of these cells are available.[3–9] Elasmobranch blood morphology can be accomplished readily using routine methods, and classification of cells into heterophils (Fig. 182.1), eosinophils (Fig. 182.2), lymphocytes (Fig. 182.3), monocytes (Fig. 182.4), and thrombocytes (Fig. 182.5) is relatively clear on the basis of cytoplasmic granule morphology and staining intensity in modified Wright-Giemsa stained smears.

A major controversy exists about the nature of the predominant granulocytic cell types found in elasmobranchs. Despite efforts to classify them as eosinophils, all functional evidence points to their being true heterophils with activities much like the neutrophil of mammals.[10] The question is complicated because both eosinophils and heterophils of the elasmobranchs that have been studied are acid phosphatase and periodic acid-Schiff (PAS) positive.[1,5] Grimaldi et al.[1] found heterophilic granulocytes to be more intensely PAS- and aliesterase-positive and weakly adenosine triphosphatase (ATPase)-positive compared with eosinophilic granulocytes, which show the presence of neutral polysaccharides in the matrix but have strongly ATPase- and acid-phosphatase–positive granules. Some phagocytic activity has been demonstrated in elasmobranch heterophils.[11] In the author's work, a cell morphologically similar to granulocytes but without cytoplasmic granules is

commonly seen in blood of some species. It is not known whether these are cells that have degranulated or have not yet developed granules, or if they represent a distinct cell type. No cytochemical staining studies have been done to elucidate the situation, and such cells are routinely grouped with heterophils in reporting differential counts.

Elasmobranchs have efficient immunosurveillance, and there is phyletic conservation of some cell mediators and regulatory products of lymphocytes and monocytes between elasmobranchs and humans.[12] Elasmobranch lymphocytes, monocytes, and thrombocytes can show weak PAS staining. Lymphocytes may also have aliesterase-positive granules, whereas monocytes occasionally show some small PAS-positive granules and weak acid phosphatase and aliesterase activities.[1] Phagocytosis has been demonstrated for elasmobranch monocytes but not for lymphocytes.[11]

Only a single thrombocyte cell type has been described in elasmobranchs. This is in contrast to similarly studied teleosts that have two morphologic thrombocyte types.[13] The thrombocytes of elasmobranchs are rounded to spindle-shaped and originate in the spleen from prothrombocytes.[14] They contain microtubules and cytoplasmic granules that seem to correspond functionally to the mammalian platelet canalicular system based on tannic acid treatment.[13,14] The cytoplasmic presence of platelet factor 4, beta-thromboglobulin, and factor VIII-related antigen has been demonstrated by immunocytochemical staining. Elasmobranch thrombocytes adhere to glass, and aggregation and degranulation can be stimulated by collagen, noradrenaline, 5-hydroxytryptamine, thrombin, or adenosine diphosphate.[14] Thrombocytes contain some peripheral granules that are PAS-positive and slightly ATPase-positive.[1]

An important methodologic problem in elasmobranch clinical pathology is the determination of serum total protein. Determinations made by refractometer return artificially high serum or plasma total protein concentrations because of the urea nitrogen concentrations elasmobranchs maintain for the purposes of osmotic regulation. Refractometer determinations are routinely 2 to 3 times higher than automated colorimetric assays for total protein, which have been reported in the range of 0.4 to 0.6 gm/dL (Table 182.3).

TABLE 182.1 Baseline Erythrocyte Indices of Elasmobranchs

Species	No.	Total RBC ($\times 10^6$/mL)	Hematocrit (%)	Hemoglobin (gm/dL)	Reference
Blue shark	14		22	6	17
Brown shark (captive)	20	0.532	20	<4	18
Lemon shark (captive)	3	0.665	20	5	18
Nurse shark (wild)	5	0.366	10	4	18
Nurse shark (captive)	7	0.35	11	<4	18
Portuguese shark	1	—	13	—	19
Sandtiger shark (captive)	9	0.276	24	6(8)	Stoskopf MK, unpublished data, 1998
Spiny dogfish	21	—	19	5	15
Torpedo	15	0.201	25	23	20

TABLE 182.2 Baseline Leukocyte Indices of Elasmobranchs

Species	No.	Total WBC ($\times 10^3$/mL)	Hetero (%)	Band (%)	Mono (%)	Lymph (%)	Eosinophil (%)	Basophil (%)	Reference
Brown shark (captive)	20	28.1	58	0	1	40	1	0	18
Lemon shark (captive)	3	25.9							18
Nurse shark (wild)	5	27.8							18
Nurse shark (captive)	7	27.2	56		1.4	30	0	0	18
Sandtiger shark (wild)	8	16.1	45		1	19	28	0	Stoskopf MK, unpublished data, 1998
Torpedo	15	43.8							20

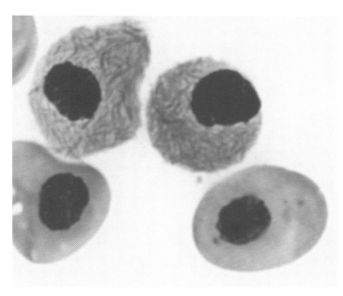

FIGURE 182.1 Two heterophils from a sandtiger shark (*Odontaspis taurus*) showing numerous elongated fusiform cytoplasmic granules and no lobation of the nucleus.

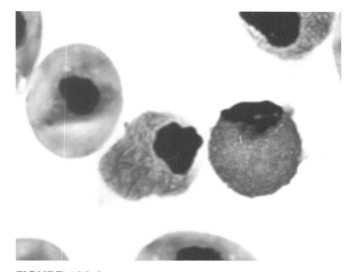

FIGURE 182.2 An eosinophil (right) and a heterophil (left) from a sandtiger shark (*Odontaspis taurus*) showing the eccentric nucleus and rounder more eosinophilic cytoplasmic granules of the eosinophil compared to the long spicular cytoplasmic granules of the heterophil.

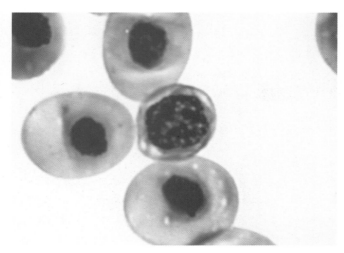

FIGURE 182.3 A small lymphocyte among erythrocytes from a sandtiger shark (*Odontaspis taurus*) showing the relatively dense central round nucleus of the lymphocyte surrounded by a thin rim of cytoplasm.

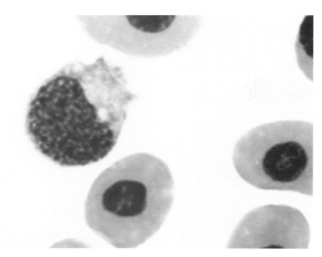

FIGURE 182.4 A monocyte from a brown shark (*Carcharhinus plumbeus*). Note the large nucleus and foamy cytoplasm of this leukocyte, which is larger than young lymphocytes.

Determination of circulating thyroid hormone concentrations in elasmobranch blood can also be problematic. Very low or undetectable levels of hormone are frequently reported if samples are routinely processed using current methods for human blood. The problem appears to be very strong binding of hormone to elasmobranch thyroid hormone binding proteins. Older methods that use more stringent methods for stripping hormone from the binding protein yield more consistent and useful values for circulating T3 and T4 (Table 182.4).

RESPONSES TO INFECTIOUS DISEASE

Elasmobranch hematologic parameters respond to infectious diseases with many of the same changes seen in mammals. Bacterial infections routinely cause marked leukocytosis usually due to heterophilia. A distinct shift to the left is difficult to demonstrate, because the mature granulocytic series of cells in elasmobranchs have less distinctly lobated nuclei than analogous cells of most mammals. This makes detection of young cells less certain.

There has been little or no experience in the hematologic changes seen with viral or protozoal diseases in elasmobranchs. Overwhelming trematode infections can be accompanied by leukocytosis, but it is difficult to know whether this is a response to trematodes, a generalized stress response, or a response to secondary bacterial infections that can accompany heavy trematode infestations.

RESPONSE TO NONINFECTIOUS DISEASE

Stress is a common factor in interpretation of elasmobranch hemograms. Confinement stress appears to cause decreased erythrocyte counts, hematocrit, and hemoglobin levels in the spiny dogfish. In addition to this nonregenerative and most likely redistributional anemia, serum glucose and the total leukocyte count increase dramatically.[15] This suggests that the stress leukogram of elasmobranchs may be difficult to differentiate from a response to bacterial septicemia. The leukocytosis in both instances is primarily due to heterophilia, and accompanying eosinopenia in the stress leukogram may not be appreciated easily.

The other reasonably well-documented apparent noninfectious cause of hematologic changes in sharks, skates, and rays is heavy metal toxicity. Copper expo-

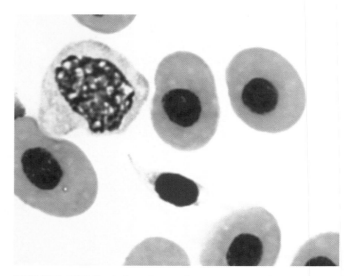

FIGURE 182.5 A thrombocyte (lower center) and a monocyte from a brown shark (*Carcharhinus plumbeus*). The thrombocyte has a typical dense nucleus and a characteristic elongated tag of cytoplasm that is not always seen. A few cytoplasmic granules are also present. The nucleus of the monocyte is more open than the example in Figure 182.4.

TABLE 182.3   Baseline Serologic Parameters of Elasmobranchs

Species	No.	Urea Nitrogen (mg/dL)	Uric Acid (mg/dL)	Creatinine (mg/dL)	Total Protein (gm/dL)	Albumin (gm/dL)	Globulin (gm/dL)	Reference
Blacktip shark (captive)	2	1015	0.3	0.5	3.3	0.5	2.8	Stoskopf MK, unpublished data, 1998
Brown shark (wild)	33	848 (34)	0.45	0.45	2.2	0.5	1.7	18
Dusky shark (wild)	5	912	0.8	0.5	1.7	0.6	1.1	18
Finetooth shark (captive)	3	983	0.4	0.4	2.4	0.4	2.0	Stoskopf MK, unpublished data, 1998
Scalloped hammerhead shark (wild)	4	880	1.0	0.4	2.5	0.4	2.1	18
Lemon shark (captive)	2	1023	1.0	0.9	3.5	0.6	2.9	18
Nurse shark (wild)	9	1147	0.2	0.4	2.6	0.6	2.2	18
Nurse shark (captive)	12	1087	0.3	0.45	2.0	0.4	1.5	18
Sharpnose shark (wild)	10	847	1.1	0.5	2.1	0.4	1.7	18
Sandtiger shark (wild)	3	1027	0.1	0.3	3.3	0.6	2.7	Stoskopf MK, unpublished data, 1998
Spinner shark (captive)	3	923	0.2	0.6	2.6	0.4	2.2	Stoskopf MK, unpublished data, 1998
Tiger shark (captive, compromised)	2	1134	0.8	1.0	4.6	0.5	4.2	18

TABLE 182.4   Baseline Serum Thyroid Parameters of Elasmobranchs

Species	No.	Total T4 (ug/dL)	T-Uptake (Units)	T3 Uptake (%)	Free T4 (Index)	Reference
Blacktip shark (captive)	2	3.3	0.13	68.2	2.2	Stoskopf MK, unpublished data, 1998
Dusky shark (wild)	5	4.5	0.12	68.4	3.1	18
Finetooth shark (captive)	3	4.4	0.10	69.0	3.0	Stoskopf MK, unpublished data, 1998
Scalloped hammerhead shark (wild)	4	2.9	0.2	65.2	1.8	18
Sharpnose shark (wild)	10	2.9	0.12	68.3	2.0	18
Spinner shark (captive)	3	3.6	0.12	68.2	2.5	Stoskopf MK, unpublished data, 1998

sure is a common problem in captive animals, and elasmobranchs are much more sensitive to this metal than most marine teleost fishes. A normochromic, normocytic anemia with decreased total erythrocyte count and hematocrit and a stable hemoglobin value has been documented in spiny dogfish exposed to physiologically compromising sublethal concentrations of copper (2 ppm for 48 hours). A leukopenia and decreased serum glucose has also been seen.[16] Exposure to higher copper levels (4, 6, 8, and 16 ppm) is fatal to spiny dogfish within 56 hours, with a similar anemia plus falling hemoglobin concentrations.[16]

Zinc exposure in spiny dogfish also causes hypochromic microcytic anemia characterized by decreased he-moglobin, but the hematocrit generally remains stable while the total erythrocyte count is increased. This toxicity is characterized by leukocytosis, in contrast to what is observed in copper exposure. Serum glucose may also be depressed in zinc toxicosis.[15]

REFERENCES

1. **Grimaldi MC, D'Ippolito S, Pica A, Della-Corte F.** Cytochemical identification of the leucocytes of Torpedoes (*Torpedo marmorate* and *Torpedo ocellata*). Basic Appl Histochem 1983;27:311–318.
2. **Parish N, Wrathmell A, Hart S, Harris JE.** The leucocytes of the elasmobranch *Scyliorhinus canicula* L. a morphological study. J Fish Biol 1986; 28:545–561.
3. **Fange R.** The formation of eosinophilic granulocytes in the oesophageal lymphomyeloid tissue of the elasmobranchs. Acta Zoologica 1968;49: 155–161.

4. **Fange R, Mattisson A.** The lymphomyeloid (hemopoietic) system of the Atlantic nurse shark, *Ginglymostoma cirratum.* Biol Bull 1981;160:240–249.
5. **Hine PM, Wain JM.** The enzyme cytochemistry and composition of elasmobranch granulocytes. J Fish Biol 1987;30:465–475.
6. **Hine PM, Wain JM.** Composition and ultrastructure of elasmobranch granulocytes. I. Dogfishes (Squaliformes). J Fish Biol 1987;30:547–556.
7. **Hine PM, Wain JM.** Composition and ultrastructure of elasmobranch granulocytes. II. Rays (Rajiformes). J Fish Biol 1987;30:557–565.
8. **Hine PM, Wain JM.** Composition and ultrastructure of elasmobranch granulocytes. III. Sharks(Lamniformes). J Fish Biol 1987;30:567–576.
9. **Morrow WJW, Pulsford A.** Identification of peripheral blood leucocytes of the dogfish (*Scyliorhinus canicula* L.) by electron microscopy. J Fish Biol 1980;17:461–475.
10. **Mainwaring G, Rowley AF.** Studies on granulocyte heterogeneity in elasmobranchs. In: Manning MJ, Tatner HF, eds. Fish immunology. London: Academic Press, 1986.
11. **Hyder SL, Cayer ML, Pettey CL.** Cell types in peripheral blood of the nurse shark (*Ginglymostoma cirratum*): an approach to structure and function. Tissue Cell 1983;15:437–456.
12. **Grogan ED, Lund R.** Reactivity of human white blood cells to factors of elasmobranch origin. Copeia 1991;2:402–408.
13. **Zapata A, Carrato A.** Ultrastructure of elasmobranch and teleost thrombocytes. Acta Zool (Copenhagen) 1980;61:179–182.
14. **Pica A, Lodate A, Grimaldi MC, Della-Corte F.** Morphology, origin and functions of the thrombocytes of Elasmobranchs. Arch Italiano Anat Embriol 1990;95(3-4):187–207.
15. **Torres P, Tort L, Planas J, Flos R.** Effects of confinement stress and additional zinc treatment on some blood parameters in the dogfish, *Scyliorhinus canicula.* Comp Biochem Physiol 1986;83C:89–92.
16. **Tort L, Torres P, Flos R.** Effects on dogfish haematology and liver composition after acute copper exposure. Comp Biochem Physiol 1987;87C:349–353.
17. **Johansson-Sjobeck M, Stevens JD.** Hematological studies on the blue shark, *Prionace glauca* L. J Mar Biol Assoc UK 1976;56:237–240.
18. **Stoskopf MK.** Clinical pathology of sharks, skates, and rays. In: Stoskopf MK, ed. Fish medicine. Philadelphia: WB Saunders, 1993;754–757.
19. **Sherburne SW.** Cell types, differential cell counts and blood cell measurements of a Portuguese shark (*Centrocymnus coelolepsis*) captured at 700 fathoms. Fish Bull 1973;71:435–439.
20. **Pica A, Grimaldi MC, Della-Corte F.** The circulating blood cells of torpedoes (*Torpedo marmorate* and *Torpedo ocellata*). Monitore Zool Italiano 1983;17:353–374.

CHAPTER 183

Normal Hematology of the Deer

• CATHERINE E. THORN

Members of the Cervidae family have erythrocytes with unique characteristics. The erythrocytes circulate in the vasculature as round cells which are slightly smaller than bovine red cells. However, shortly after phlebotomy, the red cells tend to assume a sickle shape (Fig. 183.1). The cells are not sickled when first removed from the body, but the shape change occurs as the blood stands at room temperature or at 4°C. This sickling phenomenon was first reported in 1875 by Gulliver.[1] The sickling effect can be prevented by acidifying the blood. At pH 7.0, few red cells are sickled; at pH 7.4, most of the red cells have a sickle shape. Sickling may be enhanced by oxygenation of the red cells. In vivo, transient alkalosis and increased oxygenation have similar effects on red cell morphology. There are at least three exceptions within the cervidae family: the erythrocytes of reindeer, caribou, and montjac deer do not assume the sickle shape when exposed to oxygen.[2]

The sickling effect is due to the formation of insoluble tactoids of variant forms of hemoglobin (Hb) in the oxygenated state. Deer erythrocytes contain several forms of Hb, each of which has different electrophoretic properties and is associated with a distinct morphologic red cell shape.[3] The number of different variant forms of Hb in a given individual deer may range from one to three. Types I and III Hb are present in approximately half the deer population. Hb type II alone or in combination with Hb types I, III, or IVb is often associated with the development of a matchstick shape, which forms subsequent to the development of sickling. Red cells that contain Hb type IVa may assume a burr shape. Other red cell shapes include the traditional crescent or holly leaf. The sickle effect does not occur if Hb type V or VII is present. The sickling phenomenon is an interesting laboratory observation but does not appear to have a deleterious effect on the deer.[4]

REFERENCE INTERVALS

Data from various species of deer are depicted in Table 183.1. Species differences in erythrocyte values, indices, and leukocyte parameters have been noted. Comparable reference intervals have been published elsewhere.[5]

White-tailed deer have red blood cell (RBC), Hb, and packed cell volume (PCV) values that are considerably higher than those found in mule deer, black-tailed deer, or chital deer. Inversely, the leukocyte count of white-tailed deer tends to be slightly lower than that reported for other species of deer. Observations on several species of deer have revealed a direct relationship between red cell size and body size in members of the Cervidae.[6] As seen in other mammals, an indirect relationship between red cell size and red cell number is also seen in deer.

INFLUENCE OF AGE

Age-related changes in hematologic patterns in deer have been reported (Table 183.2). A distinct pattern of increases in RBC, Hb, and PCV with age is evident regardless of sex or species.[7,8] Newborn animals have lower red cell values and higher reticulocyte counts than juveniles and adults. Increases in RBC and hematocrit (HCT) by 40 to 60% from birth to age 10 months were noted in chital deer.[8] Red cell values tend to be lower in juveniles than in adults. Similar findings have been reported for chital deer, captive reindeer, and fallow deer.[8–10] The total white cell count in neonatal chital deer

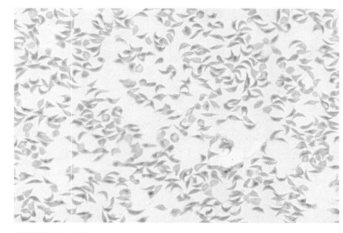

FIGURE 183.1 Sickle-shaped, or drepanocytes, deer red cells. (Courtesy of Dr. Stuart Porter.)

TABLE 183.1 Hematologic Values in Members of the Cervidae Family

Reference	Animal	No., Age, Sex	RBC (× 10⁶/μL)	Hb (g/dL)	PCV (%)	MCV (fL)	MCH (pg)	MCHC (%)	WBC (× 10³/μL)	Neutrophils	Lymphocytes	Monocytes	Eosinophils	Basophils
17	Blacktail[a] (Vancouver)	26 females, 2–21 days	5.5 ± 0.3	10.3 ± 0.3	33.8 ± 1.4	—	—	—	5.04 ± 0.43	41 ± 1.8	39 ± 2.0	15.8 ± 1.1	2.1	0.8
	Blacktail[a] (Vancouver)	23 males, 2–21 days	5.5 ± 0.3	9.8 ± 0.4	35.1 ± 1.7	—	—	—	5.52 ± 0.45	—	—	—	—	—
	Blacktail[b] (Vancouver)	11 males and females, 24–57 days	11.6 ± 0.7	14.2 ± 0.2	36.8 ± 3.5	—	—	—	5.52 ± 0.40	37 ± 3.5	57 ± 2.6	5.9 ± 1.7	0	0.2
	Blacktail[b] (Alaska)	9 males and females, 40–45 days	10.4 ± 0.6	14.0 ± 0.2	36.2 ± 1.2	—	—	—	5.45 ± 0.44	34 ± 1.9	60 ± 1.9	4.0 ± 0.5	0	0.7
	Blacktail[b] (California)	16 males and females, 65–117 days	14.2 ± 0.6	15.7 ± 0.2	43.0 ± 1.2	—	—	—	4.42 ± 0.29	41 ± 1.7	52 ± 1.8	4.0 ± 4.0	0.1	0.4
	Mule deer	8 males and females, 23–68 days	8.8 ± 0.7	13.5 ± 0.3	34.1 ± 1.4	—	—	—	5.83 ± 0.70	49 ± 3.2	45 ± 2.7	4.0 ± 0.3	0.1	0.4
18	Mule deer	368 males and females, mature	10.1	17.0	44.8	—	—	—	—	—	—	—	—	—
19	Mule deer	8 males and females, 1–6.5 yr	5.2–12.7 (9.19)	10.2–16.5 (12.8)	32.1–45.7 (39.6)	—	—	—	1.8–5.0 (3.3)	—	—	—	—	—
20	Mule deer	170–175 males and females, 1–162 mo	8.8 ± 0.2	16.4 ± 0.3	46.7 ± 0.6	—	—	—	3.0 ± 0.1	40.6 ± 1.2	43.4 ± 1.1	6.2 ± 0.5	8.3 ± 0.6	0.4 ± 0.1
21	Whitetail (Florida)	>500 males and females, >1 yr	17.0–20.0	17–21	55–61	—	—	—	1.5–3.0	30–35	55–70	2	2–15	0–2
22	Whitetail (Michigan)	126 males and females, birth to 6 mo	16.9 ± 0.4	17.5 ± 0.4	46.3 ± 0.8	30.2 ± 0.5	11.1 ± 0.1	35.8 ± 0.3	3.7 ± 0.1	—	—	—	—	—
	Whitetail (Michigan)	258 males and females, 7 mo–5 yr	17.0 ± 0.2	20.8 ± 0.1	56.3 ± 0.4	33.0 ± 0.4	12.2 ± 0.1	37.2 ± 0.2	3.2 ± 0.1	—	—	—	—	—
23	Whitetail (Minnesota)	18 males, >1 yr	10.8 ± 1.9	13.5 ± 1.9	40.0 ± 5.7	—	—	—	—	—	—	—	—	—
	Whitetail (Minnesota)	33 females, >1 yr	11.2 ± 1.6	14.7 ± 2.6	44.0 ± 7.4	—	—	—	—	—	—	—	—	—

[a]Wild animals.
[b]Captive animals revealed higher RBC parameter than wild animals.

TABLE 183.2   Changes in Blood Components with Growth of Suckling Black-Tailed Deer (*Odocoileus hemionus columbianus*) (Mean ± Standard Error and Range)[a]

Parameter	Sex	1–9 Days	10–29 Days	30–89 Days	90–139 Days	>140 Days	Probability Value[b]
RBC (× 10⁶/µL)	M	7.51 ± 1.22 (15)[c] (5.52–10.02)	7.79 ± 1.00 (18) (6.36–9.66)	9.67 ± 1.54 (23) (8.00–12.96)	10.60 ± 1.39 (9) (6.01–12.35)	10.46 ± 1.80 (15) (6.52–13.28)	***
	F	7.32 ± 0.85 (20) (5.85–9.03)	7.10 ± 0.52 (16) (6.30–8.30)	9.65 ± 1.26 (24) (7.47–12.16)	10.03 ± 1.62 (13) (8.12–13.82)	8.96 ± 1.25 (32) (7.20–11.56)	***
		NS[d]	*	NS	NS	**	
Hb (g/dL)	M	9.33 ± 0.93 (15) (8.10–11.00)	11.32 ± 1.45 (18) (8.20–14.40)	13.45 ± 2.17 (23) (8.80–18.10)	14.04 ± 1.08 (9) (12.70–15.80)	15.43 ± 2.63 (15) (10.80–22.00)	***
	F	9.38 ± 1.08 (20) (9.30–12.70)	10.93 ± 1.13 (16) (9.30–12.70)	13.73 ± 1.42 (24) (10.10–16.20)	13.44 ± 1.06 (13) (12.30–16.40)	12.90 ± 1.29 (32) (9.90–15.20)	***
		NS	NS	NS	NS	**	
PCV (%)	M	29.7 ± 3.5 (15) (24.0–37.0)	32.2 ± 3.7 (18) (26.0–40.0)	37.4 ± 5.9 (23) (25.0–50.0)	38.7 ± 2.9 (9) (34.0–42.0)	42.1 ± 7.4 (15) (31.0–61.0)	**
	F	29.1 ± 3.7 (20) (21.0–35.0)	32.3 ± 2.9 (16) (28.0–37.0)	37.9 ± 3.6 (24) (30.0–44.0)	37.6 ± 2.8 (13) (35.0–45.0)	35.4 ± 3.4 (32) (29.0–44.0)	***
		NS	NS	NS	NS	**	
MCV (fL)	M	39.9 ± 4.0 (15) (32.7–47.1)	41.6 ± 4.7 (18) (35.8–49.0)	38.9 ± 6.0 (23) (31.0–59.9)	36.8 ± 3.6 (9) (32.4–43.8)	40.8 ± 5.9 (15) (32.5–49.2)	NS
	F	40.1 ± 3.4 (20) (33.9–46.5)	45.6 ± 3.0 (16) (40.6–49.7)	39.6 ± 2.7 (24) (34.6–44.6)	38.0 ± 3.7 (13) (30.3–43.1)	39.8 ± 3.6 (32) (32.0–45.8)	*
		NS	**	NS	NS	NS	

TABLE 183.2 Changes in Blood Components with Growth of Suckling Black-Tailed Deer (*Odocoileus hemionus columbianus*) (Mean ± Standard Error and Range)[a] (continued)

Parameter	Sex	1–9 Days	10–29 Days	30–89 Days	90–139 Days	>140 Days	Probability Value[b]
MCHC (%)	M	31.7 ± 1.7 (15) (27.4–34.3)	35.2 ± 1.45 (18) (31.5–37.6)	36.1 ± 1.5 (23) (34.1–39.7)	36.3 ± 0.8 (9) (35.3–37.6)	36.1 ± 2.5 (15) (28.1–39.0)	**
	F	32.4 ± 1.5 (20) (30.9–36.2)	33.8 ± 1.0 (16) (32.2–35.2)	36.3 ± 1.2 (24) (33.7–38.8)	35.7 ± 0.6 (13) (34.9–36.4)	36.5 ± 1.1 (32) (34.2–38.3)	***
		NS	**	NS	NS	NS	
MCH (pg)	M	12.6 ± 1.4 (15) (10.8–14.7)	14.6 ± 1.6 (18) (12.3–17.6)	14.1 ± 2.5 (23) (10.9–23.5)	13.4 ± 1.3 (9) (11.7–15.9)	15.0 ± 2.1 (15) (11.6–17.8)	*
	F	13.0 ± 1.3 (20) (10.8–16.1)	15.4 ± 1.1 (16) (13.6–17.3)	14.3 ± 1.1 (24) (12.8–16.7)	13.6 ± 1.3 (13) (10.9–15.3)	14.5 ± 1.3 (32) (12.0–16.9)	**
		NS	NS	NS	NS	NS	
Protein (g/dL)	M	6.1 ± 0.6 (15) (5.4–7.5)	5.8 ± 0.6 (18) (5.0–7.0)	5.8 ± 0.5 (23) (4.9–6.4)	6.1 ± 0.3 (9) (5.7–6.5)	6.6 ± 0.5 (15) (5.4–7.5)	*
	F	6.0 ± 0.3 (20) (5.6–6.6)	6.0 ± 0.4 (16) (5.2–6.5)	6.0 ± 0.4 (24) (5.5–6.8)	6.0 ± 0.3 (13) (5.6–6.5)	6.7 ± 0.5 (32) (5.7–8.0)	*
		NS	NS	NS	NS	NS	
Fibrinogen (g/dL)	M	0.3 ± 0.15 (15) (0.1–0.6)	0.29 ± 0.12 (18) (0.1–0.5)	0.28 ± 0.14 (23) (0.1–0.6)	0.27 ± 0.11 (9) (0.1–0.4)	0.27 ± 0.12 (15) (0.1–0.5)	NS
	F	0.25 ± 0.14 (20) (0.1–0.6)	0.37 ± 0.20 (16) (0.1–0.7)	0.32 ± 0.17 (24) (0.1–0.9)	0.25 ± 0.10 (13) (0.1–0.4)	0.23 ± 0.11 (32) (0.1–0.6)	NS
		NS	NS	NS	NS	NS	
WBC (× 10³/µL)	M	5.3 ± 1.8 (15) (3.2–9.3)	5.0 ± 2.5 (18) (2.7–10.5)	4.5 ± 2.4 (23) (1.3–11.1)	2.8 ± 1.1 (9) (1.2–4.5)	3.6 ± 8.6 (15) (1.9–5.3)	**
	F	5.1 ± 2.2 (20) (2.4–12.5)	4.4 ± 1.1 (16) (2.7–5.9)	4.1 ± 9.7 (24) (2.3–6.1)	3.7 ± 1.0 (13) (2.6–5.7)	5.0 ± 1.7 (32) (2.7–9.3)	**
		NS	NS	NS	NS	***	

[a]From Dr. Nadine K. Jacobsen, unpublished observations.
[b]Probability value of unbalanced, one-way ANOVA by sex class. NS = nonsignificant difference, * = <0.05, ** = <0.01, *** = <0.001.
[c]Number in parentheses = number of deer.
[d]Probability value of unpaired *t*-test of differences between sexes within an age class.

was significantly greater than that of juveniles or adults, largely due to increased numbers of neutrophils and a neutrophil:lymphocyte ratio of 2:1.[8] In adults, lymphocytes predominate.[8]

INFLUENCE OF SEX

Gender-related changes in hematologic patterns have been reported for most deer species (Table 183.2).[11] Differences are not apparent in neonates or juveniles but are significant in adults. Males have higher red cell values than females after 140 days of age. An indirect relationship between red cell size and number, as reported for other mammals, is also seen in deer. Red cell parameters were 15 to 22% higher in chital stags than in chital hinds, but the erythrocyte indices were lower in the stags than in the hinds. The total white blood cell (WBC) count was significantly higher in stags.[8] Similar patterns have been noted in male and female rusa deer and farmed fallow deer.[10,12]

INFLUENCE OF REPRODUCTIVE STATUS

The annual rutting period of the stag is characterized by altered differential leukocyte counts.[8,13] In red deer, the stags had their lowest mean RBC during their rutting period.[10] Pregnancy results in significant increases in Hb, RBC, HCT, and mean corpuscular volume (MCV), with a decrease in mean corpuscular hemoglobin concentration (MCHC). The total white cell count also increases due to increased numbers of lymphocytes. Red cell numbers may be lower during lactation.[10]

INFLUENCE OF STRESS AND HANDLING

Deer are easily excitable as a species, which is often reflected in the hematologic parameters. Red cell values are significantly higher in excited deer than in resting deer, likely as a result of splenic contraction.[7] Erythrocyte and leukocyte parameters differ between the sexes in response to handling and restraint. This effect is most appreciable in females, resulting in significantly greater increases in PCV and red and white cell numbers than seen in males.[8] Little or no difference in WBC may be seen between excited and resting males. No significant difference in the WBC was seen between farmed male and female wild deer.[7] Periodic handling of hinds decreased the Hb, RBC, and HCT 10 to 20% over time. Hematologic parameters were thought to be reduced due to a reduction in stress.[8] Stags did not show distinct erythron changes over time with handling[7,8] but had an altered differential leukocyte count during initial sampling periods. The annual male reproductive cycle may have confounded alterations in the blood associated with adaptation of the stags to handling.

RESPONSE TO DISEASE

The hematologic response in deer has been evaluated in response to experimental infection with numerous infectious agents such as epizootic hemorrhagic disease virus, bluetongue virus, and *Yersinia pseudotuberculosis*.[14-16] Lymphopenia is a common response.

REFERENCES

1. **Gulliver G.** Observations on the sizes and shapes of the red corpuscles of the blood of vertebrates. Proc Zool Soc Lond 1875;474.
2. **Jain NC.** Hematology of laboratory and miscellaneous animals. In: Schalm's veterinary hematology. 4th ed. Philadelphia: Lea & Febiger, 1986;321–325.
3. **Kitchen H, Putnam FW, Taylor WJ.** Hemoglobin polymorphism: its relation to sickling of erythrocytes in white-tailed deer. Science 1964;144:1237.
4. **Kitchen H, Taylor WJ.** The sickling phenomenon of deer erythrocytes. In: Brewer GJ, ed. Hemoglobin and red cell structure and function. New York: Plenum Press, 1972;325–336.
5. **Kitchen H.** Hematological values and blood chemistries for a variety of artiodactylids. In: Fowler ME, ed. Zoo and wild animal medicine. 2nd ed. Philadelphia: WB Saunders, 1978;1003–1017.
6. **Hawkey CM, Hart MG.** Normal haematologic values of axis deer (Axis), Pere David's deer (*Elaphus davidianus*) and barasingha (*Cervus duvauceli*). Res Vet Sci 1985;39:247–248.
7. **Maede Y, Yamanaka Y, Sasaki A, Suzuki H, Ohtaishi N.** Hematology in sika deer (*Cervus nippon yesoensis* Heude, 1884). Jpn J Vet Sci 1990;52:35–41.
8. **Chapple RS.** The biology and behaviour of chital deer in captivity. PhD thesis. Sydney, Australia: The University of Sydney, 1989.
9. **Cately A, Kock RA, Hart MG, Hawkey CM.** Haematology of clinically normal and sick captive reindeer (*Rangifer tarandus*). Vet Rec 1990;126:239–241.
10. **Zomborszky Z, Horn E, Tuboly S, Gyodi P.** Some haematological and immunological parameters of farmed deer in Hungary. Acta Vet Hungarica 1997;45:75–84.
11. **Rawson RE, DelGiudice GD, Dziuk HE, Mech LD.** Energy metabolism and hematology of white-tailed deer fawns. J Wildl Dis 1992;28:91–94.
12. **Audige L.** Haematological values of rusa deer (*Cervus timorensis russa*) in New Caledonia. Aust Vet J 1992;69:265–268.
13. **Chapple RS, English AW, Mulley RC, Lepherd EE.** Haematology and serum biochemistry of captive unsedated chital deer (*Axis axis*) in Australia. J Wildl Dis 1991;27:396–406.
14. **Quist CF, Howerth EW, Stalknecht DE, Brown J, Pisell T, Nettles VF.** Host defense responses associated with experimental hemorrhagic disease in white-tailed deer. J Wildl Dis 1997;33:584–599.
15. **Howerth EW, Green CE, Prestwood AK.** Experimentally induced bluetongue virus infection in white-tailed deer: coagulation, clinical pathologic, and gross pathologic changes. Am J Vet Res 1988;49:1906–1913.
16. **Cross JP, Mackintosh CG, Griffin JFT.** The haematology of acute bacterial infection in farmed red deer *Cervus elaphus*: *Yersinia pseudotuberculosis*. Comp Haem Int 1994;4:86–95.
17. **Cowan I McT, Bandy PJ.** Observations on the haematology of several races of black-tailed deer (*Odocoileus hemionus*). Can J Zoo 1969;47:1021.
18. **Rosen MN, Bischoff AI.** The relation of hematology to condition in California deer. Transactions, 17th North American Wildl Conf 1952;482–496.
19. **Bowman LG, Sears HS.** Erythrocyte values and alimentary pH values in a Colorado mule deer population. J Mammal 1955;36:474.
20. **Anderson AE, Mendin DE, Bowden DC.** Erythrocytes and leukocytes in a Colorado mule deer population. J Wildl Manage 1970;34:2.
21. **Kitchen H, Pritchard WR.** Physiology of blood. Proceedings of the 1st National White-tailed Deer Disease Symposium, Athens, GA, 1962;109–111.
22. **Johnson HE, Youatt WG, Fay LD, Harte HD, Ullrey DE.** Hematological values of Michigan white-tailed deer. J Mammal 1968;49:749.
23. **Seal US, Erickson AW.** Hematology, blood chemistry and protein polymorphisms in the white-tailed deer (*Odocoileus virginianus*). Comp Biochem Physiol 1969;30:695–713.

CHAPTER 184

Hematology of Camelid Species: Llamas and Camels

• DAVID M. MOORE

BLOOD COLLECTION

Blood may be collected from three main venipuncture sites in Bactrian and dromedary camels: the jugular veins, the medial volar metacarpal veins of the fore legs, and the dorsal metatarsal veins of the hind legs. Jugular venipuncture should be attempted only when the camel is sitting or sedated, because the standing camel may be more likely to kick and severely injure the clinician. The jugular veins can be found ventral to the transverse cervical vertebrae in the lower two-thirds of the neck. The vessels can be dilated by applying either digital pressure caudal to the venipuncture site or by using the neck rope to apply pressure to the vessel near the thoracic inlet. When dilated, the jugular veins can be up to 5 cm in diameter.[1] The medial volar metacarpal vein is found on the medial aspect of the carpus of the fore leg. The dorsal metatarsal vein runs between the extensor tendons along the craniolateral aspect of the metatarsal bone of the hind leg. Both vessels are prominent and easily accessible but should be used with caution to avoid being kicked during blood collection.

Jugular venipuncture is the primary means of blood collection in llamoid species (llamas, alpacas, vicunas, and guanacos). However, a number of protective mechanisms have evolved within the animals' necks to prevent exsanguination from bite wounds by males during fighting; this may complicate localization of the vessels.[2] A jugular furrow is absent in llamoids, and the vessels lie along the ventrolateral surface of the trachea, underneath the sternomandibularis muscle, and medial to the ventral surface of the transverse processes of the cervical vertebrae. The carotid artery lies very close to the jugular vein, posing the risk of arterial puncture during blood collection. The jugular vein is more superficial in the upper portion of the neck, and the carotid artery does not lie as close to the vein at that location, but the skin is thicker in this area and visualization of the vessel can be problematic. The skin is thinner over the lower neck, but visualization is hampered by a thicker coat of fleece, and the carotid artery is more closely associated with the jugular vein in this region. Alternate venipuncture

locations include the saphenous vein (visible on the medial aspect of the stifle of the hind limb), the coccygeal vein (along the ventral surface of the tail), ear veins (along the margin of the pinna), and the brachial vein (along the cranial aspect of the fore limb).

Total blood volumes (expressed as ml/kg of body weight) for llamoid species in South America were determined to be 62.5 ± 4.1 for llamas, 72.0 ± 5.3 for alpacas, and 86.6 ± 2.1 for vicunas.[2] The total blood volume in the camel was reported to be 93 ml/kg of body weight.[3]

MORPHOLOGY AND INDICES OF PERIPHERAL BLOOD CELLS

Werney et al.[4] have published a color atlas that is useful for identifying camelid blood cells. Hematologic values for camels and llamoid species held outside their traditional geographic settings seem to correlate with values obtained from animals in native environments, but clinicians must assess results thoroughly by considering the animal's age, sex, existing climatic and geographic conditions, genetic variation in the population, and the likely effects of the sampling procedures (i.e., with or without sedation).[1] Tables 184.1 and 184.2 provide referenced erythrocyte and leukocyte parameters of llamoid species and Tables 184.3 and 184.4 provide referenced parameters for camels.

Erythrocytes

As would be expected, camelidae living at high altitudes have a relatively high erythrocyte count. The erythrocytes of llamas and other camelids are quite thin when viewed in cross-section ($\sim$1.1 μm),[4,5] and their small ellipsoid shape (measuring $6.48 \pm 0.47 \times 3.32 \pm 0.21$[6]) allows the cells to become densely packed during centrifugation, giving the impression of a lower packed cell volume (PCV) when compared to other domestic species.[7] In contrast, nucleated erythrocytes and reticu-

TABLE 184.1 Referenced Erythrocyte Parameters of Llamoid Species

Reference	Species	Gender	RBC (× 10⁶/mm³) Mean	RBC (× 10⁶/mm³) Range	PCV (%) Mean	PCV (%) Range	Hb (g/dl) Mean	Hb (g/dl) Range	MCV (μ^3) Mean	MCV (μ^3) Range	MCH ($\mu\mu g$) Mean	MCH ($\mu\mu g$) Range	MCHC (%) Mean	MCHC (%) Range
19, 20	Alpaca (SA)	NS	13.96	7.98–21.39	35.55	24–45	14.25	9.5–20.5	25.45	17.32–32.31	10.6	7.69–13.43	39.69	33.33–48.43
	Vicuna (SA)	NS	14.5	11.78–19.06	37.2	31–43	14.29	11–18.5	25.83	21.64–29.36	9.81	8.26–11.15	38.38	35.36–44.04
17	Guanaco	NS	10.4	8.9–11.7	—	—	16.4	14.6–19.2	—	—	—	—	—	—
	Llama	NS	9.91	8.3–12.5	—	—	12.8	11.6–14.5	—	—	—	—	—	—
	Vicuna	NS	10.3	9.4–11.5	—	—	12.2	9.8–14.8	—	—	—	—	—	—
6	Llama (SA)	NS	13.7 ± 0.59	—	38.1 ± 1.21	—	15.1 ± 0.45	—	28.0 ± 0.37	—	10.8 ± 0.4	—	39.7 ± 0.52	—
	Alpaca (SA)	NS	14.4 ± 0.37	—	35.5 ± 0.86	—	13.8 ± 0.27	—	24.8 ± 0.3	—	9.5 ± 0.3	—	38.8 ± 0.4	—
	Vicuna (SA)	NS	13.1 ± 0.34	—	36.0 ± 0.85	—	13.5 ± 0.51	—	27.4 ± 0.57	—	10.2 ± 0.3	—	37.5 ± 0.52	—
18	Llama (NA)	NS	12.22 ± 1.99	—	32.58 ± 5.74	—	13.76 ± 2.26	—	27.23 ± 4.47	—	11.9 ± 1.97	—	43.81 ± 1.54	—
21	Guanaco	NS	15.5	12.1–17.8	—	31–45	17.3	13.2–20.5	—	—	—	—	—	—
7	Llama (NA)	NS (<1 mo)	—	9.6–15.2	—	24–35	—	10.1–14.9	—	22.2–26.1	—	9.0–11.1	—	39.4–44.1
	Llama (NA)	NS (2–6 mo)	—	11.4–17.2	—	28–42.5	—	12.7–18.1	—	21.5–29	—	9.4–11.9	—	39.7–44.9
	Llama (NA)	NS (6–18 mo)	—	10.0–16.1	—	25.5–38.5	—	11.1–16.7	—	22.4–28	—	9.5–11.9	—	39.3–45.5
	Llama (NA)	M (adult)	—	10.5–17.1	—	27–45	—	11.7–19.1	—	22.5–29.1	—	10.3–12.5	—	39.9–48.7
	Llama (NA)	F (adult)	—	10.6–17.2	—	27.5–45	—	12.5–19.2	—	22.9–30.2	—	10.0–12.7	—	40.0–46.7
16	Llama	NS (adult)	—	11.3–16.9	—	28–39	—	12.6–17.8	—	20.1–27.5	—	—	—	43.3–46.5
22	Llama	NS (adult)	—	11.3–17.6	—	29–39	—	12.8–17.6	—	21–28	—	—	—	43.2–46.6

SA, South American location; NS, not specified; NA, North American location.

TABLE 184.2 Referenced Leukocyte Parameters of Llamoid Species

Reference	Species	Gender	WBC (× 10³/mm³) Mean	WBC (× 10³/mm³) Range	Neutrophils (%) Mean	Neutrophils (%) Range	Lymphocytes (%) Mean	Lymphocytes (%) Range	Eosinophils (%) Mean	Eosinophils (%) Range	Basophils (%) Mean	Basophils (%) Range	Monocytes (%) Mean	Monocytes (%) Range
19, 20	Alpaca (SA)	NS	15.79	5.68–28.48	52.24	25.5–86.0	36.21	11.8–69.0	8.24	0–28	—	—	1.5	0–9.8
	Vicuna (SA)	NS	12.76	8.08–22.76	55.16	41–67	28.81	17.5–42.5	8.49	0.5–22.5	—	—	6.85	1.0–26.8
17	Guanaco	NS	8.82	6.4–17.0	—	14–35	—	15–27	—	4.0–16.5	—	1–2	—	0.5–2.5
	Llama	NS	16.2	8.9–22.0	—	22–48	—	15–59	—	3.5–6.0	—	0.5–3	—	0.5–2.0
	Vicuna	NS	11.7	6.4–19.2	—	25–55	—	11–40	—	5.5–18	—	0.5–3	—	0–0.5
6	Llama (SA)	NS	11.7 ± 1.2	—	59.0 ± 3.9	—	27.7 ± 4.3	—	10.0 ± 2.9	—	—	—	3.3 ± 0.5	—
	Alpaca (SA)	NS	11.6 ± 0.85	—	58.5 ± 3.9	—	33.5 ± 4.2	—	5.0 ± 1.1	—	—	—	3.0 ± 0.6	—
	Vicuna (SA)	NS	12.2 ± 0.81	—	46.8 ± 3.1	—	33.8 ± 3.0	—	14.6 ± 2.2	—	—	—	2.4 ± 0.3	—
18	Llama (NA)	NS	13.9 ± 2.9	—	—	56–87	—	3–22	—	0–20	—	0–2	—	1–10
21	Guanaco	NS	12.6	8.6–79	64	57–76	24	16–30	5	3–8	—	0–0.5	3	2–3.5
7	Llama (NA)	NS (<1 mo)	—	7.1–19.4	—	15.9–75.0	—	23.9–24.3	—	0–5.6	—	0–0.8	—	0–7.3
	Llama (NA)	NS (2–6 mo)	—	9.1–22.9	—	47.2–62.3	—	33.5–46.6	—	0.9–12.3	—	0–1	—	1.7–6.1
	Llama (NA)	NS (6–18 mo)	—	10.2–23.6	—	41.4–54.9	—	18.4–32.5	—	2.9–29.4	—	0–1.6	—	0–6
	Llama (NA)	M (adult)	—	7.9–23.6	—	58.5–68.5	—	12.4–20.8	—	10–17.8	—	0–1.4	—	0–4
	Llama (NA)	F (adult)	—	8.3–19.2	—	61.5–73.7	—	7.8–24.7	—	7.3–28.7	—	0–1.4	—	1.4–5.2
22	Llama	NS (adult)	—	7.5–21.5	—	61.3–74.4	—	13.3–34.9	—	0–15.3	—	0–1.9	—	0.7–3.7

SA, South American location; NS, not specified; NA, North American location.

TABLE 184.3   Referenced Erythrocytes Parameters of Camels

Reference	Species	Gender/Age	RBC (× 10⁶/mm³) Mean	RBC (× 10⁶/mm³) Range	PCV (%) Mean	PCV (%) Range	Hb (g/dl) Mean	Hb (g/dl) Range	MCV (μ³) Mean	MCV (μ³) Range	MCH (μμg) Mean	MCH (μμg) Range	MCHC (%) Mean	MCHC (%) Range
1	C. dromedarius	NS	—	7.6–11	—	24–42	—	11.4–14.2	—	27.5–29.4	—	12.1–13.7	—	42.1–49.6
	C. bactrianus	NS	—	8.5–13.4	—	25–39	13.1	11.1–17.4	—	25.3–31.6	—	10.6–14.3	—	37–47
10	C. dromodarius	NS	7.24	6.1–9.3	27	20–33	13.1	10.6–15.1	—	—	—	—	—	—
23	C. dromodarius	NS	8.2	3.8–12.6	—	—	15.5	10.6–20.3	—	—	—	—	—	—
24	C. dromodarius	M	9.1	—	32	—	14	—	—	—	—	—	—	—
		F	3	—	29.6	—	12	—	—	—	—	—	—	—
25	C. dromodarius	M	8.8	7.0–11.5	—	—	12.6	11–14	—	—	—	—	—	—
26	C. dromodarius	M/F	6.7 ± 0.2	—	—	—	11.1 ± 0.3	—	—	—	—	—	—	—
27	C. dromodarius	NS	—	7.22–11.6	—	25–35	—	7.8–15.9	—	35–60	—	17–22	—	36.5–50.9
4	C. bactrianus	NS (<6 mo) r	10.5	—	28.8	—	13.6	—	27.4	—	—	—	—	—
	C. bactrianus	NS (2–12 yr)	—	10.2–13.2	—	36.5–42.7	—	11.72–13.68	—	28.8–39.0	—	—	—	—
4	C. dromedarius	NS (<6 mo) r	—	7.4–10.0	—	24–31	—	10.4–13.9	—	29.6–35.1	—	—	—	—
	C. dromedarius	NS (<6 mo) nr	—	3–6	—	14–35	—	7–13	—	—	—	—	—	—
	C. dromedarius	NS (6–24 mo) r	—	6.5–9.0	—	20–28	—	8.5–12.0	—	30–34	—	—	—	—
	C. dromedarius	NS (6–24 mo) nr	—	4–12	—	27–31	—	7–15	—	—	—	—	—	—
	C. dromedarius	NS (2–12 yr) r	—	7.5–12.0	—	26–38	—	12–15	—	26–34	—	—	—	—
	C. dromedarius	NS (2–12 yr) nr	—	7.1–10.9	—	23.8–31.3	—	10.1–14.5	—	27–59	—	—	—	—

TABLE 184.4 Referenced Leukocyte Parameters of Camels

Reference	Species	Gender/Age	WBC (× 10³/mm³) Mean	WBC (× 10³/mm³) Range	Neutrophils (%) Mean	Neutrophils (%) Range	Lymphocytes (%) Mean	Lymphocytes (%) Range	Eosinophils (%) Mean	Eosinophils (%) Range	Basophils (%) Mean	Basophils (%) Range	Monocytes (%) Mean	Monocytes (%) Range
1	C. dromedarius	NS	—	2.9–9.7	—	33–70	—	21–62	—	0–4	—	0–3	—	0–7
	C. bactrianus	NS	—	8.6–16.5	—	55–79	—	18–33	—	0–9	—	0–4	—	0–4
10	C. dromedarius	NS	18.1	10.5–28.3	50.6	30–60	40	33–58	6.5	2–17.5	0.05	0–0.5	3	1.5–6.0
23	C. dromedarius	NS	20.1	12.9–27.2	38.7	21.1–56.3	46	26.5–65.4	9.5	0–18.9	—	0–1	5.7	0–12.3
24	C. dromedarius	M	22	—	43	—	49.3	—	3.3	—	0.2	—	4.5	—
	C. dromedarius	F	17.5	—	50	—	43.8	—	1.2	—	0.3	—	2.8	—
25	C. dromedarius	M	10.5	6.5–13.6	27	23–34	51	43–59	9	5–11	1.9	1–3	13	7–18
26	C. dromedarius	M/F	10.6 ± 0.4	—	44.7 ± 1.4	—	47.5 ± 1.4	—	7.2 ± 0.4	—	—	—	1.2 ± 0.1	—
27	C. dromedarius	NS	—	11.5–16.5	50	—	40	—	—	0–4	—	0–4	—	0–4
4	C. bactrianus	NS (<6 mo)	20.6	—	51.2	28–83	37	19–56	1	—	0.1	—	8	—
	C. bactrianus	NS (2–12 yr)	—	10.0–15.8	—	—	—	—	—	0–18	—	0–3	—	0–7
4	C. dromedarius	NS (<6 mo) r	—	11.5–18.5	—	53–68	—	20–44	—	0.3–2.5	—	0.2–2.4	—	0.5–10
	C. dromedarius	NS (<6 mo) nr	—	13–24	—	53–74	—	12–39	—	1.0–3.2	—	0–1	—	1–4
	C. dromedarius	NS (6–24 mo) r	—	9.5–14.0	—	50–60	—	30–45	—	1.0–2.5	—	0–1	—	0.3–7.0
	C. dromedarius	NS (6–24 mo) nr	—	11–19	—	56–59	—	33–37	—	2.5–2.6	—	1.0–1.3	—	3.4–4.0
	C. dromedarius	NS (2–12 yr) r	—	6.0–13.5	—	50–60	—	30–45	—	0–6	—	0–2	—	2–8
	C. dromedarius	NS (2–12 yr) nr	—	10.2–21.5	—	35–60	—	29–55	—	2–12	—	0–2	—	2–5

NS, not specified; r, racing camel; nr, non-racing camel.

locytes are more rounded in shape.[8] Thread-like Cabot's rings are found in normal Bactrian camel erythrocytes and are thought to be artifacts representing denatured membrane protein.[4] The erythrocytes of dromedary camels measure approximately 7.7 × 4.2 μm,[9] whereas the size of erythrocytes in the two-humped Bactrian camel are smaller, measuring about 7.2 × 3.5 μm.[10] The Bactrian camel has a higher total erythrocyte count than does the dromedary, perhaps compensating for the smaller size of its erythrocytes. Camelid erythrocytes orient themselves along their long axis in the blood stream, making it easier for them to pass through small capillaries, minimizing the likelihood of sludging when the viscosity of blood increases during dehydration.[2,11,12] The erythrocytes of camels do not easily sediment or produce rouleaux.[8] Dacrocytes, erythrocytes whose cytoplasm has elongated to form a tail giving them a teardrop shape, may be found in all camelidae.[4] Nucleated red blood cells (RBCs) occur with greater frequency in dromedaries than in any of the other camelids. An increase in nucleated RBCs above 1% of the total erythrocyte count is indicative of blood loss or chronic anemia.[4]

Hemoglobin levels in llamoid erythrocytes are higher than those in cattle, but are similar to those of thoroughbred horses.[13] The mean corpuscular volume (MCV) in llamas is approximately half that of horses and cattle; the mean corpuscular hemoglobin concentration (MCHC) levels are higher than for the domestic species, but the MCH is slightly lower in llamoids than in horses and cattle.[7] A low MCHC in llamoids is associated with hypochromic anemia.[2]

The osmotic fragility of erythrocytes in camelidae is greatly reduced in comparison with other artiodactylids, an evolutionary advantage for desert species, for whom the ability to withstand lower ionic concentrations during water loading is of greater physiologic importance.[14] This characteristic of the camel erythrocyte may be associated with its membrane structure.[15]

Thrombocytes

Platelets in camelids are small (2 to 3.5 μm in diameter, 0.5 to 0.7 μm thick), round to irregular-shaped cells with a pinkish cytoplasm containing azurophilic granules arranged in groups or clusters. The estimated number of platelets in adult llamas was found to be in a range between 200 and 600 × 10³/μl of blood.[16] Platelet counts in dromedary racing camels of different ages were reported as 375 to 820 × 10³/μl for animals up to 6 months of age, 350 to 450 × 10³/μl for animals from 6 months to 24 months of age, and 200 to 700 × 10³/μl in animals 2 to 12 years of age.[4] Platelet counts in non-racing dromedary camels were reported in a range of 240 to 310 × 10³/μl for animals 2 to 12 years of age.[4]

Leukocytes

Neutrophils in dromedary camels have indistinct nuclear lobulation and an agranular cytoplasm. Female sex chromatin was observed in neutrophils of guanacos,

manifested as a "drumstick" lobe on the nucleus.[17] Drumsticks may be observed in the nuclei of 1 to 5% of neutrophils in other camelid species.[4] The nuclei of neutrophils in Bactrian camels are distinctly lobulated and hypersegmented, and may occasionally be observed in a ring form.

Llamoid species were found to have a higher leukocyte count that the values observed in cattle and horses, while the neutrophil:lymphocyte ratio, with neutrophils predominating, more closely resembled that in horses.[7] The neutrophil:lymphocyte ratio was found to be 1.54:1 in llamoids and 1.45:1 in camels.[2] As in other species, camelids have both large and small lymphocytes. The somewhat rounded nuclei of lymphocytes are surrounded by a thin band of cytoplasm.

Eosinophils in camelids are approximately the same size as neutrophils. Their nuclei may be band-shaped, lobulated, or dumbbell-shaped with hypersegmentation, and their cytoplasm contains red staining granules.

BONE MARROW CYTOLOGY

Bone marrow aspirates can be obtained from the sternum of a llama. A higher ratio of myeloid cells to erythrocytes (1:2) is observed in the bone marrow of llamas, in contrast to the 2:1 ratio of myeloid cells to erythrocytes demonstrated in most other mammalian species. This may be attributed to the shorter life span of llamoid erythrocytes and the need for replacement of cells.[18]

OTHER HEMATOLOGIC VALUES

The erythrocyte sedimentation rate for dromedary camels was reported as 0 to 1.0 mm/hr.[1,10]

REFERENCES

1. **Higgins A.** The camel in health and disease. London: Bailliere Tindal, 1986.
2. **Fowler ME.** Medicine and surgery of South American camelids—llama, alpaca, vicuna, guanaco. Ames, IA: Iowa State University Press, 1998.
3. **Metcalfe J, Parer JT, el-Yassin D, Oufi J, Bartels H, Riegel K, Kleihauer E.** Cardiodynamics of the dromedary camel (*Camelus dromedarius*) during phencyclidine analgesia. Am J Vet Res 1968;29:2063–2066.
4. **Werner U, et al.** Color atlas of camelid hematology. Berlin: Blackwell-Wiesenschafts-Verlag, 1999.
5. **Jain NC, Keeton KS.** Morphology of camel and llama erythrocytes as viewed with a scanning electron microscope. Br Vet J 1974;130:287.
6. **Reynafarje C, Faura J, Paredes A, Villavicencio D.** Erythrocytes in high-altitude-adapted animals (llama, alpaca, and vicuna). J Appl Physiol 1968;24:93–97.
7. **Fowler ME, Zinkl JG.** Reference ranges for hematologic and serum biochemical values in llamas (*Lama glama*). Am J Vet Res 1989;50:2049–2053.
8. **Hawkey CM.** Comparative mammalian hematology. London: William Heinemann, 1975.
9. **Kohli RN.** Cellular micrometry of camel's blood. Indian Vet J 1963;40:134.
10. **Banerjee S, et al.** Hematological studies in the normal adult Indian camel (*Camelus dromedarius*). Am J Physiol 1962;203:1185.
11. **Smith JE, Mohandas N, Shohet SB.** Variability in erythrocyte deformability among various animals. Am J Physiol 1979;236:H725–H730.
12. **Smith JE, Mohandas N, Clark MR, Greenquist AC, Shohet SB.** Deformability and spectrin properties in three types of elongated red cells. Am J Hematol 1980;8:1–13.
13. **Schalm OW, Jain NC, Carroll EJ.** Veterinary hematology. 3rd ed. Philadelphia: Lea & Febiger, 1975.
14. **Perk K.** The camel's erythrocyte. Nature 1963;200:272.
15. **Eitan A, Aloni B, Livine A.** Unique properties of the camel erythrocyte

membrane. II. Organization of membrane proteins. Biochim Biophys Acta 1976;426:647–658.

16. **Van Houten D, Weiser MG, Johnson L, Garry F.** Reference hematologic values and morphologic features of blood cells in healthy adult llamas. Am J Vet Res 1992;53:1773–1775.

17. **Kraft H.** Untersuchungen uber das blutbild der cameliden. Munch Tierarztl Wschr 1957;70:371.

18. **Fowler ME.** Camelids. In: Fowler ME, ed. Zoo and wild animal medicine. 2nd ed. Philadelphia: WB Saunders, 1986.

19. **Copaira B.** Hematologic studies in South American camelids. Rev Fac Med Vet (Lima) 1949;4:49.

20. **Copaira B.** Hematologic studies in South American Camelids. Fac Med Vet Zootec (Lima) 1953;5:78.

21. **Jain NC.** Schalm's veterinary hematology. 4th ed. Philadelphia: Lea & Febiger, 1986.

22. **Weiser MG, et al.** Characterization of erythrocytic indices and serum iron values in healthy llamas. Am J Vet Res 1992;53:1776.

23. **Soni BK, Aggarwala AC.** Studies in the physiology of the camel (*Camelus dromedarius*). Indian Vet J 1958;35:209.

24. **Nassar SM, et al.** Influence of sex on the normal blood picture of adult Egyptian camel (*Camelus dromedarius*). Assiut Vet Med J 1977;4:43.

25. **Kahn AA, Kohli IS.** A note on some haematological studies on male camel (*Camelus dromedarius*) before and during rut. Indian J Anim Sci 1978; 48:325.

26. **Majeed MA, et al.** Effects of sex and season on 10 haematological values of normal adult one-humped camel. Rev Elev Med Vet Pays Trop 1980;33:135.

27. **Abdelgadir SE, et al.** A note on the haematology of adult Sudanese dromedaries. In: Cockrill WR, ed. The camelid—an all purpose animal. Uppsala, Sweden: Scandinavian Institute of African Studies, 1984.

CHAPTER 185

Hematology of the Elephant

• SUSAN K. MIKOTA and MARC J. KAHN

There are two species of elephants alive today, the African elephant (*Loxodonta africana*) and the Asian elephant (*Elephas maximus*). Both species are endangered, largely due to human overpopulation, diminishing habitat, and poaching. Elephants are intelligent and powerful animals. Adult Asian elephants weigh 3000 to 5000 kg, and adult African elephants weigh up to 6000 kg. Elephants should be approached with caution and respect. It is essential to have an experienced handler present when working with elephants. Elephants that have been properly conditioned will readily permit blood sampling.

BLOOD COLLECTION

There are three primary blood collection sites in elephants. The auricular veins are probably the most common venipuncture sites. Although the auricular veins may be accessed with the animal standing, they are more prominent when the elephant is in lateral recumbency. The external pinnae plays a major role in thermoregulation, particularly in the African elephant.[1,2] Consequently, auricular veins may dilate in warm ambient temperatures and constrict in cold weather. Placing elephants in lateral recumbency and applying warm compresses or dry heat (using a hair dryer) promotes vasodilatation and facilitates venipuncture in cold weather. Elephants can be bled from the cephalic vein, located on the proximal medial forelimb, while standing. The saphenous vein, on the lower medial aspect of the hindlimb, can be approached with the elephant standing, in a stretched position, or in lateral recumbency. The cephalic and saphenous vessels are deeper than they appear. Winged infusion sets permit the operator to move with the animal and are useful for blood collection in elephants.

BLOOD VOLUME

A blood volume of 112.6 L was measured in an Asian elephant weighing 3216 kg. The blood volume was calculated to be 3.5% of body weight.[3]

RED BLOOD CELLS

The elephant erythrocyte is the largest of any mammal, with a mean diameter of 8.8 to 10.6 μm.[1,4-7] The sedimentation rate is the fastest of any mammalian species examined.[4,5,8] Both Asian and African elephant red blood cells demonstrate rouleaux formation (Fig. 185.1).[4,6] Reticulocytes are rarely observed.

The total number of red cells is relatively low compared with other mammals.[4,8-10] Pregnancy may cause a decrease in the total erythrocyte count and hematocrit but an increase in the sedimentation rate.[5] Total erythrocyte values for young free-ranging African elephants (1 to 5 years) are higher than for adults, but mean corpuscular hemoglobin and mean corpuscular volume are lower.[11] Total red blood cell counts in free-ranging African elephants may differ seasonally.[11] Values for hemoglobin, mean corpuscular hemoglobin, and mean corpuscular hemoglobin concentration are higher in the dry season for free-ranging African elephants, but mean corpuscular volume is lower.[11] Reference ranges for red blood cell indices for captive Asian and African elephants are given in Tables 185.1 and 185.2.

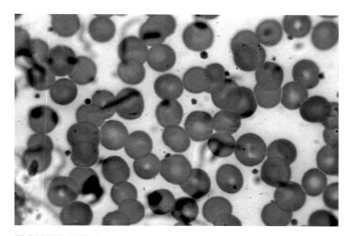

FIGURE 185.1 Normal peripheral smear from a healthy Asian elephant showing normal platelets and erythrocytes with rouleaux formation.

TABLE 185.1	Red Blood Cell Reference Ranges for Captive Asian Elephants in North America: Both Sexes and All Ages Combined				
Test	**Mean**	**Standard Deviation**	**Range**	**Sample Size**[a]	**Animals**[b]
RBC ($10^6/\mu L$)	3.11	0.53	1.78–5.15	1157	144
Hbg (g/dL)	13.3	2.2	6.8–22.7	1219	153
Hct (%)	37.7	6.0	23.0–58.0	1472	159
MCV (fL)	122.4	13.9	58.2–213.2	1148	144
MCH (pg/cell)	43.4	4.5	16.6–63.2	1130	143
MCHC (g/dL)	35.3	3.4	16.9–68.6	1188	151
Platelets ($10^3/\mu L$)	474	172	127–1085	335	58
nRBC (/100 WBC)	1	1	0–3	77	33
Reticulocytes (%)	0.0	0.0	0.0–0.1	7	4
Sedimentation rate (mm/hr)	98	32	53–130	7	4

From International Species Information System, 12101 Johnny Cake Ridge Road, Apple Valley, MN 55124.
[a] Number of samples used to calculate reference range.
[b] Number of individuals contributing to the reference values.

TABLE 185.2	Red Blood Cell Reference Ranges for Captive African Elephants in North America: Both Sexes and All Ages Combined				
Test	**Mean**	**Standard Deviation**	**Range**	**Sample Size**[a]	**Animals**[b]
RBC ($10^6/\mu L$)	3.18	0.38	2.10–4.80	1299	102
Hbg (g/dL)	13.8	1.5	8.5–23.7	1337	104
Hct (%)	39.9	4.5	28.0–56.0	1718	111
MCV (fL)	125.7	7.7	91.1–190.0	1287	101
MCH (pg/cell)	43.3	2.8	34.8–65.6	1282	100
MCHC (g/dL)	34.6	1.9	28.3–47.3	1322	104
Platelets ($10^3/\mu L$)	423	205	11–1031	148	39
nRBC (/100 WBC)	0	1	0–3	35	19
Reticulocytes (%)	0.0	0.0	0.0–0.0	7	4
Sedimentation rate (mm/hr)	27	0	27–27	1	1

From International Species Information System, 12101 Johnny Cake Ridge Road, Apple Valley, NM 55124.
[a] Number of samples used to calculate reference range.
[b] Number of individuals contributing to the reference values.

Polycythemia (packed cell volume greater than 66%) and anemia (packed cell volume less than 33%) have been reported in African elephants.[11] Lower packed cell volumes have been associated with chemical immobilization in free-ranging Asian and African elephants.[4,6] Based on electrophoresis patterns, the structure of Asian and African elephant hemoglobin differs.[12]

WHITE BLOOD CELLS

The nuclei of elephant granulocytes are poorly segmented.[6] Basophils are rare.[4,8] Two types of monocytes have been observed: one with a bilobed (Fig. 185.2) or trilobed nucleus, and the other with a nonsegmented nucleus. Although some researchers have classified the bilobed and trilobed cells as lymphocytes, the presence of peroxidase-positive cytoplasmic granules supports classification of these cells as monocytes.[6] It is therefore common for the monocyte to be reported as the most numerous leukocyte in normal elephant blood.

Although the total white blood cell (WBC) count has

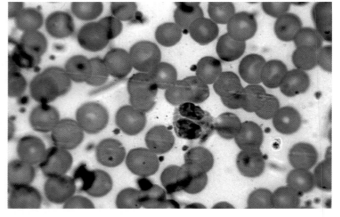

FIGURE 185.2 Normal peripheral smear from a healthy Asian elephant showing a characteristic bilobed monocyte.

been reported to be higher in the Asian elephant,[14,15] the ranges given for both species overlap.[13,16–19] Reference values for WBC indices for captive Asian and African elephants are given in Tables 185.3 and 185.4.

Increased total WBC counts have been reported in young Asian and African elephants.[5,11] Increased neutrophils, decreased lymphocytes, and decreased eosinophils were seen in pregnant captive Asian elephants.[5] Free-ranging male African elephants had lower total WBC counts than females in one study[8]; however, other authors have reported no difference between the genders of either species.[7,18] Seasonal differences may occur in WBC counts in free-ranging African elephants.[11]

Platelets and Coagulation

Coagulation can be divided into primary hemostasis and secondary hemostasis. Primary hemostasis refers to the ability of platelets to adhere to an injured endothelial surface. Secondary hemostasis refers to the sequence of coagulation reactions that results in the formation of a fibrin clot. These two processes do not occur independently, and many of the coagulation reactions require an aggregated platelet surface to proceed.

Platelets are the cells responsible for primary hemostasis. Elephants have a relatively high platelet count

(Fig. 185.1), with a mean of $637 \times 10^9/L$ for Asian elephants[20] and ranges of 46 to $644 \times 10^9/L$ for African elephants.[21] Mammalian platelets occur in two forms. One platelet type exhibits irreversible aggregation when stimulated by a low-dose agonist such as platelet activating factor, whereas others are able to aggregate and disaggregate reversibly on stimulation and recovery.[22] Platelets from the Asian elephant have been shown to aggregate reversibly, much like bovine platelets.[23] Morphologically, it has been shown that platelets from Asian elephants lack a well-developed cannicular system and contain many granules.[24] This is in contrast to other mammalian platelets. A canicular system is important for both secretion of platelet reactants into the surrounding medium and for transport of extracellular substances into the platelet.[25] Consequently, it has been suggested that activation of platelets from Asian elephants requires the movement of granules to the outer platelet membrane for secretory processes to occur. In addition, platelets from Asian elephants lack pseudopods, which assist with platelet adherence and spreading in other animal species. Platelets become activated when exposed to pressure changes.[26] Large animals such as elephants exhibit great postural blood pressure changes on rising. One can infer that the elephant platelet has adapted to accommodate this high pressure environment. Similar platelet characteristics have been seen in

TABLE 185.3	White Blood Cell Reference Ranges for Captive Asian Elephants in North America: Both Sexes and All Ages Combined				
Test	Mean	Standard Deviation	Range	Sample Size[a]	Animals[b]
WBC (10^3 μL/mL)	14.78	4.53	6.35–33.30	1383	153
Neutrophils (10^3 μL/mL)	5.095	3.038	0.291–23.90	1138	132
Lymphocytes (10^3 μL/mL)	5.687	3.303	0.196–22.20	1142	132
Monocytes (10^3 μL/mL)	3.209	2.838	0.000–9.983	935	128
Eosiniphils (10^3 μL/mL)	0.523	0.653	0.000–5.145	846	120
Basophils (10^3 μL/mL)	0.164	0.114	0.000–0.508	105	46
Bands (10^3 μL/mL)	1.211	2.006	0.000–11.40	274	72

From International Species Information System, 12101 Johnny Cake Ridge Road, Apple Valley, MN 55124.
[a] Number of samples used to calculate reference range.
[b] Number of individuals contributing to the reference values.

TABLE 185.4	White Blood Cell Reference Ranges for Captive African Elephants in North America: Both Sexes and All Ages Combined				
Test	Mean	Standard Deviation	Range	Sample Size[a]	Animals[b]
WBC (10^3 μL/mL)	10.55	2.602	4.500–22.10	1281	101
Neutrophils (10^3 μL/mL)	3.021	1.698	0.000–11.80	971	90
Lymphocytes (10^3 μL/mL)	5.087	3.148	0.022–64.40	980	92
Monocytes (10^3 μL/mL)	1.387	1.619	0.000–8.639	931	87
Eosiniphils (10^3 μL/mL)	0.238	0.313	0.000–3.450	737	73
Basophils (10^3 μL/mL)	0.044	0.077	0.000–0.525	446	32
Bands (10^3 μL/mL)	0.856	0.743	0.000–3.960	566	62

From International Species Information System, 12101 Johnny Cake Ridge Road, Apple Valley, MN 55124.
[a] Number of samples used to calculate reference range.
[b] Number of individuals contributing to the reference values.

other animals exposed to high barometric pressures during diving, such as killer whales.[27]

In many species, platelet activation via an agonist results in the liberation of arachidonic acid from the platelet that is subsequently converted into thromboxane (TXA2), which serves as a potent platelet agonist.[28] Platelets of Asian elephants have been shown to be unresponsive to arachidonic acid.[29] As a result, unlike other species, elephants are resistant to the effects of aspirin.

Secondary hemostasis is important to prevent major blood loss during traumatic injury. Secondary hemostasis is initiated by the conversion of factor VII to activated factor VIIa when tissue factor is expressed on damaged endothelial surfaces.[30] Factor VIIa is then able to convert factor X to Xa, and using factor V as a cofactor, factor Xa is able to convert prothrombin to thrombin. Thrombin allows for the conversion of fibrinogen to fibrin. This pathway is sometimes known as the extrinsic pathway, and the integrity of this system is reflected in the prothrombin time (PT). In a study of Asian elephants, it was determined that elephants have a mean PT of 9.6 seconds when Simplastin was used and 10.3 seconds when recombinant tissue factor was used in the assay.[31] In the same study, levels of factor VII were found to be 1.15 μ/mL, similar to human plasma. Fibrinogen and factor X levels were also similar to human values, with mean levels of 4.61 g/L and 0.91 μ/mL, respectively.

Once thrombin is generated, it can activate factor XI, which can in turn activate factor IX to IXa.[32] Factor IXa can activate factor X to Xa using factor VIIIa as a cofactor.[33] This system is referred to as the intrinsic system, and its integrity is measured by the activated partial thromboplastin test (aPTT). A wide range of values for aPTT has been found for Asian elephants, with values ranging from 52 to 83 seconds.[31] Factor IX levels in elephants are similar to human values (0.88 μ/mL), whereas factor VIII levels are approximately twice that of humans.[34]

To prevent excess fibrin formation, coagulation is modulated by several inhibitors, including circulating antithrombin.[35] Antithrombin levels for Asian elephants have been found to be similar to human levels (1.07 μ/mL).[31]

Hematologic Diseases

There are few reports of parasitic infections of the blood in elephants. The earliest report is an occurrence of a trypanosome similar to *Trypanosoma brucei* in an African elephant.[36] Trypanosomes have also been described in an Asian elephant, but the species was not identified.[37] Babesia species have been described within the erythrocytes of a sick African elephant.[38] Asian elephants infected with unsheathed microfilaria that were different from *Dipetalonema gossi* and *D. loxodontis* have been reported.[39] More recently, anemia has been described in an Asian elephant infected with the liver fluke, *Fasciola jacksoni*.[40] Hemorrhagic septicemia has been described in three African elephants in Sri Lanka and one in Ceylon.[41,42]

Atherosclerotic Disease

Atherosclerotic disease can be thought of as an arterial coagulation abnormality. Arterial disease has been the subject of a number of field studies in elephants conducted in the 1960s and 1970s. Sikes examined the aortas and selected arteries from 40 African elephants living in grassland, scrubland, and montane habitats in Kenya and Uganda.[43] Calcium deposition (associated with constriction of the aortic lumen) was more prevalent in grassland than scrubland animals and was not observed in any animals from montane habitat. Associated clinical signs included decreased mobility, lethargy, head drooping, and emaciation.

Sikes suggests that environmental factors are contributory to the development of arterial disease. Citing historical evidence that the forest is the natural and preferred habitat of wild African elephants, she maintains that grassland and scrubland are stressed habitats used because of confinement pressures from encroaching human populations. Possible mechanisms for the development of atherosclerosis include a lack of arboreal food items (resulting in a mineral deficiency affecting calcium metabolism), restricted movement (causing overcrowding and preventing access to previously available salt licks), and increased exposure to sunlight (resulting in hypervitaminosis D, known to be associated with the aortic calcium deposition in other mammals).[44,45]

The term "atherosclerosis" is one of at least three types of arteriosclerotic disease. Atherosclerosis, as defined by the World Health Organization is, "a variable combination of changes of the arterial intima consisting of the focal accumulation of lipids, complex carbohydrates, blood and blood products, fibrous tissue and calcium deposits, and associated with medial changes." Atherosclerosis affects the intima of the aorta and larger arteries. Arteriosclerosis signifies diffuse, hyperplastic sclerosis of small arteries. Medial or Mönckeberg's sclerosis affects the muscular arteries.[46]

McCullagh and Lewis[47] examined the hearts and aortas of 415 elephants culled in Uganda and Kenya. They observed gross lesions in 298 aortas (72%) and 29 coronary arteries (27%). Two types of lesions were noted. Atherosclerotic lesions occurring in the intima were characterized by fibrous tissue proliferation and the presence of fat and cholesterol, and in advanced lesions, calcification. Lesions in the media showed extensive fibrosis and calcification and resembled Mönckeberg's sclerosis in humans.

In contrast to humans, atherosclerotic lesions in African elephants are most severe in the aorta and least severe in the coronary arteries. The distribution of aortic lesions is similar, however, with both species demonstrating more severe lesions in the abdominal than the thoracic aorta. There is no apparent correlation between the levels of cholesterol, phospholipids, triglycerides, or free fatty acids and the severity of the atherosclerotic lesions in elephants.[48,49] Arterial disease is not unique to wild elephants and has also been reported in a limited number of captive elephants.[50,51]

REFERENCES

1. **Sikes SK.** The natural history of the African elephant. New York: Elsevier, 1971.
2. **Buss IO, Estes JA.** The functional significance of movements and position of the pinnae of the African elephant, *Loxodonta africana.* J Mammal 1971;52:21–27.
3. **Shoshani J, et. al.** On the dissection of a female Asian elephant (*Elephas maximus maximus* Linnaeus, 1758) and data from other elephants. Elephant 1982;2:3–93.
4. **Young E, Lombard CO.** Physiologic values of the African elephant (*Loxodonta africana*). Veterinarian 1967;4:169–172.
5. **Nirmalan G, Nair SG, Simon KJ.** Hematology of the Indian elephant (*Elephas maximus*). Can J Physiol Pharmacol 1967;45:985–991.
6. **Silva ID, Kuruwita VY.** Hematology, plasma, and serum biochemistry values in free-ranging elephants in Sri Lanka. J Zoo Wildl Med 1993;24:434–439.
7. **Silva ID, Kuruwita VY.** Hematology, plasma and serum biochemistry values in domesticated elephants (*Elephas maximus ceylonicus*) in Sri Lanka. J Zoo Wildl Med 1993;24:440–444.
8. **Debbie JG, Clausen B.** Some hematological values of free-ranging African elephants. J Wildl Dis 1975;11:79–82.
9. **Simon KJ.** Haematological studies on elephants. Indian Vet J 1961;38:241–245.
10. **Schmidt MJ.** Elephants. In: Fowler ME, ed. Zoo and wild animal medicine. Philadelphia: WB Saunders, 1986;884–923.
11. **White PT, Brown IRF.** Haematological studies on wild elephants. *Loxodonta africana.* J Zool (Lond) 1978;185:491–503.
12. **Schmitt J.** Haematological studies in elephants. Vet Med Rev Leverkusen 1964;2:87–95.
13. **Gromadzka-Ostrowska J, Jakubow K, Zalewska B, Kryzywicki Z.** Haematological and blood biochemical studies in female domesticated Indian elephants (*Elephus maximus* L.) Comp Biochem Physiol [A] 1988;89:313–315.
14. **Dhindsa DS, Sedgwick CJ, Metcalfe J.** Comparative studies of the respiratory functions of mammalian blood. VIII. Asian elephant (*Elephas maximus*) and African elephant (*Loxodonta africana africana*). Respir Physiol 1972;14:332–342.
15. **Wallach JD, Boever WJ.** Perissodactyla (equids, tapirs, rhinos), Proboscidae (elephants), and Hippopotamidae (hippopotamus). In: Wallach JD, Boever WJ, eds. Diseases of exotic animals. Philadelphia: WB Saunders, 1983;761–829.
16. **Allen JL, Jacobson ER, Harvey JW, Boyce W.** Hematologic and serum chemical values for young African elephants (*Loxodonta africana*) with variations for sex and age. J Zoo Anim Med 1985;16:98–101.
17. **Jainudeen MR, Jaysinghe JB.** Hemogram of the domesticated Asiatic elephant (*Elephas maximus*). J Zoo Anim Med 1971;2:5–11.
18. **Niemuller C, Gentry PA, Liptrap RM.** Longitudinal study of haematological and biochemical constituents in blood of the Asian elephant (*Elephas maximus*). Comp Biochem Physiol [A] 1990;96:131–134.
19. **Bechert U.** Morphology and physiology. Anim Keepers' Forum 1993;20:111–115.
20. **Lewis JH.** Comparative hematology: studies on elephants, Elephas maximus. Comp Biochem Physiol [A] 1974;49:175–181.
21. **Brown PT, White PT.** Elephant blood haematology and chemistry. Comp Biochem Physiol [B] 1980;65:1–12.
22. **Gentry PA.** The mammalian platelet: its role in hemostasis, inflammation, and tissue repair. J Comp Pathol 1992;107:243–270.
23. **Cheryk LA, Gentry PA, Bast T, Yamashiro S.** Alterations in blood platelet morphology during aggregate formation in the Asian elephant. J Zoo Wildl Med 1998;29:177–182.

24. **Gentry PA, Cheryk LA, Yamashiro S.** Absence of pseudopod formation in activated elephant platelets. Thromb Hemost 1995;73:1071.
25. **Escolar G, White JG.** The platelet open cannicular system: a final common pathway. Blood Cells 1991;17:467–485.
26. **Murayama M.** Compression inhibits aggregation of human platelets under high hydraulic pressure. Thromb Res 1987;45:729–738.
27. **Patterson WR, Dalton LM, McGlasson DL, Cissik JH.** Aggregation of killer whale platelets. Thromb Res 1993;70:225–231.
28. **Smith JB.** Formation of prostaglandins and thromboxanes. In: Holmsen H, ed. Platelet responses and metabolism. Boca Raton, FL: CRC Press, 1986;2:287–299.
29. **Gentry PA, Niemuller C, Ross ML, Liptrap RM.** Platelet aggregation in the Asian elephant is not dependent on thromboxane B2 production. Comp Biochem Physiol 1989;94A:47–51.
30. **Nemerson Y.** The tissue factor pathway of blood coagulation. Semin Hematol 1992;29:170–176.
31. **Gentry PA, Ross ML, Yamada M.** Blood coagulation profile of the Asian elephant (*Elephas maximus*). Zoo Biol 1996;15:413–423.
32. **Broze GJ, Gailand D.** The role of factor XI in coagulation. Thromb Hemost 1993;70:72–74.
33. **Davie EW, Fujikawa K, Kisiel W.** The coagulation cascade: initiation, maintenance, and regulation. Biochemistry 1991;30:10363–10370.
34. **Lewis JH.** Comparative hematology: studies on elephants, *Elephas maximus.* Comp Biochem Physiol 1974;49A:175–181.
35. **Bauer KA, Rosenberg RD.** Role of antithrombin III as a regulator of in vivo coagulation. Semin Hematol 1991;28:10–18.
36. **Bruce D, Hamerton AE, Bateman HR, Mackie FP.** A note on the occurrence of a trypanosome in the African elephant. Proc Royal Soc London [B] Biol Sci 1909;81:414–416.
37. **Evans GH.** Elephants and their diseases. Rangoon: Government printing, 1910.
38. **Brocklesby DW, Cambell H.** A babesia of the African elephant. East Africa Wildl J 1963:1:119.
39. **Seneviratna P, Hayasinghe JB, Jainudeen MR.** Filariasis in elephants in Ceylon. Vet Rec 1967;81:716–717.
40. **Caple IW, Jainudeen MR, Buick TD, Song CY.** Some clinico-pathologic findings in elephants (*Elephas maximus*) infected with *Fasciola jacksoni.* J Wildl Dis 1978;14:110–115.
41. **Wickremasuriya UGJS, Kenderagama KWT.** A case report of haemorrhagic septicaemia in a wild elephant. Sri Lankan Vet J 1982;30:24.
42. **De Alwis MCL, Thambithurai V.** Haemorrhagic septicaemia in a wild elephant in Ceylon. Ceylon Vet J 1965;23:17–19.
43. **Sikes SK.** Observations on the ecology of arterial disease in the African elephant (*Loxodonta africana*) in Kenya and Uganda. Proc Zool Soc Lond 1968;21:251–273.
44. **Sikes SK.** Habitat and cardiovascular diseases, observations made on elephants (*Loxodonta africana*) and other free-living animals in East Africa. Trans Zool Soc Lond 1969;32:1–104.
45. **Sikes SK.** Habitat stress and arterial disease in elephants. Oryx 1968;9:286–292.
46. **French JE.** Atherosclerosis. In: Florey H, ed. General pathology. London: Loyd-Luke, 1964;418–446.
47. **McCullagh K, Lewis MG.** Spontaneous arteriosclerosis in the wild African elephant. Its relation to the disease in man. Lancet 1967;2:492–495.
48. **McCullagh KG.** Arteriosclerosis in the African elephant. I. Intimal atherosclerosis and its possible causes. Atherosclerosis 1972;16:307–335.
49. **Dillman JS, Carr WR.** Observations on arteriosclerosis, serum cholesterol and serum electrolytes in the wild African elephant. J Comp Pathol 1970;80:91–87.
50. **Lindsay S, Skahen R, Chaikoff IL.** Arteriosclerosis in an elephant. Arch Pathol 1956;61:207–218.
51. **Finlayson R.** Spontaneous arterial disease in exotic animals. J Zool Lond 1965;147:239–343.

CHAPTER 186

Hematology of Reindeer

• KURT A. HENKEL

The blood cells of reindeer (*Rangifer tarandus*; family Cervidae, order Artiodactylia), also known as caribou, in may ways resemble those of the bovidae. Hematologic morphology, parameters, and responses for reindeer have recently been investigated (Table 186.1).[1,2]

ERYTHROCYTES

The erythrocytes of reindeer are apparently discoid and approximately 5 μm in diameter as viewed on a standard peripheral blood smear (Figs. 186.1A, F, K, P, U and 186.2). Central pallor, although present, is generally indistinct. A mild amount of anisocytosis is present, with erythrocytes ranging from 3 to 7 μm in diameter.

Polychromatophils are rare, and an occasional Howell-Jolly body is found. Mild to moderate crenation (echinocytosis) is often present on a variable percentage of erythrocytes. Erythrocytes do not sickle as is seen in some other Cervidae, such as white-tailed deer.[3] Rouleaux formation is not a common feature. An organism resembling *Anaplasma* sp. has been identified on reindeer red blood cells (RBCs) (KA Henkel, in preparation). Reference ranges for adult reindeer erythrocytes are shown in Table 186.1. Age- and sex-related changes to the erythron have been noted. Newborns have lower packed cell volume (PCV) and RBC counts.[4] PCV, RBC, and hemoglobin (HGB) increase in juveniles up to 18 months of age, and adult values have been reported to be slightly lower than juveniles.[5] Seasonal changes have been reported in adult females, with PCV and HGB

TABLE 186.1   Complete Blood Count Data From Four Reindeer

Analyte	Reindeer					Published Reference Values[a]	
	A	B	C	D	Mean	Range	Mean ± SD
Total solids (g/L)	NA	64	60	68	64	48–106	66[b]
RBC (× 10¹²/L)	8.88	6.61	8.73	10.77	8.75	7.9–12.3	9.37 ± 1.17
HGB (g/L)	139	109	139	177	141	139–217	163 ± 22
HCT (%)	0.380	0.281	0.370	0.462	0.373	0.34–0.54	0.42 ± 0.05
MCV (fL)	42.1	42.6	42.3	42.9	42.5	41.6–50.8	42.2 ± 2.6
MCH (pg)	15.6	16.5	15.9	16.4	16.1	15.7–19.1	17.3 ± 1.0
MCHC (g/L)	370	386	376	382	378.5	357–435	384 ± 17
RDW (%)	14.4	15.3	14.0	17.6	15.3	NA	NA
HDW (g/L)	18.4	19.1	18.4	20.9	19.2	NA	NA
Platelets (× 10⁹/L)	650	493	353	311	452	140–675	323 ± 127
MPV (fL)	5.7	5.7	5.2	6.4	5.8	NA	NA
WBC (× 10⁹/L)	9.07	7.24	6.37	10.41	8.27	3.1–12.0	5.2 ± 2.0
Segmented neutrophils (× 10⁹/L)	3.05	3.61	2.33	6.91	3.975	1.4–4.6	2.6 ± 1.0
Band neutrophils (× 10⁹/L)	0	0	0	0	0.000	NA	NA
Lymphocytes (× 10⁹/L)	4.08	2.59	3.48	2.95	3.275	0.7–5.3	1.6 ± 1.0
Monocytes (× 10⁹/L)	0.12	0.07	0.18	0.18	0.140	0.0–0.4	0.1 ± 0.0
Eosinophils (× 10⁹/L)	1.13	0.76	0.33	0.25	0.618	0.0–2.9	0.8 ± 0.7
Basophils (× 10⁹/L)	0.69	0.21	0.05	0.12	0.268	0.0–0.9	0.2 ± 0.0

[a]Results from adult male reindeer (n = 85) except where indicated; adapted from Catley et al., 1990.[2]
[b]Results from 224 reindeer; adapted from McEwan and Whitehead, 1969.[8]
NA, not available.

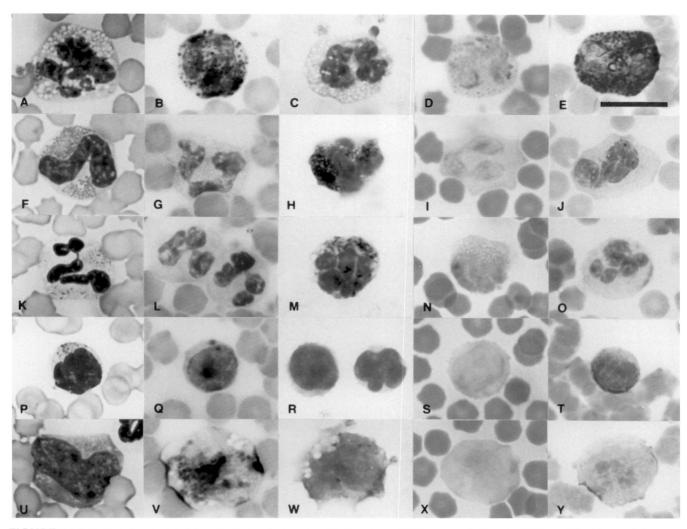

FIGURE 186.1 Cytochemical staining of reindeer leukocytes. (**A**) Grey basophil, Romanowsky's stain. (**B**) Basophil, alpha-naphthyl butyrate esterase (α-NBE). (**C**) Basophil, Sudan black B (SBB). (**D**) Basophil, chloroacetate esterase (CAE). (**E**) Basophil, alkaline phosphatase (ALP). (**F**) Eosinophil, Romanowsky's stain. (**G**) Eosinophil, α-NBE. (**H**) Eosinophil, SBB. (**I**) Eosinophil, CAE. (**J**) Eosinophil, ALP. (**K**) Neutrophil, Romanowsky's stain. (**L**) Neutrophil, α-NBE. (**M**) Neutrophil, SBB. (**N**) Neutrophil, CAE. (**O**) Neutrophil, ALP. (**P**) Lymphocyte, Romanowsky's stain. (**Q**) Lymphocyte, α-NBE. (**R**) Lymphocyte, SBB. (**S**) Lymphocyte, CAE. (**T**) Lymphocyte, ALP. (**U**) Monocyte, Romanowsky's stain. (**V**) Monocyte, α-NBE. (**W**) Monocyte, SBB. (**X**) Monocyte, CAE. (**Y**) Monocyte, ALP. Scale bar = 10 μm. (Reprinted with permission from Henkel KA, Swenson CL, Richardson B, Common R. Morphology, cytochemical staining and ultrastructural characteristics of reindeer (*Rangifer tarandus*) leukocytes. Vet Clin Pathol 1999;28:8–15.)

being lower in the spring and higher in the autumn.[2,5] Observed changes to the erythron due to disease processes have included anemia with inflammatory diseases and microcytosis with malnutrition.[2] Moderate increases in erythrocytes have been associated with stress.[6]

PLATELETS

The platelets of reindeer are relatively small and greatly resemble those of bovines (Figs. 186-2D [lower left and

upper right adjacent to eosinophil] and 186.6 [lower left]). Ultrastructurally there appears to be an open canalicular system.

LEUKOCYTES

Extensive work on the morphology, cytochemistry, and ultrastructure of reindeer leukocytes has been done.[1] The morphology of reindeer leukocytes generally resembles that of the cow (Figs. 186.1 and 186.2), except

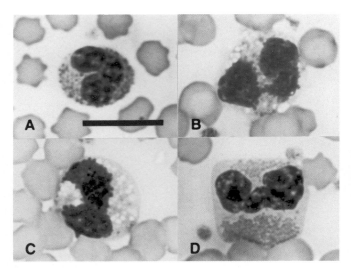

FIGURE 186.2 Comparison of a dark basophil (**A**) with grey basophils (**B, C**) and an eosinophil (**D**) from reindeer blood. The dark basophil granules are similar to basophil granules in other ruminants. Romanowsky's stain. Scale bar = 10 μm. (Reprinted with permission from Henkel KA, Swenson CL, Richardson B, Common R. Morphology, cytochemical staining and ultrastructural characteristics of reindeer (*Rangifer tarandus*) leukocytes. Vet Clin Pathol 1999;28:8–15.)

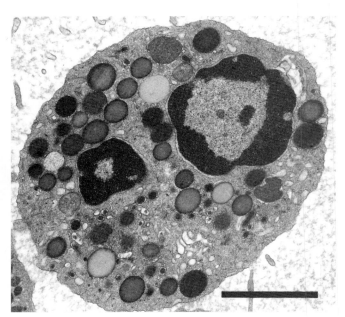

FIGURE 186.3 Electron micrograph, reindeer basophil. Scale bar = 2 μm. (Reprinted with permission from Henkel KA, Swenson CL, Richardson B, Common R. Morphology, cytochemical staining and ultrastructural characteristics of reindeer (*Rangifer tarandus*) leukocytes. Vet Clin Pathol 1991;28:8–15.)

TABLE 186.2   Comparison of Cytochemical Staining Patterns in Mammalian Leukocytes

Cell Type	Staining Technique	Reindeer	Cow[a]	Sheep[a]	Goat[a]	Horse[a]	Dog[a]	Cat[a]	Human[b]
Neutrophil	α-NBE	−	−	−	±	±	−	−	±
	SBB	+	+	+	+	+	+	+	+
	CAE	+	+	+	+	+	+	+	+
	ALP	−	+	+	+	+	−	−	+
Lymphocyte	α-NBE	±	±	±	±	±	±	±	±
	SBB	−	−	−	−	−	−	−	−
	CAE	−	±	−	−	±	−	−	−
	ALP	−	−	−	−	−	−	−	−
Monocyte	α-NBE	+	±	±	+	±	±	±	+
	SBB	±	±	−	±	±	±	±	±
	CAE	±	±	±	±	+	−	−	±
	ALP	−	−	−	−	−	−	−	−
Eosinophil	α-NBE	−	±	−	±	+	−	−	±
	SBB	+	+	+	+	+	+	−	+
	CAE	−	−	−	−	−	−	−	−
	ALP	−	+	−	−	+	±	+	−
Basophil	α-NBE	+*	NK	NK	NK	NK	−	−	−
	SBB	+*	NK	NK	NK	NK	NK	NK	NK
	CAE	+	NK	NK	NK	NK	NK	+	±
	ALP	+	±	NK	NK	−	NK	±	−

[a]Adapted from Jain, 1986.[9]
[b]Adapted from Parmley, 1988.[10]
α-NBE, alpha-naphthyl butyrate esterase; *SBB*, Sudan black B; *CAE*, chloroacetate esterase; *ALP*, alkaline phosphatase; −, negative staining; ±, positive or negative staining; +, positive staining; *, faintly staining; *NK*, not known.

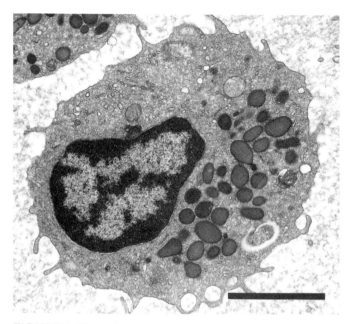

FIGURE 186.4 Electron micrograph, reindeer eosinophil, Scale bar = 2 μm. (Reprinted with permission from Henkel KA, Swenson CL, Richardson B, Common R. Morphology, cytochemical staining and ultrastructural characteristics of reindeer (*Rangifer tarandus*) leukocytes. Vet Clin Pathol 1999;28:8–15.)

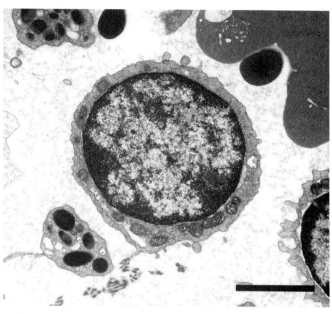

FIGURE 186.6 Electron micrograph, reindeer lymphocyte. Scale bar = 2 μm. (Reprinted with permission from Henkel KA, Swenson CL, Richardson B, Common R. Morphology, cytochemical staining and ultrastructural characteristics of reindeer (*Rangifer tarandus*) leukocytes. Vet Clin Pathol 1999;28:8–15.)

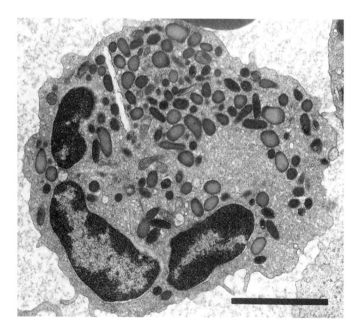

FIGURE 186.5 Electron micrograph, reindeer neutrophil. Scale bar = 2 μm. (Reprinted with permission from Henkel KA, Swenson CL, Richardson B, Common R. Morphology, cytochemical staining and ultrastructural characteristics of reindeer (*Rangifer tarandus*) leukocytes. Vet Clin Pathol 1999;28:8–15.)

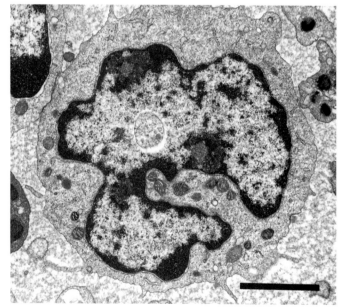

FIGURE 186.7 Electron micrograph, reindeer monocyte. Scale bar = 2 μm. (Reprinted with permission from Henkel KA, Swenson CL, Richardson B, Common R. Morphology, cytochemical staining and ultrastructural characteristics of reindeer (*Rangifer tarandus*) leukocytes. Vet Clin Pathol 1999;28:8–15.)

that reindeer neutrophils have a few basophilic cytoplasmic granules, and reindeer basophil granules stain variably, ranging from nonstaining or clear (gray basophil) to moderately dark staining even within the same sample. The cytochemical staining has been compared with that of other mammalian species (Fig. 186.1 and Table 186.2). Lymphocytes have the same cytochemical profile as those of other mammals, monocytes the same as humans and goat, eosinophils the same as sheep, and neutrophils are similar to those of the dog and cat. The transmission electron microscope ultrastructure of reindeer leukocytes is shown in Figures 186.3 through 186.7.

Concentrations of white blood cells, neutrophils, and lymphocytes may be higher in adult females than adult males, and seasonal leukocyte increases may occur toward summer and autumn in adult females.[7,8] Leukocyte responses have been reported to be similar to those of other ruminants.[2] Lymphocyte concentration was reportedly higher in juveniles than in adults.[2] Eosinophilia is found with subclinical parasitism; stress response includes leukocytosis, neutrophilia, and lymphopenia; and inflammation causes neutrophilia, left shift, eosinophilia, and basophilia.[5]

REFERENCES

1. **Henkel KA, Swenson CL, Richardson B, Common R.** Morphology, cytochemical staining and ultrastructural characteristics of reindeer (*Rangifer tarandus*) leukocytes. Vet Clin Pathol 1999;28:8–15.
2. **Catley A, Kock RA, Hart MG, Hawkey CM.** Haematology of clinically normal and sick captive reindeer (Rangifer tarandu). Vet Rec 1990;126:239–241.
3. **Jain NC.** Essentials of veterinary hematology. Philadelphia: Lea & Febiger, 1993;66–67.
4. **Timisjrvi J, Niemenen M, Saari E.** Hematological values for reindeer. J Wildl Mgmt 1981;45:976–981.
5. **Nieminen M, Timisjarvi J.** Blood composition of the reindeer I. Haematology. Rangifer 1981;1:10–26.
6. **Rehbinder C, Edqvist L-E.** Influence of stress on some blood constituents in reindeer (Rangifer tarandus). Acta Vet Scand 1981;22:480–492.
7. **Chapman DI.** Haematology of the deer. In: Archer RK, Jeffcott LB, eds. Comparative clinical haematology. Oxford: Blackwell Scientific, 1977;345–364.
8. **McEwan EH, Whitehead PE.** Changes in the blood constituents of reindeer and caribou occurring with age. Can J Zool 1969;47:557–562.
9. **Jain NC.** Schalm's veterinary hematology. 4th ed. Philadelphia: Lea & Febiger, 1986.
10. **Parmley RT.** Mammals. In: Rowley AF, Ratcliffe NA, eds. Vertebrate blood cells. Cambridge: Cambridge University Press, 1988;337–424.

CHAPTER 187

Ratite Hematology

• ROBERT A. GREEN and ALICE BLUE-McLENDON

Evaluation of the ratite hemogram has become increasingly important in the veterinary care of diseased birds. The usefulness of ratite hematology is limited by technical difficulties similar to other avian species having nucleated erythrocytes and thrombocytes. However, their large blood volume means that ample blood can be obtained easily for evaluation. The value of the hemogram in confirming health and evaluating disease is well established in most domestic species. Unfortunately, wide laboratory-to-laboratory differences in reference ranges and sparse clinical information concerning hematologic changes expected with specific ratite diseases frustrate interpretation of ratite hematology.

In the past 5 years, the focus of ratite medicine has shifted from individual care of extremely expensive breeding stock to one concerned primarily with flock-oriented production. This economic shift has limited the use of rather expensive hematologic procedures. Although a full hemogram is quite useful in the diagnosis of or therapy for an individual sick ratite, partial automated hemograms can also provide useful clinical information in screening for the presence of disease in a flock. To this end, the development of automated laser-based hematologic analyzers provides an inexpensive way to perform hematologic screening of ratite flocks. The authors' experience with the Abbott CELL-DYN 3500 Hematology Analyzer (Santa Clara, California) is that it accurately determines the hematocrit (based on mean corpuscular volume [MCV] and red blood cell [RBC] count) and the absolute heterophil count. The instrument has difficulty separating the similar-sized ratite small lymphocytes from thrombocytes. However, once a specific disease problem is identified in a flock, knowing the status of heterophils and hematocrit in individual birds can be quite useful in the treatment and evaluation of the disease in the flock. As their accuracy improves, the automated hematologic analyzers of the future may prove increasingly useful in efficient, economic evaluation of flock problems.

SAMPLE COLLECTION

In larger ratites, blood is commonly collected from the cutaneous ulnar vein located on the ventral surface of the wing. In smaller ratites and ostrich chicks, the medial metatarsal vein is a commonly used blood collection site. Blood collection is facilitated by using a 21-gauge butterfly needle attached to a 12-inch flexible plastic infusion set. This allows some movement of the minimally restrained patient after venipuncture without dislodging the needle and causing hematoma formation. After sufficient blood has been aspirated into the syringe, any bubbles in the infusion line are cleared and the needle is inserted into appropriate Vacutainer tubes. Blood is allowed to flow into the Vacutainer tube without pressure on the syringe. The use of head hoods to facilitate restraint in ratites may be necessary but is often associated with some degree of excitement or struggling, which compromises interpretation of the hemogram values.

The preferred anticoagulant in ratite blood is citrate (blue top Vacutainer tube). When comparing citrate values to other values, the effect of 1:9 citrate dilution must be considered. Heparin interferes with staining and causes marked heterophil clumping.[1] There is increased scatter of the ostrich heterophil population collected in heparin compared with the rather homogeneous heterophil population when collected in citrate (Fig. 187.1). Ethylenediamine tetraacetic acid (EDTA) adversely affects blood from some ratites, causing severe hemolysis or poor cell preservation. It is recommended that blood smears be made immediately after collection for optimal morphology of ratite blood cells. Some laboratories have found that smears made by the coverslip method have fewer smudge cells.[2]

The same laboratory hemogram techniques are used with ratite blood as with other avian species and will not be repeated here.[3] If automated hematology analyzers can accurately determine the absolute heterophil count in ratites, then that count along with the manual differential could be used to establish the white blood cell (WBC) count. This would replace the inaccurate and labor-intensive absolute granulocyte count using the eosinophil Unopette (Becton-Dickinson, Rutherford, NJ) and the hemocytometer. Of course, the variable spectrophotometric effects of avian erythrocyte nuclei invalidate automated hemoglobin measurement.

REFERENCE RANGE VALUES

Reference range values for ratites are sparse and vary considerably from laboratory to laboratory (Tables 187.1

and 187.2). In part, this reflects the high laboratory error inherent in manual granulocyte count and the common 100-cell count differential, which are used to estimate the total WBC count. Automated hematology analyzers have greatly improved the accuracy of counting and sizing ratite RBCs.

Because ratite hematocrits are similar to other species, there is an inverse relationship between their large RBC size (MCV greater than 175 fL) and their low RBC counts (less than $2 \times 10^6/\mu L$). There are age-related differences in reference range values, particularly with respect to erythrocyte parameters. Ostrich chicks (1 to 3 months of age) have hematocrits of about 30%, whereas adult ostriches have hematocrits of about 40%.[4] Despite the

lower MCV of juvenile ostriches, their higher RBC count makes their hematocrit approach that of adult ostriches. In contrast to reports suggesting that the presence of a nucleus in the avian erythrocyte causes lowered mean corpuscular hemoglobin concentration (MCHC), most ratite reference range MCHC determinations appear quite similar to those of mammals (Tables 187.1 and 187.2).[5] In ratite patients, the presence of lipemia or incomplete removal of erythrocyte nuclei causes spuriously increased hemoglobin values (which also increase MCH or MCHC). It is noted that the WBC count of juvenile ostriches is higher than that of adults, so heterophilic leukocytosis must be interpreted with caution in young ratites.[2,4] Some reference ranges show higher lymphocyte and basophil counts in young ostriches than in adults.

CELL-DYN 3500
(AVIAN WBC DIFFERENTIATION)
CITRATE VS HEPARIN EFFECTS

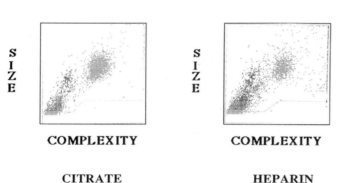

| CITRATE | HEPARIN |

FIGURE 187.1 CELL-DYN 3500 outputs of ostrich blood collected in either sodium citrate or heparin anticoagulants. Note the uniformity of the (orange-colored) heterophil population in citrate compared with the scattered, more diffuse heterophil population when collected in heparin.

COMMENTS ON SPECIFIC BLOOD CELL MORPHOLOGY

Erythrocyte Morphology

The ratite erythrocyte is an oval nucleated cell that is much larger (MCV, greater than 200 fL) than most other avian species (MCV, 125 to 179 fL) or common domestic animals (MCV, 40 to 70 fL). It has a centrally placed compressed oval nucleus with uniformly clumped chromatin which becomes progressively more condensed as cells age. The nucleus of the ostrich erythrocyte varies in shape from an elongated oval to teardrop-shape. The erythrocyte cytoplasm has a uniform orange-pink color when stained with most Wright's stains.

Young polychromatophilic ratite erythrocytes normally comprise approximately 1 to 2% of the total erythrocyte population and reflect the status of marrow erythrocyte production. Immature ratite erythrocytes have a more round shape than mature erythrocytes, and their

TABLE 187.1	Ostrich Reference Ranges									
Species	**Ostrich**		**Ostrich**				**Ostrich**			
Reference	**Fudge 1995**[2]		**Green 1999**[9]				**Levi 1989**[4]			
Age	**Adults**		**Adults (>5 yrs)**		**5–6 Months**		**1–6 yrs**		**9 Months**	
	Mean	*Range*	*Mean*	*SD*	*Mean*	*SD*	*Mean*	*SD*	*Mean*	*SD*
WBC × 10³	18.65	10–24	19.8	6.9	29.2	7.4	5.20	1.60	7.5	1.5
Heterophils × 10³/μL	13.60	10.8–16.6	15.3	6.6	21.6	6	3.31	0.24	4.57	4.77
Lymphocytes × 10³/μL	4.51	2.2–7.6	3.1	0.7	4.8	2.4	1.41	0.24	2.66	2.03
Monocytes × 10³/μL	0.49	0–0.7	0.7	0.4	1.3	1.2	0.10	0.05	0.25	0.11
Basophils × 10³/μL	0.04	0–0.4	0.3	0.2	0.8	0.5	0.01	0.02	0.01	0.02
Eosinophils × 10³/μL	0.01	0–0.4	0.2	0.2	0.3	0.3	0.01	0.02	0.015	0.03
RBC × 10⁶/μL	1.80		1.5	0.2	1.7	0.1	1.5	0.2	2.1	0.3
Hematocrit %	45	41–57	35	3.6	33.8	2.8	40	4	37	3
Hemoglobin g/dL	16.9		11.7	1.4	10.8	0.9	13.8	3	12.7	2.1
MCV fL	212		219	5.3	192	8	193	52	164	16
MCHC %	37.65		33	2.6	32	0.01	37	4	35	6
RDW %	11.11		11.1	1.3	12.1	0.7	—	—	—	—

RDW = RBC distribution width determined by Abbott CELL-DYN 3500 analysis.

TABLE 187.2   **Ratite Reference Ranges**

Species	Emu		Cassowary		Rhea	
Reference	Fudge 1995[2]		Stewart 1994[10]		Green 1999[9]	
Age	Adults		Not given		1 year	
	Mean	Range	Mean	SD	Mean	SD
WBC × 10³	14.87	8–21	18	4.50	13.6	3.3
Heterophils × 10³/μL	11.72	8.0–13.1	13.99	4.64	8.1	2.7
Lymphocytes × 10³/μL	2.94	1.5–6.5	3.546	1.87	4.3	1
Monocytes × 10³/μL	0.01	0–0.2	0.432	0.43	0.5	0.5
Basophils × 10³/μL	0.03	0–0.2			0.5	0.4
Eosinophils × 10³/μL	0.38	0–0.9			0.2	0.2
RBC × 10⁶/μL					2.25	0.1
Hematocrit %					41.6	1.9
Hemoglobin g/dL					13.4	0.45
MCV fL					185	5.9
MCHC %					32	0.01
RDW %					12.6	0.6

RDW = RBC distribution width determined by Abbott CELL-DYN 3500 analysis.

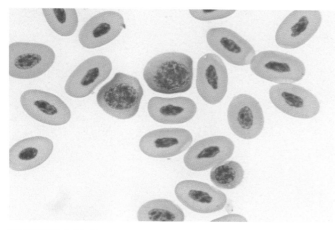

FIGURE 187.2 Diff-Quik stain of emu blood showing immature erythrocytes. Note the two larger rubricytes and the smaller metarubricyte having blue-gray (polychromatophilic) cytoplasm with nuclei that are more round and have less condensed nuclear chromatin than the mature erythrocytes.

cytoplasmic color ranges from blue to gray-purple (Fig. 187.2). Their nucleus is also more round and much less condensed than the mature erythrocyte nucleus. Reticulocyte counts are uncommonly performed on ratite blood but can be used in quantifying regenerative responses similar to other avian species. Using Wright's stains, reticulocytes tend to be slightly larger and bluer (polychromatophilic macrocytes) than mature erythrocytes. The new methylene blue stain reveals variable numbers of dark blue staining RNA aggregates that surround the reticulocyte nucleus. Both punctate and aggregate reticulocytes are present in ratites, but only the aggregate forms are counted in performing a reticulocyte count (similar to the evaluation of feline reticulocytes).[3]

Thrombocyte Morphology

The ratite thrombocyte is a nucleated cell that is about half the size of their erythrocytes. It has a round to oval shape, with a dense pyknotic round nucleus and a moderate amount of clear, somewhat reticulated cytoplasm. The cytoplasm often has several reddish granules and may have several clear spaces or vacuoles (which are more commonly noted in partially activated thrombocytes) (Figs. 187.3A and 187.4). Thrombocytes often tend to aggregate in clusters of reactive thrombocytes on blood smears, which makes estimating the thrombocyte count difficult. Although not well established in ratites, normal thrombocyte counts range from 20,000 to 30,000/μL or 10 to 15 per 100 erythrocytes on blood smears. A qualitative thrombocyte count is often determined during blood smear evaluation and is usually reported as decreased, adequate, or increased. Adequate thrombocyte numbers are usually associated with finding 5 to 10 thrombocytes per 5 oil immersion fields on a blood smear. Immature thrombocytes are occasionally noted on smears, indicating enhanced thrombocyte production. Their size is somewhat larger than mature thrombocytes (approaching the size of a large lymphocyte). Their nuclear shape is round, with a condensed clumped chromatin pattern; their cytoplasm is lightly basophilic with increased numbers of small, round, red granules, similar to those found in mature thrombocytes (Fig. 187.3C).

Recent studies using aspirin to inhibit normal thrombocyte aggregation in whole blood from ostriches suggested that prostaglandin-dependent mechanisms play a role in thrombocyte activation, similar to mammalian platelets.[6] Agonists causing irreversible whole blood thrombocyte aggregation included platelet-activating factor and collagen, but not adenosine diphosphate (ADP). Hemorrhagic diseases of ratites caused by abnormal thrombocyte function are uncommon; however,

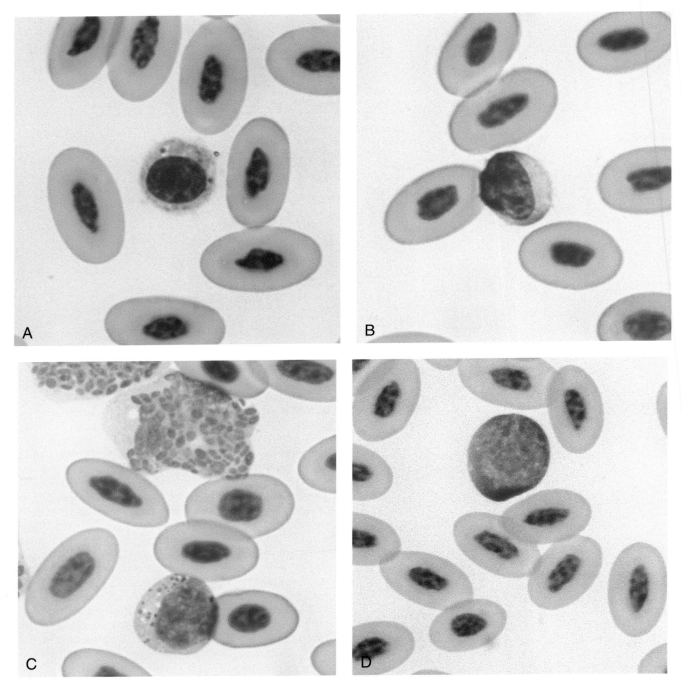

FIGURE 187.3 (A) Typical ostrich thrombocyte showing a few red granules in its cytoplasm with a centrally located, highly condensed oval nucleus. (B) Small ostrich lymphocyte showing a less condensed, indented eccentric nucleus with light blue cytoplasm. (C) A heavily granulated heterophil (top) with an immature thrombocyte (bottom) having granules similar in appearance to the mature thrombocyte and a slightly enlarged, moderately condensed oval nucleus. Alternatively, this cell may be a granulated lymphocyte, although its granule and nuclear characteristics seem more consistent with a thrombocyte classification. (D) A plasma cell (or reactive lymphocyte) characterized by a round eccentric nucleus with dark blue cytoplasm and a prominent Golgi zone adjacent to the nucleus.

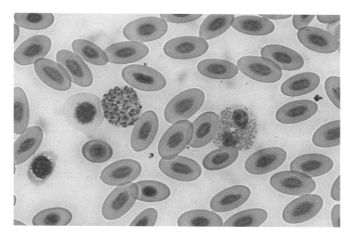

FIGURE 187.4 Comparison of the Diff-Quik stain appearance of the ostrich eosinophil (right) having a bilobed nucleus and numerous small round red granules with that of a heavily granulated heterophil (center). A thrombocyte (lower left) with a centrally located oval nucleus and several perinuclear clear zones is also present.

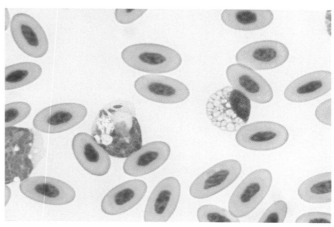

FIGURE 187.5 Diff-Quik stain of ostrich blood showing a basophil (right) with an eccentric nucleus and a vacuolated appearance due to lysis of its granules. Compare this cell with the toxic heterophil (left of center) characterized by cytoplasmic hypogranularity and vacuolization.

thrombocyte dysfunction may be responsible for a high incidence of hemorrhage noted in emus with hereditary gangliosidosis.[7]

Granulocyte Morphology

Heterophils are the most numerous WBCs in ratite blood and have similar functions to those of neutrophils in mammalian blood. The mature heterophil is a round cell with a segmented nucleus that is often partially occluded by numerous round to fusiform granules that have a red-orange color (Figs. 187.3C and 187.4). The background cytoplasm is clear in the mature heterophil. Immature heterophils are uncommon in normal ratite blood, and their stage of maturation is based on nuclear shapes, similar to other species. The cytoplasm of immature heterophils is slightly more basophilic than that of mature heterophils.

The granulation of immature heterophils ranges from early cells with moderate numbers of basophilic round (primary) granules, to intermediate cells having mostly round eosinophilic granules, to mature cells having mostly orange fusiform granules. Increased immature heterophils in blood (called a left shift) imply increased demand for heterophils, often associated with inflammatory diseases of ratites. In diseases associated with toxicity, it is common to see abnormal heterophil granulation characterized by cells that are poorly granulated or retain the round primary granules of early precursors (Fig. 187.5). In severe toxicity, heterophils may partially degranulate, nuclear swelling occurs, and their cytoplasm becomes more basophilic.[3] An Abbott CELL-DYN output from an ostrich with septicemia shows the effect of increased immature heterophils by causing the heterophil population pattern to be extended upward compared with the control (Fig. 187.6). Inflammatory

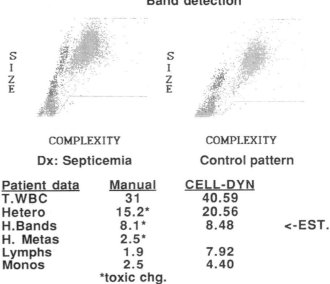

CELL-DYN 3500 (WBC DIFFERENTIATION)
Ostrich #656803
Band detection

Patient data	Manual	CELL-DYN	
T.WBC	31	40.59	
Hetero	15.2*	20.56	
H.Bands	8.1*	8.48	<-EST.
H. Metas	2.5*		
Lymphs	1.9	7.92	
Monos	2.5	4.40	
	*toxic chg.		

FIGURE 187.6 CELL-DYN 3500 patterns for WBC collected from a normal ostrich (right) and from an ostrich with septicemia (left). Note the orange-colored heterophil population is shifted upward and to the left, indicating the presence of immature (larger, less complex) heterophils in the septicemic ostrich. Monocytes are indicated by purple, lymphocytes by blue, and background erythrocytic debris with thrombocytes by red. The CELL-DYN analysis of ratite lymphocyte populations is consistently overestimated because of interference from similar-sized thrombocytes. Toxic heterophils (noted on the blood smear) featured hypogranularity that also produced a leftward shift in the CELL-DYN heterophil population. The heterophil band population was estimated (est.) by the CELL-DYN analysis and appears to correlate well with the left shift noted in the manual count.

diseases of ratites associated with heterophilic left shifts and toxic changes are usually associated with a poor prognosis.

Eosinophils are found in low numbers in blood from normal ratites, and their function is uncertain. The emu reference range suggests slightly higher levels of eosinophils in emus than ostriches (Table 187.2). Eosinophils often have a bilobed nucleus with abundant small, round, red-to-pink granules and light blue cytoplasm (Fig. 187.4). The granules of eosinophil precursors are larger, and primary granules may also be present in their cytoplasm. Parasitism appears to induce eosinophilia less commonly in ratites than in mammals or certain other avian species (particularly raptors).

Basophils are found in low numbers in normal ratite blood (although they are more common than eosinophils in juvenile ostriches). The ratite basophil is slightly smaller than the heterophil and has an eccentric round to oval, nonsegmented nucleus. The basophil cytoplasm is moderate in amount and often has a distinct purple hue. The numerous dark metachromatic granules of the basophil commonly dissolve with routine Wright's stains, leaving the cytoplasm with a vacuolated or reticulated appearance (Fig. 187.5). A few remnant basophilic granules are often present to assist cell classification. Although basophil function is unclear in ratites, basophilia is occasionally noted in hypersensitivity reactions and chronic respiratory diseases.

Lymphocyte Morphology

Lymphocytes are the second most common WBC in normal ratites, and lymphopenias are commonly associated with diseases causing increased stress. Lymphocyte morphology is similar to that of other avian species, with cells varying in size from small lymphocytes (which may be difficult to differentiate from thrombocytes) to intermediate or large lymphocytes (which may become reactive and appear similar to monocytes). The nuclear shape of small lymphocytes is round with a lacy chromatin pattern. Their cytoplasm varies in amount from scant to moderate and is usually lightly basophilic (Fig. 187.3B). This feature is quite helpful in distinguishing small lymphocytes from activated thrombocytes having clear cytoplasm. Lymphocytes are often found abutting adjacent erythrocytes, which makes their shape appear rectangular. Degenerate lymphocytes may have scant cytoplasm or cytoplasmic blebs. Occasionally, larger lymphocytes are noted with a few azurophilic granules, similar to those found in killer lymphocytes of mammals. Plasmacytoid or reactive lymphocytes may be seen in ratites, particularly during convalescent immune responses (Fig. 187.3D). These plasma cell-like lymphocytes have an eccentric round nucleus, dark basophilic cytoplasm, and a pale perinuclear Golgi zone. Mild lymphocytosis is also associated with immune stimulation, noted particularly during convalescence. Marked lymphocytosis of either small or larger lymphoid cells is suggestive of lymphocytic leukemia in ratites.[8]

Monocyte Morphology

Monocytes are found in low numbers in ratite blood, and their morphology is quite similar to mammalian monocytes. They are large cells with moderate amounts of blue-gray cytoplasm that occasionally has small discrete vacuoles. Their nuclei are pleomorphic with a chromatin pattern that is lacy and somewhat less condensed than lymphocytes. Distinct cytoplasmic granules are uncommon in ratite monocytes, although faint, dust-like eosinophilic granules are noted commonly. Differentiating monocytes from enlarged reactive lymphocytes can be challenging in ratite blood smears. Monocytosis is associated with various chronic granulomatous diseases of ratites, including mycoses, and diseases in which marked tissue necrosis occurs.

CONCLUSIONS

In the 1980s when individual ratites were valued at several thousand dollars, it was easy to justify veterinary care and extensive laboratory evaluation of individual birds. Despite this, there is a paucity of veterinary literature available concerning hematologic changes expected with ratite diseases. The present economics of ratite production are so marginal that it is difficult to justify minimal veterinary care for diseased birds. On the other hand, this industry is cyclic, and should the economic factors improve, hematologic evaluation will again provide useful information with respect to medical evaluation of diseased ratites.

REFERENCES

1. **Campbell TW.** Hematology. In: Ritchie BW, Harrison GJ, Harrison LR, eds. Avian medicine: principles & application. Lake Worth: Winger's Publishing, 1994.
2. **Fudge AM.** Clinical hematology and chemistry of ratites. In: Tully TN, Shane SM, eds. Ratite management, medicine, & surgery. Malabar: Kreiger, 1996.
3. **Campbell TW.** Avian hematology. In: Campbell TW, ed. Avian hematology & cytology. Ames, IA: Iowa State University Press, 1995.
4. **Levi A, Perelman B, Waner T, Van Grevenbroek M, Van Creveld C, Yagil R.** Haematological parameters of the ostrich (Struthio camelus). Avian Pathol 1989;18:321–327.
5. **Van der Heyden N.** Evaluation & interpretation of the avian hemogram. Avian Exotic Vet Med 1994;3:5–13.
6. **Thomas JS, Blue-McLendon A.** The effects of in vitro incubation with acetylsalicylic acid on thrombocyte aggregation in whole blood from normal ostriches. Comp Haematol Intern 1998;8:137–141.
7. **Bermudez AJ, Freischütz B, Yu RK, Nonneman D, Johnson GS, Boon GD, Stogsdill PL, Ledoux DR.** Heritability and biochemistry of gangliosidosis in emus (Dromaius novaehollandiae). Avian Dis 1997;41:838–849.
8. **Gregory CR, Latimer KS, Mahaffey EA, Doker T.** Lymphoma and leukemic blood picture in an emu (Dromaius novaehollandiae). Vet Clin Pathol 1996;25:136–139.
9. **Green RA.** Reference range for normal ostriches & rheas. Veterinary clinical pathology laboratory. Texas A & M University Teaching Hospital, 1999.
10. **Stewart J.** Hematologic and biochemical values for ratites. In: Ritchie BW, Harrison GJ, Harrison LR eds. Avian medicine: principles & application. Lake Worth: Winger's Publishing, 1994;1347.

CHAPTER 188

Hematology of the American Bison
(*Bison bison*)

• DAVID M. MOORE

BLOOD COLLECTION

Venipuncture sites for blood collection in the American Bison (*Bison bison*) include the jugular vein and coccygeal (tail) vein, using the same techniques that would be used in domestic cattle. Blood collection can be accomplished in an unanesthetized animal when restrained within a squeeze chute.

MORPHOLOGY AND INDICES OF PERIPHERAL BLOOD CELLS

Reported hematologic values for American Bison are provided in Tables 188.1 and 188.2. The morphology of erythrocytes, leukocytes, and platelets in bison is comparable to that observed in domestic cattle (*Bos taurus*).[6]

Bison are capable of prolonged running, facilitated by the comparatively great oxygen-carrying capacity and low oxygen affinity of their erythrocytes. Average oxygen-carrying capacity was 22.2 mL/100 mL blood from adult blood and 17.0 mL/100 mL from calf blood; hemoglobin in one group of animals averaged 17.1 g/dL in adults and 13.6 g/dL in calves.[10]

The average packed cell volume (PCV) in bison is approximately 47% (range, 24 to 61%). Compared with reported values for domestic cattle, sheep, and goats,[11] the following parameters were found to be higher in bison: total erythrocyte count, PCV, and hemoglobin. Bison calves have significantly higher erythrocyte counts than do adult bison, which is also the case with calves of domestic cattle.[11] The average hemoglobin in bison is about 16.8 g/dL (range, 8.2 to 23.0 g/dL). Bison raised/maintained under ranch conditions comparable to those used in beef cattle operations had similar hematologic values as free-ranging bison living on range

lands or in national parks.[7] However, an increase in PCV was seen in free-ranging wild bison that had been impounded for 24 hours before blood collection.[4]

The following parameters in bison were found to be comparable with reported parameters[11] in domestic cattle, sheep, and goats: total white blood cell count, neutrophil count, lymphocyte count, eosinophil count, and monocyte count. Lymphocytes outnumber neutrophils in both bison and domestic cattle. This is in contrast to earlier reports that indicated that the neutrophil:lymphocyte ratio in bison was opposite to that observed in cattle.[2,7] The average total leukocyte count for all ages and sexes of bison is $8.0 \times 10^6/mm^3$ (range, 1.0 to $18.4 \times 10^6/mm^3$).

REFERENCES

1. **Marler RJ.** Some hematologic and blood chemistry values in two herds of American bison in Kansas. J Wildl Dis 1975;11:97–100.
2. **Mehrer CF.** Some hematologic values of bison from five areas of the United States. J Wildl Dis 1976;12:7–13.
3. **Keith EO, Ellis JE, Phillips RW, Benjamin MM.** Serologic and hematologic values of bison in Colorado. J Wildl Dis 1978;14:493–500.
4. **Hawley AWL, Peden DG.** Effects of ration, season and animal handling on composition of bison and cattle blood. J Wildl Dis 1982;18:321–338.
5. **Clemens ET, Meyer KL, Carlson MP, Schneider NR.** Hematology, blood chemistry and selenium values of captive pronghorn antelope, white-tailed deer, and American bison. Comp Biochem Physiol 1987;87C:167–170.
6. **Miller LD, Thoen CO, Throlson KJ, Himes EM, Morgan RL.** Serum biochemical and hematologic values of normal and Mycobacterium bovis-infected American bison. J Vet Diagn Invest 1989;1:219–222.
7. **Sikarskie JG, Schillhorn van Veen TW, van Selm G, Kock MD.** Comparative blood characteristics of ranched and free-ranging American bison (*Bison bison*). Am J Vet Res 1990;51:955–957.
8. **Vestweber JG, Johnson DE, Merrill GL, Staats JJ.** Hematological and blood chemistry profiles of American bison grazing on Konza Prairie of Kansas. J Wildl Dis 1991;27:417–420.
9. **Zaugg JL, Taylor SK, Anderson BC, Hunter DL, Ryder J, Devine M.** Hematologic, serologic values, histopathologic and fecal evaluations of Bison from Yellowstone Park. J Wildl Dis 1993;29:453–457.
10. **Haines H, Chichester HG, Landreth HF Jr.** Blood respiratory properties of *Bison bison*. Respir Physiol 1977;30:305–310.
11. **Jain NC.** Schalm's veterinary hematology. 4th ed. Philadelphia: Lea & Febiger, 1986.

TABLE 188.1 Referenced Erythrocyte Parameters of the American Bison (*Bison bison*)

Reference	Age	Gender	RBC (×10⁶/mm³) Mean	RBC (×10⁶/mm³) Range	PCV (%) Mean	PCV (%) Range	Hb (g/dL) Mean	Hb (g/dL) Range	MCV (μ³) Mean	MCV (μ³) Range	MCH (μμg) Mean	MCH (μμg) Range	MCHC (%) Mean	MCHC (%) Range
1	<2 yrs	NS	—	—	49.8 ± 1.3	—	16.6 ± 1.3	12.5–19.0	—	—	—	—	—	—
	Adult	NS	—	—	50.0 ± 4.5	42.6–61.1	17.2 ± 1.5	14.2–21.0	—	—	—	—	—	21.47–51.86
2	All	M/F	10.08 ± 1.43	6.53–13.9	47.11 ± 4.06	37–57	16.99 ± 1.43	12.24–19.19	59.74 ± 8.76	41.01–87.29	19.79 ± 4.4	11.42–29.38	35.92 ± 6.21	—
	All	F	10.33 ± 1.45	—	47.2 ± 4.46	—	16.93 ± 1.47	—	45.69 ± 9.41	—	16.39 ± 4.53	—	35.87 ± 5.34	—
	1–2 yr	F	10.14 ± 1.41	—	46.95 ± 4.99	—	17.06 ± 1.6	—	46.3 ± 7.56	—	16.82 ± 2.96	—	36.34 ± 3.29	—
	3–4 yr	F	10.01 ± 1.67	—	48.52 ± 3.29	—	16.97 ± 1.04	—	48.47 ± 8.63	—	16.95 ± 3.63	—	34.97 ± 4.56	—
	>5 yr	F	10.97 ± 1.12	—	46.14 ± 4.03	—	16.52 ± 1.49	—	42.06 ± 8.97	—	15.06 ± 3.97	—	35.8 ± 4.99	—
	All	M	9.97 ± 1.32	—	46.9 ± 3.73	—	16.72 ± 1.34	—	47.0 ± 9.73	—	16.77 ± 4.38	—	35.65 ± 4.71	—
	1–2 yr	M	9.64 ± 1.28	—	46.17 ± 4.27	—	16.51 ± 1.58	—	47.89 ± 8.43	—	17.17 ± 3.59	—	35.76 ± 4.87	—
	3–4 yr	M	9.93 ± 1.28	—	47.63 ± 3.49	—	16.93 ± 1.24	—	47.97 ± 7.56	—	18.15 ± 4.13	—	35.54 ± 3.96	—
	>5 yr	M	11.24 ± 0.92	—	42.44 ± 8.47	—	17.0 ± 0.85	—	42.44 ± 8.47	—	15.13 ± 4.53	—	35.63 ± 5.11	—
3	Winter	M/F			43 ± 4	—	15.8 ± 1.1	—						
	Spring	M/F			41.7 ± 2.5	—	15.2 ± 0.6	—						
	Summer	M/F			26.8 ± 3.1	—	16.7 ± 1.4	—						
	Fall	M/F			51.4 ± 4.2	—	18.6 ± 1.3	—						
4	Ranched	NS	8.5 ± 0.5	—	46.8 ± 2.6	—	17.5 ± 0.9	—	55.1 ± 1.6	—	20.2 ± 0.4	—	36.5 ± 0.8	—
	Park 1 Juvenile	NS	8.7 ± 0.5	—	44.1 ± 2.0	—	16.7 ± 0.8	—	50.8 ± 2.7	—	18.7 ± 0.8	—	36.7 ± 0.6	—
	Park 1 Adult	NS	7.9 ± 0.6	—	45.9 ± 4.1	—	16.6 ± 1.4	—	58.5 ± 4.7	—	20.7 ± 2.3	—	35.3 ± 3.6	—
	Park 2 Juvenile	NS	7.9 ± 1.2	—	39.7 ± 6.4	—	14.8 ± 1.5	—	48.7 ± 2.6	—	19.0 ± 1.4	—	37.8 ± 2.1	—
	Park 2 Adult	NS	7.6 ± 0.8	—	41.3 ± 3.9	—	15.8 ± 1.5	—	53.3 ± 1.9	—	21.1 ± 0.7	—	38.0 ± 1.8	—
5	NS	NS	—	—	47.3 ± 1.3	—	—	—	—	—	—	—	—	—
6	1–2 yr	M/F	—	—	51.3 ± 3.2	28–59	18.6 ± 1.0	10.3–23.0	—	—	—	—	—	—
7	Ranched All	M/F	10.19 ± 1.87	—	44.65 ± 3.93	—	17.04 ± 1.62	—	—	—	—	—	—	—
	Ranched Calf (<185 kg)	M/F	11.67 ± 1.24	—	46.3 ± 3.69	—	17.59 ± 1.58	—	—	—	—	—	—	—
	Ranched Adult (>185 kg)	M/F	8.72 ± 0.84	—	43.0 ± 3.2	—	16.49 ± 1.36	—	—	—	—	—	—	—
8	<6 mo	M/F	11.94 ± 0.25	—	50.77 ± 1.11	—	17.94 ± 0.38	—	42.97 ± 1.07	—	15.04 ± 0.44	—	35.35 ± 0.21	—
	7–23 mo	M/F	9.64 ± 0.21	—	50.48 ± 0.92	—	17.92 ± 0.31	—	52.37 ± 0.89	—	18.6 ± 0.37	—	35.5 ± 0.18	—
	>24 mo	M/F	9.12 ± 0.14	—	51.75 ± 0.61	—	18.36 ± 0.21	—	56.86 ± 0.59	—	20.35 ± 0.24	—	35.49 ± 0.11	—
9	<1 yr	M/F	9.27 ± 0.23	5.86–11.38	42.26 ± 1.42	28–61	16.34 ± 0.42	9.9–20.9	—	—	—	—	—	—
	Adult	M	8.62 ± 0.19	5.23–20.7	45.55 ± 1.21	25–62	15.91 ± 0.37	8.3–20.7	—	—	—	—	—	—
	Adult	F	8.29 ± 0.14	5.47–11.13	42.85 ± 0.68	24–59	15.41 ± 0.25	8.2–21.2	—	—	—	—	—	—

NS, not specified.

TABLE 188.2 Referenced Leukocyte Parameters of the American Bison (*Bison bison*)

Reference	Age	Gender	WBC (×10³/mm³) Mean	WBC (×10³/mm³) Range	Neutrophils (%) Mean	Neutrophils (%) Range	Lymphocytes (%) Mean	Lymphocytes (%) Range	Eosinophils (%) Mean	Eosinophils (%) Range	Basophils (%) Mean	Basophils (%) Range	Monocytes (%) Mean	Monocytes (%) Range
1	<2 yrs	NS	8.0 ± 2.4	4.0–14.2	34 ± 10	7–55	56 ± 5	31–93	7 ± 5	1–22	0	0–1	2 ± 2	1–4
	Adult	NS	6.99 ± 2.1	4.2–13.1	46 ± 13	22–74	42 ± 12	22–74	10 ± 5	2–23	0	0–1	1 ± 1	0–3
2	All	Both	8.03 ± 1.41	4.67–10.74	63.77 ± 7.95	40–83	24.86 ± 6.4	12–44	3.98 ± 3.31	0–20	0.77 ± 1.01	0–10	6.34 ± 4.17	0–36
	All	F	7.83 ± 1.6	—	64.03 ± 8.21	—	24.47 ± 6.08	—	4.21 ± 3.81	—	0.77 ± 1.09	—	6.67 ± 4.39	—
	1–2 yr	F	7.75 ± 1.69	—	62.67 ± 9.83	—	25.16 ± 6.97	—	4.98 ± 4.79	—	0.86 ± 1.12	—	6.28 ± 5.51	—
	3–4 yr	F	8.03 ± 1.39	—	64.14 ± 6.01	—	24.71 ± 5.99	—	3.52 ± 1.94	—	0.31 ± 0.8	—	7.29 ± 2.59	—
	>5 yr	F	7.8 ± 1.69	—	66.9 ± 5.8	—	22.95 ± 3.96	—	3.38 ± 2.67	—	1.0 ± 1.22	—	5.71 ± 2.65	—
	All	M	8.11 ± 1.14	—	63.18 ± 8.1	—	25.35 ± 7.18	—	3.41 ± 2.42	—	0.77 ± 0.97	—	6.64 ± 4.05	—
	1–2 yr	M	8.09 ± 1.28	—	64.23 ± 6.64	—	24.14 ± 6.8	—	3.73 ± 2.33	—	0.93 ± 0.91	—	5.33 ± 3.04	—
	3–4 yr	M	8.13 ± 1.22	—	59.96 ± 8.96	—	27.81 ± 7.71	—	2.93 ± 2.74	—	0.41 ± 0.75	—	8.93 ± 4.7	—
	>5 yr	M	8.1 ± 1.18	—	68.4 ± 6.0	—	22.0 ± 4.08	—	3.7 ± 1.34	—	1.2 ± 1.4	—	5.1 ± 2.6	—
3	Winter	Both	8.57 ± 0.25	—	44 ± 8.9	—	50.78 ± 7.8	—	3.7 ± 2.1	—	0	—	2.7 ± 0.6	—
	Spring	Both	8.47 ± 1.85	—	43 ± 9	—	53.3 ± 8.1	—	2.0 ± 1.7	—	0	—	2.0 ± 1.7	—
	Summer	Both	6.43 ± 0.89	—	50.2 ± 12.8	—	37.8 ± 11.3	—	8.6 ± 3.0	—	0.3 ± 0.5	—	4.5 ± 2.6	—
	Fall	Both	6.2 ± 0.64	—	48.2 ± 4.6	—	40.8 ± 4.9	—	8.0 ± 4.2	—	0.2 ± 0.4	—	2.6 ± 0.9	—
4	Ranched	NS	6.6 ± 1.2	—	—	—	—	—	—	—	—	—	—	—
	Park 1 Juvenile	NS	9.1 ± 1.5	—	—	—	—	—	—	—	—	—	—	—
	Park 1 Adult	NS	7.9 ± 1.9	—	—	—	—	—	—	—	—	—	—	—
	Park 2 Juvenile	NS	11.3 ± 1.8	—	—	—	—	—	—	—	—	—	—	—
	Park 2 Adult	NS	8.4 ± 2.2	—	—	—	—	—	—	—	—	—	—	—
5	NS	NS	—	—	44.2 ± 3.6	—	46.1 ± 3.1	—	10.8 ± 1.7	—	0	—	2.6 ± 0.6	—
6	1–2 yr	M/F	7.72 ± 1.7	3.4–18.4	43.3	—	51.2	—	3.6	—	0.27	—	0.75	—
7	Ranched All	M/F	10.56 ± 3.62	—	43.8 ± 15.46	—	44.0 ± 16.38	—	6.6 ± 5.31	—	0	—	0.65 ± 0.75	—
	Ranched Calf (<185 kg)	M/F	9.64 ± 2.99	—	36.2	—	53.2	—	5.2	—	0	—	4.8	—
	Ranched Adult (>185 kg)	M/F	11.48 ± 3.78	—	51.4	—	34.8	—	9.1	—	0	—	4.5	—
	Free-ranging All	M/F	—	—	41.75 ± 11.47	—	50.8 ± 11.66	—	4.1 ± 2.67	—	0	—	3.25 ± 3.91	—
8	<6 mo	M/F	8.45 ± 0.94	—	29	—	65.7	—	0.95	—	0	—	4	—
	7–23 mo	M/F	9.38 ± 0.79	—	42	—	49.4	—	3.4	—	0.4	—	4.3	—
	>24 mo	M/F	10.59 ± 0.52	—	49	—	43.9	—	3.7	—	0.3	—	3	—
9	<1 yr	M/F	4.9 ± 0.42	1.2–11.8	29.91 ± 3.56	13–49	54.55 ± 4.14	34–81	4.18 ± 1.31	0–11	0.18 ± 0.12	0–1	1.73 ± 0.47	0–5
	Adult	M	4.22 ± 0.35	1.5–14.1	36.53 ± 5.33	0–78	44.44 ± 4.45	11–86	3.56 ± 0.8	0–10	0	0	3.31 ± 0.71	0–8
	Adult	F	4.43 ± 0.22	1.0–11.13	31.54 ± 2.61	12–76	48.61 ± 3.83	8–86	2.96 ± 0.49	0–11	0.14 ± 0.07	0–1	1.71 ± 0.34	0–6

NS, not specified.

CHAPTER 189

Hematology of the Rat (*Rattus norvegicus*)

• DAVID M. MOORE

BLOOD COLLECTION

Moore[1] described and illustrated several methods for blood collection from rats, which are applicable to other rodent species as well (i.e., mice, hamsters, gerbils, and guinea pigs). Blood is commonly collected from rats either from the retroorbital venous plexus or by cardiac puncture, preferably while the animal is anesthetized. The technique for blood collection from the orbital sinus requires skill, expertise, and training to obtain the necessary quantities of blood successfully and without causing undue injury or distress to the animal. Both Pasteur pipettes and microhematocrit tubes have been used to penetrate the orbital venous plexus or sinus, but it is important that the tip of the tube used not be broken off to form a jagged, cutting edge. A jagged edge will cause excessive trauma to structures and tissues within the orbit, whereas the normal smooth tip can bluntly dissect through the conjunctival tissues, minimizing tissue damage. Heparinized microhematocrit tubes, with an internal diameter of 1.1 to 1.2 mm, 75 mm in length, and a wall thickness of 0.2 ± 0.02 mm are ideal for orbital blood collection. The expiration date on the container should be checked before use of the tubes. The microhematocrit tube should be handled along its middle, because contact with either tip by the technician's fingers will initiate the clotting cascade when the rat's blood contacts that surface, causing the blood to coagulate within the tube. The anesthetized animal is restrained using the thumb and forefinger to retract the upper and lower eyelids, and a microhematocrit tube is then inserted into the medial canthus (the corner of the eye nearest the nose) at an angle of 30 to 45° with respect to the plane of the lateral aspect of the face. The tube should be rotated back and forth between the fingers during insertion to aid in blunt dissection through the conjunctiva. The tube is inserted until it contacts the back of the bony orbit, at which time the tube is withdrawn slightly to allow the blood to flow from the venous plexus/sinus. As blood begins to fill the tube, the rat should be rotated so that the tube is pointing downward, allowing the blood to flow not only by capillary action but also with gravity. Blood will drop from the tip of the tube into the collection vessel, and one must take care not to touch the tip of the tube to the vessel, as this will also initiate the clotting cascade, and foil collection attempts. An experienced technician can obtain 3 mL of blood by this method within approximately 10 seconds.

Once the appropriate quantity of blood is obtained, the microhematocrit tube is removed from the orbit. As the eye retracts into the socket, the pressure provides some measure of hemostasis; however, additional slight pressure should be applied to the closed eyelids for about 10 seconds to assure that bleeding has stopped. This method does not pose the same risk of death to the animal as does cardiac puncture, but if done inappropriately, can lead to loss of blood supply to the eye with subsequent blindness or atrophy of the eye. Serial samples should be taken by alternating the site of collection (from the opposite orbital sinus each time) and preferably not more frequently than once every 5 to 7 days from each eye.

Cardiac puncture, performed by a skilled individual, can quickly and safely yield 3 mL of blood from an adult rat. The animal should be anesthetized with either an injectable agent or an inhalant gas anesthetic (i.e., halothane, metofane, isoflurane, or a brief exposure to carbon dioxide). The injectable anesthetics produce a prolonged recovery period that may impact the ongoing study, affecting metabolism and food consumption (adverse factors that can be avoided with the use of shorter-acting gas anesthetics). Animals removed from a bell jar or other gas anesthetic induction chambers/devices will quickly awaken from the anesthetic, within 10 to 20 seconds, leaving little time for error; therefore, this should not be the method used by unskilled individuals. Before blood collection, the technician should palpate the xiphoid process of the sternum, a cartilaginous flap located along the ventral midline, identifying the area known as the left cardiac notch, where the hypodermic needle will be inserted. The area of the insertion site should be swabbed with an appropriate disinfectant solution. Using a 3- or 5-mL syringe fitted with a 1-inch

22- or 23-gauge needle, the technician should insert the needle cranially into the left cardiac notch somewhat parallel to the ventral midline, at approximately a 25° angle. The needle will penetrate the skin, the diaphragm, and ultimately the left ventricle. Once the needle has penetrated into the thoracic cavity, the technician should begin slowing withdrawing the plunger (creating a negative pressure within the needle) and continue insertion until blood flows into the needle hub. He or she should then stop insertion and continue blood withdrawal. The plunger should not be withdrawn too quickly, because this will create excessive negative pressure, causing tissue to be drawn into the bevel of the needle, occluding blood flow. Should blood flow into the syringe erratically, the technician can very gently and slowly rock the needle up and down or side to side to free the bevel from the heart wall. Excessive motion of the needle may slash or traumatize the heart, so great care should be exercised. Cardiac puncture, even in skilled hands, can lead to the death of an animal from shock (hypovolemia and hypotension) as a result of hemorrhage from the site of myocardial penetration into the thorax (hemothorax) or into the pericardial sac (producing cardiac tamponade). Multiple cardiac punctures for serial samples can weaken the heart muscle through scar formation, altering cardiovascular dynamics and predisposing the heart to arrhythmias. Another technique for cardiac puncture involves palpation of the thorax for the location of the strongest detectable heartbeat, with insertion of a hypodermic needle between the ribs over that site. Penetration of and trauma to the lungs will likely occur using this method.

Alternate blood collection sites for rats include the anterior vena cava, jugular vein,[2] saphenous vein, lateral tail veins,[3] and dorsal metatarsal vein. Blood can be collected into a capillary tube or syringe and needle from the saphenous vein, lateral tail veins, and dorsal metatarsal vein following puncture of the vessel with a sterile lancet or a hypodermic needle. Warming the tail in warm water, using a warm compress or heating pad, or placing the rat in a 40°C chamber for 10 to 15 minutes will all facilitate vasodilation and blood collection. Terminal blood collection in anesthetized rats can be accomplished by opening the thoracic or abdominal cavities and collecting blood from the heart or posterior vena cava. To minimize or eliminate the effects of anesthetics on enzyme systems within tissues and body fluids collected at the time of euthanasia, rats can be decapitated, using a guillotine, to facilitate collection of large quantities of mixed venous and arterial blood. The AVMA Panel on Euthanasia recommends that, whenever possible, the animal(s) be sedated or lightly anesthetized to avoid struggling by the animal and injury to the handler, because the fingers of the restraining hand are perilously close to the guillotine blades.[4]

Hematologic values may vary depending on the site and method of blood withdrawal/collection. Packed cell volume (PCV), hemoglobin, and total leukocyte counts are generally higher in blood samples taken from the tail vein versus blood collected directly from the heart.[5]

The blood volume in a rat was reported as being between 5.0 and 7.1 mL/100 g of body weight,[5,6] although it was more recently determined to be 7.2 ± 1.19 mL/100 g of body weight using a different technique.[7] It has been suggested that approximately 5.5 mL/kg of blood can be withdrawn safely from the rat during a single collection.[8] However, Scipioni et al.[9] demonstrated that collection of up to 40% of blood volume in 13 serial samples taken within a 24-hour period did not lead to an increase of morbidity or mortality, that body weight gain was not affected, and that hematologic values returned to control levels within 2 weeks after the blood was collected.

MORPHOLOGY AND INDICES OF PERIPHERAL BLOOD CELLS

Reported hematologic values for three stocks/strains of laboratory rats (*Rattus norvegicus*) are provided in Tables 189.1 through 189.6. Literature references on hematology of the rat may be consulted for additional data.[6,8,10–15]

Erythrocytes

Rat erythrocytes are biconcave disks, with an average diameter of 6.2 μm (range, 5.7 to 7.0 μm).[16] Rat red blood cells (RBCs) are smaller than those of guinea pigs and rabbits. Marked anisocytosis of rat erythrocytes is common, with more variation in size than in shape, and the diameter of some cells may be observed to be about one-third that of the average diameter listed above.[16] Polychromatic erythrocytes may be found in a range from 1 to 18% to the total erythrocyte count;[8] along with the large number of polychromatic cells, a large number of reticulocytes may also be found, accounting for 2 to 5% of the counts in adults and 10 to 20% in young rats.[16] Polychromatic cells have a grayish coloration and lack the full complement of hemoglobin. It has been reported that "diseased" rats have a more pronounced polychromatophilia and anisocytosis than is observed in healthy animals.[17] Although normoblasts may be observed occasionally in adults (approximately 0.12 to 2.0% of red cells), they are observed with greater regularity in neonatal and postweanling rats.[16] Erythrocyte counts in rats reach adult levels at approximately 4 months of age, with slightly lower counts in females than in males.[8] The life span of erythrocytes in rats is approximately 45 to 68 days.[5]

Hemoglobin levels may vary between inbred strains and outbred stocks of rats and may be affected by gender, age, and health status.[6] Hemoglobin levels in male rats (range, 13.4 to 15.8 g/dL; mean, 14.6 g/dL) are higher than those observed in female rats (range, 11.5 to 16.1 g/dL; mean, 13.8 g/dL).[8] The hematocrit of rats is approximately three times the hemoglobin value,[6] with hematocrit values ranging from 39 to 54%. Between 66 and 121 weeks of age, the number of circulating reticulocytes in rats increases, while the mean corpuscu-

TABLE 189.1 Erythrocyte Parameters and Plasma Composition in Sprague–Dawley Rats—Sex and Age Influence (Means and 1 SD)[a]

No. of Rats	Sex	Age	PCV (%)	RBC (×10⁶/µL)	Hb (g/dL)	MCV (fL)	MCHC (%)	MCH (pg)	Reticulocytes (%)	Icterus Index Units	Plasma Proteins (g/dL)	Fibrinogen (g/dL)
22	Male	25–35 days	36.6 ± 2.4	5.15 ± 0.57	10.8 ± 0.8	71.2 ± 3.8	29.4 ± 0.9	20.9 ± 1.1	16.2 ± 7.5	2.0 ± 2.0	5.7 ± 0.4	0.27 ± 0.05
28	Male	50–77 days	46.6 ± 1.8	7.04 ± 0.50	14.6 ± 0.6	66.6 ± 5.0	31.3 ± 0.9	20.9 ± 1.6	4.6 ± 3.1	5.0 ± 2.0	7.0 ± 0.4	0.21 ± 0.08
29	Male	3 mo	48.7 ± 2.2	7.95 ± 0.49	15.4 ± 1.1	61.3 ± 2.3	31.6 ± 1.5	19.4 ± 1.2	2.8 ± 1.8	4.6 ± 1.9	7.1 ± 0.4	—
29	Male	4–6 mo	48.1 ± 1.9	8.53 ± 0.47	15.3 ± 0.6	56.4 ± 2.4	31.8 ± 0.9	17.9 ± 1.0	2.3 ± 1.6	4.4 ± 2.2	7.3 ± 0.4	—
67	Male	7–12 mo	47.1 ± 2.6	8.20 ± 0.56	15.0 ± 0.9	57.6 ± 3.4	31.9 ± 1.2	18.3 ± 1.1	2.1 ± 1.3	4.0 ± 2.2	7.3 ± 0.5	0.28 ± 0.08
26	Male	13–15 mo	46.5 ± 1.6	8.28 ± 0.59	15.1 ± 1.0	56.3 ± 3.3	32.4 ± 1.6	18.3 ± 1.6	2.1 ± 0.7	3.3 ± 1.8	7.9 ± 0.5	0.37 ± 0.06
20	Female	25–35 days	37.4 ± 2.0	5.19 ± 0.61	11.0 ± 0.8	72.5 ± 5.3	29.5 ± 1.3	21.4 ± 1.7	16.2 ± 8.1	3.0 ± 2.0	5.7 ± 0.3	0.20 ± 0.06
24	Female	50–77 days	45.6 ± 1.6	7.05 ± 0.38	14.8 ± 0.6	64.9 ± 3.5	32.3 ± 0.9	21.0 ± 1.4	2.5 ± 1.5	4.0 ± 1.5	7.2 ± 0.3	0.25 ± 0.05
12	Female	3 mo	45.3 ± 2.0	7.14 ± 0.63	14.7 ± 0.7	63.8 ± 4.8	32.4 ± 1.0	20.7 ± 1.7	3.4 ± 1.5	4.0 ± 2.0	7.3 ± 0.5	0.17 ± 0.06
30	Female	4–6 mo	46.0 ± 1.5	7.60 ± 0.34	15.2 ± 0.7	60.4 ± 2.3	33.0 ± 1.1	19.9 ± 0.9	2.8 ± 1.2	3.0 ± 1.7	7.7 ± 0.5	—
67	Female	7–12 mo	45.1 ± 1.8	7.46 ± 0.43	14.5 ± 0.7	60.4 ± 2.4	32.1 ± 0.9	19.5 ± 0.9	2.4 ± 1.0	2.6 ± 2.0	8.1 ± 0.5	0.17 ± 0.06
29	Female	13–15 mo	44.7 ± 2.2	7.27 ± 0.40	14.5 ± 0.8	61.5 ± 2.4	32.5 ± 0.8	20.0 ± 0.9	2.6 ± 1.1	3.7 ± 2.4	8.6 ± 0.5	0.20 ± 0.09
42	Both	25–35 days	37.0 ± 2.2	5.18 ± 0.59	10.9 ± 0.8	71.8 ± 4.6	29.4 ± 1.1	21.2 ± 1.5	16.2 ± 7.8	2.7 ± 1.9	5.7 ± 0.4	0.24 ± 0.06
52	Both	50–77 days	46.2 ± 1.8	7.04 ± 0.45	14.7 ± 0.6	65.7 ± 4.5	32.0 ± 1.0	20.9 ± 1.5	3.6 ± 2.7	4.5 ± 2.1	7.1 ± 0.4	0.23 ± 0.07
41	Both	3 mo	47.7 ± 2.6	7.71 ± 0.65	15.2 ± 1.0	62.0 ± 3.4	31.8 ± 1.4	19.8 ± 1.5	3.0 ± 1.7	4.3 ± 2.0	7.1 ± 0.4	0.17 ± 0.06
59	Both	4–6 mo	47.0 ± 2.0	8.06 ± 0.62	15.2 ± 0.7	58.4 ± 3.1	32.4 ± 1.2	19.0 ± 1.4	2.6 ± 1.5	3.7 ± 2.1	7.5 ± 0.5	—
134	Both	7–12 mo	46.1 ± 2.5	7.83 ± 0.62	14.8 ± 0.8	59.0 ± 3.2	32.5 ± 1.1	18.9 ± 1.2	2.2 ± 1.2	3.4 ± 2.2	7.7 ± 0.7	0.23 ± 0.09
55	Both	13–15 mo	45.5 ± 2.1	7.75 ± 0.70	14.8 ± 1.0	59.0 ± 3.9	32.5 ± 1.3	19.2 ± 1.5	2.3 ± 1.0	3.5 ± 2.2	8.3 ± 0.6	0.26 ± 0.12

[a] Heart blood collected under ether anesthesia.
From Jain NC. Schalm's veterinary hematology. 4th ed. Philadelphia: Lea & Febiger, 1986.

TABLE 189.2 Leukocyte and Platelet Counts in Sprague–Dawley Rats—Sex and Age Influence (Means and 1 SD)[a]

| | | | | Differential Leukocyte Count (%) | | | | | | |
| | | | | Neutrophils | | | | | | |
No. of Rats	Sex	Age	WBC/μL	Band	Mature	Lymphocytes	Monocytes	Eosinophils	Basophils	Platelets (×10³/μL)
22	Male	25–35 days	8377 ± 2896	0.14 ± 0.43	14.4 ± 4.5	81.9 ± 5.5	2.9 ± 1.7	0.4 ± 0.7	0.02 ± 0.10	1173 ± 261
28	Male	50–77 days	12,457 ± 3506	0.02 ± 0.09	13.7 ± 3.9	83.6 ± 4.1	2.0 ± 1.3	0.7 ± 0.7	0.04 ± 0.13	1051 ± 278
29	Male	3 mo	15,255 ± 3536	0.12 ± 0.28	16.0 ± 5.6	81.5 ± 5.7	1.5 ± 1.4	0.8 ± 0.7	0.05 ± 0.15	998 ± 183
29	Male	4–6 mo	11,983 ± 3111	0.07 ± 0.21	20.1 ± 5.6	77.3 ± 6.0	1.4 ± 1.0	1.0 ± 0.9	0.13 ± 0.24	1031 ± 201
67	Male	7–12 mo	11,585 ± 2269	0.06 ± 0.20	25.3 ± 7.3	70.6 ± 8.0	2.3 ± 1.8	1.6 ± 1.2	0.10 ± 0.31	1108 ± 193
26	Male	13–15 mo	15,076 ± 13,280	0.10 ± 0.30	31.3 ± 6.4	61.9 ± 6.9	5.0 ± 2.7	1.3 ± 0.9	0.04 ± 0.13	1179 ± 257
20	Female	25–35 days	7430 ± 2963	0	14.2 ± 4.9	82.3 ± 5.4	3.2 ± 2.2	0.3 ± 0.5	0	1038 ± 254
24	Female	50–77 days	12,479 ± 2689	0.08 ± 0.19	15.4 ± 6.0	82.0 ± 6.6	1.5 ± 1.4	0.9 ± 0.5	0.06 ± 0.17	1135 ± 202
12	Female	3 mo	11,458 ± 2567	0.04 ± 0.14	12.1 ± 6.8	84.8 ± 8.3	2.0 ± 2.5	1.1 ± 0.9	0	1112 ± 135
30	Female	4–6 mo	9810 ± 1789	0.02 ± 0.09	15.4 ± 4.5	81.3 ± 5.1	2.3 ± 1.6	1.2 ± 1.1	0.08 ± 0.19	1139 ± 258
67	Female	7–12 mo	8366 ± 2011	0.04 ± 0.16	23.6 ± 8.6	71.6 ± 9.3	2.8 ± 2.1	1.8 ± 1.4	0.05 ± 0.23	980 ± 187
29	Female	13–15 mo	7417 ± 1624	0.05 ± 0.27	28.4 ± 7.2	66.4 ± 7.5	3.0 ± 1.5	1.9 ± 1.5	0.17 ± 0.35	1120 ± 220
42	Both	25–35 days	7926 ± 2966	0.07 ± 0.32	14.3 ± 4.6	82.1 ± 5.6	3.1 ± 1.8	0.4 ± 0.6	0.01 ± 0.07	1111 ± 266
52	Both	50–77 days	12,467 ± 3156	0.05 ± 0.15	14.5 ± 5.1	82.9 ± 5.4	1.8 ± 1.4	0.8 ± 0.6	0.05 ± 0.15	1089 ± 194
41	Both	3 mo	14,143 ± 3709	0.10 ± 0.25	14.9 ± 6.2	82.5 ± 6.7	1.7 ± 1.8	0.9 ± 0.8	0.04 ± 0.13	1026 ± 179
59	Both	4–6 mo	10,878 ± 2750	0.04 ± 0.16	17.7 ± 5.6	79.3 ± 5.9	1.9 ± 1.5	1.1 ± 1.0	0.11 ± 0.21	1085 ± 237
134	Both	7–12 mo	9975 ± 2680	0.05 ± 0.18	24.5 ± 8.0	71.1 ± 8.7	2.5 ± 2.0	1.7 ± 1.3	0.08 ± 0.28	1043 ± 200
55	Both	13–15 mo	10,963 ± 9882	0.09 ± 0.29	29.8 ± 7.0	64.3 ± 7.6	4.0 ± 2.2	1.6 ± 1.3	0.11 ± 0.28	1148 ± 239

[a] Heart blood collected under ether anesthesia.
From Jain NC. Schalm's veterinary hematology. 4th ed. Philadelphia: Lea & Febiger, 1986.

TABLE 189.3 Erythrocyte Parameters and Plasma Composition in Long–Evans Rats—Sex and Age Influence (Means and 1 SD)[a]

No. of Rats	Sex	Age	PCV (%)	RBC (×10⁶/μL)	Hb (g/dL)	MCV (fL)	MCHC (%)	MCH (pg)	Reticulocytes (%)	Icterus Index Units	Plasma Proteins (g/dL)	Fibrinogen (g/dL)
10	Male	26–30 days	37.7 ± 2.1	5.40 ± 0.32	11.5 ± 0.9	69.9 ± 2.3	30.3 ± 0.8	21.2 ± 0.8	21.1 ± 9.8	2.3 ± 2.2	5.6 ± 0.4	—
23	Male	37–75 days	46.1 ± 2.6	7.25 ± 0.93	14.3 ± 1.0	64.2 ± 5.9	31.1 ± 0.9	19.9 ± 1.5	5.8 ± 3.1	3.3 ± 2.4	6.6 ± 0.5	0.20 ± 0.04
11	Male	3 mo	47.1 ± 5.9	8.57 ± 0.57	15.6 ± 0.9	57.2 ± 3.9	31.9 ± 1.0	18.3 ± 1.4	2.6 ± 1.6	3.7 ± 2.8	7.0 ± 0.5	0.26 ± 0.11
41	Male	4–6 mo	48.2 ± 3.6	8.46 ± 0.61	15.1 ± 1.6	57.6 ± 3.1	31.5 ± 1.4	17.8 ± 1.8	2.2 ± 1.1	3.7 ± 2.3	7.1 ± 0.4	0.25 ± 0.08
70	Male	7–12 mo	48.2 ± 2.0	8.69 ± 0.50	15.3 ± 0.7	54.8 ± 6.4	31.6 ± 1.1	17.6 ± 1.1	1.7 ± 1.2	4.6 ± 2.2	7.2 ± 0.4	—
21	Male	13–15 mo	47.1 ± 2.1	8.49 ± 0.37	14.8 ± 0.8	55.4 ± 1.9	31.5 ± 1.0	17.5 ± 0.9	2.0 ± 1.0	2.7 ± 2.9	7.6 ± 0.5	—
10	Female	26–30 days	39.0 ± 2.3	5.54 ± 0.29	11.8 ± 0.8	70.4 ± 3.1	30.1 ± 0.9	21.2 ± 1.0	17.6 ± 5.0	2.4 ± 1.8	5.6 ± 0.4	—
25	Female	37–82 days	45.5 ± 2.7	6.85 ± 0.61	14.3 ± 1.1	66.6 ± 3.3	31.5 ± 0.9	21.0 ± 0.7	5.0 ± 2.6	2.9 ± 2.4	6.7 ± 0.6	0.19 ± 0.05
13	Female	3 mo	46.7 ± 2.0	7.46 ± 0.35	15.0 ± 0.6	62.7 ± 2.2	32.1 ± 0.6	20.1 ± 0.8	2.4 ± 1.3	4.7 ± 2.7	6.8 ± 0.3	—
36	Female	4–6 mo	47.7 ± 1.7	7.74 ± 0.58	15.4 ± 0.6	61.9 ± 5.2	32.3 ± 0.8	20.0 ± 1.6	2.6 ± 1.2	4.6 ± 2.0	7.5 ± 0.5	0.18 ± 0.07
75	Female	7–12 mo	46.7 ± 2.2	7.85 ± 0.50	15.1 ± 0.7	59.6 ± 3.1	32.3 ± 1.0	19.2 ± 1.0	2.9 ± 1.4	4.0 ± 2.0	7.7 ± 0.5	0.16 ± 0.07
6	Female	13–15 mo	46.5 ± 2.1	7.92 ± 0.39	14.5 ± 0.8	58.7 ± 1.7	31.2 ± 1.0	18.4 ± 1.0	4.3 ± 1.4	3.3 ± 4.0	8.3 ± 0.5	—
20	Both	26–30 days	38.6 ± 2.3	5.47 ± 0.31	11.6 ± 0.8	70.2 ± 2.8	30.2 ± 0.8	21.2 ± 0.9	19.4 ± 8.0	2.4 ± 2.0	5.6 ± 0.4	—
48	Both	37–82 days	45.8 ± 2.7	7.04 ± 0.81	14.3 ± 1.1	65.4 ± 4.9	31.3 ± 0.9	20.5 ± 1.3	5.6 ± 2.9	3.1 ± 2.4	6.6 ± 0.5	0.20 ± 0.05
24	Both	3 mo	46.9 ± 4.3	7.98 ± 0.72	15.3 ± 0.8	60.2 ± 4.1	32.0 ± 0.8	19.3 ± 1.5	2.5 ± 1.5	4.3 ± 2.8	6.9 ± 0.4	0.25 ± 0.11
77	Both	4–6 mo	47.9 ± 2.9	8.13 ± 0.70	15.2 ± 1.3	59.6 ± 4.7	31.8 ± 1.3	18.9 ± 2.0	2.4 ± 1.1	4.1 ± 2.2	7.3 ± 0.5	0.23 ± 0.08
145	Both	7–12 mo	47.4 ± 2.2	8.26 ± 0.65	15.2 ± 0.8	57.3 ± 5.6	32.0 ± 1.1	18.5 ± 1.3	2.4 ± 1.5	4.3 ± 2.1	7.5 ± 0.5	0.16 ± 0.07
27	Both	13–15 mo	47.0 ± 2.1	8.36 ± 0.44	14.8 ± 0.8	56.2 ± 2.3	31.4 ± 1.0	17.7 ± 1.0	2.5 ± 1.5	2.8 ± 3.2	7.7 ± 0.6	—

[a] Heart blood collected under ether anesthesia.
From Jain NC. Schalm's veterinary hematology. 4th ed. Philadelphia: Lea & Febiger, 1986.

TABLE 189.4 Leukocyte and Platelet Counts in Long–Evans Rats—Sex and Age Influence (Means and 1 SD)[a]

| | | | | Differential Leukocyte Count (%) | | | | | | |
| | | | | Neutrophils | | | | | | |
No. of Rats	Sex	Age	WBC/μL	Band	Mature	Lymphocytes	Monocytes	Eosinophils	Basophils	Platelets (×10³/μL)
10	Male	26–30 days	4000 ± 944	0	16.1 ± 8.2	78.8 ± 7.7	4.2 ± 2.9	0.9 ± 0.7	0.1 ± 0.20	1099 ± 145
23	Male	37–75 days	8543 ± 2231	0.02 ± 0.10	16.6 ± 5.7	78.3 ± 7.1	3.4 ± 2.5	1.5 ± 1.9	0.6 ± 2.70	923 ± 294
11	Male	3 mo	8809 ± 2342	0.09 ± 0.19	21.3 ± 5.6	74.6 ± 5.7	2.2 ± 1.2	1.7 ± 1.5	0.1 ± 0.30	840 ± 155
41	Male	4–6 mo	10,249 ± 2794	0.05 ± 0.24	20.1 ± 5.4	75.9 ± 5.9	1.8 ± 1.5	2.1 ± 1.5	0.06 ± 0.20	882 ± 173
70	Male	7–12 mo	9591 ± 1961	0.07 ± 0.30	26.6 ± 7.8	66.8 ± 9.1	3.1 ± 2.2	3.4 ± 2.4	0.1 ± 0.24	953 ± 194
21	Male	13–15 mo	9595 ± 3433	0.07 ± 0.20	35.3 ± 7.8	56.0 ± 7.6	5.2 ± 3.3	3.1 ± 2.1	0.2 ± 0.60	980 ± 193
10	Female	26–30 days	3800 ± 865	0.20 ± 0.60	13.4 ± 4.3	82.5 ± 5.5	3.7 ± 2.0	0.3 ± 0.4	0.05 ± 0.15	1089 ± 123
25	Female	37–82 days	7100 ± 2423	0.04 ± 0.20	15.3 ± 5.7	80.9 ± 5.7	1.6 ± 1.0	2.1 ± 2.4	0.04 ± 0.14	949 ± 149
13	Female	3 mo	8315 ± 1868	0.04 ± 0.13	17.9 ± 6.1	77.5 ± 5.9	2.5 ± 1.6	2.0 ± 1.2	0.04 ± 0.13	969 ± 156
36	Female	4–6 mo	8478 ± 3126	0.10 ± 0.23	18.5 ± 6.8	76.3 ± 8.9	1.3 ± 1.5	3.7 ± 3.4	0.08 ± 0.25	1016 ± 196
75	Female	7–12 mo	7079 ± 2045	0.09 ± 0.40	23.2 ± 7.4	69.8 ± 8.9	2.9 ± 2.4	3.9 ± 3.6	0.07 ± 0.20	984 ± 175
6	Female	13–15 mo	6983 ± 1293	0.17 ± 0.40	22.7 ± 9.4	69.2 ± 9.6	2.8 ± 1.4	5.3 ± 6.0	0	1038 ± 136
20	Both	26–30 days	3900 ± 911	0.10 ± 0.40	14.8 ± 6.7	80.6 ± 7.0	3.9 ± 2.5	0.6 ± 0.7	0.08 ± 0.20	1093 ± 133
48	Both	37–82 days	7792 ± 2442	0.03 ± 0.20	15.9 ± 5.7	79.7 ± 6.5	2.5 ± 2.1	1.8 ± 2.2	0.3 ± 1.90	936 ± 234
24	Both	3 mo	8542 ± 2113	0.06 ± 0.20	19.4 ± 6.1	76.2 ± 6.0	2.3 ± 1.5	1.9 ± 1.4	0.06 ± 0.20	907 ± 169
77	Both	4–6 mo	9421 ± 3084	0.07 ± 0.20	19.4 ± 6.1	76.1 ± 7.4	1.6 ± 1.5	2.8 ± 2.7	0.07 ± 0.20	946 ± 196
145	Both	7–12 mo	8309 ± 2365	0.08 ± 0.30	24.9 ± 7.6	68.3 ± 9.1	3.0 ± 2.3	3.6 ± 3.1	0.08 ± 0.20	969 ± 185
27	Both	13–15 mo	9015 ± 3274	0.09 ± 0.30	32.5 ± 9.7	58.9 ± 9.8	4.7 ± 3.2	3.6 ± 3.5	0.17 ± 0.50	993 ± 183

[a] Heart blood collected under ether anesthesia.
From Jain NC. Schalm's veterinary hematology. 4th ed. Philadelphia: Lea & Febiger, 1986.

TABLE 189.5   Erythrocyte Parameters of F344 Rats[6,18]

Gender (Age)	No.	RBC (×10⁶/mm³)	PCV (%) Mean	PCV (%) Range	Hb (g/dL) Mean	Hb (g/dL) Range	MCV (μ) Mean	MCV (μ) Range	MCH (μμg) Mean	MCH (μμg) Range	MCHC (%) Mean	MCHC (%) Range	Reticulocytes (%) Mean	Reticulocytes (%) Range
F (2 wks)	24	4.3 ± 0.1	34 ± 0.1	32–35	10.8 ± 0.5	9.7–11.8	78.7 ± 2.7	73.8–82.7	25.2 ± 1.1	22.8–26.9	32.0 ± 1.0	30.7–34.7	16.5 ± 6.1	8.0–36.0
F (4 wks)	15	6.1 ± 0.3	41 ± 0.2	38–44	12.9 ± 0.6	11.8–13.8	67.6 ± 2.3	64.1–71.4	21.2 ± 0.7	20.2–22.5	31.5 ± 0.3	30.8–32.0	2.2 ± 2.0	0.3–7.8
F (8 wks)	17	7.3 ± 0.4	47 ± 0.1	44–49	15.3 ± 0.6	14.2–15.9	64.0 ± 2.6	60.2–69.2	20.9 ± 0.7	19.8–21.9	32.6 ± 0.6	31.5–33.6	1.4 ± 1.1	0.2–3.8
F (20 wks)	17	7.4 ± 0.3	47 ± 0.1	45–49	15.4 ± 0.3	15.0–16.0	62.9 ± 2.2	59.6–68.1	20.7 ± 0.7	19.7–22.0	32.9 ± 0.5	32.0–33.9	0.6 ± 0.5	0.1–2.0
M (26 wks)	NS	9.17	48.1		17.5		52.6				36.5		1.66	
F (26 wks)	NS	9.03	49.3		16.9		54.6				34.4		0.81	
M (52 wks)	NS	9.13	47.2		16.2		51.8				34.3		0.46	
F (52 wks)	NS	8.41	46.8		15.7		55.9				33.5		1.69	
F (66 wks)	14	7.7 ± 0.4	47 ± 0.1	45–49	15.1 ± 0.4	14.5–16.0	61.0 ± 3.6	55.2–68.2	19.7 ± 1.2	17.5–21.8	32.4 ± 0.6	31.3–33.3	1.6 ± 0.8	0.5–3.3
M (78 wks)	NS	9.60	54.5		18.9		56.8				34.7		1.99	
F (78 wks)	NS	8.32	46.7		16.3		56.3				35.1		1.80	
M (104 wks)	NS	9.26	57.8		19.5		62.4				33.7		3.08	
F (104 wks)	NS	8.20	45.8		15.1		55.9				32.9		1.25	
F (121 wks)	13	7.5 ± 0.8	45 ± 0.5	36–58	14.3 ± 1.5	11.7–17.8	60.3 ± 2.4	57.5–64.0	19.2 ± 1.0	17.5–20.9	31.7 ± 0.8	30.4–33.0	5.3 ± 3.7	0.2–12.7

NS, not specified.

TABLE 189.6   Leukocyte Parameters of F344 Rats

Gender (Age)	No.	WBC (×10³/mm³) Mean	WBC (×10³/mm³) Range	Neutrophils (%) Mean/Range	Lymphocytes (%) Mean/Range	Eosinophils (%) Mean/Range	Basophils (%) Mean/Range	Monocytes (%) Mean/Range
F (2 wks)[18]	24	2.3 ± 0.8	1.0–3.6	23.9	73.9	0	0	0
F (4 wks)[18]	15	2.8 ± 0.7	1.8–4.4	25.7	82.9	0.7	0.4	0
M (6–8 wks)[25]	20	6.4	3.1–9.7	17 (3–32)	78 (63–93)	1 (0–2)	0 (0–2)	4 (0–8)
F (6–8 wks)[25]	20	5.5	1.7–9.3	14 (0–28)	83 (67–99)	1 (0–2)	0 (0–2)	3 (0–6)
F (8 wks)[18]	17	2.3 ± 1.0	1.0–4.8	21.3	77	0.4	0	0.4
M (16 wks)[6]	NS	10.2		23.8	73.4	0.9	0	2.3
F (16 wks)[6]	NS	13.8		31.7	66	0.5	0	1.8
F (20 wks)[18]	17	2.0 ± 0.6	0.8–3.1	25.5	74	0.5	0	0.5
M (19–21 wks)[25]	20	8.2	5.2–11.2	30 (14–46)	68 (52–84)	1 (0–2)	0 (0–2)	1 (0–2)
F (19–21 wks)[25]	20	8.3	6.3–10.3	43 (25–61)	52 (38–66)	1 (0–2)	0 (0–2)	5 (1–9)
M (32–34 wks)[25]	20	4.7	3.4–6.0	52 (40–60)	46 (28–64)	1 (0–2)	0 (0–2)	2 (0–4)
F (32–34 wks)[25]	20	6.9	4.1–9.7	38 (24–52)	56 (41–71)	1 (0–2)	0 (0–2)	4 (0–8)
F (66 wks)[18]	14	2.2 ± 1.0	1.0–4.1	32.3	72.3	1.8	0	2.7
F (121 wks)[18]	13	4.5 ± 1.6	1.7–7.0	39	59.3	0.6	0	0

NS, not specified.

lar hemoglobin concentration (MCHC) is observed concurrently to decrease.[18]

Thrombocytes

Observed ranges of numbers of circulating platelets in rats have been reported in several references: 430 to 840 × 10³/mm³;[16] 121 to 460 × 10³/mm³;[8] 685 to 1244 × 10³/mm³ in Long-Evans rats, and 793 to 1436 × 10³/mm³ in Sprague-Dawley rats;[15] 694 to 1412 × 10³/mm³ (pooled males and females), 694 to 1158 × 10³/mm³ (males), and 695 to 1412 × 10³/mm³ (females);[19] and 1126 ± 32 × 10³/mm³ (orbital sinus collection) and 1213 ± 31 × 10³/mm³ (posterior vena cava collection).[20] The numbers of platelets in rats is considerably larger than the numbers observed in guinea pigs and rabbits. The number of circulating platelets in rats increases by 11.5% between 4 weeks and 36 weeks of age (645.5 × 10³/mm³ at 4 weeks, and 720 × 10³/mm³ at 36 weeks).[21]

Leukocytes

Neutrophils account for between 12 and 38% of circulating white blood cells (WBCs) in normal rats. The average diameter of the rat neutrophil is 11 μm, and its nucleus is highly segmented, coiled, or ribbon-like and has numerous indentations. The cytoplasm of neutrophils contains fine, diffuse granules. The cytoplasm of eosinophils contains densely packed, round eosinophilic granules, and the nucleus is a ribbon-like annular structure. Eosinophils, which comprise 1 to 4% of the total WBC count in normal rats, are slightly smaller than neutrophils. Circulating basophils are rare and when present may, in fact, be tissue basophils from subcutaneous tissue released during compression

of tissues in the tail during tail vein blood collection.[16] "Blood" basophils are not larger than typical granulocytes, and their nuclei are segmented or lobulated. In contrast, the "tissue" basophil is much larger, with a small, round, bright nucleus, and its cytoplasm is densely packed with round dark-blue granules. Lymphocytes are the predominant leukocyte in rats, accounting for 60 to 75% of the total WBC count. Two size classes can be identified—small and large lymphocytes, with the latter having a diameter of up to 15 μm, and the former being found in greater numbers with a diameter of about 6 μm.[16] The cytoplasm of large lymphocytes may be scant to abundant and varies from deep blue to pale blue.[6] The small lymphocytes are only slightly larger than the erythrocytes, and the cytoplasm of some cells contain azurophilic granules. The nucleus of the rat monocyte is markedly convoluted or kidney-bean-shaped and surrounded by a broad zone of cytoplasm, which may contain some azurophilic or reddish-purple granules. Monocytes may account for 1 to 6% of the total WBC count.

Excitement/stress associated with blood collection in an unanesthetized rat can dramatically alter white blood cell counts, causing an immediate leukocytosis and an increase in circulating lymphocytes by up to 12%.[16] Additional factors including gender (including intact or castrated animals), age, and dietary constituents may also result in significant changes in leukocyte counts.[8] Postpubertal females exhibit changes in the numbers and types of circulating leukocytes during their estrous cycle, with a leukocytopenia observed during estrus and a decrease in the number of circulating neutrophils noted during the diestrus phase of the cycle. Removal of the ovaries and/or uterus in female rats (ovariectomy, ovariohysterectomy, or hysterectomy) results in an increase in the number/percentage of circulating T and B lymphocytes.[22]

BONE MARROW CYTOLOGY

Rat bone marrow accounts for approximately 3% of total body weight.[16] The cellular constituents of the bone marrow of rats is presented in Table 189.7. The myeloid to erythroid (M:E) ratio in normal bone marrow from rats is between 1.16 and 1.36:1.[23]

TABLE 189.7	Bone Marrow Constituents in Rats[23]
Erythrocyte series	
Proerythrocytes	0.6%
Erythroblasts	11.8%
Normoblasts	16.2%
Other cells	
Lymphocyte	21.1%
Monocyte	1.8%
Plasma cell	0.8%
Megakaryocytes	0.4%
Granulocytic Series	
Myeloblast	2.2%
Promyelocyte	1.3%
Myelocyte (neut)	6.7%
Metamyelocyte (neut)	2.5%
Neutrophil	4.1%
Eosinophil	4.2%
Basophil	0.4%
M:E ratio = 1.16–1.36:1	

TABLE 189.8	Observed Coagulation Values in Rats	
Parameter	**Mean ± SD**	**Reference**
Bleeding time	120	6
(sec)	210 ± 60[a]	26
Clotting time	120–300	16
(sec)	240 ± 48[b]	26
	180 ± 18[a]	26
Prothrombin	10.8 ± 0.4	16
time (sec)	10.5 (range 8–14)	27
	13.5 (range 12.6–14.4) [pooled][a]	19
	13.5 (range 12.6–14.4) [males][a]	19
	13.5 (range 12.7–14.3) [females][a]	19
	15.4 ± 0.5[c]	20
	12.7 ± 0.1[d]	20
	15.3 ± 2.1[b]	26
	10.1 ± 0.1[a]	26
Partial thrombo-	21.1 ± 3.7	28
plastin time	14.3 (range 8.9–28.1) [pooled][a]	19
(sec)	14.3 (range 9–28.1) [males][a]	19
	14.4 (range 8.9–22.5) [females][a]	19
	63.2 ± 12.2[c]	20
	16.3 ± 1.4[d]	20
	180 ± 24[b]	26
	85 ± 5.8[a]	26

[a] Sprague–Dawley (SD) rats.
[b] Wistar rats.
[c] From orbital venous plexus.
[d] From posterior vena cava.

OTHER HEMATOLOGIC VALUES

Reported coagulation values for rats are provided in Table 189.8. The sedimentation rate for normal rat blood, characterized as being extremely slow, was reported by a number of authors: 0.7 mm/hr in males, and 1.8 mm/hr in females;[16] 1.0 to 2.5 mm/hr (mean, 1.5 mm/hr) in males;[24] and 0.68 to 1.76 mm/hr (mean, 1.22 ± 0.27 mm/hr) in males, and 0.58 to 1.62 mm/hr (mean, 1.10 ± 0.26 mm/hr) in females.[8]

REFERENCES

1. **Moore DM. Rats. In: Rollin BE, Kesel ML, eds.** The experimental animal in biomedical research. Boca Raton, FL: CRC Press, 1995;2.
2. **Archer RK, Riley J.** Standardized methods for bleeding rats. Lab Anim 1981;15:25–28.
3. **Conybeare G, Leslie GB, Angles K, Barrett RJ, Luke JSH, Gask DR.** An improved simple technique for the collection of blood samples from rats and mice. Lab Anim 1988;22:177–182.
4. **Andrews EJ, Bennett BT, Clark JD, Houpt KA, Pascoe PJ, Robinson GW, Boyce JR.** 1993 report of the AVMA panel on euthanasia. J Am Vet Med Assoc 1993;202:229–249.
5. **Harkness JE, Wagner JE.** The biology and medicine of rabbits and rodents. 4th ed. Baltimore: Williams & Wilkins, 1995.
6. **Ringler DH, Dabich L.** Hematology and clinical chemistry. In: Baker HJ, et al. The laboratory rat. New York: Academic Press, 1979;1.
7. **Argent NB, Liles J, Rodham D, Clayton CB, Wilkinson R, Baylis PH.** A new method for measuring blood volume of the rat using [113m]indium as a tracer. Lab Anim 1994;28:172–175.
8. **Mitruka BJ, Rawnsley HM.** Clinical biochemical and hematological reference values in normal experimental animals and normal humans. 2nd ed. New York: Masson, 1981.
9. **Scipioni RL, Diters RW, Myers WR, Hart SM.** Clinical and clinicopathological assessment of serial phlebotomy in the Sprague Dawley rat. Lab Anim Sci 1997;47:293–299.
10. **Johnson-Delaney CA.** Exotic companion medicine handbook. Lake Worth, FL: Wingers Publishing, 1996.
11. **Hillyer EV, Quesenberry KE.** Ferrets, rabbits, and rodents–clinical medicine and surgery. Philadelphia: WB Saunders, 1997.
12. **Archer RK.** Haematology of conventionally-maintained Lac:P outbred Wistar rats during the 1st year of life. Lab Anim 1982;16:198.
13. **Burns KF, Timmons EH, Poiley SM.** Serum chemistry and hematological values for axenic (germfree) and environmentally associated inbred rats. Lab Anim Sci 1971;21:415–419.
14. **Harris C, Burke WT.** The changing cellular distribution in bone marrow of the normal albino rat between one and fifty weeks of age. Am J Pathol 1957;33:931.
15. **Jain NC.** Schalm's veterinary hematology. 4th ed. Philadelphia:, Lea & Febiger, 1986.
16. **Schermer S.** The blood morphology of laboratory animals. Philadelphia: FA Davis, 1967.
17. **Godwin KO, et al.** Hematological observations on healthy (SPF) rats. Br J Exp Pathol 1964;45:514.
18. **Turton JA, Hawkey CM, Hart MG, Gwynne J, Hicks RM.** Age-related changes in the haematology of female F344 rats. Lab Anim 1989;23:295–301.
19. **Leonard R, Ruben Z.** Hematology reference values for peripheral blood of laboratory rats. Lab Anim Sci 1986;36:277–281.
20. **Dameron GW, Weingand KW, Duderstadt JM, Odioso LW, Dierckman TA, Schwecke W, Baran K.** Effect of bleeding site on clinical laboratory testing of rats: orbital venous plexus versus posterior vena cava. Lab Anim Sci 1992;42:299–301.
21. **Weisse VI, Knappen F, Frolke W, Guenard J, Kollmer H, Stotzer H.** Blutewerte der ratte in abhangigkeit van alter und geschlect. Arzneim Forsch 1974;24:1221–1225.
22. **Kuhn G, Hardegg W.** Quantitative studies of haematological values in long-term ovariectomized, ovariohysterectomized and hysterectomized rats. Lab Anim 1991;25:40–45.
23. **Hulse EV.** Quantitative cell counts of the bone marrow and blood and their secular variations in the normal adult rat. Acta Haematol 1964;31:50–63.
24. **Zingg W, Morgan CD, Anderson DE.** Blood viscosity, erythrocyte sedimentation rate, packed cell volume, osmolality, and plasma viscosity of the Wistar rat. Lab Anim Sci 1971;21:740–742.
25. **Charles River Laboratories.** Baseline hematology and clinical chemistry values for Charles River Fischer344 rats as a function of sex and age. Wilmington, MA: Charles River Labs, 1984.
26. **Lewis JH.** Comparative hemostasis in vertebrates. New York: Plenum Press, 1996.
27. **Hardy J.** Hematology of rats and mice. In: Cotchin E, Roe FJC, eds. Pathology of laboratory rats and mice. Philadelphia: Davis, 1967.
28. **Tschopp TB, Zucker MB.** Hereditary defect in platelet function in rats. Blood 1972;40:217–226.

CHAPTER 190

Hematology of the Mouse (*Mus musculus*)

• DAVID M. MOORE

BLOOD COLLECTION

Moore[1] listed several methods for blood collection in mice including orbital venous plexus collection (described in Chapter 189 "Hematology of the Rat"), cardiac blood collection, and tail vein collection. Additional blood collection methods include aseptically cutting/amputating approximately 2 mm of the tip of the tail, decapitation, or following anesthesia, incising the brachial vessels or collection from the posterior vena cava after opening the abdominal cavity. An alternate means of blood collection from the lateral tail vein of mice has been described.[2] It requires that the mouse's tail be placed in ~45°C water or the animal be placed in a commercially available forced air warming chamber at 40°C for 10 to 15 minutes to facilitate vasodilation. The mouse is placed in a rigid plastic restrainer, and then a 21-gauge butterfly catheter needle is used for venipuncture. Blood is collected as it drips from the catheter, which was previously trimmed to a length of ~3 mm.

Arterial blood collected from mice had both lower erythrocyte and leukocyte counts compared with values observed following blood collection from tail veins.[3] Blood obtained from the lateral tail vein of mice was found to have higher hemoglobin levels than samples obtained from the orbital venous plexus or posterior vena cava.[2] Blood collected from the orbital venous plexus of mice had slightly lower total erythrocyte counts compared with the posterior vena cava.[2]

The mean total blood volume in mice, using the ^{51}Cr method, was calculated to be 5.85 mL/100 g of body weight, and the mean plasma volume was found to be 3.15 mL/100 g.[4] Other dilution methods yielded a range of total blood volume values from 5 to 12 mL/100 g of body weight[5] and 7 to 8 mL/100 g of body weight.[6] Schermer[3] reported that the total blood volume in mice was 5.4 to 8.2% (average, 6.6%) of body weight.

MORPHOLOGY AND INDICES OF PERIPHERAL BLOOD CELLS

Reported hematologic values for laboratory mice (*Mus musculus*) are provided in Tables 190.1 through 190.4,

and reported values for other mouse species are provided in Table 190.5. Differences in hematologic values, in particular total leukocyte counts, may be noted between various inbred strains and outbred stocks of mice.[5]

Erythrocytes

The mouse erythrocyte is a biconcave disc, nonnucleated, with a mean cell diameter in adults of between 5 and 7 μm and a cell thickness of 2.1 to 2.13 μm.[3,5] Anisocytosis and pronounced polychromasia of mouse erythrocytes is common. Howell-Jolly bodies are frequently seen in mouse erythrocytes.[5] Reticulocytes may account for 1 to 6% of total counts.[7] Total erythrocyte counts in mice reported in the literature range from 6.14 to 11.5 × 10^6/mm^3.[3] Kunze[8] reported an increase in average erythrocyte counts for mice from birth to adulthood: 3.7 × 10^6/mm^3 at birth, 4 × 10^6/mm^3 at 4 days of age, 5.18 × 10^6/mm^3 after 10 days of age, 5.9 × 10^6/mm^3 after 14 days of age, and 9.34 × 10^6/mm^3 at 2 to 3 months of age. The average packed cell volume (PCV) in adult mice is usually between 35 and 44%. The average life span of mouse red blood cells was reported as being between 38 and 42 days,[9] 40 and 50 days,[5] and 40 and 47 days.[10]

Unlike humans, neonatal mice have slightly lower hemoglobin and hematocrit values than do adults, have larger erythrocyte diameters (approximately 10 to 11 μm),[3] a higher mean corpuscular volume (MCV), and greater morphologic variation and polychromasia. The MCV decreases rapidly within the first week of life, reaching adult size about the time of weaning (i.e., 21 days).[11] Hemoglobin levels fall during the first few days of life, before rebounding around 2 weeks of age and reaching adult levels soon after weaning.[12] Reticulocytes in circulation were observed to total 40% at birth in mice, 20% at 14 days of age, and 5% by 6 weeks of age.[3]

Thrombocytes

Mouse platelets are about 1 to 3 μm in diameter[13] and have a life span of approximately 4 to 5 days in the

TABLE 190.1 Referenced Erythrocyte Values in the Mouse (*Mus musculus*)—Gender and Strain/Stock Not Specified

Reference	RBC (×10⁶/mm³) Mean	RBC (×10⁶/mm³) Range	PCV (%) Mean	PCV (%) Range	Hb (g/dL) Mean	Hb (g/dL) Range	MCV (μ³) Mean	MCV (μ³) Range	MCH (μμg) Mean	MCH (μμg) Range	MCHC (%) Mean	MCHC (%) Range
3	9	6–12	—	—	—	—	—	—	—	—	—	—
27	8.6	—	45	—	14.2	—	51	—	17	—	33	—
28	7.85 ± 2.12	—	41.0 ± 2.13	—	11.9 ± 0.94	—	—	—	—	—	—	—
25	—	7–11	—	35.45–40.0	—	10–20	—	—	—	—	—	—
26	—	8.7–10.5	44	42–44	13.4	12.2–16.2	—	—	—	—	—	—
10	—	7.0–12.5	—	39–49	—	10.2–16.6	—	—	—	—	—	—
19	—	7.0–12.5	—	36–49	—	10.2–18	—	—	—	—	—	—
6	—	7.9–10.1	—	37–46	—	11.0–14.5	—	—	—	—	—	—

TABLE 190.2 Referenced Leukocyte Values in the Mouse (*Mus musculus*)—Gender and Strain/Stock Not Specified

Reference	WBC (×10³/mm³) Mean	WBC (×10³/mm³) Range	Neutrophils (%) Mean	Neutrophils (%) Range	Lymphocytes (%) Mean	Lymphocytes (%) Range	Eosinophils (%) Mean	Eosinophils (%) Range	Basophils (%) Mean	Basophils (%) Range	Monocytes (%) Mean	Monocytes (%) Range
3	10	7–15	—	10–60	—	35–90	—	0–7	—	0–1	—	0–3
27	9.2	—	20	—	80	—	0.9	—	0	—	0.2	—
25	—	4–12	—	5–40	—	30–90	—	0–5	—	0–1	—	0–10
26	8.4	5.1–11.6	17.9	6.7–37.2	69	63–75	2.1	0.9–3.8	0.5	0.0–1.5	1.2	0.7–2.6
10	—	6–15	—	10–40	—	55–95	—	0–4	—	0–0.3	—	0.1–3.5
19	—	6–15	—	10–40	—	55–95	—	0–4	—	0–0.3	—	0.1–3.5

TABLE 190.3   Referenced Erythrocyte Values in the Mouse (*Mus musculus*)—by Strain/Stock and Age

Reference	Strain/ Stock	Gender/ Age	RBC (×10⁶/mm³) Mean	RBC (×10⁶/mm³) Range	PCV (%) Mean	PCV (%) Range	Hb (g/dL) Mean	Hb (g/dL) Range	MCV (μ³) Mean	MCV (μ³) Range	MCH (μμg) Mean	MCH (μμg) Range	MCHC (%) Mean	MCHC (%) Range
16	ICR	M	9.3 ± 1.2	6.9–11.7	41.5 ± 4.2	33.1–49.9	11.3 ± 0.1	11.1–11.5	49.0 ± 0.75	47.5–50.5	12.2 ± 0.25	11.7–12.7	27.2 ± 2.0	23.2–31.2
16	ICR	F	9.1 ± 1.12	6.86–11.3	42.1 ± 1.2	39.7–44.5	10.9 ± 0.1	10.7–11.1	49.5 ± 1.25	47–52	11.98 ± 0.42	11.1–12.7	25.9 ± 1.8	22.3–29.5
18	ICR	M < 1 yr	9.11 ± 0.697	—	42.6 ± 3.22	—	15.4 ± 1.05	—	46.8 ± 1.82	—	17.0 ± 0.79	—	36.3 ± 1.26	—
	ICR	F < 1 yr	8.74 ± 0.689	—	41.0 ± 3.23	—	15.0 ± 0.9	—	46.9 ± 1.86	—	17.3 ± 0.9	—	36.7 ± 1.59	—
	ICR	M > 1 yr	8.27 ± 0.884	—	37.5 ± 4.14	—	13.5 ± 1.42	—	45.3 ± 2.72	—	16.5 ± 1.0	—	36.2 ± 0.71	—
	ICR	F > 1 yr	7.46 ± 0.927	—	34.5 ± 3.87	—	12.4 ± 1.36	—	46.3 ± 2.76	—	16.7 ± 1.11	—	36.0 ± 1.01	—
24	ICR	M/F	—	6.86–11.7	—	33.1–49.9	—	10.7–11.5	—	47–52	—	11.1–12.7	—	22.3–31.2
15	B6D2F1	NS	6.74 ± 0.47	—	42 ± 3	—	14.5 ± 0.8	—	—	—	—	—	—	—
29	CD-1®(ICR)	M (6–8 wk)	7.6	7.2–8.0	42	36–48	14.4	12.6–16.2		—		—	35	33–37
	CD-1®(ICR)	F (6–8 wk)	5.61	4.7–6.5	43	38–48	14.8	13.0–16.6		—		—	35	31–39
	CD-1®(ICR)	M (19–21 wk)	7.0	6.4–7.6	40	36–44	11.2	8.2–14.2		—		—	35	31–39
	CD-1®(ICR)	F (19–21 wk)	5.41	4.3–6.4	40	35–46	13.5	11.9–15.1		—		—	34	31–37
	CD-1®(ICR)	M (32–34 wk)	7.2	6.9–7.5	44	40–48	12.6	9.9–15.3		—		—	34	32–36
	CD-1®(ICR)	F (32–34 wk)	5.41	4.5–6.3	39	33–45	13.4	11.4–15.4		—		—	34	31–37
30	BALB/c	M (1–3 mo)	9.5 ± 0.8	—	45.2 ± 2.7	—	15.7 ± 1.2	—	48.1 ± 1.8	—	16.7 ± 1.2	—	35.0 ± 2.3	—
	BALB/c	F (1–3 mo)	9.5 ± 0.5	—	45.3 ± 2.1	—	15.9 ± 1.0	—	48.5 ± 1.0	—	17.2 ± 0.9	—	35.8 ± 1.6	—
	BALB/c	M (6–12 mo)	9.8 ± 0.9	—	44.0 ± 2.9	—	16.0 ± 1.1	—	44.4 ± 1.5	—	16.5 ± 1.0	—	36.7 ± 1.6	—
	BALB/c	F (6–12 mo)	9.7 ± 0.7	—	41.2 ± 2.9	—	15.3 ± 0.7	—	42.4 ± 1.0	—	16.1 ± 0.5	—	38.4 ± 2.2	—
	BALB/c	M (12–18 mo)	10.0 ± 0.8	—	44.2 ± 5.6	—	14.9 ± 1.0	—	44.4 ± 1.4	—	15.0 ± 1.1	—	35.3 ± 1.7	—
	BALB/c	F (12–18 mo)	9.3 ± 0.7	—	40.7 ± 7.0	—	14.3 ± 1.1	—	42.3 ± 1.9	—	15.1 ± 2.1	—	35.3 ± 4.2	—
	BALB/c	M (>18 mo)	9.1 ± 1.0	—	38.9 ± 3.9	—	14.7 ± 1.7	—	43.0 ± 2.1	—	16.5 ± 1.3	—	38.1 ± 2.7	—
	BALB/c	F (>18 mo)	9.3 ± 0.7	—	38.9 ± 6.4	—	14.9 ± 1.1	—	41.3 ± 1.4	—	16.2 ± 1.5	—	38.9 ± 3.2	—
31	BALB/c	F	7.11 ± 0.41	—	41.4 ± 1.77	—	14.8 ± 0.66	—		—		—		—
30	C57BL/6	M (1–3 mo)	9.1 ± 1.1	—	42.7 ± 2.6	—	14.7 ± 1.2	—	47.7 ± 1.1	—	16.5 ± 0.7	—	34.7 ± 1.6	—
	C57BL/6	F (1–3 mo)	9.1 ± 0.9	—	43.1 ± 3.5	—	14.7 ± 1.4	—	48.1 ± 1.2	—	16.5 ± 0.6	—	34.6 ± 1.3	—
	C57BL/6	M (6–12 mo)	9.6 ± 0.5	—	42.0 ± 2.3	—	14.8 ± 0.6	—	48.3 ± 1.3	—	15.7 ± 0.4	—	35.6 ± 0.7	—
	C57BL/6	F (6–12 mo)	9.2 ± 0.5	—	40.4 ± 2.2	—	14.5 ± 0.5	—	44.1 ± 1.0	—	16.1 ± 0.5	—	36.0 ± 1.1	—
	C57BL/6	M (12–18 mo)	8.9 ± 0.7	—	38.6 ± 4.1	—	13.7 ± 1.2	—	43.7 ± 1.4	—	15.7 ± 0.7	—	35.3 ± 1.5	—
	C57BL/6	F (12–18 mo)	8.8 ± 1.0	—	38.8 ± 3.7	—	13.8 ± 1.0	—	44.0 ± 1.5	—	15.8 ± 0.9	—	35.4 ± 2.0	—
	C57BL/6	M (>18 mo)	8.1 ± 0.6	—	34.1 ± 3.1	—	13.1 ± 1.1	—	42.6 ± 2.2	—	16.6 ± 0.8	—	38.7 ± 1.3	—
	C57BL/6	F(>18 mo)	8.5 ± 0.6	—	35.9 ± 6.0	—	13.2 ± 1.1	—	42.1 ± 1.5	—	15.9 ± 1.0	—	37.1 ± 2.7	—
32	C57BL/6J	M (8–10 mo)	—	—	51.7 ± 2.8	46–58	—	—	—	—	—	—	—	—
	C57BL/6J	M (25–28 mo)	—	—	45.3 ± 4.6	28–52	—	—	—	—	—	—	—	—
31	Swiss Webster	M	6.5 ± 0.7	—	38.05 ± 3.94	—	12.25 ± 1.14	—	58.5 ± 2.06	—	18.78 ± 0.28	—	32.17 ± 0.9	—
	Swiss Webster	F	6.29 ± 0.62	—	37.31 ± 2.84	—	12.44 ± 0.64	—	59.3 ± 1.98	—	20.16 ± 1.59	—	34.2 ± 2.27	—

NS, not specified.

TABLE 190.4 Referenced Leukocyte Values in the Mouse (*Mus musculus*)—by Strain/Stock and Age

Reference	Strain/Stock	Gender/Age	WBC (×10³/mm³) Mean	WBC (×10³/mm³) Range	Neutrophils (%) Mean	Neutrophils (%) Range	Lymphocytes (%) Mean	Lymphocytes (%) Range	Eosinophils (%) Mean	Eosinophils (%) Range	Basophils (%) Mean	Basophils (%) Range	Monocytes (%) Mean	Monocytes (%) Range
16	ICR	M	14.2 ± 0.87	12.5–15.9	17.4 – 2.1	13.2–21.6	72.6 ± 5.1	62.4–82.8	2.09 ± 0.36	1.37–2.81	0.52 ± 0.15	0.22–0.82	2.35 ± 0.06	2.22–2.47
	ICR	F	12.9 ± 0.42	12.1–13.7	17.1 ± 0.7	15.7–18.5	71.9 ± 2.98	65.9–77.9	2.41 ± 0.18	2.05–2.77	0.49 ± 0.18	0.13–0.85	2.04 ± 0.03	0.98–1.11
18	ICR	M <1 yr	8.0 ± 3.2	—	19 ± 8.9	—	77 ± 11	—	1.0 ± 1.0	—	0	—	2.0 ± 1.9	—
	ICR	F <1 yr	6.0 ± 2.53	—	16 ± 9.2	—	80 ± 9.6	—	1.0 ± 1.1	—	0 ± 0.1	—	2.0 ± 2.0	—
	ICR	M >1 yr	9.3 ± 4.97	—	32 ± 11.1	—	63 ± 13.8	—	0 ± 0.8	—	0	—	5 ± 4.2	—
	ICR	F >1 yr	6.7 ± 4.26	—	32 ± 12.4	—	62 ± 13.4	—	0 ± 0.5	—	0	—	4 ± 2.3	—
24	ICR	M/F	—	12.1–15.9	—	13.2–21.6	—	62.4–82.8	—	1.37–2.77	—	0.13–0.85	—	0.98–2.47
29	CD-1®(ICR)	M (6–8 wk)	9.0	8.9–9.1	25	10–40	70	52–86	1	0–2	0	0–2	4	0–8
	CD-1®(ICR)	F (6–8 wk)	3.0	1.0–5.0	27	11–43	68	50–86	4	0–8	0	0–2	2	0–5
	CD-1®(ICR)	M (19–21 wk)	12.0	9.7–14.3	25	8–40	72	52–92	1	0–3	0	0–2	4	0–8
	CD-1®(ICR)	F (19–21 wk)	9.6	5.2–14.0	19	10–28	75	63–87	2	0–4	0	0–2	4	0–8
	CD-1®(ICR)	M (32–34 wk)	12.9	5.5–20.3	27	10–45	70	50–85	1	0–3	0	0–2	2	0–6
	CD-1®(ICR)	F (32–34 wk)	8.7	4.1–13.3	29	15–43	66	49–84	2	0–4	0	0–2	3	0–6
30	BALB/c	M (1–3 mo)	3.2 ± 2.0	—	—	—	—	—	—	—	—	—	—	—
	BALB/c	F (1–3 mo)	3.5 ± 1.8	—	—	—	—	—	—	—	—	—	—	—
	BALB/c	M (6–12 mo)	2.9 ± 1.2	—	—	—	—	—	—	—	—	—	—	—
	BALB/c	F (6–12 mo)	2.3 ± 0.9	—	—	—	—	—	—	—	—	—	—	—
	BALB/c	M (12–18 mo)	2.7 ± 1.5	—	—	—	—	—	—	—	—	—	—	—
	BALB/c	F (12–18 mo)	2.6 ± 1.0	—	—	—	—	—	—	—	—	—	—	—
	BALB/c	M (>18 mo)	2.9 ± 1.6	—	—	—	—	—	—	—	—	—	—	—
	BALB/c	F (>18 mo)	2.9 ± 1.6	—	—	—	—	—	—	—	—	—	—	—
31	BALB/c	F	6.93 ± 0.92	—	15.4 ± 5.06	—	83.5 ± 4.95	—	0.3 ± 0.48	—	0	—	0.7 ± 0.48	—
30	C57BL/6	M (1–3 mo)	3.0 ± 1.0	—	—	—	—	—	—	—	—	—	—	—
	C57BL/6	F (1–3 mo)	3.7 ± 1.6	—	—	—	—	—	—	—	—	—	—	—
	C57BL/6	M (6–12 mo)	2.5 ± 0.7	—	—	—	—	—	—	—	—	—	—	—
	C57BL/6	F (6–12 mo)	3.0 ± 0.8	—	—	—	—	—	—	—	—	—	—	—
	C57BL/6	M (12–18 mo)	2.3 ± 1.1	—	—	—	—	—	—	—	—	—	—	—
	C57BL/6	F (12–18 mo)	2.8 ± 1.0	—	—	—	—	—	—	—	—	—	—	—
	C57BL/6	M (>18 mo)	2.5 ± 1.3	—	—	—	—	—	—	—	—	—	—	—
	C57BL/6	F (>18 mo)	3.1 ± 1.2	—	—	—	—	—	—	—	—	—	—	—
32	C57BL/6J	M (8–10 mo)	9.7 ± 3.3	4–18	10.5	2.5–27.8	78.7	—	1.34	—	—	—	5.9	—
	C57BL/6J	M (25–28 mo)	11.2 ± 4.3	4–28	17.2	12.5–46.4	67.9	—	2.5	—	—	—	8.7	—
31	Swiss Webster	M	3.0 ± 1.0	—	6.9 ± 3.04	—	91.3 ± 3.16	—	1.77 ± 0.34	—	0	—	3.78 ± 0.51	—
	Swiss Webster	F	3.26 ± 0.81	—	9.5 ± 3.17	—	89.3 ± 3.82	—	1.73 ± 0.22	—	0	—	3.22 ± 0.41	—

TABLE 190.5   Referenced Hematologic Values for Two Wild Mouse Species[16]

Parameter	Multimammate Mouse (*Mastomys natalenis*) Range	Deer Mouse (*Peromyscus maniculatus*) Range
Total erythrocytes ($\times 10^6$/mm^3)	7.05–8.73	10.2–12.0
PCV (mL%)	35.1–49.0	43.3–53.3
Hemoglobin (g/dL)	11.0–14.8	11.8–15.4
MCV (μ^3)	46.6–60.3	34.8–45.7
MCH ($\mu\mu$g)	15.3–20.2	11.4–12.8
MCHC (%)	31.3–35.3	29.1–32.1
Platelets ($\times 10^3$/mm^3)	208–446	190–340
Total leukocytes ($\times 10^3$/mm^3)	5.4–10.6	6.91–12.9
Neutrophils (%)	8–48	8.25–40.8
Lymphocytes (%)	57–93	62–90
Eosinophils (%)	0–0.5	0.1–0.93
Basophils (%)	0–0.5	0–0.5
Monocytes (%)	0–7	0.0–5.4

peripheral circulation.[14] Platelets have a bluish cytoplasm that contains violet inclusions. Observed ranges of numbers of circulating platelets in mice have been reported in several references: 100 to 400 $\times$ 10^3/mm^3 (mean, 200 $\times$ 10^3/mm^3);[3] 421 $\pm$ 179 $\times$ 10^3/mm^3;[15] 232 $\pm$ 80 $\times$ 10^3/mm^3 (range, 157 to 412 $\times$ 10^3/mm^3) in males, and 250 $\pm$ 77 $\times$ 10^3/mm^3 (range, 170 to 410 $\times$ 10^3/mm^3) in females;[16] 592 to 2897 $\times$ 10^3/mm^3;[17] 1199 $\pm$ 199.9 $\times$ 10^3/mm^3 in males younger than 1 year of age, and 1071 $\pm$ 178.4 $\times$ 10^3/mm^3 in females younger than 1 year of age;[18] 1300 $\pm$ 224.5 $\times$ 10^3/mm^3 in males older than 1 year of age, and 912 $\pm$ 182 $\times$ 10^3/mm^3 in females older than 1 year of age;[18] 160 to 410 $\times$ 10^3/mm^3;[19] 600 to 1200 $\times$ 10^3/mm^3;[6] and 800 to 1100 $\times$ 10^3/mm^3.[10] Platelet counts are low in newborn mice but reach adult levels soon after weaning.[12]

Leukocytes

A diurnal fluctuation in total leukocytes has been reported, and it has been recommended that serial samples taken over several days be collected at the same time of day throughout the study to minimize variability.[20]

White blood cell (WBC) counts are somewhat lower in neonatal mice, with levels declining during suckling period but increasing again around weaning, to reach adult levels by 6 to 7 weeks of age.[5] Reported total WBC counts were 4.5 $\times$ 10^3/mm^3 at birth, 7.8 $\times$ 10^3/mm^3 at 5 days of age, 8.7 $\times$ 10^3/mm^3 at 5 months of age, and greater than 9.0 $\times$ 10^3/mm^3 at 1 year of age.[16] Normal total leukocyte counts could range as high as 12 to 20 $\times$ 10^3/mm^3 after 1 year of age.[16]

The nucleus of the mouse neutrophil fills most of the cell and appears ring-shaped with numerous irregular indentations, broken-ring-shaped, or segmented/multilobulated with the segments connected by thin fibers. Alternating highly pyknotic and pale areas may be observed in the nucleus.[3] The sparse cytoplasm of neutrophils appears to be pale pink and contains small, discrete dust-like pink granules. Mouse neutrophils do not show alkaline phosphatase activity.[21] Neutrophils account for between 20 and 30% of the total leukocyte count. Neutrophil counts in male mice are usually higher than those observed in females.

Lymphocytes are the predominant type of WBCs, accounting for between 70 and 80% of the total leukocyte count in adults and more than 80% in young mice. Both large and small lymphocytes are observed, occurring in a ratio of 1:3 respectively.[3] Small lymphocytes are characterized by a round, slightly indented, highly pyknotic nucleus, surrounded by a very thin band of uniformly dark blue cytoplasm. Large lymphocytes have a larger, less pyknotic nucleus, with a broader and brighter band of cytoplasm[3]; some may have scattered azurophilic granules in the cytoplasm.[17]

Eosinophils may account for 0 to 7% of the total leukocyte count. The nucleus of the mouse eosinophil is typically annular, forming a U-shaped broad band or more commonly a ring-like shape, and is less pyknotic than the nucleus of the neutrophil.[3] The cytoplasm is basophilic and contains scanty, clumped acidophilic granules that seem almost to fuse and are thus blurred.

Monocytes, found at 0 to 2% of the total leukocyte count, are the largest of the WBCs of mice, with diameters up to 17 μm.[3] The nucleus of the mouse monocyte is slightly pyknotic, amoeboid, indented or lobulated/convoluted, and surrounded by a grey-blue, reticular or slightly granulated cytoplasm (azurophilic granules), which usually contains vacuoles.[3]

Circulating basophils are only rarely seen in mice, accounting for 0 to 1% of the total leukocyte count. Large deep purple cytoplasmic granules often obscure the nucleus of the basophil. As is the case in rats, basophils can be seen following collection of blood from the tails of mice and may, in fact, be tissue basophils that enter the sample when the tail is compressed/"milked" to facilitate collection of blood.[3]

TABLE 190.6 Observed Coagulation Values in Mice

Parameter	Mean ± SD	Reference
Bleeding time (sec)	50–60	3
Clotting time (sec)	120–180	3
	120–600	5
	120–600	26
Prothrombin time (sec)	7–19	5
	7–19	26
	13 ± 1 (11.5–16.5)	33
Partial thromboplastin time (sec)	55–110	5
	55–110	26
	25.2 ± 3.4 (18.5–33.4)	33

BONE MARROW CYTOLOGY

The bone marrow in the femur and vertebral column occupies between 90 and 96% of the available medullary space.[22] The cells of the bone marrow of the mouse resemble those found in the rat, although annular nuclei are more prominently observed in mice. The granulocyte is the most prevalent medullary cell. The myeloid:erythroid (M:E) ratio in mouse bone marrow was found to range from 0.8 to 2.4:1.0 (mean, 1.49 ± 0.47:1.0).[23]

OTHER HEMATOLOGIC VALUES

Reported coagulation values for mice are provided in Table 190.6. The sedimentation rate for normal mouse blood was reported by a number of authors: 0.0 to 0.91 mm/hr;[24] 0.45 ± 0.23 mm/hr (range, 0.0 to 0.91 mm/hr) in males, and 0.43 ± 0.22 mm/hr (range, 0.0 to 0.87 mm/hr) in females;[16] and 1 to 2 mm/hr.[25]

REFERENCES

1. **Moore DM.** Mice. In: Rollin BE, ed. The experimental animal in biomedical research Boca Raton, FL: CRC Press, 1995;2.
2. **Conybeare G, Leslie GB, Angles K, Barrett RJ, Luke JSH, Gask DR.** An improved simple technique for the collection of blood samples from rats and mice. Lab Anim 1988;22:177–182.
3. **Schermer S.** The blood morphology of laboratory animals. Philadelphia: FA Davis, 1967.
4. **Pinkerton PH, Bannerman RM, Doeblin TD, Benisch BM, Edwards JA.** Iron metabolism and absorption studies in the X-linked anaemia of mice. Br J Hematol 1970;18:211–228.
5. **Bannerman RM.** Hematology. In: Foster HL, et al., eds. The mouse in biomedical research. Normative biology, immunology, and husbandry. New York: Academic Press, 1983;3.
6. **Hillyer EV, Quesenberry KE.** Ferrets, rabbits, and rodents—clinical medicine and surgery. Philadelphia: WB Saunders, 1997.
7. **Brodsky I, Dennis LH, Kahn SB, Brady LW.** Normal mouse erythropoiesis. I. The role of the spleen in mouse erythropoiesis. Cancer Res 1966;26:198–201.
8. **Kunze H.** Die erythropoese bei einer erblicken anamie rontgenmutierti mause. Folia Hematol 1954;72:392.
9. **Horky J, Vacha J, Znajil V.** Comparison of lifespan of erythrocytes in some inbred strains of mouse using ^{14}C-labelled glycine. Physiol Bohemoslov 1978;27:209–217.
10. **Harkness JE, Wagner JE.** The biology and medicine of rabbits and rodents. 4th ed. Baltimore: Williams & Wilkins, 1995.
11. **Grewal MS.** A sex-linked anemia in the mouse. Genet Res 1962;3:238–247.
12. **Rugh R, Somogyi C.** Pre- and postnatal normal mouse blood cell counts. Proc Soc Exp Biol Med 1968;127:1267–1271.
13. **Zucker-Franklin D.** The ultrastructure of megakaryocytes and platelets. In: Gordon AS, ed. Regulation of hematopoiesis. New York: Appleton, 1970;2.
14. **Odell TT, McDonald TP.** Peripheral counts and survival of blood platelets in mice. Fed Proc Fed Am Soc Exp Biol 1960;19:63.
15. **Harrison SD, Burdeshaw JA, Crosby RG, Cusic AM, Devine P.** Hematology and clinical chemistry reference values. Cancer Res 1978;38:2636–2639.
16. **Mitruka BJ, Rawnsley HM.** Clinical biochemical and hematological reference values in normal experimental animals and normal humans. 2nd ed. New York: Masson, 1981.
17. **Jain NC.** Schalm's veterinary hematology. 4th ed. Philadelphia: Lea & Febiger, 1986.
18. **Wolford ST, Schroer RA, Gohs FX, Gallo PP, Brodeck M, Falk HB, Ruhren R.** Reference range data base for serum chemistry and hematology values in laboratory animals. J Toxicol Environ Health 1986;18:161–188.
19. **Johnson-Delaney CA.** Exotic companion medicine handbook. Lake Worth, FL: Wingers Publishing, 1996.
20. **Plata EJ, Murphy WH.** Growth and hematologic properties of the BALB/wm strain of inbred mice. Lab Anim Sci 1972;22:712–720.
21. **Eng LL.** Alkaline phosphatase activity of the leukocytes in animals. Nature 1964;204:191–192.
22. **Endicott KM, Gump H.** Hemograms and myelograms of healthy female mice of the C57 brown and CFW strains. Blood 1950;1:60.
23. **Quittner H, et al.** The effect of massive doses of cortisone on the peripheral blood and bone marrow of the mouse. Blood 1951;6:345.
24. **Mitruka BJ, Rawnsley HM.** Clinical biochemical and hematological reference values in normal experimental animals and normal humans. 1st ed. New York: Masson, 1977.
25. **Wallach JD, Boever WJ.** Diseases of exotic animals—medical and surgical management. Philadelphia: WB Saunders, 1983.
26. **Jacoby RO, Fox JG.** Biology and diseases of mice. In: Fox JG, et al., eds. Laboratory animal medicine. Orlando: Academic Press, 1984.
27. **Melby EC Jr, Altman NH.** Handbook of laboratory animal science. Cleveland: CRC Press, 1976.
28. **Loeb WF, Harrison SD, Burdeshaw JA, Crosby RG, Cusic AM, Devine P.** Hematologic disorders. In: Benirschke KE, et al. Pathology of laboratory animals. New York: Springer-Verlag, 1978;1.
29. **Charles River Laboratories.** Baseline hematology and clinical chemistry values as a function of sex and age for Charles River outbred mice: Crl: CD-1® (ICR)BR. Wilmington, MA: Charles River Labs, 1999.
30. **Frith CH, Suber RL, Umholtz R.** Hematologic and clinical chemistry findings in control BALB/c and C57BL/6 mice. Lab Anim Sci 1980;30:835–840.
31. **Taconic Farms, Inc.** Hematology values for several strains/stocks of mice. Germantown, NY: Taconic Farms, 1999.
32. **Finch CE, Foster JR.** Hematologic and serum electrolyte values of the C57BL/6J male mouse in maturity and senescence. Lab Anim Sci 1973;23:339–349.
33. **Abildgaard CF, Lewis JP, Harrison J.** Quantitative coagulation studies in mice. Lab Anim Sci 1972;22:99–101.

SECTION XV
Case Studies
Joseph G. Zinkl

Case Studies

The purpose of this section is to demonstrate basic principles in the responses of the different domestic animals to disease as revealed in blood and bone marrow. The brief histories and summaries of clinical findings, complete hemograms, and suggestions for interpretation provide a means whereby typical situations can be discussed in greater depth than wass possible in the general text.

For the most part, the title for each case suggests the principal feature to be demonstrated.

A LISTING OF CASES BY ANIMAL SPECIES

CASE 1 (DOG). METHEMOGLOBIN REDUCTASE DEFICIENCY

Animal	Hematocrit	Methemoglobin (%)	MR (IU/g Hb)
Affected female	57.6	21.6	5.5
Offspring	48.1	0	8.8
Sire of offspring	53.9	0.4	12.1
Control dog	46.7	0.8	11.1
Reference range	37–54	0–1.1	8.3–13.9

MR, methemoglobin reductase; *IU*, international units; *Hb*, hemoglobin.

Case 1 (Dog). Methemoglobin Reductase Deficiency

JOHN W. HARVEY

A 3.5-year-old female Pomeranian dog was presented to a private veterinary hospital for ovariohysterectomy. Her hematocrit was 53% and total plasma protein was 6.6 g/dL. During the operation, the blood in the surgical site appeared dark and brownish. The animal was placed on 100% oxygen, but the blood remained dark, suggesting the presence of methemoglobinemia. The mucous membranes appeared "muddy" and the tongue appeared "cyanotic" the next morning. The methemoglobin content was 31.3% and the dog was treated with N-acetyl cysteine for a possible toxic methemoglobinemia. The appearance of tongue and mucous membranes did not improve. With the exception of cyanotic-appearing tongue and mucous membranes, the animal appeared normal when examined for suture removal 10 days later. The methemoglobin content was 31.5% at that time. Blood samples from the affected female dog, a male offspring, the sire of the male offspring, and a control Labrador Retriever were submitted to the University of Florida for methemoglobin reductase enzyme assays 1.5 weeks later. The results are given above.

Interpretation

The methemoglobinemia was present before elective surgery but was not appreciated until dark-brownish blood was seen in the surgical site. As expected for methemoglobinemia, the discoloration remained even though the arterial pO_2 was undoubtably high following oxygen therapy. The lack of clinical signs, persistence of methemoglobinemia, and slight erythrocytosis were more consistent with an inherited methemoglobinemia than a toxic methemoglobinemia. The hematocrit may be slightly increased in dogs with methemoglobin reductase deficiency, because of increased erythropoietin production in response to the decreased oxygen content in blood. In contrast, the hematocrit is usually decreased with toxic methemoglobinemia, because of concomitant Heinz body hemolytic anemia. From enzyme assay results, it is clear that the affected dog had methemoglobinemia due to a deficiency in the erythrocyte methemoglobin reductase enzyme. Neither of the other Pomeranians had methemoglobinemia. The enzyme activity in erythrocytes from the male offspring of the affected female was midway between values from his parents, and at the low end of the reference range. This may indicate that the male offspring is an obligate carrier for this defect, but enzyme activity assays may not unambiguously identify carriers.

CASE 2 (DOG). RELAPSING AUTOIMMUNE HEMOLYTIC ANEMIA

	Day 1	Day 10	Day 13	1 mo.	5 mos.	6 mos.
Erythrocytes						
PCV (%)	11.1	15.6	17.8	40.9	11.3	35.6
RBC ($\times 10^6/\mu$L)	1.66	2.08	2.16	5.44	1.45	4.76
Hemoglobin	4.0	5.1	6.1	14.1	3.9	13.7
MCV (fL)	66.9	74.9	82.2	75.2	77.9	74.8
MCHC (%)	36.0	32.7	34.3	34.5	34.5	38.5
Reticulocytes (%)	1	4.6	21.8	1.2	35.2	5.6
Nucleated RBC (%)	0	0	5	0	14	0
Anisocytosis	+++	+++	+++	−	+	+
Polychromasia	+	++	++	−	+++	++
Spherocytes	+	+	+	−	+	+
Autoagglutination	+	−	−	−	−	−

(Continued)

CASE 2 (DOG). RELAPSING AUTOIMMUNE HEMOLYTIC ANEMIA *(continued)*

	Day 1	Day 10	Day 13	1 mo.	5 mos.	6 mos.
Leukocytes						
WBC/μL	13,000	18,200	35,100	6,400	57,500	5,800
Metamyelocytes (/μL)	780	182	351	0	2300	0
Neutrophils (/μL)	10,790	14,014	31,239	4224	48,875	4466
Lymphocytes (/μL)	650	910	702	640	1725	812
Monocytes (/μL)	390	2730	2808	704	3458	290
Eosinophils (/μL)	390	364		768	1150	232
Basophils (/μL)	0	0	0	0	0	0
Platelets/μL	350,000	347,000	206,000	464,000	43,000	21,000
Immunologic tests						
Direct antiglobulin test	IgG, C3	IgG	–	–	IgG	–
Direct enzyme-linked antiglobulin test	IgG, IgM, IgA, C3	IgG, IgM, C3	IgM, C3	–	IgG, IgM	IgG

−, not observed; +, occasional; ++, moderate; +++, many.

Case 2 (Dog). Relapsing Autoimmune Hemolytic Anemia

ROBERT N. BARKER

A 3-year-old, female Afghan Hound was referred with a history of pyrexia and severe lethargy over the previous week. The dog was vomiting occasionally, and the referring veterinarian had reported anemia with autoagglutination of the red blood cells (RBCs). There was no history or evidence of blood loss. Following hospitalization, the dog was given 30 mg/day (2 mg/kg) oral prednisolone, and 10 days later a concurrent course of cyclophosphamide was started at 30 mg (2 mg/kg or approximately 50 mg/M²) every other day. Within 1 month, the dog was discharged on a reducing dose of prednisolone. However, there was a relapse 5 months later, and the dog was readmitted with depression and petechial hemorrhages on the gingival and vulval mucous membranes. On this occasion, the response to prednisolone and cyclophosphamide was poor and it was necessary to give a blood transfusion 15 days later. The condition undulated over the next few months, and the dog was euthanized at the owner's request 11 months after it was first presented.

Interpretation

1. At hospitalization the dog was diagnosed as having autoimmune hemolytic anemia (AIHA). This case is one of the significant minority of dogs with AIHA in which there is initially poor erythroid regeneration, with no increase in reticulocytes or mean corpuscular volume (MCV). The lack of re-

sponse can often be attributed to the physiologic lag of 4 to 5 days before erythroid production can increase after acute hemolysis. However, in this case hemograms did not reveal marked reticulocytosis for nearly 2 weeks, suggesting that erythropoiesis may have been suppressed by the anti-RBC autoantibodies. The neutrophilia and monocytosis that accompanied the eventual erythroid regeneration are features of a stress response.

2. If canine AIHA does not respond to high doses of glucocorticoids, the cytotoxic drugs cyclophosphamide or azathioprine are indicated. In this case, there was a good response to the introduction of cyclophosphamide treatment during the first period of hospitalization.

3. AIHA developed again some 5 months after initial resolution of the disease. Because such relapses occur occasionally, the long-term prognosis for AIHA is guarded even when the response to treatment appears to be favorable. The relapse was also associated with thrombocytopenia, perhaps due to the development of concurrent antiplatelet autoantibodies or to platelet consumption. Other autoimmune phenomena are often seen in AIHA, and the case demonstrates that these associations may be due to diversification of autoantibody specificity over time.

4. Transfusion should be reserved for cases with life-threatening anemia because it can suppress the erythroid response or provoke a hemolytic crisis. The AIHA failed to respond to medical treatment after the relapse and, with the PCV falling below 11%, a transfusion was necessary to stabilize the dog. Unless comparable blood is used, repeated

(Continued)

administration of blood may provoke a transfusion reaction.

5. This case illustrates the limitations of the direct antiglobulin test (DAT). The DAT was negative on two occasions when a more sensitive assay (the direct enzyme-linked antiglobulin test) revealed antibody on the RBC surface. The DAT was also unable to detect sensitization with multiple immunoproteins in the first sample. Although the DAT is the standard method for detecting RBC-bound immunoproteins in AIHA, the test can often give false-negative results due to its insensitivity.

CASE 3 (DOG). IRON DEFICIENCY ANEMIA

Parameter	October 4	May 23	Reference Range
Erythrocytes			
RBC count ($10^6/\mu$L)	15.2	6.55	5.5–8.5
Hemoglobin (g/dL)	1.8	12.6	12.0–18.0
Hematocrit (%)	7	36	37–54
MCV (fL)	46	55	62–74
MCHC (%)	26	35	32–36
MCH (pg)	12	19	22–27
Reticulocytes ($\times 10^3/\mu$L)	52	40	<80
Hypochromasia	4+	Slight	None
Poikilocytosis	2+	Slight	None
Leukocytes			
Leukocytes ($\times 10^3/\mu$L)	15.2	7.6	6.0–17.0
Band neutrophils	0	0.1	0–0.3
Neutrophils	14.0	5.2	3.0–11.5
Lymphocytes	0.3	1.1	1.0–4.8
Monocytes	0.9	1.0	0.1–1.3
Eosinophils	0	0.2	0.1–1.2
Basophils	0	0	<0.1
Other tests			
Plasma proteins (g/dL)	5.2	6.7	6.0–7.8
Fibrinogen (mg/dL)	100	100	100–400
Icterus index (units)	<5	<5	<5
Platelets ($\times 10^3/\mu$L)	342	250	160–430
Iron (mg/dL)	17	—	84–233
TIBC (mg/dL)	357	—	284–572
Saturation (%)	4.8	—	19.6–59.3

Case 3 (Dog). Iron Deficiency Anemia Secondary to Chronic Hemorrhage

JOHN W. HARVEY

A 7-year-old, female golden retriever dog presented with a history of episodes of vomiting with anorexia and weight loss for several months. The dog was examined 5 weeks earlier for anorexia and depression. The hematocrit at that time was 21%. Diarrhea with stools that were sometimes dark began 2 weeks previously. The dog was treated with intravenous fluids and glucocorticoids on the day of referral. On examination at the veterinary medical teaching hospital, the dog was depressed, weak, and ataxic. She exhibited a rapid respiratory rate and a rapid heart rate with soft murmur. Her mucous membranes were pale.

A fecal flotation revealed a few *Trichuris* ova, and a fecal sample was strongly positive for occult blood. Results of the urinalysis were normal. Bone marrow smears were cellular, with a myeloid:erythroid (M:E) ratio of 1.6. No stainable iron was observed. A gastrointestinal barium series revealed an intestinal mass. Two blood transfusions were given, and oral iron therapy was initiated. The mass was surgically

(Continued)

excised, and an intestinal anastomosis was performed. The surgical pathology diagnosis was a jejunal adenocarcinoma.

Eight months later the dog was presented with a history of emesis and abdominal distention of 3 weeks duration. An exploratory laparotomy revealed a non-resectable regrowth of the adenocarcinoma.

Interpretation

1. The presence of a severe microcytic hypochromic anemia indicates the presence of chronic iron deficiency. The low serum iron, normal serum TIBC, low iron saturation, and lack of stainable iron in the bone marrow support the diagnosis of iron deficiency.
2. Iron deficiency is almost always the result of blood loss in adult animals. The low hematocrit and low plasma protein concentration are consistent with blood loss, most likely from the gastrointestinal tract, as indicated by the history of dark stools and the positive fecal occult blood test.
3. The absolute reticulocyte count is not increased, indicating that decreased iron availability is limiting the bone marrow response to the anemia.
4. A majority of dogs with iron deficiency anemia have thrombocytosis, but the platelet count is normal in this animal.
5. The neutrophilia, lymphocytopenia, and eosinopenia are likely the result of glucocorticoid treatment before referral.
6. Eight months is sufficient time for the microcytic anemia to resolve with appropriate iron therapy. Consequently, the presence of a slight microcytic anemia when examined during the second hospitalization indicates that either iron therapy was not continued long enough to replenish iron stores or additional hemorrhage is occurring with recurrence of the tumor.

CASE 4 (CAT). PRIMARY ERYTHROCYTOSIS

	June 20	June 21	June 24	Reference Range	Other Data
PCV %	71	61	65	30–45	*Arterial blood gas analysis:* pO$_2$ 85
Hb g/dL	23.1	21.3	20.8	8.0–15.0	mm Hg, O$_2$ saturation 97%
RBC × 10^6/µL	18.8	16.5	16.2	5–10	
MCV fL	43	41	40	39–55	*Bone marrow aspirate:* sample was
MCHC g/dL	32.0	35.0	32.0	30.0–36.0	hypercellular. Mature and imma-
MCH pg	19	17	14	13–17	ture megakaryocytes were promi-
Reticulocytes/µL	—	—	65,000		nent. Myeloid and erythroid
Platelets	Adequate	Clumped	Clumped	—	lines showed normal maturation,
WBC/µL	23,000	19,000	16,700	5500–19,500	no atypical cells, and M:E ratio
Neutrophils/µL	21,800	17,600	13,600	2500–12,500	of 1:1.
Lymphocytes/µL	500	400	1,300	1500–7000	
Monocytes/µL	700	400	1,000	0–800	
Eosinophils/µL	0	600	800	0–800	
TPP g/dL	7.7	6.8	7.5	6.0–8.0	

Case 4 (Cat). Erythrocytosis (Polycythemia)

A.D.J. WATSON

A 12-year-old male domestic shorthair cat had been polyuric/polydipsic, lethargic, and losing weight for 7 months. Two episodes of ataxia, dilated pupils, panting, tachypnea, and foaming at the mouth had been observed. A high packed cell volume (PCV) had been present for at least 1 month. When referred for investigation, the cat was lethargic and dehydrated and its mucous membranes were dark red. Along with erythrocytosis, mild azotemia, hyperalbuminemia, and inappropriately dilute urine (specific gravity 1.022) were found. Azotemia corrected with intravenous fluid therapy but erythrocytosis persisted.

Thoracic radiographs disclosed no evidence of cardiopulmonary disease, and arterial blood gas analyses excluded hypoxemia. Abdominal ultrasonic examination ruled out renal mass lesions and nonre-

(Continued)

nal tumors but showed diffuse hyperechogenicity in both renal cortices. Renal biopsy findings indicated glomerulonephritis and pyelonephritis; *Escherichia coli* was isolated from urine.

The presumptive diagnosis was primary erythrocytosis and unrelated bacterial pyelonephritis. A serum sample was submitted for erythropoietin assay. Treatment commenced with sulfadiazine-trimethoprim for pyelonephritis, phlebotomy (200 mL removed in 4 aliquots reduced PCV to 45% in 6 days), and hydroxyurea 100 mg orally twice daily.

While under treatment the cat experienced two episodes of leukopenia and/or anemia which necessitated discontinuation of hydroxyurea. Eventually a maintenance dose of 100 mg thrice weekly was found to maintain PCV at 40 to 55% without adverse effects.

Interpretation

1. Marked erythrocytosis was evident in the initial hemogram and persisted despite intravenous fluid therapy. Leukocyte changes in the first few days were indicative of response to stress.
2. Bone marrow cytology suggested increased activity of all cell lines, although this was not reflected by peripheral blood cell counts. Erythroid hyperplasia has been the main marrow finding in some cases of primary erthrocytosis. In general, bone marrow cytology may not be of great diagnostic use in such cases, neither to confirm erythrocytosis nor to identify possible causes.
3. The absence of hypoxemia indicated that cardiac and/or pulmonary disease could be excluded as causes. Normal thoracic radiographs supported this conclusion.
4. Inappropriate secondary erythrocytosis (ISE) was considered unlikely as physical and ultrasonic examinations excluded renal mass lesions and tumors elsewhere. Some nephropathies have the potential to cause ISE, but this is very rare. Pyelonephritis was believed to be coincidental in this case. The presumptive diagnosis of primary erythrocytosis was supported by a finding of low serum erythropoietin concentration (<9 U/L; reference range, 10–30).
5. Initial phlebotomy and drug therapy may have been unnecessarily vigorous in this cat. An alternative would have been to forgo phlebotomy and begin hydroxyurea at 500 mg orally every 7 days, maintaining or lengthening the interval subsequently as needed to keep PCV at 40 to 45%. Potential complications with hydroxyurea are neutropenia, hypoplastic anemia, hemolytic anemia, and methemoglobinemia, but successful long-term management is feasible with appropriate hematologic monitoring.

CASE 5 (DOG). INTERNAL HEMORRHAGE IN A DOG WITH HEMANGIOSARCOMA

	Dec. 28		Dec. 29		Dec. 30		Reference Range	Units
RBC	4.10		3.55		2.90		5.50–8.63	$\times 10^6/\mu L$
HGB	11.6		9.27		8.51		13.0–20.5	gm/dL
HCT	31.6		27.6		25.2		37.3–62.0	%
MCV	77		81		86		58–83	fL
MCH	26.3		22.2		22.1		22.2–26.2	pg
MCHC	36.7		31.5		29.4		31.6–36.5	%
Reticulocyte	1.0		1.5		3.0		0.0–1.0	%
Total reticulocytes	41,000		53,250		87,000		40,000–80,000	/μL
Nucleated RBC	2		4		2			/100 WBC
Anisocytosis					Modest			
Polychromasia					Modest			
Hypochromasia								
Poikilocytosis								
WBC		18,000		19,200		18,500	5400–16,600	/μL
Myelocytes	0%	0	0%	0	1%	185		/μL
Band neutrophils	0%	0	1%	192	2%	370	0–200	/μL
Segmented	88%	15,840	87%	16,704	59%	10,915	32,000–10,700	/μL
Lymphocytes	3%	540	4%	768	32%	5920	800–5600	/μL
Monocytes	9%	1620	8%	1536	4%	740	0–1100	/μL
Eosinophils	0%	0	0%	0	2%	370	0–2400	/μL
Platelets	230		190		165		179–473	$10^3/\mu L$
Plasma protein	6.1		5.8		5.9		6.0–7.5	g/dL

Case 5 (Dog). Internal Hemorrhage in a Dog With Hemangiosarcoma

DONALD PRATER AND JOHN L. ROBERTSON

A 9-year-old, spayed, female Vizsla was presented because of acute collapse, inability to rise, and labored breathing. A physical examination revealed hyperpnea, cyanosis, cold extremities, and a palpable abdominal mass. Peripheral pulses were weak, and the heart rate was 140/min. The dog was clinically stable for approximately 48 hours, then experienced acute cardiovascular failure.

Serial hemograms show initial normocytic, normochromic anemia and leukocytosis characterized by neutrophilia, lymphopenia, and monocytosis (stress leukogram). Frequently, in dogs with hemangiosarcoma there is intermittent bleeding into the abdominal or thoracic cavity associated with rupture of primary or metastatic tumor nodules. Blood components (erythrocytes, leukocytes, plasma) are lost in approximately equal proportions, with subsequent absorption back into peripheral circulation. As a consequence, the hematocrit and plasma protein remain nearly normal. Transient anemia or hypoproteinemia may be observed shortly after an episode of internal hemorrhage. Plasma proteins are absorbed rapidly; however, during the absorption process, the cell membrane of erythrocytes is often altered, making them more susceptible to phagocytosis by splenic macrophages. Additionally, erythrocyte damage can occur as a result of increased turbulence during blood flow through neoplastic channels, contributing to accelerated phagocytic removal.

The second hemogram continues to reflect normocytic, normochromic anemia and a stress leukogram.

The third hemogram displays slightly macrocytic, normochromic anemia as there is an increased reticulocyte response (corrected reticulocytosis, 1.6%) with a noticeable anisocytosis and polychromasia. Nucleated red blood cells are metarubricytes in this case. Dogs with hemangiosarcoma may have none or a variable number of incidents of compensated internal hemorrhage, with some animals having a terminal bleeding event, as in this case. Significant loss of blood from a ruptured primary or metastatic nodule into the abdomen or thorax results in hypovolemia and rapid, fatal cardiovascular decompensation.

Necropsy findings were hemoperitoneum, multiple splenic nodules, and numerous dark red, peritoneal masses including a large, multiloculated nodule in the pelvic region which had ruptured and was covered with loosely adherent strands of clotted blood. Histologically, the splenic nodules and peritoneal masses were composed of multiple blood-filled channels lined by atypical endothelial cells and locally extensive areas of necrotic tissue. The endothelial cells had large, angular, and hyperchromatic to open vesicular nuclei with mitoses observed at a frequency of 0 to 1 per high-power field. These cells were seen exfoliating singly from the capsular surface. No evidence of pulmonary or hepatic metastasis was observed.

Hemangiosarcoma is a tumor of blood vessels most commonly seen in the dog. Typical visceral sites are spleen, right atrium, and liver. This is a highly malignant and metastatic neoplasm commonly metastasizing to lung, liver and omentum. Disseminated abdominal metastases are observed in this case. Dogs with this neoplasm have a poor prognosis with mean survival time of approximately 4 months following diagnosis.

CASE 6 (DOG). PERIOPERATIVE TREATMENT AND RESPONSE

	vWF:Ag	BMBT
Pretreatment	5%	>15 minutes
Post cryo 1 (4 U[a])	35%	4.7 minutes
Post DDAVP	35%	3.8 minutes
Pre cryo 2	22%	Not determined
Post cryo 2 (2.5 U[a])	40%	Not determined
24-hr post cryo 2	14%	Not determined

[a]One unit cryo prepared from 200 mL of fresh frozen plasma.

Case 6 (Dog). Perioperative Management of von Willebrand Disease

MARJORY BROOKS

A 7-month-old, 34.5-kg, male, Doberman pinscher with von Willebrand disease (vWD) was scheduled for elective castration. The dog was first examined at 3 months of age because of prolonged bleeding from the gingiva as deciduous teeth were shed. At that time, platelet count and coagulation panel (aPTT, PT, fibrinogen) were within reference ranges; however, plasma von Willebrand factor (vWF) concentration was low (vWF:Ag, 5%; reference range, 70 to 180%) and buccal mucosa bleeding time (BMBT) was prolonged (>12 minutes; reference range, 2 to 4 minutes). Gingival hemorrhage was controlled with application of topical tissue adhesive, after the dog was sedated. Over the course of the next 3 months, repeated episodes of gingival hemorrhage and prolonged bleeding from a minor cutaneous laceration were treated with topical wound care.

To prevent hemorrhagic complications from the

(Continued)

castration surgery, the dog was transfused preoperatively and 6 hours postoperatively with cryoprecipitate. Desmopressin (DDAVP; 1 ug/kg SQ) was given 30 minutes preoperatively as an adjunct to transfusion. Plasma vWF:Ag and BMBT were measured to monitor response to transfusion and hormone therapy. No signs of abnormal bleeding were noted intraoperatively or postoperatively, and the hematocrit was stable (Hct, 47% preoperatively and 45% postoperatively). The dog was released to the owner's care 24 hours after surgery.

He was reevaluated approximately 24 hours later because of bleeding from the cutaneous incision. The dog was transfused with cryoprecipitate (2.5 U) and confined with cage rest for 24 hours. After this treatment, he was released to the owner's care and healed uneventfully.

Interpretation

1. On the basis of abnormal gingival mucosal bleeding, low plasma vWF concentration, and long BMBT, a diagnosis of vWD was made. Although there is a high breed prevalance of vWD in Doberman pinschers, evaluation of platelet count and coagulation panel were appropriate to rule out acquired hemostatic defects.
2. This dog's repeated episodes of abnormal bleeding in response to tooth eruption and minor trauma indicated that he was at risk for hemorrhage at

surgery. Perioperative transfusion will prevent this complication, which the owner requested. Cryoprecipitate is the best transfusion product for replacement of vWF. It is used without risk of red cell sensitization or volume overload. Fresh frozen plasma is an alternate component if cryoprecipitate is not available.
3. An initial high dose of cryoprecipitate was given to attain maximal levels of plasma vWF at the time of surgery. A lower dose was given postoperatively to sustain vWF levels during the initial wound healing period.
4. Desmopressin administration did not increase plasma vWF concentration in this dog; however, bleeding time was slightly shortened. This type of response has been described in type 1 vWD-affected Doberman pinschers. Dogs having mild clinical expression of type 1 vWD may be treated preoperatively with desmopressin, with transfusion given only if signs of abnormal bleeding are noted. Although there are no reports of adverse effects of desmopressin, more rigorous evaluation of its efficacy are needed.
5. Delayed bleeding might have been prevented by prescribing a longer period of cage confinement or by administering a third dose of cryoprecipitate at 24 hours postoperatively. Medical management (confinement, suture, tissue adhesive) may have controlled the rebleed. Cryoprecipitate, however, was highly effective.

CASE 7 (CAT). MYELODYSPLASTIC SYNDROME (MDS-EXCESS BLASTS)

	Admission Hemogram	Reference Limits	Bone Marrow Evaluation	% ANC[a]
HCT (%)	5	25–45		
Hemoglobin (g/dL)	1.6	8.4–15.0	Erythroid cells	14
RBC ($10^6/\mu$L)	0.9	5.5–10.3	Myeloblasts	10
MCV (fL)	57	41–51	Differentiating neutrophils	69
MCH (pg)	18	13–18	Eosinophils	7
MCHC (g/dL)	32	32–36	M:E = 5.4	
RDW (%)	21	14.8–20.0	Lymphocytes = 73/300 hemopoietic cells	
Retic (%)	0	0–1	Dysplastic changes in erythroid cells, neutrophils, and megakaryocytes	
WBC ($10^3/\mu$L)	10.0	6.1–21.1		
Neutrophils (/μL)	9000	2600–13,600		
Lymphocytes (/μL)	500	1300–9100		
Monocytes (/μL)	300	0–700		
Eosinophils (/μL)	200	200–4300		
Basophils (/μL)	0	0–200		
Platelets ($10^3/\mu$L)	1365	215–760		
Protein (g/dL)	7.6	5.9–7.5		

[a]ANC, all nucleated hemopoietic cells.

Case 7 (Cat). Myelodysplasia With Excess Blasts (MDS-EB) and Myelofibrosis

JOANNE B. MESSICK

An 11-month-old spayed female DSH cat was presented with a history of listlessness, weight loss, and poor appetite for about 10 days. The cat was stuporous during physical examination. Rectal temperature was subnormal (98.4°F), and heart and respiratory rates were increased. Mucous membranes were very pale, and a heart murmur heard during auscultation was attributed to anemia. No evidence of ill health had been recognized when the cat was spayed 7 weeks earlier. An ELISA test for feline leukemia virus (FeLV) was positive at that time. A hemogram and clinical chemistry profile were performed at admission to the hospital. Hemogram results indicated severe macrocytic normochronic anemia, normal leukocyte count with lymphopenia, and thrombocytosis. Neither aggregate nor punctate reticulocytes were found in blood, consistent with severe anemia from markedly depressed erythropoiesis. Clinical chemistry results were within reference limits except for moderate increases in ALT and AST activity, which were attributed to hypoxic liver injury. Large, firm, white particles of marrow were aspirated from the femur. Examination of smears showed densely cellular particles with little fat. The differential count was 300 marrow cells. The erythroid series was markedly reduced, and most of the cells in this series were rubriblasts and prorubricytes. A few megaloblastic rubricytes were present. Myeloid blast cells were 10% of all hemopoietic cells. There were giant metamyelocytes, band neutrophils, and segmented neutrophils mixed with cells of more normal size. Eosinophils were increased but had normal morphologic features. Megakaryocyte number was not appreciably increased but many were large, monolobed cells. Mature lymphocytes composed approximately 24% of marrow cells. Myelodysplasia with excess blasts (MDS-EB) was diagnosed from the pattern of hematologic abnormalities. The cat was euthanized and a necropsy was performed. There were no gross abnormalities. Sections of femoral marrow were markedly cellular and contained multiple lymphoid nodules. A network of coarse argyophilic fibers, assessed as grade 2 myelofibrosis, was apparent in a section stained with Gomori's silver stain. There was centrilobular hepatic necrosis; liver, spleen, and lymph nodes were unremarkable.

Interpretation

1. Hemopoietic neoplasia is the most likely cause of severe macrocytic, poorly regenerative anemia in an FeLV-positive cat. Intense reticulocytosis in strongly regenerative anemias can raise the MCV quite high but does not account for macrocytosis in this patient since its CBC revealed reticulocytopenia. Lingering macrocytosis from an earlier regenerative response (postregenerative macrocytosis) is unlikely because of present anemia. Hemolytic and blood loss anemias can be ruled out by other findings, such as absence of regenerative response, hyperbilirubinemia, hypoproteinemia, and hypovolemia. Deficiencies of vitamin B_{12} and folate, potential causes of macrocytosis, are extremely rare in domestic animals and do not cause anemia this severe. Severe nonregenerative anemia in cats can result from immune-mediated suppression of erythropoiesis, as in pure red cell aplasia and immune-mediated ineffective erythropoiesis, but such anemias are usually normocytic. Bone marrow must be examined to distinguish between neoplastic and nonneoplastic disorders of hemopoiesis.
2. Although most cats with myelodysplasia are thrombocytopenic, some have increased platelet counts.
3. Examination of bone marrow smears provided ample evidence of a myelodysplastic syndrome in the form of increased myeloid blast cells and the morphologic evidence of dysplastic maturation in all three cell lines. Acute myeloid leukemia was ruled out by a blast cell count of less than 30%. Because the M:E ratio was greater than 1, rubriblasts were not included in the blast cell count. The diagnosis was MDS-EB.
4. Myelofibrosis and lymphoid nodules in bone marrow are secondary abnormalities found in some cats with MDS and AML. Myelofibrosis can frustrate attempts to collect a diagnostic sample of marrow by aspiration. In such cases, a core biopsy should be performed and impression smears prepared before fixing the tissue.
5. The absence of infiltrates of hemopoietic cells in spleen, liver, and lymph nodes is typical of all forms of MDS except chronic myelomonocytic leukemia.

Case 8 (Dog). Febrile Transfusion Reaction Due to Contamination of the Transfer Blood

ANN HOHENHAUS

A 5-kg, 17-year-old, spayed poodle was referred for diagnostic evaluation and treatment of gingival hemorrhage, grade 5 periodontal disease with pyorrhea, and thrombocytopenia (platelet count, 46,000/μL; reference range, 180,000–500,000/μL). A complete blood count obtained by the referring veterinarian demonstrated anemia (hematocrit, 20.8%; reference range, 37–55%; RBC count, 3.19 $\times$ 10^6/μL; reference range, 5.5–8.5 $\times$ 10^6/μL), mild leukocytosis (17,500/μL; reference range, 6000–17,000/μL), and a left shift (neutrophil band forms 525/μL (reference range, 0–300/μL). The prothrombin time and activated partial thromboplastin time were within the reference ranges. The owner reported blood-tinged urine in the past 24 hours. Physical examination revealed multiple petechiations, epistaxis, and brisk gingival hemorrhage. At the time of hospital admission, the packed cell volume had fallen to 14% and the decision was made to administer packed red blood cells.

A crossmatch was performed, and a compatible unit of packed red blood cells was identified. The packed red blood cells were diluted with 0.9% sodium chloride to facilitate administration. Before transfusion, the dog's rectal temperature was 101°F. Three hours after the initiation of the transfusion, the dog had a rectal temperature of 104.8°F. The dog was restless and panting, and had vomited one time. The transfusion was discontinued, and an investigation into the cause of the fever was initiated. The intravenous line was maintained with an infusion of 0.9% sodium chloride.

The label on the blood bag was checked to confirm that the blood transfused was from a canine blood donor and that the unit administered was the compatible unit determined by the crossmatch. The color and consistency of the unit of blood was normal. Samples of the recipient dog's blood and blood from the blood bag were obtained for culture. A sample of the sodium chloride used to dilute the packed red blood cells was cultured. A second sample of the transfused blood was placed in an EDTA tube to allow a repeat crossmatch, and a third sample of the transfused blood was Gram-stained and microscopi-

cally evaluated. Blood from the transfusion recipient was submitted for a packed cell volume, examination of the plasma color, and Coombs' testing.

Results

Review of the crossmatch procedure and the blood bag label indicated the correct unit of blood had been administered. The packed cell volume was 15% and the plasma was red. The Coombs' test was negative, and the repeat crossmatch indicated compatibility. The Gram stain of the blood in the blood bag showed Gram-negative rods and the culture grew *Enterococcus sp.* The blood culture of the recipient dog grew *Pseudomonas aeruginosa.* Bacterial culture of the saline was negative.

Interpretation

Febrile transfusion reactions are defined as a 1°C rise in temperature during or up to 2 hours following the completion of a blood transfusion. They most commonly result from an interaction of recipient antibodies to donor leukocytes. When fever occurs without hemolysis, a febrile nonhemolytic transfusion reaction should be suspected. Discontinuation of the transfusion in febrile nonhemolytic transfusion reactions is the only therapy necessary. When fever occurs with hemolysis, as in this dog, red blood cell incompatibility or transfusion of an infectious agent should be suspected.

This case study illustrates the diagnostic evaluation indicated when a febrile, hemolytic transfusion reaction occurs. An acute hemolytic reaction, due to red blood cell incompatibility, would be expected to show an incompatible crossmatch and a positive Coombs' test. Identification of an infectious agent by microscopic examination or culture, as occurred in this case, confirmed the etiology of the transfusion reaction.

This dog experienced a transfusion reaction due to contamination of the transfused blood with bacteria. The reaction is not mediated by the transfusion recipient's immune system, but is a result of the endotoxin produced by the Gram-negative bacteria in the transfused blood. The *Pseudomonas aeruginosa* bacteremia was attributed to hematologic spread of an oral infection and was believed to be the cause of the dog's illness.

CASE 9 (COW). HYPERPROTEINEMIA, HYPOALBUMINEMIA, AND HYPERFIBRINOGENEMIA IN PYELONEPHRITIS

CBC	Patient Value	Reference Range
RBC (×10⁶/μL)	6.44	5.0–10.0
Hemoglobin (g/dL)	10.0	8–15
PCV (%)	28.3	24–46
MCV (fL)	43.9	40–60
MCHC (g/dL)	35.3	30–36
Plasma Protein (g/dL) (refractometer)	10.2	6.5–8.5
Fibrinogen (mg/dL)	1200	300–700
WBC/μL	5900	4000–12000
Segmented neutrophils	2537	600–4000
Band neutrophils	0	0–120
Lymphocytes	3186	2500–7500
Monocytes	177	25–840
Eosinophils	0	0–2400
Platelet estimate	Adequate	
Chemistry profile (heparinized plasma)		
Blood urea nitrogen (mg/dL)	48	4–23
Creatinine (mg/dL)	5.0	0.6–1.6
Serum protein electrophoresis		
Albumin (g/dL)	1.8	3.0–4.2
α-Globulins (g/dL)	1.5	0.79–0.93
β-Globulins (g/dL)	3.7	0.84–1.16
γ-Globulins (g/dL)	2.5	1.84–2.35
A:G ratio	0.23	0.8–0.9
Urinalysis (voided sample)		
Specific gravity	1.018	
pH	8.0	
Occult blood	+++ (large amount)	
Protein	++++ (>2000 mg/dL)	

Case 9 (Cow). Hyperproteinemia, Hypoalbuminemia, and Hyperfibrinogenemia in Pyelonephritis

JENNIFER S. THOMAS

A 4-year-old mixed breed cow had been losing weight for 2 to 3 weeks. No other animals in the herd were affected. Physical examination revealed a thin cow with normal hydration status. Body temperature was 102.7°F, pulse rate was 90/min, and respiratory rate was 35/min. On rectal palpation, the left kidney felt moderately enlarged with multiple, soft, fluctuant areas. Ultrasound per rectum revealed a greatly enlarged left kidney with multiple fluid pockets throughout. Rectal examination confirmed that the cow was approximately 70 days pregnant. Voided urine was red colored. *Escherichia coli* was isolated following urine culture.

Interpretation

1. The fibrinogen concentration was elevated. This occurs with inflammation or with dehydration.

The calculated protein:fibrinogen ratio was 7.5. In cattle ratios less than 10 indicate a selective increase in fibrinogen secondary to inflammation. The leukogram was within references limits; however, it is not unusual for cattle with inflammatory disease to have elevated fibrinogen concentrations and normal leukocyte counts. Elevated firbinogen concentrations are common in cattle with renal disease.

2. The cow had azotemia as indicated by the elevated blood urea nitrogen (BUN) and creatinine concentrations. Although a prerenal component could not be ruled out, the azotemia in conjunction with the isosthenuric urine was consistent with renal dysfunction. The physical findings, ultrasound findings, and urine culture results were consistent with pyelonephritis.

3. The cow had hypoalbuminemia, hyperglobulinemia, and a decreased A:G ratio. Likely causes for the hypoalbuminemia included decreased production secondary to hyperglobulinemia as part of the acute phase response and selective loss of protein by the kidneys. Due to the hematuria in the urine, it was not possible to quantitate the protein loss in the urine. Decreased liver produc-

tion of albumin could not be ruled out but was not supported by other laboratory findings. The elevated globulin levels consisted of increased α, β and γ globulins. Increased α and β fractions occur as part of the acute phase response associated with inflammation. Elevated γ globulins indi-

cate in creased immunoglobulin production secondary to chronic antigenic stimulation. In this cow, the elevations were most likely secondary to chronic septic inflammation.

4. The hematuria and proteinuria were likely secondary to the renal lesion.

CASE 10 (DOG). HYPERPROTEINEMIA AND HYPERGLOBULINEMIA IN COCCIDIOIDOMYCOSIS

CBC	Patient Value	Reference Range
RBC ($\times 10^6/\mu L$)	5.58	5.8–8.5
Hemoglobin (g/dL)	11.3	12–18
PCV (%)	33.7	37–55
MCV (fL)	60.4	60–77
MCHC (g/dL)	33.5	30–36
Reticulocytes (%)	0.4	
Plasma protein (g/dL) (refractometer)	10.9	6.0–8.0
WBC/μL	12800	6000–17000
Segmented neutrophils	9856	3000–11500
Band neutrophils	0	0–300
Lymphocytes	1536	1000–48000
Monocytes	512	150–1350
Eosinophils	896	100–1250
Platelet estimate	adequate	
Serum protein electrophoresis		
Albumin (g/dL)	2.3	2.1–3.3
α_1-globulins (g/dL)	0.3	0.21–0.51
α_2-globulins (g/dL)	1.1	0.31–1.13
β-globulins (g/dL)	3.4	1.3–2.7
γ-globulins (g/dL)	4.2	0.92–2.26
Total protein (g/dL)	11.3	5.6–7.9
A:G ratio	0.26	0.6–1.1

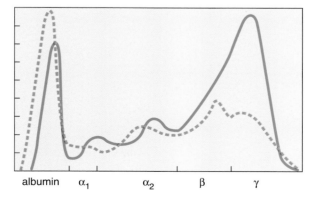

FIGURE A.1 Electrophoretograms of a dog with cuccidioidomyeosis and a normal dog. —— = patient, ---- = normal dog.

Case 10 (Dog). Hyperproteinemia and Hyperglobulinemia in Coccidioidomycosis

JENNIFER S. THOMAS

A 2-year-old female spayed Dachshund was lethargic and had intermittent fever and shifting leg lameness of 6 months duration. On physical examination, the dog stood with an arched back and hindlimbs tucked under. Palpation of left carpal, tarsal, and coxofemoral joints elicited pain. The left axillary lymph node was enlarged as were both popliteal lymph nodes. Body temperature was 103.7°F, pulse rate was 150/minute, and the respiratory rate was 30/minute.

Hyperproteinemia was the only abnormality on a serum biochemical profile. Antinuclear antibody (ANA) titer, rheumatoid factor test, and lupus erythematosus (LE) preparation were negative. Serology was negative for *Ehrlichia canis* and for lyme disease. Radiographs revealed a lytic lesion in the dorsal spinous process of the tenth thoracic vertebrae and a lytic lesion in one rib. Cytologic examination of material aspirated from the vertebral lesion revealed pyogranulomatous inflammation but no organisms were ob-

served. Histologic examination of tissue surgically excised from the vertebrae revealed pyogranulomatous inflammation with intralesional organisms consistent with *Coccidioides immitis*.

Interpretation

1. The dog had hyperproteinemia consisting of normal albumin concentration, hyperglobulinemia, and a decreased A:G ratio. Serum protein electrophoresis documented a polyclonal gammopathy associated with elevated β and γ globulins. Polyclonal gammopathies are associated with chronic antigenic stimulation. In dogs, common causes include chronic infections (bacterial, fungal, rickettsial, or parasitic), neoplasia, or immune-mediated disorders. In this case, the gammopathy was due to coccidioidomycosis.

2. There was a mild, normocytic, normochromic anemia that was nonregenerative. The most likely cause was the anemia of chronic disorders. Bone marrow examination was not performed to investigate other potential causes of depressed erythroid production.

CASE 11 (CAT). FELINE IMMUNODEFICIENCY VIRUS (FIV) INFECTION

Parameter	Initial Presentation	6 years later
Packed cell volume	31	20
Hemoglobin	10.4	7.0
RBC ($\times 10^6$)	5.01	4.15
WBC/μL	5500	1500
Band neutrophils	200	200
Segmented neutrophils	3900	300
Lymphocytes	1200	700*
Monocytes	200	300
Eosinophils	0	0
Reticulocytes	0	0.2
Anisocytosis	Slight	Slight
Plasma protein	6.5	6.0
Comments[a]		*lymphoblasts observed
FeLV/FIV test	FIV positive	

Case 11 (Cat). Feline Immunodeficiency Virus (FIV) Infection

DEBRA ZORAN

A 6-year-old, neutered domestic short hair cat was presented with a 1-week history of a draining lesion on his right hip that was not healing. The cat primarily

lived indoors but was allowed to go outside and occasionally got into fights with neighborhood cats. His vaccinations (FVRCP, rabies, feline leukemia virus) were up-to-date. Physical examination revealed a thin cat with a rectal temperature of 103.8°F, a pulse of 180 beats per min, respirations of 40 breaths per min, moderate gingivitis and stomatitis (despite minimal

(Continued)

tartar accumulation on the teeth), and an open, 1-cm draining wound at midshaft femur on the right hip. Impression smears of the exudate revealed a few coccoid bacteria, many neutrophils (both degenerate and nondegenerate), and a few macrophages with engulfed bacteria. The presumptive diagnosis was a cat fight abscess. The wound was flushed and cleaned with dilute chlorhexidene solution, antibiotics (amoxicillin) were dispensed, and the cat was sent home. One week later at a follow-up examination, the wound was smaller but not completely healed, and a second wound had appeared distal to the area. The physical examination was essentially unchanged otherwise, with a persistent low-grade fever (temperature 103.5°F) and moderate gingivitis and stomatitis present in the oral cavity. Due to failure of the abscess to heal as expected, further evaluation of this cat included hematology, an FeLV-FIV test, radiographs of the affected area, and culture of the lesion. The cat was anesthetized to debride and clean the wound surgically, a Penrose drain was placed, and the wound was sutured closed. Results of the hematologic examination and viral testing are shown in the table. There was no bony invasion at the site of the lesion, and only mild soft tissue swelling could be visualized. Culture of the wound revealed both *Pasteurella multocida* and *Staphylococcus spp.* that were sensitive to amoxicillin-clavulonic acid, cephalexin, enrofloxacin, and potentiated sulfa drugs. The cat was discharged with a 2-week supply of amoxicillin-clavulonic acid, and the owners were instructed to keep the cat indoors only. Over the next 7 to 10 days, the wound healed, the cat's temperature returned to normal, and the stomatitis and gingivitis resolved to a large degree. However, once the antibiotics were stopped, the gingivitis and stomatitis returned. A dental prophylaxis was performed, viral isolation for calici and herpes virus were submitted, and a mucosal biopsy specimen was submitted at the time of the dental procedure. The biopsy results revealed a lymphoplasmacytic stomatitis and gingivitis with no evidence of neoplastic disease. The calici virus isolation test was positive, suggesting that the cause of

the chronic oral inflammation was a combination of the effects of FIV and calici virus. The cat's oral signs were controlled with oral chlorhexidene gel application, frequent dental prophylaxis, and antibiotics as needed.

Over the succeeding years the cat had several bouts of otitis externa, cystitis, and recurrent stomatitis that were managed routinely. At age 12, approximately 6 years after the cat was found to be FIV-positive, he was presented for reduced appetite, lethargy, and weight loss of several days duration. A routine hematology and serum chemistry profile were performed. The results of the hematology profile are presented in the table (the chemistry profile was within normal limits). A bone marrow examination revealed normal platelet and monocyte precursors, but reduced red cell precursors and lymphoid dysplasia with a maturation arrest and numerous atypical blast cells in the marrow sample. A diagnosis of lymphoblastic leukemia was made. The owners elected not to pursue further treatment, and the cat was humanely euthanized. Postmortem examination confirmed the lymphoblastic leukemia, anemia due to chronic disease, chronic gingivitis due to Calicivirus, and FIV infection.

Interpretation

1. Cats with FIV may live relatively disease free for long periods after the initial diagnosis is made, as long as appropriate supportive care and husbandry are maintained.
2. The presentation of a chronic, nonhealing abscess and persistent gingivitis-stomatitis both were suggestive of a tentative diagnosis of FIV infection.
3. Lymphopenia and neutropenia are not diagnostic but are consistent with FIV infection and secondary bacterial infection.
4. Few FIV-positive cats (<10%) develop the AIDS syndrome, but many in the late stages of the disease will develop lymphoreticular neoplasms, chronic wasting syndromes, or degenerative neurologic disorders instead.

Case 12 (Cat). Hereditary Factor XII (Hageman Trait) Deficiency

W. JEAN DODDS

A 9-month-old, female Oriental shorthair cat was admitted for routine ovariohysterectomy. On physical examination, the veterinarian noted that the cat was in estrus. The owner was advised that elective surgery

is generally not recommended during estrus, but the owner wanted the procedure performed because the cat was cycling frequently, and her vocalization behavior was annoying. During surgery, the veterinarian noted excessive oozing of blood from the incision site and, on further inspection, saw that the abdomi-

(Continued)

nal fat and areas in and around the ovarian pedicle ligatures and uterine stump appeared bruised. When this progressed to frank bleeding, blood samples were obtained for diagnostic evaluation of hemostasis, routine complete blood counts, and chemistry profile. Fresh whole blood (950 mL) was administered after the donor and patient bloods were found to be compatible on a rapid cross-match. The bleeding stopped following the transfusion.

Results of the diagnostic laboratory tests revealed mild anemia and hypoproteinemia, presumably from blood loss; normal white cell and differential counts and blood chemistries; negative FeLV, FIP, hemobartonella, and FIV tests; moderate thrombocytopenia (72,000/μL); normal PT and slightly elevated fibrinogen level (450 mg/dL); negative fibrinogen degradation d-dimer level (less than 250 mg/dL); and markedly prolonged APTT (greater than 120 seconds). After consulting with a clinical pathology specialist at the clinic's reference laboratory, factor XII deficiency was suspected based on the history and

species involved. (Additional questioning of the owner revealed that the cat had received a combination vaccination booster 5 days earlier.) Further specific coagulation factor testing was recommended.

Results of repeat testing at that time confirmed a severe intrinsic coagulation factor defect; the platelet count had returned to normal. Specific coagulation factor assays were all within the reference laboratory's normal limits for cats, with the exception of factor XII activity which was only 1.2%. The diagnosis of factor XII deficiency was thus confirmed.

This case illustrates what can happen when an animal having an unrecognized congenital coagulopathy, not usually associated with abnormal bleeding (i.e., factor XII deficiency), is subjected to elective surgery while in estrus, because of the relative impairment of platelet function that accompanies elevated estrogen levels. Hemostasis was likely to have been compromised further by the recent vaccination, which could explain the low platelet count (during the viremic period 3 to 10 days after vaccination).

Case 13 (Dog). Perioperative Management of Otterhound Thrombasthenia

JAMES L. CATALFAMO and W. JEAN DODDS

A 6-year-old, 35-kg, female Otterhound affected with thrombasthenia presented with a round, 6-cm in diameter cutaneous mass on her left forelimb. Its surface appeared ulcerated and necrotic. The buccal mucosa bleeding time (BMBT) was greater than 15 minutes (reference range, 2 to 4 minutes), and platelet count, coagulation panel (APTT, PT, fibrinogen), and plasma von Willebrand factor (vWF) were within normal limits. Evaluation of this dog's platelet function revealed absent platelet aggregation in response to ADP, collagen, and thrombin as well as abnormal clot retraction. Aperture closure times for both the epinephrine and ADP/collagen agonists were infinite (>300 seconds) (reference range epinephrine/collagen, 68 to 184 seconds; ADP/collagen 47 to 119 seconds). Platelet membrane glycoproteins IIb and IIIa were undetectable using flow cytometry. An excision biopsy of the mass was scheduled. The dog's preoperative hematocrit was 53% (reference range, 39 to 57%); blood chemistry values were within reference ranges, platelet count was 186,000/μL (reference range, 179 to 510,000/μL); and MPV was 10.6 fL (reference range, 7.6 to 11.6 fL). The dog's blood type was DEA 1.2.

To prevent hemorrhagic complications during the excision biopsy, the dog was transfused preoperatively with 300 mL of platelet-rich plasma (PRP) over the course of 1 hour. PRP was obtained from a DEA 1.1-negative donor and banked at room temperature 24 hours beforehand. The platelet count in the donor PRP was 269,000/uL. A second 300-mL transfusion of donor PRP was given for 1.5 hours during the surgery and postoperatively. In the immediate postoperative period, the patient's BMBT was greater than 12 minutes. No signs of abnormal bleeding were noted intra- or postoperatively, and the dog's hematocrit (45%) remained within the reference range. The wound was sutured using multilayer closure, and a pressure wrap was applied. The bandage was changed daily for one week and then sutures were removed. Results of the mass biopsy indicated multiple trichoepitheliomas.

Interpretation

1. Laboratory results that included abnormal BMBT, normal platelet number, normal plasma vWF, normal coagulation screening assays, markedly abnormal platelet aggregation, abnormal clot retraction, and undetectable levels of membrane GPIIb/IIIa supported a diagnosis of Glanzmann's thrombasthenia, which is the most common plate-

(Continued)

let defect encountered in Otterhounds. The dog's long-term platelet dysfunction and the functional and biochemical features characterizing the platelet defect rule out acquired platelet defects.
2. Perioperative transfusion of PRP was effective in preventing bleeding complications associated with the excision biopsy surgery.
3. The blood type of the Otterhound was DEA 1.2-positive. Since erythrocytes are present in PRP, blood from a DEA1.1-negative donor dog was used. This precaution is particularly relevant to animals with inherited platelet defects because they are more likely to receive multiple platelet transfusions.

4. Two transfusions of PRP, one delivered preoperatively and the other administered intra- and postoperatively, were given to attain maximal levels of functional platelets at a time when the patient was at greatest risk for bleeding. It is noteworthy that despite achieving a level of hemostatic function that resulted in no excessive intra- or postoperative bleeding, the BMBT remained outside the reference range. Correction of the BMBT would appear not to be predictive of the level of hemostatic coverage afforded by perioperative platelet transfusion support.

CASE 14 (BIRD). REACTIVE LYMPHOCYTOSIS

	Hyacinth Macaw	Reference Range
PCV (%)	43	35–55
Anisocytosis	0.5%	<2.5%
Polychromasia	2%	<5%
Hypochromasia	0	None
Poikilocytosis	0	<2.5%
Erythroplastids	0	<0.5%
Leukocytes		
WBC (/μL)	26,000	8000–20,000
Heterophils (/μL)	10,100 (39%)	4000–11,000
Lymphocytes (/μL)	14,600 (56%)	1500–8000
Monocytes (/μL)	1000 (4%)	0–700
Eosinophils (/μL)	0 (0%)	0–400
Basophils (/μL)	300 (1%)	0–400
Leukocyte morphology	Reactive lymphocytes and large vacuolated monocytoid cells	
Thrombocytes		
Estimated number	Adequate	1–5/1000× field
Morphology	Normal, clumped	
Plasma protein (refractometry) (gm/dL)	5.3	3.0–5.0

Case 14 (Bird). Reactive Lymphocytosis: Possibly Chlamydia Infection

TERRY W. CAMPBELL

An 11-year old Hyacinth macaw (*Anodrohychus hyacinthinus*) was presented with a 10-day history of anorexia. The bird had been doing poorly for 3 months, with periodic episodes of anorexia and lethargy. The bird's urates were yellow, suggesting bilirubinuria associated with hepatobiliary disease. Radiographs revealed a large abdominal mass that was displacing other structures. The mass was presumed to be a greatly enlarged spleen.

Interpretation

The erythrocyte parameters were within the reference range. There is mild leukocytosis with marked lymphocytosis. The plasma protein measured by refractive index suggests slight hyperproteinemia. The lymphocytosis may be reactive or proliferative. No immature lymphocytes were found in the peripheral blood that would support a proliferative lymphocytosis; however, their absence does not rule out that possibility. The presence of reactive lymphocytes in the peripheral blood is supportive of a persistent lymphocytosis associated with chronic marked antigenic

(Continued)

stimulation as seen with chronic infections. The vacuolated monocytes are indicative of reactive monocytes and suggest severe bacterial infection or septicemia.

The bird died 24 hours later. The necropsy confirmed the marked splenomegaly. The spleen had ruptured, most likely triggering the sudden death. A mild air sacculitis and hepatomegaly were also found. Many plasma cells were found on the microscopic examination of the spleen. These are typical necropsy findings for chlamydiosis in psittacine birds; however, no etiologic agent was found.

CASE 15 (DOG). GLOMERULONEPHRITIS

	May 3		May 10		May 11		May 12	
RBC ($\times 10^6/\mu$L)	5.18		4.35		4.30		4.24	
Hemoglobin (g/dL)	12.4		10.8		9.9		10.0	
PCV (%)	37.0		31.0		29.0		29.0	
MCV (fL)	71.4		71.2		67.4		68.3	
MCH (pg)	23.9		24.8		23.0		23.5	
MCHC (%)	33.5		34.8		34.1		34.4	
Icterus index	2		2		2		2	
Plasma proteins (g/dL)	5.2		5.0		5.1		4.6	
Fibrinogen (g/dL)	0.7		0.9		1.0		1.0	
Reticulocytes (%)	—		0		0.2		0	
Anisocytosis	slight		slight		slight		slight	
Polychromasia	none		none		none		none	
WBC/μL	10,900		6,100		8,100		24,400	
		%		%		%		%
Band neutrophils	109	1.0	671	11.0	648	8.0	749	3.5
Segmenters	9,374	86.0	4,331	71.0	5,751	71.0	18,932	88.0
Lymphocytes	545	5.0	854	14.0	729	9.0	107	0.5
Monocytes	763	7.0	244	4.0	972	12.0	1,712	8.0
Eosinophils	109	1.0	0	0.0	0	0.0	0	0.0
Blood urea nitrogen (mg/dL)	181.5		135		122		104	
Creatinine (mg/dL)	3.8		3.8		—		3.0	
Urine specific gravity	1.017		—		—		1.017	
Urine protein	4+[a]		—		—		2+	
Blood calcium (mg/dL)	7.9		—		—		—	
Blood phosphorus (mg/dL)	17.6		—		—		—	

[a]Urine protein on May 7 = 1.2 g/24 hr. An immune panel of Coombs' test, antinuclear antibody test, and LE cell test, also conducted on May 7, was negative.

Case 15 (Dog). Hypoproteinemia and Hyperfibrinogenemia in Glomerulonephritis

A 6-year-old Shetland sheepdog had been vomiting for 3 weeks and had lost weight over a period of 6 months. Physical examination revealed a thin, apprehensive dog in a fair state of hydration. Body temperature was 100.8°F, pulse rate was 160/min, and respiration was 16/min. The owner stated that polydipsia had been noted over a period of a few weeks.

Initial laboratory data indicated a diagnosis of chronic nephritis, possibly glomerulonephritis. Therapy was directed toward increasing urine flow and reducing the level of blood urea nitrogen. Fluid therapy was administered daily, mannitol diuresis was conducted twice, and peritoneal dialysis was carried out daily from May 8 through May 12. Prednisolone, approximately 0.5 mg/pound of body weight b.i.d., was initiated on May 9. Antibiotics and other therapeutics were also given daily. The effects of fluid therapy, dialysis, and prednisolone administration are reflected in the sequential hemograms and the BUN determinations. Therapy did not bring sufficient

(Continued)

improvement to recommend its continuation. The owner requested that the dog be destroyed.

Necropsy. The kidneys were swollen and pale. The capsule peeled easily. On cut surface, the cortex bulged, and glomeruli were prominent. There was intercostal mineralization. Microscopic examination revealed relatively avascular and diffusely hyalinized glomeruli. Bowman's capsules were thickened, and diffusely hyalinized and presented numerous adhesions. Cortical tubules were moderately dilated and lined with somewhat atrophic epithelium. There were perivascular accumulations of neutrophil leukocytes and mononuclear cells in the interstitial tissues, particularly in the lower cortical area. The pelvis of the kidney appeared essentially normal.

Interpretation

1. In chronic nephritis with uremia, the following findings are common in the hemogram: anemia, elevated plasma fibrinogen, and absolute lymphopenia.

2. RBC, Hb, and PCV were at their minimum normal levels in the first hemogram. The existence of a moderate anemia became apparent as hemoconcentration was reduced by fluid therapy. The anemia was normocytic-normochromic, indicating that it was the result of depression of erythrogenesis. This was further substantiated by the absence or very low level of reticulocytes in peripheral blood.

3. Hyperfibrinogenemia is a common finding in chronic nephritis, and the hypoalbuminemia results from loss of albumin into the urine. The loss of albumin into the urine was significant, as demonstrated by 1.2 g/24-hour urine sample on May 7.

4. Dysfunction of the kidneys was demonstrated by a BUN of 181.5 mg/dL of serum, creatinine of 3.8 mg/dL, a marked retention of phosphorus, and a compensatory decrease in serum calcium, leading to the intercostal mineralization noted at necropsy.

CASE 16 (DOG). REGENERATIVE LEFT SHIFT IN PYOMETRA

	October 28 (Admission Date)		November 1 (2nd Day Postsurgery)	
Erythrocytes				
RBC (×10⁶/μL)	6.10		6.00	
Hemoglobin (g/dL)	13.2		13.6	
PCV (%)	41.0		43.0	
MCV (fL)	67.0		71.6	
MCHC (%)	32.2		31.6	
Anisocytosis	slight		slight	
Polychromasia	slight		slight	
Leukocytes		%		%
WBC/μL	59,500		66,000	
Myelocytes	298	0.5	330	0.5
Metamyelocytes	7,438	12.5	1,320	2.0
Band neutrophils	17,850	30.0	7,260	11.0
Neutrophils	23,800	40.0	46,860	71.0
Lymphocytes	3,272	5.5	1,320	2.0
Monocytes	5,950	10.0	6,270	9.5
Eosinophils	892	1.5	330	0.5
Degenerated cells	0	0.0	2,310	3.5
Toxic signs	Neutrophils are large with basophilic, foamy cytoplasm			
Plasma				
Protein (g/dL)	8.3		8.0	
Blood urea nitrogen (mg/dL)	29.8		46.2	

Case 16 (Dog). Regenerative Left Shift in Pyometra

A female weimaraner, 9 years old, was presented with a complaint of urinary incontinence associated with polydipsia. She had given birth to her last litter some 5 years earlier. According to the owner, the dog had shown signs suggestive of estrus about 1 month before. There had been no history of vomiting.

Physical Examination. The dog was obese and presented a distended, painful abdomen. The rectal temperature was 103°F, pulse 172/min, and respiration was rated as fast. The conjunctivae were congested, and there was evidence of dehydration.

Radiographic Examination. Both uterine horns were very much enlarged.

Interpretation

1. A borderline anemia that commonly accompanies pyometra was probably masked by some hemoconcentration. The above-normal plasma protein concentration was possibly both relative (from hemoconcentration) and absolute (from increase in production of globulins in response to the suppurative inflammatory process).

2. The marked leukocytosis with left shift indicates that the bone marrow has adjusted to accelerated granulopoiesis in response to continual heavy demands for neutrophils. The signs of "toxicity" in neutrophils suggest exposure to metabolic and bacterial toxins produced in conjunction with pyometra. The initial hemogram can be distinguished from the leukocytosis and left shift of an acute disease process, such as leptospirosis, by the persistence of lymphocytes and eosinophils. These latter cell types have become diminished in the second hemogram as a result of the stress of surgery. The monocytosis of the level seen here is common to pyometra.

3. The elevated blood urea nitrogen is referable to the decomposition of body protein associated with the suppurative process within the uterus and also to the dehydration.

4. An increase in WBC, due to an increase in the neutrophil leukocytes, is a common finding during the first days after surgery for pyometra.

CASE 17 (DOG). DEGENERATIVE LEFT SHIFT IN PYOMETRA

	October 24		October 28		November 5	
Erythrocytes						
RBC ($\times 10^6/\mu$L)	6.95		5.90		6.70	
Hemoglobin (g/dL)	6.0		12.5		13.9	
PCV (%)	46.0		42.0		44.0	
MCV (fL)	66.2		71.2		65.7	
MCHC (%)	34.8		29.7		31.6	
Nucleated RBC/100 WBC	0		0		0.5	
Anisocytosis	slight		slight		slight	
Leukocytes		%		%		%
WBC/μL	14,800		17,000		33,200	
Metamyelocytes	814	5.5	0	0.0	1,826	5.5
Band neutrophils	3,700	25.0	935	5.5	11,122	33.5
Neutrophils	8,066	54.5	12,155	71.5	12,118	36.5
Lymphocytes	1,628	11.0	2,380	14.0	2,324	7.0
Monocytes	444	3.0	1,360	8.0	4,482	13.5
Eosinophils	74	0.5	85	0.5	0	0.0
Unclassified cells	74	0.5	0	0.0	332	1.0
Degenerated cells	0	0.0	85	0.5	996	3.0
Toxic signs in neutrophils	basophilic cytoplasm		none		slight basophilia of the cytoplasm	
Plasma						
Protein (g/dL)	8.0		7.9		7.5	
Blood urea nitrogen (mg/dL)	6.3		—		6.8	

Case 17 (Dog). Degenerative Left Shift in Pyometra

A female miniature poodle, 3 years old, was presented with a complaint of anorexia, depression, and polydipsia. The owner stated that the dog had exhibited signs of estrus 3 weeks previously. Rectal temperature was 104°F, pulse 118, hydration appeared to be good, and a mass about the size of a golf ball could be palpated in the abdomen. No diarrhea or vomiting had been observed.

Radiographic Examination. Enlarged uterine horns were demonstrated.

Therapy. The record indicates that treatment was limited to antibiotics administered twice daily between October 25 and 31, after which the dog was permitted to go home, with antibiotic therapy to be continued by the owner. The patient was returned November 5 for removal of the uterus. Three hemograms were obtained covering the period from first entry to return for surgery.

Interpretation

1. The plasma proteins were at the maximum and above maximum normal concentrations. Since pyogenic bacteria are often associated with pyometra, an absolute increase in plasma proteins may develop as a result of hyperglobulinemia. Serum protein fractionation would be required to demon-strate this occurrence. Plasma proteins also increase relatively in hemoconcentration. However, the low blood urea nitrogen and lack of signs of dehydration on physical examination suggested that the dog was in water balance.
2. The left shift without significant elevation in total neutrophils reflected a state of toxemia with some depression of granulopoiesis. This depression of maturation of neutrophils is further demonstrated by the persistence of basophilia (bluish staining) of the cytoplasm.
3. Administration of antibiotics appeared to lessen the toxemia, for the left shift was receding and the signs of toxicity in neutrophils had disappeared in the second hemogram. However, the improvement in general well-being did not persist for long. On Nov. 5 a leukocytosis was demonstrated in which immature neutrophils outnumbered the mature neutrophils (degenerative left shift) pointing to a demand for neutrophils that could not be met by the bone marrow. This is generally interpreted as a poor prognostic sign.
4. Lymphocytes remaining within the normal range despite signs of systemic stress is a common finding in chronic suppurative diseases.
5. A monocytosis is a characteristic feature of pyometra. However, this feature did not express itself until the third hemogram. Perhaps the initial toxemia depressed production of monocytes as well as of granulocytes.

CASE 18 (DOG). CHRONIC PERITONITIS

	November 5		November 15		November 19	
Erythrocytes						
RBC ($\times10^6/\mu$L)	4.10		3.9		3.75	
Hemoglobin (g/dL)	10.6		8.6		8.4	
PCV (%)	29.0		25.0		25.0	
MCV (fL)	70.7		64.1		66.6	
MCHC (%)	36.6		34.4		33.6	
Nucleated RBC/100 WBC	0		0		0	
Reticulocytes (%)	0.2		1.0		—	
Anisocytosis	slight		slight		slight	
Polychromasia	rare		slight		slight	
Leptocytosis	moderate		moderate		moderate	
Leukocytes		%		%		%
WBC/μL	26,800		104,000		61,400	
Myeloblasts	rare		rare		rare	
Progranulocytes	268	1.0	rare		rare	
Myelocytes	402	1.5	1,040	1.0	307	0.5
Metamyelocytes	2,814	10.5	23,400	22.5	6,140	10.0
Band neutrophils	4,556	17.0	36,920	35.5	20,569	33.5
Neutrophils	8,978	33.5	38,480	37.0	26,402	43.0
Lymphocytes	2,412	9.0	1,560	1.5	4,298	7.0

(Continued)

CASE 18 (DOG). CHRONIC PERITONITIS (continued)

	November 5		November 15		November 19	
Monocytes	7,236	27.0	2,600	2.5	2,456	4.0
Eosinophils	0	0.0	0	0.0	0	0.0
Unclassified cells	134	0.5	0	0.0	1,228	2.0

Leukocyte morphology: The cytoplasm is blue to gray and somewhat granular in metamyelocytes and most band neutrophils. These are signs of toxic interference with maturation. An occasional neutrophil presents a double nucleus. This reflects failure of the cell to divide after division of the nucleus. It is an additional indication of toxemic disease.

Plasma

Protein (g/dL)	7.5	6.9	6.9

Urine

Specific gravity	1.007	—	1.002

Case 18 (Dog). Leukemoid Reaction in Chronic Peritonitis

A spayed female mixed-breed terrier, 5 ½ years old, had exhibited polydipsia, polyuria, and severe incontinence for 2 months. On arrival, the temperature was 101.9°F, pulse 160/minute, and respiration approximately 60/minute. The palpable lymph nodes were of normal size, the mucous membranes were somewhat pale, and the abdomen was distended. An attempt at fluid aspiration from the peritoneal cavity was unsuccessful. The hemograms revealed increasing leukocytosis with left shift, pointing to the possibility of suppuration. An exploratory laparotomy revealed an extensive granulomatous peritonitis involving all serous surfaces in the abdominal cavity. Infection was suspected but not verified. The patient died on the seventh day after surgery. Necropsy findings failed to elucidate the cause of the peritonitis.

Interpretation

1. The first hemogram directed attention to the possibility of a chronic infection with associated normocytic-normochromic anemia from toxic depression of erythropoiesis. The marked left shift without significant elevation of total leukocyte numbers indicated toxic depression of granulopoiesis.
2. The very marked increase in total leukocyte count in the second hemogram, with immature neutrophils outnumbering the mature neutrophils, without an apparent significant change in the physical condition of the dog, caused some thought to be given to the possibility of a granulocytic leukemia. However, the evidence of toxemic disease as revealed by basophilia and double nuclei in neutrophils continued to support the original conclusion that the disease was of inflammatory nature.
3. The progressive anemia, marked leukocytosis, "toxic" neutrophils, and immature neutrophils in excess of mature forms called for an unfavorable prognosis.

CASE 19 (DOG). POLYCYTHEMIA VERA

	March 23	March 30	April 9	April 17	April 24
Erythrocytes					
RBC ($\times 10^6/\mu$L)	13.78	12.94	13.92	7.30	7.07
Hemoglobin (g/dL)	29.6	28.0	27.6	14.5	14.8
PCV (%)	83.0	80.0	80.0	43.0	45.0
MCV (fL)	60.2	61.8	57.5	58.9	63.6
MCHC (%)	35.6	35.0	34.5	33.7	32.9
MCH (pg)	21.4	21.6	19.9	19.9	20.9
Nucleated RBC/100 WBC	0	2	0	0	0

(Continued)

CASE 19 (DOG). POLYCYTHEMIA VERA   *(continued)*

	March 23		March 30		April 9		April 17		April 24	
Reticulocytes (%)	—		0.8		—		0.8		—	
Anisocytosis	slight		slight		slight		slight		slight	
Polychromasia	slight		slight		slight		slight		slight	
Leukocytes		%		%		%		%		%
WBC/μL	9,900		8,600		10,300		9,300		10,300	
Band neutrophils	0	0.0	172	2.0	0	0.0	0	0.0	0	0.0
Neutrophils	5,940	60.0	5,504	64.0	5,099	49.5	5,766	62.0	5,459	53.0
Lymphocytes	2,673	27.0	2,150	25.0	4,120	40.0	2,371	25.5	3,039	29.5
Monocytes	693	7.0	688	8.0	618	6.0	558	6.0	463	4.5
Eosinophils	594	6.0	86	1.0	463	4.5	605	6.5	1,287	12.5
Basophils	0	0.0	0	0.0	0	0.0	0	0.0	51	0.5
Plasma										
Total plasma proteins (g/dL)	7.0		6.8		6.7		4.6		6.7	
Fibrinogen (g/dL)	0.2		0.2		0.2		0.1		0.3	
Thrombocytes/μL	94,000		90,000		—		—		352,000	

Case 19 (Dog). Polycythemia Vera

An intact female Old English sheepdog, 14 months old, was referred with a tentative diagnosis of polycythemia vera. Laboratory data accompanying the dog indicated a PCV of 80.3% and a WBC of 19,500/μL of blood.

On admission, the body temperature was 101.2°F, and the pulse rate was 100/min. The conjunctival and oral mucous membranes were intensely red, the result of engorgement of the blood vessels. The dog weighed 21.8 kg.

Hemograms. The admission hemogram agreed with the accompanying laboratory data in that the PCV was 83%, Hb was 29.6 g/dL; RBC count was 13.78 $\times 10^6$/μL; WBC was 9,900/μL; and a modest thrombocytopenia of 94,000/μL was present. Numerous hemograms were made on this dog to follow results of phlebotomy. Five representative hemograms are presented.

Radiography revealed hypervascularity of lung fields, hepatomegaly, and possibly a minor degree of right heart enlargement. Cardiac evaluation results were within normal limits.

Blood gas values were Po$_2$ 90.0 mmHg; Pco$_2$, 24.5 mmHg; pH, 7.60; CO$_2$CT, 19.3 mM/L; and HCO$_3^-$, 18.7 mEq/L.

Blood volume studies with Evans blue and ^{51}Cr gave plasma volume of 54.0 mL/kg, RBC volume of 106.0 mL/kg, and total blood volume of 160.0 mL/kg. Normal blood volume is usually 80 to 90 mL/kg.

Erythrocyte fragility test was normal, with beginning hemolysis at 0.55% and complete hemolysis at 0.30% buffered NaCl solution.

Erythrocyte kinetics. Erythrocyte ^{51}Cr T½ = 56 days. ^{59}Fe transfer rate was 8.88 mg/100 mL/day.

Treatment. Reduction of erythrocyte volume was accomplished by periodic phlebotomy. Beginning on April 10 and continuing through April 16, 300 mL of blood was withdrawn on six separate occasions. On April 13 and 16, blood was removed both in the morning and again in the afternoon. The PCV was reduced from 83.0% to 45.0%. The dog was discharged on April 29. The referring veterinarian reported an increase in PCV to 57% on May 13 and to 72% by June 29. By the periodic removal of 500 mL of blood, the PCV was maintained at 40% to 52%. A lapse of 6 to 8 weeks between phlebotomies resulted in the elevation of the PCV to 70%.

Interpretation

1. A marked polycythemia was evident in the initial hemogram. Leukocytosis and thrombocytosis, however, were not present as is commonly the case in polycythemia vera of humans.

2. The arterial O$_2$ tension was normal (Po$_2$ = 90 mmHg) indicating that the polycythemia was primary and not due to a lowered O$_2$ tension secondary to lung or cardiac disease. The normal radiographic and cardiovascular findings confirmed the absence of lung or cardiac disease.

3. The erythrocyte and plasma volume studies indicated an absolute increase in RBC and total blood volume characteristic of polycythemia vera.

4. The erythrocyte fragility was normal, although the erythrocyte half-life of 56 days was somewhat longer than normal. The ^{59}Fe transfer rate indicated

a marked acceleration of erythropoiesis, which further characterizes polycythemia vera.
5. The accelerated rate of erythrocyte production in the presence of a normal arterial O_2 tension and an increased red cell mass support the diagnosis of polycythemia vera.
6. In addition, blood erythropoietin levels can be

measured to determine the erythropoietin-independent nature of primary polycythemia vera.
7. The hypoproteinemia on April 17 was the result of circulatory loss as well as hemodilution in response to repeated phlebotomy between April 13 and 16.

CASE 20 (DOG). POLYCYTHEMIA DUE TO TETRALOGY OF FALLOT

	Dec. 16, 1968		Jan. 24, 1969		Feb. 27, 1969[a]		April 16, 1969		July 9, 1969	
Erythrocytes										
RBC ($\times 10^6/\mu$L)	13.06		13.26		7.49		12.81		14.52	
Hemoglobin (g/dL)	28.2		26.6		14.8		21.6		20.3	
PCV (%)	83		83		49		69[b]		68	
MCV (fL)	63.5		62.6		65.4		53.9		46.8	
MCH (pg)	21.6		20.0		19.7		16.1		13.9	
MCHC (%)	34.0		32.0		30.2		31.3		29.9	
Nucleated RBC/100 WBC	2		1		0		0		0	
Anisocytosis	slight		slight		slight		slight		slight	
Polychromasia	slight		slight		slight		slight		slight	
Leukocytes		%		%		%		%		%
WBC/μL (corrected)	11,862		8,700		22,000		7,400		7,200	
Band neutrophils	0	0.0	261	3.0	330	1.0	74	1.0	72	1.0
Neutrophils	10,319	87.0	6,699	77.0	17,820	81.0	3,848	52.0	4,896	68.0
Lymphocytes	1,186	10.0	783	9.0	990	4.5	1,332	18.0	864	12.0
Monocytes	0	0.0	783	9.0	2,640	12.0	592	8.0	576	8.0
Eosinophils	355	3.0	174	2.0	220	1.0	1,554	21.0	792	11.0
Plasma										
Plasma proteins (g/dL)	9.5		7.2		6.9		7.8		8.2	
Fibrinogen (g/dL)	0.5		0.3		0.5		0.3		0.4	
Blood urea nitrogen (mg/dL)	31.8		30.0		—		39.0		—	
Urine										
Specific gravity	1.008		1.010		—		1.028		—	
Protein	1+		1+		—		2+		—	

[a]After withdrawal of 1,100 mL of blood and corrective surgery (blood withdrawn over 10-day period).
[b]After withdrawal of 1,100 mL of blood between April 18 and 25, PCV was 44% on April 29.

Case 20 (Dog). Secondary Polycythemia Due to Tetralogy of Fallot

A 4-year-old intact English bulldog, weighing 20 kg, was presented with the complaint of dyspnea, cyanosis, polyphagia, polydipsia, and polyuria. Body temperature was normal.

Physical Examination. Dyspnea was not noticeable at rest, but cyanosis due to engorgement of blood vessels was marked. The pulse rate was 150/min,

and respiratory rate was 29/min and of the abdominal type. There was a grade-2 systolic heart murmur heard over the left chest at the fourth interspace. The dog would walk only a few steps and then rest. An initial hemogram revealed a PCV of 83%, RBC of $13.06 \times 10^6/\mu$L and Hb of 28.2 g/dL.

Cardiac Angiography. Multiple films were taken at 0.5-sec intervals after injection of a contrast medium through a catheter placed into the right ventricle. The

(Continued)

findings were consistent with the presence of a right-to-left shunt through a septal defect with marked holdup of the contrast medium within the pulmonary artery. The changes were compatible with tetralogy of Fallot.

Blood Volume. Plasma volume based on Evans blue was 62.5 mL/kg. The RBC volume was determined with ^{51}Cr to be 100.5 mL/kg. Total blood volume was 163.0 mL/kg. Normal blood volume is usually reported to be 80 to 90 mL/kg. Arterial blood oxygen saturation was 65% and 69% in two blood gas studies.

Other Findings. The dog developed a persistent ulcer of the right cornea, and urinalysis indicated continuous mild proteinuria associated with blood urea nitrogen levels of 23.2 to 48.6 mg/dL. Erythrocyte osmotic fragility test was normal, and ^{51}Cr T½ was 28 days.

Treatment. Phlebotomies were performed as follows: Feb. 10, 200 mL; Feb. 11, 250 mL; Feb. 13, 400 mL; and Feb. 19, 250 mL. The dog was hydrated on Feb. 14 with 500 mL of lactated Ringer's solution b.i.d. and 500 mL on Feb. 15, s.i.d. On Feb. 25, corrective surgery was attempted; the left pulmonary artery was anastomosed to the descending aorta. Temporary improvement followed, but polycythemia developed again, with PCV attaining a value of 69% by April 16. Periodic phlebotomy was employed to maintain the PCV between 50% and 60%. The dog collapsed and died on the following Jan. 28, 1 hour after a routine phlebotomy.

Interpretation

1. Compensatory polycythemia developed as a result of the right-to-left shunt of blood, which allowed a portion of venous blood to bypass the lungs, resulting in hypoxemia. The low arterial oxygen saturation of 65% and 69% reflected the failure of all blood to circulate through the lungs.
2. The increase in erythrocyte number and total volume to compensate for the induced hypoxemia was reflected in the congested and cyanotic mucous membranes.
3. Erythrocyte size (MCV) was minimum normal and microcytic at times. This possibly reflected a compensating effect due to the markedly increased numbers of erythrocytes. MCHC and MCH decrease in parallel with repeated blood withdrawal, suggesting some depletion of body iron stores.
4. Total leukocyte count was mostly in the low normal range, with persistent lymphopenia. The stress pattern of neutrophilia, monocytosis, and lymphopenia was manifested in the hemogram of Feb. 27, taken 2 days after the attempt at corrective surgery.

CASE 21 (DOG). HEMANGIOSARCOMA

	Jan. 22		Jan. 28		Jan. 30	
Erythrocytes						
RBC (×10⁶/µL)	1.83		2.30		1.08	
Hemoglobin (g/dL)	4.5		5.9		2.5	
PCV (%)	18.0		20.0		11.0	
MCV (fL)	98.3		87.0		102.0	
MCHC (%)	25.0		29.5		22.7	
Reticulocytes (%)	24.8		20.2		33.2	
Nucleated RBC/100 WBC	8.5		24.5		15.5	
Anisocytosis	marked		marked		marked	
Polychromasia	marked		marked		marked	
Howell-Jolly bodies	few		few		few	
Leptocytes (macrocytic)	many		moderate		moderate	
Leukocytes		%		%		%
WBC/µL (corrected)	28,700		14,100		28,500	
Band neutrophils	1,004	3.5	141	1.0	2,280	8.0
Neutrophils	22,099	77.0	10,716	76.0	22,800	80.0
Lymphocytes	1,722	6.0	2,044	14.5	570	2.0
Monocytes	3,875	13.5	1,199	8.5	2,280	8.0
Eosinophils	0	0.0	0	0.0	0	0.0
Degenerated cells	0	0.0	0	0.0	570	2.0
Plasma						
Protein (g/dL)	8.1		7.7		6.7	
Icterus index units	10		10		7.5	

(Continued)

CASE 21 (DOG). HEMANGIOSARCOMA *(continued)*

Rib marrow at necropsy

Rubriblasts	4	0.8%
Prorubricytes	11	2.2
Basophilic rubricytes	53	10.6
Mitotic rubricytes	2	0.4
Polychromatic rubricytes	219	43.8
Mitotic polychromatic rubricytes	4	0.8
Metarubricytes	10	2.0
Total erythrocytic cells	303	60.6
Myeloblasts	1	0.2
Progranulocytes	4	0.8
Myelocytes, neutrophilic	23	4.6
Myelocytes, eosinophilic	1	0.2
Metamyelocytes, neutrophilic	31	6.2
Band neutrophils	30	6.0
Band eosinophils	2	0.4
Neutrophils	24	4.8
Total granulocytic cells	116	23.2
Metarubricyte nuclei	9	1.8
Lymphocytes	0	0.0
Plasma cells	1	0.2
Monocytes	1	0.2
Other free nuclei	9	1.8
Degenerated cells	61	12.2
Total other cells	81	16.2

Myeloid:erythroid ratio = 0.38:1.0

Case 21 (Dog). Acute Internal Blood Loss in Hemangiosarcoma

A male cocker spaniel, 7 years old, was presented because of abdominal enlargement of 1 week's duration. Appetite was normal. The dog was less active than usual but not listless. The mucous membranes were pale; there was an inspiratory dyspnea, the temperature was 102.4°F, pulse 126/min. The distended abdomen was not painful on palpation and did not appear on first examination to contain an excess of fluid. The first hemogram, however, demonstrated a well-advanced macrocytic hypochromic anemia with intense erythrogenesis. This directed attention to the likelihood of blood loss into the abdominal cavity. An attempt at paracentesis produced 5 mL of blood fluid (Jan. 23) that compared favorably with peripheral blood with respect to erythrocyte content. The dog's condition deteriorated during the following week. Finally, on Jan. 30 an exploratory laparotomy was performed. Numerous blood-filled, pea- to grape-size tumor implants were found throughout the peritoneal cavity. Euthanasia was performed.

Necropsy. In addition to the extensive distribution of tumor implants in the peritoneal cavity, tumor implants were scattered throughout the lungs and were associated with bleeding into the thoracic cavity. Neoplastic foci were present also in the hepatic and sternal lymph nodes. The spleen and liver were not involved. The primary site was not definitely established.

Interpretation

1. The very intense bone marrow response to compensate for the continuing escape of erythrocytes into the body cavities and tissues was reflected in the massive movement of reticulocytes into the circulation. This movement was reflected in the stained blood film by the macrocytic leptocytes, many of which stained blue or gray as a result of incomplete hemoglobin synthesis. Bone marrow taken from a rib at necropsy further exhibited the intense erythrogenesis in the M:E ratio of 0.38:1.0. It is of interest that most of the cells were in the polychromatic rubricyte stage, and a few were in the final nucleated metarubricyte stage. This indicates that under the intense demand for erythrocytes in peripheral blood, the cells were released primarily as polychromatophilic erythrocytes and bypassed the metarubricyte stage.

(Continued)

2. A neutrophilia with left shift of magnitudes far greater than that seen here may be anticipated in association with intensification of erythrogenesis of the degree displayed.
3. The progressive loss of blood is also reflected in the falling plasma proteins.
4. The final hemogram reflects the crisis of Jan. 30 in the extremely low RBC, PCV, and hemoglobin concentration. The severe systemic stress was also expressed in the frank lymphopenia.
5. Despite the very large loss of erythrocytes into the body cavities and tissues, the icterus index remained low. The urine gave a very strong reaction for bile pigment. Thus, much of the conjugated bilirubin from hemoglobin degradation was escaping into the urine.

CASE 22 (DOG). GASTROINTESTINAL HEMORRHAGE

	Admission Hemogram		Other Data
Erythrocytes			
RBC ($\times 10^6/\mu$L)	2.04		
Hemoglobin (g/dL)	4.6		
PCV	17.0		
MCV (fL)	83.3		
MCHC (%)	27.1		
Reticulocytes (%)	32.0		Many thrombocytes seen on blood film
Nucleated RBC/100 WBC	10.5		Coombs' test: negative
Anisocytosis	moderate		
Polychromasia	moderate		Fecal examination: Blackish-green (tarry) color; no parasitic
Hypochromasia	moderate		ova seen; occult blood test = 4+
Leptocytosis	marked		
Howell-Jolly bodies	few		
Leukocytes		%	
WBC/μL (corrected)	17,800		
Band neutrophils	356	2.0	
Neutrophils	12,282	69.0	
Lymphocytes	1,513	8.5	GI tract barium series: detected a mass occluding the as-
Monocytes	3,204	18.0	cending duodenum
Eosinophils	445	2.5	Histopathology: a leiomyoma with ulcerated bleeding surface
Plasma			
Plasma proteins (g/dL)	6.4		
Fibrinogen (g/dL)	0.7		
Blood urea nitrogen (mg/dL)	23.2		

Case 22 (Dog). Blood Loss From Gastrointestinal Hemorrhage

An intact male beagle, 11 years old, was referred with the accompanying history: The dog was treated with antibiotics for a cough considered to be due to bronchitis. The coughing disappeared in 1 week, but later the owner noticed that the dog was very weak. The consulting veterinarian found the dog to be anemic and noticed some blood in its stool. Over a period of 3 weeks, iron, vitamin B_{12}, and three whole-blood transfusions were administered. There was no vomiting or diarrhea, and the dog seemed to improve. For 3 days before admission, however, the dog had been anorectic and unable to walk.

Interpretation

1. The hemogram was representative of blood loss due to a bleeding intestinal tumor. The significant findings were an advanced anemia in remission, as indicated by macrocytic hypochromic erythrocytes, accompanied by active reticulocytosis (32.0%) and the occurrence of nucleated eryth-

(Continued)

rocytes in peripheral blood. In addition, the stained film revealed moderate anisocytosis and polychromasia.
2. Total plasma proteins of 6.4 g/dL further substantiated blood loss. The normal value for an 11-year-old dog would be 7.5 g/dL or greater.

3. The presence of a significant lesion was indicated by the elevated fibrinogen.
4. The nature of the feces further indicated bleeding. Existence of a neoplasm was verified by the barium series. The dog made an uneventful recovery after removal of the tumor.

Case 23 (Dog). Disseminated Intravascular Coagulation

An urgent consultation was requested for a patient in the intensive care unit. A 7-year-old, mixed breed, spayed female had returned from surgery following an extensive bowel resection for carcinoma. Over a 24-hour period she had received 3 units of blood as treatment for mild preoperative anemia and extensive blood loss during surgery. She had received 2 of these 3 units during the 30 minutes immediately following surgery. Oozing was noted from the abdominal drain tube following surgery and following venipuncture. There was no previous history of bleeding, and a coagulogram performed 24 hours before surgery was normal. Petechiae and purpura were noted on the lower limbs.

Laboratory values included: hemoglobin, 11 g/dL; WBC, 15,500/μL with 80% neutrophils, 15% lymphocytes, and 3% monocytes; platelet count, 25,000/μL; bleeding time, not performed; prothrombin time (PT), 23 sec (control 12 sec); partial thromboplastin time (PTT), 48 sec (control 21 sec); thrombin time (TT) 19 sec (control 12 sec); and fibrin and fibrinogen degradation products (FDPs), >40 μg/mL (control, <10 μg/mL). Chest radiographs suggested no abnormalities, and blood culture was negative.

Interpretation

1. Based on the patient's history, clinical signs, and laboratory test results, disseminated intravascular coagulation (DIC; consumption coagulopathy) was diagnosed.
2. Common laboratory abnormalities in DIC include a profound thrombocytopenia, mild anemia, prolonged coagulation screening tests (PT, PTT, and TT), elevated FDPs, and fractured red cells known as schistocytes.
3. A bleeding time was not performed in this patient because of the thrombocytopenia. Thrombocytopenia always prolongs the bleeding time. It should be noted that the petechiae and purpura present on the lower hind limbs resulted from the severe thrombocytopenia.
4. DIC is never a primary event; it is always secondary to a primary or inciting event. In this case, several inciting events are suggested. These include tumor, surgical trauma, and perhaps transfusion hemolysis.
5. Treatment of DIC is complex. The basic therapeutic principles include removal or mitigation of the primary or inciting cause, establishing microvascular blood flow through fluid administration, inhibiting hemostasis through the use of aspirin (platelet prostaglandin inhibition) and heparin (activation of the circulatory inhibitor antithrombin III), and blood transfusion.

Case 24 (Dog). Hemophilia B

A 9-month-old male golden retriever was presented because of a swollen, painful left knee joint of 1 day's duration. The dog's owners related previous problems with joints and occasional hematuria. There was no history of epistaxis, gastrointestinal bleeding, purpura, polydipsia, or polyuria. Physical examination was normal other than abnormalities noted in association with the left knee. Aspiration of the joint revealed frank blood (hemarthrosis).

Laboratory findings included: hemoglobin, 10.5 g/dL with normocytic-normochromic red cell indices; platelet count, 175,000/μL; bleeding time, 5 min (normal to 9 min); prothrombin time (PT), 13 sec (control 12 sec); partial prothrombin time (PTT), 60

(Continued)

sec (control 32 sec); and thrombin time (TT), 12 sec (control 12 sec).

Interpretation

1. A mild normocytic-normochromic anemia may be seen in disorders of hemostasis when bleeding is infrequent and of a lesser magnitude. The bleeding in this case was associated with defective hemostasis from a coagulation protein (factor) disorder, as was evident from the normal platelet count and bleeding time. Platelet functional disorders will also prolong the bleeding time.
2. A prolonged PTT with normal PT and TT indicates an intrinsic pathway defect. Results of all screening coagulation factor tests must be compared to values established within individual laboratories or to control values derived from similar animals, i.e., matched by age, weight, and sex. When a patient's value exceeds a control value by a ratio of more than 1:1.3, the prolongation is considered significant. In this case, the ratio was 1:1.88.
3. A defect of intrinsic pathway includes factors XII, XI, IX, and VIII. Factor XII (Hageman factor) deficiency, while causing prolonged PTTs, does not cause bleeding problems as activation of factor XI occurs through a contact activation similar to that of factor XII. Hence factor XII deficiency may be eliminated. Although factor XI deficiency has been reported in the dog, it is rare. Factor VIII (factor VIII:C) deficiency (hemophilia A) is the most common, and factor IX deficiency (hemophilia B) is the second most common sex-linked coagulation protein deficiency. However, in order to establish which factor is the cause of prolonged PTT, factor XI, IX, and VIII:C analyses must be performed.
4. A factor analysis revealed the patient had less than 15% of the normal factor IX concentration, indicating a diagnosis of hemophilia B.

Case 25 (Dog). Circulating Inhibitor of Coagulation

A 2-year-old Doberman, known to have factor VIII deficiency (hemophilia A) was presented because of right hind leg pain of sudden onset. He had been treated with cryoprecipitate by the owners. Recently, however, this therapy had no obvious beneficial effect. During the past few hours the intensity of pain had increased and the leg was carried in a flexed position. A tender mass was palpated in the right iliac fossa.

Laboratory findings included: hemoglobin, 11.5 g/dL; platelet count, 300,000/μL; bleeding time, <5 min; partial prothrombin time (PTT), 66 sec (control 22 sec); factor VIII assay, 1% (normal 70–120%).

A dose of cryoprecipitate calculated to produce a factor VIII:C concentration of 50% was infused. Twenty minutes later, the PTT was 60 sec (control 22 sec), and PTT performed with equal parts of normal and patient plasma was 61 sec.

Interpretation

1. Hemophilia A was evident from the factor VIII concentration of 1%.
2. The history of bleeding despite infusion of cryoprecipitate and failure of cryoprecipitate infusion to normalize PTT suggested the possibility of a plasma inhibitor (antibody) active against factor VIII:C. This was further substantiated by the persistence of prolonged PTT in a mixing study in which normal plasma added to the patient plasma did not correct PTT as expected. The PTT exhibits normal time when factor concentrations are ≥20%; in the present case assuming the normal plasma had 100% of the normal factor VIII:C concentration and the patient had a 1% concentration, the resultant mixture should have approximated 50% of normal concentration and resulted in normal PTT.
3. Some inhibitors may be time-dependent; hence mixing studies are often conducted over several hours. Equal parts of patient and control plasma are mixed and a PTT is performed. A normal result suggests a true factor deficiency or the presence of a time-dependent inhibitor. The mixture is then incubated at 37°C for several hours. During this period PTT is performed at 30-minute intervals. Any prolongation of the PTT by more than a few seconds suggests a time-dependent coagulation protein inhibitor.
4. Although immunosuppressive therapy has been attempted to suppress the inhibitor concentration, this form of therapy offers only transient relief, and most patients succumb at an early age.
5. The normal bleeding time suggests normal platelet function, thus von Willebrand's disease could be tentatively eliminated as a second or concurrent disease.

CASE 26 (DOG). EARLY IMMUNE-MEDIATED HEMOLYTIC ANEMIA

	Jan. 25		Jan. 27		Jan. 28		Jan. 31[a]		Feb. 3[b]	
Erythrocytes										
RBC ($\times 10^6/\mu$L)	1.86		2.05		1.75		1.69		2.82	
Hemoglobin (g/dL)	4.0		4.8		3.6		3.9		7.0	
PCV (%)	12		13		12		12		25	
MCV (fL)	64.5		63.4		68.5		71.0		88.6	
MCHC (%)	33.3		36.9		30.0		32.5		28.0	
MCH (pg)	21.5		23.4		20.6		23.1		24.8	
Reticulocytes (%)	none		none		0.4		22.4		24.6	
Nucleated RBC/100 WBC	none		none		0.5		17		7.5	
Anisocytosis	slight		slight		moderate		marked		marked	
Polychromasia	rare		none		rare		marked		marked	
Other	no aggluti-nation		moderate leptocytes		some macro-cytes		few H-J		—	
Spherocytes	moderate		moderate		some		few		rare	
Leukocytes		%		%		%		%		%
WBC/μL	24,500		43,500		48,600		32,300		34,800	
Metamyelocytes	735	3.0	435	1.0	486	1.0	0	0.0	0	0.0
Bands	2,695	11.0	5,438	12.5	5,103	10.5	2,099	6.5	2,784	8.0
Neutrophils	15,680	64.0	30,667	70.5	34,263	70.5	25,194	78.0	24,708	78.0
Lymphocytes	3,553	14.5	2,610	6.0	1,458	3.0	646	2.0	1,218	3.5
Monocytes	1,837	7.5	4,350	10.0	6,804	14.0	4,361	13.5	5,916	17.0
Eosinophils	0	0.0	0	0.0	486	1.0	0	0.0	0	0.0
Basophils	0	0.0	0	0.0	0	0.0	0	0.0	174	0.5
Platelets/μL	—		—		331,000		—		271,000	
Plasma										
Icterus index units	hemolyzed		50		15		—		2	
Plasma protein (g/dL)	7.8		7.3		6.3		—		6.3	
Fibrinogen (g/dL)	0.8		0.7		0.6		—		0.5	
Coombs test	negative		—		—		—		—	

[a]Excessive EDTA.
[b]Feb. 1: PCV 17%; reticulocytes, 19%.

Case 26 (Dog). Early Immune-Mediated Hemolytic Anemia

A female Pomeranian, 4 years old, was seen early, perhaps within 24 hours of the beginning of a hemolytic crisis. The dog had no history of a previous illness. It was a closely watched house pet. The dog was seldom permitted outside. The owners noticed that the dog seemed to be weak on Jan 24. It was taken to a veterinarian, who found the PCV to be 12%. He suggested that the dog be taken to the university clinic. On arrival on Jan. 25, the dog was calm and in generally good condition with the following findings: pale and icteric mucous membranes, PCV 12%, rectal temperature 104.5°F, rapid respiration, and enlarged spleen. After the first hemogram, 130 mL of whole blood was administered. No additional blood was given throughout the course of hospitalization. Prednisolone therapy IM was begun at 1 mg/lb total daily dose (7.5 mg given b.i.d.). On Jan 29, the dose was increased to 10 mg b.i.d.

Interpretation

1. This patient was seen in the beginning state of immune mediated hemolytic anemia (IMHA). The diagnosis was in doubt at the time of the first hemogram because of a negative direct Coombs' test. It was necessary to make the diagnosis on the basis of the spherocytes. Gross agglutination of erythrocytes was not present.

2. The neutrophilia with left shift and monocytosis were characteristic of IMHA, but the high normal absolute lymphocyte number was not consistent with an acute stress response. The significantly increased neutrophil and monocyte numbers in response to the steroid therapy was as anticipated (Jan. 27 through Feb. 3), but the absolute lymphocyte number did not fall to lymphopenic levels until after the fourth day on steroid therapy.

(Continued)

3. A reticulocytosis failed to develop during the first 4 days of therapy. The clinician in charge decided to increase the dose of steroid on the fifth day. At that time (Jan. 29), however, a blood film stained with new methylene blue revealed beginning reticulocytosis, and by Jan. 31, reticulocytosis was a prominent feature of the stained blood film.

4. The 5-day-delay in appearance of reticulocytes in peripheral blood indicated that the first hemogram was representative of the earliest stage of hemolytic crisis in IMHA. It requires 4 to 5 days for a significant reticulocytosis to develop after an initial massive blood loss or erythrocyte destruction from any cause.

5. The dog was released to the owners on Feb. 3 with directions for gradual reduction of the steroid dose to a maintenance level to be administered every 48 hours.

CASE 27 (DOG). IMMUNE-MEDIATED HEMOLYTIC ANEMIA

	June 19		June 23 Preoperative (Blood transfusion given)		June 23 Postoperative (Blood transfusion given)		June 25		June 29	
Erythrocytes										
RBC ($\times 10^6/\mu L$)	1.22		1.10		3.48		4.05		3.10	
Hemoglobin (g/dL)	3.1		3.6		8.8		9.9		8.5	
PCV (%)	13		15		30		33		29	
MCV (fL)	106.5		136.4		86.2		81.5		93.5	
MCHC (%)	23.8		24.0		29.3		30.0		29.3	
MCH (pg)	25.4		32.7		25.3		24.4		27.4	
Reticulocytes (%)	25.2		54.4		11.2		23.5		2.18	
Nucleated RBC/100 WBC	24.0		14.5		25.5		11.5		20.5	
Anisocytosis	marked		marked		moderate		marked		marked	
Polychromasia	marked		marked		marked		marked		moderate	
Spherocytes	present		present		present		prominent		present	
Leukocytes		%		%		%		%		%
WBC/μL (corrected)	71,500		63,500		27,000		46,200		23,600	
Metamyelocytes	357	0.5	1,588	2.5	405	1.5	0	0.0	0	0.0
Band neutrophils	2,145	3.0	8,255	13.0	2,160	8.0	924	2.0	118	0.5
Neutrophils	60,060	84.0	42,228	66.5	19,980	74.0	33,264	72.0	16,756	71.0
Lymphocytes	0	0.0	952	1.5	945	3.5	1,155	2.5	1,062	4.5
Monocytes	8,937	12.5	10,478	16.5	3,510	13.0	10,857	23.5	5,664	24.0
Eosinophils	0	0.0	0	0.0	0	0.0	0	0.0	0	0.0
Platelets	adequate		adequate		adequate		adequate		adequate	
Plasma										
Proteins (g/dL)	7.6		7.4		7.0		7.0		6.7	
Icterus index units			10		10					
	hemolyzed		(hemolyzed)		(hemolyzed)		10		5 (hemolyzed)	
Other										
Coombs' test	+		—		—		+		+	

Case 27 (Dog). Immune-Mediated Hemolytic Anemia

A spayed beagle terrier female, 5 years old, was referred with the following brief medical history: On May 22, she was listless, exhibiting pharyngitis and a temperature of 104°F. Treatment consisted of antibiotics and B-complex vitamins. The dog had displayed anorexia, and on May 27 it was noted that she was eating a little. At that time, the temperature was 102.5°F. On June 18, the condition worsened; anorexia, vomiting, listlessness, evidence of severe anemia, and red urine were all noted. The hematocrit was 11.0%. Antibiotics and iron were administered intramuscularly. The next day, the dog was referred for diagnosis and treatment.

On arrival, the dog was depressed and pale and exhibited a fast, thready pulse and a temperature

(Continued)

of 102°F. The initial hemogram (June 19) revealed advanced anemia in remission, with evidence of spherocytes. A urinalysis revealed a reddish-brown color, 4+ albumin, and 4+ hemoprotein. Coombs' test was positive. Blood from six donor dogs was submitted for crossmatch, and only one was found suitable for transfusion.

Treatment. Oral prednisolone was given twice daily beginning with 20 mg/dose on June 20 through June 24; the dose was continued twice daily but was reduced to 10 mg through June 28; thereafter, 5 mg of prednisolone was administered twice daily. This dose was to be continued by the owner after release of the patient. The dog was bright and active when released to the owner on July 3.

Interpretation

1. In IMHA, the erythrocytes become coated with specific IgG antibody and/or C3b and are consequently destroyed intravascularly or through phagocytosis in the mononuclear phagocyte system or by both processes. Partial erythrophagocytosis results in formation of spherocytes. Spherocytes appear smaller and more darkly stained than normal erythrocytes. Spherocytes are inflexible cells that become trapped in the microcirculation of the spleen, where they are destroyed.

2. The centers of erythrogenesis are responsive to the hemolytic anemia. Within a few days of initial massive destruction of erythrocytes, the blood picture is typical of anemia in remission, as seen in the admission hemogram of this patient (MCV 106.5 fL, reticulocytes 25.2%, and marked anisocytosis and polychromasia).

3. The neutrophilia and monocytosis are responses to immune mediated destruction of erythrocytes with subsequent release of mediators such as GM-CSF and G-CSF. This occurs because of enhanced mononuclear phagocytic activity destroying antibody-coated erythrocytes.

CASE 28 (DOG). MICROCYTIC HYPOCHROMIC ANEMIA

	Jan. 3		Jan. 17		Jan. 28		Jan. 30	
Erythrocytes								
RBC (×10⁶/μL)	4.10		5.35		6.25		7.25	
Hemoglobin (g/dL)	4.6		10.3		11.8		13.2	
PCV (%)	18		35		38		41	
MCV (fL)	43.9 (microcytic hypochromic)		65.4 (normocytic hypochromic)		60.8 (normocytic normochromic)		56.5 (microcytic normochromic)	
MCHC (%)	25.5		29.4		31.1		32.2	
MCH (pg)	11.2		19.2		18.8		18.2	
Reticulocytes (%)	7.3		0.2		2.0		—	
Nucleated RBC/100 WBC	1		0		0		0	
Anisocytosis	moderate		slight		slight		moderate	
Polychromasia	moderate		slight		slight		slight	
Poikilocytosis	moderate		slight		slight		none	
Leptocytosis	marked		marked		marked		moderate	
Hypochromasia	prominent		moderate		slight		none	
Leukocytes		%		%		%		%
WBC/μL	17,500		5,000		5,200		5,600	
Neutrophils	13,038	74.5	2,125	42.5	2,418	46.5	2,632	47.0
Lymphocytes	2,100	12.0	1,875	37.5	1,300	25.0	1,568	28.0
Monocytes	1,487	8.5	700	14.0	546	10.5	644	11.5
Eosinophils	787	4.5	300	6.0	936	18.0	728	13.0
Basophils	0	0.0	0	0.0	0	0.0	28	0.5
Degenerated cells	0	0.0	0	0.0	0	0.0		
Unclassified cells	88	0.5	0	0.0	0	0.0		
Plasma								
Total protein (g/dL)	5.6		6.6		6.4		6.7	
Icterus index units	2		2		2		5	

(Continued)

CASE 28 (DOG). MICROCYTIC HYPOCHROMIC ANEMIA (*continued*)

			(Jan. 23)	(Feb. 1)
Fecal Examination				
Occult blood test	4+	3+	fresh blood	4+

Bone marrow evaluation, aspiration from iliac crest on Jan. 3 (500 cells differentiated)

Rubriblast	1.0%	Myeloblast	0.8%	Lymphocytes	8.4%
Prorubricyte	2.6	Progranulocyte	0.6	Monocytes	2.2
Basophilic rubricyte	16.6	Neutrophilic myelocyte	1.6	Plasma cells	0.6
Polychromatic rubricyte	8.8	Eosinophilic myelocyte	0.6	RE nuclei	2.0
Metarubricyte	16.0	Neutrophilic metamyelocyte	5.0	Degenerated	2.8
Mitotic figure	0.6	Neutrophilic band cells	6.4	Total other	16.0
Total erythrocytic	45.6	Neutrophils mature	22.6	cells	
		Eosinophils	0.8		
M:E ratio = 0.84:1.0		Total granulocytic	38.4		

Case 28 (Dog). Microcytic Hypochromic Anemia in Chronic Blood Loss

A male English pointer, 4 years old, was presented with a complaint of loss of blood in the stools for the past 3½ years. The initial hemogram verified the existence of an advanced anemia in which erythrocyte morphology was typical of iron-deficiency anemia. Fresh blood was present in the stools. The condition was diagnosed as a case of ulcerative colitis. Treatment consisted of daily administration of a hematinic and salicyl-azosulfapyridine from Jan. 4 through Feb. 6. The bleeding was controlled and the anemia corrected.

Interpretation

1. In chronic blood loss leading to iron deficiency, hemoglobin synthesis is delayed, leading to buildup of metarubricytes in the bone marrow and production of microcytic hypochromic erythrocytes. In the dog, MCV is less than 60 fL, MCHC is less than 30%, and MCH is less than 15 pg.
2. Peripheral blood contained about 7% reticulocytes, thereby indicating active erythrogenesis. Early fragmentation of erythrocytes was reflected in the presence of poikilocytes in the initial hemograms.
3. The less-than-normal plasma protein concentration was as expected in continuous blood loss.
4. The effect of therapy was dramatic. Blood loss was gradually reduced and, within 2 weeks the hemoglobin concentration had more than doubled. By the end of the fourth week, all values of the hemogram were within the normal range, with the exception of the leukocyte count. A leukopenia was evident from January 17 onward and was due essentially to a neutropenia. It was speculated that this was a direct result of the daily administration of salicylazosulfapyridine.

CASE 29 (DOG). PLASMA CELL MYELOMA AND GLOMERULONEPHRITIS

	Jan. 19	Jan. 26	April 12
Erythrocytes		(postsplenectomy)	
RBC (×10⁶/μL)	2.86	5.05	2.65
Hb (g/dL)	7.3	11.3	5.1
PCV (%)	20	35	17
MCV (fL)	69.9	69.3	64.1
MCH (pg)	25.5	22.3	19.2
MCHC (%)	36.5	32.2	30.0
Reticulocytes (%)	10.8	5.2	2.5
Nucleated RBC/100 WBC	4	0	5
Anisocytosis	moderate	slight	moderate
Polychromasia	moderate	slight	slight

(*Continued*)

CASE 29 (DOG). PLASMA CELL MYELOMA AND GLOMERULONEPHRITIS *(continued)*

	Jan. 19		Jan. 26		April 12	
Leukocytes		%		%		%
WBC/μL (corrected)	10,800		23,600		7,100	
Band neutrophils	324	3.0	1,062	4.5	284	4.0
Mature nutrophils	7,938	73.5	17,818	75.5	4,118	58.0
Lymphocytes	1,134	10.5	1,298	5.5	2,201	31.0
Monocytes	1,296	12.0	3,422	14.5	426	6.0
Eosinophils	0	0.0	0	0.0	71	1.0
Plasma cells	108	1.0	0	0.0	0	0.0
Platelets	56,000		—		24,000	
Plasma						
Protein (g/dL)	14.1		7.8		14.9	
Fibrinogen (g/dL)	0.1		0.2		<0.1	

Serum Protein Fractionation (g/dL)

	Jan. 19	Jan. 29	April 12 (see Fig. A.2)
Total protein	13.9	6.8	14.7
Albumin	1.9	3.6	1.93
Globulin	12.0	3.2	12.77
alpha-1	0.2	0.7	0.13
alpha-2	0.3	—	0.09
beta-1	0.9	0.1	} 0.44
beta-2	0.6	0.7	
gamma-1	5.3	0.6	} 12.11
gamma-2	4.7	1.1	
A:G ratio	0.16:1.0	1.12:1.0	0.15:1.0

Case 29 (Dog). Plasma Cell Myeloma and Glomerulonephritis

A 6-year-old male Scottish terrier was presented on Jan. 19 with the complaint of vomiting and difficulty in walking. The dog was unable to hold its head in a central position and appeared to be weak and unbalanced. Palpation detected a mass in the middle left abdomen. An exploratory laparotomy revealed an enlarged spleen with infarction, hematoma, and massive intra-abdominal hemorrhage. Splenectomy was performed. Histopathologic examination of the splenic tissue revealed large areas of hemorrhage and accumulations of round cells, with vesicular nuclei and prominent nucleoli, resulting in separation and compression of splenic follicles. Numerous megakaryocytes and extramedullary hemopoiesis were evident.

After removal of the spleen, the dog's condition improved and there was gain in weight, but a slight head tilt to the left persisted. On April 12, the dog was readmitted to the hospital with a history of poor appetite, polydipsia, and polyuria for the preceding 2 weeks and vomiting for the preceding 2 days. Laboratory findings were similar to those of the first admission. On the basis of all available data, multiple myeloma was suspected, and a skeletal survey was made. Decreased bone density was noted in the proximal right tibia, distal right femur, and dorsal spine of the second lumbar vertebra. The dog was euthanized.

Necropsy. The liver was somewhat enlarged, the kidneys were small and pale with atrophic cortices, and the mesenteric and colonic lymph nodes were slightly enlarged. On histopathologic examination of selected tissues, plasma cells were observed in the myocardium, liver, and bone marrow. There were several myeloma cell foci in the cortex of the kidney, and, in addition, many glomeruli were small with thickened tufts and some clumps of amyloid. A diagnosis of plasma cell myeloma and glomerulonephritis was made.

Interpretation

1. On first admission (Jan. 19), an anemia in remission was in evidence. The low plasma fibrinogen concentration and thrombocytopenia gave rise to speculation of internal bleeding due to disseminated intravascular coagulation. This concept was supported by the observation of infarction and massive hematoma of the spleen.

(Continued)

2. The most significant feature of the initial laboratory study was the demonstration of a dysproteinemia due to marked elevation of γ-globulin. The finding of a proliferation of abnormal and immature cells in the spleen pointed to the existence of a neoplastic, globulin-secreting plasma cell population, as supported by subsequent findings.

3. Removal of the spleen and the transfusion of whole blood during surgery led to an increase in erythrocyte number, PCV, and hemoglobin and a decrease in total plasma proteins, as demonstrated in the hemogram of Jan. 26 and the protein fractionation pattern on Jan. 29.

4. The improvement in health was temporary; in 2 months, the dog was exhibiting signs of general poor health. Laboratory studies on April 12 revealed advanced nonresponsive anemia and marked dysproteinemia characterized by a monoclonal gammopathy. A bone scan by radiography indicated decreased density of several bones, thereby lending support to a diagnosis of multiple myeloma.

5. The anemia and thrombocytopenia of April 12 may be attributed to replacement of normal marrow cells by malignant cells. The low plasma fibrinogen may be explained by the extensive infiltration of the liver by malignant plasma cells. Protein fractionation revealed a monoclonal gammopathy (Fig. A.2).

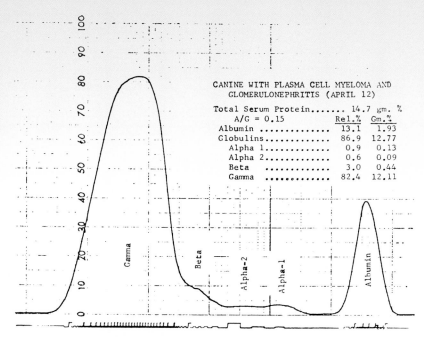

CANINE WITH PLASMA CELL MYELOMA AND
GLOMERULONEPHRITIS (APRIL 12)

Total Serum Protein		14.7 gm. %	
A/G = 0.15		Rel.%	Gm.%
Albumin		13.1	1.93
Globulins		86.9	12.77
Alpha 1		0.9	0.13
Alpha 2		0.6	0.09
Beta		3.0	0.44
Gamma		82.4	12.11

FIGURE A.2 Protein fractionation demonstrating a monoclonal gammopathy in a dog with plasma cell myeloma.

CASE 30 (CAT). ABNORMAL GRANULOPOIESIS

	April 27	May 1
Erythrocytes		
RBX (×10⁶/μL)	8.30	6.95
Hemoglobin (g/dL)	10.1	10.8
PCV (%)	36.0	32.0
MCV (fL)	43.4	46.0
MCHC (%)	28.0	33.7
Anisocytosis	slight	slight
Heinz bodies	rare	rare

(Continued)

CASE 30 (CAT). ABNORMAL GRANULOPOIESIS   (*continued*)

	April 27		May 1	
Leukocytes		%		%
WBC/μL	41,200		27,300	
Progranulocytes	206	0.5	0	0.0
Myelocytes	618	1.5	0	0.0
Metamyelocytes	1,442	3.5	0	0.0
Band neutrophils	8,034	19.5	0	0.0
Neutrophils	28,016	68.0	22,796	83.5
Lymphocytes	2,678	6.5	3,549	13.0
Monocytes	206	0.5	273	1.0
Eosinophils	0	0.0	410	1.5
Basophils	0	0.0	136	0.5
Unclassified cells	0	0.0	136	0.5
Neutrophil morphology	Large cells, many with bizarre coiled nuclei and basophilic, granular crytoplasm		Essentially normal in size and appearance. Cytoplasm has the normal dust-like, pinkish granulation with only an occasional tiny bluish granule	

Case 30 (Cat). Abnormal Granulopoiesis in Acute Toxemic Disease

A male seal-point Siamese, 5 years old, was presented exhibiting signs of dyspnea, increased vesicular sounds, depression, dehydration, and a temperature of 103.6°F. Antibiotics and multivitamins were administered daily. Recovery was rapid and uneventful. The hemograms are of interest in view of the change in the leukogram within a 4-day period.

Interpretation

1. The cat occasionally expresses the severity of a disease process in changes in the morphology of the neutrophil granulocyte. In toxemic diseases, there may be complete depression of granulopoiesis, initially, leading to leukopenia, followed by remission with a marked left shift and "toxic" neutrophils. The toxic state is shown in increased size of neutrophils, bizarre nuclear patterns, sometimes giant forms, and basophilia of the cytoplasm. The cytoplasm is very granular and diffusely bluish. As the toxemia decreases, the succeeding generations of neutrophils are more normal in size, and the cytoplasm presents its normal pinkish granularity with residual deposits of angular to round bluish structures called Döhle bodies.

2. Changes in neutrophil morphology occur rapidly as the toxemia is brought under control. Examination of the stained blood film taken daily from capillary blood of the ear is a rapid and practical means for evaluation of the progress in toxemic diseases of the cat.

CASE 31 (CAT). MARKED LEUKOPENIA

	October 24	October 26	October 30
Erythrocytes			
RBC ($\times 10^6$/μL)	9.25	7.4	5.75
Hemoglobin (g/dL)	12.7	12.4	10.0
PCV (%)	34	34	28
MCV (fL)	36.7	45.9	48.7
MCHC (%)	37.3	36.5	35.7
Icterus index units	—	2	—
Nucleated RBC/100 WBC	0	0	2.5
Anisocytosis	slight	slight	moderate
Heinz bodies	few	rare	none
Polychromasia	none	none	moderate

(Continued)

CASE 31 (CAT). MARKED LEUKOPENIA (*continued*)

	October 24		October 26		October 30	
Leukocytes		%		%		%
WBC / μL (corrected)	1,300		5,200		22,900	
Progranulocytes	0	0.0	52	1.0	0	0.0
Myelocytes	0	0.0	26	0.5	0	0.0
Metamyelocytes	0	0.0	26	0.5	0	0.0
Band neutrophils	0	0.0	260	5.0	229	1.0
Neutrophils	312	24.0	1,716	33.0	16,259	71.0
Lymphocytes	806	62.0	1,430	27.5	5,611	24.5
Monocytes	169	13.0	1,066	20.5	458	2.0
Eosinophils	13	1.0	312	6.0	229	1.0
Basophils	0	0.0	0	0.0	0	0.0
Unclassified cells	0	0.0	208	4.0	0	0.0
Degenerated cells	0	0.0	104	2.0	114	0.5
Neutrophil morphology	Larger than normal; blue, granular cytoplasm		Larger than normal with basophilic cytoplasm		Essentially normal	

Case 31 (Cat). Marked Leukopenia with Rapid Remission

A castrated male seal-point Siamese, 3½ years old, was presented exhibiting signs of anorexia, nausea characterized by bile-stained vomitus, and bloody diarrhea. One popliteal lymph node was enlarged. There was evidence of dehydration, and the temperature was 102.6°F. The cat had been vaccinated against panleukopenia virus at 2 months of age. Therapy consisted of antibiotics, multivitamins, and fluids. A total of 150 ml of 5% dextrose was given between Oct. 24 and Oct. 27. The cat was considerably improved by October 28, and it was able to go home on the seventh day from admission.

Bone marrow aspiration on Oct. 26 revealed a nearly complete absence of mature neutrophils. The cells of the granulocytic series were large, with many metamyelocytes appearing as large as the progranulocytes. The impression gained was that maturation of the nucleus proceeded directly from the progranulocyte stage without division of the cell. Thus the cells were large and the cytoplasm remained basophilic.

There was a distinct lack of cells within the erythrocytic maturation series.

Interpretation

1. The disease produced a depression of all leukocyte types as well as cells of the erythrocytic maturation series. The bone marrow and blood findings on Oct. 26 were typical of the cellular patterns to be seen during the early recovery stage from panleukopenia virus infection.
2. Marrow suppression of erythropoiesis was not reflected as frank anemia because of the considerably long life span of red cells compared to that of the neutrophils, which can be depleted within a few days of inhibition of granulopoiesis. The rebound of the erythrocytic series followed a few days later. There was evidence of red blood cell production and release to peripheral blood on Oct. 30.
3. This sequence of hemograms clearly reveals the speed with which neutrophilic granulocytes of the cat enter a remission phase after a marked neutropenia in an acute disease process.

CASE 32 (CAT). ADENOCARCINOMA

	August 8	September 19	October 15	October 17
Erythrocytes				
RBC (×10⁶/μL)	8.10	9.00	5.05	3.65
Hemoglobin (g/dL)	13.8	15.1	7.3	6.0
PCV (%)	41.0	41.0	22.0	18.0
MCV (fL)	50.6	45.5	43.6	49.3
MCHC (%)	33.6	36.8	33.2	33.3

(Continued)

CASE 32 (CAT). ADENOCARCINOMA (*continued*)

	August 8		September 19		October 15		October 17	
Nucleated RBC/100 WBC	0		0		4.5		0	
Icterus index units	—		—		—		15	
Reticulocytes (%)	—		—		—		none seen	
Anisocytosis	slight		slight		Slight to moderate variation in cell size, with many erythrocytes presenting "punched-out" centers. No polychromasia.			
Polychromasia	none		none					
Other	—		Heinz bodies distinctly observable in Wright-Leishman-stained film.					
Heinz bodies	few		numerous, very large		numerous		numerous, large	
Leukocytes		%		%		%		%
WBC/μL	20,300		18,100		16,900		22,300	
Band neutrophils	0	0.0	452	2.5	85	0.5	112	0.5
Neutrophils	15,225	75.0	14,752	81.5	12,590	74.5	20,404	91.5
Lymphocytes	2,741	13.5	1,900	10.5	3,251	19.0	1,561	7.0
Monocytes	812	4.0	91	0.5	507	3.0	0	0.0
Eosinophils	1,320	6.5	724	4.0	507	3.0	223	1.0
Basophils	102	0.5	0	0.0	0	0.0	0	0.0
Degenerated cells	102	0.5	181	1.0	0	0.0	0	0.0

Case 32 (Cat). Progressive Anemia in Adenocarcinoma of the Small Intestine

A female seal-point Siamese cat, 11½ years old, was first presented on August 7 with a complaint of vomiting sporadically over a period of 2 weeks. An essentially normal hemogram (Aug. 8) was observed. The cat was treated as an outpatient, but vomiting started again about 3 weeks later, and by September 19 hardly any food could be retained. The cat entered the clinic again on Oct. 14. The 2-hour film after barium administration exhibited a dilatation of the small intestine anterior to a narrow band of intestinal constriction. The cat died on Oct. 20.

Necropsy Report. Adenocarcinoma of the intestine causing incomplete obstruction was present. There was a mild nephrosis, and the liver and spleen contained extensive deposits of hemosiderin.

Interpretation

1. The hemogram of September 19 revealed Heinz bodies in profusion and of such large size to be readily visible in the Wright-Leishman-stained blood film. Thereafter, a progressive anemia developed with no evidence of remission. The pathologist's report indicated extensive deposits of hemosiderin in the liver and spleen from erythrocyte destruction in macrophages. It would appear that destruction of the erythrocytes containing large Heinz bodies enhanced the development of anemia of chronic disease. Heinz body anemia is typically hemolytic and regenerative. Reticulocytopenia and absence of polychromasia indicate inability of the bone marrow to respond. In the presence of depressed erythropoiesis, the anemia persists and becomes progressively more severe.
2. The progressive fall in eosinophils with terminal neutrophilia and lymphopenia were an expression of a marked systemic stress.

CASE 33 (CAT). LYMPHOMA

	February 28		April 8		April 12		April 15	
Erythrocytes								
RBC ($\times 10^6/\mu$L)	6.25		4.01		3.95		3.45	
Hemoglobin (g/dL)	10.5		7.4		5.9		5.0	
PCV (%)	32		22		18		15	
MCV (fL)	51.2		54.8		45.5		43.5	
MCHC (%)	32.8		33.6		32.8		33.3	
Nucleated RBC/100 WBC	1		1		2		1	
Reticulocytes (NMB stain)	none seen		none seen		none seen		none seen	
Heinz bodies (NMB stain)	moderate number		moderate number		moderate number		moderate number	
Anisocytosis	slight		slight		slight		slight	
Polychromasia	none		slight		none		none	
Poikilocytosis	few		few		few		few	
Leukocytes		%		%		%		%
WBC/μL	6,900		1,600		3,300		1,800	
Band neutrophils	0	0.0	16	1.0	33	1.0	72	4.0
Neutrophils	5,279	76.5	960	60.0	2,046	62.0	1,260	70.0
Lymphocytes	1,000	14.5	528	33.0	858	26.0	252	14.0
Monocytes	517	7.5	48	3.0	132	4.0	162	9.0
Eosinophils	35	0.5	32	2.0	0	0.0	0	0.0
Unclassified cells	0	0.0	16	1.0	165	5.0	36	2.0
Degenerated cells	69	1.0	0	0.0	66	2.0	18	1.0

Case 33 (Cat). Anemia and Leukopenia in Lymphoma

A male domestic shorthair cat, 9 months old, was presented with a complaint of lethargy and some loss of appetite of 1 week's duration.

Physical Examination. Temperature of 103.5°F, enlarged lymph nodes, tenderness of abdominal area, some palpable nodules in the abdomen, and a dry, nonproductive cough were noted. An initial hemogram at this time revealed a low total leukocyte count mainly due to a well-advanced lymphopenia. Antibiotics were administered, and there appeared to be an immediate improvement. However, 5 weeks later, the cat returned to the clinic exhibiting coughing, weakness, anorexia, and a body temperature of 104°F. The patient was hospitalized for observation and treatment. Body temperature dropped to 102.6°F for a few days and then increased to between 104° and 106°F. Death came on the tenth day of hospitalization (April 18).

Necropsy. Lymphoma involved all layers of the intestine in the region of the jejunum, producing a constriction and dilatation. The contents were dark and tarry from hemorrhage originating in the area of dila-

tation. Neoplastic nodules were present in the spleen liver, and the lymph nodes.

Interpretation

1. Progressive anemia was associated with the formation of Heinz bodies in the erythrocytes. These bodies were of sufficient size to cause destruction of the erythrocytes. The pathologist's comment concerning the presence of macrophages filled with hemosiderin supports the opinion that the spleen or mononuclear phagocyte system was destroying erythrocytes. There was no evidence of remission of the anemia.
2. Progressive nonregenerative anemia and marked lymphopenia are common findings in feline lymphoma.
3. Proliferation of neoplastic lymphocytes in the bone marrow may cause development of progressive anemia and neutropenia.
4. This case illustrates the difficulty often encountered in diagnosis of lymphosarcoma from blood examination only. Lymphopenia may be seen in as many as 50% of the cats and 25% of the dogs with lymphoma.

CASE 34 (CAT). FELINE INFECTIOUS ANEMIA

	November 14		November 15		November 19	
Erythrocytes						
RBC ($\times 10^6/\mu$L)	4.20		3.40		3.20	
Hemoglobin (g/dL)	7.20		6.60		5.60	
PCV (%)	23.0		20.0		18.0	
MCV (fL)	54.8		58.8		56.3	
MCHC (%)	31.3		33.0		31.1	
Nucleated RBC/100 WBC	2.5		4.0		2.0	
Anisocytosis	Slight		Slight		Moderate	
Polychromasia	Slight		Slight		Moderate	
Haemobartonella felis	None seen		None seen		Few ring forms	
Leukocytes		%		%		%
WBC/μL (corrected)	4,680		4,368		13,328	
Band neutrophils	0	0.0	0	0.0	133	1.0
Neutrophils	2,761	59.0	1,791	41.0	6,397	48.0
Lymphocytes	1,778	38.0	2,446	56.0	5,864	44.0
Monocytes	94	2.0	131	3.0	600	4.5
Eosinophils	23	0.5	0	0.0	133	1.0
Unclassified cells	23	0.5	0	0.0	200	1.5

Case 34 (Cat). Feline Infectious Anemia (Hemobartonellosis)

A male domestic shorthair cat, 7 months old, was referred for diagnosis and treatment of anemia. The referring veterinarian had administered a blood transfusion 2 weeks previously, and vitamin B_{12} and iron had been given at weekly intervals.

Physical Examination. The cat appeared normal except for pale mucous membranes. The temperature was 101.4°F on admission, and during the 6 days of hospitalization it was 101.7–102.4°F. Three hemograms were obtained over a 6-day period. The first two verified the existence of an anemia in which the erythrocytes were bordering on being macrocytic. The third hemogram was diagnostic for *Hemobartonella felis.*

Interpretation and Remarks

1. This series of hemograms clearly demonstrates the difficulty of diagnosis of feline infectious anemia in the chronic state on the basis of demonstration of *Hemobartonella felis* in the stained blood film. Often several sequential hemograms are necessary before the parasite is observed in peripheral blood.
2. Moderate anisocytosis and polychromasia on November 19 indicated beginning remission of the anemia. The marked increase in absolute lymphocyte count at this time reflected the decrease in systemic stress.

CASE 35 (HORSE). NEONATAL ISOERYTHROLYSIS IN A FOAL

	Aug. 1, 1977 (3 days old)	Aug. 3	Aug. 8	Aug. 10
Erythrocytes				
RBC ($\times 10^6/\mu$L)	3.86	5.55	5.32	4.7
Hemoglobin (g/dL)	5.7	9.2	8.9	7.7
PCV (%)	16	26	27	24
MCV (fL)	41.5	46.8	50.8	51.1
MCHC (%)	35.6	35.4	32.9	32.1
MCH (pg)	14.8	16.6	16.7	16.4
Anisocytosis	Slight	Slight	Slight	Slight
Crenation				Marked

(Continued)

CASE 35 (HORSE). NEONATAL ISOERYTHROLYSIS IN A FOAL (*continued*)

	Aug. 1, 1977 (3 days old)		Aug. 3		Aug. 8		Aug. 10	
Leukocytes								
WBC/μL	12,500	%	15,500	%	3,100	%	6,800	%
Band neutrophils	688	5.5	310	2.0	0	0.0	0	0.0
Neutrophils	7,500	60.0	13,098	84.5	589	19.0	3,298	48.5
Lymphocytes	1,687	13.5	1,627	10.5	2,325	75.0	2,992	44.0
Monocytes	2,625[a]	21.0	465	3.0	186	6.0	510	7.5
Platelets/μL	Present		Present		Present		Present	
Plasma								
Icterus index (units)	>100		50		50		75	
Total protein (g/dL)	5.7		5.8		4.0		3.5	
Fibrinogen (g/dL)	0.4		0.4		0.3		0.3	
Total bilirubin (mg/dL)	28.8		18.8					

[a]Rare cell with phagocytosed RBC.

Case 35 (Horse). Neonatal Isoerythrolysis in a Foal

A 3-day-old male foal was presented with the chief complaints of weakness and slight icterus the previous night and marked icterus, dark urine, and loose yellow feces on the day of presentation. The foal was listless and too weak to stand. Its temperature was 103°F, pulse 130/min, and respiration 40/min. Initial CBC showed PCV 16%, total plasma protein 5.7, and icterus index > 100 units. A diagnosis of neonatal isoerythrolysis (NI) was made.

Therapy consisted of administering 4 L of dextrose-saline, washed red cells from 2 L of mare's blood, phenylbutazone, antibiotics, and dexamethasone. One liter of mare's milk was fed by stomach tube on the first day of hospitalization. The foal's condition improved by the next day, and it began to nurse. However, it developed diarrhea and became febrile again on Aug. 4, with body temperature ranging between 103 and 104.6°F until Aug. 6. Clinical dehydration was not observed. With continued antibiotic therapy, gradual improvement occurred after Aug. 7, although mucous membranes were still orangish on Aug. 11. A transfusion of 900 mL of plasma was given on Aug. 11, and the foal was sent home on Aug. 12. The foal was normal on Aug. 25.

Interpretation

1. Marked anemia and icterus during the first few days of life are suggestive of neonatal isoerythrolysis (NI). An icterus index of 50 to 100 units with red cell values within the normal range is to be anticipated in newborn foals as a result of their inability to conjugate and excrete bilirubin because of immaturity of the liver.
2. The increase in PCV on Aug. 3 is an effect of blood transfusion. Adequate survival of mare's red cells, as expected, is reflected in stabilization of PCV in subsequent hemograms.
3. A gradual increase in MCV indicates accelerated effective erythropoiesis in response to anemia. In the absence of reticulocyte response in the horse, such changes in MCV can be a valuable aid in assessing response to anemia.
4. Although increases in icterus index values usually parallel elevations in serum bilirubin concentrations, the degree of bilirubinemia cannot be assessed accurately from a subjective reading of the icterus index, particularly when it has reached its maximum (100 units). Total bilirubin content, and if possible direct and indirect bilirubin, should be determined for proper evaluation.
5. The finding of a rare monocyte with a phagocytosed red cell in the circulation signifies immune-mediated destruction of red cells by the mononuclear phagocyte system. Spherocyte formation follows partial erythrophagocytosis and may be encountered occasionally in NI. Similarly, indications for intravascular hemolysis are hemoglobinemia and hemoglobinuria, which may be observed in cases of NI.
6. Hypoproteinemia is anticipated in a newborn even after colostrum consumption. Marked decreases in total plasma protein concentrations on Aug. 8 and 10 seem to be related primarily to protein loss associated with diarrhea and to some extent inanition.
7. Leukopenia, primarily from neutropenia, on Aug. 8 probably indicates endotoxemia developing in association with diarrhea from intestinal infection. Monocytopenia in the horse is considered an expression of stress effect from an acute disease such as endotoxemia. The increase in neutrophils on Aug. 10 was a favorable sign.

CASE 36 (HORSE). COMBINED IMMUNE DEFICIENCY IN AN ARABIAN FOAL

Erythrocytes
RBC ($\times10^6/\mu$L)	8.66
Hemoglobin (g/dL)	11.7
PCV (%)	36
MCV (fL)	41.6
MCHC (%)	32.5
MCH (pg)	13.5
Anisocytosis	Slight

Leukocytes
WBC/μL	12,300	%
Neutrophils	11,316	92
Lymphocytes	rare, seen on scanning	
Monocytes	984	8
Eosinophils	0	0
Platelets/μL	Present in adequate numbers	

Plasma
Icterus index (units)	5
Total protein (g/dL)	6.6
Fibrinogen (g/dL)	0.8
Serum IgG (mg/dL)	355
Serum IgM (mg/dL)	0

Case 36 (Horse). Combined Immune Deficiency in an Arabian Foal

A male Arabian foal, about 2 weeks old, was presented with a 1 week history of respiratory distress and nasal discharge. The foal did not suckle colostrum until about 8 hours after birth. Physical examination revealed cyanotic mucous membranes, abnormal inspiratory and expiratory sounds, with both rales and rhonchi present. Temperature was 102°F, pulse 150/min, and respiration 50/min. Increased pulmonary densities, compatible with bronchopeumonia, were seen on radiologic examination of the chest.

Cytologic examination of the tracheal wash revealed many neutrophils, rarely with intracellular bacilli and cocci, and occasional macrophages. *E. coli* and *Actinobacillus* were cultured from the tracheal wash. Serologic examination demonstrated absence of IgM and 355 mg/dL of IgG. Results of the hematologic examination are shown in the table. A diagnosis of combined immune deficiency (CID), with a partial failure of passive transfer based on the low IgG levels, was made. Virus isolations and indirect immunofluorescence tests were negative for equine herpesvirus 1 and adenovirus.

Because of its acute condition, the foal was placed under intensive care and given oxygen, fluids, hyperalimentation, antibiotics (potassium penicillin and gentamicin) and aminophylline. However, because of its progressively deteriorating condition, the foal was euthanized the next day.

Necropsy. All lymph nodes appeared smaller than normal, were difficult to locate, and showed absence of differentiation between cortex and medulla on cut surface. The thymus weighed 15 g, was almost gelatinous, and showed marked interlobular edema. The spleen was very meaty and lacked obvious follicles on cut surface. Histopathologic examination of various lymphoid organs such as the thymus, lymph nodes, and spleen revealed mainly reticular stroma and total absence of lymphocytic elements. The respiratory system showed lesions of severe, acute, patchy bronchopneumonia and severe, necrotizing diffuse bronchitis and bronchiolitis. Histologic changes were compatible for an adenovirus infection, although virologic examination for it was negative. The liver showed moderate, multifocal necrosis and diffuse hepatocellular lipidosis. Diffuse nonsuppurative enteritis was also present. Cryptosporidiosis and *Pneumocystis carinii*, common to CID in human and animals, were not observed in this foal.

Interpretation

1. Foals with CID generally develop complications from secondary bacterial, viral, and/or protozoan infections within a few weeks to a few months of birth.
2. The clinical history and signs and the breed and age of the animal indicated a tentative diagnosis of CID.
3. Severe absolute lymphopenia and absence of IgM were consistent with a diagnosis of CID, and this was further substantiated by necropsy findings of marked lymphoid hypoplasia.
4. A history of delayed colostrum consumption coupled with <400 mg/dL of serum IgG levels suggest the possibility of a partial failure of passive transfer of immunoglobulins. However, some consideration should be given to catabolic disappearance of maternal IgG over the 2 weeks of life of the foal, which would tend to reduce its serum IgG level from that attained after colostral consumption. The diagnosis of partial or complete failure of transfer of immunoglobulins generally entails measuring IgG concentrations in serums collected within the first 24-48 hours of birth.
5. The elevated fibrinogen concentration and neutrophilia were indicative of response to acute inflammation from secondary infection. Absence of left shift indicated that the foal was able to meet the increased functional demand for neutrophils without depletion of body reserves of mature neutrophils.
6. Red cell parameters were within the normal range for a foal less than 1 month old.

CASE 37 (HORSE). FIBRINOUS PERICARDITIS AND BRONCHITIS

	September 30		October 2		October 7	
Erythrocytes						
RBC ($\times 10^6/\mu$L)	7.05		6.05		6.50	
Hemoglobin (g/dL)	11.5		9.5		10.1	
PCV (%)	35.0		29.0		30.0	
MCV (fL)	49.6		47.9		46.1	
MCHC (%)	32.8		32.7		33.7	
Leukocytes		%		%		%
WBC/μL	23,900		18,400		17,900	
Band neutrophils	359	1.5	92	0.5	0	0.0
Neutrophils	22,705	95.0	16,744	91.0	16,916	94.5
Lymphocytes	597	2.5	644	3.5	447	2.5
Monocytes	239	1.0	644	3.5	268	1.5
Eosinophils	0	0.0	92	0.5	0	0.0
Basophils	0	0.0	184	1.0	268	1.5
Neutrophil morphology	Hypersegmented		Hypersegmented		Cytoplasm slightly blue, indicating beginning of "toxic" signs	
Plasma						
Proteins (g/dL)	7.5		7.7		8.3	
Icterus index units	20		25		30	

Case 37 (Horse). Severe Lymphopenia Associated with Fibrinous Pericarditis and Bronchitis

A female Standardbred horse, 15 years old, had been sick for 2 weeks with signs of coughing, diarrhea, and weight loss. Upon examination, the rectal temperature was 100°F, pulse 61/min, and respiration 24/min. There was ventral edema to the thickness of about 3 inches and fluid in the thoracic cavity. The latter was tapped and 2 gallons of reddish fluid removed. A jugular pulse was evident that diminished upon removal of the 2 gallons of fluid. The horse was hospitalized and treated daily with antibiotics. Since no improvement resulted, permission was obtained to destroy the horse.

Necropsy. The epicardium was completely covered with a fibrinous exudate. The pericardium was thickened and coarsely granular. The lung tissues revealed patchy consolidation oriented about bronchioles.

Interpretation

1. A normocytic-normochromic anemia was evident by Oct. 2. The anemia was due in part to the loss of red blood cells into the thoracic cavity as indicated by the reddish color of the removed fluid. Inflammatory diseases of this type commonly depress erythrogenesis, which in turn enhances the development of anemia. Furthermore, the anemia was possibly more advanced than demonstrated since there was clinical evidence of a disturbance in water balance.

2. The icterus index increased progressively, and in the terminal stages, it exceeded normal values for the PCV. An above-normal icterus index is difficult to evaluate in the horse, since retention of bilirubin occurs readily in this species when food and water intake is significantly reduced. In the present case, the above-normal icterus index values, may have resulted in part, from destruction of red blood cells escaping into the fluid accumulating in the thoracic cavity.

3. A marked neutrophilia and marked lymphopenia that persisted despite antibiotic therapy were grave signs. Hypersegmentation of neutrophil nuclei indicated a retention of the neutrophil leukocyte in peripheral blood for a longer period than normal. It is conjectured that this is one of the effects of corticosteroids of stress whereby diapedesis of neutrophil leukocytes is partially prevented and the cells continue to age within the circulation.

4. It was surprising that plasma protein concentration was not found to be higher than 7.5–8.3 g/dL. The loss of protein into the thoracic cavity may have masked an anticipated absolute increase in protein in response to the extensive inflammatory process.

CASE 38 (HORSE). HYPERGLOBULINEMIA IN CHRONIC DERMATITIS

	February 13		February 20		February 27		March 11	
Erythrocytes								
RBC ($\times 10^6/\mu$L)	6.85		7.00		7.35		7.70	
Hemoglobin (g/dL)	9.8		10.5		10.0		11.1	
PCV (%)	33.0		32.0		32.0		33.0	
MCV (fL)	48.2		45.7		43.5		42.9	
MCHC (%)	29.7		32.8		31.3		33.6	
Leukocytes		%		%		%		%
WBC/μL	21,200		12,500		13,600		13,200	
Band neutrophils	424	2.0	0	0.0	0	0.0	0	0.0
Neutrophils	14,946	70.5	8,375	67.0	8,500	62.5	6,468	49.0
Lymphocytes	4,452	21.0	3,688	29.5	4,353	32.0	5,808	44.0
Monocytes	848	4.0	250	2.0	272	2.0	66	0.5
Eosinophils	318	1.5	125	2.0	272	2.0	528	4.0
Basophils	212	1.0	0	0.0	68	0.5	132	1.0
Degenerated cells	0	0.0	63	0.5	136	1.0	198	1.5
Plasma								
Protein (g/dL)	11.6		9.7		9.5		8.3 (March 4)	
Serum proteins (g/dL) (biuret)	10.0		—		—		8.1	
Albumin	1.2		—		—		1.7	
Globulin	8.8		—		—		6.4	
γ globulin	5.7		—		—		3.9	
A:G ratio	0.14:1.0		—		—		0.27:1.0	

Case 38 (Horse). Hyperglobulinemia in Chronic Dermatitis

A female quarter horse was under treatment for dermatitis characterized by alopecia, eczema, and pruritus. Examination of skin scrapings for bacteria, fungi, and parasites failed to reveal specific agents. No cause could be established from histologic study of skin biopsy material. Several hemograms were developed during the period of treatment. They were of interest from the point of view of increase in plasma proteins due to production of γ-globulin.

Interpretation

1. The circulating erythrocyte volume as reflected in RBC and PCV values remained at the minimum normal level. Hemoglobin concentration was below the minimum normal. A borderline normocytic hypochromic anemia existed initially as an anemia of chronic disease.
2. In the first hemogram, the plasma protein concentration was 11.6 g/dL. In chronic suppurative diseases in the horse, globulins often increase markedly, as in this case. The albumin fraction becomes reduced as a protective mechanism to maintain osmotic pressure of blood plasma within limits. The albumin:globulin ratio approximates 1.0:1.0 in health but becomes significantly less than unity (below 0.5:1.0) when hyperglobulinemia develops. Plasma protein concentrations increase in dehydration, but under conditions of hemoconcentration, the A:G ratio is not significantly altered.
3. Serum protein concentration determined by the biuret method on Feb. 13 was found to be 10.0 g/dL, and protein fractionation demonstrated the A:G ratio to be 0.14:1.0. This finding demonstrated that the hyperproteinemia was absolute and not the result of hemoconcentration.
4. A total leukocyte count of 20,000 + is a significant leukocytosis in the horse. The first hemogram demonstrated a significant neutrophilia, with other leukocyte types remaining in the normal range, which probably reflected a response to an established inflammatory lesion.

CASE 39 (HORSE). LEUKOCYTOSIS WITH MULTIPLE ABSCESSES

	Sept. 26		Oct. 9		Dec. 7		Aug. 10	
Erythrocytes								
RBC ($\times 10^6/\mu$L)	6.3		6.4		7.75		6.60	
Hemoglobin (g/dL)	11.3		10.2		13.8		10.6	
PCV (%)	30		29		39		30	
MCV (fL)	47.6		45.3		50.3		45.5	
MCHC (%)	37.6		35.2		35.4		35.3	
Leukocytes		%		%		%		%
WBC/μL	51,500		21,400		13,100		12,400	
Band neutrophils	1,030	2.0	0	0.0	0	0.0	0	0.0
Neutrophils	46,608	90.5	16,050	75.0	8,253	63.0	8,370	67.5
Lymphocytes	1,802	3.5	4,280	20.0	4,061	31.0	3,348	27.0
Monocytes	2,060	4.0	642	3.0	458	3.5	558	4.5
Eosinophils	0	0.0	321	1.5	262	2.0	124	1.0
Basophils	0	0.0	107	0.5	66	0.5	0	0.0

Neutrophil morphology: No evidence of toxic changes, but the neutrophils appeared to be somewhat larger than normal on Sept. 26 and to be hypersegmented.

	Sept. 26	Oct. 9	Dec. 7	Aug. 10
Plasma				
Plasma proteins (g/dL)	10.4	8.3	7.8	7.1
Blood urea nitrogen (mg/dL)	24.1	22 (Oct. 2)	—	—
Serum proteins (g/dL)	8.8	—	7.0	6.3
Icterus index units	5	2	5	10
Albumin:globulin ratio	0.17:1.0	—	0.89:1.0	0.75:1.0
Urine				
Specific gravity	1.020	1.010	1.024	1.018
Proteinuria	3+	1+	negative	negative
Occult blood	3+	trace	negative	negative
WBC/high-power field	50–100	none	none	none
RBC/high-power field	numerous	5	none	none

Case 39 (Horse). Extreme Leukocytosis Associated With Multiple Abscesses

A pregnant Arabian mare, 15 years old, had had a problem with abscesses over the chest and abdomen. Currently, her urine contained fresh blood. Rectal examination revealed a pregnancy of about 50 days' duration. The bladder felt normal to palpation, but a large mass in the area of the left kidney was detected. These findings were reported on Sept. 26. Treatment consisted of 3 million units of penicillin and 5 g of streptomycin repeated several times at daily intervals. The mare gained weight, and the urine was grossly normal by Oct. 4. She was discharged Oct. 10 as clinically improved. Blood and urine were rechecked on Dec. 7 and again in August of the following year.

Interpretation

1. Leukocytosis of 51,500 in the horse is an extremely high count and is typical of a localizing suppurative inflammatory process. The lymphopenia and eosinopenia were referable to systemic stress, and the monocytosis suggests chronicity.

2. Total proteins in plasma and serum were elevated, principally by hyperglobulinemia in response to the suppurative inflammatory process. With convalescence, the albumin:globulin ratio returned to the low normal range.

3. Marked improvement was reflected in near normal urine on Oct. 9 and the return of lymphocytes in large numbers to peripheral blood. The reduction in monocytes and reappearance of eosinophils and basophils also verified the relief from systemic stress. A significant neutrophilia persisted on Oct. 9.

4. A borderline anemia of chronic inflammatory disease was evident in slightly below normal values for RBC, PCV, and hemoglobin in the Sept. 26 and Oct. 9 hemograms.

5. The final hemogram, developed 1 year after the onset of the disease, revealed a fall in circulating erythrocyte volume that perhaps was due to the recent termination of gestation with a normal foal. The mare, however, had been losing weight during the month before the last hemogram.

CASE 40 (HORSE). PERFORATION OF THE RECTUM

	April 25		April 29		May 2		May 3	
Erythrocytes								
RBC ($\times 10^6/\mu$L)	10.25		10.00		10.30		10.50	
Hemoglobin (g/dL)	21.2		18.3		18.9		18.9	
PCV (%)	57.0		56.0		53.0		53.0	
MCV (fL)	55.6		56.0		51.5		50.5	
MCHC (%)	37.2		32.7		35.6		35.6	
Leukocytes		%		%		%		%
WBC/μL	3,400		6,700		13,000		9,300	
Progranulocytes	0	0.0	0	0.0	0	0.0	47	0.5
Myelocytes	68	2.0	0	0.0	0	0.0	0	0.0
Metamyelocytes	102	3.0	167	2.5	65	0.5	325	3.5
Band neutrophils	714	21.0	1,440	21.5	2,405	18.5	2,186	23.5
Neutrophils	1,938	57.0	3,116	46.5	7,410	57.0	4,510	48.5
Lymphocytes	408	12.0	1,374	20.5	3,120	24.0	2,139	23.0
Monocytes	136	4.0	502	7.5	0	0.0	93	1.0
Eosinophils	34	1.0	0	0.0	0	0.0	0	0.0
Basophils	0	0.0	33	0.5	0	0.0	0	0.0
Degenerated cells	0	0.0	67	1.0	0	0.0	0	0.0
Neutrophil morphology:			Cytoplasm of the immature neutrophils was blue and granular; the cytoplasm of the mature cell presented a bluish background in which a variable number of pink granules were interspersed.					
Plasma								
Protein (g/dL)	—		8.3		8.3		7.7	
Icterus index units	50		50		25		10	

Case 40 (Horse). Degenerative Left Shift with "Toxic" Neutrophils in Perforation of the Rectum

A 14-year-old female horse of mixed breeding was presented with a history of perforation of the rectum. The condition under which the perforation occurred was not stated. The horse was received on April 23 and died on May 4. The first hemogram was not obtained until 48 hours after the perforation had occurred.

Necropsy. A tear about 4 inches long was found in the wall of the rectum. A large organized pocket occurred at the site of the rent, and there were massive adhesions between the peritoneum and intestines. The liver was enlarged and of normal color, and thrombi were present in the portal veins. A large thrombus containing strongyle larvae was present at the origin of the iliac artery.

Interpretation

1. The initial PCV of 57% and hemoglobin concentration of 21.2 g/dL were due to hemoconcentration from dehydration and, perhaps, splenic contraction as a result of extreme stress. Some improvement in water balance appeared to be evident in subsequent hemograms.
2. The elevated icterus index of the first two hemograms is a common finding in the horse in diseases leading to anorexia and reduced water intake.
3. The leukopenia, marked left shift, and "toxic" neutrophils of the first hemogram indicated the extremely serious nature of the disease. Although leukocyte numbers increased, including both neutrophils and lymphocytes, perhaps as a response to antibiotic therapy, the persistence of "toxic" cells called for a continuing grave prognosis.

CASE 41 (HORSE). ACUTE SALMONELLOSIS

	April 28	April 29	May 1	May 2	May 3	May 4	May 5	May 8
RBC ($\times 10^6/\mu$L)	11.0	8.89	10.20	9.74	13.14	14.80	13.06	8.92
Hb (g/dL)	16.9	13.7	14.4	16.3	19.5	21.1	19.2	14.4
PCV (%)	45	38	44	45	56	62	51	39
MCV (fL)	40.9	42.7	43.1	46.2	42.6	41.9	39.1	43.7
MCHC (%)	37.5	36.0	32.7	36.2	34.8	34.0	37.6	36.9
MCH (pg)	15.4	15.4	14.1	16.7	14.8	14.3	14.7	16.1
Icterus index units	100	50	50	75	75	50	75	10 slightly lipemic
Protein (g/dL)	6.9	6.2	7.1	7.1	8.0	8.7	7.7	5.8
Fibrinogen (g/dL)	0.4	0.2	0.6	0.8	1.2	1.4	1.3	0.8
WBC/μL	12,900	8,900	2,500	1,800	4,200	3,600	5,900	11,100
Myelocytes	0	0	25[a]	90[a]	126[a]	36[a]	0	0
Metamyelocytes	0	0	125[a]	270[a]	870[a]	396[a]	472[a]	0
Bands	387	0	1,450[a]	486[a]	756[a]	936[a]	1,298[a]	610
Neutrophils	10,385	6,898	150[a]	0	252[a]	0	1,180[a]	6,105
Lymphocytes	1,935	1,735	550	918	2,142	2,196	2,950	2,886
Monocytes	193	178	200	36	42	36	0	1,332
Eosinophils	0	89	0	0	0	0	0	167
Unclassified	0	0	0	0	42	0	0	0
Na (mEq/L)	141	—	135	125	120	131	133	134
K (mEq/L)	2.8	—	2.9	3.8	4.5	3.8	3.6	3.3
Cl (mEq/L)	105	—	100	95	90	94	101	101
pH	—	—	7.40	7.42	7.34	7.35	7.35	7.38
P$_{CO_2}$	—	—	37.5	33.0	32.5	35.0	37.5	42.0
HCO$_3^-$ (mEq/L)	—	—	22.7	21.1	21.0	18.7	20.3	24.0
CO$_2$Ct (mmole/L)	—	—	23.6	21.9	21.8	19.6	21.3	25.0
Base excess (mEq/L)	—	—	−1	−2	−1	−5	−4	0

[a] Toxic cells.

Case 41 (Horse). Acute Salmonellosis

A thoroughbred female, 3 years old, was a nervous filly that had to be tranquilized for training. She was exhibiting signs of colic at 5 a.m. April 28. Upon admission to the teaching hospital, her temperature was 100°F, and her pulse was 50/min, steady and strong. There were reduced gut sounds. Passage of a stomach tube released foul-smelling gas. Mucous-covered feces were in the rectum. Clinical dehydration was not apparent. Initial therapy consisted of a combination of dihydrostreptomycin and procaine penicillin G. On April 29, the filly appeared normal until 6:30 p.m., when profuse diarrhea was noted. However, the feces were formed again the next morning. At this time, there appeared to be a loss of appetite. By noon on April 30, she was kicking at her abdomen. An indwelling catheter was placed in the left jugular, and 9 liters of lactated Ringer's solution was administered over a 2-hour period. Profuse diarrhea was present on May 1 and persisted throughout a 5-day period. Diarrhea began to recede on May 6, with the first formed feces on May 9. Therapy from May 1 through May 5 consisted of IV fluids, 8 to 12 liters b.i.d., basically lactated Ringer's fortified with

potassium and sodium as needed to maintain electrolyte levels. In addition, fluids were given by stomach tube and fortified with NaCl, dextrose, and furazolidone. Group B *Salmonella* organisms in moderate numbers were isolated from the feces on May 1. Considerable improvement was noted on May 10, although some weight loss was evident and weakness was apparent.

Interpretation

1. The colicky signs noted on April 29 were probably due to the beginning enteritis from *Salmonella* infection.
2. Although the combination of dihydrostreptomycin and procaine penicillin G was the only treatment administered initially, the horse appeared to be clinically normal the following day. This improved clinical state was also reflected in the near normal blood picture. Lymphopenia and bilirubinemia were the only abnormalities noted, but the icterus index was reduced somewhat from the high level of the previous day.

(*Continued*)

3. Profuse diarrhea leading to dehydration was apparent on May 1 through May 5. The dehydrating effect of the diarrhea was partially controlled by massive fluid therapy given orally and by intravenous infusion. The peak of dehydration was on May 4, when the PCV was 62% and the plasma protein concentration was 8.7 g/dL. A comparison of these data with those of May 8, when convalescence was in evidence, reveals the severity of water loss despite the daily administration of more than 30 liters of fluids consisting of lactated Ringer's solution fortified with electrolytes for intravenous infusion and water fortified with NaCl and dextrose given by stomach tube.

4. Loss of the electrolytes, sodium and chlorine, was greatest on May 3, and blood pH dropped to its lowest level of 7.34 at that time. The massive fluid therapy contributed significantly to success in maintaining blood pH within reasonable limits.

5. Blood gas evaluation indicated a mild metabolic acidosis that was greatest on May 4 when dehydration was at its peak. Loss of the base HCO_3^- into the gut was compensated for by reduction of carbonic acid through removal of CO_2 by increased respiration. This was reflected in the below-normal concentration of P_{CO_2} and CO_2Ct (CO_2 content) in the blood.

6. Plasma fibrinogen increased from 0.2 to 1.4 g/dL between April 29 and May 4, indicating a marked response of the liver to the acute enteritis.

7. Leukopenia due to decrease of all leukocyte types has been a constant feature of acute salmonellosis in the horse. Most spectacular was the marked suppression of granulopoiesis with exhaustion of the bone marrow pool of mature neutrophils. On May 2, no mature neutrophils were seen in the peripheral blood, and the total leukocyte count was at its lowest level of 1,800/μL.

8. Circulating leukocyte numbers started to increase on May 3, due mainly to a significant rise in lymphocytes. Since the increase in lymphocytes to more than 2,000/μL persisted through the following days, it is conjectured that this may have been the first sign of beginning improvement despite the apparent worsening of the state of hydration and the marked hyponatremia and hypochloremia on May 3 and the acidosis on May 4.

CASE 42 (COW). ACUTE MASTITIS

Date	July 16[a]	July 17[a]	July 18	July 19	July 20	July 23
Body temp. (°F)	—	—	107	102.7	104.1	102.6
WBC/μL	9,400	2,850	800	1,500	1,700	8,500
Myelocytes	0	0		0	187	127
Metamyelocytes	0	0		0	391	2,082
Band neutrophils	0	0	too few cells	30	102	1,700
Neutrophils	2,538	342	for valid	90	85	1,062
Lymphocytes	5,358	1,995	differential	1,170	799	2,762
Monocytes	1,128	399	count	195	0	467
Eosinophils	188	144		15	51	85
Basophils	188	0		0	0	56
Degenerated cells	0	0		0	85	159
"Toxic" neutrophils	—	—	—	—	4+	4+

[a]Cow was normal on this day.

Case 42 (Cow). Leukopenia and Left Shift in Acute Mastitis

A Holstein cow was near the end of her first lactation when once-daily milking was practiced for a 2-week period followed by abruptly stopping further milk removal. All mammary quarters were normal at that time. Since the cow was part of a small herd established for research purposes, the plan was to follow blood morphology on a daily basis to note if the abrupt cessation of milk removal would be reflected in a stress pattern in peripheral blood. The last milking was on the morning of July 16. *Escherichia coli* was present in the milk of the right front gland at this time, but little attention was given to this finding for it was assumed to be an extraneous contaminant. However, the hemogram of the following day, July 17, indicated the cow to be sick, although the milker had not noticed any significant change in her attitude. Body temperature was 107°F on the morning of July 18, but the mammary glands were not swollen. *E. coli* was isolated from the secretions of three of the mammary quarters. By July 20, the cow was recumbent and refused to rise. The two rear mammary quarters were swollen at this time. However, by July 23, the cow was well on the way to recovery. No therapy had been administered; therefore, the sequential hemograms reveal the typical leukocytic patterns to be anticipated in acute coliform mastitis followed by recovery.

Interpretation

1. Coliform organisms multiply rapidly in cell-free milk within the mammary gland. Eventually, the presence of the multiplying bacterial population brings on an exudation of neutrophils into the milk. The neutrophils participate in the destruction of the coliform bacteria. Death of the Gram-negative bacteria leads to release of endotoxin, which in turn precipitates the local and systemic signs of acute mastitis.

2. The movement of neutrophils in large numbers from blood to milk results in neutropenia. The bone marrow pool of mature neutrophils is also soon exhausted, and, therefore, a marked left shift is commonly seen in the cow in response to a developing inflammatory process. Endotoxin absorbed into the circulation may temporarily depress granulopoiesis, and then a severe neutropenia may persist for several days. Other leukocyte types also become reduced in numbers in blood in response to corticosteroids of stress. Thus the cow has no other way to respond to a developing acute inflammatory process but by almost complete disappearance of all leukocyte types from peripheral blood. New generations of neutrophils become available to peripheral blood by the fourth or fifth day from original stimulus. A delay in granulopoietic response may take place, as in this case, if the bone marrow cells have been injured by circulating toxin.

CASE 43 (COW). JOHNE'S DISEASE

Hemogram		Serum Protein Fractionation	
RBC ($\times 10^6/\mu$L)	4.80	Total protein (g/dL)	5.9
Hb (g/dL)	7.5	Albumin	1.0
PCV (%)	24	Globulin	4.9
Icterus index units	2	alpha	1.1
WBC/μL	12,700	beta	0.7
Band neutrophils	131	gamma	3.1
Neutrophils	7,112	A:G ratio	0.2 (normal =
Lymphocytes	3,933		0.86–1.18)
Monocytes	1,524		

Case 43 (Cow). Johne's Disease

In a herd of dairy cattle, there was a history of illness characterized by anorexia, scouring, weight loss, and eventual death. Cows ranging in age from heifers to older cows were affected, and 25 cattle had been lost. An 8-year-old pregnant Guernsey cow in poor condition and in the fourth month of lactation was admitted to the clinic for diagnostic tests. Physical examination revealed a rough hair coat, pale mucous membranes, and grossly normal rectal mucosa from which acid-fast bacilli were cultured. A johnin skin test was positive. A urine sample was cloudy with a specific gravity of 1.018 and a 1+ test for protein.

The cow was euthanized, and necropsy revealed a disseminated interstitial nephritis and an infarct in the kidney. The intestinal wall was thickened, and the mucosa had a corrugated appearance throughout. There was obstruction of the lymphatics of the small intestine with an accumulation of giant cells in the submucosal lymphatics.

Interpretation

The hemogram reflected a chronic disease problem, as indicated by a PCV at the low normal level, a hemoglobin concentration below normal, and a differential leukocyte count indicating neutrophilia and monocytosis. There was a marked hypoalbuminemia from loss of protein into the intestine, but a fairly good level of total protein was maintained by a modest hyperglobulinemia, which was possibly a reflection of an immunologic response.

CASE 44 (SHEEP). HAEMONCHOSIS

Erythrocytes ($\times10^6/\mu$L)	3.3		
Hemoglobin (g/dL)	2.9		
PCV (%)	11.5		
MCV (fL)	34.7		
MCHC (%)	25.2		
Icterus index units	<5		
Reticulocyte count (%)	5.7		
Nucleated erythrocytes	1/100 WBC		
Anisocytosis	moderate to marked	Basophilic stippling	marked
Poikilocytosis	moderate to marked	Polychromasia	moderate to marked
Hypochromasia	moderate to marked	H-J bodies	occasional

Leukocytes/μL	7,100	%
Bands	71	1.0
Neutrophils	2,698	38.0
Lymphocytes	3,905	55.0
Monocytes	177	2.5
Eosinophils	213	3.0
Degenerated cells	35	0.5

Fecal examination: McMaster count—84,000 eggs per gram, most of which were *Haemonchus contortus.*

Case 44 (Sheep). Haemonchosis

A 1-year-old male Suffolk sheep had been showing edema of head and throat for 2 days. On physical examination, the following were observed: temperature 102.5°F, pulse 136/min, respiration 28/min, mucous membranes pale, pupils dilated, moderate degree of nasal exudate, and marked depression.

Interpretation

1. *Haemonchus contortus* is a bloodsucking parasite of the abomasum.
2. A macrocytic hypochromic anemia with active erythrogenesis is anticipated in acute blood loss from heavy infection with *H. contortus*, whereas a normocytic normochromic or hypochromic anemia develops in chronic infections. In the present case, the normocytic hypochromic anemia indicates a chronic rather than acute blood loss, while reticulocytosis, moderate to marked polychromasia, and basophilic stippling indicate active but inadequate red cell production. Together, these findings probably suggest a transitional phase of anemia from acute to chronic stage in which iron deficiency is setting in with diminution of erythropoiesis from progressive heavy parasitism.
3. The occurrence of many poikilocytes seems to be an expression of the inability of the newly formed erythrocytes to withstand the stress of circulation. This is common to anemia associated with iron deficiency from chronic blood loss. Thus anemia in this sheep may have resulted from both blood loss and shortened life span of newly formed erythrocytes.
4. Although plasma protein concentration was not determined in this case, the presence of edema of head and throat are most likely a manifestation of hypoproteinemia (hypoalbuminemia) associated with haemonchosis.